Brief Contents

CRITICAL CARE NURSING

A Holistic Approach

9th Edition

Patricia Gonce Morton, RN, PhD, ACNP, FAAN

Professor, Associate Dean for Academic Affairs, and Co-coordinator of
the Acute Care Nurse Practitioner and Clinical Nurse Specialist Master's
Program in Trauma, Critical Care, and Emergency Nursing
University of Maryland School of Nursing
Baltimore, Maryland

Dorrie K. Fontaine, RN, PhD, FAAN

Dean, School of Nursing, University of Virginia
Sadie Heath Cabaniss Professor of Nursing
Charlottesville, Virginia
Past-President, American Association of Critical-Care Nurses (AACN)

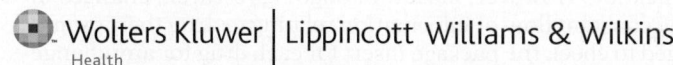

Wolters Kluwer | Lippincott Williams & Wilkins
Health

Philadelphia · Baltimore · New York · London
Buenos Aires · Hong Kong · Sydney · Tokyo

Acquisitions Editor: *Elizabeth Nieginski*
Development Editor: *Melanie Cann*
Senior Production Editor / Production: *Tom Gibbons*
Art Director, Design: *Joan Wendt*
Art Director, Illustration: *Brett MacNaughton*
Manufacturing Coordinator: *Karin Duffield*
Compositor: *Circle Graphics*
Indexer: *Alexandra Nickerson*

9th Edition

9 8 7 6 5 4 3 2 1

Printed in China.

Library of Congress Cataloging-in-Publication Data

Critical care nursing : a holistic approach / [edited by] Patricia Gonce Morton, Dorrie Fontaine. — 9th ed.
    p. ; cm.
    Includes bibliographical references and index.
    ISBN 978-0-7817-6829-0 (cloth : alk. paper) 1. Intensive care nursing. 2. Holistic nursing. I. Morton, Patricia Gonce, 1952- II. Fontaine, Dorrie.
    [DNLM: 1. Critical Care. 2. Holistic Nursing. WY 154 C9328 2009]
    RT120.I5C744 2009
    616.02'8—dc22
                                                        2008031747

Care has been taken to confirm the accuracy of the information presented and to describe generally accepted practices. However, the authors, editors, and publisher are not responsible for errors or omissions or for any consequences from application of the information in this book and make no warranty, expressed or implied, with respect to the currency, completeness, or accuracy of the contents of the publication. Application of this information in a particular situation remains the professional responsibility of the practitioner; the clinical treatments described and recommended may not be considered absolute and universal recommendations.

The authors, editors, and publisher have exerted every effort to ensure that drug selection and dosage set forth in this text are in accordance with the current recommendations and practice at the time of publication. However, in view of ongoing research, changes in government regulations, and the constant flow of information relating to drug therapy and drug reactions, the reader is urged to check the package insert for each drug for any change in indications and dosage and for added warnings and precautions. This is particularly important when the recommended agent is a new or infrequently employed drug.

Some drugs and medical devices presented in this publication have Food and Drug Administration (FDA) clearance for limited use in restricted research settings. It is the responsibility of the health care provider to ascertain the FDA status of each drug or device planned for use in his or her clinical practice.

LWW.COM

In memory of my parents, Charles and Dorothy Gonce, my brother William C. Gonce, and my brother-in-law Raymond Tamberino. Thanks for the many years of love, support, and laughter. To my husband John, for his help, encouragement, and love throughout my career. And to Dorrie Fontaine, my best friend and colleague.

—TRISH

To Barry and Sumner, for their constant love and support and to Trish Morton, extraordinary friend. I dedicate this book to my parents who received compassionate nursing care.

—DORRIE

To Carolyn Hudak and Bobbie Gallo who had the vision to create the first edition of this book and the commitment to write six additional editions of the book. Thanks for all you have done to support critical care nurses.

—TRISH AND DORRIE

Contributors

Susan E. Anderson, RN, MSN
Senior Quality Assurance Specialist
U.S. Army Graduate Program in
Anesthesia Nursing
Fort Sam Houston, Texas

Sue Apple, PhD, RN
Assistant Professor
Department of Professional Nursing
Georgetown University
School of Nursing and Health Studies
Washington, District of Columbia

Carla A. Aresco, CRNP, MS, RN
Neurotrauma Nurse Practitioner
R. Adams Cowley Shock Trauma Center
Baltimore, Maryland

Mona N. Bahouth, MSN, CRNP
Nurse Practitioner, Neurology
Director, Clinical Programs and Research
The Maryland Brain Attack Center
University of Maryland Medical Center
Baltimore, Maryland

Kathryn S. Bizek, MSN, CNS-BC, CCRN
Nurse Practitioner, Cardiac Electrophysiology
Henry Ford Heart and Vascular Institute
Henry Ford Health System
Detroit, Michigan

Nancy Blake, RN, MN, CCRN, CNAA
Director, Critical Care Services and Education
Children's Hospital Los Angeles
Los Angeles, California

Kay Blum, PhD, CRNP
Nurse Practitioner
Visiting Assistant Professor
University of Maryland School of Nursing
Baltimore, Maryland

Eileen M. Bohan, RN, BSN, CNRN
Senior Program Coordinator
The Johns Hopkins University
Baltimore, Maryland

Garrett K. Chan, APRN, BC-PCM, PhD, CEN
Lead Advanced Practice Nurse
Clinical Decision Area/Emergency Department
Stanford Hospital and Clinic
Assistant Clinical Professor
Schools of Nursing and Medicine,
University of California, San Francisco
San Francisco, California

Donna Charlebois, RN, MSN, ACNP-CS
Lung Transplant Coordinator
University of Virginia
Charlottesville, Virginia

Mary Ciechanowski, RN, MSN, APRN, BC, CCRN
Stroke Advanced Practice Nurse
Christiana Care Health Systems
Newark, Delaware

JoAnn Coleman, RN, MS, ACNP, AOCN
Acute Care Nurse Practitioner and Coordinator
Pancreas Multidisciplinary Cancer Clinic
Sidney Kimmel Comprehensive Cancer Center at
Johns Hopkins
Baltimore, Maryland

Vicki J. Coombs, PhD, RN
Executive Director
The Midatlantic Cardiovascular Foundation
Baltimore, Maryland

Joan M. Davenport, RN, PhD
Assistant Professor, Nursing
University of Maryland
Baltimore, Maryland

Marla J. De Jong, PhD, RN, CCNS, CCRN
Executive Director of Research
Wilford Hall Medical Center
Lackland Air Force Base, Texas

Nancy Kern Feeley, RN, MS, CRNP, CNN
Nephrology Adult Nurse Practitioner
The Johns Hopkins University
Baltimore, Maryland

Charles Fisher, RN, MSN, CCRN, ACNP-BC
Outcomes Manager
University of Virginia Health System
Charlottesville, Virginia

Barbara Fitzsimmons, RN, MS, CNRN
Nurse Educator
Department of Neuroscience Nursing
The Johns Hopkins Hospital
Baltimore, Maryland

Conrad Gordon, RN, MS, ACNP
Assistant Professor
University of Maryland School of Nursing
Baltimore, Maryland

Christine Grady, RN, PhD
Head, Section on Human Subjects Research
Department of Bioethics
Clinical Center
National Institutes of Health
Bethesda, Maryland

Debby Greenlaw, MS, CCRN, ACNP
Acute Care Nurse Practitioner
Hospitalist Group, Providence Hospital
Columbia, South Carolina

Thomasine D. Guberski, PhD, CRNP
Associate Professor
University of Maryland School of Nursing
Baltimore, Maryland

Kathy A. Hausman, RN, C, PhD
Assistant Professor
University of Maryland School of Nursing
Baltimore, Maryland

Jan M. Headley, RN, BS
Director, Clinical Marketing and
Professional Education
Edwards Lifesciences
Irvine, California

Janie Heath, PhD, APRN-BC, FAAN
Associate Dean Academic Affairs
Medical College of Georgia School of Nursing
Augusta, Georgia

Kiersten N. Henry, MS, APRN-BC, CCNS, CCRN-CMC
Cardiovascular Nurse Practitioner
Montgomery General Hospital
Olney, Maryland

Gennell D. Hilton, PhD, CRNP
Nurse Practitioner, Trauma Services
Adjunct Faculty, Life Sciences Department, Santa
Rosa Junior College
San Francisco, California

Dorene M. Holcombe, RN, MS, ACNP, CCRN
Nephrology Acute Care Nurse Practitioner
The Johns Hopkins University
Baltimore, Maryland

Christina Hurlock-Chorostecki, RN, MScN, APN
Advanced Practice Nurse
Cardiac Surgery Intensive Care
London, Ontario, Canada

Karen L. Johnson, PhD, RN
Assistant Professor
University of Maryland School of Nursing
Director of Nursing Research
University of Maryland Medical Center
Baltimore, Maryland

Dennis W. Jones, MS, RN, NREMT-P
Critical Care Flight Nurse
Nurse Clinician III
The Johns Hopkins Hospital
Baltimore, Maryland

Kimmith Jones, RN, MS, CCNS
Advanced Practice Nurse
Critical Care and Emergency Center
Sinai Hospital of Baltimore
Baltimore, Maryland

Roberta Kaplow, PhD, RN, CCNS, CCRN
Clinical Nurse Educator
Innovex
Parsippany, New Jersey

Jane Kapustin, PhD, CRNP
Assistant Professor of Nursing
Assistant Dean for Masters Studies
Adult Nurse Practitioner Program Director
University of Maryland School of Nursing
Baltimore, Maryland

Susan N. Luchka, RN, MSN, CCRN, ET
Director of Clinical Education
Memorial Hospital
York, Pennsylvania

Christine N. Lynch, RN, MS, CCRN, CRNP
Acute Care Nurse Practitioner, Surgical Critical Care
Union Memorial Hospital
Baltimore, Maryland

Cathleen R. Maiolatesi, RN, MS
Case Manager GYN/OB
The Johns Hopkins Hospital
Baltimore, Maryland

Sandra W. McLeskey, RN, PhD
Professor
University of Maryland School of Nursing
Baltimore, Maryland

Alexander R. McMullen, III, RN, JD, MBA, BSN
Attorney/Principal
McMullen and Drury
Towson, Maryland

Patricia C. McMullen, PhD, JD, CRNP
Associate Provost for Academic Administration
The Catholic University of America School of Nursing
Washington, District of Columbia

Paul K. Merrel, MSN, RN
Outcomes Manager
Advanced Practice Nurse 1
University of Virginia Health System
Charlottesville, Virginia

Sandra A. Mitchell, CRNP, MScN, AOCN
Predoctoral Fellow and Oncology Nurse Practitioner
National Institute of Health
Rockville, Maryland

Patricia A. Moloney-Harmon, RN, MS, CCNS, CCRN, FAAN
Advanced Practice Nurse/Clinical Nurse Specialist
Children's Services
Sinai Hospital of Baltimore
Baltimore, Maryland

Donna Mower-Wade, RN, MS, CNRN, APRN
Trauma Clinical Nurse Specialist
Christiana Care Health System
Newark, Delaware

Nancy Munro, RN, MN, CCRN, ANCP
Acute Care Nurse Practitioner
Critical Care Medicine Department
National Institutes of Health
Bethesda, Maryland

Angela C. Muzzy, RN, MSN, CCRN
Clinical Nurse Specialist
University Medical Center
Tucson, Arizona

Colleen Krebs Norton, PhD, RN, CCRN
Associate Professor and Director
of the Baccalaureate Program
Georgetown University School of Nursing and
Health Studies
Washington, District of Columbia

Dulce Obias-Manno, RN, BSN, MHSA
Coordinator, Cardiac Arrhythmia Device Clinic
Medstar/Washington Hospital Center
Washington, District of Columbia

Mary O. Palazzo, RN, MS
Director of Nursing, Heart Institute
St. Joseph Medical Center
Towson, Maryland

Suzanne Prevost, RN, PhD, COI
Associate Dean for Practice and Community
Engagement
University of Kentucky, College of Nursing
Lexington, Kentucky

Kim Reck, RN, MSN, CRNP
Adult Nurse Practitioner
Clinical Program Manager, CRNP
Division of Cardiology
University of Maryland Medical Center
Baltimore, Maryland

Kathryn P. Reese, RN, BSN, CCRN
Element Chief/Staff Nurse,
Cardiac Intensive Care Unit
Edwards Air Force Base, California

Michael V. Relf, PhD, RN, ACNS-BC, AACRN, FAAN
Associate Professor and Assistant Dean
for Undergraduate Education
Duke University School of Nursing
Durham, North Carolina

Kenneth J. Rempher, PhD, RN, MBA, CCRN, APRN, BC
Director, Professional Nursing Practice
Sinai Hospital of Baltimore
Baltimore, Maryland

Barbara Resnick, PhD, CRNP, FAAN, FAANP
Professor
University of Maryland
Baltimore, Maryland

Caleb A. Rogovin, CRNA, MS, CCRN, CEN
Staff Nurse Anesthetist
Temple University Hospital
Philadelphia, Pennsylvania

Valerie K. Sabol, MSN, ACNP-CS
Co-Director and Assistant Professor
Trauma, Critical Care, and Emergency Nursing
Acute Care
Nurse Practitioner and Clinical Nurse
Specialist Program
University of Maryland School of Nursing
Baltimore, Maryland

Eric Schuetz, BS Pharm
Certified Specialist in Poison Information
Maryland Poison Center
Baltimore, Maryland

Julie Schuetz, CRNP
Nurse Practitioner
Department of Radiation Oncology
University of Maryland Medical Center
Baltimore, Maryland

Brenda K. Shelton, MS, RN, CCRN, AOCN
Clinical Nurse Specialist
The Sidney Kimmel Comprehensive Cancer Center
at Johns Hopkins
Baltimore, Maryland

Jo Ann Hoffman Sikora, RN, MS, CRNP
Nurse Practitioner, Cardiac Surgery
University of Maryland Medical Center
Baltimore, Maryland

Kara Adams Snyder, RN, MS, CCRN, CCNS
Clinical Nurse Specialist, Critical Care
University Medical Center
Tucson, Arizona

Debbi S. Spencer, RN, MS
Deputy Commander Nursing
10th Combat Support Hospital
Fort Carson, Colorado

Allison G. Steele, BSN, MSN, CRNP
Nurse Practitioner
Division of Hepatology and Gastroenterology
University of Maryland
Baltimore, Maryland

Louis R. Stout, RN, MS, CEN
Lieutenant Colonel, United States Army Nurse Corps
United States Army Medical Department
Fort Sam Houston, Texas

Lieutenant Colonel Mary E. Tenhet
Chief, Medical-Surgical Nursing Section
Womack Army Medical Center
Fort Bragg, North Carolina

Sidenia S. Tribble, RN, MSN, APRN-BC, CCRN
Acute Care Nurse Practitioner
Page Memorial Hospital
Luray, Virginia

Terry L. Tucker, RN, MS, BA CCRN, CEN
Critical Care Nurse Specialist
Baltimore Veterans Administration Health Center
Veterans Administration Maryland
Health Care System
Baltimore, Maryland

Jeffrey S. Upperman, MD, FAAP, FACS
Associate Professor of Surgery
Pediatric Surgery
Director, Trauma Program
Director, Disaster Resource and Training Center
Children's Hospital Los Angeles
Keck School of Medicine
University of Southern California
Los Angeles, California

Mary van Soeren, RN, PhD
Consultant
Canadian Health Care Innovations
Guelph, Ontario, Canada

Kathryn T. VonRueden, RN, MS, FCCM
Assistant Professor, Trauma, Critical Care,
ED Program
University of Maryland School of Nursing
Clinical Nurse Specialist
R Adams Cowley Shock Trauma Center
University of Maryland Medical Center
Baltimore, Maryland

Janet Armstead Wulf, MS, RN, CNL
Staff RN
Union Memorial Hospital
Adjunct Laboratory Instructor
University of Maryland School of Nursing
Baltimore, Maryland

Karen L. Yarbrough, MS, CRNP
Director
Programs and Clinical Research
University of Maryland Stroke and Brain Attack
Center, ACNP
University of Maryland Medical Center
Baltimore, Maryland

Elizabeth Zink, RN, MS, CCRN, CNRN
Clinical Nurse Specialist
Neurosciences Critical Care Unit
The Johns Hopkins Hospital
Baltimore, Maryland

Reviewers

Susan J. Appel, PhD, APRN, BC
Associate Professor
Acute and Continuing Care Nurse Practitioner
Option Facilitator
School of Nursing, University of Alabama
Birmingham, Alabama

Elizabeth A. Archer, EdD, RN
Associate Professor, Nursing
Baptist College of Health Sciences
Memphis, Tennessee

Alyce S. Ashcraft, PhD, RN, CS, CCRN
Associate Professor
Texas Tech University Health Sciences Center
Lubbock, Texas

Jeanie Krause-Bachand, BSN, MSN, EdD, RN BC
Associate Professor, Department of Nursing
York College of Pennsylvania
York, Pennsylvania

Valerie O'Toole Baker, APRN, BC
Assistant Professor
Villa Maria School of Nursing
Gannon University
Erie, Pennsylvania

Kristi Beam, MSN, RN
Nursing Instructor
Jacksonville State University
Jacksonville, Alabama

Renea L. Beckstrand, PhD, RN, CCRN
Associate Professor
Brigham Young University College of Nursing
Provo, Utah

Mary Spitak Bilitski, MSN, RN, CVN
Instructor of Nursing
The Washington Hospital School of Nursing
Washington, Pennsylvania

Wanda J. Borges, PhD, MSN, CNS-BC
Assistant Professor
New Mexico State University School of Nursing
Las Cruces, New Mexico

Debbie Bradford, MSN, ANP, RNCS-BC
Internal Medicine Specialty Nurse Leader
Harvard Vanguard Medical Associates
Quincy, Massachusetts
Instructor
MGH Institute of Health Professions
Boston, Massachusetts

Diane Breckenridge, PhD, RN
Associate Professor, School of Nursing
and Health Sciences
La Salle University
Philadelphia, Pennsylvania
Associate Research Director, Nursing Department
Abington Memorial Hospital
Abington, Pennsylvania

Roberta M. Bumann, RN, MSN
Assistant Professor, Nursing
Winona State University—Rochester
Staff RN, Intensive Care Unit
Mayo Clinic—Rochester
Rochester, Minnesota

Nita Jane Carrington, EdD, MSN, RN, ANP
Associate Professor
Hawaii Pacific University, School of Nursing
Honolulu, Hawaii

Karen Chandra, RN, MSN, MBA
Instructor
Harper College
Palatine, Illinois

Tammy Chapin, RN, MSN
Academic Staff/Lecturer
University of Wisconsin Oshkosh College of Nursing
Oshkosh, Wisconsin

Pamela J. Chapman, MSN, RN, CCRN
Assistant Professor
La Roche College
Pittsburgh, Pennsylvania

Dawn Clyens, RN, MN
Sessional Professor BScN Program
Mohawk College of Applied Arts and Technology
Hamilton, Ontario, Canada

Glenn Donnelly, RN, ENC(C), BScN, MN, PhD
Associate Professor
College of Nursing, University of Saskatchewan
Saskatoon, Saskatchewan, Canada

Margaret Downey, RN, PhD, CCRN, AHN-BC
Associate Professor
Boise State University Department of Nursing
Boise, Idaho

Judith B. Dyne, MS, RN, ARNP, BC
Assistant Professor of Nursing
Adult Nurse Practitioner—Cardiology
Utica College
Utica, New York

Mary Fabick, MSN, MEd, CEN
Associate Professor of Nursing
Milligan College
Milligan College, Tennessee

Teresa Faykus, MSN, CRNI
Instructor of Nursing
West Liberty State College
West Liberty, West Virginia

Toni J. Galvan, RN, CNS, MSN, CCRN, CEN
Staff Nurse, Surgical Intensive Care Unit
University Medical Center
Lubbock, Texas

Mary Gipson, MSN, ARNP
Assistant Professor
Jacksonville University
Jacksonville, Florida

Sandra Goldsworthy, RN, BScN, MSc, CNCC (C)
Coordinator, Critical Care Hub of Excellence
Nursing Professor
Durham College
Oshawa, Ontario, Canada

Karen Toby Haghenbeck, PhD, APRN, FNP, RN-BC, CCRN
Assistant Professor
Pace University
Lienhard School of Nursing
Pleasantville, New York

Jenny Hamner, RN, DSN
Assistant Dean and Associate Professor
Auburn University
Auburn, Alabama

Peggy Kalowes, RN, PhD, CNS
Director, Center for Women's Cardiac
Health and Research
Heart and Vascular Institute
Long Beach Memorial Hospital
Long Beach, California

Catherine T. Kelly, PhD, MA, RN, CEN, FAEN
Assistant Professor—Nursing
State University of New York at New Paltz
New Paltz, New York

Kristine M. L'Ecuyer, RN, MSN, CCNS
Associate Professor of Nursing
Saint Louis University School of Nursing
St. Louis, Missouri

R. Shelly Lancaster, MSN, RN
Instructor/Lecturer
University of Wisconsin
Oshkosh, Wisconsin

Will Lanman, RN, BSN
Critical Care Clinical Educator
Norton Hospital
Louisville, Kentucky

Sharon Little-Stoetzel, RN, MS
Associate Professor of Nursing
Graceland University
Independence, Missouri

Karen S. March, PhD, RN, CCRN, APRN-BC
Associate Professor of Nursing
York College of Pennsylvania
York, Pennsylvania

Caron Martin, MSN, RN
Associate Professor
School of Nursing and Health Professions
Northern Kentucky University
Highland Heights, Kentucky

Pamela S. Merida, RN, MS, CMSRN
Visiting Assistant Professor
Purdue University
West Lafayette, Indiana

Sheri R. Noviello, RN, PhD
Associate Professor
Columbus State University
Columbus, Georgia

Chris Orton, PhD, FNP-BC
Assistant Professor
Armstrong Atlantic State University
Savannah, Georgia

Efrosini A. Papaconstantinou, RN, MSc, PhD(c)
Sessional Assistant Professor
York University
Toronto, Ontario, Canada

Rebecca B. Parnell, RN, MNSc, CS
Assistant Professor of Nursing
Southern Arkansas University
Magnolia, Arkansas

Eva Peisachovich, RN, BScN, MScN
Faculty, Lecturer
York University
Toronto, Ontario, Canada

Deborah Pool, MS, RN, CCRN
Residential Faculty Department of Nursing
Glendale Community College
Glendale, Arizona

Mercy Mammah Popoola, PhD, RN, CNS, CFCN, FWACN
Nursing Program Director
Herzing College Atlanta
Atlanta, Georgia

Kathryn Wirtz Powell, PhD, RN, FNP
Associate Chief Nurse for Education and Research
Jesse Brown VA Medical Center
Clinical Assistant Professor, College of Nursing
University of Illinois at Chicago
Chicago, Illinois

Gail B. Rea, PhD, RN, CNE
Assistant Dean, Pre-Licensure Programs
Barnes-Jewish College
St. Louis, Missouri

Shirley Retzlaff, MSN, RN
Assistant Professor
BryanLGH College of Health Sciences
Lincoln, Nebraska

Catherine J. Rose, RN, MS
Nursing Faculty/Senior Chairperson
St. Joseph School of Nursing
North Providence, Rhode Island

Melanie Rush, MSN, RN
Nursing Instructor
Washington Hospital School of Nursing
Washington, Pennsylvania

Eileen Shackell, RN, MSN, CCNC(C)
Faculty, Critical Care Nursing
British Columbia Institute of Technology
Burnaby, British Columbia, Canada

Lynn C. Simko, PhD, RN, CCRN
Associate Professor
Duquesne University
Pittsburgh, Pennsylvania

Linda Slater-MacLean, RN, MN, CNCC(C)
Clinical Nurse Specialist
General Systems Intensive Care Unit,
University of Alberta Hospitals
Edmonton, Alberta, Canada

Carol S. Smith, PhD(c), MSN, RN
Assistant Professor
Lansing School of Nursing and Health Sciences
Bellarmine University
Louisville, Kentucky

Cynthia Lee Terry, RN, MSN, CCRN, EdD
Associate Professor
Health Sciences Division
Lehigh Carbon Community College
Schnecksville, Pennsylvania
Outdoor Emergency Care Instructor
National Ski Patrol
Blue Mountain Ski Area
Palmerton, Pennsylvania

Lori Thomas, PhD, ARNP, ACNP-BC/ANP-BC
Assistant Professor
Acute Care Nurse Practitioner Track Coordinator
University of Florida College of Nursing
Gainesville, Florida

Ronald S. Ulberg, MSN, RN, CCRN
Assistant Professor
College of Nursing
Brigham Young University
Provo, Utah

JoAlice Vecchio, RN, MSN, CCM, CSN, CNS
Associate Professor of Nursing
Community College of Allegheny County
Pittsburgh, Pennsylvania

Karen Vuckovic, RN, APRN-BC, CCRN, MS
Department of Medical-Surgical Nursing
Clinical Faculty
University of Illinois
Chicago, Illinois

Laura Jean Waight, MSN, RN
Instructor of Nursing
West Texas A&M University
Canyon, Texas

Sharon Wallace, MSN, RN, CCRN
Assistant Dean Senior Level, Instructor
Thomas Jefferson University
Jefferson College of Health Professions
Jefferson School of Nursing
Philadelphia, Pennsylvania

Susan A. Walsh, MN, RN, CCRN
Assistant Professor
School of Nursing
Clayton State University
Morrow, Georgia

Valerie Watters-Burke, DNSc, MSN, FNP-BC, PNP-BC
Chair of Graduate Nursing Program
Associate Professor
Union University
Germantown, Tennessee
Hanissian Health Care
Collierville, Tennessee

M. M. West, DNSc, CNE, RN
Assistant Dean and Associate Professor
Thomas Jefferson University
Jefferson School of Nursing
Nursing Education Center
Geisinger Medical Center
Danville, Pennsylvania

Trish Whelan, RN, BScN, MHS, ENC(C)
Nursing Instructor
Grant MacEwan College
Edmonton, Alberta, Canada

Diane E. White, RN, CCRN, PhD
Chair Department of Nursing
Associate Professor
Georgia Perimeter College
Clarkston, Georgia

Linda Wilson, RN, PhD, CPAN, CAPA, BC, CNE
Assistant Professor
Drexel University College of Nursing and Health Professions
Philadelphia, Pennsylvania

Preface

Carolyn Hudak and Barbara (Bobbie) Gallo were early pioneers in critical care nursing and in 1973 wrote the first edition of *Critical Care Nursing: A Holistic Approach*. Their text became a classic in the field of critical care nursing, and they continued to publish updated editions over the next several decades.

The ninth edition of the text represents a new beginning for the book. Carolyn and Bobbie have now retired, and we are proudly carrying on their legacy. Our goal is to remain true to their commitment to excellence by providing critical care nurses and nursing students with the most up-to-date information needed to care for patients and their families using a holistic framework.

Today's critical care nurse is expected to be able to care for critically ill patients in a variety of settings—no longer is critical care strictly "unit-based." Also, today's critically ill patient is liable to be older and even more critically ill than ever before. Advances in nursing, medicine, and technology; the rapidly changing health care climate; and the shortage of nursing staff and faculty are other factors that have come together to effect great changes in the practice of critical care nursing. A healthy work environment also is essential if critical care nurses are to make their optimal contribution to care of patients and families.

Critical care nurses, more than ever before, must possess an extensive body of knowledge in order to provide competent and compassionate care to critically ill patients and their families. Some of this knowledge can be gained through formal education and textbooks, like the one you hold in your hand. The rest can only be gained through experience. It is our goal, with this ninth edition of *Critical Care Nursing: A Holistic Approach*, to assist readers on their journey by providing a comprehensive, up-to-date resource and reference.

As in past editions, the goal of this text is to promote excellence in critical care nursing. Presenting theory and principles within the context of practical application helps the reader to gain competence and confidence in caring for critically ill patients and their families. As always, the patient as the center of the health care team's efforts is emphasized throughout. In the highly specialized and complicated technical environment of critical care, knowing when to merely be present with patients by sitting with them and demonstrating caring behaviors is just as important as knowing how to operate complex equipment and perform difficult procedures.

• AN OVERVIEW OF CRITICAL CARE NURSING: A HOLISTIC APPROACH, 9e

Critical Care Nursing: A Holistic Approach, Ninth Edition, consists of 13 parts. The following is a brief overview of those parts and the information they contain.

PART 1: THE CONCEPT OF HOLISM APPLIED TO CRITICAL CARE NURSING PRACTICE

The six chapters that make up Part 1 introduce the student to the concept of holistic care, as it applies in critical care practice. In Chapter 1, the student is introduced to critical care nursing practice. Chapters 2 and 3 review the psychosocial effects of critical illness on the patient and the family, respectively. These chapters also describe the effect of the critical care environment on the patient and review actions the nurse can take to help reduce environment-induced stress and promote healing. Chapter 4 emphasizes the role of patient and family education in critical care. Chapter 5 focuses on strategies for relieving pain and promoting comfort. We conclude the part with Chapter 6, which concentrates on end-of-life and palliative care.

PART 2: PROFESSIONAL PRACTICE ISSUES IN CRITICAL CARE

This part consists of three chapters that are of concern to the nursing profession. In Chapters 7 and 8, ethical and legal issues are explored. Chapter 9 describes characteristics of critical care nurses, delineates aspects of nursing professionalism, and defines critical attributes of nursing excellence.

PART 3: SPECIAL POPULATIONS IN CRITICAL CARE

The four chapters in this part focus on the special needs of certain groups of people who are critically ill. Chapters 10, 11, and 12 focus on the pediatric patient, the pregnant patient, and the elderly patient, respectively. Chapter 13 describes the role of the nurse in caring for the patient who is recovering from anesthesia.

PART 4: SPECIAL SITUATIONS IN CRITICAL CARE

This section opens with a chapter that focuses on the care of the patient who is being transported within or between facilities. The second chapter in this section is new and describes the role of the critical care nurse in disaster management.

PART 5: CARDIOVASCULAR SYSTEM

This part, the first of eight organ system–based parts, focuses on the care of the patient with a cardiovascular disorder. Each organ system–based part begins with a chapter that reviews the anatomy and physiology of the organ system under discussion (Chapter 16). The part then continues with a chapter on patient assessment (Chapter 17), general patient management (Chapter 18), and common disorders (Chapter 19). In Part 4, heart failure and acute myocardial infarction are each given their own chapters (Chapters 20 and 21, respectively). The unit concludes with a discussion of the most recent developments in cardiac surgery (Chapter 22). Throughout the unit, the latest diagnostic tests (such as cardiac serum markers), the newest medications for treating cardiovascular disorders, and updates on technologies (such as the left ventricular assist device, the implantable cardioverter defibrillator, and the cardiac pacemaker) are discussed.

PART 6: RESPIRATORY SYSTEM

In this part, current assessment technologies (such as end tidal carbon dioxide monitoring) and the newest modes of ventilation for patients in respiratory failure are discussed. Evidence-based treatment strategies for respiratory disorders such as pneumonia, pleural effusion, and chronic obstructive pulmonary disease are described. Chapter 27 is devoted to the latest developments in the assessment and management of the patient with acute respiratory distress syndrome (ARDS).

PART 7: RENAL SYSTEM

In this edition of the text, Part 7 includes a more in-depth discussion of the assessment and management of fluids, electrolytes, and acid-base balance. Updates on laboratory and diagnostic tests are included. The newest dialysis technologies and the latest drugs are discussed in Chapter 30. Chapter 31 focuses on common renal disorders, including recent developments in the care of the patient with renal failure.

PART 8: NERVOUS SYSTEM

This part offers updates on neurological diagnostic studies and the newest approaches to treating the patient with increased intracranial pressure. The latest drugs for treating neurological disorders and the most recent developments in neurosurgery are addressed. Separate chapters are devoted to care of the patient with a head injury and spinal cord injury.

PART 9: GASTROINTESTINAL SYSTEM

In Part 9, the latest diagnostic tests for evaluating patients with gastrointestinal disorders are discussed. The management of patients with gastrointestinal disorders has been updated to include the newest drugs, the latest developments in the use of enteral and parenteral nutrition, and recent trends in the treatment of common disorders such as liver failure and hepatitis.

PART 10: ENDOCRINE SYSTEM

In this edition, Part 10 includes an assessment chapter covering multiple components of the endocrine system. The content is organized by the major gland, and for each gland addressed in the chapter, the reader is given information on the history, laboratory tests, and diagnostic tests. The most current information on the treatment of endocrine disorders, especially glycemic control and diabetic emergencies, is included in Chapter 44.

PART 11: HEMATOLOGICAL AND IMMUNE SYSTEMS

This part continues to be a unique feature that is not included in many critical care texts. The numerous recent developments in organ and hematopoietic stem cell transplant are described in Chapter 47. Chapter 48 addresses up-to-date information on the assessment and management of critically ill patients with HIV/AIDS as well as those with oncological emergencies. The latest trends in the treatment of patients with hematological disorders such as disseminated intravascular coagulation are included in Chapter 49.

PART 12: INTEGUMENTARY SYSTEM

This part includes three chapters not covered in other critical care texts: the anatomy and physiology of the integumentary system, assessment of the integumentary system, and management of integumentary disorders, respectively. Evidence-based assessment and management of wounds are addressed. In addition, care of the critically ill burn patient is covered in Chapter 53.

PART 13: MULTISYSTEM DYSFUNCTION

In Chapter 54, hypoperfusion states such as shock, systemic inflammatory response syndrome (SIRS), and multiple organ dysfunction syndrome (MODS) are discussed. The latest understanding of the pathophysiologic process is described, as well as how this knowledge guides the selection of the most recent interventions. Chapter 55 reviews care of the trauma patient, including the latest trends in the management of these complex patients. Chapter 56 reviews care of the patient with a drug overdose or poisoning, a problem that is becoming more common in the critical care setting.

APPENDIX

An appendix completes the textbook; it contains updated ACLS guidelines.

• Features

The features of the ninth edition of *Critical Care Nursing: A Holistic Approach* have been designed to assist readers with practice as well as learning.

PRACTICE-ORIENTED FEATURES

▶ **Considerations for the Older Patient boxes.** Older adults constitute the fastest growing part of our population. As a result, the number of critically ill patients who are older is also increasing. These boxes highlight the special needs of this patient population.

▶ **Red Flag boxes.** These boxes alert readers to risk factors, signs and symptoms, side effects, and complications that the critical care nurse must be vigilant for.

▶ **Health History boxes.** These boxes summarize key areas that should be covered and relevant information that may be revealed during the health history.

▶ **Nursing Diagnoses and Collaborative Problems boxes.** Critical care nurses work both independently and collaboratively when caring for critically ill patients. These boxes summarize common nursing diagnoses and collaborative problems for particular conditions.

▶ **Collaborative Care Guides.** These boxes describe how the health care team works together to manage a patient's illness and minimize complications. The information is presented in a tabular format, with outcomes in the first column and interventions in the second.

▶ **Nursing Intervention Guides.** These boxes present guidelines for carrying out certain key nursing interventions.

▶ **Teaching Guides.** These boxes help the nurse to prepare patients and family members for procedures, assist patients and family members with understanding the illness they are dealing with, and explain postprocedure or postoperative activities.

▶ **Discharge Planning Guides.** These boxes, which were formerly called "Considerations for Home Care" boxes, outline what the nurse needs to consider when preparing a patient for discharge from the hospital.

▶ **Drug Therapy tables and boxes.** These tables and boxes summarize information related to the administration and monitoring of drug therapy.

▶ **Evidence-Based Practice Highlights.** These boxes help the reader to understand the importance of research-based practice.

▶ **Internet Resources.** Each part begins with a list of key websites of interest that direct the reader to sources of additional information and patient education materials.

PEDAGOGICAL FEATURES

▶ **Chapter Outlines and Learning Objectives.** Each chapter begins with an outline of the chapter and a list of learning objectives. These give the reader an overview of the chapter and help to focus his or her reading.

▶ **Clinical Applicability Challenges.** Each chapter concludes with a Clinical Applicability Challenge section. In the introductory chapters (Chapters 1 through 9) and the anatomy and physiology chapters (Chapters 16, 23, 28, 32, 42, 45, and 50), the Clinical Applicability Challenge consists of 3 to 5 **short-answer questions** and 5 to 10 **multiple-choice questions.** In the remaining chapters, the Clinical Applicability Challenge consists of a **case study** followed by 3 to 5 short-answer questions, and 5 to 10 multiple-choice questions. Answers with rationales to the multiple-choice questions are provided on thePoint.

▶ **References.** A list of current references cited in the chapter is given at the end of each chapter.

▶ **Other Selected Readings.** A bibliography is provided at the end of each chapter to encourage further reading of key sources relevant to the chapter.

• ANCILLARY PACKAGE

▶ **Instructor's Resource CD-ROM.** The instructor's resource CD contains the following items:
  ▶ A thoroughly revised Test Generator, featuring several hundred questions
  ▶ An Image Bank, containing illustrations from the book in formats suitable for printing and incorporating into PowerPoint presentations and Internet sites
  ▶ PowerPoint Presentations for each chapter
  ▶ Guided Lecture Notes for each chapter
  ▶ Concepts in Action Animations
  ▶ Monographs of 100 Commonly Prescribed Drugs
▶ **Interactive Front-of-Book CD-ROM.** Packaged with the textbook at no additional charge, this CD contains a wealth of resources for the student:
  ▶ Concepts in Action Animations
  ▶ Monographs of Most Commonly Prescribed Drugs
  ▶ NCLEX Alternative Item Format Tutorial
  ▶ Spanish-English Audio Glossary
▶ **ThePoint.** ThePoint (http://thepoint.lww.com) is a web-based course and content management system that provides every resource instructors and students need in one easy-to-use site. Advanced technology and superior content combine at thePoint to allow instructors to design and deliver on-line and off-line courses, maintain grades and class rosters, and communicate with students. Students can visit thePoint to access supplemental multimedia resources to enhance their learning experience, check the course syllabus, download content, upload assignments, and join an on-line study group. ThePoint . . . where teaching, learning, and technology click!

It is with great pleasure that we introduce these resources—the textbook and the ancillary package—to you. One of our primary goals in creating these resources has been to promote excellence in critical care nursing practice so that nurses can help patients and families cope with the consequences of critical illness. It is our intent that these resources will provide aspiring and currently practicing critical care nurses the tools to make their optimal contribution to the care of critically ill patients and their families and to the nursing profession. We hope that we have succeeded in that goal, and we welcome feedback from our readers.

Patricia Gonce Morton, RN, PhD, ACNP, FAAN
Dorrie Fontaine, RN, PhD, FAAN

• ACKNOWLEDGMENTS

This project required the help and cooperation of many people. First we want to thank our many colleagues who contributed to the text, either by authoring a chapter or by sharing their expertise as a reviewer. Our publisher through all editions of this book, Lippincott Williams & Wilkins, remains committed to producing the best text possible. We especially want to thank Melanie Cann, Senior Developmental Editor; Jane Velker, Director of Development—Nursing Education; and Elizabeth Nieginski, Executive Acquisitions Editor, for their support, humor, and words of positive encouragement as they cheered us on to the finish line with the project. Special thanks also to Laura Scott, Editorial Assistant, for her assistance with preparing the manuscript for Production; Tom Gibbons, Senior Production Editor, for his oversight of the production process; and Season Evans, Ancillary Editor, for her oversight of the ancillary package.

We also wish to express our thanks to Regina Mabrey, who compiled and checked all the websites that appear in the beginning of each part of the text. Her hours of work were an enormous help to us. And finally, we wish to express a word of thanks to our families and nursing colleagues who endured the time we took to complete this project.

Tricia and Dorrie

Contents

The Concept of Holism Applied to Critical Care Nursing Practice

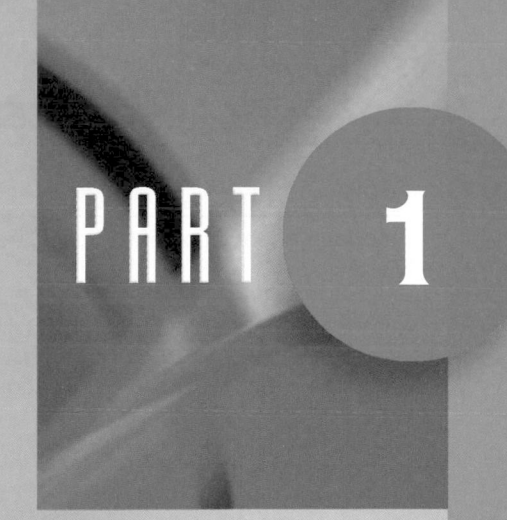

PART 1

INTERNET RESOURCES

Topic	Web Page Address
American Association of Critical Care Nurses	www.aacn.org
Americans for Better Care of the Dying	www.abcd-caring.org
American Holistic Nurses Association (AHNA)	www.ahna.org
American Pain Foundation	www.painfoundation.org
American Society of Pain Management Nurses	www.aspmn.org
Before I Die: Medical Care and Personal Choices	www.wnet.org/archive/bid
Canadian Association of Critical Care Nurses	www.caccn.ca
Center of Advanced Palliative Care	www.capcmssm.org
End of Life Nursing Education Center	www.aacn.nche.edu/elnec
Family Caregiver Alliance	www.caregiver.org
Growth House (Web-based resource for end-of-life care)	www.growthhouse.org
Healing Touch International, Inc.	www.healingtouch.net
Hospice Foundation of America	www.hospicefoundation.org
Hospice and Palliative Nurses Association	www.hpna.org
Institute for Family Centered Care	www.familycenteredcare.org
National Center for Complementary and Alternative Medicine	www.nccam.nih.gov
National Family Caregivers Association	www.nfcacares.org
National Hospice Organization	www.nho.org
National Hospice and Palliative Care Organization	www.nhpco.org
National MultiCultural Institute	www.nmci.org
Palliative Care Nursing Web site	www.palliativecarenursing.net
The Patient Education Institute	www.patient-education.com
Promoting Excellence in End-of-Life Care	www.promotingexcellence.org
Rand/Center to Improve Care of the Dying (CICD)	www.medicaring.org
Transcultural Nursing Society	www.tcns.org

Critical Care Nursing Practice: Promoting Excellence Through Caring, Competence, and Commitment

Roberta Kaplow • Michael Relf

Value of Certification
Value to the Patient and Family
Value to Employers
Value to Nurses

Evidence-Based Practice in Critical Care Nursing
Barriers to Implementation
Strategies to Promote Implementation

Healthy Work Environments
Skilled Communication
True Collaboration
Effective Decision Making
Appropriate Staffing
Meaningful Recognition
Authentic Leadership

The Synergy Model
Future Challenges in Critical Care Nursing

Objectives

Based on the content in this chapter, the reader should be able to:

❶ Describe the value of certification in critical care nursing.

❷ Describe the value of evidence-based practice in caring for critically ill patients.

❸ Discuss the value of collaborative practice in critical care.

❹ Provide examples of how the Synergy Model can promote positive patient outcomes.

❺ Discuss future issues facing critical care nursing practice.

As the health care delivery system continues to evolve and transform, so too does the discipline of nursing and the specialty of critical care nursing. Today, the care of critically ill patients occurs not only in the traditional setting of the hospital intensive care unit (ICU) but also on the progressive care unit, the medical unit, and the surgical unit, as well as in the subacute facility, the community, and the home. Since the first critical care unit opened in the late 1960s, significant technological, procedural, and pharmacological advances have occurred, accompanied by a knowledge explosion in critical care nursing. Consequently, critical care nurses of the 21st century are routinely caring for the complex, critically ill patient, integrating sophisticated technology with the accompanying psychosocial challenges and ethical conflicts associated with critical illness while addressing the needs and concerns of the family.

In response to the ever-changing delivery system, critical care nurses are championing the needs of the patient and the family and developing healthy work environments that yield quality clinical outcomes while optimizing professional collaboration and nursing practice. During the past several decades, critical care nurses have experienced first hand what nurse scientists have consistently demonstrated—critical illness is not only a physiological alteration but also a psychosocial, developmental, and spiritual process as well as a threat to the individual and his or her family. Through specialty certification by the American Association of Critical-Care Nurses (AACN), professional nurses voluntarily demonstrate their breadth and depth of knowledge of critical care nursing. Furthermore, as health care becomes increasingly technological, the concurrent need for humanization is increasingly essential. Compatible with the need for "humanized" health care is the necessity of providing effective interventions that are based on evidence instead of being steeped in tradition.

This chapter describes select aspects of the critical care environment. These include the value of certification, evidence-based practice, healthy work environments, and the AACN Synergy Model for Patient Care. Each of these, when implemented, helps promote optimal outcomes for acute and critically ill patients and their families who are being cared for in a complex health care environment.

• Value of Certification

"Certification is a process by which a nongovernmental agency validates, based on predetermined standards, an individual nurse's qualification and knowledge for practice in a defined functional or clinical area of nursing."[1] Certification promotes continuing excellence in the critical care nursing profession, helping nurses achieve and maintain an up-to-date knowledge base of critical care nursing.[2,3] In addition, it validates their knowledge of the acute and critically ill to patients and families, to employers, and to themselves. A white paper, *Safeguarding the Patient and the Profession*, published in 2003 by the AACN, demonstrated and recognized the value of specialty certification.[2]

VALUE TO THE PATIENT AND FAMILY

Consumers are increasingly frightened of the health care system, and this lack of trust is universal. Certification provides patients and families with validation that the nurses caring for them have demonstrated experience and knowledge. This knowledge exceeds that which is assessed in entry-level licensure examinations.[2]

As research has suggested, nurses who have had their knowledge validated through a certification examination make decisions with greater confidence.[4] Although "failure to rescue" a patient in trouble cannot always be avoided, experienced and knowledgeable nurses are able to recognize signs and symptoms and respond accordingly. This can be critical to ensuring optimal outcomes. In addition, nurses who are certified in a specialty have demonstrated commitment to continual learning. This is an attribute that is needed to care for patients with complex multisystem problems.

VALUE TO EMPLOYERS

Certification allows the employer to know that the nurses working for them have the knowledge and experience to work efficiently to promote optimal patient outcomes. Nurses who take the initiative to become certified have demonstrated their commitment to quality and the profession. It can be assumed that if a nurse has taken the time to become certified in a specialty, the nurse intends to remain employed in an area where he or she can apply the knowledge. As such, certification sends a message of commitment to the employer. It has been suggested that organizations that support and recognize the value of certification may experience improved turnover and retention rates.[5] Certification is also a means for hospitals to distinguish themselves from competitors and to demonstrate to health care consumers that they have recruited and retained knowledge-validated nurses.[2]

As health care organizations apply to achieve Magnet designation by the American Nurses Credentialing Center (ANCC), certification is one of the many important factors considered and is of considerable significance for the organization.[6] In addition, hospital administrators must demonstrate to the Joint Commission (formerly the Joint Commission for Accreditation of Healthcare Organizations [JCAHO]) that nurses are competent to provide care. Certification is a clear demonstration of knowledge competency.[7]

VALUE TO NURSES

Certification provides nurses with a sense of professional pride and achievement.[1] A survey by AACN revealed that most nurses who sat for certification examinations did so for personal fulfillment and commitment to excellence in practice.[8] Certification demonstrates to the employer that the nurses are taking personal responsibility for their own professional development, and it may give nurses a competitive edge when seeking promotion or new career opportunities. Certified nurses have a greater sense of confidence.

In addition, certified nurses can anticipate increased recognition from peers and employers. An anonymous certificant stated that "getting certified has given me the recognition I expected from my hospital and my profession" (meaningful recognition and its value are discussed later in this chapter). One of the world's largest insurance brokers offers a discount on malpractice premiums to nurses who are certified in critical care.[2] A survey reported that 77% of respondents reported that certification enabled them to experience personal growth and that 67% felt more satisfied as professional nurses.[4] Some hospitals recognize certification with a salary differential. The average full-time annual income of certified nurses is reportedly almost $10,000 higher than that of noncertified nurses.[8]

Researchers have found that certified nurses had higher perceptions of empowerment. They have suggested that the enhanced empowerment may improve work effectiveness.[5] Other investigators have found that more than 90% of certified nurses agreed or strongly agreed that certification resulted in feelings of personal accomplishment and satisfaction. These nurses believed that certification validated knowledge of their specialty, enhanced their professional growth, and demonstrated professional commitment and credibility.[9]

• Evidence-Based Practice in Critical Care Nursing

Evidence-based practice (EBP) is the use of the best available research data from well-designed studies, coupled with experiential knowledge and patient preferences in clinical practice in order to support clinical decision making.[10] Nursing practice changes on almost a daily basis, partly because of advances in nursing research.[11] EBP is essential to help optimize patient outcomes in today's dynamic health care environment.

Although knowledge regarding effectual nursing interventions continues to increase, practice lags behind the available evidence. The use of research findings in clinical practice is essential to promote optimal outcomes and to ensure that nursing practice is both cost-efficient and effective.[12] Practice based on intuition or information that does not have a scientific basis is not in the best interest of patients and families and should be discouraged when care decisions are being made. Efforts by individuals, groups, and organizations to implement EBP are essential.

BARRIERS TO IMPLEMENTATION

Despite the perceived value of EBP, transfer of evidence is a multifaceted process.[13] It takes an average of 17 to 20 years for research findings to be translated into clinical practice.[14,15] As identified in the literature, the numerous barriers to the implementation of EBP include lack of knowledge, lack of skills/resources, changing behavior, and lack of organizational support and management commitment. Researchers classified barriers to incorporating EBP into the clinical setting by the user.[16] Specifically, they identified individual practitioners, the clinical team, the practice setting, and organizational factors.

In two surveys of nurses regarding knowledge of EBP, 86% of respondents had not heard of the term, and 43% were unaware of sources of information and resources for EBP.[17] A recently conducted survey of randomly selected nurses nationwide found that approximately 50% of the nurses had not heard of EBP.[18] Although just over 25% had been taught to use electronic databases for information searches, most of the respondents reported that they did not use such databases to obtain information on practice issues.

Other investigators noted that nurses also reported lack of time, lack of relevant skills, and poor teamwork as barriers.[19] A report has corroborated the existence of some of these barriers.[20] However, in another study, researchers found that 42% of nurses did feel adequately prepared to evaluate research.[21] Fewer than 33% of these nurses believed they had the competency necessary to conduct scientific research studies. Some nurses believed they were able to access and review data but were less confident about their ability to change practice.[20]

As previously mentioned, another part of the complexity of implementing an EBP model is the challenge associated with changing provider behavior.[13] Data from one study indicated a lack of support and management commitment to EBP in the participating organization.[21] Nurses in another study reported lack of support, authority, and incentives as barriers to embracing an EBP culture.[19]

STRATEGIES TO PROMOTE IMPLEMENTATION

Various articles have proposed several strategies to help enhance incorporating evidence into clinical practice. Use of protocols, clinical pathways, and algorithms is one approach to bringing evidence-based standards to the bedside.[16] Some investigators have recommended use of interventions to improve knowledge, access, and implementation of EBP for nurses working in clinical settings.[17] Other researchers have suggested using educational interventions.[21] They have proposed increasing clinicians' awareness of available resources and that these clinicians be educated and mentored when carrying out EBP activities.

One report described formation of a critical care research utilization committee.[12] Organizers sought representatives from each of the adult ICUs, the emergency department, and the postanesthesia care unit. The tasks of the committee members included review and revision of each policy and procedure based on the best available evidence. As a result, the committee generated research questions based on identified gaps in the literature, and this led to enhanced staff utilization of research.

Another author has suggested using multifaceted interventions to assist with implementation.[13] Similarly, others have recommended strategies such as identifying EBP champions, incorporating EBP activities into nurses' roles, allocating time and money to the process, and developing an organizational culture that promotes EBP.[22] Part of the organizational culture may include promotion of multidisciplinary collaboration among researchers and practitioners.

Several resources are available for clinician use to facilitate adoption of an EBP culture. Several databases are available, including PubMed, CINAHL, and MEDLINE. Many practice settings subscribe to UpToDate, a website designed to assist clinicians confronting daily clinical challenges by offering real-time evidenced-based recommendations for patient care. The Cochrane Library, a website containing high-quality, independent evidence to inform health care decision making, is also a valuable tool to obtain evidence-based information.

In addition, professional nursing organizations may have research-based practice suggestions posted on their websites. For example, AACN has a Practice Alerts section that is available to members as well as to the public.[23] Examples of Practice Alerts that are currently available include Noninvasive Blood Pressure Monitoring, Severe Sepsis, Deep Vein Thrombosis Prevention, Preventing Catheter-Related Bloodstream Infections, Verification of Feeding Tube Placement, Dye in Enteral Feedings, Family Presence During CPR and Invasive Procedures, ST Segment Monitoring, Dysrhythmia Monitoring, Pulmonary Artery Pressure Monitoring, and Ventilator Associated Pneumonia.

• Healthy Work Environments

The current health care climate and the nursing shortage call for major change in the workplace. A healthy work environment (HWE) can lead to positive patient outcomes. In addition, nurses gravitate to facilities that have optimal work conditions. Conversely, unhealthy work environments play a role in errors, ineffective care, and moral distress.

In 2001, AACN affirmed that the best way to address the nursing shortage was to focus on HWEs. After conducting an extensive literature search, the AACN helped develop the HWE initiative, which is based on data indicating that harmful health care working environments exist nationwide and that these environments result in medical errors, poor health care delivery, and dissatisfaction among health care providers. A nine-person expert panel was chaired by a past president of the AACN, Connie Barden. The HWE standards are based on analysis of several focus groups, interviews, and workplace observations. After the standards were delineated, a 50-person national expert review panel validated the standards and the critical elements within them. AACN made the six standards public at a national briefing in Washington, D.C., in January 2005.

The HWE initiative focuses on barriers to employee and patient safety and identifies six essential standards: skilled communication; true collaboration; effective decision making; appropriate staffing; meaningful recognition; and authentic leadership (Box 1-1).[24] The six elements discussed encompass the aspects that are most important as nurses strive to provide patients with optimal care.[25] Boxes 1-2 through 1-7 list the critical elements inherent in the respective standards.

Box 1-1 • Essential Elements of a Healthy Work Environment

- *Skilled Communication.* Nurses must be as proficient in communication skills as they are in clinical skills.
- *True Collaboration.* Nurses must be relentless in pursuing and fostering true collaboration.
- *Effective Decision Making.* Nurses must be valued and committed partners in making policy, directing and evaluating clinical care, and leading organizational operations.
- *Appropriate Staffing.* Staffing must ensure the effective match between patient needs and nurse competencies.
- *Meaningful Recognition.* Nurses must be recognized and must recognize others for the value each brings to the work of the organization.
- *Authentic Leadership.* Nurse leaders must fully embrace the imperative of a healthy work environment, authentically live it, and engage others in its achievement.

From http://www.aacn.org/aacn/pubpolcy.nsf.

Box 1-2 • Standard 1: Critical Elements of Skilled Communication

Nurses must be as proficient in communication skills as they are in clinical skills.

- The health care organization provides team members with support for and access to education programs that develop critical communication skills including self-awareness, inquiry/dialogue, conflict management, negotiation, advocacy, and listening.
- Skilled communicators focus on finding solutions and achieving desirable outcomes.
- Skilled communicators seek to protect and advance collaborative relationships among colleagues.
- Skilled communicators invite and hear all relevant perspectives.
- Skilled communicators call on goodwill and mutual respect to build consensus and arrive at common understanding.
- Skilled communicators demonstrate congruence between words and actions, holding others accountable for doing the same.
- The health care organization establishes zero-tolerance policies and enforces them to address and eliminate abuse and disrespectful behavior in the workplace.
- The health care organization establishes formal structures and processes that ensure effective information sharing among patients, families, and the health care team.
- Skilled communicators have access to appropriate communication technologies and are proficient in their use.
- The health care organization establishes systems that require individuals and teams to formally evaluate the impact of communication on clinical, financial, and work environment outcomes.
- The health care organization includes communication as a criterion in its formal performance appraisal system, and team members demonstrate skilled communication to qualify for professional advancement.

From http://www.aacn.org/aacn/pubpolcy.nsf/Files/ExecSum/$file/ExecSum.pdf.

Box 1-3 • Standard 2: Critical Elements of True Collaboration

Nurses must be relentless in pursuing and fostering true collaboration.

- The health care organization provides team members with support for and access to education programs that develop collaboration skills.
- The health care organization creates, uses, and evaluates processes that define each team member's accountability for collaboration and how unwillingness to collaborate will be addressed.
- The health care organization creates, uses, and evaluates operational structures that ensure the decision-making authority of nurses is acknowledged and incorporated as the norm.
- The health care organization ensures unrestricted access to structured forums, such as ethics committees, and makes available the time needed to resolve disputes among all critical participants, including patients, families, and the health care team.
- Every team member embraces true collaboration as an ongoing process and invests in its development to ensure a sustained culture of collaboration.
- Every team member contributes to the achievement of common goals by giving power and respect to each person's voice, integrating individual differences, resolving competing interests, and safeguarding the essential contribution each must make in order to achieve optimal outcomes.
- Every team member acts with a high level of personal integrity.
- Team members master skilled communication, an essential element of true collaboration.
- Each team member demonstrates competence appropriate to his or her role and responsibilities.
- Nurse managers and medical directors are equal partners in modeling and fostering true collaboration.

From http://www.aacn.org/aacn/pubpolcy.nsf/Files/ExecSum/$file/ExecSum.pdf.

Box 1-4 • Standard 3: Critical Elements of Effective Decision Making

Nurses must be valued and committed partners in making policy, directing and evaluating clinical care, and leading organizational operations.

- The health care organization provides team members with support for and access to ongoing education and development programs focusing on strategies that ensure collaborative decision making. Program content includes mutual goal setting, negotiation, facilitation, conflict management, systems thinking, and performance improvement.
- The health care organization clearly articulates organizational values, and team members incorporate these values when making decisions.
- The health care organization has operational structures in place that ensure the perspectives of patients and their families are incorporated into every decision affecting patient care.
- Individual team members share accountability for effective decision making by acquiring necessary skills, mastering relevant content, assessing situations accurately, sharing fact-based information, communicating professional opinions clearly, and inquiring actively.
- The health care organization establishes systems, such as structured forums involving all departments and health care disciplines, to facilitate data-driven decisions.
- The health care organization establishes deliberate decision-making processes that ensure respect for the rights of every individual, incorporate all key perspectives, and designate clear accountability.
- The health care organization has fair and effective processes in place at all levels to objectively evaluate the results of decisions, including delayed decisions and indecision.

From http://www.aacn.org/aacn/pubpolcy.nsf/Files/ExecSum/$file/ExecSum.pdf.

SKILLED COMMUNICATION

Dr. Dennis O'Leary, President of the Joint Commission, was a featured speaker at the press conference that unveiled the HWE standards. He noted that "communication is the most common problem underlying medical errors."[26] Skilled communication is essential to prevent errors as well as to recruit and retain health care providers. Almost 70% of sentinel events reported to the Joint Commission in 2005 were related to communication issues. This is an increase from 65% in 1995 to 2004.[26]

AACN partnered with VitalSmarts to conduct a study of conversations that do not occur in hospitals, to the detriment of patient safety and provider well-being. The "Silence Kills" study used focus groups, interviews, observations in the workplace, and surveys of nurses, physicians, and administrators in urban, rural, and suburban hospitals nationwide.[27] Overwhelming data indicated that poor communication and collaboration were prevalent among health care providers.

In this report,[27] more than 92% of practitioners surveyed witnessed disruptive behavior by physicians, and 77% reported that they work with some who are condescending, rude, or verbally abusive. A pharmacist reported letting incorrect orders "slide" if the physician is a "jerk" and the incorrect dose was not going to make the patient sicker. Another pharmacist reported filling an incorrect prescription without question because of the hostility experienced when challenged in the past. Several physicians in this study stated that they worked with peers who were incompetent, but they did not confront them. Rather, they avoided scheduling sicker patients when the incompetent physician was scheduled to work. Another physician reported leaving a practice because of another's poor work ethic. In this case, the physician would delay patient issues until the next morning. The data further suggested that physicians are equally as

Box 1-5 • Standard 4: Critical Elements of Appropriate Staffing

Staffing must ensure the effective match between patient needs and nurse competencies.

- The health care organization has staffing policies in place that are solidly grounded in ethical principles and support the professional obligation of nurses to provide high quality care.
- Nurses participate in all organizational phases of the staffing process from education and planning—including matching nurses' competencies with patients' assessed needs—through evaluation.
- The health care organization has formal processes in place to evaluate the effect of staffing decisions on patient and system outcomes. This evaluation includes analysis of when patient needs and nurse competencies are mismatched and how often contingency plans are implemented.
- The health care organization has a system in place that facilitates team members' use of staffing and outcomes data to develop more effective staffing models.
- The health care organization provides support services at every level of activity to ensure nurses can optimally focus on the priorities and requirements of patient and family care.
- The health care organization adopts technologies that increase the effectiveness of nursing care delivery. Nurses are engaged in the selection, adaptation and evaluation of these technologies.

From http://www.aacn.org/aacn/pubpolcy.nsf/Files/ExecSum/$file/ExecSum.pdf.

Box 1-6 • Standard 5: Critical Elements of Meaningful Recognition

Nurses must be recognized and must recognize others for the value each brings to the work of the organization.

- The health care organization has a comprehensive system in place that includes formal processes and structured forums that ensure a sustainable focus on recognizing all team members for their contributions and the value they bring to the work of the organization.
- The health care organization establishes a systematic process for all team members to learn about the institution's recognition system and how to participate by recognizing the contributions of colleagues and the value they bring to the organization.
- The health care organization's recognition system reaches from the bedside to the board table, ensuring individuals receive recognition consistent with their personal definition of meaning, fulfillment, development, and advancement at every stage of their professional career.
- The health care organization's recognition system includes processes that validate that recognition is meaningful to those being acknowledged.
- Team members understand that everyone is responsible for playing an active role in the organization's recognition program and meaningfully recognizing contributions.
- The health care organization regularly and comprehensively evaluates its recognition system, ensuring effective programs that help to move the organization toward a sustainable culture of excellence that values meaningful recognition.

From http://www.aacn.org/aacn/pubpolcy.nsf/Files/ExecSum/$file/ExecSum.pdf.

Box 1-7 • Standard 6: Critical Elements of Authentic Leadership

Nurse leaders must fully embrace the imperative of a healthy work environment, authentically live it, and engage others in its achievement.

- The health care organization provides support for and access to educational programs to ensure that nurse leaders develop and enhance knowledge and abilities in skilled communication, effective decision making, true collaboration, meaningful recognition, and ensuring resources to achieve appropriate staffing.
- Nurse leaders demonstrate an understanding of the requirements and dynamics at the point of care and within this context successfully translate the vision of a healthy work environment.
- Nurse leaders excel at generating visible enthusiasm for achieving the standards that create and sustain healthy work environments.
- Nurse leaders lead the design of systems necessary to effectively implement and sustain standards for healthy work environments.
- The health care organization ensures that nurse leaders are appropriately positioned in their pivotal role in creating and sustaining healthy work environments. This includes participation in key decision-making forums, access to

essential information, and the authority to make necessary decisions.
- The health care organization facilitates the efforts of nurse leaders to create and sustain a healthy work environment by providing the necessary time and financial and human resources.
- The health care organization provides a formal co-mentoring program for all nurse leaders. Nurse leaders actively engage in the co-mentoring program.
- Nurse leaders role-model skilled communication, true collaboration, effective decision making, meaningful recognition, and authentic leadership.
- The health care organization includes the leadership contribution to creating and sustaining a healthy work environment as a criterion in each nurse leader's performance appraisal. Nurse leaders must demonstrate sustained leadership in creating and sustaining a healthy work environment to achieve professional advancement.
- Nurse leaders and team members mutually and objectively evaluate the impact of leadership processes and decisions on the organization's progress toward creating and sustaining a healthy work environment.

From http://www.aacn.org/aacn/pubpolcy.nsf/Files/ExecSum/$file/ExecSum.pdf.

unlikely to confront a peer as a nurse or other health care provider. This study also stated that 88% of physicians reported working with people with persistent poor clinical judgment, causing deleterious complications.

Nurses described working with peers who are imprecise and negligent. In one case, instead of confronting their colleague, other nurses reviewed her work and rechecked her patients. Only 7% of the nurses surveyed reported having spoken with their peers. According to the report, 48% of surveyed nurses worked with health care providers whose consistent poor clinical decisions had harmful results.[27] Seventy-seven percent of nurses were concerned about the disrespect they experience. They reported being treated discourteously or abusively at least 25% of the time. Researchers found a significant correlation between the frequency of being mistreated and the intent to resign from the job. The study concluded that health care providers repeatedly observe errors, breaking of rules, and dangerous levels of incompetence. Yet they do not speak up; rather, they consider leaving their respective units because of their concerns. These viewpoints play a role in ongoing medication errors and lack of staff retention.

TRUE COLLABORATION

Collaboration is a multifaceted concept, which has been defined as working together to accomplish a common goal.[28] One researcher has identified collaboration as both a process and an outcome in which an issue is addressed by multiple stakeholders.[29] It involves a blending of different points of view to better comprehend a difficult issue. The collaborative outcome is the integration of solutions contributed by more than one person.[29] According to this same researcher, there are 10 lessons in collaboration. The lessons include (1) know thyself; (2) learn to value and manage diversity; (3) develop constructive conflict resolution skills; (4) use personal power to create win–win situations; (5) master interpersonal and process skills; (6) recognize that collaboration is a journey; (7) leverage all multidisciplinary forums; (8) appreciate that collaboration can occur spontaneously; (9) balance autonomy and unity in collaborative relationships; and (10) remember that collaboration is not required for all decisions.[29] Other investigators have suggested that collaboration is defined through five concepts: sharing, partnership, power, interdependency, and process.[30]

Ninety percent of all AACN members have reported that collaboration with physicians and administrators is among the most important elements in creating an HWE. Results of several studies have supported a high correlation between nurse–physician collaboration and positive patient outcomes.[31–35] There is a relationship between collaboration and a decreased incidence of medication errors.[36] One researcher has reported a direct relationship between nurse–physician collaboration and efficiency of health care workers.[31] Others have addressed the importance of collaborative relationships between physicians and pharmacists.[37]

Interprofessional collaboration is a vital aspect of plans designed to increase the effectiveness of delivery of health care.[30,38,39] Despite the reported benefits of collaboration, it is not practiced often enough.[29] A number of barriers exist that preclude its existence in health care organizations. The lack of an agreed-upon definition and variation in how collaboration is conceptualized, the lack of time for communication, and the complexity of the skills required to ease the process are daunting.[29,30] Other barriers include issues related to autonomy, contrasting insight with decision making, role confusion, and power issues.[40]

In the book *Internal Bleeding—The Truth Behind America's Terrifying Epidemic of Medical Mistakes*, the authors reported that despite the fact that nurses and physicians have worked closely together, "there is still little understanding and appreciation for each others' roles."[41] Collaboration requires each member of the health care team to listen to and respect others' perspectives. The question of "why is collaboration so hard to embrace when the evidence supports better outcomes when there is communication and collaboration?" requires an answer.[41]

Researchers conducted a meta-analysis to determine the effectiveness of interventions developed to enhance nurse–physician collaboration relating to patient satisfaction and effectiveness and efficiency of health care.[42] Although numerous strategies to enhance collaboration (e.g., joint workshops, meetings, team system development, and training in collaboration) have been suggested, no studies measured the efficacy of these interventions on the delineated outcomes. The authors suggested that more research is needed to assess efficacy of interprofessional collaboration and patient outcomes.

EFFECTIVE DECISION MAKING

Clinical decision making is an essential component of nursing responsibilities in an effort to promote quality patient outcomes. Researchers do not agree about the role of knowledge in decision making. Some have suggested that it entails application of knowledge learned in the classroom and through readings. Others have proposed that clinical decision-making skills involve experiential knowledge and intuition.[43] Yet, as described in the *AACN Standards for Establishing and Sustaining Healthy Work Environments*, "a significant gap often exists between what nurses are accountable for and their ability to participate in decisions that affect those accountabilities."[44] The standards also note that only a small percentage of physicians acknowledge nurses as part of the decision-making team.

In a study of nurses working in medical, surgical, and critical care units, investigators found that the majority of nurses made clinical decisions related to direct patient care on a regular basis.[45] Nurses working in the ICU reported commonly making decisions in emergency situations and deciding to change patient medication. Medical and surgical nurses only made these types of decisions on an occasional basis. The amount of clinical experience correlated with frequency of decision making.

Other researchers conducted a study that explored the relationship between interdisciplinary teamwork and nurse autonomy on patient and nurse outcomes and nurse-assessed quality of care.[46] Results supported a positive correlation among nursing autonomy, control over resources, relationship with physicians, emotional exhaustion, and decision making. These variables also correlated with nurse-assessed quality of care and nurse satisfaction. Furthermore, a positive relationship was reported between nursing autonomy and better perceptions of the quality of care delivered and higher levels of job satisfaction. Higher teamwork scores were associated with higher levels of nurse-assessed quality of care and perceived quality improvement. Nurses with higher teamwork scores had higher levels of autonomy and were more involved in decision making. Finally, data from this study suggest a strong association between teamwork and autonomy.

To promote quality patient outcomes, nurses must monitor patients and prevent and recognize problems promptly. Part of their role is to work with a multidisciplinary team to identify complex patient problems, a role with high levels of accountability. A high degree of responsibility and autonomy is necessary. If hospitals are going to continue to retain nurses and if quality patient outcomes are to result, methods that encourage nurses to participate in decision making must be consistent and successful. Because the health care environment mandates that nurses be accountable for their practice, they must be able to participate in effective decision making.

APPROPRIATE STAFFING

Using traditional models, adequacy of staffing has been based primarily on the number of staff assigned to a unit on a given shift. Appropriate staffing must consider the competencies of the staff assigned in relation to the needs of the patient and family during that shift. When the needs of patients and families are matched with the competencies of the assigned nurse, optimal outcomes may be achieved.

In 2002, a study indicated that when the nurse/patient ratio was 1:8, the patient's risk for death was 31% higher than when the nurse/patient ratio was 1:4 or lower. After the fourth patient, each surgical patient added to a nurse's assignment resulted in a 7% increase in chance of patient death within 30 days of hospital admission and a 7% increase in failure to rescue. In addition, nurses working in hospitals with higher nurse/patient ratios were more likely to develop burnout and job dissatisfaction.[47]

Other researchers found significant relationships between nurse staffing and adverse patient events.[48] In this case, the incidence of pneumonia and the probability of developing a pressure ulcer both increased

and were associated with an increased length of stay (and increased medical costs). The hospital mortality rate was greater in patients who developed pneumonia, wound infection, or sepsis. The authors concluded that appropriate nurse staffing is an important consideration. Other studies cited in the literature have supported a relationship between nurse staffing and hospital mortality.[49]

Investigators have reported a higher risk for respiratory complications in patients undergoing abdominal aortic surgery in ICUs with higher nurse/patient ratios.[50] Researchers found that a lower in-hospital mortality rate of patients who sustained acute myocardial infarction was associated with higher nursing staff levels,[51] thus corroborating these findings. These authors further reported a higher mortality rate in hospitals with higher licensed practical nurse staffing. According to the Joint Commission, staffing levels were a root cause of 24% of the sentinel events in their database from 1995 to 2004 that resulted in death, injury, or permanent loss of function.[26]

In its report, *Keeping Patients Safe: Transforming the Work Environment of Nurses,* the Institute of Medicine acknowledged the relationship between nurse staffing and quality of care.[52] Nurse staffing levels and the knowledge and skill level of the nursing staff have an impact on both patient outcomes and safety. The Institute further acknowledged that the temporary fixes implemented by health care organizations such as mandatory overtime or leaving units understaffed are ineffective, contributing to errors; these solutions are counterproductive to the nation's efforts to recruit and retain nurses and reduce medical errors.

In her Presidential Address at the National Teaching Institute in 2004, Dorrie Fontaine stated, "Nurses are a hospital's most precious resource; one that is in shortest supply. Would you expect a precious resource to go chasing after urinals and linen? Yet hospitals seem willing to spend hundreds of thousands of dollars recruiting new nurses, instead of addressing solvable systems errors that will retain nurses in the first place."[53] It is unrealistic to expect to monitor patient health status, perform therapeutic interventions, integrate patient care to avoid health care gaps, and promote optimal patient outcomes properly with inadequate numbers of nurses who lack the required competencies.

MEANINGFUL RECOGNITION

Effective recognition programs are important to retain high-performing nurses, to engage them actively in providing patient satisfaction, to use scarce nursing resources appropriately, and to enhance nursing accomplishment. Employee recognition can have a significant effect on job satisfaction. The recognition may be modest in scale but must represent genuine caring and appreciation.[54] Monetary rewards may not be feasible in the current health care climate, but verbal and written praise may suffice. However, according to an AACN report, most nurses are disappointed with the recognition they receive from their employer.[44]

Meaningful employee recognition may mean more than acknowledgment for high performance. Because of generational differences, employees today want more out of a job than a big salary.[55] Researchers have suggested that to recruit and retain staff, employers need to recognize staff expectations. Specifically, staff want to lead balanced lives, enjoy partnership with their employers, receive opportunities for personal and professional growth, be able to make a meaningful contribution to the world through their work, and experience opportunities to socialize at work.

There seems to be universal agreement that to retain staff during a critical shortage, in addition to monetary rewards when possible, expression of understanding, recognition for excellent performance, and appreciation are part of the strategy.[56-59] The American Organization of Nurse Executives has corroborated this conclusion.[60] Demonstrating the value of nurses' contributions to the quality of health care is among the recommendations for ensuring an adequate workforce in the future.

AUTHENTIC LEADERSHIP

People are drawn to places that provide a positive work environment. Nursing leaders are essential to create a health care environment that is conducive to promoting quality patient outcomes and health for staff.[61-64] According to the Joint Commission, leadership was a root cause of approximately 14% of the sentinel events in their database from 1995 to 2004 that resulted in death, injury, or permanent loss of function. The percentage increased to greater than 30% for sentinel events in 2005.[26] According to 2006 data, leadership was the root cause of almost 50% of sentinel events reported to the Joint Commission.

Researchers have described authentic leadership as "the 'glue' needed to hold together a healthy work environment."[65] A recent article delineated the five attributes of an authentic leader that are essential for establishing and maintaining an HWE: genuineness, trustworthiness, reliability, compassion, and believability.[66] Descriptors of an authentic leader include "an individual in a position of responsibility who is genuine, trustworthy, reliable, and believable," one who is "confident, hopeful, optimistic, resilient, and high on moral character," and one who "create[s] lasting organizational value that extends well beyond bottom-line success."[66-68]

One report has identified five evidence-based processes that are always essential in a health care environment: (1) balancing the tension between production and efficiency, (2) creating and sustaining trust throughout the organization, (3) actively managing the process of change, (4) involving workers in decision making pertaining to work design and work flow, and (5) using knowledge management to establish the organization as a learning organization.[66] It is essential that nurse leaders translate these evidence-based processes to the bedside. The researcher concluded by noting that authentic leadership may be essential to establish and sustain HWEs and may hold promise in creating lasting organizational and professional value.

• The Synergy Model

The Synergy Model developed by the AACN has served as the foundation for certified practice since the late 1990s.[69-71] Developed based on the results of a think tank commissioned by the AACN, the model describes nursing practice on the basis of the needs and characteristics of patients. The underlying premises of the Synergy Model are as follows: (1) patients' characteristics are of concern to nurses; (2) nurses' competencies are important to patients; (3) patients' characteristics drive nurses' competencies; and (4) when patients' characteristics and nurses' competencies match and synergize, outcomes for the patient are optimal.[69,70]

Eight patient characteristics and eight nurse competencies that constitute nursing practice form the basis of the model (Fig. 1-1; Boxes 1-8 and 1-9). The eight patient characteristics are resiliency, vulnerability, stability, complexity, resource availability, participation in care, participation in decision making, and predictability. These characteristics range in intensity and are expressed as level 1, 3, or 5. The level can change from one minute to the next.

The eight nurse competencies are clinical judgment, clinical inquiry, facilitation of learning, collaboration, systems thinking, advocacy/moral agency, caring practices, and response to diversity. Like the patient characteristics, the nurse competencies exist on a continuum and are also expressed as level 1, 3, or 5. The level can vary based on level of expertise of the nurse in a given clinical situation.

The Synergy Model is also used to determine outcomes. Optimal outcomes are evaluated based on those derived from the patient, the nurse, and the health care system. Patient-derived outcomes may include functional change, behavioral change, trust, satisfaction, comfort, and quality of life. Nurse-derived outcomes may include physiological changes, presence or absence of complications, and extent to which care or treatment objectives are attained. Health care system–derived outcomes may include recidivism, costs, and resource utilization.

Since its development, the Synergy Model has been used in a variety of clinical settings as a basis for nursing career ladders based on levels of expertise in caring, clinical practices, and leadership; job descriptions; and performance appraisals.[71] For example, the Clarian Health System in Indianapolis, Indiana, uses the model to facilitate organizational change.[72] Job descriptions at this health system are based on the eight nurse characteristics. The model facilitates differentiation of various levels of expertise, including competent, proficient, and expert clinical

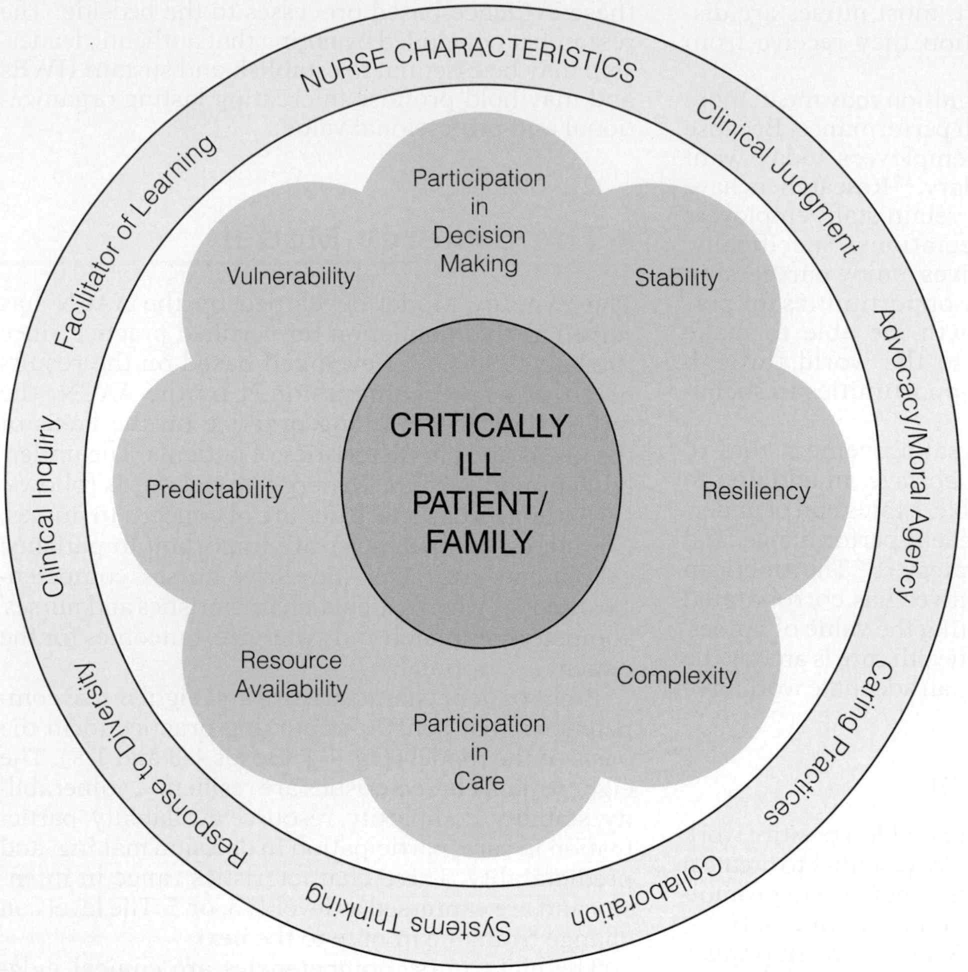

Figure 1-1 • The relationship between the patient/family and the nurse in the Synergy Model.

practice and leadership.[73] Baylor Hospital in Dallas, Texas, has implemented the Synergy Model. In this facility, the model is the foundation for evaluation of nursing orientation. In addition, the model is the basis for Baylor's professional nursing advancement program. The model also has an effect in other areas such as shift report; curriculum design; and nurse manager job analysis (managers use the eight nurse competencies to evaluate the state of their units). Their most recent development, in progress, is classifying educational offerings based on the Synergy Continuing Education Recognition Point (CERP) methodology.

In addition, the Synergy Model serves as the conceptual model for undergraduate and graduate curricula. For example, the graduate nursing curriculum at Duquesne University in Pittsburgh, Pennsylvania is based on the model. Similarly, Georgetown University in Washington, D.C., has adapted its Values Based Model for Nursing incorporating the elements of the Synergy Model. The resulting integrated model serves as the conceptual guide for the undergraduate and graduate programs and is being used as the basis for the development of the Doctor of Nursing Practice (DNP) program at this institution. Like the certification programs offered by the Certification Corporation of AACN, the HIV/AIDS Nursing Certification Board uses the Synergy Model when developing its specialty certification for Advanced HIV/AIDS Nursing Practice.[74] As the Synergy Model gains popularity and more hospitals seek Magnet designation, integration of this intuitive nursing model is likely to expand.

• Future Challenges in Critical Care Nursing

Because health care, nursing, and the world in which we live are dynamic, critical care nursing must continue to evolve and adapt. As the United States becomes increasingly diverse, nursing must increase its ability to deliver evidence-based interventions that are also culturally congruent and relevant. With a growing Hispanic population, it will become increasingly critical for health care systems and nurses to have multilingual, culturally diverse staffs. This requires not only the need to recruit and retain diverse professionals into critical care nursing but also the need to retrain and expand the skill set of today's already experienced critical care nurses.

Box 1-8 • Characteristics of Patients, Clinical Units, and Systems of Concern to Nurses

- **Resiliency**—the capacity to return to a restorative level of functioning using compensatory/coping mechanisms; the ability to bounce back quickly after an insult
  - *Level 1: Minimally resilient.* Unable to mount a response; failure of compensatory/coping mechanisms; minimal reserves; brittle
  - *Level 3: Moderately resilient.* Able to mount a moderate response; able to initiate some degree of compensation; moderate reserves
  - *Level 5: Highly resilient.* Able to mount and maintain a response; intact compensatory/coping mechanisms; strong reserves; endurance
- **Vulnerability**—susceptibility to actual or potential stressors that may adversely affect patient outcomes
  - *Level 1: Highly vulnerable.* Susceptible; unprotected, fragile
  - *Level 3: Moderately vulnerable.* Somewhat susceptible; somewhat protected
  - *Level 5: Minimally vulnerable.* Safe; out of the woods; protected, not fragile
- **Stability**—the ability to maintain a steady-state equilibrium
  - *Level 1: Minimally stable.* Labile; unstable; unresponsive to therapies; high risk of death
  - *Level 3: Moderately stable.* Able to maintain steady state for limited period of time; some responsiveness to therapies
  - *Level 5: Highly stable.* Constant; responsive to therapies; low risk of death
- **Complexity**—the intricate entanglement of two or more systems (e.g., body, family, therapies)
  - *Level 1: Highly complex.* Intricate; complex patient/family dynamics; ambiguous/vague; atypical presentation
  - *Level 3: Moderately complex.* Moderately involved patient/family dynamics
  - *Level 5: Minimally complex.* Straightforward; routine patient/family dynamics; simple/clearcut; typical presentation
- **Resource Availability**—extent of resources (e.g., technical, fiscal, personal, psychological, and social) the patient/family/community bring to the situation

- *Level 1: Few resources.* Necessary knowledge and skills not available; necessary financial support not available; minimal personal/psychological supportive resources; few social systems resources
- *Level 3: Moderate resources.* Limited knowledge and skills available; limited financial support available; limited personal/psychological supportive resources; limited social systems resources
- *Level 5: Many resources.* Extensive knowledge and skills available and accessible; financial resources readily available; strong personal/psychological supportive resources; strong social systems resources
- **Participation in Care**—extent to which patient/family engages in aspects of care
  - *Level 1: No participation.* Patient and family unable or unwilling to participate in care
  - *Level 3: Moderate participation.* Patient and family need assistance in care
  - *Level 5: Full participation.* Patient and family fully able to participate in care
- **Participation in Decision Making**—extent to which patient/family engages in decision making
  - *Level 1: No participation.* Patient and family have no capacity for decision making; requires surrogacy
  - *Level 3: Moderate participation.* Patient and family have limited capacity; seek input/advice from others in decision making
  - *Level 5: Full participation.* Patient and family have capacity and make decisions
- **Predictability**—a characteristic that allows one to expect a certain course of events or course of illness
  - *Level 1: Not predictable.* Uncertain; uncommon patient population/illness; unusual or unexpected course; does not follow critical pathway, or no critical pathway developed
  - *Level 3: Moderately predictable.* Wavering; occasionally noted patient population/illness
  - *Level 5: Highly predictable.* Certain; common patient population/illness; usual and expected course; follows critical pathway

From the American Association of Critical-Care Nurses Certification Corporation.

As new and emerging infectious diseases present, as severe acute respiratory syndrome (SARS) illustrated, health care systems, including critical care nurses, must be prepared to identify, manage, and treat unknown threats. Similarly, Hurricane Katrina clearly demonstrated the impact that natural disasters have on health care systems and professionals. Furthermore, in the era after 9/11, health care systems and critical care units must be prepared to handle any actual or potential bioterrorism threat.

Finally, as critical care continues to evolve and becomes increasingly technologically sophisticated, critical care nurses must continue to expand their repertoire of skills and evidence-based interventions to address not only the physiological needs but also, simultaneously, the psychosocial, spiritual, ethical, and advocacy needs of multicultural patients and families. With implementation of advances in technology, the critical care unit will continue to require caring, competent, and knowledgeable critical care nurses who can also foster interdisciplinary collaboration, navigate complex delivery and reimbursement systems, and facilitate patient/family learning while responding to diverse communities that are vulnerable with complex needs. These are the exciting challenges awaiting today's and tomorrow's critical care nurse—challenges that critical care nurses will overcome with commitment, dedication, and grace!

Box 1-9 • Nurse Competencies of Concern to Patients, Clinical Units, and Systems

- **Clinical Judgment**—clinical reasoning, which includes clinical decision making, critical thinking, and a global grasp of the situation, coupled with nursing skills acquired through a process of integrating formal and informal experiential knowledge and evidence-based guidelines

    Level 1: Collects basic-level data; follows algorithms, decision trees, and protocols with all populations and is uncomfortable deviating from them; matches formal knowledge with clinical events to make decisions; questions the limits of one's ability to make clinical decisions and delegates the decision making to other clinicians; includes extraneous detail

    Level 3: Collects and interprets complex patient data; makes clinical judgments based on an immediate grasp of the whole picture for common or routine patient populations; recognizes patterns and trends that may predict the direction of illness; recognizes limits and seeks appropriate help; focuses on key elements of case, while sorting out extraneous details

    Level 5: Synthesizes and interprets multiple, sometimes conflicting, sources of data; makes judgment based on an immediate grasp of the whole picture, unless working with new patient populations; uses past experiences to anticipate problems; helps patient and family see the "big picture"; recognizes the limits of clinical judgment and seeks multidisciplinary collaboration and consultation with comfort; recognizes and responds to the dynamic situation

- **Advocacy and Moral Agency**—working on another's behalf and representing the concerns of the patient/family and nursing staff; serving as a moral agent in identifying and helping to resolve ethical and clinical concerns within and outside the clinical setting.

    Level 1: Works on behalf of patient; self-assesses personal values; aware of ethical conflicts/issues that may surface in clinical setting; makes ethical/moral decisions based on rules; represents patient when patient cannot represent self; aware of patients' rights

    Level 3: Works on behalf of patient and family; considers patient values and incorporates in care, even when differing from personal values; supports colleagues in ethical and clinical issues; moral decision making can deviate from rules; demonstrates give and take with patient's family, allowing them to speak/represent themselves when possible; aware of patient and family rights

    Level 5: Works on behalf of patient, family, and community; advocates from patient/family perspective, whether similar to or different from personal values; advocates ethical conflict and issues from patient/family perspective; suspends rules—patient and family drive moral decision-making; empowers the patient and family to speak for/represent themselves; achieves mutuality within patient/professional relationships

- **Caring Practices**—nursing activities that create a compassionate, supportive, and therapeutic environment for patients and staff, with the aim of promoting comfort and healing and preventing unnecessary suffering. Includes, but is not limited to, vigilance, engagement, and responsiveness of caregivers, including family and health care personnel

    Level 1: Focuses on the usual and customary needs of the patient; no anticipation of future needs; bases care on

standards and protocols; maintains a safe physical environment; acknowledges death as a potential outcome

    Level 3: Responds to subtle patient and family changes; engages with the patient as a unique patient in a compassionate manner; recognizes and tailors caring practices to the individuality of patient and family; domesticates the patient's and family's environment; recognizes that death may be an acceptable outcome

    Level 5: Has astute awareness and anticipates patient and family changes and needs; is fully engaged with and sensing how to stand alongside the patient, family, and community; caring practices follow the patient and family lead; anticipates hazards and avoids them, and promotes safety throughout patient's and family's transitions along the health care continuum; orchestrates the process that ensures patient's/family's comfort and concerns surrounding issues of death and dying are met

- **Collaboration**—working with others (e.g., patients, families, health care providers) in a way that promotes/encourages each person's contributions toward achieving optimal/realistic patient/family goals. Involves intradisciplinary and inter-disciplinary work with colleagues and community

    Level 1: Willing to be taught, coached, and/or mentored; participates in team meetings and discussions regarding patient care and/or practice issues; open to various team members' contributions

    Level 3: Seeks opportunities to be taught, coached, and/or mentored; elicits others' advice and perspectives; initiates and participates in team meetings and discussions regarding patient care and/or practice issues; recognizes and suggests various team members' participation

    Level 5: Seeks opportunities to teach, coach, and mentor and to be taught, coached, and mentored; facilitates active involvement and complementary contributions of others in team meetings and discussions regarding patient care and/or practice issues; involves/recruits diverse resources when appropriate to optimize patient outcomes

- **Systems Thinking**—body of knowledge and tools that allow the nurse to manage whatever environmental and system resources exist for the patient/family and staff, within or across health care and non-health care systems

    Level 1: Uses a limited array of strategies; limited outlook—sees the pieces or components; does not recognize negotiation as an alternative; sees patient and family within the isolated environment of the unit; sees self as key resource

    Level 3: Develops strategies based on needs and strengths of patient/family; able to make connections within components; sees opportunity to negotiate but may not have strategies; developing a view of the patient/family transition process; recognizes how to obtain resources beyond self

    Level 5: Develops, integrates, and applies a variety of strategies that are driven by the needs and strengths of the patient/family; global or holistic outlook—sees the whole rather than the pieces; knows when and how to negotiate and navigate through the system on behalf of patients and families; anticipates needs of patients and families as they move through the health

---

Box 1-9 • Nurse Competencies of Concern to Patients, Clinical Units, and Systems (Continued)

care system; utilizes untapped and alternative resources as necessary

- **Response to Diversity**—the sensitivity to recognize, appreciate, and incorporate differences into the provision of care. Differences may include, but are not limited to, cultural differences, spiritual beliefs, gender, race, ethnicity, lifestyle, socioeconomic status, age, and values.

    Level 1: Assesses cultural diversity; provides care based on own belief system; learns the culture of the health care environment

    Level 3: Inquires about cultural differences and considers their impact on care; accommodates personal and professional differences in the plan of care; helps patient/family understand the culture of the health care system

    Level 5: Responds to, anticipates, and integrates cultural differences into patient/family care; appreciates and incorporates differences, including alternative therapies, into care; tailors health care culture, to the extent possible, to meet the diverse needs and strengths of the patient/family

- **Facilitation of Learning**—the ability to facilitate learning for patients/families, nursing staff, other members of the health care team, and community. Includes both formal and informal facilitation of learning

    Level 1: Follows planned educational programs; sees patient/family education as a separate task from delivery of care; provides data without seeking to assess patient's readiness or understanding; has limited knowledge of the totality of the educational needs; focuses on a nurse's perspective; sees the patient as a passive recipient

    Level 3: Adapts planned educational programs; begins to recognize and integrate different ways of teaching into delivery of care; incorporates patient's understanding into practice; sees the overlapping of educational plans from different health care providers' perspec-

tives; begins to see the patient as having input into goals; begins to see individualism

    Level 5: Creatively modifies or develops patient/family education programs; integrates patient/family education throughout delivery of care; evaluates patient's understanding by observing behavior changes related to learning; is able to collaborate and incorporate all health care providers' and educational plans into the patient/family educational program; sets patient-driven goals for education; sees patient/family as having choices and consequences that are negotiated in relation to education

- **Clinical Inquiry (Innovator/Evaluator)**—the ongoing process of questioning and evaluating practice and providing informed practice. Creating practice changes through research utilization and experiential learning

    Level 1: Follows standards and guidelines; implements clinical changes and research-based practices developed by others; recognizes the need for further learning to improve patient care; recognizes obvious changing patient situation (e.g., deterioration, crisis); needs and seeks help to identify patient problem

    Level 3: Questions appropriateness of policies and guidelines; questions current practice; seeks advice, resources, or information to improve patient care; begins to compare and contrast possible alternatives

    Level 5: Improves, deviates from, or individualizes standards and guidelines for particular patient situations or populations; questions and/or evaluates current practice based on patients' responses, review of the literature, research and education/learning; acquires knowledge and skills needed to address questions arising in practice and improve patient care. (The domains of clinical judgment and clinical inquiry converge at the expert level; they cannot be separated.)

From http://www.certcorp.org/certcorp/certcorp.nsf/vwdoc/SynModel.

• Clinical Applicability Challenges

Short-Answer Questions

1. Describe a patient care situation that exemplifies use of the Synergy Model.
2. Identify a problem in your area of practice that needs change based on evidence in the nursing scientific literature.
3. Describe a situation in which collaboration with other members of the health care team enhanced patient outcomes.

Review Questions

1. Evidence-based practice strongly supports which element of the Synergy Model?
   a. Caring practices
   b. Systems thinking
   c. Facilitator of learning
   d. Clinical inquiry

2. A new drug has been approved to treat cardiac dysrhythmias. Before the introduction of the drug in the clinical environment, a critical care nurse educator conducts a series of in-service classes about the drug's dosing and side effects as well as related nursing interventions. This is an example of
   a. collaboration.
   b. advocacy/moral agency.
   c. facilitator of learning.
   d. clinical judgment.

3. When a critical care nurse works as a patient advocate and moral agent, it is important that the nurse promote
   a. patient autonomy.
   b. justice.
   c. paternalism.
   d. collaboration.

4. A critical care nurse is collaborating with a physician colleague to discuss changes in the treatment plan. During this skilled communication interaction, it is critical that the nurse
   a. invite and hear all relevant perspectives.
   b. advocate for the patient.
   c. focus on recognizing all team members for their contributions to the treatment plan.
   d. utilize organizational values to guide the interaction.

5. The integration of evidence-based nursing interventions in health care
   a. results in improved clinical outcomes.
   b. is easy to implement.
   c. requires physician review and approval.
   d. is dependent on the cost of the intervention.

References

1. American Association of Critical Care Nurses Certification Corporation: General information regarding certification. Retrieved June 30, 2006, from http://www.certcorp.org/certcorp/certcorp.nsf/

2. American Association of Critical Care Nurses: Safeguarding the patient and the profession: The value of critical care nurse certification—white paper. Am J Crit Care 12:154–164, 2003

3. Byrne M., Valentine W, Carter, S: The value of certification—a research journey. AORN J 79(4):831–835, 2004

4. Cary AH: Certified registered nurses: Results of a study of the certified workforce. Am J Nurs 10(1):44–52, 2001

5. Piazza IM, Donahue M, Dykes PC, et al: Differences in perceptions of empowerment among nationally certified and noncertified nurses. J Nurs Admin 36(5):277–283, 2006

6. Shirey MR: Celebrating certification in nursing: Forces of magnetism in action [The pull of magnetism: The what, why, and where of achieving and sustaining Magnet status]. Nurs Admin Q 29(3):245–253, 2005

7. O'Neale M, Kurtz S: (2001). Certification: Perspectives on competency assurance. Semin Perioper Nurs 10(2):88–92, 2001

8. The many benefits of certification. Crit Care Nurse 29(Suppl): 63–44, 2006

9. Gaberson KB, Schroeter K, Killen AR, et al: The perceived value of certification by certified perioperative nurses. Nurs Outlook 51(6):272–276, 2003

10. Melnyk BM, Fineout-Overholt E: Evidence-Based Practice in Nursing and Healthcare: A Guide to Best Practice. Philadelphia: Lippincott Williams & Wilkins, 2005

11. Pape TM: Evidence-based nursing practice: To infinity and beyond. J Contin Educ Nurs 34(4):154–161, 2003

12. Hodge M, Kochie LD, Larsen L, et al: Clinician-implemented research utilization in critical care. Am J Crit Care 12(4): 361–366, 2003

13. Davies BL: Sources and models for moving research evidence into clinical practice. J Obstet Gynecol Neonat Nurs 31(5): 558–562, 2002

14. Balas EA, Boren SA: Managing clinical knowledge for healthcare improvements. In Schattauer V (ed): Yearbook of Medical Informatics. Stuttgart, Germany: Schattauer Publishing, 2000, pp 65–70

15. Ervin NE: Evidence-based nursing practice: are we there yet? J N Y State Nurses Assoc 33(2):11–16, 2002

16. Thomson P, Angus NJ, Scott J: Building a framework for getting evidence into critical care education and practice. Intensive Crit Care Nurs 16(3):164–174, 2000

17. Mott B, Nolan J, Zarb N, et al: Clinical nurses' knowledge of evidence-based practice: Constructing a framework to evaluate a multifaceted intervention for implementing EBP. Contemp Nurse 19(1–2):96–104, 2005

18. Pravikoff DS, Pierce ST, Tanner A: Evidence-based practice readiness study supported by academy nursing informatics expert panel. Nurs Outlook 53:49–50, 2005

19. Sitvia J: Barriers to research utilisation: The clinical setting and nurses themselves. Intensive Crit Care Nurs 18(4):230–243, 2002

20. Gerrish K, Clayton J: Promoting evidence-based practice: an organizational approach. J Nurs Manage 12(2):114–123, 2004

21. Bucknall T, Copnell B, Shannon K, et al: Evidence based practice: Are critical care nurses ready for it? Aust Crit Care 14(3): 92–98, 2001

22. Fineout-Overholt E, Levin RF, Melnyk BM: Strategies for advancing evidence-based practice in clinical settings. J N Y State Nurses Assoc 35(2):28–32, 2004–2005

23. American Association of Critical-Care Nurses. Available at: http://www.aacn.org

24. American Association of Critical-Care Nurses: AACN's healthy work environment initiative backgrounder. Retrieved June 25, 2006, from http://www.aacn.org/AACN/pubpolcy.nsf

25. Brinker D: Healthy work environments. RN 68(5):9, 2005

26. Joint Commission on Accreditation of Healthcare Organizations. Retrieved June 15, 2006, from http://www.jointcommission.org/NR

27. Maxfield D, Grenny J, McMillan R, et al: Silence kills: The seven crucial conversations for healthcare. Available at: http://www.aacn.org/aacn/pubpolcy.nsf

28. Powers J: APNs are essential in promoting collaboration. AACN News 20(1), 2003

29. Gardner DB: Ten lessons in collaboration. Online J Issues Nurs 10(1):2, 2005

30. D'Amour D, Ferrada-Videla M, San Martin Rodriguez L, et al: The conceptual basis for interprofessional collaboration: Core concepts and theoretical frameworks. J Interprof Care 19(Suppl 1):116–131, 2005

31. Aiken LH: Evidence-based management: Key to hospital workforce stability. J Health Adm Educ special issue: 117–125, 2001

32. Baggs JG, Schmitt MH, Mushlin AI, et al: Association between nurse-physician collaboration and patient outcomes in three intensive care units. Crit Care Med 27(9):1991–1998, 1999

33. Gitell JH, Fairfield KM, Bierbaum B, et al: Impact of relational coordination on quality of care, postoperative pain and functioning, and length of stay: A nine-hospital study of surgical patients. Med Care 38(8):807–819, 2000

34. Horak BJ, Pauig J, Keidan B, et al: Patient safety: A case study in team building and interdisciplinary collaboration. J Healthc Qual 26(2):6–13, 2004

35. Wheelan SA, Burchill CN, Tilin F: The link between teamwork and patients' outcomes in intensive care units. Am J Crit Care 12:527–534, 2003

36. Sim TA, Joyner J: A multidisciplinary team approach to reducing medication variance. Jt Comm J Qual Improv 28(7): 403–409, 2002

37. McDonough RP, Doucette WR: Dynamics of pharmaceutical care: Developing collaborative working relationships between pharmacists and physicians. J Am Pharm Assoc 41(5):682–692, 2001

38. Daly G: Understanding the barriers to multiprofessional collaboration. Nurs Times 100(9):78–79, 2004

39. Zwarenstein M, Bryant W: Interventions to promote collaboration between nurses and doctors. Cochrane Database Syst Rev 2:CD000072, 2000

40. Corser WD: The contemporary nurse-physician relationship: Insights from scholars outside the two professions. Nurs Outlook 48:263–268, 2000

41. Wachter RM, Shojania K: Internal Bleeding—The Truth Behind America's Terrifying Epidemic of Medical Mistakes. New York: Rugged Land, LLC, 2004

42. Zwarenstein M, Bryant W, Bailie R, et al: Meta-analysis of the Cochrane Collaboration. Promoting collaboration between nurses and physicians. Assist Inferm Ric 19(2):97–99, 2000

43. American Association of Critical-Care Nurses: AACN Standards for Establishing and Sustaining Healthy Work Environments: A Journey to Excellence. Aliso Viejo, CA: AACN, 2005

44. Rashotte J, Carnevale FA: Medical and nursing clinical decision making: A comparative epistemological analysis. Nurs Philos 5(2):160–174, 2004

45. Bakalis NA, Watson R: Nurses' decision-making in clinical practice. Nurs Standard 19(23):33–39, 2005

46. Rafferty AM, Ball J, Aiken LH: Are teamwork and professional autonomy compatible, and do they result in improved hospital care? Qual Healthc 10:32–37, 2001

47. Aiken LH, Clarke SP, Sloane DM, et al: Hospital nurse staffing and patient mortality, nurse burnout, and job dissatisfaction. JAMA 288:1987–1993, 2002

48. Cho SH, Ketefian S, Barkauskas VH, et al: The effects of nurse staffing on adverse events, morbidity, mortality, and medical costs. Nurs Res 52(2):71–79, 2003

49. Needleman J, Buerhaus P: Nurse staffing and patient safety: Current knowledge and implications for action. Int Soc Qual Healthc 15:275–277, 2003

50. Pronovost PJ, Dang D, Dorman T, et al: Intensive care unit nurse staffing and the risk for complications after abdominal aortic surgery. Effect Clin Practice 4(5):199–206, 2001

51. Person SD, Allison JJ, Kiefe CI, et al: Nurse staffing and mortality for Medicare patients with acute myocardial infarction. Med Care 42(1):4–12, 2004

52. Institute of Medicine: Keeping Patients Safe: Transforming the Work Environment of Nurses. Washington, DC: National Academies Press, 2003

53. Fontaine D: Rising Above. Presidential address at the National Teaching Institute. Delivered on May 17, 2004. Available at: http://www.aacn.org/AACN/nti04.nsf/Files/PresidentSpeech

54. Freed DH: Fifty-two effective, inexpensive ways to reward and recognize hospital employees. Healthc Manager 18(1):20–28, 1999

55. Izzo JB, Withers P: Winning employee-retention strategies for today's healthcare organizations. Healthc Financ Manage 56(6):52–57, 2002

56. Collins SK, Collins KS: Employee retention: An issue of survival in healthcare. Radiol Manage 26(4):52–55, 2004

57. Gering J, Conner J: A strategic approach to employee retention. Healthc Financ Manage 56(11):40–44, 2002

58. Lamberth B, Comello RJ: Identifying elements of job satisfaction to improve retention rates in healthcare. Radiol Manage 27(3):34–38, 2005

59. Randolph DS: Predicting the effect of extrinsic and intrinsic job satisfaction factors on recruitment and retention of rehabilitation professionals. J Healthc Manage 50(1):49–60, 2005

60. Reid Ponte P: The American health care system at a crossroads: An overview of the American Organization of Nurse Executives monograph. Online J Issues Nurs 9(2), 2004. Available at: http://www.nursingworld.org/ojin/topic24

61. Disch J: The nurse executive: Healthy work environments for all nurses. J Prof Nurs 16(2):75, 2000

62. Hawkins AL, Kratsch LS: Troubled units: Creating changes. AACN Clin Issues 15:215–221, 2004

63. Heath J, Johanson W, Blake N: Healthy work environments: A validation of the literature. J Nurs Admin 34:524–530, 2004

64. Whiley K: The nurse manager's role in creating a healthy work environment. AACN Clin Issues 12:356–365, 2001

65. McCauley K: President's note: All we needed was the glue. AACN News 22:2, 2005

66. Shirey MR: Authentic leaders creating healthy work environments for nursing practice. Am J Crit Care 15(4):256–267, 2006

67. Avolio BJ, Gardner WL, Walumbwa FO, et al: Unlocking the mask: A look at the process by which authentic leaders impact follower attitudes and behaviors. Leadersh Q 15:801–823, 2004

68. George B: Authentic Leadership: Rediscovering the Secrets to Creating Lasting Value. San Francisco: Jossey-Bass, 2003

69. American Association of Critical-Care Nurses Certification Corporation: The AACN Synergy Model for Patient Care. Retrieved June 15, 2006, from http://www.certcorp.org/certcorp/certcorp.nsf/vwdoc/SynModel

70. Hardin SR, Kaplow R: Synergy for Clinical Excellence: The AACN Synergy Model For Patient Care. Sudbury, MA: Jones & Bartlett, 2005

71. Reed KD, Cline M, Kerfoot KM: Implementation of the synergy model in critical care. In Kaplow R, Hardin SR (eds): Critical Care Nursing: Synergy for Optimal Outcomes. Sudbury, MA: Jones & Bartlett, 2007

72. Kerfoot K: Multihospital system adapts AACN Synergy Model—In Our Unit—Clarian Health Partners chooses patient care model. Crit Care Nurse 23(5):88, 2003

73. Kerfoot KM, Cox M: The Synergy Model: The ultimate mentoring model. Crit Care Nurs Clin North Am 17:109–112, 2005

74. Relf MV, Berger B, Crespo-Fierro M, et al: The value of certification in HIV/AIDS nursing. J Assoc Nurses AIDS Care 15(1):60–64, 2004

2

The Patient's Experience With Critical Illness

Kathryn S. Bizek • Dorrie K. Fontaine

Objectives

Based on the content in this chapter, the reader should be able to:

❶ Explore relationships among stress, response to illness, and anxiety.

❷ Explore the role of the nurse in controlling environmental stressors to promote healing.

❸ Compare and contrast techniques that the patient and family can learn in an effort to manage stress and anxiety.

❹ Describe strategies to promote sleep in critically ill patients.

❺ Develop nursing interventions that foster the ability of patients to draw strength from their personal spirituality.

❻ Discuss alternatives to the use of physical restraint in the intensive care unit.

The patient's experience in an intensive care unit (ICU) has lasting meaning for the patient and his or her family members and significant others. Although actual painful memories are blurred by drugs and the mind's need to forget, attitudes that are highly charged with feelings about the nature of the experience survive. These attitudes shape the person's beliefs about nurses, physicians, health care, and the vulnerability of life itself.

This chapter describes specific measures that nurses use to support patients in managing the stressors associated with critical illness and injury. It is the caring and emotional support given by the nurse that will be remembered and valued.

• Perception of Critical Illness

Admission to an ICU may signal a threat to the life and well-being of the patient who is admitted. Critical care nurses perceive the unit as a place where fragile lives are vigilantly scrutinized, cared for, and preserved. However, patients and their families frequently perceive admission to critical care as a sign of impending death, based on their own past experiences or the experiences of others. Understanding what critical care means to patients may help nurses care for their patients. However, effective communication with critically ill patients is often challenging and frustrating.[1-4] Barriers to communication may relate to the patients' physiological status; the existence of endotracheal tubes, which inhibit verbal communication; medications; or other conditions that alter cognitive function.

A number of authors have sought to study and describe patients' experiences related to their ICU stay. In a review of 26 studies, Stein-Parbury and McKinley noted that between 30% and 100% of patients studied could recall all or part of their stay in the ICU.[5] Although many of the patients recalled feelings that were negative, they also recalled neutral and positive experiences. Negative experiences were related to fear, anxiety, sleep disturbance, cognitive impairment, and pain or discomfort. Positive experiences were related to feelings of being safe and secure. Often, these positive feelings were attributed to the care provided by nurses. The need to feel safe and the need for information were predominant themes in other research studies.[2,6,7] Nurses' technical competence and effective interpersonal skills were cited by patients as promoting their sense of security and trust.[6,8]

• Stress

Stress has been defined as a situation that exists when an organism is faced with any stimulus that causes disequilibrium between psychological and physiological functioning. Patients admitted to the ICU are subject to multiple physical, psychological, and environmental stressors. Stimulation of the body's stress response involves activation of the hypothalamic–pituitary–adrenal axis. The resultant increase in catecholamine, glucocorticoid, and mineralocorticoid levels leads to a cascade of physiologic responses.

ACUTE STRESS RESPONSE

Critical injury or illness can initiate the first phase of the stress response. This phase is characterized by the body's efforts to survive and involves the stimulation of the sympathetic nervous system and activation of multiple neuroendocrine responses. This "ebb phase" results in increased heart rate and contractility, vasoconstriction, and increase in blood pressure. Blood flow is redirected to vital organs. Pain sensations are temporarily attenuated. Body temperature and nutrient consumption fall. A sensation of thirst may be prominent. Other physiological effects include increase in minute ventilation and respiratory rate, hyperglycemia, insulin resistance, and coagulopathies. This initial phase is deeply catabolic as protein stores are mobilized to respond to the threat and begin to repair the injury. If this phase is prolonged, it can result in impaired oxygen delivery and nutrients to tissues secondary to alterations in microcirculatory blood flow. Table 2-1 summarizes the effects of hormones released in response to major stress.[9–12]

The second phase of the stress response, or the "flow phase," is a hyperdynamic state that results as the body compensates for the oxygen deprivation. This phase is also characterized by multiple hormonal influences. Pain and discomfort are now prominent. Movement is minimized to conserve metabolic costs.

Table 2-1 • Major Stress-Related Hormones and Effects

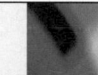

Stress Hormones	Source	Major Effects
Adrenocorticotropic hormone	Anterior pituitary	Stimulates adrenal cortex to release cortisol
Catecholamines	Adrenal medulla and the sympathetic nervous system	Increases overall strength, blood flow to vital organs, glyconeogenesis
Epinephrine		Increases myocardial contractility (inotropic effect), heart rate (chronotropic effect), venous return to the heart and cardiac output
Norepinephrine		Constricts smooth muscle in all blood vessels, increases blood pressure, dilates pupils, inhibits gastrointestinal activity
Cortisol	Adrenal cortex (following stimulation by adrenocorticotropic hormone from the anterior pituitary)	Gluconeogenesis; hyperglycemia; decreases protein synthesis, immunoglobulin synthesis, number of lymphocytes, and leukocytes (at inflammatory site); promotes muscle and lymphoid tissue catabolism; delays healing; suppresses cell-mediated immune response
Antidiuretic hormone	Posterior pituitary	Increases water retention
Aldosterone	Adrenal cortex	Increases sodium and water retention
Growth hormone (somatotropin)	Anterior pituitary	Increases immune function; levels are increased during stress
Prolactin	Anterior pituitary	β-Cell activation and differentiation; levels are reduced during stress
Testosterone	Testis	Regulates male secondary characteristics; levels are decreased during chronic stress
Endorphins	Anterior pituitary	Endogenous opiates, elevated during stress, down-regulate pathways to the stress response
Enkephalins	Adrenal medulla	Endogenous opiates, elevated during stress, down-regulate pathways to the stress response

From: Lusk B, Lash AA: The stress response, psychoneuroimmunology, and stress among ICU patients. DCCN 24(1):25–31, 2003.

Prolonged activation of the stress response can lead to immunosuppression, hypoperfusion, tissue hypoxia, and eventual death. Treatment is directed at eliminating the stressors and providing supportive care in the form of nutrition, oxygenation, pain management, control of anxiety, and specific measures directed at the cause of illness or injury.[9–12]

ENVIRONMENTAL STRESSORS IN THE INTENSIVE CARE UNIT

The ICU is a stressful environment for patients and caregivers.[13] Walk into any ICU and you will find the following common physical features: blinking monitors, ventilators, intravenous (IV) pumps, noise from equipment and the many practitioners talking at the bedside, bright lights, and a hurried pace in a crowded space. Intra-aortic balloon pumps, extracorporeal membrane oxygenation machines, and other sophisticated technologies are increasingly commonplace. Critical care nursing was invented to flourish in this setting, where the most acutely ill and injured receive concentrated nursing care to enhance survival. In the early ICUs of the 1950s, nurses were confronted daily with pain, suffering, and death, while caring for patients in a confined open space.[14] These ICUs were often a few beds carved out of existing wards in older hospitals that brought the sickest patients to one area. The most distinctive feature of the first ICUs was this concentration of nursing care, and the specialty of intensive care nursing was born. The design of ICUs has changed over the decades and provides a rationale for why care needs for the patient and family have also evolved. The concept of

healing environments in hospitals emerged as one where the environment can make a difference in how quickly the patient recovers.[15]

Table 2-2 summarizes the key design features of ICUs from the 1950s to an envisioned future.[16] Common to all these designs is the notion of close observation and rapid intervention. Meeting patient needs through continuous monitoring is the hallmark of all critical care. However, the close monitoring has led to patient complaints of noise, lighting with no day–night distinction, and frequent interruptions of sleep and rest. Intensive care beds were often so close to each other that patients could hear everything happening to the critically ill patient in the next bed. Lack of privacy and fears related to overheard procedures and conversations in the unit created undue anxiety and the potential for physiological instability in vulnerable patients.

The evolution of ICUs has demonstrated increasing use of the precepts of family-focused care. Early units typically had no space for family to visit, and visits were not encouraged. Emphasis today is on how the design of the ICU can best meet the needs of patients and families as a unit, despite the important life-sustaining technology. The shift to family-focused care is a good example of how the structure and function of ICUs has changed.[17] Signs that welcome family and visitors to the ICU often suggest the philosophy of the hospital and the culture of the unit. The more welcoming the ICU is to visitors, the more likely the environment is to offer a healing culture of care and support. Does the sign on the door read "Stop, Do Not Enter" or "Welcome to the ICU"?

Patients experience a positive outcome in an environment that incorporates natural light, elements of

Table 2-2 • Intensive Care Unit (ICU) Designs

	First Generation (1950s)	Second Generation (1970s)	Third Generation (1980s–Present)	Fourth Generation–Future
Characteristics	Open unit/ward. No partitions except curtains or screens. Nurses' station/desk in center or at the foot of beds. Unit lighting control often on one switch.	Individual rooms or walled cubicles. Rooms often on either side of a hall containing an open nursing station or surrounding an open nursing station on three to four sides (square configuration). Central monitoring. Some units without external patient room windows (increased incidence of delirium). Patient room lighting with separate switch(es) from nursing station. Calendars and clock in patient rooms.	Individual rooms. Folding or sliding glass doors. Rooms often arranged on a semicircle or circle with the nursing station in the center. Some units configured with decentralized nursing stations. Patient room windows with external views/lighting. Increased control of patient room lighting levels.	Individual rooms. Folding or sliding glass doors with privacy curtains/blinds. Circular/pod-shaped floor plan. Increased noise reduction design. Patient windows with a view of outdoors (natural or contrived). Patient-controlled lighting—artificial and natural. Planned areas for family in patient rooms. Increased use of color and texture in wall, floor, and ceiling coverings.
Advantages	Increased nurses' proximity to patients	Increased patient privacy. Better control of lighting, noise, and infection.	Increased nursing access during high-intensity activities.	Nursing access and availability of high-tech care in a more homelike environment.
Disadvantages	Lack of privacy. Inability to control noise or light. Infection control issues.	Less direct patient access/observation. Less than optimal control of noise and lighting.	Glass doors reduce patient privacy.	

From Fontaine DK, Prinkey Briggs L, Pope-Smith B: Designing humanistic critical care environments. Crit Care Nurs Q 24(3):21–34, 2001, with permission.

nature, soothing colors, meaningful and varied stimuli, peaceful sounds, and pleasant views.[15] In fact, research demonstrates less pain medication is needed and a faster recovery may occur when careful attention is given to providing a soothing environment. Hospitals that combine creative design elements with an emphasis on family-focused care are the leaders in creating healing spaces for recovery.

Noise

Despite third-generation unit design and architecture, the problems of noise and bright lighting have remained a challenge. Beds surrounded by noisy machines and equipment are intimidating to patients, family, and novice nurses in critical care. Noise is an environmental hazard that creates discomfort in a patient. Consequences of noisy environments include disrupted sleep, impaired wound healing, and activation of the sympathetic nervous system. Moderate noise levels may produce vasoconstriction. Hyperarousal due to noise can occur over many days to even weeks for patients with prolonged ICU stays.

Patient complaints include listening to banging noises, alarms going off at all times, water sounds (such as the bubbling of chest tubes), and doors opening and closing. Sources of noise include equipment, alarms, telephones, televisions, ventilators, and staff conversations. Health care providers are often unaware of the loudness of their conversations and the irritation they may create in the minds of patients. People differ in their perceptions of noise as irritating; therefore, nurses should perform an objective assessment of the environment.

Noise is measured in decibels using a logarithmic scale. An increase of 10 decibels makes a sound seem twice as loud. Sleep occurs best below 35 decibels. The Environmental Protection Agency recommends unit noise be less than 45 decibels during the day and 35 decibels at night. Numerous studies measuring noise levels in the ICU demonstrate consistent elevations as high as 80 to 90 decibels. New technology can be an additional source of noise, although several manufacturers attempt to provide equipment that lowers the total unit volume of sound.

Decades of studies consistently point to noise as a key aspect of the ICU environment. Noise was measured in two ICUs using a sound meter placed at the head of a patient's bed.[18] More than 50% of the noise in the environment was attributed to human behavior, with a mean sound level in the medical ICU of 84 decibels. Television and talking were some of the most frequent disruptive sounds for patients. Another study investigated the perceptions of 203 patients who filled out a questionnaire on discharge from the ICU and found that noise from talking and alarms was the most disruptive to sleep.[19] Sound peaks greater than 80 decibels are common in ICUs and are directly related to arousals from sleep.[20] Noise levels in ICUs have remained fairly unchanged despite the evolution of unit design. Newer thinking suggests that noise is not the only culprit in limiting sleep in the ICU, although it remains an important one.[21]

Lights and Color

Light is a powerful zeitgeber, or environmental synchronizer, that assists in entraining sleep by promoting the normal circadian cycle of sleep and wakefulness. Many critical care settings could benefit from more natural lighting and lights that are lowered during normal sleep times. In addition to natural lighting, providing a soothing view for the patient to look on instead of the ceiling or a hospital curtain may foster recovery. A classic study found that when a patient had a view of natural scenery and the outdoors, as opposed to viewing a brick wall, less pain medication was used and the hospital stay was shorter.[22] Other studies have demonstrated that impaired cognition occurs more often in windowless units than in those with windows.[23]

In the hospital setting, artificial light is provided by fluorescent bulbs and tubes. This creates a harsh type of light that leads to visual fatigue and headaches, if unshielded. Glare can occur when light is reflected off environmental surfaces such as glass, shiny metal, mirrors, and enameled or polished finishes. Any glare is especially troublesome to elderly patients. Bright lights may be left on for many hours in ICUs, even when no direct patient care is being performed. Lack of control over artificial lighting is a source of frustration to critical care patients.

Interruptions in normal light–dark patterns can disrupt normal physiological processes. For example, artificial light exposure for as little as 20 minutes during a normal sleep cycle caused a drop in melatonin levels.[24] In addition, constant lighting and high-intensity light can lead to a complete disruption of the normal melatonin concentration rhythm. This has important implications in the critical care setting because melatonin facilitates sleep and modulates corticosteroid and thyroid hormone levels.[25]

The ideal ICU environment has windows with natural views, soothing artwork, and calm colors.[26] The nurse and other health care providers have access to work and computer stations with glass soundproof partitions that permit proximity to the patient (for easy observation) while shielding the patient from noise. Equipment is selected for its low noise level. Stress created by unnecessary noise and light is diminished for the good of the patients, family, and staff. This vision may already be a reality in some institutions. For example, muted colors of beige, blue, and green were used to design a holistic nursing unit in a Minnesota Hospital.[27] Art on the walls depicts many different cultures and the peacefulness of nature. The goal of a more peaceful, healing ICU environment is possible to attain.

• Anxiety

CAUSES OF ANXIETY

Anxiety may be defined as an emotional state of apprehension in response to a real or perceived threat associated with motor tension, increased sympathetic activity, and hypervigilance. Any stressor that threatens a person's sense of wholeness, containment, security, and control can cause anxiety. Illness and injury are such stressors. Other common causes of anxiety include feelings of increased vulnerability and decreased security, such as occurs when patients admitted to ICUs perceive a loss of control, a sense of isolation, and fear of death or loss of functionality. Anxiety, pain, and fear can all initiate or perpetuate the stress response. Left untreated or undertreated, anxiety can contribute to the morbidity and mortality of critically ill patients.

Anxiety occurs when people experience the following:

▶ Threat of helplessness
▶ Loss of control
▶ Sense of loss of function and self-esteem
▶ Failure of former defenses
▶ Sense of isolation
▶ Fear of dying

ASSESSMENT OF ANXIETY

Assessment of anxiety is challenging in the critical care population because of the severity of illness, barriers to communication, and altered cognitive states. However, most critical care nurses believe that assessment of anxiety is important.[28] Multiple-item, self-report scales of anxiety may be used, but they have specific drawbacks in critical care areas, especially for patients on mechanical ventilators because of communication barriers.[29] According to many critical care nurses, the top five physiological and behavioral indicators of anxiety are agitated behavior, increased blood pressure, increased heart rate, verbalization of anxiety, and restlessness.[28] Monitoring of these patient parameters is useful, but there is still a need for a reliable and comprehensive anxiety assessment tool.[28,30] Examples of nursing diagnoses associated with critical illness and injury can be seen in Box 2-1.

Box 2-1	Examples of Nursing Diagnoses and Collaborative Problems for the Patient With Critical Illness or Injury

- Anticipatory Grieving
- Anxiety
- Body Image Disturbance
- Communication, Impaired Verbal
- Coping, Ineffective
- Denial, Ineffective
- Fear
- Hopelessness
- Risk for Loneliness
- Powerlessness
- Self-Esteem Disturbance
- Sleep Deprivation
- Spiritual Distress
- Potential for Enhanced Spiritual Well-Being

• Nursing Interventions

In caring for the critically ill patient, the nurse helps the patient manage a multitude of stressors. Stress management includes not only physical and environmental stressors but also psychological stressors. This complex and labor-intensive process requires use of advanced assessment skills, adept manipulation of a variety of highly technological treatment strategies, and creativity in care and compassion.[31]

CREATING A HEALING ENVIRONMENT

Florence Nightingale is considered the founder of modern nursing. She often wrote about the nurse's role in creating an environment to allow healing to occur.[32] She emphasized holism in nursing—that is, caring for the whole person. In today's technological age, critical care nurses are challenged to create an environment of healing. These environments must allow critically ill patients to have their psychological needs as well as physical needs met. Manipulating the milieu may involve timing interventions to allow adequate sleep and rest, providing pain-relieving medication, playing music, or teaching deep-breathing exercises. As previously discussed, the physical environment of the ICU can be altered to create a more healing and restful environment.

PROMOTING REST AND SLEEP

Sleep Assessment

Promotion of sleep and rest for critically ill patients begins with an understanding of sleep, the major environmental disruptions, and a sleep assessment. Sleep is composed of two very distinct types of brain activity: rapid eye movement (REM) sleep and non-REM sleep. A description of these sleep stages can be found in Box 2-2. Healthy adults progress through sleep stages in a specific order, from a light stage to a deeper stage, in 90-minute cycles. REM sleep increases later in the normal nighttime sleep patterns of most people, with morning naps containing primarily REM sleep. Specific sleep stages have a circadian rhythm and are controlled by brainstem mechanisms.[33]

Although sleep patterns are very individual, most patients can tell when they feel rested and have had a "good night's sleep." Unfortunately, this is a rare occurrence in the hospital. Sleep, once thought to be a quiescent state, actually involves physiological activation while the brain and body rejuvenate themselves. Sleep is often appreciated only when it has been "lost" and is typically taken for granted by health care providers, who often do not make sleep a priority for patients. In the ICU, sleep is often severely fragmented and nonconsolidated,[34] with those on mechanical ventilation experiencing some of the worst sleep disruption.[35]

Sleep deprivation in patients in ICUs can have cumulative effects and lead to altered cognition, confusion, impaired wound healing, and the inability to

Box 2-2 • Stages and Characteristics of Sleep

Stage 1. Transitional stage between wakefulness and
sleep
Relaxed state where person is somewhat
aware of surroundings
Involuntary muscle jerking that may waken
the person
Normally lasts only minutes
Easily aroused
Constitutes only about 5% of total sleep
Stage 2. Beginning of sleep
Arousal occurs with relative ease
Constitutes 50% to 55% of sleep
Stage 3. Depth of sleep increased and arousal increas-
ingly difficult
Constitutes about 10% of sleep
Stage 4. Greatest depth of sleep (*delta sleep*)
Arousal from sleep difficult
Physiological changes in the body—slow brain
waves on electroencephalogram; decreased
pulse and respiratory rates; decreased blood
pressure; relaxed muscles; slow metabolism
and low body temperature
Constitutes about 10% of sleep
Stage REM Sleep with vivid dreaming (REM)
Rapid eye movement, fluctuating heart and
respiratory rates, fluctuating blood pressure
Skeletal muscle tone lost
Most difficult to arouse
Duration of REM sleep increased with each
cycle and averages 20 minutes
Constitutes about 20%–25% of sleep

*Adapted from Taylor C, Lillis C, LeMone P: Fundamentals of Nursing: The Art and
Science of Nursing Care, 6th ed. Philadelphia: Lippincott Williams & Wilkins, 2008.*

wean from the ventilator due to muscle fatigue and carbon dioxide retention. The clinical significance is not fully appreciated because the relationship between poor sleep and recovery is unknown.[34] However, promotion of sleep for patients is not only a humanistic intervention but may also be a life-sustaining one.

The complex brain biology that enables sleep to occur is not fully understood. Melatonin, synthesized from tryptophan, is secreted by the pineal gland, and this is inhibited by light and stimulated by darkness. It is easy to see how melatonin secretion could be out of normal rhythm in an ICU setting. In fact, septic patients in an ICU are likely to have disrupted melatonin secretion not linked to the normal circadian pattern.[36] Many drugs interrupt sleep in critically ill patients.[37]

Sleep in patients with critical illness is greatly disrupted. Over four decades, researchers have noted that patients in ICUs have frequent awakenings, little to no REM sleep, shorter total sleep time than at home, and perceived poor quality of sleep.[38–40] Care interventions, including unnecessary baths between the hours of 2 and 5 a.m., have disturbed the sleep of critically ill patients on a routine basis.[41] A poor sleep pattern is characteristic of all age groups, from elderly to pediatric patients.[42] The impact of sleep disruption on the clinical outcome of ICU patients is not fully known. However, patients often report that sleep disruption is one of the most unpleasant aspects of their illness.

The patient's own report of sleep quality is the best measure of sleep adequacy, although this is inherently difficult when the patient is receiving mechanical ventilation. Similar to pain assessment, only the person can make the assessment: "I slept well" or "I didn't sleep at all." Monitoring brain waves by polysomnography is the gold standard for measuring patient sleep, but is not feasible as a standard measure in the ICU. If self-report of sleep is unobtainable, systematic observation of patients by nurses has been shown to be somewhat valid and reliable.[43] In addition, a visual analog scale is recommended for select patients at high risk for sleep disruption owing to extended stay in the ICU.[44] Wrist actigraphy is used as a research tool to continuously monitor activity and rest but may overestimate sleep in sedentary and elderly people.[33]

Promoting Sleep

Despite four decades of research into reasons why patients do not sleep in the ICU, little is done to facilitate what patients often rate as their number-one priority after pain relief: sleep. Box 2-3 outlines strategies that are most often recommended to promote sleep. The challenging environment dictates that the nurse first is sensitive to the patient's needs and attuned to the environment, and then has the tools and resources to implement sleep promotion. An old idea is the 5-minute backrub. The concept of using back massage to ease patients to sleep seems intuitive; however, until recently, it has never been systematically studied. In a study of 69 patients in an ICU, a 5-minute slow back massage (or *effleurage*) promoted increased sleep by 1 hour, compared with a control group.[45] If back massage were a hypnotic medication, it would be routinely ordered for ICU patients. The effective backrub was not the cold application of lotion and a quick one-handed massage while holding the patient on his side with the other hand, but rather a soothing, slow-stroke massage, in which the nurse first became centered and truly present with the patient.

The role of the nurse as a gatekeeper to protect patient sleep time will be more difficult to fulfill as patient/nurse ratios escalate but must remain a priority.[46] According to the 2002 clinical practice guidelines for sedatives and analgesics in the critically ill adult, now under revision by a multidisciplinary team of physicians, pharmacists, and nurses, sleep promotion should include optimization of the environment and nonpharmacologic methods to promote relaxation, with adjunctive use of hypnotics.[47] One intervention is to implement a sleep protocol that institutionalizes the importance of sleep,[48] blocks sleep times, and truly controls the environment. In one study, having a "quiet time" helped improve the

Box 2-3 • NURSING INTERVENTIONS for Promoting Sleep

- Provide large clocks and calendars.
- Block sleep times.
- Provide a quiet time.
- Have the patient use earplugs.
- Assess sleep time and quality of sleep by asking the patient when possible.
- Provide opportunity for music therapy.
- Provide a 5-minute backrub before sleep.
- Consider using white noise or ocean sounds.
- Eliminate pain.
- Position patient for comfort with pillows.
- Stop the practice of bathing patients in the middle of the night for the convenience of the nursing staff.
- Titrate environmental stimuli: turn down lights, turn down alarms, and decrease noise from television and talking.
- Evaluate the need for nursing care interruptions.
- At bedtime, provide information to lower anxiety. Do a review of the day and remind patient of progress made toward recovery, then add what to expect for the next day.
- Institute "PM Care" back to basics, brushing teeth, washing face before "bedtime."
- Allow family to be with the patient.
- Use relaxation techniques and guided imagery.
- Ensure patient privacy: close door or pull curtains.
- Post sign at designated times: "Patient Sleeping."

opportunity for sleep.[49] Another innovation in sleep promotion, which decreased noise and promoted sleep, involved moving all routine chest radiographs from 3 a.m. to 10 p.m.[50] Although this increased the workload of the radiology department on the evening shift, patient and nurse satisfaction rose dramatically.

Sleep of the health care provider is also an important aspect of the healing dyad in the ICU. Nurses who work nights are routinely sleep deprived and may have young children to care for at home or school to attend when the next day begins. The growing interest in patient safety makes the work patterns of nurses, including 12-hour shifts and overtime, a focus of study.[51] Nurses' vigilance to patient needs is threatened with longer work hours and increased risk for error.[51] Antidotes for working at night include scheduling of shifts to phase-advance the sleep cycle (i.e., going from days to evenings to nights), eating healthy snacks, using bright lights during a shift away from patient rooms, and obtaining regular exercise.[51] Compassionate caring includes the nurse caring for self to meet better the demands of patients, families, and colleagues.

FOSTERING TRUST

Almost every nurse in critical care can relate stories of special bonds that formed with individual patients and families. They can describe special situations where a trusting relationship developed and they made a difference in the patient's recovery or even dignified death. In contrast, research has shown that when patients mistrust their caregivers, they are more anxious and more vigilant of staff behaviors and lack the feeling of safety and security. The goals, then, are to display a confident, caring attitude, demonstrate technical competence, and develop effective communication techniques that will foster the development of a trusting relationship. Communication can be especially difficult with mechanically ventilated and intubated patients. Use of nonverbal signals, writing pads, or commercial communication boards can help make communication of basic needs easier.[4]

PROVIDING INFORMATION

Besides the need to feel safe, critically ill patients identify the need for information as having a high priority. This need to know involves all aspects of the patients' care. They need to know what is happening at the moment. They also need to know what will happen to them, how they are doing, and what they can expect. Many patients also need frequent explanations of what happened to them. These explanations reorient them, sort out sequences of events, and help them distinguish real events from dreams or hallucinations.[52] Anxiety can be greatly relieved with simple explanations. Consider the patient, for example, who was being weaned from the ventilator who just needed reassurance that if he did not breathe, the machine would do it for him. Families, too, have identified the need for information as a high priority. This is followed closely by the need to have hope. Most families identify physicians as the primary source for information. It is important for nurses to be mindful of patient confidentiality issues when speaking to family members. Nurses should have the patient's permission before giving confidential medical information to family members. If that is not possible because of the patient's condition, a family spokesperson should be identified as the person who may receive confidential information. This information should be recorded in the patient's medical record.[53]

ALLOWING CONTROL

Nursing measures that reinforce a sense of control help increase the patient's autonomy and reduce the overpowering sense of a loss of control. The nurse can help the patient exert more control over his or her environment in the following ways:

► Providing order and predictability in routines
► Using anticipatory guidance
► Allowing the patient to make choices whenever possible

▶ Involving the patient in decision making

▶ Providing information and explanation for procedures

Providing order and predictability allows the patient to anticipate and prepare for what is to follow. Perhaps it creates only a mirage of control, but anticipatory guidance keeps the patient from being caught off-guard and allows the mustering of coping mechanisms. Allowing small choices when the patient is willing and ready increases the patient's feeling of control over the environment. Would the patient prefer to lie on his or her right or left side? In which arm should the IV line be placed? What height is preferred for the head of the bed? Does the patient want to cough now or in 20 minutes after pain medication? Any decisions that afford the patient a certain amount of control and predictability are important. These small choices may also help the patient accept lack of control during procedures that involve little choice.

PRACTICING CULTURAL SENSITIVITY

Interventions for individual patients must be contextually based and culturally sensitive. Transcultural nursing refers to a formal area of study and practice that focuses on providing care that is compatible with the cultural beliefs, values, and lifestyles of people. A cultural assessment includes the patient's usual response to illness as well as his or her cultural norms, beliefs, and world views. Because individual responses and values may vary within the same culture, the patient should be recognized as an individual person within the cultural context. Exploring the meaning of the critical event with the patient, family members, and significant others may give clues to the patient's perception of what is happening. In addition, the nurse may ask if there is a particular ethnic or religious group with which the patient identifies and if there is anything the nurses may do to provide care that is sensitive to individual values or norms while the patient is hospitalized. Awareness and acceptance are the heart of cultural competence.[54] Incorporating complementary therapies that are culturally based may have a role in a person's treatment plan. Careful exploration of traditional or complementary therapies needs to be performed before implementation to avoid any harm due to interaction of therapies. This is especially true with use of herbal therapies or nutritional supplements that may have multiple ingredients with unknown or undesired side effects or interactions.[55]

PRESENCING AND REASSURANCE

Presence, or just "being there," can in itself be a meaningful strategy for alleviating distress or anxiety in the critically ill patient. Presencing is the therapeutic use of self, adopting a caring attitude, and paying attention to a person's needs. However, this presence implies more than just physical presence. It means giving one's full attention to the person, focusing on the person, and practicing active listening. When a nurse uses presence, the focus is not on a task or outside thoughts. Energy and attention are directed at the patient and his or her needs or feelings. This means one makes a conscious effort to use all of one's capacity, including eyes, voice, energy, and touch, in a more intentionally healing way.[56] Reassurance can be provided to the patient in the form of presencing and caring touch. Reassurance can also be verbal. Verbal reassurance can be effective for patients if it provides realistic encouragement or clarifies misconceptions. However, verbal reassurance is not valuable if it prevents a patient from expressing his or her emotions or stifles the need for further dialogue. Reassurance is intended to reduce fear and anxiety and evoke a calmer, more passive response. It is best directed at patients expressing unrealistic or exaggerated fears.

COGNITIVE TECHNIQUES

Techniques that have evolved from cognitive theories of learning may help anxious patients and their families. They can be initiated by the patient and do not depend on complex insight or understanding of one's own psychological makeup. They can also be used to reduce anxiety in a way that avoids probing into the patient's personal life. Furthermore, the patient's friends and family members can be taught these techniques to help them and the patient reduce tension.

Internal Dialogue

Highly anxious people are most likely giving themselves messages that increase or perpetuate their anxiety. These messages are conveyed in one's continuously running "self-talk," or internal dialogue. The patient in the ICU may be silently saying things such as, "I can't stand it in here. I've got to get out." Another unexpressed thought might be, "I can't handle this pain." By asking the patient to share aloud what is going on in this internal dialogue, the nurse can bring to awareness the messages that are distracting the patient from rest and relaxation. Substitute messages should be suggested to the patient. It is important to ask the patient to substitute rather than delete messages because the internal dialogue is continuously operating and will not turn off, even if the patient wills it to do so. Therefore, asking the patient to substitute constructive, reassuring comments is more likely to help the patient significantly reduce his or her tension level. Comments such as, "I'll handle this pain just one minute at a time" or "I've been in tough spots before, and I am capable of making it through this one!" automatically reduce anxiety and help the patient shape coping behaviors accordingly. Any message that enhances the patient's confidence, sense of control, and hope and puts him or her in a positive, active role, rather than the passive role of victim, increases the patient's sense of coping and well-being.

The nurse helps the patient develop self-dialogue messages that increase:

▶ Confidence
▶ Sense of control
▶ Ability to cope
▶ Optimism
▶ Hope

External Dialogue

A similar method can be applied to the patient's external conversation with other people. By simply requiring patients to speak accurately about themselves to others, the same goals can be accomplished. For example, patients who exclaim, "I can't do anything for myself!" should be asked to identify the things that they are able to do, such as lifting their own bodies, turning to one side, making a nurse feel good with a rewarding smile, or helping the family understand what is happening. Even the smallest movement in the weakest of patients should be acknowledged and claimed by the patient. This technique is useful in helping patients correct their own misconceptions of themselves and the way others see them. This reduces patients' sense of helplessness and therefore their anxiety.

Cognitive Reappraisal

This technique asks the patient to identify a particular stressor and then modify his or her response to that stressor. In other words, the patient reframes his or her perception of the stressor in a more positive light so that the stimulus is no longer viewed as threatening. The patient is given permission to take personal control of responses to the stimulus. This technique may be combined with guided imagery and relaxation training.

GUIDED IMAGERY AND RELAXATION TRAINING

These two useful techniques can be taught to the patient to help reduce tension. The nurse can encourage the patient to imagine either being in a very pleasant place or taking part in a very pleasant experience. The patient should be instructed to focus and linger on the sensations that are experienced. For example, asking the patient questions such as, "What colors do you see?", "What sounds are present?", "How does the air smell?", "How does your skin feel?", or "Is there a breeze in the air?" helps increase the intensity of the fantasy and thereby promotes relaxation through mental escape.

Guided imagery also can be used to help reduce unpleasant feelings of depression, anxiety, and hostility. Patients who must relearn life-sustaining tasks, such as walking and feeding themselves, can use imagery to prepare mentally to meet the challenge successfully. In these instances, patients should be taught to visualize themselves moving through the task and successfully completing it. If this method seems trivial or silly to the patients, they can be reminded that this method demands concentration and skill and is commonly used by athletes to improve their performance and to prepare themselves mentally before an important event. Guided imagery is a way of purposefully diverting or focusing the patients' thoughts and has been shown to empower patients, improving their satisfaction and well-being.[31,57]

The nurse can also use techniques that induce deep muscle relaxation to help the patient decrease anxiety. Deep muscle relaxation may reduce or eliminate the use of tranquilizing and sedating drugs. In progressive relaxation, the patient is first directed to find as comfortable a position as possible and then to take several deep breaths and let them out slowly. Next, the patient is asked to clench a fist or curl toes as tightly as possible, to hold the position for a few seconds, then to let go while focusing on the sensations of the releasing muscles. The patient should practice this technique, beginning with the toes and moving upward through other parts of the body—the feet, calves, thighs, abdomen, chest, and so on. This procedure is done slowly while the patient gives nonverbal signals (e.g., lifting a finger) to indicate when each new muscle mass has reached a state of relaxation. Extra time and attention should be given to the back, shoulders, neck, scalp, and forehead because many people experience physical tension in these areas.

Once a state of relaxation is achieved, the nurse can suggest that the patient fantasize or sleep as deeply as the patient chooses. The patient must be allowed to select and control the depth of relaxation and sleep, especially if the fear of death is prominent in the patient's mind. A moderately dark room and a soft voice facilitate relaxation. Asking the patient to relax is frequently nonproductive compared with directing the patient to release a muscle mass actively, let go of tension, or imagine tension draining through the body and sinking deeply into the mattress. Again, the patient is assisted to take an active rather than passive role by the nurse's careful use of language. In addition, a number of commercially available recordings can be used to assist in guided imagery and relaxation.[56–58]

DEEP BREATHING

When acutely anxious, the patient's breathing patterns may change, and the patient may hold his or her breath. This could be physically and psychologically detrimental. Teaching diaphragmatic breathing, also called abdominal breathing, to the patient may be useful as both a distraction and a coping mechanism. Diaphragmatic breathing can be taught easily and quickly to the preoperative patient or to a patient experiencing acute fear or anxiety. The patient may be asked to place a hand on the abdomen, inhale deeply through the nose, hold briefly, and exhale through pursed lips. The goal is to have the patient push out his own hand to demonstrate the deep breath. The nurse may demonstrate the technique and perform it along with the patient, until the patient is comfortable with the technique and is in control. The mechanically ventilated patient may be able to modify this technique by concentrating on breathing and on pushing out the hand. However, a mechanically ventilated patient experiencing severe agitation may not be able to respond to this technique.

MUSIC THERAPY

Music therapy has been used in the critical care environment as a strategy to reduce anxiety, provide distraction, and promote relaxation, rest, and sleep.[31,57] The patient is provided with a choice of specially recorded audiotapes and a set of headphones. Usually, music sessions are 20 to 90 minutes long, once or twice daily. Music selections may vary by individual taste, but the most commonly used selections have a tempo of 60 to 70 beats; a simple, direct musical rhythm; and a low-pitched sound with primarily a string composition. Most patients prefer music that is familiar to them. Many ICUs maintain a CD library with a variety of genres to satisfy patient choices. This intervention has proved effective for relaxing mechanically ventilated patients.[56–63]

HUMOR

A good belly laugh produces positive physiological and psychological effects. Laughter can increase the level of endorphins, the body's natural pain relievers, which are released into the bloodstream. Laughter can relieve tension and anxiety and relax muscles. Humor is a universal emotion that can help patients cope with stressful experiences. The use of humor by nurses in critical care, which can be spontaneous or planned, can help reduce procedural anxiety or provide distraction. Once again, the humor must be compatible with the context in which it is offered and with the person's cultural perspective. Many nurses report using humor cautiously after they have established a rapport with the individual. Nurses also report that they are able to take cues from the patient and visitors regarding the appropriate use of humor. Patients have reported that nurses who have a good sense of humor are more approachable and easier to talk with. Humor that is lighthearted, witty, and, of course, timed just right, is the most well received by adults.

Humor therapy has been used successfully in a variety of treatment settings, including pediatrics, surgery, oncology, and palliative care.[64–69] In an effort to incorporate the positive effects of humor into health care settings, some institutions have developed humor resource rooms or mobile humor carts. These provide patients with a variety of lighthearted reading materials, videotapes, and audiotapes. Also included on the cart may be games, puzzles, and magic tricks. Some nurses have created their own portable therapeutic humor kits, comic strips, jokes, or humorous stories to which their patients can relate.

In summary, use of humor by patients may help them reframe their anxiety and channel their energy toward feeling better. Some patients link humor with spirituality, noting that humor helped them cope better with serious illness and develop a closer relationship with God.[70] In addition, appropriate use of humor can relieve stress among critical care nurses who work in complex, challenging environments with significant economic pressures.

MASSAGE, AROMATHERAPY, AND THERAPEUTIC TOUCH

Massage is the purposeful stroking and kneading of muscles with the goal of providing comfort and promoting relaxation.[31,32,57] Nurses have traditionally used effleurage for backrubs for patient comfort. Effleurage uses slow, rhythmic strokes from distal to proximal areas of long muscles such as the back or extremities. Consistent, firm, yet flexible hand pressure is applied with all parts of the hand to conform to body contours. Lotion may be used to decrease friction and add moisture. Massage has been effective at reducing anxiety and promoting relaxation.[31] Patient selection is an important consideration when electing massage as a therapeutic intervention. Patients who are hemodynamically unstable, for example, would not be appropriate candidates. In addition, nurses require additional training in massage therapy to effectively incorporate more advanced massage techniques such as pétrissage or pressure points into plans of care for critically ill patients.

Massage can be combined with aromatherapy, in which massage is carried out with scented oils or lotions.[31,32] Some scents have been associated with specific beneficial effects. For example, lavender oil and other floral scents are said to be relaxing, citrus oils to be positive mood enhancers, and peppermint oils to be promoters of mental stimulation. Aromatherapy can also be accomplished with use of scented bath water or unlit scented candles placed in the room.[31,32]

Therapeutic touch is a set of techniques in which the practitioner's hands move over a patient in a systematic way to rebalance the patient's energy fields. An important component of therapeutic touch is compassionate intent on the part of the healer. Therapeutic touch as a complementary therapy has been used successfully in acute care settings to decrease anxiety and promote a sense of well-being. It is a foundational technique of healing touch. Healing touch involves a number of full-body and localized techniques to balance energy fields and promote healing. Implementation of healing touch therapy involves a formal educational program for healers, and its potential benefits are under active investigation.[57]

MERIDIAN THERAPY

Complementary and alternative medicine describes an array of nontraditional healing approaches. Meridian therapy refers to therapies that involve an acupoint, such as acupuncture, acupressure, and the activation of specific sites with electrical stimulation and low-intensity laser.[54] Meridian therapy originates from traditional Chinese medicine. Meridians are complex energy pathways that integrate into intricate patterns. These pathways contain sensitive energy points that are amenable to stimulation to relieve blockages that affect various physiological functions. Research has demonstrated the effectiveness of meridian therapy for pain relief, postoperative nausea, and other functions. Currently, research is underway to validate acupoint sites. Meridian therapy should be performed only by professionals with specialized training.

ANIMAL-ASSISTED THERAPY

The human–animal bond has been well documented. Pet ownership has been linked to higher levels of self-esteem and physical health. Pet therapy (or, more broadly, animal-assisted therapy) has had measurable benefits for schoolchildren and residents of nursing homes. More recently, this concept has been introduced to the acute and critical care settings with positive results. Some hospitals have developed guidelines for pet visitation; a patient's leashed pet may be brought to the hospital to visit with the patient. This type of program has been well received by patients and staff. However, it does require coordination between staff and family members. Pets must in good health, have up-to-date vaccinations, and be well-behaved in unfamiliar environments. The handler must be familiar with the pet and agree to follow hospital guidelines regarding time limits (generally 20 to 30 minutes per visit). A private patient room or visiting room is required. It is recommended that pets be leashed and wear a "shirt," which reduces shedding and identifies the pet. In some hospitals, a formal program exists in which volunteer owner–dog teams visit patients in the hospital on a variety of units. In addition, one hospital reported patients' delight in having fish aquariums placed in their rooms while they were awaiting heart transplantation.[32,56,58]

FOSTERING SPIRITUALITY AND HEALING

Caring in nursing includes recognition and support of the spiritual nature of human beings. Spirituality refers to the realm of invisible and intangible factors that influence our thoughts and behaviors. This includes not only religious beliefs, but goes beyond them. When people sense power and influence outside of time and physical existence, they are said to be experiencing the metaphysical aspects of spirituality.

Spirituality, which includes one's system of beliefs and values, can be defined "as the manner by which persons seek meaning in their lives and experience transcendence-connectedness to that which is beyond the self. . . ."[71] Intuition and knowledge from unknown sources and origins of unconditional love and belonging typically are viewed as spiritual power. A sense of universal connection, personal empowerment, and reverence for life also pertains to the existence of spirituality. These elements also may be viewed as benefits of spirituality. Spirituality includes the following:

- Religion
- Beliefs and values
- Intuition
- Knowledge from the unknown
- Unconditional love
- A sense of belonging
- A sense of connection with the universe
- Reverence for life
- Personal empowerment

Critical care patients and their families frequently find strength in prayer, which is used by people of many faiths. Research on prayer and health has demonstrated prayer to be a powerful tool to help patients cope with difficult situations, chronic illnesses, and impending death.[72–77] Nursing goals related to spirituality include the recognition and promotion of patients' spiritual sources of strength. By allowing and supporting patients to share their beliefs about the universe without disagreement, nurses help patients recognize and draw on their own sources of spiritual courage. Recognition of the unique spiritual nature of each patient is thought to assist personal empowerment and healing.

Nurses who find their own spiritual values in religion must acknowledge and respect that nonreligious people may also be spiritual and experience spirituality as a life force. Regardless of personal views, the nurse is obligated to assess patients' spiritual belief systems and assist them to recognize and draw on the values and beliefs already in existence for them.

Furthermore, critical illness may deepen or challenge existing spirituality. Patients have reported deeper faith after coping with critical illness.[72] During these times, it may be useful for the nurse or family to call on a spiritual or religious leader, hospital chaplain, or pastoral care representative to help the patient make meaningful use of the critical illness experience. Patients may also gain support from members of their congregation or family. It is important for nurses to assess and recognize the spiritual nature of their patients, to allow time for spiritual and religious practices, and to make referrals when needed. Referrals may be made to the hospital chaplain or to a clergy person of the patient's choice.

• Restraints in Critical Care

PHYSICAL RESTRAINTS

Physical restraints include any device that is used to restrict the patient's mobility and normal access to his or her body. These may include limb restraints, mittens with ties, vests or waist restraints, geriatric chairs, and side rails. Side rails are considered a restraint if used to limit the ability of the patient to get out of bed rather than to help him or her sit or stand up.

Historically, physical restraints have been used for patients in critical care to prevent potentially serious disruptions in patient care through accidental dislodgment of endotracheal tubes or lifesaving IV lines and other invasive therapies. Other reasons that have been cited for use of restraints include the prevention of falls, behavior management, and avoidance of liability suits due to patient injury. However, research related to restraint use, especially in elderly patients, has demonstrated that these reasons, although well intentioned, often are not valid.[78–82] Patients who are restrained have been shown to have more serious injuries secondary to falls as they "fight" the device that limits their freedom. In addition, there are reportedly a greater number of lawsuits related to improper restraint use than to injuries sustained when restraints were not used. Critically ill, intubated patients have been known to self-extubate despite the use of soft wrist restraints.

The forced immobilization that results from restraining a patient can prolong a patient's hospitalization by contributing to skin alterations, loss of muscle tone, impaired circulation, nerve damage, and pneumonia. Restraints have been implicated in accelerating patients' levels of agitation, resulting in injuries such as fractures or strangulation.

Standards on physical restraint use are published and monitored by the Joint Commission (formerly known as the Joint Commission on Accreditation of Healthcare Organizations) and the Centers for Medicare and Medicaid Services (formerly known as the Health Care Financing Administration). A summary of these standards is given in Box 2-4. These standards may be viewed on the websites of the respective agencies. Many hospitals have revised their policies, procedures, and documentation of the use of restraints to comply with the most recent revision of these standards, effective January 2001. Clinical practice guidelines have been published by the Society of Critical Care Medicine.[79]

CHEMICAL RESTRAINT

Chemical restraints refer to pharmacological agents that are given to patients as discipline or to limit disruptive behavior. Medications that have been used for behavior control include, but are not limited to, psychotropic drugs such as haloperidol, sedative agents such as benzodiazepines (e.g., lorazepam, midazolam), or the anticholinergic antihistamine, diphenhydramine. This definition does not apply to medications that are given to treat a medical condition. The use of sedative, analgesic, and anxiolytic medications is an important adjunct in the care of the critically ill patient.

Care must be taken to provide adequate comfort for patients experiencing life-threatening illnesses and a variety of noxious interventions. It is desirable to use the least amount of medication as feasible to achieve the goals of patient care because all medications have potential side effects and adverse reactions. Patients must be continually assessed for adequacy of comfort. Behaviors that seem to indicate pain may actually indicate a change in the patient's physiological status. Agitation, for example, may be a sign of hypoxemia. Caution must be exercised when using as-needed (PRN) medications to reduce pain and promote comfort. Without consistency in assessment, goal setting, and administration, PRN dosing may inadvertently lead to overmedication or undermedication in the critically ill patient. In addition, these medications can have rebound effects if abruptly withdrawn. Weaning a patient from analgesic or sedative medication may be as important as weaning a patient from a mechanical ventilator. Many ICUs incorporate assessment tools for patient comfort on their daily flow sheets.

ALTERNATIVES TO RESTRAINTS

What, then, is the well-meaning nurse to do when a patient is experiencing confusion or delirium and is pulling at his or her lifesaving devices and tubes?[83] Remember that physical restraint is the last resort, to be used only when the patient is a danger to himself or others and when other methods have failed. Restraints may actually potentiate the dangerous behavior. Rather, the nurse should attempt to identify what the patient is feeling or experiencing. What is the meaning behind the behavior? Is the patient cold? Does the patient itch? Is the patient in pain? Does the patient know where he or she is and why he or she is there? Sometimes addressing the patient's needs or concerns and reorienting the patient is all that is needed to calm him or her. Other interventions may include modifying the patient's environment, providing diversionary activities, allowing the patient more control or choices, and promoting adequate

---

Box 2-4 • Summary of Care Standards Regarding Physical Restraints

Initiating Restraints
- Restraints require the order of a licensed independent practitioner who must personally see and evaluate the patient within specified time periods.
- Restraints are used only as an emergency measure or after treatment alternatives have failed. (Treatment alternatives and patient responses are documented.)
- Restraints are instituted by staff who are trained and competent to use restraints safely. (A comprehensive training and monitoring program must be in place.)
- Restraint orders must be time limited. (A patient must not be placed in a restraint for longer than 24 hours, with reassessment and documentation of continued need for restraint at more frequent intervals.)
- Patients and families are informed about the reason/rationale for the use of the restraint.

Monitoring Patients in Restraints
- The patient's rights, dignity, and well-being are to be protected.
- The patient will be assessed every 15 minutes by trained and competent staff.
- The assessment and documentation must include evaluation of adequate nutrition, hydration, hygiene, elimination, vital signs, circulation, range of motion, injury due to the restraint, physical and psychological comfort, and readiness for discontinuance of the restraint.

Box 2-5 • Alternatives to Physical Restraints

Modifications to Patient Environment
- Keep the bed in the lowest position.
- Minimize the use of side rails to what is needed for positioning.
- Optimize room lighting.
- Activate bed and chair exit alarms where available.
- Remove unnecessary furniture or equipment.
- Ensure that the bed wheels are locked.
- Position the call light within easy reach.

Modifications to Therapy
- Frequently assess the need for treatments and discontinue lines and catheters at earliest opportunity.
- Toilet patients frequently.
- Disguise treatments, if possible (e.g., keep intravenous [IV] solution bags behind patient's field of vision, apply loose stockinette or long-sleeved gown over IV sites).
- Meet physical and comfort needs (e.g., skin care, pain management, positioning wedges, hypoxemia management).
- When possible, guide the patient's hand through exploration of the device or tube, and explain the purpose, route, and alarms of the device or tube.
- Mobilize the patient as much as possible (e.g., consider physical therapy consult, need for cane or walker, reclining chairs, or bedside commode).

Involvement of the Patient and Family in Care
- Allow patient choices and control when possible.
- Family members or volunteers can provide company and diversionary activities.
- Consider solitary diversionary activities (e.g., music, videos or television, books on tape).
- Ensure that the patient has needed glasses and hearing aids.

Therapeutic Use of Self
- Use calm, reassuring tones.
- Introduce yourself and let the patient know he or she is safe.
- Find acceptable means of communicating with intubated or nonverbal patients.
- Reorient patients frequently by explaining treatments, devices, care plans, activities, and unfamiliar sounds, noises, or alarms.

sleep and rest (Box 2-5).[84,85] Some hospitals have instituted restraint protocols and decision trees to help nurses with assessment and care of patients in restraints.[80–82,86]

• Clinical Applicability Challenges

Short-Answer Questions

1. You are the nurse caring for a patient who is scheduled for a cardiac catheterization in the morning. In report, you are told the patient has been "acting out all day—crying and very emotional." Explore the possible meaning behind the patient's behavior. Formulate an action plan, including additional data that may be needed.

2. You observe an elderly African-American woman clutching her Bible to her chest with her eyes tightly shut. She is moving her lips as if in animated prayer. Formulate a nursing plan to provide spiritual support for this patient.

Review Questions

1. Anxiety occurs when patients
   a. are occupied with internal dialogue.
   b. are overly dependent on the nurse.
   c. have a long-term recovery ahead.
   d. perceive a threat to their well-being.

2. The best way to help patients handle anxiety is to
   a. reassure them that they will receive the best possible care.
   b. assist them to talk about their fears and concerns.
   c. be direct and honest with them.
   d. limit visitors' time with them.

3. The nurse can help provide a sense of control in patients by
   a. controlling external stimuli.
   b. limiting choices to avoid confusion.
   c. including the patient in decision making.
   d. organizing items on the bedside table.

4. Cognitive reappraisal is a technique that allows the patient to
   a. identify the stressor and alter the response to it.
   b. ignore a threatening stimulus.
   c. use guided imagery and progressive muscle relaxation.
   d. use distraction as a coping mechanism.

5. A positive effect of laughter is
   a. reduced catecholamines.
   b. a psychological sense of well-being.
   c. increased muscle tension.
   d. an alteration in mental status.

6. Reassurance will not be valuable for the patient if it
   a. calms excessive fears.
   b. ceases expression of emotions.
   c. decreases respiratory rate.
   d. is combined with presencing.

7. Sleep deprivation in patients who are critically ill is most often attributed to
   a. bed baths during the evening shift.
   b. untreated pain and anxiety.
   c. family visiting.
   d. altered melatonin levels.

8. ICU design should consider which one of the following?
   a. Bright, overhead lighting
   b. Waiting rooms to keep family members out of the patient's room
   c. Thick carpets to muffle sound
   d. Soft, calm colors

References

1. Claesson A, Mattson H, Idvall E: Experiences expressed by artificially ventilated patients. J Clin Nurs 14:116–117, 2005
2. Doering LV, McGuire AW, Rourke D: Recovering from cardiac surgery: What patients want you to know. Am J Crit Care 11(4):333–343, 2002
3. Nelson JE, Meier DE, Oei EJ, et al: Self-reported symptom experience of critically ill cancer patients receiving intensive care. Crit Care Med 29(2):277–282, 2001
4. Thomas L: Clinical management of stressors perceived by patients on mechanical ventilation. AACN Clinical Issues 14(1):73–81, 2003
5. Stein-Parbury J, McKinley S: Patients' experiences of being in an intensive care unit: A select literature review. Am J Crit Care 9(1):20–27, 2000
6. McKinley S, Nagy S, Stein-Parbury J, et al: Vulnerability and security in seriously ill patients in intensive care. Intensive Crit Care Nurs 18(1):27–36, 2002
7. McKinney AA, Deeny P: Leaving the intensive care unit: A phenomenological study of the patient's experience. Intensive Crit Care Nurs 18:320–331, 2002
8. Rotondi AJ, Chelluri L, Sirio C, et al: Patients' recollections of stressful experiences while receiving prolonged mechanical ventilation in an intensive care unit. Crit Care Med 30(4):746–752, 2002
9. Buchman TG: Stress and the biology of the responses. In Albert RK, Slutsky AS, Ranieri VM, et al (eds): Clinical Critical Care Medicine. Philadelphia, Mosby Elsevier, 2006
10. Caine RM: Psychological influences in critical care: Perspectives from psychoneuroimmunology. Crit Care Nurse 23(2):60–70, 2003
11. Hadley JS, Hinds CJ: Anabolic strategies in critical illness. Curr Opin Pharmacol 2(6):700–707, 2002
12. Lusk B, Lash AA: The stress response, psychoneuroimmunology, and stress among ICU patients. DCCN 24(1):25–31, 2005
13. Donchin Y, Seagull FJ: The hostile environment of the intensive care unit. Curr Opin Crit Care 8:316–320, 2002.
14. Fairman J, Lynaugh J: Critical Care Nursing: A History. Philadelphia, University of Pennsylvania Press, 1998
15. Stichler JF: Creating healing environments in critical care units. Crit Care Nurs Q 24(3):1–20, 2001
16. Fontaine DK, Prinkey Briggs L, et al: Designing humanistic critical care environments. Crit Care Nurs Q 24(3):21–34, 2001
17. Henneman EA, Cardin S: Family-centered care: A practical approach to making it happen. Crit Care Nurse 22(6):12–19, 2002
18. Kahn DM, Cook TE, Carlisle CC, et al: Identification and modification of environmental noise in an ICU setting. Chest 114:535–540, 1998
19. Freedman NS, Kotzer N, Schwab RJ: Patient perception of sleep quality and etiology of sleep disruption in the intensive care unit. Am J Respir Crit Care Med 159(4 Pt 1):1155–1162, 1999
20. Aaron JN, Carlisle CC, Carskadon MA, et al: Environmental noise as a cause of sleep disruption in an intermediate respiratory care unit. Sleep 19:707–710, 1996
21. Gabor JY, Cooper AB, Crombach SA, et al: Contribution of the intensive care unit environment to sleep disruption in mechanically ventilated patients and healthy subjects. Am J Respir Crit Care Med 167:706–715, 2003.
22. Ulrich RS: View through a window may influence recovery from surgery. Science 224:420–421, 1984
23. Stein-Parbury J, McKinley S: Patients' experiences of being in an intensive care unit: A select literature review. Am J Crit Care 9:20–27, 2000
24. Vinall PE: Design technology: What you need to now about circadian rhythms in healthcare design. J Healthc Design 9:141–144, 1997
25. Holtzclaw BJ: Thermal balance. In Kinney MR, Dunbar SB, Brooks-Brunn JA, et al (eds): AACN Clinical Reference for Critical Care Nursing, 4th ed. St. Louis, Mosby, 1998
26. Jastremski CA: ICU bedside environment: A nursing perspective. Crit Care Clin 16(4):723–734, 2000
27. Horrigan B: Region's hospital opens holistic nursing unit. Alt Ther Health Med 6(4):92–93, 2000
28. Frazier SK, Moser DK, Riegel B, et al: Critical care nurses' assessment of patients' anxiety: Reliance on physiological and behavioral parameters. Am J Crit Care 11(1):57–64, 2002
29. Chlan L: Description of anxiety levels by individual differences and clinical factors in patients receiving mechanical ventilatory support. Heart Lung 32(4):275–282, 2003
30. McKinley S, Dean L: Assessment and reduction of anxiety in mechanically ventilated patients. Connect World Crit Care Nurs 4(2):1, 2005
31. Keegan L: Therapies to reduce stress and anxiety. Crit Care Nurs Clin N Am 15(3):321–327, 2003
32. Molter NC: Creating a healing environment for critical care. Crit Care Nurs Clin N Am 15(3):295–304, 2003
33. Lee KA: Impaired sleep. In Carrieri-Kohlman V, Lindsey AM, West CM (eds): Pathophysiological Phenomena in Nursing: Human Responses to Illness. St. Louis: Saunders, 2003, pp 363–383
34. Weinhouse GL, Schwab R: Sleep in the critically ill patient. Sleep 29(5):707–716, 2006
35. Reishtein JL: Sleep in mechanically ventilated patients. Crit Care Nurs Clin N Am 17:251–255, 2005
36. Mundigler G, Delle-Karth G, Koreny M, et al: Impaired circadian rhythm of melatonin secretion in sedated critically ill patients with severe sepsis. Crit Care Med 30:536–540, 2002
37. Bourne RS, Mills GH: Sleep disruption in critically ill patients—pharmacological considerations. Anaesthesia 59:374–384, 2004
38. Gabor JY, Cooper AB, Crombach SA, et al: Contribution of the intensive care unit environment to sleep disruption in mechanically ventilated patients and healthy subjects. Am J Respir Crit Care Med 167:706–715, 2003
39. Parthasarathy S, Tobin MJ. Sleep in the intensive care unit. Intensive Care Med 30:197–206, 2004
40. Redeker NS: Sleep in acute care settings: An integrative review. J Nurs Scholarsh 32:31–38, 2000
41. Tamburri LM, DiBrienza R, Zozula R, Redeker NS: Nocturnal care interactions with patients in critical care units. Am J Crit Care 13:102–115, 2004
42. Cureton-Lane RA, Fontaine DK: Sleep in the pediatric ICU: An empirical investigation. Am J Crit Care 6:56–63, 1997
43. Edwards GB, Schuring LM: Pilot study: Validating staff nurses' observations of sleep and wake states among critically ill patients using polysomnography. Am J Crit Care 2:125–131, 1993
44. Richardson SJ: A comparison of tools for the assessment of sleep pattern disturbance in critically ill adults. Dimens Crit Care Nurs 16:226–239, 1997
45. Richards KC: Effect of a back massage and relaxation intervention on sleep in critically ill patients. Am J Crit Care 7(4):288–299, 1998
46. Dracup K, Bryan-Brown CW: To work: Perchance to sleep. Am J Crit Care 9:224–226, 2000
47. Jacobi J, Fraser GL, Coursin DB, et al: Clinical practice guidelines for the sustained use of sedatives and analgesics in the critically ill adult. Crit Care Med 30:119–141, 2002
48. Edwards GB, Schuring LM: Sleep protocol: A research-based practice change. Crit Care Nurse 13(2):84–88, 1993
49. Olson DM, Borel CO, Laskowitz DT, et al: Quiet time: A nursing intervention to promote sleep in neurocritical care units. Am J Crit Care 10:74–78, 2001
50. Cmiel CA, Karr DM, Gasser DM, et al: Noise control: A nursing team's approach to sleep promotion. Am J Nurs 104(2):40–48, 2004

51. Scott LD, Rogers AE, Hwang WT, Zhang Y: Effects of critical care nurses' work hours on vigilance and patients' safety. Am J Crit Care 15:30–37, 2006

52. Roberts B, Chaboyer W: Patients' dreams and unreal experiences following intensive care unit admission. Nurs Crit Care 9(4):173–180, 2004

53. Jansen MPM, Schmitt NA: Family-focused interventions. Crit Care Nurs Clin N Am 15(3):347–354, 2003

54. Snyder M, Niska K: Cultural related complementary therapies: Their use in critical care units. Crit Care Nurs Clin N Am 15(3):341–346, 2003

55. Lu Y: Herb use in critical care: what to watch for. Crit Care Clin N Am 15(3):313–319, 2003

56. Brenner ZR, Krenzer ME: Using complementary and alternative therapies to promote comfort at end of life. Crit Care Nurs Clin N Am 15(3) 355–362, 2003

57. McCaffrey R, Taylor N: Effective anxiety treatment prior to diagnostic cardiac catheterization. Holist Nurs Pract 19(2): 70–77, 2005

58. Floyd JP, Fernandes JH: Making a place for CAM in the ICU. RN 66(7):44–47, 2003

59. Almerud S, Petersson K: Music therapy: A complementary treatment for mechanically ventilated intensive care patients. Intensive Crit Care Nurs 19(1):21–30, 2003

60. Bally K, Campbell D, Chesnick K, Tranmer JE: Effects of patient-controlled music therapy during coronary angiography on procedural pain and anxiety distress syndrome. Crit Care Nurse 23(2):50–59, 2003

61. Chan MF, Wong OC, Chan HL, et al: Effects of music on patients undergoing a C-clamp procedure after percutaneous coronary interventions. J Adv Nurs 53(6):669–679, 2006

62. Hanser SB, Mandel SE: The effects of music therapy in cardiac healthcare. Cardiol Rev 13(1):18–23, 2005

63. White JM: State of the science of music interventions: critical care and perioperative practice. Crit Care Nurs Clin N Am 12(2):219–225, 2000

64. Christie W, Moore C: The impact of humor on patients with cancer. Clin J Oncol Nurs 92:211–218, 2005

65. Dean RAK, Gregory DM: More than trivial: Strategies for using humor in palliative care. Cancer Nurs 28(4):292–300, 2005

66. Dowling JS: Humor: A coping strategy for pediatric patients. Pediatr Nurs 28(2):123–129, 2002

67. Greenberg M: Therapeutic play: Developing humor in the nurse-patient relationship. J N Y State Nurses Assoc 34(1):25–31, 2003

68. Hoare J: The best medicine: When we laugh, the ensuing endorphin rush makes us feel better. Nurs Standard 19(14–16): 18–20, 2004

69. Vagnoli L, Caprilli S, Robiglio A, Messeri A: Clown doctors as a treatment for preoperative anxiety in children: A randomized, prospective study. Pediatrics 116(4):e563–e567, 2005

70. Johnson P: The use of humor and its influences on spirituality and coping in breast cancer survivors. Oncol Nurs Forum 29(4):691–695, 2002

71. Smith AR: Using the synergy model to provide spiritual nursing care in critical care settings. Crit Care Nurs 26(4):41–47, 2006

72. Pargament KI, Koenig HG, Tarakeshwar N, Hahn J: Religious coping methods as predictors of psychological, physical and spiritual outcomes among medically ill elderly patients: A two year longitudinal study. J Health Psychol 9(6):713–730, 2004

73. Johnson KS, Elbert-Avila KI, Tulsky JA: The influence of spiritual beliefs and practices on the treatment preferences of African-Americans: A review of the literature. J Am Geriatr Soc 53(4):711–719, 2005

74. Narayanasamy A: Spiritual coping mechanisms in chronic illness: A qualitative study. J Clin Nurs 13(1):116–117, 2004

75. Kelly J: Spirituality as a coping mechanism. DCCN 23(4): 162–168, 2004

76. Puchalski CM, Dorff E, Hendi IY: Spirituality, religion, and healing in palliative care. Clin Geriatr Med 20(4):689–714, 2004

77. Scobie G, Caddell C: Quality of life at end of life: Spirituality and coping mechanisms in terminally ill patients. Internet J Pain Symptoms Control Palliat Care 4(1):36, 2005

78. Kielb C, Hurlock-Chorostecki C, Sipprell D: Can minimal patient restraint be safely implemented in the intensive care unit? Dynamics 16(1):16–19, 2005

79. Maccioli GA, Dorman T, Brown BR, et al: Clinical practice guidelines for the maintenance of patient physical safety in the intensive care unit: Use of restraining therapies. American College of Critical Care Medicine Task Force 2001–2002. Crit Care Med 31(11):2665–2676, 2003

80. Martin B: Restraint use in acute and critical care settings: Changing practice. AACN Clin Issues Adv Pract Acute Crit Care 13(2):294–306, 2002

81. Martin B, Mathisen L: Use of physical restraints in adult critical care: A bicultural study. Am J Crit Care 14(2):133–142, 2005

82. Mion LC, Fogel J, Sandhu S, et al: Outcomes following physical restraint reduction programs in two acute care hospitals. Jt Comm J Qual Improv 27(11):605–618, 2001

83. Marshall MC, Soucy MD: Delirium in the intensive care unit. Crit Care Nurs Q 26(3):172–178, 2003

84. Honkus VL: Sleep deprivation in critical care units. Crit Care Nurs Q 26(3):179–192, 2003

85. Richards K, Nagel C, Markie M, et al: Use of complementary and alternative therapies to promote sleep in critically ill patients. Crit Care Nurs Clin N Am 15:329–340, 2003

86. Vance DL: Effect of a treatment interference protocol on clinical decision making for restraint use in the intensive care unit: a pilot study. AACN Clin Issues Adv Pract Acute Crit Care 14(1):82–91, 2003

The Family's Experience With Critical Illness

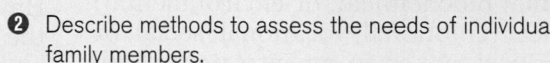

Colleen Norton

Objectives

Based on the content in this chapter, the reader should be able to:

❶ Describe the impact of a critical illness and the critical care environment on the family.

❷ Describe methods to assess the needs of individual family members.

❸ Describe nursing behaviors that help families cope with crisis.

❹ Discuss palliative care issues in the critical care environment that have an impact on the family.

❺ Define the components of the critical care family assistance program.

❻ List items to include in a plan of care that reflect the needs of the family.

Nurses who strive to deliver consistent quality critical care from a holistic perspective need to recognize the importance of also caring for patients' families. The interaction between the family/support system and the patient in the critical care environment, and the needs that result from this interaction, remain a challenge and responsibility of the contemporary critical care nurse.

The *Oxford English Dictionary* defines family as "a group of persons consisting of the parents and their children whether actually living together or not; in a wider sense, the unity formed by those who are nearly connected by blood and affinity." For the purpose of this chapter, *family* is defined as any people who share intimate and routine day-to-day living with the critically ill patient. Anyone who is a significant part of the patient's normal lifestyle is considered a family member. The term family describes the people whose social homeostasis and well-being are altered by the patient's entrance into the arena of critical illness or injury. To provide family-centered care, a philosophy that acknowledges that patients are part of a larger "whole" or family is essential to provide the best possible care to the patient and family.[1]

This chapter addresses the family in crisis, stressors in the critical care environment, coping mechanisms, and the family and the nursing process. The evolution of the Critical Care Family Assistance Program and palliative care are also discussed.

• Stress, Critical Illness, and the Impact on the Family

A critical illness is a sudden, unexpected, and often life-threatening occurrence for both the patient and the family that threatens the steady state of internal equilibrium usually maintained in the family unit. It can be an acute illness or trauma, an acute exacerbation of a chronic illness, or an acute episode of a previously unknown problem. A family member's entrance as a participant in the life–death sick role of a loved one threatens the well-being of the family and can trigger a stress response in both the patient and the family. Family members of patients in the critical care unit (CCU) may experience stress, disorganization, and helplessness, which may ultimately result in difficulty in mobilizing appropriate coping resources, thus leading to anxiety.[2] The family enters this unplanned situation with its unexpected outcomes and often is forced into the role of decision maker. The astute critical care nurse recognizes that the fear and anxiety demonstrated by the patient and family is an expected consequence of activation of the stress response, a somewhat protective, adaptive mechanism initiated by the neuroendocrine system in response to stressors. The stress response of family members is varied.

Studied initially by Selye in 1956,[3] *stress* has been defined as a specific syndrome that was nonspecifically induced. Selye also discussed the role of stressors, the stimuli that produced tension and could contribute to disequilibrium. Stressors can be physiological (trauma, biochemical, or environmental) and psychological (emotional, vocational, social, or cultural). The critical care environment is rich in both physiological and psychosocial stressors that threaten the state of well-being of the patient and family.

In response to a stressor, the fight-or-flight mechanism is activated, releasing the catecholamines norepinephrine and epinephrine through the sympathetic nervous system. These hormones are responsible for the increased heart rate, increased blood pressure, and vasoconstriction that make up the physiological response to the *alarm stage*, the initial stage of the general adaptation syndrome to stress described by Selye. The alarm stage is followed by the *stage of resistance*, which attempts to maintain the body's resistance to stress. According to Selye's theory, all people move through the first two stages many times and become adapted to the stressors encountered during ordinary life. If the person is unsuccessful at adaptation, or if the stressor is too great or prolonged, alarm and resistance are followed by the *stage of exhaustion*, which can lead to death, the result of a wearing down of the human body. It is a challenge to the critical care nurse to assist both the patient and family through this stress response, resulting in an adaptation to the critical care environment. Helping the patient's family resolve the crisis response and facilitate successful coping by creating a safe passage is an identified competency of the contemporary critical care nurse.[4] Family members expect nurses to intervene and meet their needs, and they have high expectations for family-centered care.[5]

After the initial fear and anxiety over the possible death of the family member, other considerations affect the family, including a shift in responsibilities and role performance; unfamiliarity with the routines of the CCU; and a lack of knowledge concerning the course and outcome of the disease. These issues can develop and persist over the duration of the patient's stay in the CCU.

Contributions to the family unit previously attributed to the patient are added to the responsibilities of others. Financial concerns are usually major, and daily activities that were of little consequence before become important and difficult to manage. Chores such as balancing a checkbook, contributing to car pools, and shopping for groceries can become critically significant if left undone. This consequence of the critical illness requires adding the responsibilities of the patient to the responsibilities of others.

The social role that the patient plays in the family is absent during the critical illness. Comforter, organizer, mediator, lover, friend, and disciplinarian are examples of important roles in family functioning that may be, under normal circumstances, fulfilled by the patient. When that role function is unfulfilled, havoc and grief may ensue.

The circumstances surrounding the nature of the patient's illness can also be a stressor for the family. In a sudden, unexpected event, such as a blunt trauma or an acute myocardial infarction, the life of the family can be brought to a halt in a matter of minutes. Having little or no time to prepare for such an event, the family is overwhelmed with a massive amount of unmanageable stress and can be thrown into crisis. The hospital CCU, in most instances an unknown entity, becomes the center of the life of the family. When allowed to visit in the CCU, the family observes sophisticated, intimidating equipment that causes additional fear. Such stress often can manifest itself as anger toward the caregiver. The caregiver, absorbed with the physical care of the patient, frequently has limited or inadequate time to respond to family members' emotional needs, unrealistic goals, and expectations of the health care staff.[6]

In other instances, the critical event is an acute exacerbation of a chronic but life-threatening illness. Such an episode brings with it a different set of stressors, reminding the family of difficult and painful times in the past when they have faced similar circumstances. Prolonged critical illness can present emotional difficulties for the family, which may increase the likelihood of crisis.

COPING MECHANISMS

Coping mechanisms can be defined as a person's response to a change in the environment; they can be positive or negative. The critical care nurse, as caregiver to both the patient and family, should be aware of the use of coping mechanisms by the family as a means of maintaining equilibrium. A sense of fear, panic, shock, or disbelief is sometimes followed by irrational acts, demanding behavior, withdrawal, perseveration, or fainting. The family attempts to obtain some sense of control over the situation, often demonstrated by refusing to leave the bedside or, alternatively, by minimizing the severity of the illness. Reactions to crisis are difficult to categorize because they depend on the different coping styles, personalities, and stress management techniques of the family. The nurse must be able to interpret the feeling that a person in crisis is experiencing, particularly when that person cannot identify the problem or the feeling to himself or herself or to others. The following are four generalizations about crisis:

► Whether people emerge stronger or weaker as a result of a crisis is based not so much on their character as on the quality of help they receive during a crisis state.

▶ People are more open to suggestions and help during an actual crisis.

▶ With the onset of a crisis, old memories of past crises may be evoked. If maladaptive behavior was used to deal with previous situations, the same type of behavior may be repeated in the face of a new crisis. If adaptive behavior was used, the impact of the crisis may be lessened.

▶ The primary way to survive a crisis is to be aware of it.

• The Family and the Nursing Process

NURSING ASSESSMENT

Nursing assessment by the critical care nurse involves primarily but not exclusively an appraisal of the patient. It is also the responsibility of the nurse to include members of the family in order to provide holistic nursing care. The nursing assessment serves as a database and an identification of strengths and concerns on which care of the patient and family can be supported. It includes not only physiological responses but also psychological, social, environmental, cultural, economic, and spiritual reactions. It involves an assessment of verbal and nonverbal behavior and requires clinical expertise. A thorough nursing assessment guides the formulation of nursing diagnoses. The standards of the American Association of Critical-Care Nurses (AACN) emphasize and support the importance of an assessment of the family and the continual involvement of the family in the nursing care of the patient.[7]

An important part of the family assessment is a history of the family. Who does the patient include in the description of his or her family? Although all patients belong to a family, the family might not include or be restricted to blood relatives. Who are the people most upset about the patient's illness? Is there a formal or informal leader identified by the group? This becomes important when communicating with the family in decision making, as well as with legal matters, such as obtaining consent and withdrawing life support. What is the coping style of the family? Does the family have a history of dealing with a critical illness? What are the relationships between the members of the family? How close is the family? Do the family members identify any unresolved issues? The family history can aid the nurse in interpreting how the family is coping with stress, how their coping mechanisms will affect the patient, and how they are adapting to the patient's illness.

Four intrinsic elements of an assessment of the family are:[8]

1. Providing a human, caring presence
2. Acknowledging multiple perceptions
3. Respecting diversity
4. Valuing each person in the context of the family

Numerous assessment tools are available to aid the nurse in determining the needs and problems the family faces. One of the initial assessment tools was developed by Molter in 1979.[9] This method includes a 45-item needs assessment tool, which became an instrument to describe the needs of critical care family members. Leske modified the tool used by Molter by adding an open-ended item and calling it the Critical Care Family Needs Inventory (CCFNI).[10] The CCFNI has been used widely during the past two decades to identify the needs of family members in the CCU. The CCFNI, after analysis, was found to contain five distinct subscales: support, comfort, information, proximity, and assurance.[11] Mendonca and Warren used the CCFNI to assess the needs of family members and the importance of these needs in the first 18 to 24 hours after admission of the adult patient to the CCU.[2] The family remains the most important social context to assess and consider when determining interventions to influence patient outcomes in a positive way.[10]

Nursing research using these tools reveals consistency in what areas are important and should be addressed with family members. These areas include but are not limited to:

1. Family satisfaction with care given
2. Explanations that the family can understand
3. The need for close proximity to the patient
4. Honest information about the patient's condition
5. An understanding of why things are done
6. Delivery of care by staff members who are courteous and show interest in how the family is doing
7. Assurance that someone will call the family with any changes

The tools also suggest assessing how comfortable the family is in the waiting room and inquiring about what things could be made better for them. Identified needs included physical needs (e.g., having comfortable furniture, having the waiting room near the patient, and having a bathroom nearby) as well as emotional needs, such as a place to be alone in the hospital and the opportunity to discuss negative feelings. In addition, families of critically ill patients have other needs, which should be addressed frequently. These needs include:[11]

▶ To feel that there is hope
▶ To feel that hospital personnel care about the patient
▶ To know the prognosis
▶ To receive information about the patient once a day
▶ To see the patient frequently

In summary, recent research has shown that the top needs of families of critically ill patients are the need for information, the need for support from hospital staff, and the need for hope.[12]

Although the needs perceived by the family may differ from those perceived by the nurse, strong communication skills, as well as an atmosphere of concern

<table>
<tr><td>

Box 3-1

Examples of Nursing Diagnoses and Collaborative Problems for the Family With Critical Illness or Injury

- Altered Family Process
- Altered Health Maintenance
- Altered Parenting
- Altered Role Performance
- Anticipatory Grieving
- Anxiety
- Caregiver Role Strain, Risk for
- Communication, Readiness for
- Confusion, Acute
- Decisional Conflict
- Denial
- Family Process: Dysfunctional
- Fatigue
- Fear
- Hopelessness
- Impaired Memory
- Ineffective Denial
- Ineffective Individual/Family Coping
- Knowledge Deficit
- Loneliness, Risk for
- Powerlessness
- Sleep Pattern Disturbance
- Spiritual Distress
- Spiritual Distress, Risk for

</td></tr>
</table>

and caring, help the nurse gather the subjective and objective assessment data and formulate the appropriate nursing diagnoses for the family. Examples of nursing diagnoses appropriate to the family members of a critically ill patient are given in Box 3-1. The nursing diagnosis guides both the nurse and the family in establishing mutual goals.

NURSING INTERVENTIONS

The time spent by the critical care nurse with the family is often limited because of the crucial physiological and psychosocial needs of the patient. Therefore, it is important to make every interaction with the family as useful and therapeutic as possible. Nursing interventions should address cognitive, affective, and behavioral domains[13] and should be designed to:

▶ Help the family learn from the crisis experience and move toward adaptation

▶ Regain a state of equilibrium

▶ Experience the normal (but painful) feelings associated with the crisis, to avoid delayed depression and allow for future emotional growth

A novel idea in the practice of family-centered care is to consider inviting a family member on daily rounds with the team in the CCU. An advantage of having a family member on rounds includes reduced stress in families because members have current information and a representative who can ask questions. A disadvantage could be that care is complex; a family member may not be well prepared to handle the information cognitively or emotionally. However, a recent study demonstrated widespread family member satisfaction with the invitation to join patient care rounds in a trauma patient population.[14] This example of including family members on rounds is just one of several ideas to improve the family's experience in critical care. Asking family members to assist in providing some aspects of basic care is also under study, but not all family members are willing participants, and thus the requests must be considered on an individual basis.[15,16]

Suggestions for nursing interventions with the family in crisis are outlined in Box 3-2. Considerations for the older patient are presented in Box 3-3.

 Box 3-2 • NURSING INTERVENTIONS for Care of the Family in Crisis

- Guide the family in defining the current problem.
- Help the family identify its strengths and sources of support.
- Prepare the family for the critical care environment, especially regarding equipment and purposes of the equipment.
- Speak openly to the patient and the family about the critical illness.
- Demonstrate a concern about the current crisis and an ability to help with the initial relationship.
- Be realistic and honest about the situation, taking care not to give false reassurance.
- Convey feelings of hope and confidence in the family's ability to deal with the situation.
- Try to perceive the feelings that the crisis evokes in the family.
- Help the family identify and focus on feelings.
- Assist the family to determine the goals and steps to take in facing the crisis.

- Provide opportunities for the patient and the family to make choices and avoid powerlessness and hopelessness.
- Assist the family in finding ways to communicate with the patient.
- Encourage the family to help with the care of the patient.
- Discuss all issues as they relate to the patient's uniqueness, avoiding generalizations.
- Help the family to set short-term goals so that progress and positive changes can be seen.
- Ensure that the family receives information about all significant changes in the patient's condition.
- Advocate the adjustment of visiting hours to accommodate the needs of the family as permitted by the situation in the unit.
- Determine whether there is space available in the hospital near the unit where the family can be alone and have privacy.
- Recognize the patient's and family's spirituality, and suggest the assistance of a spiritual advisor if there is a need

Box 3-3 • CONSIDERATIONS FOR THE OLDER PATIENT: Providing Care for the Critically Ill Older Patient

- Respect the dignity, intelligence, privacy, and maturity of the patient at all times.
- Maintain the patient's right to make decisions as long as possible.
- Avoid the use of paternalism in patient care.
- Integrate the physiological and cognitive changes of aging with the assessment and care of the patient.
- Allow the family to share in the care of their family member.
- Provide active participation and a sense of control for the patient and family.
- Ascertain that the patient remains the focus of care and that interventions are performed for the good of the patient.
- Assess the impact that medical and nursing interventions have on quality of life and sense of well-being.
- Determine family burden resulting from the critical illness.

VISITATION ADVOCACY

Policies regarding the use and provision of visiting hours should be evaluated periodically. Research has demonstrated that novel approaches to visitation, such as allowing children who are accompanied by an adult to visit a relative in the CCU and the use of animal-assisted therapy in the CCU, can have positive effects on the patient, including increased feelings of happiness and calmness and reduced feelings of loneliness.[17]

Visiting hours in CCUs were restricted for many years, with the rationale that rest, quiet, and an undisturbed environment were all therapeutic nursing interventions. Families often interpreted these restrictions as being denied access to their loved ones. As early as 1978, Dracup and Breu reported that satisfying the needs of the families of patients was improved by relaxing a policy of restricted visiting hours and initiating set communication with patients' spouses.[18] Increased visiting time was seen as a strategy to improve coping skills and strengthen the relationship between nurses and the family members of patients.[19] Over time, many units began the policy of unrestricted visiting hours. Such interventions were designed to strengthen the relationship between the family and health care provider as well as foster adaptation to the crisis on the part of the family. Through nursing research, family presence at the bedside has also been shown to decrease the patient's intracranial pressure, decrease patient and family anxiety, increase social support for the patient, and give the patient some sense of control over the situation. These findings support the need for less restrictive and individualized visiting policies for patients and families. The focus should be on what proves best for the patient, not on what is dictated by tradition or nurse preference.

Critical care nurses must take the responsibility for revising visiting hours to meet the needs of patients and families. When choosing a less restrictive policy, the physical layout of the unit must be considered. Smaller units may not be appropriate for unrestricted visiting hours with unlimited visitors. The effectiveness of changes in visiting hours must also be evaluated. Additional nursing research is needed to determine the effect of changes in visiting hours on the needs of patients and families.

The nurse must prepare family members for the initial visit to the CCU because it can be an overwhelming environment. The functions of monitors, intravenous drips, ventilators, and other technologies, as well as the meaning of alarms, should always be explained before and during the family visits. The names, roles, and responsibilities of all members of the health care team should be identified to both the patient and family. The nurse, by example, can demonstrate the value of communication and touch to the family. Encouraging family members to provide direct care to the patient, if they are interested, can help decrease anxiety and provide the family with some control. Direct care activities for the family to perform may include brushing teeth, combing hair, helping with a meal, providing skin care, or giving a bath.

Allowing children to visit a CCU may require special arrangements on the part of the staff. Visits should include short, simple explanations to the child concerning the patient's condition. Answering the child's questions in terms that he or she can understand helps reduce possible fears. The person who is escorting the child into the CCU should be aware that invasive monitoring and other equipment might upset a youngster. If a visit from the child is not possible, arrangements can be made for a telephone visit.

A phenomenon in both emergency departments and critical care settings is the presence of family members during invasive procedures and resuscitation. Research has demonstrated that although it remains highly controversial, the experience has positive benefits for family members. When family members were interviewed, 97.5% believed that family presence was a right, 100% said they would repeat family presence in the same situation again, 95% believed that their presence helped the patient, even if the patient was unconscious, and 95% said it helped them realize the seriousness of the patient's case.[20]

USE OF THE NURSE–FAMILY RELATIONSHIP

Initiating nursing interventions and establishing a meaningful relationship with the family tends to be easier during crisis than at other times. People in crisis are highly receptive to an interested, caring, and empathetic helper. When first meeting the patient's family, the nurse must demonstrate the desire and ability to help. Help that is specific to the family's needs at that time demonstrates the nurse's interest in their comfort and well-being. Deciding who is to be notified of the patient's status and validating that contact person's telephone number can be an overwhelming family decision. Assisting the family to determine immediate priorities is essential in the early phase of crisis intervention. The existence of advanced directives, a living will, and power of attorney should be determined. In the absence of these documents, support and methods to obtain them should be given to the family.

With this type of timely involvement, the family will begin to trust and depend on the nurse's judgment. This process then allows family members to believe the nurse when the nurse conveys feelings of hope and confidence in the family's ability to cope with whatever is ahead of them. It is important to avoid giving false reassurance; rather, the reality of the situation should be expressed in a kind, supportive fashion.

PROBLEM-SOLVING WITH THE FAMILY

As the relationship between the nurse and the family develops, the nurse begins to understand the dynamics of the problem facing the family. Problem-solving with the family takes into consideration items such as:

▶ The meaning the family has attached to the event

▶ Other crises with which the family may be coping

▶ The adaptive and maladaptive coping behaviors previously used in time of stress

▶ The normal support systems of the family, which might include friends, neighbors, clergy, and colleagues

Using the information collected and recorded in the assessment base, the nurse is able to help the family deal with the stress. Areas to include in interventions are defining the problem, identifying support, focusing on feelings, and identifying steps.

Defining the Problem

A vital part of the problem-solving process is to help the family clearly state the immediate problem. Often people are overwhelmed and immobilized by the anxiety or panic caused by acute stress. Being able to state the problem and acknowledge the difficulty or threat it poses reduces the family's anxiety by helping family members realize that they have achieved some sort of an understanding of what is happening. Defining the problem is a way of delimiting its parameters. Simply asking the family what constitutes the greatest concern for them at this time helps in problem definition. In addition, the family's response helps the nurse to clarify his or her understanding of what the family needs.

Defining and redefining problems can occur many times before the problem is solved. Stating the problem clearly helps the family assign priorities and direct needed actions. Goal-directed activities help decrease anxiety.

Identifying Support

Under high levels of stress, some people expect themselves to react differently. Rather than turning to the resources they use daily, they become reluctant to involve them. Asking people to identify the person to whom they usually turn when they are upset, and encouraging them to seek assistance from that person now, helps direct the family back to the normal mechanisms for handling stressful issues. Few families are truly without resources; rather, they only have failed to recognize and call on them.

Defining and redefining the problem may also help put the problem in a different light. It is possible in time to view tragedy as a challenge and the unknown as an adventure. The process of helping the family view a problem from a different perspective is called reframing.

The nurse can also help the family call on its own inherent strengths. What is it as a family that they do best? How have they handled stress before? Encouraging the family members to capitalize on their strengths as a family unit is well worth the effort.

Focusing on Feelings

A problem-solving technique emphasizing choices and alternatives helps the family achieve a sense of control over part of their lives. It also reminds them, and clarifies for them, that they are ultimately responsible for dealing with the event and that they will live with the consequences of their decisions.

Helping the family focus on feelings is extremely important to avoid delayed grief and protracted depression in the future. The reflection of feelings or active listening is necessary throughout the duration of the crisis. Valuing the expression of feelings might help the family avoid the use of unhealthy coping mechanisms, such as alcohol or excessive sleep. In difficult and sad times, the critical care nurse can promise the family, with some certainty, that things will become easier with the passage of time. Adaptation takes time. Providing valid assurance (e.g., that a patient will eventually be weaned from a ventilator, or that a tube feeding is a temporary measure) can give the family a sense of trust in the caregiver.

During the difficult days of the critical illness, the family may become dependent on the judgment of professionals. The family may have some difficulty identifying the appropriate areas in which to accept the judgments of others. It is important that the nurse acknowledges the family's feelings and recognizes the complexity of the problem, while emphasizing the responsibility each member of the family has for his or her feelings, actions, and decisions. Encouraging family members to focus on things they can change helps to give them a sense of control. For example, if the patient is experiencing pain, the family can be encouraged to advocate for the patient by requesting that the physician evaluate the patient's pain control.

Identifying Steps

Once the problem has been defined and the family begins goal-directed activities, the nurse may help further by asking the family members to identify the steps that they must take. Such anticipatory guidance may help reduce the family's anxiety. However, the nurse must recognize moments when direction is vital to health and safety. It is often necessary to direct families, for example, to return home to rest. This can be explained by stating that by maintaining their own health, family members will, at a later date, be as helpful to the patient as possible. To make each interaction more meaningful and therapeutic, the nurse should focus on the crisis situation and avoid involvement in long-term chronic problems.

COLLABORATIVE MANAGEMENT

The health care providers who most often meet the needs of family members are generally thought to be nurses and physicians. Additional help comes in the form of written materials, other family members, the patient, and other hospital sources. In some cases, nurse-coached hospital volunteer programs have proved effective.[21] These programs consist of an inservice program taught by nurses and followed by the assignment of a nurse mentor to the volunteer. Some families benefit by a referral to a mental health clinical specialist, a social worker, a psychologist, or a chaplain. A nurse can best encourage the family to accept help from others by acknowledging the difficulty and complexity of the problem and providing several names and phone numbers. It may be appropriate for the nurse to set up the first meeting, with follow-up meetings coordinated between the family and the consultant. Many CCUs have such resources on a 24-hour on-call basis to ensure prompt interventions. An objective professional with experience in critical illness and its impact on the family can be an excellent resource.

A new concept for improving family-centered care in critical care is the Patient-Family Advisory Council.[22] An advisory council composed not just of nurses and other health care providers but also of past patients and family members represents the needs of family members. Driven by the consumer movement, the concept of the advisory council has the potential to provide new insights leading to improved family care. In one institution, clinical nurse specialists served as the facilitators, and the council worked on assessing how well the unit was doing in several categories with plans for improvement.[22]

• Palliative Care Issues in Critical Care

According to the World Health Organization, palliative care is an "approach that improves the quality of life of patients and their families facing the problem associated with life-threatening illness, through the prevention and relief of suffering by means of early identification and impeccable assessment and treatment of pain and other problems, physical, psychosocial, and spiritual." Important components of palliative care are the inclusion of the family in decision making and the provision of patient care. Families are faced with complex palliative care decisions that must be made in the unfamiliar environment of the CCU. These decisions can be made easier with the involvement of the nurse in facilitating and guiding the decision-making process. The focus of palliative nursing care should be the entire family. This is often difficult in acute care units with time and space constraints. Nurses' personal issues, such as previous experiences with the death of their own family members, have the potential either to enhance or threaten assessment and intervention. Family meetings with the critical care nurse and the palliative care team help to ensure that the wishes and concerns of the family are heard.

Caring for a patient's family at any point during the dying process encompasses three major areas: access, information and support, and involvement in caregiving activities. Family members of dying loved ones should be allowed more liberal access in both visiting hours and number of visitors allowed. Ensuring that a family can be with their critically ill loved one will be a source of comfort. Information has been identified as a crucial component in the family's coping, and support in the form of the nurse's caring behaviors is influential in shaping the critical care experience for both the patient and family. Honesty and truth telling are important skills in this emotionally charged time. Finally, family involvement in caregiving, in tasks as simple as being physically present to those as complex as assisting with postmortem care, may help families work through their grief. Facilitation of family involvement is a practical nursing intervention.[23] See Chapter 6 for further discussion of end-of-life and palliative care issues in the critical care setting.

• The Critical Care Family Assistance Program

Several hundred research studies during the past 20 years have focused on the environmental and social issues of anxious families awaiting the outcome of a family member's stay in the CCU, demonstrating that attending to the needs of these family members cannot be ignored.[24] Additionally, a crucial initiative of the AACN, established in 1969, has focused on the establishment of respectful, healing, and humane nursing care environments. As a result of collaboration between the Chest Foundation and Eli Lilly and Company Foundation, the Critical Care Family Assistance Program (CCFAP) was developed as an example of a renewed awakening to the concepts of family-centered care.[1] The objectives of the CCFAP are:[24]

▶ To better prepare a multidisciplinary team to meet the needs of families

▶ To increase families' satisfaction with the care and treatment of critically ill patients

▶ To improve families' comprehension of, and satisfaction with, the information provided by caregivers

► To identify common formats for providing information and financial resources

► To improve a hospital's ability to respond to family needs within a structured feedback model

► To increase the medical team's knowledge and understanding of the CCFAP model

► To increase knowledge about the CCFAP and foster the dissemination within the medical and lay community

► To compare and contrast specific levels of family needs across various models of care

Needs assessments completed at the original CCFAP sites validated the findings of decades of research. Commonly noted gaps in supporting the families of patients included:

► Discrepancies in the viewpoint with regard to the sharing of information

► The need of the family to involve more family members in decision making

► A lack of resources and services offered during this time of crisis

Because of shortened lengths of stay and nursing shortages, family members are increasingly more active participants in the care of their loved ones. Family-centered care focuses on better integration of the family into the care planning process. Engaging family members early and encouraging them to work in partnership with the nursing staff can make a difference. Box 3-4 lists the components of the CCFAP model. It is hoped that with expanded use of this model, quality of critical care delivered will increase, whereas cost of critical care delivery will decrease.

Box 3-4 • Components of the Critical Care Family Assistance Program (CCFAP)

Communication
Example: "ICU Navigators," weekly group family sessions that provide information about equipment, medical procedures, and assertiveness skills

Environmental Changes
Examples: expanding the waiting area, brightening the look of the room, new and more comfortable furniture

Educational Materials
Example: Publications that are up to date and written in nontechnical language

Information Kiosk
Examples: Electronic messaging system, Internet access, CCFAP family satisfaction surveys

Hospitality Programs
Examples: Hotel discounts, meals for families

Other Services
Examples: music therapy, pet therapy

• Cultural Issues Related to Critical Illness

Nursing interventions for the critically ill patient include recognition and appreciation of the cultural uniqueness of each person. In today's diverse society, culture affects the nursing care of patients in many ways—from pain control and visitation expectations to care of the body after death. Critical care nurses must recognize the uniqueness of each person and the ways in which that uniqueness affects the care of the patient and the needs of the family.

Health care providers in Western medicine often address a critical illness as a disease process and focus on the physical symptoms, the pathology of organ function, or injury to a body part. The patient and family, having a different cultural perspective, may view the illness in a more psychophysiological manner, focusing on the physical, psychological, personal, and cultural ramifications of the illness. In other cultures, the patient's critical illness may be viewed as a curse or disharmony in the universe. Culture serves as an important influence in the patient's attitudes about approach to suffering, beliefs about life-prolonging treatments, palliative care, and advanced directives and health care proxies.[25]

Cultural competence is a reflection of one's attitudes, knowledge base, acquired skills, and behavior. Although it is unrealistic to expect that the nurse should know the customs and beliefs of all critically ill patients he or she cares for, it is not unreasonable to expect some degree of cultural competence. Glass and colleagues make the following suggestions:[26]

► Be aware of one's own ethnocentrism.

► Assess the family's beliefs about illness and treatment.

► Consistently convey respect.

► Request that the family and patient act as guides for cultural preferences.

► Ask for the patient's personal preference.

► Respect cultural differences regarding personal space and touch.

► Note appropriate complementary and alternative medical practices, and allow their use if possible.

► Incorporate the patient's cultural healing practices into the plan of care.

► Be sensitive to the need for a translator.

Cultural characteristics such as language, values, behavioral norms, diet, and attitudes toward disease prevention, death and dying, and management of illness vary from culture to culture. Critical illness may be viewed by the family from a religious or spiritual perspective. Astuteness and sensitivity on the part of the critical care nurse ensure that the beliefs of the highly technologic, illness-focused health care system will not clash with cultural beliefs in folk medicine, rituals, religious healing, and medicine men.

• Clinical Applicability Challenges

Short-Answer Questions

1. Mrs. J. is a critically ill patient with multiple trauma who has been admitted to your unit. She is not expected to survive her injuries. Mrs. J.'s husband, her two children ages 6 and 10, and her parents have just arrived on your unit. Formulate a plan of care that reflects sensitivity to the issues that will assist the patient's family in dealing with the probable death of their loved one.

2. Mr. E. is a 73-year-old man admitted to your unit after resuscitation. He has a long-standing history of cardiac disease and collapsed at home after what has been interpreted as a life-threatening rhythm disturbance. Although he received cardiopulmonary resuscitation, he was unconscious for 10 minutes before the rescue team arrived. His older daughters are fighting over the maintenance of ventilatory support. Discuss how you would help his daughters at this difficult time.

3. Mr. and Mrs. P. are the parents of a critically ill child on your unit. They are Indian and speak very little English. Describe the criteria you would use to assess their degree of stress and anxiety. How could you be certain that the cultural needs of the family are met while the child is a patient in your unit?

Review Questions

1. To help the family develop a sense of control, the nurse may
   a. offer reassurance that the patient is receiving the best possible care.
   b. refer family members to a grief counselor or clergy.
   c. offer choices for the family whenever possible.
   d. offer visiting privileges every 3 hours.

2. Assisting the family members to define or state a problem associated with a crisis is useful because it
   a. decreases their sense of understanding of the problem.
   b. implies parameters or limits of the problem.
   c. denies family members a sense of cognitive mastery.
   d. directs nursing interventions.

3. The family enters a crisis under several conditions. Identify the condition most likely to increase the probability that the family will enter a crisis.
   a. An event has short-term consequences for a family.
   b. A family's ability to problem-solve is inadequate.
   c. The equilibrium of the family is undisturbed.
   d. A family spokesperson is appointed by the family.

References

1. Henneman EA, Cardin S: Family-centered critical care: A practical approach to making it happen. Crit Care Nurse 22(6):12–19, 2002

2. Medacona D, Warren N: Perceived and unmet needs of critically ill family members. Crit Care Nurse Q 21(1):58–67, 1998

3. Selye H: The Stress of Life. New York, McGraw-Hill, 1956

4. Curley M: Critical Care Nursing of Infants and Children. New York, Elsevier Science, 1996

5. Fox-Wasylyshyn S, El-Masri M, Williamson K: Family perceptions of nurses' roles toward family members of critically ill patients: A descriptive study. Heart Lung 34:335–344, 2005

6. Warren NA: Critical care family members' satisfaction with bereavement experiences. Crit Care Nurs Q 25:54–60, 2002

7. American Association of Critical-Care Nurses: Standards for Acute and Critical Care Nursing Practice, 3rd ed. Aliso Viejo, CA, AACCN, 2000

8. Hartrick G, Lindsey AE, Hills M: Family nursing assessment: Meeting the challenge of health promotion. J Adv Nurs 20:85–91, 1994

9. Molter NC: Needs of relatives of critically ill patients. Heart Lung 8:332–339, 1979

10. Leske J: Internal psychometric properties of the Critical Care Family Needs Inventory. Heart Lung 20:236–244, 1991

11. Kosco M, Warren NA: Critical care nurses' perceptions of family needs as met. Crit Care Nurs Q 23:60–72, 2002

12. Holden J, Harrison L, Johnson M: Families, nurses and intensive care patients: A review of the literature. J Clin Nurs 11:140–148, 2002

13. Naebel B, Fothergill-Bourbonnais F, Dunning J: Family assessment tools: A review of the literature from 1978–1997. Heart Lung 29:196–209, 2000

14. Schiller WR, Anderson BF: Family as a member of the Trauma Rounds: A strategy for maximized communication. J Trauma Nurs 10(4):93–101, 2003

15. Azoulay E, Pouchard F, Chevret S, et al: Family participation in care to the critically ill: Opinions of families and staff. Intensive Care Med 29:1498–1504, 2003

16. Eldredge D: Helping at the bedside: Spouses' preferences for helping critically ill patients. Res Nurs Health 27:307–321, 2003

17. Gavaghan S, Carroll D: Families of critically ill patients and the effect of nursing interventions. Dimens Crit Care Nurs 21(2):64–71, 2002

18. Dracup KA, Breu CS: Using nursing research to meet the needs of grieving spouses. Nurs Res 27:212–216, 1978

19. Stillwell SB: Importance of visiting needs as perceived by family members of patients in the intensive care unit. Heart Lung 13:238–242, 1984

20. Meyers TA, Eichhorn DJ, Guzzetta CE, et al: Family presence during invasive procedures and resuscitation: The experience of family members, nurses and physicians. Am J Nurs 100:32–34, 2000

21. Appleyard M, Gavaghan S, Gonzalez C, et al: Nurse-coached interventions for the families of patients in critical care units. Crit Care Nurse 20(3):40–48, 2000

22. Halm MA, Sabo J, Rudiger M: The patient-family advisory council: Keeping a pulse on our customers. Crit Care Nurse 26(5):58–67, 2006.

23. Davies B: Supporting families in palliative care. In Ferrell B, Coyle N (eds): Textbook of Palliative Nursing. Oxford, UK, Oxford University Press, 2001

24. Lederer M, Goode T, Dowling J: Origins and development: The critical care family assistance program. Chest 128(3):65S–75S, 2005

25. Davidson JE, Powers K, Hedayat KM, et al: American College of Critical Care Medicine Task Force 2004-2005, Society of Critical Care Medicine. Clinical practice guidelines for support of the family in the patient-centered intensive care unit: American College of Critical Care Medicine Task Force 2004-2005. Crit Care Med 35:605–622, 2007

26. Glass E, Cluxton D, Rancour P: Principles of patient and family assessment. In Ferrell B, Coyle N (eds): Textbook of Palliative Nursing. Oxford, Oxford University Press, 2001

Other Selected Readings

Azoulay E, Pochard F, Cheveret S, et al: Meeting the needs of intensive care unit patient's families: A multidisciplinary study. Am J Respir Crit Care Med 163(1):135–139, 2001

Baystate Medical Center: A quality improvement approach to meeting the needs of critically ill patients and their families. Dimens Crit Care Nurs 19(1):30–34, 2000

Benner P: Death as a human passage: Compassionate care for persons dying in critical care units. Am J Crit Care 10(5):355–359, 2001

Bijttebier P, Vanoost S, Delva D, et al: Needs of relatives of critical care patients: Perceptions of relatives, physicians, and nurses. Intens Care Med 27(1):160–165, 2001

Bisaillon S, Li-James S, Mulcahy V, et al: Family partnership in care: Integrating families into the coronary care unit. Can J Cardiovasc Nurs 8(4):43–46, 1997

Board R, Ryan-Winger N: State of the science on parental stress and family functioning in pediatric intensive care units. Am J Crit Care 9(2):106–122, 2000

Burr G: The family and critical care nursing: A brief review of the literature. Aust Crit Care 10(4):124–127, 1997

Copstead L, Banasik J: Pathophysiology: Biological and Behavioral Perspectives. Philadelphia, WB Saunders, 2000

Coyle MA: Meeting the needs of the family: The role of the specialist nurse in management of brain death. Intens Crit Care Nurse 16(1):45–51, 2000

Curtis JR, Patrick DL, Shannon S, et al: The family conference as a focus to improve communication about end of life care in the intensive care unit: Opportunities for improvement. Crit Care Med 29:N26–N33, 2001

Dowling B, Wang B: Impact on family satisfaction: The critical care family assistance program. Chest 128(3):76S–80S, 2005

Dowling J, Vender J, Guilianelli S, Wang B: A model of family centered care and satisfaction predictors. Chest 128(3):81S–92S, 2005

Dowling J, Lederer M: Emergent models of implementation and communication. Chest 128(3):93S–98S, 2005

Fox S, Jeffrey J: The role of the nurse with families of patients in ICU: The nurse's perspective. Can J Cardiovasc Nurs 8(1):17–23, 1997

Gentling S, Grady R, Mattox K: Hospital administrator's perspective. Chest 128(3):103S–105S, 2005

Jastremski C, Harvey M: Making changes to improve the intensive care unit experience for patients and their families. New Horiz 6(1):99–109, 1998

Johnson D, Wilson M, Cavanaugh B, et al: Measuring the ability to meet family needs in an intensive care unit. Crit Care Med 26(2):266–271, 1998

Lissman I: Maintaining confidentiality and information giving in intensive care. Crit Care Nurs 5(4):187–193, 2000

Medina J: A natural synergy in creating a patient-focused environment: The Critical Care Family Assistance Program and critical care nursing. Chest 128(3), 99S–102S, 2005

Miracle V: Strategies to meet the needs of families of critically ill patients. Dimens Crit Care Nurse 25(3):121–125, 2006

Offord RJ: Should relatives of patients with cardiac arrest be invited to be present during cardiopulmonary resuscitation? Intens Crit Care Nurse 14(6):288–293, 1998

Pryzby B: Effects of nurse caring behaviors on family stress responses in critical care. Intens Crit Care Nurs 21(1):16–23, 2005

Quinn S, Redmond K, Begley C: The needs of relatives visiting adult critical care units as perceived by relatives and nurses: Part one. Intens Crit Care Nurs 12(3):168–172, 1996

Roland P, Russell J, Richards K, et al: Visitation in critical care: Processes and outcomes of a performance improvement initiative. J Nurs Care Q 15(2):18–26, 2001

Snyder M, Brandt CL, Tseng YH: Use of presence in the critical care unit. AACN Clin Issues 11(1):27–33, 2000

Tin M, French P, Leung K: The needs of the family of critically ill neurosurgical patients: A survey of nurses' and patients' perceptions. J Neurosci Nurs 31(6):348–356, 1999

Waters CM: Professional nursing support for culturally diverse family members of critically ill adults. Res Nurs Health 22(2):107–117, 1999

Wesson JS: Meeting the informational, psychosocial and emotional needs of each ICU patient and family. Intens Crit Care Nurse 13(2):111–118, 1997

Patient and Family Education in Critical Care

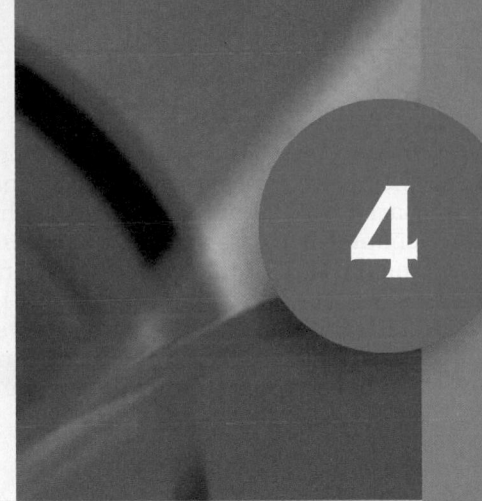

4

Mary O. Palazzo

Objectives

Based on the content in this chapter, the reader should be able to:

❶ Describe the barriers to learning that are unique to the critical care setting.

❷ Describe and differentiate between the concepts of education and learning.

❸ Identify the three domains of learning.

❹ Identify the six principles of adult learning.

❺ Describe the assessment of learning in the critical care environment.

In the critical care setting, it is always a challenge to meet the educational needs of patients and families because of the life-threatening nature of critical illness. Patient and family education is a vital component of nursing care. The nurse must deal with the anxiety and fear that is associated with a diagnosis of critical illness, while trying to teach difficult concepts in an environment that is poorly suited to learning.

Health care is no longer solely defined in terms of sound clinical decision making; now, it also encompasses prudent use of resources and financial accountability. Information about the quality of care provided by a facility is now more readily available to consumers, with public access to clinical outcomes and mandatory reporting of quality indicators to insurers and regulatory agencies. Soon reimbursement for care will be based on hospital performance against quality measures. Many of the quality indicators include patient and family education components. This change in the health care climate necessitates clear evidence of nursing involvement in patient and family instruction and quantification of nursing care.

In addition, the financial constraints of managed care have resulted in an overall decrease in length of hospital stays and the subsequent discharge of patients and families, sometimes before they are ready to learn. Today, it is not unusual for a patient to be discharged home from an intensive care unit (ICU), placing even greater responsibility on the patient and family to provide for high-intensity care at home. The critical care nurse not only manages the hemodynamic instability that often accompanies critical illness but also prepares the patient and family for the likelihood of early discharge from the hospital.

At the same time, hospitals are facing an ongoing shortage of critical care nurses. ICUs that were once reserved for the most experienced nurses are now training grounds for the newly graduated nurse. The novice nurse must focus on learning how to manage the myriad of technological devices used to support the critically ill patient while understanding the pathophysiology of multisystem illness. For the new nurse, it may be very difficult to move beyond the essential nursing tasks that are an integral part of patient care to address the educational needs of the patient and family. In addition, the expanded use of contract nurses to meet the demands of a variable patient census or to fill staff vacancies can also have a negative impact on patient and family education. A nurse working only one or two shifts a week may not develop a relationship with the patient and family or be able to follow up and validate learning. Difficulties mount when there is little or no continuity of care to assess learning needs and promote education.

These are just a few examples of the realities of health care. The fragmentation of patient care across the health care system presents many obstacles and barriers to patient education. The purpose of this chapter is to assist students and nurses in developing the skills and tools needed to meet the challenge of patient and family education in the presence of critical illness. Nurses who understand the learning barriers that are unique to the critical care setting are better prepared to address the learning needs of patients and families.

• Barriers to Learning

CRITICAL ILLNESS AND STRESS

Typically, the patient and family enter an ICU quite unexpectedly because of a life-threatening event. The onset of illness signals the beginning of a physical and emotional crisis for all involved. Altered metabolic responses, exposure to general anesthesia, use of cardiopulmonary bypass, episodes of hypoxia, and marked sleep deprivation are common events for the critically ill. Each of these factors can compromise mental acuity and decrease a person's learning capacity and recall. In addition, combating a severe illness consumes most of the patient's energy, leaving him or her with a limited ability to learn.

The patient experiences not only the physical effects related to the disease process but also emotional and spiritual distress. When facing serious illness, patients express feelings of helplessness, loss of control, and fear of death. In a qualitative study by Hupcey, patients expressed an overwhelming need to feel safe within a critical care setting, and they found that relatives, health care providers, and religion provided some measure of that desired security.[1] Nurses can play a beneficial role. The vigilant critical care nurse who recognizes a patient's fear and anxiety and offers the patient guidance through the unfamiliar course of illness, treatment, and recovery can support the patient's need for safety. Clear explanation and reassurances further support reducing the patient's anxiety before invasive procedures, discussions about treatment options, or major events such as transfer to another unit or level of care. These are special opportunities for patient education despite the extreme stress of critical illness.

However, in the critical care setting, it is not unusual for the focus of education to quickly shift away from the patient and be redirected to meet the learning needs of the family members. An emotional and physical toll is exacted on the family members of critically ill patients, with stress levels peaking within 72 hours of admission to the unit.[2] The descriptive study by Halm and colleagues demonstrates changes in the sleeping and eating patterns of family members, as well as an increased use of cigarettes, over-the-counter medications, alcohol, and prescription drugs, while coping with the crisis of a critically ill patient.[2] Stress can also manifest in hypervigilant behaviors such as repetitive questions, frequent telephone calls, and numerous visits. Intense anxiety and the fear of death evoked by critical illness may cause families to forget much of the information that has been given to them. Often, the critical care nurse must repeat the same information and answer identical questions repeatedly. Nursing interventions aimed at reducing family anxiety and supporting the family throughout the course of critical illness are important for improving the mental health, both in the short term and in the long term. Research has shown that the incidence of post-traumatic stress disorder is higher in families following an ICU event.[3] The following case study demonstrates how the interventions of the critical care nurse are used to support the educational and emotional needs of a family in crisis.

Case Study: A Patient and Family in Crisis

The electronic doors to the cardiovascular intensive care unit (CVICU) swing open, and John and Margaret enter their 40-year-old daughter's room. Mary Ann has just returned to the CVICU after a mitral valve replacement and a tricuspid valve repair. Unfortunately, the valve replacement was complicated, and she had a prolonged course on cardiopulmonary bypass. Her heart was quite weak before the surgery, and now she requires an intra-aortic balloon pump and multiple medications to support her cardiac output. She has also developed a coagulopathy related to the extended time on cardiopulmonary bypass and continues to bleed. Her vital signs are stable, but she requires a continuous infusion of blood products to keep up with the blood loss from her chest tubes.

John and Margaret are shocked by their daughter's appearance. Her pale, edematous face and lifeless expression are certainly not what they expected to see. There is little about their daughter that resembles the person they know and love. Equipment surrounds her bed and supports nearly every bodily function. Visibly shaken, they look at each other with tears in their eyes, wondering how a seemingly routine valve operation could turn out this way.

Suzanne, the critical care nurse caring for Mary Ann, greets John and Margaret, her patient's parents, and begins to talk about their daughter's appearance. She carefully explains the purpose of all the bedside equipment as she cares for their daughter. Suzanne tells the worried parents what she is doing and why she is performing each procedure. It is the nurse's calm and caring approach that engenders a sense of hope for their daughter's eventual recovery. The parents begin to relax a little and start to ask questions about what to expect in the next few hours.

This brief example illustrates the unpredictability of illness and just how quickly a crisis can develop. In this scenario, the bedside nurse initiates family education through an informal discussion of the patient's status. The initial interaction with family members is extremely important because it helps establish a foundation of trust and respect between the nurse and family.[4] In the course of talking with the parents, the nurse is continually assessing their learning needs and developing an understanding of their coping mechanisms. She is helping the family to deal with the crisis phase of this illness by providing consistent and accurate information about the condition of their loved one. Research has demonstrated that up-to-date information is the highest priority for family members who are coping with critical illness.[5] The critical care nurse teaches families about the pathophysiology of the illness, the diagnostic studies that are performed, and the treatment plan that is underway. The primary education goal for most families is to learn all that they can about their loved one.

PROLONGED ILLNESS AND STRESS

Frequently, the period of illness extends well beyond the initial crisis phase and creates additional burdens for the patient and the family. The critically ill patient may experience a slow and unpredictable course with periods of organ system compromise or failure over time. Recovery is tedious and is measured in small changes that occur over days and weeks. Families are forced to balance their home and work schedules with time spent at the hospital, often evoking feelings of guilt and anxiety. Over time, it may become increasingly difficult for the family to obtain information and patient status reports from the health care team. Often, physician schedules are unpredictable and do not mesh with family visits. This further underscores the vital role that the critical care nurse plays as a link to the family. With protracted critical illness, many families struggle to keep the lines of communication open to the extended family, creating opportunities for conflict and misinformation.

As a patient and family advocate, the nurse provides accurate information and shares the plan of care with the family. Additional interventions such as a patient care or ethics conference may be arranged by the critical care nurse to give the family an opportunity to discuss the case with the entire health care team. Patient care conferences afford open communication with the family and may be a therapeutic method for dispelling misinformation and misconceptions about the patient's progress.

As the patient's condition improves and plans for transfer to step-down status are discussed with the health care team, the critical care nurse must prepare the patient and family for the eventual discharge from the unit. This milestone in recovery is typically viewed by the patient and family in one of two ways. If the patient and family believe that the patient's condition has improved sufficiently and that the intensity of critical care is no longer necessary, then this step is viewed in a positive light. However, if they believe that the depth of nursing support and level of monitoring on the floor are inadequate to meet the needs of the patient, there may be resistance to the transfer process. If the critical care nurse spends time educating the patient and family about the floor routine,

staffing patterns, and visiting hours before making the transfer, it helps mitigate some of the negative feelings and anxiety associated with the change.[6]

Once the transfer has been made, it is important that the receiving step-down nurse further assist the patient and family with "settling" into the new routine. The nurse should begin by acknowledging the normal anxiety that accompanies the transfer process. He or she should establish trust and allay fears by explaining the changeover in care in transitioning from ICU to step-down status, emphasizing that the transition to step-down is a positive stage in the recovery process. The nurse should also reassure the patient and family that even though the intensity of treatment has changed, the step-down staff are trained to anticipate each patient's recovery needs and will respond appropriately to changes in the patient's status. Once the patient and family's initial anxiety diminishes, the nurse can begin to set new self-care goals and expectations based on his or her assessment.

Clearly, nursing plays a vital role in helping the patient and family cope with the crisis of critical illness and the transitions in care by providing education from admission to discharge.

ENVIRONMENTAL STRESS

Ringing telephones, chiming call lights and pagers, overhead announcements, equipment alarms, staff conversations, banging automatic doors, and pneumatic tubes are just a few examples of the sounds that fill the air of a typical ICU. It is easy for nurses to become desensitized to these familiar noises because they are an integral part of the work environment. However, taking a moment to listen to the background sounds from a patient's bedside quickly reminds a person how stressful noise can be. Patients and families are not accustomed to the normal sounds of an ICU. Yet, as difficult as it may be, nurses ask patients and families to learn in this setting.

A typical ICU setting is hardly an optimal learning environment. Ideally, a quiet moment is spent with the patient and family using comfortable chairs arranged to optimize discussion and with audiovisual aids, if possible. However, common measures can help reduce the environmental stress and enhance the success of learning. The simple act of closing the door to the patient's room or placing a comfortable chair at the bedside can reduce the background noise sufficiently and enhance the learner's attention span. Reducing the alarm volumes on bedside equipment while the nurse is talking with the patient or family helps minimize the number of interruptions and may improve the learner's ability to focus on the topic of a teaching session.

Ensuring privacy while sensitive or confidential information is being exchanged can markedly reduce the anxiety of a patient or family member. Often, strangers witness the emotional outbursts and intimate interactions of families who are agonizing over the illness of a loved one. Health care providers are not always mindful of their surroundings when discussing confidential details of a patient's case. Critical care nurses can direct health care team members and families to a quiet room away from the general waiting area to afford privacy when discussing specific patient information.

This regard for the patient also applies to teaching rounds or patient care rounds that are held in the halls of an ICU. Patients should be treated with respect, and they often wish to be included in bedside presentations. The health care team should make a concerted effort to provide the patient with privacy. Members of the team should make appropriate introductions and give clear explanations of the medical jargon used in the course of rounds.

CULTURAL AND LANGUAGE BARRIERS

As the U.S. population changes, the patients and families that nurses care for in hospitals and critical care settings are becoming increasingly diverse. The U.S. Census Bureau estimates that ethnic minorities will make up 50% of the population by the year 2050.[7] Beliefs about health and illness are deeply rooted in culture. How a patient or family member responds to the diagnosis or a proposed treatment and education may be strongly influenced by his or her values and culture.[8] Although the nursing literature readily acknowledges the importance of providing culturally sensitive patient care, in practice there is little evidence of cultural awareness in the nurse's daily assessments and interactions with patients and families. Culturally competent nursing care is defined as being sensitive to issues related to culture, race, gender, sexual orientation, social class, and economic situation.[9] In addition, culturally competent nursing also considers the family structure and gender role as it relates to the patient. For example, in the Asian culture, important health care decisions should be discussed with the family. An individual person would not make an independent decision because the family is considered to be the smallest decision-making unit.[10]

Successful education of culturally diverse patients and families requires more than just basic knowledge regarding ethnic groups. Critical care nurses must recognize their own individual biases and examine their personal values and beliefs about health and nursing care. Many of our health beliefs are based on commonly held Euro-American values such as belief in individualism, belief in informed consent, orientation toward clock time, and belief in God as the most powerful being.[10] Other shared beliefs also exist, such as the belief that technology and science will improve the overall human condition.[10] The imposition of these Euro-American values on other cultures may impede communication between the nurse and patient and hinder the education process. Although critical care nurses do not have the time to complete a thorough cultural assessment, several key pieces of information should be obtained. This information is outlined in Box 4-1.

Language barriers also pose a major obstacle to patient and family education, especially in the stressful critical care environment. Every effort should be

---

Box 4-1 • Key Pieces of Information to Obtain as Part of the Cultural Assessment

- Place of birth
- Length of time in this country
  - Does the patient live in an ethnic community?
  - Who are the patient's major support people?
- Primary and secondary languages (speaking and reading ability)
- Religious practices
- Health and illness beliefs and practices
- Communication practices (verbal and nonverbal)
- How decisions are made in the context of the patient and family

Adapted from Lipson JG: Culturally competent nursing care. In Lipson JG, Dibble SL, Mainarik PA (eds): Culture and Nursing Care: A Pocket Guide. San Francisco, UCSF Nursing Press, 2005, pp 1–6.

---

made to provide an interpreter to translate information for the non–English-speaking patient and family. Although it is convenient for health care providers to rely solely on a family member or friend to translate complex medical information and terminology that is likely to be unfamiliar, it may be difficult for the family member or friend to keep personal bias from entering the context of the conversation. In many cultures, decision making is assumed by the eldest member of the family, and asking a child to interpret medical information disrupts the social order of the family.[11] In addition, the information that may be exchanged between the health care provider and the patient may be personal or embarrassing to either the patient or to the family member who is pressed into service. Box 4-2 offers some suggestions for communicating

---

Box 4-2 • Guidelines for Communication Using an Interpreter

- Before the session, meet with the interpreter to give background information and explain the purpose of the session.
- If possible, have the interpreter meet with the patient or family to determine their educational level, health care beliefs, and health care attitudes to plan the depth of information needed.
- Speak in short units of speech and avoid long explanations and use of medical jargon, abbreviations, and colloquialisms.
- When communicating to the patient or family, look directly toward the person and not at the interpreter. Watch the patient's and family members' body language and nonverbal communication response.
- Be patient. Interpreted interviews take a long time to complete and may become tiresome for the patient.
- Have the patient and family members validate the information given to them through the interpreter, to make sure that they understand the instructions or message that has been given.

with a patient and his or her family through an interpreter. Written instructions should also be translated and reviewed in the presence of an interpreter so that any questions can be addressed immediately. Printed instructions in several languages should be readily available for use in the ICU.

SENSORY BARRIERS

Effective education for deaf and hearing-impaired patients and families necessitates planning and additional resources. The Americans with Disabilities Act prohibits discrimination against people with disabilities, including those who are deaf or hearing impaired.[12] Under the law, these disabled people must be able to communicate with hospital staff, and the medical facility must be ready to meet that requirement. Deaf or hearing-impaired patients or family members should indicate their preferred mode of communication such as sign language, written notes, lip reading, oral interpreters, or other assistive devices.[12] To ensure that deaf or hearing-impaired patients or family members can communicate effectively, an oral interpreter should be used in the critical care setting for the discussion of treatment options; informed consent for procedures, blood administration, or surgery; and discharge instructions. These types of decisions typically require extended discussions and free-flowing communication that is best supported with an interpreter.

• Education and Learning

It is important to discriminate between education and learning. Many times these terms are used interchangeably, but there is a difference between these two concepts. Education is an activity, initiated by one or more persons, that is designed to effect changes in the knowledge, skill, and attitudes of people, groups, or communities.[13] Education places more emphasis on the person facilitating the learning, whereas learning itself is a phenomenon of internal change. The learner experiences a flash of insight that results in behavioral changes.[13] The key concept in learning is changing to a new state of mind.[14] The focus shifts from the role of the educator to that of the person who experiences the change.

THREE DOMAINS OF LEARNING

Three domains of human behavior or learning to consider when developing an education plan are the cognitive domain, the affective domain, and the psychomotor domain. Keeping these domains in mind while assessing and developing a teaching plan can assist the nurse in selecting suitable teaching methods.

The cognitive domain of learning involves the development of insight or understanding that provides a basis or guideline for behavior.[14] In this domain,

knowledge expands, and teaching–learning material is organized from simple to complex. Learning is enhanced when information builds on previous knowledge. Therefore, the basic ideas should be well introduced before attempting to teach the hard-to-remember facts. As an example, cognitive learning occurs when a family member learns to assess wound healing. The critical care nurse provides basic information about the normal healing process and the appearance of a healthy incision. Once the family member understands how a healed incision should look, the nurse can explain the signs and symptoms of infection and when to call the physician. Once prepared, the family member should then be able to apply the learned principles to provide appropriate home care for the patient.

The affective domain pervades all spheres of learning because it encompasses the patient's values, attitudes, and feelings.[14] Attempting to modify an attitude or emotional response requires a safe and trusting relationship between the patient and the nurse. When formulating a teaching plan, the nurse should take a nonthreatening approach to assessing what the patient considers important enough to learn. A helpful teaching strategy may be the interactive group learning that is typical of a smoking cessation class. In this situation, the teacher demonstrates behaviors that the learner wants to imitate and provides positive feedback to the participants to encourage them to stop smoking cigarettes. If the learning experiences are satisfying and the patient associates positive feelings with the experience, it may help influence the change in behavior.

The psychomotor domain involves motor skills that are composed of an ordered sequence of movement that must be learned.[14] To learn a particular skill, the patient must have a neuromuscular system that is able to perform the skill and the capacity to form a mental image of the act.[14] A mental image is created when the learner watches a demonstration while the teacher points out the relevant steps that are required to successfully complete the task. The nurse may use a written, step-by-step guide as a reference while demonstrating the skill and allowing the patient to ask questions. Learning to inject insulin is an example of psychomotor learning. It takes practice for the patient or family member to become proficient at performing the task. The thought of learning a new skill is intimidating to many adults; therefore, it is important that the nurse provide praise and encouragement with each teaching session.

Teaching methods that are based on the three domains of learning are displayed in Figure 4-1.

ADULT LEARNING PRINCIPLES

The principles of adult learning are based on multiple learning theories that originate in many different disciplines, such as developmental psychology, sociology, philosophy, and education. Adult learning is a relatively new field (about 40 years old),

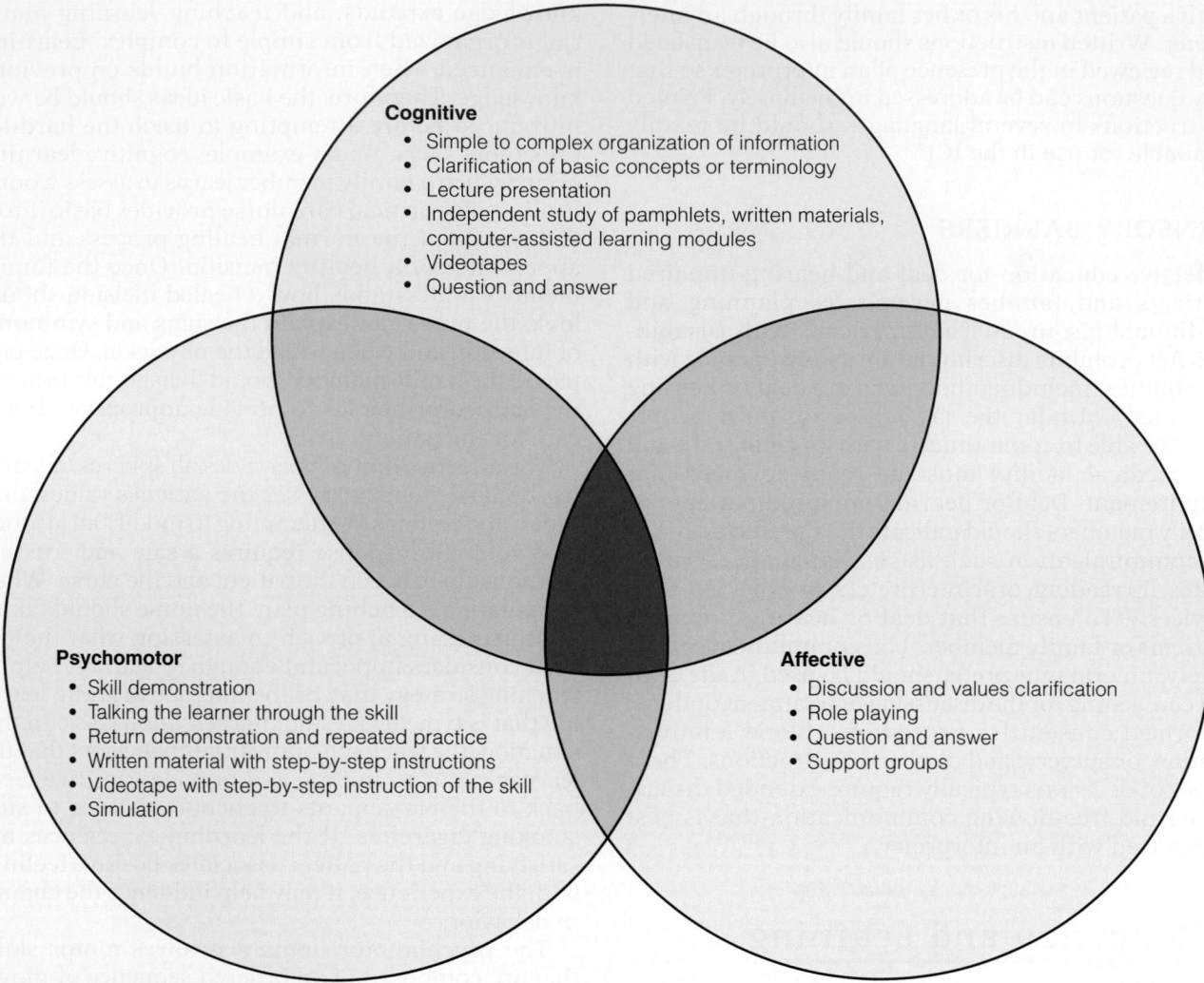

Cognitive
- Simple to complex organization of information
- Clarification of basic concepts or terminology
- Lecture presentation
- Independent study of pamphlets, written materials, computer-assisted learning modules
- Videotapes
- Question and answer

Psychomotor
- Skill demonstration
- Talking the learner through the skill
- Return demonstration and repeated practice
- Written material with step-by-step instructions
- Videotape with step-by-step instruction of the skill
- Simulation

Affective
- Discussion and values clarification
- Role playing
- Question and answer
- Support groups

Figure 4-1 • Teaching methods based on the domains of learning.

with the fundamental principles grounded in child-hood learning and education. A new conceptual framework known as the andragogical model emerged from research studies that identified some of the unique characteristics of adult learners.[13] The core principles of the andragogical model of adult learning are as follows:

1. *The need to know.* Adults need to understand why they need to learn something before they are willing to commit the energy and time to learn it. It is important for the learner to understand and be aware of the "need to know." To raise the learner's level of awareness, the facilitator may need to use real or simulated experiences to help the learner discover the lack of knowledge.

2. *The learner's self-concept.* Adults are self-directed and responsible for their own decision making. In general, adults resent the feeling that others are making choices for them. Adult educators need to create learning situations that are more self-directed and independent.

3. *The learner's life experience.* Adults have lived longer and accumulated more life experiences than chil-

dren. Life experience defines and shapes adult beliefs, values, and attitudes. Adult education methods emphasize experiential techniques such as case method, simulation, and problem-solving exercises. In addition, adults learn well from their peers, making group learning an effective teaching method.

4. *Readiness to learn.* Adults are ready to learn the things they need to know. The information should be applicable to real-life situations.

5. *Orientation to learning.* Adults are motivated to learn if the information will help them to perform useful tasks or to deal with problems in their life.

6. *Motivation to learn.* Adults are more motivated by internal forces such as improved quality of life, increased job satisfaction, and improved self-esteem. External factors such as job promotion or increased salary are less likely to sustain learning.[13]

An example of how the critical care nurse might use adult learning principles in the practice setting is presented in the following scenario.

Case Study: A Patient Who Is Motivated to Learn

Mr. Jones underwent a coronary artery bypass graft procedure 2 days ago. He questions the nurse about a breakfast tray that contains scrambled eggs and ham, while explaining that the eggs contain too much cholesterol and that he has been told to avoid all high-cholesterol foods. The nurse replies that the scrambled egg is an egg substitute product that is actually part of a heart-healthy diet. Mr. Jones is demonstrating his readiness to learn and is attempting to apply the new knowledge to alter his eating habits. His learning motivation stems from an intrinsic desire to change that is now focused on his overall quality of life and improving his health. His question affords the nurse an opening to discuss other heart-healthy activities and lifestyle changes that will help the patient achieve wellness in his recovery.

The critically ill patient and family are highly motivated to learn because a life-threatening event has triggered an intense need for information. Successful teaching plans should incorporate adult learning principles and relevant information that readily apply to real life and assist with recovery from critical illness.

• The Process of Adult Education

The process of patient and family education entails more than just providing an educational brochure or turning on an instructional videotape; it is an interactive process based on a therapeutic relationship. The fundamentals used in patient and family education include assessment, diagnosis, goals, intervention, and evaluation.[11,14] Frequently, the nursing process is used informally by critical care nurses because teaching is so highly integrated into routine nursing care and family interactions. Just as the bedside nurse uses clinical judgment to recognize and treat the hemodynamic instability that often accompanies critical illness, he or she also diagnoses and intervenes to meet the learning needs of the patient and family. As nurses advance in practice, learning assessment becomes more refined and focuses on meeting the educational goals. Each learning session enhances the knowledge of the patient and family and offers the nurse a chance to evaluate the success or failure of what he or she has taught.

ASSESSING LEARNING NEEDS IN A TIME OF CRISIS

The critical care nurse must be very sensitive to the heightened anxiety that accompanies an admission to the ICU. Anxiety markedly reduces the ability of the patient and family to concentrate. Therefore, the nurse should avoid long explanations or tedious questions.

The first step in the assessment process is to get to know the patient and family. This often begins with a simple introduction. Taking a few minutes to learn the family names and their relationship to the patient signifies respect and begins to build a therapeutic and trusting relationship. It gives the nurse a chance to orient the patient and family to the ICU as well as to teach them about some of the equipment used in the care of the patient.

Understanding the learning needs of patients and families does not need to entail a protracted interview or use of formal assessment tools with overly generic questions about health beliefs and learning styles.[15] It is better to use an informal and open-ended dialogue between the nurse and the family to establish the "need to know." Use of open-ended questions such as "What is your understanding of your mother's condition?" or "What did the physician tell you about the surgery?" gives the nurse a starting point for teaching the family. It also validates whether the patient or family member clearly understands previous explanations given by other members of the health care team.

Informal assessment often provides the nurse with a baseline evaluation of literacy and the person's level of education. Literacy assessment can be very difficult and requires sensitivity because most adults with a reading difficulty spend a lifetime hiding it.[14] Nonthreatening questions such as, "Do you prefer to learn new information by reading or watching a program on television?" may give the nurse a clue about a patient or family member's level of literacy. With about 20% of the U.S. population considered to be functionally illiterate, it is very likely that the educational brochures or the operative consent forms that are given to patients or families are beyond their reading level.[14] Every day, critical care nurses assume that the consent forms are clearly understood when they are returned signed and unquestioned. Written educational material should always be in the active voice and targeted for a fifth- to eighth-grade reading level.[16] In addition, the nurse should verbally review any written material with the patient or family in case they are unable to read the document and are too embarrassed to admit it.

Further assessment may reveal that a patient or family has a low level of health literacy. This term describes "the degree to which individuals have the capacity to obtain, process and understand basic health information and services needed to make appropriate health decisions."[17] Within the context of critical care, patients and families with low health literacy often struggle with the urgency and the abstract concepts that health care decisions demand.[18] For example, a physician explains the risks and benefits of a tracheostomy for a patient who has been intubated for 3 weeks and cannot be weaned from mechanical ventilation. To fully comprehend the assignment of risk, it is necessary to have a basic understanding of the concept of percentages as applied to the probability of complications. In this situation, a family member may have difficulty making an informed decision because the risks and benefits are not meaningful, and they are fearful of "cutting a hole into a loved one's neck." Such an emotional reaction should signal to the critical care nurse the need to bridge the knowledge gap between the physician's explanation and the family's negative perception of the procedure. To accomplish this, it helps to use more concrete methods such as the phrase "most people experience few complications following this procedure" to illustrate the risk for complications instead of using percentages to quantify the risk. In addition, using familiar words, showing a picture of a tracheostomy, and giving family members time to talk about the procedure may dispel further misconceptions and reduce their anxiety, thus enabling them to reach a decision about the surgery.

Assessment is a dynamic and ongoing process, providing the critical care nurse with many opportunities to assist patients and families to cope with the stress and anxiety associated with critical illness while meeting their learning needs. It also entails knowing when the patient or family is unable to learn. For example, patients who are experiencing pain are not able to focus on learning a new skill such as insulin administration without first having adequate pain control. A family member who has just learned that a loved one has suffered a cardiac arrest is not likely to be able to assimilate the intricate details of myocardial ischemia. Setting unrealistic educational goals hinders learning and frustrates both the nurse and the learner. The teaching plan must be continually evaluated. If it is ineffective, poorly timed, or not meeting the learner's needs, it should be altered.

INTERVENTION: EFFECTIVE TEACHING STRATEGIES IN CRITICAL CARE

Teachable Moments

Teachable moments are those instances when the nurse and learner together recognize the need for education and the learner is open to hearing information and learning new problem-solving skills.[11] Life-threatening illness often stimulates changes in unhealthy behavior patterns, only then igniting a patient's interest in learning. Much of the learning required of a patient who is recovering from critical illness involves behavior changes that require alterations in lifestyle. Smoking cessation, dietary restrictions, and activity limitations are the types of lifestyle changes that patients frequently struggle to achieve and maintain. Teachable moments often occur in the course of routine patient care. Therefore, the nurse should be ready to incorporate teaching while providing care. For example, the nurse can review postoperative incision care in a brief teaching session while performing skin assessment. The review can include the signs and symptoms of infection, proper wound cleansing, and a description of a healthy healing incision. Teaching pertinent information about the indications or side effects of medications, while giving them to the patient, is another way to reinforce learning. Both of these examples highlight the importance of focusing on a single concept, especially considering the limited attention span that is typical of

a patient who is recovering from a critical illness. Learning is best accomplished when the message is consistent and the knowledge progresses from simple to more complex concepts.

The Family Connection

Often the critical care nurse recognizes the limitations of the patient's ability to comprehend information and then turns to the family to provide instruction. Most patients forget 80% of the information they receive, and nearly half of what they remember is incorrect.[19] It is likely that retention of information by critically ill patients is much worse. Therefore, family participation in teaching sessions helps ensure the success of the teaching plan. In addition, providing written materials that patients can review after discharge from the hospital helps bridge the retention gap. Guidelines for developing printed materials that are appropriate for use with older patients are presented in Box 4-3.

Another effective teaching strategy for the adult learner is group learning. For example, postoperative cardiac surgical patients can benefit from a class on posthospital care. A group teaching session allows patients the chance to share common experiences and concerns about recovery with each other. Including families in the group may stimulate questions and allow them to express concerns about potential complications and fears about taking care of a loved one at home. Many times families are fearful of caring for a loved one who has recovered from a life-threatening illness. They are afraid that they will miss an important symptom or that something will go wrong and their loved one will become ill again or even die. The critical care nurse should acknowledge these feelings and provide the family with emotional support while giving the tools and information to ensure safe care at home. The family interaction also provides the nurse with an assessment of potential home health care needs. It may become apparent that a home health care consultation is indicated for further teaching, and reinforcement of newly learned skills may be needed to facilitate a safe transition from the hospital to home.

Box 4-3 • CONSIDERATIONS FOR THE OLDER PATIENT: Guidelines for Printed Educational Materials

- Font should be 12 points or greater.
- Serif type is preferred over sans-serif type.
- Avoid script or stylized types.
- Avoid the use of all uppercase letters for body type.
- Line lengths should be no longer than 5 inches.
- Paper with a glossy finish should be avoided because the glare makes reading difficult. Use matte-finish paper instead.
- Legibility is enhanced when black ink is printed on white or off-white paper.
- Avoid printing over a designed or customized background.

EVALUATING THE LEARNING PROCESS

Evaluation is a measurement of the critical learning elements established in the teaching plan. It provides evidence about patient accomplishments or skills that may need further development.[20] Evaluation also reinforces correct behavior on the part of learners and helps teachers determine the adequacy of their instruction.[20] Questions provide the teacher and learner with immediate feedback and validate the learner's grasp of the information presented. The nurse should avoid using leading questions to achieve a desired answer. True evaluation is based on the learner's responses, which indicate whether additional reinforcement of the key concepts is needed. Direct observation of newly learned skills or procedures should also be part of the evaluation. Because adults do not want to appear awkward or clumsy when performing a task, it is important to have a relaxed, positive learning environment where the teacher and student have a good rapport before asking a patient or family member to demonstrate a new task or skill. The learner should be able to successfully answer or perform 94% of all the critical elements outlined in the teaching plan.[20] Often the success or failure of patient and family education influences the discharge plans. Patients who are unable reliably to perform new tasks need supervision and further practice to learn the new skill. Therefore, adequate evaluation of the learning process is an essential component of the health care continuum.

There are many ways to develop a patient and family teaching plan. Given a homogeneous population, standardized patient teaching plans and records can be used. Plans should include information that is essential for most patients but can also be flexible enough to accommodate individual needs. Teaching plans include nursing diagnoses, outcome criteria, and interventions. A sample teaching plan for a patient who has experienced a myocardial infarction is given in Box 4-4.

The nursing diagnosis assists the nurse to identify the appropriate content to teach. It also helps formulate the outcomes that are used to evaluate the progress of the patient and family and the effectiveness of the teaching plan. The outcomes should be stated in measurable terms, and the teaching should be outlined in a logical sequence. Each nursing intervention should include the content, method, and media used for teaching. In addition, the patient's barriers to learning should be addressed, and the nursing interventions are aimed at meeting those personal needs. In critical care, families are often included in the teaching plans because of the limited learning ability of the patient.

• The Standards of Patient and Family Education

There is great emphasis on patient and family education that stems from the Joint Commission (formerly the Joint Commission on Accreditation of Healthcare Organizations [JCAHO]) patient care standards. These standards serve to promote overall patient care quality in health care organizations. Hospitals voluntarily participate in Joint Commission surveys to ensure that the patient care provided meets or exceeds the criteria set forth in the standards. Some examples of Joint Commission standards related to patient and family education include the following:

▶ "The hospital plans, supports, coordinates activities and resources for patient and family education."

▶ "The patient receives education and training specific to the patient's assessed needs, abilities, learning preferences and readiness to learn as appropriate to the care and services provided by the hospital."[21]

The goal of these educational standards is to guide hospitals to create an environment in which both the patient and the health care team members are responsible for teaching and learning. The medical record should reflect an interdisciplinary approach toward patient education throughout the hospital stay. This begins on admission with the initial assessment of the patient's current health problems, based on socioeconomic status, cultural and religious practices, motivation and ability to learn, family support, and current knowledge base.[22] The Joint Commission educational assessment guidelines are detailed in Box 4-5. Teaching records should illustrate documentation of the information taught and how it relates to specific illness, medications, safe and effective use of medical equipment, restraint/seclusion, pain management, and available community resources.[22]

Finally, the teaching record should also reflect an evaluation of how well the patient and family absorbed the information. The details of teaching record documentation are outlined in Box 4-6. A sample patient education record is shown in Figure 4-2.

How do these standards affect patient education in the critical care setting? It may be difficult for critical care nurses to think in terms of teaching plans and interdisciplinary learning because critically ill patients have so much instability and require great vigilance just to maintain physiological function. However, remember that much of the patient teaching is informal and may not be clearly visible at first glance. Nurses are taught to explain each procedure, medication, intervention, or diagnostic test to the patient beforehand. This is patient education. For example, the nurse who explains that the medication she is hanging is an antibiotic that is given through the intravenous line to fight the patient's abdominal wound infection is teaching. Yet, many nurses would not recognize this action as patient education, and they would not document it in the teaching record. Nonetheless, this type of informal instruction meets the Joint Commission standard for patient education. Critical care nurses teach patients and families routinely, but often the patient education record is left blank because "there isn't enough time to teach." If critical care nurses would only remember to note each informal teaching session, the patient's educational records would be filled with entries after just one day in the unit.

Box 4-4 • COLLABORATIVE CARE GUIDE for Educating a Patient About Myocardial Infarction

Mr. Chang is a 50-year-old married Asian man who was admitted to the hospital after experiencing chest pain while at work. He had mild elevation in his cardiac enzymes and was taken to the cardiac catheterization laboratory within a few hours of the onset of the chest pain. The interventional cardiologist found two arteries 50% occluded. He was able to perform an angioplasty, place a stent in the arteries, and suc-cessfully restore the blood flow to the affected myocardium. The morning after his procedure, Mr. Chang spoke with the cardiac rehabilitation nurse, who reviewed his cardiac risk factors. He is 30 pounds overweight, his cholesterol level is 250 mg/dL, and he smokes two packs of cigarettes per day. After this procedure, Mr. Chang is anxious to learn ways to reduce his risk for myocardial infarction.

NURSING DIAGNOSES	OUTCOMES	INTERVENTIONS
Knowledge Deficit	Patient will be able to state content presented.	• Plan teaching sessions for a period of time with minimal interruptions. • Include patient's wife and family in teaching sessions. • Provide written information to reinforce the verbal information. • Review the diagnosis of myocardial infarction and the therapies used to prevent further damage to the heart muscle. • Review cardiac risk factors for this patient and identify those risk factors that he can control. • Consult the dietitian for weight reduction and meal planning. • Discuss the sodium content of foods related to Asian cuisine. • Discuss the target cholesterol level for this patient and the medications and dietary changes needed to reduce the risk for myocardial infarction. • Discuss tobacco use related to myocardial oxygen demand and the vasoactive effects of nicotine. • Offer information about smoking cessation programs and medical options available to assist him with stopping smoking. • Refer the patient to a formal cardiac rehabilitation program after discharge from the hospital.
Knowledge, Readiness for Enhanced	Patient will participate in goal setting for weight loss, decreased tobacco consumption, and cholesterol targets and will participate in an exercise program, lose weight, reduce tobacco use, and decrease cholesterol according to his personal goals.	• Plan and set goals with the patient for weight loss, reduction in tobacco use, and target cholesterol levels. • Have the patient identify appropriate menu selections and portion control to achieve weight loss. • Have the patient identify the triggers for tobacco use and steps that he might find useful to reduce or stop smoking. • Refer the patient to a weight loss and a smoking cessation support group. • Have the patient identify appropriate exercises after myocardial infarction.
Coping, Ineffective	Patient will begin to demonstrate effective coping mechanisms.	• Discuss the patient's feelings about multiple lifestyle changes and the diagnosis of myocardial infarction. • Discuss the patient's feelings about participating in both a weight loss and smoking cessation program. • Mobilize the patient's resources for support. • Help the patient to design a chart to use to map his progress with weight loss, smoking cessation, and cholesterol targets. • Acknowledge all questions and concerns that the patient expresses as meaningful.

Box 4-5 • Joint Commission on Accreditation of Healthcare Organizations (JCAHO) Guidelines for Patient and Family Education Assessment

- Cultural background
- Religious beliefs and values
- Family support
- Literacy level
- Primary language
- Ability to read and comprehend information
- Barriers to learning
- Physical limitations such as visual or hearing impairment
- Emotional barriers
- Preferred learning methods
- Motivation to learn

Adapted from Iacono J, Campbell A: Patient and Family Education: The Compliance Guide to the JCAHO Standards, 2nd ed. Marblehead, MA, Opus Communication, 2000, pp 25–36.

Box 4-6 • Components of Teaching Documentation

- Participants (Who was taught?)
- Content (What was taught?)
- Date and time (When was it taught?)
- Patient status (What was the patient's condition at the time?)
- Evaluation of learning (How well was the information absorbed?)
- Teaching methods (How was the patient taught?)
- Follow-up and learning evaluation (If teaching was incomplete, what was the reason? What additional education needs does the patient have?)

KEY

Barriers to Learning	Learners	Tools/Method	Level of Learning (LOL)
1. No barrier 2. Language/Communication/Literacy 3. Cultural/Religious Practices 4. Cognitive/Sensory Impairment 5. Severity of illness/pain 6. Motivation 7. Physical limitation	P = patient F = family/significant other O = other	C = Class/group D = Demonstration A = Audiovisual L = Literature T = Translator TV = Video/ed channel M = Model 1:1 One to one	8. Needs further reinforcement 9. Demonstrates partial skill or knowledge 10. Demonstrates skill with minimal assistance 11. Demonstrates competent skill and knowledge

EDUCATION	Content	Date	Barrier	Learner	Tool	LOL	Initials
Outcome Criteria **Discharge Plan of Care** • Identifies disease process • Cause • Signs and symptoms • Risk factors • Prevention							
Medications/ Food and Drug Interactions • Identifies purpose of medications • States side effects of medications • Demonstrates administration of medications • Reviews food–drug interactions							
Activity • Verbalizes activity restrictions after discharge • Identifies need for assistive apparatus as needed • Identifies safety precautions							
Equipment • States purpose • Demonstrates correct use of equipment • Identifies safety measures							
Treatments • States the purpose of the treatment • Demonstrates correct technique • Identifies findings that should be reported to health care provider							
Follow-up Care and Community Resources							

Figure 4-2 • Example of a patient education record. (Adapted from Georgetown University Hospital: Interdisciplinary Patient Education. Washington, DC, author, 2000.)

• Clinical Applicability Challenges

Short-Answer Questions

1. Discuss nursing interventions that have effectively reduced patient and family anxiety in a clinical situation that you have encountered.

2. Discuss when patient and family anxiety would preclude all learning.

Review Questions

1. Following admission to a critical care unit, which nursing intervention is most effective in reducing family member/significant other anxiety?
   a. Providing frequent information updates on the patient status
   b. Orienting the family member/significant other to the critical care unit
   c. Providing unlimited visiting to the family member/significant other
   d. Limiting visits to 10 minutes only

2. Evaluation of learning effectiveness should include all of the following *except* that
   a. the patient demonstrates at least 94% of all critical elements of the teaching plan.
   b. the patient defers all questions to a family member to answer.
   c. learning evaluation should avoid embarrassing the patient if they are unable to perform a newly learned skill correctly.
   d. effective learning should involve the patient and family/significant other to enhance success.

3. Which of the following principles of adult learning should the critical care nurse assess?
   a. The need to know
   b. Readiness to learn
   c. Motivation to learn
   d. All of the above

References

1. Hupcey JE: Feeling safe: The psychosocial needs of ICU patients. J Nurs Scholar 32(4):361–367, 2000
2. Halm MA, Titler MG, Kleiber C, et al: Behavioral responses of family members during critical illness. Clin Nurs Res 2:414–437, 1993
3. Cuthbertson BH, Hull A, Strachan M, et al: Post-traumatic stress disorder after critical illness requiring general intensive care. Intensive Care Med 30(3):450–455, 2004
4. Leske JS: Treatment for family members in crisis after critical injury. AACN Clin Issues 9(1):129–139, 1998
5. Verhaeghe S, Defloor T, Van Zuuren F, et al: The needs and experiences of family members of adult patients in an intensive care unit: a review of the literature. J Clin Nurs 12:501–509, 2005
6. Pattison N: Psychological implications of admission to critical care. Br J Nurs 14(13):708–714, 2005
7. U.S. Census Bureau: US interim projections by age, sex, race, and Hispanic origin: March 18, 2004. Available at: http://www.census.gov/ipc/www/usinterimproj/
8. Ersek M, Kagawa-Singer M, Barnes D, et al: Multicultural considerations in the use of advance directives. Oncol Nurs Forum 25:1683–1690, 1998
9. Meleis A, Isenberg M, Koerner J, et al: Diversity, marginalization, and culturally competent health care: Issues in knowledge development. Washington, DC, American Academy of Nursing, 2000
10. Lipson JG, Dibble SL (eds): Culture and Clinical Care: A Pocket Guide. San Francisco, UCSF Nursing Press, 2005
11. Rankin SH, Stallings KD, London F: Patient Education in Health and Illness, 5th ed. Philadelphia, Lippincott, Williams and Wilkins, 2005, pp 224–250
12. Michigan Association for Deaf, Hearing, and Speech Services: Hospitals' responsibilities to the deaf under the ADA. Retrieved November 1, 2006, from http://www.deaf-talk.com/pdf/hospitalresponsibilites.pdf
13. Knowles MS, Holton EF, Swanson RA: The Adult Learner, 5th ed. Houston, TX, Gulf Publishing, 1998, pp 35–72
14. Redman BK: The Practice of Patient Education: A Case Study Approach, 10th ed. St. Louis, Mosby Elsevier, 2007, pp 1–26
15. Palazzo MO: Teaching in crisis: Patient and family education in critical care. Crit Care Nurs Clin North Am 13(1):83–92, 2001
16. Fisher E: Low literacy levels in adults: Implications for patient education. J Contin Educ Nurs 30:56–61, 1999
17. U.S. Department of Health and Human Services: Healthy People 2010, 2nd ed. With understanding and improving health and objectives for improving health. Washington, DC, US Government Printing Office, November 2000
18. Riley JB, Cloonan P, Norton C: Low health literacy: A challenge to critical care. Crit Care Nurs Q 29(2):174–178, 2006
19. Kessels RPC: Patients' memory for medical information. J Royal Soc Med 96:219–222, 2003
20. Redman BK: The Practice of Patient Education: A Case Study Approach, 10th ed. St. Louis, Mosby Elsevier, 2007, pp 56–73
21. Joint Commission on Accreditation of Healthcare Organizations: CAMH Comprehensive Accreditation Manual for Hospitals: The Official Handbook. Oakbrook Terrace, IL, Joint Commission, 2006, pp 1–12
22. Iacono J, Campbell A: Patient and Family Education: The Compliance Guide to the JCAHO Standards, 2nd ed. Marblehead, MA, Opus Communication, 2000, pp 25–36

Relieving Pain and Providing Comfort

5

Suzanne S. Prevost

Objectives

Based on the content in this chapter, the reader should be able to:

❶ Differentiate between acute and chronic pain.

❷ Identify factors that exacerbate the experience of pain in the critically ill.

❸ Prepare patients for the common sources of procedural pain in intensive care.

❹ Compare and contrast tolerance, physical dependence, and addiction.

❺ Discuss national guidelines and standards for pain management.

❻ Identify appropriate analgesics for high-risk critically ill patients.

❼ Describe nonpharmacological interventions for alleviating pain and anxiety.

Pain is one of the most common experiences and stressors in critically ill patients.[1,2] Many interventions and procedures in the critical care unit increase pain,[3] which is also a coexisting symptom of critical illness.[4] Even though pain management has become a national priority in recent years, pain continues to be misunderstood, poorly assessed, and undertreated in intensive care units (ICUs) and many other health care settings.[5] Uncontrolled pain triggers physical and emotional stress responses, inhibits healing, increases the risk for other complications, and increases the length of ICU stay. Critical care nurses need a clear understanding of concepts related to pain assessment and management to achieve effective pain control. This chapter provides an overview of key concepts related to the management of acute pain and comfort in the critically ill adult patient.

• Pain Defined

Pain is a complex, subjective phenomenon. It is a protective mechanism, causing one either to with-draw from or avoid the source of pain and seek assistance or treatment. The International Association for the Study of Pain defined pain as "an unpleasant sensory and emotional experience associated with actual or potential tissue damage or described in terms of such damage."[6] McCaffery provides an operational definition of pain that considers the subjectiveness and individuality of the pain experience and is based on the premise that the individual experiencing the pain is the true authority: "Pain is whatever the experiencing person says it is, existing whenever he or she says it does."[7]

The pain most ICU patients experience is classified as *acute* because it has an identified cause and is expected to resolve within a given time frame. For example, the pain experienced during endotracheal suctioning or a dressing change can be expected to end when the treatment is completed. Similarly, pain at an incision or area of injury is expected to cease once healing has occurred. In contrast, *chronic* pain is caused by physiological mechanisms that are less well understood. Chronic pain differs from acute pain in terms of etiology and expected duration. It may last for an indefinite period and may be difficult, if not impossible, to treat completely.[8]

• Pain in the Critically Ill

Critical illness is painful. Consider the most common illnesses or injuries treated in the ICU: myocardial infarction, thoracic and neurosurgery, multiple trauma, and extensive burns. All are associated with severe pain. Nearly all ICU patients experience acute pain; but many, particularly those who are elderly, suffer with the combination of both acute and chronic pain. For some of these patients, the pain is considered continuous because it persists for more than half of each day.[9] Previously it was thought that critically ill patients were unable to remember their painful experiences due to the acute nature of the illness or injury. More recent research demonstrates that ICU patients do remember painful experiences, and they frequently describe their pain as being moderate to severe in intensity.[3]

Multiple factors inherent in the ICU environment affect the patient's pain experience: anxiety, sleep deprivation, unfamiliar and unpleasant surroundings, loss of control, and separation from family or significant others. The effects of each of these factors increase when they are experienced together. For example, pain and anxiety act in a synergistic and cyclical fashion to exacerbate each other. See Box 5-1 for a list of physical, psychosocial, and environmental factors that contribute to pain and discomfort in the critically ill.

PROCEDURAL PAIN

Efforts to provide pain relief and comfort measures are complicated by the fact that critical care nurses must continuously perform procedures or treatments that cause pain to the patient. Procedures such as chest tube insertion and removal, endotracheal suctioning, and wound débridement are obviously painful. Additionally, simple procedures, such as turning, can also cause considerable pain.

A national, multicenter research study supported by the American Association of Critical Care Nurses, referred to as the Thunder Project II, examined procedural pain in 5,957 critically ill adults.[3] The investigators documented the patients' responses to six procedures that are frequently performed on critically ill patients: central venous catheter placement, femoral sheath removal, tracheal suctioning, turning, wound care, and wound drain removal. The most painful and least painful procedures are noted in Table 5-1.

Researchers also asked the patients in the study to use words to describe the pain they felt before and after each procedure. The patients used the word "aching" most frequently to describe pain before a procedure and the word "sharp" during and after the procedure.[10] In addition, the Thunder II investigators also discovered that very few of the patients (less than 20%)

Box 5-1 • Factors Contributing to Pain and Discomfort in the Critically Ill

Physical
- Symptoms of critical illness (e.g., angina, ischemia, dyspnea)
- Wounds—post-trauma, postoperative, or postprocedural
- Sleep disturbance and deprivation
- Immobility, inability to move to a comfortable position because of tubes, monitors, restraints
- Temperature extremes associated with critical illness and the environment—fever, hypothermia

Psychosocial
- Anxiety and depression
- Impaired communication, inability to report and describe pain
- Fear of pain, disability, or death
- Separation from family and significant others
- Boredom or lack of pleasant distractions

Intensive Care Unit Environment or Routine
- Continuous noise from equipment and staff
- Continuous or unnatural patterns of light
- Awakening and physical manipulation every 1–2 h for vital signs or positioning
- Continuous or frequent invasive, painful procedures
- Competing priorities in care—unstable vital signs, bleeding, dysrhythmias, poor ventilation—may take precedence over pain management

---

received opioid analgesics before their procedures. Many of the patients even reported that they were in pain before the procedure and still did not receive an analgesic to control their pain during the procedure.[11]

Before undergoing procedures known to be associated with pain, patients should be premedicated, and the procedure should be performed only after the medication has taken effect. Critical care nurses must be attuned to the pain the patient is experiencing before the procedure in order to provide the best interventions to help the patient during the procedure. In

---

Table 5-1 • Thunder Project II: Procedures Causing Pain in the Critically Ill Adults*

Procedure	Degree of Pain
Femoral sheath removal	Least painful
Central venous catheter placement	Painful
Tracheal suctioning	Painful
Wound care	Painful
Wound drain removal	More painful
Turning	Most painful

*Ranked from least to most painful.
From Puntillo KA, Morris A, Thompson C, et al: Pain behaviors observed during six common procedures: Results from Thunder Project II. Crit Care Med 32(2): 421–427, 2004.

addition to providing preprocedural analgesic medication, the nurse can educate patients to help them prepare and plan for procedures.

During procedures, intravenous (IV) opioids, such as morphine or fentanyl, are usually used for analgesia. The IV bolus dose of morphine is individualized and depends on the age, weight, pain intensity, and type of procedure. The patient's response must be monitored during the procedure with additional doses given as needed for breakthrough pain. Anxiolytic medications, such as midazolam or propofol, can be given to relieve anxiety during the procedure; however, these agents should be used as *adjuncts* because they only provide sedation and do not relieve the pain associated with the procedure. In addition, the nurse can use interventions such as imagery, distraction, and family support during procedures.

• Consequences of Pain

Pain produces many harmful effects that inhibit healing and recovery from critical illness. The autonomic nervous system responds to pain by causing vasoconstriction and increased heart rate and contractility. Pulse, blood pressure, and cardiac output all increase. This increases myocardial workload and oxygen use, both of which can cause or exacerbate myocardial ischemia in the already compromised critically ill person. Respiratory alterations resulting from pain include splinting, decreased respiratory effort, and reduced pulmonary volume and flow. Pulmonary complications, such as atelectasis and pneumonia, can result. In the gastrointestinal system, gastric emptying and intestinal motility decrease, which can result in impaired function and ileus. Pain also negatively affects the musculoskeletal system by causing muscle contractions, spasms, and rigidity. Because movement increases pain, the patient is hesitant to move, cough, or breathe deeply. Unrelieved pain suppresses the immune functions, predisposing the patient to pneumonia, wound infections, and sepsis. Patients who have a high level of uncontrolled pain during an acute hospitalization are at risk for delayed recovery and development of chronic pain syndromes after discharge.[12]

Patients who are pain free have better outcomes than those stressed by unrelieved pain. In a classic study, patients whose pain was controlled with epidural anesthesia and epidural analgesia had shorter ICU stays, shorter hospital stays, and half as many complications as patients receiving standard anesthesia and analgesia.[13] The benefits of effective pain relief are summarized in Table 5-2.

• Barriers to Effective Pain Control

Pain continues to be undertreated in many settings, even though the negative consequences of uncontrolled pain and the benefits of pain relief have been

Table 5-2 • Benefits of Effective Pain Relief

System	Benefit
Cardiovascular	Decreased pulse, blood pressure, and myocardial workload
Pulmonary	Enhanced respiration, oxygenation, and decreased incidence of pulmonary complications
Neurologic	Decreased anxiety and mental confusion, enhanced sleep
Gastrointestinal, nutritional	Enhanced gastric emptying, promotion of positive nitrogen balance
Musculoskeletal	Earlier ambulation, reducing complications of immobility
Economic	Decreased length of stay, decreased costs, enhanced patient satisfaction with care

well documented.[5] Pain relief is often relegated to a low priority because of the life-threatening nature of the patient's illness and the other lifesaving interventions that are required. Critical care nurses are often concerned that analgesic administration may create problems, such as hemodynamic and respiratory compromise, oversedation, or drug addiction.

The fear of addiction is one of the greatest concerns and impediments associated with analgesia and pain control. This fear causes anxiety for patients and their families as well as health care providers. Critical care nurses must have a clear understanding of the differences between, and implications of, addiction, tolerance, and dependence. Patients who require long-term analgesic medication for pain control can develop tolerance or physical dependence. However, these scenarios should not be confused with addiction, which is characterized by behaviors such as impaired control, compulsive use, and continued use despite serious negative physical or social consequences.[14] Table 5-3 clarifies these concepts.

• Resources to Promote Effective Pain Control

During the past decade, government agencies, professional organizations, health care institutions, and pain management experts have focused their attention on improving pain management across the United States. These efforts have produced abundant resources to support nurses in their efforts to provide effective pain management.

CLINICAL PRACTICE GUIDELINES

Early in the 1990s, the Agency for Health Care Policy and Research (AHCPR), now known as the Agency for Healthcare Research and Quality (AHRQ), intro-

Table 5-3 • Tolerance, Physical Dependence, and Addiction

	Definition	Implication
Tolerance	A state of adaptation in which exposure to a drug induces changes that result in a diminution of one or more of the drug's effects over time.	Increase dose by 50% and assess effect. Tolerance to side effects, such as respiratory depression, increases as the dose requirement increases.
Physical dependence	A state of adaptation that is manifested by a drug class–specific withdrawal syndrome that can be produced by abrupt cessation, rapid dose reduction, decreasing blood level of the drug, and/or administration of an antagonist.	Gradually taper opioid dosage to discontinuation to avoid withdrawal symptoms.
Addiction	A primary, chronic, neurobiological disease, with genetic, psychosocial, and environmental factors influencing its development and manifestations. It is characterized by behaviors that include one or more of the following: impaired control over drug use, compulsive use, continued use despite harm, and craving.	Rarely seen in critical care patients, unless patient is admitted for drug overdose or other sequelae of illicit drug use

Definitions from American Pain Society: Definitions related to the use of opioids for the treatment of pain. Retrieved August 25, 2007, from http://www.ampainsoc.org/advocacy/opioids2.htm.

duced the concept of clinical practice guidelines. These guidelines were intended to serve as nationwide standards of care for specific clinical problems. This concept arose from the recognition that in the midst of a rapidly expanding body of health care research and literature, there were still wide variations in opinions and practice patterns regarding the best interventions for common clinical problems. The AHCPR convened multidisciplinary panels of national experts to review the research, provide expert opinions, summarize current knowledge, and make recommendations for practice for each targeted clinical problem. Acute pain management was the topic of the first guideline that this agency published and disseminated.

Over the next few years, several national agencies, including the American Association of Critical-Care Nurses (AACN), the American College of Cardiology, and the Society of Critical Care Medicine (SCCM), assembled their own panels of experts to develop clinical practice guidelines for their target populations. In 1996, the AHRQ discontinued its support for the production of clinical practice guideline documents and instead entered into a collaborative relationship with the American Medical Association and the American Association of Health Plans to sponsor the web-based National Guideline Clearinghouse.[15] This website currently contains more than 1,000 practice guidelines developed by a variety of organizations. Pain management guidelines have been disseminated throughout the United States and have served as a catalyst for several improvements in pain management over the past decade. These guidelines are also used as legal documents representing the national standard of care for pain management in medical liability cases.

One practice guideline that is particularly useful to critical care nurses and physicians is the guideline published jointly by the SCCM and the American Society of Health-System Pharmacists on *Sustained Use of Sedatives and Analgesics in the Critically Ill Adult*.[16] Table 5-4 includes information about this and other important guidelines and standards for pain management.[15,17]

INTERNET RESOURCES

The Internet is one of the most important sources of information and resources for pain management. Table 5-5 lists websites containing pain management information that may be useful to critical care nurses, patients, and families.

• Pain Assessment

The failure of health care providers to assess pain and pain relief routinely is one of the most common reasons for unrelieved pain in hospitalized patients.[18] Assessment of pain is as important as any method of treatment. The patient's pain is assessed at regular intervals to determine the effectiveness of therapy, the presence of side effects, the need for dose adjustment, or the need for supplemental doses to offset procedural pain. Pain is reassessed at an appropriate interval after pain medications or other interventions have been administered, for example 30 minutes after an IV dose of morphine. In critical care, a number of conditions may exist, making assessment of the patient's pain and subsequent treatments difficult. These conditions include the following:

▶ Acuity of the patient's condition
▶ Altered levels of consciousness
▶ Inability to communicate pain
▶ Restricted or limited movement
▶ Endotracheal intubation

A common misconception among health care professionals is that they are the most qualified to determine the presence and severity of the patient's pain. Absence of physical signs or behaviors is often incorrectly interpreted as the absence of pain. To perform an effective pain assessment, the critical care nurse must attempt to elicit a self-report from the patient. Behavioral observation and changes in

Table 5-4 • National Standards and Guidelines Related to Pain Management

Agency or Source	Standard or Guideline	Content Highlights
Society of Critical Care Medicine (SCCM) and the American Society of Health-System Pharmacists (ASHP)	Clinical Practice Guidelines for the Sustained Use of Sedatives and Analgesics in the Critically Ill Adult (2002)[16]	Developed by a national panel of experts in critical care medicine, critical care nursing, and pharmacy. Includes summaries and recommendations of recent research related to analgesia and sedation specifically in the critically ill population. The summary contains 28 explicit recommendations targeted to the critically ill, including the following: • Patient report is the most reliable standard for pain assessment. • Scheduled doses or continuous infusions of opioids are preferred over PRN or "as-needed" regimens. • Fentanyl, hydromorphone, and morphine are the drugs of choice for intravenous opioid analgesia. • Fentanyl is preferred for rapid onset of analgesia in acutely distressed patients. • Sedation of agitated patients should be provided only after providing adequate analgesia. • Lorazepam is recommended for sedation of most patients via intermittent IV or continuous infusion. • Midazolam or diazepam should be used for rapid sedation of acutely agitated patients. • Haloperidol is the preferred agent for treatment of delirium (pp. 119–141).[16]
American Geriatric Society	The Management of Persistent Pain in Older Persons[17]	This guideline, originally published in 1998, was revised in 2002 by an interdisciplinary panel of geriatric experts. Major recommendations include: • All older persons should be screened for persistent pain on admission to any health care facility. • The verbal 0 to 10 scale is a good first choice for assessment of pain intensity; however, other scales such as word descriptor scales or pain thermometers may be more appropriate for some older patients. • For patients with cognitive impairment, assessment of behaviors and family observations are essential. • Acetaminophen should be the first drug to consider in the treatment of mild to moderate musculoskeletal pain. • Opioid analgesic drugs are effective, with a low potential for addiction, and may have fewer long-term risks than other analgesic drugs.[17]
American College of Cardiology/ American Heart Association Task Force on Practice Guidelines	Guidelines for Cardiovascular Disease Management[15]	This joint task force has published multiple practice guidelines that are relevant to painful conditions experienced by critically ill patients, including: • Patients with chronic stable angina • Patients with unstable angina • Patients with peripheral arterial disease • Patients with ST-elevation myocardial infarction • Guideline update for coronary artery bypass graft surgery These guidelines are available from the National Guideline Clearinghouse at http://www.guidelines.gov/[15]

physiological parameters should be considered along with the patient's self-report.

PATIENT SELF-REPORT

Because pain is a subjective experience, the patient's self-report is considered to be the foundation of pain assessment; however, family members and caregivers are often used as proxies for patient self-reports, especially in situations such as critical illness, which can pose significant communication barriers.[18] A self-report or proxy assessment of pain should be obtained not only at rest, but also during routine activity, such as coughing, deep breathing, and turning. Critical care nurses are frequently more attuned to objective indicators of pain than to the patient's self-report. If the patient can communicate, the ICU nurse must accept the patient's description of pain as valid. In the conscious and coherent patient, behavioral cues or physiological indicators should never take precedence over the patient's self-report of pain. Behavioral and physiological manifestations of pain are extremely individualized and may be minimal or absent, despite the presence of significant pain.

Table 5-5 • Internet Resources	
Website	**Resources Provided**
American Chronic Pain Association: http://www.theacpa.org	Offers information and support for people with chronic pain
American Pain Foundation: http://www.painfoundation.org	Resource center for people with pain, their families, friends, caregivers, the media, legislators, and the general public
American Society of Pain Management Nurses: http://www.aspmn.org	Information about society membership, conferences, resources, guidelines and position statements
City of Hope Pain/Palliative Care Resource Center: http://www.cityofhope.org/prc/	Resources to assist others in improving pain management and end of life care; a source for assessment tools, patient education materials, quality assurance materials, end of life resources, and research instruments
National Guideline Clearinghouse: http://www.guidelines.gov	Multiple evidence-based clinical practice guidelines for pain and various other clinical problems; sponsored by the Agency for Healthcare Research and Quality

In assessing pain quality, the nurse should elicit a specific verbal description of the patient's pain, such as "burning," "crushing," "stabbing," "dull," or "sharp," whenever possible. These terms help pinpoint the cause of the pain.

Pain scales and rating instruments based on the patient's self-report provide a simple but consistent measure of pain trends over time. Numerical rating scales and visual analog scales are used to measure pain intensity. With these scales, the patient is asked to choose a number, word, or a point on a line that best describes the amount of pain he or she is experiencing. The SCCM clinical practice guideline suggests that the numerical rating scale is the preferred type of scale for use in critical care units.[16] With this type of scale, the patient is asked to rate the pain, with 0 being no pain and 10 being the worst possible pain imaginable (Fig. 5-1).

Pictures or word boards can also facilitate communication about the patient's pain. The board should include open-ended questions, such as "Do you have pain?" "Where is the pain located?" "How bad is your pain?" and "What helps your pain?" Developing a simple system of eye movements ("blink once for yes and twice for no") or finger movements can be effective for the patient who cannot speak or move his or her hands.[9]

Pain assessment and subsequent treatment are dilemmas if the patient is unable to use any of the above methods to verbalize or indicate that he or she is in pain. In this situation, it is appropriate to observe for the behavioral cues or physiological indicators discussed in the next section. However, the absence of physiological indicators or behavioral cues should *never* be interpreted as absence of pain. If the procedure, surgery, or condition is believed to be associated with pain, the presence of pain should be assumed and treated appropriately.

OBSERVATION

Recent research has demonstrated that ICU nurses can rely on behavioral and physiological indicators of pain in critically ill patients who cannot provide a verbal self-report.[19,20] Protective behaviors, such as guarding, withdrawal, and avoidance of movement, protect the patient from painful stimuli. Attempts by the patient to seek relief, such as touching or rubbing the area and changing positions, are palliative behaviors. Crying, moaning, and screaming are affective behaviors and reflect an emotional response to pain. Facial expressions such as frowning, grimacing, clenching the teeth, tight closure of the eyes, and tears can indicate pain.

Patients who are unable to speak may use eye or facial expressions or movement of hands or legs to communicate their pain. Restlessness, agitation, and muscular bracing may be seen in the nonverbal patient. Because nonverbal cues can be difficult to interpret as indicators of pain, input from family members or other caregivers is helpful in interpreting specific behavioral manifestations of pain based on their knowledge of the patient's behavior before hospitalization.

PHYSIOLOGICAL PARAMETERS

Critical care nurses are skilled in assessing the patient's physical status in terms of changes in blood pressure, heart rate, or respirations. Therefore, the observation of the physiological effects of pain assists in pain assessment. Unfortunately, the physiological response to pain is highly individualized. Vital signs, such as heart rate, blood pressure, and respiratory rate, may increase or decrease in the presence of pain.[19] With critically ill patients, it can be difficult to attribute these physiological changes specifically to pain rather than to other causes. For example, an unexpected increase in the severity and intensity of the patient's pain associated with hypotension, tachycardia, or fever must be evaluated immediately. These findings may signal the development of life-threatening complications, such as wound dehiscence, infection, or deep venous thrombosis.

Pain assessment is an ongoing process. In addition to the initial pain assessment, assessment after

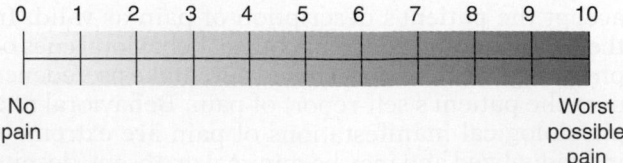

0	1	2	3	4	5	6	7	8	9	10

No pain   Worst possible pain

Figure 5-1 • Numerical rating scale for pain assessment.

pain management interventions and before procedures is essential. After pharmacological therapy, pain reassessment should correspond to the time of onset or peak effect of the drug administered and the time the analgesic effect is expected to dissipate. Response to therapy is best measured as a change from the patient's baseline pain level. Occasionally, there may be discrepancies between the patient's self-report and behavioral and physiological manifestations. For example, one patient may report pain as 2 out of 10, while being tachycardic, diaphoretic, and splinting with respirations. Another patient may give a self-report of 8 out of 10 while smiling. These discrepancies can be due to the use of diversionary activities, coping skills, beliefs about pain, cultural background, fears of becoming addicted, or fears of being bothersome to the nursing staff. When these situations occur, they should be discussed with the patient. Any misconceptions or knowledge deficits should be addressed and the pain treated according to the patient's self-report. Box 5-2 lists common nursing diagnoses for the patient in pain.

• Pain Intervention

The nurse plays an important role in providing pain relief. Although pharmacological intervention is the most commonly used strategy, nursing management of pain also includes physical, cognitive, and behavioral measures. In addition to administering medications or providing alternative therapies, the nurse's role involves measuring the patient's response to those therapies. Because pain may diminish or the pain pattern may change, therapy adjustments may be needed before improvements are seen. General guidelines for nursing interventions are listed in Box 5-3.

PHARMACOLOGICAL INTERVENTIONS

In general, the ideal method of analgesia should allow adequate serum drug levels to be achieved and maintained quickly and easily. Medications should be titrated based on the patient's response, and the drug should be quickly eliminated when analgesia is no longer needed. Most clinicians agree that when using a numerical scale for assessment, pain medications should be titrated according to the following goals:

▶ The patient's reported pain score is less than his or her own predetermined pain management goal (e.g., 3 on a scale of 1 to 10).

▶ Adequate respiration is maintained.

The efficacy of analgesia depends on the presence of an adequate and consistent serum drug level. Regardless of the method being used, scheduled opioid doses or continuous infusions are preferred over "as needed" (PRN) administration.[16] The traditional PRN analgesic order is a major barrier to effective pain control in all patient populations. The PRN order suggests that the nurse should administer a dose of analgesic only when the patient requests it and only after a certain time interval has elapsed since the previous dose. Invariably, a delay occurs between the time of the request and the time the medication is actually administered. In some cases, this delay can be up to an hour. The PRN order poses another problem when the patient is asleep. As serum drug levels decrease, the patient is suddenly awakened by severe pain, and a greater amount of the drug is needed to achieve adequate serum levels.

Nonopioid Analgesics

Ideally, analgesic regimens should include a nonopioid drug, even if the pain is severe enough to also require an opioid.[2] In many patient populations, nonsteroidal anti-inflammatory drugs (NSAIDs) are the preferred choice for the nonopioid component of analgesic therapy. NSAIDs decrease pain by inhibiting the synthesis of inflammatory mediators (prostaglandin, histamine, and bradykinin) at the site of injury and effectively relieve pain without causing sedation, respiratory depression, or problems with bowel or bladder function. When NSAIDs are used in combination with opioids, the opioid dose can often be reduced and still produce effective analgesia. This decreases the incidence of opioid-related side effects.

Many NSAIDs are supplied only in oral forms, and this is not satisfactory for critically ill patients whose oral intake is restricted. Ketorolac is available in parenteral form, but it can cause renal impairment if administration exceeds 5 days; therefore, it must be used with caution in patients with renal insufficiency or in those receiving dialysis. Indomethacin is available in suppository form and can be combined with opioids to provide effective pain relief.[21]

In addition to the concerns about route of administration, a major concern associated with NSAID use is the potential for adverse effects, including gastrointestinal bleeding, platelet inhibition, and renal insufficiency. Second-generation NSAIDs, such as celecoxib and rofecoxib, are more selective in their site of action and therefore do not cause these harmful adverse effects, but their slow onset of action may decrease their utility in critically ill patients. Long-term use of these agents can increase the risk for developing cardiovascular disease.[16]

Acetaminophen is commonly used in critical care. When it is used in combination with opioids, it produces a greater effect than opioids alone. In addition to mild analgesia, acetaminophen is an effective antipyretic; however, it does have the potential to cause hepatic damage. Dosages should be limited to a maximum of 2,400 mg/day if patients have a history of, or high potential for, liver impairment. Nonopioid analgesics that are commonly used in critical care and their recommended doses are listed in Table 5-6.

Opioids

Opioids are the pharmacological cornerstone of postoperative pain management. They provide pain relief by binding to various receptor sites in the spinal cord, central nervous system (CNS), and peripheral nervous system, thus changing the perception of pain.

Opioids are selected based on individual patient needs and the potential for adverse effects. Commonly used opioids are compared in Table 5-7. According to the SCCM, morphine sulfate, fentanyl, and hydromorphone are the preferred agents when IV opioids are needed.[16] Other opioids used in critical care include codeine, oxycodone, and methadone.

Meperidine is the least potent opioid and is administered in the largest doses. For example, to produce a level of analgesia comparable to 10 mg of morphine every 4 hours, 100 to 150 mg of meperidine every 3 hours would be needed. Meperidine is commonly underdosed and given at intervals too infrequent to be effective. Even though meperidine continues to be widely used in some settings, national experts and national practice guidelines consider it to be dangerous and do not recommend it for most patients.[16,22] Rationales for not using this drug are summarized in Box 5-4.

Dosing Guidelines

Equianalgesia means approximately equal analgesia. This term is used when changing a patient's regimen from one analgesic to another. Morphine, 10 mg intramuscularly, is generally considered the gold standard dose for comparison. Dosing guidelines for opioid analgesics are presented in Table 5-7.

Opioid dosage varies depending on the individual patient, the method of administration, and the pharmacokinetics of the drug. Adequate pain relief occurs once a minimum serum level of the opioid has been achieved. Each patient's optimal serum level is different, and this level can change as pain intensity

Table 5-6 • Nonopioid Analgesic Drugs

Drug	Adult Dose	Usual Pediatric Dose	Comments
Acetaminophen	650–975 mg q4h	10–15 mg/kg q4h	Available in liquid form, lacks anti-inflammatory action. Doses exceeding 4,000 mg/day increase the risk for hepatic toxicity.
Aspirin	650–975 mg q4h	10–15 mg/kg q4h	Can cause gastrointestinal or postoperative bleeding
Celecoxib (Celebrex)	100–400 mg bid		Less adverse effects than other NSAIDs, considerably more expensive
Ibuprofen (Motrin)	200–400 mg q4–6h	10 mg/kg q6–8h	Available in liquid form
Indomethacin (Indocin)	25 mg q8–12h		Available in rectal and IV forms, but high incidence of side effects
Ketorolac (Toradol)	30–60 mg IM initially; then 30 mg IV q6h or 15–30 mg IM q6h; or 10 mg PO q6–8h		Available in parenteral form, limit use to 5 days, contraindicated with renal insufficiency
Naproxen (Naprosyn)	500 mg initially; then 250 mg q6–8h	5 mg/kg q12	Available in liquid form

All doses are oral, unless noted otherwise.

Table 5-7 • Opioid Analgesic Drugs

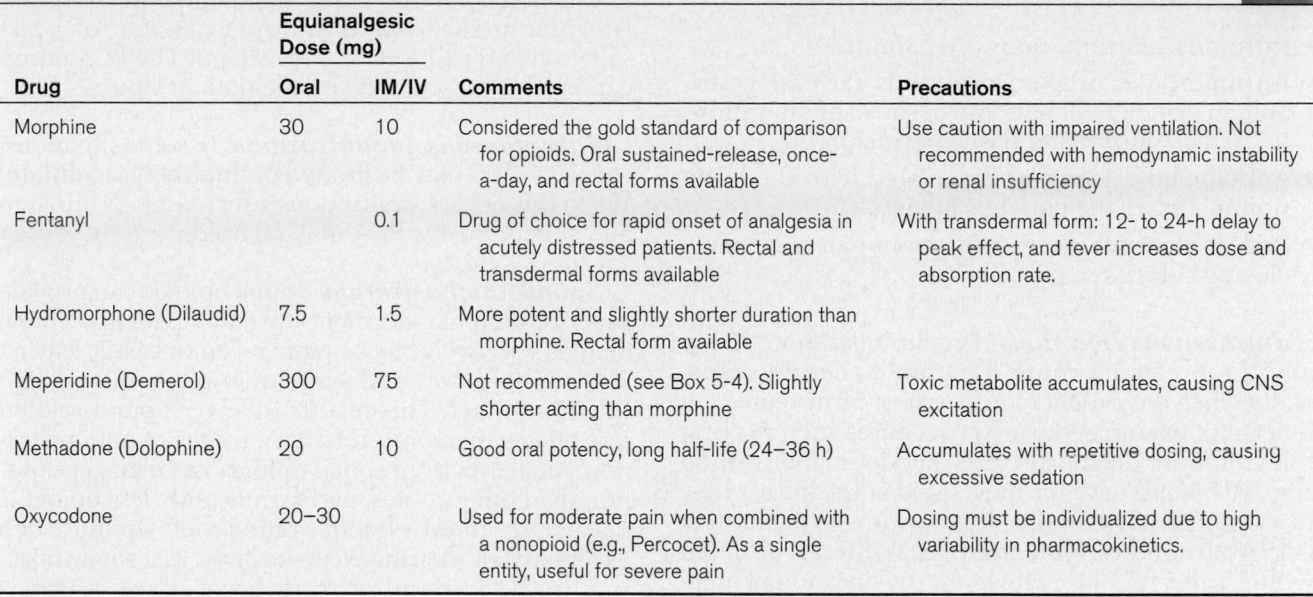

Drug	Equianalgesic Dose (mg) Oral	IM/IV	Comments	Precautions
Morphine	30	10	Considered the gold standard of comparison for opioids. Oral sustained-release, once-a-day, and rectal forms available	Use caution with impaired ventilation. Not recommended with hemodynamic instability or renal insufficiency
Fentanyl		0.1	Drug of choice for rapid onset of analgesia in acutely distressed patients. Rectal and transdermal forms available	With transdermal form: 12- to 24-h delay to peak effect, and fever increases dose and absorption rate.
Hydromorphone (Dilaudid)	7.5	1.5	More potent and slightly shorter duration than morphine. Rectal form available	
Meperidine (Demerol)	300	75	Not recommended (see Box 5-4). Slightly shorter acting than morphine	Toxic metabolite accumulates, causing CNS excitation
Methadone (Dolophine)	20	10	Good oral potency, long half-life (24–36 h)	Accumulates with repetitive dosing, causing excessive sedation
Oxycodone	20–30		Used for moderate pain when combined with a nonopioid (e.g., Percocet). As a single entity, useful for severe pain	Dosing must be individualized due to high variability in pharmacokinetics.

changes. Therefore, the dosing and titration of opioids must be individualized, and the patient's response and any undesirable effects, such as respiratory depression or oversedation, must be closely assessed. If the patient has previously received an opioid (e.g., before surgery), doses should be adjusted above the previous required dose to achieve an optimal effect. Factors such as age, individual pain tolerance, coexisting diseases, type of surgical procedure, and the concomitant use of sedatives warrant consideration as well. Older patients are often more sensitive to the effects of opioids; therefore, decreasing the initial opioid dose and slow titration are recommended for older patients.

Methods of Administration

Oral Administration Oral administration is simple, noninvasive, and inexpensive, and it provides effective analgesia. Oral is the preferred route for patients with cancer and chronic nonmalignant pain. However, the oral route is used infrequently in the ICU setting because many patients are unable to take anything by mouth. Serum drug levels obtained after oral administration of opioids are variable and difficult to titrate. In addition, the transformation of oral opioids by the liver causes a significant decrease in serum levels.

Rectal Administration Morphine and hydromorphone are available in a rectal form. This provides an alternative for patients who cannot take anything by mouth. Unfortunately, this mechanism has many of the same disadvantages as oral administration, including variability in dosing requirements, delays to peak effect, and unstable serum drug levels.

Transdermal Administration Fentanyl is available in a transdermal patch format. This form is used primarily to control chronic cancer pain because it takes 12 to 16 hours to obtain substantial therapeutic effects and up to 48 hours to achieve stable serum concentrations. If used for acute pain, such as post-operative pain, high serum concentrations may remain after the pain has subsided, putting the patient at risk for respiratory depression.[22]

Box 5-4 • RED FLAG: Precautions and Concerns Associated with Meperidine Use

Meperidine is a dangerous analgesic that continues to be used in some settings. It is not recommended for the following reasons:

- Low potency—requires unusually high doses
- Produces toxic metabolite—normeperidine
- Can cause CNS excitation, anxiety, tremors, seizures
- IM administration produces fibrosis
- Contraindicated in patients with compromised renal function
- Contraindicated in elderly patients
- Should not be used for more than 48 h
- Dose should not exceed 600 mg/24 h
- Should not be used for chronic pain treatment
- Use in patients with sickle cell disease creates high risk for seizures
- Coadministration with monoamine oxidase inhibitors can be lethal

Adapted from American Pain Society: Principles of Analgesic Use in the Treatment of Acute Pain and Cancer Pain, 4th ed. Glenview, IL: Author, 1999; and Latta K, Ginsberg B, Barkin R: Meperidine: A critical review. Am J Ther 9(1):53–68, 2002

Intramuscular Injections   Intramuscular injections should not be used to provide acute pain relief for the critically ill patient for several reasons:

▶ Intramuscular injections are painful.

▶ Intramuscular drug absorption is extremely variable in critically ill patients because of alterations in cardiac output and tissue perfusion.

▶ Anticipated discomfort associated with the injection increases the patient's anxiety.

▶ Repeated intramuscular injections can cause muscle and soft tissue fibrosis.

Intravenous Injections   IV administration is usually the preferred route for opioid therapy, especially when the patient requires short-term acute pain relief—for example, during procedures such as chest tube removal, diagnostic tests, suctioning, or wound care. IV opioids have the most rapid onset and are easy to administer. With morphine, the time to peak effect is 15 to 30 minutes; for fentanyl, peak effect is achieved within 1 to 5 minutes. However, the duration of analgesia is shorter with intermittent IV injections, and this can cause serum drug levels to fluctuate.

Continuous IV administration has many benefits for critically ill patients, especially those who have difficulty communicating their pain because of an altered level of consciousness or an endotracheal tube. Continuous IV infusions are easily initiated and maintain consistent serum drug levels. For continuous IV opioid infusions, fentanyl and morphine are commonly used because of their short elimination half-life (compared with other available opioids). Before starting a continuous IV infusion, an initial IV loading dose is given to achieve an optimal serum level. Appropriate dosing and titration must be individualized, and this can be difficult because many critically ill patients have hepatic or renal dysfunctions that result in decreased metabolism of the opioid. A disadvantage of continuous IV infusions is that pain occurring during painful procedures may not be managed unless additional IV bolus injections are given.

Patient-controlled analgesia (PCA) is an effective method of pain relief for the critically ill patient who is conscious and able to participate in the pain management therapy. The patient-controlled method of opioid administration produces good-quality analgesia, stable drug concentrations, less sedation, less opioid consumption, and fewer adverse effects.[16] Effective use of PCA is based on the assumption that the patient is the best person to evaluate and manage his or her pain. PCA individualizes pain control therapy and offers the patient greater feelings of control and well-being.

With PCA, the patient self-administers small, frequent IV analgesic doses using a programmable infusion device. Most often, morphine sulfate or fentanyl is used. The PCA device limits the opioid dose within a specific time period, thus preventing oversedation and respiratory depression. If the patient is physically or cognitively unable to use "conventional" PCA, other adaptations can be made. For example, the PCA pump can be activated by a designated family member. This family member needs thorough education in terms of how to assess for the presence of pain, how to administer the medication, and how to assess for oversedation and respiratory depression. The PCA pump can be also be activated by the patient's nurse.

Subcutaneous Administration   In some situations, venous access may be limited or impossible to obtain. When this occurs, continuous subcutaneous infusion and subcutaneous PCA may be used.

Spinal Administration   Spinal opioids can provide superior pain management for many patients. Spinal opioids selectively block opioid receptors while leaving sensation, motor, and sympathetic nervous system function intact. This results in fewer opioid-related side effects than oral, IM, or IV routes of administration. Analgesia from spinal opioids has a longer duration than other routes, and significantly less opioid is needed to achieve effective pain relief. Opioids such as fentanyl or morphine can be given as a single injection in the epidural or intrathecal space, as intermittent injections, as continuous infusions through an epidural catheter, or through epidural PCA.

Epidural analgesia is noted for providing effective pain relief and improved postoperative pulmonary function. This method is especially beneficial for critically ill patients after thoracic, upper abdominal, or peripheral vascular surgery, rib fractures, or orthopedic trauma, or for postoperative patients with a history of obesity or pulmonary disease. With epidural analgesia, opioids are administered through a catheter inserted in the spinal canal between the dura mater and vertebral arch. Opioids diffuse across the dura and subarachnoid space and bind with opioid receptor sites.

Intermittent injections may be given before, during, or after a surgical procedure. For more sustained pain relief, continuous epidural infusions are recommended. For patient-controlled epidural analgesia (PCEA), the same parameters are used as with IV PCA, except that smaller opioid doses are used. Contraindications to epidural analgesia include systemic infection or sepsis, bleeding disorders, and increased intracranial pressure.

Preservative-free morphine and fentanyl are most commonly used for epidural analgesia because preservatives can be neurotoxic and may cause severe spinal cord injury. Morphine is more water soluble than fentanyl and thus is more likely to accumulate in the cerebrospinal fluid and systemic circulation. With increased accumulation, side effects are more likely. Fentanyl diffuses more quickly to the opioid receptors and causes fewer opioid-related side effects. The most serious adverse effect of epidural analgesia is respiratory depression. Although the incidence of serious respiratory depression is extremely low with epidural analgesia, respiratory assessments should be performed hourly during the first 24 hours of therapy and every 4 hours thereafter.

Because epidural analgesia is more invasive than the other methods discussed, the patient must be closely monitored for signs of local or systemic infections. The insertion site is covered with a sterile dressing, and the catheter is taped securely. To avoid accidental injection of preservative-containing medications, the epidural catheter, infusion tubing, and pump should be clearly marked.

With intrathecal analgesia, the opioid is injected into the subarachnoid space, located between the spinal cord and dura mater. Intrathecal opioids are significantly more potent than those given epidurally; therefore, less medication is needed to provide effective analgesia. The intrathecal method is usually used to deliver a one-time dose of analgesic, such as before surgery, and is infrequently used as a continuous infusion because of the risk for CNS infection.

With epidural or intrathecal analgesia, a local anesthetic, such as bupivacaine, can be added to the continuous opioid infusion. Local anesthetics block pain by preventing nerve cell depolarization. They act synergistically with intraspinal opioid and have a dose-sparing effect. Less opioid is needed to provide effective analgesia, and the incidence of opioid-related side effects is decreased. This combination is more commonly administered by the epidural route.

Side Effects

Opioids cause undesirable side effects, such as constipation, urinary retention, sedation, respiratory depression, and nausea. These side effects represent a major drawback to their use. Opioid-related side effects are best managed in the following ways:

▶ *Decreasing the opioid dose:* This is the most effective strategy because it is directed at the cause of the side effect. Side effects are usually seen with excessively high serum levels of the drug. Decreasing the opioid dose can alleviate the side effect while still providing effective pain relief.

▶ *Avoiding PRN dosing:* When opioids are administered on a PRN basis, fluctuating serum drug levels occur, causing a greater tendency toward sedation and respiratory depression. Around-the-clock administration of analgesics, including opioids, is recommended.

▶ *Adding an NSAID to the pain management plan:* Using an NSAID in addition to an opioid can decrease the amount of opioid needed, still provide effective pain relief, and decrease opioid-related side effects.

Medications can be given to minimize or alleviate some side effects (e.g., stool softeners for constipation, antihistamines for pruritus, and antiemetics for nausea). However, medications commonly prescribed to treat the opioid-related adverse effects can actually cause other adverse effects. For example, promethazine, a commonly prescribed antiemetic, can cause hypotension, restlessness, tremors, and extrapyramidal effects in the older patient.

Respiratory depression, a life-threatening complication of opioid administration, is often a concern for nurses and physicians. The incidence of true opioid-induced respiratory depression is low in most patients. In some cases, a respiratory rate as low as 10 may not be significant, if the patient is still breathing deeply. Patients most at risk for respiratory depression are infants, elderly people who have not recently used opioids, and patients with coexisting pulmonary, renal, or hepatic disease.

Opioid Antagonists

If serious respiratory depression does occur, naloxone (Narcan), a pure opioid antagonist that reverses the effects of opioids, can be administered. The dose of naloxone is titrated to effect—which means reversing the oversedation and respiratory depression, not reversing analgesia. This usually occurs within 1 to 2 minutes. After giving naloxone, the nurse continues to observe the patient closely for oversedation and respiratory depression because the half-life of naloxone (1.5 to 2 hours) is shorter than that of most opioids.

Naloxone should be diluted (0.4 mg in 10 mL of saline) and given intravenously, very slowly. Giving the drug too quickly or giving too much can precipitate severe pain, withdrawal symptoms, tachycardia, dysrhythmias, and cardiac arrest. Patients who have been receiving opioids for more than a week are particularly at risk.

Sedation and Anxiolysis

Acute pain is frequently accompanied by anxiety, and anxiety can increase the patient's perception of pain. When treating acute pain, anxiolytics can be used to complement analgesia and improve the patient's overall comfort. This is an important consideration, especially before and during painful procedures. Table 5-8 provides a comparison of sedatives commonly used in critical care.[21]

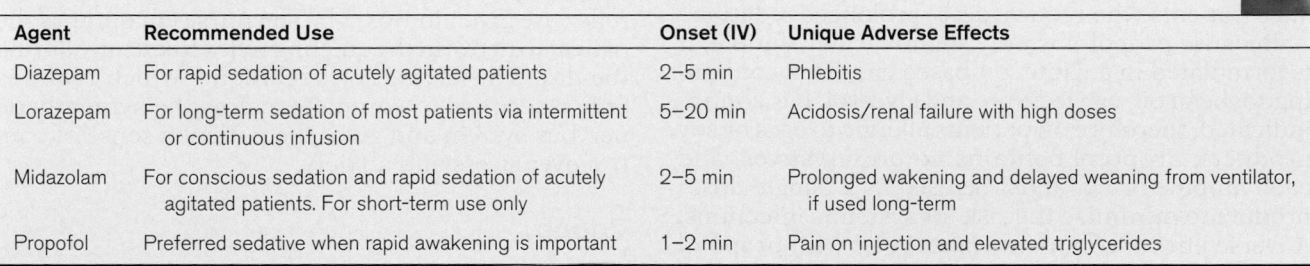

Table 5-8 • Comparison of Sedatives Commonly Used in Critical Care

Agent	Recommended Use	Onset (IV)	Unique Adverse Effects
Diazepam	For rapid sedation of acutely agitated patients	2–5 min	Phlebitis
Lorazepam	For long-term sedation of most patients via intermittent or continuous infusion	5–20 min	Acidosis/renal failure with high doses
Midazolam	For conscious sedation and rapid sedation of acutely agitated patients. For short-term use only	2–5 min	Prolonged wakening and delayed weaning from ventilator, if used long-term
Propofol	Preferred sedative when rapid awakening is important	1–2 min	Pain on injection and elevated triglycerides

Adapted from Jacobi J, Fraser, G, Coursin D, et al: Clinical practice guidelines for the sustained use of sedatives and analgesics in the critically ill adult. Crit Care Med 30(1):119–141, 2002.

Benzodiazepines

Benzodiazepines, such as midazolam, diazepam, and lorazepam, can control anxiety and muscle spasms and produce amnesia for uncomfortable procedures. In the ICU, benzodiazepines may be given intravenously as an intermittent bolus or by continuous infusion and titrated according to the patient's response. Because these medications have no analgesic effect (except for controlling pain caused by muscle spasm), an analgesic must be administered concomitantly to relieve pain. If an opioid and benzodiazepine are used together, the doses of both medications should usually be reduced because of their synergistic effects. The patient should also be closely monitored for oversedation and respiratory depression.

Midazolam is recommended for conscious sedation and short-term relief of anxiety because of its rapid onset (1 to 5 minutes with IV administration) and its short half life (1 to 12 hours). Another advantage is its retrograde amnesia effect, which is particularly beneficial during procedures. The duration of effect of midazolam can be longer in older or obese patients and those with liver disease.[16]

A major advantage of benzodiazepines is that they are reversible agents. If respiratory depression occurs because of benzodiazepine administration, flumazenil can be administered intravenously. Flumazenil is a benzodiazepine-specific reversal agent that reverses the sedative and respiratory depressant effects without reversing opioid analgesics. The dosing of flumazenil should be individualized and titrated so that only the smallest effective amount is used. After prolonged benzodiazepine therapy, flumazenil should be used with caution because of the potential for stimulating withdrawal symptoms.[21]

Critically ill patients who are receiving repeated doses or continuous infusions of sedatives are given a break from sedation at least once per day. Administration should be interrupted until the patient is fully awake. This helps prevent oversedation, which can inhibit weaning from mechanical ventilation.

Propofol

Propofol is a rapid-acting sedative-hypnotic agent that has no analgesic properties and minimal amnesic effects. With appropriate airway and ventilatory management, propofol can be an ideal agent for patients requiring sedation during painful procedures. Because of its ultrashort half-life, it is reversible simply by discontinuing the infusion, and patients awaken within a few minutes. Propofol can also be used as a continuous infusion for mechanically ventilated patients who require deep, prolonged sedation.

Because propofol is only slightly water soluble, it is formulated in a white, oil-based emulsion containing soybean oil, egg lecithin, and glycerol. It is contraindicated, therefore, in patients allergic to eggs or soy products. Propofol contains no preservatives, and each ampule or vial must be used as a "single-dose" product to minimize the risk for systemic infections. Adverse effects commonly associated with propofol include respiratory depression, hypotension, elevated triglycerides, and pain and stinging at the injection site.

NONPHARMACOLOGICAL COMFORT MEASURES

Research has shown that the combination of nonpharmacologic and pharmacologic interventions provides better pain control, with less use of opioid analgesics, decreased incidence of anxiety, and increased patient satisfaction.[23,24] These nonpharmacologic approaches, which include interventions such as distraction, relaxation, music, therapeutic touch, and massage, can be challenging to provide in the critical setting.

Environmental Modification

In critical care, the most basic and logical nonpharmacologic intervention is environmental modification. The excessive noise and light in ICUs can disrupt sleep and increase anxiety and agitation, in turn contributing to pain and discomfort. Care should be preplanned to minimize noise and disruptions during normal sleeping hours and to create a pattern of light that mimics normal day–night patterns. Earphones, with music of the patient's choice, and earplugs have also been recommended for use in the ICU.[23,25]

Distraction

Distraction helps patients direct their attention away from the source of pain or discomfort toward something more pleasant. Patients, families, and nurses often use distraction routinely without giving it much consideration. Initiating a conversation with the patient during an uncomfortable procedure, watching television, and visiting with family are all excellent sources of distraction.

Relaxation Techniques

Relaxation exercises involve repetitive focus on a word, phrase, prayer, or muscular activity, and a conscious effort to reject other intruding thoughts. Relaxation can give the patient a sense of control over a particular body part. Most relaxation methods require a quiet environment, a comfortable position, a passive attitude, and concentration. Each of these can be challenging to achieve in an ICU.

Breathing exercises have been used with much success in childbirth. They can also be used successfully in the critically ill patient. The quieting reflex is a breathing and relaxation technique that reduces stress and can easily be taught to the conscious and coherent patient. Instructions regarding the quieting reflex are given in Box 5-5. The nurse encourages the patient to perform the quieting reflex frequently during the day. This relaxation technique, which requires only 6 seconds to complete, calms the sympathetic nervous system and gives the patient a sense of control over stress and anxiety.

Touch

Historically, one of the greatest contributions nurses have made is the comfort and caring of presence and

Box 5-5 • TEACHING GUIDE:
The Quieting Reflex

1. Inhale an easy, natural breath.
2. Think "alert mind, calm body."
3. Smile inwardly (with your internal facial muscles).
4. As you exhale, allow your jaw, tongue, and shoulders to go loose.
5. Allow a feeling of warmth and looseness to go down through your body and out through your toes.

touch. These contributions still have an important place in today's highly technological ICUs. Nurses may feel that touching is too simple to be effective. However, few medical advances can replace the benefits of warm and caring touch. The need for touch is thought to intensify during times of high stress and cannot be totally met by other forms of communication. Nurses, when using touch, are usually trying to convey understanding, support, warmth, concern, and closeness to the patient. Touching not only contributes to the patient's sense of well-being but also promotes physical recovery from disease. It has a positive effect on perceptual and cognitive abilities and can influence physiological parameters, such as respiration and blood flow. Touch represents a positive therapeutic element of human interaction.

The effects of touch in the clinical environment are far reaching. Touch has played a major part in promoting and maintaining reality orientation in patients prone to confusion about time, place, and personal identification. Nursing touch may be most helpful in situations in which people are experiencing fear, anxiety, depression, or isolation. It may also be beneficial for patients who have a need for encouragement or nurturing, who have difficulty verbalizing needs, or who are disoriented, unresponsive, or terminally ill. Patients often feel that the desire for touch increases with the seriousness of the illness.

Massage

Superficial massage initiates the relaxation response and has been shown to increase the amount of sleep in ICU patients.[26] Although the back is the most common location used for massage, backs are often difficult to access in ICU patients. Hands, feet, and shoulders are also good sites for massage. Massage is an excellent intervention for family members to use in their attempts to provide comfort to the critically ill.

PATIENT EDUCATION

To educate the patient about pain and pain relief, the critical care nurse must be familiar with the patient's pain management plan and therapy being used. Communication between the nurse and patient is essential. During the course of therapy, the nurse periodically reinforces any information that has been presented previously and encourages the patient to verbalize

any questions or concerns. The nurse includes family members in discussions whenever possible.

It is necessary to talk about plans for pain management with patients when they are most able to understand, such as before surgery rather than during recovery. Emphasis is on prevention of pain because it is easier to prevent pain than to treat it once it becomes severe.

Patients need to know that most pain can be relieved and that unrelieved pain may have serious consequences for physical and psychological well-being and may interfere with recovery. The nurse helps patients and families understand that pain management is an important part of their care and that the health care team will respond quickly to reports of pain.

The nurse also gives patients instructions about nonpharmacological interventions and traditional methods to minimize pain. Splinting the incisional area with a pillow while coughing or ambulating is a traditional pain relief measure.

The potential for drug addiction or overdosage is often a major concern for the patient and family. It is important to address and clarify these issues because they create a barrier to effective pain relief. The patient also needs a clear understanding of any specialized pain management technology, such as PCA to alleviate the fear of overdosage. Box 5-6 summarizes key points about pain management that should be covered with the patient and his or her caregiver before discharge.

• Pain Management in Special Populations

Some critically ill populations create unique pain management challenges. Special considerations for elderly patients are noted in Box 5-7. Another population that is particularly challenging is patients who are known to be dying. Pain is a primary concern for patients and their families at the end of life. Recent initiatives to promote high-quality palliative and end-of-life care[27, 28] have contributed to the diligence of health care providers in their efforts to understand and control pain in dying patients.

Box 5-6 • DISCHARGE PLANNING GUIDE:
Pain Management at Home

- Teach family caregivers to assess the impact of analgesics on pain and respiratory status.
- Encourage the use of prophylactic medications, such as stool softeners, to prevent opioid-induced constipation.
- Help caregivers to understand the difference between tolerance and addiction.
- Ensure that fears of addiction do not impede necessary analgesic administration.
- Reinforce the importance of preventing pain before it occurs or becomes severe.

> **Box 5-7 • CONSIDERATIONS FOR THE OLDER PATIENT:** Pain
>
> - Painful chronic diseases often compound the acute pain of critical illness in older patients.
> - Arthritis, the most common cause of chronic pain in older patients, often affects the back, hips, knees, and shoulders, increasing the pain of turning in the ICU.
> - Some older patients can experience acutely painful conditions, such as myocardial infarction or appendicitis, without the presence of pain.
> - Older patients often use words such as "aches" or "tenderness," rather than "pain."
> - Family caregivers can help assess pain in older patients with cognitive or language impairments.
> - Older patients are particularly sensitive to opioids, achieving higher peak concentrations and longer duration.
> - Meperidine, pentazocine, propoxyphene, and methadone should not be used to treat pain in older adults.[21]
> - Older patients often have an increased need for meaningful touch during episodes of crisis.

Progression toward death is often marked by decreased cardiac output, decreased perfusion, and failure of major organ systems. This can create problems with excessive accumulation of analgesics and their metabolites owing to limited hepatic and renal function. In such cases, hydromorphone, oxycodone, and fentanyl are preferred agents because of their short half-lives. If pain or dyspnea becomes uncontrollable despite aggressive analgesic administration, high doses of sedatives may also be used. In such cases, the goal of sedation is comfort and relief of suffering, and the common byproduct is end-stage unconsciousness.[29]

• Clinical Applicability Challenges

Case Study

Mr. B., a 28-year-old man, is admitted to the intensive care unit (ICU) with multiple orthopedic and abdominal injuries sustained in a motorcycle accident. During his third day in the ICU, he continues to describe his pain as "intolerable" and says it is not relieved by the combination of oxycodone and acetaminophen that he receives every 4 hours. He is grimacing and continuously asking for more medication before the scheduled dosage interval. The medical resident is frustrated by Mr. B.'s frequent requests and has advised the nurses to be conservative in medicating him because of his history of drug and alcohol abuse.

1. As a nurse caring for Mr. B., what are your major concerns or fears?

2. How would you advocate for Mr. B.?
3. How would you determine whether Mr. B. was seeking drugs for illicit purposes rather than for relief of pain?
4. What arguments could you use to convince the resident to consider a different analgesic regimen?

Review Questions

1. Mr. Smith is a 54-year-old patient in the transitional care unit. On the third day after his lobectomy, the nurse collects information from several sources during her morning assessment. Which of the following is the best description of Mr. Smith's current pain?
   a. The night nurse reported that Mr. Smith's pain has subsided because he was able to sleep through the night without requesting additional medication.
   b. After early morning rounds, the surgeon documented that Mr. Smith's pain was well-controlled and that he was resting comfortably.
   c. Mrs. Smith says that she can tell her husband has much less pain today because he can get out of bed independently.
   d. Mr. Smith tells the nurse that his pain is an "8" on a scale of 0 to 10 this morning.

2. Which of the following is the most accurate statement related to procedural pain management in the critically ill patient?
   a. Noninvasive procedures, such as turning, cause less pain than invasive procedures such as central line placement or femoral sheath removal.
   b. Pain associated with nursing procedures, such as wound care, is insignificant to patients who have experienced major surgery or trauma.
   c. Intravenous opioids, such as morphine or fentanyl, are appropriate medications to prepare the patient for nursing procedures such as suctioning or turning.
   d. Recent research demonstrates that critically ill patients usually receive analgesics before painful nursing procedures.

3. Which of the following physical signs would the nurse expect to see in a patient with uncontrolled pain?
   a. Tachycardia
   b. Hypotension
   c. Coughing
   d. Decreased cardiac output

4. After 10 days in the intensive care unit, the nurse discontinues Mrs. Perry's morphine infusion to prepare her for transfer to the stepdown unit. Before transfer, the nurse notices that Mrs. Perry is restless, diaphoretic, and experiencing muscle spasms in her legs. This patient is most likely demonstrating symptoms of:
   a. tolerance.
   b. physical dependence.
   c. addiction.
   d. overdose.

5. Mr. Jones is a 75-year-old patient who has been hospitalized with advanced cirrhosis and upper gastrointestinal bleeding. Which of the following medications would be the best choice for treating his back pain due to osteoarthritis?
   a. Acetaminophen
   b. Aspirin
   c. Celecoxib
   d. Demerol

References

1. Pasero C: Pain in the critically ill patient. J Perianesth Nurs 18(6):422–425, 2003
2. Stanik-Hutt JA: Pain management in the critically ill. Crit Care Nurse 23(2):99–103, 2003
3. Puntillo KA, Morris AB, Thompson CL, et al: Pain behaviors observed during six common procedures: Results from Thunder Project II. Crit Care Med 32(2):421–427, 2004
4. Li DT, Puntillo K: A pilot study on coexisting symptoms in intensive care patients. Appl Nurs Res 19(4):216, 2006
5. O'Malley P: The undertreatment of pain: Ethical and legal implications for the clinical nurse specialist. J Adv Nurs Pract 19(5):236, 2005
6. International Association for the Study of Pain: Pain Terminology. Retrieved August 28, 2007, from http://www.iasp-pain.org/AM/Template.cfm?Section=Home&template=/CM/HTMLDisplay.cfm&ContentID=3088#Pain
7. McCaffery M: Nursing Practice Theories Related to Cognition, Bodily Pain and Man-Environment Interaction. Los Angeles: University of California at Los Angeles, 1968
8. St. Marie B: Core Curriculum for Pain Management Nursing. Philadelphia, WB Saunders, 2002
9. Pasero C, McCaffery M: Pain in the critically ill. Am J Nurs 102(1):59–60, 2002
10. Puntillo KA, White C, Morris AB, et al: Patients' perceptions and responses to procedural pain: Results from Thunder Project II. Am J Crit Care 10(4):238–251, 2001
11. Puntillo KA, Wild LR, Morris AB, et al: Practices and predictors of analgesic interventions for adults undergoing painful procedures. Am J Crit Care 11(5):415–429; quiz, 430–431, 2002
12. Swope E: Benefits of proper pain management. In: St Marie B (ed): Core Curriculum for Pain Management Nursing. Philadelphia: WB Saunders, 2002, pp 55–66
13. Yeager MP, Glass DD, Neff RK, et al: Epidural anesthesia and analgesia in high-risk surgical patients. Anesthesiology 66(6):729–736, 1987
14. American Pain Society: Definitions related to the use of opioids for the treatment of pain. Retrieved August 25, 2007, from http://www.ampainsoc.org/advocacy/opioids2.htm
15. Agency for Healthcare Research and Quality: National Guideline Clearinghouse. Retrieved August 25, 2007, from http://www.guideline.gov/
16. Jacobi J, Fraser G, Coursin D, et al: Clinical practice guidelines for the sustained use of sedatives and analgesics in the critically ill adult. Crit Care Med 30(1):119–141, 2002
17. American Geriatric Society: The management of persistent pain in older persons. J Am Geriatr Soc 50(6 Suppl):S205–224, 2002
18. National Cancer Institute: Pain (PDQ). Retrieved September 1, 2007, from http://www.cancer.gov/cancertopics/pdq/supportivecare/pain/HealthProfessional/page1
19. Gelinas C, Fillion L, Puntillo KA, et al: Validation of the critical-care pain observation tool in adult patients. Am J Crit Care 15(4):420–427, 2006
20. Gelinas C, Johnston C: Pain assessment in the critically ill ventilated adult: Validation of the critical-care pain observation tool and physiologic indicators. Clin J Pain 23(6):497–505, 2007
21. Lehne R: Pharmacology for Nursing Care, 5th ed. St. Louis, WB Saunders, 2004
22. American Pain Society: Principles of Analgesic Use in the Treatment of Acute Pain and Cancer Pain, 4th ed. Glenview, IL: Author, 1999
23. Pellino TA, Gordon DB, Engelke ZK, et al: Use of nonpharmacologic interventions for pain and anxiety after total hip and total knee arthroplasty. Orthop Nurs 24(3):182–190; quiz, 191–192, 2005
24. Simkin P, Bolding A: Update on nonpharmacologic approaches to relieve labor pain and prevent suffering. J Midwifery Women's Health 49(6):489–504, 2004
25. Bally K, Campbell D, Chesnick K, Tranmer JE: Effects of patient-controlled music therapy during coronary angiography on procedural pain and anxiety distress syndrome. Crit Care Nurse 23(2):50–58, 2003
26. Beezley M: Massage: is there a place for it in the ICU? Aust Crit Care 19(4):154, 2006
27. Tuog RD, Meyer EC, Burns JP: Toward interventions to improve end-of-life care in the pediatric intensive care unit. Crit Care Med 34(11 Suppl):S373–379, 2006
28. Fineberg IC, Wenger NS, Brown-Saltzman K: Unrestricted opiate administration for pain and suffering at the end of life: Knowledge and attitudes as barriers to care. J Palliat Med 9(4):873–883, 2006
29. Panke JT: Difficulties in managing pain at the end of life. Am J Nurs 102(7):26–33; quiz 34, 2002

Other Selected Readings

Berry L, Morrissey B: Content validity of the Cognitively Impaired Adult pain assessment tool. Am J Crit Care 16(3):302, 2007
Chanques G, Jaber S, Barbotte E, et al: Impact of systematic evaluation of pain and agitation in an intensive care unit. Crit Care Med 34(6):1691–1699, 2006
Ferrell B, Coyle N (eds): Textbook of palliative nursing, 2nd ed. New York: Oxford University Press, 2006
Gelinas C, Fillion L, Viens C, Puntillo K: Management of pain in cardiac surgery ICU patients: Have we improved over time? Am J Crit Care 16(3):311, 2007
Gelinas C, Fortier M, Viens C, et al: Pain assessment and management in critically ill intubated patients: A retrospective study. Am J Crit Care 13(2):126–135, 2004
Hamill-Ruth RJ: Managing pain and agitation in the critically ill—are we there yet? Crit Care Med 34(6):1838–1839, 2006
Mair H, Sodian R, Daebritz S: Modern drainage techniques for pain reduction during chest tube removal. Heart Lung 36(3):232–233, 2007
McMahon S, Koltzenburg M: Wall and Melzack's Textbook of Pain, 5th ed. Philadelphia: Elsevier, 2006
Puntillo K: Pain assessment and management in the critically ill: Wizardry or science? Am J Crit Care 12(4):310–316, 2003
Puntillo K: Part 1: Managing pain in the ICU patient. Crit Care Nurs 27(2 Suppl):S8–10, 2007
Puntillo K, Ley SJ: Appropriately timed analgesics control pain due to chest tube removal. Am J Crit Care 13(4):292–301; discussion, 302; quiz, 303–304, 2004
Wegman DA: Tool for pain assessment. Crit Care Nurse 25(1):14–15, 2005

6

End-of-Life Issues in Critical Care

Garrett K. Chan

Objectives

Based on the content in this chapter, the reader should
be able to:

❶ List at least three end-of-life issues related to
critical care nursing.

❷ List at least three components of palliative care.

❸ Describe how palliative care can be integrated into
curative or disease-modifying care.

❹ Identify at least three symptoms commonly
experienced at the end of life.

❺ Recognize the importance of flexible visiting hours
for a patient at the end of life.

❻ Describe activities by the nurse in preparing for
and coordinating a family conference.

❼ Identify strategies for self-care of the nurse.

About 2 million people die in the United States every year. Although some people die in peace and comfort, others die in severe distress and suffering. Over the past decade, nurses in the acute care setting have been increasingly concerned about how people die. Thoughts about critical care have slowly shifted; clinicians now recognize that death may be inevitable and that the use of technology to prevent death is limited. Critical care nurses are well positioned to help patients and families during this difficult transitional period. "Being with" patients and families in addition to "doing things to" them enables critical care nurses to provide the holistic care that is central to nursing.[1]

• Need for Quality End-of-Life Care in the Critical Care Setting

In the early 20th century, the average life expectancy was 50 years. Common causes of death included infection, accidents, and childhood mortality.[2] Few life-extending measures were available, and death occurred after hardly any interventions. The focus was on caring for the dying person by family members, who witnessed the death.

However, in the mid to late 20th century, medical interventions such as antibiotics, cardiopulmonary resuscitation (CPR), mechanical ventilation, dialysis, intra-aortic balloon pumps, and pulmonary artery catheters were discovered and routinely used to combat morbidity and mortality. These technologies, combined with other public health initiatives such as improved sanitation, carried the promise of treating the causes of death and therefore extending life. By the year 2000, the average life expectancy had been extended to 77 years.

Critical care nurses became focused on these life-extending procedures, and critical care units were developed to house seriously ill patients in one area of a hospital and closely monitor their response to curative, lifesaving, and aggressive treatments.[3] Increasingly, people died in the hospital setting surrounded by health care practitioners rather than their families. Over the course of the years of technological advancement, nurses increasingly viewed patients in terms of disease processes or technologies. The concept that the patient lying in the bed was a person who experienced physical, emotional, psychological, social, and spiritual suffering was lost.[4]

Recently there has been an increased awareness and effort to improve care for people who are near the end of their lives. It is important to recognize that people approach death in a variety of ways. Therefore, instituting these caring practices from the moment the patient reaches the critical care environment is vital to providing good care.

UNDERSTANDING HUMAN DEATH

Over the past decade, there has been an increase in understanding the human experience of dying in the acute care setting. In 1995, a major study titled the *Study to Understand Prognoses and Preferences for Outcomes and Risks of Treatment* (SUPPORT) was published.[5] This study, conducted in five major academic medical centers across the United States, involved more than 9,000 seriously ill patients. The goal was to improve end-of-life decision making and reduce the frequency of mechanically supported, painful, and prolonged death. Despite use of an intervention designed to communicate preferences among providers, patients, and families, such wishes were often unknown, and aggressive treatment was common. Physicians were not aware that their patients preferred to avoid CPR. In addition, nearly 40% of patients who died spent at least 10 days in an intensive care unit (ICU), and 50% of family members of conscious patients reported that the patients were in moderate to severe pain at least half the time.

After publication of the SUPPORT study, the Institute of Medicine (IOM) released a report titled *Approaching Death: Improving Care at the End of Life.*[6] The IOM group of experts listed seven recommendations to improve end-of-life care (Box 6-1). These recommendations are important for critical care nurses because it is estimated that about 20% of deaths in the United States occur while patients are using ICU services.[7] Critical care nurses play an important role in recognizing opportunities for interventions that support patients, families, and other staff members

---

Box 6-1 • Recommendations to Improve End-of-Life Care

1. People with advanced, potentially fatal illnesses and those close to them should be able to expect and receive reliable, skillful, and supportive care.
2. Physicians, nurses, social workers, and other health professionals must commit themselves to improving care for dying patients and to using existing knowledge effectively to prevent and relieve pain and other symptoms.
3. Because many deficiencies in care reflect system problems, policymakers, consumer groups, and purchasers of health care should work with health care providers and researchers to:
   a. Strengthen methods for measuring the quality of life and other outcomes of care for dying patients and those close to them
   b. Develop better tools and strategies for improving the quality of care and holding health care organizations accountable for care at the end of life
   c. Revise mechanisms for financing care so that they encourage rather than impede good end-of-life care and sustain, rather than frustrate, coordinated systems of excellent care
   d. Reform drug prescription laws, burdensome regulations, and state medical board policies and practices that impede effective use of opioids to relieve pain and suffering
4. Educators and other health professionals should initiate changes in undergraduate, graduate, and continuing education to ensure that practitioners have the relevant attitudes, knowledge, and skills to care well for dying patients.
5. Palliative care should become, if not a medical specialty, at least a defined area of expertise, education, and research.
6. The nation's research establishment should define and implement priorities for strengthening the knowledge base for end-of-life care.
7. A continuing public discussion is essential to develop a better understanding of the modern experience of dying, the options available to dying patients and families, and the obligations of communities to those approaching death.

Adapted from Field MJ, Cassel CK: Approaching Death: Improving Care at the End of Life. Washington, DC: Institute of Medicine, 1997.

---

during this difficult transition in life. Although technology, urgency, uncertainty, and conflict are common in critical care practice, these characteristics may inhibit or fragment a coordinated effort that aims to provide good end-of-life care.[1]

PALLIATIVE CARE

The introduction of palliative care principles into critical care can provide a framework to address these end-of-life issues. Palliative care originated from hospice care, which was designed to improve the quality of death and dying for patients and their families by addressing aspects of care that are unrelated to disease-specific treatments, cure, or rehabilitation.[8] According to the World Health Organization[9] and the IOM,[6] palliative care from an interdisciplinary perspective includes the following core principles: symptom management; advanced care planning; family-centered care; emotional, psychological, social, and spiritual care; facilitating communication; awareness of ethical issues, and caring for the caregiver. These principles should be addressed and incorporated into the total care of the patient, even when disease-modifying or curative therapies are used. In critical care nursing, it is vital that these core palliative care principles are incorporated in the daily plan of care of patients using an interdisciplinary approach.[10] Figure 6-1 illustrates how palliative care can be incorporated throughout the patient's illness.

According to von Gunten and Lupu,[11] there are three levels of palliative care:

1. Primary palliative care is the responsibility of all nurses and includes a basic understanding of interventions to relieve suffering and improve the quality of life for the whole person.

2. Secondary palliative care is provided by specialists in hospital or hospice consult services or hospice programs. Secondary palliative care assists the providers of primary palliative care.

3. Tertiary palliative care is found primarily in academic medical centers that conduct research to discover new knowledge. In addition, the new knowledge is disseminated through educational programs.

Palliative care services in critical care have demonstrated an improvement in symptom management, family support, reduction in length of hospital stay, increased discharges to home with hospice referrals, and reduced costs.[12] The American Association of Critical-Care Nurses (AACN) has developed protocols for critical care practice in palliative and end-of-life care.[13] These protocols provide a good overview of core issues and clinical recommendations for critical care nurses. Resources to assist nurses in addressing issues surrounding the end-of-life phase are given in Table 6-1.

A particular therapeutic intervention may be either curative or palliative depending on its intent. For example, a packed red blood cell transfusion may be curative in a patient with an acute hemorrhage or palliative in a patient with chronic anemia and severe fatigue following chemotherapy. Whether an intervention attempts to cure or to palliate determines whether it is curative or palliative. Additional examples of treatments that can be either curative or palliative are surgeries that resect the bowel to remove a tumor that is causing an intestinal obstruction or administering furosemide in a patient who has severe pulmonary edema. If the treatment relieves the patient's suffering, then it is considered palliative.

• Symptom Management

In critical care, patients experience a wide range of symptoms from their diseases as well as from the therapies that are used to treat those diseases. Common symptoms at the end of life include pain, dyspnea, anxiety and agitation, depression, delirium, and nausea and vomiting. The nurse assesses for the presence and severity of each of these symptoms. Interventions appropriate for the symptoms and an evaluation of those interventions are crucial in providing good end-of-life care.

PAIN

Pain is the most prevalent symptom in critical care units and is distressing to patients and families.[5] Diseases, procedures, and interventions such as turning, suctioning, and wound care can be sources of painful stimuli.[14] Assessing for the presence of pain and intervening to prevent or treat it using pharmacological and nonpharmacological interventions should be incorporated into every patient's care plan. Including a bowel regimen to prevent constipation is crucial

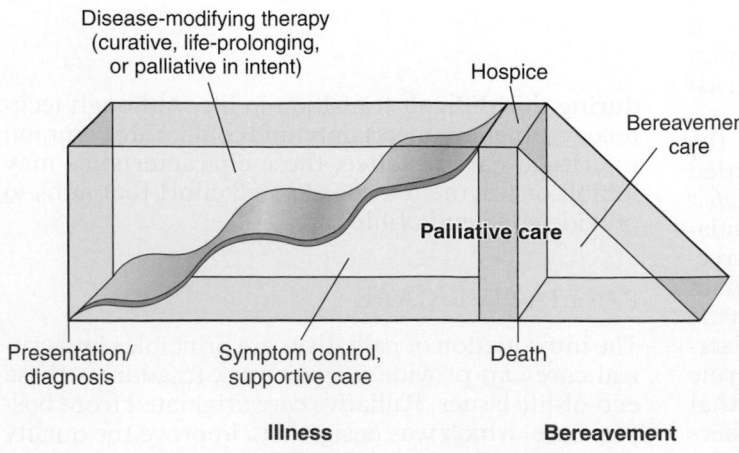

Figure 6-1 • The continuum of care. (Adapted from Emanuel L, von Gunten C, Ferris F, Hauser JM [eds]: The Education in Palliative and End-of-Life Care [EPEC] Curriculum: © The EPEC Project. Chicago: Author, 2003.)

Table 6-1 • End-of-Life Care Resources

Organization	Website
End-of-Life Nursing Education Consortium (ELNEC)	http://www.aacn.nche.edu/elnec/
Education in Palliative and End-of-Life Care (EPEC)	http://www.epec.net
End-of-Life/Palliative Education Resource Center (EPERC)	http://www.eperc.mcw.edu
City of Hope Pain & Palliative Care Resource Center	http://www.cityofhope.org/prc/
National Hospice and Palliative Care Organization	http://www.nhpco.org
Nursing Leadership Academy on End-of-Life Care	http://www.palliativecarenursing.net
Center to Advance Palliative Care (CAPC)	http://www.capc.org
National Consensus Project for Quality Palliative Care (NCP)	http://www.nationalconsensusproject.org
Hospice and Palliative Nurses Association (HPNA)	http://www.hpna.org
American Association of Critical-Care Nurses (AACN)	http://www.aacn.org
Emergency Nurses Association (ENA)	http://www.ena.org
Association of Organ Procurement Organizations	http://www.aopo.org

in the management of pain. Chapter 5 describes, in detail, the assessment of pain and nursing interventions that can be used to treat it.

DYSPNEA

It is estimated that dyspnea is present in 21% to 90% of all patients with a life-threatening illness.[15] Causes of dyspnea can include the underlying disease pathology (e.g., chronic obstructive pulmonary disease, pulmonary embolism, pleural effusion); anxiety; or family, spiritual, or social issues. Investigation for the source of the dyspnea directs the nurse to the appropriate intervention. Common interventions used for dyspnea include oxygen, opioids, and anxiolytics. Nonpharmacological interventions such as reducing the room temperature (but not chilling the patient), reducing the number of people in the room at one time, keeping an unobstructed line of sight between the patient and the outside environment, and using a fan to blow gently across the face (not directly into mucous membranes) have all been found to be effective in decreasing dyspnea.[16]

ANXIETY AND AGITATION

Patients and families who face life-threatening illnesses commonly experience anxiety.[16] Anxiety can be related to any number of physical, emotional, psychological, social, practical, and spiritual issues. Assessment of anxiety can be complex, and an interdisciplinary approach, including nursing, social services, psychology, and chaplaincy, may be needed to evaluate the patient accurately and treat the anxiety properly. Nonpharmacological interventions may include counseling, taking care of practical matters (e.g., arranging for the care of a pet), and arranging for spiritual concerns to be addressed (e.g., arranging for a visit from a clergy member). If medication

is needed, short- or long-acting benzodiazepines and atypical antidepressants may be helpful. Additional interventions for anxiety are discussed in Chapter 2.

DEPRESSION

When confronted with a serious illness, many patients experience intense sadness and anxiety accompanied by depressive symptoms such as anhedonia (loss of pleasure); loss of self-esteem; pervasive despair; thoughts of suicide; or feelings of helplessness, hopelessness, or worthlessness.[16] These are natural feelings and are usually present for only a short time. It is a myth that depression is "normal" at the end of life. If these feelings of depression persist, appropriate treatment needs to be initiated using a multidimensional approach such as supportive psychotherapy, cognitive-behavioral therapy, and antidepressants.

DELIRIUM

Delirium is an acute change in awareness or cognitive status that may manifest as agitation, withdrawal, or confusion. "Confusion" is an all-inclusive term that refers to inappropriate behavior, disorientation, or hallucinations. Terminal delirium is common in patients near death and may manifest as day–night reversal.[16] Management of delirium during the end-of-life phase is focused more on symptom control and relief of the distress of the patient and family than on the diagnosis and treatment of the underlying cause of the delirium. Benzodiazepines or neuroleptics (e.g., haloperidol) are helpful in managing this symptom.

NAUSEA AND VOMITING

Nausea is very common in patients with advanced disease. Nausea can be acute, delayed, or anticipatory. It can be exhausting, debilitating, and frustrating for the patient and the family. The pathophysiology of nausea and vomiting is complex and can vary based on the underlying etiology. Causes of nausea and vomiting may include physiological factors such as gastrointestinal causes (e.g., intestinal obstruction, constipation, pancreatitis); metabolic causes (e.g., hypercalcemia, uremia); central nervous system causes (e.g., increased intracranial pressure); emotional factors; treatment-related factors (e.g., chemotherapy); and vestibular disturbances.

A careful assessment and investigation of the source of nausea and vomiting is important in determining the appropriate treatment course. Drug classes that are commonly used to treat nausea and vomiting are serotonin (5-HT) receptor agonists (e.g., ondansetron), anticholinergics (e.g., hyoscine hydrobromide), antihistamines (e.g., dimenhydrinate), phenothiazines (e.g., prochlorperazine), steroids (e.g., dexamethasone), prokinetic agents (e.g., metoclopramide), butyrophenones (e.g., haloperidol), and benzodiazepines (e.g., lorazepam). A nasogastric tube may be used, but it may cause discomfort. To relieve persistent nausea and vomiting, surgery to resect an intestinal obstruction may be appropriate. If a patient has an unresectable intestinal obstruction, a draining percutaneous endoscopic gastrostomy tube may also be placed. Lastly, patients should be positioned to avoid any aspiration of emesis.

END-OF-LIFE SEDATION

End-of-life sedation, also known as terminal sedation, may be considered when all interventions have failed to control the symptoms. End-of-life sedation is used when the patient (1) is experiencing unbearable and unmanageable pain or other symptoms, and (2) is approaching the last hours or days of his or her life.[16] The goal of end-of-life sedation is to produce a level of obtundation sufficient to relieve suffering without hastening death.[16] Before end-of-life sedation is considered, specialists in pain or palliative care are consulted, and it is verified that all therapies have been attempted without success. In addition, other disciplines such as social services, chaplaincy services, and psychology should be consulted to investigate other potential causes of suffering before resorting to end-of-life sedation.

• Advanced Care Planning

Advanced care planning involves deciding how a patient would like to be treated in the event that he or she becomes unable to make decisions or communicate his or her wishes regarding care.[6] Advanced care planning involves more than just advance directives—it also involves issues such as determining health care proxies as well as trying to discover from the patient or the health care proxy the preferences for the goals of care during the end-of-life phase.

The critical care nurse communicates with the patient's primary care provider, who may have a long-standing relationship with the patient and know the patient's preferences regarding end-of-life treatment. The primary care provider may have had conversations with the patient on this subject. It is important to note that some patients want aggressive treatment despite a poor prognosis, whereas other patients want to forego any aggressive treatment despite the treatment's probable success. Patients are allowed, by federal law, to refuse treatment.

ADVANCE DIRECTIVES

Advance directives are written or oral instructions about future medical care that are to be followed in the event that the person loses the capacity to make decisions.[17] Types of advance directives include living wills and health care proxies (durable powers of attorney for health care). Each state regulates the use of advance directives differently. Advance directives are not "set in stone." They can be revised, orally or in writing, at any time.

A health care proxy is a person who has been designated to make decisions in the event that the patient cannot make decisions for himself or herself. The designation of a person as a health care proxy must be in written form and should always be up to date. The proxy should know the preferences of the patient and be able to communicate and adhere to those preferences. He or she should not confuse his or her own wishes and desires with those of the patient. Health care proxies are also known as "surrogate decision makers" or "health care agents."

DO NOT RESUSCITATE AND DO NOT ATTEMPT RESUSCITATION ORDERS

The standard of care for patients who suffer a cardiac or respiratory arrest is to initiate CPR. Do not resuscitate (DNR) or do not attempt resuscitation (DNAR) orders are orders placed by a physician, most often with the consent of the patient or the health care proxy, to alert other caregivers that if the patient has a cardiac or pulmonary arrest, no attempts to restore cardiac or pulmonary function should occur.[6,18]

Although resuscitation efforts should not be initiated for a patient with a DNR or DNAR order, the patient should continue to receive appropriate care. In one study of critically ill cancer patients in a surgical ICU, researchers noted that the patients with a DNR or DNAR order received less medical care than other patients.[19] However, supportive nursing care remained unchanged. It is important to recognize that DNR and DNAR do not mean "do not give appropriate care."

• Family-Centered Care

Family-centered care is a cornerstone of palliative care. In palliative care, the patient is recognized as being part of a larger social network. Serious illness and death affects not only the patient but also the family. Four core issues form the basis for family-centered care at the end of life: family presence during resuscitation, visitation, family conferences, and bereavement care.

When the patient can communicate, according to Stannard,[20] the ideal definition of family is whomever the patient defines as his or her family. When a patient is unable to communicate, the practical definition of family is anyone who shares a history and a future with the patient. The legal definition of family is based on blood relations and is purposefully narrow and limiting to clearly distinguish who may have authority over the patient should the patient lose decision-making capacity.

FAMILY PRESENCE DURING RESUSCITATION

In a critical review of the literature, Halm[21] noted that research has found that families have a right to be present during resuscitation; in addition, families report that being present during resuscitation was helpful during the bereavement process. Family members who have been present during resuscitations have not experienced more anxiety, depression, grief, intrusive imagery, or avoidance behavior compared with family members who did not witness resuscitations. In addition, there is no evidence to substantiate that the presence of family members invites litigation.

However, research studies do report that many health care providers are uncomfortable with family presence. Nurses who have less experience with resuscitation report more discomfort with family presence than nurses who have more such experience. In addition, the staff surveyed expressed concern that family members may take time and attention away from the patient. The AACN recommends that hospitals should have policies and procedures about how family presence during resuscitation is to be handled in their institutions.[22] It has been suggested that a successful family presence program depends on having a dedicated staff member attend to the family witnessing the resuscitative efforts.

VISITATION

To the greatest extent possible, families should be free to visit a patient who is near death, to allow for coping during this period. Family members may communicate with and touch the patient, which may reassure both the patient and family. During this period of closure, cultural or spiritual ceremonies may also take place. Staff who have developed a relationship with the family should continue to work with the patient and family to the greatest extent possible. The extended visiting hours provide a continuity of care that is invaluable to families and helps cultivate a trusting relationship to reassure families that the nurses are working for the benefit of the patient.

It is important to be aware of the dynamics of each individual family. For example, if there is tension among certain family members, a visiting schedule may need to be established to allow family members to see the patient without crossing paths. In addition, the nurse should be alert to any signs from the patient that a particular family member is unwelcome. The patient may exhibit signs of agitation when that person is in the room. The nurse acts as an advocate to uphold the patient's wishes. Visitation advocacy as it relates to families and the critical care environment is discussed in more detail in Chapter 3.

FAMILY CONFERENCES

The family conference is a mechanism for sharing information in an organized way among clinicians and family members. During the family conference, the health care team (1) provides information about the condition of the patient and the patient's prognosis, and (2) reviews recommendations from the primary and consult services. Family conferences also serve as a forum for exploring future care preferences with the family—how family members may wish to participate in determining the goals of care for the patient.[23] Cultural or religious beliefs may influence how these conversations develop and how the family reacts to the information.

Careful planning should occur before the family conference. Curtis and colleagues[23] describe the nurse's role before and after the family conference (Box 6-2). Box 6-3 describes how to facilitate a family conference. Encouraging the family to be active participants during the family conference increases their level of satisfaction and improves the quality of communication among providers and families.[24]

BEREAVEMENT CARE

The death of a patient can affect the family members and the staff in different ways. Previous coping skills, cultural and spiritual beliefs, and the circumstances surrounding the death influence the grief experience. A multidisciplinary team consisting of other nurses, social workers, chaplains, physicians, and volunteers can assist family members and staff with managing their grief. Critical care nurses should be familiar with the bereavement information and support services available within their institutions for both family members and themselves. Bereavement support includes providing family members with information regarding what to do after the death and who can be contacted at the hospital if questions arise.

Critical care staff should do everything possible to allow the family sufficient time to go through their leave-taking rituals. Bed shortages can make this difficult. However, not allowing family members the chance to say goodbye can complicate the grieving process. Survivors have reported that they remember unsatisfactory interactions with staff for a very long time. Sensitivity must be exercised during this potentially traumatic period.

Box 6-2 • The Nurse's Role Before and After the Family Conference

Before the Conference
- Explain to the family about the patient's medical equipment and therapies.
- Tell the family what to expect during their conference with the health care team members.
- Talk with the family about their spiritual or religious needs and take actions to address the unmet spiritual or religious needs.
- Talk with the family about specific cultural needs and take actions to address unmet cultural needs.
- Talk with the family about what the patient valued in life.
- Talk with the family about the patient's illness and treatment.
- Talk with the family about their feelings.
- Reminisce with the family about the patient.
- Tell the family it is all right to talk to and touch their loved one.
- Discuss with the family what the patient might have wanted if he/she were able to participate in the treatment decision-making process.
- Locate a private place or room for the family to talk among themselves.

After the Conference
- Talk with the family about how the conference went.
- Talk with any other health care team members who were present at the conference about how the conference went.
- Ask the family if they had any questions following the conference.
- Talk with the family about their feelings.
- Talk with the family about any disagreement among the family concerning the plan of care.
- Talk with the family about changes in the patient's plan of care as a result of the conference.
- Support the decisions the family made during the conference.
- Assure the family that the patient will be kept comfortable.
- Tell the family it is all right to talk to and touch their loved one.
- Locate a private place or room for the family to talk among themselves.

From Curtis JR, Patrick DL, Shannon SE, et al: The family conference as a focus to improve communication about end-of-life care in the intensive care unit: Opportunities for improvement. Crit Care Med. 29(2 Suppl):N26–N33, 2001.

• Emotional, Psychological, Social, and Spiritual Care

Patients nearing the end of their lives may experience emotional, psychological, social, and spiritual crises. Critical care nurses play a vital role in helping patients identify these concerns. An interdisciplinary team can attend to these potential feelings of loss, isolation, fear, and existential distress. At times, these crises can manifest as physical symptoms such as pain, dyspnea, and fatigue. To assist patients at the end of life, assessment and interventions by social services, chaplaincy, psychologists, and volunteers may be necessary.

• Facilitating Communication

Communication among the health care team, the patient, and family is the most important aspect of caregiving in critical care, especially at the end of life. Through good communication, all people involved in the patient's care have a better understanding of how to care for the patient and family through this hospitalization. In addition, good communication facilitates a healing environment that supports the physical and psychosocial needs of the patient, family, and providers. Three significant communication issues that surface frequently in end-of-life care include establishing treatment goals and priorities, ensuring interdisciplinary communication, and delivering bad news.

ESTABLISHING TREATMENT GOALS AND PRIORITIES

Establishing goals and treatment priorities is essential to facilitating decision making with regard to care. The way in which options are presented can influence the decisions the patient and family make. For example, if a nurse asks the family, "Do you want the health care team to do everything for your loved one," it sets the family up for a "yes" answer. In the family's mind, the opposite of "everything" is "nothing." So, if the family answers "no" to the question, they may feel as if they are abandoning their loved one. In addition, it is important that nurses avoid ambiguous language and clearly define terms to ensure a shared knowledge. For example, the critical care nurse's understanding of "everything" commonly means intubation, CPR, defibrillation, and other aggressive procedures, whereas the family's understanding of "everything" may include only those interventions that might be helpful and calling a spiritual leader.

Emanuel and colleagues[16] suggest a seven-step approach to help negotiate goals for care for patients:

1. Create the proper setting. Sit down, ensure privacy, and allow adequate time.
2. Determine what the patient and family know. Clarify the current situation and the context in which decisions about goals of care should be made. For example, if the family thinks that the renal failure is transient, yet the nurses believe the kidneys are beyond recovery, the determination of goals of care must be delayed until everyone has agreed about the clinical situation.
3. Explore what the patient and family are expecting or hoping for, such as asking the family what they hope will happen during this last hospitalization, or asking the family what outcomes they think will be attained while in the ICU. Understanding these hopes and expectations will assist the nurse in tailoring communication and reorienting families to what is or might be possible. Focus on what you will do to achieve those expectations and hopes. As appropriate, identify those things that you cannot

Box 6-3 • Facilitating a Family Conference

Making preparations before an ICU family conference about end-of-life care
- Review previous knowledge of the patient and/or family.
- Review previous knowledge of the family's attitudes and reactions.
- Review your knowledge of the disease—prognosis, treatment options.
- Examine your own personal feelings, attitudes, biases, and grieving.
- Plan the specifics of location and setting: a quiet, private place.
- Discuss with the family in advance about who will be present.

Holding an ICU family conference about end-of-life care
- Introduce everyone present.
- If appropriate, set the tone in a nonthreatening way: "This is a conversation we have with all families. . ."
- Discuss the goals of the specific conference.
- Find out what the family understands.
- Review what has happened and what is happening to the patient.
- Discuss prognosis frankly in a way that is meaningful to the family.
- Acknowledge uncertainty in the prognosis.
- Review the principle of substituted judgment: "What would the patient want?"

- Support the family's decision.
- Do not discourage all hope; consider redirecting hope toward a comfortable death with dignity if appropriate.
- Avoid temptation to give too much medical detail.
- Make it clear that withholding life-sustaining treatment is not withholding caring.
- Make explicit what care will be provided including symptom management, where the care will be delivered, and the family's access to the patient.
- If life-sustaining treatments will be withheld or withdrawn, discuss what the patient's death might be like.
- Use repetition to show that you understand what the patient or family is saying.
- Acknowledge strong emotions and use reflection to encourage patients or families to talk about these emotions.
- Tolerate silence.

Finishing an ICU family conference about end-of-life care
- Achieve common understanding of the disease and treatment issues
- Make a recommendation about treatment.
- Ask if there are any questions.
- Ensure basic follow-up plan and make sure the family knows how to reach you for questions.

From Curtis JR, Patrick DL, Shannon SE, et al:. The family conference as a focus to improve communication about end-of-life care in the intensive care unit: Opportunities for improvement. Crit Care Med. 29(2 Suppl):N26–N33, 2001.

do, perhaps because they will not help achieve the goals or because they are not possible.

4. Suggest realistic goals. To assist with decision making, share your knowledge about the patient's illness, its natural course, the experience of patients in similar circumstances, and the effects that contemporary health care may have. After sharing this information, suggest realistic goals (e.g., comfort, peace, closure, loving care, withdrawal of interventions) and how they can be achieved. Work through unreasonable or unrealistic expectations.

5. Respond empathically to the emotions that may arise.

6. Make a plan and follow through with it.

7. Review and revise the goals and treatments as appropriate.

ENSURING INTERDISCIPLINARY COMMUNICATION

A clear and a unified communication process is important to minimize confusion and distress among patients, families, and the health care team.[25] Critical care nurses should explore their understandings and beliefs about prognosis, goals, and plans of care and share these understandings with other health care providers to develop a unified message before dis-

cussing these issues with the families. An interdisciplinary approach in which all nurses are giving the same information consistently is ideal. Consensus among providers is an important step in deciding how treatment choices are presented.[25] Providing conflicting information creates confusion for everyone involved and may lead families to request non-beneficial interventions. Being asked to provide care that is not helpful for the patient can create moral distress in nurses. Other disciplines such as social services, chaplaincy, and the bioethics committee can assist in clarifying issues and values among patients, families, and providers.

DELIVERING BAD NEWS

Despite the best efforts of the health care team, patients may not respond positively to interventions. Keeping an honest and open line of communication is essential to preserve the trust of the patient and family. For this reason, it is important that critical care nurses practice strategies for delivering bad news. Such news can range from reporting that an antibiotic is not reducing an infection or a vasopressor medication is not maintaining an acceptable blood pressure to telling a family member that a patient has died. Because nurses are at the bedside 24 hours a day, communicating with families early that a patient is not doing well may help avoid a "surprise" announcement that the patient has died. Critical care nurses must remember that family members are not health care professionals. The health care system requires that patients and their proxy decision makers be active in making decisions about health care treatment. However, at times, the health care team tries to place the responsibility of making a crucial decision such as withdrawing mechanical ventilation on the family because clinicians may fear a threat of legal retaliation and may try to abdicate responsibility for the decision. A better approach would be to help the family understand the benefits and drawbacks of continuing mechanical ventilation and making the decision jointly. Even if family members are health care professionals, they are family members first and health care professionals second, and they may make decisions based more on their relationship with their loved one than on sound medical or nursing decisions.

Simple strategies for communicating bad news may include phrases such as:

▶ "The blood pressure is worrisome given the amount of medication that we are giving your sister. We have reached the limit of how much we can safely give, and her blood pressure is not responding."

▶ "The ventilator alarm keeps ringing. It is letting me know that your father's lungs are becoming more resistant to mechanical ventilation. This is not a good sign."

▶ "I have noticed that your mother's kidneys have not been working well for the past couple of days. We have been trying to reverse her disease. However, now it seems that her heart and lungs are having difficulty as well."

Phrasing bad news in this way clearly indicates that the patient is not doing well but that the health care team is doing its best to help the patient. If discussions regarding withholding or withdrawing life-sustaining measures become necessary, the family may be more receptive because they see what the nurses are seeing.

Notifying the family members that the patient has died is a special case of delivering bad news. The manner that the nurse uses to deliver the bad news has a significant impact on how the family members remember the last moments of the patient's life. An excellent resource to help nurses learn more about how to communicate bad news to families is the book by Dr. Kenneth Iserson, *Grave Words: Notifying Survivors About Sudden, Unexpected Deaths.*[26] This book recommends that nurses divide death notification into four stages: prepare, inform, support, and afterwards.

1. In the preparation stage, the nurse gathers all the facts surrounding the death of the patient in order to answer any questions that might come up. Family members try and make sense of the death and request information.

2. In the inform stage, the nurse uses the person's name instead of "the patient" or "the deceased."

3. In the support stage, the nurse is available to the family members to answer any questions.

4. In the afterwards stage, the nurse provides information for the family, such as the names of funeral homes, medical examiner/coroner's office information, and who to contact at the hospital if the family has any questions.

Many more interventions and how to discuss these issues with the family are found in Dr. Iserson's book. Using clear, unambiguous language is important when delivering the bad news. Supporting the family members after the notification is essential. Becoming comfortable with the wording of the message (e.g., by practicing phrases before they are needed) allows the nurse to focus on the family and their reaction to the message, instead of the message itself and how that message is delivered.

• Ethical Issues

Ethical issues affect how nurses work and provide care in the critical care environment. Ethical and legal issues are discussed in general terms in Chapters 7 and 8, respectively. Four ethical issues with special significance when talking about end-of-life care are the principle of double effect, moral distress, the withdrawal of life-sustaining technology, and organ and tissue donation.

PRINCIPLE OF DOUBLE EFFECT

The principle of double effect is an ethical principle that distinguishes between consequences a person intends and consequences that are unintended but foreseen and may be applicable in various situations where an action has two effects, one good and one bad.[27] The principle of double effect is most commonly applied to the administration of pain medications to patients who are dying. Opioids are used to relieve pain and other symptoms of suffering (i.e., the good effect). However, opioids also may cause respiratory and cardiovascular depression that may, if left untreated, lead to death (i.e., the bad effect). If the primary intention is to relieve pain and suffering with the recognition that the patient may die, it is morally and legally permissible to administer the opioid. If the primary intention is to cause death, it is not morally or legally permissible to administer the opioid.

The End-of-Life/Palliative Education Resource Center (EPERC) has created Fast Facts, which are quick step-by-step instructions about how to deal with a variety of end-of-life issues (see Table 6-1).

MORAL DISTRESS

Moral distress occurs when nurses cannot turn moral choices into moral action.[28, 29] This distress occurs when the nurse knows the proper course of action to take, but institutional or interpersonal constraints make it nearly impossible to pursue it.[28] For example, nurses tend to recognize when therapies are no longer beneficial or helpful to a patient sooner than family members. For families, it is difficult to realize that therapies may no longer be helpful. Moral distress can arise when the family's understanding about the utility of therapy differs from that of the nurse.

The AACN has identified moral distress as a key issue affecting the work environment. To produce a more healthy occupational environment, the AACN has developed a resource for nurses to use to address this issue.[30] This resource, *The Four A's to Moral Distress*, provides a framework for nurses to address their moral distress and find avenues for its resolution. The four A's are ask, affirm, assess, and act, which facilitates change, thus creating a healthier nursing environment. Copies of this resource are available to AACN members or by contacting the AACN office (see Table 6-1). In addition, hospital bioethics or ethics committees are available to staff to help work through situations in which moral distress is a factor.

WITHHOLDING OR WITHDRAWING LIFE-SUSTAINING MEASURES

When it becomes clear to both the nurse and family that additional treatment will not be beneficial, the decision may be made to withdraw life-support methods. Mechanical ventilation is one intervention that is often withdrawn in such circumstances. Other life-sustaining measures that may be stopped include implantable cardiac defibrillators or pacemakers and hemodialysis.

When the decision is made to withdraw a therapy, special considerations are taken to reduce the suffering of the patient and to minimize the exhibition of distress to the family members. In the case of withdrawing mechanical ventilation, the decision is first made jointly with the family. In the case of extubation, opioids and sedatives are administered to the patient to reduce the pain and discomfort. In addition, the alarms to both the ventilator and the cardiac monitor are silenced to focus the family on the patient rather than the technology. Many of the Fast Facts on the EPERC website relate to withdrawal of therapies, including mechanical ventilation and tube feeding (see Table 6-1).

ORGAN AND TISSUE DONATION

Organs and tissues can be procured after cardiac death or brain death. Federal law (Public Law 99-5-9; section 9318), Medicare, and the Joint Commission (formerly the Joint Commission on Accreditation of Healthcare Organizations) all require that (1) hospitals have written protocols regarding organ and tissue donation and (2) these institutions give the surviving family members the chance to authorize donation of their family member's tissues and organs.[31] When organ or tissue procurement is an issue, it is important that all family members are given the information they need to make a decision with which they are comfortable and that their grief is respected. In some cases, family members have initiated the conversation with their health care providers independently.

The local organ procurement organization (OPO) can provide additional resources. To find the OPO in your area, see Table 6-1.

• Caring for the Nurse

Some deaths affect some people significantly. The death of a child, the death of a friend or colleague, mass casualties, or a particularly horrific, traumatic death can have a profound effect on the nurse. Colleagues must be supportive and explore ways to support each other rather than dismissing the impact the death has on a colleague. According to Badger,[32] some self-care strategies to cope with the event include asking to be relieved from care responsibilities and to take a break; discussing the experience with a colleague, friend, or a nurse leader; taking a moment to reflect on one's feelings after the event; focusing on what was done right; and following basic health principles such as physical exercise, meditation, humor, music, eating properly, and obtaining adequate rest.

Working in a critical care unit is demanding physically, intellectually, and emotionally. Dealing with death on a consistent basis can take its toll on the nurse's well-being.[32] In the critical care setting, nurses caring for the patient may delay attending to their own grief because the demands of the unit and the needs of the family members may take precedence. It is important to be vigilant in recognizing signs and symptoms of unexpressed grief, burnout, and post-traumatic stress. Symptoms may include an increase in the number of sick days; indecision; difficulty with problem solving; isolation or withdrawal; behavioral outbursts; denial and shock; fixation on a single detail; immobilization; a feeling of extreme serenity; emotionally numbing responses such as withdrawal, pessimism, or a diminished capacity for experiencing pleasure; and intrusive responses such as unwanted or unpleasant recollections or flashbacks.[32] To maintain emotional health, it is important to seek assistance in dealing with these issues. Nurse leaders and human resources representatives can provide resources to assist with the stresses of working in critical care.

Clinical Applicability Challenges

Case Study

You are caring for Mrs. M., a 35-year-old woman who was in a motor vehicle crash. She sustained a subdural hematoma, bilateral pulmonary contusions, blunt cardiac injury, a liver laceration, a splenic laceration, a severe pelvic fracture, and bilateral femur fractures. By hospital day 16, she has received more than 80 units of blood and blood products and is now exhibiting early signs of disseminated intravascular coagulation. Her peak inspiratory and plateau pressures on the mechanical ventilator are increasing, and it is becoming difficult to ventilate her. Furthermore, her intra-abdominal pressures are increasing, and the trauma surgery team is considering taking her back to the operating room to perform an exploratory laparotomy.

1. When the surgeons arrive to discuss their treatment plan with Mrs. M.'s family, they ask, "Do you want us to do everything if her heart stops beating?" The family looks puzzled at the question. As a nurse, what should you do?

2. While the team is discussing helpful options for Mrs. M. with the family, the social worker arrives. The patient has a cardiopulmonary arrest. The family is present during the cardiopulmonary resuscitation (CPR) and receives support from the social worker. While CPR is in progress, the family asks the health care team to stop their resuscitation efforts. After turning off all the machines and monitors, what should you do to facilitate bereavement care of the family?

Review Questions

1. A 65-year-old woman with end-stage congestive heart failure is admitted to the intensive care unit for respiratory failure. She is intubated, mechanically ventilated, and sedated but is arousable. While the nurse assesses the patient, the patient complains of continued dyspnea and pain in her throat from the endotracheal tube. The patient has coarse lung sounds (rales) in all lung fields. Which intervention incorporates palliative care principles into the plan of care?
   a. The nurse reassures the patient that the endotracheal tube and the ventilator will help her breathing.
   b. The nurse reviews the medication order sheet, and if no diuretic or opioid has been ordered, the nurse contacts the physician to request an order for both a diuretic and opioid.
   c. The nurse raises the head of the bed to 90 degrees.
   d. The nurse increases the rate and the tidal volume on the mechanical ventilator.

2. A 25-year-old man has been in the coronary care unit for the past 2 months awaiting a heart transplantation. His last echocardiogram showed an ejection fraction of 10% despite maximal vasopressor therapy. The cardiology team wants to decide on goals of care and is thinking of inserting a left ventricular assist device (LVAD). The critical care clinical nurse specialist is going to moderate the family conference and asks the nurse to be present.

As the nurse caring for this patient, what can you do to be prepared for the family conference?
   a. Carefully memorize and report the patient's hemodynamic values such as blood pressure, cardiac output/cardiac index, ejection fraction, left ventricular end diastolic pressure, and systemic vascular resistance.
   b. Point out to the patient that the LVAD is a great technology and attempt to convince him that he should consent to the LVAD placement.
   c. Discuss with other staff nurses the prognosis for a patient awaiting a heart transplantation and being placed on an LVAD.
   d. Discuss with the patient and family their understanding of the disease, their values and concerns, and their goals for the family conference.

3. The patient in Question 2 decides to not have the left ventricular assist device (LVAD) and to withdraw the vasopressor therapy. The family agrees to the plan. What can the nurse do to prepare for this last phase of the patient's life?
   a. Discuss with social services how to try to persuade the family to consent to the LVAD placement and discuss the prognosis for patients with a heart transplant.
   b. In an effort to reverse the patient's decision, educate the family about how dying from cardiogenic shock will appear.
   c. Secure a do not attempt to resuscitate order, ensure that the orders for analgesia and sedation are appropriate for the patient, allow for flexible visiting hours for the family, turn off monitors or alarms, and be present with the family to answer any questions they might have.
   d. Call chaplaincy services to provide the last rituals to prepare for the imminent death.

References

1. Rushton CH, Williams MA, Sabatier KH: The integration of palliative care and critical care: One vision, one voice. Crit Care Nurs Clin North Am 14:133–140, 2002
2. Ariès P: The Hour of Our Death. New York: Knopf, 1981
3. Luce JM, Prendergast TJ: The changing nature of death in the ICU. In Curtis JR, Rubenfeld GD (eds): Managing Death in the Intensive Care Unit. The Transition from Cure to Comfort. New York: Oxford University Press, 2001, p 388
4. Benner P, Kerchner S, Corless IB, Davies B: Attending death as a human passage: Core nursing principles for end-of-life care. Am J Crit Care 12(6):558–561, 2003
5. SUPPORT Investigators: A controlled trial to improve care for seriously ill hospitalized patients. The study to understand prognoses and preferences for outcomes and risks of treatments (SUPPORT). The SUPPORT Principal Investigators [see comments] [published erratum appears in JAMA 275(16):1232, 1996]. JAMA 274(20):1591–1598, 1995
6. Field MJ, Cassel CK: Approaching Death: Improving Care at the End of Life. Washington, DC: Institute of Medicine, 1997
7. Angus DC, Barnato AE, Linde-Zwirble WT, et al: Use of intensive care at the end of life in the United States: An epidemiologic study. Crit Care Med 32(3):638–643, 2004
8. Egan KA, Labyak MJ: Hospice care: A model for quality end-of-life care. In Ferrell BR, Coyle N (eds): Palliative Nursing. New York: Oxford University Press, 2001, pp 7–26
9. World Health Organization: Cancer Pain Relief and Palliative Care. Geneva, Switzerland: Author, 1990

10. Puntillo KA: The role of critical care nurses in providing and managing end-of-life care. In Curtis JR, Rubenfeld GD (eds): Managing Death in the ICU: The Transition From Cure to Comfort. New York: Oxford University Press, 2001, pp 149–164

11. von Gunten CF, Lupu D: Development of a medical subspecialty in palliative medicine: Progress report. J Palliat Med 7(2): 209–219, 2004

12. Campbell ML: Palliative care consultation in the intensive care unit. Crit Care Med 34(11 Suppl):S355–S358, 2006

13. Medina J, Puntillo KA: AACN Protocols for Practice: Palliative Care and End-of-Life Issues in Critical Care. Sudbury, MA: Jones & Bartlett, 2006

14. Puntillo KA, White C, Morris AB, et al: Patients' perceptions and responses to procedural pain: Results from Thunder Project II. Am J Crit Care 10(4):238–251, 2001

15. Zeppetella G: Palliation of dyspnea in terminal disease. Am J Hospice Palliat Care 15(6):322–330, 1998

16. Emanuel L, von Gunten C, Ferris F, Hauser JM (eds): The Education in Palliative and End-of-Life Care (EPEC) Curriculum: © The EPEC Project. Chicago: Author, 2003.

17. National Institute on Aging: Long Distance Caregiving. Chapter 19: What is the difference between an advance directive and a living will? Retrieved October 20, 2006, from http://www. nia.nih.gov/HealthInformation/Publications/LongDistanceCare giving/chapter19.htm

18. Burns JP, Edwards J, Johnson J, et al: Do-not-resuscitate order after 25 years. Crit Care Med 31(5):1543–1550, 2003

19. Keenan CH, Kish SK: The influence of do-not-resuscitate orders on care provided for patients in the surgical intensive care unit of a cancer center. Crit Care Nurs Clin North Am 12(3):385–390, 2000

20. Stannard D: Family care. In Schell HM, Puntillo KA (eds): Critical Care Nursing Secrets. St. Louis: Mosby Elsevier, 2006, pp 767–772

21. Halm MA: Family presence during resuscitation: A critical review of the literature. Am J Crit Care 14(6):494–512, 2005

22. American Association of Critical-Care Nurses: Family presence during CPR and invasive procedures. Practice alert. Retrieved October 20, 2006, from http://www.aacn.org/AACN/practice Alert.nsf/Files/FP/$file/Family%20Presence%20During%20CP R%2011-2004.pdf

23. Curtis JR, Patrick DL, Shannon SE, et al: The family conference as a focus to improve communication about end-of-life care in the intensive care unit: Opportunities for improvement. Crit Care Med 29(2 Suppl):N26–N33, 2001

24. McDonagh JR, Elliott TB, Engelberg RA, et al: Family satisfaction with family conferences about end-of-life care in the intensive care unit: Increased proportion of family speech is associated with increased satisfaction. Crit Care Med 32(7): 1484–1488, 2005

25. Curtis JR, Patrick DL: How to discuss dying and death in the ICU. In Curtis JR, Rubenfeld GD (eds): Managing Death in the Intensive Care Unit. New York: Oxford University Press, 2001, pp 85–102

26. Iserson KV: Grave Words: Notifying Survivors About Sudden, Unexpected Deaths. Tucson, AZ: Galen Press, 1999

27. Williams G: The principle of double effect and terminal sedation. Med Law Rev 9:41–53, 2001

28. Jameton A: Nursing Practice: The Ethical Issues. Englewood Cliffs, NJ: Prentice Hall, 1984

29. Rushton CH: Defining and addressing moral distress. Tools for critical care nursing leaders. AACN Adv Crit Care 17(2): 161–168, 2006

30. American Association of Critical-Care Nurses: The four A's to rise above moral distress. Retrieved October 20, 2006, from http://www.aacn.org/AACN/practice.nsf/Files/4as/$file/ 4A's%20to%20Rise%20Above%20Moral%20Distress.pdf

31. Campbell ML, Zalenski R: The emergency department. In Ferrell BR, Coyle N (eds): Textbook of Palliative Care, 2nd ed. New York: Oxford University Press, 2006, pp 861–869

32. Badger JM: Understanding secondary traumatic stress. Am J Nurs 101(7):26–32, 2001

Other Selected Readings

Campbell ML: Forgoing Life-Sustaining Therapy. Aliso Viejo, CA: American Association of Critical-Care Nurses, 1998

Campbell ML: End-of-life care in the ICU: Current practice and future hopes. Crit Care Nurs Clin North Am 14:197–200, 2002

Curtis JR, Rubenfeld GD (eds): Managing Death in the Intensive Care Unit: The Transition From Cure to Comfort. New York: Oxford University Press, 2001

Ferrell BR, Coyle N: Textbook of Palliative Nursing, 2nd ed. New York: Oxford University Press, 2006

Hallenbeck JL: Palliative Care Perspectives. New York: Oxford University Press, 2003

Lunney JR, Lynn J, Hogan C: Profiles of older Medicare decedents. J Am Geriatr Soc 50:1108–1112, 2002

Matzo ML, Sherman DW: Palliative Care Nursing: Quality Care to the End of Life. New York: Springer, 2001

President's Commission for the Study of Ethical Problems in Medicine and Biomedical and Behavioral Research: Deciding to Forgo Life-Sustaining Treatment. Publication 0 425-748. Washington, DC: U.S. Government Printing Office, 1983

Puntillo KA, Benner P, Drought T, et al: End-of-life issues in intensive care units: A national random survey of nurses' knowledge and beliefs. Am J Crit Care 10:216–229, 2001

Schell HM, Puntillo KA (eds): Critical Care Nursing Secrets. St. Louis: Mosby Elsevier, 2006

Professional Practice Issues in Critical Care

PART 2

INTERNET RESOURCES

Topic	Web Page Address
Agency for Healthcare Research and Quality (AHRQ)	www.ahrq.gov
American Association of Critical-Care Nurses	www.aacn.org
American Association of Legal Nurse Consultants	www.aalnc.org
American Association of Nurse Attorneys	www.taana.org
American Hospital Association	www.aha.org/aha/about
American Medical Association	www.ama-assn.org
American Nurses Association	www.nursingworld.org
Canadian Association of Critical Care Nurses	www.caccn.ca
Canadian Bioethics Society	www.bioethics.ca
The Center for Ethics and Human Rights	www.nursingworld.org/ethics/
The Center for Health Design	www.healthdesign.org
Centers for Medicare and Medicaid Services (CMS)	www.cms.hhs.gov
Cochrane Collaboration	www.cochrane.org
The ICN Code of Ethics for Nursing	www.icn.ch/icncode.pdf
Institute for Healthcare Improvement	www.ihi.org
Joanna Briggs Institute	www.joannabriggs.edu.au
Joint Commission on Accreditation of Health Care Organizations (JCAHO)	www.jcaho.org
National Guideline Clearinghouse	www.guidelines.gov
The National League for Nursing	www.nln.org
Nursing Ethics	www.nursingethics.ca/
Sarah Cole Hirsh Institute	http://fpb.cwru.edu/HirshInstitute/
Sigma Theta Tau International Honor Society of Nursing	www.nursingsociety.org
Society of Critical Care Medicine	www.sccm.org
U.S. National Library of Medicine and NIH	http://medlineplus.gov
World Medical Association	www.wma.net

Ethical Issues in Critical Care Nursing

Christine Grady

7

Ethics and the Nurse
The Tools of Ethics
   Approaches to Ethics
   Principles of Bioethics and the Ethics of Care
Ethical Decision Making Within
a Nursing Process Model
   Gather the Relevant Facts
   Identify the Problem
   Analyze the Problem Using Ethical Principles
    and Rules
   Analyze Alternatives and Act
   Evaluate and Reflect
Bioethics Resources and Services
   Ethics Committees and Consultation Services
   Professional Nursing Organizations

Objectives

Based on the content in this chapter, the reader should be able to:

❶ Explain the way ethics assists nurses and other clinicians in resolving moral problems.

❷ Recognize the applicability of the *Code of Ethics for Nurses* of the American Nurses Association to everyday practice.

❸ Name and describe the ethical principles most frequently appealed to in clinical ethics.

❹ Describe steps in the process of ethical decision making.

❺ Identify resources available to nurses to resolve ethical dilemmas.

❻ Discuss an example of an ethical issue confronted by critical care nurses in practice and how applying ethical principles may assist in its resolution.

Mechanical replacement of kidney function was once science fiction. Now we routinely replace kidney function through dialysis and replace kidneys through transplantation, and soon we will be able to predict who is at genetic risk for kidney failure. The incorporation of sophisticated technology into the clinical arena has made the once simpler questions of life and death increasingly complex. Although advancements in health care technology and information provide indisputable benefits, these same advancements also raise profound ethical, legal, economic, and social challenges and dilemmas.

Questions regarding the appropriate use of technology and information abound in critical care. In the complex arena of the intensive care unit (ICU), crucial decisions about life and health are made with striking frequency and urgency. Nurses make moral choices constantly in everyday practice. Sometimes the choices are difficult and create feelings of uncertainty or distress. Ethics helps to clarify and illuminate moral issues and obligations and provides systematic methods for reaching resolutions.

Identifying a problem as a source of moral uncertainty, distress, or dilemma begins the process of reasoning through the complexity. According to Jameton,[1] moral uncertainty results from being unable to clearly identify a moral conflict within a situation while experiencing the troublesome feeling that "something is not quite right." Moral dilemmas occur if two or more conflicting principles or alternatives exist, and choosing one would involve violating or compromising the other. Moral distress occurs when the nurse believes he or she knows the ethically correct action to take in a situation, but a different action is taken because of institutional protocol, disagreement between members of the health care team, or professional rules or lines of authority. The American Association of Critical-Care Nurses (AACN) initiative to address moral distress recognizes that moral distress is one of the key issues affecting the work environment of critical care nurses. The AACN proposes implementation of the "four As"—ask, affirm, assess, act—as essential to promoting the optimal practice of critical care nurses to best serve patients and families.[2]

Nurses can reason through most moral conflicts in the clinical environment with the help of ethics education, interdisciplinary dialogue, collaboration, communication, consultation with institutional ethics committees, and the use of institutional ethics policies, professional codes of ethics, and other ethics resources. Ethical analysis helps the nurse to clarify moral issues and principles involved in a situation, examine his or her responsibilities and obligations, and provide an ethically adequate rationale for any decision or action taken. This chapter presents an overview of ethics, some principles and guidelines for nursing ethics, and a process by which to apply them clinically.

• Ethics and the Nurse

The American Nurses Association (ANA) *Code of Ethics for Nurses* begins with the statement "Ethics is an integral part of the foundation of nursing."[3] But what exactly is ethics, and how does it form part of the foundation of nursing?

Ethics refers to a set of principles of right conduct, a theory or a system of moral values, and the study of both the general nature of moral choice and values and the specific moral choices that people make. Ethical inquiry allows us to think reasonably about, to question, to critique, and ultimately to try to understand the dimensions of moral conduct. Specifically, ethics helps us answer questions about what is right or good, what ought to be done in specific situations, and what kind of people—and what kind of nurses—we ought to be, and why.

Sometimes the term *ethics* refers to the formal beliefs or practices of a particular group of people, such as "business ethics." Most professional groups have formal codes of ethics for their members; the nursing profession is guided by the ANA *Code of Ethics for Nurses With Interpretive Statements* (Box 7-1).[3] Other professional associations, such as the AACN, support the ANA code. The International Council of Nurses (ICN) also has a *Code of Ethics for Nurses* that serves as a standard for nursing worldwide.[4]

Bioethics is the study of ethical issues and judgments made within the biomedical sciences, including care of patients, the delivery of health care, public health, and biomedical research. Bioethics takes into account the difficult and practical realities found in the clinical care of people with illnesses. Some argue that there is little morally unique to nursing, that nursing ethics is just a subset of bioethics. As such, nursing ethics is the ethical analysis of judgments made by nurses, and the same moral issues emerge whether one is the nurse, physician, or patient.[5] Others contend that nursing ethics is a separate and unique field of inquiry built on an understanding of the nature and philosophy of nursing and the nurse–patient relationship.[6] In either case, nursing ethics encompasses the nurse's specific professional roles and responsibilities and the relationships the nurse has with patients, other health care providers, the institutions with which he or she is affiliated, and society. A nurse

Box 7-1 • The American Nurses Association's (ANA) Code of Ethics for Nurses

1. The nurse, in all professional relationships, practices with compassion and respect for the inherent dignity, worth, and uniqueness of every individual, unrestricted by considerations of social or economic status, personal attributes, or the nature of health problems.
2. The nurse's primary commitment is to the patient, whether an individual, family, group, or community.
3. The nurse promotes, advocates for, and strives to protect the health, safety, and rights of the patient.
4. The nurse is responsible and accountable for individual nursing practice and determines the appropriate delegation of tasks consistent with the nurse's obligation to provide optimum patient care.
5. The nurse owes the same duty to self as to others, including the responsibility to preserve integrity and safety, to maintain competence, and to continue personal and professional growth.
6. The nurse participates in establishing, maintaining, and improving health care environments and conditions of employment conducive to the provision of quality health care and consistent with the values of the profession through individual and collective action.
7. The nurse participates in the advancement of the profession through contributions to practice, education, administration, and knowledge development.
8. The nurse collaborates with other health professionals and the public in promoting community, national, and international efforts to meet health needs.
9. The profession of nursing, as represented by associations and their members, is responsible for articulating nursing values, for maintaining the integrity of the profession and its practice, and for shaping social policy.

Reprinted with permission from American Nurses Association, Code of Ethics for Nurses with Interpretive Statements, © 2001 American Nurses Publishing, American Nurses Foundation/American Nurses Association, Washington, DC.

never practices in isolation. Decision making, conflict resolution about ethical issues, and ethical practice are accomplished through communication and collaboration with patients, peers, and colleagues on the health care team.

Answers to questions such as "What are the obligations and responsibilities of nurses?", "What makes a good nurse?", and "What goals or ends ought nursing to seek?" guide our everyday practice. Codes of professional ethics, bioethical principles, and ethical theories all provide nurses with guidance for addressing these questions and for making judgments about individual clinical cases.

The ANA *Code of Ethics for Nurses* reflects the expanded and increasingly complex role of nurses in our current health care environment and describes desired behaviors for nurses. It also clearly delineates the commitments and obligations of professional nurses to society.[3] The ICN Code, revised most recently in 2006, describes multiple responsibilities for ethical nursing practice and acknowledges that the need for nursing is universal.[4]

• The Tools of Ethics

Resolving moral conflicts can be difficult. Systematically applying the tools of ethics, basic moral principles, and professional guidelines can help us identify our ethical obligations and systematically decide which "right" actions can help us meet them. Multidisciplinary collaboration and dialogue and, when appropriate, consultation with ethics committees or other experts are also critical to satisfactorily resolving ethical problems.

Ethical decision making does not promise absolute answers, however. Ethical dilemmas are dilemmas precisely because compelling reasons exist for taking each of two or more opposing actions. Decisions about which action to take should be analyzed and justified using available codes of ethics and bioethical principles. Careful ethical reflection and analysis do not preclude the possibility that reasonable people may disagree or that a nurse may be disappointed in decisions made. However, the value of thoughtful debate and reflection in making ethical judgments cannot be overestimated.

APPROACHES TO ETHICS

Several general approaches to ethics are used to determine what is right or wrong. Consequentialism includes theories that determine actions to be right or wrong on the basis of their consequences. Utilitarianism, a familiar form of consequentialism, asserts that the right action is that which offers the greatest possible benefit with the least amount of burden for all affected. A second general approach, a deontological or nonconsequentialist approach, includes theories that judge an action right or wrong on the basis of features other than consequences, such as conformity of the action to moral rules. Principlism, an approach that depends on a specific set of principles to identify, discuss, and analyze the ethics of a situation, is widely used in bioethics and in nursing. Virtue ethics, another approach, emphasizes that what matters is not only what agents do but also how their actions reflect their virtues. Faced with an ethical problem, persons of good character, virtue, and judgment provide direction for what is best rather than applying rules or calculating consequences. An ethics of care approach emphasizes the salience and characteristics of caring relationships between people as essential in determining right actions. Sympathy, compassion, trust, solidarity, fidelity, collaboration, and discernment are emphasized over rules and principles.

Ethical principles, professional guidelines, personal values, emotions, and judgment help guide our particular actions and decisions. How we feel about an issue is a manifestation of our moral convictions that should not be ignored. We should strive, though, to reach ethical decisions by allowing reason to temper emotions and emotions to tutor reason. Nurses are dedicated to serving the needs of patients but must be allowed to practice in a manner that maintains their own sense of self-respect while maintaining the dignity of their patients.

In specific situations, awareness of differences in professional and personal values and obligations can provide insight into sources of interprofessional or interpersonal ethical conflict. Nursing practice takes place within a team of health care professionals, reflecting a multiplicity of values and views that can be in conflict. Differing personal, professional, and institutional values can compound moral conflict, yet all voices should be considered. Ideally, competing values are weighed and assigned priority in light of the ethical norms that guide us.

PRINCIPLES OF BIOETHICS AND THE ETHICS OF CARE

Four widely accepted bioethical principles are often applied to ethical problems in health care and nursing practice: nonmaleficence, beneficence, respect for autonomy, and justice (Box 7-2).[7] Fidelity and veracity are two other principles often cited as relevant to nursing practice. Fidelity is the duty to be faithful to others by keeping promises and fulfilling contracts and commitments. It is the moral covenant between people in a relationship, such as the nurse–patient relationship. Veracity is the duty to tell the truth and not to lie or deceive others. All these principles stipulate *prima facie* obligations (i.e., obligations that are binding unless superseded by another obligation of equal or stronger claim).

The complex, human dimensions of real cases sometimes make a principle-based approach to ethical problem solving seem too abstract. An ethic of care adds an important dimension, especially for nursing. The care ethic is built on the understanding that people are unique, that relationships and their value are crucial in moral deliberations, and that emotions and character traits play a role in moral judgment. Caring is considered essential to nursing and has been long valued in the nurse–patient relationship. In caring for patients, nurses are committed to promoting the health and welfare of patients and respecting human dignity. Caring has been called a central art and moral virtue of nursing practice.[7] The AACN describes its "mission, vision and values as framed within an ethic of care and ethical principles."[8]

Box 7-2 • Principles of Bioethics

Nonmaleficence: An obligation to never deliberately harm another

Beneficence: An obligation to promote the welfare of others, to maximize benefits and minimize harms

Respect for autonomy: An obligation to respect, and not to interfere with, the choices and actions of autonomous individuals (i.e., those capable of self-determination)

Justice: An obligation to be fair in the distribution of burdens and benefits and in the distribution of social goods, such as health care or nursing care

Veracity: An obligation to tell the truth

Fidelity: An obligation to keep promises and fulfill commitments

Nonmaleficence and Beneficence

The principle of nonmaleficence says that we have an ethical duty not to inflict harm or evil. Foundational to our society, the duty not to harm others bears more weight than the duty to benefit others. Citing the Hippocratic Oath and the words of Florence Nightingale, Jameton (p. 93) says that "it is more important to avoid doing harm than it is to do good."[1] Nonmaleficence is a strong *prima facie* principle. However, in nursing, avoiding harm is not enough. Beneficence involves taking deliberate steps to benefit another person by preventing and removing harm and making decisions based on carefully balancing benefits and harms, such as when weighing the side effects of a drug against its therapeutic actions.[7] The following scenario illustrates a situation in which appeal to the principles of nonmaleficence and beneficence may facilitate decision making:

> **BALANCING RISKS AND BENEFITS**
>
> Mr. E., a 59-year-old man with a history of previous myocardial infarction, came into the emergency department with ventricular tachycardia (VT). He had been experiencing dizziness and chest pain for the past couple of days. He was given amiodarone, but the cardiac monitor showed continued VT. After successful cardioversion, he was admitted to the coronary care unit. Over the next 30 hours, he required multiple cardioversions for recurrent VT and, at one point, cardiopulmonary resuscitation (CPR) for sustained symptomatic VT. Laboratory work indicated a massive myocardial infarction, and an echocardiogram showed an ejection fraction of 25%. His cardiologist planned electrophysiology studies, with a possible implantable cardiac defibrillator (ICD) when Mr. E. became stable.
>
> On day 14 of his hospital stay, Mr. E. went into congestive heart failure and sustained VT, requiring CPR and multiple defibrillations. The cardiologist continued to be optimistic that Mr. E. could benefit from an ICD. Tired and sometimes confused, Mr. E. began to seek frequent reassurance from the nurses that he would live long enough for the ICD insertion. He expressed fear about the frequent cardioversions and the discomfort they caused him. The nurses began to question what kind of long-term benefit such treatment would offer this severely compromised patient.

This scenario illustrates the difficulty of weighing the possible benefits and risks of ICD implantation for recurrent VT compared with repeated cardioversion in a patient who has sustained severe cardiac damage. A risk–benefit analysis includes the following questions:

▶ What are the benefits and risks of recurrent cardioversions for this patient?
▶ At what point do the risks exceed the possible benefits?
▶ What are the long-term benefits of ICD implantation?
▶ What are the overall goals for the patient, and how are they best achieved?
▶ Are there reasonable alternatives to ICD implantation for the patient?
▶ Does the benefit of avoiding sudden cardiac death always outweigh the risks for physical and emotional harm caused by repeated cardioversions and defibrillations while the patient awaits ICD implantation?
▶ Has everything been done to reduce the discomforts associated with these treatments?

Clinicians who work in the ICU frequently use aggressive treatment to attempt to stabilize patients and keep them alive. It is important to step back to assess the complex factors that contribute to suffering and comfort for an individual patient. Sometimes clinicians forget that relief of suffering is a fundamental goal in health care. The desire to prevent harm by postponing death is shaped by beneficence. However, physical and psychological suffering caused by aggressive treatment, especially treatment of questionable or slight benefit, sometimes constitutes a greater harm than death, and less aggressive treatment and more comfort may be a more beneficent course. It is crucial to involve the patient or surrogate in discussions and decisions about goals and the risks and benefits of the various treatment and care options. Respect for the patient's considered opinions, preferences, and decisions based on and guided by the principle of respect for autonomy can be very helpful in deciding appropriate action in a situation like the one involving Mr. E.

Respect for Autonomy

Respect for autonomy involves respecting the capacity of a person to be self-determining, to deliberate about actions and life choices, and to act on those deliberations without interference from others. Informed consent is an application of the principle of respect for autonomy in the health care setting. The nurse helps to ensure that the patient receives adequate information, has the capacity to understand available options, and can deliberate and make a health care decision. Promoting respect for autonomy includes being honest with the patient and family, protecting the patient's privacy and confidentiality, and helping the patient make important decisions. Respect for autonomy is part of a more encompassing principle of respect for persons.

In the ICU, patients frequently have compromised autonomy and are unable to make decisions for themselves for two reasons: (1) their clinical status, and (2) the possible effects of the treatments they are receiving. The nurse frequently and carefully assesses the patient's ability to understand treatment options and make decisions. If a patient is incapable of making an informed decision about a treatment or intervention, a legally authorized surrogate is asked to consent for the patient. A surrogate decides for the patient in a way that is consistent with what the patient would want, if known, or that is consistent with the patient's best medical interests. The surrogate is usually a spouse, parent, adult child, or someone previously designated by the patient as having the durable power of attorney for health care. Most important, the surrogate should be someone who knows and can represent the preferences and interests of the patient regarding treatment options.

The patient or surrogate needs all the information a "reasonable person" would need to make a particular decision. Sometimes, because of age, physical condition, educational level, position, language, culture, emotional stress, or other factors, the health care team may need to spend additional time and care providing information and ensuring that the patient or surrogate understands. Health care providers are responsible for presenting information in an understandable and sensitive manner and for assessing the patient's or surrogate's understanding.

Consistent with respect for autonomy, consent given should be voluntary. The patient should not be subject to coercion, fraud, or deceit. An informed, freely consenting patient has a right to make an autonomous decision, regardless of whether it corresponds with what others think he or she should do, as long as it does not harm others.

In the case of Mr. E., respect for his autonomy calls for talking with him when he is not confused about his goals and preferences, seeking his opinion about the benefits and burdens of the treatment options, and then planning care accordingly. The nurse and other members of the health care team might also respectfully engage Mr. E. in a process of advance care planning, including the preparation of an advance directive, if he is interested.

Making Treatment and Care Decisions Historically, health care professionals and hospitals have occasionally sought to override the autonomy of the patient by giving the patient treatment or continued treatment that the patient did not want but that health professionals deemed necessary for the patient's benefit. In most cases, according to both ethical and legal standards, the wishes of the patient or surrogate take priority. The right to refuse treatment is similar to the right to informed consent and is grounded in the principle of respect for autonomy. The famous words of former Supreme Court Justice Cardozo articulate this respect for a patient's decision to refuse treatment: "Every human being of adult years and sound mind has a right to determine what shall be done with his body. . . ."[9] The *Code of Ethics for Nurses* (section 1.4) states that "patients have the moral and legal right to determine what will be done with their own person, to be given adequate, complete, and understandable information in a manner that facilitates an informed judgment, to be assisted in weighing the benefits, burdens, and available options in their treatment, including the option of no treatment; to accept, refuse, or terminate treatment without deceit, undue influence, duress, coercion, or penalty; and to be given necessary support throughout the decision making and treatment process."[3]

Advance Care Planning Some patients are concerned about the possibility of being forced to endure an existence supported by machines without hope of a meaningful life and without the ability to have a say in the decision. The Patient Self-Determination Act of 1990 requires all health care facilities that receive federal funds to provide written information to patients about their rights to make decisions about medical care, including the right to accept or refuse care and the right to formulate a health care advance directive.

All states in the United States and the District of Columbia have statutes regarding advance directives for health care. There are two main types of advance directives, instructional directives and designation of surrogate decision makers, and some people have both. A living will or instructional advance directive allows a person to specify any preferences regarding treatment and care for such time that he or she may lose the capacity to make decisions. A durable power of attorney for health care designates a surrogate or proxy decision maker who is familiar with the person's treatment preferences, to make decisions in the event of the person's incapacity. Advance care planning is a process that offers the person an opportunity to deliberate about and express any preferences and values for treatment and care in advance of such time when he or she can no longer deliberate or make decisions. Encouraging people to reflect on preferences, talk to loved ones and health care providers, and implement a durable power of attorney for health care or a living will is a demonstration of respect for their autonomy.

The ANA *Code of Ethics for Nurses* (section 1.4) reminds us, though, that "support of autonomy in the broadest sense also includes recognition that people of some cultures place less weight on individualism and choose to defer to family or community values in decision making. Respect not just for the specific decisions but also for the patient's method of decision making is consistent with the principle of autonomy."[3] Honoring expressed preferences and wishes, including those found in a patient's advance directive, is also a demonstration of respect. Unfortunately, despite efforts to encourage advance care planning, a remarkably small number (less than 25%) of even seriously ill patients have written advance directives,[10] perhaps because people generally do not want to think about death or incompetence. Unfortunately, even when an advance directive exists, a copy is not always available, the language can be vague, or the surrogate and team may be unsure what instructions apply or may even disagree as to what the patient actually wants.

A DIFFICULT SURROGATE

Ms. A., a 28-year-old woman with end-stage human immunodeficiency virus disease, was admitted to the ICU for complications associated with chemotherapy for central nervous system lymphoma. In an advance directive, Ms. A. designated her aunt as her surrogate decision maker. Ms. A.'s aunt is very protective, does not trust the ICU staff, and regularly and angrily accuses them of not taking good care of Ms. A. Before her admission to the ICU, Ms. A.'s nurse had thoroughly discussed advance directives with her. The nurse, surprised when her patient chose her aunt instead of her husband as her surrogate decision maker, talked with Ms. A. about this, but she was clear and adamant about her choice, and her husband was fully supportive.

Ms. A. has now spent more than a month in the ICU. Based on previous discussions with Ms. A. and statements she made in her advance directive, the care team believes it would be appropriate and consistent with Ms. A.'s wishes to take Ms. A. off the respirator. Her aunt disagrees and refuses to discuss it. The ICU staff asks the ethics consultant if there are grounds for bypassing Ms. A.'s aunt and asking her husband to make a decision. The ethics consultation group meets with the team as well as with Ms. A.'s aunt and husband, together and separately. They recommend that a designated member of the team establish a regular time to update Ms. A.'s aunt about Ms. A.'s clinical status and treatment options and discuss how best to respect Ms. A.'s wishes. Respect for Ms. A.'s autonomous decision calls for both respecting her choice of surrogate decision maker and respecting her previously specified preferences. Reconciling apparent conflicts between these two courses of action requires sensitivity and patience.

Withholding and Withdrawing Treatment, Especially at the End of Life In some cases, a patient or surrogate may decide to withhold or withdraw a treatment, especially at the end of life. *Withholding* refers to never initiating a treatment, whereas *withdrawing* refers to stopping a treatment once started. The distinction between not starting a treatment and stopping it is not itself of ethical significance; what matters most is whether the decision is consistent with the patient's interests and preferences. Health care professionals may find it emotionally more difficult to withdraw a treatment than to withhold it in the first place, yet starting a treatment may allow evaluation of its effectiveness, confirmation of a diagnosis, or time for the patient or family to deliberate and make often-difficult decisions. The Hastings Center's *Guidelines on the Termination of Life-Sustaining Treatment and Care of the Dying* states that "there is strong reason to prefer stopping treatment over not starting it in some cases. . . . There is often uncertainty about the efficacy of a proposed treatment, or the burdens and benefits it will impose on the patient. It is better to start the treatment and later stop if it is ineffective than not to start treatment for fear that stopping will be impossible."[11]

Ending treatment for sound moral reasons does not violate professional obligations. When the patient or surrogate decides in good faith that a proposed treatment will impose undue burdens and refuses such treatment, it is morally correct for the health care professional to respect that decision. If the patient or surrogate decides that a treatment in progress and the life it provides have become too burdensome, then the treatment may permissibly be stopped. Imposing harmful or futile treatment against the patient's wishes violates the autonomous patient's right to self-determination. Respecting a patient's wish to stop treatment acknowledges his or her autonomous right to refuse treatment and to determine what constitutes "benefit." It also acknowledges the principle of nonmaleficence, or not harming the patient's dignity and quality of life by forcing unwanted, painful, or futile treatment on him or her. Even when the patient's wishes are not known or cannot be known, continued aggressive treatment can sometimes violate the nonautonomous patient's best interests. Because withdrawing an intervention can be difficult and emotional for the nurse, the physician, and other members of the health care team, communication and mutual support are critically important. Family members and others also need accurate information and emotional support.

One familiar example of a decision to withhold treatment is the decision not to attempt CPR in the event of an arrest, recorded as a "do not resuscitate" or "do not attempt resuscitation" (DNR or DNAR) order. The original intent of CPR was to resuscitate or revive patients suffering specific types of sudden cardiac or pulmonary arrest: victims of drowning, electric shock, untoward effects of drugs, anesthetic accidents, heart block, and acute myocardial infarction. CPR is now a routine medical intervention extended to almost all patients suffering cardiac or pulmonary arrest, no matter what the underlying disease process. Although CPR has proved dramatically effective for certain limited groups of patients, it is of little, if any, benefit for many others.

The immediate, reflexive intervention to preserve life without the express consent of the patient is supported by the principle of beneficence. Health care personnel assume that a "reasonable person" would wish to be resuscitated and act on the assumption that death is undesirable to the patient. Therefore, CPR is initiated unless there is a DNR order. In some cases, however, CPR could be predictably unsuccessful or could be more harmful than beneficial. Patients can request that resuscitation not be attempted or that other aggressive, possibly futile or harmful procedures not be performed, especially when death is imminent and inevitable.

To presume to understand the needs of a patient and act against the patient's expressed wishes (or to avoid ascertaining what those wishes might be) can be paternalistic. Paternalism is the act of overriding another's autonomous actions or requests to bring about what is believed to be the best outcome for that person; it violates respect for the patient's autonomy. To ensure respect for patient self-determination, discussion about treatment preferences, including CPR, should ideally occur when the patient is alert and has a reasonably clear sensorium. Before making a voluntary and informed decision to accept or to refuse CPR (or any treatment, including life-sustaining treatments), the patient or surrogate should understand what the treatment entails and how it will most likely affect the disease process and future quality of life.

The ANA *Code of Ethics for Nurses* (section 1.3) acknowledges that "Nurses are leaders and vigilant advocates for the delivery of dignified and humane care. Nurses actively participate in assessing and assuring responsible and appropriate use of interventions in order to minimize unwarranted or unwanted treatment and patient suffering. The acceptability and importance of carefully considered decisions regarding resuscitation status, withholding or withdrawing life-sustaining treatment, forgoing medically provided nutrition and hydration, aggressive pain and symptom management and advance directives are increasingly evident."[3] Wright and colleagues state, "All critical care nurses are expected to master the skills necessary for assisting patients and families through the harrowing experience of life-threatening illness . . . [and] must assume responsibility . . . [for] working through the ethical issues which often include end-of-life decisions and organ donation."[12] Decisions about treatment at the end of life are often difficult[13] and best made after careful presentation of accurate information about realistic outcomes and possible interventions and discussions between the health care professional and the patient or surrogate. The nurse ensures that the patient or surrogate understands the information by clarifying technical terms, helping the patient weigh treatment options, and providing an opportunity to discuss personal choices about end-of-life care. The nurse might also help by calling on other resources, including palliative care, spiritual care, social work, ethics, and others to assist the patient in making these difficult decisions. Ideally, the patient considers his or her own values and wishes in the context of prognoses and realistic options and makes a decision; such decisions should be supported by the nurse and other members of the health care team.

Critical care nurses may have a limited role in some decisions about end-of-life care.[14] In some cases, the nurse may have a personal moral conviction contrary to a certain decision or may believe that the particular decision is against the patient's best interests or wishes. The nurse is morally permitted to refuse to participate in withholding or withdrawing treatment from a patient as long as the patient's care is assumed by someone else. As stated in section 5.4 of the ANA *Code of Ethics for Nurses*, "Where a particular treatment, intervention, activity, or practice is morally objectionable to the nurse, whether intrinsically so or because it is inappropriate for the specific patient, or where it may jeopardize both patients and nursing practice, the nurse is justified in refusing to participate on moral grounds. . . . The nurse . . . must communicate the decision in appropriate ways. . . . The nurse is obliged to provide for the patient's safety, to avoid patient abandonment and to withdraw only when assured that alternative sources of nursing care are available to the patient."[3]

Limits to Treatment and "Futility" In contrast to cases in which health care workers want to treat patients against their wishes, sometimes a patient, family member, or surrogate wants treatment that physicians, nurses, or other members of the health care team feel is inappropriate or even futile. Providing care perceived as "excessive," especially for dying patients, is a source of great concern among care providers, especially nurses and critical care nurses.[15–17]

Critical care nurses and others who provide care find that they experience inappropriate moral distress, emotional exhaustion, burnout, and concern about compromised integrity.[17–20]

A landmark case of this type involved Helga Wanglie, an 86-year-old woman in a persistent vegetative state who had been on a ventilator in the ICU for more than 1 year. The health care team treating her believed that continued treatment was futile, but her husband disagreed. The state court upheld the right of Mr. Wanglie to act as surrogate decision maker for his wife.[21] Another famous case involved a hospital's request to withhold ventilator treatment from Baby K., an anencephalic baby. Again, the court upheld the wishes of the baby's mother for continued ventilation and treatment. These and other cases stimulated a great deal of discussion among ethicists, health care professionals, and patients' rights groups about when, if ever, a patient's request for treatment can be denied because of futility. However, lack of consensus on a definition of, or criteria for, futility, plus concern about whether health care providers can be objective enough to make these determinations, have led to seemingly irresolvable disagreements. Futility is a complex concept that can be understood in at least one of two different ways: (1) when an intervention would be ineffective at producing its intended effect (e.g., CPR in the setting of cardiac rupture), and (2) more broadly, when an intervention might be physiologically effective but is unlikely to provide meaningful benefit (e.g., ventilation in a terminally ill patient who has lost the ability to breathe on his own). In the latter sense of futility, the treatment might achieve the patient's goals, but clinicians perceive these goals to be of little value; Veatch argues that clinicians should provide these treatments.[22]

Because health care providers have no particular expertise in deciding what goals and benefits patients find important, patients and families need accurate information about the chances of benefit from any particular intervention and may need assistance in determining how much benefit is acceptable and at what costs. The Council on Ethical and Judicial Affairs of the American Medical Association recommends that institutions adopt a policy that follows a "fair process approach" to determine futility of interventions.[23] Most such policies require deliberation by multidisciplinary committees, such as ethics committees, rather than unilateral decisions by a physician, and require genuine attempts to transfer the patient's care.[24] Some institutions allow a physician, under carefully delineated circumstances and after consultation with others, to write a DNR order or withhold certain treatments without the consent of the patient.

Advocacy Nurses promise to act in their patients' best interests, respect their autonomy, and advocate for them. The AACN policy sheet *Role of the Critical Care Nurse* describes the critical care nurse as a patient advocate.[25] Communicating honestly with patients and their significant others, discussing and respecting their wishes regarding treatment and care, convening patient care conferences for all involved parties when indicated, and facilitating advance care planning discussions and the use of advance directives are all important methods of fulfilling these obligations, as the following case study illustrates.

RESPECTING AND ADVOCATING FOR THE PATIENT

Ms. C. is a 44-year-old woman with severe and persistent pain from metastatic cancer. After a stay in the ICU marked by slow deterioration, Ms. C., who was weak, short of breath, anasarcic, and in considerable pain, confided to her primary care nurse that she was ready to die and did not want any life-sustaining treatments. The nurse knew that Mr. C. had not accepted his wife's prognosis, was hoping for a miracle, and insisted on aggressive treatment to extend his wife's life, and she dreaded the impending conflict between the unit's aggressive oncologist, the patient with no hope of a life without pain, and the husband who was not ready to let his wife die.

The primary nurse had worked to develop a trusting relationship with Ms. C. and her husband and felt it was her responsibility to act as her patient's advocate. She was aware that Ms. C. trusted her to facilitate communication about her wishes to the physician and the rest of the health care team and to help ensure that they were followed. Accordingly, she set up a family conference to discuss the plan of care with Ms. C. and her husband, the physician, the nursing staff, and the social worker. She hoped they could discuss Ms. C.'s prognosis and desires and come to an agreement on current goals of treatment and care that would be of benefit to Ms. C. and consistent with her wishes.

Justice

Justice is a principle of fairness. In health care, the most frequent appeal is to distributive justice, which requires a fair or equitable distribution of burdens and benefits. Justice is appealed to when determining how health care should be distributed in society; whether people are entitled to receive health care, regardless of their ability to pay; and whether they should receive a similar amount (e.g., type, quality) of health care. Fairness requires that decisions about the distribution of health care be based on morally significant characteristics, and not on factors such as race, ethnicity, gender, social standing, or religious beliefs. Substantive criteria useful for making distribution decisions for social goods, such as health care, might stipulate equal access to health care for everyone, or that health care should be distributed according to need, contribution, or free market exchange.[7]

Criteria such as these are also useful for decisions about allocation of limited resources, treatments, and even time and attention among patients. Every time a decision is made to transplant a kidney into one person and not another, to respond to one patient's need before another's, or to admit one patient to the ICU instead of another, a decision is made about distribution of resources using criteria such as those listed previously. Some egalitarians argue that because ab-

solute equality is not possible in the distribution of health care goods, the only fair methods of deciding how to distribute goods are random selection or "first come, first served," thereby avoiding the use of any criteria that make distinctions between people. Allocation decisions are ordinarily made independent of the wishes of the patient or family and usually require balancing potential harms and benefits *between* people. Allocation decisions can be very difficult, and not everyone will be happy with decisions made; hence the need for well-thought-out and carefully applied criteria. Two important examples of difficult allocation decisions involve organs for transplantation and beds in the ICU.

Allocation of Organs for Transplantation Despite great technological successes in the transplantation of organs such as kidneys, hearts, pancreata, and other organs, the need for organs is greater than the available supply. In great part, this is because people do not donate organs even when they can. Critical care nurses may be at the bedside of a patient pronounced brain-dead when discussions with the family about procuring organs are initiated. Usually, a procurement coordinator from the nearest Organ Procurement Organization works with hospital staff to discuss with the patient's family the option of donating organs. When a donation occurs, difficult distribution decisions are also made about who receives the organs that are available. Many factors influence the likelihood of an individual patient receiving a transplanted organ. In the United States, the Organ Procurement and Transplantation Network maintains a national registry for organ matching.[26] All patients put onto a transplant center's waiting list are registered with the United Network for Organ Sharing (UNOS) Center. When an organ becomes available, information is entered into a computerized organ-matching system. The computer program generates a list of potential recipients according to objective criteria agreed on by UNOS. Distribution criteria have been delineated for allocating different organs; specific criteria include factors such as blood type, human leukocyte antigen type, size of the organ, time on the waiting list, medical urgency, and distance between donor and recipient, but not ethnicity, gender, or financial status.[27] However, the criteria used for deciding whether someone who needs an organ is put on a transplant center waiting list in the first place are less transparent.

Allocation of Intensive Care Unit Beds Sometimes when a patient requires care in the ICU, either all the beds are already filled with critically ill patients or admitting another patient would endanger the care of patients already in the ICU because of limits on available staffing. Decisions about admitting or discharging patients from the ICU often involve some sort of triage to maximize the effective and efficient use of resources. Triage decisions are usually based on considerations of medical utility; that is, a comparative judgment about the probability of success of ICU care for the individual patients involved.

Beauchamp and Childress argue that "principles and rules of justice mandate attention to medical utility followed by the use of chance or queuing for scarce resources when medical utility is roughly equal for eligible patients."[7] Truog and colleagues recognize that bedside practitioners engage in several types of rationing and argue that allocation decisions justified by clinical judgment ". . . deserve particular scrutiny because they may mask unethical prejudices or bias."[28]

Zoloth-Dorfman and Carney[29] discuss the case of James Ramsey, a young patient with acquired immun-odeficiency syndrome (AIDS) admitted through the emergency department in acute respiratory distress and diagnosed with *Pneumocystis carinii* pneumonia. Unable to obtain a bed in the ICU, the emergency department physician transferred Mr. Ramsey to an AIDS ward where despite the valiant efforts of the evening nurses and the house staff, his condition continued to worsen. The resident was told that there were "no available beds" in the ICU but later found out that one bed was being reserved for a "code." The patient continued to deteriorate throughout the night, and developed acute respiratory distress and hypotensive shock; eventually a code was called, but the patient died in transit to the ICU.

ICU staff believed that intensive care in this case was futile, and bed space was limited. However, AIDS unit staff believed that the patient had been discriminated against because he had AIDS and worried about the appeal to "futility" as an excuse. Perhaps institutional clarification of ICU admitting criteria, including when the bed saved for "codes" could be used, would have helped in this case.

Increasingly, decisions about allocation of health care resources, such as ICU care, are influenced by the number of available qualified nurses. Given the current nursing shortage and the personnel cutbacks that have been made by many hospitals, this is a growing problem. Studies show that higher patient-to-nurse ratios are associated with higher mortality rates and more complications among surgical patients, as well as with higher burnout and job dissatisfaction among nurses.[30]

The Joint Commission requires hospitals and other health care institutions to have policies and procedures that ensure fair and equitable standards for admissions, care, discharge, and billing.[31] Ethical principles applied to some organizational business practices are important in helping a health care organization meet its obligations as a business while maintaining its commitment to the ethical care of patients. Nurses, as members of the multidisciplinary team and as an essential but scarce resource, have a valuable and critical perspective to bring to the development and ongoing review of these organizational and societal policies.

Health Care in the United States   Justice also applies to the distribution of health care services in the country. Health care in the United States has been described as fragmented, inefficient, and unjust. The United States spends approximately 16% of its gross national product on health care, and costs have continued to escalate in recent years.[32] Nonetheless, more than an estimated 45,000,000 people in the United States, most of them poor, have no health insurance.[33,34] In addition, eligibility, coverage, and reimbursement provided by different health plans, including Medicaid, vary dramatically. With the goal of reducing waste and controlling costs, much of health care in the United States is managed care, in which health insurance companies, industrial health care plans, or groups of patients contract with health care providers to provide a specified level of health care services at a predetermined cost. The ANA is committed to the principle that all people are entitled to ready access to affordable, quality health care services.[35] The ANA *Agenda for Health Care Reform*, introduced in 1991, represents a solid and ethical proposal for equitable and appropriate care.[35] The ANA recognizes that fundamental reform is even more necessary today because the health care system remains in a state of crisis, with costs of care and the number of uninsured continuing to rise and questions about the safety and quality of available care continuing to be raised.[35] In 2006, Massachusetts passed the Massachusetts Health Care Reform Plan designed to provide nearly universal health care coverage to state residents.[36] Continued changes in the structure and payment of health care delivery in the United States are likely to occur.

• Ethical Decision Making Within a Nursing Process Model

Ethical decisions should take into consideration the patient's best interest, the health care providers' professional and personal values, institutional values, personal feelings, moral principles, and legal issues. At first glance, it might seem impossible to integrate these into anything other than an incoherent mass of conflicting possible actions, but with careful reflection and deliberation, acceptable resolutions can usually be achieved. The ANA *Code of Ethics for Nurses* (section 5.2) states that "nurses are required to have knowledge relevant to the current scope and standards of nursing practice, changing issues, concerns, controversies, and ethics."[3]

Ethical decision-making models provide a process for systematically and thoughtfully examining a conflict, ensuring that participants consider all important aspects of a situation before taking action. The steps of ethical analysis and evaluation are much like the steps of the nursing process and, as such, are a skill that can be learned. Both provide an orderly approach to problems. There are usually five steps to resolution of an ethical problem in the clinical setting (Box 7-3).

GATHER THE RELEVANT FACTS

The first step is to identify information needed to understand the situation fully. What are the medical facts (i.e., diagnoses, prognoses, treatment

---

Box 7-3 • Model for Ethical Decision Making

Analysis of an ethical problem in the clinical setting usually involves the following five steps:
1. Gather the relevant facts and identify the decision maker(s) and the stakeholders.
2. Identify the ethical problem(s). Involve others in the process and use consultation resources as appropriate.
3. Analyze the problem using ethical guidance and resources.
4. Deliberate about the action alternatives in light of guidance; choose one and justify the choice.
5. Evaluate and reflect.

---

alternatives)? Who are the principal agents involved, including the decision makers and the stakeholders? Are the patient's values and goals for treatment and care clear? How do the values, interests, and relationships of others involved affect the problem? Are cultural, religious, or other aspects relevant to the case? It is important to understand the physiological, psychosocial, and legal dimensions of the situation. Are there legal ramifications, institutional policies, or economic factors to consider?

IDENTIFY THE PROBLEM

The next step is to identify the ethical problem or problems. Is it truly a problem involving a question about or conflict between ethical principles or values, or is it primarily a legal or organizational issue or a communication problem? Ethical problems are often complicated by communication problems and legal restrictions; however, some problems can be resolved simply through better communication or legal counsel without ethical analysis.

ANALYZE THE PROBLEM USING ETHICAL PRINCIPLES AND RULES

It is essential to identify the person or people who have the responsibility and authority to make a decision. Is the patient competent, fully informed, and free to make a choice (respect for autonomy)? Is there a designated surrogate or family member able to speak to the best interests of a comatose patient (beneficence) or a designated person with durable power of attorney for health care who knows the patient's wishes (respect for autonomy)? How is the family involved? Are there vested interests to consider?

Consider ethical principles. Is harm being avoided or minimized? What are the anticipated benefits from actions being considered, and who will benefit? What are the risks, and who will be harmed? Are rights being protected? Have the patient's wishes and interests been articulated? Has adequate information been provided? Have promises been made? Have all the relevant voices been heard? Has fairness been considered? Which principles are most applicable to the case? How can the principles be specified to pro-

vide guidance in the particular situation? Consider the role of care and compassion. There may be competing claims, all of which are reasonable and justifiable, and conflicting principles. There may also be conflicts between principles and legal or institutional requirements. These should be clearly articulated.

ANALYZE ALTERNATIVES AND ACT

Identify all the possible and reasonable alternatives, and evaluate each of them on their conformity to principles and rules and their compatibility with care and compassion for the patient and the patient's preferences and interests. Which option most promotes respect for the patient? How will each proposed action and its outcome benefit or harm those involved? Which of the possible alternatives seems fairest in terms of process, outcome, or both? Will the action strengthen or jeopardize patient–professional bonds and reaffirm society's expectations of health care professionals? After reflection and careful reasoning, which option is most consistent with sound ethical analysis? The nurse may not be the primary decision maker, but as an integral member of the health care team, it is important that she or he contribute to the dialogue, facilitate communication, articulate relevant personal views and values, and cooperate in implementing the course of action. The nurse's role may also include planning a multidisciplinary conference or arranging for an ethics consultation.

EVALUATE AND REFLECT

After the action has been taken, the ethical problem, the process of resolution, and the outcome are further analyzed. The outcome should be compared with what was hoped for or intended. How can a similar situation be handled with greater sensitivity or wisdom in the future? Evaluation is especially helpful if it is undertaken in a nonjudgmental and nonthreatening atmosphere conducive to reflection and constructive change.

• Bioethics Resources and Services

Informed clinicians and clear organizational policies and support help to prevent and resolve ethical dilemmas in health care organizations. Many health care organizations have an ethics committee or an ethics consultation service that provides education, policy development, and consultation at the bedside for ethical problems that arise in patient care.

ETHICS COMMITTEES AND CONSULTATION SERVICES

Institutional ethics committees are usually multidisciplinary and usually include representatives from various patient care professions and disciplines (e.g., nursing, medicine, social work, spiritual care).

Committees frequently include one or more member of the lay community, as well as lawyers, ethicists, or clergy, as committee members or ad hoc consultants.

Ethics committee members may offer education to the professional staff and community on issues related to clinical ethics and serve as an institutional resource for policy studies and the drafting of institutional policies concerning ethical issues. The Joint Commission requires policy statements and guidelines on the process of addressing ethical issues, informed consent, use of surrogate decision makers, decisions about care and treatment at the end of life, and confidentiality of information. Well-thought-out and articulated policies about these issues offer useful guidance to clinicians in often-difficult situations.

Ethics consultation through an initial bedside consultation by one or more trained consultants may be sufficient to provide the education, clarification, or dialogue necessary to assist decision makers in resolving an ethical problem. In some more complicated cases or when conflict exists among decision makers, consultation by the entire ethics committee may be appropriate. Some committees aim to make a single recommendation for the resolution of the ethical problem, whereas others attempt to frame the morally acceptable options and assist key decision makers in choosing a course of action. Limited data show that physicians and nurses find ethics consultation helpful in difficult situations.[37] Nurses should be aware of what resources are available to them, what they have to offer, and how to access such resources. One study found that nurses often lack awareness of the ethics consultation service or how to request a consult, but also exhibited "moral courage" when they took steps to request an ethics consultation.[38]

In addition to services provided by an ethics committee or consultant service, other resources are sometimes available to nurses. Some institutions have nursing ethics committees, which, although possibly coordinated with an existing institutional ethics committee, can function independently. These committees are designed to meet the needs of nurses in the institution by providing education and addressing issues unique to nursing, such as refusal of assignment, staffing patterns, or allocation of beds. Some institutions sponsor periodic ethics rounds, which may be general, unit based, or specific to nursing, and serve primarily an educational function. Pastoral care, quality assurance, and peer support activities are other examples of institutional resources that may facilitate the resolution of ethical problems.

PROFESSIONAL NURSING ORGANIZATIONS

Professional nursing organizations also address ethical issues of concern to nursing practice. The ANA addresses professional issues and moral dilemmas common to all nurses in the United States. In addition to the aforementioned ANA *Code of Ethics for Nurses,* the ANA's Center for Ethics and Human Rights publishes position statements and guidelines on many issues for which nurses seek ethical guidance. The AACN also has an active ethics committee, which develops policy statements and position papers that set standards for ethical behavior and decision making for critical care nurses. The AACN's ethics committee works closely with other professional nursing organizations and interfaces with other professional organizations, such as the Society of Critical Care Medicine, to examine issues shared by both professions.

• Clinical Applicability Challenges

Short-Answer Questions

1. You believe that cardiopulmonary resuscitation is inappropriate for your patient, who is terminally ill with metastatic cancer. Construct plans for proceeding. Identify the people with whom you would talk and in what order you would speak to them. Structure arguments you would make to support your position.

2. A patient in your unit has severe and intractable pain, which you believe is being inadequately managed. Consider whether this is an ethical issue, and state why or why not. Explain what you would do to resolve the problem. Defend your position by using the American Nurses Association's *Code of Ethics for Nurses.*

3. You receive a call from the emergency department regarding a patient with sepsis who needs to be admitted to your unit. However, at the time of the call, your unit is full. Explain the criteria you would use to determine whether there is a patient who could be moved to another unit to accommodate the patient from the emergency department. Determine who would make this decision, and construct how the decision would be made. Describe the ethical principle relevant to this situation.

Review Questions

1. An ethic of care is primarily based on
   a. acknowledgment of the history of nurses providing care to patients.
   b. recognition of the uniqueness of people, the value of relationships, and the importance of emotions in moral judgments.
   c. expectations of the American Nurses Association.
   d. extra efforts for those one cares about.

2. Ethical analysis helps people resolve moral dilemmas by
   a. clarifying the moral issues and principles and providing an ethically adequate rationale for a decision.
   b. helping a person avoid his or her responsibilities to patients.
   c. defending a specific general ethical theory.
   d. consulting with institutional lawyers.

3. A nurse believes that the medical treatment being given a particular patient is ethically inappropriate and refuses to give the patient care, abruptly leaving the workplace that day to avoid being involved in the situation. This is an example of
   a. a nurse standing up for his or her right not to participate in morally objectionable care.
   b. a violation of the principles of beneficence and fidelity through patient abandonment.
   c. a nurse's support for the principle of nonmaleficence (noninfliction of harm).
   d. the exercise of professional nursing judgment.

4. Respect for a patient's autonomy encompasses
   a. providing accurate information and choice for a patient's informed consent.
   b. withholding life-sustaining treatment when it seems futile.
   c. allocating intensive care units beds fairly.
   d. preventing harm by monitoring interventions.

References

1. Jameton A: Nursing Practice: The Ethical Issues. Englewood Cliffs, NJ, Prentice-Hall, 1984
2. Rushton CH: Defining and addressing moral distress: Tools for critical care nursing leaders. AACN Adv Crit Care 17(2):161–168, 2006
3. American Nurses Association: Code of Ethics for Nurses With Interpretive Statements. Washington, DC, American Nurses Publishing, 2001. Retrieved July 30, 2006, from http://www.nursingworld.org/ethics/ecode.htm
4. International Council of Nursing: Code of Ethics for Nurses, April 2006. Retrieved July 29, 2006, from http://www.icn.ch/icncode.pdf
5. Veatch R, Fry S: Case Studies in Nursing Ethics, 2nd ed. Sudbury, MA, Jones & Bartlett, 2000
6. Fry S: Toward a theory of nursing ethics. Adv Nurs Sci 11(4):9–22, 1989
7. Beauchamp T, Childress J: Principles of Biomedical Ethics, 5th ed. New York, Oxford University Press, 2001
8. American Association of Critical-Care Nurses: Key Statements, beliefs, and philosophies behind the AACN. An ethic of care. Retrieved July 30, 2006, from http://www.aacn.org
9. Schloendorff v. Society of N.Y. Hospital, 211 N.Y. 125, 105 N.E. 92, 93, 1914
10. The Hastings Center: Improving end of life care: Why has it been so difficult? Hastings Center Special Report 35(6), 2005
11. The Hastings Center: Guidelines on the termination of life-sustaining treatment and care of the dying. Briarcliff Manor, NY, The Hastings Center, 1987
12. Wright F, Cohen S, Caroselli C: How culture affects ethical decision making. Crit Care Nurs Clin North Am 9(1):63–73, 1997
13. Stroud R: The withdrawal of life support in adult intensive care: An evaluative review of the literature. Nurs Crit Care 7(4):176–184, 2002
14. Miller P, Forbes S, Boyle D: End-of-life care in the intensive care unit: A challenge for nurses. Am J Crit Care Nurs 10(5):369, 2001
15. Beckstrand R, Callister L, Kirchhoff K: Providing a "good death": Critical care nurses' suggestions for improving end of life care. Am J Crit Care 15(1):38–45, 2006
16. Beckstrand R, Kirchhoff K: Providing end of life care to patients: Critical care nurses' perceived obstacles and supportive behaviors. Am J Crit Care 14(5):395–403, 2005
17. Meltzer L, Huckabay L: Critical care nurses' perceptions of futile care and its effect on burnout. Am J Crit Care 13(3)202–208, 2004
18. Heland M:. Fruitful or futile: Intensive care nurses' experiences and perceptions of medical futility. Aust Crit Care 19(1):25–31, 2006
19. Palda V, Bowman K, McLean R, Chapman M: "Futile" care: do we provide it? Why? A semistructured Canada-wide survey of intensive care doctors and nurses. J Crit Care 20(3):207–213, 2005
20. Hamric A, Blackhall L: Nurse–physician perspectives on the care of dying patients in intensive care units: Collaboration, moral distress, and ethical climate. Crit Care Med 35(2):422–429, 2007
21. Lomasky LE: Ventilating issues of life and death: The case of Helga Wanglie. Public Affairs Q 8(2):153–168, 1994
22. Veatch R: Terri Schiavo, Son Hudson, and "nonbeneficial" medical treatments. Health Affairs 24(4):976–979, 2005
23. Council on Ethical and Judicial Affairs, American Medical Association: Medical futility in end-of-life care. JAMA 281:937–941, 1999
24. Helft P, Siegler M, Lantos J: The rise and fall of the futility movement. N Engl J Med 343:293–296, 2000
25. American Association of Critical Care Nurses: Policy statement: Role of the critical care nurse. Retrieved July 28, 2006, from http://www.aacn.org/AACN/pubpolicy.nsf
26. The Organ Procurement and Transplantation Network: About transplantation. Retrieved July 28, 2006, from http://www.optn.org/about/transplantation
27. The Organ Procurement and Transplantation Network: Organ distribution and allocation. Retrieved August 1, 2006, from http://www.optn.org/policiesAndBylaws/policies.asp
28. Truog R, Brock D, Cook D, et al, for the Task Force on Values, Ethics, and Rationing in Critical Care (VERICC): Rationing in the intensive care unit. Crit Care Med 34(4):958–963, 2006
29. Zoloth-Dorfman L, Carney B: The AIDS patient and the last ICU bed: Scarcity, medical futility, and ethics. QRB–Qual Re Bull 17(6):175–181, 1991
30. Aiken L, Clarke S, Sloane D, et al: Hospital nurse staffing and patient mortality, nurse burnout, and job dissatisfaction. JAMA 288(16):1987–1993, 2002
31. Marsee V: Ethical perspectives of reimbursement under economic pressures. Crit Care Nurs Clin North Am 12(3):365–372, 2000
32. National Coalition on Health Care. Retrieved August 15, 2007, from http://www.nchc.org/facts/cost/shtml
33. Committee on the Consequences of Uninsurance: Care Without Coverage: Too Little, Too Late. Washington, DC, National Academy of Sciences, 2002
34. U.S. Department of Health and Human Services Office of the Assistant Secretary for Planning and Evaluation: Overview of the uninsured in the United States: An analysis of the 2005 Current Population Survey. Retrieved August 8, 2007, from http://aspe.hhs.gov/health/reports/05/uninsured-cps/index.htm#Insurance
35. American Nurses Association. ANA's Health Care Agenda 2005. Washington, DC. American Nurses Association. Available at http://nursingworld/MainMenuCategories/Healthcareandpolicyissues/HSR/HealthCareAgenda.as
36. Kaiser Communication of Key Facts: Massachusetts Health Care Reform, April 2006. Retrieved August 1, 2006, from http://www.kff.org/uninsured/upload/7494.pdf
37. Schneiderman L, Gilmer T, Teetzel H: Impact of ethics consultation in the intensive care setting: A randomized, controlled trial. Crit Care Med 28(12):3920–3924, 2000
38. Gordon E, Hamric A: The courage to stand up: Cultural politics of nurses' access to ethics consultation. J Clin Ethics 17(2):231–254, 2006

Legal Issues in Critical Care Nursing

Patricia C. McMullen • Alexander R. McMullen

Objectives

Based on the content in this chapter, the reader should be able to:

❶ Describe major areas of the law that affect critical care nursing practice.

❷ Define the four elements of malpractice (professional negligence).

❸ Delineate allegations commonly made against nurses.

❹ Explain types of vicarious liability.

❺ Apply knowledge of advance directives to patient care situations.

Because society seems to be more litigious than ever, legal issues involving critical care are of increasing concern. The number of malpractice suits that name or involve nurses is increasing. Issues such as refusal and termination of treatment have been widely discussed and addressed in the literature. Even legislators have become involved by enacting so-called living will statutes in their jurisdictions.

This chapter begins with a discussion of the major areas of law that may have an impact on the practice of nursing. After this discussion, the legal principle of negligence is reviewed, and pertinent critical care case examples are provided. The chapter then proceeds to identify and address certain current legal issues most applicable to the critical care nurse.

• An Overview of Major Areas of the Law

There are three areas of the law that affect the practice of the critical care nurse: administrative law, civil law, and criminal law.

ADMINISTRATIVE LAW

Administrative law exists as a consequence of state and federal laws and regulations related to the practice of nursing. In all states, the legislatures have enacted nurse practice acts. Within each of these acts, the practice of nursing is defined, and powers are delegated to a state agency, usually the State Board of Nursing. These agencies develop regulations that dictate how the nurse practice act is to be interpreted and implemented.

Practicing nurses are expected to know the provisions of the nurse practice act in their state and any regulations dealing with the practice of nursing. If a nurse is unfamiliar with the nurse practice act, it is important that he or she contact the State Board of Nursing to request and review a copy of this act. Copies of the nurse practice act are also available in state statutes. Law libraries in every state maintain copies of their state statutes, and many public libraries have state statutes as well. A number of state boards of nursing also place their nurse practice act and regulations on a website.

State government is charged with protecting the health, safety, and well-being of the citizens in each state. If a citizen feels that he or she has not received reasonable nursing care, the citizen may contact the State Board of Nursing and file a complaint against the nurse or nurses involved in the care. The state is then responsible for conducting an investigation to determine whether the patient's claim has merit. The National Council of State Boards of Nursing has excellent information on filing a complaint.[1]

Under the Fifth Amendment of the U.S. Constitution, all citizens are afforded the right to due process before any property can be taken by a state or federal government. Case law indicates that a nurse's license is a form of property because it helps a person earn a living. Because due process rights are attached to a nursing license, certain due process requirements must be met before a State Board of Nursing can revoke, discipline, or place conditions on a nursing license. First, the nurse is entitled to a notice that someone has filed a claim on his or her license. Next, the nurse must be given an opportunity to answer any charges that are alleged. This opportunity usually takes the form of a hearing before the State Board of Nursing. Usually, the nurse will want to attend the hearing with an attorney to make sure all rights are respected.

At the hearing, the investigators for the State Board of Nursing present the complaint that was filed and any investigation that was performed. The nurse may call witnesses who have knowledge of facts surrounding the complaint. These witnesses may include the person who filed the complaint, any witnesses to the incident, and people who supervised the nurse. At this hearing, the nurse, either directly or through legal counsel, can question witnesses and introduce evidence or testimony to refute the allegations in the complaint. Based on these presentations, the State Board of Nursing makes a determination as to whether reasonable nursing care was given and what, if any, discipline is warranted. Typically, the decision of the State Board of Nursing is final, and unless there were violations of the nurse's due process rights, a court upholds the State Board's findings.

Although the nurse's right of due process cannot be abridged, state boards of nursing have the right to temporarily suspend a nurse's license immediately for acts the Board deems dangerous to the welfare of the general public. When the state immediately suspends a nursing license, it must afford the nurse a right to a hearing within a prescribed short time from the date of suspension.

CIVIL LAW

Civil law is the second area of the law that affects the practice of nursing. One specific area of civil law, tort law, forms the foundation of most civil cases involving nurses. Torts are civil wrongs. The torts of negligence, malpractice, assault, and battery are addressed later in this chapter. The civil concepts of vicarious liability and product liability also are discussed.

CRIMINAL LAW

The third area of the law relevant to nursing practice is criminal law. Unlike civil law, whereby private parties sue one another, criminal law encompasses cases in which the local, state, or federal government has filed a lawsuit against a nurse. Criminal cases include criminal assault and battery, negligent homicide, and murder. Criminal cases are extremely rare in nursing situations. An example of a criminal case is presented with the case studies given later in this chapter.

• Nursing Negligence in Critical Care

The legal responsibility of the registered nurse in critical care settings does not differ from that of the registered nurse in any work setting. The registered nurse adheres to five principles for the protection of the patient and the practitioner (Box 8-1). The most common lawsuits against nurses and their employers are based on the legal concept of malpractice, known as negligence by a professional. The following discussion emphasizes the major elements of malpractice and provides some case examples for clarification.

DUTY AND BREACH OF DUTY

A duty is a legal relationship between two or more parties. Several different kinds of situations can create this type of duty. In most nursing cases, duty arises out of a contractual relationship between the patient and the health care facility. That is, when a patient receives health care, an implied contract arises. The patient, the insurer, or both agree to pay for any health care services the patient receives; in return, the health care facility agrees to supply "reasonable care." A nurse who cares for a patient is legally responsible for providing reasonable care under the circumstances present at the time of the incident. The critical care nurse who fails to provide reasonable care under the circumstances has breached (violated) his or her duty toward the patient.

Many different methods are used to determine whether the nurse complied with reasonable standards of care that existed at the time of the incident.

Box 8-1 • Five Legal Responsibilities of the Registered Nurse

- Performs only those functions for which he or she has been prepared by education and experience
- Performs those functions competently
- Delegates responsibility only to personnel whose competence has been evaluated and found acceptable
- Takes appropriate measures as indicated by observations of the patient
- Is familiar with policies of the employing agency

The following factors can be used to determine whether the care of the critical care nurse was reasonable:

▶ Testimony from experts in critical care
▶ Agency procedure and protocol manuals
▶ Nursing job descriptions
▶ Nursing texts, professional journals, medication books
▶ Professional organization standards (Advanced Cardiac Life Support [ACLS] and Certified Critical Care Registered Nurse [CCRN] standards)
▶ Equipment manufacturers' instructions

Once duty is established, a breach of that duty is required; that is, the nurse must have been negligent. Negligence is found or refuted by a comparison of the nurse's conduct with the standard of care. In general, negligence is either ordinary or gross. Ordinary negligence implies professional carelessness, whereas gross negligence suggests that the nurse willfully and consciously ignored a known risk for harm to the patient. Most cases involve ordinary negligence, but gross negligence can be present if the nurse ignored sound nursing advice or harmed a patient while under the influence of drugs or alcohol.

CAUSATION

Malpractice law also requires that there be a causal relationship between the conduct of the critical care nurse and the injury to the patient, and that the injury that the patient suffers must be reasonably anticipated. For example, if a critical care nurse administered digoxin to a cardiac patient who had a pulse of 30 beats/minute and the patient suffered a cardiac arrest, it is likely that the critical care nurse would be found to have caused the patient's arrest; that is, the wrongful administration of the digoxin will be deemed to be the "proximate cause" of the arrest. However, if the patient had a pulse of 70 beats/minute when the digoxin was administered, and the patient suffered a totally unanticipated seizure, it is probable that the nurse would not be found to have caused the seizure. In this case, the seizure was not caused by the digoxin, and the nurse would normally be exonerated because seizures are not an expected complication of digoxin administration.

INJURY

The intent of the law is to make "the injured patient whole." That is, the law attempts to return the plaintiff to a position he or she would have been in had an injury not been suffered. Unfortunately, injuries sustained usually cannot be undone. As such, most court awards attempt to give monetary damages to compensate for the injuries sustained by a plaintiff.

In a malpractice suit, the plaintiff has to show that some type of injury or harm occurred as a result of the nurse's actions or inaction. The law allows several different types of monetary damages. These are grouped under the broad headings of economic and noneconomic damages.

Economic damages relate to those damages that can be calculated within a degree of certainty. Medical costs and lost wages are the two major types of economic damages. Attorneys have a special type of accountant, called an actuary, to estimate how much an injured patient was likely to earn over the course of a normal life expectancy and how the injury has affected this earning capacity. This monetary amount constitutes the "lost wages" part of the award. Similarly, the actuary is able to use past figures and inflation factors to estimate how much present and future medical expenses will cost the plaintiff.

Noneconomic damages are somewhat more difficult to calculate. These damages include pain and suffering and loss of consortium (services) that occurred as a result of the malpractice. Many state and federal governments place monetary limits on the amount a patient can recover for pain and suffering, regardless of the amount that may be awarded by a jury. Loss of consortium damages include such issues as the patient's inability to perform household tasks or loss of marital relations.

In a number of cases, the spouse and minor children of a patient may also be able to recover both economic and noneconomic damages that they suffer as a consequence of injuries to the patient. When a minor child is the plaintiff, it is not unusual for the parents to file for noneconomic losses due to the loss of society and affection of their child. On the economic side, a parent can sue for his or her own lost wages due to a need to care for the child.

Many types of malpractice complaints are lodged against critical care nurses. The following cases illustrate reasons nurses are often named in malpractice suits.

FAILURE TO COMPLY WITH REASONABLE STANDARDS OF CARE

Mr. S., a 46-year-old man with a history of ventricular tachycardia, was prescribed flecainide acetate (Tambocor) for his heart condition. One evening he reported his heart "started feeling funny" and had a friend take him to the emergency department. An electrocardiogram on admission to the emergency department revealed he was experiencing ventricular tachycardia.

Mr. S. told a nurse and a physician in the emergency department that he did not want cardioversion. The emergency department physician, in telephone consultation with a cardiologist, ordered 5 mg of verapamil. Within 2 minutes, Mr. S.'s blood pressure crashed, and he seized and went into cardiac arrest. Because of the arrest, Mr. S. suffered brain damage and was forced to reside in a nursing home because of lack of any independent motor function and inability to speak.

The emergency department nurse, physician, and hospital were sued for several reasons, including malpractice. During deposition, the nurse testified that she was ACLS certified and admitted to knowing that verapamil was contraindicated in patients with ventricular tachycardia. She related that she had serious questions about administering the verapamil but acceded to the physician's orders.

The court found that the standard of reasonable nursing care required the nurse to intervene to prevent complications and that failure to intervene was a violation of the nursing standard of care. In addition, the court determined that the standard of nursing care requires a nurse to exercise independent nursing judgment if he or she believes that an order may have adverse consequences for the patient.[2]

IMPROPER MEDICATION ADMINISTRATION

Baby M., a 26- to 28-week premature female infant, was brought to the local hospital when she was unexpectedly delivered at home. This hospital arranged to have the infant transported to a hospital that had a neonatal intensive care unit. A registered nurse and respiratory therapist accompanied the infant during transport. During the course of the transport, she received an overdose of heparin, which caused a cerebral hemorrhage, resulting in brain damage and physical and mental impairments.

Baby M.'s parents sued the transport nurse, the respiratory therapist, and the transport system for malpractice. The defendants in the case claimed the transport was for emergency services and that they should be absolved from liability under the state's Good Samaritan statute, which provides immunity from suit for responding to certain types of emergencies. The court found that the infant's medical assistance coverage had paid for the transport services, so that the Good Samaritan statute was not applicable. A trial was ordered on the malpractice suit.[3]

In this case, an overdose of heparin was the alleged cause of malpractice. Such medication errors often form the basis of malpractice suits against critical care nurses.

CRIMINAL LIABILITY IN CRITICAL CARE

Mr. D., an 86-year-old man, was admitted to the hospital with abdominal pain. He was diagnosed with a perforation in the proximal duodenum, causing diffuse peritonitis. The day after his surgery, he was found to have a serum potassium level of 3.2 mEq/L, below the normal level of 3.3 to 5.5 mEq/L. The intensive care unit (ICU) nurse administered an ordered dose of potassium chloride elixir through his nasogastric tube. However, subsequent laboratory tests showed this had not been well absorbed.

Mr. D.'s physician ordered the ICU nurse to run in an intravenous (IV) bag with 40 mEq of potassium chloride in 100 mL of saline. After the nurse informed the physician that the potassium chloride would need to be infused over the course of 1 hour, the physician ordered the nurse to draw up a syringe of 40 mEq of potassium chloride in 30 to 50 mL of saline. The nurse drew up the syringe but refused to administer it, knowing that this was dangerous. Another ICU nurse was also present and informed the physician

that it was contrary to hospital policy to administer a maximum dosage of 40 mEq of potassium chloride over 1 hour. The physician then took the syringe from the nurse and administered the potassium chloride directly. During the injection, Mr. D. stopped breathing, and efforts at cardiopulmonary resuscitation were unsuccessful.

The physician's failure to use reasonable standards of medical care and total disregard of the cautions given by the ICU nursing staff resulted in criminal liability. A court convicted the physician of involuntary manslaughter, "the unlawful killing of a human being without malice in the commission, without due caution and circumspection, of a lawful act which might produce death." The sentence was 5 months' imprisonment, 36 months' supervised parole, a $100 assessment, and a $25,000 fine.[3] The U.S. Court of Appeals for the 10th Circuit upheld the criminal conviction.[4]

VICARIOUS LIABILITY

In some cases, a person or institution can be held liable for the conduct of another. This is called vicarious liability. There are various types of vicarious liability, including respondeat superior, corporate liability, negligent supervision, and rule of personal liability.

Respondeat Superior

The doctrine of respondeat superior is translated as "let the master answer for the sins of the servant." This is the major legal theory under which hospitals are held liable for the negligence of their employees. Respondeat superior is a public policy type of legal doctrine. The philosophy behind respondeat superior is based on the idea that because a hospital typically generates profits from the patients seeking care, the hospital should pay for some of the damages caused by hospital personnel if negligence occurs. This doctrine applies only when hospital employees act within the scope of their employment.

In some situations, respondeat superior is not applicable. For instance, hospitals are not usually responsible for temporary agency personnel because they are usually employees of the agency, not the hospital. Physicians, unless they are employed by the hospital, do not typically come within the sphere of this doctrine. Actions by hospital nurses who cause malpractice outside of their employment rarely fall into the respondeat superior category.

Because hospitals may be held liable for nursing activities conducted by their employees, they carry professional liability insurance for the activities of their employees. Usually, a hospital will defend a nurse named in a malpractice case. However, many nurses also carry their own malpractice insurance for off-the-job nursing activities and in order to retain independent counsel in the event they are sued.

Corporate Liability

Another type of vicarious liability is called corporate liability. Corporate liability occurs when a hospital is found liable for its own unreasonable conduct. For example, if it is found that a unit is chronically understaffed and a patient suffers an injury as a result of short staffing, the hospital can be held accountable. It is reasonable to expect any hospital that has an ICU or an emergency department to take precautionary measures to ensure that it is adequately staffed or that beds or admissions are reduced. Failure to ensure adequate staffing can lead to payment of monetary damages under the theory of corporate liability.

Corporate liability may also occur within "floating" situations. A nurse working in a critical care setting must be competent to make immediate nursing judgments and to act on those decisions. If the nurse does not possess the knowledge and skills required of a critical care nurse, he or she should not be rendering critical care. A nurse who is not well versed in critical care should notify the charge nurse or nursing supervisor of this fact. The nurse needs to clearly state which nursing care activities he or she can and cannot implement. The supervisor and charge nurse must then delegate the remaining nursing duties to staff members with adequate education, training, and experience. Box 8-2 addresses issues of concern to the floating nurse.

Negligent Supervision

A third type of vicarious liability is negligent supervision. Negligent supervision is claimed when a supervisor fails to reasonably supervise people under his or her direction. For example, if a nurse is rotated to an unfamiliar unit and informs the charge nurse that she has never worked in critical care, it would be unreasonable for the charge nurse to ask her to perform invasive monitoring. If the charge nurse did assign such responsibilities to the floater and a patient injury resulted, the charge nurse could be held accountable to the patient for negligent supervision.

Captain of the Ship Doctrine

Finally, a fourth type of vicarious liability is known as the captain of the ship doctrine. At one time, the physician was viewed as the captain of the ship. Therefore, any order by the physician was expected to be implemented by the nurse. This doctrine has largely been replaced by a legal concept known as the rule of personal liability; that is, nurses are expected to make sound decisions by virtue of their specialized education, training, and experience. If they are unsure about the propriety of a physician's order, they should seek clarification from the physician or, if needed, from their supervisor.

ESTABLISHMENT OF PROTOCOLS

If the critical care nurse is required to perform medical acts and is not under the direct and immediate supervision of a delegating physician, the activities must be based on established protocols. These protocols should be created by the medical and nursing departments and should be reviewed for compliance with state nurse practice acts. They must be reviewed

---

Box 8-2 • Commonly Asked Questions When Rotating to an Unfamiliar Unit

1. If I am asked to go to another unit, must I go?
   Usually, you will be required to go to the other unit. If you refuse, you can be disciplined under the theory that you are breaching your employment contract or that you are failing to abide by the policies and procedures of the hospital. Some nursing units negotiate with hospitals to ensure that only specially trained nurses rotate to specialty units.

2. If I rotate to an unfamiliar unit, what types of nursing responsibilities must I assume?
   You will be expected to carry out only those nursing activities that you are competent to perform. In some instances, this will be the performance of basic nursing care activities, such as blood pressures, and uncomplicated treatments. If you are unfamiliar with the types of medications used on the unit, you should not be administering them until you are thoroughly familiar with them. Consider the medication cards the student completes in nursing school. They were assigned because a reasonable, prudent nurse does not give medications without knowledge of their pharmacology, dosage, method of administration, side effects, and interactions with other medications. The same reasoning applies for any other type of critical care monitoring.

3. What should I do if I feel unprepared when I get to the unit?
   Suggest that you assist the unit with basic nursing care requirements and that specialized activities (e.g., invasive monitoring, cardiac monitoring, or the administration of unfamiliar drugs) be performed by staff who are adequately prepared. Do not feel incompetent because you are not familiar with all aspects of nursing care. After all, when is the last time you saw the neurologist go to labor and delivery and perform a cesarean birth?

4. What if the charge nurse orders me to do something I am not able to do safely?
   You are obligated to say you are unqualified and request that another nurse carry out the task. The charge nurse also needs to remember that she could be held liable for negligent supervision if she orders you to do an unsafe activity and a patient injury results.

---

frequently so that health care professionals can determine whether they reflect current medical and nursing standards of care. In the event of a malpractice suit, the critical care protocols and procedures can be introduced as evidence to help establish the applicable standard of care. Although it is important that protocols provide direction, excessive detail restricts the critical care nurse's flexibility when selecting a proper course of action.

THE QUESTIONABLE MEDICAL ORDER

In addition to protocols, a policy statement should exist (in procedures or by directive) that indicates the manner of resolving the issue of the "questionable" medical order. This is important for all medical orders, but particularly for those given for critically ill patients because of the unusual doses of medication that are frequently ordered. The nurse who questions a particular order should express his or her specific reasons for concern to the physician who wrote the order. This initial approach frequently results in an explanation of the order and a medical justification for the order in the patient's medical record. If this approach is unsuccessful, many hospitals require that the attending physician or the nursing supervisor be notified; others have a policy that the chief of the service must be consulted about questionable orders. If these options are unavailable or are unsuccessful, a critical care nurse or any other nurse can refuse to give a medication.

As was demonstrated in the case of Mr. D. described earlier, an order that is patently wrong can harm the patient if it is followed. A secondary consequence can be liability for the physician, the nurse, and the hospital (as the employer) if the patient suffers harm as a direct result of the order.

LIABILITY FOR DEFECTIVE MEDICAL EQUIPMENT

A medical device, defined as virtually anything used in patient care that is not a drug, includes intricate pieces of equipment (e.g., intra-aortic balloon pumps, endotracheal tubes, pacemakers, defibrillators), along with less complicated ones, such as bedpans, suture materials, patient restraints, and tampons. Before 1976, medical devices were unregulated; since 1976, medical devices have been regulated by the U.S. Food and Drug Administration (FDA). Before November 1991, hospitals, their employees, and staffs were permitted, but not required, to report device malfunctions to the device manufacturer or to the FDA.

On November 28, 1991, the Safe Medical Devices Act of 1990 (Fl 10 1-629) became effective just after proposed regulations (called the Tentative Final Rule) were published for comment. This act requires user facilities (which include hospitals and ambulatory surgery facilities, but not physician offices) to report to the manufacturer medical device malfunctions that result in serious illness, injury, or death to a patient. They are also required to report to the FDA those that result in a patient's death. A serious illness or injury includes not only a life-threatening injury or illness but also an injury that requires "immediate medical or surgical intervention to preclude permanent impairment of a body function or permanent damage to a body structure."[5] Therefore, the rupture of an intra-aortic balloon pump that requires that the balloon-dependent patient immediately be transported to the operating room for removal and replacement of the device is a reportable event.

Nursing and other staff must now participate in reporting device malfunctions, including those associated with user error, to a designated hospital department. Personnel in that area are usually responsible for determining which malfunctions engender an

obligation to report and to whom they should be reported.

More recently, the FDA has implemented a new tracking system in which hospitals must participate. As of March 1, 1993, facilities that implant certain devices (e.g., pacemakers, heart valves, or silicone breast implants) must notify the manufacturer when the devices are implanted. They must also maintain files that the hospital can use to determine the identities and certain other information about patients in whom the devices have been implanted.[6]

There is a duty not to use equipment that is patently defective. If the equipment suddenly ceases to do what it was intended to do, makes unusual noises, or has a history of malfunction and has not been repaired, the hospital could be liable for damage caused by it. Likewise, the nurses could be liable if they know or should know of these problems and use the equipment anyway. The following cases involved liability for defective equipment.

DEFECTIVE EQUIPMENT AND PATIENT INJURIES

In one recent case, Mr. T. underwent a partial right nephrectomy for renal cancer. Postoperatively, an ICU nurse noted a "skin tear" on his coccyx. A dressing was applied to the area, and he was subsequently discharged home. Ten days after discharge, he was evaluated at a wound center, where the ostomy wound nurse reported that the area was "suspicious for a burn." Burn ointment was prescribed, and the patient was referred to a burn center for evaluation. The physician at the burn center diagnosed a "nonhealing wound to bilateral buttocks, probable third-degree." He was admitted for 3 weeks because of a secondary staphylococcal and herpes simplex infection at the wound site.

The patient sued the hospital that performed his nephrectomy, alleging that he was burned by the cautery machine during his surgery and that the nurses had failed to adequately evaluate and treat his wound during the initial hospitalization. The hospital and nurses contended that his wound was due to a decubitus ulcer. Both the trial and appeals courts found that there was insufficient evidence of negligence and dismissed the case against the hospital and nurses.[7]

DEFECTIVE EQUIPMENT AND NEGLIGENCE

Baby K. suffered a cardiac arrest during surgery and was treated after surgery with a hypothermia machine. Although the nurse knew that the continuous-readout thermometer often malfunctioned, she did not check it with a glass thermometer. After the infant's temperature did not decrease, the nurse did not use other methods to lower body temperature, nor did she call a physician. The infant had a seizure and required mechanical ventilation. The nurse noticed poor air exchange but did not correct a kink in the ventilator tubing. The infant suffered permanent neurologic damage. The court held that the injury was proximately caused by the negligence of the hospital's employees and by the defective equipment used in the ICU.[8]

THE NEED FOR CONSENT

In most instances, the law requires that the patient be given enough information before a treatment to make an informed, intelligent decision. However, in some situations, such consent is not required. For example, an emergency situation does not require informed consent, and a patient can waive informed consent by stating that he or she does not want information about a proposed treatment or procedure. In addition, some courts allow a physician to avoid full disclosure if the information disclosed might lead to further patient harm. This exception is known as therapeutic privilege.

Usually, obtaining informed consent from the patient or the family is the responsibility of the physician, but the nurse is frequently asked to witness signing of the consent form. In these cases, the nurse is attesting that the signature on the consent form is the patient's or the family member's. When the nurse actually witnesses the physician's explanation concerning the nature of the proposed treatment, the risks and benefits of the treatment, alternative treatments, and potential consequences if the patient decides to do nothing, the nurse may want to place a note on the consent form or in the nurse's notes stating "consent procedure witnessed." This information may be vital in the rare case in which the patient or family sues the physician for lack of informed consent.

• Issues That Involve Life-Support Measures

Several basic issues regarding refusal and termination of treatment can involve the critical care nurse. Do not resuscitate (DNR) orders, refusal of treatment for religious reasons, advance directives, and withdrawal of life support are all complex topics that fall into this category.

DO NOT RESUSCITATE (DNR) ORDERS

CPR success rates for those receiving in-hospital care are quite variable and are affected by patient environment and resuscitative factors.[9] However, CPR is not appropriate for all patients who experience a cardiac arrest because it is highly invasive and may constitute a "positive violation of an individual's right to die with dignity." Furthermore, CPR may not be indicated when the illness is terminal and irreversible and when the patient can gain no benefit.

Prestigious authorities (e.g., the President's Commission for the Study of Ethical Problems in Medicine and Biomedical and Behavioral Research; hereafter "the President's Commission") have recommended that hospitals have an explicit policy on the practice of writing and implementing DNR orders.[10] Most hospitals and medical societies, and some states, have published DNR policies.[11]

Whether to resuscitate any patient is a decision that is made by the attending physician, the patient,

and the family, although critical care nurses and other nurses often have substantial input into the decision. However, in general, the consent of a competent patient should be required when a DNR order is written. If the patient is incompetent, the physician and family members make the decision. The situation can be more complex, and the physician and the family or patient can disagree.

Once the DNR decision has been made, the order should be written, signed, and dated by the responsible physician. It should be reviewed periodically; hospital policies may require review every 24 to 72 hours. The more informal methods of designating patients with whom CPR is not to be undertaken can lead to errors if an arrest occurs. For example, the wrong patient can be allowed to die.

If an arrest occurs in an emergency department or in another situation in which a formal DNR decision has not been made and written, the presumption of the medical and nursing staffs should be in favor of life, and a code should be called. A "slow code" (in which the nurse takes excessive time to call or the health care team takes its time responding) is never permissible. Either CPR is indicated, or it is not.

Courts may be involved in DNR decisions. In 1978, a Massachusetts appellate court ruled that an attending physician may lawfully write a DNR order for an incompetent patient for whom there is no lifesaving or life-prolonging treatment.[12] In a 1984 case, a New York grand jury investigated a hospital that indicated DNR decisions by using purple dots stuck to nursing cards that were discarded after the death of the patient. Nurses from the hospital complained that the decals could be stuck to the wrong patient's card; in one case, a card had two dots affixed to it. The grand jury found that the dot system "virtually eliminated professional accountability, invited clerical error and discouraged physicians from obtaining informed consent from the patient or his family."[13]

DECISIONS CONCERNING VENTILATOR DISCONTINUATION

Mrs. L., a 64-year-old woman with diabetes, was admitted to the hospital with complaints of weakness, a low-grade fever, a nonproductive cough, frequent urination, anorexia, and malaise. On admission, her blood glucose was low and she was indeed febrile. Her attending physician placed her on ampicillin sodium/sulbactam sodium (Unasyn), a broad-spectrum antibiotic, and adjusted her insulin dosage. The day after Mrs. L.'s admission, she suffered a respiratory arrest, was resuscitated, and had her cardiac function restored. She was intubated and placed on mechanical ventilation. During the arrest she sustained severe neurologic damage.

Two days after her arrest, Mrs. L. remained unresponsive, with fixed, dilated pupils and no purposeful movements, and did not respond to external stimuli. The chief of neurology consulted with the family, suggesting that no significant recovery was possible. The neurologist proposed that the patient be removed from mechanical ventilation and placed on patient-assisted ventilation. If she had no brain function, she would not breathe and would die. Her family was aware that if she could not assist with ventilation she would die.

Mrs. L. was removed from the mechanical ventilator and died shortly after being placed on patient-assisted ventilation. She did not have a living will, health care proxy, or notation concerning her wishes regarding life support. Further, she had never made her wishes known to her family. The family subsequently sued the physicians and the hospital, alleging medical malpractice on the grounds that the physicians neither acted according to the state statute pertaining to continuation or removal of life support systems nor followed hospital protocol.

After review of applicable state law and the hospital's policies, the trial court concluded that brain death was not necessary in order to place Mrs. L. on assisted ventilation. The lawsuits against the physicians and hospital were dismissed. This dismissal was upheld on appeal.[14]

Unfortunately, it is estimated that as few as 4% to 24% of Americans have an advance directive.[15–17] An advance directive can help with troublesome decisions such as those that were faced by both the family and the health care team in this case. The case was unclear as to whether Mrs. L. received advance directive information at the time of her admission, but this certainly would have been helpful. It is also important for patients to speak with their families and their attending physician concerning end-of-life decisions. Relevant references on the ethical issues surrounding advance directives are found in the works cited previously.

REFUSAL OF TREATMENT FOR RELIGIOUS REASONS

LIFESAVING TRANSFUSION FOR A JEHOVAH'S WITNESS

Ms. W., a 32-year-old Jehovah's Witness and the single mother of two young children, was admitted to the emergency department after an accident; she suffered from internal bleeding. The physician ordered an immediate blood transfusion and surgery, stating that with it she would most likely recover, but without it she would likely die. The patient refused the transfusion for religious reasons. When she refused the transfusion, the charge nurse and physician notified hospital counsel immediately. They were concerned because the woman was the sole guardian of her two young children. A court authorized the blood transfusion. The patient received the transfusion and survived the accident.[18]

The courts are divided as to whether blood transfusions violate the religious rights of the patient or family. For example, in one case, the Connecticut Supreme Court found that a hospital cannot "thrust unwanted medical care on a patient who . . . compe-

tently and clearly denied that care." Consequently, ICU nurses need to consult the hospital's risk management department or legal counsel in such situations to ensure proper handling of these types of legal issues.[19]

ADVANCE DIRECTIVES: LIVING WILLS AND POWERS OF ATTORNEY

A living will is a written directive from a competent patient to family and health care team members concerning the patient's wishes in the event the patient is unable to express these wishes. One difficulty associated with a living will is its limited applicability. In most states, a living will becomes effective only if the patient is terminally ill or permanently comatose. Consequently, when the patient is critically ill or temporarily unable to make health care decisions, the living will is not operative.

To provide broader coverage, many patients opt for a durable power of attorney for health care. A durable power of attorney allows the patient to appoint a surrogate decision maker, known as a health care agent or proxy, who has authority to make treatment and health care decisions in the event that the patient is not able to do so. This type of document allows a trusted friend or relative to "stand in the shoes of the patient" when the patient is not able to make health care decisions.

Many savvy patients elect to combine the living will and the durable power of attorney for health care into one document, commonly called an advance directive. An advance directive allows the patient to communicate his or her wishes in the event of terminal illness or a permanently comatose state. It also names an agent who assists in decision making. Many advance directives give the health care agent specific instructions concerning health matters. For example, the advance directive may provide instructions concerning artificial nutrition and hydration, or it may outline specific treatments, such as a "no code" status under specified circumstances.

In response to federal law,[20] all 50 states have statutes that allow patients to execute living wills, durable powers of attorney for health care, and advance directives. However, each state may place unique requirements on the drafting of these documents. Some states require that the directive be notarized. Other states mandate that the patient be counseled by a state-appointed ombudsman who outlines the pros and cons associated with the advance directive. Witness requirements also vary from state to state. Consequently, it is important to know the laws concerning advance directives that apply in your state. An excellent starting point is the living wills/advance directive web page of the American Association of Retired Persons. This group provides lay people and health care providers with up-to-date information on laws applicable in their state.

In most states, it is likely that a recent living will would be taken as evidence of what the patient would have wanted had he or she been competent when the decision was presented. Although there have not been any cases concerning a written living will, there have been several involving patients who had expressed wishes orally about life-sustaining measures.

RECENT LEGAL DEVELOPMENTS

In the matter of *Schiavo v. Schiavo,*[21] the United States was drawn into a legal and emotional battle over the issue of the right to die and, barring advance directives, who may speak for an unconscious patient. Theresa (Terri) Schiavo was in a vegetative state for 13 years. In 2003, Ms. Schiavo's husband, Michael, petitioned to cease his wife's feeding and hydration over the objections of her parents and brother.

In response, Terri's parents, Robert and Mary Schindler, led a battle before the Florida State Courts, the U.S. Courts of Appeal, the Florida State Legislature and Executive Branch, the U.S. Congress, the White House and, eventually, the U.S. Supreme Court.[22] Aside from the legal activities, the parties to the action also tried Terri's circumstances and future before the court of public opinion.

This legal process occurs with greater frequency than the general public believes. When a disabled person is unable to coherently understand or speak on his or her own behalf, the law requires that health care providers first obtain the patient's personal advance directives, documents that are familiar to most health care providers. Often, however, no advance directives were executed before the patient's disability; for this reason, many states have enacted laws allowing family members to act on behalf of the patient. These laws often give one relative priority over decision making. Thus, a spouse may have more authority than the patient's parents, or a family member may have more authority than a good friend of the patient. Courts have repeatedly struggled over who should make decisions about the disabled patient's care when relatives cannot agree on the appropriate plan of care for the patient, such as occurred in the Schiavo case.

The Schiavo case is representative of a typical guardianship action. The petitioner (e.g., Michael Schiavo) petitioned the court to act on behalf of the alleged disabled (e.g., his wife, Terri). Notice of the proposed order to name Mr. Schiavo as Terri's guardian was given to all interested persons, including any known relatives, such as Mr. and Mrs. Schindler.[21] In addition, courts also appoint a *temporary* guardian ad litem, who was charged with the duty to represent the interests of the alleged disabled. The temporary guardian ad litem, usually an attorney, is an independent, disinterested party whose responsibilities are to review the medical records, interview all medical providers, interview the petitioner (i.e., Mr. Schiavo) and any interested persons, and most importantly, interview the alleged disabled as to his or her mental and physical capacity. The temporary guardian ad litem reports independently to the court on his or her findings of the status of the alleged disabled.

A custodial hearing was held allowing the petitioner, witnesses, and any other interested persons to testify as to (1) the competency of the alleged disabled, (2) whether the alleged disabled would be best served with a guardianship, and (3) who would be best to act as *permanent* guardian ad litem. In deciding these issues, the courts place great weight on the findings of the temporary guardian ad litem.

Michael Schiavo prevailed in maintaining his position as permanent guardian ad litem of Terri.[22] After her tube feeding was discontinued, she eventually died as a consequence of dehydration and malnutrition. As a result of this and other cases, families throughout the nation may be faced with the awful possibility of being pitted emotionally, legally, and monetarily against each other when advance directives are not executed.

Nurses, particularly those working in critical care areas, are frequently confronted with patients who are incompetent to understand the nature of their care. Nurses are instrumental in educating patients, families, friends, and society about the importance of understanding and executing advance directives. From an attorney's perspective, the consensus is, "Pay me a little now to prepare a valid advance directive, or pay me dearly when we need to litigate guardianship and end-of-life issues."

PATIENT SELF-DETERMINATION ACT

On December 1, 1991, the Patient Self-Determination Act went into effect.[20] This federal statute is applicable to facilities that receive Medicare reimbursement for patient care. As a condition of reimbursement, the law requires that hospitals, nursing facilities, home health care services, hospice programs, and certain health maintenance organizations provide information to adults about their rights concerning decision making in that state. For hospitals, this information must be provided to every adult on admission regardless of diagnosis and regardless of whether the person is eligible for Medicare coverage. The material distributed must include information about the types of advance directives that are legal in that state. Documentation that the patient has received this information must be placed in the medical record. If the patient is incapacitated on admission, the information must be provided to a family member, if available. However, this action does not relieve the hospital of its duty to provide information to the patient once he or she is no longer incapacitated.

WITHDRAWAL OF LIFE-SUPPORT MEASURES

What constitutes life support, when these measures must be used, and when they may be terminated are issues that have been raised in many court cases. However, the law in these areas is still developing and will continue to do so as each state creates its own guidelines.

Given the regularity with which life-support decisions must be made in health care facilities, it is remarkable that it was not until 1976 that the first case, *In re Quinlan,* focused national attention on the "right to die" controversy. The cases concern competent minors and adults who have a disease or condition that would eventually be terminal. States have not been consistent in their decisions, even when the situations are arguably similar. For example, the New Jersey court in the case of Karen Ann Quinlan, a 21-year-old woman in a persistent vegetative state, held that the decision about treatment is in the hands of the patient's guardian in consultation with the hospital ethics committee.[23] However, Massachusetts rejected the New Jersey approach in favor of judicial review of decisions made by physicians and family members.[24] The President's Commission stated (p. 6) that judicial review of these decisions should be reserved for occasions when "adjudication is clearly required by state law or when concerned parties have disagreements that they cannot resolve over matters of substantial import."[10]

RIGHT TO REFUSE TREATMENT

Ms. B. was a 28-year-old woman who suffered from severe cerebral hemorrhage. Although mentally competent, she was a quadriplegic. She was a patient at a public hospital and was totally dependent on the care of others. Eventually, her physical condition deteriorated to the point that she required nasogastric tube feedings. Ms. B. requested that the hospital remove the nasogastric tube and resort only to those feedings that she could tolerate orally. The trial court concluded that physically she tolerated the nasogastric tube and that it was not a great physical discomfort. The California Court of Appeals, Second District reversed the trial court and ordered that the hospital remove Ms. B.'s nasogastric tube and that clinicians not replace it or aid in replacing it without her express consent.[25]

RIGHT TO RESTRICT FOOD AND FLUIDS

Nancy Cruzan, a young woman who suffered anoxic brain damage in an automobile accident, remained in a persistent vegetative state in Missouri and was fed by gastrostomy. After rehabilitation was unsuccessful, Ms. Cruzan's parents (as co-guardians) requested withdrawal of the feeding tube. After the employees of the residential rehabilitation center where Ms. Cruzan was receiving care refused to withdraw the feedings, her parents sought judicial review of their request. After testimony, the trial court approved the parents' request.

On appeal, the Missouri Supreme Court reversed the lower court. First, it held that Missouri law does not permit surrogate decision making in decisions of this importance. For a person to exercise the right to terminate artificial feeding in Missouri, that person must have previously expressed his or her wishes, either orally or in writing. Evidence of those wishes had to meet a relatively high evidentiary standard, a standard that the court held had been met in the lower court proceeding.

This case was appealed to the U.S. Supreme Court, and in 1990, it was affirmed on constitutional grounds.[26] After the decision was issued, the Cruzans returned to the Missouri lower court and presented further evidence (through additional witnesses) about what their daughter had expressed while competent. The lower court found that they had presented clear and convincing evidence and affirmed the rights of the co-guardians to authorize withdrawal of the feeding tube. After withdrawal of the tube, Nancy Cruzan died on December 26, 1990.

It is important to note that although the Cruzan case is still applicable law, the way in which this landmark case has been interpreted and implemented has been extremely variable at state court levels. Although this case received much publicity, it did not change the law in any state but Missouri. Most states continue to permit surrogate decision making by relatives and require a lower evidentiary standard than that required in Missouri. Also note that, unlike the Schiavo case described previously, family members were all in agreement that Ms. Cruzan's artificial nutrition and hydration should be discontinued.

RIGHT TO TERMINATE TREATMENT

In the case *In re the Conservatorship of Wanglie,* Mrs. W., who was ventilator dependent and competent, had a cardiopulmonary arrest. After this event, she remained in a persistent vegetative state. Pursuant to the wishes of the family, she was nourished by feeding tube and treated aggressively for recurrent pneumonia. Hospital staff disagreed with the family in this case, and intervention by the hospital ethics committee did not resolve the conflict. Therefore, the hospital filed an application for a non–family member guardian to decide for the patient. The state court instead appointed Mr. W., her husband, as guardian, determining that he was in the best position to know his wife's wishes. The court found that the hospital had requested the appointment of a non–family member not because Mr. W. was incompetent to be guardian but because he disagreed with hospital staff.[27]

In recent years, as health care providers have become more comfortable recommending termination of treatment in selected cases, they have met resistance from some families who wish to continue treatment no matter what its chance of success. Although no law or legal principle requires that extraordinary, but clearly futile, treatment be provided, it is probably also true that health care providers have no legal recourse against families who refuse to withdraw life support, that is, unless the patient has left written indications of his or her wishes before incompetence.

In most states, problems of terminating treatment need not be resolved in court. Decisions regarding treatment or nontreatment that meet accepted medical standards and with which the patient concurs are made virtually every day in health care settings. If the patient is not competent to decide, usually family members may do so, although they may not refuse therapy that would benefit the patient. Finally, a distinction should be made between termination of treatment and termination of care. Even patients who are not being treated for their terminal condition require competent and sensitive nursing and medical care so that their final days are as comfortable as possible. The families of these patients may also require information along with sensitive emotional support. The need for good nursing care does not end with the decision not to treat.

For an excellent review of all the issues concerning advance directives, right to refuse treatment, and restriction of patient treatments, refer to Beauchamp and Walters' book, *Contemporary Issues in Bioethics.*[11]

BRAIN DEATH

In 1968, the Harvard criteria established standards for determining brain death. The criteria have been found quite reliable. Some states adopted the Harvard criteria by statute, whereas other states enacted legislation defining brain death in broader, less restrictive terms.

The President's Commission published *Defining Death* in July 1981. The Commission recommended a uniform statute defining death; it recommended that the statute address "general physiological standards rather than medical criteria and tests, which will change with advances in biomedical knowledge and refinements in technique."[28] All states have laws addressing the definition of death in the state. Some states use brain death as the sole criterion; other states rely on a number of factors, such as response to pain and cessation of cardiac function. It is important that the nurse know the legal definition of death in any state where he or she is practicing, although such a determination typically rests with the patient's attending physician and may also require the concurrence of other consulting physicians.

A patient who is brain-dead is legally dead, and there is no legal duty to continue to treat him or her. It is not necessary to obtain court approval to discontinue life support on a patient who is brain-dead. Furthermore, although it can be desirable to obtain family permission to discontinue treatment of a brain-dead patient, there is no legal requirement. However, before terminating life support, physicians and nurses should be sure that organs are not intended for transplantation purposes.

ORGAN DONATION

Every state in the United States has a law based on the Uniform Anatomical Gift Act. The statutes establish the legality of organ donation by people and their families and set procedures for making and accepting the gift of an organ. Every state also has some provision to enable people to consent to organ donation using a designated place on a driver's license. More recently, many states have enacted "required request" laws. These laws attempt to increase the supply of organs for transplantation by requiring hospital personnel to ask patients' families about an organ gift at the time of the patient's death.

• Clinical Applicability Challenges

Short-Answer Questions

1. You are the charge nurse in the ICU on night shift. One of the nurses on your shift reports to work smelling of alcohol. What should you do? What legal principles may be applicable if you allow this nurse to care for patients and a patient is subsequently injured?

2. Mr. M. is a patient on your unit. He has chronic obstructive pulmonary disease and suffers a respiratory arrest. He has not drafted any type of advance directive, but you are aware that he has spoken to his family about his wishes in the event he is no longer able to make his desires known concerning extraordinary care. As a nurse caring for Mr. M., what legal issues do you feel are of relevance? Whom can you turn to concerning this dilemma?

Review Questions

1. The doctrine of respondeat superior is the legal theory under which
   a. a hospital is directly liable for its corporate hiring decisions.
   b. a health care provider is personally liable for acts of negligence.
   c. an employer is vicariously liable for the negligent acts of its employees as long as they act within the scope of employment.
   d. a hospital is liable for injuries to its employees.

2. The Patient Self-Determination Act went into effect in 1991. This federal law requires that hospitals, nursing homes, and certain other providers
   a. provide patients with information about advance directives and require them to execute at least one type of advance directive.
   b. provide patients with information about living wills only.
   c. provide patients with information about all types of advance directives applicable in that state.
   d. provide patients with information about all types of advance directives, regardless of whether the information is applicable in that state.

3. A living will is applicable under which of the following circumstances?
   a. The patient is incapacitated and is terminally ill.
   b. The patient is incapacitated and has a life-threatening but curable illness.
   c. The patient is competent to express his or her wishes, has a desire to be treated, and has subsequently become incapacitated.
   d. The patient is competent but wants his or her grown children to make the health care decisions.

References

1. National Council of State Boards of Nursing: Complaints. Available at https://www.ncsbn.org

2. Las Collinas Medical et al v. Bush, 122 SW3d 835 (TX App 2nd Dist), 2003

3. Martin v. The Fulton-DeKalb Hospital Authority d/b/a Grady Memorial Hospital d/b/a Grady Health System et al, 2001 Ga. App. LEXIS 762, 1 Fulton County DR 2168, 2001

4. U.S. v. Wood, 207 F.3d 1222; 2000 U.S. App. LEXIS 5475, 2000 Colo J. C.A.R. 1645, 2000

5. U.S. Department of Health and Human Services, Food and Drug Administration: Medical devices: Medical device, user facility, distributor, and manufacturer reporting, certification and registration. Federal Register 56:64004–64182, December 6, 1991

6. U.S. Department of Health and Human Services, Food and Drug Administration: Medical devices: Device tracking. Federal Register 57:22971–22981, May 29, 1992

7. Carter v. Anderson Memorial Hospital, 325 S.E.2d 78 (S.C. App.), 1985

8. Rose v. Hakim, 335 F. Supp. 1221 (DDC) 1971, affirmed in part, reversed in part, 501 F.2d 806 (DC Cir), 1974

9. Dumot JA, Burval DJ, Sprung J, et al: Outcome of adult cardiopulmonary resuscitations at a tertiary referral center including results of "limited" resuscitations. Arch Intern Med 161(14):1751–1758, 2001

10. President's Commission for the Study of Ethical Problems in Medicine and Biomedical and Behavioral Research: Deciding to forego life-sustaining treatment. Washington, DC, U.S. Government Printing Office, March 1983

11. Beauchamp TL, Walters L: Contemporary Issues in Bioethics, 5th ed. Belmont, CA, Wadsworth, 1999

12. Matter of Dinnerstein; 380 NE2d 134, Massachusetts, 1978

13. Panel accuses hospital of hiding denial of care. New York Times, March 21, 1984

14. Law v. Camp et al, 116 F. Supp. 2d 295 (CT), 2000

15. Center for Bioethics: Advanced directives. Retrieved March 1, 2004, from http://www.bioethics.umn.edu/resources/topics/advance_directives.shtml

16. Huffman GB: Benefits of discussing advance directives with patients. Retrieved March 1, 2004, from http://www.aafp.org/afp/20010715/tips/4.html

17. Ackermann RJ: Withholding and withdrawing life-sustaining treatment. Retrieved March 1, 2004, from http://www.aafp.org/afp/20001001/1555.html

18. Novak v. Cobb County Kennestone Hospital Authority, No 94-8403 (11th Cir), February 14, 1996

19. Stamford Hosp. v. Vega, 646 (CT), 1996

20. Omnibus Budget Reconciliation Act of 1990. Pub. L. No. 101-508 §§4206, 4751 (codified in scattered sections of 42 USC, particularly §§1395cc, 1396a) (West Supp), 1991

21. Michael Schiavo, as Guardian of the person of Theresa Marie Schiavo, v. Jeb Bush, Governor of the State of Florida, and Charlie Crist, Attorney General of the State of Florida, Florida Circuit Court Civil Case No. 03-008212-CI-20 (2004).

22. Schiavo v. Schiavo, DC CV-05-00530-T, U.S. 11th Circuit Court of Appeals, 2005. See also, Bush v. Schiavo, Case No. SC04-925, Supreme Court of Florida. The U.S. Supreme Court denied the Schindlers' petition for a stay of action without any further opinion, thus allowing the removal of Terri's tube feeding (S Ct Order 04A825), March 24, 2005

23. In re Quinlan, 70 NJ 10, 355 A2d 647, New Jersey, 1976

24. Superintendent of Belchertown State School v. Saikewicz, 373 Mass. 728, 370 NE2d 417, Massachusetts, 1977

25. Bouvia v. Superior Court, 225 Cal Rptr 297 (Cal App 2 Dist), 1986

26. Cruzan v. Director, Missouri Department of Health et al, III L Ed2d 224, 110 S Ct 2841, 1990

27. In re the Conservatorship of Wanglie, No. PX-91-283 (Minn Dist Ct, Probate Ct Division), July 1991

28. President's Commission for the Study of Ethical Problems in Medicine and Biomedical and Behavioral Research: Defining death. Washington, DC, U.S. Government Printing Office, July 1981, p 1

Building a Professional Practice Model for Excellence in Critical Care Nursing

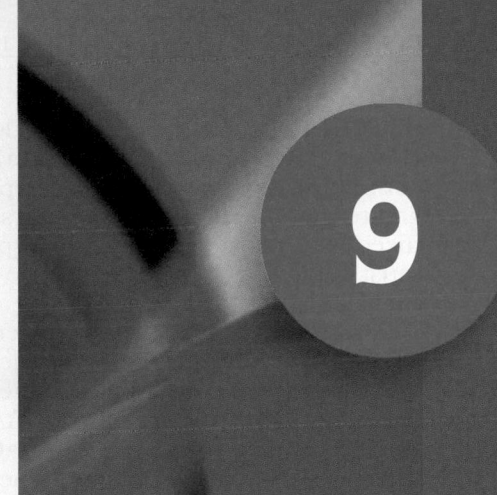

9

Janie Heath

Objectives

Based on the content in this chapter, the reader should be able to:

❶ Discuss nursing professionalism and nursing excellence.

❷ Recognize characteristics of professional development.

❸ Explore personal and professional attributes to build a professional practice model of critical care nursing excellence.

In today's fast-paced critical care environment, nurses respond to the needs of patients and families who have entered a chaotic and frightening world of illness, trauma, and pain. Often, finding the time for professional growth can be challenging. Building a professional practice of excellence requires a "passion" to profoundly affect the lives of patients and families. At the same time, it requires advancing the critical care nursing profession through evidence-based practice, best practice models of care, or both. This chapter discusses how a professional practice for excellence in critical care nursing can be built with the attributes of values, vision, mastery, passion, action, and balance as the framework.

• Defining the Critical Care Nurse

Like their patients and patients' families, critical care nurses are an exceptional and diverse group of people. Knowledgeable, highly skilled, and caring are a few of the professional attributes that can be applied to critical care nurses. However, the term *nursing professionalism* may bring to mind different images, especially to health care consumers. To some, nursing professionalism still means wearing a crisp, clean, white uniform, whereas to others, regardless of the uniform, it means demonstrating a high level of intellectual, interpersonal, ethical, and clinical skills. Kalisch and Kalisch first reported on the image of nursing in the early 1980s. They found that "90% of the public thought nurses were nice ladies who help doctors."[1]

Critical care nurses know all too well that responding to lethal dysrhythmias, administering blood products, and weaning patients from ventilators is more about having a specialized body of knowledge, competent skills, and clinical experience in holistic nursing than just "helping doctors." For both the novice and the experienced critical care nurse, the journey of nursing professionalism and nursing excellence goes beyond the bedside skills required to take care of the sickest and most vulnerable patients and families. Critical care nursing started being recognized as a specialty when the first intensive care units (ICUs) emerged in the 1950s, yet Buresh and Gordon have found increasing evidence of a large communication gap between the profession and the greater public.[2] If critical care nursing is to be recognized as a respected and valued profession, nurses must boldly speak up to define who they are and what they do.

A starting point to define who critical care nurses are can be found in the annual demographic membership survey conducted by the American Association of Critical-Care Nurses (AACN), the world's largest specialty nursing organization.[3] Since 1969, the AACN has been serving the needs of more than 400,000 nurses who care for critically ill patients and their families. With a steady membership of approximately 65,000 nurses, the majority of members (55%) are between the ages of 40 and 49 years of age and have a Bachelor of Science in Nursing (Fig. 9-1A).[3] With an average income between $55,000 and $74,999 per year, the majority of members (25%) have been in critical care practice for more than 20 years (see Fig. 9-1B).[3] Although the profession continues to be predominantly female (90%), the number of men in critical care is increasing (10%), according to the AACN membership survey.[3] The largest ethnic background represented was white (82%), followed by Asian (10%), African American (4%), Hispanic (2%), and Native American (1%).[3] Of interest, the AACN

membership data are consistent with the average findings of today's 2.9 million registered nurses (RNs) reported by the 2004 National Sample Survey of Registered Nurses.[4]

It is important to evaluate such data because this helps drive decision making and determine trends, issues, and policy and advocacy implications that affect critical care nursing practice, patients and families, and systems. Currently, 83% of the AACN membership surveyed work full time. Of these members, the majority (17%) work in combined ICU and coronary care unit (CCU) settings, 15% work in ICU settings, 7% work in CCU, 6% work in progressive care and telemetry stepdown units, 5% work in surgical ICU settings, 4% work in medical ICU settings, and 4% work in emergency department settings. The remaining top categories make up less than 4% of the total and include the recovery room, pediatric ICU, medical-surgical ICU, catheterization laboratory, trauma unit, cardiovascular-surgical ICU, and neuro-neurosurgical ICU (Fig. 9-2A).[3] Most of the AACN members surveyed (66%) have positions providing direct care as staff nurses (see Fig. 9-2B). The AACN membership data are consistent with the average findings of Kirchhoff and Dahl's national survey of facilities and units that provide critical care.[5] Their study revealed that 74% of the facilities participating in the study were nongovernment, not-for-profit organizations with a mean of 217 operating beds and 13,000 admissions per year.[5]

• Defining Nursing Professionalism

The struggle to define nursing professionalism expands beyond critical care environments. For many years there has been an ongoing dialogue about whether nursing is a true profession. Kelly emphasized that the status of nursing as a profession is important because it reflects the value society places on the work of nurses.[6] However, some think that because entry into nursing practice does not require a baccalaureate degree, it is, at best, an emerging profession that requires new models of nursing education.[7] Such new models, the clinical nurse leader and doctorate of nursing practice, are believed to help ensure quality patient outcomes and patient safety.[7,8] However, others believe that the nursing profession has made adequate progress to meet full-fledged professional status with current models of nursing education.[9]

One of the first definitions of professionalism came from Abraham Flexner, who wrote the classic Flexner Report in the early 1900s to reform medical education.[10] Flexner defines professionalism as a process by which an occupation achieves professional status. Although other professions have developed their own criteria, Flexner's work remains the benchmark and foundation for many. Kelly (1981) was the first to expand his work for the nursing profession by providing a theoretical framework from which pro-

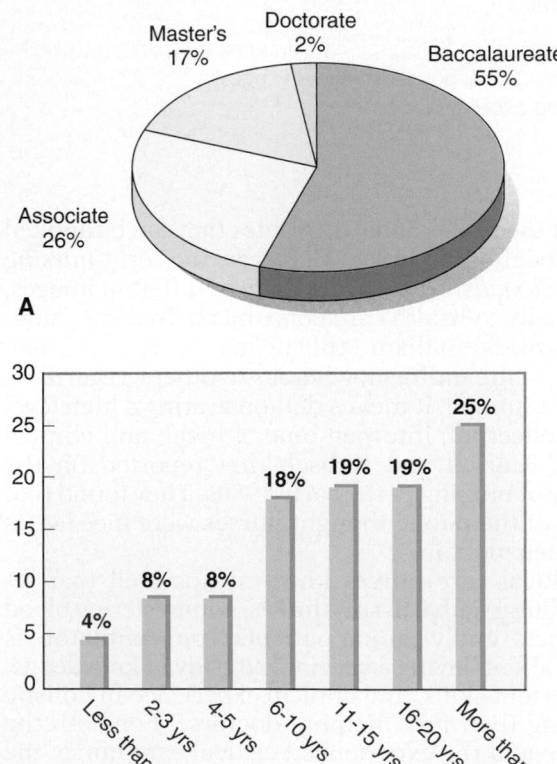

Figure 9-1 • Mastery of the profession. **A:** The nursing degrees earned by critical care nurses. **B:** Years of experience in critical care nursing. (From American Association of Critical-Care Nurses: 2005 Demographics. Retrieved August 1, 2006, from http://www.aacn.org.)

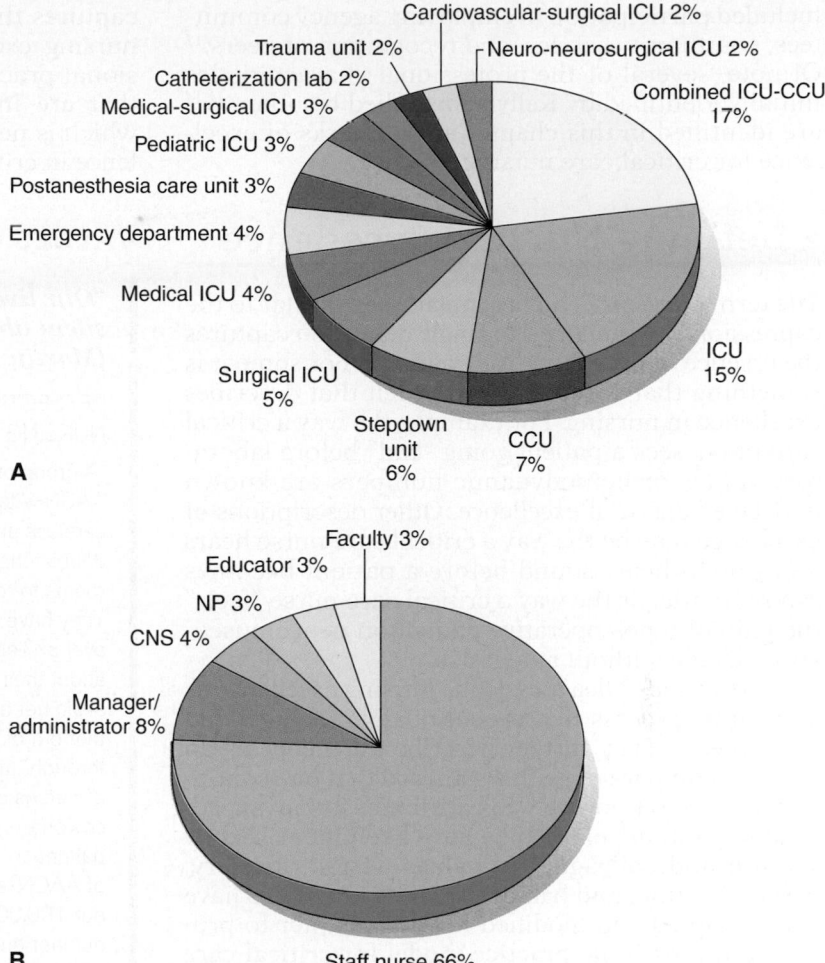

Figure 9-2 • Who are critical care nurses? **A:** Practice settings for critical care nurses. **B:** The positions held by critical care nurses. (From American Association of Critical-Care Nurses: 2005 Demographics. Retrieved August 1, 2006, from http://www.aacn.org.)

fessional nursing characteristics are defined today[6] (Box 9-1).

To a great extent, the criteria addressed by Flexner and Kelly are only as good as the person who takes personal responsibility and accountability for committing to a professional role. One legendary nurse leader, Margretta Styles, argued that professionalism

of nursing can only be achieved through the "professionhood" of its members.[7] Like Kelly, Styles believes there must be a sense of social significance, commitment to the ultimacy of professional performance, and appreciation of collegiality and collectivity.[7] However, as Styles approached the end of her nursing career, she proposed a new term to phrase the work of nurses: *professionalist.*[7] In her words, "professionalists strive to build a solid foundation for their calling—an ethical, academic, political, and socioeconomic foundation to serve as the underpinning for a strong profession to evolve and serve."[7(p 89)]

Researchers have investigated how to describe professionalism among critical care nurses as well. In 1994, Holl investigated such critical care nursing characteristics as professional beliefs, decision making, level of education, membership of professional nursing organization, and certification.[11] Holl found that nurses who continue their education and belong to professional organizations are more likely than others to be independent thinkers and to participate in creative problem solving.[11] In a similar study, Heath and colleagues found that there was a high level of "passion about nursing and promoting the profession" and that self-motivation was the leading influential factor for fostering individual professional development among critical care nurses.[12] Other professional development characteristics evaluated included participation in employing agency committees, community service, and recognition of peers.[12] Of note, several of the professional characteristics initially identified by Kelly and studied by others[13,14] are identified in this chapter as hallmarks of excellence for critical care nursing practice.

• Defining Nursing Excellence

The term *excellence* can be a misnomer similar to the expression *best practice*. No single definition captures the essence of excellence for everyone. For some it is something that is seen, heard, or felt that describes excellence in nursing. For example, the way a critical care nurse sees a patient going "bad" before laboratory values or hemodynamic numbers are known may be evidence of excellence. Other descriptions of excellence may be the way a critical care nurse hears an S_3 or S_4 heart sound before a patient becomes symptomatic, or the way a critical care nurse "feels" the pain of a postoperative patient on neuromuscular blockade without analgesics.

Weston and colleagues define nursing excellence as a dynamic process that is continually redefined and reinforced.[15] They further describe excellence as an ongoing comparison with a standard that one continuously tries to improve.[10] Six attributes for advanced-practice nursing excellence have been identified by Weston and colleagues as values, vision, mastery, passion, action, and balance.[15] These attributes have been adopted and modified for this chapter to propose a professional practice model for critical care nursing (Fig. 9-3). The foundation for this model consists of strong values and a vision. The supporting structures of the model are composed of mastery, passion, action, and balance. The top of the model captures the essence of the structure: critical care nursing excellence. Each structure of the professional practice model has defining characteristics that are instrumental for ongoing self-reflection, which is necessary to develop and commit to excellence in critical care nursing.

VALUES

"Our lives begin to end the day we become silent about things that matter."
(Martin Luther King Jr.)[16]

REFLECTION ON "VALUES" FOR CRITICAL CARE NURSING EXCELLENCE

"A group of nurses, participating in a focus group for the AACN-VitalSmarts Silence Kills Study, describe a peer as careless and inattentive. Instead of confronting her, they double check her work—sometimes running into patient rooms to retake a blood pressure or redo a safety check. They have 'worked around' this nurse's weaknesses for over a year. The nurses resent her but never talk to her about their concerns, nor do any of the physicians who also avoid her and compensate for her."[17(p 2)] Further data reveal that out of 1,700 health care providers and administrators throughout U.S. hospitals, 84% of physicians and 62% of nurses and other clinical care providers have seen coworkers taking shortcuts that could be dangerous to patients.[17] Kathy McCauley, RN, PhD, FAAN, past president of AACN, said, "This research (Silence Kills) validates what our 100,000 constituents have communicated to us as the number one barrier hindering optimal care for patients. Too often, improving workplace communications is seen as a 'soft' issue—the truth is, we must build environments that support and demand greater candor among staff if we are to make a demonstrable impact on patient safety."[18]

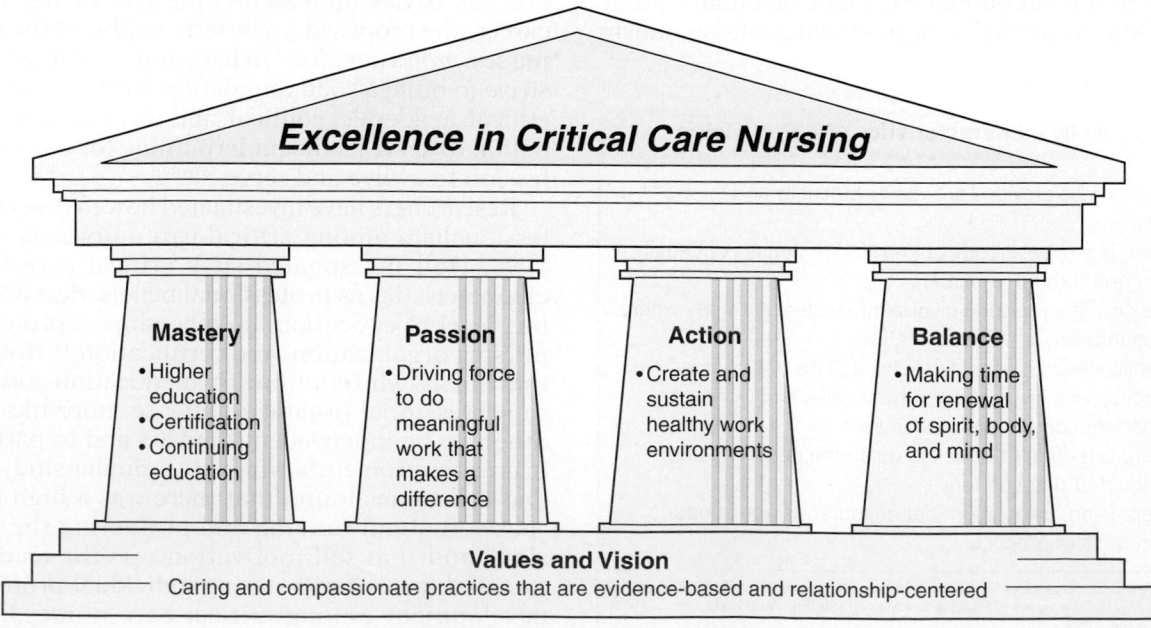

Mastery
• Higher education
• Certification
• Continuing education

Passion
• Driving force to do meaningful work that makes a difference

Action
• Create and sustain healthy work environments

Balance
• Making time for renewal of spirit, body, and mind

Excellence in Critical Care Nursing

Values and Vision
Caring and compassionate practices that are evidence-based and relationship-centered

Figure 9-3 • A professional practice model for critical care nursing.

Do you value communication about competence and accountability? Do you value having a healthy work environment where skilled communication protects patients and fosters collaborative relationships? What are your values to foster critical care nursing excellence?

True excellence is seen when professionals reflect their core values. The values of one's profession, the values of one's employing organization, and one's own personal values are the behaviors that guide professional practice for excellence. The unique contributions that critical care nurses bring to the bedside are often a reflection of an inner core value of caring. It is this deep and personal connection to caring that brings many into the nursing profession. The word *nursing* is derived from the Latin word *nutrire,* which means "to nourish." The term *nurturing* describes an ability to care for, sustain, and provide for another. Critical care nurses are privileged to care for individuals who face life-threatening conditions during the most vulnerable and private times of their lives. It is through this value of altruism (the desire to help others) that critical care nurses have the ability to creatively bridge high-tech and high-touch with everyday practice.

The everyday busyness of critical care nursing is labor intensive, but taking the time to share joyful, painful, and tearful experiences with complex patients and families is the core of critical care nurses' existence. The art of nursing is probably what dominates the image of nursing for the public. Six times since 1999, Gallup polls have reported that the public rates nursing as the most honest and ethical profession.[19] In their book, *From Silence to Voice,* Buresh and Gordon reported that the Gallup poll results about nurses reflect a paradox.[2] As non-nurse authors, they discuss how the public holds nurses in the highest regard, even though the public has limited information about the science that nurses really practice.[2]

There is power in the nursing profession when nurses articulate not only the core values of caring but also evidence-based practice, advocacy, accountability, autonomy, and collaboration. It is now well established that nurses have been silent for too long and that the days of "It is just my job" or " I am just a nurse" need to come to an end.[2,17,20] Campaigns such as AACN's "Bold Voices: Fearless and Essential," "Rising Above," "Live Your Contribution," and "Engage and Transform" help empower nurses to make their voice heard for their patients, families, and profession.[21–24] Strong personal and professional core values at AACN (Box 9-2) inspired a nine-person panel to develop the AACN Healthy Work Environment Standards to help address work environments that tolerate ineffective interpersonal relationships resulting in medical errors, ineffective delivery of care, and conflict and stress among health professionals.[20] Creating and sustaining healthy work environments ensure safe patient care and set a path toward the AACN core value to "commit to quality and excellence."[25]

Box 9-2 • Core Values: American Association of Critical-Care Nurses (AACN)

- **Be accountable** to uphold and consistently act in concert with ethical values and principles.
- **Advocate** for organizational decisions that are driven by the needs of patients and families.
- **Act with integrity** by communicating openly and honestly, keeping promises, honoring commitments, and promoting loyalty in all relationships.
- **Collaborate** with all essential stakeholders by creating synergistic relationships to promote common interest and shared values.
- **Provide leadership** to transform thinking, structures, and processes to address opportunities and challenges.
- **Demonstrate stewardship** through fair and responsible management of resources.
- **Embrace lifelong learning,** inquiry, and critical thinking to enable each to make optimal contributions.
- **Commit to quality and excellence** at all levels of the organization, meeting and exceeding standards and expectations.
- **Promote innovation** through creativity and calculated risk taking.
- **Generate commitment and passion** to the organization's causes and work.

From American Association of Critical-Care Nurses: Core values. Retrieved June 1, 2006, from http://www.aacn.org.

VISION

"There is no power greater than a community discovering what it cares about." (Margaret Wheatley)[16]

REFLECTION ON "VISION" FOR CRITICAL CARE NURSING EXCELLENCE

"Why did I come to work here? Because of the nurse manager. When she interviewed me, she asked me what kind of support I would need from her. The openness of her question impressed me, so I told her. She said she could meet my expectations—not just try. Our manager is respectful of the nurses, of our knowledge, and of what we do. Day after day, her words and actions show that she believes that each of us is very valuable. At unit meetings, she is the one who reminds us that what nurses know is different, but just as important, as what physicians know. She has earned my trust and respect, and I know I have earned hers. That's why I'm here and why I'll stay."[20(p 40)] Debbie Brinker, RN, MSN, CCRN, CCNS, past president of AACN, said, "In order for hospitals and healthcare systems to be truly transformed—to live up to what we call the preferred future—we must be leaders in redesigning our systems to produce outstanding results in patient care and in the experience of those who care for patients. We must reinvent the cumbersome systems we work in and often work around."[24]

Do you have a vision to create a healthy work environment and live that vision in all of your actions? Do you have a vision to develop a culture in which people hold themselves and others accountable to professional standards and collaborative relationships? What is your vision to foster critical care nursing excellence?

A clear vision, based on core values, is essential to building a professional practice model of critical care nursing excellence. It requires envisioning the future's possibilities and then taking the challenge of making the vision a reality. In 2001, the AACN made a strategic decision to promote the creation of healthy work environments that embrace a culture of excellence when taking care of acute and critically ill patients.[20] Based on the escalating evidence from the Institute of Medicine and the Joint Commission on Accreditation of Healthcare Organizations about unhealthy work environments and how they contribute to medical errors, the AACN had a vision to propose solutions to improve patient safety.[26–28] Through a partnership with VitalSmarts, a national study was conducted to evaluate communication and collaboration challenges among hospital providers of care. The findings of the study resulted in the need to develop standards addressing six essential areas: skilled communication, true collaboration, effective decision making, appropriate staffing, meaningful recognition, and authentic leadership.[20]

As risk takers and agents for change, today's critical care nurses are making history by embracing the AACN Healthy Work Environment Standards. Winston Churchill once said, "The pessimist sees difficulty in every opportunity and the optimist sees the opportunity in every difficulty."[16] It is challenging to create and sustain work environments of excellence, especially when there are concerns about nurse-to-patient ratios, mandatory overtime, unionization, nursing recruitment, and retention. It is also difficult to provide critical care nurses with the tools, resources, and support they need to meet patient and family needs effectively and at the same time enhance their own professional growth, learning, and satisfaction. Nursing has a long tradition of taking "bumpy" roads to make a vision reality. No matter how many times nurses fall down and get bruised on the way to reach a vision, they maintain their resilience by having the courage to listen, learn, and act for themselves, their patients, and their professional practice.

MASTERY

"Education is our passport to the future for tomorrow belongs to the person who prepares for today." (Malcolm X)[16]

REFLECTION ON "MASTERY" FOR CRITICAL CARE NURSING EXCELLENCE

"At 3:30 a.m. in a busy ICU, a nurse prepares to give insulin to a patient with an elevated blood sugar level. The sliding scale doses of insulin on the medication sheet are unclear, and the physician's order sheet is difficult to read. From past experience, the nurse knows how late night calls to this physician often result in verbal outbursts and demeaning slurs, no matter how valid the inquiry. Needing to act but not wanting another harassing encounter with the physician, she makes a judgment of the appropriate dose and administers the insulin. Two hours later, she finds the patient completely unresponsive. To treat the critically low blood sugar level, she administers concentrated injections of glucose and calls for additional emergency help. Despite all attempts to restore the patient's brain to consciousness, he never awakens and his brain never functions normally again."[20(p 10)] Connie Barden, RN, MSN, CCNS, CCRN, past president of AACN, said, "Nurses must be as proficient at handling personal communication as they are in clinical skills. A culture of safety and excellence requires that individual nurses and healthcare organizations make it a priority to develop communication skills that are on par with expert clinical skills."[18]

What mastery of knowledge and skills have you achieved to stop verbally abusive behavior in the workplace? What mastery of knowledge and skills have you achieved to seek solutions that preserve a nurse's personal integrity and ensure a patient's safety? What are you mastering to foster critical care nursing excellence?

Studer, author of *Hardwiring Excellence*, believes that excellence in health care occurs when "employees feel valued, physicians feel their patients are getting great care, and patients feel the service and quality they receive are extraordinary."[29(p 45)] Studer further believes that creating and sustaining a culture of excellence requires the willingness to take individual ownership (be an owner, not a renter of an organization) of problems and opportunities.[29] To value lifelong learning and to have a vision for personal mastery is essential to building a professional practice model for critical care nursing excellence (see Fig. 9-3). There are many pathways for personal mastery. Weston and colleagues believe that seeking feedback and peer review for self-improvement is one of the most effective pathways for building mastery.[15] Other pathways for personal mastery include seeking a degree in higher education, making a commitment to ongoing continuing education, and demonstrating competence through certification. The rewards of mastery often go beyond these pathways. Mastery combines expert professional skills with leadership and interpersonal and organizational proficiency and often leads to the most coveted role of all, the role of mentoring.

The importance of demonstrating personal mastery of knowledge and skills can also be seen in the mounting evidence about how poor communication and lack of collaboration among health care professionals contributes to medical errors and staff turnover.[17,26,27] The Silence Kills Study revealed that 88% of physicians and 48% of nurses and other providers work with people who show poor clinical judgment, and unfortunately, fewer than 10% of them confront their colleagues about their concerns.[17] Avoiding crucial conversations about incompetent or inappropriate practices such as observing violation of infection standards or verbal abuse impairs patient safety and impedes quality care. It is essential that critical care nurses achieve the personal mastery of knowledge and skills that promote high-quality health care delivery and patient safety.

To emphasize the importance of validating clinical competency, on December 11, 2002, AACN released a compelling white paper on the benefits that specialty certification brings to the public, employers, and nurses.[28] The document, *Safeguarding the Patient and the Profession: The Value of Critical Care Nurse Certification,* raises awareness about the responsibility nurses have to honor and validate the public's trust for patient safety. The AACN believes that certification validates competency of knowledge, skills, and experience for quality patient care.[28] Consumers of nursing services must be able to recognize the contributions critical care nurses make to ensure high-quality and competent care to patients and families.

Barden (2003) believes that there should be two types of critical care nurses at the bedside: (1) those who are certified, and (2) those who are in the process of becoming certified.[30] Certification is a process of achieving the highest recognition of excellence. It is more than "another initial"[31]; it is a mark of excellence that can be referred to as "the Good Housekeeping Seal of Approval." Credentials on name badges, such as CCRN (critical care registered nurse), PCCN (progressive care certified nurse), or CCNS (clinical nurse specialist in acute and critical care), make personal mastery visible to the consumer and ensure public protection.

Since 1975, the AACN Certification Corporation has promoted and enhanced mastery of patient health and safety by certifying and recertifying nurses in the care of acute and critically ill patients.[32] Throughout the United States and Canada, nurses have received more than 410,000 certifications in 134 specialties. A total of 67 different certifying bodies granted these certifications and use at least 95 different credentials.[33] Currently, there are more than 40,000 certified critical care nurses with the credentials of CCRN, PCCN, CCNS, CMC (cardiac medicine certification), or CSC (cardiac surgery certification).[32]

Achieving a culture of excellence requires meaningful recognition of achievements such as mastery of certification.[20,28] Cary reported four avenues through which certification status can be recognized: public acknowledgment, financial compensation, career advancement, and retention.[33] In addition, Cary's study revealed that there is a perception, especially among newly certified nurses, that certification gives autonomy, enhances collaboration with other health care providers, allows control over practice, and results in higher patient satisfaction ratings.[33] Similarly, Kirchhoff and Dahl found that 42% of CCUs provided public acknowledgment of certification and that 25% provided financial compensation with a certification bonus.[5] Ulrich and colleagues reported less support for an initial certification bonus (13.8%) and slightly higher support for certification recognition (45%).[34]

PASSION

> *"Perpetual optimism is a force multiplier." (General Colin Powell, U.S. Army, retired, and former Secretary of State)*[16]

REFLECTION ON "PASSION" FOR CRITICAL CARE NURSING EXCELLENCE

On May 30, 2005, Suzanne Burns, RN, MSN, RRT, ACNP, CCRN, FAAN, FCCM, FAANP, past board of director of AACN and advanced practice nurse at Virginia Health System's Medical ICU in Charlottesville, VA, had a vision to recognize and reward colleagues at her institution who she believed were passionate about excellence in acute and critical care nursing practice. She submitted and/or mentored six nurses for the AACN Circle of Excellence Awards Program. Awards were given in the areas of Excellent Nurse Manager, Excellence in Leadership, Excellence in Patient Safety (two recipients), Excellent Clinical Nurse Specialist, and Excellent Nurse Practitioner. The passion and commitment to recognize meaningful and purposeful work for critical care nursing excellence paid off; all six nurses she cited for excellence received national awards at AACN's 2006 National Teaching Institute and Critical Care Exhibition in Anaheim, CA. Six national awards were the most awarded to one institution by AACN.[35]

Do you have a passion to recognize team members for their contributions and the value they bring to your organization? Do you have a passion to follow and/or lead evidence-based and relationship-centered initiatives at your organization? What are you passionate about to foster critical care nursing excellence?

Just as a link is seen between values, vision, and mastery, passion is the essential thread to link together all the professional practice attributes for critical care nursing excellence (see Fig. 9-3). Passion involves enthusiastically striving for what is best for ourselves and those we serve. In *You Are the Leader You've Been Waiting for,* Klein described how to enjoy high performance and high fulfillment at work by being passionate about your calling or purpose.[36] He stated, "When your values, gifts, and calling operate in unison your work has a sense of inner congruence and outer effectiveness. You are clear about who you are and enjoy the ways in which you bring your gifts to life through your work."[36(p 119)] Similarly, others believe passion fuels results so that there is a "flywheel" effect, building in momentum with every step, action, decision, and turn.[36,37]

Weston and colleagues stated that "passion involves ardently striving for the best, even when repeated efforts seem tedious or appear exceedingly strenuous."[15(p 310)] The truly passionate critical care nurse is not satisfied with providing less than the highest-quality care possible to patients and families.

Achieving this goal often requires going beyond an 8- or 12-hour shift. Acts of passion for critical care nursing excellence can be seen in bringing the latest research findings to the bedside, revising unit policy and procedure books with the most up-to-date procedures, and teaching coworkers the most effective therapies to produce the best outcomes for patients and families. Acts of passion for critical care nursing excellence can be seen when people take ownership to become engaged and transform work environments so that they are respectful, healing, and humane.

Passion can be felt in critical care nursing not only at the bedside but throughout the profession. Nursing leaders in critical care are partnering with interdisciplinary groups and talking to legislators to improve patient safety issues such as the workforce shortage, computerized physician and provider order entry, intensivist models of practice, evidence-based practice, and appropriate staffing. Being passionate about something requires time, energy, and commitment. The journey to excellence for healthy work environments started in 2001 for AACN because leadership was passionate about its mission of providing the highest-quality resources to maximize nurses' contribution to caring and improving the health care of critically ill patients and their families.[20]

In *Good to Great,* Collins describes why some organizations make the leap and sustain the leap from being a good organization to a great organization.[37] He challenges people and organizations to pick up their rocks and look at the "ugly squiggly things" underneath them, rather than putting the rocks back down and covering them up. Using resources from AACN, critical care nurses are picking up their rocks and addressing the "ugly squiggly things" in their workplace environments that impede quality patient care. Acts of passion for healthy work environments are taking place as the AACN standards for skilled communication, true collaboration, effective decision making, appropriate staffing, meaningful recognition, and authentic leadership are established.[20]

ACTION

"We are what we repeatedly do. Excellence then is not an act but a habit." (Aristotle)[16]

REFLECTION ON "ACTION" FOR CRITICAL CARE NURSING EXCELLENCE

"On Tuesday, November 1, 2005, the President and Board of Directors of the Greater Washington Area Chapter (GWAC) of the AACN and its premier partner, Georgetown University Hospital, 'engaged' over 300 nursing leaders representing 30 hospital affiliations in the Washington D.C. greater metropolitan area to 'transform' critical care practice. At this dinner event, entitled the 'Beacons of Leadership: In Pursuit of Healthy Work Environments,' GWAC promoted the AACN Healthy Work Environment Standards and launched an AACN Beacon Award Challenge for Critical Care Excellence. By attending the event, each of the 30 affiliated hospitals was eligible for a one-

time $500 gift contribution to use toward the AACN Beacon Award application fee. This is a 5-year budget commitment by GWAC for $15,000 to encourage local hospitals and units to participate. In addition, the GWAC Board of Directors created a new board position and the Beacon Committee, which includes ambassadors to mentor nurses in the Beacon application process. On November 1, 2005, members of GWAC 'engaged' its critical care community by planting seeds for nursing excellence to 327 attendees. Now the fruit is already being reaped as critical care units show evidence of becoming 'transformed.' This truly was a chapter membership–driven effort to engage the hospitals with the AACN Healthy Work Environment Standards and transform the critical care units into Beacons of Excellence."

AACN Circle of Excellence Awards 2006
President's Award for Chapters
GWAC President, Heather Russell RN, MSN, CCRN
Director Critical Care Services
Fairfax Inova Hospital, Fairfax, VA

What action have you taken to participate in creating healthy work environments? What action have you taken to ensure safety becomes the norm and excellence the goal? What action will you take to foster critical care nursing excellence?

Florence Nightingale once said, "one's feelings waste themselves in words, they ought all to be distilled into action which brings results."[38(p 44)] In other words, part of professionalism in critical care nursing is "to walk the talk" for excellence. As values, vision, mastery, and passion for critical care nursing excellence build, the attribute of action (see Fig. 9-3) becomes another essential pillar for the framework and one that resonates well for tangible results in critical care. Recognizing that so many vulnerable patients' lives are at risk and the invaluable contributions that nurses make, the AACN leadership decided it was time to act deliberately and definitively.[39] In 2003, AACN launched the Beacon Award for Critical Care Excellence, an award specifically designed to recognize the leading critical care units in the United States.[39] Currently, more than 45 critical care units have received the Beacon Award for demonstrating high-quality standards, exceptional care of patients and families, and healthy work environments.[40]

Dorrie Fontaine, RN, PhD, FAAN, president of the AACN when the awards were launched, defined a *beacon* as "a source of light, an inspiration, or signal of guidance." She went on to say that "AACN believes every critical care unit can be a Beacon unit."[39] The 42-item Beacon application addresses innovation, excellence, or both in six categories: recruitment and retention; education, training and mentoring; evidence-based practice and research; patient outcomes; creating and promoting healing environments; and leadership and organizational ethics. In addition, the Beacon Award provides a mechanism for individual and collective critical care units to measure progress against evidence-based initiatives and national criteria for performance, learn and refine their processes and systems, and be recognized for their achievements.[40] What bolder action or stronger message can be conveyed to the public and the patients whom critical care nurses serve than to validate excellence in practice?

Seeking opportunities and partnerships to further extend action to ensure optimal health outcomes for people experiencing acute and life-threatening illness requires a relentless and fearless voice by critical care nurses. These nurses have been using their innate gift of inquiry for decades to tackle patient care issues. However, Nightingale is perhaps nursing's most famous leader who first used research to change practice.[38] Even though she lacked the theoretical bases that are known today, she had a core set of values, a vision, the mastery, and a passion to improve England's hospital care in the mid-19th century. Today critical care nurses are seeing "sacred cows" that were once revered being thrown out of practice. For example, nursing research has well demonstrated that using dye in enteral feeding, restricting family presence during cardiopulmonary resuscitation, and restricting visitation hours in ICUs need to be eliminated from practice.

Even though new models of nursing education are evolving, it does not take a doctorate-prepared critical care nurse to raise questions and put a plan in place for collecting, analyzing, and reporting patient and family outcomes. Outcome-based practice is the responsibility of all nurses, whether one is actually doing the research, disseminating the research to the bedside, or reporting the research findings. In addition, it is important for all nurses to celebrate and showcase high-quality nursing outcomes, no matter what nursing specialty provided the body of knowledge. Focusing on quality indicators and performance improvement in acute and critical care settings as daily practice is a bold and powerful action for improving patient care.

This is the commitment and voice that needs to be heard about critical care nursing. Practice alerts from AACN are another example of efforts to prevent and minimize infection, reduce complications from critical illness, promote patient safety, and establish best practices. First launched in 2004, the AACN practice alerts are succinct dynamic directives that are well supported with current authoritative evidence to ensure best practice. There are more than a dozen practice alerts that (1) bridge the gap between practice and research, (2) provide guidance, (3) standardize care, and (4) identify and inform new trends and provide information about them.[41] A few recent practice alerts include oral care in the critically ill, noninvasive blood pressure monitoring, and severe sepsis.[41] Because critical care nurses have a great opportunity to promote the science of nursing through the AACN practice alerts, it is helpful to remember that "the public cannot protect a social resource that it does not know and understand; only nurses can give the public the knowledge and understanding necessary to protect human caregiving."[2(p 42)]

BALANCE

> ### "Balance isn't either/or, it's AND." (Steven Covey)[16]
>
> #### REFLECTION ON "BALANCE" FOR CRITICAL CARE NURSING EXCELLENCE
>
> "It seemed like a routine day in the progressive care unit, but Mr. T. was anything but routine. He was a very demanding patient who had an abdominal aortic aneurysm repair with a complicated recovery. He was on total parenteral nutrition and intravenous antibiotics, and had a large abdominal incision. When I walked into the room, Mr. T. demanded that I remove his staples. I checked the incision; six staples were intact but with redness, swelling and increased heat in the area. I said I would check with the surgeon. He started yelling, so I looked at him and said, 'You can yell all you want; I am looking out for your best interests, and I will do nothing that is unsafe.' He immediately calmed down and apologized. Later, Mr. T. called me to his room complaining of diarrhea. I discovered there was drainage from the incision. I called the surgeon, told him what I had seen and that the patient was now having pain after being pain-free for days. When the surgeon arrived he opened the incision with his gloved fingers and stool flew everywhere, as Mr. T. groaned in pain. As the surgeon left the room yelling orders, I asked him for an order for IV pain medication and asked another nurse to help me. The patient's scan revealed a perforated bowel and he was taken back to surgery. As he left he whispered that he was scared and asked me to pray for him. As I held his hand I realized that my demanding patient was gone, replaced with a scared man who needed a nurse's touch."
>
> *Marva D. Pharis, RN, BSN, PhD, PCCN, RNBC*
> *AACN Circle of Excellence Awards 2006*
> *Excellence in Clinical Practice, Non-traditional Setting*
> *Lee Memorial Health System, La Belle, FL*
>
> What balance have you put in your life for renewal? What balance can you give as a gift to yourself and others? How will you start balancing your life to foster critical care nursing excellence?

Balance is the final component of the professional practice model for critical care nursing excellence (see Fig. 9-3). Balance can bring renewal to the spirit, which often breaks down in our busy personal and professional lives. Taking the time to care for one's self is essential to keeping the body and mind in balance. Otherwise, it can be difficult to keep perspectives clear. Today, nurses are increasingly blurring the lines between home and work and work and leisure. The lines of communication are continuously open because of the proliferation of pagers, cell phones, facsimile machines, text messages, e-mail, and voicemail. It is time to say "no" to being "supernurse" and "supermom" or "superdad" and find the time to take care of oneself. Nurses do not do their patients, their families, or themselves any good if they consistently place the needs of others above their own. Critical care nurses listen to patients and families 24 hours a day, 7 days a week. They must also have time to listen to their own minds and hearts and those who love them most.

In *You Are the Leader You've Been Waiting for,* Klein stresses the importance of letting go.[36] He believes letting go of the old can make space for something new. It is during a time of transformation that he believes one should not act but be still.[36] Nurses cannot stop the beeps, alarms, and phone calls at work, but when the shift is over, it is time to "let go." As difficult as it may be, it is time for nurses to let go of the complex, vulnerable, and unstable patients who were in their hands during their shift. It is a time to be "still"; nurses may turn the television off and read to the children, take a leisurely walk with a pet, or sit quietly listening to the sounds of life. The minds and hearts of nurses need time to renew and be recharged for the next day of taking care of critically ill patients and their families. When nurses are balanced, it is easier not to give in to the cynicism and frustration that abound in the workplace or home. To be truly engaged and energized requires nurturing oneself first and then empowering others to do the same. Look around your unit today and ask yourself some questions. Who are the critical care nurses who reach out to others the most? Who are the critical care nurses who smile the most? Who are the critical care nurses who say "thank you" and give compliments the most? You may find that your answer is with nurses who have discovered how to make balance a priority in their personal and professional lives.

• Conclusion

In today's fast-paced critical care environment, finding the time for professional growth can be challenging. Building a professional practice of excellence requires a passion to profoundly affect the lives of those who trust critical care nurses most: complex, unstable, and vulnerable patients and their families. At the same time, it requires advancing the critical care nursing profession through a healthy work environment that is patient centered, collaborative, interdisciplinary, and evidence based. The desire and commitment for critical care nursing excellence requires self-reflection about the values, vision, mastery, passion, action, and balance in one's practice (see Fig. 9-3). Critically ill patients and their families expect and deserve nothing but the best care.

Building a professional practice model of excellence can give critical care nurses the confidence to use their bold voice and presence to make significant contributions for improving the delivery of care to the patients and families who have entered a chaotic and frightening world of illness, trauma, and pain. Even in the fastest-paced critical care environments of today, finding the time for professional growth is challenging but, as evidence demonstrates, essential. For the profession of critical care nursing to advance, nurses must acquire the necessary clinical experience and competencies to provide best practice models of care for critically ill patients and their families. Whether it is participating on a patient safety hospital committee

▨ CLOSING THOUGHTS ON CRITICAL CARE NURSING EXCELLENCE

REMEMBER . . . Ready or not, someday it will all come to an end

There will be no more sunrises, no shift work, no change of report

All the things you valued, whether treasured or forgotten, will pass to someone else

It will not matter what you owned or what you were owed

Your challenges, frustrations, and disappointments will finally disappear

So too your hopes, ambitions, and plans

What will matter is not your success, but your significance

What will matter is not what you learned, but what you taught

What will matter is every act of integrity, compassion, courage or sacrifice that enriched, empowered or encouraged others to emulate your example of critical care nursing excellence

Living a life that matters doesn't happen by accident

It's not a matter of circumstance but of choice

Live your contribution and choose to live a life that matters

Become engaged and transformed for a healthy work environment

Modified from Josephson M: What will matter. Retrieved August 1, 2006, from http://www.charactercounts.org.

or recruiting youth to critical care nursing, endless opportunities exist for building a professional practice of excellence. The days of landmark studies reporting that nursing is a silent and unknown profession[42,43] will soon come to an end as more bold and committed voices are heard about excellence in critical care nursing practice.

• Clinical Applicability Challenges

Short Answer Questions

1. If more critical care nurses were prepared at the Baccalaureate of Nursing degree level or higher, how would that influence the nursing profession (or would it)?

2. How would requiring mandatory certification for critical care nursing influence the profession (or would it)?

3. As a critical care nurse, what is one issue that you would commit to address in order to create or sustain a healthy work environment and advance professional nursing practice? How would you implement this?

Review Questions

1. A novice critical care nurse observed a coworker fail to wash her hands before donning gloves and

performing a wound care procedure. She was concerned that the patient might develop a secondary infection and spoke up about the importance of proper handwashing before starting the wound care procedure. The coworker laughed and said, "You're young—just wait, and you'll learn some shortcuts too." Which American Association of Critical-Care Nurses value do you think best describes why the novice critical care nurse spoke up?

a. Innovation
b. Passion
c. Collaboration
d. Advocation

2. A certified critical care nurse (CCRN) was concerned about the increasing number of critically ill patients in her intensive care unit with poorly controlled glycemic levels. She knew that physicians were not writing insulin orders that were in accordance with evidence-based practice recommendations. When she told a coworker that the practice council should develop a collaborative Intensive Insulin Therapy Protocol with members of the multidisciplinary team, the coworker said, "You're a CCRN; can't you just write it yourself?" What would be the best response for a nurse trying to build a professional practice of critical care nursing excellence?

a. "No, that's not my job."
b. "Yes, I can, but I think it would be good experience for you to participate as well."
c. "Thank you for that confidence, but to optimally meet the needs of patients and families, I think collaborative work that is evidence-based will give us our best outcome."
d. "Thank you for that confidence. I think I will, since my CCRN validates the knowledge, skills, and experience necessary to ensure high-quality and competent care."

3. Which of the following attributes (as discussed in this chapter) serve as the foundation to build a professional practice model for critical care nursing excellence?

a. Values and vision
b. Mastery and passion
c. Action and balance
d. Mission and drive

4. All of the following would be examples of the type of culture that could receive a Beacon Award for Critical Care Excellence except

a. a culture where critical care nurses are as proficient in communication skills as they are in clinical skills.
b. a culture where critical care nurses are valued and committed partners in making decisions related to patient care.
c. a culture where critical care nurses are trained how to tolerate and compensate for verbal abuse and inappropriate staffing.
d. a culture where critical care nurses receive meaningful recognition for the value each brings to his or her organization.

5. Which of the following best demonstrates a critical care nurse who follows a professional practice model of excellence?

a. One who is certified in more than one specialty area of critical care nursing
b. One who is educated at the baccalaureate of nursing level or higher and obtains more than the annual minimum continuing education requirements
c. One who is published with research in nursing and provides scholarly presentations at the regional, national, and international level
d. One who is continually self-assessing his or her inner core values about how to bring the best critical care nursing performance to patients, families, and the profession

References

1. Kalisch P, Kalisch B: Working together for nursing. Focus Crit Care 10:12–14, 1983
2. Buresh B, Gordon S: From Silence to Voice: What Nurses Know and Must Communicate to the Public. Ottawa, Canada, Canadian Nurses Association, 2000
3. American Association of Critical-Care Nurses: 2005 Membership Demographics. Retrieved August 1,2006, from http://www.aacn.org/AACN/Memship.nsf/Files/MembDemographics/$file/MembDemographics.pdf
4. Division of Nursing, Bureau of Health Professionals in the Health Resources and Services Administration, U.S. Department of Health and Human Services: 2004 National Sample Survey of Registered Nurses. Retrieved August 1, 2006, from http://bhpr.hrsa.gov/healthworkforce/reports/rnpopulation/preliminaryfindings.htm
5. Kirchhoff K, Dahl N: American Association of Critical-Care Nurses' national survey of facilities and units providing critical care. Am J Crit Care 15(1):13–27, 2006
6. Kelly L: Dimensions of Professional Nursing. New York, Macmillan, 1981
7. Styles M: Professionalists, all. J Contin Educ Nurs 31(2):88–89, 2000
8. Bartels J, Bednash G: Answering the call for quality nursing care and patient safety: A new model for nursing education. Nurs Adm Quart 29(1):5–13, 2005
9. Dracup A, Cronenwett L, Meleis A, Benner P: Reflections on the doctorate of nursing practice. Nurs Outlook 53(6):177–182, 2005
10. Flexner A: A Medical Education in the United States and Canada: A Report to the Carnegie Foundation for the Advancement of Teaching. Bethesda, MD, Science & Health Publications, 1910
11. Holl R: Characteristics of the registered nurse and professional beliefs and decision making. Crit Care Nurs Q 17:60–66, 1994
12. Heath J, Andrews J, Graham-Garcia J: Assessment of professional development of critical care nurses: A descriptive study. Am J Crit Care 10(1):17–22, 2001
13. Manojlovich M: Predictors of professional nursing practice behaviors in hospital settings. Nurs Res 54(1):41–47, 2005
14. Wynd C: Current factors contributing to professionalism in nursing. J Prof Nurs 19(5):251–261, 2003
15. Weston M, Buchda V, Bergstrom D: Creating excellence in practice. In Stanley, J (ed): Advanced Practice Nursing: Emphasizing Common Roles. Philadelphia, FA Davis, 2005, pp 395–411
16. Famous Quotations Network. Retrieved August 1, 2006, from http://www.famous-quotations.com
17. Maxfield D, Grenny J, McMillan R, et al: Silence kills: The seven crucial conversations for healthcare. VitalSmarts L.C. 2005. Retrieved May 1, 2006, from http://www.silencekills.com

18. American Association of Critical-Care Nurses and VitalSmarts Press Release: New study finds U.S. hospitals must improve workplace communication to reduce medical errors, enhance quality of care. Washington, DC, January 26, 2005

19. Jones J: Nurses remain at top of honesty and ethics poll. The Gallup Organization, December 5, 2005. Retrieved August 1, 2006, from http://poll.gallup.com/content/?ci=20254

20. American Association of Critical-Care Nurses: AACN Standards for Establishing and Sustaining Healthy Work Environments: A Journey to Excellence. Aliso Viejo, CA, AACN, 2005

21. Barden C: Bold voices: Speak up for a new tomorrow. AACN News 20(7):2, 2003

22. Fontaine D: Rising above: New questions, new possibilities. AACN News 21(6):2, 2004

23. McCauley K: Live your contribution: Our quest for excellence. AACN News 22(6):2, 2005

24. Brinker D: Engage and transform: Achieving our preferred future. AACN News 23(6):2, 2006

25. American Association of Critical-Care Nurses: Core values. Retrieved May 1, 2006, from http://www.aacn.org

26. Institute of Medicine: Crossing the quality chasm: A new health system for the 21st century. Washington, DC, National Academy Press, 2001

27. Joint Commission on Accreditation of Healthcare Organizations: Root causes of sentinel events. Retrieved May 1, 2006, from http://jcaho.com/accredited+organizations/ambulatory+care/sentinel+events/root+causes+of+sentinel+event.htm

28. American Association of Critical-Care Nurses and AACN Certification Corporation: Safeguarding the patient and the profession: The value of critical care nurse certification. Retrieved May 1, 2006, from http://www.aacn.org/AACN/mrkt.nsf/Files/CertWhitePaper/$file/CertWhitePaper.pdf

29. Studer Q: Hardwiring Excellence: Purpose, Worthwhile Work, Making a Difference. Gulf Breeze, Fla, Fire Starter Publishing, 2004

30. Barden C: Certification: Good for whom? AACN News 20(2):2, 2003

31. Mason D: What's in a letter. Am J Nurs 101(1):7, 2001

32. American Association of Critical-Care Nurses Certification Corporation: AACN Certification Corporation Fact Sheet. Retrieved June 1, 2006, from http://www.certcorp.org

33. Cary AH: Certified registered nurses: Results of the study of the certified workforce. Am J Nurs 101(1):44–52, 2001

34. Ulrich B, Lavandero R, Hart K, et al: Critical care nurses' work environments: A baseline status report. Crit Care Nurse 26(5):646–657

35. American Association of Critical-Care Nurses: AACN Circle of Excellence 2006 Award Recipients. Retrieved August 1, 2006, from http://www.aacn.org/AACN/Memship.nsf/vwdoc/COE2006Rec

36. Klein E: You Are the Leader You've Been Waiting for: Enjoying High Performance and High Fulfillment at Work. Encinitas, Calif, Wisdom Heart Press, 2006

37. Collins J: Good to Great. New York, Harper Collins, 2001

38. Nightingale F: Notes on Nursing: What It Is, and What It Is Not. London, Harrison and Sons, 1859

39. American Association of Critical-Care Nurses: AACN Launches Beacon: Award Recognizes Critical Care Excellence Press Release. Retrieved August 1, 2006, from http://www.aacn.org/AACN/mrkt.nsf/Files/BeaconRelease/$file/BeaconRelease.doc

40. American Association of Critical-Care Nurses: Beacon Application Facts. Retrieved August 1, 2006, from https://www.aacn.org/AACN/ICURecog.nsf/vwdoc/toc

41. American Association of Critical-Care Nurses: Practice Alerts. Available at http://www.aacn.org

42. Buresh B, Gordon S, Bell N: Who counts in news coverage of health care. Nursing Outlook 39(5):204–208, 1991

43. Sigma Theta Tau International: The Woodhull Study on Nursing and the Media: Health Care's Invisible Partner. Indianapolis, Ind, Author, 1998

Special Populations in Critical Care

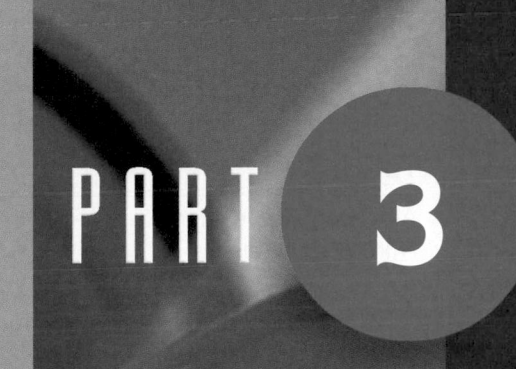

PART 3

INTERNET RESOURCES

Topic	Web Page Address
American Association of Nurse Anesthetists	www.aana.com
American College of Obstetricians and Gynecologists	www.acog.org
American Geriatrics Society	www.americangeriatrics.org
American Society of Perianesthesia Nurses	www.aspan.org
Association of periOperative Registered Nurses	www.aorn.org
Association of Women's Health, Obstetric and Neonatal Nurses	www.awhonn.org
Congenital Heart Information Network	www.tchin.org/index.htm
Gerontological Society of America	www.geron.org
Malignant Hyperthermia Association of the United States	www.mhaus.org
National Association of Pediatric Nurse Practitioners, Inc.	www.napnap.org
National Association of Professional Geriatric Care Managers	www.caremanager.org
National Family Caregivers Association	www.nfcacares.org
National Gerontological Nurses Association	www.ngna.org
National Institute on Aging	www.nih.gov/nia/
Pediatric Critical Care Medicine	www.pedsccm.org
Society of Pediatric Nurses	www.pedsnurses.org
The Universe of Women's Health	www.obgyn.net
World Federation of Pediatric and Intensive Critical Care Societies	www.wfpiccs.org

The Critically Ill Pediatric Patient

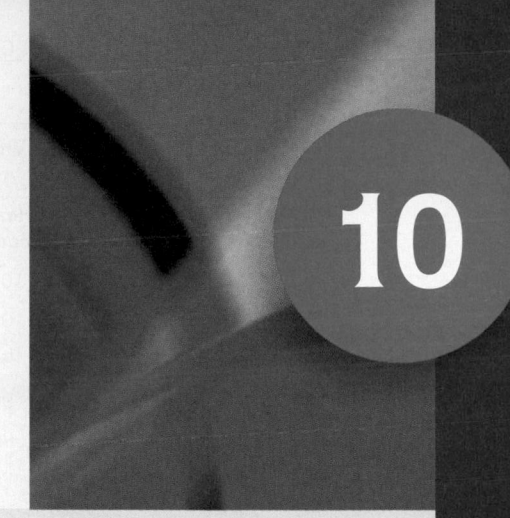

10

Patricia A. Moloney-Harmon

Prominent Anatomical and Physiological Differences and Implications
Vital Signs
Neurological System
Cardiovascular System
Respiratory System
Gastrointestinal System
Renal System
Endocrine System
Immune System
Integumentary System
Selected Pediatric Challenges
Ventilatory Issues
Medication Administration
Pain Management
Interaction With Children and Families

Objectives

Based on the content in this chapter, the reader should be able to:

❶ Analyze anatomical and physiological differences in the infant and child that necessitate the modification of physical assessment parameters and intervention techniques.

❷ Describe special considerations in ventilatory management and medication administration for the critically ill child.

❸ Evaluate pain assessment tools that can be used for the critically ill child.

❹ Examine important aspects of interaction with the critically ill child and family that will enhance interventions.

Many critical care clinicians feel ill equipped to care for children seen in adult intensive care units (ICUs), emergency departments, procedural suites, and recovery rooms. To facilitate smooth and optimal care of the critically ill child, it is wise to adopt a framework for the modification of the adult critical care practice to include the pediatric patient. A comprehensive framework is beyond the scope of this chapter, but readers are referred to the PEDS framework, discussed in more detail elsewhere.[1] This chapter highlights prominent anatomical and physiological differences and related implications, equipment selection, recognition of the decompensating child, and unique challenges in caring for the pediatric patient in a critical care environment.

• Prominent Anatomical and Physiological Differences and Implications

VITAL SIGNS

Infants and young children have an age-appropriate, but higher, heart rate and respiratory rate than adults. The higher heart and respiratory rates assist in meeting the need for a higher cardiac output, despite a smaller stroke volume and a higher basal metabolic rate. Blood pressure in children is lower than that of adults. Vital signs (Table 10-1), although important parameters, should not be evaluated in isolation, but rather in a trending fashion.

Tachycardia is a nonspecific response to a variety of entities, such as anxiety, fever, shock, and hypoxemia. Although the child is predisposed to bradycardia, tolerance is poor. Persistent bradycardia produces significant changes in perfusion because cardiac output is heart rate dependent. Bradycardia is most often caused by hypoxemia, but any vagal stimuli, such as suctioning, nasogastric tube insertion, and defecation, may precipitate an event.

As for respiratory rate, an infant or child increases his or her respiratory rate to compensate for an increased oxygen demand. Tachypnea is often the first sign of respiratory distress. A slow respiratory rate in a sick child often indicates impending respiratory arrest. Associated conditions, such as fever and seizure activity, which further increase the metabolic rate, also increase oxygen requirements. These conditions can cause rapid deterioration in an already compromised child.

Table 10-1 • Pediatric Vital Signs

Age	Heart Rate (beats/min)	Respirations (breaths/min)	Systolic Blood Pressure (mm Hg)
Newborn	100–160	30–60	50–70
1–6 wk	100–160	30–60	70–95
6 mo	90–120	25–40	80–100
1 y	90–120	20–30	80–100
3 y	80–120	20–30	80–110
6 y	70–110	18–25	80–110
10 y	60–90	15–20	90–120
14 y	60–90	15–20	90–130

Unlike the adult, the child's blood pressure is the last parameter to fall in the face of shock. Children can compensate for up to a 25% blood loss before the systolic blood pressure falls. A normal blood pressure should never discourage interventions for the child showing signs of circulatory failure. The pulse pressure is often a more reliable indicator for assessing the adequacy of perfusion. Hypertension is uncommon unless the child has renal disease.

NEUROLOGICAL SYSTEM

Brain growth occurs at a rapid rate during the first few years of life. Because brain growth is rapid during this time, measurement of head circumference is important in the child until 2 years of age. The circumference of the child's head is related to intracranial volume and estimates the rate of brain growth.

The child's cranial sutures are not completely fused until 18 to 24 months of age. The posterior fontanel closes by 3 months of age, and the anterior fontanel closes by 9 to 18 months of age. The fontanels provide a useful assessment tool in the infant. The characteristics of the fontanels can be used to assess hydration status or the presence of increased intracranial pressure (ICP). Bulging fontanels may indicate increased ICP or fluid overload. Sunken fontanels may be seen with fluid deficit.

Like adults, infants and children have protective reflexes (e.g., the cough and gag reflexes). There are also several newborn reflexes (i.e., the Moro, rooting, grasp, and Babinski reflexes), which differ from adult reflexes. For example, the Babinski reflex is present until 9 to 12 months of age or until the child starts walking. A positive Babinski reflex response (fanning of the toes and dorsiflexion of the big toe when the lateral aspect of the sole of the foot is stroked) is expected in an infant, yet is considered an abnormal finding in an older child or adult. In-depth discussion of these reflexes is beyond the scope of this chapter; the reader is referred to a developmental anatomy text for further information.

An infant's or child's mental status is assessed the same way as an adult's, by noting the level of consciousness, interaction with the environment, and appropriateness of behavior for age. Level of consciousness is assessed by noting whether the child is arousable and oriented. This can be done by observing for spontaneous arousability or by providing verbal, tactile, or noxious stimuli. Even though the assessment is the same, the assessment techniques must be age appropriate. Specific techniques are provided in the section in this chapter on interaction. An important difference to note when interacting with the child is paradoxical irritability (i.e., the inability of the child to be calmed with normal comfort measures, such as cuddling). Paradoxical irritability, when present with meningeal irritability, nuchal rigidity, and positive Brudzinski's and Kerning's signs, may indicate meningitis.

Infants and young children are at high risk for ineffective thermoregulation, resulting in physiological instability, due to a variety of maturational and environmental factors.[2] Close monitoring of body temperature and providing a temperature-controlled environment help manage temperature regulation. The temperature is measured at regular intervals, and external factors affecting body temperature should be controlled.

CARDIOVASCULAR SYSTEM

Decreased perfusion to the skin is an early and reliable sign of shock. Because a child's skin is thinner than an adult's, skin characteristics change easily and rapidly with changes in perfusion. Skin color, texture, and temperature and capillary refill are of great significance during assessment of the child. Before assessing the skin, it is important to note the room temperature because some findings may be a normal response to the environment (such as mottling in a drafty operating room). Mottling in a bundled infant or warm environment is reason for further investigation. The nurse assesses skin temperature and the line of demarcation between extremity coolness and body warmth. Coolness or the progression of coolness toward the trunk may be a sign of diminishing perfusion.

Peripheral cyanosis is normal in newborns but abnormal in young children and adults. Central cyanosis (circumoral) is always abnormal. Capillary refill time is normally recorded in seconds rather than as "brisk, normal, or slow" and normally is no longer than 2 seconds. Estimated blood volume varies with age; despite a higher volume per kilogram of body weight in children, the overall total circulating volume is small. A small amount of blood loss can be significant in a child.

RESPIRATORY SYSTEM

The infant's or child's large head (in proportion to body size); weak, underdeveloped neck muscles; and lack of cartilaginous support to the airway lead to an easily compressible or obstructed airway. The nurse must avoid overextending or overflexing the neck because the airways are easily collapsible. Head and neck position alone can facilitate a patent airway. Ideal positioning for the decompensating child is in a neutral ("sniffing") position and can be accomplished by placing a small roll horizontally behind the shoulders (Fig. 10-1). Infants, until 6 months of age, are obligate nose-breathers, so any obstruction of nasal passages can produce significant airway compromise and respiratory distress. Secretions, edema, inflammation, poorly taped nasogastric tubes, or occluded nasal cannulas can cause obstructed nasal passages in an infant. The infant's and young child's airways are smaller in diameter and in length, thus requiring smaller artificial airways. Airway compromise can be caused by the slightest amount of inflammation or edema of the natural airway or from a mucus plug in either the natural or artificial airway. The narrowest part of the child's airway (until approximately 8 years of age) is at the level of the cricoid ring, as opposed to the glottic opening in the adult.

The young child's thin, compliant chest wall allows for easy assessment of air entry. Air entry is assessed by observing the rise and fall of the child's chest with adequate ventilatory efforts. Unequal chest movement may indicate the development of a pneumothorax or atelectasis but also may indicate endotracheal tube obstruction or displacement into the right mainstem bronchus. The child's flexible rib cage and poorly developed intercostal muscles offer little stability to the chest wall; therefore, suprasternal, sternal, intercostal, and subcostal retractions may be seen during respiratory distress. The presence and location of retractions should be noted. Accessory muscles also are poorly developed, so an infant or child may use the abdominal muscles to assist with breathing. This gives the appearance of "seesaw" breathing, a paradoxical movement of the chest and abdomen. Seesaw breathing becomes more exaggerated with respiratory distress. As in the adult, the major muscle of respiration is the diaphragm. However, the child is more diaphragm dependent.

Because of the thin chest wall, breath sounds are more audible than in the adult. In addition, obstructed airways often produce sounds that are easily heard during assessment. The nurse listens for expiratory grunting, inspiratory and expiratory stridor, and wheezing. Expiratory grunting is a sound produced in an attempt to increase physiological positive end-expiratory pressure to prevent small airways and alveoli from collapsing. The infant's and child's thin chest wall may allow breath sounds to be heard over an area of pathology when sounds are actually being referred from another area of the lung. The nurse listens for changes in the breath sounds as well as for their presence or absence.

GASTROINTESTINAL SYSTEM

Children normally have a protuberant abdomen; however, there are numerous causes of abnormal abdominal distention. A nasogastric or orogastric tube should be inserted early rather than later in a critically ill child to minimize the risk for distention. Abdominal distention can interfere with respiratory excursion and may even cause respiratory arrest. Active removal of air with a syringe may be necessary if distention is not relieved by putting the tube to straight drainage. In addition, the abdominal girth is measured every shift or more often if there is a concern about abdominal distention.

Stomach capacity varies with the age of the child. A newborn's stomach capacity is 90 mL, a 1-month-old's is 150 mL, a 12-month-old's is 360 mL, and an adult's is 2,000 to 3,000 mL. Because stomach capacity is smaller, care is taken when formula and other fluids are instilled into the abdomen. Bolus feedings are of an appropriate amount, consistent with the child's stomach capacity.

The infant and young child have a gastric emptying time of 2.5 to 3 hours, which increases to 3 to 6 hours in the older child. An appropriate amount of time to allow for absorption of formula is taken into account when measuring residuals. If the child is receiving chest physiotherapy, the amount of time between therapy and feeding is considered, or the gastric contents are checked to avoid problems with reflux and aspiration.

RENAL SYSTEM

Infants have less ability to concentrate urine and therefore have a normal urine output of 2 mL/kg/h. For children and adolescents, normal urine output is 1 mL/kg/h and 0.5 mL/kg/h, respectively. Because of the infant's limited ability to concentrate urine, a low specific gravity does not necessarily mean that the infant

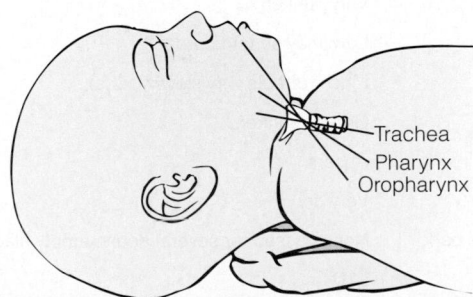

Figure 10-1 • The neutral ("sniffing") position can improve airflow in a decompensating child by aligning the oropharynx, pharynx, and trachea with the mouth.

Table 10-2 • Calculation of Maintenance Fluid

Body Weight (kg)	Fluid Requirements per Day	Fluid Requirements per Hour
<10	100 mL/kg	4 mL/kg
10–20	1,000 mL + 50 mL/kg for each kg above 10	2 mL/kg for each kg above 10
>20	1,500 mL + 20 mL/kg for each kg above 20	1 mL/kg for each kg above 20

From Roberts KE: Fluid and electrolyte regulation. In Curley MAQ, Moloney-Harmon PA (eds): Critical Care Nursing of Infants and Children, 2001, pp 369–392, with permission of Elsevier Science.

is adequately hydrated. The immaturity of the child's kidney means that the child may not process fluid as efficiently as the adult and is less able to handle sudden large amounts of fluid, leading to fluid overload.

Infants and young children have a larger body surface area in relation to body weight. Maintenance fluid requirements are determined based on body weight (Table 10-2). Children have a higher percentage of total body water, most of which is composed of extracellular fluid (ECF), compared with adults. The ECF makes up 50% of the body weight in infants but 20% in adults. In addition, children have a higher insensible water loss because of a higher basal metabolic rate, higher respiratory rate, and larger body surface area. The child's higher percentage of total-body water and higher insensible water loss increase the risk for dehydration. Sudden weight loss or gain may indicate fluid imbalance. Children should be weighed daily at the same time using the same scale.

Signs of dehydration include dry mucous membranes, decreased urine output, increased urine concentration, sunken fontanels and eyes, and poor skin turgor (Table 10-3). The severity of dehydration varies with the degree of dehydration and the child's fluid and electrolyte status. Circulatory compromise accompanies severe dehydration. Treating a child's dehydration in an adult ICU requires pediatric consultation.

Fluid overload is manifested by bulging fontanels, taut skin, edema (usually periorbital and sacral), hepatomegaly, and other signs of congestive heart failure.

ENDOCRINE SYSTEM

Infants and young children have smaller glycogen stores and increased glucose demand because of their larger brain-to-body size ratio. The smaller stores and increased demand predispose infants and young children to the development of hypoglycemia. Blood glu-

Table 10-3 • Clinical Assessment of Severity of Dehydration

	Mild Dehydration	Moderate Dehydration	Severe Dehydration
Physical appearance			
Infants and young children	Thirsty, alert, restless	Thirsty, restless, or lethargic but irritable to touch or drowsy	Drowsy, limp, cold, sweaty, cyanotic extremities, may be comatose
Older children and adults	Thirsty, alert, restless	Thirsty, alert, postural hypotension	Usually conscious, apprehensive, cold, sweaty, cyanotic extremities, wrinkled skin of fingers and toes, muscle cramps
Radial pulse	Normal rate and strength	Rapid and weak	Rapid, feeble, sometimes impalpable
Respiration	Normal	Deep, may be rapid	Deep and rapid
Anterior fontanel	Normal	Sunken	Very sunken
Systolic blood pressure	Normal	Normal or low	Low, may be unrecordable
Skin elasticity	Pinch retracts immediately	Pinch retracts slowly	Pinch retracts very slowly (>2 s)
Eyes	Normal	Sunken (detectable)	Grossly sunken
Tears	Present	Absent	Absent
Mucous membranes	Moist	Dry	Very dry
Urine output	Normal	Reduced amount and dark	None passed for several hours, empty bladder
Body weight loss (%)	3–5	6–9	≥10
Estimated fluid deficit (mL/kg)	30–50	60–90	≥100

Data from Adelman RD, Solhaug MJ: Pathophysiology of body fluids and fluid therapy. In Behrman RE (ed): Nelson Textbook of Pediatrics, 16th ed. 1999, pp 211–215, with permission from Elsevier Science.

cose levels are closely monitored, especially when the infant or child is not permitted to have anything by mouth and numerous adjustments are being made to nutritional support.

IMMUNE SYSTEM

Immunological differences in infants and small children may predispose them to infection. The skin of newborns is thinner; therefore, it provides less of a barrier to outside pathogens. Because infants and young children have fewer stored neutrophils, they are less able to repeatedly replenish white blood cells in the face of an overwhelming infection. The complement levels are lower, which affects the chemotactic activity of phagocytes and the opsonization of bacteria. There is also a relative deficiency of immunoglobulins, making infants and young children more susceptible to infections caused by viruses, *Candida* species, and acute inflammatory bacteria. In addition, infants may not demonstrate fever and leukocytosis in response to an infection. It is important to observe for subtle signs, such as changes in feeding behaviors, altered glucose metabolism, and hypothermia.

INTEGUMENTARY SYSTEM

Expected differences in the skin, hair, nails, and glands depend on the age of the child. Infants and children, without exposure to the sun or wind, are expected to have smooth-textured skin without coarse adult terminal hair. Infants, up to about 14 days of age, may be covered with lanugo, a fine, silky-textured hair. Infants also have less developed hypodermal fat and, as a result, are at risk for hypothermia. The sweat glands do not begin to function until 1 month of age and are not fully functional until adolescence.

In the young child, the most noticeable variation may be that of bruising as the child increases activity and play becomes more aggressive. It is very important to attend to bruising seen in the child because it may be associated with abusive situations. The nurse notes the location and color changes of bruising indicating the stage of healing. Bruising is more common and not unexpected on the lower legs and the face. Bruising on the upper arms, buttocks, and abdomen occurs less often and may be indicative of abuse.

In the adolescent, the sweat glands and sebaceous glands become fully functional. The adolescent may be expected to experience body odor, increasing axillary perspiration, and acne. The development of axillary and pubic hair is expected related to the increasing levels of circulating androgen levels in both male and female adolescents.

• Selected Pediatric Challenges

VENTILATORY ISSUES

The most common cause of cardiopulmonary arrest in children is respiratory in nature. This fact mandates that respiratory distress and failure be recog-

nized early and that airway management interventions be immediate (Table 10-4). Signs of respiratory decompensation include diminished level of consciousness, tachypnea, minimal or no chest movement with respiratory effort, evidence of labored respirations with retractions, seesaw breathing, minimal or no air exchange noted on auscultation, and the presence of nasal flaring, grunting, stridor, or wheezing.

The initial intervention for respiratory decompensation is positioning the child to open the airway. If the child does not respond to position alone, manual ventilation with 100% oxygen using a bag-mask device is initiated. There are several sizes of pediatric manual resuscitation bags; the correct size is determined by noting the child's tidal volume and deciding whether the bag is capable of delivering 1.5 times the child's tidal volume. Even though a pressure manometer may assist in minimizing pressure, the true indicator of delivery of an adequate tidal volume is a clinical one. The adequate amount of tidal volume delivered during a manual resuscitation breath is the amount that causes rise and fall of the child's chest.

If bag-mask ventilation is not successful in restoring the child's ventilatory status, endotracheal intubation is required. Numerous sizes of endotracheal tubes are available for infants and children. To estimate the correct size of endotracheal tube, the size of the child's little finger or the following formula can be used:

$$\text{Internal diameter} = (16 + \text{age in years})/4$$

A cuffed tube can be used safely in the in-hospital setting.[3] For cuffed endotracheal tubes, the formula used to estimate the internal diameter is:

$$\text{Internal diameter} = (\text{age in years}/4) + 3$$

Because these are both estimations of endotracheal tube size, tubes one-half size smaller and larger should be available for immediate use. Table 10-5 provides information regarding endotracheal tube sizes and other equipment issues.

Monitoring the patient during intubation is critical to assess for desaturation or bradycardia. Once the child is intubated, observation of chest movement and auscultation of the lungs help determine correct placement. A radiograph is used to confirm proper placement. When placement is confirmed, the tube is securely taped to avoid accidental displacement. In addition, soft restraints should be used to prevent the child from removing the tube. Adequate sedation and analgesia are provided to increase the child's comfort and manage anxiety while intubated.

MEDICATION ADMINISTRATION

Because a child may differ in weight significantly from the average child in the associated age group, medications are prescribed on a microgram, milligram, or milliequivalent per kilogram of body weight basis rather than on a standard dose according to age. Confirming the weight (in kilograms) that is being used to determine drug dosages is important. This same weight should be used during the child's entire hospitalization unless there is a significant change in

Table 10-4 • Quick Examination of a Healthy Versus Decompensating Child

Assessment	Healthy Child	Decompensating Child
Airway		
Patency	Child requires no interventions; child verbalizes and is able to swallow, cough, gag.	Child self-positions and requires interventions, such as head positioning, suctioning, adjunct airways. Unmaintainable airway requires intubation.
Breathing		
Respiratory rate	Breathing is within age-appropriate limits.	Breathing is tachypneic or bradypneic compared with age-appropriate limits and conditions.* Note: Warning parameter: >60 breaths/min
Chest movement (presence)	Chest rises and falls equally and simultaneously with abdomen with each breath.	Child has minimal or no chest movement with respiratory effort.
Chest movement (quality)	Child has silent and effortless respirations.	Child shows evidence of labored respirations with retractions. Asynchronous movement (seesaw) is observed between chest and abdomen with respiratory efforts.
Air movement (presence)	Air exchange is heard bilaterally in all lobes.	Despite movement of the chest, minimal or no air exchange is noted on auscultation.
Air movement (quality)	Breath sounds are of normal intensity and duration.	Nasal flaring, grunting, stridor, and/or wheezing are noted.
Circulation		
Heart rate (presence)	Apical beat is present and within age-appropriate limit.*	Heart rate is absent; bradycardia or tachycardia occurs as compared with age-appropriate limits.* Note: Warning parameters: Infant: <80 beats/min; Child <5 y: >180 beats/min; Child >5 y: >150 beats/min
Heart rate (quality)	Heart rate is regular with normal sinus rhythm.	Heart rate is irregular, slow, or very rapid; common dysrhythmias include supraventricular tachycardia, bradyarrhythmias, and asystole.
Skin	Extremities are warm, pink with capillary refill ≤2 s; peripheral pulses are present bilaterally with normal intensity.	Child has pallor, cyanosis, or mottled skin color and cool-to-cold extremities. Capillary refill time is ≥2 s; peripheral pulses are weak or absent; central pulses are weak.
Cerebral perfusion	Child is alert to surroundings, recognizes parents or significant others, is responsive to fear and pain, and has normal muscle tone.	Child is irritable, lethargic, obtunded, or comatose; has minimal or no reaction to pain; and/or has loose muscle tone (floppy).
Blood pressure	Blood pressure is within age-appropriate limits.	Blood pressure falls from age-appropriate limits,* a late sign of decompensation. Note: A fall of 10 mm Hg systolic pressure is significant. Lower systolic blood pressure limit: Infant ≤1 mo, 60 mm Hg; Infant ≤1 y, 70 mm Hg; Child, 70 mm Hg + (2 × age in years)

*All vital signs are interpreted within the context of age, clinical condition, and other external factors, such as the presence of fever.
Adapted from Moloney-Harmon PA, Rosenthal CH: Nursing care modifications for the child in the adult ICU. In Stillwell S (ed): Mosby's Critical Care Nursing Reference, pp 588–670, 1992, with permission from Elsevier Science.

the child's weight. Because pediatric dosages may be unfamiliar to the adult clinician, precalculated emergency drug sheets are helpful. The emergency drug sheet should include the recommended resuscitation medication dosages, medication concentration, and final medication dose and volume the individual child is to receive. The recommended dosages should reflect the American Heart Association's Pediatric Advanced Life Support standards.

An important recommendation for medication administration in the pediatric patient is the single-dose system. The single-dose system involves preparing one syringe to contain only the prescribed medication dose. The syringe should be properly labeled with the drug name and dose. The nurse administers the entire volume of the syringe to ensure that the prescribed dose has been given. The single-dose system prevents overmedication or undermedication of the child.

Medication errors have received increased attention since the 2000 Institute of Medicine report, "To Err Is Human." The most common reason for harm to pediatric patients, medication errors result in a higher risk for death.[4] The prescribing phase is associated with the most errors (dosing errors), and the administration phase results in the second most errors.[5] Nurses are the last potential barrier between an occurrence and an adverse outcome; they are most likely to intercept the error. Preventing medication errors is especially important in children because there is a much smaller margin for error in this patient pop-

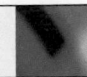

Table 10-5 • Recommended Resuscitation Equipment for Infants and Children

	Child's Weight						
	4–8 kg (8.8–17.6 pounds)	8–11 kg (17.6–24.2 pounds)	11–14 kg (24.2–30.8 pounds)	14–18 kg (30.8–39.6 pounds)	18–24 kg (39.6–52.8 pounds)	24–32 kg (52.8–70.4 pounds)	32+ kg (70.4+ pounds)
Oxygen mask	Newborn	Pediatric	Pediatric	Pediatric	Pediatric	Adult	Adult
Oral airway	Infant	Small child	Child	Child	Child	Small adult	Small adult
Resuscitation bag	Infant	Child	Child	Child	Child	Adult	Adult
Laryngoscope blade	0–1 straight	1 straight	2 straight or curved	2 straight or curved	2 straight or curved	2–3 straight or curved	3 straight or curved
Endotracheal tube (mm)	2.5 preterm; 3.0–3.5 term infant	4.0 uncuffed	4.5 uncuffed	5.0 uncuffed	5.5 uncuffed	6.0 cuffed	6.5 cuffed
Endotracheal tube (cm at the tip)	10–10.5	11–12	12.5–13.5	14–15	15.5–16.5	17–18	18.5–19.5
Stylet	Small	Small	Small	Small	Large	Large	Large
Suction catheter	6–8	8	8–10	10	10	10–12	12–14
Nasogastric tube (F)	5–8	8–10	10	10–12	12–14	14–18	18
Urinary catheter	5–8	8–10	10	10–12	10–12	12	12
Chest tube (F)	10–12	16–20	20–24	20–24	24–32	28–32	32–40
Blood pressure cuff	Newborn or infant	Infant or child	Child	Child	Child	Child or adult	Adult
IV catheter (G)	22–24	22–24	20–22	18–22	18–20	18–20	16–20
Butterfly catheter	23–25	23–25	21–23	21–23	21–23	20–22	18–21
Vascular catheter	3.0 F 5–12 cm	3.0–4.09 F 5–12 cm	3.0–4.0 F 5–12 cm	4.0–5.0 F 5–25 cm	4.0–5.0 F 5–25 cm	4.0–5.0 F 5–25 cm	5.0–8.0 F 5–30 cm
Guide wire (mm)	0.46	0.46–0.53	0.53–0.89	0.53–0.89	0.53–0.89	0.53–0.89	0.89

Data from Hazinski M: PALS Provider Manual. Dallas, American Heart Association, 2002; Slota M: AACN Core Curriculum for Pediatric Critical Care Nursing, Philadelphia, WB Saunders, 2006.
From the AACN Pediatric Critical Care Pocket Reference Card. © 1998 American Association of Critical-Care Nurses (AACN). Adapted with permission of the publisher.
Reprinted from Dimens Crit Care Nurs 20(1):23, 2001, with permission.

ulation. Safety strategies such as ensuring staff competency and computerized physician order entry should be evaluated and implemented.[6]

PAIN MANAGEMENT

Because of the nature of the environment and associated procedures, the critically ill child is at high risk for pain. The first step in assessing pain in children is to understand the child's response to, and communication of, pain. This is based on a variety of factors, including the child's developmental level, past and present experience with pain, cultural aspects, personality, parental presence, and age, as well as the nature of the illness or injury.[7] For instance, critically ill children may be in severe pain but may be unable to communicate because of sedation, paralytic agents, mechanical ventilation, or coma.

Pain assessment is multidimensional. Synthesis of a variety of parameters provides information that can be used to make a decision about the level of the child's pain and the most appropriate intervention. Assessment of pain by nurses is influenced by factors such as educational level, skills, experience, personal beliefs, and different strategies adopted

for assessment.[8] Infants and young children cannot communicate verbally, which makes pain assessment challenging. This inability to communicate is also an issue in the sedated or chemically paralyzed child. This requires that the nurse use different cues for assessment of pain, which include physiological and behavioral changes.[9]

Physiological parameters used in pain assessment include heart rate, respiratory rate, blood pressure, and oxygen saturation. Other parameters described by Anand and Carr[10] include sweating, increased muscle tone, and skin color changes. These parameters return to normal as physiological adaptation occurs. This adaptation can actually occur within minutes, and the nurse must realize that the child may still be in pain. The physical signs are not necessarily specific for pain but may be the only parameter available to the nurse caring for the critically ill child.

Behavioral responses may be helpful for pain assessment, especially in the child who cannot communicate. The next section on interaction with children and families discusses the continuum of responses related to pain and comfort.

Another dimension of pain assessment is self-report. Many tools are available. However, these often require

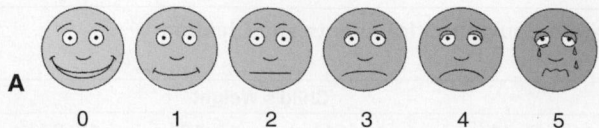

A

0   1   2   3   4   5

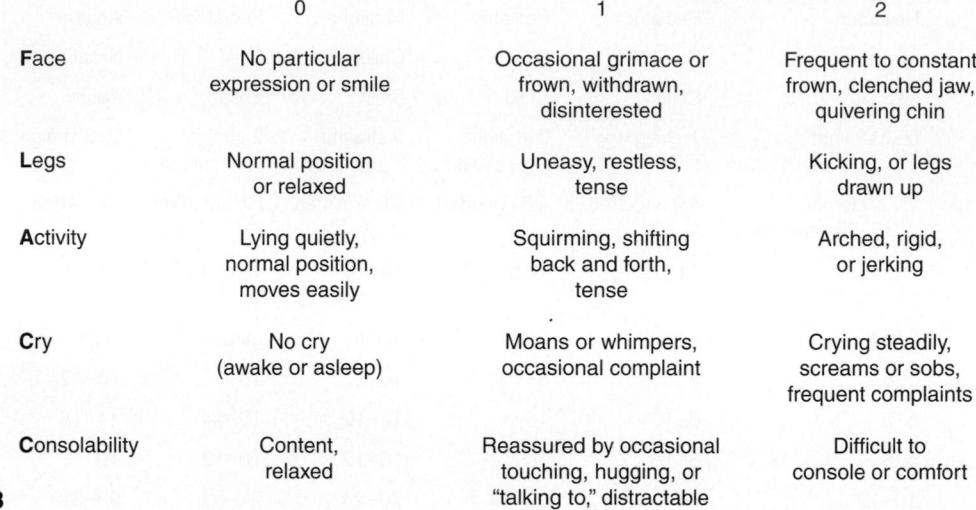

	0	1	2
Face	No particular expression or smile	Occasional grimace or frown, withdrawn, disinterested	Frequent to constant frown, clenched jaw, quivering chin
Legs	Normal position or relaxed	Uneasy, restless, tense	Kicking, or legs drawn up
Activity	Lying quietly, normal position, moves easily	Squirming, shifting back and forth, tense	Arched, rigid, or jerking
Cry	No cry (awake or asleep)	Moans or whimpers, occasional complaint	Crying steadily, screams or sobs, frequent complaints
Consolability	Content, relaxed	Reassured by occasional touching, hugging, or "talking to," distractable	Difficult to console or comfort

B

Figure 10-2 • Tools for assessing pain in children. **A:** The FACES scale. This scale may be used in children 3 years and older. Explain that FACE 0 is a very happy face because there is no pain. FACE 1 hurts just a little bit. FACE 2 hurts a little bit more. FACE 3 hurts even more. FACE 4 hurts a whole lot. FACE 5 hurts very much; the pain can make you cry. Ask the child to choose the face that best describes the pain he or she is feeling. **B:** The FLACC (face, legs, activity, cry, consolability) scale. This scale can be used with children younger than 3 years. To use the FLACC scale, assess the child in each category, assigning a score between 0 and 2. Total the score, and then evaluate the total using the 0–10 pain scale parameters. (**A** from Wong DL, Hockenberry-Eaton M, Wilson D, et al: Wong's Essentials of Pediatric Nursing, 7th ed. St Louis, Mosby, 2005, p 1259. Copyrighted by Mosby, Inc. Reprinted by permission. **B** from Merkel SI, Voepel-Lewis T: The FLACC: A behavioral scale for scoring post-operative pain in young children. Pediatr Nurs 23[3]:293–297, 1997. Reprinted by permission.)

children to interact or use their hands and are not usually helpful in the critical care setting. Examples of self-report tools include the numerical rating scale (see Chapter 5, Fig. 5-1), the FACES scale (Fig. 10-2), and the color scale. If the child is unable or unwilling to give a report, the parent's report of pain is often helpful. Multidimensional scales, such as the COMFORT, Modified Motor Activity Assessment, and FLACC (face, legs, activity, cry, consolability) scales (see Fig. 10-2), are helpful because they combine dimensions of behavioral and physiological distress and do not require interaction or use of the hands.

Pain management interventions are multidimensional whenever possible, including nonpharmacological and pharmacological approaches. However, pharmacological intervention is never withheld when it is appropriate. Opioids are usually the first-line drugs for pain management in the critically ill child. A variety of pharmacological agents are available, and the choice of drug depends on the child's response and the practitioner's preference. Nursing responsibilities include assessing the child's need for the drug, administering the appropriate dose, and monitoring the child's response. Sedation and analgesia are part of the daily management of the critically ill child. However, inherent in the use of these agents is the risk for adverse responses. The nurse is responsible for vig-

ilant monitoring and for implementing changes based on the child's response and recommendations by the multidisciplinary team.[11]

Other methods of pain control include intravenous patient-controlled analgesia (PCA) and epidural analgesia. PCA helps the child maintain a steady state of pain relief and also gives the child some control over pain. Epidural analgesia is also helpful for a variety of children. Epidural narcotics provide selective analgesia but do have associated side effects, including respiratory depression, nausea and vomiting, pruritus, and urinary retention.

Nurses may consider the use of nonpharmacological methods, such as distraction, relaxation, massage, and hypnosis, in conjunction with pharmacological agents. The method must be age appropriate, and parental presence is considered. Whatever methods are used, a critical determinant of their effectiveness is the child's response.

• Interaction With Children and Families

Interacting with children demands familiarity with their developmental capabilities and psychosocial needs. Categorization of children into groups according to physical and cognitive age can assist the nurse in predicting the child's expected social, cognitive, and physical capabilities. Developmental and psychosocial assessment is beyond the scope of this chapter; therefore, the reader should consult an appropriate growth and development reference. Although each age group of children has common developmental capabilities, tasks, and fears, it is helpful to recognize the common fears of all children despite their age. These fears include loss of control, threat of separation, painful procedures, and communicated anxiety.[12]

Unlike the adult patient, the young child does not consciously screen most behavior and spoken words. The young child subconsciously communicates behaviorally through verbal, nonverbal (body language, behaviors), and abstract (play, drawing, story telling) cues. Although the child's behavior is more natural in a familiar environment, the cues available to the clinician can suggest how a child is feeling or perceiving an event or the presence of a person. In general, the child's behavior is more activity oriented and more emotional than that of adults.[12] These qualities of a child's behavior should be expected as the norm of average, healthy children and may be used as parameters against which to contrast the behavior of the critically ill child (Table 10-6).

Behavioral responses are particularly helpful during the assessment of pain or comfort. The infant or child may display body movement that spans the entire activity continuum from minimal movement, such as rigidity and guarding, to high activity, such as thrashing and kicking. Assessing various behavioral responses (e.g., gestures, posture, movement, and facial expression) and examining the congruency between these responses are particularly helpful.

Interaction with pediatric patients and their families is also facilitated by the appreciation of the child's significant others. The philosophy of family-centered care is essential to the optimal care of the pediatric patient. Gone are the days when parents dropped their children for care at the entrance of the hospital. Although there are several components of family-centered care, the salient concept is to value, recognize, and support the family in the care of their child. The family is the constant in the child's life and is ultimately responsible for responding to the child's emotional, social, developmental, physical, and health care needs. Appropriate support and incorporation of parents may buffer the threats of the ICU environment on the child. Parents may assist or influence the child's cognitive appraisal of the environment, personnel, and events. The child often uses the reactions of the parent as a barometer in interpreting events in ways ranging from threatening to beneficial.[13]

The tone and manner in which the clinician approaches the bedside of a pediatric patient and his or her family are important. Communicated anxiety refers to the anxious feelings conveyed to the child

Table 10-6 • Contrasting Nonverbal Behavioral Cues of the Healthy and the Critically Ill Child

Healthy	Critically Ill
Posture	
Moves, flexes	May be loose, flaccid
	May prefer fetal position or position of comfort
Gestures	
Turns to familiar voices	Responds slowly to familiar voices
Movement	
Moves purposefully	Exhibits minimal movement, lethargy
Moves toward new, pleasurable items	Shows increased movement, irritability (possibly indicating
Moves away from threatening items, people	cardiopulmonary or neurological compromise, pain, or sleep deprivation)
Reactions/Coping Style	
Responds to parent(s) coming, leaving	Exhibits minimal response to parent presence, absence
Responds to environment and equipment	Exhibits minimal response to presence or absence of transitional objects
Cries and fights invasive procedures	Displays minimal defensive responses
Facial Expressions	
Looks at faces and makes eye contact	May not track faces, objects
Changes facial expressions in response to interactions	Avoids eye contact or has minimal response to interactions
Responds negatively to face wash	Minimally changes facial expression during face wash
Blinks in response to stimuli	Exhibits increased or decreased blinking
Widens eyes with fear	Avoids eye contact
Is fascinated with own mouth	Avoids or dislikes mouth stimulation
Holds mouth "ready for action"	Drools or displays loose mouth musculature
	Sucks intermittently or weakly

Taken from Moloney-Harmon P, Rosenthal CH: Nursing care modifications for the child in the adult ICU. In Stillwell S (ed): Critical Care Nursing Reference Book, 1992, p 590, with permission from Elsevier Science.

> **Box 10-1   Examples of Nursing Diagnoses and Collaborative Problems for the Critically Ill Pediatric Patient**
>
> - Airway Clearance, Ineffective related to obstructed airway
> - Anxiety related to environment
> - Risk for Imbalanced Body Temperature
> - Interrupted Family Processes related to shift in health status of a family member
> - Deficient Fluid Volume related to active fluid volume loss, failure of regulatory mechanisms
> - Delayed Growth and Development related to separation from significant others

by the parents, the health care team members, or both. Interventions to relieve the anxiety of parents and fellow health care team members have a direct impact on the child's well-being. Interventions may include assisting parents and staff in anticipating the child's responses to therapy and illness and guiding parents and staff in therapeutic communication techniques.[14]

Parents depend on nurses to humanize the critical care experience for their child. A recent study examined parents' perceptions of nurses' caring practices in the pediatric ICU. Parents reported that nurses used behaviors that demonstrated affection, caring, watching, and protecting. Parents stated that the most desirable nursing behaviors were those that complemented the parental role, which preserved family integrity during a time of crisis.[15]

Examples of nursing diagnoses and collaborative problems for the pediatric patient in the ICU are given in Box 10-1.

• Clinical Applicability Challenges

Case Study

J. is an 18-month-old, 12-kg girl who is admitted for respiratory distress. On admission, her vital signs are as follows: heart rate, 160 beats/minute; respiratory rate, 52 breaths/minute; blood pressure, 100/60 mm Hg; axillary temperature, 100.4°F (38°C); and oxygen saturation, 94%. Physical examination reveals an agitated, irritable, and crying young girl with intercostal and substernal retractions and nasal flaring. Her expiratory wheezing can be heard across the room. The child's respiratory rate is slightly high for her age, although tachypnea is to be expected for her clinical condition. She has a low-grade fever and is anxious, which may also account for the tachypnea. The anxiety, agitation, and increased work of breathing increase the oxygen demand while the lower airway obstruction decreases oxygen transport. The warning parameters of

mild tachypnea, nasal flaring, retractions, and wheezing indicate a child with respiratory distress who is at risk for respiratory failure.

Initial management priorities include having J. assume a position of comfort and administering oxygen while assessing her response. Albuterol, an inhaled β_2-agonist, is administered. After these interventions, her vital signs are as follows: heart rate, 150 beats/minute; respiratory rate, 42 breaths/minute; blood pressure, 105/62 mm Hg; and oxygen saturation, 98% on 40% oxygen by face mask.

One hour later, J.'s vitals signs are as follows: heart rate, 90 beats/minute; respiratory rate, 22 breaths/minute; blood pressure, 92/52 mm Hg; and oxygen saturation, 90%. Retractions are more pronounced, and wheezing is not audible by auscultation. She is extremely lethargic and is not responding to her parents. Arterial blood gases reveal the following: pH, 7.25; $PaCO_2$, 56 mm Hg; PaO_2, 80 mm Hg; and HCO_3^-, 27 mEq/L on a fraction of inspired oxygen of 0.5. The child is demonstrating signs of fatigue and respiratory failure. Warning parameters include an unmaintainable airway, bradypnea, worsening retractions, lethargy, no air movement (indicated by lack of wheezing), and failure to recognize her parents. Management priorities at this time include bag-mask ventilation and intubation.

Treatment is directed toward ensuring oxygenation and ventilation while reversing bronchospasm. Medications include inhaled bronchodilators and corticosteroids. Mechanical ventilation is also provided until J. shows improvement, as demonstrated by arterial blood gases, vital signs, and clinical condition.

1. What are the signs of impending respiratory failure in J.?
2. What are the management priorities for J.?
3. What would you assess to determine J.'s response to interventions?

Review Questions

1. A 1-month-old infant is admitted to the intensive care unit. She has a history of vomiting for the past 24 hours. She is lethargic and cool to touch; her mother reports that she has had no wet diapers for the past 12 hours. She has a temperature of 100.4°F (38°C); a heart rate of 170 beats/minute; a respiratory rate of 40 breaths/minute, with shallow respirations; and a blood pressure of 50 mm Hg by palpation. Her peripheral pulses are weak and thready, her capillary refill time is 4 seconds, and she is mottled and cool to the touch. Based on her history and assessment findings, you determine that the category of shock is
   a. septic.
   b. cardiogenic.
   c. hypovolemic.
   d. distributive.

2. Consider the child described in question 1. The most appropriate initial intervention is to administer
  a. 5% dextrose in water.
  b. normal saline (0.9% NaCl).
  c. clear fluids orally.
  d. packed red blood cells.

3. You are caring for a 3-year-old, 15-kg boy who presents with grunting, nasal flaring, and retractions. You note that he has both inspiratory and expiratory wheezing. His oxygen saturation is 91% on room air. Your initial intervention is to
  a. administer oxygen.
  b. begin an inhalation bronchodilator.
  c. intubate.
  d. begin a terbutaline infusion.

4. A 5-year-old boy comes to the emergency department after being hit by a car. He is unconscious and showing signs of acute respiratory distress and hypotension. He has a heart rate of 85 beats/minute and a respiratory rate of 6 breaths/minute. The first priority for his resuscitation is to
  a. insert an intravenous line but restrict the fluids to 10 mL/kg.
  b. insert an intravenous line and begin fluids at 20 mL/kg.
  c. send the child for a magnetic resonance imaging.
  d. intubate the child and begin artificial ventilation.

5. A 5-year-old, 18-kg girl has been admitted for dehydration. Once she is rehydrated, how much maintenance fluid should she receive in 24 hours?
  a. 1000 mL
  b. 1200 mL
  c. 1400 mL
  d. 2000 mL

References

1. Moloney-Harmon P, Rosenthal CH: Nursing care modifications for the child in the adult ICU. In Stillwell S (ed): Critical Care Nursing Reference Book. St. Louis, Mosby-Year Book, 1992, pp 588–670
2. Rupp LA, Day MW: Children are different: Pediatric differences and the impact on trauma. In Moloney-Harmon PA, Czerwinski SJ (eds): Nursing Care of the Pediatric Trauma Patient. Philadelphia: W. B. Saunders, 2003, pp 35–52
3. American Heart Association: Pediatric advanced life support. Circulation 112(24):N-167-N–187, 2005
4. Kohn LT, Corrigan JM, Donaldson MS (eds): To Err Is Human: Building a Safer Health System. Washington, DC, National Academy Press, 2000
5. American Academy of Pediatrics: Prevention of medication errors in the pediatric inpatient setting. Pediatrics 112(2):431–436, 2003
6. Cohen H: Pediatric medical errors. Part 3: Safety strategies. Pediatr Nurs 30(4):334–335, 2004
7. Oakes LL: Caring practices: Providing comfort. In Curley MAQ, Moloney-Harmon PA (eds): Critical Care Nursing of Infants and Children. Philadelphia, WB Saunders, 2001, pp 547–576
8. Van Hulle VC: Nurses' knowledge, attitudes, and practices: Regarding children's pain. MCN Am J Matern Child Nurs 30(3):177–183, 2005
9. Byers JF, Thornley K: Cueing into infant pain. MCN Am J Matern Child Nurs 29(2):84–89, 2004
10. Anand KJS, Carr DB: The neuroanatomy, neurophysiology, and neurochemistry of pain, stress, and analgesia in newborns and children. Pediatr Clin North Am 36(4):795–821, 1989
11. Sorce LR: Adverse responses: Sedation, analgesia and neuromuscular blocking agents in critically ill children. Crit Care Nurs Clin North Am 17(4):441–450, 2005
12. Smith J, Martin SA: Caring practices: Providing developmentally supportive care. In Curley MAQ, Moloney-Harmon PA (eds): Critical Care Nursing of Infants and Children. Philadelphia, WB Saunders, 2001, pp 17–46
13. Slota M, Shearn D, Potersnak K, Haas L: Perspectives on family-centered, flexible visitation in the intensive care unit setting. Crit Care Med 31(Suppl 5):362–366, 2003
14. Curley MAQ, Meyer EC: Caring practices: The impact of the critical care experience on the family. In Curley MAQ, Moloney-Harmon PA (eds): Critical Care Nursing of Infants and Children. Philadelphia, WB Saunders, 2001, pp 47–67
15. Harbaugh BL, Tomlinson PS, Kirschbaum M: Parents' perceptions of nurses' caring behaviors in the pediatric intensive care unit. Issues in Comprehens Pediatr Nurs 27(3):163–178, 2004

Other Selected Readings

Haut C: Oncological emergencies in the pediatric intensive care unit. AACN Clin Issues 16(2):232–245, 2005
Jenkins T: Sickle cell anemia in the pediatric intensive care unit: Novel approaches for managing life-threatening complications. AACN Clin Issues 13(2):154–168, 2002
Kimberly A: Caring for adolescents in the adult intensive care unit. Crit Care Nurse 22(2):80–99, 2002
Kline AM: Pediatric catheter-related bloodstream infections: Latest strategies to decrease risk. AACN Clin Issues 16(2):185–198, 2005
Knapp J: Hyperosmolar therapy in the treatment of severe head injury in children: Mannitol and hypertonic saline. AACN Clin Issues 16(2):199–211, 2005
Marcoux KK: Current management of status asthmaticus in the pediatric ICU. Crit Care Nurs Clin North Am 17(4):417–430, 2005
Marcoux KK: Management of increased intracranial pressure in the critically ill child with an acute neurological injury. AACN Clin Issues 16(2):212–231, 2005
Moloney-Harmon PA: Pediatric sepsis: The infection unto death. Crit Care Nurs Clin North Am 17(4):417–430, 2005
Oakes L: Assessment and management of pain in the critically ill pediatric patient. Crit Care Nurs Clin North Am 13(2):281–296, 2001
Rice BA, Nelson C: Safety in the pediatric ICU: The key to quality outcomes. Crit Care Nurs Clin North Am 17(4):431–440, 2005
Roberts KE: Pediatric fluid and electrolyte balance: Critical care case studies. Crit Care Nurs Clin North Am 17(4):261–374, 2005
Ware L: Inhaled nitric oxide in infants and children. Crit Care Nurs Clin North Am 14(1):1–6, 2002
Wedekind C, Fidler B: Compatibility of commonly used intravenous infusions in a pediatric intensive care unit. Crit Care Nurse 21(4):45–51, 2001

11

The Critically Ill Pregnant Woman

Physiological Changes in Pregnancy
    Cardiovascular Changes
    Respiratory Changes
    Renal Changes
    Gastrointestinal and Metabolic Changes
    Hematological Changes
    Fetal and Placental Development Considerations
Critical Care Conditions in Pregnancy
    Severe Preeclampsia
    HELLP Syndrome
    Disseminated Intravascular Coagulation
    Amniotic Fluid Embolism
    Acute Respiratory Distress Syndrome
    Trauma
Providing Emotional Support

Objectives

Based on the content in this chapter, the reader should be able to:

❶ Summarize normal physiological changes that occur in the cardiovascular, respiratory, renal, and hematological systems during pregnancy.

❷ Differentiate the signs and symptoms of preeclampsia and severe preeclampsia.

❸ Explain the pathophysiology of severe preeclampsia.

❹ Describe parameters of nursing assessment of a severely preeclamptic patient on intravenous magnesium sulfate.

❺ Name three obstetrical conditions that predispose a woman to development of disseminated intravascular coagulation.

❻ Describe the initial care of an obstetrical trauma patient.

❼ Summarize the psychosocial support needed for an obstetrical patient in the intensive care unit (ICU).

Most women experience a normal pregnancy. However, a small percentage of women experience life-threatening complications that may result from the pregnancy itself or develop as a result of a preexisting (comorbid) condition. Such critically ill pregnant women provide a unique challenge to nurses. The physical assessment of these patients includes the interaction between the maternal host and the fetus. Critical care nurses are not expected to have the knowledge and skills associated with fetal heart rate monitoring, and perinatal nurses may not possess the knowledge and skills required for patients needing ventilator support or hemodynamic monitoring. It is important when a critically ill pregnant woman is in the ICU that a collaborative approach be used to provide care.[1]

The general principles of diagnosis and management are similar to those used for other ICU patients. However, physiological changes inherent in pregnancy must be considered to decrease mor-

bidity and mortality.[2] Critical care nurses caring for these patients must understand the physiological changes that occur as the body adapts to pregnancy and distinguish normal from abnormal responses. Table 11-1 outlines these changes.

• Physiological Changes in Pregnancy

CARDIOVASCULAR CHANGES

Normal cardiovascular changes that occur during pregnancy affect pulse, blood pressure, cardiac output, and blood volume (see Table 11-1). Maternal blood volume increases 40% to 50% above baseline. This increase, which is mostly plasma, begins in the first trimester and continues throughout pregnancy. The increase is necessary to provide adequate blood flow to the uterus, fetus, and changing maternal

Table 11-1 • Physiological Changes in Pregnancy

	Change	Pregnancy Levels
Cardiovascular Changes		
Blood volume	>40%–50%	1,260–1,625 mL
Red blood cells	>20%	250–450 mL
Blood pressure		
Systolic	<5–12 mm Hg	
Diastolic	<10–20 mm Hg	
Cardiac output	>30%–50%	6–7 L/min
Heart rate	>10%–30%	Increased by 15–20 beats/min
Systemic vascular resistance	<20%–30%	$1,210 \pm 266$ dynes/s/cm^{-5}
Pulmonary vascular resistance	<34%	78 ± 22 dynes/s/cm^{-5}
Colloid osmotic pressure	<10%–14%	$<22.4 \pm 0.5$
Respiratory Changes		
Functional residual capacity	<10%–21%	1343–1530
Tidal volume	>30%–35%	600 mL
Renal Changes		
Renal blood flow	>25%–50%	1,500–1,750 mL/min
Glomerular filtration rate	>50%	140–170 mL/min
Creatine clearance	>50%	100–150 mL/min

tissues and to accommodate blood loss at birth. Red blood cell volume increases by 20% and is disproportionate to the plasma increase, resulting in maternal physiological anemia. Heart rate increases 10 to 15 beats/minute as early as 7 weeks' gestation and returns to the prepregnancy level by 6 weeks postpartum.[2] Changes in blood volume and heart rate lead to an increase in cardiac output of 30% to 50% (6 to 7 L/minute) during pregnancy.[3] Cardiac output increases slightly more intrapartum as a result of the shunting of blood from the placental–fetal unit. Immediately after birth, a larger increase in cardiac output (59% to 80%) occurs when the empty uterus contracts and shunts approximately 1,000 mL of blood back into the systemic circulation[3] (Table 11-2). A woman loses approximately 500 mL of blood during a vaginal birth and approximately 1,000 mL of blood during a cesarean birth. This is usually well tolerated.

Development of the uteroplacental unit provides a low-resistance network for the expanded blood volume, which reduces cardiac afterload.[4] The pulmonary vascular resistance, or right afterload, also decreases in response to increased blood volume and vasodilation. Under hormonal influence, smooth muscles and vascular beds relax, lowering systemic vascular resistance. Blood pressure decreases during the first and second trimesters and returns to prepregnancy levels by the third trimester. Blood pressure during pregnancy is affected by maternal position more so than in the nonpregnant state. Supine hypotension occurs when the mother remains in a flat position. The side-lying position is recommended,

Table 11-2 • Cardiac Output Changes in Pregnancy and Labor and Delivery

Stage of Pregnancy, Labor, or Delivery	Cardiac Output
By 8 weeks' gestation	22%–30% increase
By 20 weeks' gestation	50% increase
Repositioned from supine to left lateral decubitus	21% increase
Early first stage of labor (dilated <3 cm)	13%–17% increase
Late first stage of labor (dilated 4–7 cm)	23% increase
Second stage labor (dilated >8 cm)	34% increase
During each contraction	11%–15% increase
Immediately after delivery (10 min)	59%–80% increase (dependent on type of anesthesia)
Within 1 h of delivery	49% increase

but if the patient must be supine, the uterus should be tilted away from the inferior vena cava by using a wedge under the hip.

RESPIRATORY CHANGES

Respiratory changes as seen in Table 11-1 occur to accommodate the enlarged uterus and the increased oxygen demands of the mother and fetus. Structural changes include the upward shift of the diaphragm, which decreases functional residual capacity, and rib cage volume displacement, which increases tidal volume by 30% to 35%.[5] Airway mucosal changes include hyperemia, hypersecretion, increased friability, and edema. These changes are significant when inserting nasogastric tubes or nasotracheal tubes because of the risk for epistaxis. Respiratory rate remains unchanged, although some women experience tachypnea or shortness of breath at some time during their pregnancy. The exact cause of dyspnea is unknown, but it may be related to hyperventilation, increased oxygen consumption, or decreased partial pressure of arterial carbon dioxide ($PaCO_2$).

Oxygen consumption increases by 15% to 20% during pregnancy and may increase by 300% during labor.[4] This results in an increased partial pressure of arterial oxygen (PaO_2) to 104 to 108 mm Hg. $PaCO_2$ decreases to 27 to 32 mm Hg and allows for the increased diffusion of carbon dioxide from the fetus to the mother.[6] Renal excretion of bicarbonate causes a slight increase in maternal pH, which is usually insignificant.

RENAL CHANGES

Changes in renal function, also outlined in Table 11-1, accommodate the increase in metabolic and circulatory requirements of pregnancy. Renal blood flow increases by 30% and glomerular filtration rate (GFR) by 50%.[4] These increases allow elevations in the clearance of many substances, such as creatinine and urea, and are reflected in lower serum levels.[5]

GASTROINTESTINAL AND METABOLIC CHANGES

Gastrointestinal changes in pregnancy occur as a result of the growing uterus. Displacement of the esophageal sphincter into the thoracic cavity allows stomach contents to enter the esophagus passively. The pregnant woman is prone to passive regurgitation and aspiration, especially when under general anesthesia or any time she may be unconscious.[5] Hormonal influences cause delayed gastric emptying and increased gastric acid secretion in the third trimester. Smooth muscle relaxation contributes to nausea, heartburn, and constipation. Pregnancy creates a diabetogenic state because the body becomes increasingly resistant to insulin and hyperinsulinemia occurs. Hepatic and maternal fasting blood glucose levels decrease owing to the constant transfer of glucose to the fetus. Whenever a pregnant woman fasts for more than 12 hours, the fetus is at risk for ketonemia.[7]

HEMATOLOGICAL CHANGES

Hematocrit laboratory values decrease because of the hemodilution effect of increased plasma volume. Normal hematocrit values are 32% to 40% during pregnancy.[4] The white blood cell count is elevated from the normal range of 5,000 to 10,000/mm[3] to 6,000 to 16,000/mm[3].[4] There is an increase in clotting factors VII through X and a decrease in factors XI and XIII, which inhibit coagulation. Fibrinogen increases to 300 to 600 mg/dL. Bleeding and clotting times and platelet counts remain the same in pregnancy.

FETAL AND PLACENTAL DEVELOPMENT CONSIDERATIONS

Clinicians must carefully balance the effects and risks of all treatment decisions on the pregnant woman and her fetus. Maternal circulation and nutrition and exposure to teratogens influence embryonic and fetal development.

There are three stages in fetal development: preembryonic (first 14 days), embryonic (day 15 through 8 weeks), and fetal (8 weeks through 40 weeks and delivery). During the embryonic stage, vital organs such as the heart and brain are in development. It is during this stage that the fetus is most vulnerable to teratogens (Fig. 11-1).

Certain medications used in treating the critically ill pregnant woman may cross the placenta and have teratogenic effects on the fetus. For this reason, the clinician must consider the risks and benefits of medication therapy. In 2001, the U.S. Food and Drug Administration revised the five risk categories for labeling drug use in pregnancy (Table 11-3).

The placenta is the organ responsible for the metabolic exchange of oxygen, nutrition, and waste removal between the pregnant woman and the fetus. In early pregnancy, the placenta produces four hormones necessary to maintain the pregnancy. The hormone human chorionic gonadotropin is the basis for pregnancy tests and preserves the function of the corpus luteum. Another hormone, human placental lactogen, stimulates maternal metabolism to supply needed nutrients for fetal growth. This hormone is responsible for the increase in insulin resistance associated with pregnancy. The hormones progesterone and estrogen are eventually produced by the placenta and are responsible for uterine growth and uteroplacental blood flow.

Placental function depends on maternal blood flow. Diseases and conditions that cause vasoconstriction, such as hypertension, cocaine use, or smoking, can diminish blood flow to the placenta and fetus. Even excessive maternal exercise can shunt blood away from the placenta and fetus.

• Critical Care Conditions in Pregnancy

During pregnancy, normal physiological changes occur to provide for growth of the fetus and prepare the mother for birth. Medical or obstetrical complications

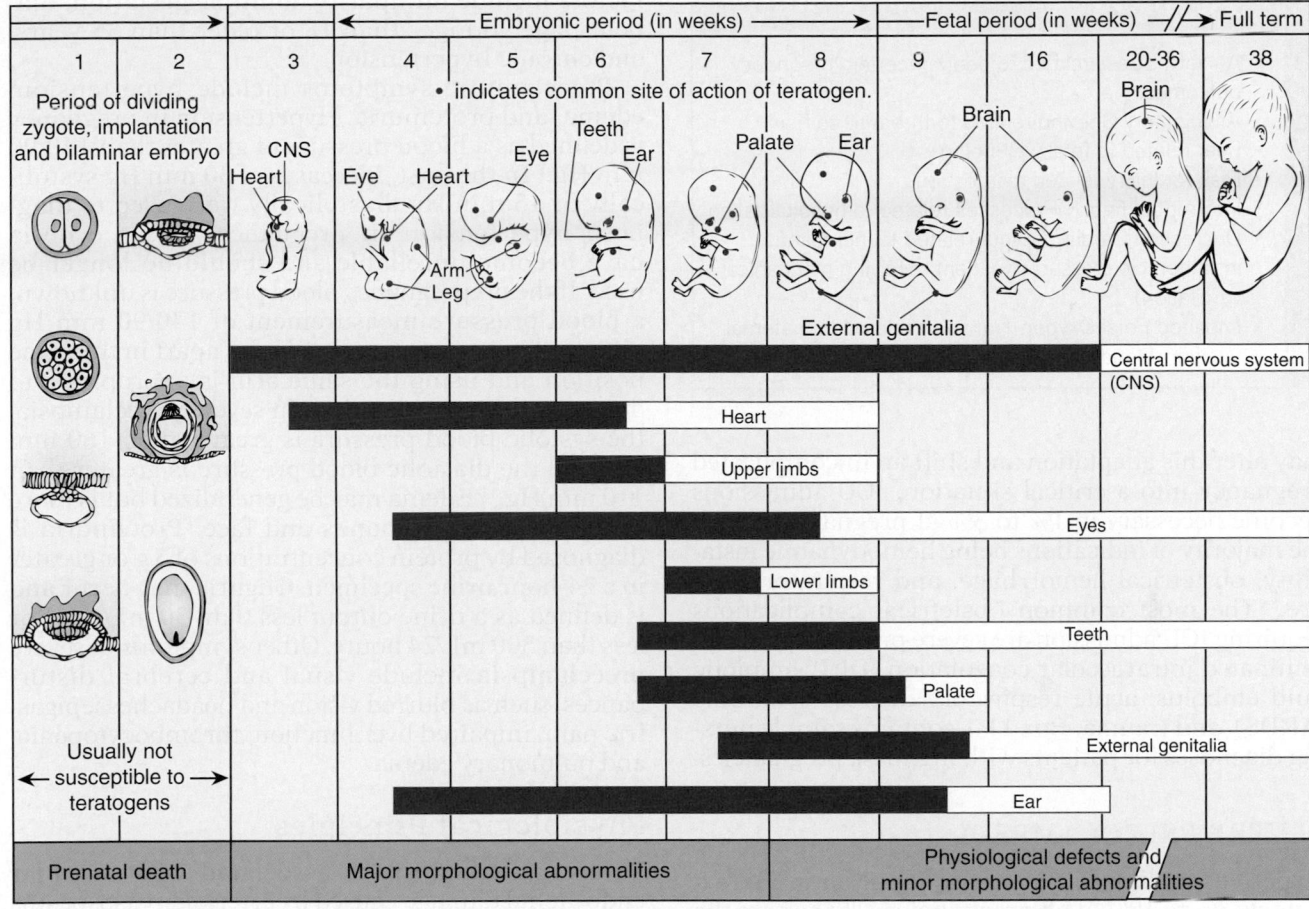

Figure 11-1 • Critical periods of development. *Red* denotes highly sensitive periods. (Reprinted with permission from Moore K: The Developing Human, 6th ed. Philadelphia, WB Saunders, 1998.)

Table 11-3 • Teratogenic Medication Risk Categories

Category	Description
A	Adequate, well-controlled studies in pregnant women have not shown an increased risk for fetal abnormalities.
B	Animal studies have revealed no evidence of harm to the fetus; however, there are no adequate and well-controlled studies in pregnant women. **OR** Animal studies have shown an adverse effect, but adequate and well-controlled studies in pregnant women have failed to demonstrate a risk to the fetus.
C	Animal studies have shown an adverse effect, and there are no adequate and well-controlled studies in pregnant women. **OR** No animal studies have been conducted and there are no adequate and well-controlled studies in pregnant women.
D	Studies, adequate well-controlled or observational, in pregnant women have demonstrated a risk to the fetus. However, the benefits of therapy may outweigh the potential risk.
X	Studies, adequate well-controlled or observational, in animals or pregnant women have demonstrated positive evidence of fetal abnormalities. The use of the product is contraindicated in women who are or may become pregnant.

may alter this adaptation and shift an uncomplicated pregnancy into a critical situation. ICU admissions become necessary in 1% to 3% of pregnancies, with the majority of indications being hemodynamic instability, obstetrical hemorrhage, and respiratory failure.[8] The most common obstetrical complications requiring ICU admission are severe preeclampsia, disseminated intravascular coagulation (DIC), amniotic fluid embolus, acute respiratory distress syndrome (ARDS), and trauma. Box 11-1 contains sample nursing diagnoses for patients with high-risk pregnancies.

SEVERE PREECLAMPSIA

Hypertensive disorders of pregnancy occur in approximately 3% to 10% of all pregnancies.[9,10] They are the third leading cause of maternal death in the United States. Terms used to describe the different types of hypertension that may occur in pregnancy are listed in Box 11-2. Preeclampsia is one hypertensive disorder

Box 11-2 • Clinical Terminology: Hypertensive Disorders During Pregnancy

- *Preeclampsia:* a pregnancy-specific syndrome observed after the 20th week of pregnancy with systolic blood pressure of ≥140 mm Hg or diastolic blood pressure of ≥90 mm Hg, accompanied by significant proteinuria. In women with preeclampsia, blood pressure usually returns to baseline within days to weeks after delivery.
- *Eclampsia:* the occurrence, in a woman with preeclampsia, of seizures that cannot be attributed to other causes. Convulsions usually occur after midpregnancy, and may occur postpartum.
- *Gestational hypertension:* a blood pressure elevation detected for the first time after midpregnancy, distinguished from preeclampsia by the absence of proteinuria.
- *Chronic hypertension:* elevated blood pressure in the mother that predated the pregnancy. It can also be diagnosed in retrospect, when preeclampsia or gestational hypertension fail to normalize after delivery.

From National Institutes of Health, National Heart Lung and Blood Institute: Report of the Working Group on Research on Hypertension During Pregnancy, April 2001.

occurring in 5% to 7% of pregnancies.[10] The etiology of preeclampsia is unknown; however, predisposing risk factors include nulliparity, multiple gestation, diabetes, age younger than 18 or older than 35 years, and chronic hypertension.

Preeclamptic symptoms include hypertension, edema, and proteinuria. Hypertension in pregnancy is defined as a blood pressure of greater than 140/90 mm Hg.[8] In the past, increases of 30 mm Hg systolically or 15 mm Hg diastolically were used to diagnose hypertension in pregnancy. These criteria have become unreliable and should no longer be used. If the prepregnancy blood pressure is unknown, a blood pressure measurement of 140/90 mm Hg obtained twice at intervals 6 hours apart in the same position and using the same arm is appropriate to diagnose this complication. In severe preeclampsia, the systolic blood pressure is greater than 160 mm Hg, and the diastolic blood pressure is greater than 110 mm Hg.[11] Edema may be generalized but is more pronounced in the hands and face. Proteinuria is diagnosed by protein concentrations of 5 g or greater in a 24-hour urine specimen. Oliguria may occur and is defined as a urine output less than 30 mL/hour or less than 500 mL/24 hours. Other symptoms of severe preeclampsia include visual and cerebral disturbances, such as blurred vision and headaches, epigastric pain, impaired liver function, thrombocytopenia, and pulmonary edema.

Physiological Principles

Severe preeclampsia is associated with vascular endothelial damage caused by arteriolar vasospasms and vasoconstriction.[9] Arterial circulation is disrupted by alternating areas of constriction and dilation. Damage to the endothelium results in leakage of plasma into the extravascular space and allows platelet aggregation to occur. Colloidal osmotic pressure decreases as protein enters the extravascular space, and the woman is at risk for hypovolemia and alteration in tissue perfusion and oxygenation.[10] Pulmonary edema may develop and can be noncardiogenic or cardiogenic. Noncardiogenic pulmonary edema develops because pulmonary capillaries become more permeable and are susceptible to fluid leakage. Cardiogenic pulmonary edema occurs because of impaired left ventricular systolic or diastolic function.[10] Symptoms of pulmonary edema include coughing, dyspnea, chest pain, tachycardia, cyanosis, and pink, frothy sputum.[6]

Arterial vasospasm and endothelial damage also decrease perfusion to the kidneys. The decreased kidney perfusion results in a decreased GFR and leads to oliguria. Oliguria may not be an indication of hypovolemia and should not be treated with diuretics. Glomerular capillary endothelial damage permits protein to leak across the capillary membrane and into the urine, resulting in proteinuria, increased blood urea nitrogen, and increased serum creatinine. If vasospasm and hypercoagulability are long lasting, ischemia occurs in the glomeruli. Complete recovery of renal function usually occurs after delivery.[9]

The liver is also affected by multisystem vasospasm and endothelial damage. Decreased perfusion to the liver can cause ischemia and necrosis. The liver may become edematous as a result of inflammatory infiltrates and obstructed blood flow.[10] Liver damage is reflected in elevated liver function study results, such as serum aspartate aminotransferase, lactate dehydrogenase, and serum alanine aminotransferase.[2]

Neurological sequelae may include seizures, cerebral edema, and cerebral hemorrhage. Symptoms associated with neurological progression are headaches, blurred vision, hyperreflexia and clonus, and changes in level of consciousness. Increased intracranial pressure and decreased perfusion can lead to hypoxia, coma, and death.[10]

Medical Management

The only cure for severe preeclampsia is delivery of the fetus. The decision to deliver the fetus versus continuing expectant management (i.e., to maintain the pregnancy and monitor changes) is individualized.[10]

Usually these patients require invasive hemodynamic monitoring, frequent blood pressure measurements, strict intake and output monitoring, laboratory report monitoring, aggressive anticonvulsant and antihypertensive drug therapy, and, if undelivered, fetal surveillance. Management is focused on preventing seizures and respiratory complications, controlling hypertension, monitoring cardiovascular status, and maintaining fluid status. If the woman does not deliver, fetal monitoring is necessary. Critical care and obstetrical staff must collaborate to provide close fetal observation. It is important that they consider the fetus to be another patient.[1]

Hemodynamic monitoring permits accurate assessments of cardiac output and fluid volume status. Normal hemodynamic values during pregnancy are listed in Table 11-4.[3] Elevated pulmonary artery wedge pressure (PAWP) and pulmonary artery pressure (PAP) values may indicate hypervolemia, thereby placing the woman at risk for cardiogenic pulmonary edema. (See Chapter 17 for a more detailed discussion of hemodynamic monitoring.) Interventions to reduce preload include restricting intravenous fluids, repositioning the patient on her side, and administering diuretics when fluid overload or pulmonary edema is present. Decreased central venous pressure, PAP, and PAWP values indicate hypovolemia, and the patient may need a fluid challenge.

Box 11-3 • Magnesium Sulfate Administration

Dose concentration: 20 g in 500 mL normal saline or D_5W = 2 g/50 mL

Loading dose: 4–6 g intravenous bolus over 10–20 min

Maintenance dose: 2–3 g/h by intravenous infusion

Drug therapy is directed at preventing seizures and hypertensive crises. Intravenous magnesium sulfate is the drug of choice for severe preeclampsia to prevent maternal seizures (Box 11-3). Magnesium sulfate blocks the reuptake of acetylcholine at the nerve end synapses and relaxes smooth muscles. Side effects include drowsiness, flushing, diaphoresis, hyporeflexia, hypocalcemia, and respiratory paralysis.[10] A therapeutic serum level of 4 to 7 mg/dL is maintained through a continuous infusion of 1 to 3 g/hour. Serum levels higher than 15 mg/dL may result in respiratory arrest.

Hydralazine hydrochloride (Apresoline) is the antihypertensive agent most commonly used during pregnancy. It causes arterial vasodilation and decreases mean arterial pressure and systemic vascular resistance. Hydralazine increases cardiac output, heart rate, and renal blood flow. Doses are commonly given in 5- to 10-mg boluses intravenously every 20 minutes until a satisfactory reduction in blood pressure is achieved.[11] Other antihypertensive agents used include nitroprusside (Nitropress), nifedipine (Procardia), and labetalol hydrochloride (Normodyne). These drugs may be used when hydralazine therapy fails.

Nursing Interventions

The nurse must assess the patient for increased risk for seizures by evaluating neurological symptoms. To reduce the risk for seizures, the nurse can decrease light and sound stimulation to the patient. Treatments and interventions are coordinated to optimize rest periods. If seizures occur, the nurse protects the patient from injury, ensures a patent airway, provides adequate oxygenation, and evaluates possible aspiration. After stabilizing the patient, uterine and fetal activity are quickly assessed. In most instances, immediate delivery of the fetus is indicated.

If the patient is receiving magnesium sulfate therapy, the nurse continuously assesses for symptoms of magnesium toxicity, such as respiratory depression and hyporeflexia. Magnesium is excreted in the urine, and prolonged oliguria allows blood levels to accumulate to toxic levels.

If the patient has delivered, magnesium sulfate therapy should be continued for 24 hours. The nurse must assess uterine bleeding. The uterus should be firm after delivery, and if not, uterine massage and oxytocin therapy are needed. Box 11-4 summarizes some of the key nursing interventions for patients with severe preeclampsia.

Table 11-4 • Hemodynamic Values in Nonpregnant and Pregnant Women		
	Nonpregnant	Pregnant
Central venous pressure	5–10 mm Hg	1.1–6.1 mm Hg
Pulmonary artery pressure		
Systolic	20–30 mm Hg	18–30 mm Hg
Diastolic	8–15 mm Hg	6–10 mm Hg
Mean	10–20 mm Hg	11–15 mm Hg
Pulmonary artery wedge pressure	6–12 mm Hg	5.7–9.3 mm Hg
Cardiac output	4.3–6.0 L/min	5.2–7.2 L/min

Box 11-4 • NURSING INTERVENTIONS for Severe Preeclampsia

Strict Bed Rest in Left Lateral Tilt
- Explain rationale and expected benefits.
- Encourage family and friends to visit and provide activities that may prevent boredom.
- Explain seizure precautions.

Medications
- Explain the action of drugs such as magnesium sulfate and hydralazine.
- Explain the frequency of laboratory tests, vital sign assessment, and urinary output measurement.

Fetal Surveillance
- Explain external fetal monitoring and tests used to monitor fetal well-being, such as the nonstress test, the biophysical profile, Doppler flow studies, and fetal pulse oximetry.

- Explain the rationale used to determine adequate uteroplacental function.

Delivery
- Prepare the patient for the possibility of cesarean delivery.
- Explain the rationale for the need to deliver.
- Explain how neonatal intensive care unit (NICU) works if unable to physically take the patient on a tour.
- Arrange for a discussion with a neonatologist, if the infant is premature or expected to be admitted to NICU.

HELLP SYNDROME

HELLP syndrome (*h*emolysis, *e*levated *l*iver enzymes, and *l*ow *p*latelets) accompanies severe preeclampsia and eclampsia in approximately 10% to 20% of diagnosed cases. Maternal mortality rates may be as high as 30%.[12] It is often considered a variation of severe preeclampsia. Women in whom HELLP syndrome develops are usually older than 27 years, white, and multiparous.[12] Patients with HELLP syndrome are at an increased risk for development of complications such as renal failure, pulmonary edema, DIC, placental abruption, ARDS, and liver hematoma and rupture.

Signs and symptoms of HELLP syndrome may be similar to those of severe preeclampsia and include epigastric pain, nausea, malaise, and right upper quadrant tenderness. Laboratory results reveal decreased platelets (<100,000/mm³) and elevated liver enzymes.

Physiological Principles

Hemolysis occurs when red blood cells pass through vasospastic vessels, producing burr cells or schistocytes.[13] Liver enzymes become elevated as liver damage occurs as a result of ischemia secondary to vasospasm.[13] Prolonged vasospasm can lead to hepatic necrosis. Platelets are consumed because of the aggregation at endothelial damage sites.

Management

As with severe preeclampsia, delivery is the treatment of choice for HELLP syndrome; however, the timing of delivery remains controversial. If the woman remains undelivered, management includes bed rest, frequent blood pressure assessments, frequent laboratory evaluation of liver function, coagulation status, and intensive fetal surveillance.[12] The patient is managed in the same manner as severe preeclampsia, and magnesium sulfate and antihypertensive agents are given as needed. Blood products may be given to correct coagulation abnormalities.[13]

HELLP syndrome may mimic other disease entities, and differential diagnosis must be made to rule out autoimmune thrombocytopenic purpura, chronic renal disease, pyelonephritis, cholecystitis, gastroenteritis, hepatitis, pancreatitis, thrombotic thrombocytopenic purpura, hemolytic–uremic syndrome, or acute fatty liver disease of pregnancy.[13]

Monitoring changes in vital signs, bleeding, pain, and laboratory values is necessary when caring for patients with HELLP syndrome. Fetal surveillance is important and should include assessments for fetal heart rate and signs and symptoms of placental abruption. Nurses must be aware of the complications that can occur in patients with HELLP syndrome. Signs of worsening pain, vascular collapse, or shock may indicate liver hematoma or rupture. Accurate monitoring of intake and output must be maintained to assess renal status.

DISSEMINATED INTRAVASCULAR COAGULATION

Several conditions predispose a pregnant woman to DIC because of changes in the coagulation and fibrinolytic systems. These conditions include preeclampsia, abruptio placentae, amniotic fluid embolus, fetal death, and sepsis.[14] Although the incidence of sepsis has decreased because of antibiotic therapy, it is responsible for 3% to 8% of the maternal deaths in the United States.[15] Sepsis during pregnancy is a result of bacterial invasion of the uterine cavity.

Immunosuppression is a normal consequence of pregnancy and thought to occur so that the fetus is not rejected by the maternal immune system. This alteration increases the susceptibility to infection and decreases the body's ability to fight infection. Septic shock may develop in a few days or several hours. Manifestations of septic shock include tachycardia, tachypnea, temperature instability, increased cardiac output, and decreased peripheral resistance.

Abruptio placentae is the premature separation of the placenta from the uterine wall and is one of the most common causes of DIC. Blood collects between the uterus and placenta, causing consumption of clotting factors. The placental unit contains high concentrations of thromboplastin. When the placenta prematurely separates, thromboplastin continues to be released systemically, activating the clotting and fibrinolytic systems throughout the body. Parallel to the activation of the fibrinolytic system, the hemostatic system initiates clot formation at the site of the separation.[16] Clinical signs of abruption include acute abdominal pain, uterine tenderness, premature contractions, and vaginal bleeding. Abruptions may be subtle, and blood may not be visible.

Intrauterine fetal death can also lead to DIC. Tissue thromboplastin is released from the dead fetus into the maternal circulation activating the procoagulant system. Coagulopathy is gradual and consistent with chronic, low-grade DIC.

Management

Management of patients with DIC includes identifying the underlying condition and initiating appropriate therapy, evaluating and monitoring the coagulation system to restore hemostasis, and preventing further hemorrhage and thrombosis. Management of DIC due to sepsis includes prompt delivery of the fetus and intravenous administration of broad-spectrum antibiotics. For abruptio placentae, prompt delivery of the fetus is necessary to control further bleeding.

Nursing care is aimed at preventing further bleeding, monitoring coagulation studies, and assessing the patient for multisystem involvement, altered tissue perfusion, and fluid volume deficits.[16] Nursing care includes monitoring respiratory status, administering intravenous fluids to prevent hypovolemia, assessing hemodynamic values, and administering and evaluating antibiotics, blood replacement products, and antipyretics.[14] (See Chapter 49 for a more detailed discussion of DIC.)

AMNIOTIC FLUID EMBOLISM

Amniotic fluid embolism (AFE), although rare, is responsible for approximately 10% of maternal deaths in the United States.[15] AFE occurs when amniotic fluid gains entry into the maternal circulation. This entry may occur during cesarean birth or uterine rupture, or through small tears in the endocervical veins during a vaginal delivery. Once amniotic fluid enters the maternal circulation, it is rapidly transported to the pulmonary vasculature, resulting in pulmonary emboli. The pulmonary response to AFE is vasospasm, which produces transient pulmonary hypertension and profound hypoxia. The maternal system becomes hemodynamically compromised, similar to anaphylactic shock, with elevated PAP and left ventricular failure.[17] Predisposing factors that may lead to AFE include preeclampsia, multiple gestation, polyhydramnios (excess amniotic fluid), low insertion of placenta, post-term pregnancy, hypertonic contractions during labor, abruptio placentae, uterine rupture, maternal seizures, and umbilical cord prolapse. Clinical manifestations of AFE include sudden onset of dyspnea, cyanosis, and hypotension, followed by cardiopulmonary arrest.

Management

Management of AFE is directed at maintaining left ventricular output and an adequate airway.[18] Interventions include intubation and ventilation with 100% oxygen, intravenous administration of vasopressors and crystalloid fluids, cardiopulmonary resuscitation (CPR), administration of blood products, and pulmonary artery catheterization. In extreme cases, extracorporeal membrane oxygenation (ECMO) may be used to provide adequate oxygenation and ventilatory support during treatment of the AFE. Potential sequelae include acute pulmonary edema, respiratory distress, DIC, hemorrhage, and multisystem failure.

The nurse must react quickly when AFE is suspected. Following the basic ABCs (airway, breathing, and circulation), the nurse can prioritize interventions needed in this stressful situation. If the patient is not intubated, oxygen must be administered using a facemask, and oxygen saturation assessed using a pulse oximeter. The nurse can anticipate that after intubation, a resuscitation bag or mechanical ventilation will be needed. To maximize venous return, the woman should be positioned on her side or a wedge placed under her hip. A large-bore intravenous line is needed to administer intravenous fluids and blood products and to correct hypotension. Assessment is focused on the cardiovascular, pulmonary, hematological, and neurological systems.

ACUTE RESPIRATORY DISTRESS SYNDROME

ARDS is characterized by progressive respiratory distress, severe hypoxemia, low lung compliance, noncardiogenic pulmonary edema, and diffuse infiltrates on chest radiography.[12] Precipitating factors of ARDS associated with pregnancy include abruptio placentae, severe preeclampsia, pyelonephritis, DIC, sepsis, AFE, aspiration, systemic infections, and fetal death in utero.[19] Maternal hypoxemia can lead to spontaneous labor and fetal hypoxia, acidosis, and death; therefore, it should be aggressively managed. Perfusion to vital organs, including the fetus, must be maintained to reduce morbidity and mortality. Adequate fetal oxygenation requires a maternal arterial oxygen saturation (SaO_2) of at least 95%.[19]

Management

Pregnant women with ARDS require cardiovascular support and mechanical ventilation using positive end-expiratory pressure (PEEP). Hemodynamic monitoring is essential for evaluating changes associated with ARDS, such as central hypovolemia and noncardiogenic pulmonary edema. Ventilator settings include a rate of 12 breaths/minute, a tidal volume of 12 to 15 mL/kg body weight, 100% oxygen, and a PEEP of 5 cm H_2O.

Nursing care of pregnant women with ARDS is primarily supportive. Interventions are directed at optimizing oxygen transport to tissues and restoring pulmonary capillary integrity.[20] A complete respiratory assessment is made, including evaluation of SaO_2 using pulse oximetry; observation of respiratory rate, character, and effort; and auscultation of lungs. The symptoms of noncardiogenic pulmonary edema are similar to cardiogenic pulmonary edema (i.e., tachypnea, tachycardia, rales, shortness of breath); however, the nurse should be aware that a decrease in PAWP and PAP (from the obstetrical normal; see Table 11–4) may indicate noncardiogenic pulmonary edema. Noncardiogenic pulmonary edema in obstetrical patients can be caused by aspiration of gastric contents, sepsis, blood transfusion reactions, DIC, and amniotic fluid embolism. Nursing interventions to improve uteroplacental blood flow include positioning the patient on her side and maintaining adequate fluid volumes.[4]

Nursing care for women who are mechanically ventilated includes psychosocial support to help relieve anxiety, fear, and separation from family. Nurses can facilitate communication between the patient and family and keep them informed about maternal and fetal conditions.

In extreme cases of ARDS in the postpartum period, ECMO may be used to provide adequate oxygenation and ventilatory support.

TRAUMA

Accidental injuries occur in 6% to 7% of all pregnancies and are associated with spontaneous abortion, preterm labor, abruptio placentae, and fetal death. Trauma is the leading cause of nonobstetrical maternal death.[21] Common types of trauma include blunt trauma from motor vehicle crashes (60%), falls and domestic violence (16% to 31%), and penetrating trauma from stab wounds or gunshots (13% to 22%).[13] Fetal survival depends on maternal survival, so immediate care and stabilization of the pregnant woman are essential.

Hemodynamic instability may not be initially apparent because of the normal physiological cardiovascular changes during pregnancy. A pregnant woman can lose up to 2,000 mL of blood before becoming hemodynamically unstable.[21]

Management

Management consists of immediate stabilization and care. Immediate stabilization of all trauma patients consists of applying the ABCs of resuscitation: establishment of airway, breathing, and circulation. First an airway is established, and oxygen is provided at a rate of 10 to 12 L/minute to produce a PaO_2 level of 60 mm Hg or higher. This PaO_2 level is necessary for optimal fetal oxygenation. A nasogastric tube should be inserted to avoid aspiration.

If CPR is necessary, the anatomical and physiological changes in pregnancy must be considered to maximize efforts. The uterus compresses major abdominal vessels and displaces abdominal contents, which decreases chest compliance. Placing a wedge under the woman's right hip displaces the uterus and decompresses the vessels (Fig. 11-2). Standard advanced cardiac life support procedures are used, including defibrillation and most drugs. The administration of vasopressors should be avoided because the vasoconstrictive action can impair uteroplacental perfusion.[21] Medical antishock trousers or pneumatic antishock garment equipment may be used, but the abdominal compartment should not be inflated.[21]

Intravenous access using large-bore catheters is needed, and aggressive intravenous infusions are used to increase stroke volume and maintain cardiac output. If hemorrhage occurs, bleeding must be controlled. A decrease in arterial blood pressure may not be an indication of hypovolemia because of low resistance in the uteroplacental system. A 30% to 35% loss can occur with severe consequence to the fetus before hypotension is noted. Fluid replacement therapy must be administered at a higher rate.[22]

Once the pregnant woman has been stabilized, her neurological status is assessed. After this assessment, a fetal assessment, including determination of life, is

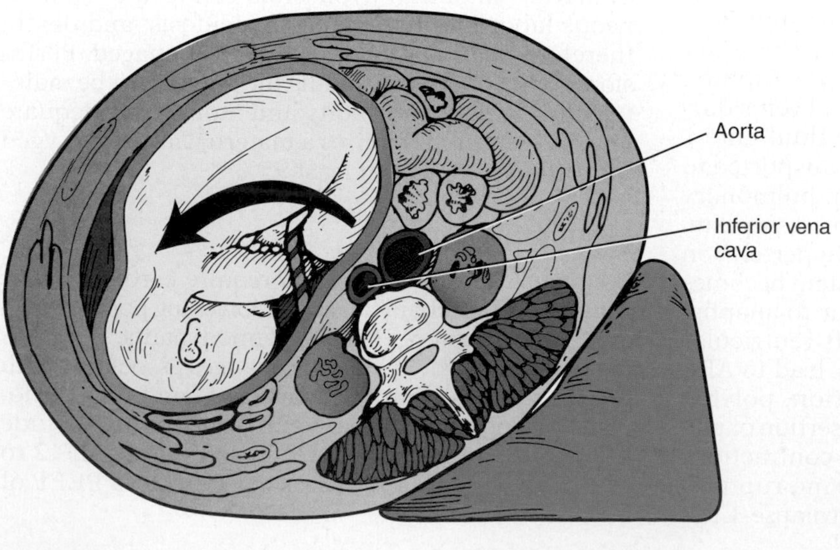

Aorta

Inferior vena cava

Figure 11-2 • Placing a wedge under the woman's right hip decompresses the major abdominal vessels, maximizing the cardiopulmonary resuscitation effort.

Table 11-5 • Arterial Blood Gas Values in Nonpregnant and Pregnant Women

	Nonpregnant	Pregnant
PaO_2	80–100 mm Hg	87–106 mm Hg
$PaCO_2$	36–44 mm Hg	27–32 mm Hg
pH	7.35–7.45	7.40–7.47
HCO_3^-	24–30 mEq/L	18–21 mEq/L

made. The fetal heart rate can be auscultated using a fetoscope, stethoscope, fetal Doppler, or ultrasound. Additional assessments can be made on arrival at the hospital or trauma center. These assessments include electrocardiography, a complete physical examination, and laboratory tests, such as arterial blood gases (Table 11-5), complete blood count, platelet count, electrolytes, blood type and crossmatch, and the Kleihauer-Betke test. Used to detect fetomaternal hemorrhage, the Kleihauer-Betke test identifies red blood cells from the fetus that have entered the maternal circulatory system. This is primarily of concern in the Rh-negative pregnant patient.[22] Assessments should include parameters such as the onset of regular contractions (indicating labor may have begun), vaginal bleeding, and leakage of fluid from the vagina (indicating ruptured membranes).

• Providing Emotional Support

Emotional support is very important to all critically ill pregnant women and their families. If the woman labors in the ICU, her coach or significant other should be allowed to remain at the bedside. When she gives birth, breast-feeding and bonding can be encouraged when feasible. The mother needs access to her newborn and family during this time. If the newborn is not able to be at the bedside, frequent updates about the newborn are important and can be provided by the staff. Providing a flexible and individualized atmosphere to a new family is a challenge in the ICU. The importance of coordinating obstetrical and critical care cannot be overemphasized. Box 11-5 outlines

Box 11-5 • Strategies for Promoting Emotional Well-Being in High-Risk Pregnancies

- Shift orientation from the health care team to family-centered care.
- Incorporate cultural beliefs into the environment. Maintain family rituals when possible.
- Understand the role of the pregnant woman and her family members and assist them with their tasks to optimize family function.
- Provide names of family support groups.
- Provide information and education to family members.
- Encourage the family when they are coping well.
- Validate the family's emotions.

strategies for promoting emotional well-being in high-risk pregnancies.

If the fetus dies as a result of maternal complications, grief support may be needed. The nurse may collaborate with Labor and Delivery staff (who may have additional grief training), psychiatric liaison nurses, social workers, psychologists, psychiatrists, or clergy to offer emotional support to a grieving mother and family.

• Clinical Applicability Challenges

Case Study

Ms. J. is a 40-year-old para 1011 (one previous full-term pregnancy, child is living, one miscarriage) admitted at 34 weeks, 5 days of gestation with complaints of vaginal bleeding, painful contractions, and nausea and vomiting. Until this time, she has received routine prenatal care, and the pregnancy has been uneventful. Before her admission to the Labor and Delivery department, she was eating lunch at work when she felt a "pop" in her abdomen; shortly afterward, her symptoms began. She states that the last time she felt fetal movement was earlier in the morning. On arrival to Labor and Delivery, an external fetal monitor and portable ultrasound detect no fetal heart tones. There is blood in the vaginal vault and no active bleeding, and her cervix is long and closed.

Ms. J. is admitted with the diagnosis of a fetal death in utero, probably due to an abruption of the placenta, and the plan is to deliver her by induction of labor. Vital signs are as follows: blood pressure (BP), 100/70 mm Hg; pulse, 92 beats/minute; and respirations, 22 breaths/minute. Blood test results are as follows: hematocrit (Hct), 32.3%; hemoglobin (Hgb), 10.8 g/dL; and platelets, 118/mm³. Shortly after admission, she complains of increasing pelvic pressure. Examination reveals that she is fully dilated, and she spontaneously delivers a stillborn male child. Delivery of the placenta, as well as a 250-mL clot, follows, confirming the diagnosis of placental abruption. Despite administration of the uterotonic drugs oxytocin (Pitocin) and methylergonovine (Methergine) (medications that assist the uterus to contract and control bleeding), Ms. J. begins to bleed steadily. Clinicians decide to transfer her to the Labor and Delivery operating room for dilation and curettage. Vital signs are as follows: BP, 90/60 mm Hg; pulse, 104 beats/minute; and respirations, 22 breaths/minute. Results of blood tests are as follows: Hct, 17.4%; Hgb, 5.7 g/dL; platelets, <100/mm³; fibrinogen, 142 mg/dL; and activated partial thromboplastin time (aPTT), 44.1 seconds. In the operating room, the anesthesiologist inserts a central line, and aggressive fluid and blood product resuscitation is initiated. The patient receives 4 units of fresh frozen plasma (FFP) and 9 units of packed red cells. Her uterus becomes well contracted, bleeding decreases, and coagulation parameters begin to improve. Her estimated blood loss is 8,000 mL.

Ms. J. begins to bleed again later that evening and is transferred again to the Labor and Delivery operating room, where a uterine artery embolization is performed. An additional unit of FFP and 7 units of platelets are administered. Vital signs are as follows: BP, 60/40 mm Hg; pulse, 140 beats/minute; and respirations, 10 breaths/minute. Ventilation becomes difficult, and she is intubated. She is transferred to the intensive care unit (ICU) for closer surveillance, ventilatory support, and fluid resuscitation. Clinicians make an additional diagnosis of disseminated intravascular coagulation. Upon arrival in the ICU, an expanding right flank hematoma is noted, and the patient is becoming hypotensive and hypothermic. Clinically important parameters are as follows: platelets, <80/mm³; aPTT, 47 seconds; and prothrombin time (PT), 14.2 seconds. Blood gas results are as follows: pH, 7.36; $PaCO_2$, 31 mm Hg; PaO_2, 128 mm Hg; and HCO_3, 17 mEq/L. She is transferred once again to the operating room, and 2 liters of blood are removed from a large right retroperitoneal hematoma. The estimated total blood loss is now 12,000 mL. She is taken back to the ICU for management. Vital signs are as follows: BP, 90/60 mm Hg; pulse, 104 beats/minute; respirations, 24 breaths/minutes; and central venous pressure (CVP), 13 mm Hg. Blood tests show Hct, 24.5%; Hgb, 8.3 g/dL; platelets, 80/mm³; aPTT, 61.8 seconds; PT, 14.2 seconds; and fibrinogen, 142 mg/dL.

Both the patient and her family grieve about the loss of the infant and the admission to the ICU. The Labor and Delivery staff provide grief counseling for the fetal loss and are able to assist the ICU staff with the emotional care of the patient and her family. The patient's husband has been allowed to stay throughout the night of days 1 and 2 in the ICU. On day 3, the patient is extubated and is hemodynamically stable, with BP of 144/60 mm Hg, pulse of 61 beats/minute, respirations of 12 breaths/minute, and CVP of 10 mm Hg. She is transferred to the progressive care unit after she is weaned from the ventilator.

In total, Ms. J. has received 33 units of packed red cells, 22 units of FFP, and 12 units of platelets. Now her central and arterial lines are removed. Her blood work improves, her vital signs remain stable, and she is transferred back to the postpartum unit on day 5. Her vital signs remain for the duration of her stay at BP, 120/70 mm Hg; pulse, 92 beats/minute; and respirations, 22 breaths/minute. On discharge, results of blood tests show Hct, 26.7%; Hgb, 9.4 g/dL; platelets, 209/mm³; PT, 10.7 seconds; aPTT, 28.1 seconds; and fibrinogen, 341 mg/dL.

1. What signs and symptoms led to the diagnosis of abruptio placentae?

2. Compare the blood work of Ms. J. (when admitted to the ICU) with that of a woman with an uncomplicated pregnancy and a woman who is not pregnant.

3. Develop a nursing care plan for Ms. J., who experienced a fetal loss.

4. What outcomes would be expected following the successful response to the therapy provided to Ms. J.?

Review Questions

1. A pregnant patient may lose how much blood before any observable signs or symptoms are present?
   a. 10%–20%
   b. 20%–30%
   c. 30%–40%
   d. 40%–50%

2. Considerations needed for enhancing uteroplacental blood flow include which of the following?
   a. Fetal monitoring and maternal hemodynamic monitoring
   b. Repositioning the patient on her left side and delivering high-flow oxygen
   c. Delivering the fetus immediately
   d. Administering vasopressors

3. Which obstetrical conditions can lead to disseminating intravascular coagulation?
   a. Amniotic fluid embolus, septic shock, stillbirth, placenta accreta, severe preeclampsia
   b. Hyperemesis gravidarum, acute respiratory distress syndrome, amniocentesis
   c. Systemic lupus erythematosus, cardiomyopathy, gestational diabetes
   d. Multiple gestations, fetal cardiac anomalies, spina bifida

4. A pregnant woman with severe preeclampsia is admitted with a blood pressure (BP) of 200/110 mm Hg. After initiation of magnesium sulfate therapy, her BP is 190/100 mm Hg. What additional drug therapy should be considered?
   a. Furosemide, hydrochlorothiazide
   b. Hydralazine, labetalol (Normodyne, Trandate), nifedipine
   c. Captopril, benazepril, enalapril
   d. Atenolol, propranolol, metoprolol

5. A pregnant undelivered patient is admitted to the intensive care unit (ICU). What is an important nursing intervention that the ICU staff should include in the plan of care?
   a. Assess the hemodynamic monitoring values at least every 2 hours.
   b. Keep the family informed of all changes, be sensitive to the patient's feelings of guilt, and explain the intradisciplinary team approach to the patient and family.
   c. Explain the strict visitation schedule to the family.
   d. Use diversion skills to keep the patient from worrying about the baby.

References

1. Simpson K: Critical illness during pregnancy: Considerations for evaluation and treatment of the fetus as the second patient. Crit Care Nurs Q 29(1):20–31, 2006

2. Dildy G, Belfort M, Saade G (eds): Critical Care Obstetrics, 4th ed. Boston, Blackwell Publishing, 2003

3. Bridges E, Womble S, Wallace M, McCartney J: Hemodynamic monitoring in high risk obstetrics patients: I. Cardiovasc Med 23(4):53–62, 2003

4. Torgenson K, Curran C: A systemic approach to the physiologic adaptations of pregnancy. Crit Care Nurs Q 29(1):2–19, 2006

5. Chesnutt A: Physiology of normal pregnancy. Crit Care Clin 20:609–615, 2004

6. Poole J, Spreen D: Acute pulmonary edema in pregnancy. J Perinat Neonat Nurs 19(4):316–331, 2005

7. Herra E: Lipid metabolism in the fetus and the newborn. Diabetes Metab Res Rev 16:202–210, 2000.

8. Keizer J, Zwart J, Meerman R, et al: Obstetric intensive care admissions: A 12-year review in a tertiary care center. Eur J Obstet Gynecol Reprod Biol 28(1–2):152–156, 2006

9. Bassam H, Sibai B: Expectant management of severe pre-eclampsia: Proper candidates and pregnancy outcome. Clin Obstet 48(2):430–440, 2005

10. Ramanathan J, Bennett K: Pre-eclampsia: Fluids, drugs and anesthetic management. Anesthesiol Clin North Am 21:146–163, 2003

11. Peters R, Flack J: Hypertensive disorders in pregnancy. J Obstet Gynecol Neonatal Nurs 33(2):209–220, 2004

12. Kidner M, Flanders-Stephen MB: A model for the HELLP syndrome: The maternal experience. J Obstet Gynecol Neonatal Nurs 33(1):44–53, 2004

13. O'Brien J, Barton J: Controversies with the diagnosis and management of HELLP syndrome. Clin Obstet Gynecol 48(2):460–477, 2005

14. Letsku E: Disseminated intravascular coagulation. Best Pract Res Clin Obstet Gynecol 15(4):623–644, 2001

15. Finkielman J, DeFeo F, Heller P, Afessa B: The clinical course of patients with septic abortion admitted to an intensive care unit. Intensive Care Med 30:1097–1102, 2004

16. Curran C: Intrapartum emergencies. J Obstet Gynecol Neonatal Nurs 32(6):802–813, 2003

17. Schoening A: Amniotic fluid embolism: Historical perspectives and new possibilities. MCN Am J Matern Child Nurs 31(2):78–85, 2006

18. Moore J, Baldisseri M: Amniotic fluid embolism. Crit Care Med 33(10):S279–S285, 2005

19. Cole D, Taylor T, McCullough D, et al: Acute respiratory distress syndrome in pregnancy. Crit Care Med 33(Suppl 10):269–278, 2005

20. Rebmann T: Severe acute respiratory syndrome: Implications for perinatal and neonatal nurses. J Perinatal Neonatal Nurs 19(4):332–345, 2005

21. Shah A, Kilcline B: Trauma in pregnancy. Emerg Med Clin North Am 21:615–629, 2003

22. Tweddale C: Trauma during pregnancy. Crit Care Nurs Q 29(1):53–67, 2006

Other Selected Readings

Arafeh J, Baird S: Cardiac disease in pregnancy. Crit Care Nurs Q 29(1):32–52, 2006

Bridges E, Womble S, Wallace M, McCartney J: Hemodynamic monitoring in high-risk obstetrics patients: II. Crit Care Nurse 23(5):52–57, 2003

Browning G, Warren N: Unmet needs of family members in the medical intensive care waiting room. Crit Care Nurs Q 29(1):86–95, 2006

Campbell P, Rudisill P: Psychosocial needs of the critically ill obstetric patient: The nurse's role. Crit Care Nurs Q 29(1):77–80, 2006

Curran C: Multiple organ dysfunction syndrome (MODS) in the obstetric population. J Perinatal Neonatal Nurs 15(4):37–55, 2002

Curran C: The effects of rhinitis, asthma, and acute respiratory distress syndrome as acute or chronic pulmonary conditions during pregnancy. J Perinatal Neonatal Nurs 20(2):147–157, 2006

Mattox K, Goetzi L: Trauma in pregnancy. Crit Care Med 33(Suppl 10):385–389, 2005

Munnar U, Bolsblanc B, Suresh M: Airway problems in pregnancy. Crit Care Med 33(Suppl 10):259–268, 2005

Murali S, Baldisseri M: Peripartum cardiomyopathy. Crit Care Med 33(Suppl 10):340–346, 2005

Robertson L, Greer J: Thromboembolism in pregnancy. Curr Opin Obstet Gynecol 17(2):113–116, 2005

Thorsen M, Poole J: Renal disease in pregnancy. J Perinatal Neonatal Nurs 15(4):13–26, 2002

Witcher P: Promoting fetal stabilization during maternal hemodynamic instability or respiratory insufficiency. Crit Care Nurs Q 29(1):70–76, 2006

12

The Critically Ill Older Patient

Barbara Resnick

Objectives

Based on the content in this chapter, the reader should be able to:

❶ Explain general physical changes that occur as a result of the normal aging process.

❷ Describe the developmental tasks of the older person.

❸ Discuss specific conditions that affect the major body systems of the older person.

❹ Explain cognitive changes that may occur in the older patient.

❺ Compare and contrast delirium and dementia in the older patient.

❻ Describe assessment indicators of potential abuse or neglect of the older person.

❼ Describe why the principle *start low, go slow* is important for the older patient in regard to the absorption, distribution, metabolism, and excretion of medications.

America is growing older. Between 2002 and 2030, the older population will more than double, increasing to 71.5 million from 35.6 million (Fig. 12-1). Almost one in five people will be 65 years of age or older,[1] and more people will seek medical care for chronic disease, the leading cause of disability among older adults. When older adults have acute exacerbations of their diseases, they often require hospitalization in an intensive care unit (ICU).

As a result, critical care nurses need to understand the many physiological changes that occur normally with aging. These alterations are progressive and usually are not apparent or pathological. However, these age-related changes put the criti-

cally ill older adult at increased risk for complications. Preventive nursing care, focusing on the avoidance of potential problems, is necessary.

The leading causes of death among older patients are heart disease, malignant neoplasms, cerebrovascular accidents, influenza, and chronic obstructive pulmonary disease. Chronic conditions (e.g., arthritis, hearing and visual deficits) are prevalent among older people. With advancing age, these conditions become more common and result in increased hospitalizations. A longer life span has been the single most important cause of the increased numbers of older patients with multiple chronic and acute illnesses.

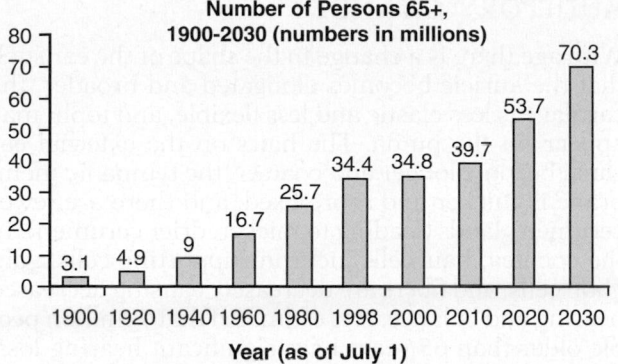

Figure 12-1 • Profile of Americans aged 65 years and older (based on data from the United States Bureau of the Census). Data from the year 1900 to present were used to predict the number of Americans aged 65 years and older in the year 2030. (From Smeltzer SC, Bare BG, Hinkle JL, Cheever KH: Brunner & Suddarth's Textbook of Medical–Surgical Nursing, 11th ed. Philadelphia, Lippincott Williams & Wilkins, 2008, p 225.)

• Normal Psychobiological Characteristics of Aging

BIOLOGICAL ISSUES

Intrinsic aging refers to characteristics and processes that occur universally with all older adults. Changes resulting from the aging process must be distinguished from those resulting from a particular disease process, disuse, or environmental factors, such as ultraviolet radiation. Extrinsic aging is composed of factors that influence aging to varying degrees in different people. Extrinsic factors include such things as lifestyle or exposure to environmental influences. Normal aging is defined as the sum of intrinsic aging, extrinsic aging, and idiosyncratic or individual genetic factors specific to each individual.[2]

In most physiological systems, the normal aging processes do not result in significant impairment or dysfunction in the absence of disease and under resting conditions. It is only in response to stress that an age-related reduction in physiological reserves causes a loss of homeostatic balance. The following are some examples of intrinsic age changes:

▶ Reduced resistance to stress

▶ Poor tolerance of extremes of heat and cold because of hypothalamic and skin changes

▶ Reduced sensory perceptions

▶ Greater fluctuation in blood pH

Aging, in one organ or the entire body, may be premature or delayed in relation to actual chronological age. The effect of aging on cellular tissues is asymmetrical. For example, the changes resulting from aging in relation to the brain, bone, cardiovascular, and lung tissues may be fairly obvious, whereas changes affecting the liver, pancreas, gastrointestinal tract, and muscle tissues are less obvious. Several organic changes that result from aging are listed in Box 12-1.

Box 12-1 • Organic Changes With Aging

- The amount of connective and collagen tissue is increased.
- Cellular elements in the nervous system, muscles, and other vital organs disappear.
- The number of normally functioning cells is reduced.
- The amount of fat is increased.
- Oxygen use is decreased.
- During rest, the amount of blood pumped is decreased.
- Less air is expired by the lungs.
- Excretion of hormones is decreased.
- Sensory and perceptual activity is decreased.
- Absorption of lipids, proteins, and carbohydrates is decreased.
- Presbyesophagus occurs.
- The arterial lumen thickens.

PSYCHOSOCIAL ISSUES

In addition to physical signs of aging, nurses caring for acutely ill older patients must be aware of the older person's normal developmental tasks and the specific dreams or wishes of a particular senior. Developmental tasks of older people are listed in Box 12-2.

The need for support and meaningful relationships continues throughout life. Support can be described as a feeling of belonging or a belief that one is an active participant in the surrounding world. The feeling of mutuality with others in the environment lends strength and helps decrease the sense of isolation. Support by family, friends, and the community can pro-

---

Box 12-2 • Developmental Tasks of the Older Person

- Deciding where and how to live for his or her remaining years
- Preserving supportive, intimate, and satisfying relationships with spouse, family, and friends
- Maintaining an adequate and satisfying home environment relative to health and economic status
- Providing sufficient income
- Maintaining a maximum level of health
- Attaining comprehensive health and dental care
- Maintaining personal hygiene
- Maintaining communication and adequate contact with family and friends
- Maintaining social, civic, and political involvement
- Initiating new interests (in addition to former activities) that increase status
- Recognizing and feeling that he or she is needed
- Discovering the meaning in life after retirement and when confronted with illness of self or spouse and death of spouse and other loved ones; adjusting to death of loved ones
- Developing a significant philosophy of life and discovering comfort in a philosophy or religion

vide an older patient with a greater sense of stability and security.

Self-worth and perceived well-being are feelings that usually coincide in older adults. The perception of well-being arises from the satisfaction of meeting an acceptable proportion of one's life goals. It can be described as an inner contentment one has in life as a whole. Related to this, a feeling of self-worth is derived not only from a sense of well-being but also from satisfaction with one's image or acceptance by others. Self-worth also reflects the quality of interactions with family and friends.

Family environment for the older adult includes, among others, dimensions of interpersonal relationships, personal growth, integrity of the family unit, and adaptation to stress. As family members age, all these areas of concern intensify because of changes in roles of family members, alterations in the family power structure, and changes in financial and decision-making dynamics. Acute illness increases the urgency for effective cooperation among all family members as the traditional family structure is suddenly challenged.

When older patients are admitted to intensive care, issues of family cohesion and adaptability often surface. Frequently, families face immediate changes in roles, with adult children and grandchildren assuming the roles of caretakers and nurturers for the older family members. The family must suddenly adjust to dramatically different demands. Frequent visits to the hospital; dialogues with nurses, physicians, and social workers; and efforts to support and communicate with the patient become primary tasks. Amid these activities, family members (particularly those who have been given power of attorney) find themselves being pressed for decisions about immediate and long-term care. At this time, the issue of the person's end-of-life care preferences, competency, and ability to be involved in treatment decisions may arise. Effective communication and a willingness to listen to and respect the wishes of the older patient become foremost. If this is achieved, the stress on families is reduced because of increased acceptance of the plan of care by all family members.

• Physical Challenges

Chronic changes in one organ system may be associated with changes in other systems. Moreover, there is individual variation in age-related changes. Therefore, each person must be evaluated based on the age-related changes actually present rather than on those that are "normal" for a particular age.

It is equally important to distinguish age-related changes from those associated with a chronic disease or acute illness and to avoid prematurely attributing some findings to age if they are caused by illness. A discussion of the effects of aging on various body systems follows; age-related changes and the clinical implications of these changes are summarized in Table 12-1.

AUDITORY CHANGES

With age there is a change in the shape of the ear such that the auricle becomes elongated and broader, the cartilage is less elastic and less flexible, and tophi may appear on the pinna. The hairs on the external ear canal become longer and coarser, the tympanic membrane is thicker and more fixed, and there are fewer cerumen glands (leading to thicker, drier cerumen). In the cochlea, hair cells, neuron-supporting cells, ganglion cells, and fibers are decreased, causing decreased hearing and balance. It is estimated that 7 million people older than 65 years have significant hearing loss, and continuation of current trends indicates that by 2010, more than 11 million people will have this problem.[3] Specifically, the aging process affects hearing in two critical ways: reduction in threshold sensitivity and reduction in the ability to understand speech. Threshold elevations that occur between 8,000 and 20,000 Hz are not detectable with a routine hearing test. Therefore, hearing loss because of aging or other factors is not documented clinically until frequencies are at or below 8,000 Hz.

Presbycusis is defined as a sensorineural hearing loss and is the most common form of hearing loss in older adults. Presbycusis is characterized by a gradual, progressive, bilateral, symmetrical, high-frequency sensorineural (perceptive) hearing loss with poor speech discrimination. Sensorineural hearing loss is due to degeneration or changes in the neural receptors in the cochlea, cranial nerve VIII (the acoustic nerve), and central nervous system. Treatment may vary dramatically from simple removal of impacted earwax to surgical removal of an auditory nerve tumor. Thirteen percent of people 65 years of age and older, if tested, would show signs of presbycusis.[3]

Conductive hearing loss is due to the blockage of sound transmission from the external ear through the tympanic membrane and small bones in the middle ear. Like presbycusis, conductive hearing loss is commonly found in older adults, and it is not unusual for older people to have both sensorineural and conductive hearing loss.

Findings on Physical Examination and Management

The ear canal of the older adult should be evaluated at regular intervals (every few months) because of the tendency to have thicker, drier cerumen, which can occlude the canal and affect hearing. The older patient may retain the ability to hear pure tones, but if these pure tones are grouped to form words, the ability to understand and perceive these sounds as intelligible speech may be lost. This loss is known as impairment of discrimination ability. The patient has increased difficulty hearing high-frequency, stimuli-sibilant sounds (-f-, -s-, -th-, -ch-, and -sh-). Noisy environments further hamper the ability to hear certain sounds. Therefore, the person may respond inappropriately to questions, withdraw, or frequently ask for the speaker to repeat what is said. Eliminating background noise, speaking lower and louder,

Table 12-1 • Summary of Age-Related Changes, Clinical Implications, and Key Nursing Interventions

System	Clinical Implications	Key Nursing Interventions
Cardiovascular • Atrophy of muscle fibers that line the endocardium • Atherosclerosis of vessels • Increased systolic blood pressure • Decreased compliance of the left ventricle • Decreased number of pacemaker cells • Decreased sensitivity of baroreceptors	• Increased blood pressure • Increased emphasis on atrial contraction with an S$_4$ heard • Increased arrhythmias • Increased risk for hypotension with position change • Valsalva maneuver may cause a drop in blood pressure • Decreased exercise tolerance	• To prevent falls related to positional hypotension, make sure the person changes position slowly and waits before ambulating.
Neurologic • Decreased number of neurons and increase in size and number of neuroglial cells • Decline in nerves and nerve fibers • Atrophy of the brain and increase in cranial dead space • Thickened leptomeninges in spinal cord	• Increased risk for neurological problems: cerebrovascular accident (CVA), parkinsonism • Slower conduction of fibers across the synapses • Modest decline in short-term memory • Alterations in gait pattern: wide based, shorter stepped, and flexed forward • Increased risk for hemorrhage before symptoms are apparent	• To compensate for the decline in short-term memory, provide more time to complete memory-associated tasks.
Respiratory • Decreased lung tissue elasticity • Thoracic wall calcification • Cilia atrophy • Decreased respiratory muscle strength • Decreased partial pressure of arterial oxygen (PaO$_2$)	• Decreased efficiency of ventilatory exchange • Increased susceptibility to infection and atelectasis • Increased risk for aspiration • Decreased ventilatory response to hypoxia and hypercapnia • Increased sensitivity to narcotics	• To prevent infection and atelectasis, encourage deep breathing and coughing.
Integumentary • Loss of dermal and epidermal thickness • Flattening of papillae • Atrophy of sweat glands • Decreased vascularity • Collagen cross-linking • Elastin regression • Loss of subcutaneous fat • Decreased melanocytes • Decline in fibroblast proliferation	• Thinning of skin and increased susceptibility to tearing • Dryness and pruritus • Decreased sweating and ability to regulate body heat • Increased wrinkling and laxity of skin • Loss of fatty pads protecting bone and resulting in pain • Increased need for protection from the sun • Increased time for healing of wounds	• To prevent damage to fragile skin, avoid shearing forces. • To counteract dryness, immerse skin in water daily and apply emollients. • To minimize pain, pad thinned areas with additional layers (e.g., extra socks for feet). • Encourage sunscreen use.
Gastrointestinal • Decreased liver size • Less efficient cholesterol stabilization and absorption • Fibrosis and atrophy of salivary glands • Decreased muscle tone in bowel • Atrophy of and decrease in number of taste buds • Slowing in esophageal emptying • Decreased hydrochloric acid secretion • Decreased gastric acid secretion • Atrophy of the mucosal lining • Decreased absorption of calcium	• Change in intake due to decreased appetite • Discomfort after eating related to slowed passage of food • Decreased absorption of calcium and iron • Alteration of drug effectiveness • Increased risk for constipation, esophageal spasm, and diverticular disease	• Encourage small, frequent meals to avoid discomfort and improve intake. • Encourage fluids and fiber to improve bowel function.
Urinary • Reduced renal mass • Loss of glomeruli • Decline in number of functioning nephrons • Changes in small vessel walls • Decreased bladder muscle tone	• Decreased glomerular filtration rate (GFR) • Decreased sodium-conserving ability • Decreased creatinine clearance • Increased blood urea nitrogen (BUN) • Decreased renal blood flow • Altered drug clearance • Decreased ability to dilute urine • Decreased bladder capacity and increased residual urine • Increased urgency	• To prevent complications from medical therapy, monitor drug clearance and alter dosing as necessary. • Monitor for urinary tract infections.
Reproductive • Atrophy and fibrosis of cervical and uterine walls • Decreased vaginal elasticity and lubrication • Decreased hormones and reduced oocytes • Decreased seminiferous tubules • Proliferation of stromal and glandular tissue • Involution of mammary gland tissue	• Vaginal dryness and burning and pain with intercourse • Decreased seminal fluid volume and force of ejaculation • Reduced elevation of the testes • Prostatic hypertrophy • Connective breast tissue is replaced by adipose tissue, making breast examinations easier	• To compensate for vaginal dryness or pain, encourage the use of lubricating creams, estrogen cream, or both. • Monitor for urinary retention in men.

(continued)

Table 12-1 • Summary of Age-Related Changes, Clinical Implications, and Key Nursing Interventions (Continued)

System	Clinical Implications	Key Nursing Interventions
Musculoskeletal • Decreased muscle mass • Decreased myosin adenosine triphosphatase activity • Deterioration and drying of joint cartilage • Decreased bone mass and osteoblastic activity	• Decreased muscle strength • Decreased bone density • Loss of height • Joint pain and stiffness • Increased risk for fracture • Alterations in gait and posture	• Encourage resistive exercises to reverse a decline in muscle strength. • Encourage exercise and intake of calcium and vitamin D. • Encourage activity and exercise.
Sensory *Vision* • Decreased rod and cone function • Pigment accumulation • Decreased speed of eye movements • Increased intraocular pressure • Ciliary muscle atrophy • Increased lens size and yellowing of the lens • Decreased tear secretion	• Decreased visual acuity, visual fields, and light/dark adaptation • Increased sensitivity to glare • Increased incidence of glaucoma • Distorted depth perception with increased falls • Less able to differentiate blues, greens, and violets • Increased eye dryness and irritation	• Provide materials with large print. • Make sure there is adequate lighting without glare. • Use contrasting colors for print material.
Hearing • Loss of auditory neurons • Loss of hearing from high to low frequency • Increased cerumen • Angiosclerosis of ear	• Decreased hearing acuity and isolation (specifically, decreased ability to hear consonants) • Difficulty hearing, especially when there is background noise, or when speech is rapid • Cerumen impaction may cause hearing loss	• Make sure to face the person; use touch and visual cues to facilitate communication. • Evaluate for cerumen impaction, and remove cerumen as necessary.
Smell • Decreased number of olfactory nerve fibers	• Inability to smell noxious odors • Decreased food intake	
Taste • Altered ability to taste sweet and salty foods; bitter and sour tastes remain		• Use alternative seasonings.
Touch • Decreased sensation	• Safety risk with regard to recognizing dangers in the environment: hot water, fire alarms, or small objects that result in tripping	• Avoid a cluttered environment.
Endocrine • Decreased testosterone, growth hormone (GH), insulin, adrenal androgens, aldosterone, and thyroid hormone • Decreased thermoregulation • Decreased febrile response • Increased nodularity and fibrosis of thyroid • Decreased basal metabolic rate	• Decreased ability to tolerate stressors such as surgery • Decreased sweating and shivering and temperature regulation • Lower baseline temperature; infection may not cause an elevation in temperature • Decreased insulin response, glucose tolerance • Decreased sensitivity of renal tubules to antidiuretic hormone (ADH) • Weight gain • Increased incidence of thyroid disease	• Monitor the temperature of the room. • Provide adequate clothing and blankets to keep the patient warm. • Closely monitor blood glucose levels of patients with diabetes.

and using multiple means of getting information across (e.g., verbal as well as written formats) can facilitate communication. These people may also have problems with balance during transfers and ambulation, and they experience frequent falls. Activity and exercise interventions should be implemented as soon as possible to strengthen muscles and bones and improve balance.

VISUAL CHANGES

Like all other body systems, the eye is affected by aging. Structural and functional changes occur slowly and gradually. Visual perception depends on the integra-

tion of various neurosensory systems and structures that age at different rates.

Normal changes associated with aging may include a loss of elasticity in the eyelids and subsequent wrinkling, ptosis (upper eyelid drooping), and "pouches" resulting from changes in the tissues beneath the eyelid skin and the subsequent formation and accumulation of fatty tissue. The conjunctiva may develop a yellowish or discolored membrane or become thickened as a result of environmental hazards, such as dust and exposure to drying and irritating pollutants. Arcus senilis, which is a white or gray ring around the limbus (junction of the cornea and sclera), may be related to a high blood level of fatty substances accumulated with advancing age. Although there is a decrease in the amount of lacrimation with age, overflow of tears may occur because of impaired drainage of the ductal system.

The iris loses its ability to accommodate rapidly to light and dark and develops an increased need for light. With age, the pupil becomes smaller and fixed. The lens becomes inflexible with less complete accommodation for near and far vision. The vitreous humor behind the lens may pull on the retina, producing holes or tears and predisposing the older person to retinal detachment. The ciliary muscle becomes stiff, which contributes to the problems of accommodating to distances. By the age of 60 years, presbyopia may develop. Presbyopia is the inability to shift focus from far to near. A possible rationale for this loss is that the older, aging lens, which is less flexible, cannot easily change shape from the action of the focusing muscle to which it is attached.

In older adults, dark–light adaptation slows as the pupillary response slows and rods degenerate. As the lens yellows with increasing age, color discrimination becomes less acute, especially in the blue-green tones. Peripheral vision may decline because of decreased extraocular muscle strength, and depth perception may decline because of a thickening lens. Therefore, time must be provided for the person to adapt when moving between dark and light environments and when getting out of bed.

In addition to normal changes in vision, there is an increased incidence of cataracts, glaucoma, senile macular degeneration, and diabetic retinopathy. These diseases must be studied in relation to normal aging of the eye structure.

A cataract is a clouding of the normally clear and transparent lens of the eye. When a cataract interferes with the transmission of light to the retina, some loss in visual acuity may result. The older patient may complain of increased sensitivity to glare, a blurring of vision, halo images, cloudiness, decreased visual acuity, and decreased contrast sensitivity. Risk factors for cataract formation include diabetes mellitus, heredity, ultraviolet-B radiation exposure, smoking, corticosteroid drugs, alcohol use, and insufficient ingestion of antioxidant vitamins. The visual changes can progress to complete loss of vision. Cataracts account for one sixth of all cases of visual impairment in the United States and mostly occur in people older than 50 years.

Glaucoma is one of the major causes of blindness and is especially prevalent in the older adult. Glaucoma is due to increased intraocular pressure. This pressure may result in compression of the optic disc of the eye and damage to cranial nerve II (the optic nerve). This results in loss of peripheral vision and visual acuity. Risk factors for glaucoma include African American race, a family history of glaucoma, ocular hypertension, advanced age, myopia, retinal vascular disturbance, corticosteroid drug use, diabetes mellitus, and vascular crisis (elevation in blood pressure). Age-related changes in the canal of Schlemm, infection, injury, swollen cataracts, and tumors are also etiological factors for glaucoma. Glaucoma is classified based on whether the angle of the anterior chamber is open or narrow and whether the glaucoma is primary or secondary. Primary, open-angle glaucoma is the most common type found in older adults. This type progresses slowly. Primary, angle-closure glaucoma is less common and is characterized by a sudden and marked increase in intraocular pressure with accompanying redness and pain in the eye, headache, nausea or vomiting, corneal edema, and decreased vision. Secondary glaucoma is characterized by an anatomical or functional blockage of the outflow channels. These types of glaucoma can be open angle (such as those that occur from corticosteroid-induced pressure increases) or closed angle (such as those caused by a swollen cataract). Early diagnosis is important because the earlier that treatment is started, the easier it is to control the disease.

Retinal degeneration, or macular degeneration, is the third major source of visual disability in the older adult. Macular degeneration is a pigmentary change of the macular area of the retina caused by small hemorrhages. People see a gray shadow in the center of the visual area but can see well at the outer border. This condition rarely results in total blindness; however, visual loss can progress to legal blindness. Early symptoms include a slight blurring of vision, followed by a blind spot. Compensation techniques include wearing sunglasses or visors, looking to the side, and using magnifiers.

Diabetic retinopathy is the leading cause of blindness in the United States. It is caused by the deterioration of the blood vessels nourishing the retina at the back of the eye. Microaneurysms and small hemorrhages in the eye may leak fluid or blood and cause swelling of the retina. If this leaking blood or fluid damages or scars the retina, the image sent to the brain becomes blurred, and the condition eventually can progress to blindness.

Findings on Physical Examination and Management

The older adult is likely to have smaller pupils, decreased visual acuity, difficulty with depth perception, decreased peripheral vision, and dry eyes. Ectropion and entropion are commonly noted with age. Ectropion is eversion of the eyelid (usually the lower lid) resulting in exposure of the lid, thickening and keratinization, and chronic irritation. Entropion is inversion of the eyelid and results in the eyelashes rubbing against and scratching the cornea. Entropion can result in corneal trauma and scarring and ultimately may result in decreased vision. When cataracts are present, there is opacity of the lens, and the red reflex may be absent during funduscopic examination. The older adult with cataracts presents with dimming of his or her vision and complains that everything appears clouded. People who have glaucoma present with complaints of blurred vision, halos around lights, or decreased peripheral vision. Funduscopic examination in these people shows cupping of the optic disc and atrophy of the optic nerve. Last, older adults with macular degeneration present with a gradual decline in vision, particularly central vision, without a change

Box 12-3 • NURSING INTERVENTIONS for Visually Impaired Patients

- Identify yourself on approach.
- Approach blind patients from the front.
- Assess impact of failing vision and patient's ability to adapt during hospitalization and after discharge.
- Assess stress level because increased stress can necessitate higher dosages of eye medication for patients with glaucoma.

- Be alert to side effects that other medications may have on the eyes (i.e., medications containing antihistamines, caffeine, and atropine-like substances).
- Provide eye lubrications when eyes are dry.
- Instill all prescribed medications.

---

in peripheral vision. Good lighting, avoiding glare, and using contrasting colors (e.g., black letters on white paper) and large print can facilitate vision. As with interventions for hearing changes, providing information in various ways is effective for facilitating vision and compensating for losses. Selected nursing interventions for people with impaired vision are listed in Box 12-3.

OTHER SENSORY CHANGES

Although hearing and vision changes are the most researched sensory changes occurring in older people, there also may be declines in other senses.

The number of taste buds is reported to decrease with age, in conjunction with a decline in the ability to taste substances. Sweet and salty substances are less detectable as one ages; therefore, many older adults complain that food tastes bitter or sour. There is very little information on smell sensation, but it is thought that a decrease in the sense of smell can result from atrophy of the olfactory organ and increased hair in the nostrils.[4] The loss of taste and smell affects the older person's ability to identify food and make odor discriminations.

The threshold of touch varies with the part of the body stimulated. There is a loss of tactile sensation as one ages, although this varies individually. Older adults may not feel the effects of lying too long in one position. A key nursing intervention is to vary the positions of the immobile older patient. The older adult also has decreased kinesthetic sense, which is the person's awareness of his or her body in space. Decreased kinesthetic sense results in postural instability and difficulty reacting to bodily changes in space.

Findings on Physical Examination and Management

With age, the lips tend to become thin and pale, and the tissue of the oral mucosa is thinner, paler, and less elastic. Small yellow sebaceous glands may be seen in the buccal mucosa. The dorsum and margins of the tongue may have decreased number and size of papillae and may be coated with a thin white film. There may also be increased fissures on the dorsal aspect of the tongue, whereas the undersurface is smooth with a bluish-purple hue from increased varicosities. Taste buds and the submaxillary, pituitary, and salivary glands atrophy. The gums are thinner and receded,

and there is decreased tooth enamel, dry and less translucent dentin, decreased dental pulp, and diminished perfusion and sensitivity of the gums. Decreased taste sensitivity (especially for sweets and salt) and increased difficulty swallowing food (due to less saliva production) may cause the older adult to present with weight loss. To facilitate taste and improve oral intake, the nurse provides frequent mouth care (before meals), offers foods in a pleasant setting using liberal seasonings to stimulate taste, and encourages the use of interventions, such as sugar-free candies, to stimulate salivation.

Older adults with decreased sensation may present with complaints of increased difficulty performing fine motor activities such as buttoning clothes or picking up objects. They may also have pressure sores and decreased balance. Frequent position changes of older patients are essential and should be instituted every 30 minutes.

SLEEP CHANGES

It is estimated that sleep disturbances occur in more than half of those older than 65 years.[5] An important aspect of the critical care nurse's assessment is to determine whether sleep problems are the result of normal aging, sleep disorders, or sleep disturbances due to the acute care environment.

Although some age-related changes in sleep patterns are the normal consequences of aging, the prevalence and potential for severe sleep disorders calls for increased clinical awareness and evaluation. Such complaints as habitual snoring, frequent awakening, nocturnal sweating, and awakening with anxiety may be signs of a genuine sleep disorder.

The loss of neurons in the brain may be responsible for the normal age changes in the sleep cycle. These include:

▶ A longer time to fall asleep
▶ Increased time spent in the lighter stages of sleep (stages 1 and 2)
▶ Decreased time spent in the deeper stages of sleep (stages 3 and 4) and in rapid eye movement sleep
▶ Increased and shorter repetitions of the sleep cycle

The amount of sleep needed for each person does not change with age. However, there is an increased tendency for older adults to sleep less at night, to be somnolent late in the day or early evening, and to awaken early in the morning. This has been referred to as the advanced sleep phase syndrome.[6] Older adults also have shortened sleep latency, resulting in daytime napping. Daytime napping further compounds the problem because it reduces the need for nighttime sleep. Common complaints (e.g., anxiety, waking up due to choking, headaches, sweating at night, nocturia, and snoring) are not normal age-related changes and should be assessed more thoroughly.

The most prevalent and most serious age-related sleep disorder is sleep apnea. There is evidence of an association between sleep apnea and circulatory disorders, including hypertension, stroke, and angina pectoris. There also may be a link between sleep apnea and reduced life expectancy. The prevalence of disordered breathing in the older patient is high. Moreover, there may be an association among habitual snoring, stroke, and angina pectoris in older men.[6]

Findings on Physical Examination and Management

Older adults with sleep disorders present with an inability to fall asleep, an inability to stay asleep, or both. They may exhibit daytime napping, and fall asleep during activities. Conversely, there may be evidence of sleep deprivation with altered mental status being the major presenting sign. Loud snoring with multiple apnea–hypopnea events is indicative of sleep apnea. These people may have daytime hypersomnolence, fatigue, irritability, and decreased cognitive function because of impaired nighttime sleep patterns.

Normal aging, chronic illness, and drug therapy increase the older person's susceptibility to insomnia. Treatment depends on the problem. Before drug therapy is considered, poor sleep hygiene habits should be addressed. Good sleep hygiene includes:

▶ Avoiding daytime naps that are longer than 30 minutes

▶ Maintaining regular bedtimes and rising times

▶ Avoiding heavy evening meals, excessive fluids, alcohol, and caffeine

▶ Increasing daytime activity, even if this is as simple as sitting up out of bed for extended periods of time

▶ Keeping the sleep environment quiet, sufficiently dark, at a comfortable temperature, and safe

▶ Maintaining a day–night schedule such that the period of time in bed for sleep is separate from daytime activities (although this is difficult in the acute care setting when the person is acutely ill; however, as recovery progresses, the person should be out of bed except for brief rest periods and sleeping at night).

Behavior modification has been used successfully for many sleep problems. The conservative use of medications may be indicated in more problematic sleep disorders, periodic movements of sleep, and dementia-related illness.[7] Drug treatment is best when accompanied by improved sleep hygiene and patient education about age-related changes in sleep.

Care should be taken in dispensing sedative-hypnotics for people with risk factors for sleep apnea. Nursing interventions include encouraging older patients with disordered breathing to sleep on their sides and to lose weight if obese. Other interventions include giving supplemental oxygen if hypoxemia, caused by chronic lung disease or hypoventilation, is present.

SKIN CHANGES

Although a variety of cutaneous changes have been associated with age, some of these changes are due to normal or intrinsic age factors, whereas others are due to chronic solar exposure.[8] Photoaging is the combined effect of repeated sun exposure and intrinsic aging on the skin, and it is the cause of what is generally associated with the clinical (and histological) changes that are consistent with "aging." With age, there is a thinning of the skin and a decrease in skin flexibility. This puts the older adult at risk for epidermal tearing from shearing forces. Likewise, there is a loss of elasticity resulting in fine wrinkling, looseness, and sagging. Over time, there is a decrease in the number of dermal blood vessels, and these blood vessels become thinner and more fragile. These changes result in the hemorrhaging (known as senile purpura) commonly seen in older adults, in impaired body temperature management and healing of wounds, and in decreased absorption of topical treatments. With age, there is decreased density and activity of the eccrine and apocrine glands and decreased sebum production.

Overall, because of a combination of skin changes in older adults, there tends to be a quicker breakdown in the skin barrier and a slower recovery of skin integrity. Common interventions to maintain skin integrity are shown in Box 12-4.

Box 12-4 • NURSING INTERVENTIONS for Maintaining Skin Integrity in the Older Adult

- Avoid shearing forces when turning the patient.
- Turn the patient frequently.
- Keep the patient appropriately covered for warmth.
- Bathe the patient daily, preferably with total immersion in water 32.2°C to 40.5°C (90°F to 105°F).

- Apply oil-based emollient to the patient's skin after bathing.
- Monitor responses from transdermal medications.
- Monitor wounds closely for healing and signs and symptoms of infection.

Findings on Physical Examination and Management

The skin of older adults tends to sag, especially on the hands and forearms, and causes underlying tissue injury. The person may appear pale and may not be able to correctly perceive surface temperature (e.g., how hot water is). The hair becomes gray and is coarser, and the nails may break and become more brittle. Additional hairs develop on the eyebrows, nose, and ears. Wound healing is prolonged, and there is increased risk for contact dermatitis due to increased skin sensitivity. Xerosis, or dry skin, is a common problem for the older adult and is the most common cause of pruritus in this group. The treatment of dry skin focuses primarily on the replacement of water, which is the major cause of dryness.

Older adults should be encouraged to do the following:

▶ Maintain a sufficient oral intake of fluid, approximately 2,000 mL of liquids daily.

▶ Increase bathing time so that there is total-body water immersion 10 minutes daily, with water temperature ranging from 90°F to 105°F (32.2°C to 40.5°C).

▶ Avoid the use of soaps.

▶ Use an emollient after bathing.

Skin lesions are more common in the older adult, and certainly any change in a skin growth or any lesion that does not heal in a reasonable time should be suspect for malignancy. Malignant lesions tend to occur in sun-exposed areas but may also be present in other areas.

CARDIOVASCULAR CHANGES

A number of cardiovascular changes occur with aging (see Table 12-1). These age-related changes, overt and occult cardiovascular disease, and reduced physical activity all affect cardiovascular function in elderly people. With age, there is a loss of myocytes in both the left and right ventricles, with a progressive increase in myocyte cell volume per nucleus in both ventricles.[9] With age, there is also a progressive reduction in the number of pacemaker cells in the sinus node, with only 10% of the number of cells at 20 years of age still remaining at 75 years of age. Aging changes in the heart have an impact on afterload, preload, contractility, diastolic function, and the cardiovascular response to exercise.

Afterload is the resistance to the ejection of blood by the left ventricle and is composed of (1) peripheral vascular resistance and (2) characteristic aortic impedance. With age, the large elastic arteries become dilated, with a reduction in compliance. Progressive thickening of the aortic media and intima is associated with aortic enlargement. There is an age-associated increase in arterial stiffness resulting from changes in the arterial media (e.g., thickening of the smooth muscle layers, increased fragmentation of elastin, an increase in the amount and characteristics of collagen,

and increased calcification). These structural changes are associated with a reduction in aortic distensibility due to increased aortic stiffness with an increase in pulse wave velocity. The reduction in arterial compliance contributes more to the age-related increase in afterload than does the loss of peripheral vascular beds.

The decrease in vessel compliance affects large and small arteries. As a result, even a small increase in intravascular volume can be accompanied by a substantial rise in aortic pressure (and, in turn, systolic blood pressure), which may lead to pressure-produced ventricular hypertrophy.[10]

Circulating levels of catecholamines increase with age, especially related to stress. Specifically, β-adrenergic vasodilation of vascular smooth muscle decreases with aging, and α-adrenergic vasoconstriction of vascular smooth muscle does not change with aging. The impaired vasodilator response to β-adrenergic stimulation with age is particularly important during exercise.

With aging there is an increase in systolic blood pressure and a widened pulse pressure. A slight reduction in diastolic blood pressure occurs after the sixth decade.[11] The increase in systolic blood pressure is due to an interaction of many factors, with age being only one of them.

Posterior left ventricular wall thickness increases (i.e., left ventricular hypertrophy develops) with age, and this is mediated by an increase in systolic blood pressure.[11] This hypertrophy is due to volume, not the number of cardiac myocytes. Fibroblasts undergo hyperplasia, and collagen is deposited in the myocardial interstitium. Increased afterload causes an increase in left ventricular systolic stress and the addition of sarcomeres. These changes result in an increased left ventricular wall thickness with a normal or decreased left ventricular chamber size and an increased relative wall thickness.

Preload is the filling volume of the left ventricle and is determined by numerous factors that influence blood return to the heart. Resting preload does not change with age,[12] although left ventricular early diastolic filling is reduced with age. With age, left ventricular stiffness is increased, left ventricular compliance is decreased, left ventricular wall thickness is increased, left ventricular relaxation is impaired, and left ventricular diastolic filling is decreased. An age-related increase in systolic blood pressure also impairs left ventricular early diastolic filling, leading to hypotension if preload is reduced. Despite this age-related reduction, preload is maintained because left atrial contraction becomes more vigorous and thereby increases late diastolic filling of the left ventricle.[12]

An age-related increase in left atrial size from increased wall stress counteracts the effects of decreased left ventricular compliance with aging. Left atrial contraction can contribute up to 50% of left ventricular filling in a poorly compliant left ventricle. Consequently, in older adults, development of atrial fibrillation may cause a marked reduction in cardiac output because of the loss of left atrial contribution to left ventricular late diastolic filling.

The intrinsic ability of the heart to generate force does not change with age, although the duration of contraction and relaxation is prolonged in older adults. There is no reduction of resting left ventricular ejection fraction or circumferential fiber shortening in healthy older adults.

Aging is associated with prolongation of isovolumic relaxation time, a reduction in early diastolic filling of the left ventricle, and augmentation of the late diastolic filling of the left ventricle.[12] Also with aging, there is a slowing of the rate at which calcium enters the sarcoplasmic reticulum after myocardial excitation, and a subsequent decrease in relaxation of the left ventricle.[13] Reduced oxidative phosphorylation and cumulative mitochondrial peroxidation occurring with aging may also impair left ventricular diastolic function.

The maximum amount of oxygen uptake (VO_2 max) decreases with age, although the degree to which oxygen uptake decreases is affected by physical conditioning, subclinical coronary artery disease (CAD), smoking, and body weight. With exercise, older adults have a decrease in heart rate, cardiac index, and left ventricular ejection fraction and increases in the left ventricular end-diastolic and end-systolic volume indices.[14]

Findings on Physical Examination and Management

In the absence of vascular disease, these changes should not interfere with normal tissue perfusion. In the older patient, however, the likelihood of atherosclerosis is increased. The narrowing of vessels, coupled with their decrease in compliance, may produce tissue ischemia. These changes, along with bed rest, contribute to tissue injury and decubitus ulcer formation.

The increased vascular stiffness of aging causes the upstroke of the arterial pulse to appear brisker than usual, potentially masking the slowly rising carotid pulse of aortic stenosis. Older adults commonly present with an early-peaking basal systolic murmur of aortic stenosis, typically accompanied by an S_4 sound at the cardiac apex as evidence of reduced ventricular compliance. These people report and demonstrate a limited ability to tolerate physical activity. Older patients may also have a greater amount of pooling in the lower extremities because of decreased muscle mass and poor venous return. If the patient is placed on bed rest, this fluid pool is redistributed and may cause an overload in the cardiovascular system. The nurse must be alert for vascular overload and congestive heart failure.

Another factor to consider is the shifting of fluids when a patient arises after having been on bed rest. The sudden shift in fluid to the lower extremities and the lowered fluid volume that results from bed rest can produce extreme lightheadedness. This is further complicated by a decrease in baroreceptor sensitivity with age. A slow progression of head elevation and dangling before moving the patient to sitting or standing is necessary to prevent syncope and possible injury from falling.

Although chest pressure is the classic symptom of angina in older adults, there is an increased incidence of silent ischemia in these people. If angina or a myocardial infarction is suspected, a comprehensive history, vital signs, and electrocardiogram (ECG) should be obtained, and a laboratory workup (including cardiac enzymes) should be sent. If at all possible, it is important to obtain a prior ECG for comparison.

About half of all older adults have abnormalities on the resting ECG, most commonly PR- and QT-interval prolongation, intraventricular conduction abnormalities, reduction in QRS voltage, and a leftward shift of the frontal plane QRS axis. Common age-related changes to the ECG are shown in Table 12-2. Elderly men more frequently have major ECG abnormalities than do elderly women, and these abnormalities increase with age.[15]

RESPIRATORY CHANGES

It is particularly difficult to distinguish age-related changes in the structure and function of the lungs from those changes caused by disease because the lungs are continually exposed to environmental stres-

Table 12-2 • Common Age-Related Changes in the Electrocardiogram (ECG)

ECG Variable	Age			
	<30 yr	30–39 yr	40–49 yr	>49 yr
R-wave amplitude (mm)	10.4	10.5	9.0	9.3
S-wave amplitude (mm)	15.2	14.2	12.2	12.4
Frontal plane axis (degrees)	48.9	48.1	36.5	38.8
PR duration (ms)	15.9	16.2	16.0	16.2
QRS duration (ms)	7.6	7.5	7.4	8.0
QT duration (ms)	37.8	37.5	37.9	39.6
T-wave amplitude (ms)	5.2	4.6	4.3	4.4

Data from Bachman S, Sparrow D, Smith LK: Age-related changes in electrocardiographic variables. Am J Cardiol 48:513, 1981.

strength of the contraction. The decrease of lean muscle mass and the loss of elasticity contribute to lost flexibility and increased stiffness.

Skeletal calcium losses are a universal concomitant of aging and reflect an imbalance of bone remodeling, with osteoclastic bony resorption exceeding osteoblastic new bone formation. After approximately 30 years of age, when peak skeletal bone mass has been achieved, resorption begins to exceed formation with subsequent skeletal calcium losses and a decline in bone density. The rate of bone loss is approximately 0.5% to 1% yearly from age 60 years onward. The bone changes that occur are likely due to a multitude of factors in addition to normal age-related changes: lack of exercise, poor nutrition, and calcium malabsorption. Known age-related changes in factors influencing bone homeostasis occur in calcium, vitamin D, and gonadal hormone status. Dietary intake of calcium, gastrointestinal absorption of calcium, and vitamin D synthesis are all decreased with age. Decreased intake of vitamin D_2 and decreased skin absorption of 7-dehydrocholesterol as a result of inadequate sunlight exposure also may contribute to vitamin D deficiency with age. The patient on bed rest may rapidly lose bone mineral concentration. The calcaneus (heel) and spine are most susceptible, with a loss of approximately 1% per week. This loss is related to lack of weight bearing.

Musculoskeletal function is dictated largely by the size of the muscle mass that is contracting, and to a lesser extent by changes in surrounding connective tissue in the joint and neural recruitment, conduction velocities, and fatigue. Sedentary people lose large amounts of muscle mass over time. Unfortunately, muscle mass cannot be maintained into old age even with habitual aerobic activities in either normal or athletic adults.[21] Only loading of muscle with weight-lifting exercise has been shown to reverse loss of muscle mass and strength in older adults.[22,23] There is also a decrease in oxidative and glycolytic enzyme capacity with age, a decrease in total number of muscle fibers, selective atrophy of type 2 (fast-twitch) fibers, and shortening of tendons and ligaments with decreased tissue elasticity. Bone changes, as evidenced by osteoporosis, present with decreased height, kyphosis, and scoliosis.

Findings on Physical Examination and Management

Older adults with osteoporosis may have spontaneous fractures, occurring simply from moving in bed. In general, older adults have a decrease in overall muscle strength and an increased tendency to have muscle cramping. Crepitus and pain with range of motion of the joints is common, particularly in the weight-bearing joints (e.g., the knee). Gait and posture changes are frequently present, and older adults tend to have a stooped posture with a slow, shuffling gait.

Forced fasting of the critically ill hospitalized patient may further accelerate muscle loss through catabolism and gluconeogenesis. The added burden of bed rest leads to a rapid loss of mobility, strength,

and energy in the older patient. Maintaining nutrition, changing position frequently, active and passive exercise, and getting out of bed as much as permitted by condition are essential to preserving strength, energy, and bone mass. If the patient is comatose or has suffered loss of function, proper positioning and splinting can help prevent permanent deformity.

ENDOCRINE CHANGES

The equilibrium concentrations of the principal hormones are not necessarily altered with age; however, for older adults, there may be a change in how hormonal equilibrium is achieved.

Therefore, with advancing age, some alterations in hormone production, metabolism, and action occur. Subtle changes are noted in pituitary dynamics, adrenal gland physiology, and thyroid function; however, the changes in glucose homeostasis, reproductive function, and calcium metabolism are more apparent.[24]

Most of the principal neuroendocrine nuclei in the hypothalamus are structurally intact in old age, although there is some loss of morphologic integrity of the suprachiasmatic nucleus. Morphometric variables associated with increased cellular functional activity have been measured in several hypothalamic nuclei. Certain neurons in the human paraventricular nuclei seem activated, and the neurons that produce arginine vasopressin (AVP) increase in size, and the number of neurons that express both AVP and corticotropin-releasing hormone increases with age.

The anterior pituitary shows unchanged output of stimulating hormones, although the peripheral levels of target hormones decrease. For example, circulating levels of daytime and nighttime thyroid-stimulating hormone and growth hormone (GH) are greatly diminished in old age.[25] In contrast, prolactin and melatonin are decreased only at night. Age-related decreases in hormonal levels are associated with a decrease in the amplitude but not the frequency of secretory pulses.

The decline in GH with age is believed to be associated with the decrease in lean body mass, increase in body fat (especially in the visceral and abdominal compartment), adverse changes in lipoproteins, and reduction in aerobic capacity commonly noted in older adults. Research is ongoing to determine whether replacement of GH in healthy older adults can reverse these changes.[25]

Normal aging is associated with insulin resistance and reduced β-cell function, but it is not known whether changes in proinsulin and the proinsulin/immunoreactive insulin ratio are also related to reduced β-cell function.[26] Glucose tolerance decreases with age. An increase in blood glucose to 200 mg/dL occurs in about half of people older than 70 years.[26] Interpretation of this glucose intolerance requires the use of age-adjusted parameters to avoid the inappropriate diagnosis and treatment of diabetes mellitus. Evaluating glycosylated hemoglobin (HbA_{1c}) or glycosylated albumin may help establish the presence or absence of diabetes mellitus in the older patient with elevated blood glucose levels. Because the renal threshold for reabsorption of glucose increases with age, higher degrees of hyperglycemia must be present before glucose spills into the urine. Therefore, monitoring for hyperglycemia with urine testing should be avoided.

Throughout life, the adrenal cortex shows significant morphogenic and steroidogenic changes. There is a subtle decline in aldosterone with age and a subtle increase in cortisol; however, the adrenal androgens dehydroepiandrosterone and dehydroepiandrosterone sulfate decline with age in a process similar to menopause. This decline is believed to aggravate some age-related diseases.[27]

The thyroid gland undergoes a progressive decrease in size with aging, although enlargement due to the presence of nodules is not uncommon. The concentration of thyroid hormones found in the blood of older adults is variable and influenced by disease. There may, however, be an alteration in the responsiveness of target tissues. Specifically, there may be an age-related reduction in the ability of aged tissues to increase receptor numbers in response to a reduction in hormone levels.[28]

Findings on Physical Examination and Management

The reduction in thyroid hormone levels with increasing age is correlated with many physiological and pathological sequelae: changes in cholesterol metabolism, heart rate, cardiac output, and strength of cardiac contraction and alterations in basal metabolic rate and thermoregulation. The symptoms of thyroid disease, such as apathy, weakness, and weight loss, may not be as pronounced in older adults as they are in younger people. Moreover, these symptoms are often attributed to old age rather than to hyperthyroidism or hypothyroidism. The older patient with hyperthyroidism is likely to present with atrial tachycardia and is more likely to be anorexic than hyperphagic; this person usually does not experience heat intolerance. The hypothyroid older adult may present with increased susceptibility to hypothermia if exposed to cold, a change in cognitive status, fatigue, dizziness, and a tendency to fall.

Being aware of the atypical presentation of thyroid disease in older adults leads the critical care nurse to recognize endocrine imbalance. Once identified, the imbalance can easily be corrected by replacing thyroid hormone or changing the dosage of thyroid replacement.

Diabetes mellitus is frequently seen in conjunction with acute illness, trauma, or surgery. The end-organ damage of diabetes mellitus is a factor in stroke, myocardial infarction, decreased renal function, and peripheral vascular disease. Long-standing non–insulin-dependent diabetes may be diagnosed only when the patient presents with a stroke or acute myocardial infarction. Therefore, it is important to distinguish among the impaired glucose tolerance of aging, a transient rise in glucose related to acute illness, and the disease process of diabetes.

Recognition of the underlying diabetes and possible end-organ damage may alter the course of the acute illness. For example, knowing that the incidence of congestive heart failure after myocardial infarction is higher in diabetic than in nondiabetic patients, the nurse can be alert for early signs of fluid retention.

Older people with diabetes are, for the most part, not insulin dependent. Therefore, even if they have extremely high blood sugars, they are rarely ketoacidotic. In fact, the coma of this age group is usually hyperglycemic, hyperosmolar, and nonketotic (HHNK). Managing this state requires a delicate balance of hydration and rapid reduction of blood sugar without massive brain edema and death. The critical care nurse must be aware that HHNK coma can be triggered by acute illness or surgery. Common problems found in older adults with diabetes, and nursing interventions to prevent these problems, are shown in Box 12-6. It should be particularly recognized that the most prevalent sign of either hypoglycemia or hyperglycemia among these people is a change in cognitive status.

IMMUNOLOGICAL CHANGES

With age there is a decline in immune function. Specifically, there is a decline in both T-cell and B-cell function, with a dramatic effect on cell-mediated immunity. The decline in B-cell function may be in-

---

 Box 12-6 • NURSING INTERVENTIONS Prevention of Problems in the Older Adult With Diabetes

Skin Alterations
- Monitor for decreased circulation and skin breakdown.
- Provide foot care to maintain skin integrity. Bathe the feet daily and apply emollient.

Hyperglycemia
- Maintain a controlled diet.
- Monitor blood glucose levels.
- Monitor for urinary frequency.
- Monitor for hyponatremia.
- Monitor for dry mouth.
- Monitor for changes in cognition.

Hypoglycemia
- Monitor for acute changes in cognition.

Hydration Status
- Monitor hydration.
- Encourage the intake of 2,000 mL of fluid daily.

End-Organ Disease
- Monitor kidney function.
- Monitor for visual changes (e.g., blurred or decreased vision).

directly related to a decline in T-cell function. The decreased numbers of B cells secreting immunoglobulin G result in a generally poor humoral immune response. With aging, the thymus gland involutes and there is a decrease in thymic hormone levels, and the number of autoantibodies increases.[29]

Findings on Physical Examination and Management

The usual symptoms of infection such as chills, fever, leukocytosis, or tachycardia may be absent or blunted in the older adult. Instead, these people may present with an acute change in cognition, function, or behavior. Delirium, for example, may be the only sign or symptom of a urinary tract infection in an older adult. The most common sites of infection in older adults are respiratory, urinary, and skin, and when subtle changes are noted in an older patient, consideration should be given to each of these areas.

• Psychological Challenges

COGNITIVE CHANGES

Cognition refers to the process of obtaining, storing, retrieving, and using information. The neuroanatomical and neurophysiological underpinnings of cognitive change are unclear. Studies[30,31] have shown that younger people have larger ventricular volumes and smaller gray and white matter volumes compared with older people. There is also greater prefrontal cortex activity in younger adults compared with older adults in the dorsolateral area during memory retrieval. These changes are believed to account for the changes in working memory[31] and executive abilities[32] associated with normal aging. As age increases, there is some decline in perceptual motor skills, concept formation, complex memory tasks, and quick-decision tasks. However, age itself is not the criterion for making decisions about a patient's cognitive functions. Each person's abilities must be judged individually rather than against a norm.

Cognitive function should be assessed and described on admission and monitored routinely over time and whenever the patient's condition changes. While assessing cognitive functions during the patient's stay in intensive care, it is important to remember that physiological deficits, some medications, and internal and external stress, such as environmental stressors, affect cognitive skills. In older adults, acute physical changes frequently initially present as changes in cognitive status. For example, an older adult with pneumonia may not have symptoms such as fever or cough. Rather, this person may present with changes in cognitive status.

A mental status questionnaire, such as Folstein's Mini-Mental State Examination (MMSE), can be used to assess cognitive function systematically. (For more information regarding the MMSE, contact the publisher: Psychological Assessment Resources, Inc., 16204 North Florida Avenue, Lutz, FL 33549.) The

MMSE has 11 questions that provide information about orientation, attention, memory, perception, and thought process, and it takes 5 to 10 minutes to complete, and the patient must be able to give oral and written responses.[33] Use of a consistent assessment tool helps the nurse compare responses and monitor results over time. The main drawback to the use of a questionnaire is that some critically ill patients may not be able to hear, see, talk, or write well enough to respond to the questions. Longer, more sensitive tools may also be more fatiguing for the critically ill older patient.

Several common syndromes cause cognitive impairment, including dementia, delirium, and depression (discussed later). Dementia is based on impairment of memory plus at least one of the following: a personality change or impairment in either abstract thinking, judgment, or higher cortical functions. Delirium is the abrupt onset of clouding of consciousness and is a medical emergency. Table 12-5 identifies factors to differentiate dementia from delirium. Reversible causes of dementia and delirium are listed in Box 12-7.

The Mental Health Toolkit is an excellent resource to use to evaluate patients for acute changes in mental health and provides appropriate interventions to manage delirium and other mental health problems. This is available at http://www.ncgnp.org. Tools to evaluate memory and differentiate between dementia and delirium are available at http://www.geronurseonline.org.

Learning

Older adults may take longer to respond to and assimilate new material. They may also be hesitant to take on new tasks. Motivation continues to be an important aspect of learning new material. If the material is irrelevant or meaningless, motivation is decreased, which is often interpreted as an inability to learn. The person's sensory and cognitive abilities are taken into account when teaching older patients. It may be necessary to present information in small segments using varied stimuli, including touching, seeing, hearing, and (if vision permits) writing. If movements are slowed, allow time for the completion of motor tasks, such as manipulating equipment or carrying out exercises.

Memory

The older person's memory decline involves short-term memory rather than long-term and remote memory. Recall of memory from the past is least impaired by age. Remote memory recall (items learned many years ago) can be a positive therapeutic strategy for older patients. Reminiscence is an adaptive mechanism that helps the nurse learn about the patient and increases the patient's feelings of self-worth and competence.

Depression

Depression disorders are among the most common complaints of older adults and the leading cause of

Table 12-5 • Summary of Differences Between Dementia and Delirium

	Dementia		Delirium
	Alzheimer's Disease (AD)	*Vascular (Multi-Infarct) Dementia*	
Etiology	Familial (genetic [chromosomes 14, 19, 21]) Sporadic	Cardiovascular (CV) disease Cerebrovascular disease Hypertension	Drug toxicity and interactions; acute disease; trauma; chronic disease exacerbation Fluid and electrolyte disorder
Risk factors	Advanced age; genetics	Preexisting CV disease	Preexisting cognitive impairment
Occurrence	50%–60% of dementias	20% of dementias	20% of hospitalized older people
Onset	Slow	Often abrupt Follows a stroke or transient ischemic attack	Rapid, acute onset A harbinger of acute medical illness
Age of onset (yr)	Early onset AD: 30s–65 Late onset AD: 65+ Most commonly: 85+	Most commonly 50–70 yr	Any age, but predominantly in older persons
Gender	Males and females equally	Predominantly males	Males and females equally
Course	Chronic, irreversible; progressive, regular, downhill	Chronic, irreversible Fluctuating, stepwise progression	Acute
Duration	2–20 yr	Variable; years	Lasts 1 day to 1 month
Symptom progress	Onset insidious. *Early*—mild and subtle *Middle and late*—intensified Progression to death (infection or malnutrition)	Depends on location of infarct and success of treatment; death due to underlying CV disease	Symptoms are fully reversible with adequate treatment; can progress to chronicity or death if underlying condition is ignored
Mood	Early depression (30%)	Labile: mood swings	Variable
Speech/language	Speech remains intact until late in disease *Early*—mild anomia (cannot name objects); deficits progress until speech lacks meaning; echoes and repeats words and sounds; mutism.	May have speech deficit/aphasia depending on location of lesion	Fluctuating; often cannot concentrate long enough to speak
Physical signs	*Early*—no motor deficits *Middle*—apraxia (70%) (cannot perform purposeful movement) *Late*—Dysarthria (impaired speech) *End stage*—loss of all voluntary activity; positive neurologic signs	According to location of lesion: focal neurologic signs, seizures Commonly exhibits motor deficits	Signs and symptoms of underlying disease
Orientation	Becomes lost in familiar places (topographic disorientation) Has difficulty drawing three-dimensional objects (visual and spatial disorientation) Disorientation to time, place, and person—with disease progression		May fluctuate between lucidity and complete disorientation to time, place, and person
Memory	Loss is an early sign of dementia; loss of recent memory is soon followed by progressive decline in recent and remote memory		Impaired recent and remote memory; may fluctuate between lucidity and confusion
Personality	Apathy, indifference, irritability *Early disease*—social behavior intact; hides cognitive deficits *Advanced disease*—disengages from activity and relationships; suspicious; paranoid delusions caused by memory loss; aggressive; catastrophic reactions		Fluctuating; cannot focus attention to converse; alarmed by symptoms (when lucid); hallucinations; paranoid
Functional status, activities of daily living	Poor judgment in everyday activities; has progressive decline in ability to handle money, use telephone, function in home and workplace		Impaired
Attention span	Distractable; short attention span		Highly impaired; cannot maintain or shift attention
Psychomotor activity	Wandering, hyperactivity, pacing, restlessness, agitation		Variable; alternates between high agitation, hyperactivity, restlessness, and lethargy
Sleep–wake cycle	Often impaired; wandering and agitation at nighttime		Takes brief naps throughout day and night

---

Box 12-7 • Reversible Causes of Dementia and Delirium

Drugs
Emotional illness (including depression)
Metabolic/endocrine disorders
Eye/ear/environment
Nutritional/neurological disorders
Tumors/trauma
Infection
Alcoholism/anemia/atherosclerosis

 Box 12-9 • Drug Groups That May Cause Depression in the Older Person

Analgesics/anti-inflammatory agents
Anticonvulsants
Antihistamines
Antihypertensives
Antimicrobials
Antiparkinsonian agents
Hormones
Immunosuppressive agents
Tranquilizers

---

suicide in later life. Symptoms of depression are listed in Box 12-8. Based on the diagnostic criteria for major depression, at least five of these symptoms should occur almost daily for at least 2 weeks. These symptoms of depression in the older adult can be masked by normal age-related changes or disease states. For example, difficulty sleeping, early morning awakening, and lethargy are common physical complaints of the normal aging person. Alternatively, depression in the older adult may more commonly present with pseudohypochondriasis, preoccupation with past life events, and changes in cognitive ability. In some patients, the dominant emotional mood may not be sadness but anger, anxiety, or irritability.

Causes of depression are multifaceted and include multiple losses associated with aging, underlying illness, or drugs. Box 12-9 lists drug groups that may cause depression. Screening tools, such as the Geriatric Depression Scale,[34] shown in Box 12-10, are useful to identify people who are depressed. Once identified, appropriate interventions, including drug therapy, behavioral modification, and counseling, can be initiated.

The nurse must also be aware of cardiovascular side effects of antidepressants. The tricyclic antidepressive drugs are less commonly used owing to the risk for side effects. For example, tricyclic antidepressants can results in ST-segment and T-wave changes, although these are not necessarily indicative of myocardial damage. Ventricular dysrhythmias and disturbances in cardiac conduction are potential serious side effects and may result in the drug being reduced or discontinued. Anticholinergic effects, especially in patients with Alzheimer's disease, benign prostatic

hypertrophy, or CAD, may also be seen. The selective serotonin reuptake inhibitors are much more commonly used now to treat depression. Side effects to monitor include changes related to sleep, appetite, personality or behavior, and blood pressure readings.

Untreated depression may result in suicide, which is a serious problem among older adults. Of all suicides committed in this country annually, 25% involve people older than 65 years of age. White men older than 85 years of age are at particular risk.[35] Because of their many losses and changes, older adults may view suicide as a means of fulfilling a fantasy of "reunion" with a dead spouse or significant other. The nurse must monitor signs and symptoms of depression, explore the causes of depression, facilitate treatment, and watch for suicide attempts or warnings.

ABUSE OF THE OLDER PERSON

Mistreatment of older people is a problem that affects more than 4% of the older adults in the United States.[36] Abuse of older adults occurs in homes and institutions and takes many forms. Abuse may be blatant or subtle; it may be physical, psychological, or material (e.g., financial). Abuse may involve neglect (by others or by self), exploitation, or abandonment. The abused older person is often physically or mentally frail and unable to report the abusive situation. Abuse can also happen to emotionally and intellectually stable older people who are unable to stop the abuse or report it because of their financial or emotional dependence on the abuser. They may also be afraid of being abandoned.

Abuse can occur because of lack of knowledge about the older person's basic needs, a lack of resources to help, or a desire to protect an inheritance. People who may or may not live with the older person may be responsible for the abuse. Caregivers who are extremely stressed may become abusive. In some situations, the abused older adult is the caretaker.

The nurse must be alert to the signs and symptoms of elder abuse as outlined in Box 12-11. Any suggestion by the patient or family that things are not well at home is pursued. A statement such as, "My son hasn't been here yet. He sometimes forgets his commitments," should open the door for further conversation.

 Box 12-8 • RED FLAG: Symptoms of Depression

- Depressed mood
- Decreased interest in activities
- Weight changes
- Sleep changes
- Psychomotor changes
- Fatigue
- Feelings of worthlessness or guilt
- Decreased concentration
- Suicidal ideation

Box 12-10 • Geriatric Depression Scale

Patient _____ Examiner _____ Date _____

Directions to Patient: Please choose the best answer for how you have felt over the past week.
Directions to Examiner: Present questions VERBALLY. Circle answer given by patient. Do not show to patient.

1.	Are you basically satisfied with your life?	yes	**no** (1)
2.	Have you dropped many of your activities and interests?	**yes** (1)	no
3.	Do you feel that your life is empty?	**yes** (1)	no
4.	Do you often get bored?	**yes** (1)	no
5.	Are you hopeful about the future?	yes	**no** (1)
6.	Are you bothered by thoughts you can't get out of your head?	**yes** (1)	no
7.	Are you in good spirits most of the time?	yes	**no** (1)
8.	Are you afraid that something bad is going to happen to you?	**yes** (1)	no
9.	Do you feel happy most of the time?	yes	**no** (1)
10.	Do you often feel helpless?	**yes** (1)	no
11.	Do you often get restless and fidgety?	**yes** (1)	no
12.	Do you prefer to stay at home rather than go out and do things?	**yes** (1)	no
13.	Do you frequently worry about the future?	**yes** (1)	no
14.	Do you feel you have more problems with memory than most?	**yes** (1)	no
15.	Do you think it is wonderful to be alive now?	yes	**no** (1)
16.	Do you feel downhearted and blue?	**yes** (1)	no
17.	Do you feel pretty worthless the way you are now?	**yes** (1)	no
18.	Do you worry a lot about the past?	**yes** (1)	no
19.	Do you find life very exciting?	yes	**no** (1)
20.	Is it hard for you to get started on new projects?	**yes** (1)	no
21.	Do you feel full of energy?	yes	**no** (1)
22.	Do you feel that your situation is hopeless?	**yes** (1)	no
23.	Do you think that most people are better off than you are?	**yes** (1)	no
24.	Do you frequently get upset over little things?	**yes** (1)	no
25.	Do you frequently feel like crying?	**yes** (1)	no
26.	Do you have trouble concentrating?	**yes** (1)	no
27.	Do you enjoy getting up in the morning?	yes	**no** (1)
28.	Do you prefer to avoid social occasions?	**yes** (1)	no
29.	Is it easy for you to make decisions?	yes	**no** (1)
30.	Is your mind as clear as it used to be?	yes	**no** (1)

TOTAL: Please sum all bolded answers (worth one point) for a total score. _____

Scores: 0–10 Normal   11–20 Moderate Depression   21–30 Severe Depression

From Yesavage JA, Brink TL: Development and validation of a geriatric depression screening scale: A preliminary report. J Psychiatr Res 17:37–49, 1983.

Box 12-11 • RED FLAG: Signs and Symptoms of Elder Abuse

- Lack of compliance with management of health problems
- Unexplained injuries, such as fractures, bruises, lacerations
- Burns
- Poor personal hygiene
- Sexually transmitted disease
- Altered mood
- Depression
- Failure to thrive (underhydration/impaired nutritional status)
- Impaired skin integrity/fungal rashes

It might uncover a mother who is worried about her son's drinking and perhaps about the way he treats her when he has been drinking. Attempts are made to compare the history given by the patient with that given by the family. Inconsistencies need to be explored further. Likewise, it is helpful to ask caretakers if they are able to give the care they feel is needed. Indications that the patient is "getting to be a handful" may be a clue to mismanaged care or a caretaker in need of support and assistance. In either situation, the nurse can provide information and support and refer the patient and caregiver to a social worker or mental health nurse for further assistance. All health care workers, including nurses, must know their responsibility under state law for reporting abuse of the older patient.

ALCOHOL ABUSE

Alcohol abuse occurs in the aging population. Clinical studies estimate that 15% of men and 12% of women are high-risk drinkers based on information provided by the National Institute on Alcohol Abuse and Alcoholism.[37] Problem drinking in older adults occurs for similar reasons as it does in younger adults. However, smaller amounts of alcohol create larger problems for older people, and they may be more susceptible to alcohol-induced disease. Differences in metabolism of alcohol in older people, the smaller volume of body water, and the decrease in lean body tissue may increase the propensity to alcoholism or alcohol problems. In addition, older adults are high consumers of psychotropic drugs and are at risk for drug–alcohol interactions.

Nursing interventions include screening the older adult for alcohol use. The HEAT screening method,[38] shown in Box 12-12, is useful for screening purposes. A positive response on any item is a reason to obtain a more detailed history of alcohol use. When alcohol abuse is suspected, the immediate goal is to stabilize physiological and psychological responses to alcohol withdrawal and determine the impact of alcohol abuse on whatever other diagnoses have resulted in the need for critical care. As soon as possible, the nurse should refer the patient to a social worker, psychiatric liaison nurse, or alcohol counselor.

• Challenges in Medication Use

The rule for giving therapeutic medications to the older patient is *start low, go slow*. In other words, be patient. Changes related to aging can have a great impact on drug response. Changes in renal function, gastrointestinal secretions and motility, and cell receptor sites and concurrent disease states can alter the absorption, distribution, and excretion of drugs. These changes are summarized in Table 12-6.

Before admission to the ICU, older patients may have been taking many different medications, including over-the-counter (OTC) medications such as vitamins, tonics, herbals (e.g., Saint John's wort, glucosamine), laxatives, antacids, and pain relievers. They may also have a history of heavy alcohol intake. Any of these drugs can cause problems if combined with medications administered in the hospital.

> **Box 12-12 • The HEAT Screening Method for Indications of Alcohol Abuse**
>
> **H**ow do you use alcohol?
> Have you ever thought you used alcohol to **E**xcess?
> Has **A**nyone else ever thought you used too much?
> Have you ever had any **T**rouble resulting from your use of alcohol?

The nurse needs to elicit a careful history of drug use from the patient and family. The family can be asked to bring in all medications the patient has been using; these include OTC medications and herbal remedies. Although alcohol use may be a sensitive topic, establishing the pattern of use can be essential in preventing untoward drug interactions and anticipating problems with liver damage or withdrawal.

Special considerations concerning administration of drugs to the older patient include knowing the drugs the patient has been taking; assessing renal, hepatic, endocrine, and digestive systems; and evaluating lean body mass. Impaired body systems may affect the absorption, metabolism, and excretion of drugs. Additional considerations are listed in Box 12-13. A decrease in lean body mass and an increase in total body fat may alter the distribution of the drug in the body.

DRUG ABSORPTION

Drug absorption is affected by the following age-related changes: decreased gastric acid, decreased gastrointestinal motility, decreased gastric blood flow, changes in gastrointestinal villi, and decreased blood flow and body temperature in the rectum. The increased pH of gastric secretions and delayed stomach emptying time can alter the degradation, and thus the absorption, of drugs. Drugs that are not stable in an acid medium can be severely reduced in bioavailability if they remain in the stomach for long periods. Drugs that are designed to be acted on in the small intestine may be affected by the higher pH of the aging stomach. A coated, pH-sensitive medication, such as erythromycin, may lose its coating in the stomach and be degraded before reaching the absorption sites in the small intestine. Coated gastric irritants may lose their coatings and cause bleeding or nausea and vomiting.

Some drugs are eliminated from the body before they enter the systemic circulation by a process called *first-pass metabolism*. In general, the enzymes responsible for this first-pass effect are decreased in the elderly so that bioavailability of drugs with high hepatic extraction may be increased with age. These drugs require dosage reduction in older adults.

DRUG DISTRIBUTION

Distribution of drugs in the body can be affected by a decrease in lean body mass, an increase in total body fat, or a decrease in total body fluid, all of which may accompany aging. Drugs that bind to muscle (e.g., digoxin) become more bioavailable as lean body mass diminishes, increasing the risk for toxicity. Fat-soluble drugs (e.g., flurazepam [Dalmane], chlorpromazine [Thorazine], phenobarbital) can be deposited in fat and result in cumulative effects of oversedation. In the presence of a volume deficit, drugs that are water soluble (e.g., gentamicin [Garamycin]) may have a higher concentration and may reach toxic levels rapidly.

Table 12-6 • Altered Drug Responses in Older People

Age-Related Changes	Effect of Age-Related Change	Applicable Medications
Absorption		
Reduced gastric acid; increased pH (less acid)	Rate of drug absorption—possibly delayed	Vitamins
Reduced gastrointestinal motility; prolonged gastric emptying	Extent of drug absorption—not affected	Calcium
Distribution		
Decreased albumin sites	Serious alterations in drug binding to plasma proteins (the unbound drug gives the pharmacologic response); highly protein-bound medications have fewer binding sites, leading to increased effects and accelerated metabolism and excretion	Selected highly protein-binding medications: Oral anticoagulants (warfarin) Oral hypoglycemic agents (sulfonylureas) Barbiturates Calcium channel blockers Furosemide (Lasix) Nonsteroidal anti-inflammatory drugs (NSAIDs) Sulfonamides Quinidine Phenytoin (Dilantin)
Reduced cardiac output	Decreased perfusion of many bodily organs	
Impaired peripheral blood flow	Decreased perfusion	
Increased percentage of body fat	Proportion of body fat increases with age, resulting in increased ability to store fat-soluble medications; this causes drug accumulation, prolonged storage, and delayed excretion	Selected fat-soluble medications: Barbiturates Diazepam (Valium) Lidocaine Phenothiazines (antipsychotics) Ethanol Morphine
Decreased lean body mass	Decreased body volume allows higher peak levels of medications	
Metabolism		
Decreased cardiac output and decreased perfusion of the liver	Decreased metabolism and delay of breakdown of medications, resulting in prolonged duration of action, accumulation, and drug toxicity	All medications metabolized by the liver
Excretion		
Decreased renal blood flow; loss of functioning nephrons; decreased renal efficiency	Decreased rates of elimination and increased duration of action; danger of accumulation and drug toxicity	Selected medications with prolonged action: Aminoglycoside antibiotics Cimetidine (Tagamet) Chlorpropamide (Diabinese) Digoxin Lithium Procainamide

From Smeltzer SC, Bare BG, Hinkle JL, Cheever KC: Brunner and Suddarth's Textbook of Medical–Surgical Nursing, 11th ed. Philadelphia, Lippincott Williams & Wilkins, 2008, p 239.

DRUG METABOLISM

The liver is the major organ for biotransformation and detoxification of medications. Drug-metabolizing reactions are classified as phase I reactions, which involve adding or unmasking a polar chemical group to increase water solubility, and phase II or conjugation reactions, which involve linking the drug to another molecule such as glucose, acetate, or sulfate. In older adults, phase I metabolism is often impaired, whereas phase II metabolism is usually unaffected. In the older patient, there may be some decrease in the metabolism of drugs requiring hepatic enzymes for transformation. This results in an increased plasma level and prolonged half-life of the drug. The benzodiazepines (e.g., diazepam [Valium], flurazepam), for example,

have a half-life increase from 20 to 90 hours in the older patient. Hepatic oxidation of these drugs can further be affected by alcohol-induced changes in the liver. There may be a decrease in drug metabolism with occasional alcohol use. In chronic alcohol use, however, drug metabolism is increased, and excretion is accelerated.

DRUG EXCRETION

The kidney is the primary excretory organ for clearing drugs. Drugs that are excreted unchanged (e.g., digoxin, cimetidine, antibiotics) or have renally excreted active metabolites require dosage reduction in the older adult to avoid accumulation and toxicity. Serum creatinine alone is not a good determinant of renal

⠿ **Box 12-13 • Considerations for Medication Use in Older People**

- Drug dosage guidelines are usually based on studies in younger people, and recommended adult dosage guidelines may not be appropriate for older patients.
- Older people may be taking numerous prescription drugs and may self-medicate with borrowed, old, and over-the-counter drugs.
- The effects of alcohol use must be considered.
- The potential for drug interactions and adverse reactions is increased because of the effects of aging on drug absorption, distribution, metabolism, and excretion.
- Drug toxicities are different from those in younger people. Fewer symptoms may be identified, and they may develop more slowly but be more pronounced once they occur.
- Behavioral side effects are more common in older people because the blood–brain barrier becomes less effective. When there is an acute change in mental status, medication should always be considered as the cause.

function in older people. A creatinine clearance study reflects a more accurate estimation for drug clearance.

• Clinical Applicability Challenges

Case Study

Mrs. F., a 92-year-old black woman, is admitted to the cardiac care unit because of an acute episode of atrial fibrillation. On admission, the emergency staff notes that the patient is in no acute distress, although she does complain of a vague fatigue and says, "I just don't feel like myself." She also notes some increased swelling of her lower extremities and feels somewhat more short of breath than her usual shortness of breath with activity. Her past medical history includes atrial fibrillation, hypertension, diabetes mellitus, degenerative joint disease, and osteoporosis. Medications include verapamil, 240 mg once per day; insulin glargine, 24 units at bedtime; sliding scale coverage 3 times per day with insulin lispro; and acetaminophen (Tylenol) for pain as needed. Drug allergies include amiodarone and sulfa, with both allergic reactions involving rashes.

On admission, Mrs. F.'s heart rate is 140 beats/minute and is irregularly irregular. She has 1+ pitting edema bilaterally to the midshin. She has bilateral crackles in both lung bases consistent with a chest radiograph that shows mild congestive heart failure. She is stabilized in the emergency room with digoxin and 40 mg of furosemide (Lasix) intravenously. Laboratory results show normal electrolytes and a blood urea nitrogen of 45 mg/100 mL. Relevant laboratory results on admission are as follows: hematocrit,

28.7%; hemoglobin, 10.0 g/100 mL; creatinine, 2.1 mg/100 mL; vitamin B_{12}, 722 pg/mL; folate, 9.5 ng/mL; Fe, 44 µg/mL; total iron binding capacity, 251 µg/mL; iron saturation, 18%; and ferritin, 331 ng/mL. Using the Modification of Diet in Renal Disease formula, Mrs. F.'s estimated glomerular filtration rate is 35 mL/min/1.73 m^2, which is indicative of stage 3 renal disease. Mrs. F. is transferred to the cardiac care unit for monitoring.

On admission, you take a comprehensive history. Mrs. F. informs you that she has been increasingly fatigued over the past few months and really does not feel like participating in her usual activities, such as going to exercise class and playing bridge at the assisted living facility where she lives. Her blood sugars have been in her usual range and are generally less than 200 mg/dL, with intermittent insulin coverage necessary during the day. Mrs. F.'s daughter is with her during the admission process, and she wants to know the results of her mother's laboratory findings and radiograph.

1. What is your immediate concern related to Mrs. F's cardiac status and underlying complaints?
2. How do you answer Mrs. F.'s daughter's questions in terms of explaining the laboratory work?
3. How would you encourage Mrs. F.'s daughter to help her mother to optimize her hospital experience and prevent complications?
4. What nursing care interventions are essential to help maintain and restore functional ability?
5. What nursing care interventions are appropriate related to cardiac status and anemia?
6. What nursing care interventions would you implement specifically related to prevention of falls?
7. What patient teaching would you initiate and how would you provide that teaching to Mrs. F. and her daughter?

Review Questions

1. Normal aging is defined as which of the following processes?
   a. One that is the sum of intrinsic aging, extrinsic aging, and idiosyncratic or individual genetic factors specific to each person
   b. One that is exclusively caused by intrinsic factors that occur universally in all people
   c. One that is exclusively caused by extrinsic factors, including factors such as lifestyle or exposure to environmental influences
   d. One that is exclusively caused by genetic factors
2. Common symptoms associated with cataracts include
   a. heightened visual acuity.
   b. photophobia.
   c. decreased sensitivity to glare.
   d. halo images.

3. Which of the following is a normal age-related sleep change?
   a. Taking less time to fall asleep
   b. Spending decreased time in the lighter stages of sleep (stages 1 and 2)
   c. Spending decreased time in the deeper stages of sleep (stages 3 and 4) and in rapid eye movement sleep
   d. Having increased and longer repetitions of the sleep cycle

4. Dementia is recognized clinically based on the following findings:
   a. An impairment of memory plus at least one of the following: a personality change or impairment in abstract thinking, judgment, or higher cortical functions
   b. An abrupt onset of clouding of consciousness, an inability to recall recent events, and impaired decision making
   c. An acute change in remote memory, impaired judgment, and abstract thinking
   d. An inability to perform simple activities of daily living

5. In older adults the optimal way to determine renal function is
   a. to use creatinine levels from recent laboratory values.
   b. to calculate an estimate of a glomerular filtration rate using the Modification of Diet in Renal Disease equation.
   c. to use the blood urea nitrogen/creatinine ratio.
   d. to calculate albumin levels based on the true lymphocyte count.

6. Differences in metabolism of alcohol in the older person are due to the following age-related changes:
   a. Increased drug resistance due to enzymatic changes
   b. Decreased drug tolerance due to fewer liver cells
   c. A decrease in lean body tissue
   d. A tendency toward hyponatremia

References

1. Federal Interagency Forum on Aging Related Statistics: Older Americans 2004: Key Indicators of Well Being. Washington, DC, U.S. Government Printing Office, November, 2004
2. Kiyokawa H: Senescence and cell cycle control. Results Probl Cell Differ 42:257–270, 2006
3. Lam BL, Lee DJ, Gomez-Marin O, et al: Concurrent visual and hearing impairment and risk of mortality: The National Health Interview Survey. Arch Ophthalmol 124(1):95–101, 2006
4. Golding M, Taylor A, Cupples L, Mitchell P: Odds of demonstrating auditory processing abnormality in the average older adult: The Blue Mountains Hearing Study. Ear Hear 27(2):129–138, 2006
5. Larsson M, Finkel D, Pederson N: Odor identification and influences of age. J Gerontol Psychosoc Behav 55:304–310, 2000
6. Bliwise DL, Ansari FP, Straight LB, Parker KP: Age changes in timing and 24-hour distribution of self-reported sleep. Am J Geriatr Psychiatry 13(12):1077–1082, 2005
7. Resnick B, Shaughnessy M, Simpson J: Sleep disorders in late life. In Mellilo K (ed): Geropsychiatric and Mental Health Nursing. Sudbury, MA, Jones & Bartlett, 2005, pp 307–320
8. Ogrin R, Darzins P, Khalil Z: Age related changes in microvascular blood flow and transcutaneous oxygen tension under basal and stimulated conditions. Gerontol A Biol Sci Med Sci 60(2):200–206, 2005
9. Terman A, Brunk UT: The aging myocardium: Roles of mitochondrial damage and lysosomal degradation. Heart Lung Circ 14(2):107–114, 2005
10. Florea VG, Henein MY, Anker SD, et al: Relation of changes over time in ventricular size and function to those in exercise capacity in patients with chronic heart failure. Am Heart J 139(5):913–917, 2000
11. Gryglewska B, Grodzicki T, Czarnecka D, et al: QT dispersion and hypertensive heart disease in the elderly. J Hypertens 18(4):461–464, 2000
12. Baldi JC, McFarlane K, Oxenham HC, et al: Left ventricular diastolic filling and systolic function of young and older trained and untrained men. J Appl Physiol 95(6):2570–2575, 2003
13. Pieske B, Maier LS, Schmidt-Schweda S: Sarcoplasmic reticulum Ca2+ load in human heart failure. Basic Res Cardiol 97(Suppl 1):I63–I71, 2002
14. Otsuki T, Maeda S, Kesen Y, et al: Age-related reduction of systemic arterial compliance induces excessive myocardial oxygen consumption during sub-maximal exercise. Hypertens Res 29(2):65–73, 2006
15. Miyajima H, Nomura M, Nada T, et al: Age-related changes in the magnitude of ventricular depolarization vector: Analyses by magnetocardiogram. J Electrocardiol 33(1):31–35, 2000
16. Bergman SA, Coletti D: Perioperative management of the geriatric patient. Part I: Respiratory system. Oral Surg Oral Med Oral Pathol Oral Radiol Endod 102(3):e1–e6, 2006
17. Watando A, Ebihara S, Ebihara T, et al: Daily oral care and cough reflex sensitivity in elderly nursing home patients. Chest 126(4):1066–1070, 2004
18. Zaugg M, Lucchinetti E: Respiratory function in the elderly. Anesthesiol Clin North Am 18(1):47–58, 2000
19. Finkelstein J, Joshi A, Hise MK: Association of physical activity and renal function in subjects with and without metabolic syndrome: A review of the Third National Health and Nutrition Examination Survey (NHANES III). Am J Kidney Dis 48(3):372–382, 2006
20. Hickson M: Malnutrition and ageing. Postgrad Med J 82(963):2–8, 2006
21. Schaap LA, Pluijm SM, Deeg DJ, Visser M: Inflammatory markers and loss of muscle mass (sarcopenia) and strength. Am J Med 119(6):526.e9–e17, 2006
22. Hikida R, Staron R, Hagerman F, et al: Effects of high intensity resistance training on untrained older men: II. J Gerontol A Biol Sci Med Sci 55(7):B347–B356, 2000
23. Cesari M, Leeuwenburgh C, Lauretani F, et al: Frailty syndrome and skeletal muscle: Results from the Invecchiare in Chianti study. Am J Clin Nutr 83(5):1142–1148, 2006
24. Haden ST, Brown EM, Hurwitz S, et al: The effects of age and gender on parathyroid hormone dynamics. Clin Endocrinol (Oxf) 52(3):329–338, 2000
25. Giannoulis MG, Sonksen PH, Umpleby M, et al: The effects of growth hormone and/or testosterone in healthy elderly men: A randomized controlled trial. J Clin Endocrinol Metab 91(2):477–484, 2006
26. Roder M, Schwartz R, Prigeon R, et al: Reduced pancreatic B cell compensation to the insulin resistance of aging: Impact on proinsulin and insulin levels. J Clin Endocrinol Metab 85(6):2275–2280, 2000
27. Dharia S, Slane A, Jian M, et al: Effects of aging on cytochrome b5 expression in the human adrenal gland. J Clin Endocrinol Metab 90(7):4357–4361, 2005
28. Morganti S, Ceda GP, Saccani M, et al: Thyroid disease in the elderly: Sex-related differences in clinical expression. J Endocrinol Invest 28(11 Suppl):101–104, 2005

29. Aspinall R, Andrew D: Thymic involution in aging. J Clin Immunol 20(4):250–256, 2000

30. Bigler ED, Neeley ES, Miller MJ, et al: Cerebral volume loss, cognitive deficit and neuropsychological performance: comparative measures of brain atrophy: I. Dementia. J Int Neuropsychol Soc 10(3):442–452, 2004

31. Jack CR Jr, Shiung MM, Weigand SD, et al: Brain atrophy rates predict subsequent clinical conversion in normal elderly and amnestic MCI. Neurology 65(8):1227–1231, 2005

32. Uekermann J, Channon S, Daum I: Humor processing, mentalizing, and executive function in normal aging. J Int Neuropsychol Soc 12(2):184–191, 2006

33. Folstein M, Folstein S, McHugh P: Mini-Mental State: A practical method for grading the cognitive state of patients for the clinician. J Psychiatr Res 12:189–198, 1975

34. Yesavage JA, Brink TL, Rose TL, et al: Development and validation of a Geriatric Screening Scale: A preliminary report. J Psychiatr Res 17(1):37–49, 1983

35. Hunt IM, Kapur N, Robinson J, et al: Suicide within 12 months of mental health service contact in different age and diagnostic groups: National Clinical Survey. Br J Psychiatry 188:135–142, 2006

36. Taylor DK, Bachuwa G, Evans J, Jackson-Johnson V: Assessing barriers to identification of elder abuse and neglect: A community wide survey of primary care physicians. J Natl Med Assoc 98(3):403–404, 2006

37. National Institute on Alcohol Abuse and Alcohol: The Physicians' Guide to Helping Patients with Alcohol Problems. NIH Publication No. 95-3769, 2004

38. Resnick B: Alcohol use in a continuing care retirement community. J Gerontol Nurs 29(10):22–29, 2003

Other Selected Readings

Adelman A: Hearing and visual impairment. In Adelman A, Daly M (eds): Geriatrics: 20 Common Problems. New York, McGraw-Hill, 2001

Black K, Osman H: Concerned about client decision-making capacity? Considerations for practice. Care Manag J 6(2):50–55, 2005

Coll P: Sleep disorder. In Adelman A, Daly M (eds): Geriatrics: 20 Common Problems. New York, McGraw-Hill, 2001

Dobbin KR, Strollo PJ: Obstructive sleep apnea: Recognition and management considerations for the aged patient. AACN Clin Issues 13(1):103–113, 2002

Durakovic Z, Misigoj-Durakovic M: Does chronological age reduce working ability? Coll Anthropol 30(1):213–219, 2006

Hall C: Special considerations for the geriatric patient. Crit Care Nurs Clin North Am 14(4):427–434, 2002

Harman SM, Blackman MR: Use of growth hormone for prevention or treatment of effects of aging. J Gerontol A Biol Sci Med Sci 59(7):652–658, 2004

Hart BD, Birkas J, Lachmann M, et al: Promoting positive outcomes for elderly persons in the hospital: Prevention and risk factor modification. AACN Clin Issues 13(1):22–22, 2002

Horner A, VanDemark M, Jensen GA: The challenge of assessing a patient with dementia and head injury. AACN Clin Issues 13(1):73–83, 2002

Juurlink DN, Mamdani MM, Kopp A, Redelmeier DA: The risk of suicide with selective serotonin reuptake inhibitors in the elderly. Am J Psychiatry 163(5):813–821, 2006

Mori H, Hirasawa H, Oda S, et al: Oral care reduces incidence of ventilator associated pneumonia in ICU populations. Intensive Care Med 32(2):230–236, 2006

Oyama H, Ono Y, Watanabe N, et al: Local community intervention through depression screening and group activity for elderly suicide prevention. Psychiatry Clin Neurosci 60(1):110–114, 2006

Pfister G, Weiskopf D, Lazuardi L, et al: Naive T cells in the elderly: Are they still there? Ann N Y Acad Sci 1067:152–157, 2006

Price R, Daly F, Pennington CR, McMurdo ME: Nutritional supplementation of very old people at hospital discharge increases muscle strength: A randomized controlled trial. Gerontology 51(3):179–185, 2005

Schretlen D, Pearlson G, Anthony J, et al: Elucidating the contributions of processing speed, executive ability, and frontal lobe volume to normal age-related differences in fluid intelligence. J Int Neuropsychol Soc 6(1):52–61, 2000

Vandeweerd C, Paveza GJ, Fulmer T: Abuse and neglect in older adults with Alzheimer's disease. Nurs Clin North Am 41(1):43–55, v–vi, 2006

Wallhagen MI, Pettengill E, Whiteside M: Sensory impairment in older adults: Part I: Hearing loss. Am J Nurs 106(10):40–48, 2006

Whiteside MM, Wallhagen MI, Pettengill E: Sensory impairment in older adults. Part 2: Vision loss. Am J Nurs 106(11):52–61, 2006

Wyatt CM, Kim MC, Winston JA: Therapy insight: How changes in renal function with increasing age affect cardiovascular drug prescribing. Nat Clin Pract Cardiovasc Med 3(2):102–109, 2006

The Postanesthesia Patient

Caleb Rogovin

13

Collaboration Between the Anesthesia Provider and Nurse
Moderate Sedation
Potential Problems in the Postanesthesia Patient
  Hypoxemia
  Hypoventilation
  Hypotension
  Hypertension
  Cardiac Dysrhythmias
  Hypothermia
  Hyperthermia
  Malignant Hyperthermia
  Nausea and Vomiting
  Postoperative Pain

Objectives

Based on the content in this chapter, the reader should be able to:

❶ Compare and contrast anesthetic options used for surgery and interventional procedures.

❷ Differentiate between anesthetic agents appropriate for the conscious patient and those appropriate for the unconscious patient.

❸ Describe nursing interventions and assessment strategies for the patient recovering from anesthesia.

❹ Summarize five potential problems encountered during the immediate postanesthetic period.

The time immediately after surgery, when the patient is taken to the postanesthesia care unit (PACU) or the intensive care unit (ICU), is the most crucial period in the patient's recovery from anesthesia. Most patients are taken to the PACU for close observation and care by a qualified PACU nurse. Others are taken directly to the ICU, where nurses must be competent in postanesthesia nursing care. Alterations in the patient's physiological condition that occur in the immediate postoperative period are the focus of this chapter.

The critical care nurse must have a basic understanding of anesthetic options available for use during the intraoperative phase. To help with this understanding, common clinical terminology related to the use of anesthesia is listed in Box 13-1.

• Collaboration Between the Anesthesia Provider and Nurse

The anesthesia provider interviews and examines the patient before surgery. From this preanesthetic examination, the anesthesia provider decides which options and techniques to use. The bases for these decisions are the patient's condition, age, surgi-cal and anesthetic history, and ongoing disease processes; the operation to be performed; and the position required for the procedure. The anesthesia provider's options range from maintaining a conscious state with the use of minimal, regional, or intravenous (IV) agents to inducing an unconscious state with the use of IV or inhalation agents. Whenever possible, the patient and family are part of the decision-making process. These options are illustrated in Table 13-1 and Figure 13-1.

What happens in the operating room may affect the patient's immediate postoperative care and overall recovery. To convey what has occurred in the operating suite, the anesthesia provider gives a detailed report to the nurse who is assuming postoperative care of the patient. Information given in the report is listed in Box 13-2.

While receiving the report from the anesthesia provider, the nurse must simultaneously assess the patient's condition and individualize the nursing plan of care. Initial assessment parameters reported by the anesthesia provider are the patient's vital signs (blood pressure, pulse, respiration, and temperature), pulse oximetry, and level of consciousness. Cardiac rhythm, hemodynamic parameters, and urine output, as well as estimated blood loss, are also indicated. Vital signs are monitored every 15 minutes or more often if the patient's condition warrants.

Box 13-1 • Clinical Terminology

Sedation: An induced state of quiet, calm, or sleep by means of a medication. The degree of sedation ranges from anxiolysis to anesthesia.

Minimal sedation: A state in which the patient responds normally to verbal stimuli. Impairment to cognition and coordination may exist.

Moderate sedation: A drug-induced depression of consciousness during which the patient responds purposefully to verbal commands either alone or in conjunction with tactile stimulation. There is some alteration of mood, drowsiness, and sometimes analgesia. The patient's protective reflexes remain intact.

Deep sedation: A drug-induced depression of consciousness during which the patient cannot be easily aroused but responds purposefully after repeated or painful stimulation. Spontaneous ventilation and the ability to maintain a patent airway may be impaired. The patient may require assistance in maintaining a patent airway.

General anesthesia: A drug-induced loss of consciousness during which a patient cannot be aroused, even by painful stimulation. The ability to independently maintain ventilatory function is often impaired. The patient may require assistance in maintaining a patent airway, and positive-pressure ventilation may be required. Cardiovascular function may be impaired.

Monitored anesthesia care (MAC): Describes a specific anesthesia service in which an anesthesia provider has been requested to participate in the care of a patient undergoing a therapeutic or diagnostic procedure. It does not describe a continuum of depth of sedation.

Regional anesthesia: This state of anesthesia produces analgesia in a specific body part. Regional anesthesia is achieved by placing local anesthetics close to appropriate nerves to achieve a conduction block.

Spinal anesthesia: In this type of anesthesia, local anesthetic is injected into the lumbar intrathecal space. The anesthetic blocks conduction in spinal nerve roots and dorsal ganglia. Analgesia occurs below the level of injection.

Epidural anesthesia: A local anesthetic is injected via a catheter into the epidural space. The effects are similar to spinal analgesia.

Peripheral nerve block: A local anesthetic is injected at a specific site to achieve a defined area of anesthesia.

Box 13-3 provides the collaborative care guidelines for the postanesthesia patient. The American Society of PeriAnesthesia Nurses, as endorsed by the American Society of Anesthesiologists and the American Association of Nurse Anesthetists, recommends that all assessment data be collected and documented on the patient's postoperative record.[1]

• Moderate Sedation

Moderate sedation is a technique that provides a drug-induced depression of consciousness during which the patient responds purposefully to verbal commands, either alone or associated with light tactile stimulation. No interventions are required to maintain airway patency or spontaneous ventilation. In addition, cardiovascular function is maintained. A patient under moderate sedation adheres to three major criteria: the ability to independently maintain a patent airway, retain protective airway reflexes, and respond to verbal and physical stimulation. If these three conditions are not met, then the patient is not receiving moderate sedation, and perhaps this is not the correct anesthetic choice for the patient or the procedure. The advantage of moderate sedation is that it allows the patient to respond to the verbal directives of the practitioner

Table 13-1 • Anesthetic Options for Surgical and Interventional Procedures

Conscious State	Sedated State	Unconscious State
Modalities		
Conscious sedation	MAC	Regional anesthesia
Monitored anesthesia care (MAC)	Local anesthesia	General anesthesia
Local anesthesia	Regional anesthesia	
Regional anesthesia		
Medications		
Local anesthetics	Local anesthetics	Local anesthetics
IV medications	IV medications	IV medications
		Inhalation anesthetics
		Muscle relaxants
Effect on Patient		
Patient cooperative	May follow commands	Unconscious
Follows commands	Usually maintains protective reflexes	Diminished or loss of protective reflexes
Maintains protective reflexes		Alterations in cardiopulmonary dynamics

IV, intravenous.

```
                                    GENERAL

                                    Inhalation
                                      Desflurane
              INTRAVENOUS              Isoflurane
                                       Nitrous oxide
                                       Sevoflurane
              Barbiturates          Muscle Relaxants
LOCAL           Methohexital        Depolarizing
ANESTHESIA      Thiopental            Succinylcholine
              Benzodiazepines       Nondepolarizing
Amides          Diazepam              Atracurium
 Bupivacaine    Lorazepam             Cisatracurium
 *EMLA          Midazolam             Pancuronium
 Etidocaine   Benzodiazepine          Rocuronium
 Lidocaine      Antagonist            Vecuronium
 Mepivacaine    Flumazenil
 Prilocaine   Nonbarbiturate
 Ropivacaine    Dexmedetomidine
Esters          Etomidate
 Chloroprocaine Ketamine
 Cocaine        Propofol
 Procaine     Narcotics
 Tetracaine     Alfentanil
                Fentanyl
                Hydromorphone
                Meperidine
                Morphine
                Remifentanil
                Sufentanil
              Narcotic Antagonist
                Naloxone
              **NSAID
                Ketorolac tromethamine
              Narcotic Agonists/
                Antagonists
                Buprenorphine
                Butorphanol
                Dezocine
                Pentazocine
                Nalbuphine
```

* EMLA, Eutectic mixture local anesthetics
** NSAID, Nonsteroidal anti-inflammatory drugs

Figure 13-1 • Medication choices for anesthetic options.

and to physical stimulation. Moderate sedation is used for certain ambulatory surgical, therapeutic, and diagnostic procedures. The regimen usually consists of an opiate, an amnestic, a sedative, and a local anesthetic.[2]

Scammon and colleagues developed the initial objectives for moderate sedation in 1985.[2] The main goal of moderate sedation is to decrease patient

---

Box 13-2 • Anesthesia Provider-to-Nurse Report: Information to Convey

Name of patient
Surgical procedure
Anesthetic options (agents and reversal agents used)
Estimated blood loss/fluid loss
Fluid/blood replacement
Vital signs—significant problems
Complications encountered (anesthetic or surgical)
Preoperative condition (e.g., diabetes, hypertension, allergies)
Considerations for immediate postoperative period (pain management, reversals, ventilator settings)
Language barrier

Ideally, the anesthesia provider should not leave the patient until the nurse is satisfied with the patient's airway and immediate condition.

---

anxiety associated with the proposed procedure. The least amount of medication to achieve sedation and comfort is the goal. In addition, moderate sedation alters the patient's mood and enhances cooperation, maintains stable vital signs, elevates the pain threshold, provides amnesia, and allows for rapid recovery.[2]

Several entities regulate standards for administration of moderate sedation. Individual State Boards of Nursing, the Joint Commission (formerly the Joint Commission on Accreditation of Healthcare Organizations [JCAHO]), and individual hospital and unit policies are available. Standards for planning and providing moderate sedation are available to practitioners and should be followed.[3]

A group of 14 nursing societies developed standards for the role of the registered nurse in managing patients receiving IV moderate sedation. These standards are published in Standards of Perianesthesia Nursing Practice[1] and include management and monitoring before, during, and after the procedure. Among the standards are the following skills required of the registered nurse who is managing the care of patients receiving IV moderate sedation:

▶ Demonstrate the required knowledge of anatomy, physiology, pharmacology, cardiac dysrhythmia recognition, and complications related to IV conscious sedation and medications.

▶ Assess total patient care requirements during moderate sedation and recovery. Physiological measurements should include, but are not limited to, respiratory rate and effort, oxygen saturation, blood pressure, cardiac rate and rhythm, and patient's level of consciousness.

▶ Understand the principles of oxygen delivery, respiratory physiology, transport, and uptake, and demonstrate the ability to use oxygen delivery devices.

▶ Anticipate and recognize potential complications of IV moderate sedation in relation to the type of medication being administered.

▶ Possess the requisite knowledge and skills to assess, diagnose, and intervene in the event of complications or undesired outcomes and to institute nursing interventions in compliance with orders (including standard orders) or institutional protocols or guidelines.

▶ Demonstrate skills in airway management.

▶ Demonstrate knowledge of the legal ramifications of administering IV moderate sedation or monitoring patients receiving IV moderate sedation, including the registered nurse's responsibility and liability in the event of an untoward reaction or life-threatening complication.

Monitored anesthesia care (MAC) describes a specific anesthesia service in which the anesthesia provider has been requested to participate in the care of a patient undergoing a therapeutic or diagnostic procedure. The main difference between moderate sedation and MAC is that the anesthesia provider deviates from the major goal of having the patient maintain his or her own airway and follow commands.

Box 13-3 • COLLABORATIVE CARE GUIDE for the Postanesthesia Patient

OUTCOMES	INTERVENTIONS
Oxygenation/Ventilation Depth and rate of respiration after extubation will be at baseline. Arterial blood gases are within preoperative normal values. Airway will be maintained with intact protective reflexes. There will be no evidence of aspiration.	• Monitor respiratory rate and breathing pattern every 15 min and PRN. • Assess weaning parameters before extubation. • Monitor end-tidal CO_2 and pulse oximetry of mechanically ventilated patients. • Encourage patient to cough and deep-breathe. • Elevate head of bed if not contraindicated. • Use jaw thrust, head tilt, or oral, oropharyngeal, or nasopharyngeal airway to maintain airway. • Stimulate patient every few minutes (e.g., call name, touch). • Administer antiemetic as indicated. • Position patient on side; suction and maintain airway if patient is vomiting.
Circulation/Perfusion Heart rate and blood pressure will return to preoperative values within 1–2 h after anesthesia. Body temperature will be within normal limits. There will be no evidence of malignant hyperthermia.	• Monitor vital signs every 15 min and PRN. • Assess pulse quality and regularity. • Monitor for dysrhythmias. • Monitor for hypotension related to bleeding. • Monitor for hypotension related to warming and vasodilation. • Administer IV solution and blood products as ordered. • Anticipate hypothermia; have warming devices readily available. • Measure temperature on admission and PRN until normal. • Warm patient at 1° to 2°C/h. • Monitor for malignant hyperthermia, and immediately notify anesthesia provider of temperature increase of 0.5°C. • Administer dantrolene, and initiate cooling measures. • Assist with malignant hyperthermia protocol.
Fluids/Electrolytes Patient will have stable blood pressure and heart rate. Urine output will be 0.5–2 mL/kg/h. There will be no evidence of hypervolemia or hypovolemia.	• Maintain patient IV. • Monitor intake and output. • Assess skin, mucous membranes for signs of hypovolemia. • Measure specific gravity if indicated. • Assess for signs of hypervolemia (e.g., pulmonary crackles, neck vein distention). • Measure serum electrolytes if indicated.
Mobility/Safety Patient will arouse easily and respond appropriately to commands. Patient will move all extremities purposefully and with normal strength.	• Assess level of consciousness every 15 min and PRN. • Monitor motor and sensory function to assess reversal of neuromuscular blockade. • Assess level of regional block, epidural, or spinal anesthesia.
Skin Integrity Skin will remain intact.	• Assess skin immediately postoperatively for pressure areas and burns.
Nutrition Nutritional intake will be reestablished without nausea or vomiting.	• Resume enteral feeding with return of bowel sounds. • Begin oral fluids with return of protective airway reflexes.
Comfort/Pain Control Pain will be less than 4 on pain scale or visual analog.	• Assess location, type, and severity of pain. • Administer opioids as indicated. • Monitor response to analgesics. • Institute nonpharmacological pain relief strategies and comfort measures. • Evaluate patient-controlled analgesia IV or epidural as postoperative pain management option.

(continued)

Box 13-3 • COLLABORATIVE CARE GUIDE for the Postanesthesia Patient (Continued)

OUTCOMES	INTERVENTIONS
Psychosocial Personal support systems will be used to reduce anxiety.	• Encourage significant other visits in early postoperative phase. • Validate patient's significant other's understanding of surgery and illness. • Initiate referrals to social services, clergy, and so forth.
Teaching/Discharge Planning Discharge from postanesthesia care phase will occur within 1–2 h. Exercises to prevent postoperative pulmonary complications will be demonstrated. Patient or significant other will state understanding of surgical procedure and outcome of surgery.	• Orient patient frequently. • Explain procedures and pain management treatment plan. • Teach coughing, deep breathing, incentive spirometer use. • Teach early mobilization. • Teach pain control strategies. • Provide information regarding the procedure, and discuss probable outcomes.

To facilitate the surgical/diagnostic procedure and experience, the patient may be rendered unconscious or apneic for a period of time. IV agents are used in conjunction with local anesthetics that are injected by the surgeon. Postoperative or postprocedural care of the patient who has received moderate sedation or MAC is similar, although the patient who has received MAC may require more intervention in the postanesthesia phase. Table 13-2 provides a comparison of moderate sedation and MAC.

• Potential Problems in the Postanesthesia Patient

There are common potential problems in the post-anesthesia patient for which the nurse must assess. They are discussed in the following sections. The initial focus on the postanesthesia care patient centers around assessment and management of cardiopulmonary parameters. While assessing and implementing interventions for the postanesthetic patient, the nurse uses the "stir-up" regimen. This regimen involves encouraging the patient to deep-breathe, cough, and move in bed, as allowed by the procedure or intervention. In addition, the nurse assesses pain levels and implements appropriate interventions to assist the patient in actively participating in the stir-up regimen. Because this routine is an integral part in recovery from anesthesia, the nurse should use it every time he or she checks a patient's vital signs. This technique also allows the nurse to identify subtle changes in the patient's condition and to intervene appropriately.

HYPOXEMIA

Hypoxemia is a common occurrence in the immediate postoperative period. Severe hypoxemia is characterized by a partial pressure of arterial oxygen (PaO_2) of less than 50 mm Hg and is life-threatening. Hypoventilation leads to hypoxia, which is difficult to diagnose because of its multiple presentations. Clinical manifestations of hypoxia may include hypotension or hypertension, tachycardia or bradycardia, cardiac dysrhythmias, dyspnea, tachypnea, hypoventilation, disorientation, agitation, decreased partial pressure of arterial carbon dioxide ($PaCO_2$), and cyanosis.

When investigating the etiology of hypoxemia related to anesthetic agents, the nurse considers the effects of a spinal or epidural block that has traveled too high, opioid use, deep sedation, use of inhalation agents, and the use of neuromuscular blocking agents, particularly if they have not been adequately reversed. Diffusion hypoxia may occur when nitrous oxide is used, but because administering 100% oxygen for 3 to 4 minutes after the nitrous oxide is discontinued may prevent this complication, diffusion hypoxemia usually is not seen in the PACU patient.

Table 13-2 • Comparison of Moderate Sedation and Monitored Anesthesia Care

	Moderate Sedation	Monitored Anesthesia Care (MAC)
Responsiveness	Purposeful response to repeated or painful verbal or tactile stimulation	May have purposeful response after stimulation
Airway	No intervention required	Intervention may be required
Spontaneous ventilation	Adequate	May be inadequate
Cardiovascular function	Usually maintained	Usually maintained

Most patients who receive a general anesthetic or sedation should receive supplemental oxygen in the immediate postoperative period. The oxygen may be weaned subsequently using pulse oximetry. Because pulse oximetry offers a noninvasive method of continuously monitoring oxygen saturation, increasing numbers of patients are receiving supplemental oxygen for 24 hours after surgery.

Reversal agents may be required while the patient is still under the effects of muscle relaxants, benzodiazepines, and opioids. Close monitoring is always indicated when reversal agents are administered. The effects of muscle relaxants (Box 13-4), benzodiazepines, and opioids may last longer than the reversal agent, resulting in hypoventilation and hypoxia at some point after the reversal agent is administered. It is important that the nurse be knowledgeable about the onset and duration of action of reversal agents as well as the drugs they are being used to reverse. This knowledge allows for appropriate intervention in the event of a change in the patient's condition.[4]

HYPOVENTILATION

Hypoventilation leading to hypercarbia may result from the following:

▶ Inadequate respiratory drive secondary to the effects of residual anesthesia (i.e., opioids, sedatives, and inhalation agents)

▶ Inadequate functioning of the respiratory muscles (the lungs may be unable to move an adequate tidal volume because of pain or inadequate reversal of neuromuscular blockade)

▶ Intrinsic lung disease, which often requires postoperative ventilatory support of the patient (e.g., chronic obstructive pulmonary disease)

▶ Laryngospasm and obstruction of the airway, which must be identified and treated promptly (Box 13-5)

The nurse institutes the stir-up regimen in the immediate postoperative phase to stimulate the patient, especially if opioids and sedatives were used during surgery. Also, the nurse considers the length of time since reversal agents were administered to antagonize neuromuscular blockade. The patient may not be fully reversed and exhibit signs of residual neuromuscular blockade. Inadequate respiratory

---

Box 13-4 • Muscle Relaxants

Depolarizing Agent
Succinylcholine (Anectine)

Nondepolarizing Agents
Atracurium (Tracrium)
Cisatracurium (Nimbex)
Pancuronium (Pavulon)
Rocuronium (Zemuron)
Vecuronium (Norcuron)

Box 13-5 • Managing Laryngospasm and Airway Obstruction

Laryngospasm
Laryngospasm is a spasm of the laryngeal musculature. The spasm is often caused by blood, mucus, or other oral secretions that irritate the vocal cords. Careful suctioning of the oropharynx before extubation helps to prevent spasm. In most cases, laryngospasm will break with the application of positive pressure with 100% fraction of inspired oxygen (FiO_2) via a bag-valve mask with a tight seal. If this does not break the spasm, a dose of depolarizing muscle relaxant (succinylcholine) may be given.

Upper Airway Obstruction
Upper airway obstruction must be identified and treated promptly and effectively. Airway obstruction may range from minimal to complete. Signs of obstruction include:

• Paradoxical breathing
• Stridor
• Lack of, or change in, breath sounds
• Alteration in vital signs
• Change in level of consciousness

Treatment to relieve obstruction must be provided in a systematic fashion.

1. Tilt head/lift chin.
2. Thrust jaw.
3. Call for assistance.
4. Insert an oropharyngeal or nasopharyngeal airway. (Bear in mind that an oropharyngeal airway may not be tolerated by the partially obtunded patient.)
5. Apply positive-pressure ventilation.
6. Administer succinylcholine.

---

effort, inability to maintain a head lift for 5 seconds, inappropriate use of chest and abdominal wall muscles, air hunger, anxiety, and tachycardia are signs that may indicate residual paralysis.[4] Neuromuscular blocking agents are summarized in Box 13-6. Hypothermia may prolong neuromuscular blockade associated with nondepolarizing muscle relaxants; therefore, the patient's temperature must be monitored. Other conditions that increase the effects of nondepolarizing muscle relaxants are listed in Box 13-7.

HYPOTENSION

Probably the most common cardiovascular complication seen in the postoperative period is hypotension. It is most often caused by a decreased circulating blood volume. Hypotension is defined as a 25% to 30% decrease in systolic blood pressure from the resting baseline value. Intervention is indicated if the pressure decreases by more than 30% of the baseline value.[5] Risk factors for postanesthesia hypotension are listed in Box 13-8.

Anesthetic agents may affect the blood pressure in various ways. Regional anesthetics, such as bupivacaine and tetracaine, may decrease blood pressure by sympathetic blockade and vasodilation. IV agents,

Box 13-6 • Neuromuscular Blocking Agents

Muscle Relaxants

- Neuromuscular blockers pharmacologically paralyze patients and provide no sedation or analgesia.
- Neuromuscular blocking agents are used to facilitate endotracheal intubation, relax muscles for surgical procedures, terminate laryngospasm, eliminate chest wall rigidity, and provide for ease of mechanical ventilation if indicated.
- There are two groups of muscle relaxants, depolarizing and nondepolarizing, that work at the myoneural junction, affecting the chemical transmitter acetylcholine.

Depolarizing Agent (succinylcholine)

- This drug combines with acetylcholine receptors at the myoneural junction and mimics the action of acetylcholine.
- Onset of action is 1–2 min and duration of action is 4–6 min.
- The enzyme pseudocholinesterase removes succinylcholine from plasma, so in conditions involving a decrease in pseudocholinesterase, the length of action of succinylcholine increases, keeping patients paralyzed for longer periods.
- Increased pseudocholinesterase enzyme may be seen in pregnancy, liver disease, malnutrition states, severe anemia, cancer, and with other pharmacological agents, such as quinidine, phospholine eye drops, and propranolol.

Nondepolarizing Agents

- Nondepolarizing agents (atracurium, cisatracurium, mivacurium, pipecuronium, vecuronium, pancuronium, doxacurium, rocuronium) compete with acetylcholine at the myoneural junction for muscle membrane receptors.
- Onset of action is within 2–3 min, depending on dose.
- Duration of action ranges from 20 min to 2 h, depending on the medication and dosage.
- May be reversed pharmacologically with anticholinesterase drugs (neostigmine, pyridostigmine, edrophonium). Duration of action of anticholinesterase is brief, so there is a chance the patient may have continued muscle weakness or respiratory depression. Anticholinesterases may induce muscarinic side effects, including bradycardia, lacrimation, defecation, and increased salivary and bronchial secretions. These side effects are counteracted with the routine administration of anticholinergic drugs (atropine, glycopyrrolate) in conjunction with the anticholinesterase.

Box 13-7 • Conditions and Medications That Increase the Effects of Nondepolarizing Muscle Relaxants

Local anesthetics
General anesthetics
Antibiotics: aminoglycosides, polypeptides, polymyxin
Antiarrhythmics: quinidine, procainamide
Furosemide
Acid–base status: respiratory acidosis, metabolic alkalosis
Electrolyte imbalance: hypokalemia, hypocalcemia, dehydration, magnesium administration
Hypothermia

Box 13-8 • RED FLAG: Risk Factors for Postanesthesia Hypotension

Anesthetic Agents

- Regional agents
- Opioids
- Tranquilizers
- Barbiturates
- Muscle relaxants
- Inhalation agents

Decreased Venous Return

- Hypovolemia (inadequate replacement, continued blood loss)
- Hypothermia
- Myocardial depression
- Third spacing
- Sepsis
- Transfusion reaction
- Tight abdominal dressing
- Increased intrathoracic pressure

Cardiac

- Dysrhythmias (supraventricular tachycardia)
- Myocardial infarction
- Congestive heart failure

Pulmonary

- Hypoxia
- Acidosis
- Pulmonary embolism
- Pneumothorax

Vasovagal Reactions

- Bradycardia
- Pain
- Bladder/abdominal distention

Technical Problems

- Blood pressure cuff size and position
- Transducer balance and calibration
- Stethoscope position

including opioids, cause vasodilation and histamine release, resulting in lowered blood pressure. Tranquilizers, especially droperidol and chlorpromazine hydrochloride, produce sympathetic blockade and subsequent decreased blood pressure. Barbiturates cause myocardial depression, as do inhalation agents such as isoflurane, enflurane, halothane, sevoflurane, and desflurane. Muscle relaxants may cause hypotension by ganglionic blockade and histamine release.

Because decreased venous return is seen with hypovolemia and myocardial depression, the nurse considers the adequacy of volume replacement, blood loss, third spacing, and excessive diuresis. The nurse evaluates the patient for orthostatic hypotension by taking vital signs with the patient supine and after raising the head of the bed 60 degrees (if not contraindicated by the surgical procedure or patient status). Cardiac dysrhythmias may cause hypotension, especially when cardiac output is decreased, as it is with supraventricular tachycardia and marked bradycardia. Other causes of early postoperative hypotension include sepsis, pulmonary embolism, and transfusion reaction.

Deliberate, controlled hypotensive anesthetic techniques are often used during specific procedures, such as neurosurgical procedures of the head and neck, shoulder arthroscopy, and some oncologic operations. The advantages of this technique are that it minimizes blood loss and the need for transfusion and decreases oozing and possible hematoma formation.

Treatment of hypotension is directed to the underlying cause. A complete report from the anesthesia provider, including the techniques used during surgery and any untoward events that occurred, helps the nurse identify the underlying cause.

Various interventions may be used to treat hypotension. A priority is to ensure adequate oxygenation and ventilation of the patient while the blood pressure is being addressed. Anesthetic drugs may require reversal, including muscle relaxant reversal with anticholinesterase and anticholinergic agents, opioid reversal with naloxone, and benzodiazepine reversal with flumazenil. The nurse may administer vasopressive agents, IV fluids, blood products, plasma expanders, and crystalloids to increase blood pressure. It is necessary to inspect dressings, drains, and surgical sites frequently for signs of hemorrhage.

An important consideration when assessing and treating the patient with hypotension is the possibility of technical rather than physiological problems. Is the blood pressure cuff the correct size, and is it positioned correctly? Is the stethoscope positioned correctly? Is the patient's position a factor? If an arterial line is present, is the patient peripherally constricted, or does peripheral vascular disease exist? Is the transducer balanced and correctly calibrated? Trouble-shooting should occur simultaneously with assessment.

HYPERTENSION

Hypertension is classified according to its degree of severity. It ranges from mild with a diastolic pressure between 90 and 104 mm Hg, to severe with a diastolic pressure between 105 and 120 mm Hg, to malignant with a diastolic pressure greater than 120 mm Hg.

The two most common causes of postoperative hypertension are a history of hypertension and pain. Hypertension may be associated with peripheral vasoconstriction and shivering. Inhalation and IV anesthetic agents may produce hypoxia and hypercarbia with a resultant increase in catecholamine release and blood pressure elevation. Ketamine, a nonbarbiturate drug, which is used as a dissociative anesthetic, stimulates the sympathetic nervous system and may cause tachycardia and hypertension. Also, if given too rapidly, naloxone may precipitate hypertension, which in turn may precipitate pulmonary edema or cerebral hemorrhage. Other causes of hypertension include hyperthermia, anxiety, urinary bladder distention, fluid overload, pain, a too-narrow blood pressure cuff, and withholding of antihypertensive therapy before surgery.

Transient hypertension may occur during induction, intubation, or positioning, when the surgical incision is made, or during postanesthesia. A vigilant anesthesia practitioner may avoid transient hypertension. Unless instructed otherwise, patients should take their antihypertensive medication up to the time of the surgical procedure.

Hypertensive patients require reassurance, close observation, and aggressive postoperative treatment. The treatment is first directed to the cause of the hypertension, if known. If the hypertension is severe, it may be necessary to order antihypertensive medications, such as short-acting peripheral vasodilators (e.g., hydralazine, nifedipine), labetalol or metoprolol, or β-adrenergic blocking agents. Continuous vasodilator drips of sodium nitroprusside or nitroglycerin bring the blood pressure within safe limits and maintain it. When hypertension accompanies emergence delirium, opioids or physostigmine, an anticholinesterase, may be required. If the patient is hypertensive because of anxiety and verbal reassurance is ineffective, benzodiazepines, such as diazepam, midazolam, and lorazepam, may be necessary. Urinary catheterization and aggressive treatment with diuretics such as furosemide may be indicated if the hypertension is a result of fluid overload during surgery.

CARDIAC DYSRHYTHMIAS

The dysrhythmias covered in this chapter are those induced by anesthetic agents and complications frequently seen in the immediate postoperative period (Table 13-3). Refer to Chapter 17 for detailed information on identifying specific cardiac dysrhythmias. Some of the most common causes of cardiac dysrhythmias in the immediate postoperative period are residual anesthetic agents, anticholinesterase drugs, electrolyte imbalances, hypoxemia, hypoventilation, hypovolemia, fluid overload, hyperthermia, hypothermia, and pain (Box 13-9).

HYPOTHERMIA

Hypothermia is present when the body temperature is less than 35°C (95°F). Heat loss during surgery occurs secondary to reduced basal metabolism when patients given muscle relaxants fail to shiver. Also, vasodilation caused by inhalation anesthetic agents, related to sympathetic blockade with inhibition of motor and sensory nerve fibers, and resulting when regional techniques are used, is a factor in hypothermia. Other intraoperative causes include heat loss through radiation, exposure, convection, and conduction because of prolonged exposure of body surface; lying under saturated drapes (especially in long procedures); use of antiseptic prepping solutions; and use of cold irrigation or IV solutions. Older, debilitated patients and newborns are more intolerant of temperature changes and thus more prone to hypothermia. Hats and other warming devices, such as fluid warmers and warming blankets, may prevent hypothermia.

Table 13-3 • Cardiac Dysrhythmias Associated With Anesthetic Options

Anesthetic Option	Dysrhythmia
Local anesthesia with epinephrine	Tachycardia
Spinal and epidural	Bradycardia secondary to vagal response; PACs, PVCs, supraventricular tachycardia, atrial fibrillation second-degree sympathetic stimulation; wandering pacemaker and heart block secondary to increased vagal tone
Barbiturates	
Pentothal	Bradycardia, AV dissociation, occasional PVCs
Nonbarbiturate etomidate	Sinus tachycardia
Opioids	
Morphine sulfate	Transient brachycardia
Meperidine hydrochloride	Transient tachycardia
Fentanyl	Bradycardia
Opioid antagonist	PVCs, ventricular tachycardia, occasional ventricular fibrillation
Neuroleptanalgesia (droperidol component)	Tachycardia
Dissociative agent	Myocardial depression, ventricular ectopy, tachycardia
Inhalation agents	
Halothane	AV dissociation, ventricular dysrhythmias if hypercarbia occurs
Halothane plus aminophylline, cocaine, lidocaine	Bradycardia
Halothane plus pancuronium	PACs and PVCs
Isoflurane	Tachycardia
Enflurane	AV dissociation
Muscle relaxants	
Succinylcholine	Sinus bradycardia, junctional rhythms, PVCs. Patients with burns, trauma, paraplegia or quadriplegia prone to ST-segment depression, peaked T waves, widening QRS complex leading to ventricular tachycardia, ventricular fibrillation, or asystole
Pipecuronium bromide	Atrial fibrillation, ventricular extrasystole
Pancuronium	Tachycardia and nodal rhythms
d-Tubocurarine	Tachycardia
Anticholinesterases	Bradycardia, slowed AV conduction, PVCs
Anticholinergics	Tachycardia

AV, atrioventricular; PAC, premature atrial contraction; PVC, premature ventricular contraction.

Box 13-9 • RED FLAG: Risk Factors That Precipitate Dysrhythmias

- Hypoxemia (sinus bradycardia, sinus tachycardia, PVCs, supraventricular tachycardia)
- Hypoventilation/hypercarbia (sinus tachycardia, PVCs, sinus bradycardia)
- Hypovolemia (sinus tachycardia)
- Fluid overload (PVCs, supraventricular tachycardia, PACs, atrial fibrillation/flutter)
- Hyperthermia (sinus tachycardia, PVCs)
- Hypothermia (sinus bradycardia, atrial fibrillation, atrioventricular nodal blocks)
- Pain (sinus tachycardia, PVCs)

PVCs, premature ventricular contractions; PACs, premature atrial contractions.

Hypothermia, with its associated vasoconstriction and initial increase in blood pressure, requires special attention in the postoperative phase. Care must be taken in rewarming because too rapid rewarming of the patient may result in an acute drop in blood pressure and other significant problems.

HYPERTHERMIA

Hyperthermia is a body temperature greater than 39°C (102.2°F). Elevated temperature may occur in the anesthetized patient secondary to thermal insulation from the surgical drapes and the administration of inhalation anesthetics. Anticholinergic drugs may also induce a pharmacological loss of thermoregulatory capacity. Most patients with an elevated temperature either arrive in the surgical suite with a fever or have a pyrogenic response from septicemia. Other possible causes of post-operative hyperthermia are allergic reactions to blood or drugs, central nervous system disorders, and infection.

Treatment of hyperthermia may include ceasing all therapies that elevate temperature, decreasing ambient room temperature (keeping in mind that direct application of cold air may precipitate shivering, which should be avoided), and using minimal layering of linen.

MALIGNANT HYPERTHERMIA

One of the most catastrophic events that can occur in the immediate postoperative period is malignant hyperthermia, a hypermetabolic syndrome. Although most cases of malignant hyperthermia occur in the operating room during the administration of a general anesthetic, the immediate 12-hour period after general anesthesia is also a critical time. Malignant hyperthermia may be triggered in susceptible individuals by commonly used anesthetic agents, including succinylcholine and the halogenated inhalation agents. Other anesthetic agents, including nitrous oxide, local anesthetics, opioids, propofol, sodium thiopental, and the nondepolarizing muscle relaxants are safe to use.

The exact mechanism of malignant hyperthermia is not well understood. Research points to a derangement in muscle contraction. The known triggering agents cause a release of calcium from muscle storage sites, leading to an elevated concentration of calcium. This high calcium level increases metabolism and causes muscle to contract and become rigid (masseter muscle rigidity). This process results in hyperthermia, acid–base imbalance, and muscle cell breakdown.

Malignant hyperthermia is a rare, inherited autosomal dominant disorder of skeletal muscle and is more prevalent in people with muscular abnormalities. Malignant hyperthermia has been linked to several other muscle disorders, including some forms of muscular dystrophy, but whether this is true malignant hyperthermia is not clear. Most experts on malignant hyperthermia do not believe that caffeine or stress precipitates malignant hyperthermia. The exact incidence of malignant hyperthermia is not known. The rate of occurrence has been estimated to be between 1 in 5,000 and as rare as 1 in 65,000. The states with the highest incidence are Michigan, West Virginia, and Wisconsin.[6]

Clinical manifestations include an increase in temperature of 0.5°C or more every 15 minutes from the time of induction of anesthesia to as high as 46°C, muscle rigidity, hypercarbia, unexplained tachycardia, sweating, and unstable blood pressure. Masseter muscle rigidity after the administration of succinylcholine is the earliest warning sign of malignant hyperthermia. Temperature elevation is quite dramatic but is not the first sign of malignant hyperthermia. If the patient's temperature increases rapidly and the anesthetic is not discontinued and treatment rapidly instituted, death may occur.

Malignant hyperthermia is treated vigorously with dantrolene sodium (Dantrium), 100% oxygen administration, correction of acid–base imbalances, and removal of triggering agents. Cooling measures, such as use of a cooling blanket, administration of cool IV fluids, and instillation of cool fluids through a nasogastric tube and Foley catheter, are used. Dantrolene sodium, 2.5 mg/kg IV, is given and may be repeated up to 10 mg/kg as necessary to control signs and symptoms. Dantrolene sodium is reconstituted with preservative-free sterile water. The administration of dantrolene is labor intensive, thus requiring assistance. Most institutions that administer anesthesia have a malignant hyperthermia kit in the operating suite. Box 13-10 lists the common contents of a malignant hyperthermia kit.

After the acute phase of the malignant hyperthermia crisis, care includes observation in a critical care unit for at least 24 hours and administration of dantrolene sodium, 1 mg/kg every 6 hours for 24 to 48 hours. Oral dantrolene may then be used with monitoring of arterial blood gases, creatinine kinase, potassium, calcium, urine, serum myoglobin, and clotting studies every 6 hours. Patients should be referred to the Malignant Hyperthermia Association of the United States (MHAUS) for support and continued education about this disorder.[6,7]

NAUSEA AND VOMITING

Nausea and vomiting occur frequently in the immediate postoperative period and may result from any of the anesthetic options. Nausea is a subjective, unpleasant experience usually leading to vomiting. Although not usually life-threatening, postoperative nausea and vomiting (PONV) leaves the patient with a lasting unpleasant memory and may have an impact on future surgical and anesthetic decisions. PONV is a major complication associated with the need for

---

Box 13-10 • Contents of Malignant Hyperthermia Kit

- Methylprednisolone
- Furosemide
- Sodium bicarbonate
- Dextrose (50%)
- Sterile water
- Insulin
- Mannitol
- Refrigerated intravenous fluids
- Dantrolene sodium
- New oxygen tubing and delivery devices
- Foley catheter tray
- Nasogastric tubes
- Blood specimen tubes
- Arterial blood gas kits
- MHAUS guidelines and contact information booklet

MHAUS, Malignant Hyperthermia Society of the United States.

admission after outpatient surgery. Frequent causes include use of preoperative and intraoperative opioids; increased gastric secretions; certain anesthetic techniques, particularly spinal anesthesia; and surgical procedures involving manipulation of eye muscles, abdominal muscles, and genitourinary muscles. Laparoscopic techniques and procedures involving the breast are also associated with an increase in postoperative nausea and vomiting.

Vomiting is controlled by the vomiting center located in the medulla. Once stimulated, efferent impulses are sent by the 5th, 7th, 9th, 10th, and 12th cranial nerves, spinal nerves, and phrenic nerves to the diaphragm, esophagus, and stomach. The vomiting center receives input directly from the gastrointestinal tract, the chemoreceptor trigger zone, the labyrinthine apparatus (motion sickness), and various cortical and visual stimuli.

The critical care nurse must be cognizant of the potential for regurgitation and aspiration in all patients who have been anesthetized. Vomiting is an active process, whereas regurgitation is passive. Adequate positioning of the unconscious patient is essential. The ideal position is on the side with the head and neck extended. If the surgical procedure precludes turning the patient on the side or the patient is unable to comply, then the patient must not be left unattended until consciousness is regained.

Antiemetics frequently are ordered in the immediate postoperative period. The critical care nurse should recognize that many antiemetics potentiate the effects of other medications, particularly opioids. Therefore, decreased doses of opioids for pain relief may be indicated.

Often, nausea and vomiting can be relieved by identifying the causative factor (e.g., gastric distention, hypotension, administration of opioids) and making the appropriate intervention.

POSTOPERATIVE PAIN

Patients normally expect to feel pain when their surgical procedure is over. The incidence of pain and its severity depend on the individual. All pain assessment in the immediate postoperative period must be individualized. A number of factors affect the severity of pain, including the site of the operation, the psychological state of the patient, and the anesthetic technique used.

If the anesthetic option chosen was use of inhalation agents without the use of opioids or local anesthetics, then the patient may have more pain than one who received some form of analgesia during surgery. Patients who have been given analgesic medication during the procedure and who then receive naloxone at the end may also experience severe pain because naloxone reverses the analgesic effects of any prior medication. Because these patients may renarcotize, the nurse must wait 15 to 45 minutes after the administration of naloxone before medicating the patient with an analgesic. Box 13-11 outlines some factors that may influence the patient's response to pain.

Box 13-11 • Factors Influencing Pain

Surgical procedure: site and nature of the operation
Anxiety level: fear of surgery, disfigurement, death, loss of control, previous experiences
Patient expectations: effectiveness of preoperative teaching, adequately prepared for outcome
Pain tolerance: prior use of medications, including analgesics, individual differences
Anesthesia technique: analgesics used during the intraoperative period, use of naloxone

Intravenous Medications

IV titration of opioids in the immediate postoperative period offers the quickest and most effective method of pain relief. Because the patient's basal metabolic rate is decreased during surgery, the uptake of intramuscular medication is difficult to predict.

Intramuscular Medications

One intramuscular medication, ketorolac tromethamine (Toradol), administered during surgery, has proved effective in the management of postoperative pain. Ketorolac tromethamine is a nonsteroidal antiinflammatory drug that exhibits analgesic, antiinflammatory, and antipyretic activity. Peak analgesia occurs in 45 to 60 minutes after intramuscular or IV injection, and the analgesic effect lasts 6 to 8 hours. The medication should not be used for more than 5 days, and no more than a 30-mg dose should be used. The medication is contraindicated in patients with active peptic ulcers, recent gastrointestinal bleeds, or renal insufficiency.[4]

Patient-Controlled Analgesia and Epidural Medications

Trends in pain control management include use of patient-controlled analgesia (PCA) devices and epidural analgesia. The use of PCA pumps has increased significantly during recent years, and it is believed that patients report less pain when they maintain autonomy by controlling the administration of opioids for their pain relief.

Epidural analgesia has proved successful in treating acute pain after surgery. Patients who receive epidural opioids are less sedated and therefore ambulate sooner and have improved respiratory function. Epidural medications may be administered as a bolus injection or by a continuous infusion. When administering continuous infusions, an infusion pump should be used. Safeguards to be taken include using preservative-free medications in the epidural infusion; using infusion sets that have no injection ports; and labeling the infusing pump, infusion bag, and infusion tubing with the word epidural. The reason for such safeguards is that accidental infusion of vasodilators, chemotherapy medications, antibiotics, and medications with any type of preservative could permanently destroy nerve tissue and paralyze or even kill the patient.

Frequently used preservative-free epidural medications include morphine, hydromorphone, meperidine, and fentanyl. The duration of sensory analgesia varies with the opioid administered. The more lipid-soluble agents penetrate the dura mater more rapidly, resulting in a more rapid diffusion away from the spinal cord and subarachnoid space and hence a shorter duration of action. The most frequently used opioids for epidural administration for which average duration times have been identified are morphine, with a duration that varies from 2 to 24 hours; hydromorphone, with an average duration of 10 to 14 hours; meperidine, with an average duration of 6 to 8 hours; and fentanyl, with an average duration of 4 to 6 hours.

Dilute local anesthetic solutions are used either in conjunction with the previously mentioned opioids or alone. Local anesthetics used alone and in conjunction with narcotics are lidocaine, mepivacaine, prilocaine, bupivacaine, and etidocaine. The most common local anesthesic used for epidural infusions is bupivacaine. The combination of local anesthetics and opioids has been used to obtain a rapid onset and prolonged duration of analgesia. The local agents work more rapidly, and the opioids have a more prolonged action. Side effects may occur with the use of opioids and anesthetic solutions in the epidural space. Nurses have the primary responsibility of recognizing and preventing side effects when caring for patients receiving epidural analgesia, as listed in Box 13-12. Adequate pain relief during the postoperative period allows the patient to cough, deep-breathe, and ambulate sooner, thus preventing complications.

Other Medication Methods

Other techniques investigated as alternatives in pain management include intrathecal and interpleural methods, transdermal patches, and transmucosal–nasal aerosol delivery systems. Intrathecal analgesia is injected, usually as a one-time dose, directly into the cerebrospinal fluid of the subarachnoid space.[7] Interpleural techniques involve administration of local anesthetics into the interpleural space. A series of injections are given, or a catheter is placed during the perioperative period, or occasionally after surgery. Continuous infusions and bolus injections may be given.

Transdermal patches of fentanyl are being used, as are transmucosal–nasal aerosol delivery systems.[1–3] Transdermal fentanyl is an excellent alternative to sustained-release morphine preparations, especially when oral medication is not possible or is contraindicated. Patches are constructed as a drug reservoir separated from the skin by a microporous rate-limiting membrane and adhesive polymer. The major disadvantages to the transdermal patches are the slow onset and the inability to change dosages rapidly in response to changing opioid requirements.

Box 13-12 • Side Effects From Epidural Analgesia

Specific protocols for epidural management are essential for each individual hospital.

Urinary retention
- Catheterize as needed.

Postural hypotension
- Give fluid (volume) replacement.
- Administer ephedrine 5 mg IV as ordered.

Pruritus (itching of face, head, and neck)
- Treat with Benadryl 25 mg PO, IM, IV.
- Treat with naloxone 0.1 mg IV.
- Treat with propofol 10 mg IV.

Nausea and vomiting
- Administer metoclopramide 10 mg IV.
- Administer scopolamine patch.
- Administer a 5HT-3 antagonist

Respiratory depression (risk increases with age)
- Assess for first signs which may include change in level of consciousness.
- Assess for occurrence up to 24 h after opioid administration and treat with naloxone 0.1 mg up to a maximum of 0.4 mg IV.
- Monitor for 30 min after naloxone administration because opioid half-life may be longer
- Have naloxone and ephedrine readily available at the bedside of patients who have received epidural opioids or anesthetics.

Oral transmucosal fentanyl citrate has been evaluated and approved for pediatric premedication and sedation. The onset of sedation is within 5 to 10 minutes, and full recovery is within 60 minutes after administration of the Fentanyl Oralet. Plasma levels rise as the patient sucks on the lozenge on a stick. These Oralets should be used only in the hospital setting where one-on-one observation of respiratory function may be measured. Side effects of oral transmucosal fentanyl citrate include nausea and vomiting and facial pruritus.

• Clinical Applicability Challenges

Case Study

Mr. K. is a 64-year-old man admitted to the surgical intensive care unit (SICU) from the operating room following a small bowel resection for colon cancer. He has a history of hypertension, inferior myocardial infarction 3 years prior, chronic obstructive pulmonary disease, and type 2 diabetes. He is extubated on 40% face-mask. The anesthesia provider's report yields the following information:

- 5 feet, 10 inches tall, weight 86 kg
- No known drug allergies

- Operating room time 3 hours, 35 minutes
- General endotracheal anesthesia without any complications noted
- Vital signs stable throughout the procedure
- Estimated blood loss of 100 mL
- Total crystalloid administered: 3,300 mL of lactated Ringer's solution
- Urine output of 1 mL/kg/h
- The patient received a total of 550 µg of fentanyl. Neostigmine and glycopyrrolate were given to antagonize vecuronium. The patient was extubated easily at the end of the case in the operating room. The patient received antibiotics before incision and had bilateral lower extremity sequential compression stockings on at all times.

1. What are the priorities of care upon Mr. K.'s arrival in the SICU?
2. What fluid therapy would the SICU nurse expect for Mr. K.?
3. What physiological alterations would the nurse expect to see in Mr. K. during the immediate postoperative period?
4. Devise a plan of care for treating Mr. K.'s postoperative pain.
5. Discuss possible postoperative complications that Mr. K. may experience.

Review Questions

1. What is the first priority of care when admitting a patient to the postanesthesia care unit?
   a. Determine that the patient has a patent airway.
   b. Attach the patient's pulse oximeter probe to the monitor.
   c. Receive report from the anesthesia provider.
   d. Obtain the patient's temperature.

2. Signs and symptoms of malignant hyperthermia that the postanesthesia care unit nurse would assess for include
   a. elevated core temperature, tachycardia.
   b. decreased carbon dioxide levels, alkalosis.
   c. decreased respiratory rate, bradycardia.
   d. muscle weakness, inability to clench teeth.

3. While assessing a patient on arrival to the postanesthesia care unit, the nurse notices that the patient's chest is rocking and the lips are blue. This may be related to
   a. an obstructed airway.
   b. incomplete reversal of nondepolarizing muscle relaxant.
   c. hypothermia.
   d. pain.

4. A 47-year-old woman who is status post laparoscopic cholecystectomy complains of nausea in the postanesthesia care unit. The nurse plans to administer which of the following drugs?

a. Ondansetron (Zofran)
b. Morphine sulfate
c. Cefazolin (Ancef)
d. Rocuronium (Zemuron)

5. Which oxygen administration device is indicated for the postoperative patient with pneumonia and an oxygen saturation of 88%?
a. Nasal cannula
b. Simple facemask
c. Nonrebreathing facemask
d. 40% Venturi mask

6. A 55-year-old man, status post left total hip replacement under spinal anesthesia, arrives in the postanesthesia care unit with a blood pressure of 82/42 mm Hg. His preoperative blood pressure was 158/89 mm Hg. On physical examination, the patient denies any pain and cannot move either of his lower extremities. The nurse expects to administer which of the following drugs?
a. Ephedrine
b. Morphine sulfate
c. Cefazolin (Ancef)
d. Ketorolac (Toradol)

References

1. American Society of PeriAnesthesia Nurses: Standards of PeriAnesthesia Nursing Practice. Thorofare, NJ: American Society of PeriAnesthesia Nurses, 2006
2. Kost M: Moderate Sedation/Analgesia: Core Competencies for Practice, 2nd ed. Philadelphia: WB Saunders, 2004
3. Steele SM: Ambulatory Anesthesia and Perioperative Analgesia. New York: McGraw-Hill Professional, 2005
4. Nagelhout J, Zaglaniczny K: Nurse Anesthesia, 3rd ed. Philadelphia: WB Saunders, 2004
5. Reich DL, Hossain S, Krol M, et al: Predictors of hypotension after induction of general anesthesia. Anesth Analg 101(3): 622–628, 2005
6. Malignant Hyperthermia Association of the United States: ABCs of managing malignant hyperthermia. 2006 Malignant Hyperthermia Association of the United States. August 4, 2007. Available at: http://medical.mhaus.org
7. Litman R, Rosenberg H: Malignant hyperthermia: Update on susceptibility testing. JAMA 293(23):2918–2924, 2005

Other Selected Readings

AORN Recommended Practices Committee: Recommended practices for the prevention of unplanned perioperative hypothermia. AORN J 85(5):972–974, 986–988, 2007
Atlee JL: Complications in Anesthesia, 2nd ed. Philadelphia: WB Saunders, 2007
Barone CP, Pablo CS, Barone GW: Postanesthetic care in the critical care unit. Crit Care Nurse 24(1):38, 2004
Bitner J, Hilde L, Hall K, Duvendack T: A team approach to the prevention of unplanned postoperative hypothermia. AORN J 85(5):921–923 925–929, 2007
Brauer A, English N, Steinmartz N, et al: Efficacy of forced air warming systems with full body blankets. Can J Anaesth 54(1): 34–41, 2007
Chang AM, Ip WY, Cheung TH: Patient-controlled analgesia versus conventional intramuscular injection: A cost effectiveness analysis. J Adv Nurs 46(5):531–544, 2004
Cornish PB, Barton J, Deacon A: The impact of regional anesthesia on outcome: A patient's perspective. Anaesthesia 59(6):613–615, 2004
Dal D, Kose A, Honca M, et al: Efficacy of prophylactic ketamine in preventing postoperative shivering. Br J Anaesth 95(2):189–192, 2007

Defazio Quinn D, Shick L: Perianesthesia Nursing Core Curriculum: Preoperative Phase I and Phase II PACU Nursing. Philadelphia: WB Saunders, 2004

Drain C: Perianesthesia Nursing: A Critical Care Approach, 4th ed. Philadelphia: WB Saunders, 2004

Ebell MH: Predicting postoperative nausea and vomiting. Am Fam Physician 75(10):1537–1538, 2007

Kranke P, Eberhart LH, Gan TJ, et al: Algorithms for the prevention of postoperative nausea and vomiting: An efficacy and efficiency simulation. Eur J Anesthesiol 24(10):856–867, 2007

Litman R, Rosenberg H: Malignant hyperthermia: Update on susceptibility testing. JAMA 293(23):2918–2924, 2005

McCarthy EJ: Malignant hyperthermia pathophysiology, clinical presentation, and treatment. AACN Clin Issues 15(2):231–237, 2004

Schechter LN: Advances in postoperative pain management: The pharmacy perspective. Am J Health Syst Pharm 61:S15–S21, 2004

Torpy J: Malignant hyperthermia. JAMA 293(23):2831, 2005

Troung L, Moran JL, Blum P: Post-anesthesia care unit discharge: A clinical scoring system versus traditional time-based criteria. Anaesth Intensive Care 32(1):33–42, 2004

Watson D, Odom-Forren J: Practical guide to moderate sedation/analgesia. Philadelphia: WB Saunders, 2005

Wax D, Doshi A, Hossain S, et al: Changing patterns of postoperative nausea and vomiting prophylaxis drug uses in an academic anesthesia practice. J Clin Anesth 19(5):356–359, 2007

White P: Prevention of postoperative nausea and vomiting: A multimodal solution to a persistent problem. N Engl J Med 350(24):2511–2512, 2007

Special Situations in Critical Care

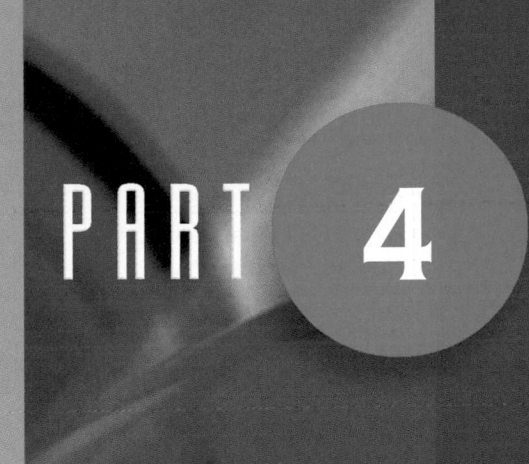

PART 4

INTERNET RESOURCES

Topic	Web Page Address
Air and Surface Transport Nurses Association	www.astna.org
American College of Emergency Physicians	www.acep.org
American Red Cross	www.redcross.org
Association of Air Medical Services	www.aams.org
Canadian Centre for Emergency Preparedness	www.ccep.ca
Center for Biosecurity, University of Pittsburgh Medical Center	www.upmc-biosecurity.org
Center for Disease Control and Prevention, Emergency Preparedness and Response	www.emergency.cdc.gov
Collaborating Agencies Responding to Disasters	www.firstvictims.org
Disaster Preparedness and Emergency Response Association	www.disasters.org
Emergency Nurses Association	www.ena.org
FEMA–Federal Emergency Management Agency	www.fema.gov
National Center for Disaster Preparedness	www.ncdp.mailman.columbia.edu
National Homeland Security	www.twotigersonline.com
National Response Center	www.nrc.uscg.mil/nrchp.html
National Response Plan	www.epa.gov/emergencies
Society of Critical Care Medicine	www.sccm.org
U.S. Dept. of Transportation	www.dotcr.ost.dot.gov/asp/emergencyprep.asp

Rapid Response Teams and Transport of the Critically Ill Patient

14

Dennis W. Jones • Christine N. Lynch

Rapid Response Teams
    Rationale for the Need
    The Role of the Rapid Response Team
Interfacility Transport
    Modes of Interfacility Transport
    Transfer Guidelines and Legal Implications
    Phases of Interfacility Transport
Intrafacility Transport

Objectives

Based on the content in this chapter, the reader should be able to:

❶ Explain the indications for a rapid response team (RRT).

❷ Discuss the role of the RRT.

❸ Describe necessary considerations before establishing an RRT system.

❹ Describe the indications for interfacility transport of the critically ill patient.

❺ Compare and contrast the advantages and disadvantages of air versus ground transport.

❻ Discuss the specific considerations and implications for care for air transport.

❼ Explain the Emergency Medical Transfer Active Labor Act (EMTALA) requirements for an appropriate interhospital transfer.

❽ Describe key factors necessary for an effective interfacility transfer plan.

❾ Analyze the role of the registered nurse in the five phases of the interfacility transport of the critically ill.

❿ Discuss the indications for intrafacility transport.

• Rapid Response Teams

The patients being cared for in hospitals today are older, sicker, and have more comorbidities. A large percentage of these patients experience an adverse event during their hospitalization. Many of these events are preceded by warning signs in the form of hemodynamic instability.[1] A system to reach these patients at the first sign of instability could prevent deterioration before cardiac arrest and improve patient outcomes. The need for early detection and rapid treatment of unstable patients led to the development of the rapid response team (RRT).

The first RRTs, called medical emergency teams (METs), were introduced at Liverpool Hospital in Australia in 1990. The METs were established to enable early identification and aggressive management of the seriously ill patient before cardiac arrest.[2]

Since 1990, RRTs have been growing in popularity not only in Australia but also around the world.

RATIONALE FOR THE NEED

The National Registry of Cardiopulmonary Resuscitation (NRCPR), the largest registry of its kind, is an American Heart Association (AHA)–sponsored, prospective, multisite, observational study of in-hospital resuscitation.[3] The NRCPR showed that despite advances in resuscitation practices and outcomes in the prehospital setting, little progress has been made with regard to improving in-hospital survival following cardiac arrest. This study found in-hospital survival following cardiac arrest to be a dismal 17%, essentially unchanged for the past 40 years.[3]

Most hospitals treat hundreds of patients each day, and there is a great deal of variability in the care provided. In addition, the level of monitoring may vary because those providing care have varying levels of skill. The performance of health care providers and of the system in which they work has a direct impact on patient care and outcomes. The variability in the care provided not only has an impact on both quality and safety, but it also contributes to the differences seen in hospital mortality rates. In a review of the literature, the Institute of Healthcare Improvement (IHI), as part of its 5 Million Lives campaign (2006), has found that three main systemic issues contribute to the differing hospital mortality rates. These include:

► Failure in planning (including assessments, treatments, and goals)

► Failure to communicate (e.g., patient-to-staff, staff-to-staff, staff-to-physician)

► Failure to recognize the deteriorating patient condition

These fundamental problems often lead to a failure to rescue.[4]

The challenge for hospitals is to create a 24-hour system to recognize the seriously ill early and respond rapidly with personnel skilled in advanced resuscitation. It has been estimated that 15% to 20% of all hospitalized patients develop serious adverse events, including cardiac arrest.[1] These adverse events are rarely sudden or unforeseen. In fact, they are usually preceded by at least one sign or symptom of physiological deterioration that occurs in the hours before the critical change in status (Box 14-1).[1]

THE ROLE OF THE RAPID RESPONSE TEAM

The RRT brings critical care expertise to the bedside. In an effort to promote the implementation of RRTs in all hospitals in the United States, the IHI has written a *Rapid Response Teams: How-To Guide* (http://www.ihi.org). The members of the RRT perform the following functions:

► Assess the patient

► Stabilize the patient using RRT protocols (Fig. 14-1)

► Collect data (e.g., vital signs, radiographic and laboratory data)

► Communicate with the health care team

Box 14-1 • Rapid Response Team Calling Criteria

- Threatened airway
- Respiratory rate < 8 breaths/min or > 28 breaths/min
- SpO_2 < 90%
- Heart rate < 40 beats/min or > 130 beats/min
- Systolic blood pressure < 90 mm Hg
- Urine output < 50 mL in 4 hours
- Acute mental status change
- Any patient about whom you are worried or concerned

► Provide education and support to the nurse initiating the call

► Assist with triage decisions

► Assist with transfer to a higher level of care, if needed[5]

The early intervention of RRTs has been shown to decrease the incidence of cardiac arrest and improve mortality rates.[5]

The RRT system is based on three major components: early recognition of the deteriorating patient, rapid response with swift provision of care by clinical staff trained in advanced resuscitation, and a means by which to measure the system. When establishing an RRT system, several factors must be considered (Boxes 14-2 and 14-3).[6]

• Interfacility Transport

With the advent of new technologies and specialty treatment centers, critically ill patients often must be transported between facilities. To ensure safe and expeditious transport, it is important to consider both the method of transport and the people involved in the transport process.

Typically, transport is indicated when the patient's need for complex diagnostic procedures or sophisticated medical and nursing expertise exceeds what can be provided at a facility. Family requests may also affect the decision to transport. For example, a family may want their family member transferred to a hospital closer to home.

Outcomes of evolving health care reform also have increased the demands for interfacility transport of critically ill patients. Third-party payers may require patients to be transported to a facility that is a member of their network. In addition, many hospitals vie for fewer patients and have developed their own transport teams to provide a flow of patients to their particular facility.

Whatever the reason for transporting a patient, a risk–benefit analysis of the transport should always be performed. Risks for the patient range from physical safety to physiological compromise to emotional distress.[7] Benefits from interfacility transport include access to life-saving assessment techniques and specialized interventions that can improve the patient's outcome. When the benefits for the patient exceed the risks, an interfacility transport is warranted. Figure 14-2 provides an algorithm for interfacility transfer.

The American College of Emergency Physicians (ACEP) has outlined physician responsibilities at this point. These responsibilities are as follows:

► The sending physician performs the patient assessment and determines the appropriate level of care during transfer.

► The receiving physician ensures that his or her facility is capable of providing necessary patient services to care for the patient.

Union Memorial Hospital	Patient Label
Rapid Response Team Protocols	

DATE	TIME	Auto fill date and time ordered	Rapid Response Team Protocols (Check all that apply.)
		1. Initiate pulse ox and cardiac monitoring. 2. Start oxygen therapy with 2L/min nasal cannula. 3. Titrate oxygen to SpO_2 92% (88 to 92% if history of COPD). May use Venturi mask if necessary. 4. ☐ ABGs ☐ EKG ☐ Portable CXR ☐ Transcutaneous pacing	
		5. ☐ Initiate Decreasing Level of Consciousness Protocol: ☐ Start IV. If hemodynamically unstable[a] or orthostatic[b] give 250 ml bolus NS. ☐ EKG ☐ CBC ☐ BMP ☐ ABGs ☐ Blood Glucose	
		6. ☐ Initiate Respiratory Distress Protocol: ☐ Start IV ☐ ABGs ☐ CBC ☐ Portable CXR ☐ Albuterol neb 2.5 mg	
		7. ☐ Initiate Chest Pain Protocol: ☐ STAT EKG ☐ Start IV ☐ Cardiac Enzymes	
		8. ☐ Initiate Seizure Protocol: ☐ Start IV ☐ Blood Glucose ☐ Pad Bedrails ☐ Anti-seizure drug level, if applicable. ☐ Page senior resident for possible anti-seizure medication order and for urgent evaluation.	
		9. ☐ Initiate GI Bleed Protocol: ☐ Large bore IV ☐ STAT, CBC, BMP, PT/INR and PTT, Type and screen if hemodynamically unstable or orthostatic ☐ Start a second large bore IV. ☐ Page senior resident for urgent evaluation. ☐ EKG ☐ Type and crossmatch for 2 units PRBCs. ☐ Page attending physician regarding desire for GI consult and/or initiation of H_2 blockers or PPI.	
		10. ☐ Initiate Hypotension Protocol: ☐ Start IV ☐ STAT CBC, BMP, PT/INR and PTT, ABGs, portable CXR. ☐ Give 500 ml bolus NS ☐ Assess surgical site. ☐ D/C any sedation and blood pressure medications.	
		Definitions: [a]Hemodynamically unstable; SBP < 90 OR HR > 130. [b]Orthostatic: 20 mm Hg drop in SBP, 10 mm Hg drop in DPB, or a 20 bpm increase in HR upon upright positioning for 3 min.	

RRT Leader Signature: _____

Date / Time: _____ Beeper: _____

Figure 14-1 • Example of rapid response team (RRT) protocols used with a nurse-led team. (Courtesy of Union Memorial Hospital, Baltimore, Maryland.)

The medical director of the critical care transportation agency provides medical direction during transport as well as all medical oversight of the transportation operation, which includes, but is not limited to, determining minimal team composition and equipment requirements, education, and practice.[8]

MODES OF INTERFACILITY TRANSPORT

Once the decision has been made to transport, the method of transport must be determined. The two primary methods of interfacility transport are ground and air. Ground transport includes ambulances and mobile intensive care units (ICUs). Air transport can

occur by either a rotary-wing vehicle (helicopter) or a fixed-wing vehicle (airplane). When selecting the mode of transport, the following factors must be considered:

► Distance
► The safety of the transport environment
► Patient "out of hospital" time
► The patient's condition and the potential for complications
► The patient's need for critical or time-sensitive intervention (e.g., rescue angioplasty)
► Traffic conditions
► Weather conditions[9]

Box 14-2 • Considerations When Implementing a Rapid Response Team (RRT) System

Gaining leadership support. The support of senior leadership is essential for the success of the proposed RRT system. Advantages of an RRT system include:
- Marketing advantage in a competitive health care environment
- Greater medicolegal protection and decreased liability
- Decreased patient and family complaints
- Improvement in identifying patients in need of palliative care
- Avoidance of unnecessary intensive care unit (ICU) admissions
- Decreased job-related stress for nurses and residents
- Decreased number of in-hospital arrests

Determining team structure. The structure of the RRT varies according to facility size, level of patient acuity, availability of resources, and the frequency of adverse events and cardiac arrest. Examples of different models include:
- ICU registered nurse (RN) and respiratory therapist (RT)
- ICU RN, RT, and nurse practitioner or physician assistant
- ICU RN, RT, and intensivist or hospitalist

Establishing communication tools and protocols. Communication tools provide the RRT leader with a template for gathering pertinent information, facilitating communication with the physician, and facilitating triage decision making. If the RRT is led by a nurse, the use of protocols is essential for the quick delivery of indicated therapies and tests (see Fig. 14-1).

Training for responders. Members of the RRT must receive the proper training. Areas to be reviewed include:
- The benefits of early rescue
- Teamwork with non–critical care staff
- Protocols available to guide RRT therapy
- Triage skills and advanced cardiac life support (ACLS) certification
- The importance of the linkage to palliative care
- What is expected of RRT members when responding to a call

- The use of communication tools such as SBAR (see Box 14-3)
- The chain of command for nurse-led teams

Training for staff. Staff members must be made aware that the RRT exists, educated about the role of the RRT, and taught how to activate the RRT system. Methods of raising staff awareness include the following:
- Formal teaching and in-service training
- Newsletters
- Posters with the RRT calling criteria
- Pocket cards and badge holder with calling criteria
- Brochures with RRT concepts and calling criteria
- Inclusion of RRT education in employee orientation sessions

Calling criteria and the mechanism for activating the RRT system. Many studies have been done to establish those physiological signs that are often displayed before an adverse event or cardiac arrest.[5] When considering the RRT calling criteria that will be used in your institution, these evidence-based data should be considered. (See Box 14-1 for examples of calling criteria.) The mechanism for activating the RRT system should be clear, quick, and easy so that the staff will use it and the team will respond rapidly.

Feedback mechanisms. Feedback promotes continued improvement of the RRT system and can be used to drive educational programs. Feedback can be obtained by:
- Tracking patient outcomes
- Conducting satisfaction surveys with the staff

Evaluation of effectiveness. A means by which to measure the success of the RRT system is imperative. Three key measures that are used include:
- Codes per 1,000 discharges
- Codes outside the ICU
- Utilization of the RRT system

Adapted from Institute for Healthcare Improvement: 5 Million Lives Campaign. Getting Started Kit. Rapid Response Teams: How-To Guide, 2006. Available at: http://www.ihi.org/IHI/Programs/Campaign/.

In addition, the advantages and disadvantages of ground versus air transport must be considered when selecting the mode of transport. Table 14-1 summarizes the advantages and disadvantages of ground versus air transport.

Air Transport

Table 14-2 summarizes the special considerations for air transport. It is important for the nurse who may be caring for a patient to have a basic understanding of these considerations. A more thorough understanding aids in preparing the patient before the arrival of the flight team and allows for a smoother transition at the bedside on arrival.

The environment in which the patient is transported differs greatly from the in-hospital setting. Because the patient is transported at a higher altitude, where the barometric pressure is reduced, the possibility of hypoxia increases. However, the degree

to which this occurs depends on the aircraft used—whether it is fixed wing or rotary wing—and the altitude. If necessary, patients transported by air receive supplemental oxygen. The flight team administers the appropriate amount of oxygen to the patient based on clinical condition and altitude. If applicable, advising the patient and family members of the need for oxygen during flight may help to allay any anxiety before departure.

Any air-filled cavity in the patient's body, such as the stomach, lungs, or containers (air splint, glass intravenous bottle), can be affected physiologically by changes in barometric pressure. The primary change that occurs is an expansion of the gas as the barometric pressure decreases. Depending on the amount of gas, the location of the gas, and the degree of barometric pressure change, the patient could suffer deleterious effects if not properly screened and managed. The flight team screens the patient carefully and takes preventive measures to ensure a safe and uneventful

---

Box 14-3 • SBAR Communication Tool

SBAR is an acronym for Situation, Background, Assessment, and Recommendation. Communication tools such as the SBAR provide the RRT leader with a template for gathering pertinent information, facilitating communication with the physician, and facilitating triage decision making.

Situation: State your name and unit.
State the name of the patient you are calling about.
State the problem for which the team was consulted.

Background: State the admission diagnosis and the date of admission.
State the pertinent medical history.
Provide a brief synopsis of the patient's hospital course.
State the code status of the patient.

Assessment: Most recent vital signs
BP: _____; pulse: _____;
respirations: _____; temp: _____
Any change from prior assessments:
Mental status:
Quality of respirations:
Pulse/rhythm change:
Pain:
Skin color:
Neurologic changes:
Nausea and vomiting, output:

Recommendation: State your triage recommendations.
For example:
Transfer to CCU
Have the physician come see the patient at this time
Arrange for specialist to see the patient now
Arrange for tests (e.g., chest x-ray, ABG, ECG, CBC)

Adapted from Duncan KD: Nurse-led medical emergency teams: A recipe for success in community hospitals. In DeVita MA, Hillman K, Bellomo R (eds): Medical Emergency Teams: Implementation and Outcome Measurement. New York, Springer, 2006, pp 122–133.

---

the patient for the presence of fear or anxiety related to flying and a history of motion sickness while in a moving vehicle. Consultation with the sending physician is indicated when any of these factors exist because treatment with an anxiolytic or antiemetic medication could aid in preventing clinical problems during the flight. The flight crew screens the patient for the presence of these factors during the preflight assessment.

TRANSFER GUIDELINES AND LEGAL IMPLICATIONS

To facilitate the appropriate transfer of patients, the ACEP has developed guidelines. These principles of appropriate patient transfer are listed in Box 14-4.

Legislation also exists that provides guidelines, regulations, and penalties for patient transfer. One such law, the Consolidated Omnibus Reconciliation Act (COBRA) of 1985, contains provisions addressing the transfer of patients from hospital to hospital. The purpose of the legislation is to prevent inappropriate transfers of patients who seek emergency department care. As a result, this legislation has become known as the "antidumping" law.

The following provisions of the COBRA legislation prevent any patient from being denied an initial screening in an emergency department or from being transferred to another hospital or discharged without receiving care:

1. Hospitals must provide screening examinations for every person who comes to the emergency department and requests care.
2. If the patient has an emergency medical condition, the hospital must provide stabilizing treatment or transfer the patient to another medical facility. The physician must document that the medical benefits outweigh the risks of the transfer.
3. The receiving medical facility agrees to accept the patient and provide appropriate medical treatment. The receiving medical facility must have adequate space and qualified personnel to care for the patient.
4. The transfer is conducted by qualified personnel and appropriate equipment needed to provide care during the transfer is available.[10]

There may be situations when a patient is not stabilized, yet conditions are appropriate for transfer. This would occur when:

1. The risks of remaining at the initial facility are outweighed by the benefits of transfer.
2. The patient or family requests the transfer.
3. A physician is not present at the initial facility but a qualified medical person certifies that the benefits outweigh the risks.
4. The transfer occurs with appropriate equipment and qualified personnel.[10]

transport. However, it is important for the sending nurse to be aware of these potential problems to assist in their prevention.

Other environmental factors affecting the patient during the transport include changes in temperature and humidity as well as the presence of noise and vibration. The degree to which each of these factors occurs depends very much on both the mode of transport—that is, whether the vehicle is a fixed-wing or rotary-wing aircraft—and the type of aircraft. The flight crew takes the necessary steps to either prevent or decrease the effects of each of these factors on the patient.

If the critically ill patient is conscious and aware of the need for air transport, the sending nurse screens

Figure 14-3 presents the requirements for evaluating a patient's suitability for transfer, as outlined

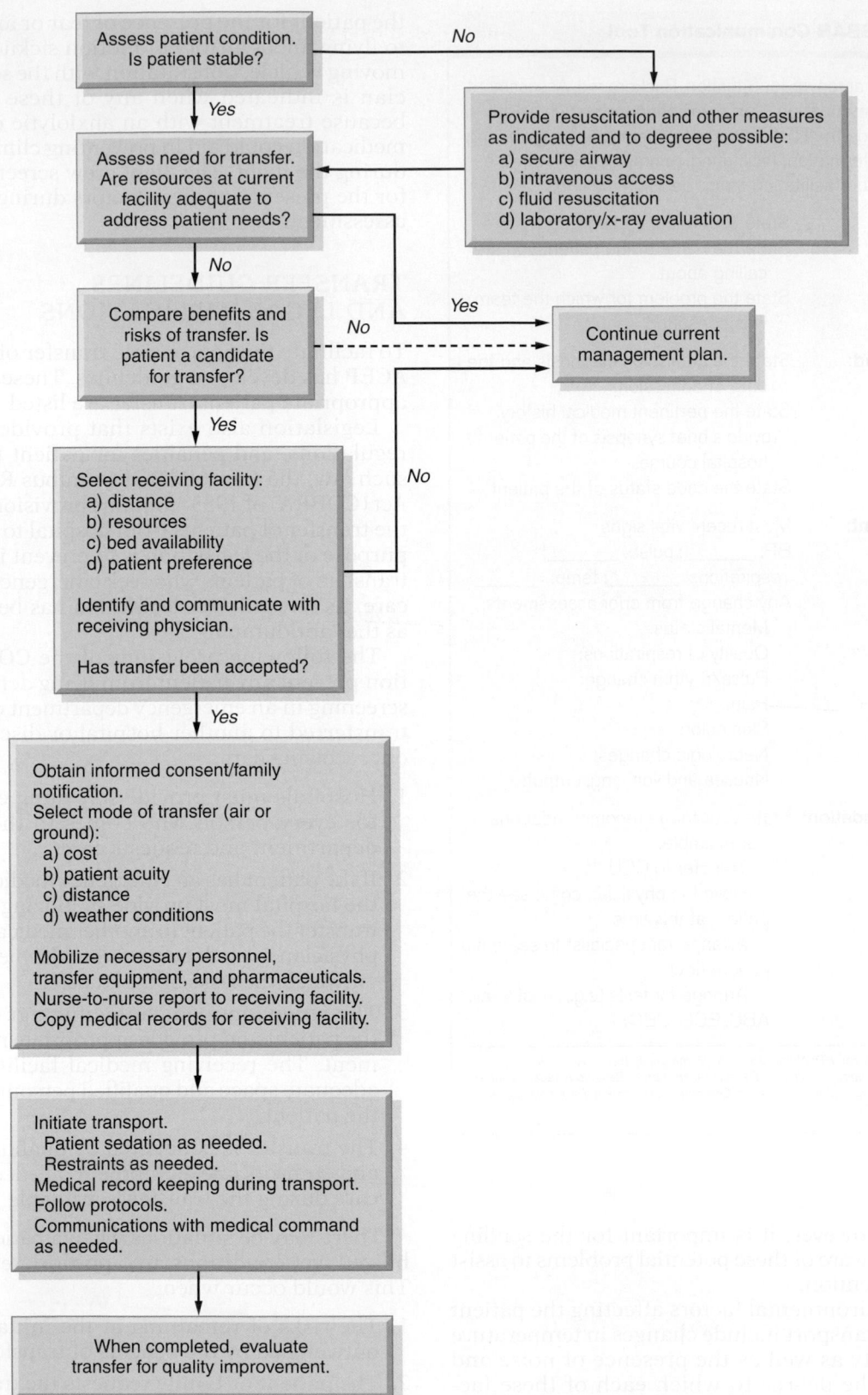

Figure 14-2 • Interfacility transfer algorithm. (From Warren J, Fromm RE, Orr RA, et al: Guidelines for the inter- and intrahospital transport of critically ill patients. Crit Care Med 32[1]:256–262, 2004.)

Table 14-1 • Advantages and Disadvantages of Ground Versus Air Transport

Mode of Transport	Advantages	Disadvantages
Ground	Adequate work space for personnel and equipment Sensitive monitoring equipment may work better No weight restrictions Adequate lighting Able to travel in most types of weather	Longer transport time Unfavorable road conditions may make transport uncomfortable for patient Interventions difficult to perform in a moving vehicle Ambulance unavailable for other calls in the community
Air	May shorten "out of hospital" time Crew generally composed of advanced-level care providers Improved communication capability Ground emergency medical services remain available in the community	Weather conditions restrict availability of the vehicle Potentially more costly Limited space (helicopters) Weight limitations Physiological impact on patient and crew Psychological impact on patient (e.g., fear of flying)

From Holleran R: Prehospital Nursing: A Collaborative Approach. St. Louis, CV Mosby, 1994.

Table 14-2 • Special Considerations for Air Transport

Stressors	Effect	Nursing Interventions
Altitude change	Hypoxia is due to the following: Decrease in the partial pressure of O_2 Decrease in the diffusion gradient for oxygen molecules to cross the alveolar membrane Decrease in oxygen availability	Provide supplemental O_2. Use pulse oximeter and end-tidal CO_2 monitor.
Barometric pressure (atmospheric pressure) change	With increasing altitude, the barometric pressure decreases and gases expand. Expansion of gases affects eardrums, sinuses, gastrointestinal tract, pleural spaces, and hollow organs. Expansion of gases affects air splints, pressure bags or cuffs, balloon cuffs on endotracheal tubes, intravenous fluid bags and bottles, pneumatic antishock garments.	Insert a nasogastric tube to decompress the stomach. If possible, fill cuffs with water or saline rather than air. Monitor equipment and decompress with higher altitudes. Vent glass bottles and wrap to protect against breakage. Apply pressure cuffs to IV solution bags.
Thermal change	As altitude increases, temperature decreases. Oxygen demand increases as the body tries to maintain warmth.	Use blankets to keep the patient warm.
Humidity change	As air is cooled, it loses moisture. Mucous membranes dry.	Humidify supplemental O_2. Provide adequate fluid intake.
Gravitational change	Gravitational change affects acceleration and deceleration forces. Transient increase in venous return occurs for patients positioned with head at the back of the aircraft. Potential exists for motion sickness.	Use a head-forward position for patients with fluid overload or increased intracranial pressure. To minimize motion sickness, provide O_2, cool cloth to face, cool air to face. Administer medications, such as transdermal scopolamine patches and promethazine.
Noise	It is difficult to monitor blood pressure, breath sounds, endotracheal tube air leak.	Explain sounds to patient. Monitor blood pressure by Doppler device. Provide continuous airway assessment. Wear head sets or ear plugs.
Vibration	Vibration may distort readings on equipment. Equipment may loosen or move.	Secure all equipment. Check equipment function frequently.

From Harrahill M: Interfacility transfer. In Kitt S, Selfridge-Thomas J, Proehl J, et al (eds): Emergency Nursing: A Physiologic and Clinical Perspective, 2nd ed. Philadelphia, WB Saunders, 1995. pp 12–18.

Box 14-4 • Principles of Appropriate Patient Transfer

- The health and well-being of the patient must be the overriding concern when any patient transfer is considered.
- Emergency physicians and hospital personnel should comply with state and federal regulations regarding patient transfer. A medical screening exam should be performed by a physician or by properly trained ancillary personnel according to written policies and procedures.
- The patient should be transferred to another facility only after medical evaluation and, when possible, stabilization.
- The physician should inform the patient or responsible party of the reasons for and the risks and likely benefits of transfer, and document this in the medical record.
- The hospital and medical staff should identify individuals responsible for transfer decisions and clearly delineate their duties regarding the patient transfer process.
- The patient should be transferred to a facility appropriate to the medical needs of the patient, with adequate space and personnel available.
- A physician or other responsible person at the receiving hospital must agree to accept the patient before transfer.

- The patient transfer should not be refused by the receiving hospital when the transfer is medically indicated and the receiving hospital has the capability and/or responsibility to provide care for the patient.
- Communication to exchange clinical information between responsible persons at the transferring and receiving hospitals must occur before transfer.
- An appropriate medical summary and other pertinent records should accompany the patient to the receiving institution.
- The patient should be transferred in a vehicle that is staffed by qualified personnel and contains appropriate equipment.
- When transfer of patients is part of a regional plan to provide optimal care of patients at specified medical facilities, written transfer protocols and interfacility agreements should be in place.

Adapted from American College of Emergency Physicians: Principles of appropriate patient transfer. Ann Emerg Med 19(3):337–338, 1990.

---

by the Emergency Medical Transfer Active Labor Act (EMTALA). In addition, the Air and Surface Transport Nurses Association (ASTNA, formerly known as the National Flight Nurses Association, or NFNA) developed nursing standards for transport of the critically ill patient by rotary-wing transport.[11]

PHASES OF INTERFACILITY TRANSPORT

Five phases of transport have been identified: (1) notification and acceptance by the receiving facility, (2) preparation of the patient by the transport team, (3) the actual transport, (4) turnover of the patient to the receiving hospital, and (5) continuous quality improvement monitoring after transport. The keys to the success of transport are a comprehensive assessment; determination of the appropriateness of the transfer; and collaboration, communication, evaluation, and education of personnel (Box 14-5).

Phase One: Notification and Acceptance by the Receiving Facility

The first phase of transport requires contacting the receiving facility to determine its willingness to accept the patient, and if accepted, determining the accepting physician and receiving patient care unit. Additionally, the mode of transport is determined at this time. Communication is an essential element in this phase of the process. The sending, transporting, and receiving personnel must have the necessary information to make the appropriate transport decision. Standards of care and protocols are necessary in order for the transport process to be carried out in an organized way. A transfer checklist is helpful to ensure that no steps in the transfer process are missed. In addition, an awareness of the policies and procedures

of the transporting agencies used in an area is needed for a smooth transport process.[7]

The identification of a responsible physician is essential so that a contact person is available for consultation while en route and on arrival. The ACEP has described medical direction for interfacility transfers as a shared responsibility. The transferring physician ensures that the transport team is composed of professionals appropriate to the needs of the patient and that an appropriate vehicle and equipment are used for transport.[8] If the local emergency medical system is not providing medical direction en route, then the responsible physician must be identified as being part of the hospital-based or private ambulance program. The Emergency Nurses Association believes that any patient transferred to another facility should be transferred at the same level of care that he or she needed in the emergency department.[3] The Commission of Air Medical Transport Services, which is the certifying body for the air medical industry, maintains the staffing standard on critical care transports; either a registered nurse (RN) or a licensed physician must be present as the primary care provider.[12] Transport teams should have standard orders and protocols if they are unable to maintain contact with a medical center physician en route. The transport flight team has practice protocols that guide their practice; however, they may also receive medical direction from the medical director of the transport program.

Once the specific transporting agency is determined, an overview of the patient's condition and specific clinical needs is communicated. Initial information provided includes the patient's name, age, diagnosis, reason for transfer, vital signs, intravenous and special monitoring lines, continuous infusion medications, airway and oxygenation or ventilation status, and special equipment needs (e.g., intra-aortic

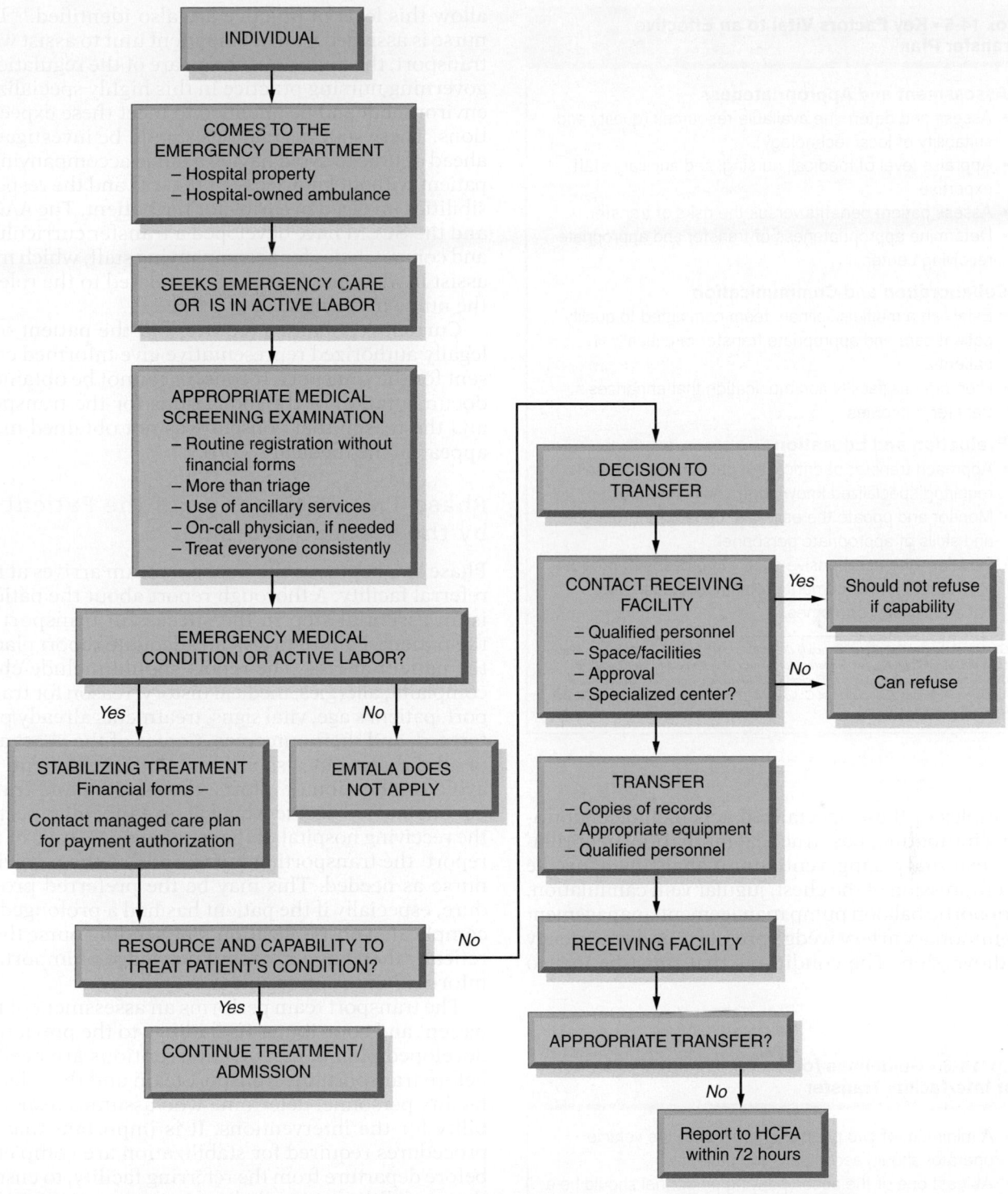

Figure 14-3 • Emergency Medical Transfer Active Labor Act (EMTALA) flow chart. HCFA (formerly Health Care Finance Administration) is now Center for Medicare and Medicaid Services. (Reprinted with permission from Lee NG: Legal Concepts and Issues in Emergency Care. Philadelphia: WB Saunders, 2001, p 140.)

balloon pump). This information assists in determining the composition of the transport team as well as the equipment and medications needed. The American Association of Critical-Care Nurses (AACN), the American College of Critical Care Medicine, and the Society of Critical Care Medicine (SCCM) offer guidelines for accompanying personnel for interfacility transfers[7] (Box 14-6). However, it is important to recognize that these are simply guidelines and may not

be followed in all cases. Therefore, it is important for the sending nurse to ascertain the credentials of the accompanying team members to ensure there is a smooth transition of care to a qualified transport team.

Individual states define the role of the nurse who may be involved in interfacility transport.[10] Some states have outlined an expanded set of specialized acts for the nurse while practicing in the prehospital setting, the interagency transport arena, or both.

Box 14-5 • Key Factors Vital to an Effective Transfer Plan

Assessment and Appropriateness

- Assess and determine available resources (quality and suitability of local technology).
- Appraise level of medical, nursing, and ancillary staff expertise.
- Assess patient benefits versus the risks of transfer.
- Determine appropriateness of transfer and appropriate receiving center.

Collaboration and Communication

- Establish a multidisciplinary team committed to quality patient care and appropriate transfer of critically ill patients.
- Promote interfacility communication that enhances transfer outcomes.

Evaluation and Education

- Approach transfer of critically ill patients as a process requiring specialized knowledge and competencies.
- Monitor and update the essential transfer knowledge and skills of appropriate personnel.
- Develop a comprehensive quality improvement program to evaluate and document problem resolution and patient transfer outcomes.

Guidelines for the Transfer of Critically Ill Patients. Prepared by the American Association of Critical-Care Nurses Transfer Guidelines Task Force and the Guidelines Committee, American College of Critical Care Medicine, Society of Critical Care Medicine. American Association of Critical-Care Nurses, Aliso Viejo, CA, 1998, p 6. Used with permission.

Examples of these specialized acts include endotracheal intubation, nasotracheal intubation, defibrillation, external pacing, ventilator management, needle decompression of the chest, jugular vein cannulation, intra-aortic balloon pump management, management of pulmonary artery wedge pressure, and emergency cardioversion. The conditions that must be met to

Box 14-6 • Guidelines for Accompanying Personnel for Interfacility Transfer

- A minimum of two people in addition to the vehicle operator should accompany the patient.
- At least one of the accompanying personnel should be a registered nurse, physician, or advanced emergency medical technician.
- When a physician does not accompany the patient, there should be a mechanism available to communicate with the physician any changes in the patient status and obtain additional orders. If an accompanying physician is not possible, advanced authorization by standing orders to perform acute life-saving interventions must be established.

Guidelines for the Transfer of Critically Ill Patients. Prepared by the American Association of Critical-Care Nurses Transfer Guidelines Task Force and the Guidelines Committee, American College of Critical Care Medicine, Society of Critical Care Medicine. American Association of Critical-Care Nurses, Aliso Viejo, CA, 1998, p 11. Used with permission.

allow this level of practice are also identified.[13] If a nurse is assigned from an inpatient unit to assist with transport, the nurse must be aware of the regulations governing nursing practice in this highly specialized environment and be qualified to meet these expectations. These state regulations should be investigated ahead of time to avoid having a nurse accompanying a patient without knowledge of the role and the responsibilities involved in caring for the patient. The AACN and the SCCM have developed a transfer curriculum and competencies for accompanying staff, which may assist in identification of issues related to the role of the nurse in the field.[7]

Current regulations require that the patient or a legally authorized representative give informed consent for the transport. If consent cannot be obtained, documentation of the indications for the transport and the reason that consent was not obtained must appear in the medical record.[7]

Phase Two: Preparation of the Patient by the Transport Team

Phase two begins as the transport team arrives at the referral facility. A thorough report about the patient is an essential step in the successful transport of the patient. Failure to give an adequate report places the patient at risk. The report should include chief complaint, allergies, medical history, reason for transport, patient's age, vital signs, treatments already performed, and their outcomes. Copies of the chart and of all radiographs also are sent with the patient. To avoid duplication of efforts, the sending and transporting nurses decide who will give the full report to the receiving hospital. If the sending nurse calls in the report, the transporting nurse updates the receiving nurse as needed. This may be the preferred procedure, especially if the patient has had a prolonged or complicated hospitalization. The sending nurse theoretically then has a broader knowledge of important information to communicate.

The transport team performs an assessment of the patient and contributes its findings to the previously developed plan of care. If interventions are needed before transport, the transport team and the referral facility personnel determine who assumes responsibility for the interventions. It is important that all procedures required for stabilization are completed before departure from the referring facility, to ensure that a well-lit, controlled environment is available to maximize safe completion of those procedures. Completion of these procedures in the less controlled transport environment increases the risk for error due to unpredictable lighting, movement, and vibration. Although resuscitation and stabilization are initiated at the referral hospital, full stabilization may not be achieved until the patient arrives at the receiving hospital.[10]

The psychosocial preparation of the patient and family for transport is an important step before transport begins. The sending nurse ensures that the patient and family understand the reason for transport, the transport mode, the time of transport, and the transport destination. Information about the family is also communicated at this time and includes identification of a family spokesperson and the family's plan for getting to the receiving hospital. If the transport team is unable to meet with the family, the sending nurse supplies information about how to contact the family. The transport team, particularly the flight team, to allay any further anxiety related to flying, explains all procedures, safety precautions, and the need for preflight medications (e.g., antiemetics) to the patient and family before departure.

Physical preparation of the patient is the next important step to ensure a safe transport. The ABCs of care (airway, breathing, and circulation) are the top priority. Adequate oxygenation and ventilation are ensured before transport begins. The need for an artificial airway is determined before leaving the sending facility so that endotracheal intubation can be performed in a more predictable environment and the endotracheal tube can be well secured. Most intubated patients are sedated to prevent them from dislodging the endotracheal tube and to decrease fear and discomfort during transport. In addition to the endotracheal tube, a nasogastric tube may be inserted to prevent aspiration of stomach contents into the airway. Because auscultation of breath sounds is difficult en route, end-tidal carbon dioxide levels and oxygen saturation are used to monitor respiratory status. If an endotracheal tube is not indicated, supplemental oxygen, as previously described, may still be used to maintain adequate oxygenation.

The patient's circulatory and hemodynamic status also are stabilized before transport. Any bleeding is controlled, and adequate intravenous access is established and well secured. For a patient with an unstable volume status, several large-bore intravenous lines are indicated. If the patient is already on intravenous drips, the transport team changes over to its own equipment and intravenous mixtures. The patient's circulatory status is also continuously assessed through cardiac monitoring during the entire transport process. Cardiac arrest medications and a defibrillator should be easily accessible.

Patients with actual or potential spinal injuries should have spinal and neck immobilization devices in place before transport. The transport team may request that the staff of the sending facility take care of this before the arrival of transport. Patients with any skeletal fractures must have the fracture immobilized before transport to prevent pain and further complications.

Pain control during transport is also addressed. The best agents for a transport patient are those with a rapid onset, short duration, and ease of administration and storage. Either transport orders or protocols dictate proper administration of pain medications.

Phase Three: The Transport Process

Phase three is the actual transport of the patient. The time spent in careful planning of the transport

and stabilization of the patient eases the transport process. The transport vehicle must contain the essential equipment needed for transporting a critically ill patient. Box 14-7 lists the minimal necessary equipment.[7]

The ABCs of care continue to be the primary focus of the transport team. Each member of the transport team must have a clear understanding of his or her role in the continuous assessment, planning, and intervention that takes place when caring for the patient. Throughout the transport, the team also provides explanations and reassures the patient because transport can be very stressful. The transport team is responsible for documenting the physical and psychosocial care provided during transport and the patient's response to the care.

Before arriving at the receiving facility, if able, the transport nurse calls either a full or updated report to the RN on the receiving unit. This report includes an estimated time of arrival at the receiving facility. The nurse also communicates any special needs, changes in patient status, and unchanged but pertinent findings. In some situations, a flight nurse may not be able to provide a patient update; therefore, an updated bedside report is provided on arrival.

Phase Four: Turnover of the Patient to the Receiving Facility

Phase four of transport involves handing over the patient to the receiving unit staff at the receiving facility. Backup plans on how to handle an acutely deteriorating patient in transit between the transport

---

Box 14-7 • Minimally Essential Equipment Necessary for Transport

- Airway and ventilatory management
  Resuscitation bag and mask of proper size and fit for the patient.
  Oral airways, laryngoscopes, and endotracheal tubes of proper size for the patient.
  Oxygen source with a quantity sufficient to meet the patient's anticipated consumption with at least 1-hour reserve in addition
  Suction apparatus and catheters
- Cardiac monitor/defibrillator/transcutaneous pacemaker
- Blood pressure cuff and stethoscope
- Materials for intravenous therapy and devices for regulation of infusion
- Drugs
  For advanced cardiac resuscitation
  For the management of acute physiological derangements
  For special needs of the patient
- Spinal immobilization devices
- Communication equipment

Guidelines for the Transfer of Critically Ill Patients. Prepared by the American Association of Critical-Care Nurses Transfer Guidelines Task Force and the Guidelines Committee, American College of Critical Care Medicine, Society of Critical Care Medicine. American Association of Critical-Care Nurses, Aliso Viejo, CA, 1998, pp 11–13. Used with permission.

vehicle and the ICU should also be identified. This plan may include stopping at the emergency department to stabilize the patient; it is essential for the emergency department staff to be aware of this possibility. Once the patient arrives safely in the receiving unit, the transport team and the receiving staff determine when the receiving staff will take over the responsibility for the patient's care. A final verbal update and all medical documents are given to the receiving staff. The written report of the transport is also completed.

Phase Five: Post-transport Continuous Quality Improvement Monitoring

The final phase of transport is very important and involves continuous quality improvement monitoring. Ideally, the referring facility, the transport team, and the receiving facility are involved in the review process. The first phase of the quality improvement monitoring involves evaluation of the current transport, including any quality indicators developed by the transporting agency. These indicators may include appropriateness of the transfer, appropriateness of the accompanying personnel, timeliness of the transfer, patient outcome, management of complications, and transfer outcome. The second phase of continuous quality improvement monitoring entails the ongoing review of the transport system. Such reviews focus on system functioning, and indicators may include complications, deaths in transport, and deaths after transport.[7]

The multidisciplinary team responsible for continuous quality improvement monitoring scrutinizes the collected data for patterns and trends, identifies solutions to patient care problems, initiates corrective action, and communicates such action to all involved in the transport process. Through a quality improvement plan, the transport process is improved and results in optimal care of the critically ill patient during the transport process.[7]

• Intrafacility Transport

The transport of a critically ill patient for diagnostic evaluation or treatment within the hospital is often necessary for optimal care. When this occurs, associated risks are involved.[14] It is imperative that the benefits of the transport outweigh the risks. Although a complete discussion regarding this topic is beyond the scope of this chapter, important factors should be considered when planning a transfer of a critically ill patient outside the ICU. One factor, for example, is the rate of adverse events that occur during intrahospital transport, which ranges from 5.9% to 70%; these events usually fall into two categories.[13] Category one involves monitoring equipment and its use (e.g., equipment failure, disconnected leads, depleted oxygen). Category two involves physiological changes in the patient, which may include changes in blood pressure, hypoxia, arrhythmias, or increased intracranial pressure.[14]

Because of the inherent risks during intrahospital transport, some hospitals are forming specially trained transport teams organized with two specific goals: to reduce risk and to improve patient safety.[14] Justification for these transport teams may be based on inadequate ICU staffing and an inability to effectively manage a clinically complex patient while out of the ICU setting.[14]

To provide safe and effective intrahospital transport of a critically ill patient, the critical care nurse prepares for the transport and communicates[5] with the receiving location when necessary. Appropriate personnel and equipment must accompany the patient. The SCCM guidelines recommend that a competent critical care nurse and at least one other person accompany the patient. The additional person may be a respiratory therapist, RN, or critical care technician. The decision should be based on the patient's needs. The SCCM strongly recommends that a physician with training in airway management, advanced cardiac life support, and critical care or equivalent accompany any unstable patient.[9] Essential equipment that must be sent with the patient includes a blood pressure monitor, a pulse oximeter, a cardiac monitor–defibrillator, airway management equipment, an oxygen source, basic resuscitation drugs, and appropriate intravenous fluids and infusion pumps.

• Clinical Applicability Challenges

Case Study

Mr. J., a 52-year-old white man, was admitted to the coronary care unit (CCU) an hour ago from the emergency department with the diagnosis of anteroseptal myocardial infarction, congestive heart failure, and cardiogenic shock. His wife and family are present. The patient is intubated and sedated; is placed on a ventilator; and is given an infusion of dopamine, dobutamine, and amiodarone. Shortly after arrival in the CCU, the cardiologist decides to insert an intra-aortic balloon catheter and place the patient on an intra-aortic balloon pump.

The hospital where Mr. J. is being treated is a large community hospital, but it does not have the capability to perform interventional cardiac procedures. The cardiologist decides to transfer the patient to the closest tertiary care facility, which is 40 miles away. Transfer is indicated for cardiac catheterization; percutaneous transluminal coronary angioplasty with possible stent placement; and the need for cardiac surgery, which cannot be performed in the facility currently treating Mr. J.

The cardiologist at the community hospital has contacted the attending cardiology interventionalist, who has agreed to accept Mr. J. This physician has agreed that Mr. J. should be transferred via air medical service. The patient will be transferred directly to the cardiac catheterization laboratory and then to the awaiting bed in the CCU. The air medical service that will be transporting Mr. J. is staffed by a critical care flight RN and paramedic. They will bring all necessary equipment for the transport, to include but not limited to a transport ventilator, intravenous infusion pump, and intra-aortic balloon pump.

The attending cardiologist for Mr. J. obtains consent for transport from Mr. J.'s wife. The consent form explains reasons for, as well as the risks and benefits associated with, the transfer.

1. What are the indications for transfer of Mr. J. to a tertiary facility?

2. Why is air medical transport indicated for Mr. J.?

3. What is the most appropriate nursing diagnosis for Mr. J.?

Review Questions

1. The nurse-led rapid response team has been called to the medical-surgical floor to evaluate a patient with a change in mental status. The primary responsibility of the team is to
   a. diagnose and treat immediately.
   b. assess, stabilize, and assist with communication and transfer.
   c. teach the nurse calling for help what he or she did wrong.
   d. order and obtain diagnostic tests.

2. The rapid response team has been called to the telemetry floor to evaluate a 59-year-old man who was admitted 1 day ago with complaints of shortness of breath and a diagnosis of congestive heart failure. The telemetry nurse reports the patient's vital signs as pulse, 90 beats/min; blood pressure, 110/70 mm Hg; respiratory rate, 28 breaths/min; and oxygen saturation, 86%. On physical examination, the patient is noted to have labored breathing with use of the accessory muscles and rales bilaterally by auscultation. The nurse responder of this team should
   a. treat the patient immediately with Lasix.
   b. intubate the patient secondary to hypoxemia.
   c. transport the patient to the intensive care unit.
   d. assess the patient and communicate findings to the nurse practitioner in charge of the patient's care using the SBAR communication tool.

3. While still at the sending facility, a patient requires additional stabilization and treatment, which the facility is capable of providing. It is best to stabilize
   a. at the sending facility, before arrival of the transport team and departure to the receiving facility.
   b. at the receiving facility because that facility is better qualified to do it.
   c. en route to the receiving facility by the specialized transport team.
   d. by the medical staff in conjunction with the transport team—at the sending facility before departure to receiving facility.

4. You are transferring a patient with an intracerebral bleed to a tertiary care center that has a neuron intensive care unit and a neurosurgeon on standby. Your patient was recently intubated and mechanically ventilated and is on a propofol drip. The transport is by ground ambulance because of weather conditions that do not allow for air transport. The transport team has arrived; however, there is no registered nurse present on the team. Based on this situation you would
   a. provide a basic patient report to the team and transfer as planned.
   b. refuse to send patient with team and send team away.
   c. consult with attending physician to remove ventilator and intravenous sedation and switch to manual ventilations and intravenous bolus of alternative medication.
   d. inform transferring physician of dilemma and advocate for need for registered nurse for transport.

References

1. Jones D, Bellomo R, Goldsmith D: General principles of medical emergency teams. In DeVita MA, Hillman K, Bellomo R (eds): Medical Emergency Teams: Implementation and Outcome Measurement. New York: Springer Press, 2006, pp 80–90

2. Kerridge RK, Saul WP: The medical emergency team, evidence-based medicine and ethics. Med J Aust 179:313–315, 2003

3. Peberdy MA, Kaye W, Ornato JP, et al: Cardiopulmonary resuscitation of adults in the hospital: A report of 14720 cardiac arrests from the National Registry of Cardiopulmonary Resuscitation. Resuscitation 58:297–308, 2003

4. Institute for Healthcare Improvement: 5 Million Lives Campaign. Getting Started Kit. Rapid Response Teams: How-To Guide, 2006. Available at: http://www.ihi.org/IHI/Programs/Campaign/

5. Buist M, Bernard S, Nguyen TV, et al: Association between clinically abnormal observations and subsequent in-hospital mortality: A prospective study. Resuscitation 62:137–141, 2004

6. Duncan KD: Nurse-led medical emergency teams: A recipe for success in community hospitals. In DeVita MA, Hillman K, Bellomo R (eds): Medical Emergency Teams: Implementation and Outcome Measurement. New York: Springer, 2006, pp 122–133

7. American Association of Critical-Care Nurses Transfer Guidelines Task Force and the Guidelines Committee, American College of Critical Care Medicine, Society of Critical Care Medicine: Guidelines for the Transfer of Critically Ill Patients. Aliso Viejo, CA, American Association of Critical-Care Nurses, 1998

8. American College of Emergency Physicians: Position Paper: Interfacility Transportation of the Critical Care Patient and Its Medical Direction, 2005. Available at: http://acep.org

9. Warren J, Fromm RE, Orr RA, et al: Guidelines for the inter- and intrahospital transport of critically ill patients. Crit Care Med 32(1):256–262, 2004

10. Glass DL, Rebstock J, Handberg E: Emergency Treatment and Labor Act (EMTALA) avoiding the pitfalls. J Perinat Neonat Nurs 18(2):104–105, 2004

11. Arndt K (ed), for the Air and Surface Transport Nurses Association. Standards for Critical Care and Specialty Rotor-Wing Transport. Lexington, KY: Myers Printing, 2003

12. Commission on Accreditation of Medical Transport Systems: Accreditation Standards: Critical Care Staffing 7th ed. Anderson, SC: Author, 2006

13. Maryland Board of Nursing: Declaratory Ruling 2004-2, Re: The Standards of Practice for the Registered Nurse When Managing and Caring for the Critically Ill Client in the Specialty Care Transport Arena (Interhospital). Baltimore: Maryland Board of Nursing, 2004

14. McClenon M: Use of a specialized transport team for intra-hospital transport of critically ill patients. Dimens Crit Care Nurs 23(5):225–229, 2004

Other Suggested Readings

Rapid Response Teams

Bellomo R, Goldsmith D, Uchino S, et al: A prospective before-and-after trial of a medical emergency team. Med J Aust 179:283–287, 2003

Braithwaite RS, DeVita MA, Mahidhara R, et al, for the Medical Emergency Response Improvement Team (MERIT): Use of medical emergency team (MET) responses to detect medical errors. Qual Saf Health Care 13:255–259, 2004

Daly M, Powers J, Orto V, et al: Innovative solutions. Leading the way: An innovative approach to support nurses on general care units with an early nursing intervention team. Dimens Crit Care Nurs 26(1):15–20, 2007

Floraida M, DeVita MA, Braithewaite RS, et al: Improving the utilization of medical crisis teams (condition C) at an urban tertiary care hospital. J Crit Care 18:87–94, 2003

Halvorsen L, Garolis S, Wallace-Scroggs A, et al: Building a rapid response team. AACN Adv Crit Care 18(2):129–140, 2007

Murray T, Kleinpell R: Implementing a rapid response team: Factors influencing success. Crit Care Nurs Clin North Am 18(4): 493–502, 2006

Schmid A, Hoffman L, Happ M, et al: Failure to rescue. J Nurs Admin 37(4):188–198, 2007

Thomas K, Force M, Rasmussen D, et al: Rapid response team: Challenges, solutions, benefits. Crit Care Nurse 27(1):20–29, 2007

Transport

Bitterman RA: Providing Emergency Care Under Federal Law: EMTALA. Dallas: American College of Emergency Physicians, 2001; Supplement, 2004

Day MW: Transport of the critically ill: The Northwest MedStar experience. Crit Care Nurs Clin North Am 17(2):183–190, 2005

DeVita M, Bellomo R, Hillman K, et al: Findings of the first consensus conference on medical emergency teams. Crit Care Med 34(9):2463–2478, 2006

Garretson S, Rauzi MB, Meister J, Schuster J: Rapid response teams: A proactive strategy for improving patient care. Nurs Stand 21(9):35–40, 2006

Mackintosh M: Transporting critically ill patients: New opportunities for nurses. Nurs Stand 20(36):46–48, 2006

McGrow KM, Roys R, Maloney RC, Xiao Y: Using wireless technologies to improve information flow for interhospital transfers of critically ill patients. Crit Care Nurse 24(2):66–72, 114, 2004

Pierce PF, Evers KG: Global presence: USAF aeromedical evacuation and critical care air transport. Crit Care Nurs Clin North Am 15(2):221–232, 2003

Strickler J: EMTALA: The basics. JONA's Healthcare Law, Ethics & Regulation 8(3):77–81, 2006

Thomas F, Hopkins RO, Handrahan DL, et al: Sleep and cognitive performance of flight nurses after 12-hour evening versus 18-hour shifts. Air Med J 25(5):216–225, 2006

Disaster Management: Implications for the Critical Care Nurse

Nancy Blake • Jeffrey S. Upperman

15

Fundamentals of Disaster Science
Response to Mass Casualty Incidents
Role of Hospital Emergency Incident
Command System
Triage
Unnatural Disasters
    Explosions and Blast Attacks
    Nuclear or Radiological Attacks
    Chemical Attacks
    Biological Attacks
Natural Disasters
Psychological Effects of Terrorism

Objectives

Based on the content in this chapter, the reader should be able to:

❶ Describe the nurse's role in mass casualty incidents.

❷ Explain the nurse's role in triage.

❸ Describe how a radiological attack can occur and how to treat patients who have experienced a radiological attack.

❹ Discuss how a chemical attack can occur and how to treat patients who have experienced a chemical attack.

❺ Describe how a biological attack can occur and how to treat patients who have experienced a biological attack.

• Fundamentals of Disaster Science

Communities rely on hospitals in times of disaster. Recent disasters and terrorist attacks in the United States have identified weaknesses of hospitals, and federal funding has become available to prepare hospitals in the event of a disaster. Hurricane Katrina affected many hospitals in 2005 and revealed how vulnerable the nation's health care system is. The Oklahoma City bombing in 1995 and the attacks on the World Trade Center and the Pentagon in 2001 alerted the nation that the United States is at risk for a major terrorist disaster that could overwhelm hospitals if hundreds or thousands of survivors need emergency treatment. With large numbers of victims, critical care units would be stretched beyond capacity.

The critical care nurse's role is crucial in the event of a disaster. The job of the critical care nurse depends on the impact of the disaster on the facility's structures, its environment, and the available staffing. For example, if the electricity is out and the generators do not operate, ventilators and monitors will not function. If patients need to be evacuated from the intensive care unit (ICU) and resources are scarce, intravenous lines may need to be capped and restarted at a later time. Vital medications may not be available or may need to be rationed; in this case, the critical care nurse will need to work closely with the physician to determine other methods or medications to use as alternatives. Because the critical care nurse is taking care of the most fragile patients, maintaining the usual level of care may be difficult, if not impossible.

In situations in which entire communities are devastated, the level of care for that community becomes dependent on the equipment, supplies, and facilities on hand. For example, if all buildings have been destroyed, patient care may take place in a tent or shelter. In these situations, the goal becomes providing the highest care possible, given the resources and equipment. Wall oxygen and suction may not be available. Portable tanks may be used as a vital oxygen source. A syringe attached to a suction catheter may provide manual suction. Portable or disposable hand-held short-term ventilators may be all that are available. In cases of severe disruption, it is important to have psychosocial resources to assist the critical care nurses because many critically ill patients may die.

Critical care nurses are a valued health resource during a disaster response. They dictate how and when patients move in the facility for internal evacuation and surge capacity (see Triage, below). Nurses perform best with adequate training and preparation; therefore, as this chapter discusses, plans must delineate the appropriate deployment of nurses during a disaster crisis and the resources needed for them to be successful.

• Response to Mass Casualty Incidents

By definition, a mass casualty incident (MCI) is characterized by large numbers of patients needing medical treatment that exceed the capabilities of local emergency and health care personnel. To be integrated as part of the community's plan for emergency preparedness in MCIs, nurses must have a basic level of education to appropriately respond and protect themselves and others, particularly during chemical, biological, radiological, nuclear, and explosive events. Critical care nurses may be the first responders to large MCIs because public health teams and the emergency medical system are overwhelmed. However, every nurse must have sufficient knowledge and skill to recognize the potential for an MCI, identify when such an incident may have occurred, and protect himself or herself while caring for victims. The trauma system in the United States is continuously improving its ability to respond to MCIs and critically ill patients who have suffered multiple traumas. Nurses perform the primary and secondary survey as with any other trauma patient. They must know how to recognize their own roles and limitations as well as where to seek additional information and resources. A group initially known as the International Nursing Coalition for Mass Casualty Education (INCMCE) has developed basic standards regarding MCIs with which all nurses should be familiar (Box 15-1). Now this group is known as the Nursing Emergency Preparedness Education Coalition.[1]

By definition, terrorism is the unlawful use of force or violence against persons or property to intimidate civilians or coerce government or a civilian population while promoting political and social objectives.[2] Terrorists aim to make people fearful. Terrorist disasters can be overwhelming to the nation's health care system.

In 2002, the American Association of Critical-Care Nurses (AACN) released a Statement of Commitment to Mass Casualty and Bioterrorism Preparedness recognizing that critical care nurses will be called on to respond to disaster and mass casualty situations. This statement includes the following:

"Bioterrorism and the potential of mass casualties is a significant public health threat facing the United States. The nation's capacity to respond to this threat depends in part on the ability of the health care professionals and public health officials to rapidly and effectively detect, manage, and communicate during an event resulting in mass casualties."[3] The AACN works closely with the Red Cross to help support critical care nurses during times of disaster.

In August, 2003, a report to the Congressional Committee from the United States General Accounting Office (GAO) regarding Hospital Preparedness for a Bioterrorist Incident was published. Some of the GAO's findings were alarming. Although most urban hospitals across the country reported that they participated in basic planning and coordination of activities for bioterrorism response, they did not have the medical equipment, especially ventilators, to handle the number of people who would likely require care following a bioterrorist incident. Most hospitals stated they lacked the necessary resources to handle a large influx of patients.[4] Because many facilities would not be prepared to handle an attack, even fewer would be able to handle a large influx of critically ill patients who needed critical care. The GAO report also recounted many projected scenarios surrounding a possible influenza pandemic suggesting that the United States would be severely short of ventilators and trained staff to care for patients on ventilators.

In 2004, a working group in Pittsburgh, Pennsylvania, made recommendations to hospital and clinical leaders regarding the delivery of critical care services in the wake of a bioterrorist attack resulting in hundreds or thousands of critically ill patients. In these situations, traditional hospital and clinical care standards in general, and critical care standards in particular, likely could no longer be maintained. The study group came up with no clinical guidelines to deal with these situations. However, it did develop the following six planning assumptions regarding the current critical care medicine response for bioterrorism:

1. Future bioterrorist attacks may be covert and could result in hundreds, thousands, or more, critically ill victims.

2. Critical care will play a key role in decreasing morbidity and mortality rates after a bioterrorist attack.

3. Mass critical care cannot be provided without substantial planning and new approaches to providing critical care.

4. A hospital has limited ability to divert or transfer patients to other hospitals in the aftermath of a bioterrorist attack.

Box 15-1 • Competencies for Entry-Level Registered Nurses Related to Mass Casualty Incidents

Core Competencies

I. Critical Thinking
1. Use an ethical and nationally approved framework to support decision making and prioritizing needed in disaster situations.
2. Use clinical judgment and decision-making skills in assessing the potential for appropriate, timely individual care during a mass casualty incident (MCI).
3. Use clinical judgment and decision-making skills in assessing the potential for appropriate, individual ongoing care after an MCI.
4. Describe at the predisaster, emergency, and post-disaster phases the essential nursing care for
   a. individuals,
   b. families,
   c. special groups (e.g., children, elderly, pregnant women), and
   d. communities.
5. Describe accepted triage principles specific to MCIs (e.g., the Simple Triage and Rapid Treatment System [START]).

II. Assessment

A. General
1. Assess the safety issues for self, the response team, and victims in any given response situation in collaboration with the incident response team.
2. Identify possible indicators of a mass exposure (i.e., clustering of individuals with the same symptoms).
3. Describe general signs and symptoms of exposure to selected chemical, biological, radiological, nuclear, and explosive (CBRNE) agents.
4. Demonstrate the ability to access up-to-date information regarding selected nuclear, biological, chemical, explosive, and incendiary agents.
5. Describe the essential elements included in an MCI scene assessment.
6. Identify special groups of patients that are uniquely vulnerable during an MCI (e.g., very young, aged, immunosuppressed patients).

B. Specific
1. Conduct a focused health history to assess potential exposure to CBRNE agents.
2. Perform an age-appropriate health assessment, including
   a. airway and respiratory assessment;
   b. cardiovascular assessment, including vital signs and monitoring for signs of shock;
   c. integumentary assessment, particularly a wound, burn, and rash assessment, and pain assessment;
   d. injury assessment from head to toe;
   e. gastrointestinal assessment, including stool specimen collection, and basic neurological assessment;
   f. musculoskeletal assessment; and
   g. mental status, spiritual, and emotional assessment.
3. Assess the immediate psychological response of the individual, family, or community following an MCI.
4. Assess the long-term psychological response of the individual, family, or community following an MCI.

5. Identify resources available to address the psychological impact (e.g., Critical Incident Stress Debriefing [CISD] teams, counselors, Psychiatric/Mental Health Nurse Practitioners [P/MHNPs]).
6. Describe the psychological impact on responders and health care providers.

III. Technical Skills
1. Demonstrate the safe administration of medications, particularly vasoactive and analgesic agents, via oral (PO), subcutaneous (SC), intramuscular (IM), and intravenous (IV) administration routes.
2. Demonstrate the safe administration of immunizations, including smallpox vaccination.
3. Demonstrate knowledge of appropriate nursing interventions for adverse effects from medications administered.
4. Demonstrate basic therapeutic interventions, including
   a. basic first aid skills,
   b. oxygen administration and ventilation techniques,
   c. urinary catheter insertion,
   d. nasogastric tube insertion,
   e. lavage technique (i.e., eye and wound), and
   f. initial wound care.
5. Assess the need for and initiate the appropriate CBRNE isolation and decontamination procedures available, ensuring that all parties understand the need.
6. Demonstrate knowledge and skill related to personal protection and safety, including the use of personal protective equipment (PPE), for
   a. level B protection,
   b. level C protection, and
   c. respiratory protection.
7. Describe how nursing skills may have to be adapted while wearing PPE.
8. Implement fluid and nutrition therapy, taking into account the nature of injuries and/or agents exposed to and monitoring hydration and fluid balance accordingly.
9. Assess and prepare the injured for transport, if required, including provisions for care and monitoring during transport.
10. Demonstrate the ability to maintain patient safety during transport through splinting, immobilization, monitoring, and therapeutic interventions.

IV. Communication
1. Describe the Incident Command System (ICS) during an MCI.
2. Identify your role, if possible, within the ICS.
3. Locate and describe the emergency response plan for the place of employment and its role in community, state, and regional plans.
4. Identify one's own role in the emergency response plan for the place of employment.
5. Discuss security and confidentiality during an MCI.
6. Demonstrate appropriate emergency documentation of assessments, interventions, nursing actions, and outcomes during and after an MCI.
7. Identify appropriate resources for referring requests from patients, media, or others for information regarding MCIs.
8. Describe principles of risk for communication to groups and individuals affected by exposure during an MCI.

(continued)

Box 15-1 • Competencies for Entry-Level Registered Nurses Related to Mass Casualty Incidents (Continued)

9. Identify reactions to fear, panic, and stress that victims, families, and responders may exhibit during a disaster situation.
10. Describe appropriate coping strategies to manage self and others.

Core Knowledge

I. Health Promotion, Risk Reduction, and Disease Prevention
  1. Identify possible threats and their potential impact on the general public, emergency medical system (EMS), and the health care community.
  2. Describe community health issues related to CBRNE events, specifically limiting exposure to selected agents, contamination of water, air, and food supplies, and shelter and protection of displaced persons.

II. Health Care Systems and Policy
  1. Define and distinguish the terms *disaster* and *MCI* in relation to other major incidents or emergency situations.
  2. Define relevant terminology, including
    a. CBRNE,
    b. WMD,
    c. triage,
    d. ICS,
    e. PPE,
    f. scene assessment, and
    g. comprehensive emergency management.
  3. Describe the four phases of emergency management: preparedness, response, recovery, and mitigation.
  4. Describe the local emergency response system for disasters.
  5. Describe the interaction between local, state, and federal emergency response systems.
  6. Describe the legal authority of public health agencies to take action to protect the community from threats, including isolation, quarantine, and required reporting and documentation.
  7. Discuss principles related to a MCI site as a crime scene (e.g., maintaining integrity of evidence, chain of custody).
  8. Recognize the impact MCIs may have on access to resources and identify how to access additional resources (e.g., pharmaceuticals, medical supplies).

III. Illness and Disease Management
  1. Discuss the differences and similarities between an intentional biological attack and that of a natural disease outbreak.
  2. Assess, using an interdisciplinary approach, the short-term and long-term effects of physical and psychological symptoms related to disease and treatment secondary to MCIs.

IV. Information and Health Care Technologies
  1. Demonstrate use of emergency communication equipment that you will be required to use in a MCI response.
  2. Discuss the principles of containment and decontamination.
  3. Describe procedures for decontamination of self, others, and equipment for selected CBRNE agents.

V. Ethics
  1. Identify and discuss ethical issues related to CBRNE events:

    a. Rights and responsibilities of health care providers in MCIs (e.g., refusing to go to work or report for duty, refusal of vaccines).
    b. Need to protect the public versus an individual's right for autonomy (e.g., right to leave the scene after contamination).
    c. Right of the individual to refuse care, informed consent.
    d. Allocation of limited resources.
    e. Confidentiality of information related to individuals and national security.
    f. Use of public health authority to restrict individual activities, require reporting from health professionals, and collaborate with law enforcement.
  2. Describe the ethical, legal, psychological, and cultural considerations when dealing with the dying and or the handling and storage of human remains in an MCI.
  3. Identify and discuss legal and regulatory issues related to
    a. abandonment of patients,
    b. response to a MCI and one's position of employment, and
    c. various roles and responsibilities assumed by volunteer efforts.

VI. Human Diversity
  1. Discuss the cultural, spiritual, and social issues that may affect an individual's response to an MCI.
  2. Discuss the diversity of emotional, psychosocial, and sociocultural responses to terrorism or the threat of terrorism on one's self and others.

Professional Role Development

1. Describe these nursing roles in MCIs:
  a. Researcher
  b. Investigator/epidemiologist
  c. EMT or First Responder
  d. Direct care provider, generalist nurse
  e. Direct care provider, advanced practice nurse
  f. Director/coordinator of care in hospital/nurse administrator or emergency department nurse manager
  g. On-site coordinator of care/incident commander
  h. On-site director of care management
  i. Information provider or educator, particularly the role of the generalist nurse
  j. Mental health counselor
  k. Member of planning response team
2. Identify the most appropriate or most likely health care role for oneself during an MCI.
3. Identify the limits to one's own knowledge, skills, abilities, and authority related to MCIs.
4. Describe essential equipment for responding to an MCI (e.g., stethoscope, registered nurse license to deter imposters, packaged snack, change of clothing, bottles of water).
5. Recognize the importance of maintaining one's expertise and knowledge in this area of practice and of participating in regular emergency response drills.
6. Participate in regular emergency response drills in the community or place of employment.

From Nursing Emergency Preparedness Education Coalition, 2002. Available at: http://www.nursing.vanderbilt.edu/incmce/competencies.html.

5. Currently deployable medical teams of the federal government have a limited role in increasing a hospital's immediate ability to provide critical care to large numbers of victims of a bioterrorist attack.

6. Hospitals may need to depend on nonfederal sources or reserves of medications and equipment necessary to provide critical care for the first 48 hours following discovery of a bioterrorist attack.[5]

• Role of Hospital Emergency Incident Command System

Hospitals respond to MCIs using the Hospital Emergency Incident Command System (HEICS), which is also referred to as the Hospital Incident Command System (HICS). HICS is an incident management system based on the Incident Command System (ICS) that assists hospitals in improving their emergency management planning as well as response and recovery capabilities for unplanned and planned events. HICS is consistent with ICS and the National Incident Management System principles, which allow for multiagency response to events. The HICS organizational chart is shown in Figure 15-1. Critical care nurses need to be aware of how they specifically fit into their hospital disaster plan; they may be called on to take on a major role in the HICS organizational system.

• Triage

Triage is a system for rationing resources in response to an overwhelming medical emergency event. Effective triage is one of the first procedures that the critical care nurse uses in responding to a disaster. In triage, patients are quickly categorized into minimal, delayed, immediate, and expectant or morgue categories (see Box 15-1).

In addition to triage occurring outside the facility, health care workers should also perform triage inside the facility and ensure that salvageable patients are appropriately categorized. As patients are triaged, personnel should send them to the area where they will receive the appropriate level of care for their triage category. The latter form of triage requires policy, education, and practice for desirable results.

An emerging concept as a result of triage is surge capacity. Surge capacity is a health care system's ability to expand quickly above and beyond normal services to meet an increased demand for medical care in the event of large-scale health emergencies. Nursing responsibility and patient care ratios will also adjust during a disaster event, and surge capacity depends on nurses caring for more patients. In some instances, disasters or surge capacity needs may require staff to move patients inside facilities to safer zones or to temporary clinical care areas.

Nurses serve as a focal point for assessing patients for movement and assembling the necessary materials for continuing the care of these patients at the new site. It is important to practice the movement of patients for internal evacuation periodically.

• Unnatural Disasters

Unnatural disasters include terrorist acts. Terrorism can take many forms.

EXPLOSIONS AND BLAST ATTACKS

Trauma injuries are usually the result of some type of blast injury; explosions and bombings are the weapons of choice for terrorists. Although some of the injuries do not result in hospital admissions, others result in critical care admissions. Many people who have sustained blast injuries require care in the ICU.

The injuries can be the result of primary, secondary, or tertiary blasts. Primary blast injuries are the result of sudden changes in atmospheric pressure caused by an explosion. Examples of primary blast injuries are:

▶ Ear injuries, such as perforated eardrums
▶ Pulmonary injuries, including hemorrhagic contusion and hemopneumothorax
▶ Gastrointestinal hemorrhage or bowel perforation or rupture

Secondary blast injury occurs when victims are struck by flying objects and debris. Tertiary blast injuries occur when the body is hurled through the air and struck by another object.

NUCLEAR OR RADIOLOGICAL ATTACKS

The medical consequences of a nuclear or radiological attack or accident are dependent on the type of device used. Radiation accidents or attacks can occur as the result of problems with nuclear reactors, industrial sources, and medical sources. It is important that clinicians understand how a radiological attack can occur and how to treat patients.

A radiological or nuclear attack can occur in one of five ways:

1. *Simple radiological device* (SRD): An SRD is a device that is designed to spread radioactive material without the use of explosives, thereby exposing many people to various levels of radiation.

2. *Radiological dispersal device* (RDD): An RDD is a device formed by combining an explosive agent with radioactive materials. The initial explosion kills or injures those closest to the bomb, and the radioactive material remains to expose and contaminate survivors and possibly emergency responders.

3. *Nuclear reactor sabotage:* This type of incident is low, because of sophisticated shielding, but it could occur with an attack on a nuclear reactor.

4. *Improvised nuclear device* (IND): An IND is any device designed to cause a nuclear detonation. It is not easy to make such a weapon detonate correctly.

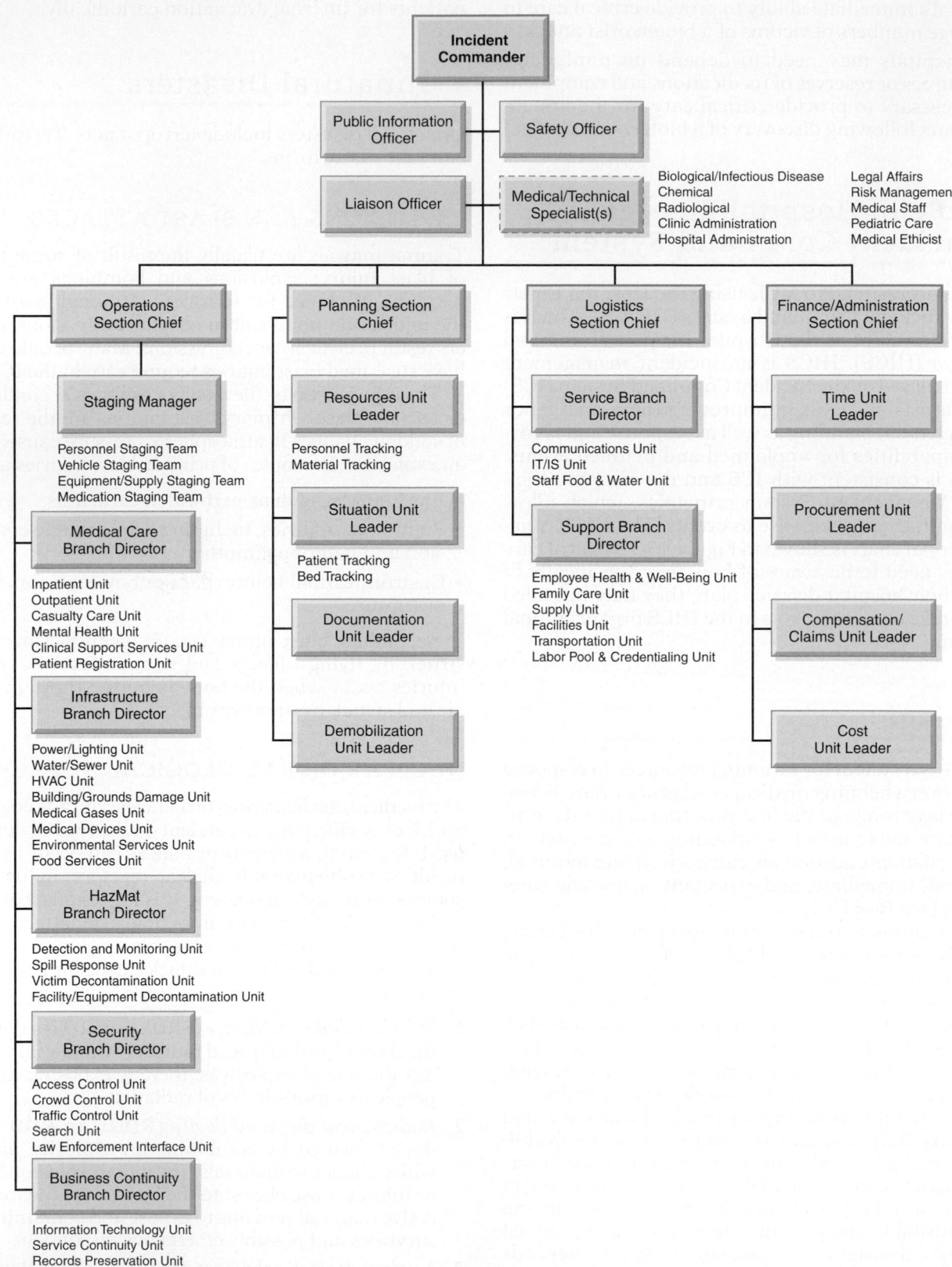

Figure 15-1 • Hospital Incident Command System organizational chart. (From the Hospital Incident Command System Training Manual. Available at: http://www.emsa.ca.gov.)

This type of incident is actually an RDD. Although an IND is unlikely because of the necessary engineering sophistication, a stolen device would generate high levels of radiation.

5. *Nuclear weapon:* This method of exposure could occur if a weapon were stolen. This is another example of a remote radiological attack, but it could happen.[6]

There are two categories of radiation incidents:

1. External exposure is irradiation from a source distant or in close proximity to the body. External irradiation can be divided into *whole-body* exposure or *local* exposure.

2. Contamination is unwanted radioactive material in or on the body.[7]

Based on the type of incident, the response is different. Most external exposures result in irradiation of the victim. Once the person is removed from the source of radiation, the irradiation ceases. A person exposed to external radiation does not become radioactive and poses no hazard to people nearby.

Contamination incidents require an entirely different approach of dealing with the victim. Caregivers and support personnel must be careful not to spread the contamination to uncontaminated parts of the victim's body, to themselves, or to the surrounding area. Internal contamination can result from inhalation, ingestion, direct absorption through the skin, or penetration of radioactive materials through open wounds. Treatment of serious or significant medical conditions should always take precedence over radiological assessment or decontamination of the patient.

After exposure to radiation, acute radiation syndrome (ARS) may develop. If exposure has been minimal and people are strong and healthy, they may not be affected. The factors that determine whether ARS occurs include exposure to high-dose radiation (minimum, 100 cGy) and rate of radiation with whole-body exposure and penetrating-type radiation. The several stages of radiation exposure are listed in Table 15-1.

Management

Treatment of a patient who has sustained a radiological attack is as follows:

1. *Treat and stabilize life-threatening injuries.* It is essential to stabilize the patient and treat life-threatening injuries first. Once that is done, a health care provider with radiological health training should perform a radiological assessment. A Geiger counter can provide radiological measurements.

2. *Prevent and minimize internal contamination.* Time is critical to prevent radioactive uptake. Administration of potassium iodide within 2 hours of contamination prevents radioiodine from accumulating in the thyroid gland (Table 15-2).

3. *Assess internal contamination and decontamination.* This information is covered in the following section on Chemical Attacks. Contaminated patients who are not seriously injured should be decontaminated before treatment.

4. *Contain contamination and decontamination.*

5. *Minimize external contamination to medical personnel.* Staff should wear personal protective clothing. Respirators are necessary if the patient is highly contaminated.

6. *Assess local radiation injuries/burns and flush them if contaminated.*

7. *Follow-up on patients with significant whole-body irradiation or internal contamination.*

8. *Counsel patient and family about the potential about long-term risks/effects.*[8]

CHEMICAL ATTACKS

Chemical warfare agents are hazardous chemicals designed to irritate, incapacitate, injure, or kill.[9] Although several of these agents are used during wartime, many of the most recent uses have been terrorist attacks. For example, the sarin gas attacks

Table 15-1 • Phases of Effects of Radiation Exposure

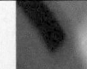

Phase	Time of Occurrence	Signs and Symptoms
Prodromal phase (presenting symptoms)	48–72 h after exposure	Nausea, vomiting, loss of appetite, diarrhea, fatigue High-dose radiation: fever, respiratory distress, increased excitability
Latent phase (a symptom-free period)	After resolution of prodromal phase; can last up to 3 wk With high-dose radiation, latent period is shorter	Decreasing lymphocytes, leukocytes, thrombocytes, red blood cells
Illness phase	After latent period phase	Infection, fluid and electrolyte imbalance, bleeding, diarrhea, shock, and altered level of consciousness
Recovery phase	After illness phase	Can take weeks to months for full recovery
or		
Death	After illness phase	Increased intracranial pressure is a sign of impending death

From Smeltzer SC, Bare BG, Hinkle JL, Cheever KH (eds): Brunner & Suddarth's Textbook of Medical-Surgical Nursing, 11th ed. Philadelphia: Lippincott Williams & Wilkins, 2008, p 2573.

Table 15-2 • Potassium Iodide (KI) Administration

Patient	KI Dose
Adults	130 mg
Women who are breastfeeding	130 mg
Children 3 to 18 years	65 mg
Infants and children 1 month to 3 years	32 mg
Newborns to 1 month	16 mg

From Pediatric Preparedness for Disaster and Terrorism: A Natural Consensus Conference. National Center for Disaster Preparedness Mailman School of Public Health, Columbus University, March 2007.

in Japan in the mid-1990s resulted in few deaths but an overwhelming influx of contaminated patients to medical facilities. Combinations of chemical attacks with explosions and blast attacks are sometimes called "dirty bombs." To have chemical contamination associated with explosions, the victims needs to be in close proximity of the explosion or blast attack.

These chemical agents pose a genuine threat. First, they are readily accessible; for example, tear gas is sold in stores. Second, they are easy to find and easy to transport without being considered unusual; for example, transport of many nerve agents occurs on a daily basis by truck or rail. By the time a chemical attack is completed, the terrorist or criminal can be gone.

These chemicals can be absorbed through the eyes, skin, airways, or a combination of these routes. A summary of the common types of chemical agents, their mechanisms of action, signs and symptoms, and treatment for exposure is listed in Table 15-3.

Types of Chemical Agents

Nerve Agents

Nerve agents are the most toxic of all weaponized military agents. Examples of these agents are tabun, sarin, soman, and VX. Nerve agents inhibit cholinesterase, and they can cause sudden loss of consciousness, seizures, apnea, and death. Diagnosis is usually made on the basis of clinical signs and symptoms.

Vesicants

Vesicants cause blistering. The most common vesicants used are sulfur mustard and lewisite. These agents injure the eyes, skin, airways, and some internal organs. These are most commonly used as a mass casualty weapon because they are potent, difficult to detect, have delayed effect, cause prolonged disability, are stable in storage, can be transported easily, and are inexpensive to produce. They can last in an area for up to 1 week. Some may have an odor of mustard or garlic.

Cyanide

Cyanide is a widely used chemical in the United States. Terrorists use cyanide in confined spaces such as subway cars, shopping centers, convention centers, and small buildings. Shortly after inhaling cyanide, victims may become anxious and hyperventilate. Inhalation of cyanide can cause convulsions, asystole, and death. Antidotes must be administered immediately.

Pulmonary Intoxicants

Pulmonary intoxicants can cause severe life-threatening lung injury after inhalation. The effects are generally delayed for several hours. Examples are phosgene,

Table 15-3 • Common Chemical Agents and Antidotes

Agent	Action	Signs and Symptoms	Decontamination and Treatment
Nerve agents: sarin, soman, organophosphates	Inhibition of cholinesterase	Increased secretions, gastrointestinal motility, diarrhea, bronchospasm	Soap and water Supportive care Benzodiazepine Pralidoxime Atropine
Blood agent: cyanide	Inhibition of aerobic metabolism	Inhalation—tachypnea, tachycardia, coma, seizures; can progress to respiratory arrest, respiratory failure, cardiac arrest, and death	Sodium nitrate Sodium thiocyanate Amyl nitrate Hydroxocobalamin
Vesicant agents: lewisite, sulfur mustard, nitrogen mustard, phosgene	Blistering agents	Superficial to partial-thickness burn with vesicles that coalesce	Soap and water Blot; do not rub dry
Pulmonary agents: phosgene, chlorine, ammonia	Separation of alveoli from capillary bed	Pulmonary edema, bronchospasm	Airway management Ventilatory support Bronchoscopy
Skin and eye irritants: mace (CN), tear gas (CS)	Local reaction to skin and eyes; may cause respiratory difficulties	Tearing of the eyes; burning of the skin; possible respiratory difficulty	Irrigate eyes—water only Soap and water to skin

From Slota M (ed): Core Curriculum for Pediatric Critical Care Nursing. St. Louis: Elsevier, 2006; and Smeltzer SC, Bare BG, Hinkle JL, Cheever KH (eds): Brunner & Suddarth's Textbook of Medical-Surgical Nursing, 11th ed. Philadelphia: Lippincott Williams & Wilkins, 2008, Table 72-3, p 2569.

perfluoroiso-butylene (PFIB), ammonia, and chlorine. In 1984, an industrial accident, not a terrorist attack, involving a pulmonary intoxicant occurred at the Union Carbide plant in Bhopal, India. The released chemicals, such as methyl isocyanate, caused great morbidity and mortality, and to this day, this industrial accident remains one of the worst incidents to occur in India. Pulmonary intoxicants are irritating to the eyes and respiratory tract. These agents can cause severe pulmonary edema of a noncardiac nature. The pathophysiology involves a permeability defect in the alveolar capillary membrane, and there may be a clinical latency period following exposure.

Riot Control Agents

Riot control agents, which have an immediate effect, irritate the eyes, nose, mouth, skin, and respiratory tract. They stimulate tear production by the lacrimal glands. The effect lasts about 30 minutes. Examples of these agents, which are routinely used by police, are chloroacetophenone (CN; Mace), oleoresin capsicum (OC; pepper spray), and chlorobenzylidenemalononitrile (CS; tear gas).[9]

Management

In the event of a chemical exposure, decontamination is necessary. Staff need to be trained to decontaminate patients appropriately and should have access to appropriate personal protective equipment (PPE). With most chemical agents, only a splash-resistant gown much like that used everyday in hospitals and an N95 mask used for respiratory isolation in hospitals are necessary. Some of the more potent chemicals also require a self-contained breathing apparatus and a chemical-resistant suit. People who use these specialty suits and breathing devices should receive training in putting on the suit and have a respiratory evaluation annually.

Hospitals should also have procedures in place to decontaminate patients if necessary; the Joint Commission (formerly the Joint Commission on Accreditation of Healthcare Organizations [JCAHO]) requires that hospitals have such a protocol. Decontamination shelters can either be a room designated at the entrance to the emergency department with the appropriate drainage and shower capability or a trailer; the latter appears to be the most popular one in the United States. Decontamination trailers are advantageous because they are mobile and can be moved to the area designated for decontamination. Decontamination shelters should:

1. Have a water connection. Most are compatible with the facility's water lines.

2. Have the ability to collect and contain large quantities of water.

3. Have something to mix with the water to remove the various chemical agents. Most chemical agents respond to soap and water.

4. Have adequate lighting in the shelter.

5. Have some connection to electricity, whether through the hospital or a generator.

6. Have a conveyor system for nonambulatory patients.

7. Allow for patient privacy.

8. Have room for about two or three personnel. These personnel are preferably not health care providers because all clinical staff will be needed to provide medical care.

9. Have sufficient room for families. It may be necessary to decontaminate parents as well as children. (Parents can also help decontaminate their children.)[10]

Decontamination of children involves some special considerations. Because children may not understand what is happening, they may be uncooperative or even combative. Size may be an issue. Children are lower to the ground, which means that they may be exposed to more of the contaminant. Children have a large surface-to-volume ratio, which places them at higher risk for absorption and exposure to the contaminant. In addition, a smaller dose may be lethal in a smaller person; it is important to decontaminate children as quickly as possible. Children are also at a higher risk for cold stress from a rapid drop in temperature or fever from exposure to very warm temperatures. It is necessary to get them into a neutral thermal environment and out of extreme heat or cold. Finally, whenever possible, it helps to keep the family unit together so that the parents can keep the smaller children safe. If the parents are not present, appropriate arrangements must be made for supervision.

BIOLOGICAL ATTACKS

A biological attack is referred to as bioterrorism or the deliberate release of microorganisms (bacteria, viruses, fungi, or microbial toxins) into a community to produce death, disease, or poisoning.[9] Humans, animals, or plants may be affected. Biological weapons are often called the "poor man's bomb" because they are relatively inexpensive to produce and disseminate. A bioterrorist attack is a real threat, as evidenced by the anthrax attacks of 2001. Letters with anthrax spores arrived by post at some media and legislative offices, closing down many post offices and federal buildings for long periods. The attack resulted in 22 cases of anthrax, 5 deaths, and a nation on high alert.

Many biological substances result in specific signs and symptoms, and every nurse should know the basics of caring for affected patients. In 1999, the Association of Professionals in Infection Control developed a template, the *Bioterrorism Readiness Plan: A Template for Healthcare Facilities*, for hospitals to follow when dealing with bioterrorism.[11] In 2002, this group made some minor modifications to this plan in 2002. Table 15-4 summarizes the diseases associated with bioterrorism and management protocols for victims of biological attacks. Many bioterrorist agents are readily accessible. For example, anthrax can be found on some farms, and terrorists can pick it up and haul it away without being noticed.

Smallpox, a viral disease, is a strong bioterrorism threat because it has a high morbidity in an otherwise healthy population. Figure 15-2 shows the smallpox

Table 15-4 • Diseases Associated With Bioterrorism

Disease	Etiology	Mode of Transmission (Route of Exposure)	Incubation Period	Clinical Features	Treatment	Prophylaxis
Anthrax	*Bacillus anthracis*	Direct contact with bacterium or spores	1 to 7 days	**Cutaneous:** itchy papular lesions that turn into vesicles and within 2 to 6 days form black eschar; lesions most often seen on head, chest, and forearms	Antibiotic therapy **Adults:** ciprofloxacin, 500 twice daily, or doxycycline, 100 mg twice daily for at least 60 days **Children:** ciprofloxacin, 15 mg/kg twice daily, or doxycycline: >8 yr & <45 kg: 100 mg twice daily >8 yr & ≤45 kg: 2.2 mg/kg twice daily ≤8 yr: 2.2 mg/kg twice daily	None
		Inhalation of spores	2 to 60 days	**Pulmonary:** nonspecific flu-like symptoms followed by the abrupt onset of respiratory failure (2 to 4 days after initial symptoms) and hemodynamic collapse	**Adults:** ciprofloxacin, 400 mg q12h *and* one or two additional microbials; switch to oral when appropriate. Ciprofloxacin, 50 mg, or doxycycline, 100 mg twice daily **Children:** Ciprofloxacin, 10 mg/kg q12h *or* doxycycline, same as for cutaneous except q12h instead of twice daily Switch to oral therapy when appropriate.	
		Ingestion of contaminated food, usually meat	1 to 7 days	**Gastrointestinal:** abdominal pain, nausea, fever, hematemesis, and bloody diarrhea		
Smallpox	Variola virus	Airborne	7 to 17 days (average, 12 days)	Nonspecific flu-like symptoms, fever, myalgia, skin lesions that progress from macules to papules to vesicles and then scab over in 1 to 2 wk	Supportive care, after 3 days can try variola immune globulin, negative isolation	Vaccination before exposure or within 3 days of exposure

Disease	Agent	Transmission	Incubation	Symptoms	Treatment	Prophylaxis
Plague	Yersinia pestis	Flea-borne (bubonic plague), airborne (pneumonic plague)	2 to 8 days (flea-borne); 1 to 2 days (airborne)	Fever, cough, chest pain, hemoptysis, mucopurulent or watery sputum with gram-negative rods on Gram stain, bronchopneumonia on x-ray	Streptomycin, 1 gm IM twice daily, or gentamycin, 5 mg/kg IM or IV daily, or 3 mg/kg loading dose followed by 1.7 mg/kg IM or IV three times a day; droplet precautions in effect until patient has completed 72 h of antimicrobial therapy	Doxycycline, 100 mg PO twice daily, or ciprofloxacin, 500 mg PO twice daily
Tularemia	Francisella tularensis	Contact with infected animals (rabbits, deer) or vectors (fleas, ticks, mosquitos); airborne	2 to 14 days	Fever, chills, headache, muscle pain, nonproductive cough, pneumonia; regional lymphadenopathy if ingested	Same as for plague	Same as for plague
Botulism	Clostridium botulinum	Foodborne (most common); airborne	**Foodborne:** 12 to 36 h **Airborne:** 24 to 72 h	Gastrointestinal symptoms, drooping eyelids, jaw clench, difficulty swallowing or speaking, descending paralysis, blurred vision, no sensory deficits	Supportive care; antitoxin may halt progression of symptoms but is unlikely to reverse them	None
Viral hemorrhagic fevers	Diverse group of viruses (e.g., Ebola virus, yellow fever)	Variable, may be person-to-person, via flea or animal bite; or airborne	2 to 22 days	Variable; usually a nonspecific illness lasting less than 1 wk with high fever and headache followed by flushing maculopapular rash and conjunctival infection, progressing to diffuse hemorrhagic disease and multiorgan system failure	Supportive care, ribavirin may be helpful in some cases	None

Data from Los Angeles County EMS and Public Health Agencies: Terrorism Agent Information and Treatment Guidelines for Clinicians and Hospitals, 2003.

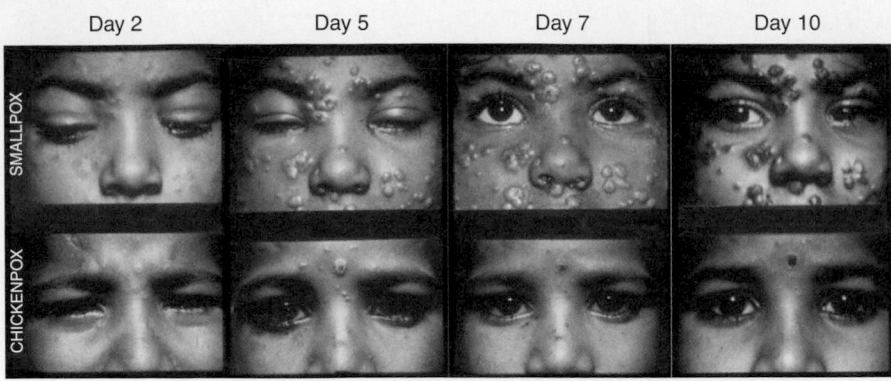

Day 2   Day 5   Day 7   Day 10

SMALLPOX

CHICKENPOX

Figure 15-2 • Progression of smallpox rash. (From World Health Organization: WHO slide set on the diagnosis of smallpox, 2001. Reproduced by permission of the World Health Organization.)

rash. In 1980, the World Health Organization declared smallpox eradicated.[9] In 2003, a smallpox vaccine became available for health care workers, but the U.S. Food and Drug Administration recalled it, and few people received the vaccine because of issues related to the exclusion criteria and the occurrence of some cardiac problems after administration of the vaccine.

Plague has a negative connotation because people still remember references to biblical times and deaths caused by bubonic plague. Animals that live in city parks and campgrounds still carry the bacteria that cause plague. Squirrels and other rodents usually carry them, and if infected animals bite humans, they can become ill.

Botulism still occurs today in developed countries. A person can contract the disease from eating food that has been infected with the botulism toxin. Treatment is available. Children who develop infantile botulism can take an antidote, commonly known as "Baby Big," if the disease is diagnosed early and verified by a laboratory approved by the Centers for Disease Control and Prevention. At the time of diagnosis, the local health department sells the hospital the necessary dosage. The main issue is that the botulism is not always diagnosed promptly enough.

One of the more common viral hemorrhagic fevers is the Ebola virus. This virus is found more commonly in Third World countries. It is treatable but does carry a negative connotation.

• Natural Disasters

A natural disaster is a result of the combination of a natural event (e.g., earthquake, extreme heat, flood, hurricane, landslide, tornado, tsunami, volcanic eruption, wildfire, winter storm) and human involvement. By definition, a natural disaster does not occur without human involvement; therefore, an earthquake that destroys an uninhabited island is technically not a natural disaster. Another important feature of a natural disaster is the notion that an unprepared or ill-prepared population is vulnerable, and therefore, a lack of preparation amplifies the unfortunate outcomes as result of a natural disaster.

Hospitals and other health care facilities play a unique role in the community because these facilities already contain an unhealthy, weak population and yet are expected to receive casualties resulting from disasters. Therefore, hospital personnel and administrators must actively prepare for any event that threatens the structure, function, and recovery of their organization and practice the appropriate responses to a hazardous event.

Some experts even consider pandemic influenza a potential natural disaster; they suggest that it is a real possibility. Public health experts are concerned that a pandemic arising from the current epidemic of avian influenza will interact with the common strain of human influenza, causing a mutation that would create a virus capable of human-to-human transmission, initiating a pandemic.[12] With most of the population potentially at risk, corporate businesses as well as the health care industry are working together to plan for this problem. Public health officials are trying to determine just when this might happen. Nurses are critical to the disaster response because they have direct patient care roles and will be present if an unforeseen event arises.

• Psychological Effects of Terrorism

It is natural to be fearful during and after a major disaster, whether or not it is a terrorist incident. People exhibit various responses to stress and stressful events such as a terrorist attack or a major natural disaster. The responses include fear, grief, and deep sadness. People may complain that they feel "sick to their stomach" and have no appetite. Their sleep pattern and conduct in daily activities may change. Several weeks to months may pass before they feel normal and stable again.

In severe cases, the psychological stress remains months after the event. Multiple factors affect how people respond. The perception of numerous losses generally has a negative impact and may be related inversely to disaster recovery. Research has found that when there are large numbers of deaths and high levels of symptoms, the presence of long-term psychiatric disorders may be quite high.[13] These people should undergo screening for post-traumatic stress disorder (PTSD). PTSD is an intense emotional and physical response to thoughts and reminders of the event that last for many weeks or months after the traumatic event. Victims of PTSD may complain of nightmares, flashbacks, and severe emotional and physical reactions to thoughts of the event.

• Clinical Applicability Challenges

Case Study

A news bulletin interrupts the local TV programming; reporters say that a mass shooting has occurred at a local elementary school. The shooter or shooters have escaped, and their whereabouts are unknown. The nursing supervisor calls the pediatric intensive care unit (ICU) and reports that the hospital may receive up to 30 patients initially and 15 transfers in the next 24 hours. The casualties arrive, and the first 10 appear to have minor flesh wounds. The next two patients need surgery, and the trauma team rushes them urgently to the operating room for emergency thoracotomies. Five other patients arrive with obvious penetrating abdominal injuries. The hospital incident commander later reports that one child died in the operating room and that one required a pneumonectomy.

1. You are the critical care nurse in charge of the pediatric ICU. What responsibilities might you have in this situation?

2. The house supervisor reports that the remaining casualties will need floor beds. The second wave of arrivals is imminent. As the critical care nurse in charge of the pediatric ICU, what should you do?

3. The second patient in the operating room dies. The 14-bed pediatric ICU is at full capacity. The labor pool calls to see if the pediatric ICU has extra staff to send to the emergency room for help with the second wave of patients. You are the critical care nurse in charge. What should you do?

Review Questions

1. Critical care nurses must be aware of what to do in a mass casualty incident (MCI) because
   a. the triage of critically ill patients is important, and first responders and the public health team may be overwhelmed.
   b. critical care nurses must have sufficient knowledge and skill to recognize the potential for an MCI, identify when such an incident may have occurred, know how to protect themselves, know how to provide immediate care for those involved, recognize their own limitations, and know where to seek additional information and resources.
   c. Red Cross does not play a role in an MCI.
   d. patients do not go to the emergency department but directly to the intensive care unit.

2. The most important treatment for a radiological attack is to
   a. treat and stabilize life-threatening injuries.
   b. administer potassium iodide.
   c. contain the contamination and decontaminate the victim.
   d. counsel the patient and family about potential for long-term risks and effects.

3. The potassium iodide dose for an adult is
   a. 130 mg.
   b. 65 mg.
   c. 32 mg.
   d. 16 mg.

4. An antidote for the chemical weapon ammonia is
   a. not required; only supportive care is needed.
   b. atropine.
   c. methemoglobin.
   d. bronchodilators.

5. The initial therapy for inhalation anthrax is
   a. ciprofloxacin, 500 mg q12h.
   b. doxycycline, 50 mg q12h.
   c. ciprofloxacin, 400 mg q12h.
   d. doxycycline, 10 to 15 mg q12h.

References

1. Stanley J: Disaster competency development and integration in nursing education. Nurs Clin North Am 40(3):453–467, 2005
2. Available at: http://www.bioterrorism.slu.edu
3. American Association of Critical Care Nurses: Statement of commitment on mass casualty and bioterrorism preparedness. Available at: http://www.aacn.org
4. General Accounting Office (GAO): Report to the Congressional Committees. Hospital preparedness: Most urban hospitals have emergency plans, but lack certain capacities for bioterrorism response. GAO-03:924, Aug 2003
5. Rubinson L, Nuzzo J, Talmor D, et al: Augmentation of hospital critical care capacity after bioterrorist attacks or epidemics: Recommendations of the Working Group in Emergency Mass Critical Care. Crit Care Med 33(10):E1–E13, 2005
6. American College of Radiology: ACR Disaster Planning Task Force—2002. Disaster Preparedness for Radiology Professional Response to Radiological Terrorism, Version 2.0.
7. American College of Radiology: ACR Disaster Planning Task Force—2002.
8. Linnemann RE: Managing Radiation Medical Emergencies. Philadelphia: Radiation Management Consultants, 2001
9. Los Angeles County EMS and Public Health Agencies: Terrorism Agent Information and Treatment Guidelines for Clinicians and Hospitals, 2003
10. Hudson T, Reilly K, Dulagh J: Considerations for chemical decontamination shelters. Disaster Management and Response 1(4):110–113, 2003
11. Association for Professionals in Infection Control and Epidemiology (APIC) and Centers for Disease Control and Prevention (CDC): Chemical-biological readiness plan: A template for healthcare facilities. ED Manag 11:1–16, 1999
12. Available at: http://.www.ca.dhs.gov/ps/dcdc/izgroup/pdf/pandemic.pdf
13. Mitchell AM, Sakraida TJ, Zalice KK: Disaster care: psychological considerations. Nurs Clin North Am 40(3):535–550, 2005

Other Selected Readings

Association for Professionals in Infection Control and Epidemiology (APIC) Bioterrorism Taskforce and Centers for Disease Control and Prevention (CDC) Hospital Infectious Program

Bioterrorism Working Group: Bioterrorism Readiness Plan: A Template for Healthcare Facilities, 2002

Bernardo LM, Kapsen P: Pediatric implications in bioterrorism: Education for healthcare providers. Disaster Management and Response 1(2):52–54, 2003

Boatright C, McGlown KJ: Homeland security challenges in nursing practice. Nurs Clin North Am 40:481–497, 2005

Bond E, Beaton R: Disaster nursing curriculum development based on vulnerability assessment in the Pacific Northwest. Nurs Clin North Am 40:441–451, 2—5

Boren D, Forbus R, Bibeau P, et al: Managing critical care casualties on the Navy's hospital ships. Crit Care Nurs Clin North Am 15(2):183–191, 2003

Bresnitz EA, DiFerdinando GT: Lessons from the anthrax attacks of 2001: The New Jersey Experience. Clin Occup Environ Med 2(2):227–252, 2002

Bridges EJ: Blast injuries: From triage to critical care. Crit Care Nurs Clin North Am 18(3):333–348, 2006

Burkle FM: Mass casualty management of a large-scale bioterrorist event: An epidemiological approach that shapes triage decisions. Emerg Med Clin North Am 20(2):409–436, 2002

Burklow T, Yu C, Madsen J: Industrial chemicals: Terrorism weapons of opportunity. Pediatr Ann 32(4):230–234, 2003

Chafee MW: Hospital response to acute onset disasters: The state of the science in 2005. Nurs Clin North Am 40:565–577, 2005

Christopher GW, Cieslak T, Pavlin JA, Eitzen EM Jr: Biological warfare: A historical perspective. JAMA 278:412–422, 1997

Cieslak T, Henretig F: Ring-a-ring-a-roses: Bioterrorism and its particular relevance to pediatrics. Pediatrics 15:107–111, 2003

Cieslak T, Henretig F: Bioterrorism. Pediatr Ann 32(3):154–165, 2003

Cox E, Briggs S: Disaster nursing: New frontiers for critical care. Crit Care Nurse 24(3):16–22, 2004

Dara SI, Ashton RW, Farmer JC: Engendering enthusiasm for sustainable disaster critical care response: Why this is of consequence to critical care professionals? Crit Care 9(1):125–127, 2005

Department of Health and Human Services, Office of Inspector General State of California: Review of Public Health Preparedness and Response for Bioterrorism Program Funds. A-09-02-1007, Aug 2003

Flowers LK, Mothershead JL, Blackwell TH: Bioterrorism preparedness II: The community and emergency medical services systems. Emerg Med Clin North Am 20(2):457–476, 2002

Jurkovich T: September 11th—the Pentagon disaster: Response and lessons learned. Crit Care Nurs Clin North Am 15(2):143–148, 2003

Karwa M, Bronzert P, Kvetan V: Bioterrorism and critical care. Crit Care Clin 19(2):279–313, 2003

Koenig KL, Kahn CA, Schultz CH: Medical strategies to handle mass casualties from the use of biological weapons. Clin Lab Med 26(2):313–327, 2006

Marklund LA: Patient care in a biological safety level-4 (BSL-4) environment. Crit Care Nurs Clin North Am 15:245–255, 2003

Mothershead JL, Tonat K, Koenig KL: Bioterrorism preparedness III: State and federal programs and response. Emerg Med Clin North Am 20(2):477–500, 2002

Newberry L (ed): Sheehy's Emergency Nursing: Principles and Practice, 5th ed. St. Louis: Mosby, 2003

Robinson L, Nuzzo J, Talmor DS, et al: Augmentation of hospital critical care capacity after bioterrorist attacks or epidemics: Recommendations of the Working Group on Emergency Mass Critical Care. Crit Care Med 33(10):E1–E13, 2005

Rotenberg J: Diagnosis and management of nerve agent exposure. Pediatr Ann 32(4):242–250, 2003

Rotenberg J: Cyanide as a weapon of terror. Pediatr Ann 32(4): 236–240, 2003

Rotenberg J, Burklow T, Selancho J: Weapons of mass destruction: The decontamination of children. Pediatr Ann 32(2):98–105, 2003

Schultz CH, Mothershead JL, Field M: Bioterrorism preparedness I: The emergency department and hospital. Emerg Med Clin North Am 20(2):437–455, 2002

Shatz DV, Wolcott K, Fairburn JB: Response to hurricane disasters. Surg Clin North Am 86(3):545–555, 2006

Slota M (ed): Core Curriculum for Pediatric Critical Care Nursing. St. Louis: Elsevier, 2006

Terrorism, mass casualty, and disaster nursing. In Smeltzer SC, Bare BG, Hinkle JL, Cheever KH (eds): Brunner & Suddarth's Textbook of Medical-Surgical Nursing, 11th ed. Philadelphia: Lippincott Williams & Wilkins, 2008

Tasota F, Henker R, Hoffman L: Anthrax as a biological weapon: An old disease that poses a new threat. Crit Care Nurse 22(5):21–35, 2002

U.S. Department of Justice: Emergency Response Guidebook for Weapons of Mass Destruction Incidents, 2001

Veenema, TG (ed): Disaster Nursing and Emergency Preparedness for Chemical, Biological and Radiologic Terrorism and Other Hazards. New York: Springer, 2003

Waeckerle JF: Domestic preparedness for events involving weapons of mass destruction. JAMA 283(2):252–254, 2000

Weiner E: A national curriculum for nurses in emergency preparedness and response. Nurs Clin North Am 40:469–479, 2005

Wheeler D, Poss WB: Mass casualty management in a changing world. Pediatr Ann 32(2):98–105, 2003

Yu C: Medical response to radiation-related terrorism. Pediatr Ann 32(3):169–176, 2003

Yu C, Burklow T, Madsen J: Vesicant agents and children. Pediatr Ann 32(4):254–257, 2003

Cardiovascular System

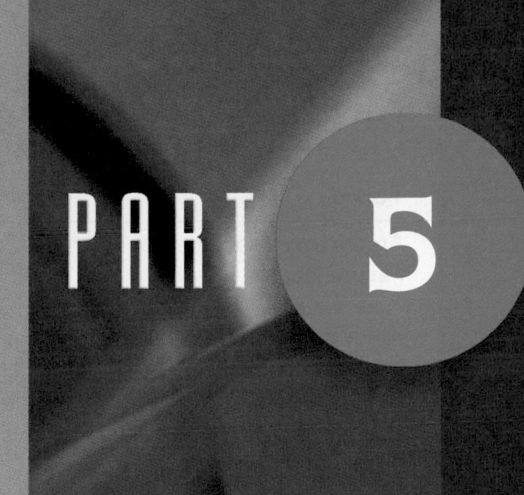

INTERNET RESOURCES

Topic	Web Page Address
American Association of Heart Failure Nurses	www.aahfn.org
American College of Cardiology	www.acc.org/
American College of Chest Physicians	www.chestnet.org
American Heart Association	www.americanheart.org
Angioplasty Website	www.ptca.org
Cardiology Resource	www.theheart.org
Cleveland Clinic	www.clevelandclinic.org
European Association for Cardio-Thoracic Surgery	www.eacts.org
Guidelines resource	www.guidelines.gov
Heart Failure Society of America	www.hfsa.org/
Heart Rhythm Society	http://www.hrsonline.org
Mayo Health Clinic	www.mayohealth.org
Medtronic Corporation (Medical Technology)	www.medtronic.com
National Heart, Lung and Blood Institute	www.nhlbi.nih.gov/
National Institute of Health	www.nih.gov
PharmWeb	www.pharmweb.net
RxList–The Internet Drug Index	www.rxlist.com
Society of Critical Care Medicine	www.sccm.org
Society of Thoracic Surgeons	www.sts.org
Society of Vascular Nursing	www.svnnet.org
St. Jude Medical (Medical Technology)	www.sjm.com
Transcatheter Cardiovascular Therapeutics	www.tctmd.com
United States Food and Drug Administration	www.fda.gov
Virtual Library Pharmacy	www.pharmacy.org
Women's Heart Foundation	www.womensheart.org

Anatomy and Physiology of the Cardiovascular System

Patricia Gonce Morton

Objectives

Based on the content in this chapter, the reader should be able to:

❶ Briefly describe the characteristics of cardiac muscle cells.

❷ Differentiate the electrical events from the mechanical events in the heart.

❸ Explain depolarization and repolarization.

❹ Describe the normal conduction system of the heart.

❺ State the formula for calculating cardiac output.

❻ Compare and contrast the role of the parasympathetic and sympathetic nervous systems in the regulation of heart rate.

❼ Explain the three factors involved in the regulation of stroke volume.

❽ Describe the coronary artery blood source for the cardiac chambers and conduction system.

❾ Explain the influence of blood volume and blood pressure on peripheral circulation.

During the 70 years in the life of the average person, the heart will pump approximately 5 quarts of blood a minute, 75 gallons an hour, 57 barrels a day, and 1.5 million barrels in a lifetime. Although the work accomplished by this organ is out of proportion to its size, for most people, the heart functions normally throughout the life span. The pumping action of the heart moves blood, a vital substance, throughout the body, supplying oxygen and nutrients to cells and removing waste. Without this action, cells die. For people in whom cardiac problems develop, the results may be dramatic and the outcome drastic. This chapter reviews the principles of cardiovascular anatomy and physiology.

• Cardiac Microstructure

Microscopically, cardiac muscle contains visible stripes, or striations, similar to those found in skeletal muscle (Fig. 16-1). The ultrastructural pattern also resembles that of striated muscle. The cells branch and connect freely and form a three-dimensional, complex network. The elongated nuclei, like those of smooth muscle, are found deep in the interior of the cells and not next to the cell membrane as they are in striated muscle.

Cardiac muscle (myocardial) cells are endowed with extraordinary characteristics, most of which belong to the cell membrane or sarcolemma. To

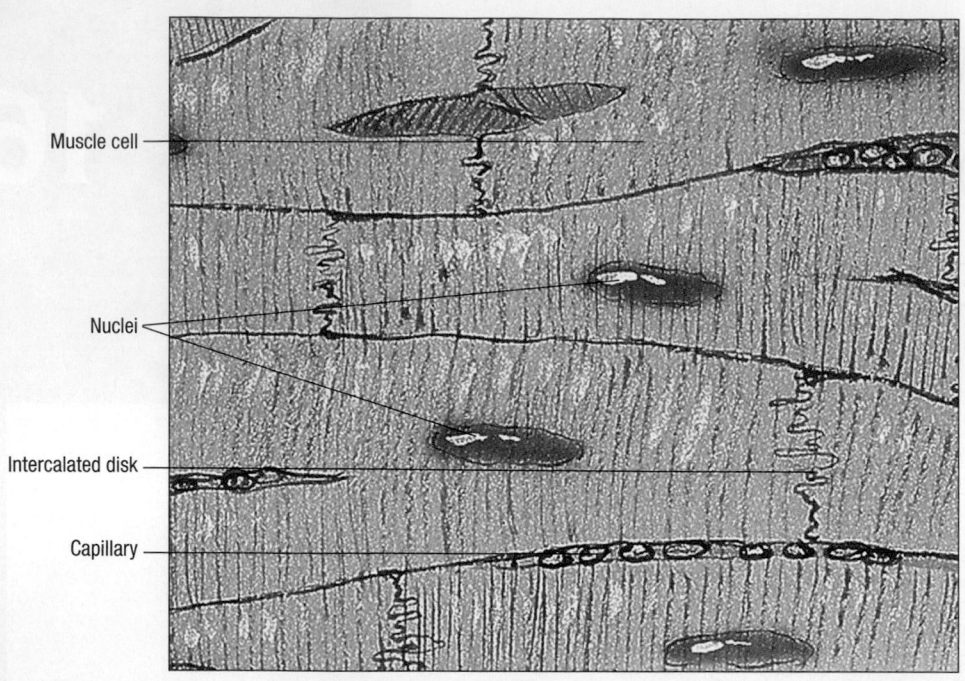

Muscle cell

Nuclei

Intercalated disk

Capillary

Figure 16-1 • Cardiac muscle fibers, showing the branching structure and intercalated disks. (From Anatomical Chart Company: Atlas of Human Anatomy. Springhouse, PA: Springhouse, 2001, p 167.)

pump effectively, the heart muscle must begin contraction as a single unit. To contract myocardial cells simultaneously, cell membranes must depolarize at the same time. The heart does this, without using much neural tissue, by rapidly conducting impulses from cell to cell through intercalated disks. At each end of every myocardial cell, adjacent cell membranes are folded elaborately and attached strongly. These areas comprise the intercalated disks, where depolarization is conducted extremely rapidly from one cell to the next[1] (see Fig. 16-1).

Another extraordinary characteristic of myocardial cells, seen mainly in cell membranes, is automaticity. Selected groups of cardiac cells are capable of initiating rhythmic action potentials, and thus waves of contraction, without any outside humoral or nervous intervention. Automaticity and other terms used to describe cardiac tissue functions are listed in Box 16-1.

Within each cardiac cell lie thousands of contractile elements, the overlapping actin and myosin filaments. Figure 16-2 illustrates these elements and the changes seen during diastole and systole. Not shown are the many cross-bridges that extend like rows of oars from the surface of the thicker myosin filaments. During diastole, these bridges are unattached to other filaments. The arrangement of actin and myosin filaments gives cardiac muscle its banded or striated appearance. One grouping of actin and myosin filaments is called a *sarcomere*.

• Mechanical Events of Contraction

Before mechanical contraction, an action potential travels quickly over each cell membrane and down into each cell's sarcoplasmic reticulum. When an action potential causes depolarization of the sarcoplasmic reticulum, calcium ions move from the sarcoplasmic reticulum into the myocardial cell cytoplasm and bind to troponin molecules on actin filaments. Calcium-bound troponin moves slightly to uncover binding sites on the actin, to which myosin filaments then attach. With a release of energy stored in adenosine triphosphate (ATP), these binding sites move so that actin and myosin slide past each other and new couplings between actin and myosin occur. Rapid, successive uncoupling of cross-bridges and their reattachment to new actin-binding sites lead to rapid and dramatic shortening of the sarcomere (see Fig. 16-2). This shortening is the essence of myocardial contraction (systole). Contraction ceases when the calcium ions return to their storage sites on the sarcoplasmic reticulum, thereby causing the binding sites on the actin filaments to be covered again. The

Box 16-1 • Terms Used to Describe Cardiac Tissue Function

Automaticity: the ability of specialized cells in the heart known as pacemaker cells to spontaneously generate an action potential, thus causing depolarization

Conductivity: the ability of cardiac cells to conduct action potentials, thus transmitting the electrical signal from one cell to another

Contractility: the ability of cardiac muscle to shorten in response to depolarization

Excitability: the ability of cardiac tissue to respond to a stimulus and generate an action potential

Rhythmicity: the ability of cardiac cells to spontaneously generate an action potential at a regular rate

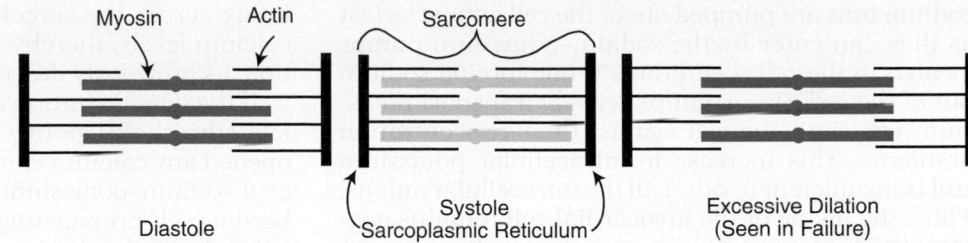

Figure 16-2 • Contractile elements lying inside a single sarcomere of a myocardial cell.

separated actin and myosin filaments then slip past each other in the reverse direction, lengthening the sarcomere to its relaxed state.

Contraction requires calcium and energy. The presence of adequate ATP stores and the movement of calcium provide the essential link between the electrical events of depolarization and the mechanical events of contraction in the heart.

• Electrical Events of Depolarization

Membranes of all the cells in the human body are charged; that is, they are polarized and therefore have electrical potentials. The charges are separated at the membrane. In humans, all cell membranes, regardless of type, are positively charged at rest, with more positively charged particles at the outer surface of the cell membrane than at the inner surface. Figure 16-3A illustrates this "resting stage."

In the depolarized state, the cell membrane is negatively charged, with more negatively charged particles at the outer surface of the cell membrane than at the inner surface. Figure 16-3B illustrates this "depolarized stage." *Excitability* is the term used to describe the ability of a cell to depolarize in response to a given stimulus.

Cardiac muscle membranes are polarized, and the electrical potential can be measured, as it can in any of the cells in the human body. The potential results from the difference between intracellular and extracellular concentrations of electrolytes. When salt compounds of various elements are dissolved in aqueous solutions, they dissociate into their charged particles, called *ions*.

In the resting myocardial cell, there are more potassium ions inside than outside the cell and more

sodium and unbound calcium ions outside than inside the cell. All three of these positively charged ions (cations) may diffuse through pores, or channels, in the cell membrane. If each ion freely obeyed the law of diffusion, however, potassium would diffuse out of the cell, whereas sodium and calcium would diffuse into it. Very soon there would be equal concentrations of each ion between the intracellular and extracellular fluids, and no resting potential would exist. It is through selective regulation of the concentrations of these ions on either side of the membrane that the resting membrane potential is maintained. Several factors contribute to this regulation. The first factor is the presence of sodium–potassium "pumps" in the cell membrane. These pumps move sodium out of the cell and potassium into the cell, with both movements occurring against the concentration gradients for each of these ions. The second factor is the active movement of calcium out of the cell against the concentration gradient in response to the passive diffusion of sodium into the cell. The third factor is the regulation of membrane channels, whereby calcium ions can enter the resting myocardial cell. The fourth factor is the presence of intracellular anions (negatively charged particles) that are too large to exit from the cell.

• Physiological Basis of the Resting Potential

The cardiac cell contains large anions that cannot exit the cell. These anions attract sodium and potassium cations, which diffuse through membrane channels into the cell. The anions would attract the calcium cation also, except that the membrane channels for the entry of this ion are closed when the cell is at rest. The potassium ions remain within the cell, but the

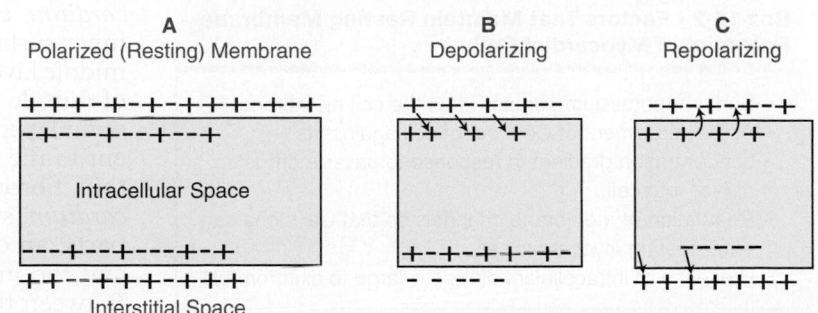

A Polarized (Resting) Membrane

B Depolarizing

C Repolarizing

Intracellular Space

Interstitial Space

Figure 16-3 • Electrical events at rest (diastolic) and preceding contraction (systolic).

sodium ions are pumped out of the cell almost as fast as they can enter by the sodium–potassium pumps located in the cell membrane. While forcing sodium out of the cell, these pumps actively transport potassium ions into the cell against their concentration gradients. This increase in intracellular potassium still is insufficient to offset all the intracellular anions. Thus, the inside of the myocardial cell remains negative with respect to the outside—as long as the pumps are operative. As a result, the resting potential is approximately –80 mV. For each molecule of an ion pumped from the cell, one molecule of ATP is required to provide the energy necessary to effect the chemical bond between ion and carrier. Maintaining a resting potential thus requires energy. Factors that maintain resting membrane potential of myocardial cells are listed in Box 16-2.

• Physiological Basis of the Action Potential

When a stimulus is applied to the polarized cell membrane, the membrane that ordinarily is only slightly permeable to sodium permits sodium ions to diffuse rapidly into the cell. This rapid diffusion occurs because of inactivation of the sodium active transport enzymes (pumps). The result is a reversal of net charges. The outer surface is now more negative than positive, and the membrane is said to be depolarized (see Fig. 16-3B).

When the sodium influx changes the polarity from –80 mV to approximately –35 mV, the electrical change opens the previously closed "calcium channels" in the myocardial cell membrane. Once opened, these channels permit the influx of calcium. The entry of this cation, together with the continued entry of sodium, is responsible for the remainder of the depolarization, which continues until the polarity of the extracellular side equals approximately +30 mV. Such a maximal depolarization inactivates sodium–potassium pumps in nearby membranes. This can cause depolarization in these areas. When the original depolarization becomes self-propagating in this way, it is termed an *action potential*. In a myocardial cell, an action potential triggers the release of intracellular calcium from its storage sites on the sarcoplasmic reticulum. This release plus the calcium

influx across the sarcolemma elevates intracellular calcium levels, thereby initiating muscular contraction, as previously described.[2]

If the depolarization remains below a certain critical (threshold) point, it dies out without having opened any calcium channel or inactivated any adjacent sodium–potassium pumps. Because it does not become self-propagating and remains localized, such a depolarization is termed a *local depolarization*.

During depolarization, the elevated intracellular sodium concentration frees potassium ions to diffuse out of the cell in accordance with their concentration gradient. Just as this potassium efflux gains some momentum, however, the sodium–potassium pumps automatically reactivate (they can be inactivated only temporarily). Once reactivated, the pumps begin to restore the original resting potential, a process termed *repolarization* (see Fig. 16-3C). During the initial phase of repolarization, the efflux of potassium and sodium ions exceeds their influx; but as the intracellular sodium ions are removed from the cell, potassium ions remain as the major cation to be electrostatically held within the cell by the intracellular anions. This halts the potassium efflux. The remainder of repolarization consists of pump activity that increases intracellular potassium and decreases intracellular sodium; thus, the resting potential is reestablished. The electrical events at the start of repolarization also reclose the calcium entry channels, thereby halting calcium influx. Intracellular calcium levels are reduced when the diffusion of sodium into the cell causes a movement of calcium out of the cell against the latter's concentration gradient.[2] The phases of the action potential are shown in Figure 16-4.

• Cardiac Macrostructure

The heart is about the size of a clenched fist and lies in the chest between the lungs in the mediastinal space of the intrathoracic cavity. The right side of the heart is almost entirely in front of the left side of the heart, and the right ventricle occupies most of the anterior cardiac surface (Fig. 16-5). Only a small portion of the left ventricle is in the frontal plane of the heart. The left ventricle forms the left lateral margin of the heart with a tapered inferior tip that is often termed the *cardiac apex*.[3]

The heart is made up four layers: the endocardium, the myocardium, the epicardium, and the pericardium. The inner layer, known as the *endocardium*, consists of endothelial tissue that lines the inner surface of the heart and the cardiac valves. The middle layer, known as the *myocardium*, is composed of muscle fibers that enable the heart to pump. The outer layer, known as the *epicardium*, is tightly adherent to the heart and the base of the great vessels. A thin, fibrous, double-layered sac, known as the *pericardium*, surrounds the heart. This structure has two parts: an outer layer called the *parietal pericardium* and the inner layer called the *visceral pericardium*. Between these two layers is a small amount of peri-

---

Box 16-2 • Factors That Maintain Resting Membrane Potential of Myocardial Cell

- Sodium–potassium pumps within the cell membrane
- Active movement of Ca^{2+} out of cell against its concentration gradient in response to passive diffusion of Na^+ into cell
- Regulation of membrane channels so that Ca^{2+} ions can enter resting myocardial cell
- Presence of intracellular anions too large to exit from cell

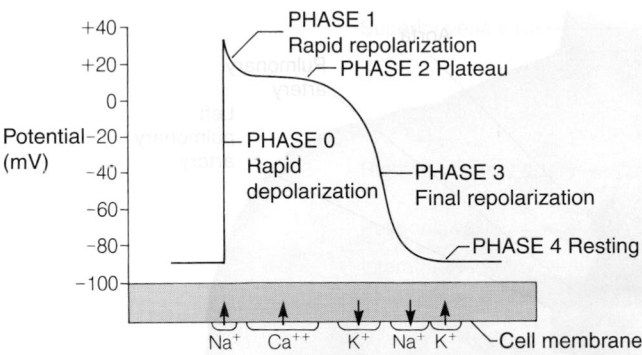

Figure 16-4 • Cardiac action potential. Phase 0 is the rapid depolarization phase. During this phase, the fast sodium channels in the cell membranes are stimulated to open, resulting in the rapid influx of sodium. Contraction of the myocardium follows depolarization. Phase 1 is the rapid repolarization phase and occurs at the peak of the action potential. This phase indicates the inactivation of the fast sodium channels with an abrupt decrease in sodium permeability. Phase 2 represents the plateau of the action potential. During this phase, potassium permeability is low, allowing the membrane to remain depolarized throughout phase 2. The influx of calcium that occurs during the plateau phase is much slower than that of sodium and lasts for a longer time. Phase 3 is the final repolarization phase and begins with the downslope of the action potential curve. During this phase, the influx of calcium and sodium ends, and there is a rapid outward movement of potassium. By the end of phase 3, sodium and potassium return to their normal resting state. Phase 4 is the resting membrane potential and corresponds to diastole. During this phase, the sodium–potassium pump is activated, resulting in the active transport of sodium out of the cell, and potassium is moved back into the cell. The *arrows* below the diagram indicate the approximate time and direction of movement of each ion influencing membrane potential. The phase of calcium moving out of the cell is not well defined but is thought to occur during phase 4.

cardial fluid (30 to 50 mL) that serves as a lubricant between the two layers.[1]

The heart consists of four chambers: right and left atria, and right and left ventricles. The atria are smaller, thinner-walled, low-pressure chambers. Approximately 30% of blood flow to the ventricles is the result of atrial contraction, also known as *atrial kick*. The remaining 70% of blood that reaches the ventricles is the result of pressure differences between the atria and the ventricles. The ventricles are larger, higher-pressure chambers with thicker walls than the atria. The walls of the left ventricle are thicker than the right ventricle because the left ventricle must generate a large amount of force to eject blood into the aorta. Deoxygenated blood enters the right atrium from the superior and inferior venae cavae. The blood passes through the tricuspid valve into the right ventricle, which then pumps the blood through the pulmonic valve into the pulmonary circulation. After gas exchange in the lungs, oxygenated blood returns to the left atrium, passes through the mitral valve, enters the left ventricle, passes through the aortic valve, and finally enters the aorta (Fig. 16-6).

The cardiac valves are composed of fibrous tissue and allow blood to flow in one direction. The valves open and close as a result of blood flow and pressure differences. The tricuspid and mitral valves are known as the *atrioventricular (AV) valves* because they are located between the atria and the ventricles. The chordae tendineae and the papillary muscles attach to the AV valves and help maintain closure and prevent eversion of the valve leaflets during ventricular contraction so that blood does not move into the atria. The pulmonic and aortic valves are known as the *semilunar valves* because each has three leaflets shaped like half-moons.

• Cardiac Conduction

To pump effectively, large portions of cardiac muscle must receive an action potential nearly simultaneously. Special cells that conduct action potentials extremely rapidly are arranged in pathways through the heart. All these cells have automaticity (see Box 16-2).

The heart chambers and specialized tissues are diagrammed in Figure 16-7. The sinoatrial (SA) node is located between the opening of the inferior and superior venae cavae in the right atrial wall. The cells of the SA node have the property of automaticity. Because the SA node normally discharges faster than any other heart cell with automaticity (60 to 100 beats/minute), this specialized tissue acts as a normal cardiac pacemaker. Atrial action potentials travel through atrial cells by intercalated disks, although some specialized conductive tissue in the atria has been discovered.

In the lower right portion of the interatrial septum is the AV node, also known as the AV junction. This tissue conducts, yet delays, the atrial action potential before it travels to the ventricles. Action potentials reach the AV node at different times. The AV node slows conduction of these action potentials until all potentials have exited the atria and entered the AV node. After this slight delay, the AV node passes the action potential all at once to the ventricular conduction tissue, allowing for nearly simultaneous contraction of all ventricular cells. This AV node delay also allows time for the atria to eject fully their load of blood into the ventricles in preparation for ventricular systole.

From the AV node, the impulse travels down the bundle of His in the interventricular septum into either a right or left bundle branch and then through one of many Purkinje fibers to the ventricular myocardial tissue itself. An action potential can traverse this conducting tissue 3 to 7 times more rapidly than it can travel through the ventricular myocardium. Thus, the bundle branches and Purkinje fibers enable a near-simultaneous contraction of all portions of the ventricle, thereby allowing a maximal unified pump action to occur.[2]

ELECTROCARDIOGRAMS

Conduction of an action potential through the heart can be shown by an electrocardiogram (ECG; Fig. 16-8). Because ECGs are extensively covered in

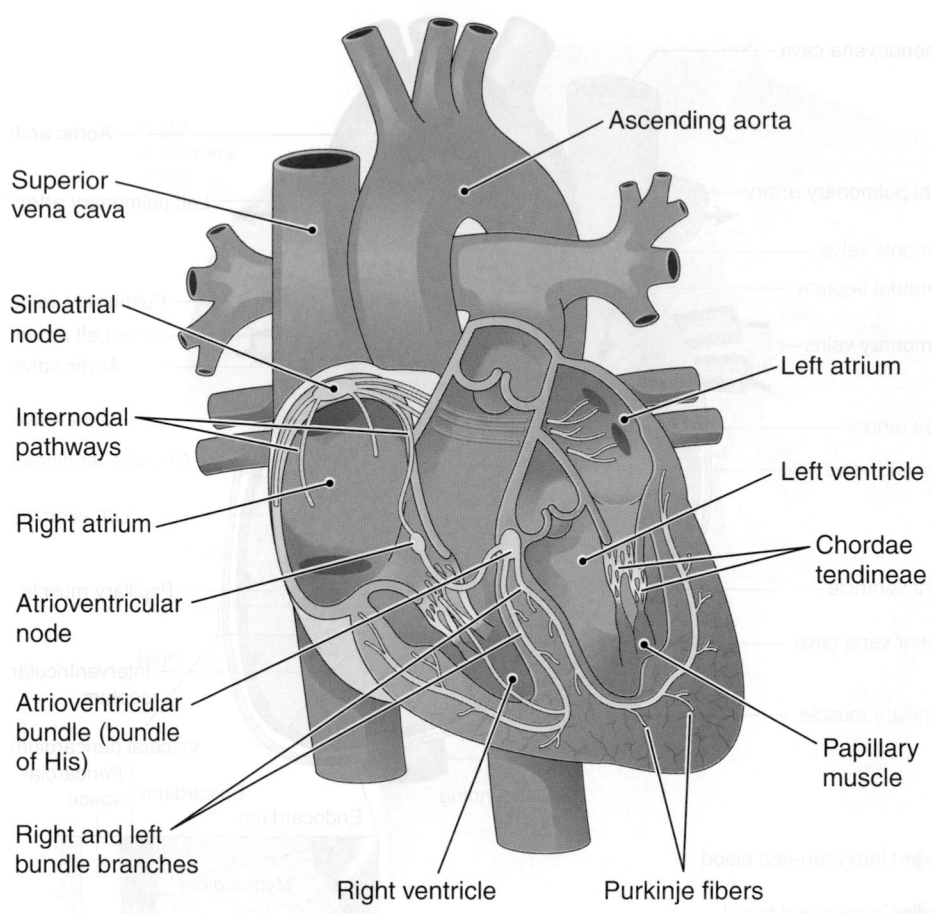

Superior vena cava

Sinoatrial node

Internodal pathways

Right atrium

Atrioventricular node

Atrioventricular bundle (bundle of His)

Right and left bundle branches

Right ventricle

Ascending aorta

Left atrium

Left ventricle

Chordae tendineae

Papillary muscle

Purkinje fibers

Figure 16-7 • The electrical conduction system of the heart begins with impulses generated by the sinoatrial node (*yellow*) and circuited continuously over the heart. (From Weber J, Kelley K: Health Assessment in Nursing, 3rd ed. Philadelphia: Lippincott Williams & Wilkins, 2007, 353.)

REGULATION OF HEART RATE

Although the heart has the ability to beat independently of any extrinsic influence, cardiac rate is under autonomic and adrenal catecholamine influence. Parasympathetic and sympathetic fibers innervate the SA and AV nodes. In addition, some sympathetic fibers terminate in myocardial tissues.

Parasympathetic stimulation releases acetylcholine near the nodal cells and decreases the rate of depolarization, thereby slowing cardiac rate. Stimulation

of sympathetic fibers causes the release of norepinephrine. This chemical increases the rate of nodal depolarization and has inotropic effects on myocardial fibers, which are discussed later. Thus, sympathetic stimulation increases heart rate (Table 16-1). The adrenal medulla also releases norepinephrine and epinephrine into the bloodstream. These circulating catecholamines act on the heart in the same way as sympathetic stimulation.

Two reflexes adjust heart rate to blood pressure: the aortic reflex and the Bainbridge reflex. In the aortic reflex (Fig. 16-9A), a rise in arterial blood pressure stimulates aortic and carotid sinus baroreceptors to fire sensory impulses to the cardioregulatory center in the medulla. The result is an increase in parasympathetic stimulation or a decrease in sympathetic stimulation to the heart. Thus, a rise in arterial blood pressure reflexively causes a slowing of cardiac rate. The decrease in heart rate results in a decrease in output, which can decrease arterial blood pressure. Conversely, a fall in arterial blood pressure, such as in shock, reflexively increases heart rate. This aortic reflex is an ongoing regulatory mechanism for homeostasis of arterial blood pressure.

The Bainbridge reflex (see Fig. 16-9B) uses receptors in the venae cavae. An increase in venous return stimulates these receptors, which then fire sensory impulses that travel to the cardioregulatory center. These reflexively cause a decrease in parasympathetic

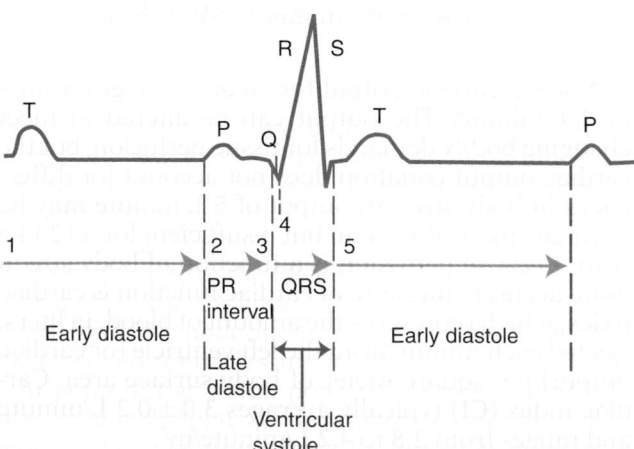

Figure 16-8 • Comparison of electrical and mechanical events during one cardiac cycle, using a normal electrocardiogram tracing.

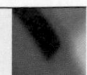

Table 16-1 • α and β Effects of Autonomic Nervous System on the Heart and Vascularity

Effector Organ	Cholinergic Impulses Response	Noradrenergic Impulses	
		Receptor Type	Response
Heart			
Sinoatrial node	Decrease in heart rate; vagal arrest	β_1	Increase in heart rate
Atria	Decrease in contractility and (usually) increase in conduction velocity	β_1	Increase in contractility and conduction velocity
Atrioventricular (AV) node and conduction system	Decrease in conduction velocity; AV block	β_1	Increase in conduction velocity
Ventricles	–	β_1	Increase in contractility and conduction velocity
Arterioles			
Coronary, skeletal muscle, pulmonary, abdominal viscera, renal	Dilation	α β_2	Constriction Dilation
Skin and mucosa, cerebral, salivary glands	–	α	Constriction
Systemic Veins	–	α β_2	Constriction Dilation

cardiac stimulation and an increase in sympathetic cardiac stimulation, thereby increasing cardiac rate. A fall in venous return causes a decrease in heart rate. Thus, the Bainbridge reflex adjusts cardiac rate to handle venous return.

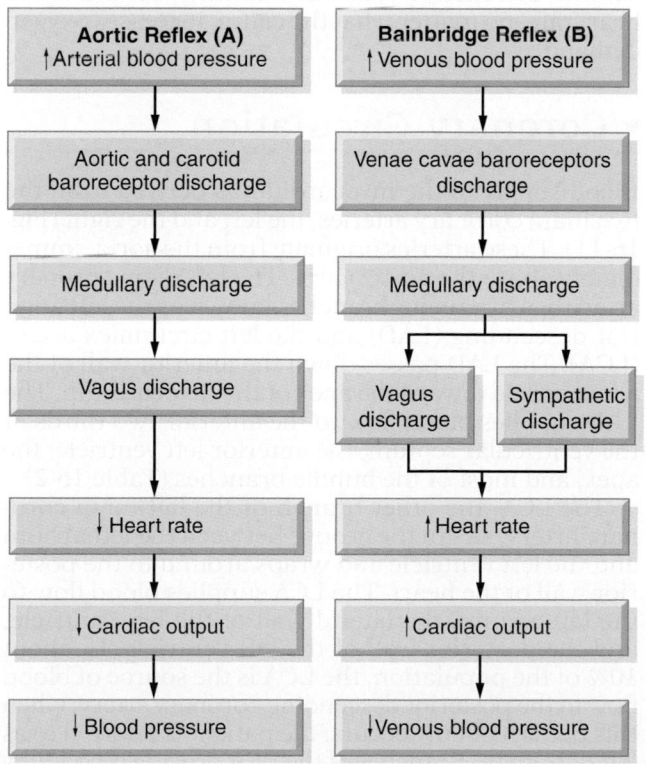

Figure 16-9 • Effects of aortic reflex (**A**) and Bainbridge reflex (**B**) on heart rate.

REGULATION OF STROKE VOLUME

Stroke volume is the amount of blood ejected by the left ventricle during systole. Normal values range from 60 to 100 mL/beat. Three factors are involved: preload, afterload (or wall tension), and inherent inotropic myocardial contractility.

Preload

Preload is the amount of stretch placed on a cardiac muscle fiber just before systole. Usually, the amount of stretch in any chamber is proportional to the volume of blood the chamber contains at the end of diastole, before systole. However, in some situations, the chamber can hold a large amount of volume with little change in pressure.

The concept of preload is related to the Frank-Starling law of the heart, which states that the force of myocardial contraction is determined by the length of the muscle cell fibers (Fig. 16-10). Within a certain range, increasing myofibril stretch increases the force of systole. Beyond optimal fibril length, it is hypothesized that too few actin–myosin binding sites overlap to provide an adequate contraction. Below optimal shortening, there is little room for filaments to slide, and cell walls limit further sliding. Also, actin filaments may have begun to overlap, decreasing the number of binding sites available to myosin fibers.

When the force of systole decreases, the chamber pumps poorly and does not empty properly. Excessive blood is left in the chamber at the end of systole. During diastole, when the chamber fills, this extra blood causes overfilling of the chamber and increases stretch. The next systole will be even weaker, as preload increases during every diastole.

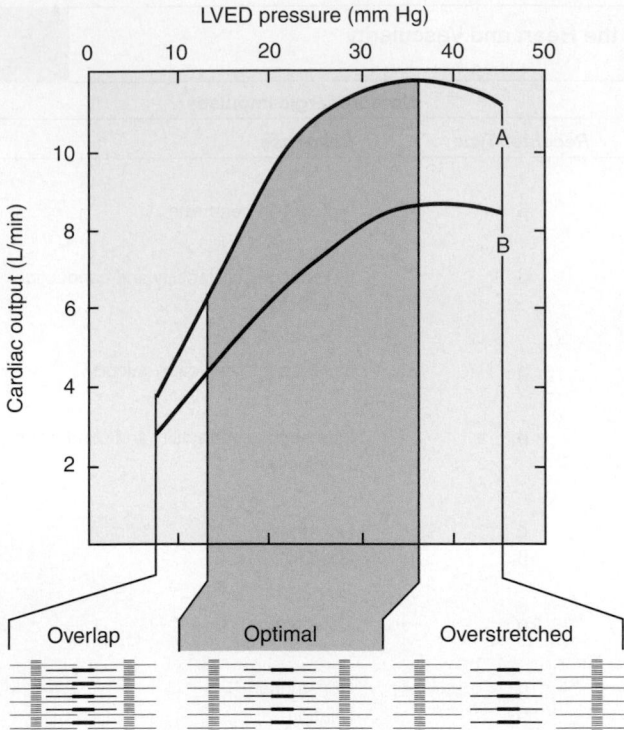

Figure 16-10 • Top: Starling ventricular function curve in normal heart. An increase in left ventricular end-diastolic (LVED) pressure produced an increase in cardiac output *(curve B)* by means of the Frank-Starling mechanism. The maximal force of contraction and increased stroke volume are achieved when diastolic filling causes the muscle fibers to be stretched about 2½ times their resting length. In *curve A,* an increase in cardiac contractility produces an increase in cardiac output without a change in LVED volume and pressure. **Bottom:** Stretching of the actin and myosin filaments at the different LVED filling pressures. (From Porth CM: Pathophysiology: Concepts of Altered Health States, 7th ed. Philadelphia: Lippincott Williams & Wilkins, 2005, p 461.)

Because preload is affected by the volume at the end of diastole, it often is equated with end-diastolic volume or pressure. Thus, left ventricular preload is represented by left ventricular end-diastolic pressure.

An example of rapid and normal adjustments to changes in preload occurs during the Valsalva maneuver. The first part of the Valsalva occurs when one holds one's breath and bears down, such as during defecation or heavy lifting. Bearing down increases intra-abdominal and intrathoracic pressures, decreasing venous return to the right atrium and ventricle. Right heart preload decreases. Bearing down also stimulates the vagus nerve, and the heart rate slows.

On exhalation, during the second part of the Valsalva maneuver, intrathoracic pressures decrease rapidly, allowing a sudden increase in venous return. Right atrial and ventricular preloads increase dramatically, stretch increases, and the right ventricular stroke volume increases. Atrial stretch receptors also signal the medulla and lead to sympathetic nervous discharge. Heart rate increases.

Afterload

Afterload is the force or pressure against which a cardiac chamber must eject blood during systole. The most critical factor determining afterload is vascular resistance, in the systemic or pulmonic vessels. Afterload often is equated with systemic vascular resistance or pulmonary vascular resistance.

Afterload affects stroke volume by increasing or decreasing the ease of emptying a ventricle during systole. A decrease in systemic vascular resistance, through vasodilation, presents the left ventricle with relatively large, open, relaxed arteries into which it can pump. Because it is easier to pump, the left ventricle empties easily, which increases stroke volume.

If systemic vascular resistance increases, for example through catecholamine-induced constriction of arteries, it takes a great deal more force for the left ventricle to pump into such a tightened vasculature. Stroke volume decreases.

Contractility

Inotropic capabilities and cardiac workload refer to contractile forces. Cardiac muscle forces change in response to neural stimuli and circulating levels of catecholamines. It is thought that through cyclic adenosine monophosphate (cAMP) mechanisms, cardiac cells change intracellular levels of calcium and ATP. These changes lead to increased inotropic actions, although the mechanisms remain unknown.

However, increased inotropic action increases the oxygen consumption of heart cells. This increased consumption also is called *increased workload* and *increased oxygen demand.*

Cardiac output depends on heart rate and stroke volume. Regardless of the initial cause of increased stroke volume (increased preload, increased afterload, or increased inotropic force), an increase in stroke volume increases workload. Similarly, an increased heart rate, no matter what the cause, increases oxygen demand.

• Coronary Circulation

Blood supply to the myocardium is derived from the two main coronary arteries, the left and the right (Fig. 16-11). These arteries originate from the aorta, immediately above the aortic valve. The left main coronary artery has two major branches known as the left anterior descending (LAD) and the left circumflex artery (LCA). The LAD passes down the anterior wall of the left ventricle toward the apex of the myocardium. The LAD supplies blood flow to the anterior two thirds of the ventricular septum, the anterior left ventricle, the apex, and most of the bundle branches (Table 16-2).

The LCA, the other branch of the left main coronary artery, sits in the groove between the left atrium and the left ventricle and wraps around to the posterior wall of the heart. The LCA supplies blood flow to the left atrium, the lateral wall of the left ventricle, and the posterior wall of the left ventricle. In about 10% of the population, the LCA is the source of blood flow to the posterior descending coronary artery; when this pattern of flow occurs, the patient is referred to as left dominant. Branches of the LCA provide blood flow to the SA node in about 45% of people and to the AV node in about 10% of people.

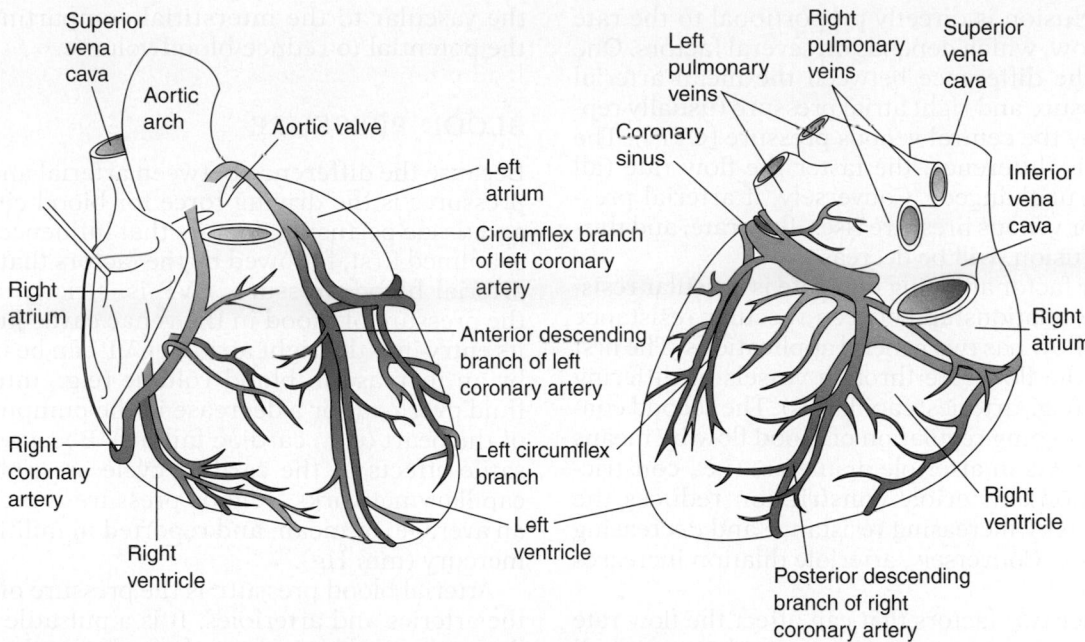

Figure 16-11 • Coronary arteries and some of the coronary sinus veins. (From Porth CM: Pathophysiology: Concepts of Altered Health States, 7th ed. Philadelphia: Lippincott Williams & Wilkins, 2005, p 540.)

The right coronary artery (RCA) also comes off the aorta and branches toward the right atrium; the anterior, lateral, and posterior regions of the right ventricle; and the posterior ventricular septum. The RCA provides blood flow to the right atrium, the right ventricle, and the inferior wall of the left ventricle. In about 90% of the population, the RCA is the source of blood flow to the posterior descending coronary artery, a pattern of flow known as right dominant. The RCA supplies oxygenated blood to the SA node in about 55% of people and to the AV node in about 90% of people.

The coronary arteries initially supply the epicardial layer of the heart and then pass deeper into the heart muscle to provide blood flow to the endocardium. As a result of this flow pattern, poor coronary blood flow initially deprives the subendocardial area of oxygenated blood. If the interruption to flow continues, the effects of decreased oxygenation expand throughout the thickness of the wall of the heart to the subepicardial surface.

Because the coronary arteries derive from the aorta (above the aortic valve) and lie between myocardial fibers, blood flow through the coronary arteries occurs when the aortic valve is closed during ventricular diastole, not systole. Therefore, anything that decreases the diastolic time (e.g., tachycardia) decreases coronary perfusion.

• Peripheral Circulation

The biological significance of the cardiovascular system is tissue perfusion. Such perfusion supplies the body's cells with oxygen and nutrients while carrying away metabolic wastes, including carbon dioxide.

Table 16-2 • Coronary Artery Blood Supply for Cardiac Muscle and Conducting System

Coronary Artery	Cardiac Muscle Supplied	Conducting Tissue Supplied
Left Main Coronary Artery		
Left anterior descending	Anterior ventricular septum Anterior left ventricle The apex	Bundle branches
Left circumflex	Left atrium Left ventricular lateral wall Left ventricular posterior wall	Sinoatrial node in 45% of hearts Atrioventricular node in 10% of hearts
Right Coronary Artery	Right atrium Right ventricle Posterior ventricular septum Inferior wall of left ventricle	Sinoatrial node in 55% of hearts Atrioventricular node in 90% of hearts

Tissue perfusion is directly proportional to the rate of blood flow, which depends on several factors. One factor is the difference between the mean arterial blood pressure and right atrial pressure (usually represented by the central venous pressure [CVP]). The greater this difference, the faster the flow rate (all else being unchanged). Conversely, if arterial pressure falls or venous pressure rises, flow rate, and thus tissue perfusion, will be decreased.

Another factor affecting flow rate is vascular resistance. The relationship between vascular resistance and blood flow has two general applications. The first describes the flow rate through vessels of differing diameters (e.g., arteries, capillaries). The second concerns the ongoing regulation of blood flow by means of adjustments in arteriole diameters (i.e., constriction, dilation). Arteriole constriction reduces the radius, thereby increasing resistance and decreasing the flow rate. Conversely, arteriole dilation increases the flow rate.

The other two factors that can affect the flow rate normally are held constant. They are the sum of all vessel lengths and blood viscosity. Because these factors do not normally change significantly, they usually are omitted from flow rate considerations. However, their relationships are obvious. The greater the length of a vessel, the more resistance and thus the slower the flow rate. Also, the more viscous the blood, the slower the rate of its flow. Blood viscosity is determined by the proportion of solvent (water) to solute and other particles, including blood cells and platelets. The less water and more particles that exist, the more viscous is the blood. The complete equation that describes all four factors is as follows:

$$\text{Flow rate} = \frac{\text{mean arterial pressure} - \text{central venous pressure}}{(\text{resistance} \times \text{viscosity} \times \text{vessel length})}$$

Because blood volume and pressure have such an important influence on tissue perfusion, the factors that alter and regulate them are examined.

BLOOD VOLUME

Urinary output and fluid input are the major normal mechanisms for regulating volume. If output is greater or fluid input is less, the volume is less—if all else is held constant. Factors that alter the volume of urine excreted every 24 hours include those that alter the glomerular filtration rate and the tubular reabsorption of water, with or without electrolytes. (For a more detailed explanation of these factors see Chapter 42, specifically the discussion of normal endocrine physiology that considers the antidiuretic hormone.) Pathological conditions that promote any type of fluid loss (e.g., burns, severe diarrhea, osmotic diuresis) or a shift of water from the vascular to the interstitial compartment have the potential to reduce blood volume.

BLOOD PRESSURE

Because the difference between arterial and venous pressures is the driving force for blood circulation and tissue perfusion, factors that influence CVP are examined first, followed by the factors that regulate arterial blood pressure. CVP is, strictly speaking, the pressure of blood in the venae cavae just before its entry into the right atrium. CVP can be increased by an increase in blood volume (e.g., intravenous fluid overload) or a decrease in the pumping ability of the heart (e.g., cardiac failure). Because the pulsatile effects of the cardiac cycle are removed by capillary networks, venous pressure is recorded as an average, or mean, and reported in millimeters of mercury (mm Hg).

Arterial blood pressure is the pressure of blood in the arteries and arterioles. It is a pulsatile pressure due to the cardiac cycle, and systolic (peak) and diastolic (trough) numbers are reported in millimeters of mercury. Average or mean arterial blood pressure can be clinically useful as an indicator of average perfusion pressures.

Arterial blood pressure is regulated by the vasomotor tone of the arteries and arterioles, the amount of blood entering the arteries per systole (i.e., cardiac output), and blood volume itself. The greater the volume or output, the greater the blood pressure, and vice versa, if vasomotor tone were held constant. The normal regulation of vasomotor tone involves neural and hormonal mechanisms.

Neural regulation is mediated by the vasomotor center of the medulla oblongata. This center consists of vasopressor and depressor subdivisions. The vasomotor center receives neural input from baroreceptors in the carotid sinuses and aorta, atrial diastolic stretch receptors, the limbic system and hypothalamus, the midbrain, and pulmonary stretch receptors. In addition, the center is directly responsive to local hypoxia or hypercapnia. Neural outputs from the vasopressor center result in increased sympathetic stimulation to arterial smooth muscle cells. This increase in sympathetic stimulation results in arterial constriction and an increase in arterial blood pressure. Stimulation of the depressor area decreases such sympathetic stimulation.

Rapid adjustments in arterial blood pressure are effected primarily by the baroreceptor reflexes. An increase in the pressure on these receptors (directly by elevated blood pressure or manual compression and indirectly by increased blood volume) reflexively stimulates the depressor area. This stimulation of the depressor area results in decreased sympathetic stimulation to major arteries and the aorta, which causes a decrease in arterial blood pressure. The decreased baroreceptor stimulation caused by a fall in arterial blood pressure reflexively stimulates the pressor area and results in increased sympathetic stimulation to arterial muscles, causing a rise in arterial blood pressure. Thus, homeostasis of arterial pressure is maintained.

In orthostatic hypotension, the baroreceptor reflex is sluggish. Because arterial pressure is not elevated rapidly enough, the postural change results in a temporary decrease in brain perfusion that leads, in extreme cases, to syncope.

Other factors may alter arterial blood pressure reflexively by their influences on the vasomotor center. Nerve fibers from the limbic system and hypothalamus are believed to mediate emotionally produced alterations in blood pressure. An example of this is fainting, caused by neurally mediated vasodilation in response to the sight of blood or very bad (or good) news. Neural inputs from the midbrain and possibly from ascending spinothalamic fibers in the medulla result in the elevation in arterial pressure that initially accompanies severe pain and in the later decrease in arterial pressure that occurs when severe pain is prolonged. Lung inflation stimulates pulmonary stretch receptors. Their input to the vasomotor center reflexively decreases arterial pressure. Hypercapnia and, to a lesser extent, hypoxia of vasomotor neurons stimulate the pressor area, reflexively causing an increase in arterial pressure. Such stimuli obviously are not part of a normal daily regulatory mechanism but can operate as a normal compensatory mechanism in certain pathological situations. Elevated intracranial pressure can promote medullary hypercapnia and hypoxia. The increase in arterial pressure reflexively produced by these stimuli (Cushing's reflex) increases medullary perfusion, which can ameliorate the medullary hypoxia, hypercapnia, or both. Hormonal regulation of arterial blood pressure is effected by adrenal medullary catecholamines and the renin–angiotensin system. In the former, adrenal medullary catecholamines mimic the action of sympathetic fibers innervating the muscle layer of arteries (tunica media), causing arterial constriction and elevating arterial pressure. The renin–angiotensin system is discussed in Chapter 28. Briefly, a decreased glomerular filtration rate, which can result, for example, from a decrease in blood volume or renal perfusion, stimulates the secretion of renin from the juxtaglomerular apparatus. This stimulation of renin leads to the production of angiotensin II, which acts directly on the tunica media to promote vasoconstriction. Thus, renin elevates arterial pressure, which increases renal perfusion and glomerular filtration.

Finally, arterial blood pressure can be influenced by alterations in the level of unbound calcium in tunica media cells. Such levels are influenced by factors that open or close calcium channels in the membranes of these muscle cells. Drugs that block calcium channels ("calcium blockers") inhibit the entry of calcium into cells. Such decreased calcium influx can lower intracellular calcium levels sufficiently to decrease muscle contractility, including contractility of the heart, thereby promoting a degree of vasodilation and lowering the arterial pressure.

• Clinical Applicability Challenges

Short-Answer Questions

1. Mr. P. has been diagnosed with 80% occlusion of his right coronary artery. Describe which anatomical walls of the heart are affected. Explain which parts of his cardiac conducting system may be affected by the occlusion.

2. Mrs. J. was brought to the hospital by her family because she has become weak and has not been eating or drinking for 3 days. Her cardiac output is 3 L/minute, and her blood pressure is 90/50 mm Hg. Discuss possible physiological causes of her decreased cardiac output and the body's response to the drop.

3. Ms. T. has been diagnosed with atrial fibrillation, a rhythm in which the atria are electrically stimulated at a rate of about 300 times per minute. The atria are not able to contract in response to such rapid stimulation; instead, the muscle merely quivers. This is known as fibrillation. What is the effect of fibrillation on blood flow in the heart?

Review Questions

1. Mr. K. had an electrophysiology study that revealed his sinoatrial (SA) node was no longer functioning. When the SA node fails to fire, what area of the heart should take over as the pacemaker site?
   a. Atrioventricular node
   b. His bundle
   c. Right bundle branch
   d. Left bundle branch

2. Mrs. D. has just returned to the progressive care unit after a cardiac catheterization. She was diagnosed with 90% occlusion of the left anterior descending (LAD) coronary artery. What area of the heart is most likely to be affected by an LAD occlusion?
   a. Right atria
   b. Right ventricle
   c. Left atria
   d. Left ventricle

3. Mr. W. is scheduled to have his mitral valve replaced. Between which two structures is the mitral valve located?
   a. Right atrium and the right ventricle
   b. Right ventricle and the pulmonary artery
   c. Left atrial and the left ventricle
   d. Left ventricle and the aorta

4. If the body experiences catecholamine-induced constriction of arteries, what is the effect on the heart?
   a. Systemic vascular resistance decreases, and afterload decreases.

b. Systemic vascular resistance increases, and afterload increases.
c. Preload increases, and heart rate decreases.
d. Preload decreases, and the heart rate increases.

5. Mr. P. has just returned from cardiac surgery and has pacemaker wires attached to the epicardial surface of the heart. The epicardial surface is the:
a. outer layer of the heart that is tightly adherent to the heart.
b. thin, fibrous double-layered sac that surrounds the heart.
c. inner layer of the heart.
d. middle layer of the heart.

References

1. Johnson LR, Bryne JH: Essential Medical Physiology, 3rd ed. St. Louis: Elsevier, 2003
2. Porth CM: Pathophysiology: Concepts of Altered Health States, 7th ed. Philadelphia: Lippincott Williams & Wilkins, 2005
3. Bickley LS: Bates' Guide to Physical Examination and History Taking, 9th ed. Philadelphia: Lippincott Williams & Wilkins, 2006

Other Selected Readings

Cohen BJ: Memmler's The Structure and Function of the Human Body, 8th ed. Philadelphia: Lippincott Williams & Wilkins, 2005
Ganong WF: Review of Medical Physiology, 22nd ed. New York: McGraw-Hill, 2005
Guyton AC, Hall JE: Textbook of Medical Physiology, 11th ed. St. Louis: Elsevier 2005
Levy M, Koeppen B, Stanton B: Berne and Levy Principles of Physiology, 4th ed. St. Louis, Elsevier, 2005
Marieb EN: Human Anatomy and Physiology, 5th ed. San Francisco: Benjamin Cummings, 2001
Scanlon V, Sanders T: Essentials of Anatomy and Physiology, 5th ed. Philadelphia: FA Davis, 2007
Thibodeau GA, Patton KT: Anatomy and Physiology, 6th ed. St Louis: Mosby, 2006
Tortora G: Principles of Human Anatomy, 10th ed. New York: Wiley, 2004

Patient Assessment: Cardiovascular System

17

Patricia Gonce Morton • Kim Reck • Terry Tucker • Kathryn Von Rueden • Jan Headley

Objectives

Based on the content in this chapter, the reader should be able to:

1. Explain the components of the cardiovascular history.
2. Describe the steps of the cardiovascular physical examination.
3. Discuss the mechanisms responsible for the production of the first, second, third, and fourth heart sounds and their timing in the cardiac cycle.
4. Explain the attributes of heart murmurs.
5. Describe the attributes of common systolic and diastolic murmurs.
6. Describe components of hematologic studies, coagulation studies, blood chemistries, and serum lipid studies.
7. Compare and contrast the usefulness of serum enzymes and myocardial proteins in diagnosing an acute myocardial infarction.
8. Describe current techniques used for diagnostic purposes in cardiology.
9. Discuss the nursing care before and after cardiac diagnostic studies.
10. Outline the patient and family teaching appropriate to prepare the patient for cardiac diagnostic studies.
11. Describe potential complications of cardiac diagnostic procedures.
12. Explain the major features of an electrocardiogram (ECG) monitoring system.
13. Explain correct electrode placement when monitoring the standard leads or the chest leads with a three-electrode and a five-electrode system.
14. Discuss steps for troubleshooting ECG monitor problems.
15. Describe the components of the ECG tracing and their meaning.
16. Explain the steps used to interpret a rhythm strip.
17. Describe the causes, clinical significance, and management for each of the dysrhythmias discussed.
18. Describe the parameters of a normal 12-lead ECG.
19. Define electrical axis, and determine the direction of the axis for a 12-lead ECG.
20. Explain the causes, clinical significance, and treatment of bundle branch blocks, atrial enlargement, and ventricular enlargement.
21. Describe the ECG changes associated with serum potassium and calcium abnormalities.

㉒ Describe the system components required to monitor hemodynamic pressures.

㉓ Analyze the characteristics of normal systemic arterial, right atrial, right ventricular, pulmonary artery, and pulmonary artery wedge pressure waveforms.

㉔ State nursing interventions that ensure accuracy of pressure readings.

㉕ Discuss the major complications that can occur with an indwelling arterial, central venous, and pulmonary artery catheter.

㉖ Identify the determinants of cardiac output.

㉗ Describe the thermodilution method of measuring cardiac output.

㉘ Describe alternative minimally invasive and noninvasive methods of obtaining hemodynamic data.

㉙ Evaluate the factors influencing oxygen delivery and consumption.

㉚ Use $\overline{S}O_2$ or $\overline{Sc}O_2$ monitoring to assess oxygen delivery and consumption.

The application of complex technology to the assessment and management of cardiovascular and cardiopulmonary conditions has increased greatly in the past several decades. Use of advanced and complex technologies is an integral part of the care of critically ill patients. Nevertheless, the value of a comprehensive cardiovascular history and physical examination should never be underestimated. The chapter begins with a discussion of the cardiac history and physical examination and then addresses laboratory and diagnostic studies, electrocardiographic monitoring, and hemodynamic monitoring.

Cardiac History and Physical Examination

The cardiovascular history provides physiological and psychosocial information that guides the physical assessment, the selection of diagnostic tests, and the choice of treatment options. During the history, the nurse asks about the patient's chief complaint and the history of the present illness, including a complete analysis of each sign and symptom. Next, the nurse asks about the patient's past health history, family history, and personal and social history. The history concludes with a review of systems that provides additional clues to the patient's health status. The information gathered during the history gives the nurse insight into risk factors and behaviors that promote or jeopardize cardiovascular health. The nurse uses this information to guide health teaching. During the process of taking a thorough history and performing a physical examination, the nurse has an opportunity to establish rapport with the patient and to evaluate the patient's general emotional status.

• History

CHIEF COMPLAINT AND HISTORY OF PRESENT ILLNESS

The nurse begins the history by investigating the patient's chief complaint, asking the patient to describe the problem or reason for seeking health care in his or her own words. The nurse then asks for more information about the present illness, using the NOPQRST format and the questions presented in Box 17-1. Answers to these questions are essential to understanding the patient's perception of the problem.

To gain a better understanding of the current illness, the nurse also asks the patient about any associated symptoms, including chest pain, nausea or vomiting, dyspnea, edema of feet or ankles, palpitations, syncope or dizziness, cough and hemoptysis, nocturia, cyanosis, and extremity pain or paresthesias.

Chest Pain

Chest pain is one of the most common symptoms of patients with cardiovascular disease. Therefore, it is an essential component of the assessment interview. Chest pain is often a disturbing or even frightening experience for a patient, so the patient may be hesitant to initiate a discussion of chest pain. The questions listed in Box 17-1 are particularly useful when assessing chest pain because the answers help determine whether the pain is cardiac in origin.

Because cardiac pain (angina pectoris) is the result of an imbalance between oxygen supply and oxygen demand, it usually develops over time. Typically, anginal pain does not start at maximal intensity. Not all chest pain is cardiac in origin, and careful reporting of the characteristics of the pain and the behaviors (or lack thereof) that precede the onset of pain is required. The nurse asks the patient about his or her normal baseline status before the symptoms developed. It is also important to ask about the onset of the symptoms to determine the date and time that the symptoms started and whether the onset was sudden or gradual. Symptoms that may accompany chest pain caused by heart disease include nausea and vomiting.

Chest pain caused by coronary artery disease is often precipitated by physical or emotional exertion, a meal, or being out in the cold. Palliative measures to relieve anginal pain may include rest or sublingual nitrates; these measures usually do not relieve the pain of a myocardial infarction (MI). The quality of cardiac chest pain is often described as heaviness, tightness, squeezing, or a choking sensation. If the pain is reported as superficial, knifelike, or throbbing, it is not likely to be anginal. Cardiac chest pain is usually located in the substernal region and often radiates to the neck, left arm, back, or jaw. Although the pain is often referred to other areas, anginal pain is visceral in origin, and most complaints include a reference to a "deep, inside" pain. When the patient is asked to point to the painful area, the painful area is about the size of a hand or clenched fist. It is unusual for true anginal pain to be localized to an area smaller than a fingertip. Using a scale of 0 to 10, with 10 being the worst pain the patient has ever experienced and 0 being the absence of pain, the patient is asked to rate the severity of the pain. When asked about time, the patient with cardiac chest pain reports the pain lasting anywhere from 30 seconds to hours.

Pain may be secondary to cardiovascular problems that are unrelated to a primary coronary insufficiency. Therefore, when obtaining the patient's history, the nurse must consider other causes. For example, if the patient reports the pain is made worse by lying down, moving, or deep breathing, it may be caused by pericarditis. If the pain is retrosternal and accompanied by sudden shortness of breath and peripheral cyanosis, it may be caused by a pulmonary embolism.

Dyspnea

Dyspnea occurs in patients with both pulmonary and cardiac abnormalities. In patients with cardiac disease, it is the result of inefficient pumping of the left ventricle, which causes a congestion of blood flow in the lungs. During history taking, dyspnea is differentiated from the usual breathlessness that follows a sudden burst of physical activity (e.g., running up four flights of stairs, sprinting across a parking lot). Dyspnea is a subjective complaint of true difficulty in breathing, not just shortness of breath. The nurse determines whether the breathing difficulty occurs only with exertion or also at rest. If dyspnea is present when the patient lies flat but is relieved by sitting or standing, it is orthopnea. If dyspnea is characterized by breathing difficulties starting after approximately 1 to 2 hours of sleep and relieved by sitting upright or getting out of bed, it is paroxysmal nocturnal dyspnea.

Edema of the Feet and Ankles

Although many other problems can leave a patient with swollen feet or ankles, heart failure may also be responsible because the heart is unable to mobilize fluid appropriately. Because gravity promotes the movement of fluids from intravascular to extravascular spaces, the edema becomes worse as the day progresses and usually improves at night after lying down to sleep. Patients or families may report that shoes do not fit anymore, socks that used to be loose are now too tight, and the indentations from sock bands take more time than usual to disappear. The nurse should inquire about the timing of edema development (e.g., immediately after lowering the extremities, only at the end of the day, only after a significant salt intake) and duration (e.g., relieved with temporary elevation of the legs or with constant elevation).

Palpitations and Syncope or Dizziness

Palpitations refer to the awareness of irregular or rapid heart beats. Patients may report the "skipping" of beats, a rushing of the heart, or a loud "thudding." The nurse asks about onset and duration of the palpitations, associated symptoms, and any precipitating events that the patient or family can remember. Because a cardiac dysrhythmia may compromise blood flow to the brain, the nurse asks about symptoms of dizziness, fainting, or syncope that accompany the palpitations.

Cough and Hemoptysis

Abnormalities such as heart failure, pulmonary embolus, or mitral stenosis may cause a cough or hemoptysis. Side effects of medications such as angiotensin-converting enzyme (ACE) inhibitors may also include a cough. The nurse asks the patient about the presence of a cough and inquires about the quality (wet or dry) and frequency of the cough (chronic or occasional, only when lying down or after exercise). If the cough produces expectorant, the nurse inquires about its color, consistency, and amount perceived by the patient. If the patient reports spitting up blood (hemoptysis), the nurse asks if the substance spit up was streaked with blood, frothy bloody sputum, or frank blood (bright or dark).

Nocturia

Kidneys that are inadequately perfused by an unhealthy heart during the day may finally receive sufficient flow during rest at night to increase their output. The nurse asks about the number of times the patient urinates during the night. If the patient takes a diuretic, the nurse also evaluates frequency of urination in relation to the time of day the diuretic is taken.

Cyanosis

Cyanosis reflects the oxygenation and circulatory status of the patient. Central cyanosis is generally distributed and best found by examining the mucous membranes for discoloration and duskiness, and reflects reduced oxygen concentration. Peripheral cyanosis is localized in the extremities and protrusions (hands, feet, nose, ears, lips) and reflects impaired circulation.

Extremity Pain or Paresthesias

Extremity pain results when the blood supply to exercising muscles is inadequate, and this type of pain is known as claudication. Usually, the cause of claudication is significant atherosclerotic obstruction to the lower extremities. The limb is asymptomatic at rest unless the obstruction is severe. Blood supply to the legs is inadequate to meet metabolic demands during exercise, and ischemic pain results. The patient describes a cramping, "charley horse," ache, or weakness in the foot, calf, thigh, or buttocks that improves with rest. The patient is asked to describe the severity of the pain and how much exertion is required to produce the pain.

PAST HEALTH HISTORY

The history includes information about the patient's past health. When assessing the patient's past health history, the nurse inquires about childhood illnesses and other previous illnesses, as well as past surgeries, previous diagnostic tests and interventions, medication use, allergies, and transfusions (Box 17-2). The nurse also asks about risk factors (Box 17-3).[1,2]

FAMILY HISTORY

The nurse asks about the age and health, or age and cause of death, of immediate family members, including parents, grandparents, siblings, children, and grandchildren. The nurse inquires about cardiovascular problems such as coronary artery disease, hypertension, diabetes mellitus, sudden cardiac death, stroke, peripheral vascular disease, and lipid disorders (see Box 17-2).

PERSONAL AND SOCIAL HISTORY

Although the physical symptoms provide many clues regarding the origin and extent of cardiac disease, the personal and social history also adds to the patient's health status. An understanding of the topics listed in Box 17-2 contributes to the nurse's knowledge of the patient as a person and guides interaction with the patient and family as well as patient education.

REVIEW OF OTHER SYSTEMS

The health history concludes with a review of relevant systems. This information gives the nurse a better understanding of the patient's total health status, and it also helps the nurse determine the impact of cardiovascular disease on the functioning of other body systems (see Box 17-2).

• Physical Examination

Cardiac assessment requires examination of all aspects of the individual, using the standard steps of inspection, palpation, percussion, and auscultation. A thorough and careful examination helps the nurse detect subtle abnormalities as well as obvious ones.

INSPECTION

General Appearance

Inspection begins as soon as the patient and nurse interact. General appearance and presentation of the patient are key elements of the initial inspection. Critical examination reveals a first impression of age, nutritional status, self-care ability, alertness, and overall physical health.

It is necessary to note the ability of the patient to move and speak with or without distress. Consider the patient's posture, gait, and musculoskeletal coordination.

Jugular Venous Distention

Pressure in the jugular veins reflects right atrial pressure and provides the nurse with an indication of heart hemodynamics and cardiac function. The height of the level of blood in the right internal jugular vein is an indication of right atrial pressure because there are no valves or obstructions between the vein and the right atrium.

The internal jugular veins are not directly visible because they lie deep to the sternomastoid muscles in the neck (Fig. 17-1). The goals of the examination are to determine the highest point of visible pulsation in the internal jugular veins, to note the level of head elevation, and to measure this point of visible pulsation as the vertical distance above the sternal angle. The patient is placed in the bed supine with the head of the bed elevated 30, 45, 60, and 90 degrees. The patient is examined at each elevation with the head slightly turned away from the examiner. The nurse

Box 17-2 • Cardiovascular Health History

Chief Complaint
- Patient's description of the problem

History of the Present Illness
- Complete analysis of the following signs and symptoms (using the NOPQRST format; see Box 17-1)
- Chest pain
- Nausea and/or vomiting
- Dyspnea
- Edema
- Palpitations
- Syncope/dizziness
- Cough and hemoptysis
- Nocturia
- Cyanosis
- Extremity pain or paresthesias

Past Health History
- Relevant childhood illnesses and immunizations: rheumatic fever, murmurs, congenital anomalies, streptococcal infections
- Past acute and chronic medical problems including treatments and hospitalizations: heart failure, hypertension, coronary artery disease, myocardial infarction, hyperlipidemia, valve disease, cardiac dysrhythmias, diabetes mellitus, endocarditis, thrombophlebitis, deep venous thrombosis, peripheral vascular disease, chest injury, pneumonia, pulmonary embolism, thyroid disease, tuberculosis
- Risk factors: age, heredity, gender, race, tobacco use, elevated cholesterol, hypertension, physical inactivity, obesity, diabetes mellitus (see Box 17-3)
- Past surgeries: coronary artery bypass grafting, valvular surgery, peripheral vascular surgeries
- Past diagnostic tests and interventions: electrocardiogram, echocardiogram, stress test, electrophysiology studies, myocardial imaging studies, thrombolytic therapy, cardiac catheterization, percutaneous transluminal cardiac angioplasty, stent placement, atherectomy, pacemaker or implantable cardioverter defibrillator implantation, valvuloplasty
- Medications, including prescription drugs, over-the-counter drugs, vitamins, herbs, and supplements: angiotensin-converting enzyme (ACE) inhibitors, anticoagulants, antihypertensives, antiplatelets, antiarrhythmics, angiotensin II receptor blockers (ARBs), β-blockers, calcium channel blockers, antihyperlipidemics, diuretics, electrolyte replacements, nitrates, inotropes, hormone replacement therapies, oral contraceptives
- Allergies and reactions to medications, foods, contrast dye, latex or other materials
- Transfusions, including type and date

Family History
- Health status or cause of death of parents and siblings: coronary artery disease, hypertension, diabetes mellitus, sudden cardiac death, stroke, peripheral vascular disease, lipid disorders

Personal and Social History
- Tobacco, alcohol, and substance use
- Family composition
- Occupation and work environment
- Living environment
- Diet: restrictions, supplements, caffeine intake
- Sleep patterns: number of pillows used
- Exercise
- Cultural beliefs
- Spiritual or religious beliefs
- Coping patterns and social support systems
- Leisure activities
- Sexual activity: use of agents for erectile dysfunction
- Recent travel

Review of Other Systems
- HEENT: retinal problems, visual changes, headaches, carotid artery disease
- Respiratory: shortness of breath, dyspnea, cough, lung disease, recurrent infections, pneumonia, tuberculosis
- Gastrointestinal: nausea, vomiting, weight loss, change in bowel habits
- Genitourinary: incontinence, erectile dysfunction
- Musculoskeletal: pain, weakness, varicose veins, change in sensation, peripheral edema
- Neurological: transient ischemic attacks, stroke, change in level of consciousness, changes in sensations
- Endocrine: thyroid disease, diabetes mellitus

---

uses tangential light to observe for the highest point of visible pulsation.[3,4]

Next, the angle of Louis is located by palpating where the clavicle joins the sternum (suprasternal notch). The examining finger is slid down the sternum until a bony prominence is felt. This prominence is known as the angle of Louis. A vertical ruler is placed on the angle of Louis. Another ruler is placed horizontally at the level of the pulsation. The intersection of the horizontal ruler with the vertical ruler is noted, and the intersection point on the vertical ruler is read.

Normal jugular venous pulsation should not exceed 3 cm above the angle of Louis. See Figure 17-2 for an illustration of the procedure for assessment of jugular venous pressure. A level more than 3 cm above the angle of Louis indicates an abnormally high volume in the venous system. Possible causes include right-sided heart failure, obstruction of the superior vena cava, pericardial effusion, and other cardiac or thoracic diseases. An increase in the jugular venous pressure of more than 1 cm while pressure is applied to the abdomen for 60 seconds (hepatojugular or abdominojugular test) indicates the inability of the heart to accommodate the increased venous return.

Chest

The chest is inspected for signs of trauma or injury, symmetry, chest contour, and any visible pulsations. The inspection may reveal the location of the point of maximal impulse (PMI). In most patients, the api-

Box 17-3 • Risk Factors for Cardiovascular Disease[1,2]

Major Uncontrollable Risk Factors

- **Age:** There is an increased incidence of all types of atherosclerotic disease with aging. More than 83% of people who die from coronary artery disease are age 65 or older. Women at older ages who have a myocardial infarction are twice as likely as men to die from it within a few weeks.
- **Heredity:** The tendency for development of atherosclerosis seems to run in families. The risk is thought to be a combination of environmental and genetic influences. Even when other risk factors are controlled, the chance for development of coronary artery disease increases when there is a familial tendency.
- **Gender:** Men have a greater risk for development of coronary artery disease than women at earlier ages. After menopause, women's death rate from myocardial infarction increases but is not as great as men's.
- **Race:** Rates of cardiovascular disease are higher for African Americans, Mexican Americans, American Indians, Native Hawaiians, and some Asian Americans.

Major Risk Factors That Can Be Modified, Treated, or Controlled

- **Tobacco smoking:** A smoker's risk for a myocardial infarction is more than twice that of nonsmokers. Smokers who have a myocardial infarction are more likely to die and die within an hour than are nonsmokers. Cigarette smoking is the greatest risk factor for sudden death. Smokers have 2 to 4 times the risk for sudden death compared with nonsmokers. Chronic exposure to environmental tobacco smoke may increase the risk for heart disease.
- **High blood cholesterol:** The risk for coronary heart disease increases as the blood cholesterol level rises. When other risk factors are present, this risk increases even more.
- **Hypertension:** Known as the "silent killer," hypertension is a risk factor with no specific symptoms and no early warning signs. Men have a greater risk for hypertension than women until the age of 55 years. The risk for development of hypertension is about the same for men and women between the ages of 55 and 75 years. After the age of

75 years, hypertension is more likely to develop in women than in men. African Americans are more likely to have hypertension than whites. Hypertension increases the risk for stroke, myocardial infarction, kidney failure, and heart failure.
- **Physical inactivity:** A lack of physical exercise is a risk factor for coronary artery disease. Moderate to vigorous regular exercise plays a significant role in preventing heart disease and blood vessel disease. Even moderate-intensity exercise is beneficial if performed regularly and long-term. Physical activity also plays a role in controlling cholesterol, diabetes, obesity, and hypertension.
- **Obesity:** People who have excess body fat, especially at the waist, are more likely to develop heart disease and stroke even if they have no other risk factors. Excess weight raises blood pressure, blood cholesterol, and blood triglyceride levels. Excess weight lowers high-density lipids and makes diabetes more likely to develop.
- **Diabetes mellitus:** Even when blood glucose levels are under control, diabetes greatly increases the risk for heart disease and stroke. If blood glucose is not well controlled, the risk is even greater. Most people with diabetes die of some form of heart or blood vessel disease. Many people with diabetes also have high blood pressure, increasing their risk even more.

Other Contributing Factors

- **Stress:** A person's response to stress may be a contributing factor to heart disease. Stress in a person's life, his or her health behaviors, and socioeconomic status may all contribute to established risk factors. For example, individuals under stress may overeat, smoke, and not exercise.
- **Excessive alcohol intake:** Drinking too much alcohol can raise blood pressure, cause heart failure, lead to stroke, contribute to high triglycerides and obesity, and produce arrhythmias. The risk for heart disease in individuals who drink moderate amounts of alcohol (an average of one drink for women and two drinks for men per day) is lower than in those who do not drink alcohol.

cal pulse is the PMI; however, in some pathological conditions, these may be two distinct areas on the chest.[3] Thrusts (abnormally strong precordial pulsations) are noted. Any depression (sternum excavatum) or bulging of the precordium is recorded.

Extremities

A close inspection of the patient's extremities can also provide clues about cardiovascular health. The extremities are examined for lesions, ulcerations, unhealed sores, and varicose veins. Distribution of hair on the extremities also is noted. A lack of normal hair distribution on the extremities may indicate diminished arterial blood flow to the area.

Skin

Skin is evaluated for moistness or dryness, color, elasticity, edema, thickness, lesions, ulcerations, and

vascular changes. Nail beds are examined for cyanosis and clubbing, which may indicate chronic cardiac or pulmonary abnormalities. General differences in color and temperature between body parts may provide perfusion clues.

PALPATION

Pulses

Cardiovascular assessment continues with palpation and involves the use of the pads of the finger and balls of the hand. Using the pads of the fingers, the carotid, brachial, radial, femoral, popliteal, posterior tibial, and dorsalis pedis pulses are palpated (Fig. 17-3). The peripheral pulses are compared bilaterally to determine rate, rhythm, strength, and symmetry. The 0-to-4 scale described in Box 17-4 is used to rate the strength of the pulse. The carotid pulses should never

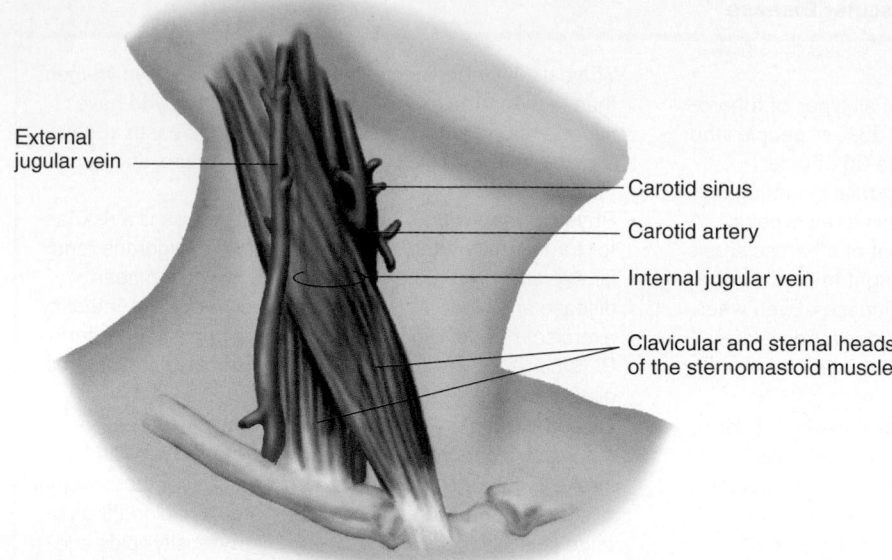

External
jugular vein

Carotid sinus

Carotid artery

Internal jugular vein

Clavicular and sternal heads
of the sternomastoid muscle

Figure 17-1 • Internal jugular veins. (From Bickley L: Bates' Guide to Physical Examination and Health History, 8th ed. Philadelphia: Lippincott Williams & Wilkins, 2003, p 32.)

be assessed simultaneously because this can obstruct flow to the brain.

Pulses can also be described according to their characteristics. For example, pulsus alternans is a pulse that alternates in strength with every other beat; it is often found in patients with left ventricular failure. Pulsus paradoxus is a pulse that disappears during inspiration but returns during expiration. To determine whether the condition is pathological, the sphygmomanometer is deflated until the pulse is heard only during expiration and the corresponding pressure noted. As the cuff continues to deflate, the point at which the pulse is heard throughout the inspiratory and expiratory cycle is noted. The second systolic pressure reading is subtracted from the first; if the difference is greater than 10 mm Hg dur-ing normal respirations, it is considered pathological. During the assessment of pulses, the nurse compares the warmth and size of the palpated areas to monitor perfusion.

Precordium

The chest wall is palpated to assess for the PMI, thrills, and abnormal pulsations. A systematic palpation sequence is used with the patient in a supine position and includes the precordial areas shown in Figure 17-4. Palpation starts with locating the PMI. In most patients, the PMI represents the point at which the apical pulse is most readily felt. Using light pressure, the nurse first uses the palmar surface of the hand to feel for pulsations and then uses the pads of the finger to palpate the apical pulse (Fig. 17-5). The PMI is palpated, noting its location, diameter, amplitude, and duration. Usually, the PMI is located in the mid-clavicular line at about the fourth or fifth intercostal space. If the pulse is difficult to palpate, it may be necessary to ask the patient to turn on the left side (left lateral decubitus position).

Next, the nurse palpates the lower left sternal border area, the upper left sternal border area, the sternoclavicular area, the right upper sternal border area, the lower right sternal border area, and finally the epigastric area. During palpation of these areas, the nurse feels for a thrill, which is a palpable vibration. A thrill usually represents a disruption in blood flow related to a defect in one of the semilunar valves.

PERCUSSION

With the advent of radiological means of evaluating cardiac size, percussion is not a significant contributor to cardiac assessment. However, a gross determination of heart size can be made by percussing for the dullness that reflects the cardiac borders.

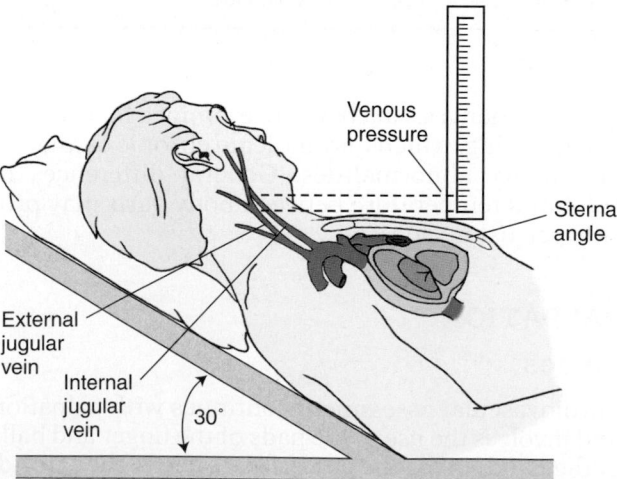

Venous pressure

Sternal angle

External jugular vein

Internal jugular vein

30°

Figure 17-2 • Assessment of jugular venous pressure. Place the patient supine in bed and gradually raise the head of the bed to 30, 45, 60, and 90 degrees. Using tangential lighting, note the highest level of venous pulsation. Measure the vertical distance between this point and the sternal angle. Record this distance in centimeters and the angle of the head of the bed.

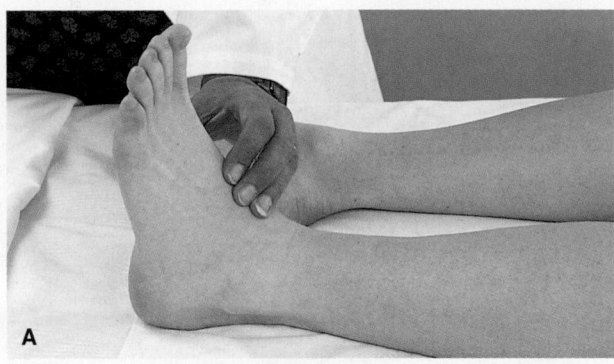
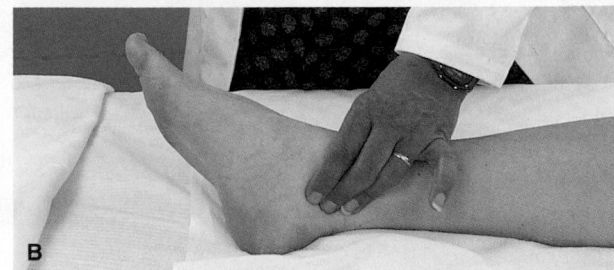

Figure 17-3 • **A:** Palpating the dorsalis pedis pulse. **B:** Palpating the posterior tibial pulse. (© B. Proud; from Weber J, Kelley J: Health Assessment in Nursing, 3rd ed. Philadelphia: Lippincott Williams & Wilkins, 2007, p 411.)

AUSCULTATION

Data obtained by careful and thorough auscultation of the heart are essential in planning and evaluating care of the critically ill patient. In this section, the following topics are discussed: the basic principles underlying cardiac auscultation; the factors responsible for the production of normal heart sounds; and the pathophysiological conditions responsible for the production of extra sounds, murmurs, and friction rubs.

To facilitate accurate auscultation, the patient should be relaxed and comfortable in a quiet, warm environment with adequate lighting. The patient should be in a recumbent position with the trunk elevated 30 to 45 degrees. To help hear abnormal sounds, the patient may be asked to roll partly onto the left side (left lateral decubitus position). This position helps bring the left ventricle closer to the chest wall. The patient also may be asked to sit up, lean forward, and exhale. In this position, it may be easier to hear murmurs caused by aortic regurgitation (Fig. 17-6).

A good-quality stethoscope is essential. The earpieces should fit the ears snugly and comfortably and follow the natural angle of the ear canals. Sound waves that travel a shorter distance are more intense and less distorted; therefore, the tubing of the stethoscope should be approximately 12 inches in length and somewhat rigid. It is best to have two tubes leading from the head of the stethoscope, one to each ear. The head of the stethoscope should be equipped with both a diaphragm and a bell on a valve system that allows the clinician to switch easily between the two components. The diaphragm is used to hear high-frequency sounds, such as the first and second heart sounds (S_1, S_2), friction rubs, systolic murmurs, and diastolic insufficiency murmurs. The diaphragm should be placed firmly on the chest wall to create a tight seal. Low-frequency sounds, such as the third and fourth heart sounds (S_3, S_4) and the diastolic murmurs of mitral and tricuspid stenosis, are best heard with the stethoscope bell, which should be placed lightly on the chest wall only to seal the edges.

The precordium should be auscultated systematically (see Fig. 17-4). Some authorities suggest the use of anatomical names for the auscultation areas (e.g., aortic and pulmonic), whereas others discourage the use of such labels because murmurs of more than one origin can be heard in a given area.[3,4] Instead, some suggest the use of anatomical landmarks such as intercostal spaces and relationship to the sternal border.[3,4]

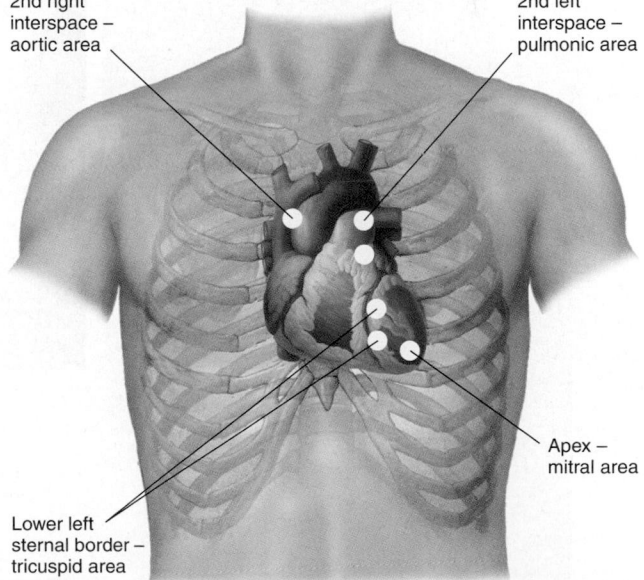

2nd right interspace – aortic area

2nd left interspace – pulmonic area

Apex – mitral area

Lower left sternal border – tricuspid area

Figure 17-4 • Areas of auscultation. I. Aortic area (second intercostal space to the right of the sternum). II. Pulmonic area (second intercostal space to the left of the sternum). III. Tricuspid area (fifth intercostal space to the left of the sternum). IV. Mitral or apical area (fifth intercostal space, midclavicular line). (From Bickley L: Bates' Guide to Physical Examination and Health History, 8th ed. Philadelphia: Lippincott Williams & Wilkins, 2003, p 278.)

Box 17-4 • Rating Scale Used for Assessing Strength of Pulses	
0	Absent
1	Palpable but thready and weak, easily obliterated
2	Normal, not easily obliterated
3	Increased
4	Bounding, cannot obliterate

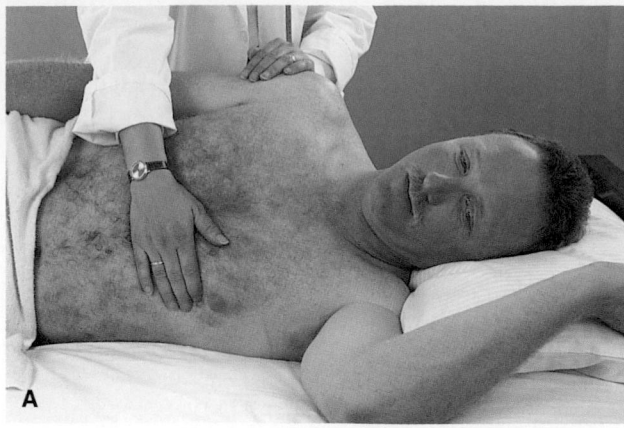 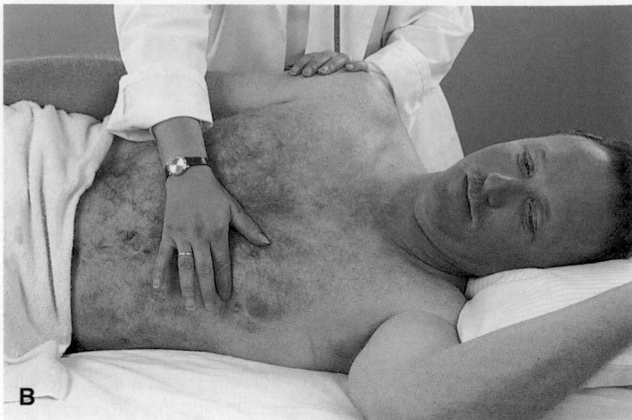

Figure 17-5 • Locate the apical impulse with the palmar surface (**A**), then palpate the apical pulse with the fingerpad (**B**). (From Weber J, Kelley J: Health Assessment in Nursing, 3rd ed. Philadelphia: Lippincott Williams & Wilkins, 2007, p 371.)

The nurse begins the examination by listening with the stethoscope diaphragm in the right second intercostal space along the sternum. This area is sometimes called the aortic area and is the place where S_2 is loudest. Next, the nurse places the stethoscope in the left second intercostal space along the sternum, which is known as the pulmonic listening area, and from there moves the stethoscope down the left sternal border between the second and fifth spaces, one intercostal space at a time. The lower left sternal border area is sometimes referred to as the tricuspid area. Finally, the nurse moves the stethoscope to the mitral area or apex of the heart, where S_1 is the loudest. This pattern is then repeated with the stethoscope bell.

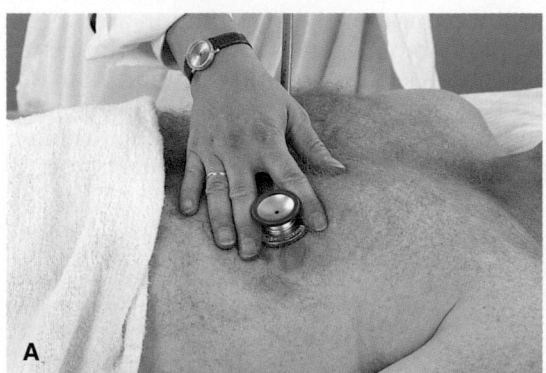

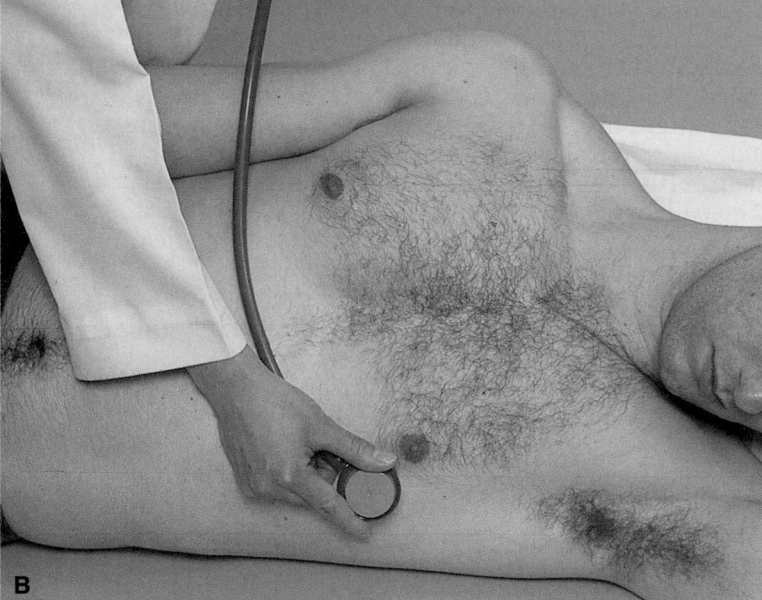

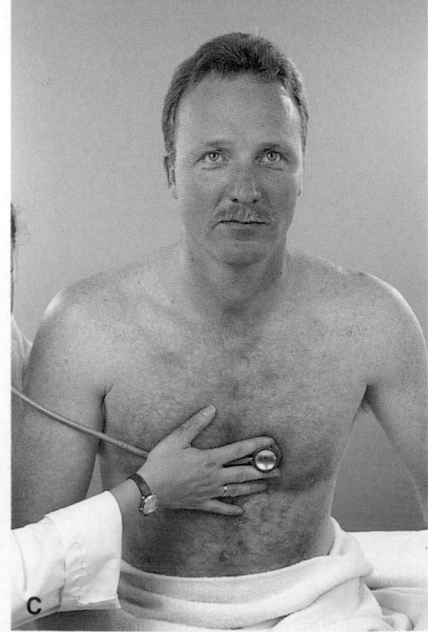

Figure 17-6 • **A:** Auscultating the heart with the patient in a recumbent position. **B:** Auscultating the heart with the patient in a left lateral decubitus position. **C:** Auscultating the heart with the patient sitting up, leaning forward, and exhaling. (**A** and **C,** From Weber J, Kelley J: Health Assessment in Nursing, 3rd ed. Philadelphia, Lippincott Williams & Wilkins, 2007, p 373–374. **B,** From Bickley L: Bates' Guide to Physical Examination and Health History, 9th ed. Philadelphia: Lippincott Williams & Wilkins, 2007, p 315.)

In each area auscultated, the nurse identifies S_1, noting the intensity of the sound, respiratory variation, and splitting. S_2 should then be identified and the same characteristics assessed. After S_1 and S_2 are identified, the presence of extra sounds is noted—first in systole, then in diastole. Finally, each area is auscultated for the presence of murmurs and friction rubs.

First Heart Sound

S_1 is timed with the closure of the mitral and tricuspid valves at the beginning of ventricular systole (Fig. 17-7). Because mitral valve closure is responsible for most of the sound produced, S_1 is heard best in the mitral or apical area. The upstroke of the carotid pulse correlates with S_1 and can be used to help distinguish S_1 from S_2.

The intensity (loudness) of S_1 varies with the position of the atrioventricular (AV) valve leaflets at the beginning of ventricular systole and the structure of the leaflets (thickened or normal). A loud S_1 is produced when the valve leaflets are wide open at the

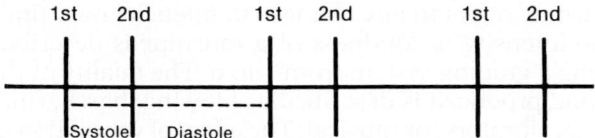

Normal: S_1 is produced by the closure of the AV valves and correlates with the beginning of ventricular systole. It is heard best in the apical or mitral area.

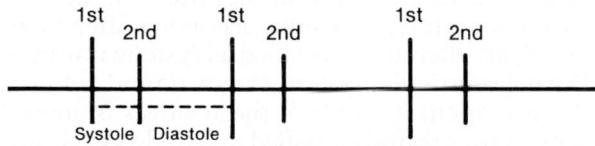

Loud First Sound: The intensity of the first heart sound may be increased when the PR interval is shortened, as in tachycardia, or when the valve leaflets are thickened, as in mitral stenosis.

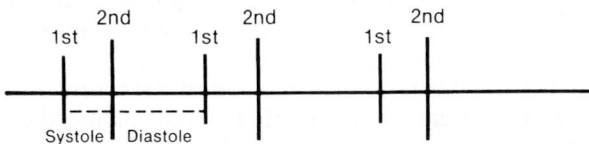

Soft First Sound: A soft S_1 is heard when the PR interval is prolonged.

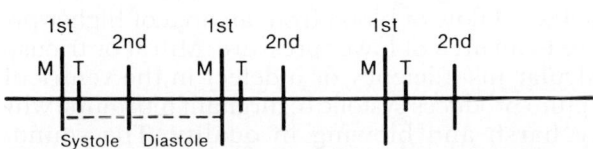

Split First Sound: A split S_1 is heard when right ventricular emptying is delayed. The mitral valve closes before the tricuspid valve and "splits" the sound into its two components.

Figure 17-7 • First heart sound.

onset of ventricular systole and corresponds to a short PR interval on the surface electrocardiogram (ECG) tracing. A lengthening of the PR interval produces a soft S_1 because the leaflets have had time to float partially closed before ventricular systole. Mitral stenosis also increases the intensity of S_1 due to a thickening of the valvular structures.

In general, S_1 is heard as a single sound. However, if right ventricular systole is delayed, S_1 may be split into its two component sounds. The most common cause of this splitting is delay in the conduction of impulses through the right bundle branch; the splitting correlates with a right bundle branch block (RBBB) pattern on the ECG. Splitting of S_1 is heard best over the tricuspid area.

Second Heart Sound

S_2 is produced by the vibrations initiated by the closure of the aortic and pulmonic semilunar valves and is heard best at the base of the heart (Fig. 17-8). This sound represents the beginning of ventricular diastole.

Like S_1, S_2 consists of two separate components. The first component of S_2 is aortic valve closure; the second component is pulmonic valve closure. With inspiration, systole of the right ventricle is slightly prolonged because of increased filling of the right ventricle. This causes the pulmonic valve to close later than the aortic valve and S_2 to become "split" into its two components. This normal finding is termed physiological splitting and is heard best on inspiration with the stethoscope placed in the second intercostal space to the left of the sternum.

The intensity of S_2 may be increased in the presence of aortic or pulmonic valvular stenosis or with an increase in the diastolic pressure forcing the semilunar valves to close, as occurs in pulmonary or systemic hypertension.

Third Heart Sound

An S_3 may be physiological or pathological (Fig. 17-9). A physiological S_3 is a normal finding in children and healthy young adults; it usually disappears after 25 to 35 years of age. An S_3 in an older adult with heart disease signifies ventricular failure.

An S_3 is a low-frequency sound that occurs during the early, rapid-filling phase of ventricular diastole. A noncompliant or failing ventricle cannot distend to accept this rapid inflow of blood. This causes turbu-

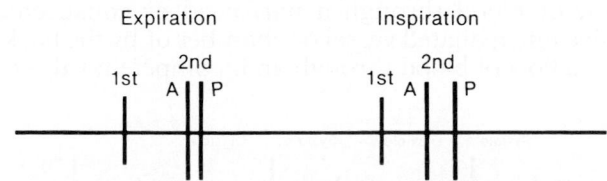

Figure 17-8 • Second heart sound. The second heart sound is produced by the closure of the semilunar valves (aortic and pulmonary). During inspiration, there is an increase in venous return to the right side of the heart, which causes a delay in the emptying of the right ventricle and the closure of the pulmonic valve. This allows the two components of the second heart sound to separate or split during inspiration.

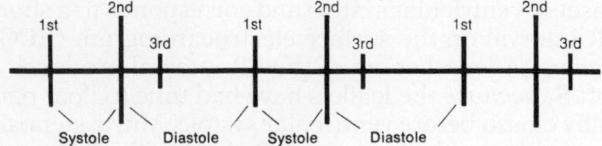

Figure 17-9 • Third heart sound. An S_3 or ventricular gallop is heard in early diastole, shortly after the second heart sound. The presence of a pathological S_3 may be indicative of heart failure.

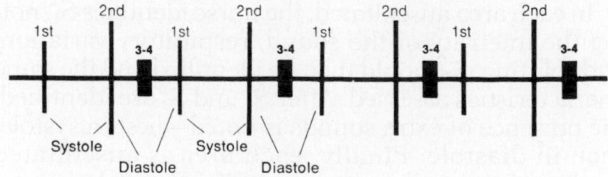

Figure 17-11 • Summation gallop. With rapid heart rates, S_3 and S_4 may become audible as a single, very loud sound that occurs in mid-diastole. This sound is a summation gallop.

lent flow, resulting in the vibration of the AV valvular structures or the ventricles themselves, producing a low-frequency sound. An S_3 associated with left ventricular failure is heard best at the apex with the stethoscope bell. The sound may be accentuated by turning the patient slightly to the left side. A right ventricular S_3 is heard best at the xiphoid or lower left sternal border and varies in intensity with respiration, becoming louder on inspiration.

Fourth Heart Sound

An S_4 or atrial gallop is a low-frequency sound heard late in diastole just before S_1. It is rarely heard in healthy patients (Fig. 17-10). The sound is produced by atrial contraction forcing blood into a noncompliant ventricle that, by virtue of its noncompliance, has an increased resistance to filling. Systemic hypertension, MI, angina, cardiomyopathy, and aortic stenosis all may produce a decrease in left ventricular compliance and an S_4. A left ventricular S_4 is auscultated at the apex with the bell of the stethoscope. Conditions affecting right ventricular compliance, such as pulmonary hypertension or pulmonic stenosis, may produce a right ventricular S_4 heard best at the lower left sternal border; it increases in intensity during inspiration.

Summation Gallop

With rapid heart rates, as ventricular diastole shortens, if S_3 and S_4 are both present, they may fuse together and become audible as a single diastolic sound. This is called a summation gallop (Fig. 17-11). This sound is loudest at the apex and is heard best with the stethoscope bell while the patient lies turned slightly to the left side.

Heart Murmurs

Murmurs are sounds produced either by the forward flow of blood through a narrowed or constricted valve into a dilated vessel or chamber or by the backward flow of blood through an incompetent valve or

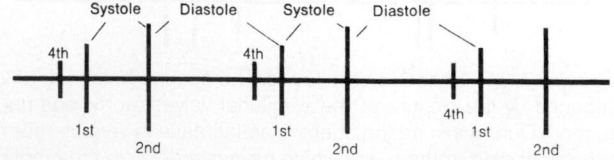

Figure 17-10 • Fourth heart sound. An S_4 is a late diastolic sound that occurs just before S_1. It is a low-frequency sound heard best with the bell of the stethoscope.

septal defect. Murmur classification is based on several attributes (Box 17-5). Timing in the cardiac cycle is an important attribute that refers to the presence of the murmur during either systole or diastole. Systolic murmurs occur between S_1 and S_2. Diastolic murmurs occur after S_2 and before the onset of the following S_1. Location of maximum intensity refers to the anatomical location on the anterior chest where the sound of the murmur is heard the loudest. Anatomical landmarks are used to describe the radiation of the sound. The pitch of the sound helps further differentiate the type of murmur. The shape of the murmur refers to any changes in intensity over time. The intensity or loudness of a murmur is described using a grading system from 1 to 6. The quality of the sound produced is described as blowing, harsh, rumbling, vibratory, or musical. The effect of ventilation or a change in body position on the murmur is another important attribute.

Systolic Murmurs

As previously described, S_1 is produced by mitral and tricuspid valve closure and signifies the onset of ventricular systole. Murmurs occurring after S_1 and before S_2 are therefore classified as systolic murmurs.

During ventricular systole, the aortic and pulmonic valves are open. If either of these valves is stenotic or narrowed, a sound classified as a mid-systolic ejection murmur is heard. Because the AV valves close before blood is ejected through the aortic and pulmonic valves, there is a delay between S_1 and the beginning of the murmur. The murmurs associated with aortic stenosis and pulmonic stenosis are described as crescendo–decrescendo or diamond shaped (Table 17-1), meaning that the sound increases and then decreases in intensity. The quality of these murmurs is harsh, and they are of medium pitch. The murmur caused by aortic stenosis is heard best in the aortic area and may radiate into the neck. The murmur of pulmonic stenosis is heard best over the pulmonic area. In severe pulmonic stenosis, S_2 may be widely split.

Systolic regurgitant murmurs are caused by the backward flow of blood from an area of higher pressure to an area of lower pressure. Mitral or tricuspid valvular insufficiency or a defect in the ventricular septum produces systolic regurgitant murmurs, which are harsh and blowing in quality. The sound is described as holosystolic, meaning that the murmur begins immediately after S_1 and continues throughout systole up to S_2 (see Table 17-1).

Mitral insufficiency produces a murmur, heard most easily in the apical area with radiation to the left

Box 17-5 • Attributes of Heart Murmurs

Timing: A systolic murmur is heard between S_1 and S_2. A diastolic murmur is heard between S_2 and S_1.
Systolic murmurs are classified into three groups:
Midsystolic murmur begins after S_1 and stops before S_2.
Pansystolic (holosystolic) murmur starts with S_1 and stops with S_2 without a gap between the murmur and the heart sound.
Late systolic murmur starts in mid to late systole and continues up to S_2.
Diastolic murmurs also are divided into three categories:
Early diastolic murmur starts right after S_2 and fades before the next S_1.
Mid-diastolic murmur starts a short time after S_2 and fades away or merges into a late diastolic murmur.
Late diastolic murmur starts late in diastole and continues up to S_1.
Location of maximal intensity: The anatomical location where the murmur is heard best. The location is identified based on intercostal space and its relation to the sternum, the apex, the mid-clavicular line, or one of the axillary lines.
Radiation or transmission from the point of maximal intensity: The nurse notes the site farthest from the location of the greatest intensity at which the sound is still heard. The farthest site is identified using anatomical landmarks as described previously.

Pitch: The terms *high, medium,* and *low* are used to describe the pitch of the murmur.
Shape: The shape of a murmur is determined by its intensity over time. A *crescendo murmur* grows louder. A *decrescendo murmur* grows softer. A *crescendo-decrescendo murmur* first rises in intensity, then falls. A *plateau murmur* has the same intensity throughout.
Intensity: A grading system is used to describe the intensity of the murmur.
Grade 1: barely audible in a quiet room, very faint; may not be heard in all positions
Grade 2: quiet, but clearly audible
Grade 3: moderately loud
Grade 4: loud with palpable thrill
Grade 5: very loud with an easily palpable thrill; may be heard when the stethoscope is partly off the chest.
Grade 6: very loud with an easily palpable thrill; may be heard with stethoscope entirely off the chest.
Quality: The terms such as *harsh, rumbling, vibratory, blowing,* and *musical* are used to describe the quality of the sound.
Ventilation and position: Note if the murmur is affected by inspiration, expiration, or a change in body position.

axilla. The type of murmur associated with tricuspid regurgitation is heard loudest at the left sternal border and increases in intensity during inspiration (see Table 17-1). Both types of regurgitant murmurs are often accompanied by a diminished S_1.

Diastolic Murmurs

Diastolic murmurs occur after S_2 and before the next S_1. During diastole, the aortic and pulmonic valves are closed while the mitral and tricuspid valves are open to allow filling of the ventricles.

Aortic or pulmonic valvular insufficiency produces a blowing diastolic murmur that begins immediately after S_2 and decreases in intensity as regurgitant flow decreases through diastole. These murmurs are described as early diastolic decrescendo murmurs (see Table 17-1).

The murmur associated with aortic regurgitation is heard best in the aortic area and may radiate along the sternal border to the apex. Pulmonic valve regurgitation produces a murmur that is loudest in the pulmonic area.

Stenosis or narrowing of the mitral or tricuspid valve also produces a diastolic murmur. The AV valves open in mid-diastole shortly after the aortic

and pulmonic valves close, causing a delay between S_2 and the start of the murmur of mitral and tricuspid stenosis. This murmur decreases in intensity from its onset and then increases again as ventricular filling increases because of atrial contraction; this is termed decrescendo–crescendo (see Table 17-1).

The murmur associated with mitral stenosis is heard best at the apex with the patient turned slightly to the left side. Tricuspid stenosis produces a murmur that increases in intensity with inspiration and is loudest in the fifth intercostal space along the left sternal border.

Friction Rubs

A pericardial friction rub can be heard when the pericardial surfaces are inflamed. This high-pitched, scratchy sound is produced by these inflamed layers rubbing together. A rub may be heard anywhere over the pericardium with the diaphragm of the stethoscope. The rub may be accentuated by having the patient lean forward and exhale. A pericardial friction rub, unlike a pleural friction rub, does not vary in intensity with respiration.

Cardiac Laboratory Studies

Knowledge of the purpose and significance of laboratory values in relation to the diagnosis and prognosis of cardiovascular disease can enhance the quality of nursing care available to patients. Laboratory studies include both routine serum analysis and special studies, such as serum and cardiac enzymes. Nurses who have a basic understanding of laboratory studies can exercise judgment in interpreting

Table 17-1 • Common Systolic and Diastolic Murmurs

Type	Possible Causes	Where to Auscultate	Radiation	Pitch	Shape	Quality	Ventilation and Position
Systolic Murmurs							
Aortic stenosis	Calcification, rheumatic fever, congenital malformation of valve cusps, degenerative process	Aortic area, right second intercostal space	Neck, upper back, right carotid, down the left sternal border to the apex	Medium	Crescendo–decrescendo, May be diminished	Harsh, may be musical at the apex	Heard best with the patient sitting and leaning forward, loudest during expiration
Pulmonic stenosis	Congenital malformation	Pulmonic area, second and third left intercostal spaces	Left side of neck, toward left shoulder	Medium	Crescendo–decrescendo	Often harsh	Loudest during inspiration
Mitral regurgitation	Chronic rheumatic fever, acute bacterial endocarditis, myocardial ischemia or infarction, calcification, dilation of valvular apparatus secondary to dilated left ventricle (e.g., heart failure), mitral valve prolapse	Mitral area, apex	Left axilla, less often to the left sternal border	Medium to high	Plateau, Diminished	Blowing, harsh	Heard best with patient in the left lateral decubitus position, does not become louder with inspiration
Tricuspid regurgitation	Right ventricular failure, dilation of valvular apparatus secondary to dilated right ventricle, bacterial endocarditis (rare)	Tricuspid area, lower left sternal border	Right sternal border, to the xiphoid area, and perhaps to the left mid-clavicular line, but not to the axilla	Medium	Plateau, Diminished	Blowing, harsh	May increase slightly with inspiration
Diastolic Murmurs							
Aortic regurgitation	Bacterial endocarditis, trauma, rheumatic fever, congenital malformation	Aortic area, right second intercostal space	Sternal border, apex	High	Decrescendo	Blowing	Heard best with the patient sitting, leaning forward, with breath held after exhalation
Mitral stenosis	Rheumatic fever, congenital malformation (rare)	Mitral area, apex	Usually none	Low	Decrescendo–crescendo, Loud	Rumbling	Best heard with the patient in a left lateral position Mild exercise and listening during exhalation also make the murmur easier to hear

results relative to other information about the patient. The ability to use this kind of judgment may well affect the patient's clinical course or prognosis.

• Routine Laboratory Studies

Appropriate assessment of normal and compromised cardiac function is essential to ensure accurate evaluation and correct diagnosis of the patient experiencing symptoms consistent with a cardiovascular disorder or coronary artery disease. Nurses can more appropriately plan the care of the patient and initiate interventions if they have an understanding of these laboratory tests and recognize their implications. Valuable information may be obtained by assessing levels of hema-

tological components, coagulation factors, electrolytes, and phospholipids. Determination of these laboratory studies may vary with institutional techniques and equipment used. Normal and abnormal assay ranges have been universally established, and a brief listing of frequently ordered laboratory studies with their normal values can be found in Table 17-2. A more extensive explanation of the effects of abnormal laboratory determinations is provided in other parts of this text and is not addressed here.

HEMATOLOGICAL STUDIES

Accurate assessment of the patient with a possible cardiac disorder merits review of hematological function. It is important for the critical care nurse to understand

Table 17-2 • Normal Reference Ranges for Laboratory Blood Tests

Blood Test	Reference Range	Blood Test	Reference Range
Hematological Studies		*Blood Chemistries (cont.)*	
Red blood cell count		Blood gases	
Men	$4.6-6.2 \times 10^6$	pH	7.35–7.45
Women	$4.2-5.4 \times 10^6$	PaO₂	80–105 mm Hg
Hematocrit		PaCO₂	35–45 mm Hg
Men	40%–50%	Bicarbonate	22–29 mEq/L
Women	38%–47%	Base excess, deficit	0±2.3 mEq/L
Hemoglobin		SaO₂	98%
Men	13.5–18.0 g/100 mL	Sv–CO₂	75%
Women	12.0–16.0 g/100 mL	Bilirubin	
Corpuscle indices		Total	0.2–1.3 mg/dL
Mean corpuscular volume	82–98 FL	Direct	0–20 mg/dL
Mean corpuscular hemoglobin	27–31 pg	Calcium	
Mean corpuscular hemoglobin concentration	32%–36%	Total	8.9–10.3 mg/dL
		Free (ionized)	4.6–5.1 mg/dL
White blood cell count		Creatinine	
Total	4,500–11,000/mm³	Men	0.9–1.4 mg/dL
Differential (in number of		Women	0.8–1.3 mg/dL
cells/mm³ blood)		Glucose (fasting)	65–110 mg/dL
Total leukocytes	5,000–10,000 (100%)	Magnesium	1.3–2.2 mEq/L
Total neutrophils	3,000–7,000 (60%–70%)	Phosphorus	2.5–4.5 mg/dL
Lymphocytes	1,500–3,000 (20%–30%)	Phosphatase, alkaline	35–148 U
Monocytes	375–500 (2%–6%)	Protein (total)	6.5–8.5 g/dL
Eosinophils	50–400 (1%–4%)	Urea nitrogen	8–26 mg/dL
Basophils	0–50 (0.1%)	Uric acid	65–110 mg/dL
Sedimentation rate	0–30 mm/h	Men	4.0–8.5 mg/dL
*Coagulation Studies**		Women	2.8–7.5 mg/dL
Platelet count	250,000–500,000/mm³	*Serum Enzymes**	
Prothrombin time	12–15 s	CK-MM	95%–100%
Partial thromboplastin time	60–70 s	CK-MB	0%–5%
Activated partial thromboplastin time	35–45 s	CK-BB	0%
		Aspartate aminotransferase	<50 U/L
Activated clotting time	75–105 s		
Fibrinogen level	160–300 mg/dL	*Myocardial Proteins*	
Thrombin time	11.3–18.5 s	Troponin-I	<0.1 ng/mL
Blood Chemistries		Troponin-T	<0.1 mcg/mL
Serum electrolytes		Myoglobin	
Sodium	135–145 mEq/L	Men	20–90 ng/mL
Potassium	3.3–4.9 mEq/L	Women	10–75 ng/mL
Chloride	97–110 mEq/L		
Carbon dioxide	22–31 mEq/L		

*Examples; regional laboratory techniques and methods may result in variations.

the role of blood cells in cardiac function and their contribution to the maintenance of healthy tissue. Blood is the transport medium for nutrients, such as oxygen and glucose, as well as electrolytes, plasma proteins, hormones, and medications. It is also the vehicle for removal of the products of metabolism. Changes in blood cell integrity and total cell count may reflect specific disorders of the cardiac system and should be considered an integral part of the laboratory assessment.

Knowledge of normal blood values is vital to understand deviations from normal that can be seen with various cardiac disruptions. It is necessary to review both the red blood cell count, which assesses cellular nutrition, and the white cell count, which assesses defensive capability against infections, when diagnosing specific insults. Table 17-2 lists the components of these helpful hematological studies.

COAGULATION STUDIES

Coagulation studies are also warranted in the laboratory assessment of patients with cardiac disease. Establishment of a baseline for coagulation function provides important information about the patient's ability to form, maintain, and dissolve blood clots. Such information may prove instrumental in patient care decisions. This is especially true in relation to the administration of anticoagulation agents, whether for long-term management, such as warfarin for the management of atrial fibrillation, or for emergency interventions, such as the use of fibrinolytic therapy during an acute MI.

BLOOD CHEMISTRIES

Mechanisms that ensure homeostatic function at the cellular and tissue level depend on the appropriate production and modulation of intracellular and extracellular electrolytes. It is important that the nurse understand normal electrolyte functions and the unique, perhaps life-threatening, situations that may occur when they are significantly abnormal. A thorough analysis of basic electrolyte chemistries is always appropriate in screening of the patient with cardiac disease, whether in the inpatient or outpatient setting. These studies are almost universally obtained during the initial clinical examination. The blood chemistries most commonly assessed are sodium, potassium, chloride, carbon dioxide, calcium, glucose, magnesium, and phosphorus. Table 17-2 provides the normal assay values for common electrolytes.

Common Electrolytes

Sodium is the most abundant cation in the body. It is essential in the maintenance of acid–base balance and osmolality of extracellular fluids as well as in the transmission of nerve impulses. It plays a pivotal role in fluid balance, and its concentration is primarily regulated by the kidneys. Significant alterations of cellular function are evident when sodium levels are lower than normal (hyponatremia) or greater than normal (hypernatremia).

Potassium is the major intracellular cation. Its role in the evaluation of cardiac patients is important because it is released when cells are damaged. It is essential for maintenance of oncotic pressure, intracellular osmolality, and acid–base balance, as well as for its role in cellular reactions. In addition, potassium is vital to the normal functioning of skeletal, smooth, and cardiac muscle. It is particularly important in the regulation of cardiac rate and force of contraction.

Chloride is another major extracellular cation. Like sodium and potassium, it plays a role in acid–base balance and is an important component in the evaluation of acid–base balance.

The carbon dioxide electrolyte is a reflection of carbon dioxide content (mainly bicarbonate), not carbon dioxide gas. In some settings, carbon dioxide is reported as bicarbonate (HCO_3^-).

Other Blood Chemistries

Calcium, like potassium, is important for cardiac function. It plays a significant role in the initiation and propagation of electrical impulses and in myocardial contractility. It is also important for blood clotting, teeth and bone formation, and intracellular energy production. Ionized calcium (free calcium) is responsible for cardiac and neuromuscular excitability. Calcium is reported as total and free (ionized) values.

Glucose levels are important to monitor with baseline laboratory studies because they reflect the nutritive status of the cell. Alterations in glucose, such as in diabetes mellitus, can provide the clinician with both diagnostic as well as prognostic information.

Magnesium is the second major intracellular cation after potassium. It is important in many metabolic processes and is necessary for the normal functioning of the neuromuscular system. It facilitates enzyme activities that help maintain protein synthesis and metabolism, carbohydrate and lipid metabolism, and nucleic acid synthesis. Alterations in normal magnesium levels are reflected in disruptions in neuromuscular activity, such as in the patient with dysrhythmia.

Phosphorus reflects levels of serum phosphate. It is controlled by the parathyroid gland and regulated in the kidneys. Phosphate is important for normal cellular function and for oxygen delivery. It is reciprocal to calcium. Abnormalities can be seen with alterations in heart rate, alterations in neuromuscular function, and reciprocal changes in serum calcium.

SERUM LIPID STUDIES

A review of serum lipid levels is a critical part of the information needed by the nurse to assess cardiovascular risk in any given patient. Patients without a history of coronary artery disease (CAD) need lipid analysis for primary prevention (i.e., prevention of the development of CAD). Patients with a new or past history of CAD need lipid analysis for secondary prevention to prevent progression of known disease after a cardiac event. Standard elements of a lipid profile are total cholesterol, low-density lipoprotein (LDL) cholesterol, very–low-density lipoprotein (VLDL) cholesterol, high-density lipoprotein (HDL) cholesterol, and triglycerides. All treatment of lipids for primary and secondary prevention is based on LDL cholesterol. In 2004, the American Heart Association (AHA) and American College of Cardiology (ACC) updated their guidelines for care of patients with a history of coronary and other atherosclerotic diseases.[1] Their guidelines, along with the National Cholesterol Education Program (NCEP) Adult Treatment Panel (ATP) III, set standards for identification and treatment of elevated cholesterol in patients with and without known coronary artery disease.[2,3] Patients who present with a suspected or confirmed acute cardiovascular or coronary event should have a lipid panel sent to a laboratory within 24 hours of presentation. The nurse is ideally positioned to advocate for this element of care.

Cholesterol, a pearly, fatlike substance, is a precursor of bile acids and steroid hormones. Most of the body's cholesterol is synthesized in the liver, but some is absorbed from the diet. The NCEP III recommends total cholesterol less than 200 mg/dL to lower the probability of CAD in patients with no history of cardiac disease, and to slow the progression of disease in patients with known CAD. Patients with known CAD should have a blood cholesterol less than 160 mg/dL.[2,3]

LDLs constitute 60% to 70% of the total cholesterol in the bloodstream. Based on numerous large-scale studies, LDL cholesterol is known to be directly correlated with the development of CAD and subsequent cardiovascular disease in susceptible individuals. The target LDL cholesterol is less than 130 mg/dL as primary prevention and less than 100 mg/dL as secondary prevention; values less than 70 mg/dL are considered reasonable.[2,3]

Triglycerides originate from VLDLs. Although VLDL cholesterol is not considered to be atherogenic, elevated levels can be a marker for a genetic form of cholesterol disorder. The NCEP ATP III recommends treatment of triglycerides above 500 mg/dL because of the association between hypertriglyceridemia and pancreatitis.[2]

Standard cholesterol tests measure only the percentages of the lipid elements mentioned previously. Particles of LDL cholesterol and HDL cholesterol come in various sizes, and accumulating data suggest that particle size affects atherogenicity. Particle sizes are measured by a test called subfraction analysis, which is used most frequently as an investigative tool and a guide for therapy in patients with known CAD. This test has become increasingly available. It costs about $100 and may not be covered by insurance unless the patient has a diagnosis of CAD.

Table 17-3 summarizes the various serum cholesterol levels, and Table 17-4 describes lipid abnormalities and associated mechanisms.

• Enzyme Studies

Enzymes are found in all living cells and act as catalysts in biochemical reactions. They are present in low amounts in the serum of healthy people. However, when cells are injured, enzymes leak from damaged cells, resulting in serum enzyme concentrations greater than the usual low levels. No single enzyme is specific to the cells of a single organ. Each organ contains a variety of enzymes, and there is considerable overlap among organs in the enzymes they contain. However, the distribution of enzymes in the cells of organs is relatively organ specific. When organ damage occurs, the presence of abnormally high levels of enzymes in the serum, their distribution, and the timing of their appearance and disappearance make the clinical use of serum enzyme studies relevant.

Cardiac enzymes are enzymes found in cardiac tissue. When cardiac injury occurs, as in acute MI, these enzymes are released into the serum, and their concentrations can be measured (Fig. 17-12). Cardiac tissue enzymes are present in other organs as well, so elevation of one or more of these enzymes is not a specific indicator of cardiac injury. However, because cardiac damage does result in above-normal serum concentrations of these enzymes, the quantification of cardiac enzyme levels, along with other

Table 17-3 • Serum Cholesterol Levels

Cholesterol Level (mg/dL)	Description
Low-Density Lipoprotein	
< 100 (<70)	Optimal (optional)
100–129	Near or above optimal
130–159	Borderline high
160–189	High
≥190	Very High
Total Cholesterol	
< 200	Desirable
200–239	Borderline high
≥240 mg/dL	High
High-Density Lipoprotein	
<40	Low
≥60	High
Serum Triglycerides	
<150	Normal
150–199	Borderline high
240–499	High
≥500	Very high

From the Third Report of the NCEP on Detection, Evaluation and Treatment of High Blood Cholesterol in Adults (ATP III). Circulation 106:3143–3421, 2002.

Table 17-4 • Lipid Abnormalities and Associated Mechanisms

Lipid Abnormality	Mechanisms
Elevated total cholesterol	High dietary intake of saturated fat and cholesterol LDL receptor deficiency or down-regulation
Elevated LDL cholesterol	LDL receptor deficiency Apoprotein B-100 genetic defect High dietary intake of saturated fat and cholesterol
Elevated triglycerides	Deficiency in lipoprotein lipase Obesity, physical inactivity, insulin resistance, glucose intolerance Excessive alcohol intake
Low HDL	Apoprotein A-1 deficiency Reduced VLDL clearance Cigarette smoking, physical inactivity Insulin resistance Elevated triglycerides Overweight and obesity Very high CHO intake (>60% total calories), certain drugs (β-blockers, anabolic steroids, progestational agents)
Increased lipoprotein remnants	
(VLDL is a surrogate marker for lipoprotein remnants when Tg is >200 mg/dL)	Defective apolipoprotein E, seen in familial combined hyper-lipidemia
Lipoprotein(a)	Level is genetically determined
Small LDL particles	Particle size is determined by level of Tg; LDL particle is denser and more atherogenic at higher levels of Tg
HDL subspecies	Low levels of HDL 2 and 3 may increase CHD risk, genetically determined vs lifestyle and other lipid levels
Apolipoprotein B	May be potential marker for all atherogenic lipoprotein
Apolipoprotein A-1	Increased CHD risk when Apo A-1 is low
Combined dyslipidemias Small, dense LDL, high triglycerides, low HDL, elevated LDL and triglycerides	Defects in VLDL and LDL receptor activities coexisting with environmental influences such as obesity, physical inactivity, diet high in saturated fat, and cigarette smoking

HDL, high-density lipoprotein; LDL, low-density lipoprotein; Tg, triglycerides; VLDL, very-low-density lipoprotein.

From Woods SL, Froelicher ESS, Motzer SU, Bridges EJ: Cardiac Nursing 5th ed. Philadelphia: Lippincott Williams & Wilkins 2005.

diagnostic tests and the clinical presentation of the patient, is routinely used for diagnosing cardiac disease, particularly acute MI.

The challenge is to identify an enzyme, or "marker", that correctly identifies cardiac cell death. In essence, a cardiac marker is a surrogate for thrombus formation in the coronary arteries. An ideal marker for cardiac injury should have several important characteristics. It should be easy to measure; be inexpensive; be cardiac specific, with a direct proportional relationship between the extent of myocardial injury and the measured level of the marker (zero blood concentration in the absence of cardiac injury); have rapid serum levels after the onset of injury; and stay in the serum long enough to be measured in patients who delay seeking treatment. No available biomarkers fit these criteria, but troponins, discussed later in this text, have several important features, making them the most useful of the biomarkers at present.

Historically, markers of cardiac injury have been pursued with the previously described criteria in mind. One of the earliest markers for cardiac cell death was the white blood cell (WBC) count. Because the WBC count is very nonspecific for cardiac tissue, its use in this setting was limited, and new markers were sought. Subsequently, total lactate dehydrogenase (LDH) and aspartate aminotransferase (AST; previously termed serum glutamic oxaloacetic transaminase [SGOT]) were used along with total creatine kinase (CK). Again, the enzymes were known to have wide tissue distribution and were therefore less useful in identifying cardiac cell death. Routine sampling of AST and LDH for the detection of acute MI is no longer recommended.

CREATINE KINASE

CK is an enzyme that stimulates transfer of high-energy phosphate groups in and out of mitochondria. It is found in heart muscle, skeletal muscle, and brain tissue. CK values vary depending on the muscle mass of the patient. Patients with low muscle mass have less ability to generate elevations in CK—an important concept to grasp when deciding whether a CK value is elevated. CK values start rising 4 to 6 hours after the onset of myocardial necrosis, typically peak at 18 to 24 hours, and return to baseline at 36 to 40 hours. To rule out an MI, samples are commonly drawn every 8 hours for 24 hours.

CK elevations are found in skeletal muscle diseases such as polymyositis and muscular dystrophy, as well as after trauma, surgery, and strenuous exercise. Seizure activity, cerebrovascular insults, heavy alcohol intake, intramuscular injections, and gastrointestinal or urologic insults can also cause significant elevations in CK levels. The noncardiac release of CK generally follows a smoother curve (e.g., elevations that both appear and disappear more slowly than those seen with myocardial necrosis).

Repeated measurement of total CK as an isolated marker for cardiac necrosis is no longer recommended based on the wide tissue distribution alone. The currently published guidelines of the ACC/AHA do not recommend serial measurements of total CK to diagnose acute MI.[1,4] However, total CK remains a relevant tool because it provides the basis for calculation of the mass of the more specific CK isoenzymes.

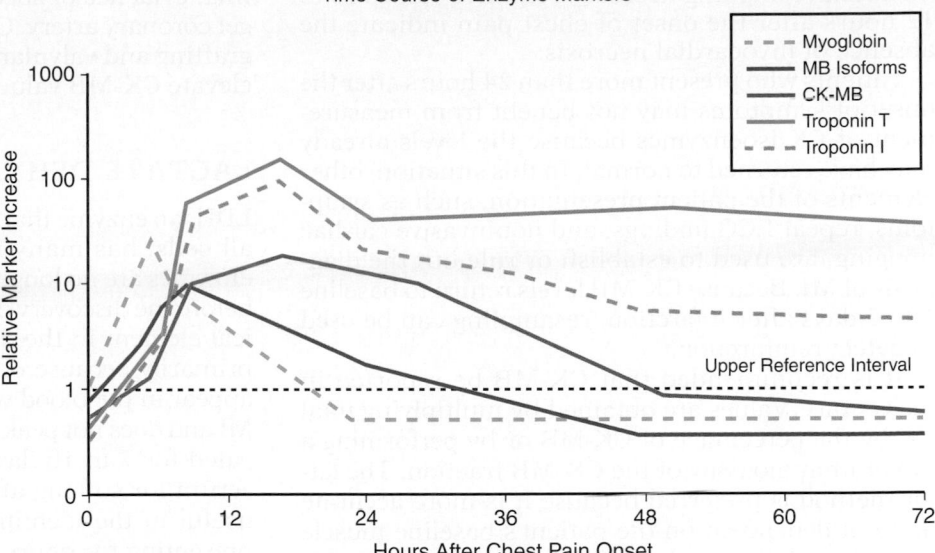

Figure 17-12 • Peak elevation and duration of serum enzymes after acute myocardial infarction. (Data from Antman EM: Acute myocardial infarction. In Braunwald E [ed]: Heart Disease: A Textbook of Cardiovascular Medicine, 5th ed. Philadelphia, WB Saunders, 1997, pp 1184–1228.)

Electrophoresis, glass bead, and radioimmunoassay are techniques used to measure CK isoenzymes. The three CK isoenzymes routinely reported are CK-MM, CK-BB, and CK-MB, which are found to the greatest extent in skeletal muscle, brain, and heart muscle, respectively. Total CK usually consists entirely of CK-MM, and neither CK-BB nor CK-MB is present. In other words, skeletal muscle accounts for the normal levels of CK found in healthy people. Normal skeletal muscle may contain up to 2% CK-MB, and values of CK-MB of as much as 5% are not necessarily considered diagnostic. The amount of CK-MB in cardiac muscle is 15% to 22%, with the remainder being CK-MM. When cardiac damage occurs, as in acute MI, total CK increases, and the percentage of CK-MB is greater than 5%. Although other organs, such as the tongue, small intestine, uterus, and prostate, contain CK-MB, the presence of CK-MB in

amounts greater than 5% generally is considered diagnostic for myocardial damage in the presence of chest pain or other symptoms believed to represent myocardial ischemia. Because the CK-MB isoform is highly specific to cardiac muscle, it has been the preferred marker for cardiac injury for many years.

Within 3 to 12 hours after the onset of infarction, CK-MB usually begins to appear in serum, and it peaks after approximately 24 hours (Table 17-5). However, the appearance and peak may be significantly earlier in patients who have a non–Q-wave infarction or who have undergone successful recannulation of the infarct-related coronary vessel by angioplasty or thrombolytic therapy. Also, because of the specific cellular distribution of the MB subunit, initial MB elevations may not appear until 12 hours after the onset of necrosis. Elevated CK-MB values return to baseline in 36 to 48 hours in patients who

Table 17-5 • Molecular Biomarkers for the Evaluation of Patients With ST-Elevation Myocardial Infarction

Biomarker	Range of Times to Initial Elevation	Mean Time to Peak Elevations (Nonreperfused)	Time to Return to Normal Range
Frequently used in clinical practice			
CK-MB	3–12 h	24 h	48–72 h
cTnI	3–12 h	24 h	5–10 d
cTnT	3–12 h	12 h–2 d	5–14 d
Infrequently used in clinical practice			
Myoglobin	1–4 h	6–7 h	24 h
CK-MB tissue isoform	2–6 h	18 h	Unknown
CK-MM tissue isoform	1–6 h	12 h	38 h

CK-MB, MB isoenzyme of creatine kinase; CK-MM, MM isoenzyme of creatine; cTnI, cardiac troponin I; cTnT, cardiac troponin T.
From Antman EM, Anbe DT, Armstrong PW, et al: ACC/AHA guidelines for the management of patients with ST-elevation myocardial infarction. Circulation; 110:e82–e293, 2004.
Copyright © 2004 American Heart Association.

do not have ongoing necrosis. Negative values 10 to 12 hours after the onset of chest pain indicate the absence of myocardial necrosis.

Patients who present more than 24 hours after the onset of symptoms may not benefit from measurement of CK isoenzymes because the levels already may have returned to normal. In this situation, other elements of the patient presentation, such as symptoms, repeat ECG findings, and noninvasive cardiac imaging, are used to establish or rule out the diagnosis of MI. Because CK-MB levels return to baseline 1 to 2 days after infarction, resampling can be used to detect reinfarction.

It is recommended that CK-MB be reported in mass units. Values are obtained by multiplying total CK by the percentage of CK-MB or by performing a direct immunoassay of the CK-MB fraction. The latter method is preferred because it is more accurate and not dependent on the patient's baseline muscle mass (i.e., ability to release CK into the bloodstream). Most laboratories report the absolute amount of each CK isoenzyme present in the serum, although some also report the percentage. Normal values for absolute amounts of each of the CK isoenzymes vary by laboratory and by the measuring technique used. The amount of CK-MB released into the serum after an acute MI offers a better correlation with infarction size than total CK because of its specificity to cardiac muscle.

Because total CK and CK isoenzymes are the cardiac enzymes whose levels become abnormal earliest after the onset of infarction, routine serial sampling for other cardiac enzymes is unnecessary. Serial analysis of CK isoenzymes is the most specific, sensitive, and cost-effective means of diagnosing acute MI. Perhaps more important, CK isoenzymes also have made it possible to "rule out" an acute MI more quickly and reliably. It no longer requires 2 to 3 days of intensive care unit (ICU) hospitalization to determine that AST or LDH enzyme levels remain normal; rather, an acute MI can be ruled out in less than 24 hours if a patient's CK isoenzyme levels do not become abnormal. Nurses and physicians are able to provide earlier reassurance to patients who are found not to have acute infarction, and patients can be discharged sooner to a less costly environment than the ICU.

Clinical presentation of the patient and the ECG usually are helpful in distinguishing patients with acute MI. Cardiac disorders other than acute MI, including pericarditis, myocarditis, and trauma, also may be associated with abnormal total CK and CK-MB levels. In addition, CK-MB values may also be elevated in a wide variety of conditions, including pericarditis, cardioversion, defibrillation, prolonged supraventricular tachycardia, myositis, hypothyroidism, alcoholism, acute cholecystitis, and collagen disorders. Further elevation in CK-MB should be expected in patients who undergo reperfusion therapy with thrombolytics or coronary angioplasty. Reperfusion therapy releases trapped CK-MB into the blood and may dramatically increase circulating values. Additional CK-MB elevations are, in this setting, evidence of successful recanalization of the target coronary artery. Cardiac surgery, including bypass grafting and valvular replacement or repair, will also elevate CK-MB values.

LACTATE DEHYDROGENASE

LDH, an enzyme that occurs in the cytoplasm of nearly all cells, has many isoenzymes. LDH or LDH isoenzymes are no longer used to diagnose MI. However, before the discovery of CK, LDH was considered a critical element in the diagnosis of myocardial necrosis primarily because of its release kinetics. It begins to appear in the blood within 24 hours after the onset of MI and does not peak for 2 to 3 days; it may remain elevated for 7 to 10 days. Because LDH persists in the serum for so long after occurrence of an MI, it was useful in the identification of patients who delayed presenting for hours to days after the onset of symptoms. That role is now played by the troponins.

• Biochemical Markers: Myocardial Proteins

Myoglobin and troponin are proteins bound within cardiac muscle. Myoglobin, the oxygen-transporting pigment of skeletal and cardiac muscle, appears in the serum less than 1 hour after the onset of symptoms of an MI and peaks in 2 to 4 hours, making it ideal for early detection of myocardial necrosis (see Table 17-5). An isolated elevated serum myoglobin within 4 to 8 hours after the onset of symptoms in a patient with no ECG changes consistent with MI is not reliable. However, because of the high sensitivity of myoglobin, a negative test in the first 4 to 8 hours after the onset of symptoms is useful in ruling out myocardial necrosis. The ACC/AHA guidelines do not include myoglobin in their early risk stratification of patients with chest discomfort.[4]

Troponins, cardiac regulatory proteins that control the calcium-mediated interaction of actin and myosin, are released into the circulation after necrosis and rupture of myocardial cells. Three subforms have been identified: cardiac troponin-I (cTnI), troponin-T (cTnT), and troponin-C (cTnC). Both cTnI and cTnT are highly specific to cardiac tissue. Because cardiac and smooth muscle share cTnC isoforms, cTnC is not useful clinically. Monoclonal antibody–based immunoassays have been developed to detect cTnT and cTnI because the amino acid sequences of the skeletal and cardiac isoforms differ sufficiently. Assays for both cTnI and cTnT have become increasingly sensitive, and very minute elevations of the troponins can be detected. Assays vary between institutions, with abnormal values set just above the upper limit of the assay for a normal healthy population. Troponin values are typically low at 0.1 to 0.4 ng/mL.

Both cTnI and cTnT have equal sensitivity and specificity in detecting myocardial necrosis. Heart failure can release troponins through myocardial strain, which occurs during extensive wall stretching, and myocyte death. Some clinicians believe that very low troponin values in the absence of CK-MB elevation indicate "minor myocardial damage" or "microinfarction." Most institutions elect to perform assays for only one of the proteins because of cost and instrumentation issues. The AHA/ACC guidelines have recommended the use of cTnI or cTnT for the diagnosis of MI.[1,4]

An increase in troponin levels is detected within 4 to 6 hours of myocardial necrosis. Again, serial testing is required. If initial levels are negative, a second set should be taken 6 to 12 hours later, with the patient under direct telemetry observation. Troponin levels generally peak within 24 hours after the onset of symptoms. Reperfusion strategies (i.e., thrombolytics or coronary angioplasty) change the timing of the peak troponin value. Troponins remain elevated for up to 10 days after the cardiac event, facilitating diagnosis of patients who delay seeking treatment (see Table 17-5). Troponin elevations have also been found to be important prognostic indicators that may guide treatment and follow-up. There is a quantitative relationship between the level of cTnI or cTnT detected and the risk for death in patients with MI.

Despite troponin's high sensitivity and specificity for detecting myocardial necrosis, other conditions can be associated with elevated troponin levels. Sepsis, hypovolemia, supraventricular tachycardias, heart failure, pulmonary embolism, myocarditis, myocardial contusion, and renal failure can be associated with elevated troponin levels. In patients with a low pretest probability of CAD, the significance of troponin elevations may be less clear, but other underlying clinical problems should be considered. Demand ischemia, or a mismatch between myocardial oxygen demand and supply, has been suggested as a cause of the higher values. Increases in myocardial oxygen demand can be seen in tachycardia, changes in cardiac loading conditions, increases in cardiac output to accommodate increased systemic oxygen consumption, myocardial depression, reduced coronary perfusion due to causes other than atherosclerosis or infarction, and decreased oxygen delivery to the heart.

In critically ill patients, troponin elevations signify a worse overall outcome. In patients with sepsis and systemic inflammatory response syndrome (SIRS), elevated troponin values are common and are associated with a fourfold increase in overall mortality. Left ventricular hypertrophy (LVH), usually a consequence of long-standing hypertension, can lead to occult subendocardial ischemia through increased oxygen demand from increased muscle mass, coupled with a decreased flow reserve due to remodeled coronary microcirculation, causing an elevation in troponins. Acute stroke is known to cause ischemic ECG changes and elevation in cardiac troponin levels. An imbalance in the autonomic nervous system, with resulting excess of sympathetic activity and

increased catecholamine effects on myocardial cells, has been implicated in this phenomenon.[5]

Between 16% and 50% of patients presenting with pulmonary embolism have troponin elevations, presumably because of right ventricular overload. This is associated with a significant increase in mortality. Pulmonary hypertension and exacerbations of chronic obstructive pulmonary disease can also increase serum troponins, and this, too, indicates a poorer overall prognosis.

In addition, renal insufficiency is an important cause of troponin elevations. Cardiac TnT is elevated more frequently than cTnI in patients with renal failure. Studies using first-generation assays for troponins showed that 71% of patients with renal failure had significant cTnT elevations, and 7% had significant cTnI elevations.[7] The origins of these elevations have been attributed to the high incidence of LVH, heart failure, and microinfarction. Awareness of the increased potential for troponin elevations in affected patients is critical because cardiovascular disease accounts for approximately 50% of deaths in patients with chronic renal failure, and the incidence of coronary disease may be as high as 73%. These patients are at higher risk for silent ischemia, and ECGs can be difficult to interpret because of underlying LVH, electrolyte disturbances, conduction abnormalities, and medications.[7]

• Neurohumoral Hormones: Brain-Type Natriuretic Peptide

When the cardiac muscle decompensates, hormones are released from extracardiac and cardiac origins. Norepinephrine and endothelin are hormones released as a peripheral response to cardiac impairment. Natriuretic peptides are neurohumoral hormones released by the heart. Atrial natriuretic peptides are secreted as a result of atrial myocardial distention, but only minute amounts are released in response to ventricular distention. Another neurohumoral hormone, brain-type natriuretic peptide (BNP), was first isolated in the porcine brain—hence the "B." Although the human brain does secrete BNP, the primary site of release is in the cardiac ventricles, with only very small amounts released in the atria. BNP is released in response to ventricular dilation and increased intraventricular pressures.[8]

BNP levels are helpful in the diagnosis of ventricular dysfunction caused by heart failure. Results of the blood test that measures endogenous levels of BNP may be available in about 30 minutes, making this test especially useful for diagnosing heart failure in the emergency department. Endogenous BNP levels accurately identify decompensated heart failure. Elevated levels of BNP provide important prognostic information for the patient with acute coronary syndromes. In acute MI and unstable angina, elevated BNP levels are predictive of a greater risk for death, postinfarction heart failure, or reinfarction.[9,10] There is an association between troponin levels and BNP, a marker for left and right ventricular wall strain.[6]

• Newer Diagnostic Markers

C-reactive protein, a newer marker of inflammation and necrosis, has been implicated as a factor that can cause disruption of fibrous cap lesions underlying acute coronary events. An acute-phase protein and marker of systemic inflammation, C-reactive protein has been shown to be elevated in patients with acute coronary syndromes. Normal values are 0 to 2 mg/dL. Serum values greater than 3 mg/dL in patients with acute coronary syndrome or greater than 5 mg/dL in

patients after a coronary interventional procedure may indicate a higher risk and merit closer monitoring or more thorough evaluation.[11]

D-Dimer is another physiological marker that may be useful in predicting the risk for cardiac events. It represents the end product of thrombus formation and dissolution that occurs at the site of active plaques in acute coronary syndromes; this process precedes myocardial cell damage and release of protein contents.[12] This marker has also been extensively studied for the diagnosis of deep venous thrombosis and pulmonary embolism. Although D-dimer can be elevated in MI and congestive heart failure, it is being used more commonly to detect other organ thromboembolic events.[13]

Cardiac Diagnostic Studies

Cardiovascular diagnostic techniques have expanded dramatically in the past few years, especially in the area of noninvasive testing. This permits a more careful screening of the population for high-risk procedures and low-risk methods for monitoring disease progression and response to treatment. In addition, many technologies are combined for a functional assessment of the patient's cardiac status so that the best treatment option can be chosen.

The critical care nurse often cares for patients who undergo one or more of these procedures. Understanding the principles on which the procedures are based enables the nurse to answer questions, incorporate diagnostic findings into the patient's plan of care, and provide high-level nursing care. The critical care nurse also can decrease the anxiety of patients and their families by providing an explanation of the procedure.

• Standard 12-Lead Electrocardiogram

The standard ECG records electrical impulses as they travel through the heart. In patients with normal conduction, the first electrical impulse for each cardiac cycle originates in the sinus node and is spread to the rest of the heart through the specialized conduction system—the intra-atrial tracts, AV node, bundle of His, and right and left bundles. As the impulse traverses the conduction system, it penetrates the surrounding myocardium and provides the electrical stimuli for atrial and ventricular contraction. The change in electrical potential in cells of the specialized conduction system as the impulse proceeds is very small and cannot be measured from electrodes outside the body. However, the change in electrical potential of myocardial cells produces an electrical signal that can be recorded from the surface of the body, as is done with an ECG.

Impulses that originate in sites other than the sinus node or impulses that are prevented from traversing

the conduction system because of disease or drugs interrupt the normal order of electrical sequences in the myocardium. An ECG may be used to record these abnormal patterns of impulse formation or conduction. A clinician then has a visual record of the abnormal pattern from which to identify the dysrhythmia.

In addition, an abnormal ECG tracing may result from diseased myocardial cells. For example, in patients with LVH, impulses traversing the enlarged muscle mass of the left ventricle produce a larger electrical signal than normal. In contrast, impulses are unable to traverse myocardial cells that are irreversibly damaged, such as in MI, and no electrical signal is present in the infarcted cells of the left ventricle.

PROCEDURE

The standard 12-lead ECG is so named because the usual electrode placement and recording device permit the electrical signal to be registered from 12 different views. The four limb and six precordial leads are attached to the patient as shown in Figure 17-13. For the limb leads, the recording device alternates the combination of electrodes that are active during recording of electrical signals from the heart (Fig. 17-14). This results in six standard views or leads (I, II, III, augmented voltage of the right arm [aVR], augmented voltage of the left arm [aVL], and augmented voltage of the left foot [aVF]) that are recorded in the heart's frontal plane. The six precordial leads (V_1, V_2, V_3, V_4, V_5, and V_6) are arranged across the chest to record electrical activity in the heart's horizontal plane (see Fig. 17-13).

Used routinely in ICU patients, ECGs assess dysrhythmias and myocardial ischemia or MI. An ECG is performed easily at the bedside, with the patient ideally placed in the supine position and the electrodes arranged as previously described. In some patients, chest bandages may preclude placement of the precordial leads. It is important that the patient remain still during the ECG recording so that skeletal muscle movement does not result in extraneous noise or arti-

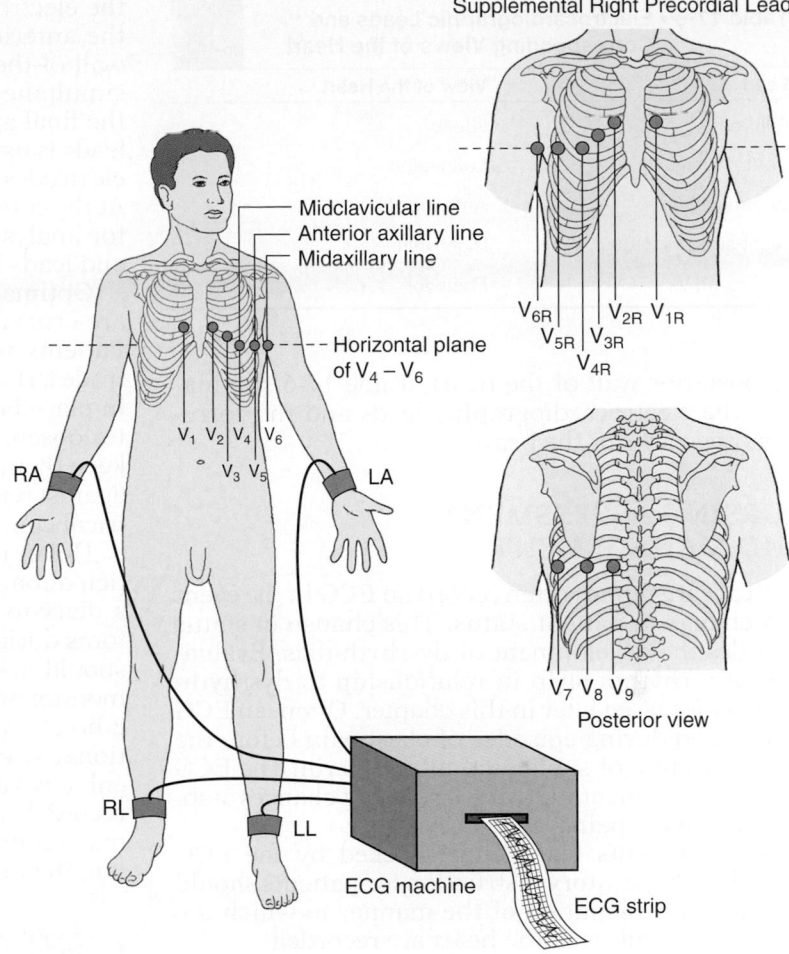

Supplemental Right Precordial Leads

Midclavicular line
Anterior axillary line
Midaxillary line

V_{6R} V_{2R} V_{1R}
V_{5R} V_{3R}
V_{4R}

Horizontal plane of $V_4 - V_6$

V_1 V_2 V_4 V_6
V_3 V_5

RA

LA

V_7 V_8 V_9
Posterior view

RL

LL

ECG machine

ECG strip

Figure 17-13 • Electrocardiogram electrode placement. The standard left precordial leads are V_1, fourth intercostal space, right sternal border; V_2, fourth intercostal space, left sternal border; V_3, diagonally between V_2 and V_4; V_4, fifth intercostal space, left mid-clavicular line; V_5, same horizontal line as V_4, anterior axillary line; V_6, same horizontal line as V_4 and V_5, mid-axillary line. The right precordial leads, placed across the right side of the chest, are the mirror opposite of the left leads. For the posterior leads, V_7 is placed at the left posterior axillary line, V_8 is placed at the left mid-scapular line, and V_9 is placed at the left border of the spine. All are placed on the same horizontal line as V_6.

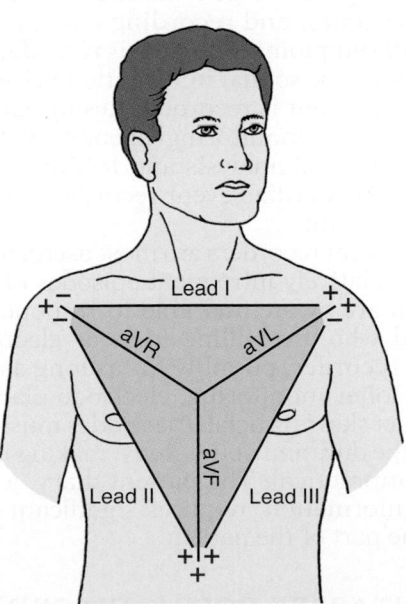

Lead I
aVR   aVL
aVF
Lead II   Lead III

Figure 17-14 • Frontal plane leads: standard limb leads, I, II, III, plus augmented leads aVR, aVL, and aVF. This allows an examination of electrical conduction across a variety of planes (e.g., left arm to leg, right arm to left arm).

fact in the electrical signal. Additional horizontal plane leads may be recorded by placing electrodes on the right side of the chest to view right ventricular activity or the back of the chest to view left ventricular posterior wall activity (see Fig. 17-13).

In the clinical setting, it is important that the nurse remember where the positive electrode is located in each of the twelve leads of the ECG. The positive electrode is like a camera and provides a view of the heart from that perspective. In lead I, the positive electrode is on the patient's left arm, giving a left lateral view of the heart. In leads II and III, the positive electrode is on the patient's left leg, resulting in an inferior view of the heart. For the augmented leads, the name of the lead corresponds with the placement of the positive electrode. In lead aVR, the view of the heart is poor because the positive electrode is far from the heart. In lead aVL, the positive electrode is on the left arm, providing a left lateral view of the heart. In lead aVF, the positive electrode is placed on the patient's left leg, resulting in an inferior view of the heart. Each of the electrodes placed on the patient's chest is a positive electrode. Therefore, V_1 through V_4 provide a view of the anteroseptal wall of the heart, and V_5 and V_6 provide a view of the left lateral wall of the heart. The right-sided chest leads V_4R through V_6R offer the best view of the right ventricle. Leads V_7 through V_9 give the best view of

Table 17-6 • Electrocardiographic Leads and Corresponding Views of the Heart	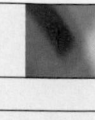
Lead	**View of the Heart**
II, III, aVF	Inferior
I, aVL, V_5, and V_6	Left lateral
V_1 through V_4	Anteroseptal
Right-sided V_4 through V_6	Right ventricle
V_7 through V_9	Posterior

the posterior wall of the heart. Table 17-6 summarizes the electrocardiographic leads and the corresponding views of the heart.

NURSING ASSESSMENT AND MANAGEMENT

Critical care nurses often record an ECG in the event of a change in patient status. This change in status includes the development of dysrhythmias. Evaluation of a rhythm strip in relationship to dysrhythmias is discussed later in this chapter. Often, an ECG is obtained during episodes of chest pain before the administration of sublingual nitroglycerin. The ECG provides documentation of ST-segment changes associated with the pain.

Some patients fear being shocked by the ECG recorder. Preparatory instruction for patients should include an explanation of the manner in which the electrical impulses of the heart are recorded.

• Electrophysiologic Studies

HOLTER OR 24-HOUR MONITORING

Holter monitoring involves the use of ECG monitoring to quantify the frequency and complexity of cardiac ectopic activity that occurs during a patient's usual activities. It is a noninvasive method of assessing for dysrhythmias, response to antiarrhythmic therapy, and development of ECG changes suggestive of ischemia. Holter monitoring is indicated for patients with syncope, near syncope, dizziness, or palpitations. It is also used to evaluate the response of patients who have undergone treatment for dysrhythmias. Patients with infrequent symptoms may not benefit from this method of gathering data because Holter monitoring is most useful in patients who are experiencing their dysrhythmias multiple times in a day. Holter monitoring is rarely used in the inpatient setting where telemetry monitoring is also available.

Holter monitoring involves placement of anterior chest electrodes that are then connected to a portable recording device, or Holter monitor. The Holter monitor is a battery-powered tape-recording device that may be worn on a belt around the patient's waist, or carried on a shoulder strap. Commonly, two leads are recorded continuously on tape through four or five electrodes placed on the patient's anterior chest; the electrodes are arranged so that one lead reflects the anterior wall and the other reflects the inferior wall of the heart. Data are collected from two leads simultaneously to minimize the effect of artifact on the final analysis. Continuous recording of the ECG leads is usually performed for 24 to 48 hours, and the electrodes must remain in place for the entire session. At the completion of the test, the recorder is returned for analysis. Some patients consider the equipment and leads involved intolerable.

Optimal skin preparation and electrode placement are crucial to obtaining high-quality ECG readings. Patients must bathe before placement of the electrodes. Bathing is prohibited while the electrodes are in place because contact with water can cause them to loosen. Fishnet placed over the electrodes helps keep them in place. It is necessary to caution patients against removal of the electrodes because loss of electrical contact can mimic dysrhythmias.

Holter monitoring requires significant patient participation. Patients receive instructions about keeping a diary to record medications, activities, and symptoms during the monitoring period. Usually, patients should maintain normal activities while wearing the monitor and record an entry in the diary at least every 2 hours. An understanding of the physical and emotional stressors, as well as the patient's symptoms, enhances analysis of the recordings. Compliance with record keeping is necessary. Hospitalized patients may require the assistance of nursing staff to maintain their diaries.

EVENT (CONTINUOUS LOOP) MONITORING

In event (continuous loop) monitoring, the patient wears electrodes and a recording device, but the device does not record continuously. Instead, the patient is required to activate the recorder when a symptom occurs, and recording can go on for the duration of symptoms. The ECG is recorded on a continuous loop tape so that information before, during, and after the event is recorded. Results can be communicated to a monitoring agency by telephone, allowing for rapid analysis and feedback to patient and caregiver. Cardiac event recorders can be worn for up to 1 month.

Cardiac event recorders are most useful for patients who have relatively infrequent episodes of dysrhythmias, who are aware and able to respond to symptoms, and who are willing to wear electrodes and carry the recorder, possibly for as long as a month. As with Holter monitoring, electrode placement on clean, intact skin is crucial. Electrodes must be kept in place for the duration of the study, making immersion bathing impractical. The patient diary, a source of detailed information, requires significant participation on the part of the patient.

IMPLANTABLE LOOP MONITORING

The implantable loop monitor (ILR) is a device that is implanted subcutaneously and provides continuous ECG monitoring for up to 14 months. ILRs were developed to provide long-term monitoring for patients with presyncope and syncope. The major limitations of the ILR are its requirement for subcutaneous implantation and cost. The use of the device requires familiarity with implantation techniques and programming. The ILR is used for patients in whom less expensive tests, such as Holter monitoring, have failed to provide a diagnosis.

Implantation of the ILR is a surgical procedure that exposes the patient to the risk for infection and bleeding. Patients undergoing ILR implantation must understand the potential risks of the procedure. They need instruction regarding postoperative site care and use of the device.

SIGNAL-AVERAGED ELECTROCARDIOGRAPHY

Signal-averaged electrocardiography (SAECG) is performed in the same manner as a resting ECG, except that the heart's electrical activity is monitored for 15 to 20 minutes. The purpose of SAECG is to filter out random noise and to allow very low levels of electrical activity, called late potentials, to be recorded. This electrical activity, which is not detected by standard ECG, is thought to be coming from the cardiac substrate. Late potentials have been shown to be useful in identifying patients at risk for lethal heart rhythms.

Historically, SAECG was used to detect late potentials in patients after MI or cardiac surgery, in patients with CAD, and in patients with unexplained syncope. Late potentials after MI are an independent risk factor that identifies patients prone to develop ventricular tachycardia (VT). SAECG can also be used to identify patients with nonsustained VT or syncope who may develop sustained VT at electrophysiology study. Currently, SAECG is rarely used, except after right ventricular MI.

SAECG must be performed by specially trained personnel in a very quiet room, with no extraneous electrical or electromagnetic signal-emitting equipment present. The patient must be cooperative and restful for the duration of the study.

DIAGNOSTIC ELECTROPHYSIOLOGY STUDY

The diagnostic electrophysiology study is a type of heart catheterization during which access to the heart is obtained through the femoral veins, or, for some more complex studies, the upper extremity (brachial, external jugular, or subclavian) veins. Multiple catheters are usually placed in one or more vessels. An arterial line is typically placed to provide continuous blood pressure monitoring during the case.

Diagnostic electrophysiology studies are performed to evaluate a broad spectrum of cardiac dysrhythmias. They can help assess the function of the sinoatrial (SA) node, the AV node, and the His-Purkinje system; determine the characteristics of reentrant dysrhythmias; map the location of dysrhythmogenic foci for potential ablation; and assess the efficacy of antiarrhythmic drugs and devices. The basic electrophysiology protocol involves measurement of baseline conduction intervals; atrial pacing to assess SA node and AV node properties; assessment of the His-Purkinje system conductivity; ventricular pacing to evaluate for retrograde conduction and ventricular dysrhythmia potentials; and drug testing.[1]

Diagnostic electrophysiology studies are very safe. The risks associated with the procedure are similar to those encountered with cardiac catheterization and include hemorrhage, thromboembolism, phlebitis, and infection. Because most diagnostic electrophysiology studies do not require arterial puncture, the risk for serious vascular damage is very low. The risk for death due to the induction of lethal dysrhythmias is close to zero, in part because the procedural setting is uniquely equipped to terminate hemodynamically unstable dysrhythmias.

The following preprocedure preparations are necessary for patients undergoing diagnostic electrophysiology studies:

▶ The physician or nurse reviews the procedure so that the patient clearly understands its purpose and nature. Appropriate personnel obtain informed consent.

▶ Because sedation is used, the patient must be NPO for 8 hours before the procedure.

▶ The ordering physician or nurse practitioner must review patient medications to be sure they are to be administered on the day of the procedure. Antiarrhythmic drugs are typically withdrawn before the procedure.

▶ Excessive anxiety can increase catecholamine release and affect sympathetic tone, so the nurse should alert the ordering physician or nurse practitioner to signs of anxiety.

Postprocedure, the following nursing care applies:

▶ The nurse checks the patient's blood pressure and heart and respiratory rates frequently according to the institution's protocols.

▶ If the diagnostic electrophysiology study failed to induce dysrhythmias, the patient may not require telemetry monitoring. If dysrhythmias were induced, the patient does need continuous telemetry monitoring.

▶ The nurse monitors venous and arterial access sites for bleeding. This monitoring may include serial complete blood counts to ensure stable hemoglobin and hematocrit counts.

TILT TABLE TESTING FOR SYNCOPE

Tilt table testing, or upright tilt table testing, refers to maintaining the patient in a head-up position for a brief period to provoke syncope, bradycardia, or hypotension. In tilt table testing, the patient is positioned on a tilt table in the supine position and tilted upright to a maximum of 60 to 80 degrees for 20 to 45 minutes. Isoproterenol may be given to provoke syncope in patients who do not become symptomatic within the testing period.

Tilt table testing is performed on patients who are suspected of having vasodepressor or vasovagal syncope. Upright posture is associated with gravitational pooling of blood, which results in a decline in central venous pressure, stroke volume, and blood pressure. These effects normally lead to activation of arterial and cardiopulmonary baroreceptor reflexes that maintain blood pressure. In people susceptible to vasovagal syncope, these reflexes are reversed, resulting in bradycardia and hypotension that leads to syncope.

The patient experience during tilt table testing can be unpleasant, particularly if the patient has syncope during the study. Patients undergoing tilt table testing need to be NPO for 8 hours before the study. They need intravenous (IV) access and should be informed that they may receive a vasoactive agent such as isoproterenol.

• Chest Radiography

Chest radiography is a routine diagnostic test used to assess critically ill patients with cardiac disease. The test can be performed easily at the bedside in patients too ill to be transported to the radiology department. The image obtained on a radiograph that allows visualization of vascular and cardiac shapes is based on the premise that thoracic structures vary in density and permit different amounts of radiation to reach the film.

Chest radiography may be used for the evaluation of cardiac size, pulmonary congestion, pleural or pericardial effusions, and position of intracardiac lines, such as transvenous pacemaker electrodes or pulmonary artery (PA) catheters. Figure 17-15 shows the structures that can be seen on a normal posteroanterior chest radiograph.

PROCEDURE

Cardiac size is evaluated best in the radiology department, where the procedure can be standardized with the patient standing and the radiograph taken from posterior and lateral views at a distance of 6 feet. Portable bedside chest radiographs usually are taken only from an anterior view with the patient lying supine or sitting erect and are not standardized.

Patients undergoing radiography of the chest are instructed not to move while the radiograph is being taken. Proper positioning of the radiographic plate behind the patient is important to ensure that thoracic structures are aligned on the film. Care is taken to remove all metal objects, including fasteners on clothing, from the field of view because metal blocks the x-ray beam. Patients usually are asked to take a deep breath and hold it when the radiograph is taken to displace the diaphragm downward; this may be uncomfortable for patients who have undergone recent thoracic surgery.

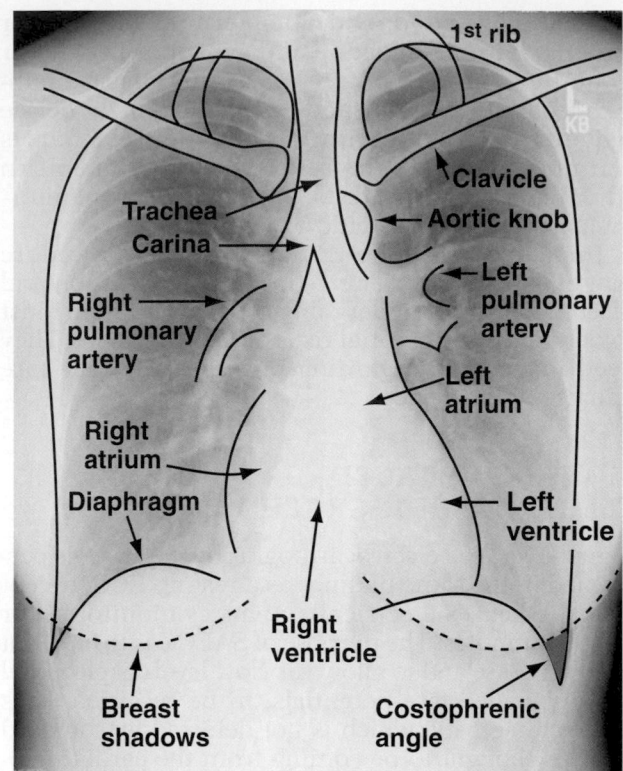

Figure 17-15 • Outline of structures visible on normal posteroanterior chest radiograph. (In Woods SL, Froelicher ESS, Motzer SU, Bridges EJ: Cardiac Nursing, 5th ed. Philadelphia: Lippincott Williams & Wilkins, 2005, p 298.)

NURSING ASSESSMENT AND MANAGEMENT

The critical care nurse's role in obtaining diagnostic thoracic radiographic films often is limited to the ICU, where portable radiographs are made. With unstable patients, the nurse must decide when the film can be taken. It is important that IV lines not become tangled or loosened while one is trying to place the radiographic plate in the proper position.

Female patients of childbearing potential should have a lead drape placed over the abdomen to protect the ovaries from any radiation scatter. For the same reason, caregivers and family members should leave the patient's room when the radiograph is taken. When caregivers cannot leave the patient's bedside, a lead apron should be worn.

• Echocardiography

Echocardiography refers to a group of tests that use ultrasound technology to provide information about cardiac structures. Ultrasound technology uses sound waves ranging from 1 to 10 million cycles/second, or 1 to 10 megahertz (MHz). Sound waves at a frequency above 20,000 cycles/second, or 20 kilohertz, are not audible to the human ear. In echocardiography, a transducer containing a rapidly vibrating piezoelectric crystal is used to generate sound waves. The piezoelectric crystal transforms electrical energy into sound energy. The resolution, or ability to see two objects that are spatially close together, with ultrasound is related to the wavelength of the sound waves being used.

In echocardiography, a transducer emits ultrasound waves and receives a signal from the reflected sound waves; it alternates periods of sound transmission and reception. As the sound waves are emitted and travel through tissues with a homogeneous density, such as when the sound waves move through the left ventricular wall, the signal travels in a straight line. When the density of the structures changes, such as when the waves move from the ventricular wall into the blood-filled left ventricle, the direction of the sound waves changes, and this difference is recorded by the receiver. These density changes are called interfaces, and they form the basis for being able to distinguish one structure from another. Ultrasound waves do not travel well through bone; thus, bony paths are avoided during the course of the examination.

Echocardiography is most often used to assess ejection fraction, wall motion and thickness, systolic and diastolic ventricular volumes, valvular function and disease, vegetations, intracardiac masses or thrombi, and pericardial fluid. It is a helpful diagnostic tool in the presence of sudden clinical deterioration in acute myocardial infarction, in which significant complications may be observed or suspected. In addition, it also may be used in the evaluation of function of all four cardiac valves, including calculation of gradients and orifice size, intracardiac tumors, and aortic dissection. Detection of intracardiac shunts is possible using echocardiography with the rapid venous infusion of an agitated bubble solution as an adjunct.

The quality and usefulness of echocardiographic studies is dependent on the relative age of the technology being used, the skill of the technologist performing the study, the habitus of the patient, and the skill of the interpreter of the study. Accuracy may decrease up to 20% in patient who are obese or who have chronic obstructive pulmonary disease or chest wall deformities. These physical features increase the distance the ultrasound waves must travel and thus increase the likelihood of artifact. Transthoracic echocardiography (TEE) is of limited usefulness in investigating the left atrium and left atrial appendage because these structures are at the back of the heart.

Echocardiography is performed in a specifically designed laboratory with dim lighting and minimal sound distraction. It can also be performed at the bedside with lighting optimized to enhance the quality of the study. Patients should be able to tolerate lying flat or nearly flat. The technician asks them periodically to change position, and they should be able to turn onto their left side for several minutes at a time. In addition, they should be able to breathe in deeply or hold their breath. They do not need to be NPO.

M-MODE ECHOCARDIOGRAPHY

Motion mode, or M-mode, echocardiography allows recording of amplitude and of the rate of motion of moving objects with great accuracy. It is often referred to as an "ice pick" view because it uses a single beam of sound that allows a small region of the heart to be visualized at any point in time. The four positions of the transducer depicted in Figure 17-16 are the typical views used during an M-mode echocardiogram. It provides rapid assessment of valvular motion and chamber wall thickness. The transmitter is placed on the anterior chest in an intercostal space or subcostal position to avoid bony structures.[2]

TWO-DIMENSIONAL ECHOCARDIOGRAPHY

Two-dimensional (2D) images of cardiac structures can be obtained by using multiple crystals to generate a cross-sectional imaging plane. The ultrasound beam is pie shaped, resulting in a "plane" of reflected echoes. Visually, 2D echocardiography creates a cross-sectional slice of the heart from parasternal, subcostal, apical, and suprasternal positions. This approach is useful for evaluating the thickness of the left ventricular wall, left ventricular wall mass, and wall motion abnormalities.[2]

THREE-DIMENSIONAL ECHOCARDIOGRAPHY

Three-dimensional (3D) echocardiography allows for the imaging and analysis of cardiac structures as they move in time and space. 3D echocardiography uses the principles of ultrasound imaging with advanced

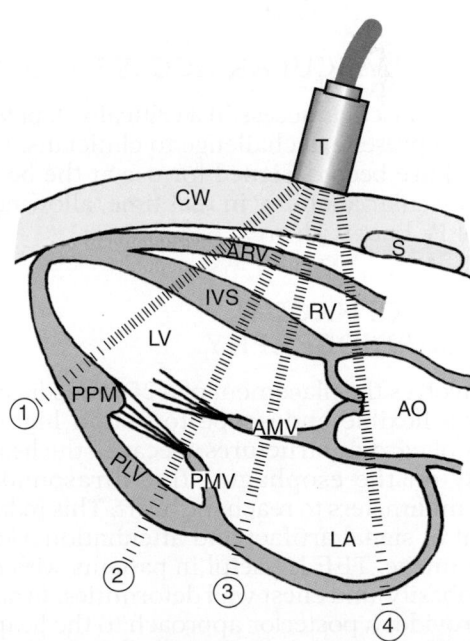

Figure 17-16 • Echocardiographic views of the heart. A cross-section of the heart shows the structures through which the ultrasonic beam passes as it is directed from the apex (1) toward the base (4) of the heart. AMV, anterior mitral valve; AO, aorta; ARV, anterior right ventricular wall; CW, chest wall; IVS, interventricular septum; LA, left atrium; LV, left ventricle; PLV, posterior left ventricular wall; PMV, posterior mitral valve; PPM, posterior papillary muscle; RV, right ventricular cavity; S, sternum; T, transducer.

real-time reconstruction capabilities to generate a more authentic representation of the heart. Early in the evolution of 3D echocardiography, the generated images required lengthy postprocedure processing, which meant that immediate results were not available. Current technology allows for real-time images, making this modality a valuable diagnostic and treatment tool.[2]

DOPPLER ECHOCARDIOGRAPHY

Doppler echocardiography superimposes Doppler techniques on either M-mode or 2D images. The direction of blood flow can be assessed by measuring echoes reflected from red blood cells as they move away from or toward the transducer. This type of study is particularly useful in patients with valvular disease. Stenotic valves cause turbulence in the forward flow of blood through the heart, and regurgitant valves cause turbulence in blood flowing retrograde through the cardiac chambers. When the direction of flow is color encoded, the study is known as a color Doppler echocardiogram. Audio signals usually are recorded during Doppler studies. Contrast material may also be used in conjunction with M-mode or 2D echocardiography. Although many agents have been used as contrast material, almost any liquid injected intravenously contains microbubbles. As the microbubbles travel through the heart, they produce multiple echoes. This technique is especially useful in identifying right-to-left intracardiac shunts because of the early appearance of the microbubble echoes on the left atrium or ventricle.

BEDSIDE VASCULAR ACCESS TESTING

Obtaining vascular access in a critically ill patient frequently represents a challenge to clinicians. Portable devices have been designed for use at the bedside to locate vascular anatomy in real time, allowing placement of IV lines with great accuracy.

TRANSESOPHAGEAL ECHOCARDIOGRAPHY

TEE involves the placement of a 2D transducer at the end of a flexible endoscope to obtain high-quality images of cardiac structures. Because the heart rests directly on the esophagus, the ultrasound signal travels millimeters to reach the heart. This reduces the amount of signal artifact and attenuation, yielding a clearer image. TEE is useful in patients with emphysema, obesity, and chest wall deformities. In addition, TEE provides a posterior approach to the heart; thus, it also allows for better imaging of the aorta, PA, valves of the heart, both atria, atrial septum, left atrial appendage, and coronary arteries.[3]

Patients undergoing TEE should be NPO for 6 hours before the study. IV sedation is given, and several staff members, including technicians, nurses, and a physician, are required throughout the study. TEE takes substantially longer than a transthora-

cic echocardiogram and can be uncomfortable for patients. There is also a risk for esophageal perforation (1 in 10,000) associated with the procedure. Table 17-7 summarizes nursing considerations for caring for the patient undergoing TEE.

INTRAVASCULAR ULTRASOUND

Intravascular ultrasound uses ultrasound technology to visualize the lumen and wall structure of the coronary arteries. It is an adjunct to cardiac catheterization and is discussed more fully in that section (see Cardiac Catheterization, Coronary Angiography, and Coronary Intervention).

• Stress Testing

Stress testing is an important tool in the evaluation of the patient with suspected ischemic cardiovascular disease. Stress testing is used to assess prognosis and to determine functional capacity. Stress testing involves monitoring physiological parameters such as blood pressure and ECG when the heart is in a resting state and again when the heart has been stressed either by exercise or by a pharmacological agent chosen to simulate exercise. A great deal more information can be obtained by also looking at images of the heart at rest and with activity. These images can be obtained by a variety of methods, including radioactive tracers and echocardiography. Boxes 17-6 and 17-7 present indications and contraindications for stress testing, respectively. These contraindications largely relate to advanced disease states; stress testing in patients with these conditions could precipitate a catastrophic event.

Fundamentally, stress testing provides information about the heart's response to activity. The heart extracts 70% of the oxygen carried by each unit of blood perfusing the myocardium. Cardiac metabolism is nearly entirely aerobic, meaning that the heart is unable to create energy in anaerobic conditions or when the oxygen supply is insufficient. Therefore, an increase in oxygen demand on the heart requires additional coronary artery blood flow to meet the new metabolic requirements. Narrowing of the coronary arteries can limit the amount of blood delivered to a portion of the myocardium, resulting in ischemia.

EXERCISE STRESS TESTING

Patients must be ambulatory to participate in exercise stress testing. Functional limitations due to orthopedic, neurological, pulmonary, or peripheral vascular issues can affect the patient's ability to complete the stress test protocol.

Procedure

In exercise stress testing, the heart rate is monitored continuously while exercise is performed on a treadmill or bicycle. The patient is exercised to a target

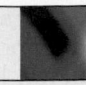

Table 17-7 • Nursing Considerations for the Patient Undergoing Transesophageal Echocardiography (TEE)

Nursing Action	Rationale
Preprocedure	
1. Evaluate patient for contraindications.	Patients with history of dysphagia or esophageal disease are not candidates for TEE.
2. Instruct patient and family about procedure.	Some discomfort may occur; patient will receive moderate sedation but will be closely monitored.
3. Ensure that documented patient history is adequate and informed consent has been signed.	Medication allergies should be noted; procedure requires consent signature.
4. Ensure that patient has been NPO for 6 h before procedure.	Aspiration precaution is vital.
5. Prepare patient for procedure.	Remove oral prosthetics, as indicated; have patient void.
6. Insert peripheral IV catheter.	IV access is required for routine medication administration; emergency vascular access line should be available.
7. Place patient on cardiac monitor with blood pressure and pulse oximetry.	Patient must be continually monitored during procedure.
8. Ensure that emergency resuscitation equipment is nearby, including medications, defibrillator, and suction apparatus.	Cardiac arrest precaution.
During Procedure	
1. Monitor cardiac rhythm, blood pressure, pulse oximetry, and airway patency per institutional policy.	Continuous observation is required after moderate sedation.
2. Assist physician with patient positioning and endoscope placement.	Allaying fears enhances patient cooperation.
3. Monitor for complications.	Vagal stimulation may occur with a resultant vasovagal reaction; transient tachycardia/bradycardia and blood pressure alterations may appear; patient may experience hypoxia or laryngospasm.
4. Reassure patient throughout procedure.	Allaying fears enhances patient cooperation.
5. Document patient response to procedures.	Per institutional protocol.
Postprocedure	
1. Assess vital signs at conclusion of procedure; document per institutional policy.	Comparison with baseline is necessary to monitor sedation recovery.
2. Assist patient to position of comfort or on one side.	Position provides comfort and patent airway support.
3. Keep patient NPO until gag reflex is assessed.	Prudent given aspiration risk.
4. If gag reflex is present, encourage patient to cough; offer lozenges or ice to soothe sore throat; keep NPO per physician order.	Interventions provide patient opportunity to clear residual secretions and obtain comfort.
5. If outpatient, instruct patient not to drive for at least 12 h.	If patient was sedated during procedure, it is best if family member or another drives patient home.
6. Instruct patient to seek care or contact physician in event of dyspnea, hemoptysis, or severe pain.	If symptoms of complications occur, patient should be reevaluated.

Box 17-6 • Indications for Stress Testing

1. Differential diagnosis of chest pain (i.e., evaluation of patients with suspected ischemic heart disease)
2. Assessment of the level of exercise at which ischemic manifestations occur in a patient with known ischemic heart disease
3. Evaluation of therapy for dysrhythmias and angina
4. Evaluation of functional disability secondary to organic heart disease (e.g., valvular heart disease)
5. Risk stratification of the asymptomatic patient with multiple risk factors for ischemic heart disease

Box 17-7 • Contraindications for Stress Testing

1. Recent myocardial infarction (4–6 wk), except when submaximal protocols are used (65% of maximum predicted heart rate or symptom-limited exercise stress testing before hospital discharge)
2. Unstable angina or angina at rest
3. Rapid ventricular or atrial dysrhythmias
4. Advanced atrioventricular block, unless chronic
5. Uncompensated congestive heart failure
6. Acute noncardiac illnesses
7. Severe aortic stenosis
8. Blood pressure greater than 170/100 mm Hg before the onset of exercise

heart rate that is 85% of the maximum predicted for that individual. By convention, the maximum predicted heart rate is calculated as 220 beats/minute for men (210 beats/minute for women) minus the patient's age in years. Attainment of maximum heart rate is a good prognostic sign.

The blood pressure, heart rate and rhythm, ECG, presence or absence of symptoms, and workload performed are monitored. Workload is determined by metabolic equivalents (METS) or by the double product (blood pressure × heart rate). METS are defined as the resting respiratory oxygen uptake for a 70-kg, 40-year-old man, and 1 MET is equivalent to 3.5 mg/minute per kilogram of body weight. Work activities are calculated in terms of METS. Stair climbing, for example, is approximately equivalent to 4 METS. A reasonable workload for most active adults is 10 METS. Although the double product correlates well with the degree of cardiovascular disease, it is less often used as a measure of workload.

Initial ECG readings are performed before exercise to document a baseline, with continuous 12-lead monitoring used throughout the study. The lead system is the same as used for the standard 12-lead ECG. However, it is necessary to move the limb leads to the torso to prevent arm or leg movement during exercise from interfering with ECG recording. Skin preparation and electrode attachment require careful attention to permit interpretable recordings during maximal exercise. It may be necessary to wrap material or fishnet over the electrodes and cables on the patient's torso to reduce movement artifact. Treadmill stress testing without a concomitant imaging modality is less reliable in females; therefore, exercise stress testing in females is typically paired with radionuclide or echocardiographic imaging. Baseline ECG abnormalities such as left bundle branch block (LBBB) make analysis of exercise-induced ECG changes more complex.

The treadmill protocol chosen should reflect the patient's physical capacity and the purpose of the test. All treadmill protocols are multistaged, using increments in time, speed, and elevation of the treadmill platform. The protocol is selected based on the condition of the patient and the purpose of the study. For example, the Ellestad protocol uses small increments in workloads of shorter duration, whereas the Bruce protocol uses larger workload increments of longer duration (Box 17-8). The Ellestad protocol may be better suited to a patient with less exercise tolerance. The Bruce protocol is among the most popular in use for reasonably functional people; a large body of diagnostic and prognostic data supports its use.

Patients who have not previously undergone exercise testing should be allowed briefly to practice walking on the treadmill or riding the bicycle. Before starting the test, a resting baseline ECG and blood pressure are obtained with the patient in sitting and standing positions. The ECG and heart rate are monitored continuously throughout the test, and blood pressure is monitored every few minutes. The monitoring continues for at least 6 to 10 minutes into recovery, or until symptoms or blood pressure and

Box 17-8 • Protocols for Exercise Stress Testing

Bruce Protocol

3 min	1.75 mph	10% grade
3 min	2.5 mph	12% grade
3 min	3.4 mph	14% grade
3 min	4.2 mph	16% grade
3 min	5.0 mph	18% grade

Ellestad Protocol

3 min	1.6 mph	10% grade
3 min	2.2 mph	10% grade
2 min	2.6 mph	10% grade
2 min	3.0 mph	10% grade
2 min	3.6 mph	10% grade

From Heger J, Niemann J, Roth R, Criley J: Cardiology, 4th ed. Philadelphia: Lippincott Williams & Wilkins, 1998, p 85.

ECG changes have resolved to document the patient's return to baseline values.

It is mandatory that emergency personnel and equipment be available in areas where exercise testing is performed. Indications of myocardial ischemia during exercise testing are the development of ST-segment depressions, chest pain or the anginal equivalent, or failure to increase blood pressure to 120 mm Hg or the sustained decrease of 10 mm Hg with progressive stages of exercise. The test is terminated for any of the following reasons:

1. The target heart rate is reached.
2. The patient is unable to continue exercising because of shortness of breath, fatigue, claudication, or severe chest pain.
3. There is ECG evidence of complete AV block, VT, or premature ventricular contractions.
4. There is ECG evidence of ST-segment changes consistent with ischemia or infarction.
5. The patient's systolic blood pressure is greater than 220 mm Hg or diastolic blood pressure is greater than 120 mm Hg during exercise, or the patient's blood pressure drops below baseline at any time during the exercise protocol.

In the absence of ECG evidence of ischemia or the development of life-threatening dysrhythmias, every effort should be made to reach the maximum predicted heart rate to improve the diagnostic accuracy of the test. When the maximum predicted heart rate is not reached, the diagnostic reliability of the study is low. Exercise stress test results are considered reliable only if patients reach the maximum predicted heart rate value (85% of their maximal predicted effort).

Nursing Assessment and Management

Adequately preparing patients for the stress test maximizes the information obtained from the study. Patients should be NPO for 4 to 6 hours before the test to minimize blood diversion to the gastrointestinal tract, which decreases available coronary blood supply. In particular, they should not drink caffeine-containing beverages because of the effect of caffeine on the heart rate. β-Blockers blunt the heart rate response to exercise and may prevent achievement of the maximum predicted heart rate, so they should be withheld on the day of the test. Digitalis may also be withheld because of its negative chronotropic effects. Badly deconditioned patients, or those with comorbidities that could affect their ability to ambulate, may not be able to complete the required exercise. Appropriate attire, including comfortable walking shoes, is necessary to maximize patient comfort and performance.

The critical care nurse may be responsible for explaining the general format of the exercise test to the patient and family. It is important that patients understand why the test is indicated and what will be expected of them. The nurse reassures patients that someone will observe them closely throughout the test and encourages them to express any concerns before, during, and after the procedure. Patients should also understand that they may have to continue exercising after the development of angina but will not be expected to exercise more than is safe.

PHARMACOLOGICAL STRESS TESTING

Pharmacological stress testing is performed in patients who are unable to bike or walk on a treadmill. Patients referred for stress testing may have limitations that prevent them from performing adequate physical exercise. This has led to the development of alternative methods of simulating the effect of exercise on the heart using adrenergic agents, such as dobutamine, or vasodilators, such as adenosine or dipyridamole. These studies require no activity on the part of the patient. There is continuous monitoring of the ECG, along with frequent blood pressure measurements. In addition, an imaging modality, such as echocardiography or nuclear imaging, is always used.

Pharmacological agents used include several drugs. Dobutamine increases myocardial oxygen demand by increasing contractility, heart rate, and systemic blood pressure. Because dobutamine has some heart rate–blunting characteristics, supplemental atropine may be required to achieve target heart rate values. With the infusion of dobutamine, coronary blood flow increases up to twofold in normal coronary arteries but less so in arteries with flow-limiting lesions. Vasodilators such as adenosine and dipyridamole also cause an increase in coronary blood flow. They simulate the effects of exercise on the heart by producing arteriolar and coronary artery vasodilation. Vasodilator agents can be used as well, but they cause symptoms that may be interpreted as cardiac related, making reported symptoms less reliable. Although information on functional capacity is not obtained during pharmacological stress testing, it is considered to provide a reasonable equivalent to that gathered during physical exercise.

ECG changes secondary to the infusion of dobutamine, adenosine, and dipyridamole have a very low sensitivity for the detection of significant CAD. There-fore, pharmacological stress testing is always accompanied by a nuclear or echocardiographic imaging modality to increase the sensitivity of the study.

NUCLEAR IMAGING WITH STRESS TESTING

Noninvasive, rapid, and accurate imaging of cardiac structure and function using radiotracers is a routine part of inpatient assessment of patients with known or suspected cardiovascular disease. Broadly speaking, this is known as radionuclide cardiac imaging. Single-photon emission computed tomography (SPECT) and positron emission tomography (PET) are both widely available types of radionuclide imaging. SPECT and PET cameras capture the photons emitted by infused radiotracers and provide information on the magnitude and location of the uptake. The images are ECG gated, or collected in synchrony with ongoing ECG monitoring, so that the final data interpretation can be presented in the context of the full cardiac cycle of contraction and relaxation. In SPECT imaging, the final result is also referred to as myocardial perfusion imaging (MPI). PET is discussed at greater length later in this chapter (see Positron Emission Tomography).

Nuclear imaging is combined with exercise or the infusion of a pharmacological agent in a variety of protocols. Protocols may involve the injection of several radiotracers over several hours, with imaging performed 24 hours later. The purpose of the protocols is to obtain information on the heart at rest and with stress. Protocols vary widely because of patient comorbidities, patient size, and available personnel and equipment. The possible elements of a nuclear cardiology study are MPI, infarct avid imaging, and radionuclide angiography.

Myocardial Perfusion Imaging

MPI uses SPECT technology to look at coronary blood flow, giving information about the location, quantity, and severity of cardiac disease. MPI uses radiopharmaceutical agents that, once injected into the venous bloodstream, accumulate in viable myocardium in proportion to the blood flow to a particular area. After injection of the tracer, the SPECT camera is used to record an image of radioactive counts from the entire myocardium. An abnormal area with decreased uptake, or "cold spot" imaging, is the type of study used to assess myocardial perfusion. An abnormal area with increased myocardial uptake, or "hot spot" imaging, is the type of study used to assess myocardial necrosis.

Perfusion studies are performed most commonly in conjunction with exercise testing so that radionuclide scans obtained at rest and with exercise can be compared. Typically, at rest, the radiotracer is spread uniformly throughout the myocardium, and the camera reads counts equally from throughout the myocardium. During exercise, a similar scan is obtained in patients without significant coronary artery stenosis because blood flow increases uniformly to meet myocardial oxygen demands.

However, in patients with significant CAD, the image obtained during exercise is altered. The amount of coronary blood flow is limited in stenotic arteries, and the quantity of tracer in myocardial segments supplied by stenotic arteries is diminished or absent compared with segments supplied by nonstenotic arteries. The presence of an area of decreased tracer uptake during exercise compared with at rest is known as a reversible perfusion defect. In patients with previous infarction, decreased uptake may be present on both the rest and exercise scans in the infarcted segments; this pattern is known as a fixed perfusion defect and usually signifies nonviable myocardium. It is possible for patients to have fixed perfusion defects in some myocardial segments, reversible defects in others, and normal perfusion in the remaining segments.

Because of the many patients who are physically unable to exercise, pharmacological agents may be used to mimic the heart's response to exercise. Vasodilating agents, such as dipyridamole, adenosine, and dobutamine, administered intravenously mimic exercise conditions in the heart by dilating nonstenotic coronary arteries. Coronary blood flow is increased preferentially through normal, nonstenosed arteries; this results in relative hypoperfusion in myocardial segments supplied by stenosed coronary arteries. A radiotracer injected during the peak action of the pharmacological agent produces images similar to those seen with exercise. As of this writing, only dipyridamole is approved by the U.S. Food and Drug Administration (FDA) for use in perfusion imaging.

Two methods—planar and tomographic—are used to record radioactive images. With the planar technique, images of the heart are obtained by the gamma camera from three views: anterior, left anterior oblique (45 degrees to the left of the anterior view), and left lateral (Fig. 17-17). Planar imaging usually is performed with the patient in the supine position, although some laboratories place patients on their right side to obtain the left lateral image. Tomographic or SPECT images are obtained by rotating the head of the camera over a 180-degree arc from the left

lateral to the anterior position while stopping to make 32 to 64 recordings of 20 to 40 seconds each. A computer uses the recorded images to reconstruct multiple slices of the heart along its short axis and both horizontal and vertical long axes. With tomographic studies, it is extremely important that the patient not move during image acquisition because computer reconstruction of the images requires the same reference points. If significant movement occurs, the entire tomographic scan may have to be repeated.

Protocols

Three radioactive tracers, thallium-201, technetium (Tc)-99m sestamibi, and Tc-99m teboroxime, are approved for perfusion imaging. Most radionuclide perfusion studies have used thallium because this agent has been available since 1974. Characteristics of the three agents differ and are responsible for the varying imaging protocols used.

Thallium Protocol The cardiac half-life of thallium is approximately 7.5 hours, meaning that 50% of the tracer still is present in myocardial cells 7.5 hours after it is administered. It also redistributes readily, so thallium in normally perfused areas moves to previously underperfused areas after the myocardial blood flow demands in that territory have decreased. The standard protocol for thallium perfusion studies begins first with the exercise portion; thallium is injected at the peak of exercise, and imaging starts within 5 minutes of injection. The rest portion is obtained 2 to 4 hours later. Because of redistribution, no additional thallium is required. However, in some patients with perfusion defects on both the rest and exercise scans, significant redistribution may not occur, and it is recommended that an additional dose of thallium be administered.

Sestamibi Protocol Perfusion imaging with sestamibi typically begins with the rest scan. Because significant uptake also occurs in the liver, imaging is delayed for approximately 60 minutes. This delay

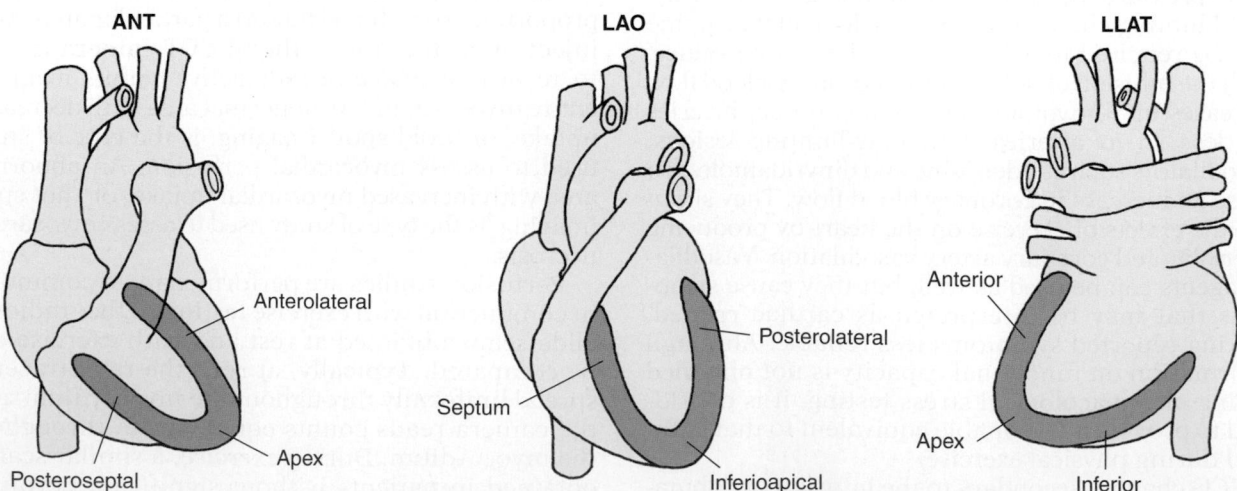

Figure 17-17 • Ventricular segments of the heart projected on radionuclide planar views. ANT, anterior; LAO, left anterior oblique; LLAT, left lateral.

allows sestamibi to be cleared from the liver but not the heart. In addition, a glass of milk or small fatty meal is taken shortly after radiotracer injection to enhance hepatic clearance. A second dose of sestamibi is administered during peak exercise, and the exercise scan is obtained 60 minutes after injection, again allowing time for hepatic clearance. Because sestamibi redistributes very slowly, the image obtained 60 minutes after peak exercise reflects the perfusion conditions at the time of injection. Initially, perfusion studies with sestamibi were performed on 2 different days, but it now is customary to complete both portions of the study in 1 day. It has been shown that exercise sestamibi myocardial perfusion SPECT can provide incremental prognostic information in patients who have not suffered a previous MI or undergone cardiac catheterization and who are determined to be at low risk.

Teboroxime Protocol Because of the very short cardiac half-life of teboroxime, two injections of the tracer are required. As with sestamibi, hepatic uptake also occurs. Redistribution is not an issue because of the short half-life. Imaging must begin within 2 to 5 minutes of injection and be completed within 15 minutes. The sequence of imaging, exercise versus rest, is not of concern, and typically the two scans are obtained 60 to 90 minutes apart. Scans may be obtained with the patient in a sitting or standing position to avoid hepatic interference.

Nursing Assessment and Management

All the directions and precautions that pertain to exercise ECG also apply to exercise radionuclide imaging. When pharmacological agents are used in place of exercise, minor side effects, such as flushing, headache, and nausea, may occur. Serious side effects due to the radiotracer are extremely rare. Medications to counteract serious side effects should be readily available. Some patients who receive sestamibi report a metallic taste several minutes after injection. Patients often are anxious about the radiation involved and the appearance of the equipment. It is important for the nurse to allay these anxieties.

Infarct Avid Imaging

Infarct or "hot-spot" imaging may be useful in patients who present to the hospital several days after MI when serum cardiac enzymes have returned to normal. Accumulation of the radiotracer in the area of myocardial necrosis compared with the surrounding normal myocardium is responsible for the hot-spot image obtained.

Tc-99m Sn-pyrophosphate, the only radiotracer currently approved by the FDA for infarct imaging, is sensitive for 1 to 5 days after onset of symptoms. Because aneurysm formation in the area of a previous infarction may result in a false-positive study, a second pyrophosphate scan may be performed 7 to 10 days after symptom onset. In patients with recent infarction, little or no radiotracer uptake is seen on the repeat scan. The diagnostic sensitivity of pyrophosphate imaging in patients with a small or nontransmural infarction is poor.

Indium-111 antimyosin is a monoclonal antibody that binds to damaged myocytes and is under investigation as an imaging agent for myocardial necrosis. Planar or tomographic images are obtained 24 to 48 hours after injection of the indium-labeled antibody. Although the study usually is performed within 1 week of an MI, a positive scan may be obtained for up to 1 year after myocardial necrosis. Initial results suggest that antimyosin is more sensitive than pyrophosphate scans for the detection of infarction. In addition, antimyosin may be useful in other clinical conditions that result in myocardial necrosis, such as myocarditis and rejection after cardiac transplantation. The pattern of radiotracer uptake is more diffuse and global in these conditions, compared with the localized pattern of uptake in infarction.

No special preparation is required for patients undergoing infarct imaging other than an explanation of the procedure. Views usually are obtained with the patient in the supine position. If an antimyosin tomographic study is to be performed, the importance of not moving during image acquisition should be reinforced. No serious side effects have been reported with either pyrophosphate or antimyosin administration.

Table 17-8 outlines some of the tests that are used to detect the presence of myocardial ischemia.

Radionuclide Angiocardiography

Radionuclide angiocardiography for the assessment of cardiac performance has been in clinical use since the 1970s. Such studies may include information about right and left ventricular ejection fractions, left ventricle regional wall motion abnormalities, ventricular volumes, and cardiac shunts. The measurement of left ventricular ejection fraction, the percentage of blood ejected with each contraction of the left ventricle, has been a key prognostic index for patients with MI or cardiac arrest.

Two approaches are used for the evaluation of cardiac performance. The technique used most commonly is known as equilibrium angiocardiography. It is performed easily at the bedside in patients too critically ill to be transported to the laboratory. The other technique, first-pass angiocardiography, likely will enjoy wider use in the future because it can use Tc radiotracers, such as teboroxime or sestamibi, and can be performed at the same time as perfusion imaging.

With equilibrium radionuclide studies, an aliquot of the patient's blood is drawn, and the erythrocytes are tagged with Tc-99m radiotracer. The blood sample is then returned intravenously to the patient. Imaging can begin within a few minutes after administration and is performed serially over a period of 4 to 6 hours because the radiotracer-tagged erythrocytes remain within the vascular system. An ECG signal from the patient is used to separate radioactive counts acquired during systole from those during diastole; imaging continues over several hundred cardiac cycles, and images are averaged for both systole and diastole to obtain a representative cardiac cycle.

Table 17-8 • Diagnostic Tests Used to Detect Myocardial Ischemia

Procedure	Abnormal Findings	Special Considerations
Standard 12-lead ECG	Transient ST-segment and T-wave changes in patients with chest pain at rest or of prolonged duration	
Holter monitoring	Transient ST-segment and T-wave changes occurring at rest or with activity	Only two ECG leads monitored
Stress echocardiogram	Segmental wall motion abnormality associated with echocardiogram obtained during exercise	May be used in patients with ventricular conduction defects Pharmacological agents may be used in patients who cannot exercise.
Exercise ECG	Transient ST-segment and T-wave changes occurring with exercise	Cannot be used in patients who are unable to exercise or who have left bundle branch block or paced rhythm Does not provide good information on the location of the coronary artery disease
Radionuclide perfusion stress study	"Cold spot" image or perfusion defect associated with scan obtained during exercise	May be used in patients with ventricular conduction defects Pharmacological agents may be used in patients who cannot exercise.
Online ischemia analysis	Myocardial ischemia dynamic analysis (MIDA)* analyzing eight leads to detect ST-segment levels indicating ischemia and QRS complex changes corresponding to infarct evolution	Noninvasive Hastens clinical decision making Graphic trends monitored online Reocclusion readily identified Helps differentiate chest pain related to ischemia from nonischemic symptoms

*MIDA CoroNet, Hewlett-Packard, Andover, MA, Product Literature

At the end of diastole, when the left ventricle is maximally filled with blood containing tagged erythrocytes, the amount of radioactivity is greatest. As the ventricle contracts during systole, blood is ejected into the aorta. The amount of blood and therefore radioactivity in the left ventricle is lowest at the end of systole. Because radioactive counts are proportional to the blood volume, the difference in counts obtained at the end of systole and the end of diastole permits the calculation of left ventricular ejection fraction. Left ventricular impairment caused by a previous infarction or cardiomyopathy usually results in a reduction in left ventricular ejection fraction from the normal values of 55% to 70%. Comparisons between ejection fractions at rest and with exercise also can be made. An inability to increase left ventricular ejection fraction by at least 5% with exercise is considered abnormal and may represent ischemic myocardium.

Left ventricular volumes and wall motion also can be assessed with equilibrium angiocardiography. By tracing the images obtained during the end of diastole and the end of systole, abnormalities in systolic or diastolic volumes can be ascertained. In addition, global versus regional impairment of ventricular function can be differentiated, including the identification of aneurysm formation after infarction. Baseline data may provide information about the etiology of the ventricular impairment, and serial measurements often are used to assess response to treatment.

First-pass radioangiocardiography also uses Tc-99m tracers; however, they are not tagged to any blood components. An image is obtained immediately after IV injection of the radiotracer as it enters the central circulation. The appearance time of the tracer in the various cardiac chambers and the right and left ventricular systolic and diastolic counts provide diagnostic information. Because the time required for the tracer to traverse the central circulation is only a few cardiac cycles, the image acquisition time is very short.

Intracardiac shunts may be diagnosed by first-pass techniques. For example, in a patient with a ventricular septal defect and right-to-left shunt, the tracer appears in the left ventricle at the same time as or before its appearance in the left atrium. In addition, this technique allows the amount of shunting to be quantified.

Right ventricular ejection fraction and volumes are measured best by first-pass angiocardiography. Because the tracer is present in the right ventricle before it appears in the left ventricle, there is no contamination of counts from the overlapping left ventricle. The methods for measuring right ventricular volumes and ejection fraction are similar to those used for the left ventricle.

Three planar views similar to those used in perfusion imaging are obtained during equilibrium angiocardiography. If exercise angiocardiography is to be performed, the patient should be instructed to wear comfortable shoes for treadmill walking or bicycle riding. As with exercise testing, emergency equipment should be readily available. Although imaging usually is performed with the patient in the supine position, semierect or erect positioning may be used. It is important that the patient not move during image acquisition for either equilibrium or first-pass studies because of the effect on systolic and diastolic images.

Nurses caring for patients who have undergone radionuclide imaging should be aware of precautions; this information is available through the radiation safety department of their institution. The length of time that any precautions may be necessary is related to the half-life of the radiotracer used. In general, nurses who are pregnant should avoid caring for patients for 24 to 48 hours after the study, and all nurses should wear gloves when handling body fluids during the 24- to 48-hour period.

STRESS ECHOCARDIOGRAPHY

There are several important advantages to the use of echocardiography as the imaging modality with stress testing. The echocardiogram identifies regional wall motion abnormalities, which are the final result of myocardium that is poorly perfused secondary to CAD. Echocardiograms can be read immediately, do not involve ionizing radiation, and are more cost effective than nuclear imaging. The disadvantages of stress echocardiography include the difficulty in obtaining quality images secondary to the experience of the technologist and because of the patient's body habitus. Images must be obtained both at rest and at peak exercise for comparison.

Stress echocardiography can be used in conjunction with exercise stress testing or pharmacological stress testing. A baseline 2D echocardiogram is performed before exercise is performed or the drug is infused. (For pharmacological stress testing, dobutamine or dipyridamole is used as the provocative agent.) The imaging is continued through and for 10 minutes after stopping the exercise or drug infusion. The echocardiogram is examined for wall motion abnormalities indicative of poor regional myocardial perfusion. A study is considered positive if, after exercise or drug infusion, new wall motion abnormalities are detected.

• Computed Tomography

Computed tomography (CT) scanning is a noninvasive technique used to evaluate the heart and its surrounding structures. CT scanning involves passing x-ray beams through a patient's body while a detector gathers and records images generated by the beams. Computers reconstruct the images into 2D or 3D images that provide strikingly detailed views of the anatomy. Cardiac CT scanning is used to detect structural diseases of the heart, including congenital anomalies and aneurysms.

Electron-beam computed tomography (EBCT) constituted the earliest form of CT-based coronary assessment. This largely outpatient-based study allowed evaluation of coronary calcium burden, which is related to coronary plaque burden. Technological limitations prevented EBCT from becoming a more useful noninvasive modality to evaluate coronary arteries, but it continues to be used in preventive cardiology. Dual-slice helical CT, which became available in 1992, provided the basis for the development of a multidetector CT (MDCT).

Early four-slice scanners were problematic because of the physiological movement related to cardiac and respiratory function. Developments in CT scanning included increasing the number of images from 16 to 64 slices (Fig. 17-18). Now 128-slice scanners are available, allowing greater detail to be captured in each reconstructed image. Currently, scanners are also ECG gated to allow imaging during specific phases of cardiac activity. Patient preparation involves the administration of β-blockers to maintain a heart rate of 55 to 65 beats/minute.

Coronary artery assessment using CT angiography (CTA) is currently most useful in the outpatient setting in patients with low to moderate risk for CAD. It involves the administration of intravascular contrast media to perform calcium scoring, assess coronary arteries, and evaluate noncoronary cardiac structures. CTA is highly accurate for detection of intracoronary lesions. Although it has not replaced coronary angiograms as the gold standard of detection and quantification of CAD, it does provide a useful diagnostic tool in specific patient circumstances.[2] With CTA, patients who are facing repeat coronary artery bypass surgery can have the exact locations and depths of their existing grafts determined to decrease surgical complications during repeat surgery.

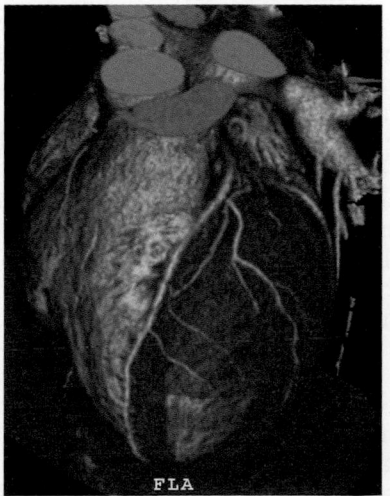

Figure 17-18 • Multislice CT image of the heart, a 64-slice cardiac computed tomography scan of the heart, frontal plane.

Patients undergoing ECG-gated CTA may need heart rate modulation. Optimal heart rates are 55 to 60 beats/minute and can be safely achieved in most patients with medications, particularly β-blockers. Patients require placement of an IV line for contrast administration. Monitoring for contrast-induced allergic reactions and renal toxicity is also necessary.

MDCT allows for precise characterization of intracardiac tumors and thrombi. Before pacemaker or intracardiac defibrillator implantation, MDCT is used to map the anatomy of the heart so that the device can be optimally positioned. Before radiofrequency ablation for atrial fibrillation, MDCT is used to map the pulmonary veins.

MDCT involves a significant amount of radiation exposure. Imaging results are suboptimal in patients with a body mass index of greater than 40 kg/m^2, heart rate greater than 65 beats/minute, existing intracoronary stents less than 3 mm in diameter, distal coronary artery bypass grafting anastomoses containing metal clips, or heavily calcified areas overlying a targeted vessel lumen.

• Magnetic Resonance Imaging

Magnetic resonance imaging (MRI) allows high-resolution assessment of cardiovascular anatomy, function, blood flow, metabolism, and perfusion. It permits assessment of cardiac structure and function at rest or during exercise or pharmacological stress testing. MRI is used in the diagnosis of CAD, coronary artery bypass graft disease, cardiomyopathy, valvulopathy, congenital heart disease, cardiac masses, intracardiac thrombi, and diseases of the pericardium. Myocardial viability studies can be performed using MRI; thus, viable or ischemic tissue can be distinguished from scarred or infarcted tissue. Centers performing electrophysiology procedures use MRI to map pulmonary veins before an atrial fibrillation pulmonary vein ablation procedure. Atrial septal defects can be characterized before the percutaneous placement of an occlusion device.[2]

Cardiovascular MRI has other advantages. It is useful in patients unable to tolerate iodine-based contrast material because of allergy or renal insufficiency. Gadolinium, the MRI contrast medium, can cause both allergic reactions and nephrotoxicity, but the frequency of both complications appears to be less than that associated with iodinated contrast material. In addition, cardiovascular MRI with a stress testing protocol is being used to provide a comprehensive evaluation of cardiac structure, wall function, valvular function, myocardial perfusion, angiography, and viability. The provocative agent used for MRI stress testing can be adenosine, dobutamine, or dipyridamole.

Coronary MRI remains challenging because of several unique issues, including the small size of coronary arteries and their nearly constant motion during respiration and cardiac cycles. MRI requires expensive equipment that may not be available at all centers.

Obesity may be a contraindication for MRI (or magnetic resonance angiography) because the patient is required to fit into a fixed-sized tunnel within the scanner. The patient must be able to lie flat and remain composed despite confinement and loud noises generated by the scanner. Non–MRI-compatible aneurysm clips, implanted devices (including implanted cardiac defibrillators and pacemakers), and other body metal are all contraindications to MRI scanning. Patients with a history of metal-working may have metal shards in their eyes, making them unsuitable for MRI scanning. Contraindications to MRI are listed in Box 17-9. Although tattoo dye may contain metallic oxides that heat up during MRI, tattoos are not contraindicated in MRI scanning. Breath holding is required to avoid breathing artifacts at intervals during MRI, so cardiac MRI scanning may not be appropriate for patients who are unable to hold their breath. An IV line is required for instilling the contrast medium. Central catheters are not used because of the high pounds per square inch injection pressure used.

• Positron Emission Tomography

PET has significantly contributed to the knowledge of cardiac physiology and metabolism. It detects coronary stenoses (perfusion) and assesses myocardial viability (metabolism). PET scanning is the gold standard for testing myocardial viability.

Rubidium-82 and nitrogen-13–labeled ammonia are tracers used in the evaluation of regional myocardial blood flow. Fluorodeoxygenase (FDG) and carbon-11–labeled acetate are used for evaluation of glucose and fatty acid metabolism, respectively. If perfusion testing with rubidium-82 and nitrogen-13 ammonia demonstrates decreased blood flow, and metabolic testing with FDG and carbon-11 acetate demonstrates absent metabolic activity, then that

---

Box 17-9 • Contraindications to Magnetic Resonance Imaging (MRI)

ABSOLUTE	RELATIVE (INDIVIDUAL ASSESSMENT REQUIRED)
Cardiac pacemaker	Prosthetic joints
Aneurysm clips	Certain foreign objects
Epicardial pacing wires	in body (e.g., dental
Metal prosthetic heart valves	braces)
Implanted cardioverter–defibrillator (ICD)	Nonmetallic prosthetic heart valves
Implanted infusion pumps	Surgical staples
Cochlear implants	Coronary stents (if
Metal intrauterine devices	recently deployed)
Metal debris (e.g., bullets, shrapnel)	

region of myocardium is considered nonviable. That is, there is a matched decrease in flow and metabolism. If, on the other hand, the flow appears reduced by the perfusion tracers but the metabolic activity is preserved, that region of myocardium is considered ischemic and viable. This would indicate a mismatch of flow and viability, and it would direct the patient's treatment to an intervention that would restore flow to a viable area of tissue.

The patient should be NPO for 6 hours before the study. Caffeinated beverages should be restricted for 24 hours before the procedure.

• Cardiac Catheterization, Coronary Angiography, and Coronary Intervention

During cardiac catheterization and related procedures, radiographic contrast is injected into the chambers of the heart and the coronary arteries under fluoroscopic guidance. These studies are commonly performed and are well established as the gold standard for evaluation of the coronary artery lumen. Intracoronary lesions may be targets for a variety of interventions, including angioplasty and stenting, or coronary artery bypass. Coronary anomalies and other disease states, including aneurysms and myocardial bridging, can also be seen. Coronary interventions are performed based on the information gained during the diagnostic cardiac catheterization.

The major limitations related to cardiac catheterization involve cost, experience of the operator, level of risk afforded, and ability to determine whether an identified lesion can cause ischemia. The cost of cardiac catheterization, which is in the thousands of dollars, is much greater than for noninvasive modalities. Extensive data indicate that the physician operator must perform at least 75 procedures annually to maintain the skills necessary to perform a safe and interpretable procedure. Although this procedure can locate blockages in the coronary arteries, more information may be required to understand the ischemic potential of a given lesion before an angioplasty is performed.

Patients undergoing cardiac catheterization require careful preprocedure evaluation, including a recent history and physical examination to identify a history of contrast media allergy as well as a recent set of laboratory studies, including a complete blood count, prothrombin and partial thromboplastin time, International Normalized Ratio (INR), and chemistry panel (serum potassium, creatinine, and blood urea nitrogen levels). Women who are premenopausal and could be pregnant must have pregnancy tests performed within 48 hours of the procedure. The patient must also be NPO for at least 8 hours before the procedure; appropriate medications may be taken with a sip of water on the morning of the procedure. Patients need IV line placement, and consideration may be given to insertion of a Foley catheter if the patient may have difficulty urinating postprocedure. Patients must be able to lie still and almost flat on a procedure table for the duration of the examination. For nursing considerations for the patient undergoing cardiac catheterization, see Box 17-10.

After the procedure, the patient requires careful monitoring of vital signs (blood pressure, heart rate, and respirations with pulse oximetry). The percutaneous entry site of the procedure needs close monitoring for signs of bleeding. Any bleeding or hematoma formation must be managed to prevent serious vascular complications, including retroperitoneal bleeding. IV fluids after the procedure promote elimination of the renal-toxic contrast media and protect the patient from hypotension due to dehydration or increased vagal tone during potentially painful portions of the recovery. Bed rest for several hours after an arteriotomy is mandatory to allow the site to stabilize and further protect the patient from vascular bleeding complications. A summary of patient teaching for patients undergoing cardiac catheterization can be found in Box 17-11.

Intravascular ultrasound (IVUS) is an adjunctive technique performed in patients undergoing cardiac catheterization. IVUS uses ultrasound technology to obtain information regarding the lumen and wall structure of the coronary artery. It permits detailed cross-sectional imaging of coronary arteries and allows for a risk assessment of individual lesions. It is frequently performed in conjunction with coronary angiograms to determine lumen measurements and characteristics, including plaque morphology and burden. The information obtained from IVUS can be used to determine the need for coronary angioplasty or stenting. It is also used to evaluate the final outcome from coronary angioplasties with and without stenting.

Coronary interventions that may be necessary include percutaneous transluminal coronary angioplasty (PTCA), which involves the displacement of intracoronary plaque or thrombus for intracoronary blockages of 70% or greater. Intracoronary stents are intraluminal scaffolds placed after PTCA to decrease the reclosure rate of angioplasty sites. In directional coronary atherectomy (DCA), the plaque is removed rather than displaced. DCA is a specialized procedure, used far less frequently than PTCA in most centers. Extraction atherectomy is performed using a transluminal extraction catheter, and uses suction to remove thrombi. A more detailed discussion of coronary interventions can be found in Chapter 18.

LEFT HEART CATHETERIZATION

Left heart catheterization provides information about the lumen of the aorta, coronary arteries, aortic and mitral valvular competencies, and wall motion of the left ventricle. Many studies also include pressure measurements in the left atrium and left ventricle, with pressure gradients measured across the aortic and mitral valves, as well as over the left ventricular outflow tract.[4]

A diagnostic left heart cardiac catheterization is typically performed percutaneously from either the

Box 17-10 • NURSING INTERVENTIONS for the Patient Undergoing Cardiac Catheterization

Preprocedure
- Explain procedure to patient and family.
- Verify that the patient has taken nothing by mouth for at least 6 h before the procedure except prescribed medications as advised by the physician.
- Ensure that ordered preoperative laboratory studies have been completed and results are available.
- Verify patient, identify allergy information; alert physician if patient is allergic to radiographic dye, medications, or specific foods.
- Ensure that informed consent has been obtained.
- Establish intravenous access per institutional protocol or physician order.
- Place patient on cardiac monitoring system with blood pressure and pulse oximetry monitoring.
- Provide supplemental oxygen as ordered/indicated.
- Premedicate patient per physician order.
- Obtain vital signs before transfer to catheterization laboratory.

During Procedure
- Continually assess patient vital signs, oxygenation, level of consciousness, and cardiac rhythm per institutional protocol.
- Alert attending physician to significant changes in vital signs, oxygenation, and presence of malignant cardiac arrhythmias (e.g., premature ventricular contractions, ventricular tachycardia, ventricular fibrillation).
- Be prepared to initiate cardiac resuscitation with emergency equipment and medications.

Postprocedure
- Ensure that patient vital signs are stable before transfer.
- Check catheterization site dressing for bleeding and integrity.
- Check distal pulses below catheterization site; if femoral site was used, check distal pulse, extremity color, capillary refill, and neurosensory status.
- Keep extremity straight and instruct patient not to bend leg or arm.
- Maintain intravenous infusion per physician order or institutional protocol.
- Maintain supplemental oxygenation support as ordered or indicated.
- Encourage oral fluids as ordered.
- Check patient's coagulation status per institutional protocol before sheath removal.
- When catheter is removed:
  Apply direct pressure over invasive site for 20 to 30 min to prevent bleeding or apply commercial hemostatic compression device per institutional protocol.
  Check distal extremity for pulse, color, capillary refill, and sensorium.
  Remind patient to lie flat for 4 to 6 h per institutional protocol.
  Check site dressing every 4 to 6 h for bleeding and integrity.

 Box 17-11 • TEACHING GUIDE:
Cardiac Catheterization

Preprocedure
- Instruct the patient not to take anything by mouth for at least 6 h before the procedure except prescription medications as advised by the physician to reduce the chance of nausea and vomiting during the procedure.
- Tell the patient that an intravenous line will be placed to allow fluid and medication administration before, during, and after the procedure.
- Tell the patient that preoperative medication will be given before transport.
- Inform the patient that only a patient gown will be worn during the procedure.
- Advise the patient that the catheterization laboratory is usually cool, and the procedure table is firm and may be uncomfortable after a prolonged time.
- Tell the patient that he may be asked to turn his head, hold his breath, or cough during the procedure.
- Advise the patient that he may experience some discomfort during the procedure but that local anesthesia will be administered to minimize pain.
- Inform the patient that he will be placed on a cardiac monitor for the duration of the procedure and for a few hours after the procedure.

- Tell the patient that he will have to lie flat for several hours after the procedure to minimize the chance of bleeding from the catheter site.
- Inform the patient that he will be encouraged to take oral fluids as tolerated after the procedure to assist in elimination of the radiographic dye.
- Encourage the patient and family to ask questions.

During Procedure
- Instruct the patient to inform the physician and team if he is experiencing chest pain.
- Remind the patient to lie still.
- Reassure the patient and allay anxiety.
- Encourage and answer the patient's questions.

Postprocedure
- Remind the patient to lie still and keep the extremity straight.
- Instruct the patient to verbalize any chest pain or shortness of breath if present.
- Tell the patient when the catheter sheath is due for removal.
- Encourage the patient to take oral fluids as ordered.
- Advise the patient that the physician will review the catheterization findings with him.

brachial or femoral artery. This procedure delineates baseline coronary anatomy, and it can identify abnormalities of the coronaries, great vessels, and cardiac chambers. Injection of the coronary vessels with radiographic contrast shows the actual lumen of the vessel and defines plaque, thrombus, and dissections that cause obstruction to blood flow. The left ventricular filling pressure is obtained as an indicator of the fluid status of the patient. A left ventriculogram, which involves rapid filling of the left ventricle with contrast media, provides the left ventricular ejection fraction as well as information regarding wall motion abnormalities and size of the left ventricle. Patients with valvular disease can have additional studies to measure valvular gradients and chamber pressures to allow for mathematical calculations of valve area and flow dynamics.

The risk profile for left heart catheterization is significant because the procedure involves cannulation of an artery and use of contrast media. The risks include bleeding at the percutaneous entry site, dissection of any of the vessels traversed during the procedure, perforation of peripheral or coronary arteries, mechanical irritation of the cardiac tissue, plaque embolization leading to MI or cerebrovascular accident, allergic reactions to the contrast media or any other drug given during the procedure, and renal compromise because of the renal toxic effects of the contrast media.

RIGHT HEART CATHETERIZATION

Right heart catheterization aids in the differentiation of left ventricular failure versus pulmonary disease as a cause of dyspnea. It is performed in patients with a history of dyspnea, valvular heart disease, and intracardiac shunts.

Diagnostic right heart cardiac catheterizations can be performed from the right or left external jugular or the femoral veins. Right heart chamber pressures and information about the pulmonic valve and pulmonary artery pressures are obtained. More commonly, the procedure may be performed through the inferior jugular vein to the superior vena cava. The goal is to sample oxygen saturations and pressures in the right atrium, right ventricle, pulmonary capillary bed, and pulmonary artery.

The most common problem during right heart catheterization is dysrhythmia resulting from stimulation of the myocardium. The dysrhythmias are self-limiting and usually do not require treatment. Postprocedure restrictions are minimal because a vein is accessed, and the risk for bleeding is low.

Electrocardiographic Monitoring

Cardiac monitoring is used in a variety of settings. Traditionally used in ICUs and operating rooms, cardiac monitors are commonly found in other inpatient units where it is necessary to monitor continuously a patient's heart rate and rhythm or the effects of a therapy. In addition, cardiac monitors are used outside the hospital in settings such as paramedic ambulances, surgical centers, outpatient rehabilitation programs, and transtelephonic monitoring clinics.

Although the type of monitor may differ in each of these settings, all monitoring systems have three basic components: a display system, a monitoring cable, and electrodes. Electrodes are placed on the patient's chest to receive the electrical current from the cardiac muscle tissue. The electrical signal is then carried by the monitoring cable to a screen, where it is magnified and displayed. The display can be obtained both at the patient's bedside and at a central station, along with displays from other patients' monitors.

The capabilities of cardiac monitors have greatly expanded since they were first introduced more than 40 years ago. Early monitoring systems were used merely for assessing the patient's heart rate and rhythm. Today's monitors have expanded capabilities that include the diagnosis of complex dysrhythmias, the detection of myocardial ischemia, and the identification of prolonged QT intervals. These expanded features are made possible through development of computerized dysrhythmia detection algorithms, ST-segment monitoring software, noise reduction features, multilead monitoring systems, and derived 12-lead ECGs with a minimum number of electrodes.[1]

• Equipment Features

Two types of cardiac monitoring equipment are in use: continuous hard-wire monitoring systems and telemetry monitoring systems.

HARD-WIRE MONITORING SYSTEMS

Hard-wire monitors, which are commonly used in ICU settings, require the patient to be linked directly to the cardiac monitor through the ECG cable. Information is displayed and recorded at the bedside along with simultaneous display and recording at a central station. Because this type of cardiac monitoring limits patient mobility, patients using this system usually are confined to bed rest or are allowed to be up at the bedside only. Hard-wire monitors operate on electricity but are well isolated so that water, blood, and other fluids do not pose an electrical hazard as long as the machine is maintained properly.

TELEMETRY MONITORING SYSTEMS

In telemetry monitoring, no direct wire connection is needed between the patient and the ECG display device. Electrodes are connected by a short monitoring cable to a small battery-operated transmitter. The ECG is then sent by radiofrequency signals to a receiver that picks up and displays the signal on an oscilloscope, either at the bedside or at a distant central recording station. Antennas are built into the receiver and may be mounted in the vicinity of the receiver to widen the range of signal pickup. Batteries are the power source for the transmitter and make it possible to avoid electrical hazards by isolating the monitoring system from potential current leakage and accidental shock. Telemetry systems are used primarily for dysrhythmia monitoring in areas where the patient is fairly mobile, such as a dysrhythmia surveillance or progressive care unit. Because the patient is mobile, stable ECG tracings often are more difficult to obtain. Some hard-wire systems have built-in telemetry capability so that patients may be switched easily from one system to another as monitoring needs change.

DISPLAY SYSTEMS

Modern electronic technology continues to make sophisticated advances in monitoring equipment, and current display systems incorporate features such as the following:

▶ Computerized storage capability that permits retrieval of dysrhythmias

▶ Automatic chart documentation, in which the ECG recorder is activated by alarms or at preset intervals

▶ Expanded alarm systems for a variety of parameters

▶ Multilead or 12-lead ECG display, which facilitates complex dysrhythmia interpretation

▶ ST-segment analysis for monitoring ischemic events

▶ Computer systems that store, analyze, and trend monitored data, allowing the information to be retrieved at any time to aid in diagnosis and to note trends in the patient's status

▶ Wireless communication devices carried by the nurse that provide data and alarms

▶ QT-interval monitoring

MONITORING LEAD SYSTEMS

All cardiac monitors use lead systems to record the electrical activity generated by cardiac tissue. Each lead system is composed of a positive or recording electrode, a negative electrode, and a third electrode used as a ground. As the heart depolarizes, the waves of electrical activity move inferiorly because the normal route of depolarization moves from the SA node and atria, downward through the AV node, His–Purkinje system, and ventricles, and to the left because the muscle mass in the left side of the heart is greater than the muscle mass of the right side of the heart. Each lead system views these waves of depolarization from a different location on the chest wall and thus produces P waves and QRS complexes of varying configuration.

The terminology used to describe lead systems can be confusing. The wires attached to the patient's chest are called leads, and the pictures produced by these wires are also called leads. A standard ECG uses 10 lead wires with electrodes at the ends (4 placed on the limbs, and 6 placed on the chest) and produces 12 electrical views of the heart, known as 12 leads.

Cardiac monitoring systems currently on the market vary from a simple three-electrode device to the more common five-electrode system. Other systems less commonly used aim to reduce the number of electrodes while monitoring all 12 leads. The discussion of monitoring in this chapter will focus on the three- and five-lead systems.

The three-electrode system produces limited selections of leads I, II, or III with only a single lead viewed on the screen at one time (single-channel recording). Five-electrode systems allow the possibility of viewing any of the 12 ECG leads and permit the nurse to view two or more leads on the monitor screen simultaneously (multichannel recording).

Three-Electrode Systems

Monitors that require three electrodes use positive, negative, and ground electrodes that are placed in the right arm (RA), left arm (LA), and left leg (LL) positions on the chest as designated by markings on the monitor cable. When the electrodes are placed appropriately, the standard leads (leads I, II, III) may be obtained by moving the lead selector on the bedside monitor to the lead I, II, or III position (Fig. 17-19). The lead selector automatically adjusts which electrode is positive, which electrode is negative, and which electrode is ground to obtain an appropriate tracing. When lead I is selected, the LA is positive, the RA is negative, and the LL is ground. For a lead II configuration, the LL is positive, the RA is negative, and the LA is ground. To obtain a lead III, the LL is positive, the LA is negative, and the RA is ground. The configuration of leads I, II, and III, known as Einthoven's triangle, is illustrated in Figure 17-20.

To obtain a chest lead on the monitor that replicates the chest lead from the 12-lead ECG, a five-wire system is needed. (See Fig. 17-13 for a review of chest lead placement.) When only three wires are available, a modified version of any of the six chest leads may be obtained. To configure a modified chest lead (MCL), the goal is to position the positive electrode in the designated chest position. For example, an MCL_1 would

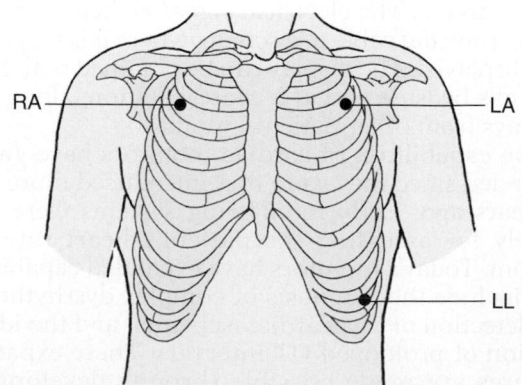

Figure 17-19 • Three-electrode monitoring system. Leads placed in this position allow the nurse to monitor leads I, II, and III. The left leg electrode must be placed below the level of the heart. LA, left arm; LL, left leg; RA, right arm.

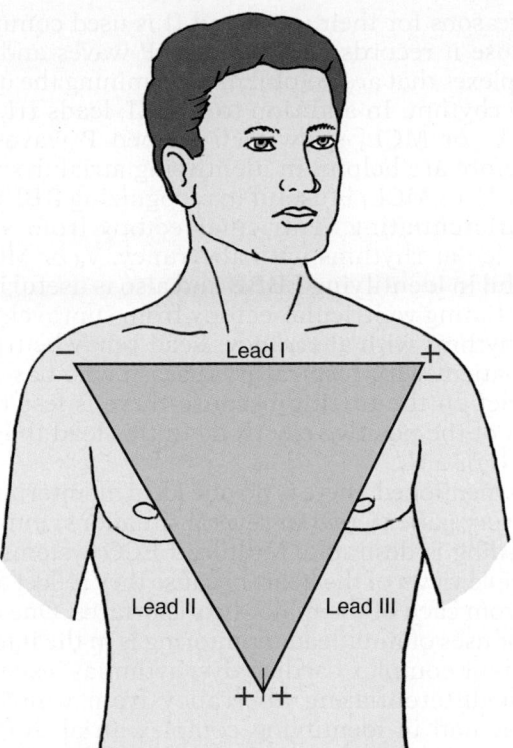

Figure 17-20 • Einthoven's triangle. Leads I, II, and III are known as the standard leads. When placed together over the chest, they form what is known as Einthoven's triangle.
Lead I: Left arm is positive, and right arm is negative.
Lead II: Left leg is positive, and right arm is negative.
Lead III: Left leg is positive, and left arm is negative.

require the positive electrode to be placed in a V_1 position (fourth intercostal space, right sternal border). The negative electrode is always positioned under the left clavicle. The ground electrode can be positioned anywhere.

To obtain an MCL_1 lead, the monitor is set to lead I (Box 17-12). By setting the monitor to lead I, the LA electrode is positive, the RA electrode is negative, and the leg wire is ground (Einthoven's triangle). The positive electrode (LA) is placed in a V_1 position (fourth intercostal space, right sternal border), and the negative electrode (RA) is positioned under the left clavicle. The ground electrode (LL) can be positioned anywhere, but if it is placed in a V_6 position, it is helpful when switching to an MCL_6 lead.

To obtain an MCL_6 lead, the goal is to place a positive electrode in a V_6 position, a negative electrode under the left clavicle, and a ground wire anywhere. By setting the monitor to lead II, the LL electrode is positive, the RA electrode is negative, and the LA electrode is ground (Einthoven's triangle). The positive electrode (LL) is placed in the V_6 position (midaxillary line, same horizontal level as V_4), and the negative electrode (RA) is placed under the left clavicle. The ground wire can be placed anywhere, but if it is placed in a V_1 position, it will be helpful when switching to an MCL_1 lead.

By arranging the electrodes as described, the nurse can monitor both MCL_1 and MCL_6 merely by

Box 17-12 • Three-Electrode System

To monitor MCL_1 using a three-electrode monitor:
1. Select lead I on the monitor.
2. Refer to Einthoven's triangle to remember that LA is positive, RA is negative, and LL is ground for lead I.
3. Place the positive electrode (LA) in a V_1 position (fourth intercostal space, right sternal border).
4. Place the negative electrode (RA) under the left clavicle.
5. Place the ground wire (LL) in the V_6 position (fifth intercostal space, left midaxillary line).

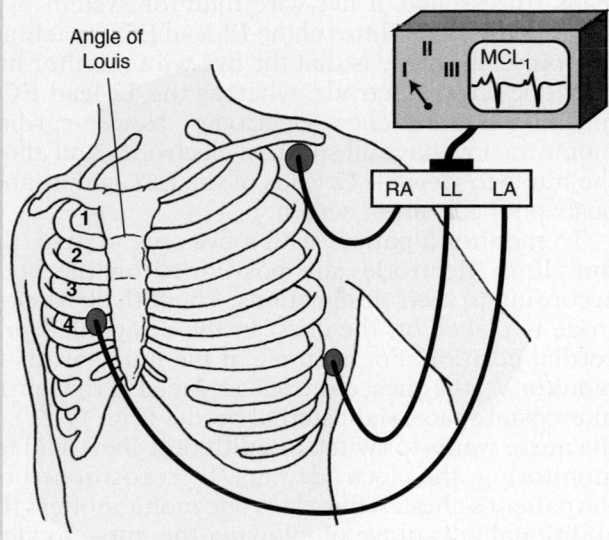

To monitor MCL_6 using a three-electrode monitor:
1. Select lead II on the monitor.
2. Refer to Einthoven's triangle to remember that LL is positive, RA is negative, and LA is ground for lead II.
3. Place the positive electrode (LL) in the V_6 position (fifth intercostal space, left midaxillary line).
4. Place the negative electrode (RA) under the left clavicle.
5. Place the ground wire (LA) in a V_1 position (fourth intercostal space, right sternal border).

Note: The electrodes are in the same position on the chest for the MCL_1 lead and the MCL_6 lead. To view the two leads, the nurse merely switches the monitor from lead I to lead II.

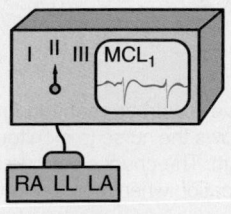

switching the monitor from a lead I to a lead II without changing the electrode placement on the patient's chest. MCL₁ and MCL₆ are ideal leads for detecting bundle branch block rhythms and for differentiating supraventricular wide-QRS tachycardias from VT.

Five-Electrode Systems

The five-electrode system increases the monitor's capability beyond the three-electrode system. (The four-electrode monitor requires a right leg electrode that is the ground for all leads described in the three-electrode system.) The five-electrode monitor adds an exploring "chest" electrode that allows one to obtain any one of the six chest leads and the six limb leads. In essence, a five-wire monitor system provides all the capabilities of the 12-lead ECG machine. The only difference is that the five-wire monitor has only one chest electrode, whereas the 12-lead ECG machine has six chest electrodes. Newer cardiac monitors now have all six chest electrodes and allow the nurse to view all 12 leads of the ECG simultaneously on the monitor screen.

To monitor a patient with a five-wire system, the four limb electrodes are positioned on the body according to their designations. The fifth chest electrode is placed on the chest in the designated precordial position. For example, if the nurse wants to monitor V₁, the chest electrode is placed in the fourth intercostal space, right sternal border (Fig. 17-21). If the nurse wants to switch to a different chest lead for monitoring, the electrode must be repositioned on the patient's chest. A five-electrode monitor offers the additional advantage of allowing the nurse to view two or more different leads simultaneously on the monitor screen.[2]

Lead Selection

No single monitoring lead is ideal for every patient. Table 17-9 summarizes the use of various leads and

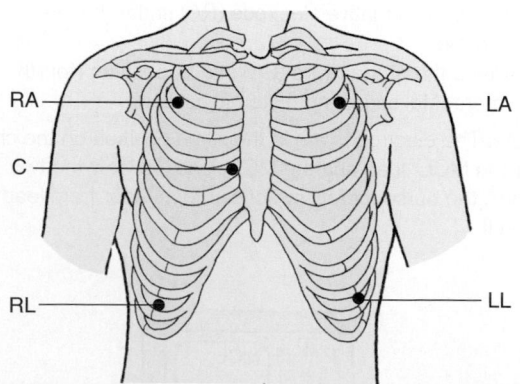

Figure 17-21 • Five-electrode monitoring system. Using a five-electrode system allows the nurse to monitor any of the 12 leads of the electrocardiogram. The chest electrode must be moved to the appropriate chest location when monitoring the precordial leads.

the reasons for their use. Lead II is used commonly because it records clear upright P waves and QRS complexes that are helpful in determining the underlying rhythm. In addition to lead II, leads III, aVF, and V₁ or MCL₁ show well-formed P waves and therefore are helpful in identifying atrial dysrhythmias. V₁ or MCL₁ is useful in recognizing RBBB and in differentiating ventricular ectopy from supraventricular rhythms with aberrancy. V₆ or MCL₆ is helpful in identifying LBBB and also is useful in differentiating ventricular ectopy from supraventricular rhythms with aberrancy. Lead I may be tried in the patient with respiratory disease who has much artifact on the tracing because there is less movement of the positive electrode in this lead than in a lead II or a V₁.

As mentioned, there is no one ideal monitoring lead for every patient, and in several situations, multilead recording is desirable. Multilead ECG systems offer multiple views of the heart because they reflect a tracing from each of the major heart surfaces. One of the major uses of multilead monitoring is in the interpretation of complex cardiac dysrhythmias, especially when differentiating aberrancy from ventricular ectopy and in identifying complex atrial dysrhythmias, uncharacteristic-looking ventricular premature beats, and fascicular blocks. Another use of multilead monitoring is in assessment of myocardial ischemia, injury, and infarction. By continuously viewing one lead from each area of the heart, episodes of anginal pain or silent ischemia can be documented. As soon as possible, these changes should be confirmed by a full 12-lead ECG.

• Procedure

ELECTRODE APPLICATION

Proper skin preparation and application of electrodes are imperative for good ECG monitoring. An adequate tracing should reflect (1) a narrow, stable baseline; (2) absence of distortion or "noise"; (3) sufficient amplitude of the QRS complex to activate the rate meters and alarm systems properly; and (4) identification of P waves.

The type of electrode currently used for ECG monitoring is a disposable silver- or nickel-plated electrode centered in a circle of adhesive paper or foam rubber. Most electrodes are pre-gelled by the manufacturer. They may have disposable wires attached to the electrodes or nondisposable wires that snap onto the electrodes. Electrodes should be comfortable for the patient. If not properly applied, undue artifact and false alarms may result.

When applying electrodes, the following procedure should be followed:

1. Select a stable site. Avoid bony protuberances, joints, and folds in the skin. Areas in which muscle attaches to bone have the least motion artifact.

2. Shave excessive body hair from the site.

Table 17-9 • Suggested Monitoring Lead Selection

Lead	Rationale for Use
II	Produces large, upright visible P waves and QRS complexes for determining underlying rhythm
V_1 or MCL_1	Helpful for detecting right bundle branch block and to differentiate ventricular ectopy from supraventricular rhythm aberrantly conducted in the ventricles
V_6 or MCL_6	Helpful lead for detecting left bundle branch block and to differentiate ventricular ectopy from supraventricular rhythm aberrantly conducted in the ventricles
III, aVF, V_1	Produce visible P waves; useful in detecting atrial dysrhythmias
I	Useful in patients with respiratory distress Left arm and right arm electrodes involved and placements less affected by chest motion compared with other leads
II, III, aVF	Helpful in detecting ischemia, injury, and infarction in the inferior wall
I, aVL, V_5, V_6	Helpful in detecting ischemia, injury, and infarction in the lateral wall
V_1 through V_4	Helpful in detecting ischemia, injury, and infarction in the anterior wall

3. Rub the site briskly with a dry gauze pad to remove oils and cellular debris. Skin preparation with alcohol may be necessary if the skin is greasy; allow the alcohol to dry completely before applying the electrode. Follow the electrode manufacturer's directions because the chemical reaction between alcohol or other skin-preparation materials and the adhesives used in some electrodes may cause skin irritation or nonadhesion to the skin.

4. Remove the paper backing and apply each electrode firmly to the skin by smoothing with the finger in a circular motion. Attach each electrode to its corresponding ECG cable wire. Sometimes it is necessary to tape over the cable wire connection or make a stress loop with the cable wire for extra stability.

5. Change electrodes every 2 to 3 days, and monitor for skin irritation.

While applying the electrodes, explain the purpose of the procedure to the patient. Reassure the patient that monitor alarm sounds do not necessarily indicate a problem with the patient's heart beat; alarms often occur when an electrode becomes loose or disconnected.

MONITOR OBSERVATION

Cardiac monitors are useful only if the information they provide is "observed," either by computers with alarms for programmed parameters or by the human eye, and appropriately acted on by competent, responsible people. Some critical care units use monitor technicians whose main responsibilities are to observe monitors, obtain chart samples, and give appropriate information to the nurse about each patient's ECG status. Those observing the monitor should know the acceptable dysrhythmia parameters for each patient and should be notified of any interruptions in monitoring, such as those caused by changing electrodes or by changing the patient to a portable monitor. The observer also should be aware of the presence of artifact from chest physical therapy or hiccups so that it may be considered in dysrhythmia diagnosis.

Regardless of the system used for monitor observation, certain practices always should be followed. If the monitor alarm sounds, the nurse evaluates the clinical status of the patient before doing anything else to see if the problem is an actual dysrhythmia or a malfunction of the monitoring system. Asystole should not be mistaken for an unattached ECG wire, nor should a patient inadvertently tapping on an electrode be misread as VT. In addition, monitor alarms always should be in the functioning mode. Only when direct physical care is being given to the patient can the alarm system safely be put on "standby." This ensures that no life-threatening dysrhythmia goes unnoticed. If the change on the monitor is not caused by an artifact or a disconnected wire, a full 12-lead ECG should be recorded to evaluate the rhythm change further.

• Troubleshooting Electrocardiogram Monitor Problems

Several problems may occur in monitoring the ECG, including baseline but no ECG trace, intermittent traces, wandering or irregular baseline, low-amplitude complexes, 60-cycle interference, excessive triggering of heart rate alarms, and skin irritation. Box 17-13 outlines the steps to follow when such problems occur.

Box 17-13 • Troubleshooting: Electrocardiogram Monitor Problem Solving

Excessive Triggering of Heart Rate Alarms
- Is the high–low alarm set too close to the patient's heart rate?
- Is the monitor sensitivity level set too high or too low?
- Is the patient cable securely inserted into the monitor receptacle?
- Are the lead wires or connections damaged?
- Has the monitoring lead been properly selected?
- Were the electrodes applied properly?
- Are the R and T waves the same height, causing both waveforms to be sensed?
- Is the baseline unstable, or is there excessive cable or lead wire movement?

Baseline but No Electrocardiogram (ECG) Trace
- Is the size (gain or sensitivity) control properly adjusted?
- Is an appropriate lead selector being used on the monitor?
- Is the patient cable fully inserted into the ECG receptacle?
- Are the electrode wires fully inserted into the patient cable?
- Are the electrode wires firmly attached to the electrodes?
- Are the electrode wires damaged?
- Is the patient cable damaged?
- Call for service if the trace is still absent.
- Is the battery dead (for telemetry system)?

Intermittent Trace
- Is the patient cable fully inserted into the monitor receptacle?
- Are the electrode wires fully inserted into the patient cable?
- Are the electrode wires firmly attached to the electrodes?
- Are the electrode wire connectors loose or worn?
- Have the electrodes been applied properly?

- Are the electrodes properly located and in firm skin contact?
- Is the patient cable damaged?

Wandering or Irregular Baseline
- Is there excessive cable movement? This can be reduced by clipping to the patient's clothing.
- Is the power cord on or near the monitor cable?
- Is there excessive movement by the patient? Are there muscle tremors from anxiety or shivering?
- Is site selection correct?
- Were proper skin preparation and application procedures followed?
- Are the electrodes still moist?

Low-Amplitude Complexes
- Is size control adjusted properly?
- Were the electrodes applied properly?
- Is there dried gel on the electrodes?
- Change electrode sites. Check 12-lead ECG for lead with highest amplitude, and attempt to simulate that lead.
- If none of the preceding steps remedies the problem, the weak signal may be the patient's normal complex.

Sixty-Cycle Interference
- Is the monitor size control set too high?
- Are there nearby electrical devices in use, especially poorly grounded ones?
- Were the electrodes applied properly?
- Is there dried gel on the electrodes?
- Are lead wires or connections damaged?

Dysrhythmias and the 12-Lead Electrocardiogram

Dysrhythmias and abnormalities of the 12-lead ECG commonly encountered in monitored patients can be recognized with a little practice. The types that occur most frequently are discussed in this chapter. Before presenting the individual dysrhythmias and 12-lead ECG abnormalities, the method for evaluating a rhythm strip is addressed.

To understand the causes, clinical significance, and treatment of dysrhythmias, knowledge of the conduction system is essential. Chapter 16 provides a review of the essential elements of the cardiac conducting system.

• Evaluation of a Rhythm Strip

ELECTROCARDIOGRAM PAPER

An ECG tracing is a graphic recording of the heart's electrical activity. The paper consists of horizontal and vertical lines, each 1 mm apart. The horizontal lines denote time measurements. When the paper is run at a sweep speed of 25 mm/second, each small square measured horizontally is equal to 0.04 second,

and a large square (five small squares) equals 0.2 second. Height or voltage is measured by counting the lines vertically. Each small square measured vertically is 1 mm, and the large square is 5 mm (Fig. 17-22). Some ECG paper also is marked by vertical slash marks across the top or bottom. The distance between two vertical markings represents 3 seconds. The distance between 6 seconds is used for rate calculation.

WAVEFORMS AND INTERVALS

During the cardiac cycle, the following waveforms and intervals are produced on the ECG surface tracing (see Fig. 17-22):

▶ P wave: The P wave is a small, usually upright and rounded deflection representing depolarization of the atria. It normally is seen before the QRS complex at a consistent interval.

▶ PR interval: The PR interval represents the time from the onset of atrial depolarization until the onset of ventricular depolarization. Included in the interval is the brief delay of the electrical signal at the AV node that allows time for the blood to move

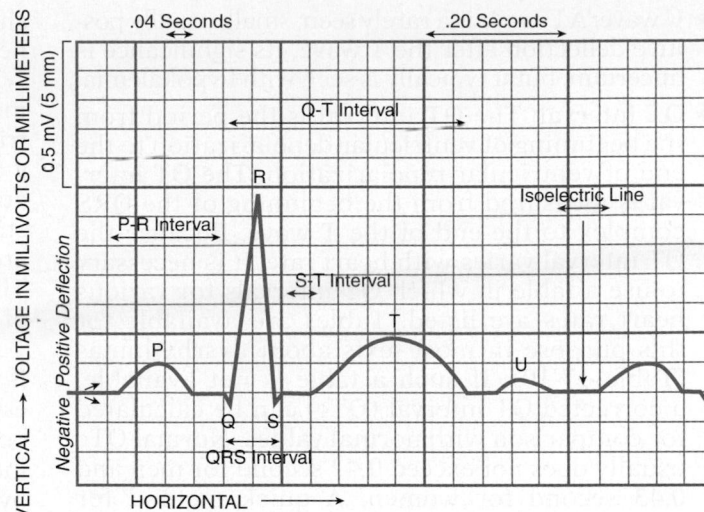

Figure 17-22 • Waveforms of the electrocardiogram. Schematic representation of the electrical impulse as it traverses the conduction system, resulting in depolarization and repolarization of the myocardium.

from the atria to the ventricles before the ventricles are depolarized. The interval is measured from the beginning of the P wave to the beginning of the QRS complex. A normal PR interval is 0.12 to 0.2 second.

▶ QRS complex: The QRS complex is a large waveform representing ventricular depolarization. Each component of the waveform has a specific connotation. The initial negative deflection is a Q wave, the initial positive deflection is an R wave, and the negative deflection after the R wave is an S wave. Not all QRS complexes have all three components, even though the complex is commonly called the QRS complex. A normal QRS complex is 0.06 to 0.11 second in width. Figure 17-23 illustrates different kinds of QRS complexes.

▶ ST segment: The ST segment is the portion of the tracing from the end of the QRS complex to the beginning of the T wave. It represents the

time from the end of ventricular depolarization to the beginning of ventricular repolarization. Normally, it is isoelectric. An isoelectric ST segment means the ST segment joins the QRS complex at the baseline. ST segments may be elevated or depressed in a variety of conditions. Elevated ST segments could indicate acute myocardial injury. Depressed ST segments may signify acute myocardial injury or myocardial ischemia. For a more detailed discussion of ST-segment abnormalities, see Chapter 21.

▶ T wave: The T wave is the deflection representing ventricular repolarization or recovery. The T wave appears after the QRS complex. The atria also have a repolarization phase. However, there is no visible wave on the ECG to represent atrial repolarization because it occurs at the same time as the QRS complex.

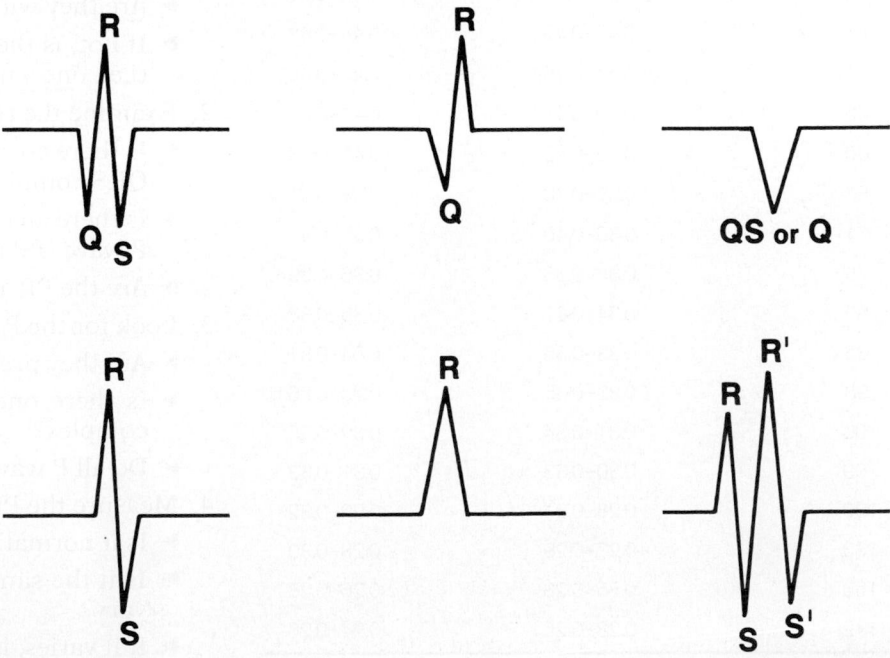

Figure 17-23 • Configurations of the QRS complex. A Q wave is a negative deflection before an R wave, an R wave is a positive deflection, and an S wave is a negative deflection after an R wave.

▶ U wave: A U wave is a rarely seen, small, usually positive deflection after the T wave. Its significance is uncertain, but it typically is seen with hypokalemia.

▶ QT interval: The QT interval is the period from the beginning of ventricular depolarization to the end of ventricular repolarization. The QT interval is measured from the beginning of the QRS complex to the end of the T wave. Because the QT interval varies with heart rate, it is necessary to use a table in which QT intervals for various heart rates are listed. Tables are available for this purpose in most texts about dysrhythmias (Table 17-10). If such a table is not available, a corrected QT interval (QTc) can be calculated for comparison with normal values. Normal QTc usually does not exceed 0.42 second for men and 0.43 second for women. A quick method for obtaining a QTc is to use half of the preceding RR interval (described later).

CALCULATION OF HEART RATE

Although cardiac monitors and ECG strips can be used to calculate heart rate, the calculated rate is merely an estimate of the number of times per minute the heart has been electrically excited. In the normal heart, each excitation should be followed by cardiac contraction. However, in some situations, electrical activity can occur without contraction, resulting in a lack of perfusion. Therefore, the heart rate obtained from the cardiac monitor or ECG strip should never be substituted for the determination of heart rate by palpating the pulse.

Both the atrial and the ventricular rates can be estimated by examining the ECG. To determine the ventricular rate, count the number of QRS complexes in a 6-second strip and multiply by 10. To estimate the atrial rate, count the number of P waves in a 6-second strip and multiply by 10. In the normal patient, the atrial and the ventricular rates should be the same. This method of rate calculation provides an estimate of heart rate for regular and irregular rhythms.

Another method of rate calculation can be used if the rhythm is regular. The ventricular heart rate is estimated by dividing 300 by the number of large boxes on the ECG paper between two R waves (the RR interval). The atrial rate is calculated by dividing 300 by the number of large boxes on ECG paper between two P waves (the PP interval).

Another quick method for estimating rate involves the use of a series of numbers. To use this method for estimating ventricular rate, the nurse first finds a QRS complex that falls directly on a dark line of the ECG paper. This dark line is the reference point. The next six dark lines of the paper are labeled 300, 150, 100, 75, 60, and 50 (Fig. 17-24). Then, the nurse finds the next QRS complex immediately after the reference point and estimates the ventricular rate using the sequence of numbers. The same method can be used for estimating atrial rate by using the P waves.

STEPS IN ASSESSING A RHYTHM STRIP

The following analysis represents a systematic approach to assessment of a cardiac rhythm strip. Whether or not this method is used, it is important to take the time to complete each step because many dysrhythmias are not as they first appear.

1. Determine the atrial and ventricular heart rates.
   ▶ Are they within normal limits?
   ▶ If not, is there a relationship between the two (i.e., one a multiple of the other)?
2. Examine the rhythm to see if it is regular.
   ▶ Is there an equal amount of time between each QRS complex (RR interval)?
   ▶ Is there an equal amount of time between each P wave (PP interval)?
   ▶ Are the PP and RR intervals the same?
3. Look for the P waves.
   ▶ Are they present?
   ▶ Is there one or more P waves for each QRS complex?
   ▶ Do all P waves have the same configuration?
4. Measure the PR interval.
   ▶ Is it normal?
   ▶ Is it the same throughout the strip, or does it vary?
   ▶ If it varies, is there a pattern to the variation?

Table 17-10 • Approximate Normal Limits for QT Intervals in Seconds		
Heart Rate per Minute	Men and Children	Women
40	0.45–0.49	0.46–0.50
46	0.43–0.47	0.44–0.48
50	0.41–0.45	0.43–0.46
55	0.40–0.44	0.41–0.45
60	0.39–0.42	0.40–0.43
67	0.37–0.40	0.38–0.41
71	0.36–0.40	0.37–0.41
75	0.35–0.38	0.36–0.39
80	0.34–0.37	0.35–0.38
86	0.33–0.36	0.34–0.37
93	0.32–0.35	0.33–0.36
100	0.31–0.34	0.32–0.35
109	0.30–0.33	0.31–0.33
120	0.28–0.31	0.29–0.32
133	0.27–0.29	0.28–0.30
150	0.25–0.28	0.26–0.28
172	0.23–0.26	0.24–0.26

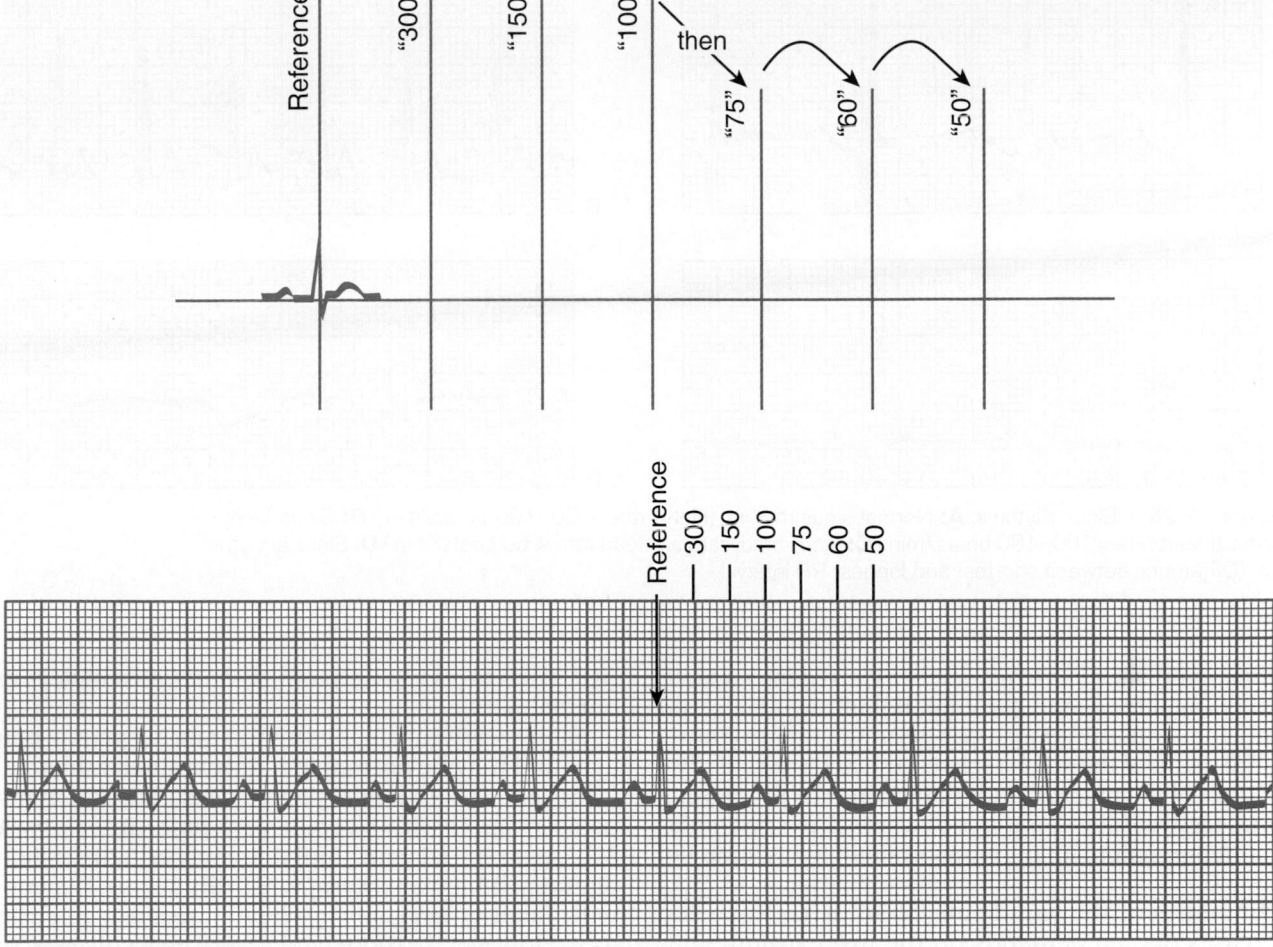

Figure 17-24 • Method for estimating heart rate. Using this method, the heart rate is approximately 85 beats/minute.

5. Evaluate the QRS complex.
   ▶ Is it normal in width, or is it wide?
   ▶ Are all complexes of the same configuration?
6. Examine the ST segment.
   ▶ Is it isoelectric, elevated, or depressed?
7. Identify the rhythm and determine its clinical significance.
   ▶ Is the patient symptomatic? (Check skin, neurological status, renal function, coronary circulation, and hemodynamic status or blood pressure.)
   ▶ Is the dysrhythmia life-threatening?
   ▶ What is the clinical context?
   ▶ Is the dysrhythmia new or chronic?

• Normal Sinus Rhythm

Normal sinus rhythm (Fig. 17-25A) is the normal rhythm of the heart. The impulse is initiated at the sinus node in a regular rhythm at a rate of 60 to 100 beats/minute. A P wave appears before each QRS complex. The PR interval is within normal limits and of equal duration (0.12 to 0.2 second), and the QRS is narrow (<0.12 second) unless an intraventricular conduction defect is present.

• Dysrhythmias Originating at the Sinus Node

Table 17-11 summarizes and compares ECG characteristics of sinus rhythms.

SINUS TACHYCARDIA

In sinus tachycardia, the sinus node accelerates and initiates an impulse at a rate of 100 times/minute or more (see Fig. 17-25B). The upper limits of sinus tachycardia extend to 160 to 180 beats/minute. All other ECG characteristics, except for heart rate, are the same as in normal sinus rhythm.

Sinus tachycardia usually is caused by factors relating to an increase in sympathetic tone. Stress, exercise, and stimulants such as caffeine and nicotine can produce this dysrhythmia. Sinus tachycardia also is associated with such clinical problems as fever, anemia, hyperthyroidism, hypoxemia, heart

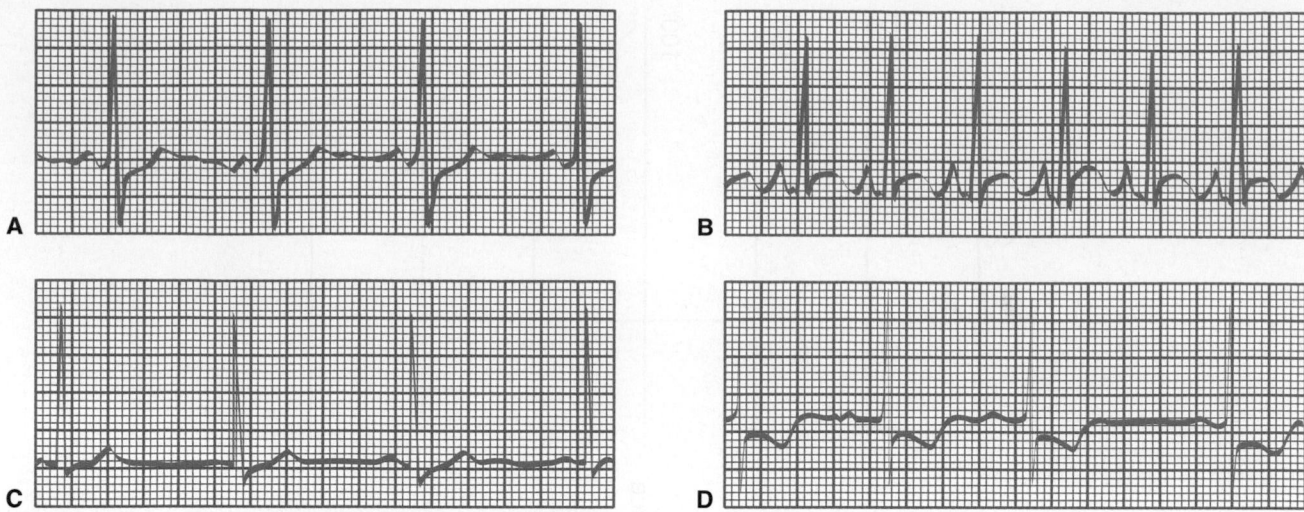

Figure 17-25 • Sinus rhythms. **A:** Normal sinus rhythm. (Heart rate = 60–100 beats/min.) **B:** Sinus tachycardia. (Heart rate = 100–180 beats/min.) **C:** Sinus bradycardia. (Heart rate < 60 beats/min.) **D:** Sinus arrhythmia. (Difference between shortest and longest RR interval.)

failure, and shock. Drugs such as atropine, which blocks vagal tone, and the catecholamines (e.g., epinephrine, dopamine) also can produce this rhythm.

The cause of the sinus tachycardia and the underlying state of the myocardium determine the prognosis. Sinus tachycardia alone is not a lethal dysrhythmia but often signals an underlying problem that should be pursued.

In addition, the rapid rate of sinus tachycardia increases oxygen demands on the myocardium and decreases the filling time of the ventricles. In people who already have depleted cardiac reserve, ischemia, or heart failure, the persistence of a fast rate may worsen the underlying condition.

Treatment of sinus tachycardia usually is directed at eliminating the underlying cause. Specific measures may include sedation, oxygen administration, digitalis, and diuretics if heart failure is present, or β-blockers if the tachycardia is caused by thyrotoxicosis.

SINUS BRADYCARDIA

Sinus bradycardia is defined as a rhythm with impulses originating at the sinus node at a rate of less than 60 beats/minute (see Fig. 17-25C). The rhythm (RR interval) is regular, and all other parameters are normal.

Sinus bradycardia is common among people of all ages and may be normal in highly trained athletes. It is present in both healthy and diseased hearts. It may be associated with sleep, severe pain, inferior wall MI, acute spinal cord injury, and certain drugs (e.g., digitalis, β-blockers, verapamil, diltiazem). In people with healthy hearts, slow heart rates are tolerated well. However, in those with severe heart disease, the heart may not be able to compensate for a slow rate by increasing the volume of blood ejected per beat. In this situation, sinus bradycardia leads to a low cardiac output.

No treatment is indicated unless symptoms are present. If the pulse is very slow and the patient is symptomatic, appropriate measures include atropine (to block the vagal effect) or cardiac pacing.

SINUS ARRHYTHMIA

Sinus arrhythmia is a disorder of rhythm (see Fig. 17-25D) that is said to be present if the RR intervals on the ECG, from the shortest RR interval to the longest, vary by more than 0.12 second. This arrhythmia is caused by an irregularity in sinus

Table 17-11 • A Comparison of the Electrocardiographic Characteristics of Sinus Rhythms				
	Normal Sinus Rhythm	Sinus Tachycardia	Sinus Bradycardia	Sinus Arrhythmia
Rate	60–100 beats/min	>100 beats/min	<60 beats/min	60–100 beats/min
Rhythm	Regular	Regular	Regular	Irregular
P waves	Present, one per QRS	Present, one per QRS	Present, one per QRS	Present, one per QRS
PR interval	<0.20 s, equal	<0.20 s, equal	<0.20 s, equal	<0.20 s, equal
QRS complex	<0.12 s	<0.12 s	<0.12 s	<0.12 s

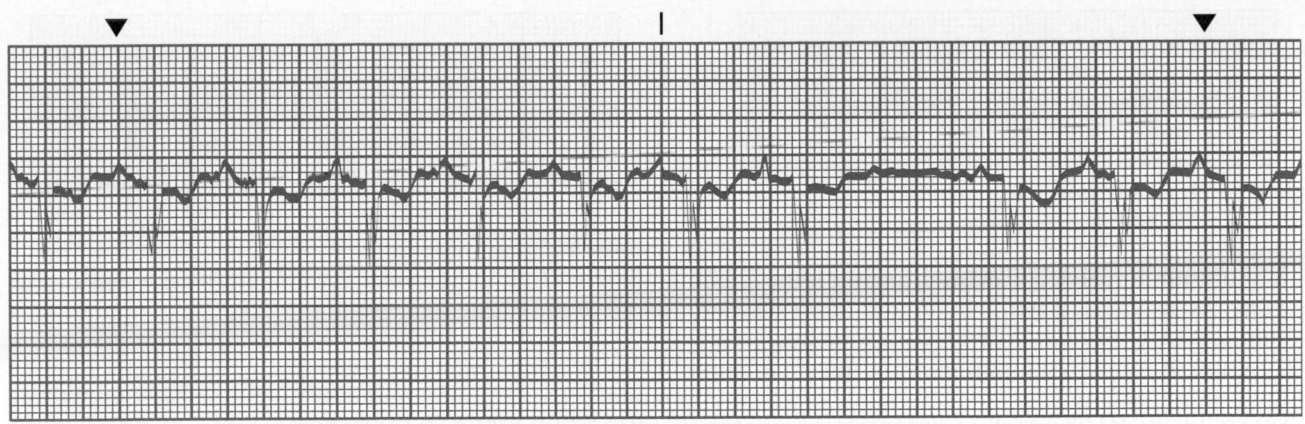

Figure 17-26 • Sinoatrial block. The pause is a multiple of the basic PP interval.

node discharge, often in association with phases of the respiratory cycle. The sinus node rate gradually increases with inspiration and gradually decreases with expiration.

Sinus arrhythmia is a normal phenomenon, seen especially in young people in the setting of lower heart rates. It also occurs after enhancement of vagal tone (e.g., with digitalis or morphine). Because it is a normal finding, sinus arrhythmia does not imply the presence of underlying disease. Symptoms are uncommon unless there are excessively long pauses between heart beats, and usually no treatment is required.

SINUS ARREST AND SINOATRIAL BLOCK

Sinus arrest is a disorder of impulse formation. The sinus node fails to form a discharge, producing pauses of varying lengths because of the absence of atrial depolarization. The P wave is absent, and the resulting PP interval is not a multiple of the basic PP interval. The pause ends either when an escape pacemaker from the junction or ventricles takes over or when sinus node function returns.

An SA block often is difficult to differentiate from sinus arrest on a surface ECG tracing. In SA block, the sinus node fires, but the impulse is delayed or blocked from exiting the sinus node. If the block is complete, the duration of the pause is a multiple of the basic PP interval (Fig. 17-26).

Both dysrhythmias may result from disruption of the sinus node by infarction, degenerative fibrotic changes, drugs (digitalis, β-blockers, calcium channel blockers), or excessive vagal stimulation. These rhythms usually are transient and insignificant unless a lower pacemaker fails to take over to pace the ventricles. Treatment is indicated if the patient is symptomatic. The goal is to increase the ventricular rate, which may require the use of atropine or, in the presence of serious hemodynamic compromise, a pacemaker.

SICK SINUS SYNDROME

Sick sinus syndrome refers to a chronic form of sinus node disease (Fig. 17-27). Patients exhibit severe degrees of sinus node depression, including marked sinus bradycardia, SA block, or sinus arrest. Often, rapid atrial dysrhythmias, such as atrial flutter or fibrillation ("tachycardia–bradycardia syndrome"), coexist and alternate with periods of sinus node depression.

Management of sick sinus syndrome requires control of the rapid atrial dysrhythmias with drug therapy and, in selected cases, control of very slow heart rates, often requiring implantation of a permanent pacemaker.

• Atrial Dysrhythmias

PREMATURE ATRIAL CONTRACTION

A premature atrial contraction (PAC) occurs when an ectopic atrial impulse discharges prematurely and, in most cases, is conducted in a normal fashion through the AV conducting system to the ventricles (Fig. 17-28). On the ECG tracing, the P wave is premature and may even be buried in the preceding T wave; it often differs in configuration from the sinus P wave. The QRS complex usually is of normal configuration. However, because of timing, the QRS complex may appear wide and bizarre if conducted with some degree of delay (aberrant PAC) or may not appear at all if the atrial impulse is blocked from being conducted to the ventricles (blocked PAC). A short pause, usually less than "compensatory," is present (see later definition of premature ventricular contraction).

People of all ages experience PACs. PACs may occur in healthy people as a result of various stimuli,

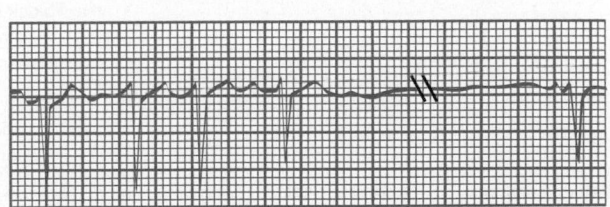

Figure 17-27 • Sick sinus syndrome. Atrial fibrillation is followed by atrial standstill. A sinus escape beat is seen at the end of the strip.

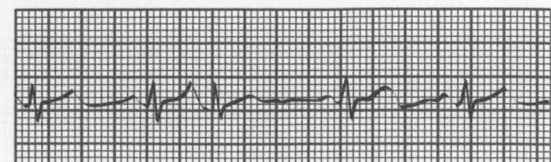

Figure 17-28 • Premature atrial contraction.

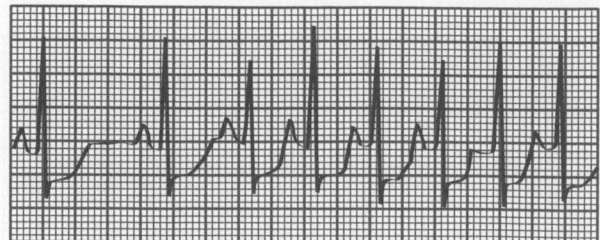

Figure 17-29 • Paroxysmal supraventricular tachycardia, which begins with a premature atrial contraction.

such as emotions, tobacco, alcohol, and caffeine. PACs also may be associated with rheumatic heart disease, ischemic heart disease, mitral stenosis, heart failure, hypokalemia, hypomagnesemia, medications, and hyperthyroidism.

Alternatively, PACs may be a precursor to an atrial tachycardia, atrial fibrillation, or atrial flutter, indicating an increasing atrial irritability. They also may indicate an underlying condition (e.g., heart failure). Patients may have the sensation of a "pause" or "skip" in rhythm when PACs are present.

No treatment is necessary in many cases. The patient should be monitored and frequency of premature beats documented. In addition, the patient should be assessed for underlying conditions and treated.

PAROXYSMAL SUPRAVENTRICULAR TACHYCARDIA

Paroxysmal supraventricular tachycardia (PSVT) describes a rapid atrial rhythm occurring at a rate of 150 to 250 beats/minute (Fig. 17-29). The tachycardia begins abruptly, in most instances with a PAC, and it ends abruptly. P waves may precede the QRS complex but also may be hidden in the QRS complex or precede the T wave at faster rates. (If some of the P waves are not followed by a QRS complex, this is referred to as PSVT with block and usually is caused by digitalis toxicity.) The P waves may be negative in leads II, III, and aVF because of retrograde conduction from the AV node to the atria. The QRS complex usually is normal unless there is an underlying intraventricular conduction problem. The rhythm is reg-

ular, and the paroxysms may last from a few seconds to several hours or even days.

The term PSVT is used to identify rhythms previously called paroxysmal atrial tachycardia and paroxysmal nodal or junctional tachycardia, rhythms similar in all respects except in their sites of origin. PSVT also is known as AV nodal reentrant tachycardia because the mechanism most commonly responsible for this dysrhythmia is a reentrant circuit or chaotic movement at the level of the AV node.

PSVT must be differentiated from other narrow QRS complex (supraventricular) tachycardias. Table 17-12 is a guide to the differential diagnosis. The following points favor the diagnosis of PSVT versus a sinus tachycardia:

► An atrial premature beat often initiates the rhythm.
► The tachycardia begins and terminates abruptly.
► The rate often is faster than a sinus tachycardia and tends to be more regular from minute to minute.
► In response to a vagal maneuver, such as carotid sinus massage, the ectopic tachycardia either is unaffected or reverts to a normal sinus rhythm; however, sinus tachycardia slows slightly in response to increased vagal tone.

Like PACs, PSVTs often occur in adults with normal hearts for the same reasons (e.g., emotions, tobacco, alcohol, caffeine). When heart disease is present, such abnormalities as rheumatic heart disease,

Table 17-12 • Differential Diagnosis of Narrow QRS Tachycardia

Type of SVT	Onset	Atrial Rate	Ventricular Rate	RR Interval	Response to Carotid Massage
Sinus tachycardia	Gradual	100–180 beats/min	Same as sinus rate	Regular	Gradual slowing
PSVT	Abrupt	150–250 beats/min	Usually same as atrial; block seen with digitalis toxicity and AV node disease	Regular, except at onset and termination	May convert to normal sinus rhythm
Atrial flutter	Abrupt	250–350 beats/min	Occurs with 2:1, 3:1, 4:1, or varied ventricular response	Regular or regularly irregular	Abrupt slowing of ventricular response; flutter waves remain
Atrial fibrillation	Abrupt	400–650 beats/min	Depends on ability of AV node to conduct atrial impulse; decreased with drug therapy	Irregularly irregular	Abrupt slowing of ventricular response; fibrillation waves remain

acute MI, and digitalis toxicity may serve as the background for a PSVT.

Often the patient has no underlying heart disease and may experience only palpitations and some lightheadedness, depending on the rate and duration of the PSVT. If the patient has underlying heart disease, dyspnea, angina pectoris, and heart failure may occur as ventricular filling time, and thus cardiac output, is decreased.

Vagal stimulation often terminates the PSVT, either through carotid massage or the Valsalva maneuver. If vagal stimulation is unsuccessful, IV adenosine may be given. Cardioversion or overdrive pacing may be required if drug therapy is unsuccessful. Long-term prophylactic therapy may be indicated.

ATRIAL FLUTTER

Atrial flutter is a rapid atrial ectopic rhythm in which the atria fire at rates of 250 to 350 beats/minute (Fig. 17-30). The AV node functions as a "gatekeeper," preventing too many impulses from reaching the ventricle. If the ventricles are stimulated 250 to 350 times per minute, they are unable to respond with effective contractions, and cardiac output is insufficient to sustain life. The AV node may allow only every second, third, or fourth atrial stimulus to proceed to the ventricles, resulting in what is known as a 2:1, 3:1, or 4:1 flutter block.

The rapid and regular atrial rate produces "sawtooth" or "picket-fence" P waves on the ECG. It is usual for a flutter wave to be partially concealed in the QRS complex or T wave. The QRS complex exhibits a normal configuration except when aberrant conduction is present.

When the ventricular rate is rapid, the diagnosis of atrial flutter may be difficult. Vagal maneuvers, such as carotid sinus massage or the administration of adenosine, increase the degree of AV block and allow recognition of flutter waves. Atrial flutter often is seen in the presence of underlying cardiac disease, including CAD, cor pulmonale, and rheumatic heart disease. If atrial flutter occurs in conjunction with a rapid ventricular rate, the ventricular chambers cannot fill adequately, resulting in varying degrees of hemodynamic compromise. Likewise, if atrial flutter is accompanied by a very slow ventricular rate, cardiac output is diminished. The loss of "atrial kick," because atrial contraction is not occurring, is also a concern. The lack of atrial kick can compromise cardiac output. Finally, without atrial contractions, thrombi can form on the walls of the atria. If these thrombi break loose, the result could be pulmonary embolus, cerebral embolus, or MI.

Treatment goals for atrial flutter are to reestablish sinus rhythm or to achieve ventricular rate control. When the ventricular rate is rapid, prompt treatment to control the rate or revert the rhythm to a sinus mechanism is indicated. Drugs may be selected to slow the conduction of the impulses through the AV node or to achieve pharmacological conversion of the rhythm. If pharmacological conversion is not successful, electrical cardioversion can be used. Synchronized cardioversion is especially useful in the prompt treatment of atrial flutter. The patient should be NPO before the procedure and receive sedation. (For a more detailed discussion of cardioversion, see Chapter 18.) If the patient has been experiencing atrial flutter for more than about 72 hours, anticoagulation may be needed before pharmacological or electrical conversion of the rhythm is attempted. Other modes of therapy may be indicated for the long-term management of atrial flutter, such as ablation, pacing, and implantable devices.

ATRIAL FIBRILLATION

Atrial fibrillation is defined as a rapid atrial ectopic rhythm, occurring with atrial rates of 350 to 500 beats/minute (Fig. 17-31). It is characterized by chaotic atrial activity with the absence of definable P waves. Instead, the P waves appear as small, quivering fibrillatory waves. Like atrial flutter, the ventricular rate and rhythm depend on the ability of the AV junction to function as a gatekeeper. If too many atrial stimuli pass through the AV junction, the ventricular response is rapid. If too few atrial stimuli pass through the AV junction, the ventricular response is slow. The ventricular rhythm is characteristically irregular.

Although atrial fibrillation may occur as a transient dysrhythmia in healthy young people, the presence of chronic atrial fibrillation is usually associated with underlying heart disease. One or both of the following are present in patients with chronic atrial fibrillation: atrial muscle disease or atrial distention together with disease of the sinus node. This rhythm commonly occurs in the setting of heart failure, ischemic or rheumatic heart disease, or pulmonary disease, and after open heart surgery. Atrial fibrillation also is seen in congenital heart disease.

The immediate clinical concern in patients with atrial fibrillation is the rate of the ventricular response. If the ventricular rate is too fast, end-diastolic filling time is decreased, and cardiac output is compromised. If the ventricular rate is too slow, cardiac output may again be decreased. As in atrial flutter, patients with

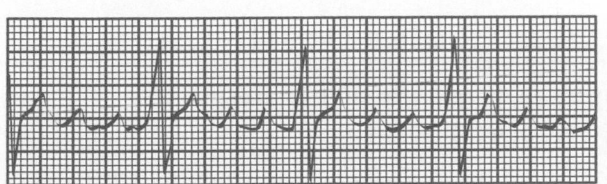

Figure 17-30 • Atrial flutter. (Atrial rate = 250–350 beats/min. P wave shows characteristic sawtoothed pattern.)

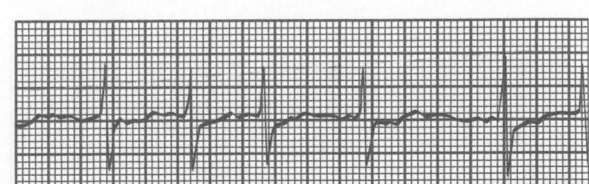

Figure 17-31 • Atrial fibrillation. (Atrial rate = 400–600 beats/min with a variable ventricular response. Characteristic atrial fibrillatory waves seen.)

atrial fibrillation have lost AV synchrony and atrial kick, resulting in a compromised cardiac output. Patients also are at risk for the formation of mural thrombi and embolic events, such as stroke, MI, and pulmonary embolus.

The treatment principles for atrial fibrillation are the same as those for atrial flutter. The goal of therapy is to achieve rate control or to convert the rhythm to sinus. If a patient has chronic atrial fibrillation, anticoagulant therapy is added to the drug regimen to prevent an embolic event. Cardioversion is indicated for rhythm control when drug therapy fails or in the setting of hemodynamic compromise. Ablation, pacing, and implantable devices are among the therapeutic options.

MULTIFOCAL ATRIAL TACHYCARDIA

Multifocal atrial tachycardia is a rapid atrial rhythm with varying P-wave morphology, resulting from the firing of three or more atrial foci (Fig. 17-32). The atrial rate exceeds 100 beats/minute, and the rhythm usually is irregular. The P waves vary in shape because of the multiple foci. The PR intervals may vary also, depending on the proximity of the focus to the AV node. The QRS complexes are normal unless an impulse is conducted with aberrancy.

This rhythm characteristically occurs in patients with severe pulmonary disease. Such patients often exhibit hypoxemia, hypokalemia, alterations in serum pH, or pulmonary hypertension. They usually manifest symptoms associated with the underlying disease rather than with the dysrhythmia itself. Treatment is directed at controlling the underlying pulmonary disease and slowing the ventricular rate if necessary.

• Junctional Dysrhythmias

JUNCTIONAL RHYTHM

A junctional rhythm, also known as a nodal rhythm, is a rhythm originating in the AV node. When the SA node fails to fire, the AV node usually takes control, but the rate is slower. The rate of a junctional rhythm ranges between 50 and 70 beats/minute. The P wave in the dysrhythmia can have one of three possible configurations.

1. The AV node fires, and the wave of depolarization travels backward (retrograde conduction) into the atria. The impulse from the AV node then moves forward into the ventricle. When this sequence

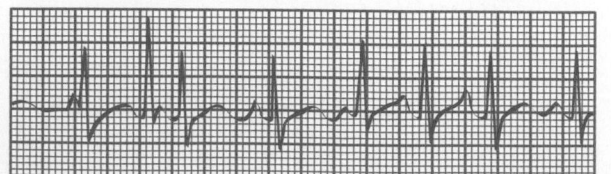

Figure 17-32 • Multifocal atrial tachycardia. (The atrial rate exceeds 100 beats/min with three or more different P-wave morphologies.)

occurs, the P wave appears as an inverted wave before a normal QRS complex (Fig. 17-33A).

2. The retrograde conduction into the atria occurs at the same time as the forward conduction into the ventricles. The resulting rhythm strip shows an absent P wave with a normal QRS complex. In reality, the P wave is not absent. Instead, it is buried inside the QRS complex (see Fig. 17-33B).

3. Forward conduction of the ventricles precedes retrograde conduction of the atria. When this sequence occurs, a normal QRS complex is followed by an inverted P wave (see Fig. 17-33C).

A junctional rhythm may be the result of hypoxia, hyperkalemia, MI, heart failure, valvular disease, drugs (digoxin, β-blockers, calcium channel blockers), or any cause of SA node dysfunction. Patients with a junctional rhythm may become symptomatic as a result of the slower rate. Hypotension, decreased cardiac output, and decreased perfusion may occur. The benefit of AV synchrony and atrial kick may be lost when the atria are stimulated with or after ventricular depolarization.

Treatment should be directed at the underlying cause. Symptomatic patients may require immediate treatment. The heart rate can be increased through the use of atropine or cardiac pacing. Interventions are also directed toward improving cardiac output.

PREMATURE JUNCTIONAL CONTRACTIONS

A premature junctional contraction (PJC) is an ectopic impulse from a focus in the AV junction, occurring prematurely, before the next sinus impulse (Fig. 17-34). As in all rhythms originating in the AV junction, the QRS complex is narrow (<0.12 second), reflecting normal AV conduction. On rare occasions, the QRS complex may be wide if the impulse is conducted aberrantly. The atria are depolarized in a retrograde fashion before, during, or after ventricular excitation, producing inverted P waves that may occur before, during, or after the QRS complex. As with PACs, PJCs may occur in healthy people or in those with underlying heart disease. Ischemia or infarction may activate an ectopic focus in the AV junction, as may stimulants, such as nicotine or caffeine, or pharmacological agents (e.g., digitalis).

Frequent PJCs may indicate increasing irritability and may be a precursor of a junctional rhythm. Although usually asymptomatic, patients may experience a "skipped beat." Treatment for PJCs is not necessary.

• Ventricular Dysrhythmias

PREMATURE VENTRICULAR CONTRACTIONS

A premature ventricular contraction (PVC) is an ectopic beat originating prematurely at the level of the ventricles (Fig. 17-35A). The beat is ventricular in

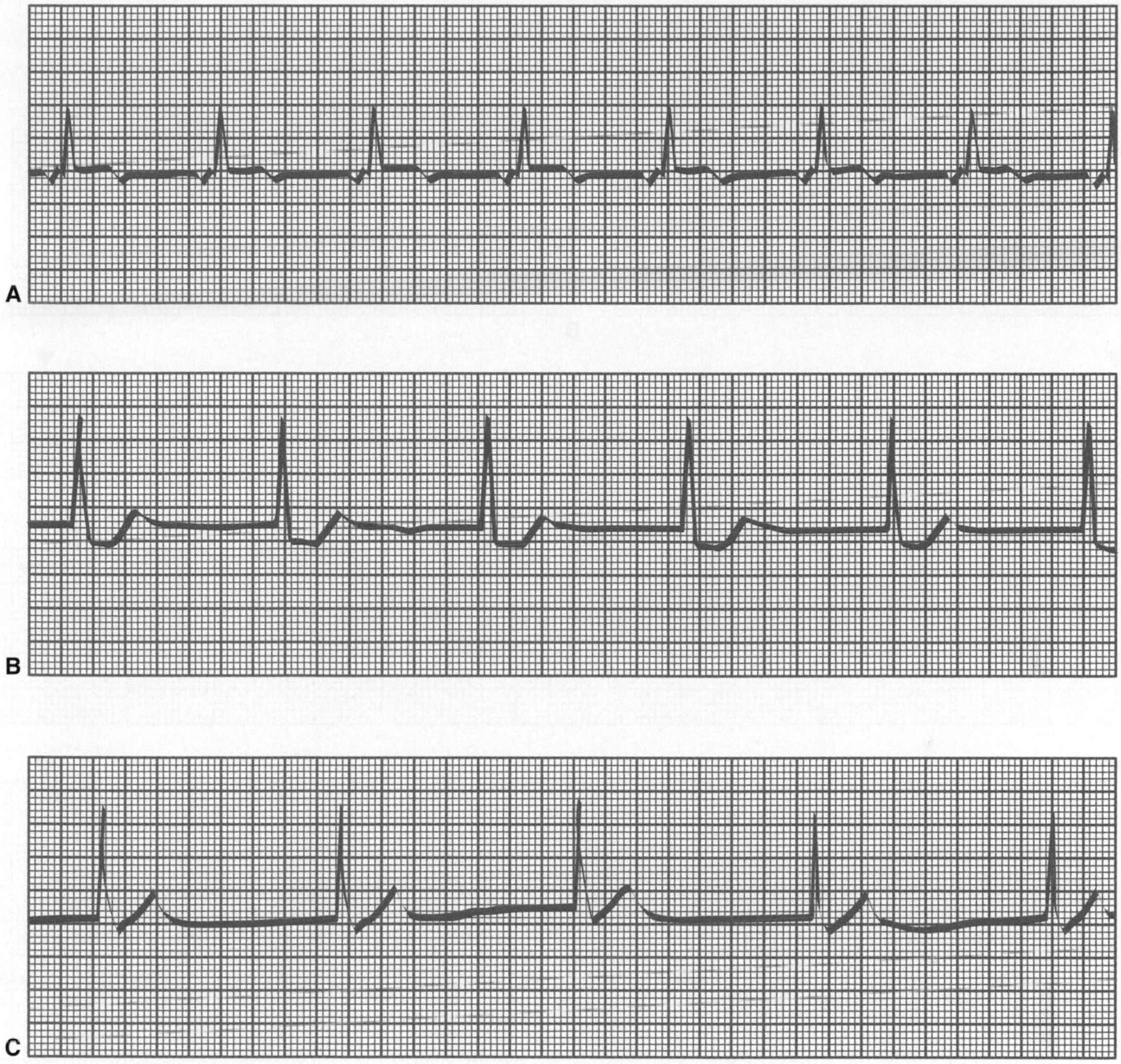

Figure 17-33 • Junctional rhythm. **A:** A junctional rhythm in which the inverted P wave appears before a normal QRS complex. **B:** A junctional rhythm in which the inverted P wave is buried inside the QRS complex. **C:** A junctional rhythm in which the inverted P wave follows the QRS complex.

origin and results in no electrical activity in the atria. As a result, no P waves appear. The ventricular depolarization does not travel through the normal rapid ventricular conduction system. Instead, ventricular conduction spreads more slowly through the Purkinje system, resulting in a wide QRS complex with a T wave that is opposite in direction to the QRS complex. A compensatory pause often follows the premature beat as the heart awaits the next stimulus from the sinus node. The pause is considered fully compensatory if the cycles of the normal and premature beats equal the time of two normal heart cycles.

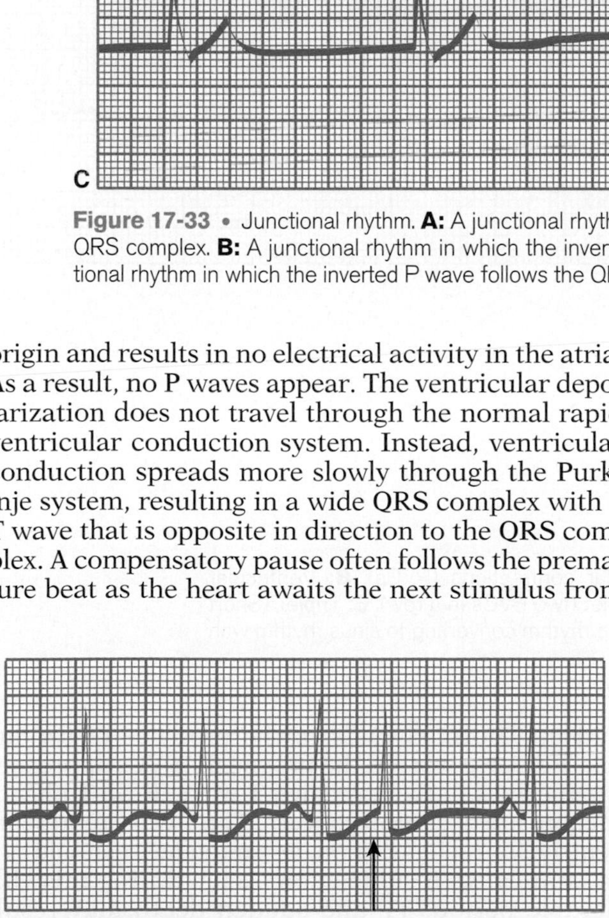

Ventricular premature beats can be described by their frequency and pattern. They can be rare, occasional, or frequent; optimally, they are described as number of PVCs per minute. If PVCs occur after each sinus beat, ventricular bigeminy is present (see Fig. 17-35B). Ventricular trigeminy is a PVC occurring after two consecutive sinus beats. When PVCs appear in only one form (from one ventricular site), they are referred to as uniformed, as opposed to multiformed, when two or more forms (from more than one ventricular site) of the QRS complex are apparent (see Fig. 17-35C). Two PVCs in a row are a couplet (see Fig. 17-35D), whereas three in a row are a triplet, which is a short run of VT (see Fig. 17-35E).

The most common of all ectopic beats, PVCs can occur with or without heart disease in any age group. They are especially common in people with myocardial disease (ischemia or infarction) or with

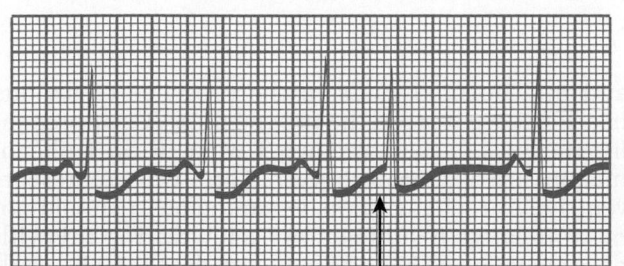

Figure 17-34 • Premature junctional contraction.

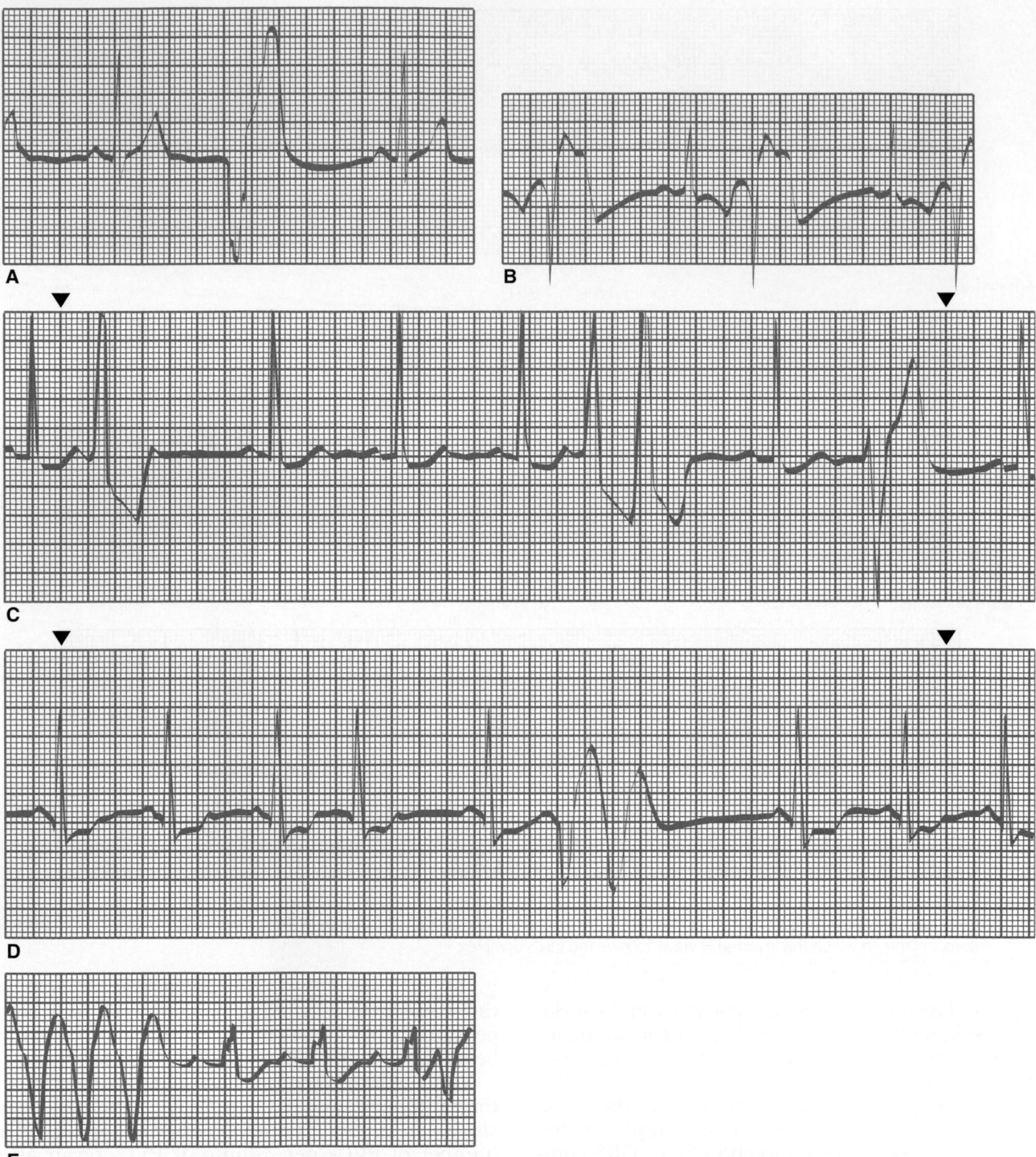

Figure 17-35 • Ventricular dysrhythmias. **A:** Premature ventricular contractions (PVCs). **B:** Ventricular bigeminy. (Every other beat is a PVC.) **C:** Multiformed PVCs. **D:** Couplet (two PVCs in a row). **E:** Triplet. (Short run of ventricular tachycardia [VT]; the first three beats are VT with the rhythm converting to sinus rhythm with first-degree heart block.)

myocardial irritability (hypokalemia, increased levels of catecholamines, or mechanical irritation with a wire or catheter). The presence of PVCs is a sign of ventricular myocardial irritability and, in some patients, may lead to VT or ventricular fibrillation (VF). The nature of the patient's underlying heart disease rather than the presence of PVCs as such determines the treatment and prognosis. Numerous

and multiformed PVCs in the presence of serious heart disease worsen the prognosis. PVCs approaching the apex of the preceding T wave (R-on-T phenomenon) are of clinical concern. The T wave represents ventricular repolarization, when the heart should not be stimulated. If stimulation occurs during this vulnerable period, VF and sudden death may result (Fig. 17-36).

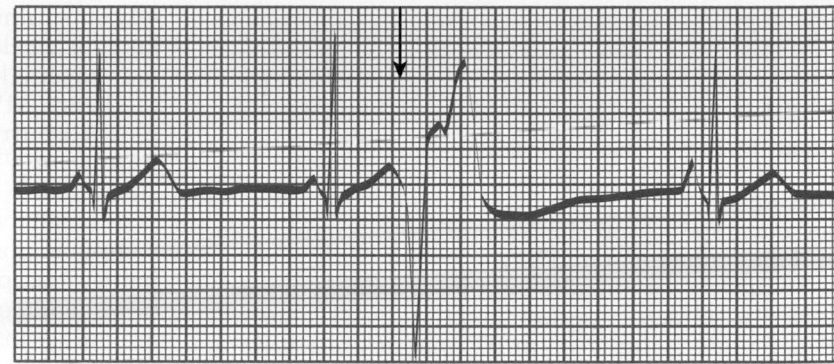

Figure 17-36 • R-on-T premature ventricular contraction. (From Huff J: ECG Workout, 4th ed. Philadelphia: Lippincott Williams & Wilkins, 2002, p 195.)

Infrequent, isolated PVCs require no treatment. Multiple or consecutive PVCs may be managed with antiarrhythmic agents. In the emergency setting, amiodarone and lidocaine are the drugs of choice. Many antiarrhythmic agents are available for chronic therapy. If serum potassium is low, potassium replacement may correct the dysrhythmia. If the dysrhythmia is caused by digitalis toxicity, withdrawal of the digitalis may correct it.

VENTRICULAR TACHYCARDIA

In the previous section, VT was defined as three or more PVCs in a row. VT is recognized by wide, bizarre QRS complexes occurring in a fairly regular rhythm at a rate greater than 100 beats/minute (Fig. 17-37). P waves usually are not seen and, if seen, are not related to the QRS complex. VT may be a short, non-sustained rhythm or longer and sustained.

In adults with normal hearts, VT is rare but is a common complication of MI. Other causes are the same as those described for PVCs. VT is a precursor of VF, and signs and symptoms of hemodynamic compromise (e.g., ischemic chest pain, hypotension, pulmonary edema, and unconsciousness) may be seen if the rate is fast and the tachycardia is sustained. Serious dysrhythmia progression depends on the underlying heart disease.

If the patient is hemodynamically stable with the dysrhythmia, lidocaine may be administered intravenously. If the patient becomes unstable, synchro-nized cardioversion (or in emergency situations, unsynchronized defibrillation) is indicated. Long-term treatment for this dysrhythmia may involve the use of an implantable cardioverter–defibrillator (ICD). See Chapter 18 for a more detailed discussion of ICDs.

TORSADES DE POINTES

Torsades de pointes ("twisting of the points") is a specific type of VT (Fig. 17-38). The term refers to the polarity of the QRS complex, which swings from positive to negative and vice versa. The QRS complex morphology is characterized by large, bizarre, polymorphous, or multiformed QRS complexes of varying amplitude and direction, frequently varying from beat to beat and resembling torsion around an isoelectric line. The rate of the tachycardia is 100 to 180 beats/minute but can be as fast as 200 to 300 beats/minute. The rhythm is highly unstable; it may terminate in VF or revert to sinus rhythm. This form of VT is most likely to develop in myocardial disease when the underlying QT interval has been prolonged.

Torsades de pointes is favored by conditions that prolong the QT interval. Examples include severe bradycardia; drug therapy, especially with type IA antiarrhythmic agents; and electrolyte disturbances, such as hypokalemia and hypocalcemia. Other factors that can precipitate this dysrhythmia include intrinsic cardiac disease, familial QT-interval prolongation, central nervous system disorders, and hypothermia. Torsades de pointes may terminate spontaneously

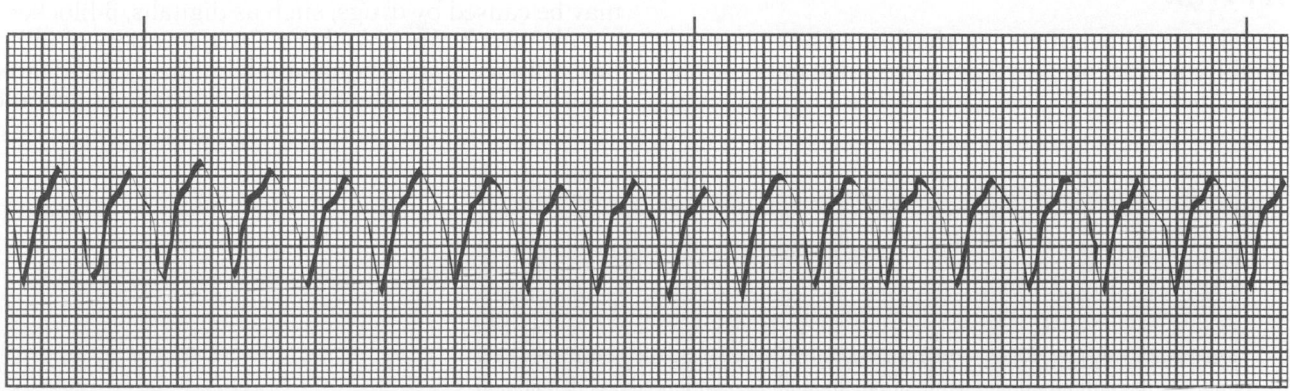

Figure 17-37 • Ventricular tachycardia. (From Huff J: ECG Workout, 4th ed. Philadelphia: Lippincott Williams & Wilkins, 2002, p 197.)

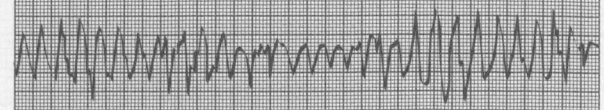

Figure 17-38 • Torsades de pointes.

and may repeat itself after several seconds or minutes, or it may transform into VF.

Treatment for torsades de pointes consists of shortening the refractory period (and thus the QT interval) of the underlying rhythm. IV magnesium sulfate, magnesium chloride, or isoproterenol is effective in suppression of the dysrhythmia. Overdrive pacing also can be used. Treatment is directed at correcting the underlying problem and may necessitate stopping the offending pharmacological agent or correcting the electrolyte imbalance. Emergency cardioversion or defibrillation is indicated if the torsades does not revert spontaneously to sinus rhythm.

VENTRICULAR FIBRILLATION

VF is defined as rapid, irregular, and ineffectual depolarizations of the ventricle (Fig. 17-39). No distinct QRS complexes are seen. Only irregular oscillations of the baseline are apparent; these may be either coarse or fine in appearance.

VF may occur in the following circumstances: myocardial ischemia and infarction, catheter manipulation in the ventricles, electrocution, prolonged QT interval, or as a terminal rhythm in patients with circulatory failure. As in asystole, loss of consciousness occurs within seconds in VF. There is no pulse and no cardiac output. VF is the most common cause of sudden cardiac death and is fatal if resuscitation is not instituted immediately.

If VF occurs, rapid defibrillation is the management of choice (see the discussion of cardiopulmonary resuscitation in Chapter 18). The patient should be supported with cardiopulmonary resuscitation and drugs if there is no response to defibrillation. An ICD may be indicated for long-term management of VF (see Chapter 18 for a discussion of ICDs).

ACCELERATED IDIOVENTRICULAR RHYTHM

Accelerated idioventricular rhythm (AIVR) is produced by a "speeding up" of ventricular pacemaker cells, which normally have an intrinsic rate of 20 to

40 beats/minute (Fig. 17-40). When the idioventricular rate accelerates above the sinus rate, the ventricular pacemaker becomes the primary pacemaker for the heart. AIVR is characterized by wide QRS complexes occurring regularly at a rate of 50 to 100 beats/minute. AIVR may last for a few beats or may be sustained.

Typically, AIVR is seen with acute MI, often in the setting of coronary artery reperfusion after thrombolytic therapy. It may occur less commonly as a result of ischemia or digitalis intoxication. Patients usually are not symptomatic. Adequate cardiac output can be maintained, and degeneration into a rapid VT is rare.

In most cases, treatment is not necessary. If a patient is hemodynamically compromised, the sinus rate is increased with atropine or atrial pacing to suppress the AIVR.

• Atrioventricular Blocks

A disturbance in some portion of the AV conduction system causes an AV block. The sinus-initiated beat is delayed or completely blocked from activating the ventricles. The block may occur at the level of the AV node, bundle of His, or the bundle branches because the AV conduction system contains all of these structures. In first- and second-degree AV block, the block is incomplete; some or all of the impulses eventually are conducted to the ventricles. In third-degree or complete heart block, none of the sinus-initiated impulses are conducted. Table 17-13 summarizes and compares heart block rhythms.

FIRST-DEGREE ATRIOVENTRICULAR BLOCK

In first-degree block, AV conduction is prolonged and equal in time. All impulses eventually are conducted to the ventricles (Fig. 17-41A). P waves are present and precede each QRS complex in a 1:1 relationship. The PR interval is constant but exceeds the upper limit of 0.2 second in duration.

First-degree heart block occurs in people of all ages and in healthy and diseased hearts. PR prolongation may be caused by drugs, such as digitalis, β-blockers, or calcium channel blockers; CAD; a variety of infectious diseases; and congenital lesions. First-degree block is of no hemodynamic consequence but should

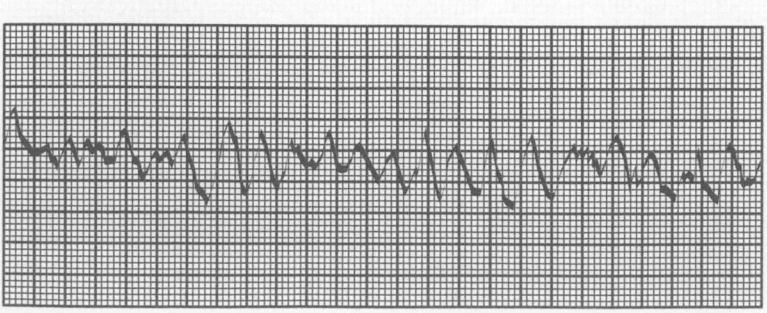

Figure 17-39 • Ventricular fibrillation.

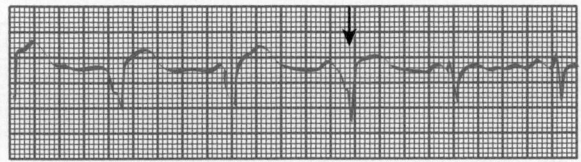

Figure 17-40 • Accelerated idioventricular rhythm. The first three beats are of ventricular origin. The fourth beat (*arrow*) represents a fusion beat. The subsequent two beats are of sinus origin.

be seen as an indicator of a potential AV conduction system disturbance. First-degree block may progress to second- or third-degree AV block.

No treatment is indicated for first-degree heart block. The PR interval should be monitored closely, watching for further block. The possibility of a drug effect also should be evaluated.

SECOND-DEGREE ATRIOVENTRICULAR BLOCK—MOBITZ I (WENCKEBACH)

Mobitz type I (Wenckebach) block occurs when AV conduction is delayed progressively with each sinus impulse until eventually the impulse is completely blocked from reaching the ventricles. The cycle then repeats itself (see Fig. 17-41B). Of the two types of second-degree block, Mobitz I (Wenckebach) and Mobitz II, Mobitz I occurs more commonly.

On the ECG tracing, P waves are present and related to the QRS complex in a cyclical pattern. The PR interval progressively lengthens with each beat until a QRS complex is not conducted. The QRS complex has the same configuration throughout the underlying rhythm.

A Mobitz type I block usually is associated with block above the bundle of His. Therefore, any drug or disease process that affects the AV node, such as digitalis, myocarditis, or an inferior wall MI, may produce this type of second-degree block.

Patients with Mobitz type I second-degree AV block rarely are symptomatic because the ventricular rate usually is adequate. Wenckebach block often is temporary, and if it progresses to third-degree block, a junctional pacemaker at a rate of 40 to 60 beats/minute usually takes over to pace the ventricles. No treatment is required for this rhythm except to discontinue a drug if it is the offending agent. The patient should be monitored for further progression of block.

SECOND-DEGREE ATRIOVENTRICULAR BLOCK—MOBITZ II

Mobitz type II block is described as an intermittent block in the AV conduction, usually in or below the bundle of His. Mobitz type II block is characterized by a fixed PR interval when AV conduction is present and a nonconducted P wave when the block occurs (see Fig. 17-41C). This block in conduction can occur occasionally or be repetitive with a 2:1, 3:1, or even 4:1 conduction pattern. Because there is no disturbance in the sinus node, the PP interval is regular. Often there is accompanying bundle branch block, so the QRS complex may be wide.

A Mobitz type II pattern is seen in the setting of an anterior wall MI and various diseases of the conducting tissue, such as fibrotic disease. A Mobitz type II block is potentially more dangerous than a Mobitz type I block. Mobitz type II block often is permanent, and it may deteriorate rapidly to third-degree heart block with a slow ventricular response of 20 to 40 beats/minute.

Constant monitoring and observation for progression to third-degree heart block are required. Medications, such as atropine, or cardiac pacing may be required if a patient becomes symptomatic or if the block occurs in the setting of an acute anterior wall MI. Permanent pacing often is indicated for long-term management.

Table 17-13 • A Comparison of the Electrocardiographic Characteristics of Heart Block Rhythms

	First-Degree Heart Block	Second-Degree Heart Block—Mobitz Type I (Wenckebach)	Second-Degree Heart Block—Mobitz Type II	Third-Degree Heart Block
Rate	Usually 60–100 beats/min	Usually 60–100 beats/min	May be slow depending on number of blocked P waves	Rate determined by ventricular focus, usually very slow
Rhythm	Regular	Irregular due to dropped QRS	Often regular but depends on pattern of block	May be regular or irregular ventricular focus
P waves	Present, one per QRS	Present, one per QRS until QRS is missed	Present, more than one P wave per QRS	Present, more than one P wave per QRS; P waves no relationship to QRS complexes
PR interval	>0.20 s, equal throughout	Progressively gets longer until QRS is missed; pattern repeats	May be normal or prolonged, equal throughout	May be normal or prolonged, unequal throughout
QRS complex	<0.12 s	<0.12 s	Usually >0.12 s	>0.12 s

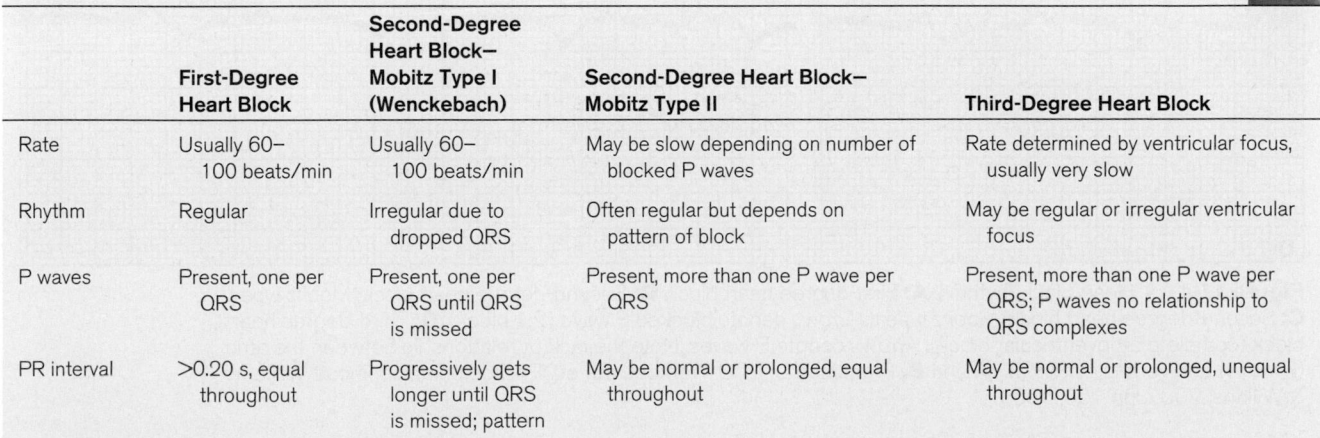

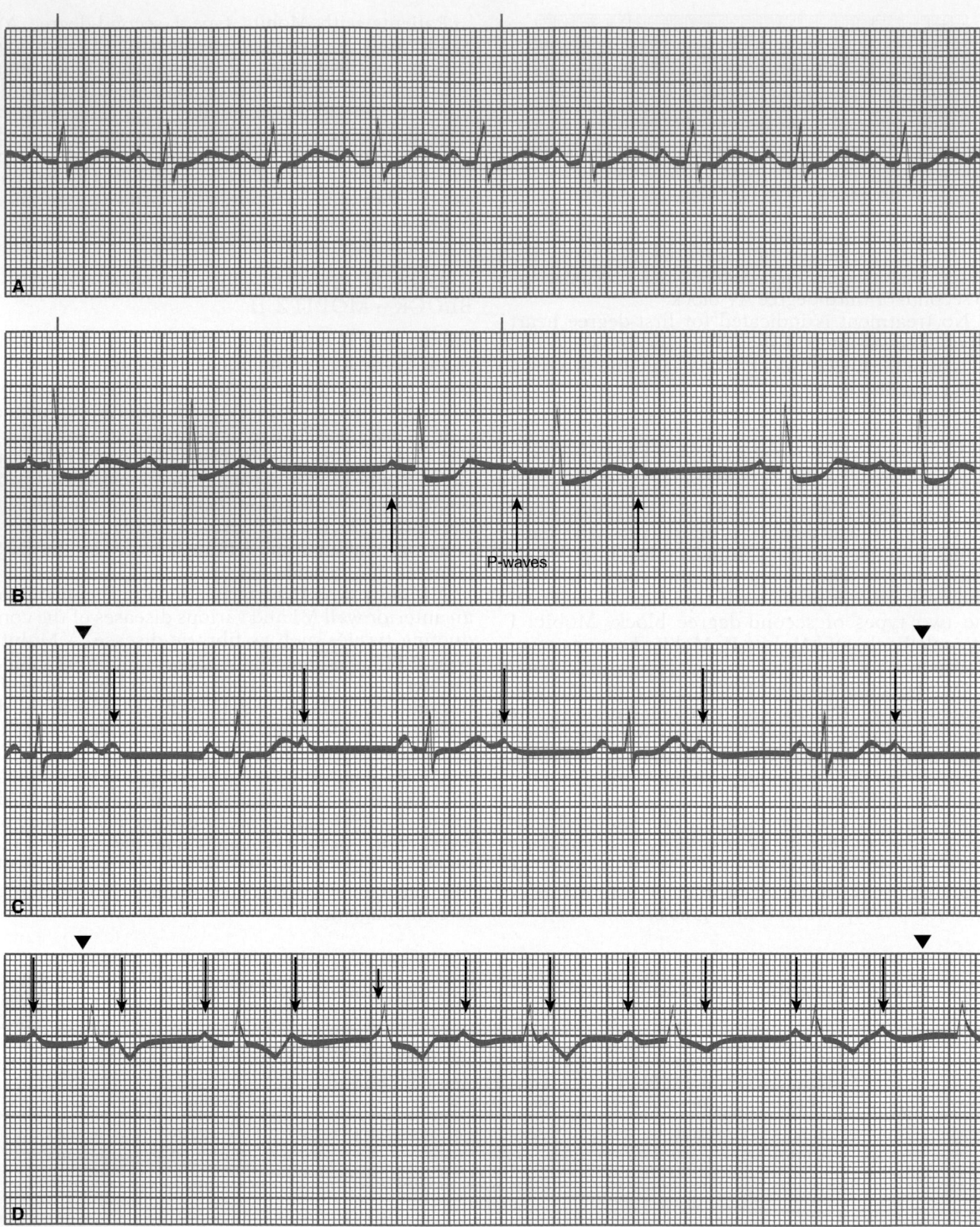

Figure 17-41 • Heart block rhythms. **A:** First-degree heart block. **B:** Second-degree heart block: Mobitz type I.
C: Second-degree heart block: Mobitz type II. *Arrows* denote blocked P wave (2:1 block). **D:** Third-degree heart
block (complete atrioventricular block). *Arrows* denote P waves. Note the lack of relationship between the atria
(P wave) and ventricles (QRS). (**A** and **B,** From Huff J: ECG Workout, 4th ed. Philadelphia: Lippincott Williams
& Wilkins, 2002, pp 150, 156.)

THIRD-DEGREE (COMPLETE) ATRIOVENTRICULAR BLOCK

In third-degree or complete heart block, the sinus node continues to fire normally, but the impulses do not reach the ventricles (see Fig. 17-41D). The ventricles are stimulated from escape pacemaker cells either in the junction (at a rate of 40 to 60 beats/minute) or in the ventricles (at a rate of 20 to 40 beats/minute), depending on the level of the AV block.

On the ECG tracing, P waves and QRS complexes are both present, but there is no relationship between the two. Therefore, complete heart block is considered one form of AV dissociation. The PP and RR intervals are each regular, but the PR interval is variable. If a junctional pacemaker paces the ventricles, the QRS complex is narrow. A pacemaker site lower in the ventricles produces a wide QRS complex.

The causes of complete heart block are the same as for lesser degrees of AV block. Complete heart block is often poorly tolerated. The rate and dependability of the ventricular pacemaker depend on its location. If the escape rhythm is ventricular in origin, the rate is slow, and the pacemaker site is unreliable. The patient may be symptomatic because of a low cardiac output. A pacemaker site high in the bundle of His may provide an adequate rate and is more dependable. The patient may remain asymptomatic if the escape rhythm supports a normal cardiac output.

A temporary pacing wire is usually inserted immediately, and when the patient is stabilized, a permanent pacemaker is implanted.

• The 12-Lead Electrocardiogram

THE NORMAL 12-LEAD ELECTROCARDIOGRAM

As previously described, the ECG provides 12 electrical views of the heart. The first three electrical views are provided by the standard leads I, II, and III.

The next three electrical views are provided by the augmented leads, aVR, aVL, and aVF. The standard and augmented leads are referred to as the limb leads and provide a view from a vertical plane. The remaining six electrical views of the heart, the precordial leads, chest leads, or V leads, V_1 through V_6, provide a horizontal plane view of the heart (Fig. 17-42).

In the normal 12-lead ECG, the P wave representing atrial depolarization is usually upright and rounded. Each component of the QRS complex (ventricular depolarization) is analyzed separately. The Q wave, the initial downward deflection of the QRS complex, should be absent or small. The R component is the tallest upright portion of the QRS complex in the limb leads except aVR. In the precordial leads, the R wave begins as a small wave in V_1 and gradually progresses to a tall wave by V_6. The S wave, the downward stroke after the R wave, is small or absent in the limb leads. The S wave begins as a deep wave in V_1 and gradually disappears by V_6 in the precordial leads. The ST segment is isoelectric but may be slightly elevated in V_1 through V_3. The T wave, representing ventricular repolarization, is usually upright, although a variety of configurations can be normal. Table 17-14 summarizes the normal 12-lead ECG.

The 12-lead ECG may be useful in determining the electrical axis of the heart and detecting abnormalities that require more than one electrical view. These abnormalities include bundle branch block; atrial or ventricular enlargement; and patterns of ischemia, injury, or infarction.

ELECTRICAL AXIS

Electrical axis refers to the general direction of the wave of excitation as it moves through the heart. In the normal heart, the flow of electrical forces originates in the SA node, spreads throughout atrial tissue, passes through the AV node, and moves throughout the ventricles. This flow of forces is normally downward and to the left, a pattern known as normal axis.

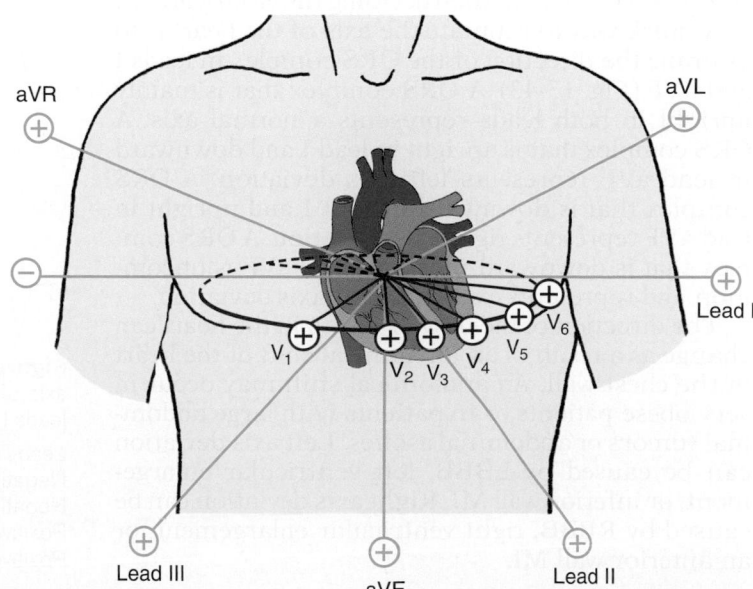

Figure 17-42 • Electrocardiographic views of the heart.

Table 17-14 • The Normal 12-Lead Electrocardiogram

Lead	P	Q	R	S	S-T	T
I	Upright	Small, 0.04 sec, or none	Dominant	< R or none	Isoelectric +1 to -0.5 mm	Upright
II	Upright	Small or none	Dominant	< R or none	+1 to -0.5 mm	Upright
III	Upright Flat Diphasic Inverted	Small or none	None to dominant	None to dominant	+1 to -0.5 mm	Upright Flat Diphasic Inverted
aVR	Inverted	Small, none, or large	Small or none	Dominant	+1 to -0.5 mm	Inverted
aVL	Upright Flat Diphasic Inverted	Small, none, or large	Small, none, or dominant	Small, none, or dominant	+1 to -0.5 mm	Upright Flat Diphasic Inverted
aVF	Upright Flat Diphasic Inverted	Small or none	Small, none, or dominant	None to dominant	+1 to -0.5 mm	Upright
V_1	Upright Flat Diphasic	None May be QS	Small	Deep	0 to +3 mm	Inverted Flat Upright Diphasic
V_2	Upright	None			0 to +3 mm	Upright Diphasic Inverted
V_3	Upright	Small or none			0 to +3 mm	Upright
V_4	Upright	Small or none			+1 to -0.5 mm	Upright
V_5	Upright	Small			+1 to -0.5 mm	Upright
V_6	Upright	Small	Tall	Small or none	+1 to -0.5 mm	Upright

The ventricles make up the largest muscle mass of the heart and therefore make the most significant contribution to the determination of the direction of the flow of forces in the heart. For this reason, the QRS complex is examined when deciding the electrical axis.

A quick way to estimate the axis of the heart is to examine the direction of the QRS complex in leads I and aVF (Fig. 17-43). A QRS complex that is mainly upright in both leads represents a normal axis. A QRS complex that is upright in lead I and downward in lead aVF represents left axis deviation. A QRS complex that is downward in lead I and upright in lead aVF represents right axis deviation. A QRS complex that is downward in leads I and aVF is uncommon and represents extreme right axis deviation.

The direction of the flow of forces in the heart can change as a result of an anatomical shift of the heart in the chest wall. An anatomical shift may occur in very obese patients or in patients with large abdominal tumors or abdominal ascites. Left axis deviation can be caused by LBBB, left ventricular enlargement, or inferior wall MI. Right axis deviation can be caused by RBBB, right ventricular enlargement, or an anterior wall MI.

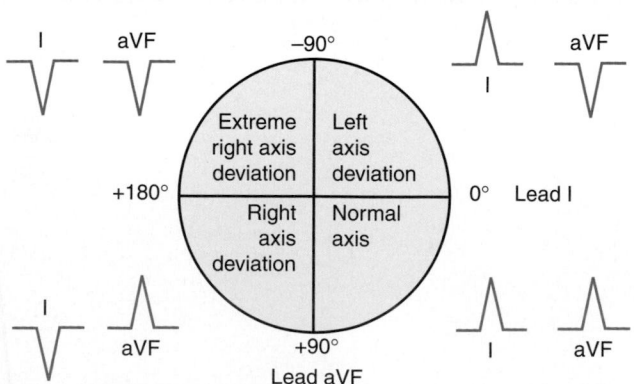

Figure 17-43 • Determining electrical axis. To determine the axis of the heart, examine the direction of the QRS complex in leads I and aVF.

Lead I	Lead aVF	Axis
Negative	Negative	Extreme right axis deviation
Negative	Positive	Right axis deviation
Positive	Negative	Left axis deviation
Positive	Positive	Normal axis

Patients with an axis shift are asymptomatic. The only way an axis shift can be detected is through a 12-lead ECG. The axis shift usually represents some underlying abnormality, and treatment is directed at the underlying cause.

BUNDLE BRANCH BLOCK

A bundle branch block develops when there is either a functional or pathological block in one of the major branches of the intraventricular conduction system. As conduction through one bundle is blocked, the impulse travels along the unaffected bundle and activates one ventricle normally. The impulse is delayed in reaching the other ventricle because it travels outside of the normal conducting fibers. The right and left ventricles are thus depolarized sequentially instead of simultaneously. The abnormal activation produces a wide QRS complex, representing the increased time it takes for ventricular depolarization (Fig. 17-44). The broad QRS complex has two peaks (RSR'), indicating

that depolarization of the two ventricles was not simultaneous.

An RBBB and LBBB are diagnosed on the 12-lead ECG but also can be identified on the bedside monitor using a V_1 or MCL_1 tracing and a V_6 or MCL_6 tracing (see section on Electrocardiographic Monitoring for description of lead selection). To identify the presence of a bundle branch block, the QRS complex duration must be prolonged to 0.12 second or longer, representing the delay in conduction through the ventricles. An RBBB alters the configuration of the QRS complex in the right-sided chest leads, V_1 and V_2. Normally, these leads have a small, single-peaked R-wave and deep S-wave configuration. With an RBBB, depolarization of the right ventricle is delayed, and the ECG pattern changes. An RBBB is evidenced by an RSR' configuration in V_1. If the initial peak of the QRS complex is smaller than the second peak, the pattern would be described as rSR'. An "r" is used to describe the first, smaller peak, and an "R" is used to describe the second, taller peak. Likewise, if the initial

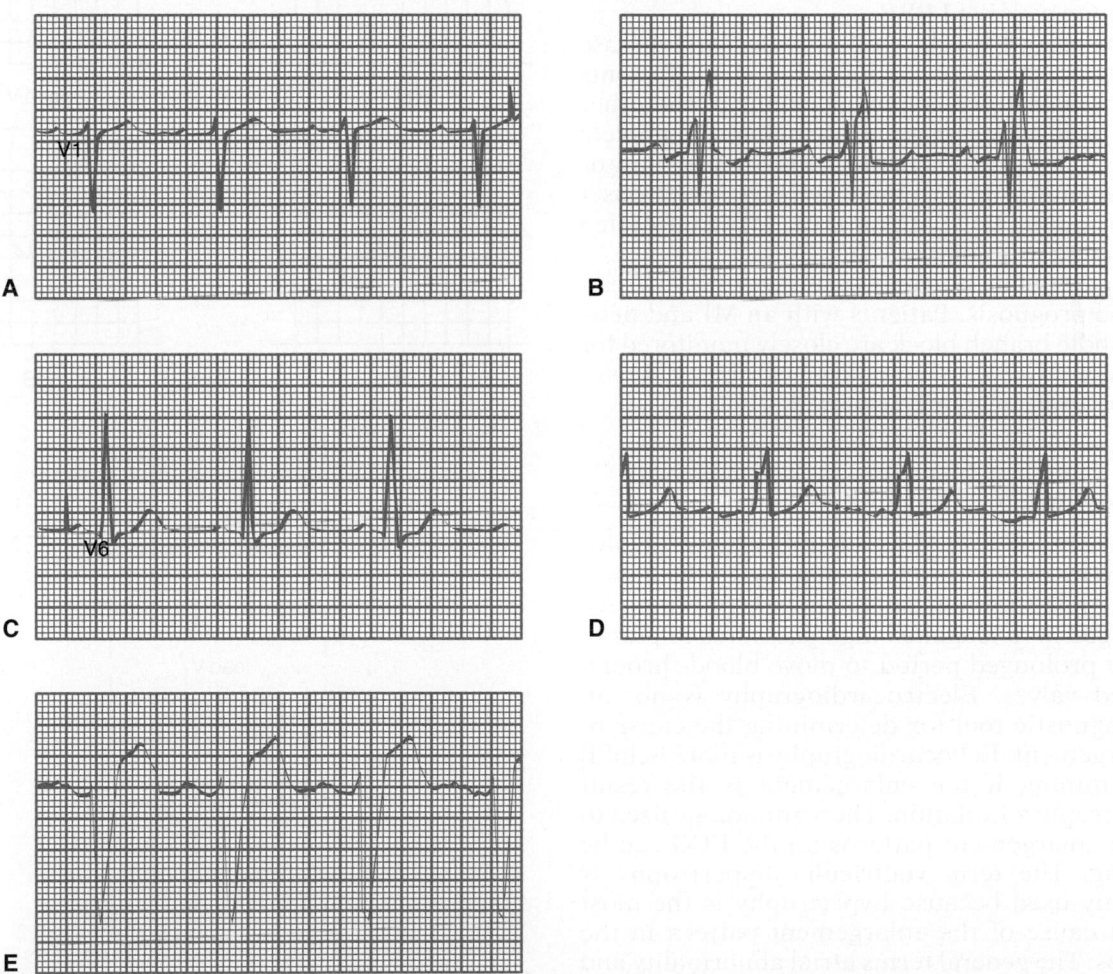

Figure 17-44 • Comparison of right versus left bundle branch block. **A:** A normal V_1 tracing. Note the small narrow R and deep narrow S wave. **B:** V_1 tracing showing the wide QRS complex and double-peaked R wave, indicating a right bundle branch block. **C:** A normal V_6 tracing. Note the tall narrow R wave and absent S wave. **D:** A V_6 tracing showing the wide QRS complex and double-peaked R wave, indicating a left bundle branch block. **E:** A V_1 tracing. Note the small narrow R and deep wide S wave, indicating a left bundle branch block.

peak of the QRS complex is taller than the second peak, the pattern is described as an RSr'. Whenever ventricular depolarization is abnormal, so is ventricular repolarization. As a result, ST-segment and T-wave abnormalities may be seen in leads V_1 and V_2 for patients with an RBBB.

An LBBB changes the QRS complex pattern in the left-sided chest leads, V_5 and V_6. Normally, these leads have a tall, single-peaked R wave and a small or absent S wave. Instead, the double-peaked RSR' pattern is noted. In addition, V_1 shows a small R wave with a widened S wave, indicating delayed conduction through the ventricles. Like RBBB, the ST segments and T waves may be abnormal in the left-sided chest leads V_5 and V_6 when the patient has an LBBB (see Fig. 17-44).

The most common causes of bundle branch block are MI, hypertension, heart failure, and cardiomyopathy. RBBB may be found in healthy people with no clinical evidence of heart disease. Congenital lesions involving the septum and right ventricular hypertrophy (RVH) are other causes of RBBB. LBBB is usually associated with some type of underlying heart disease. Long-term cardiovascular disease in the older patient is a common cause of LBBB.

Bundle branch block signifies underlying disease of the intraventricular conduction system. Patients should be monitored for involvement of the other bundles or fascicles or for progression to complete heart block. Progression of block may be very slow or rapid, depending on the clinical setting. A new-onset LBBB in conjunction with an acute MI is associated with a higher mortality rate.

The underlying heart disease determines treatment and prognosis. Patients with an MI and new-onset bundle branch block are closely monitored for progression to a type of complete heart block. A temporary pacemaker may be inserted.

ENLARGEMENT PATTERNS

Enlargement of a cardiac chamber may involve hypertrophy of the muscle or dilation of the chamber. The most common causes include pumping for a prolonged period against high pressures or pumping for a prolonged period to move blood through narrowed valves. Electrocardiography is not an ideal diagnostic tool for determining the cause of the enlargement. Echocardiography is more helpful in determining if the enlargement is the result of hypertrophy or dilation. The terminology used to describe enlargement patterns on the ECG can be confusing. The term ventricular hypertrophy is commonly used because hypertrophy is the most frequent cause of the enlargement pattern in the ventricles. The general terms atrial abnormality and atrial enlargement are often used rather than the specific terms atrial hypertrophy or atrial dilation because atrial changes on the ECG may result from a variety of causes, including atrial dilation, hypertrophy, or other conditions.

Right Atrial Enlargement

When the atria enlarge, changes are seen in the P wave because the P wave represents atrial depolarization. Right atrial enlargement is noted on the ECG by the presence of tall, pointed P waves in leads II, III, and aVF. The P wave in V_1 may show a diphasic wave with an initial upstroke that is larger than the downstroke (Fig. 17-45B).

The right atrium is more likely to enlarge as a result of pressures created by pulmonary causes, such as pulmonary hypertension and chronic obstructive pulmonary disease. For this reason, right atrial enlargement is often referred to as P pulmonale. Right atrial enlargement is often associated with RVH.

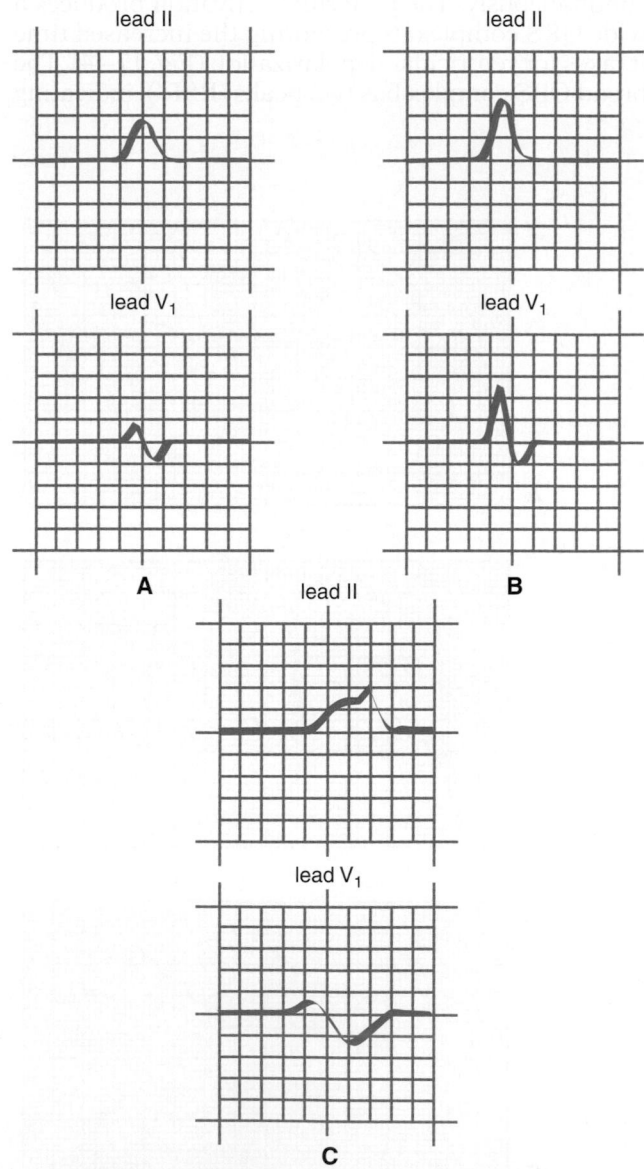

Figure 17-45 • Right versus left atrial enlargement. **A:** The normal P wave in leads II and V_1. **B:** Right atrial enlargement. Note the increased amplitude of the early, right atrial component of the P wave in V_1 and the tall, pointed P wave in lead II. **C:** Left atrial enlargement. Note the increased amplitude and duration of the P wave in V_1 and the broad, notched P wave in lead II.

Treatment is directed at the underlying cause. Often, however, the underlying cause may be a chronic condition that cannot be cured.

Left Atrial Enlargement

Left atrial enlargement is noted on the ECG by the presence of broad, notched P waves in leads I, II, and aVL. The P wave in V_1 may show a diphasic wave with a terminal downstroke that is larger than the initial upstroke (see Fig. 17-45C).

The left atrium is more likely to enlarge because of increased pressures created by trying to pump blood through a stenotic mitral valve. For this reason, left atrial enlargement is often referred to as P mitrale. When a left atrial enlargement pattern is noted on the ECG, the patient should be evaluated for the presence of mitral stenosis. An echocardiogram is a helpful diagnostic tool in addition to cardiac auscultation. Treatment is directed at the underlying cause. A valve replacement may be necessary.

Right Ventricular Hypertrophy

RVH may exist without clear evidence on the ECG because the left ventricle normally is larger than the right and can mask changes in the size of the right ventricle. ECG evidence suggestive of RVH includes right atrial enlargement and right axis deviation. In addition, the normal QRS complex pattern across the precordial leads is reversed. Normally, R waves are small in V_1 and gradually grow tall by V_6. With RVH, the R wave is tall in V_1 and progresses to small by V_6. Precordial S waves persist rather than gradually disappear.

The presence of RVH is most likely an indicator of a chronic pulmonary condition, most likely chronic obstructive pulmonary disease, pulmonary hypertension, or pulmonic stenosis. Right atrial enlargement is usually seen with an accompanying RVH. Treatment is directed at the underlying pulmonary disease.

Left Ventricular Hypertrophy

Numerous criteria exist for the detection of LVH on the ECG. The simplest criterion involves remembering the number "35." LVH is determined by adding the deepest S wave in either V_1 or V_2 to the tallest R wave in either V_5 or V_6. If the sum is 35 mm or more and the patient is older than 35 years of age, LVH is suspected. In addition, the T waves in V_5 and V_6 may be asymmetrically inverted, and a left axis shift is likely.

Usually, LVH is the result of chronic systemic hypertension, a chronic cardiovascular problem, or aortic stenosis. LVH may result in a displacement of the point of maximal impulse when palpating the apical pulse. Treatment of LVH is directed at the underlying condition.

ISCHEMIA, INJURY, AND INFARCTION PATTERNS

The 12-lead ECG can be very useful in detecting evidence of myocardial ischemia, injury, or infarction. Ischemia is seen on the ECG by ST-segment depressions and T-wave inversions. Acute patterns of injury are noted by ST-segment elevations. The presence of significant Q waves indicates an MI. For a more detailed discussion of patterns of ischemia, injury, and infarction, see Chapter 21.

Effects of Serum Electrolyte Abnormalities on the Electrocardiogram

Maintenance of adequate fluid and electrolyte balance assumes high priority in the care of patients in any medical, surgical, or coronary ICU. Patients being treated for renal or cardiovascular diseases are especially vulnerable to electrolyte imbalances. The cure may well be worse than the disease if electrolyte abnormalities go undetected or ignored because they frequently are caused by the treatment rather than by the disease itself.

Diuresis can very quickly cause major shifts in electrolytes. Certainly, the often insidious drop of serum potassium levels in the patient with cardiac disease who has been taking digitalis and then starts diuretics is well known. Diuretics also are used frequently as part of the medical regimen for the control of hypertension. Any addition, deletion, or change in diuretic therapy warrants close monitoring of serum electrolytes. A history of any of these problems should

alert the nurse to check the patient's serum electrolytes on an ongoing basis.

Potassium and calcium are probably the two most important electrolytes involved in the proper function of the heart. Because of their effects on the electrical impulse in the heart, an excess or insufficiency of either electrolyte frequently causes changes in the ECG (Table 17-15). The nurse who is aware of and able to recognize these changes may well suspect electrolyte abnormalities before laboratory findings or clinical symptoms appear and hazardous dysrhythmias occur.

However, it is necessary to remember that just as a patient who sustains MI may not have chest pain, the patient with electrolyte abnormalities may not exhibit any of the ECG changes described in the following sections. The ECG manifestations are valuable primarily in arousing suspicion of electrolyte abnormalities. Not one of them even approaches being diagnostic.

Table 17-15 • Electrocardiographic Changes Associated With Electrolyte Imbalances

Hyperkalemia	Tall, narrow, peaked T waves; flat, wide P waves; widening QRS complex	Sinus bradycardia; sinoatrial block; junctional rhythm; idioventricular rhythm; ventricular tachycardia; ventricular fibrillation
Hypokalemia	Prominent U waves; ST segment depression; T-wave flattening or inversion	Premature ventricular beats; supraventricular tachycardia; ventricular tachycardia; ventricular fibrillation
Hypercalcemia	Shortened QT interval	Premature ventricular contractions
Hypocalcemia	Lengthened QT interval; T-wave flattening or inversion	Ventricular tachycardia

• Potassium

Potassium is the primary intracellular cation found in the body. Inside the cardiac cell, potassium is important for repolarization and for maintaining a stable, polarized state.

HYPERKALEMIA

The earliest sign of hyperkalemia on the ECG is a change in the T wave. It usually is described as tall, narrow, and "peaked" or "tented" in appearance (Fig. 17-46). As the serum potassium level increases, the P-wave amplitude decreases and the PR interval is prolonged. Atrial asystole occurs, along with a widening of the QRS complex. At high,

near-lethal potassium levels, the widened QRS complex merges with the T wave and starts to resemble a sine wave. Various dysrhythmias may occur during this time, with progression to VF and asystole. Clinically, the described changes in T waves begin to appear at serum levels of 6 to 7 mEq/L, and QRS complex widening is seen at serum levels of 8 to 9 mEq/L. Vigorous treatment must be instituted to reverse the condition at this point because sudden death may occur at any time after these levels are reached.

The ECG changes in hyperkalemia also may be associated with other conditions. Tall, peaked T waves may be a normal finding or may occur in the early stages of MI. QRS complex widening may be seen with quinidine and procainamide toxicity.

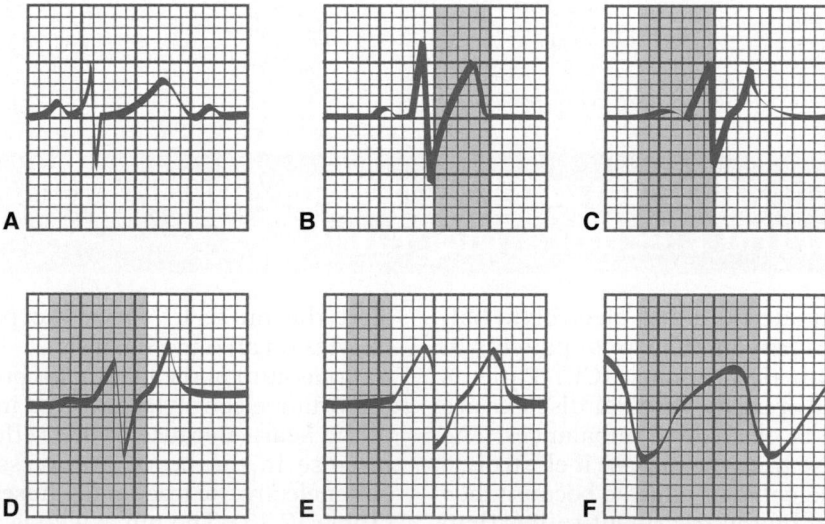

Figure 17-46 • The effect of hyperkalemia on an electrocardiogram. **A:** This waveform is produced when the serum potassium level falls within the normal range—usually considered to be 3.5 to 5 mEq/L. **B:** When the serum potassium level rises above 5.5 mEq/L, the T wave begins to peak (see highlighted area). The P wave and QRS complex are normal. **C:** When the potassium level exceeds 6.5 mEq/L, the P wave grows wider, and its amplitude falls. The QRS complex also widens (see highlighted area) as intraventricular conduction velocity diminishes. **D:** When the potassium level reaches 10 mEq/L, the P wave becomes almost indiscernible; the QRS complex is slurred and widened (see highlighted area). **E:** When the potassium level ranges from 10 to 12 mEq/L, the P wave is undetectable (see highlighted area) because the atria are no longer excitable. **F:** When the potassium level exceeds 12 mEq/L, the QRS complex is no longer identifiable. The waves are known as sine waves (see highlighted area). Ventricular fibrillation and cardiac arrest follow. (From Springhouse: ECG Interpretation: Clinical Skillbuilders. Springhouse, PA: Author, 1990, p 113.)

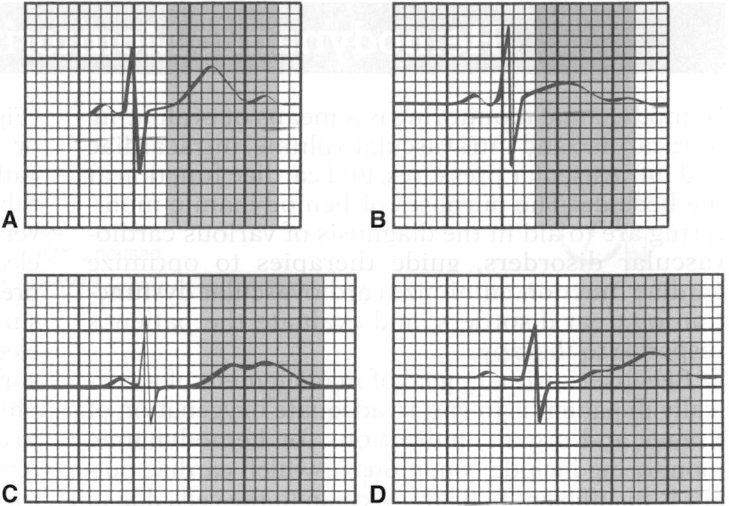

Figure 17-47 • The effect of hypokalemia on an electrocardiogram. **A:** When the potassium level is normal—usually considered to be 3.5 to 5 mEq/L—the T wave is much higher than the U wave (see highlighted area). **B:** When the potassium level falls to 3 mEq/L, the T wave and U wave are almost the same height (see highlighted area). **C:** When the potassium level falls to 2 mEq/L, the U wave starts rising above the T wave (see highlighted area). **D:** As the potassium level reaches 1 mEq/L, the U wave starts to resemble a T wave (see highlighted area). The duration of the QT interval remains the same, but it cannot be measured because the two waves are fusing. (From Springhouse: ECG Interpretation: Clinical Skillbuilders. Springhouse, PA: Author, 1990, p 114.)

HYPOKALEMIA

Hypokalemia is associated with the appearance of U waves. Although the presence of U waves may be normal in many people, these waves also may be an early sign of hypokalemia (Fig. 17-47). Usually easily recognized (best seen in lead V_3), a U wave may encroach on the preceding T wave and go unnoticed. The T wave may look notched or prolonged when it is hiding the U wave, giving the appearance of a prolonged QT interval. With increased potassium depletion, the U wave may become more prominent as the T wave becomes less so. The T wave becomes flattened and may even invert. The ST segment tends to become depressed, somewhat resembling the effects of digitalis on the ECG. Only at very low serum levels is there reasonable correlation between ECG changes and serum potassium concentrations.

The changes seen in hypokalemia also are observed in other conditions. The U wave may be accentuated in association with digitalis, LVH, and bradycardia.

Untreated hypokalemia enhances instability in the myocardial cell. Ventricular premature beats are the most common manifestation of this imbalance, but supraventricular dysrhythmias, conduction problems, and eventually VT and VF may occur. Hypokalemia also increases the sensitivity of the heart to digitalis and its accompanying dysrhythmias, even at normal serum levels. The severity of the dysrhythmias associated with hypokalemia requires early recognition of this problem.

• Calcium

Like potassium, calcium is important in normal cardiac function. It is essential for the initiation and propagation of electrical impulses and for myocardial contractility. Abnormal calcium levels are not commonly seen unless they are associated with an underlying disease, and therefore they are not as common as serum potassium abnormalities.

HYPERCALCEMIA

On an ECG, the major finding associated with hypercalcemia is shortening of the QT interval (Fig. 17-48). Because the QRS complex and T wave usually are unaffected by changes in serum calcium levels, the shortened QT interval is a result of shortening of the ST segment. QT-interval shortening also is seen in patients taking digitalis. In addition, ST-segment depression occasionally occurs, and T-wave inversion may be seen.

HYPOCALCEMIA

On an ECG, low serum calcium levels prolong the QT interval because of a lengthening of the ST segment (see Fig. 17-48). The T wave itself is not prolonged but may be inverted in some cases. The prolongation of the QT interval in hypocalcemia should not be mistaken for a prolonged QTU interval seen in hypokalemia. In patients with chronic renal failure, hypocalcemia may be associated with decreased potassium levels.

QT interval prolongation also may be seen in cerebral vascular disease and after cardiac arrest. Several antiarrhythmic agents produce prolonged QT intervals and always should be considered when evaluating an ECG for hypocalcemic changes.

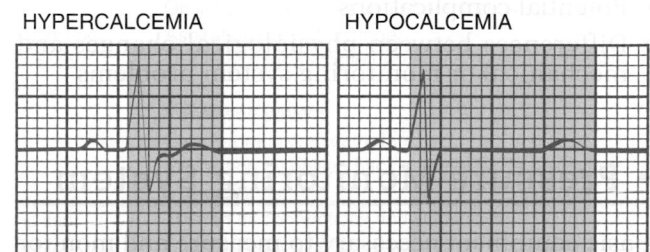

Figure 17-48 • The effects of hypercalcemia and hypocalcemia on an electrocardiogram. Changes in serum calcium levels are reflected in phase 2 of the action potential. Hypercalcemia shortens the QT interval, whereas hypocalcemia lengthens it (see highlighted areas). (From Springhouse: ECG Interpretation: Clinical Skillbuilders. Springhouse, PA: Author, 1990, p 115.)

Table 17-16 • Troubleshooting Pressure Monitoring Systems and Measurements (Continued)

Problem	Cause	Prevention	Intervention
3. Underdamped waveforms; whip or ringing	Excessive movement of catheter Air bubbles in tubing	Correct catheter placement. Use appropriate catheter size for vessel. Eliminate excessive length of pressure tubing. Check for very rigid pressure tubing.	Try different catheter tip position. Eliminate excessive tubing. Change tubing. Eliminate excessive stopcocks.
4. False low readings	Leveling or zero reference (transducer) is too high	Check level periodically. Level air–fluid interface of stopcock nearest the transducer to the phlebostatic axis.	Re-level transducer air–fluid interface to phlebostatic axis.
	Improper zeroing	Check monitor settings. Observe waveforms.	Re-zero monitor.
	Overdamped waveforms	Perform square-wave test.	Optimize length of pressure tubing.
5. False high readings	Leveling or zero reference (transducer) is too low	Check level periodically. Level air–fluid interface of stopcock nearest the transducer to the phlebostatic axis.	Re-level transducer air–fluid interface to phlebostatic axis.
	Improper zeroing	Check monitor settings. Observe waveforms.	Re-zero monitor.
	Overdamped waveforms	Perform square-wave test.	Remove excessive length of pressure tubing.
6. Inappropriate pressure waveform	Incorrect catheter position		Reposition patient. Obtain chest x-ray. Reposition catheter.*
	Migration of pulmonary artery catheter into mechanical wedge position	Establish optimal position carefully during the insertion process, ensuring use of 1.25 to 1.5 mL air for proper balloon inflation volume for obtaining a PAWP tracing.	Observe waveforms and confirm with initial insertion tracings. If right ventricular tracing is observed from PAC distal tip, slowly inflate balloon to allow PAC to "float" into pulmonary artery. If PAWP tracing is observed with balloon deflated, withdraw catheter slightly while observing waveforms. Stop withdrawing as soon as a pulmonary artery tracing is observed.
7. Bleed back into pressure tubing or transducer	Loose connections Stopcocks not returned to proper position Pressure bag not at 300 mm Hg	Ensure all connections are tight. Return stopcocks to proper positions. Maintain 300 mm Hg of pressure.	Tighten connections. Ensure stopcocks are in correct position Check pressure device.

*Repositioning the PAC usually is done by a physician or advanced practice nurse such as a nurse practitioner and varies with hospital policies.
PAC, pulmonary artery catheter; PAWP, pulmonary artery wedge pressure.

dynamic response of the system. In addition, the nurse ensures proper leveling of the air–fluid interface and zeroing of the transducer to optimize the system.

Square-Wave Test: Dynamic Response Testing

For a rapid bedside assessment of the dynamic response of the system, a simple evaluation of dynamic response can be obtained by performing a square-wave test and observing the resultant oscillations. Checking the dynamic response of the system determines the natural frequency and damping coefficient. Factors affecting the response of the system include the natural frequency of the system itself, the pressure tubing quality, number of stopcocks, and other components such as blood sampling systems. The steps required to measure the natural frequency and damping coefficient accurately are complex and time

consuming. Other references describe the steps for performing this process.

To perform a square-wave test, a flush device that can be activated and released rapidly is required. Activating the flush device opens the internal restrictor and increases the fluid flow through the system. The nurse observes the bedside monitor for the increase in pressure. The waveform sharply rises and "squares off" at the top of the scale. After the flush device is released, the restrictor closes. The nurse observes the waveform as it returns to baseline, counts the number of oscillations, and observes the distance between them.

In an ideal system, also called optimally damped, the square wave has a straight vertical upstroke from the baseline, a straight horizontal component, and more importantly, a straight vertical downstroke back to the baseline with approximately one and one-half to two sharp oscillations. The distance between the

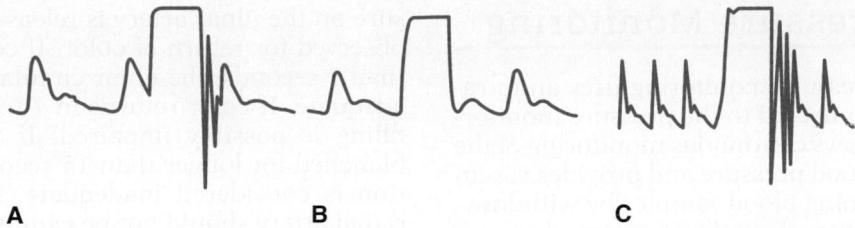

A   **B**   **C**

Figure 17-50 • Steps to perform a square wave test include:
1. Activate the snap or pull tab of the flush device.
2. Observe the square wave generated on the bedside monitor.
3. Count the oscillations after the square wave.
4. Observe the distance between the oscillations.
    A. Optimally damped system: Activation of the fast flush device generates a sharp vertical upstroke, horizontal line, and straight vertical downstroke ending with 1.5 to 2 oscillations close together before returning to baseline.
    B. Overdamped system: Activation of the fast flush device generates a slurred upstroke and downstroke with less than 1.5 oscillations above or below the baseline. Causes include system leaks, blood clots, or large air bubbles in the tubing or transducer. Systolic pressures read erroneously low, diastolic pressures occasionally read low.
    C. Underdamped system: Activation of the fast flush device generates more than 2 to 3 oscillations above and below the baseline. Causes include small air bubbles in the system, very rigid pressure tubing, and additional length of tubing. Systolic pressures read erroneously high, diastolic pressures read erroneously low.
(Courtesy of Edwards Lifesciences LLC.)

oscillations is also close.[1,2] Figure 17-50 depicts a normal square wave and examples of square waves from nonoptimized hemodynamic monitoring systems. Overdamped systems produce lower than actual systolic pressures and potentially loss of dicrotic notch identification. Underdamped systems produce artificially high systolic pressures and low diastolic pressures. By performing a square-wave test, the bedside clinician can quickly assess if the abnormal waveform tracing is a result of the patient's physiology or a less-than-optimal system.[3,4]

Leveling and Zeroing

After a square-wave test is performed, the system is leveled to an external landmark and then zeroed to atmospheric pressure to ensure accurate pressure monitoring. Typically, the stopcock nearest the transducer is used as the air–fluid interface for leveling and zeroing; however, any stopcock port in the system can be used as long as it is leveled to the phlebostatic axis. The phlebostatic axis is best described as the bisection of the fourth intercostal space and the midpoint of the anterior-posterior chest diameter (see Fig. 17-49); it is often called the zero reference point. Zeroing the transducer is the action of opening the pressure system to atmospheric air and observing a reading of zero on the bedside monitor. With the stopcock turned off to the patient and opened to air, the influence of hydrostatic pressure is negated from the fluid-filled pressure system. Subsequent pressures recorded on the monitor now reflect those generated by the patient, not external forces. Bedside monitor manufacturers vary; however, most have a function key to ensure that the zeroing process has been successful. Newer disposable transducers come from the manufacturer precalibrated and do not require adjustment to an electronic zero. The term zeroing is used, however, when referencing to atmospheric pressure.

Once the zero reference point is established, the patient's chest is marked to ensure consistent leveling when other practitioners obtain subsequent pressure readings. With the patient placed in the supine position, a carpenter-type level or laser-light level device is used to align the air–fluid interface with the phlebostatic axis. Further pressure measurements are taken with the patient in the supine position.

If the alignment of the air–fluid interface changes after initial leveling and zeroing, an inversely related error of approximately 2 mm Hg for every inch misaligned occurs. For example, if the transducer air–fluid interface is raised from initial leveling, the values displayed will be about 2 mm Hg too low, and if lowered from initial leveling, the values recorded will be erroneously too high.

The head of the bed may be elevated as much as 60 degrees, provided that the air–fluid interface is re-leveled after any changes in patient position. Lateral or side-lying positions may be used if the external landmark is properly identified. Because some patients respond differently to head of bed elevation and side-lying positions, their hemodynamic values should be compared from supine.[3,4]

After the level and zero is verified, the only way to determine whether the pressures displayed on the monitor are accurate is to apply a known value to the transducer. Steps to accomplish this involve attaching a piece of sterile 12-inch extension tubing to the stopcock port on the transducer, turning the stopcock to fill the tubing with flush solution, and holding the tubing straight up so as to apply a column of water on the transducer. The 12-inch column of water height displays 22 mm Hg on the bedside monitor (±2 mm Hg) if the transducer is accurate. Some transducer manufacturers provide a device that applies a known pressure to the transducer for rapid determination of accurate pressure recordings.

• Arterial Pressure Monitoring

Invasive arterial pressure monitoring uses an intra-arterial catheter connected to the pressure monitoring system. This allows continuous monitoring of the systemic arterial blood pressure and provides vascular access for obtaining blood samples by withdrawing blood from a stopcock or closed system device in the system. Indications for intra-arterial blood pressure monitoring include monitoring patients with vasoactive IV infusions; cardiovascular instability; and fluctuating, unstable blood pressures.

ARTERIAL LINE INSERTION

The most common sites for arterial catheter insertions are the radial, brachial, and femoral arteries. Alternative and less frequent sites include the axillary and dorsalis pedis arteries in adults and the temporal and umbilical arteries in neonates. The following factors are considered for selecting the artery for cannulation:

▶ Size of the artery in relation to the size of the catheter; the artery should be large enough to accommodate the catheter without occluding or significantly impeding flow.

▶ Accessibility of the site; the chosen site should be easily accessible and free from contamination by body secretions.

▶ Blood flow to the limb distal to the insertion site; there should be adequate collateral flow in the event that the cannulated artery becomes occluded.

The radial artery, which satisfies these criteria, is the most frequent site for an arterial catheter. It is superficially located and therefore easy to palpate. Cannulation of this artery also usually poses the least limitation on the patient's mobility.

Before a catheter is inserted into the radial artery, the presence of adequate collateral circulation to the hand by the ulnar artery is assessed by performing Allen's test (Fig. 17-51). Both the ulnar and radial arteries are occluded. The patient then clenches and unclenches the fist until the hand is blanched. Pressure on the ulnar artery is released, and the hand is observed for return of color. If color returns in less than 7 seconds, the ulnar circulation to the hand is adequate. If color returns in 7 to 15 seconds, ulnar filling is possibly impaired. If the hand remains blanched for longer than 15 seconds, ulnar circulation is considered inadequate, in which case the radial artery should not be cannulated. Use of ultrasound devices for assessing blood flow in place of the Allen's test is becoming more common.

Regardless of the site chosen for arterial catheter placement, the insertion is performed using sterile technique. The pressure monitoring system is assembled and flushed, and the transducer is leveled and zeroed before the catheter is inserted. Once the catheter is in place, it should be secured and the site dressed according to institutional policy.

ARTERIAL PRESSURE WAVEFORM

The normal arterial waveform should have a rapid upstroke, a clear dicrotic notch, and a definite end-diastole, as shown in Figure 17-52. The mechanical activity of systole and diastole follows the electrical activity of depolarization and repolarization, respectively. The initial sharp upstroke of the waveform results partly from the rapid ejection of blood from the left ventricle into the aorta. On a dual-channel tracing of both the ECG and arterial waveforms, the QRS complex precedes the rapid rise in arterial pressure. The dicrotic notch reflects a slight backflow of blood in the aorta, reflecting closure of the aortic valve or may be a reflective wave from the periphery.

OBTAINING ARTERIAL PRESSURES

The value measured at the peak of the waveform is the systolic pressure. A normal arterial systolic pressure is typically 90 to 140 mm Hg. The dicrotic notch typically indicates the end of ventricular systole and the beginning of diastole. As blood flows to the periphery, the pressure in the arterial system decreases. The lowest point of the waveform is the diastolic pressure, which is normally between 60 and 90 mm Hg.

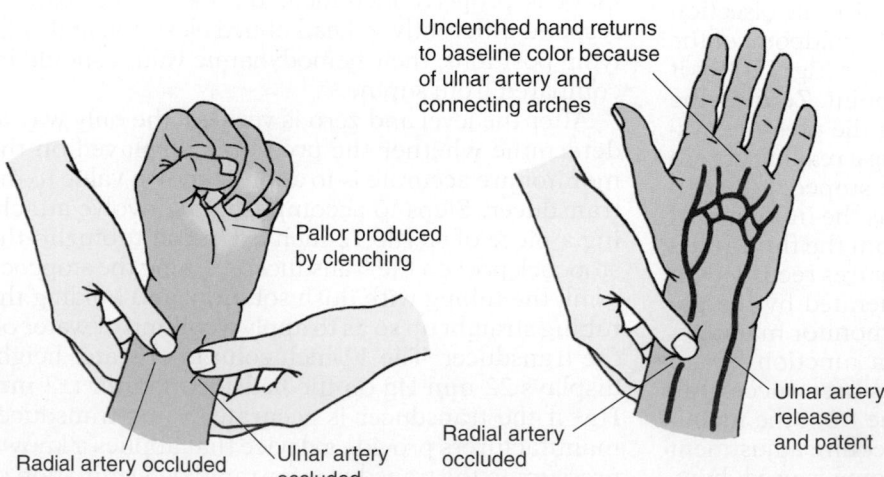

Unclenched hand returns to baseline color because of ulnar artery and connecting arches

Pallor produced by clenching

Radial artery occluded

Ulnar artery occluded

Radial artery occluded

Ulnar artery released and patent

Figure 17-51 • Modified Allen's test.

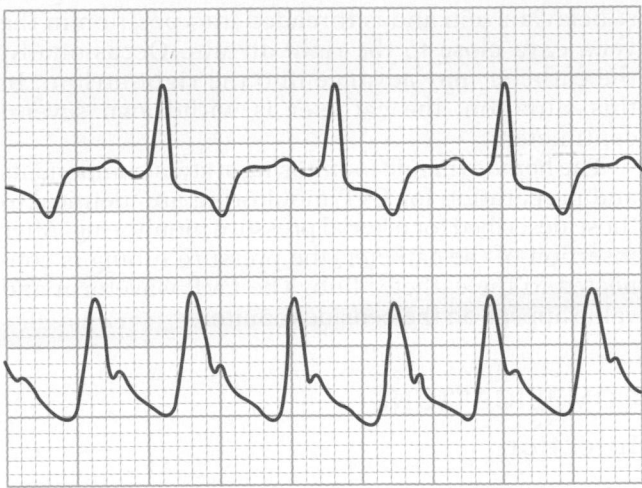

Figure 17-52 • Normal relationship of electrocardiogram and arterial pressure waveform.

Mean arterial pressure (MAP) is used to evaluate perfusion of vital body organs. Normal MAP is 70 to 105 mm Hg. The MAP calculation incorporates the impact of diastolic time being approximately 2 times longer than systole during a cardiac cycle. Therefore, MAP = diastolic pressure + ⅓ pulse pressure, or

$$\frac{Systolic\ pressure + \left(Diastolic\ pressure \times 2\right)}{3}$$

Most bedside monitors automatically calculate and continuously display the MAP. Algorithms to determine MAP may vary from manufacturer to manufacturer; however, most incorporate assessment of the area under the full arterial waveform rather than a mathematical model.

The difference between the systolic and diastolic pressure is the pulse pressure. This value more closely reflects the stroke volume from the ventricle. Stroke volume is proportional to pulse pressure and inversely related to the aortic compliance. Bedside monitors do not automatically display this valuable parameter. Clinicians who want to assess the patient's volume status should include pulse pressure in their assessment because it is an indirect reflection of the stroke volume. The range of pulse pressure may be as wide as 30 to 100 mm Hg at the far ends of the spectrum. A wide pulse pressure occurs typically with elevated systolic pressures resulting from aortic regurgitation and some vascular conditions. A narrow pulse pressure may result from hypovolemic states when the diastolic pressure rises.[4]

COMPLICATIONS

Infection

Proper attention to sterile technique during catheter insertion; care of the insertion site; blood sampling; and maintenance of a sterile, closed monitoring system reduce the risk for infection. The following should be performed according to institution policy: assessment of insertion site for signs of infection; use of sterile technique when changing dressings, tubing, and flush solution; and maintenance of the integrity of the system. Opening the pressure system to air for either zeroing or blood sampling provides opportunity for infection. Applying sterile nonvented or "dead-ender" caps to the stopcock ports helps eliminate contamination. Closed systems for blood sampling help reduce the potential for open stopcock infections and assist with managing potential blood loss.

Accidental Blood Loss

Accidental blood loss from an arterial catheter can be catastrophic and often can be prevented. All connections in the system should use a Luer-Lok–type connector. The extremity in which the catheter is placed may be immobilized (e.g., placing the wrist on an arm board). If some type of patient self-protective device is used, it should not be placed over the insertion site. Easy access to the insertion site and connections is imperative.

Impaired Circulation to Extremity

Circulation to the extremity in which the arterial line is placed must be monitored frequently. Initial assessment of color, sensation, temperature, and movement of the extremity is made after insertion of the arterial catheter and as frequently as the institution policy states. Any indication of impaired circulation may be an indication for catheter removal and is reported immediately.

NURSING CONSIDERATIONS

Blood pressures obtained by an intra-arterial catheter and with an optimal pressure monitoring system are most accurate. Values are very similar in normotensive patients, with the intra-arterial pressures higher by about 5 to 10 mm Hg than the pressures obtained using a cuff. Indirect methods tend to overestimate direct measurements in hypotensive patients and underestimate them in hypertensive patients. Variations as wide as 20 to 60 mm Hg occur, depending on specific patient conditions.

Comparisons between intra-arterial and cuff pressures may be misleading because the methods of measurement reflect different physiological events and are therefore not truly comparable.[4] Direct or invasive monitoring measures pressure, and indirect cuff measurements are based on flow. For interventions when accurate values are important for therapeutic decisions, intra-arterial pressures remain the gold standard. Using a trend value from one source is often more helpful than comparing values obtained between different technologies. Documenting the site of pressure measurements and what type of technique used is key.

Patient safety measures include the proper setting and activation of all alarms on the bedside physiological monitor. Bedside monitor alarms provide warning that a change has occurred either in the system or in the patient's physiological status. Alarms are set either around a patient's specific parameter or according to institution policy. Typically, high and low alarms are set for systolic, diastolic, and mean pressures and within 10 to 20 mm Hg of the patient's blood pressure. The alarms must be visible and audible to the caregiver for the specific patient environment. Troubleshooting steps for an alarm are listed in Table 17-16.

General steps to ensure accurate pressures from invasive lines include assessing the patient first, then checking the pressure monitoring system, and then inspecting the monitor itself. Assess the insertion site: Is the catheter kinked? Are there any blood clots? Is there any sign of bleeding? Next, evaluate the pressure system: Are any stopcocks turned the wrong way? Is there sufficient pressure in the pressure bag (i.e., does the pressure read 300 mm Hg)? Are there any air bubbles? Is the bedside monitor functioning properly? Are the alarms set correctly?

If catheter patency is in question, blood and fluid are aspirated from the blood-drawing port or stopcock in an attempt to remove a blood clot (if present), and then the system is flushed using the fast flush device. The system should not be flushed with a syringe. No additional IV solution or medication should be administered through the arterial pressure monitoring system at any time.

• Central Venous Pressure Monitoring

Central venous pressure (CVP) is typically measured in the superior vena cava near the right atrium via a catheter placed in the jugular or subclavian vein. It therefore reflects the pressure of blood in the right atrium and provides information about intravascular blood volume, right ventricular end-diastolic pressure (RVEDP), and right ventricular function. To a limited degree in persons with normal pulmonary vasculature and left ventricular function, the CVP indirectly reflects left ventricular end-diastolic pressure (LVEDP) and function because the left and right sides of the heart are linked by the pulmonary vascular bed. Alterations in intravascular volume status or ventricular function usually are associated with abnormally high or low CVP measurements.

CATHETER INSERTION

The CVP catheter is long and flexible. It is inserted under sterile conditions with a chlorhexidine site preparation. The physician uses a sterile field with a full sterile drape, sterile gloves and gown, and a mask and cap. Those assisting the physician also should wear a cap and mask and sterile gloves if near the catheter or insertion site. The catheter is inserted into an antecubital, jugular, femoral, or subclavian vein and is threaded into position in the vena cava close to the right atrium. Occasionally, the catheter may advance into the right atrium. In this situation, the catheter is withdrawn several centimeters.

The hemodynamic monitoring system components and preparation for CVP monitoring are identical to those described for arterial pressure monitoring. After insertion of the catheter, the pressure tubing is connected to the catheter hub. The CVP waveform and value appear on the bedside monitor.

COMPLICATIONS
Infection

Infection may occur within the catheter or around the insertion site. Central venous catheter–associated bloodstream infection is diagnosed and verified by blood cultures. Occasionally after catheter removal, the tip is cut off with sterile scissors and sent to the microbiology laboratory. Signs and symptoms of infection include erythema at the insertion site, fever, or elevated white blood cell count. Primary measures to prevent infection include routine dressing and IV fluid tubing changes, as outlined by the Centers for Disease Control and Prevention and hospital policy, as well as adherence to sterile technique during catheter insertion and dressing changes. When catheters are left in place for an extended period of time, antibiotic-impregnated catheters may be used to reduce the risk for infection.

Thrombosis

Thromboses occasionally form and may vary in size from a thin fibrin sheath over the catheter tip to a large thrombus. A small thrombus may be flushed away without causing harm, but a larger thrombus occluding the catheter and vein should not be flushed into the venous circulation. A large thrombus may be detected by loss of hemodynamic waveform and inability to infuse fluid or withdraw blood from the catheter. The patient may have edema of the arm closest to the catheter site, varying degrees of neck pain (which may radiate), and jugular vein distention. A large thrombus is classified as an emergency because it may impair circulation to a limb. A nurse may attempt to aspirate this clot if hospital policy permits. Frequently, hospitals also have protocols to administer small doses of thrombolytic agents to dissolve the clot. At the very least, the nurse is responsible for reporting suspected catheter occlusion to a physician.

Air Embolism

Air embolism occurs as a result of air entering the system and traveling through the vena cava to the right ventricle. Usually, air entry into the catheter is associated with disconnection of the catheter from the IV tubing. Changes in intrathoracic pressure with inspiration and expiration draw air into the catheter and vena cava. Sudden hypotension may be the first indicator of this sometimes lethal problem.

Approximately 10 to 20 mL of air must enter the venous system before the patient becomes symptomatic. Signs of such an emergency may include confusion, lightheadedness, anxiety, and unresponsiveness. The physiological event is the creation of foam in the ventricle with each heart contraction and loss of stroke volume due to air instead of blood in the ventricle, causing a sudden decrease in cardiac output. Cardiac arrest may occur.

If this problem is suspected, turning the patient on the left side in the Trendelenburg position may allow the air to rise to the wall of the right ventricle and improve blood flow. Oxygen should be started unless contraindicated.

Strategies to prevent disconnections include having Luer-Lok connections on all central line catheters and tubings, careful manipulation of catheter and tubing during dressing changes, and routine monitoring of the connections. There is no substitute for close observation by skilled and educated nursing staff.

NURSING CONSIDERATIONS

Ensuring the integrity of the monitoring system, obtaining and documenting accurate data, and monitoring trends in CVP data are critical to the interpretation and utilization of information to assess a patient's cardiovascular function and response to interventions.

Normal CVP is less than 8 mm Hg. Low CVP indicates a hypovolemic state often requiring fluid administration. The anticipated response to fluid therapy is an increase in the CVP. Similarly, diuretic therapy reduces intravascular volume, and its administration is expected to be associated with a decrease in the CVP. Vasodilation from sepsis or vasodilating drugs may also lead to a low or decreasing CVP; both create a relative hypovolemia because blood volume has not changed. Rather, the intravascular space has become greater relative to the patient's blood volume.

Increased CVP may be caused by a number of complex and interrelated factors, each of which requires scrutiny. Two of the more common causes of increased CVP are right ventricular failure and mechanical ventilation. Rarely is intravascular volume overload and hypervolemia alone a cause of increased CVP.

Mechanical ventilation increases intrathoracic pressure, which is transmitted to the pulmonary vasculature, heart, and great vessels. This pressure may directly affect CVP, which may increase as well, because intrathoracic pressure compresses the pulmonary vessels, creating resistance to blood flow from the right side to the left side of the heart and causing blood to "back up" in the right ventricle, right atrium, and vena cava. In extreme cases, the increased intrathoracic pressure associated with mechanical ventilation causes significant right ventricular dysfunction, and the CVP is elevated because of reduced forward blood flow into the pulmonary vasculature, resulting in increased volume and pressure of the blood in the right atrium and vena cava.

Increased CVP is associated with right ventricular failure due to coronary artery disease or left ventricular failure. The inability of the right ventricle to pump blood through the pulmonary vasculature because of injured or infarcted myocardium results in increased volume and pressure in the right atrium and vena cava. Left ventricular failure may increase CVP as the pressure of blood volume congests the pulmonary vasculature and impairs flow from the right ventricle, causing right ventricular dilation and subsequent failure. Again, the increased pressure is reflected backward to the right atrium and vena cava. In these instances, interventions are directed toward facilitating forward blood flow by improving ventricular contractility and reducing the intravascular blood volume. A decrease in the CVP is an indication of the effectiveness of therapy.

CVP is always interpreted in conjunction with other clinical observations, such as auscultation of breath sounds, heart and respiratory rate, ECG, neck vein distention, and urine output. For example, increased CVP associated with pulmonary basilar crackles and decreased urine output is often indicative of left ventricular failure. Distended neck veins but clear breath sounds and a high CVP might be caused by increased intrathoracic pressure from mechanical ventilator effects. Patients who are septic may have a low CVP that is associated with fever, elevated white blood cell count, tachycardia, and tachypnea, whereas patients who are taking vasodilating agents may have a low CVP that is associated with an increased heart rate but none of the other aforementioned clinical signs. A CVP value alone is meaningless, but when used in conjunction with other clinical data, it is a valuable aid in managing and predicting the patient's clinical course.

• Pulmonary Artery Pressure Monitoring

The PAC has made possible the assessment of right ventricular function, pulmonary vascular status, and, indirectly, left ventricular function. Right atrial, right ventricular, and PA pressures, as well as pulmonary artery wedge pressure (PAWP), are measured using a PAC. PACs with a thermistor have the capability of determining cardiac output. The pressures and cardiac output obtained allow the clinician to calculate derived parameters and facilitate diagnosis of cardiovascular and cardiopulmonary dysfunction, determine the therapy needed, and evaluate the effectiveness of the interventions.

PULMONARY ARTERY CATHETERS

Several types of flow-directed, balloon-tipped PACs are available in different sizes. The type of catheter used is determined by the parameters to be monitored and additional requirements governed by the patient's condition. The 7.5- or 8-French (F; a measure of catheter size) thermodilution catheter is the size most commonly used (Fig. 17-53). All PACs have several external ports or lumen hubs corresponding to internal lumens and lumen openings into the right side of the heart and PA. A typical PAC has four lumens with external hubs or ports: the proximal hub and lumen, distal hub and lumen, balloon inflation valve and lumen, and thermistor connector and lumen.

The proximal or right atrial lumen opens into the right atrium; in smaller patients, the location might be in the superior or inferior vena cava, depending on insertion location. The lumen is used for infusion of fluids and is often connected to a transducer to provide right atrial pressure measurements and display of the right atrial pressure waveform. The right atrial lumen port also is used as the injectate port for measuring cardiac outputs.

The distal or PA lumen hub is always attached to a transducer and a continuous flush system. The PA waveform is displayed continuously, as are the PA systolic, diastolic, and mean pressures. The PA port is used for the withdrawal of mixed venous blood, which is necessary for venous oxygen saturation, oxygen extraction, oxygen consumption, and intrapulmonary shunt measurements. Use of the PA distal port for fluid or medication administration is not recommended.

The balloon inflation port and lumen enable inflation of the balloon near the catheter tip with a small volume of air to measure the PA occlusion pressure, known as the PAWP. The balloon capacity of most PACs is 1.5 mL, and the balloon should not be inflated with more than this amount of air. Fluid is never inserted into the balloon inflation port.

The tip of the PAC also contains a thermistor. A cable to the bedside monitor or to a cardiac output computer connects to the external thermistor port. The thermistor permits measurement of the patient's temperature in the PA (core temperature), and it detects the blood temperature change when solution is injected through the right atrial port to obtain a cardiac output.

Specialty PACs include the previously described components and additional features and lumens.

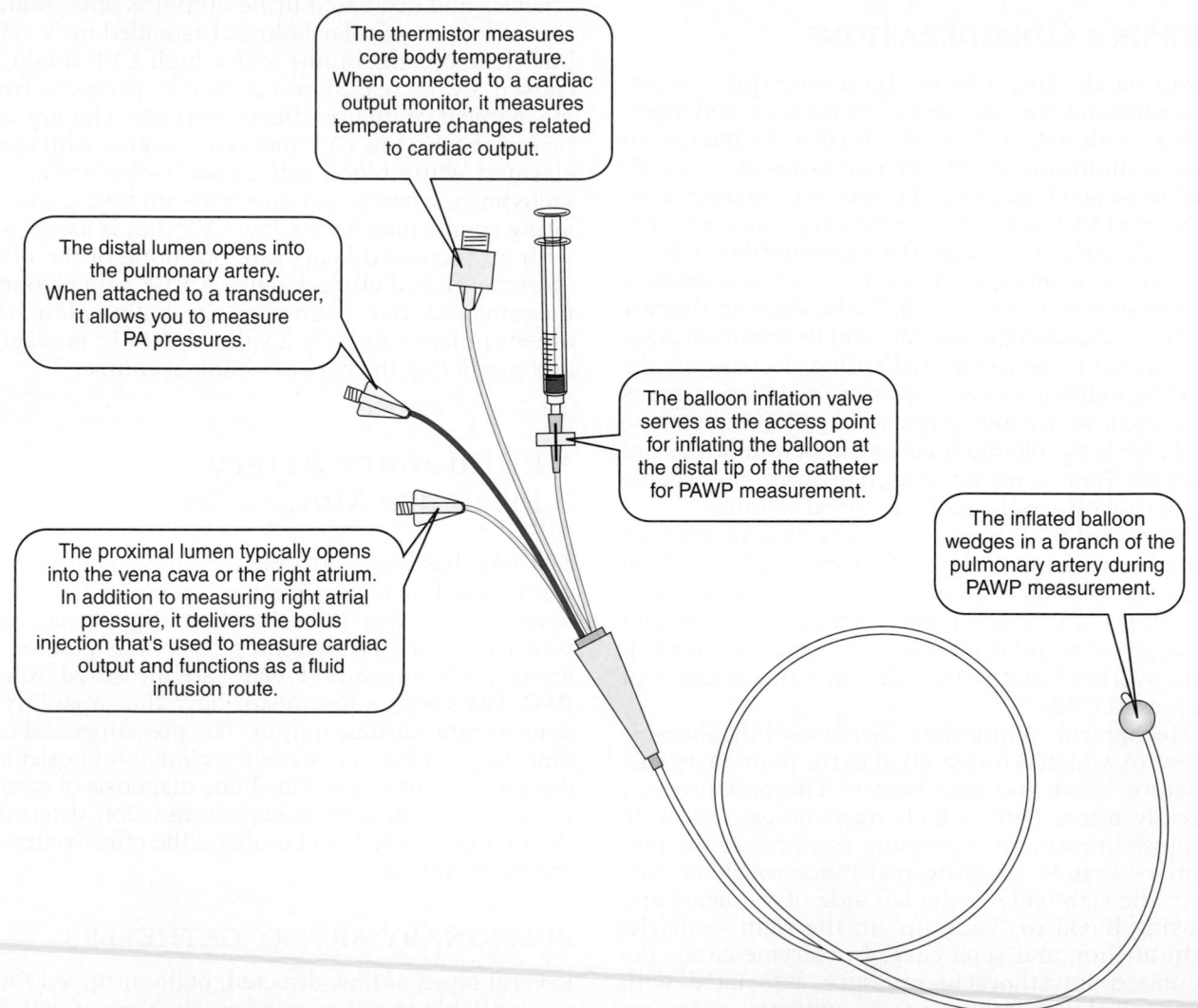

Figure 17-53 • Pulmonary artery catheter. PA, pulmonary artery; PAWP, pulmonary artery wedge pressure. (Courtesy of Edwards Lifesciences, LLC.)

Some of the features include additional lumens in the right atrium, right ventricle, or both for added infusion. A distal lumen containing fiberoptic filaments allows continuous measurement of mixed venous oxygen saturation (S$\overline{\text{v}}$O$_2$). The external optic connecting cable is attached to an optics module and then special oximetry monitor. Catheters modified with a thermal filament and combined with a thermal filament connector and special monitor provide and display cardiac output on a continuous basis. Other advanced catheters with advanced monitor algorithms determine right ventricular ejection fraction and additional derived parameters such as end-diastolic volume. Figure 17-54 shows various types of PACs.

Specially designed catheters may also be used for temporary pacing. There are PACs that house pacing electrodes for both atrial and ventricular pacing as well as PACs with lumens in the right atrium and right ventricle for placing of special probes for pacing.

PULMONARY ARTERY CATHETER INSERTION

Before the PAC is inserted, all necessary equipment should be assembled and prepared according to institution policies. The flushed pressure monitoring system is placed at the zero reference point, leveled, and zeroed. Each lumen of the PA catheter is flushed with sterile solution from the flush system. (Note that fiberoptic $\overline{\text{S}}$O$_2$ monitoring catheters must be calibrated in the calibration cup housed in the sterile tray package before flushing the PA lumens.) The balloon lumen is inflated with air to ensure proper inflation and to check for leaks; it is then deflated before insertion. The PA port is then connected to the prepared pressure tubing, and the other lumens are connected to either a pressure monitoring system or an IV solution.

Strict sterile technique, including a full sterile drape, is required for the insertion procedure. The clinician performing the procedure wears a cap,

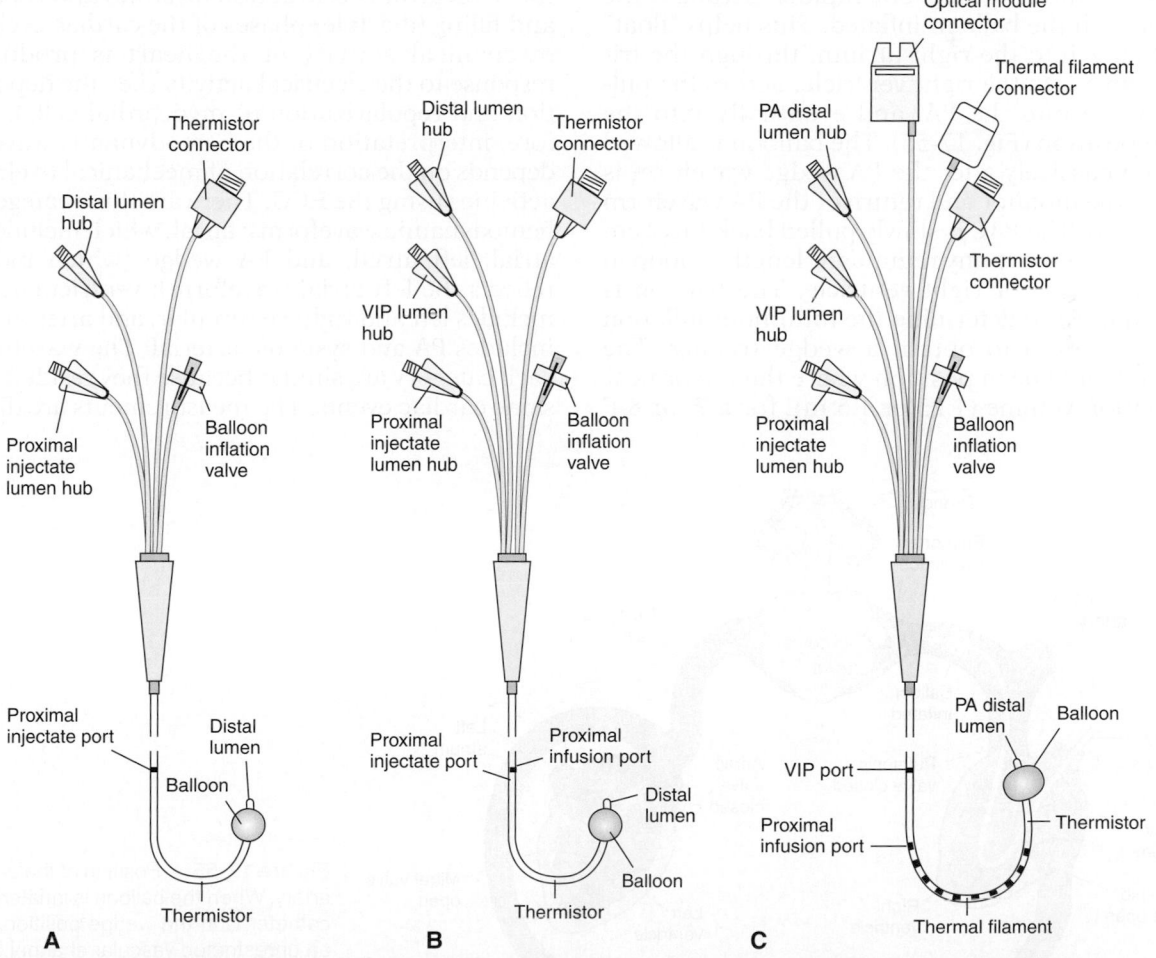

Figure 17-54 • Types of pulmonary artery catheters. **A:** Four-lumen catheter. **B:** Five-lumen catheter that includes an additional venous infusion port (VIP) into the right atrium. **C:** Seven-lumen catheter that includes a VIP port and two additional lumens for continuous cardiac output (CCO) and thermal filament, and continuous mixed venous oxygen saturation (SvO$_2$) monitoring (optical module connector). An additional option is to combine use of the CCO filament and the thermistor response time to calculate end-diastolic volume monitoring. (Courtesy of Edwards Lifesciences, LLC.)

mask, gown, and gloves. The nurse assisting wears a cap and mask and, if manipulating the catheter, gloves. The PAC is inserted into a large vein through an introducer catheter, which is usually placed by a percutaneous approach. The most common insertion sites are the right internal jugular, right or left subclavian, and femoral veins. Occasionally, the antecubital vein is used; this requires a venous cutdown.

Determination of the catheter tip location is established by monitoring the waveform and pressures on the bedside monitor as the catheter passes through the heart chambers and vessels. Black catheter markings occur every 10 cm, with a heavier black line at the 50-cm and 100-cm points. Distances are identified from the distal tip (i.e., the proximal lumen exits 30 cm from the distal tip). These marking are also used during the insertion procedure to assist with catheter tip placement. When the catheter tip is approximately 15 cm into the introducer, the tip has typically exited the sheath and lies in the vena cava and right atrial junction. Waveforms on the monitor show respiratory excursions.

At this time, the balloon is inflated with the recommended balloon inflation volume of 1.5 mL air or CO_2. The clinician gently but rapidly advances the catheter with the balloon inflated. This helps "float" the catheter into the right atrium, through the tricuspid valve into the right ventricle, across the pulmonic valve into the PA, and eventually into the wedged position (Fig. 17-55). The balloon is allowed to deflate passively after the PA wedge waveform is noted on the monitor and return of the PA waveform is confirmed. The PAC is slowly pulled back 1 to 2 cm to reduce or remove any redundant length or loop in the right atrium or right ventricle. The balloon is then reinflated to determine the minimum inflation volume required to obtain a wedge tracing. The catheter should be in position where the full or near full inflation volume (1.25 or 1.5 mL for a 7- or 8-F

PAC) is required to obtain a wedge pressure tracing. Again, the balloon is passively deflated, and return of the PA tracing is observed. The PAC is made of a material that softens in vivo. This additional step during insertion helps decrease distal migration of the PAC after it has been placed. The PAC is then secured, and a sterile dressing is placed over the insertion site. Catheter position is also verified with a chest radiograph after the insertion.

Nursing responsibilities during the insertion procedure include ensuring use of sterile technique, monitoring the changes in hemodynamic waveforms, recording the pressures in each chamber of the heart as the catheter is passed through, and monitoring the patient for complications. Ventricular dysrhythmias are the most common complication during PAC insertion (see section on Complications). Therefore, it is advisable to have a lidocaine bolus and defibrillator available for the insertion procedure.

WAVEFORM INTERPRETATION

All hemodynamic pressures and waveforms are generated by pressure changes in the heart caused by the myocardial contraction (systole) and relaxation and filling (diastole) phases of the cardiac cycle. This mechanical activity of the heart is produced in response to the electrical activity (i.e., the depolarization and repolarization of myocardial cells). Therefore, interpretation of the hemodynamic waveforms depends on the correlation of mechanical to electrical activities using the ECG. There are three categories of hemodynamic waveforms: atrial, which includes right atrial, left atrial, and PA wedge (which indirectly reflects the left atrial waveform); ventricular, which includes left and right ventricular; and arterial, which includes PA and systemic arterial. The waveforms in each category are similar because they result from the same cardiac events. The measurements are different

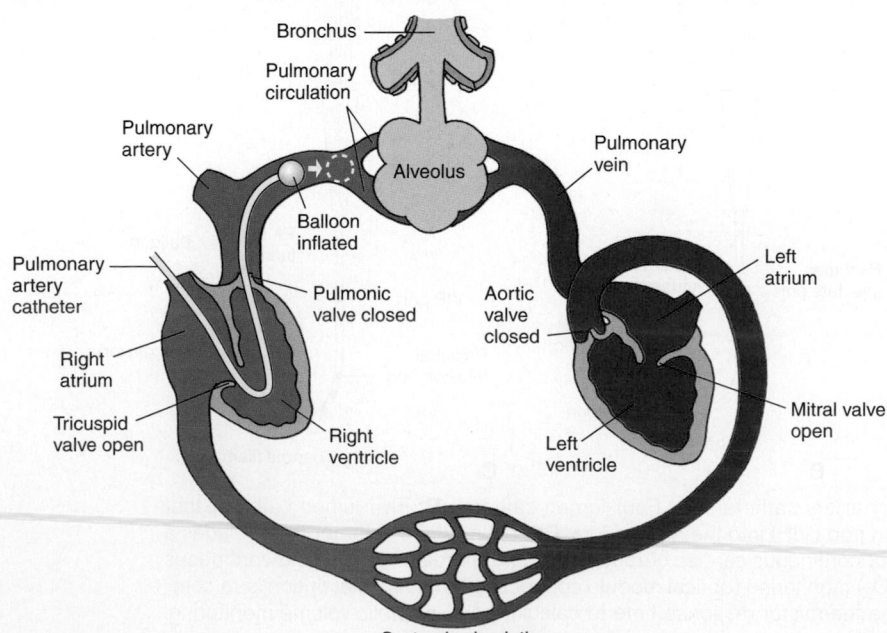

Figure 17-55 • Position of the pulmonary artery. When the balloon is inflated and the catheter is in the wedge position, there is an unrestricted vascular channel between the tip of the catheter and the left ventricle in diastole. Pulmonary artery wedge pressure thus reflects left ventricular end-diastolic pressure, an important indicator of left ventricular function. (Courtesy of Philips.)

because the pressures generated in the right side compared with the left side of the heart differ.

Right Atrial Pressure

The right atrium is a low-pressure chamber, receiving blood volume passively from the vena cava. The normal pressure is 2 to 6 mm Hg. Atrial waveforms have three positive waves: a, c, and v. The a wave reflects the increase in atrial pressure during atrial systole. The c wave results from a small increase in pressure associated with closure of the atrioventricular valve and early atrial diastole. It may be a distinct wave or a notch on the a wave. The v wave represents atrial diastole and reflects the increase in pressure caused by filling of the atrium with blood. It also occurs during ventricular systole. Figure 17-56 shows the right atrial waveform.

Accurate identification of the a, c, and v waves requires correlation of the waveform with the ECG. On the ECG, the P wave represents discharge of the sinoatrial node and atrial depolarization, which causes right atrial and left atrial contraction. Therefore, the a wave occurs after the P wave and usually in the PR interval. The QRS complex represents ventricular depolarization and causes ventricular contraction. Simultaneously, the atria relax and fill with blood. The v wave generated by these events thus falls after the QRS complex and in the T-to-P interval.

Atrial pressure tracings also have two primary negative waves or descents: x and y. The x descent follows the a or c wave if present and represents a decrease in pressure caused by atrial relaxation at the beginning of atrial diastole. The y descent follows the v wave and represents the initial, passive atrial emptying into the ventricle as the atrioventricular valve opens.[1,2]

Right Ventricular Pressure

The right ventricle is a low-pressure chamber. RVEDP is usually 0 to 8 mm Hg. When the tricuspid valve is open, the right atrial pressure and the RVEDP are similar. Right ventricular systolic pressure is normally 20 to 30 mm Hg because the right ventricle must generate only enough pressure to open the pulmonic valve and move blood through the low-pressure pulmonary vasculature.

As the PAC is advanced from the right atrium into the right ventricle, or if the PAC has a right ventricular lumen and is being transduced, the waveform has

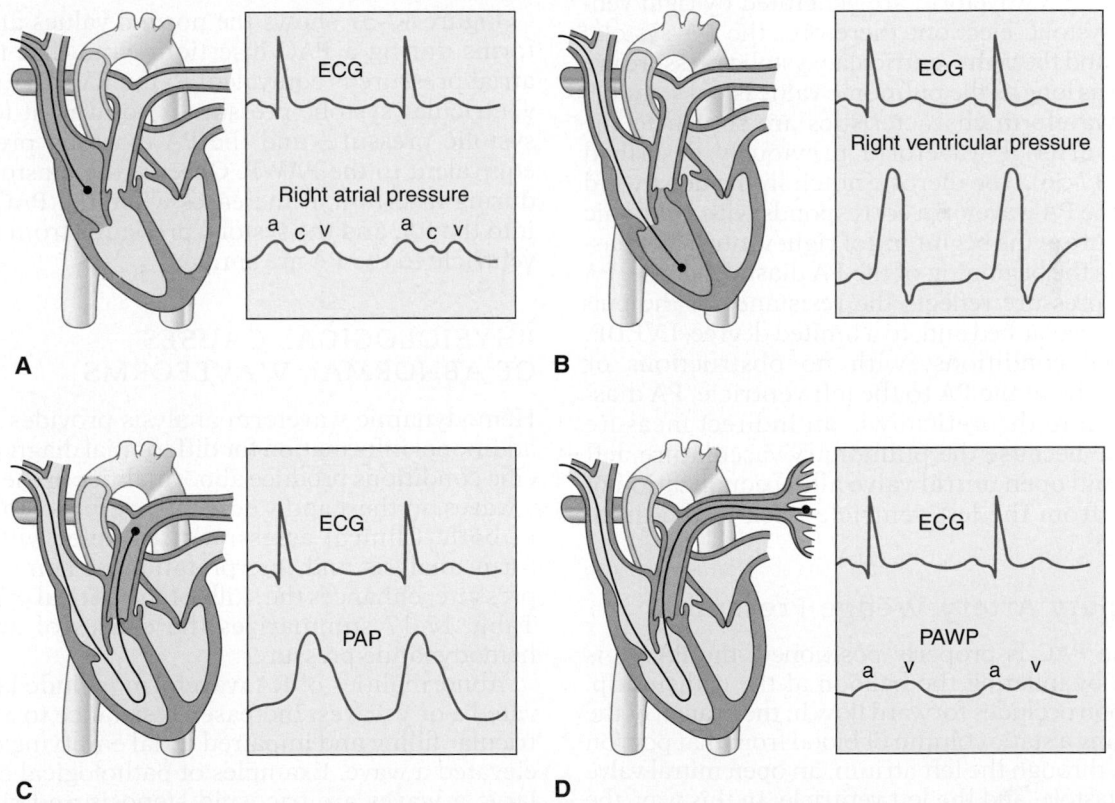

Figure 17-56 • Normal pulmonary artery (PA) waveforms. During PA insertion, the waveforms change as the catheter advances through the heart. **A:** When the catheter enters the right atrium (RA), a waveform with three small upright waves appears. The a waves represent the right atrial systole; the v waves, right atrial filling. **B:** When the catheter reaches the right ventricle, a waveform with sharp systolic upstrokes and lower diastolic dips appears. **C:** When the catheter "floats" into the PA, a PA pressure (PAP) waveform appears. Note that the upstroke is smoother than on the right ventricle waveform. The dicrotic notch indicates pulmonic valve closure. **D:** When the catheter "floats" into a distal branch of the pulmonary artery, the balloon wedges where the vessel becomes too narrow for it to pass, and a pulmonary artery wedge pressure (PAWP) waveform, with two small upright waves, appears. The a wave represents left atrial systole; the v wave, left atrial filling. ECG, electrocardiogram. (Courtesy of Edwards Lifesciences, LLC.)

a distinctive "square root" configuration. Figure 17-56 shows the right ventricular waveform. The initial rapid increase in right ventricular pressure represents isovolumetric contraction, which follows the QRS complex of the ECG. The right ventricular pressure continues to increase as the tricuspid and pulmonic valves are closed until the ventricular force generated exceeds the PA pressure. Rapid ejection occurs when the pulmonic valve opens. After ventricular systole, the pulmonic valve closes, and the right ventricular pressure rapidly decreases, creating a diastolic dip. Next in the cardiac cycle, the tricuspid valve opens and the right ventricle passively fills with blood from the right atrium. Right ventricular diastole occurs within the period from the T wave to the next Q wave on the ECG. The point on the waveform just before the rapid increase in pressure represents RVEDP.[1,2]

Pulmonary Artery Pressure

The pulmonary vasculature is a relatively compliant low-resistance, low-pressure system in healthy people. Normal PA systolic pressure is 20 to 30 mm Hg. Normal diastolic PA pressure is 8 to 15 mm Hg, with a mean of 10 to 20 mm Hg. Systolic PA pressure and the peak of the PA waveform are generated by right ventricular systolic ejection; therefore, the PA systolic pressure and the right ventricular systolic pressure are the same as long as the pulmonic value is not stenotic. The PA waveform characteristics are similar to the systemic arterial waveform previously described (see Fig. 17-56). The dicrotic notch in the downward slope of the PA waveform corresponds with pulmonic valve closure at the beginning of right ventricular diastole and is the beginning of the PA diastolic phase. PA diastolic pressure reflects the resistance of the pulmonary vascular bed and, to a limited degree, LVEDP. In normal conditions, with no obstructions or resistance from the PA to the left ventricle, PA diastolic pressure theoretically is an indirect measure of LVEDP because the pulmonary vasculature, left atrium, and open mitral valve allow equalization of pressure from the left ventricle back to the tip of the PAC.[1,2]

Pulmonary Artery Wedge Pressure

When the PAC is properly positioned, the PAWP is obtained by inflating the balloon at the catheter tip. The balloon occludes forward flow in the branch of the PA, creating a static column of blood from that portion of the PA through the left atrium, an open mitral valve during diastole, and the left ventricle. In this way, the PAWP reflects LVEDP. Normal PAWP is 8 to 12 mm Hg. The PAWP more closely measures left atrial pressure and LVEDP than the PA diastolic pressure because balloon inflation halts blood flow past the catheter tip, thereby decreasing the influence of pulmonary vascular resistance on the pressure reading.

Inflation of the PA balloon causes the PA waveform on the monitor to become a PAWP tracing. No more than 1.5 mL of air is used to inflate the balloon.

If less than 1 to 1.25 mL of air generates a PAWP tracing, the PAC has migrated distally and needs to be withdrawn slightly. Depending on institution policies, a physician or advanced practice clinician performs this procedure.

A left atrial tracing has a, c, and v waves and x and y descents. The electrical and mechanical events of the heart generating these waves are identical to those of the right atrial waveform. The a wave corresponds to left atrial contraction, and the v wave corresponds to left atrial filling and left ventricular contraction. With a direct left atrial line, the c wave is typically visible as in a right atrial tracing. The c wave is rarely visible on the PAWP tracing because the slight increase in pressure from backward bulging of the mitral valve is difficult to observe.

The ECG may be correlated with the PAWP waveform just as with the right atrial waveform. The primary difference between the PAWP and the right atrial waveforms is the slight delay of a and v waves in PAWP relative to the ECG because of the distance from the left side of the heart over which these pressures are transmitted. The a wave now falls more closely in line with the QRS complex, although it may be within the PR interval. The v wave correlates with the T-to-P interval.[1,2]

Figure 17-57 shows the normal values and waveforms during a PAC insertion. Note that the right atrial pressure is equivalent to the RVEDP, the right ventricular systolic pressure is equivalent to the PA systolic pressure, and the PA diastolic pressure is equivalent to the PAWP. Observe the diastolic value during insertion; it increases when the PAC "floats" into the PA, and the systolic pressures from the right ventricle to the PA are similar.

PHYSIOLOGICAL CAUSES OF ABNORMAL WAVEFORMS

Hemodynamic waveform analysis provides valuable additional information for differential diagnosis. Specific conditions produce abnormalities in the a, c, and v waves, in the x and y descents, or in a combination of both. Clinical assessment, coupled with waveform analysis and interpretation of hemodynamic pressure, enhances the skills of the critical care nurse. Table 17-17 summarizes the causes of abnormal hemodynamic pressures.

Abnormalities of RA waveform include large, elevated a or v waves. Increased resistance to right ventricular filling and impaired atrial emptying cause an elevated a wave. Examples of pathological causes of large a waves are tricuspid stenosis and right ventricular failure. Elevated v waves are related to regurgitant flow from the ventricle back into the atrium during ventricular contraction. Examples of pathological causes of large v waves are tricuspid valve insufficiency and right ventricular failure. Elevations in either the a or v wave cause the mean right atrial pressure to be higher.

Increased PA pressures may be systolic or diastolic. Because PA systolic pressure is a reflection of right

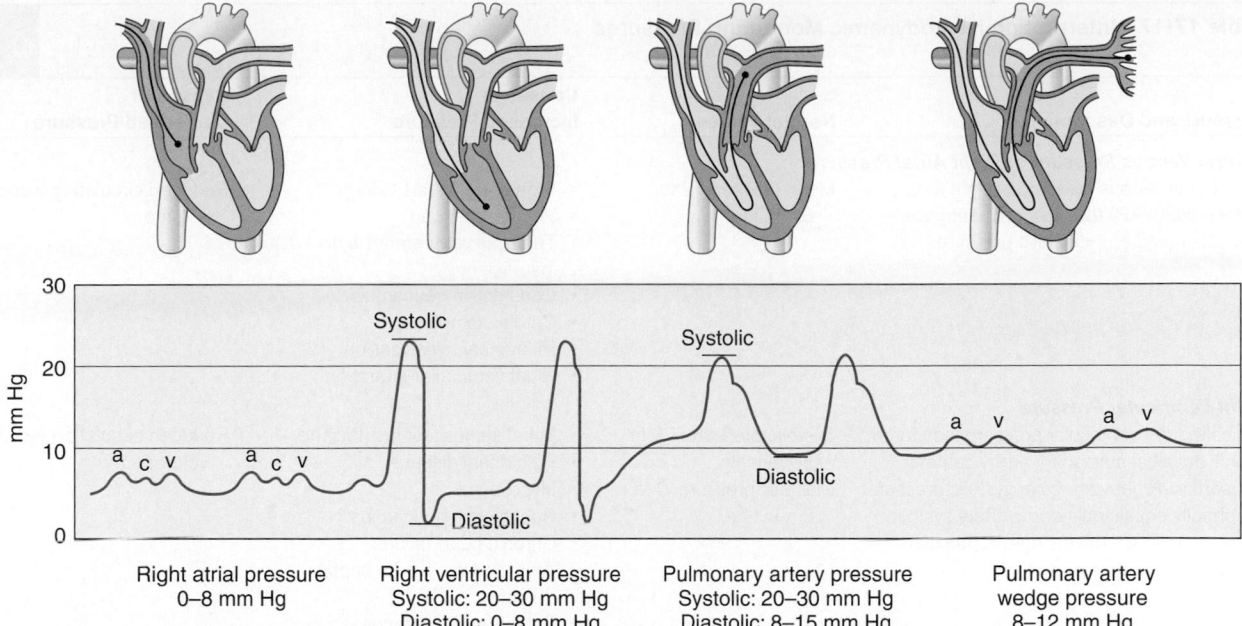

Figure 17-57 • Normal values and wave configurations produced by the pulmonary artery catheter.

ventricular systolic pressure, factors that increase right ventricular pressures such as increased pulmonary vascular resistance, hypervolemia, left ventricular failure, and mechanical ventilation can produce an increased PA systolic pressure. Left ventricular failure, hypervolemia, and increased pulmonary vascular resistance cause increased PA diastolic pressure. Increased pulmonary vascular resistance may result from acute respiratory distress syndrome, primary pulmonary hypertension, or pulmonary embolus.

Left ventricular dysfunction and mitral valve disease occur more frequently than right ventricular or tricuspid valve disorders, and therefore abnormal PAWP waveforms are more common than abnormal right atrial waveforms. Abnormalities of the PAWP waveform usually are large, elevated a or v waves. Increased resistance to left ventricular filling and impaired atrial emptying cause elevated a waves. Examples of pathological causes of large a waves are mitral stenosis and left ventricular failure. Elevated v waves relate to regurgitation from an incompetent mitral valve, allowing blood to flow from the ventricle back into the atrium during ventricular contraction. In both these valvular diseases, the PAWP does not accurately reflect LVEDP. Left ventricular failure usually causes elevation of both the a and v waves and significantly increases the PAWP because of reduced contractility and forward blood flow. Except for the higher pressure reading, the PAWP waveform configuration is usually normal.

Elevated PAWP frequently is due to left ventricular dysfunction or hypervolemia. In some cases, such as in acute respiratory distress syndrome or with mechanical ventilator settings that generate extremely high intrathoracic pressure, PAWP is elevated because of noncardiogenic causes. In these cases, the PA diastolic pressure is greater than the

PAWP and widens the normal PA diastolic pressure/PAWP gradient by 1 to 4 mm Hg. Such a widened pressure gradient is a differential diagnostic sign of pulmonary hypertension or increased pulmonary vascular resistance.

COMPLICATIONS

Generally, most complications that occur with use of the PAC relate to the process of percutaneous central venous access. The other complications such as infection, thrombus, and air embolus are discussed in the earlier section on central venous pressure.

Pneumothorax

Pneumothorax is a complication from vessel access through the subclavian vein. Anatomical factors can make placement of a PAC difficult, particularly if the patient is obese or has torturous subclavian veins. The needle or introducer sheath may pass through the vessel wall and puncture the lung during insertion, causing an apical pneumothorax. Signs and symptoms of a pneumothorax and routine post-insertion chest radiograph are used to diagnose this complication.

Infection

Systemic infection and sepsis are caused by contamination of the PAC, insertion site, or pressure monitoring system. Careful attention to sterile technique during pressure tubing assembly, insertion, and dressing changes helps prevent infection. Protocols for changing the PAC and monitoring system should be followed carefully. Diagnosis of PAC-related sepsis is based on blood cultures, white blood

Table 17-17 • Interpreting Hemodynamic Monitoring Pressures

Pressure and Description	Normal Values	Causes of Increased Pressure	Causes of Decreased Pressure
Central Venous Pressure or Right Atrial Pressure			
The central venous pressure or right atrial pressure (RAP) reflects right ventricular function and end-diastolic pressure.	Mean pressure: 2 to 8 mm Hg	• Right-sided heart failure • Volume overload • Tricuspid valve stenosis or insufficiency • Constrictive pericarditis • Cardiac tamponade • Pulmonary hypertension • Right ventricular infarction	Reduced circulating blood volume
Right Ventricular Pressure			
Typically, right ventricular pressure monitored only on initial pulmonary artery catheter insertion. Right ventricular systolic pressure normally equals pulmonary artery systolic pressure; RAP reflects right ventricular end-diastolic pressure.	Systolic pressure: 20 to 30 mm Hg Diastolic pressure: 0 to 8 mm Hg	• Mitral stenosis or insufficiency • Pulmonary disease • Hypoxemia • Constrictive pericarditis • Chronic heart failure • Atrial and ventricular septal defects • Patent ductus arteriosus	Reduced circulating blood volume
Pulmonary Artery Systolic Pressure			
Pulmonary artery systolic pressure results from right ventricular systolic pressure and reflects right ventricular function.	Systolic pressure: 20 to 30 mm Hg Mean pressure: 8 to 15 mm Hg	• Left-sided heart failure • Increased pulmonary blood flow (left or right shunting, as in atrial or ventricular septal defects) • Any condition causing increased pulmonary arteriolar resistance (such as pulmonary hypertension, volume overload, mitral stenosis, or hypoxia)	Reduced circulating blood volume
Pulmonary Artery Diastolic Pressure			
Pulmonary artery diastolic pressure is an indirect reflection of left ventricular end-diastolic pressure in a patient without significant pulmonary artery disease.	Diastolic pressure: 8 to 12 mm Hg	• Any condition causing increased pulmonary arteriolar resistance (such as pulmonary hypertension, volume overload, mitral stenosis, or hypoxia)	Reduced circulating blood volume
Pulmonary Artery Wedge Pressure or Left Atrial Pressure			
Pulmonary artery wedge pressure (PAWP) indirectly reflects left atrial and left ventricular end-diastolic pressures, unless the patient has obstructions from the tip of the pulmonary artery catheter to the left ventricle. Changes in PAWP reflect changes in left ventricular filling pressure.	Mean pressure: 8 to 12 mm Hg	• Left-sided heart failure • Mitral stenosis or insufficiency • Pericardial tamponade	Reduced circulating blood volume
Pulse Pressure			
Pulse pressure is the difference between systolic and diastolic pressure. Pulse pressure can be used to assess the patient's stroke volume.	Normal range: 40 to 60 mm Hg with a wider range of 30 to 100 mm Hg	• Increased stroke volume • Decreased vascular resistance • Peripheral vascular disease • Aortic insufficiency	Decreased stroke volume Severe vasodilation in conditions such as late sepsis, various shock states

Modified from Springhouse: Critical Care Made Incredibly Easy. Springhouse, PA: Author, 2004, p 170.

cell count, and fever in the absence of other sources of infection.

Ventricular Dysrhythmias

Ventricular dysrhythmias may occur during the insertion of a PAC. As the catheter passes through the right ventricle, it may irritate the endocardium and cause premature ventricular complexes and occasionally ventricular tachycardia. The dysrhythmias typically resolve when the catheter is advanced into the PA. After the PAC is in proper position, it may become dislodged if it is not well secured, and the tip may "fall back" into the right ventricle. The patient may experience dysrhythmias, and the hemodynamic pressures and waveform reflect those of the right ventricle. Usually in this situation, because of potential contamination at the insertion site, the catheter is withdrawn or occasionally by inflating the balloon, the catheter may "refloat" into the PA. It is essential to have ready access to emergency drugs and equipment in case the ventricular dysrhythmias persist. Many introducer kits contain sterile sheaths; when placed over the PAC, they provide additional protection from contamination.

Pulmonary Artery Rupture or Perforation

A rare but very serious and potentially fatal complication is rupture or perforation of the PA. Perforation of the PA may occur during insertion or manipulation of the PAC. Patients with friable PAs may be at some risk. However, proper advancement of the catheter with the balloon fully inflated with 1.5 mL of air and avoidance of advancing the catheter too far into a small artery minimize the chance of PA perforation. Rupture of the PA is associated with overinflation of the balloon, particularly if the catheter has migrated distally into a small PA. Close observation of the PA waveform as the balloon is inflated and filling the balloon only with the amount of air necessary to obtain a PAWP tracing prevent overdistending a small PA. As previously stated, the catheter should become wedged when inflated with 1.25 to 1.5 mL of air. If less air is required to obtain the PAWP waveform, the catheter has migrated out of proper position.

NURSING CONSIDERATIONS

Nursing care of the patient undergoing PA pressure monitoring is complex. Critical care nurses must be able to interpret waveforms and pressure data as well as be alert to potential complications. It is necessary to ensure accurate readings and minimize operator error. Consistency of leveling and measurement techniques is especially important because small variations in the zero reference point elicit large and erroneous changes in the pressures observed. Table 17-16 outlines problems and troubleshooting strategies associated with hemodynamic pressure monitoring.

Measurement of all hemodynamic pressures is most accurate when obtained at the end of expiration in the respiratory cycle. In the healthy person, intrathoracic pressure at end expiration is about equal to atmospheric pressure. During the end-expiration period, there is minimal airflow and little variation in pleural pressures that influence cardiac pressures. Thus, end expiration provides a standard reference point for obtaining measurements. Spontaneous breathing causes negative intrathoracic pressure during inspiration, which produces a decline in the waveform. The waveform used for measurement is the last clear wave occurring just before the inspiratory dip. Mechanical ventilation causes increased intrathoracic pressure during inspiration, which produces an inspiratory "push" or rise in the waveform. The end-expiratory wave used for measurement is the last clear wave occurring just before the inspiratory rise (Fig. 17-58).

Closely set alarm parameters alert the nurse to potential physiological or technical complications. For example, one indication of a pulmonary embolus is an acute increase in PA pressures. Distal migration of the PAC may cause the catheter to wedge spontaneously without balloon inflation, and PA pressures may decrease to that of a PAWP. With properly set alarms, conditions such as these are detected.

• Determination of Cardiac Output

Cardiac output is the volume of blood ejected from the heart per minute, expressed in liters per minute. Normally, cardiac output is 4 to 8 L/minute at rest. Cardiac output is a function of heart rate and stroke volume. The left ventricle must generate enough pressure in systole to overcome aortic pressure and systemic vascular resistance (SVR) and eject sufficient blood volume to perfuse the organs of the body. The determination of cardiac output and assessment of its determinants are important adjuncts to the care of critically ill patients. Routine evaluation of cardiac output is essential when technology such as a PAC is used.

Cardiac index relates cardiac output to body size. Normally, the cardiac index is 2.5 to 4 L/minute/m^2. To obtain it, the cardiac output is divided by the patient's body surface area (BSA). Two common formulas, Dubois or Boyd, incorporate the patient's height and weight to determine BSA. Both formulas require obtaining of accurate patient height and

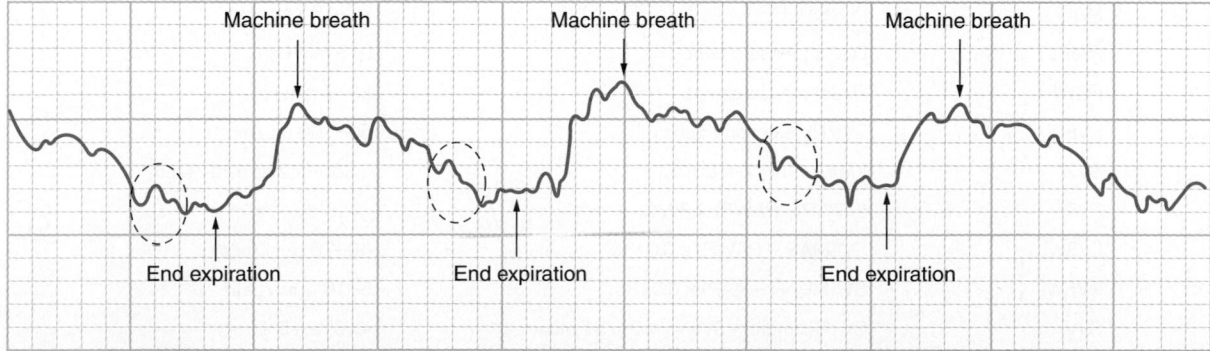

Figure 17-58 • Pulmonary artery wedge pressure (PAWP) tracing showing respiratory variation from positive pressure mechanical ventilation. Measurement of PAWP is made at the last clear tracing before the inspiratory rise as identified by the open circles.

weight. Standard bedside monitors and cardiac output computers automatically calculate the cardiac index when the patient's height and weight are entered. The BSA is also used to index other valuable hemodynamic parameters (Table 17-18).

FACTORS THAT DETERMINE CARDIAC OUTPUT

Cardiac output should include analysis of its determinants, heart rate and stroke volume. An increased or decreased cardiac output provides global information only and needs to be evaluated in light of the components affecting it.[5] For example, an increase in heart rate can produce an increase in cardiac output; however, this may be a compensatory physiological response to a decreased stroke volume. The increase in heart rate increases myocardial oxygen demands and may place a compromised patient at risk for myocardial ischemia. Tachycardia may decrease cardiac output because of shortened diastole and decreased filling time of the ventricles. A patient with bradycardia may be symptomatic because of low cardiac output and blood pressure.

Stroke volume, the volume of blood ejected by each ventricular contraction, is influenced by preload, afterload, and contractility (see Chapter 16 for detailed discussion). Preload is the amount of stretch on the myocardial muscle fibers at end-diastole and is determined by ventricular filling (end-diastolic) volume. Within physiological limits, increases in end-diastolic volume cause stretch of the myofibrils and increase the force of the next ventricular contraction (Frank-Starling law of the heart). Preload is primarily influenced by total blood volume. Because the PAC measures pressure, not volume, assumptions are made that volume and pressure can be equated.

Many factors alter the pressure–volume relationship; therefore, the use of pressures to evaluate preload must be considered in light of these. A specialized PAC is able to provide right ventricular ejection fraction and volumetric data. Indirect assessment of preload uses the right atrial pressure or CVP for the right ventricular preload, and the PA diastolic pressure, left atrial pressure, and PAWP for the left ventricular preload.

Afterload is often defined as the impedance or resistance to ejection of blood from the ventricles. Primary factors affecting afterload are semilunar valve conditions and vascular resistance. Pulmonary vascular resistance (PVR) is a clinical assessment of right ventricular afterload. Left ventricular afterload is clinically evaluated by calculating SVR. PVR and SVR can be indexed to body size using the patient's BSA (see Table 17-18).

Contractility is an inherent property of the heart. It is not affected by preload or afterload and cannot be directly measured. Indices used to assess contractility include determining stroke volume and calculating the stroke work index for both the left and right ventricles. Myocardial oxygen supply and demand balance, electrolytes, and minerals (e.g., calcium) influence myocardial contractility.

OBTAINING CARDIAC OUTPUT VALUES

Several methods for evaluating cardiac output are available. These include invasive, minimally invasive, and noninvasive technologies. All techniques have certain assumptions and limitations that need to be considered to provide an understanding of the indications and applications of each. This section discusses the more common methods of cardiac output monitoring used in the critical care areas.

Table 17-18 • Calculation of Cardiac Hemodynamic Parameters

Parameter	Formula	Normal Values
CO	Heart rate × SV	4–8 L/min
CI	CO/body surface area	2.5–4 L/min/m²
SVI	CI/heart rate	33–47 mL/beat/m²
MAP	[Systolic BP + (diastolic BP × 2)]/3	70–105 mm Hg
RAP	Direct measurement	0–8 mm Hg
PAWP	Direct measurement	8–12 mm Hg
RVEDVI	SVI/RV ejection fraction	60–100 mL/m²
SVRI	[(MAP − RAP) × 80]/CI	1,360–2,200 dyne/s/cm⁻⁵
PVRI	(MPAP − PAWP) × 80/CI	<425 dyne/s/cm⁻⁵
LVSWI	SVI(MAP − PAWP) × 0.0136	40–70 g-m²/beat
RVSWI	SVI(MPAP − RAP) × 0.0136	5–10 g-m²/beat
SVV	SV maximum − SV minimum/SV mean	<10%–15%

CO, cardiac output; CI, cardiac index; SVI, stroke volume index; RAP, right atrial pressure; RVEDVI, right ventricular end-diastolic volume index; SVRI, systemic vascular resistance index; PVRI, pulmonary vascular resistance index; MAP, mean arterial pressure; MPAP, mean pulmonary artery pressure; LVSWI, left ventricular stroke work index; RVSWI, right ventricular stroke work index; SVV, stroke volume variation; SV, stroke volume.

Fick Method for Cardiac Output Determination

The Fick method, originally developed in the 1800s by Adolf Fick, is the historical laboratory gold standard. The Fick method is based on the principle that the uptake or release of a substance by an organ divided by the arterial and venous concentration of that substance is the product of flow or cardiac output. The classical method of determining cardiac output uses oxygen as the substance and the lungs as the organ. In order for this relationship to be valid, simultaneous samples of arterial and venous blood must be obtained and accurately measured. In addition, inspired and expired oxygen concentration must be measured by indirect calorimetry to determine the oxygen consumption. Other technologies use these principles; however, they use CO_2 as the measured substance.

Indicator-Dilution Methods for Cardiac Output Determination

Stewart proposed the principles of the indicator-dilution method, and Hamilton further refined them. The Stewart-Hamilton equation is based on use of a known indicator as a signal and determination of the dilution rate of that signal over a given period of time. Three indicators in clinical use are dye, thermal, and small doses of lithium. The indicator is injected into the venous system, and a time–concentration curve is generated from a blood sample obtained from the arterial system. Analysis of the curve allows cardiac output calculation.[1,2]

Thermodilution is the most common method used to measure cardiac output and is considered the clinical gold standard. Cold or room temperature solution is the indicator and is injected into the right atrial port of the PAC. A thermistor near the end of the catheter continuously measures the temperature of blood flowing past it. A dilution curve is generated by the change in blood temperature after indicator injection. Based on this curve, cardiac output is calculated by the computer.

Determination of cardiac output through thermodilution is obtained either on an intermittent or continuous basis. Intermittent cardiac output requires the injection of a known amount of "cooler than blood" injectate, and a single cardiac output curve is produced. Specialty catheters house thermal filaments and, with a dedicated thermal cable and computer, emit energy as the indicator. The "warmer than blood" signal is measured at the thermistor, and thermodilution curves are produced on a 30- to 60-second frequency for continuous cardiac output assessment.

Procedure for Intermittent Thermodilution Cardiac Output Determination

A computation constant, based on the catheter size, volume, and temperature of the injectate, as well as injection method, is set on the computer or programmed into the bedside cardiac output module. Five or 10 mL of sterile D_5W or normal saline is used as the injectate solution and volume. The injectate syringe used is usually part of a closed system that remains intact and attached to the right atrial port by a stopcock (Fig. 17-59). Iced (0°C to 4°C) or room-temperature solution may be used. A temperature difference between the patient's blood temperature and the injectate of at least 10°C improves accuracy. In most conditions, room-temperature injectate with a 10-mL volume provides accurate results. With hypothermia or very low cardiac output states, iced solution and a 10-mL injectate volume provide a greater signal and increased accuracy.

Steps for performing a manual cardiac output determination vary according to bedside monitor or cardiac output computer manufacturer. See specific operations manuals for directions for use. General steps include:

► Ensuring the accurate amount of injectate volume in the syringe
► Injecting the volume in a smooth and rapid manner, in less than 4 seconds
► Waiting approximately 1 minute between injections to allow the catheter thermistor to return to baseline

When injected, the solution passes a temperature probe in the closed system and flows through the right atrium and right ventricle, past the thermistor at the tip of the PAC. A curve is produced and used for determining the cardiac output. The average of several cardiac output determinations is required to obtain a final measurement. Serial measurements and averaging are necessary because of the number of physiological variables and the performance of the technical procedure. Three or more consecutive measurements are usually necessary. Measurements included in the averaging process should be within 10% to 15% of the mean, and each one should be associated with a normal cardiac output curve. Abnormal curves are eliminated from the cardiac output averaging process.

Interpretation of Cardiac Output Curves

Many bedside monitors and cardiac output computers are equipped with a means of visualizing the cardiac output curves. Normal cardiac output curves have a smooth upstroke from the rapid injection followed by a gradual decline (Fig. 17-60). The area under the curve is inversely proportional to the cardiac output. Curves associated with a high cardiac output have a small area under the curve, with a steeper upstroke and more rapid return to baseline, and curves associated with a low cardiac output have a greater area under the curve, with a more sloped upstroke and slower return to baseline.

Arterial Pressure- and Waveform-Based Cardiac Output Determinations

Use of arterial pressures, arterial waveforms, or both is another method for determining cardiac output and stroke volume. Otto Frank first proposed the concept of using the arterial pulse for determining flow, or cardiac output, in the late 1890s. Other researchers and advances in technology provided

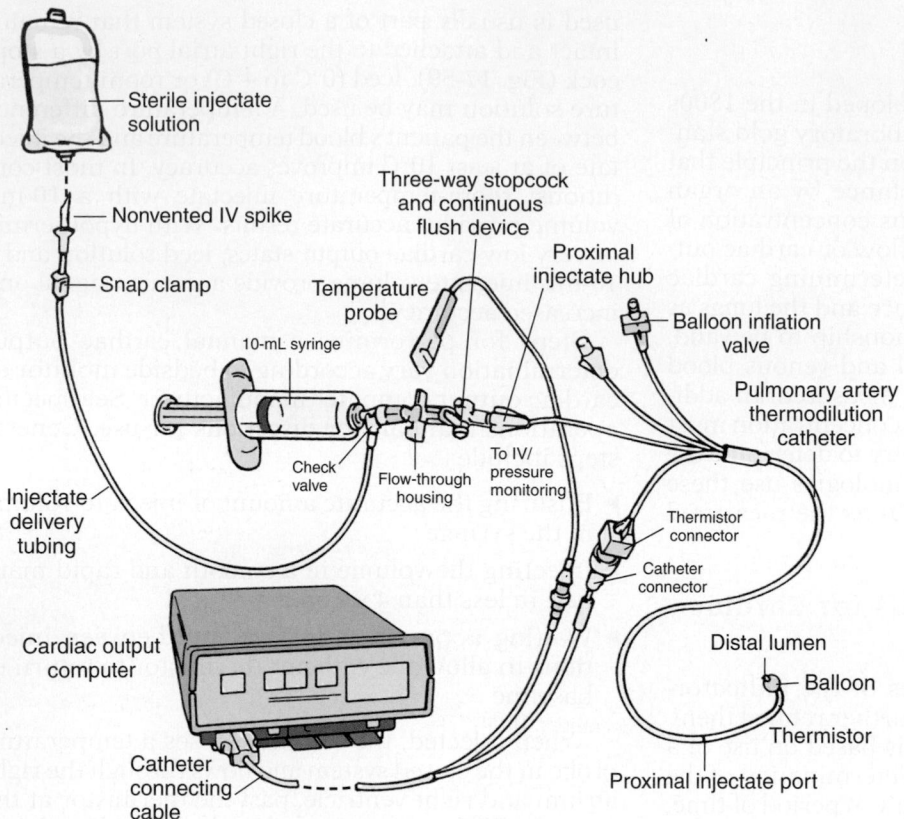

Figure 17-59 • A closed room-temperature injectate system for measurement of cardiac output.

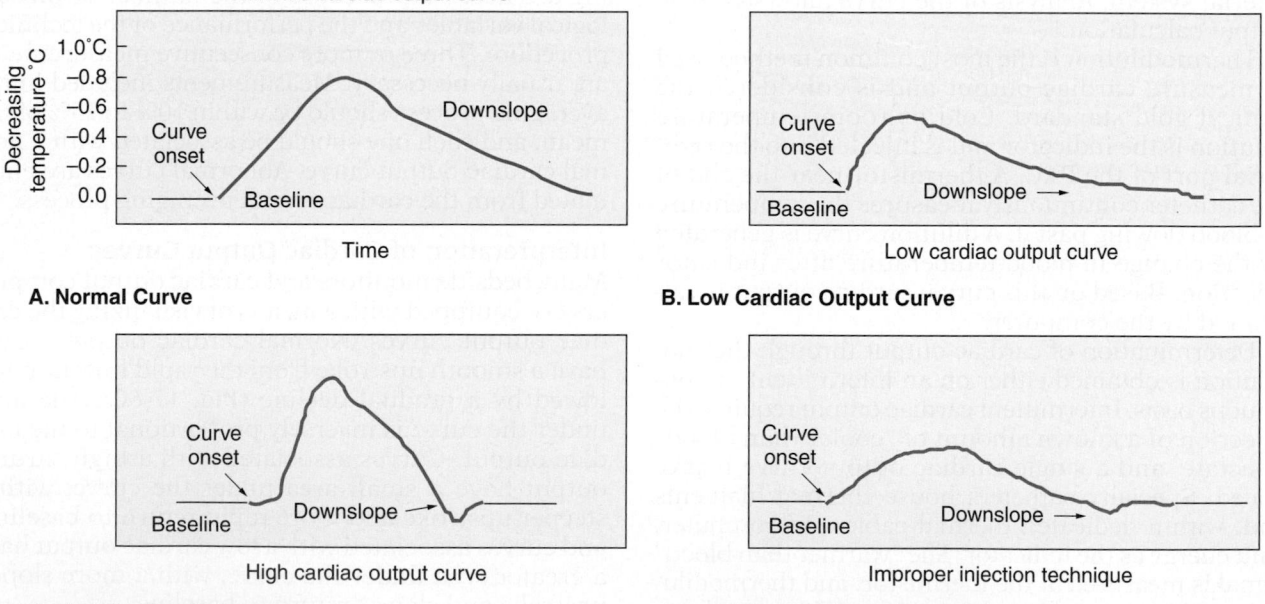

Figure 17-60 • Examples of thermodilution curves observed on a bedside monitor or strip chart recorder. **A:** Normal curve with smooth upstroke and gradual decline to baseline. Note that the temperature change is actually lower than patient baseline temperature; however, the graph is shown in an upright orientation. **B:** Low cardiac output produces a greater area under the curve. The upstroke is normal with a more gradual decline. **C:** A high cardiac output has a smaller area under the curve. The upstroke is more rapid with a faster return to baseline. **D:** Irregular curve shows an erroneously low cardiac output probably due to irregular or uneven emptying of the injectate syringe. (Courtesy of Edwards Lifesciences LLC.)

refinement for clinical application of Frank's concepts. The basic premise relates to the proportionality relationship of pulse pressure to stroke volume and the inverse relationship of pulse pressure to aortic compliance. Other factors considered for use of this method are factors and conditions that change vascular tone: larger vessel compliance and peripheral vessel resistance.

General components required for this method are an existing arterial line placed in the patient, a special sensor, and specific monitor that uses a unique algorithm for the stroke volume and cardiac output determinations. Some systems use the shape of the arterial wave to determine the dicrotic notch location, which signifies the end of systole. This method is referred to as pulse contour. The area under the curve then represents the amount of volume ejected into the arterial vascular bed and reflects stroke volume. Other systems assess the systolic and diastolic pressure to obtain a mean value to arrive at stroke volume. This method is described as pulse power. Another method samples the full waveform for pressures and uses waveform characteristics for cardiac output determinations. This method is termed arterial pressure–based cardiac output. External calibration with either thermodilution or lithium is required for both the pulse contour and pulse power methods. The arterial pressure–based cardiac output method does not require external calibration. Once the stroke volume is determined, the pulse rate, assessed by the arterial waves, reflects the heart rate; stroke volume times heart rate equals cardiac output. All the technologies, regardless of the specific algorithm used to determine the cardiac output value, use the arterial pressure. This requires obtaining of accurate values and ensuring optimal waveforms.

Other parameters obtained with an arterial pressure system include stroke volume variation or its surrogate, pulse pressure variation, and systolic pressure variation. These parameters evaluate the difference between the maximum and minimum values of systolic pressure, pulse pressure, or stroke volume during a respiratory cycle and are predictors of fluid responsiveness in the critically ill. A natural phenomenon occurs during the respiratory cycle in which the arterial pressure falls during inspiration and rises during expiration. The variation is a result of changes in intrathoracic pressure during respiration; a negative pressure during inspiration results in a fall in systolic pressure, and a relatively higher intrathoracic pressure during expiration causes a rise in systolic pressure. The normal variation during a respiratory cycle is 5 to 10 mm Hg. When the difference is greater, the condition is termed *pulsus paradoxus*. Reverse pulsus paradoxus is the same phenomenon that occurs during controlled mechanical ventilation. The mechanics are opposite of spontaneous breathing in that arterial pressure rises during inspiration and falls during expiration.[6,7]

Nursing Considerations

Alterations in cardiac output are caused by changes in heart rate, preload, afterload, and contractility. Therefore, analysis of these parameters is essential in directing interventions to address the underlying pathophysiological process. One strategy to consider is to evaluate cardiac output, then systematically assess the determinants of heart rate, then stroke volume with preload first, afterload second, and finally contractility.

Decreased cardiac output may be related to either tachycardia or bradycardia. An elevated heart rate is frequently a compensatory response to external stimuli or a hypovolemic state. If the elevated heart rate is due to external stimuli, identify the cause and direct interventions to eliminate or decrease the stimuli. Conditions to assess for are pain, fever, stress, and hypermetabolic states. Hypovolemia or decreased venous return associated with mechanical ventilation and elevated intrathoracic pressures causes decreased preload. Patient assessment includes assessing for pulsus paradoxus that occurs during cardiac tamponade, obstructive lung diseases, and hypovolemic states. A stroke volume variation greater than 10% to 15% has a high level of sensitivity and specificity for determining the need for fluid and in predicting preload responsiveness. Limitations to using variation parameters relate to factors that cause changes in intrathoracic pressure and those that affect ventricular filling time. Any cardiac dysrhythmia can affect the overall value because of irregular ventricular responses. Intravascular volume resuscitation increases preload, which in turn increases cardiac output.

Vasoconstriction causes elevated afterload and has several causes. Increased SVR may be a compensatory response to hypovolemia caused by vasoconstriction to maintain cardiac output in this state. An increase in afterload occurs with some medications, hypothermia, and the compensatory vascular response to cardiogenic shock. This increase in afterload may also be accompanied by a decrease in cardiac output and an increase in oxygen demand and myocardial work. A decrease in afterload due to vasodilation reduces resistance to ejection of blood, thus increasing cardiac output. Vasodilating medications, septic states, and allergic and anaphylactic reactions are all causes of vasodilation and thus increased cardiac output.

Reduction in contractility decreases cardiac output. Examples include insufficient oxygen delivery to the myocardium, causing myocardial ischemia and infarction; medications, such as β-blocking agents; or metabolic imbalances, such as low serum levels of calcium, phosphorus, or magnesium. Positive inotropic agents or correction of impaired myocardial oxygenation or metabolic derangements may cause enhanced contractility, most often resulting in increased cardiac output.

Impedance Cardiography for Cardiac Output Determination

Impedance cardiography (ICG), or thoracic electrical bioimpedance, is a noninvasive method of cardiac output monitoring. Impedance (Z), or resistance to flow, of an electrical current is decreased in the presence of fluid. The ICG device uses a very small electrical current injected through external electrodes placed at the

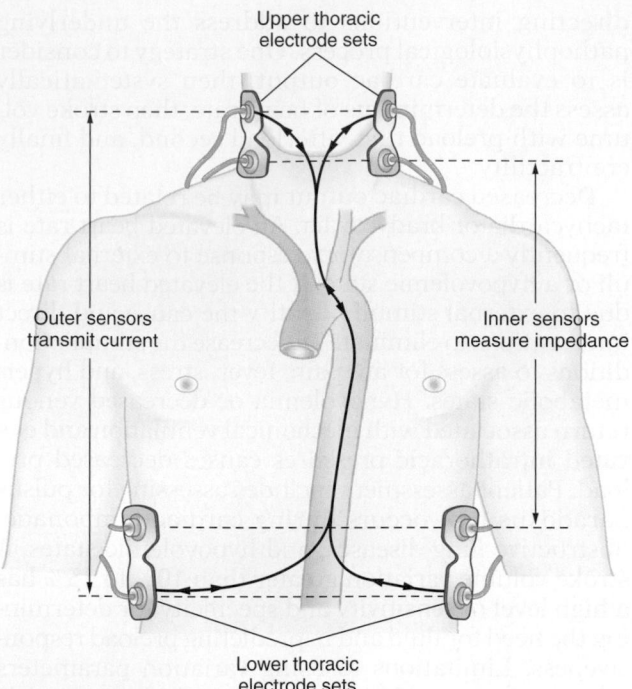

Figure 17-61 • Placement of thoracic impedance sensors. (Courtesy of Cardiodynamic International.)

base of the neck and the lower thorax (Fig. 17-61). These electrodes also sense the change in impedance due to pulsatile blood flow in the descending aorta during systole and diastole. The change in impedance over time (dZ/dt) directly reflects left ventricular contractility (Fig. 17-62). This dZ/dt change is mathematically converted into stroke volume and cardiac output values using an algorithm. Other hemodynamic parameters are either measured or calculated from the ICG data and are provided on a continuous, real-time basis (Table 17-19).

ICG provides traditional hemodynamic determinations such as cardiac output, stroke volume, and SVR, if a blood pressure and CVP or right atrial pressure is entered into the monitor. Because aortic blood flow causes the change in impedance, ICG provides more direct indices of left ventricular contractility that are not available from a PAC. ICG also is used to measure systolic time intervals that are valuable in determining the contractile function of the left ventricle.

Nursing Considerations

Because ICG is a noninvasive technology, nurses in any inpatient or outpatient setting can initiate this type of hemodynamic monitoring. Thus, the clinical applications are broad. For example, ICG parameters are used to evaluate patients with heart failure, hypertension, and permanent pacemakers in the emergency department, outpatient clinic, or physician office.

Because electrical impedance is reduced in the presence of fluid, the baseline impedance reflects all of the fluid in the thorax (interstitial, intravascular, or intracellular). The thoracic fluid content measurement is therefore useful in the differential diagnosis of heart failure or chronic obstructive pulmonary disease as well as in the assessment and management of patients with heart failure who may have pulmonary congestion or pulmonary edema. Adjustment in diuretics, inotropic agents, and ACE inhibitor or angiotensin-receptor blockers can be fine-tuned based on ICG parameters. Similarly, patients with chronic and resistant hypertension can be managed more closely and more aggressively on an outpatient basis using ICG hemodynamic parameters as opposed to using blood pressure alone to adjust or add various medications. ICG cardiac output and hemodynamic parameters are also used to optimize the settings of atrial-ventricular (A-V) sequential cardiac pacemakers, specifically adjusting the time for A-V delay to allow appropriate ventricular filling to achieve optimal stroke volume and cardiac output.[8]

Esophageal Doppler Monitor for Cardiac Output Determination

An esophageal Doppler monitor (EDM) is a minimally invasive hemodynamic monitoring device that incorporates a Doppler transducer into a nasogastric

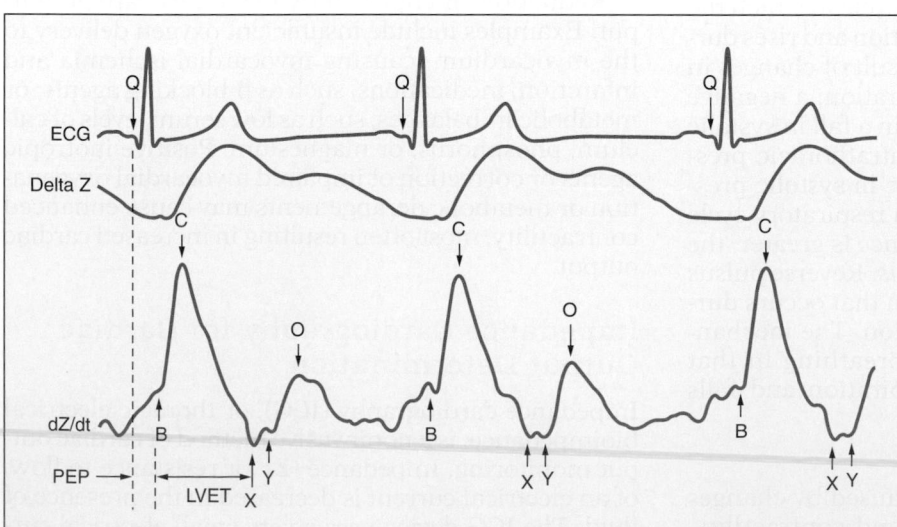

Figure 17-62 • Electrocardiogram and normal change in impedance over time (dZ/dt) waveform. Q, start of ventricular depolarization; B, opening of aortic and pulmonic valves; C, maximum deflection of dZ/dt (dZ/dt$_{max}$); X closure of aortic valve; Y, closure of pulmonic valve; O, mitral opening snap and early ventricular diastolic filling. (Courtesy of Cardiodynamics International, Inc.)

Table 17-19 • Additional Hemodynamic Indices from Impedance Cardiography

Change in impedance/time (dZ/dt)	Magnitude and rate of impedance change Direct reflection of force of left ventricular contraction	0.8–2.5 ohms/s
Velocity index (VI)	Peak velocity of blood flow in the aorta Direct reflection of force of left ventricular contraction	33–65/1000 s
Acceleration contractility index (ACI)	Direct reflection of myocardial contractility Initial acceleration of blood flow in the aorta	Males: 70–150/100 s^2 Females: 90–170/100 s^2
Preejection period (PEP)	Systolic time interval, measuring length of time for isovolumetric contraction	0.05–0.12 s
Ventricular ejection time (VET)	Systolic time interval, measuring the length of time for left ventricular ejection	0.25–0.35 s (depends on heart rate, preload, and contractility)
Thoracic fluid content status (Zo)	Base thoracic impedance The electrical conductivity of the chest cavity, which is primarily determined by the intravascular, intra-alveolar, and interstitial fluids in the thorax Lower Zo indicates a greater volume of thoracic fluid.	Males, 20–30 ohms Females, 25–35 ohms (Normal ranges may vary slightly by manufacturer.)
Thoracic fluid content (TFC)	The inverse of Zo (1/Zo × 1000) Electrical conductivity of the chest cavity, which is primarily determined by the intravascular, intra-alveolar, and interstitial fluids in the thorax Reflects intravascular, interstitial, alveolar, and intracellular fluid Higher TFC indicates greater thoracic fluid volume.	Males: 30–50/k ohms Females: 21–37/k ohms (Normal ranges may vary slightly by manufacturer.)

tube. When placed in the esophagus, the EDM provides monitoring of descending aortic blood flow velocity (Fig. 17-63). The pulsatile velocity waveform directly reflects left ventricular contractility as well as the patient's intravascular volume status (preload). Continuous cardiac output and stroke volume determinations are calculated from the Doppler waveform through an algorithm based on the Doppler waveform configuration and the patient's height, weight, and age.

The EDM provides hemodynamic data in real time relative to changes in blood flow. These include traditional parameters such as cardiac output, stroke volume, and SVR, if a blood pressure and CVP or right atrial pressure is entered into the monitor. EDM parameters also include peak velocity, which is measured from the amplitude of the waveform. Peak velocity is an indicator of myocardial contractility.

The width of the base of the waveform, flow time corrected, reflects systolic ejection time and thus intravascular volume and changes in preload.

Nursing Considerations

A valuable aspect of the EDM is use of the waveform shape to determine changes in myocardial contractility and intravascular volume (preload) because the waveform displayed on the monitor reflects the volume and velocity of blood in the aorta. The normal waveform is triangular, consisting of the beginning of systole, peak systole, and end-systole (Fig. 17-64). As flow from the left ventricle increases, the shape of the waveform changes, becoming a larger, higher, and wider triangle. Conversely, decreased contractility is reflected in a smaller waveform; hypovolemia causes the waveform to become more narrow at the

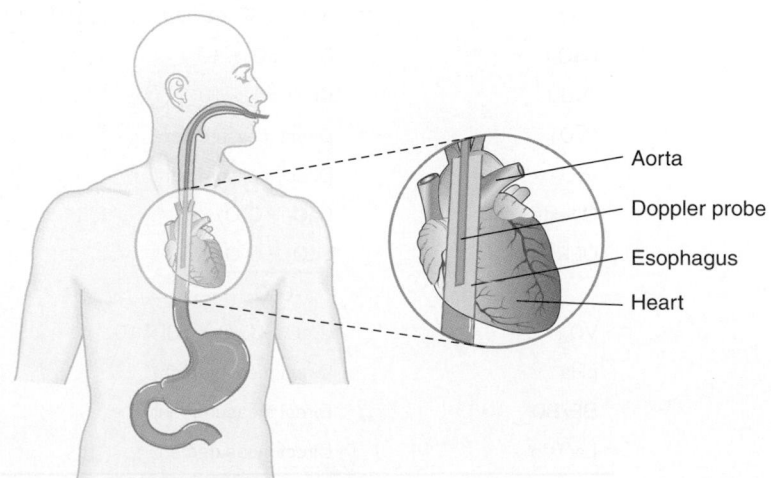

Aorta

Doppler probe

Esophagus

Heart

Figure 17-63 • Location of the esophageal Doppler probe in the esophagus in relation to the heart and descending aorta. (Courtesy of Deltex Medical, Inc.)

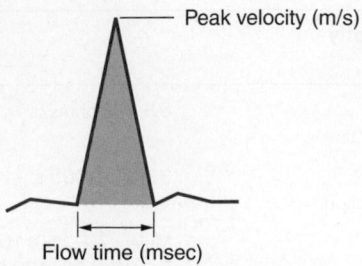

Figure 17-64 • Esophageal Doppler waveform showing peak velocity and flow time. (Courtesy of Deltex Medical, Inc.)

base. The baseline shape of the waveform, as well as changes in response to therapy, can significantly contribute to hemodynamic assessment.

EDM is most often used in the critical care unit, the operating room and postanesthesia care unit, and the emergency department. Patients who may benefit from less invasive EDM include the elderly, critically ill patients with unstable or questionable hemodynamic status, and patients at risk for hypoperfusion or fluid overload due to impaired left ventricular function. EDM is useful in patients for detecting subtle hemodynamic changes (e.g., covert hypovolemia) that are not detectable using physical signs and symptoms in the early phases because of normal compensatory mechanisms. The EDM data can guide the clinician in evaluating the patient's response to fluid administration and titration of vasopressors and inotropes.[9]

• Evaluation of Oxygen Delivery and Demand Balance

One of the primary objectives of hemodynamic monitoring is to apply the data in the evaluation of oxygen delivery or transport and the consumption of oxygen by the tissues and organs. Adequate oxygen delivery to the body's organs is essential for maintenance of cellular, tissue, and ultimately organ function. Insufficient oxygen delivery and consumption to meet the cellular requirements for oxygen, or oxygen demand, result in hypoxia and the accumulation of an oxygen deficit. Persistent oxygen deficit causes cell and organ dysfunction and eventually leads to cell death and organ failure. Table 17-20 lists the parameters that are used to evaluate oxygen delivery and demand balance, the formulas, and normal values.

DETERMINANTS OF OXYGEN DELIVERY

Arterial oxygen delivery (DaO_2) is the amount of oxygen transported to the tissues. DaO_2 depends on arterial oxygen content and cardiac output.

Oxygen Content

Oxygen content is the total amount of oxygen in the blood that is available to the cells. Most of the available oxygen in arterial blood (more than 95%) is reversibly bound to hemoglobin in the form of oxyhemoglobin and is measured by arterial oxygen saturation (SaO_2). A very small amount of oxygen (less than 5%) is dissolved in plasma and measured as PaO_2. A sufficient amount of hemoglobin is required to ensure adequate oxygen-carrying capacity. The two primary determinants of oxygen content are hemoglobin and oxygen saturation.

Cardiac Output

Cardiac output is required to deliver oxygenated blood to the cells of the body. DaO_2 is assessed by evaluating the adequacy of cardiac output and arterial oxygen content. In nonstressed states, normal DaO_2 is 1,000 mL O_2/minute, or indexed to BSA, 600 mL O_2/

Table 17-20 • Oxygen Utilization Variables		
Parameter	**Formula**	**Normal Values**
CaO_2	$(Hb \times 1.37 \times SaO_2) + (0.003 \times PaO_2)$	20 mL O_2/dL
CvO_2	$(Hb \times 1.37 \times S\bar{v}O_2) + (0.003 \times PvO_2)$	15 mL O_2/dL
DaO_2l	$CI \times CaO_2 \times 10$	500–600 mL O_2/min/m²
DvO_2l	$CI \times CvO_2 \times 10$	375–450 mL O_2/min/m²
$S\bar{v}O_2$	Direct measurement	60%–80%
PvO_2	Direct measurement	35–45 mm Hg
O_2 extraction	$CaO_2 - CvO_2$	3–5 mL O_2/dL
OER	$\dfrac{CaO_2 - CvO_2}{CaO_2}$	22%–30%
VO_2l	$(CaO_2 - CvO_2) \times CI \times 10$	120–170 mL/min/m²
pHa	Direct measurement	7.35–7.45
BE/BD	Direct measurement	−2 to +2
Lactate	Direct measurement	0.5–2.2 mmol/L

OER, oxygen extraction ratio; VO₂l, oxygen consumption index; pHa, arterial pH; BE/BD, base excess/base deficit; CaO₂, arterial oxygen content; Hb, hemoglobin; CvO₂, venous oxygen content; DaO₂l, arterial oxygen delivery index; DvO₂l, venous oxygen delivery index.

minute/m². Increases in the body's oxygen demand associated with injury or illness are initially and primarily met by a compensatory increase in cardiac output. Deficiencies of hemoglobin, arterial saturation, or cardiac output decrease DaO_2 to cells and threaten the adequacy of cellular oxygenation.[10]

DETERMINANTS OF OXYGEN CONSUMPTION

Oxygen consumption ($\dot{V}O_2$) is the amount of oxygen used by the tissues of the body. The primary determinants of $\dot{V}O_2$ are the cellular demand for oxygen, the delivery of adequate amounts of oxygen, and the extraction of oxygen from the blood for use by the cells.

Oxygen Demand

Oxygen demand is the requirement of cells for oxygen and is not directly measurable. Any stress increases the oxygen demand (e.g., surgery, infection, mobilization, pain, anxiety). Reduced oxygen demands are associated with lower metabolic rates (e.g., hypothermia, sedation, pharmacological paralysis). Oxygen demands are met through adequate delivery of oxygen and cellular extraction of oxygen.

Oxygen Delivery

Cellular use of oxygen depends on an adequate supply of oxygen. This is termed delivery-dependent oxygen consumption (Fig. 17-65). As oxygen delivery increases, oxygen consumption also increases to meet the oxygen demand. When the requirement for oxygen is met, further increases in oxygen delivery do not increase consumption. The level of critical oxygen delivery is the point at which a decrease in oxygen delivery results in decreased $\dot{V}O_2$ because of an insufficient oxygen supply.

Oxygen Extraction

Oxygen extraction ($CaO_2 - C\bar{v}O_2$) is the amount of oxygen removed from the blood for use by the cells.

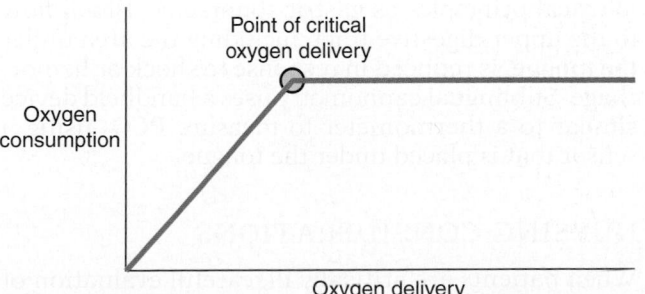

Figure 17-65 • Delivery-dependent oxygen consumption curve reflecting the change in oxygen consumption related to oxygen delivery. At the point of critical oxygen delivery, oxygen delivery is sufficient to meet oxygen demand, and oxygen consumption does not increase further. However, any decrease in oxygen delivery from this point results in a decrease of oxygen consumption due to an inadequate supply of oxygen.

It is measured by comparing the arterial oxygen content to venous oxygen content. Like arterial oxygen content, venous oxygen content ($C\bar{v}O_2$) is primarily determined by the amount of hemoglobin that is saturated with oxygen. Venous saturation is obtained by withdrawing a mixed venous blood gas sample from the distal port of the PAC, or by using an $S\bar{v}O_2$ or $ScvO_2$ monitoring PAC or central venous catheter, as discussed later in this section.

In normal circumstances, provided that oxygen is supplied in adequate amounts, the cells extract the oxygen they need to support tissue and organ function. Increased demand for oxygen results in a compensatory increase in oxygen extraction as more oxygen is "unloaded" from the hemoglobin for cellular use. The decreased amount of oxygen in venous blood means that the $CaO_2 - C\bar{v}O_2$ difference is larger. Conversely, as oxygen demands decrease, less oxygen is required and extracted from the blood, and the $CaO_2 - C\bar{v}O_2$ difference becomes smaller.[9]

OXYGEN SUPPLY AND DEMAND IMBALANCE

An imbalance of oxygen supply and demand occurs whenever oxygen delivery is inadequate to meet cellular demand or the cells are unable to extract sufficient quantities of oxygen. Specific threats to the balance of oxygen supply and demand are decreased cardiac output, hemoglobin, or arterial saturation; impaired cellular extraction of oxygen; or oxygen demands that are so great that they cannot be met by increased oxygen delivery or extraction.

Metabolic Indicators of Oxygen Delivery and Utilization Imbalance

Inadequate oxygen consumption causes an anaerobic state and cellular hypoxia. Cells deprived of oxygen begin to acquire an oxygen debt. Over time, oxygen debt accumulation becomes irreversible, cell damage is irreparable, and cell death results. Oxygen debt is a major cause of multisystem organ dysfunction and failure. If oxygen debt accumulation is identified before irreversible cell injury has occurred, the oxygen deficit may be reversed by increasing oxygen availability.

Several metabolic parameters can be measured to evaluate oxygen debt. When these indicators of oxygen debt are used in conjunction with hemodynamic monitoring of oxygen delivery and consumption, therapies may be more specifically directed to achieve a balanced oxygen supply and demand.

Because hypoxia and oxygen debt are associated with anaerobic metabolism, the byproducts of anaerobic metabolism can be used to assess the presence of an oxygen deficit. Lactic acid accumulation causes a metabolic acidosis in an oxygen debt state. Therefore, laboratory measurement of lactate levels, serum pH, and base deficit/excess are means to evaluate oxygen debt. Serum pH and base deficit/excess are routinely measured and reported with blood gas analysis. Elevated lactate levels (>2.2 mm/L) or metabolic acidosis (pH < 7.35 with normal $PaCO_2$) correlate with oxygen debt, particularly when the patient has a low or even normal level of DaO_2 and $\dot{V}O_2$. As with all assessment parameters, lactate levels, pH, and base deficit should not be viewed in isolation; they should be evaluated in conjunction with other assessment parameters.[9]

Monitoring of Mixed Venous and Central Venous Oxygen Saturation

Mixed venous oxygen saturation ($S\bar{v}O_2$) is measured using a PAC and reflects the level of oxyhemoglobin in desaturated blood returning to the right ventricle and PA. Venous oxygen saturation can also be measured in the superior vena cava ($ScvO_2$) through a central venous catheter. Both $S\bar{v}O_2$ and $ScvO_2$ are useful to evaluate the global balance of oxygen supply, oxygen utilization, and oxygen demand. The $S\bar{v}O_2$ or $ScvO_2$ is significantly lower than arterial saturation because of the extraction of oxygen by the cells and the unloading of oxygen from hemoglobin.

$S\bar{v}O_2$ or $ScvO_2$ is influenced by the degree of arterial saturation, the quantity of hemoglobin, the cardiac output (the determinants of oxygen delivery), and the amount of oxygen extracted and consumed by the cells. Under normal conditions of oxygen delivery, oxygen consumption, and oxygen demand, approximately 25% of the available oxygen is extracted and used to meet demand. In this situation, the $S\bar{v}O_2$ or $ScvO_2$ is in the normal range of 60% to 80%. If oxygen delivery is reduced by a decrease in arterial saturation, hemoglobin, or cardiac output, then more oxygen is extracted from the blood to meet cellular demand. The blood returning to the right side of the heart and PA has had a greater quantity of oxygen removed and is more desaturated, which is reflected by a decrease in $ScvO_2$ or $S\bar{v}O_2$. Similarly, if oxygen demand increases but oxygen delivery does not increase to meet this requirement, additional oxygen is extracted from the blood and consumed by the cells. Therefore, oxyhemoglobin is reduced in the venous blood, decreasing $S\bar{v}O_2$ or $ScvO_2$. Persistently low $S\bar{v}O_2$ or $ScvO_2$ is a warning that cellular hypoxia and an oxygen debt may be developing because of inadequate oxygen delivery or a high oxygen demand not met by the oxygen supply.

Three general conditions result in increasing $S\bar{v}O_2$ or $ScvO_2$:

▶ An oxygen delivery that is much greater than the oxygen demand; only a small percentage of the delivered oxygen is extracted, causing $S\bar{v}O_2$ or $ScvO_2$ to increase.

▶ A low metabolic rate and oxygen demand; the need for oxygen is reduced, and less oxygen is extracted and consumed. $S\bar{v}O_2$ or $ScvO_2$ reflects the decrease in extraction as greater amounts of oxyhemoglobin are returned to the right side of the heart.

▶ Pathological states in which the cells cannot extract oxygen from the blood or in which tissue beds are not well perfused with oxygenated blood; oxygen is not extracted from the blood despite the cellular oxygen demand. The $S\bar{v}O_2$ or $ScvO_2$, returning to the right side of the heart and PA, is therefore higher because of the decreased oxygen consumption.

Although the $S\bar{v}O_2$ or $ScvO_2$ may be in the normal range, cells in the body may not use or receive the oxygen they require. In these instances, cells become reliant on anaerobic metabolism because of the reduced cellular oxygen extraction or the shunting of oxygenated blood past tissue beds. Thus, a normal $S\bar{v}O_2$ or $ScvO_2$ may be misleading when viewed in isolation.

As mentioned previously, $S\bar{v}O_2$ or $ScvO_2$ can be continuously measured at the bedside by specialized central venous catheters or PACs containing fiberoptic filaments in one of the lumens ending at the distal end. The venous blood in the superior vena cava and PA is desaturated venous blood. An infrared light is emitted that reflects off the red blood cells that are saturated with oxygen. The percentage of saturated hemoglobin compared with the total hemoglobin is calculated by the $S\bar{v}O_2$ monitoring computer to yield the venous saturation value. The information is updated every few seconds; thus, a continuous $S\bar{v}O_2$ or $ScvO_2$ reading is obtained.

Regional Tissue Perfusion Monitoring

Lactate, base deficit and excess, and $S\bar{v}O_2$ or $ScvO_2$ are measures of global tissue oxygenation status. Gastric tonometry and sublingual CO_2 monitoring are methods to evaluate perfusion of specific tissue beds that have early susceptibility to hypoperfusion.[11,12] In early shock or shock states, compensatory diversion of blood flow from the splanchnic bed and digestive tract to vital organs causes the gastric mucosa and upper gastrointestinal tract to be underperfused. Anaerobic metabolism produces increased amounts of CO_2 and lactate; thus, measuring the CO_2 level or pH of these tissue beds provides an early indicator of oxygen supply and demand mismatch.

Gastric tonometry uses a nasogastric tube with a gas-permeable balloon near the distal end. CO_2 diffuses from the gastric wall into the balloon. Sampling the contents allows measurement of the PCO_2 and gastric mucosal pH. Normal gastric mucosal pH is 7.35 to 7.45, and normal gastric mucosal PCO_2 is 35 to 45 mm Hg. Decreasing gastric mucosal pH or an increasing gastric PCO_2 out of the normal range suggests hypoperfusion and is an indication that oxygen delivery and consumption should be analyzed and optimized.

Sublingual capnometry is based on the same physiological principles as gastric tonometry. Blood flow to the upper digestive tract, including the area under the tongue, is reduced in response to shock or hemorrhage. Sublingual capnometry uses a handheld device similar to a thermometer to measure PCO_2 using a sensor that is placed under the tongue.

NURSING CONSIDERATIONS

When patients are critically ill, careful evaluation of the adequacy of oxygen delivery, oxygen extraction, and consumption with respect to oxygen demand is paramount. Scrutiny of each determinant of cardiac output (heart rate, preload, afterload, and contractility parameters), oxygen content (arterial saturation and hemoglobin), oxygen consumption (DaO_2

and $CaO_2 - CvO_2$), and oxygen debt (lactate, pH, base deficit and excess, $S\bar{v}O_2$ or $ScvO_2$) is important to critical care nursing.

Numerous interventions are used to enhance oxygen delivery. Measures to increase cardiac output include the addition of intravascular volume to increase preload as well as the administration of positive inotropic agents to improve contractility and vasodilating agents to reduce afterload. Interventions that may increase oxygen content include changes in mechanical ventilator settings; chest physiotherapy; positioning and mobilization; and, in nonmechanically ventilated patients, coughing and deep-breathing exercises. All these techniques improve arterial oxygenation. Administration of packed red blood cells increases hemoglobin and oxygen-carrying capacity. In all cases, it is necessary to manage both the treatment modalities and patient response to therapy.

Many of the interventions used to decrease oxygen demand and increase oxygen consumption are important tenets of nursing care. For example, appropriate management of the environment, pain, and anxiety reduces stress, thus decreasing the demand for oxygen. Maintaining normothermia by control of the patient's temperature may decrease oxygen requirements associated with fevers and facilitate impaired perfusion and oxygen consumption associated with hypothermia.

$S\bar{v}O_2$ or $ScvO_2$ monitoring may be a helpful guide in nursing interventions. For example, endotracheal suctioning may cause a temporary decrease in arterial oxygenation and increase discomfort and anxiety. Monitoring $S\bar{v}O_2$ or $ScvO_2$ allows the nurse to judge the impact of this activity on the patient's oxygen supply and demand. A decreasing $S\bar{v}O_2$ or $ScvO_2$ during suctioning is usually caused by increased oxygen demand and decreased arterial oxygenation. Hyperoxygenating and hyperventilating before, during, and after suctioning helps lessen the negative effects on oxygen demand and arterial oxygenation. Before proceeding to another activity such as repositioning, the nurse should monitor the $S\bar{v}O_2$ or $ScvO_2$ and wait until the value normalizes, thereby avoiding an additional stressor and further increase on oxygen demand.

• Clinical Applicability Challenges

Case Study: Hemodynamic Monitoring

Ms. J., a 68-year-old woman, collapsed in her garden. She was subsequently admitted to the coronary care unit. She has a 10-year history of coronary artery disease and is taking propranolol, digoxin, and nitroglycerin ointment. On admission, she appears pale, diaphoretic, lethargic, and disoriented. Heart sounds S_1, S_2, S_3, S_4 are audible. Her electrocardiogram (ECG) shows Mobitz II, premature ventricular contractions (PVCs), and ST elevation in V_3, V_4, and aVL. Vital signs are: heart rate, 90 beats/minute; blood pressure, 90/50 mm Hg; and respiratory rate,

24 breaths/minute. Arterial blood gas measurements are: PaO_2, 73 mm Hg; $PaCO_2$, 25 mm Hg; SaO_2, 96%; and pH, 7.35.

Initial interventions include control of anginal pain, supplemental oxygen, and a lidocaine infusion. Because of Ms. J.'s age and history, a pulmonary artery catheter is inserted. One hour after admission, the following hemodynamic data are obtained:

- Right atrial pressure: 10 mm Hg
- Pulmonary artery systolic/diastolic pressure: 35/20 mm Hg
- Pulmonary artery wedge pressure: 19 mm Hg
- Cardiac index:1.3 L/min/m²
- Systemic vascular resistance: 1688 d/s/cm⁻⁵
- $S\bar{v}O_2$: 48%

Interventions to improve Ms. J.'s cardiac function and organ perfusion include lidocaine infusion at 1 mg/minute, nitroglycerin infusion at 10 µg/minute, dobutamine infusion at 7 µg/min, morphine for pain, IV, PRN; oxygen, 4 L/min by nasal cannula; intra-aortic balloon counterpulsation, 1:1; and standby pacemaker insertion. Therapeutic goals are stabilized cardiac conduction, enhanced myocardial contractility at the least cost to the heart by reducing preload and afterload, and improved oxygen supply to the myocardium. The combination of drugs and supplemental oxygen serves to achieve these goals. Intra-aortic balloon pumping primarily decreases afterload but also augments coronary perfusion.

Several hours later, assessment shows that Ms. J. is still pale but has improved capillary refill and is oriented to person, place, and time. Audible heart sounds are S_1, S_2, and S_4. ECG shows rare premature ventricular contractions with ST elevation and T inversion in V_3, V_4, and aVL. Vital signs are: heart rate, 85 beats/min; blood pressure, 100/50 mm Hg; respiratory rate, 18 breaths/minute. Arterial blood gas measurements are: PaO_2, 138 mm Hg; $PaCO_2$, 31 mm Hg; SaO_2, 99%, and pH, 7.44. At this time, hemodynamic data are:

- Right atrial pressure: 9 mm Hg
- Pulmonary artery systolic/diastolic pressure: 33/17 mm Hg
- Pulmonary artery wedge pressure: 15 mm Hg
- Cardiac index: 2.6 L/min/m²
- Systemic vascular resistance: 1014 d/s/cm⁻⁵
- $S\bar{v}O_2$: 60%

The results of the interventions are improved left ventricular function, which reduced the backward failure; loss of S_3; and improved arterial oxygenation. The Mobitz II conduction defect resolves as coronary perfusion increases. The metabolic acidosis also appears to be resolving due to improved oxygen delivery to the organs as evidenced by normalization of both the $PaCO_2$ and pH.

1. What are the main concerns associated with the initial assessment findings?

2. What is the significance of the first set of hemodynamic data?

3. How did the interventions affect Ms. J.'s hemodynamic status and oxygen delivery?

Review Questions

1. Risk factors for cardiovascular disease are classified as controllable and uncontrollable. Which of the following factors is considered controllable?
   a. Age and gender
   b. Hypertension
   c. Heredity
   d. Race

2. You are listening to your patient's heart sounds and hear both the S_1 and the S_2 sounds. S_1 is best heard in what area of the chest?
   a. Mitral area, the apex
   b. Tricuspid area, the left sternal border
   c. Aortic area, the second right intercostal space
   d. Pulmonic area, the second left intercostal space

3. You see on the patient's record that he has a mid-systolic heart murmur. This means that
   a. the murmur starts with S_1 and stops with S_2 without a gap between the murmur and the heart sound.
   b. the murmur starts in mid to late systole and continues up to S_2.
   c. the murmur starts just after S_2 and fades before the next S_1.
   d. the murmur begins after S_1 and stops before S_2.

4. Mrs. D. is a 67-year-old woman with a history of past (and current) cigarette smoking, hypertension, chest pain, and type 2 diabetes mellitus. Her low-density lipoprotein (LDL) cholesterol is 160 ng/mL, and she asks if she should be treated for high cholesterol. Her situation is described as
   a. low risk for heart disease, with normal LDL cholesterol.
   b. high risk for heart disease, with high LDL cholesterol.
   c. low risk for heart disease, with high LDL cholesterol.
   d. high risk for heart disease, with low LDL cholesterol.

5. In a patient with myocardial infarction, the serum markers for myocardial injury most likely to be elevated within the first 24 hours of infarct are
   a. creatine kinase (CK), CK-MM, and troponin-I.
   b. CK, CK-MB, and B-type natriuretic peptide (BNP).
   c. troponin-T, BNP, and lactate dehydrogenase.
   d. CK, CK-MB, and troponin-T.

6. Troponin-I and troponin-T elevations are most likely to be seen in
   a. myocardial necrosis only.
   b. myocardial necrosis, renal failure, and sepsis.
   c. myocardial necrosis and advanced osteoporosis.
   d. chest pain, renal failure, and advanced osteoporosis.

7. Mr. S. is 63-year-old man who has been admitted after an extensive myocardial infarction. He has developed heart failure as a result of the myocardial infarction and is being sent for testing to determine the extent of the heart failure. The diagnostic study most likely to give information regarding the status of his left ventricular function is
   a. exercise stress test with myocardial perfusion imaging.
   b. signal-averaged electrocardiogram.
   c. Holter monitoring.
   d. transthoracic echocardiogram.

8. Tracey is an 18-year-old woman who presents complaining of a fluttering sensation in her chest. She has had three episodes in the past 6 months. The duration of the episodes varies, but when they last more than a minute, she becomes dizzy and feels faint. The episodes are also unpredictable in timing and frequency. The test most likely to identify any cardiac cause of the episodes is
   a. tilt table study.
   b. continuous loop monitoring.
   c. Holter monitoring.
   d. electrophysiology testing.

9. Mrs. C. is an 82-year-old woman with advanced heart failure, with known mitral and aortic stenosis. She presents in stable condition from home for transesophageal echocardiography. Preprocedure care for Mrs. C. would include
   a. NPO for 6 hours, intravenous (IV) line in place, and electrocardiogram (ECG) within the previous 24 hours.
   b. NPO for 6 hours, arterial line in place for continuous blood pressure monitoring, and continuous ECG monitoring.
   c. IV line in place, continuous ECG monitoring, and intubation.
   d. NPO for 6 hours, IV line in place, and continuous ECG monitoring.

10. Pharmacological stress testing always includes
    a. myocardial perfusion imaging.
    b. serum measurements of markers for myocardial injury.
    c. treadmill walking or stationary biking.
    d. Holter monitoring.

11. You have decided to monitor your patient using a modified version of chest lead V_1 (MCL_1). To achieve this electrical view of the heart, you would turn the monitor to lead I and place the lead wires in which of the following positions?
    a. Negative below the left clavicle and positive in the left midaxillary line, fifth intercostal space
    b. Negative below the right clavicle and positive in the left midclavicular line below lowest rib
    c. Negative below the right clavicle and positive below the left clavicle
    d. Negative below the left clavicle and positive in the fourth intercostal space, right sternal border

12. You have decided to monitor your patient using lead I. Based on Einthoven's triangle, where are the positive and negative leads located?
    a. The positive is the left arm and the negative is the right arm.
    b. The positive is the right arm and the negative is the left arm.
    c. The positive is the left leg and the negative is the right arm.
    d. The positive is the left leg and the negative is the left arm.

13. The P wave represents
    a. contraction of the atria.
    b. repolarization of the atria.
    c. depolarization of the atria.
    d. depolarization of the ventricles.

14. You are analyzing your patient's rhythm strip and note the following: rate is 62 beats/minute; rhythm is irregular; P waves are present; and there is one P wave for each QRS complex. What is the name of this rhythm?
    a. Normal sinus rhythm
    b. Atrial fibrillation
    c. Sinus arrhythmia
    d. Sinus bradycardia

15. Patients in atrial flutter are at increased risk for thromboembolism. The reason for this is that
    a. the contents of the atria are not sufficiently expelled, allowing thrombi to form.
    b. atrial flutter is often accompanied by platelet aggregation.
    c. atrial flutter so diminishes cardiac output that patient's inactivity results in thrombus formation in the lower legs and pelvic regions.
    d. atrial flutter is nearly always a symptom of underlying valvular heart disease, a common site of thrombus formation.

16. If the PR interval were prolonged,
    a. the sinoatrial node would probably be malfunctioning.
    b. conduction through the atrioventricular node would be delayed.
    c. conduction through the ventricle would be delayed.
    d. conduction would be blocked at the left bundle branches.

17. Which criterion below is most important in deciding when sinus bradycardia should be treated?
    a. Whether the patient is symptomatic from the bradycardia
    b. The rate; if the rate is less than 50 beats/minute, it should be treated
    c. Ventilatory status; if the bradycardia is due to inadequate ventilations, atropine is indicated
    d. The stability of the ventricular focus

18. Mrs. Smith develops a sinus tachycardia at a rate of 140 beats/minute. Although her heart rate is rapid, she may still have inadequate cardiac output because of
    a. the loss of atrial kick.
    b. the decreased systolic filling time.
    c. the decreased diastolic filling time.
    d. the increased afterload.

19. Second-degree atrioventricular block, Mobitz II is characterized by
    a. a PR interval of more than 0.20 seconds and equal.
    b. more than one P wave per QRS and unequal PR intervals.
    c. more than one P wave per QRS and equal PR intervals.
    d. a progressive lengthening of the PR interval.

20. Hypokalemia may cause which of the following changes on the electrocardiogram?
    a. Tall, peaked T waves
    b. U wave
    c. Prolonged QT interval
    d. Shortened QT interval

21. Hypercalcemia produces which of the following changes on the electrocardiogram?
    a. Prolonged QT interval
    b. Shortened QT interval
    c. Prominent U waves
    d. Tall, peaked T waves

22. The nurse notes a change in the arterial line pressure waveform and a decrease in the patient's blood pressure. The appropriate first action is to
    a. conduct a square wave test.
    b. re-level the transducer.
    c. place the patient in Trendelenburg position.
    d. notify the physician of the decrease in blood pressure.

23. A patient with a history of a myocardial infarction has a pulmonary artery wedge pressure that increased from 8 mm Hg to 14 mm Hg in the past 4 hours. This may be an indication of
    a. reduced blood volume and decreased left ventricular preload.
    b. left ventricular failure and decreased forward blood flow.
    c. pulmonary embolus and decreased left ventricular preload.
    d. right ventricular failure and venous congestion.

References

Cardiac History and Physical Examination

1. American Heart Association: Risk Factors and Coronary Heart Disease. Retrieved January 18, 2008, from http://www.AHA.org
2. American Heart Association: Heart and Stroke Facts. Retrieved January 18, 2008, from http://www.AHA.org
3. Bickley L: Bates' Guide to Physical Examination and Health History, 9th ed. Philadelphia: Lippincott Williams & Wilkins, 2007
4. Weber J, Kelley J: Health Assessment in Nursing, 3rd ed. Philadelphia: Lippincott Williams & Wilkins, 2007

Cardiac Laboratory Studies

1. Antman EM, Anbe DT, Armstrong PW, et al: ACC/AHA guidelines for the management of patients with ST-elevation myocardial infarction. Executive summary: A report of the American College of Cardiology/American Heart Association task force on practice guidelines (Committee to revise the 1999 guidelines for the management of patients with acute myocardial infarction). Circulation 110:588–636, 2004
2. Third Report of the NCEP on Detection, Evaluation and Treatment of High Blood Cholesterol in Adults (ATP III). Circulation 106:3143–3421, 2002

3. Grundy SM, Cleeman JI, Merz N: Implications of recent clinical trials for the National Cholesterol Education Program Adult Treatment Panel III Guidelines. Circulation 110:227–239, 2004
4. ACC/AHA Guidelines for the Management of Patients with Unstable Angina/non-ST Segment Myocardial Infarction: A report of the ACC/AHA Task Force on Practice Guidelines. Circulation 116:803–807, 2007
5. Homma S, Grahame-Clarke C: Editorial comment-myocardial damage in patients with subarachnoid hemorrhage. Stroke 35:552, 2004
6. Logeart D, Beyne P, Cusson C, et al: Evidence of cardiac myolysis in severe nonischemic heart failure and the potential role of increased wall strain. Am Heart J 141:24
7. Freda B, Tang W, Van Lente F, et al: Cardiac troponins in renal insufficiency, review and clinical implications. J Am Coll Cardiol 40:2065–2071, 2002
8. de Lemos JA, Morroq DA, Bentley JH, et al: The prognostic value of B-type natriuretic peptide in patients with acute coronary syndromes. N Engl J Med 345:1014–1021, 2001
9. Doust JA, Tietrazak E, Dobson A, Glasziou P: How well does B-type natriuretic peptide predict death and cardiac events in patients with heart failure? A systematic review. BMJ 330:625, 2005
10. Wang TJ, Larson MG, Levy D, et al: Plasma natriuretic peptide levels and the risk of cardiovascular events and death. N Engl J Med 350:655, 2004
11. Sabatine MS, Morrow DA, Jablonski KA, et al: Prognostic significance of the Centers for Disease Control/American Heart Association high-sensitivity C-reactive protein cut points for cardiovascular and other outcomes in patients with stable coronary artery disease. Circulation 115:1528, 2007
12. McCullough PA, Nowak RM, Foreback C, et al: Performance of multiple cardiac biomarkers measured in the emergency department in patients with chronic kidney disease and chest pain. Acad Emerg Med 9:1389, 2002
13. Paneesha S, Cheyne E, French K, et al: High D-dimer levels at presentation in patients with venous thromboembolism is a marker of adverse clinical outcomes. Br J Haematol 135(1): 85–90, 2006

Cardiac Diagnostic Tests

1. Blancher S: Cardiac electrophysiology procedures. In Woods SL, Froelicher ESS, Motzer SU, Bridges EJ (eds): Cardiac Nursing, 5th ed. Philadelphia: Lippincott Williams & Wilkins, 2005, pp 425–430
2. Albert N, Massaro L, Morley M, Overman K: Cardiac diagnostic testing: Past, present, and future. Crit Care Nurse 1–13, 2006
3. Marchiondo K: Transesophageal imaging and interventions: Nursing implications. Crit Care Nurse 27(2):25–35, 2007
4. Deelstra MH, Jacobson C: Cardiac catheterization. In Woods SL, Froelicher ESS, Motzer SU, Bridges EJ (eds): Cardiac Nursing, 5th ed. Philadelphia: Lippincott Williams & Wilkins, 2005, pp 459–477

Electrocardiographic Monitoring

1. Drew BJ, Califf RM, Funk M, et al. Practice standards for electrocardiographic monitoring in hospital settings: An American Heart Association scientific statement from the Councils on Cardiovascular Nursing, Clinical Cardiology, and Cardiovascular Disease in the Young. Circulation 110: 2721–2746, 2004
2. Huff J: EKG Workout: Exercises in Arrhythmia Interpretation, 5th ed. Philadelphia: Lippincott Williams & Wilkins, 2006

Hemodynamic Monitoring

1. Darovic G: Hemodynamic Monitoring: Invasive and Noninvasive Clinical Application, 3rd ed. Philadelphia: WB Saunders, 2002
2. Daily E: Hemodynamic waveform analysis. J Cardiovasc Nurs 15(2):6–22, 2001
3. AACN Practice Alert Pulmonary Artery Pressure Monitoring 2004. Retrieved June 6, 2006, from http://www.aacn.org
4. McGhee B, Bridges E: Monitoring arterial blood pressure: What you may not know. Crit Care Nurse 22(2):60–79, 2002
5. Adams K: Hemodynamic assessment: The physiologic basis for turning data into clinical information. AACN Clin Issues 15(4):535–546, 2004
6. Headley JM: Arterial Pressure-Based Technologies: A New Trend in Cardiac Output Monitoring. Crit Care Nurs Clin N Am 18:179–187, 2006
7. Michard F: Changes in arterial pressure during mechanical ventilation. Anesthesia 103(2):419–428, 2005
8. Albert N: Bioimpedance cardiography measurements of cardiac output and other cardiovascular parameters. Crit Care Nurs Clin N Am 18(2):195–202, 2006
9. Turner MA: Doppler-based hemodynamic monitoring: A minimally invasive alternative. AACN Clin Issues 14(2):220–231, 2003
10. Vary T, McLean B, Von Rueden KT: Shock and multiple organ dysfunction syndrome. In McQuillan K, Von Rueden K, Hartsock R, et al (eds): Trauma Nursing: Resuscitation Through Rehabilitation, 3rd ed. Philadelphia: WB Saunders, 2002, pp 173–200
11. Boswell S, Scalea TM: Sublingual capnometry: An alternative to gastric tonometry for the management of shock resuscitation. AACN Clin Issues 14:176–184, 2003
12. Ruffolo D, Headley J: Regional carbon dioxide monitoring: A different look at tissue perfusion. AACN Clin Issues 14:166–175, 2003

Other Selected Readings

Cardiac Laboratory Studies

Casey PE: Markers of myocardial injury and dysfunction. AACN Clin Issues 15(4):547–557, 2004
Chizner MA: Clinical Cardiology Made Ridiculously Simple, 2nd ed. Miami: Medmaster, 2007
Lin W, Cook DJ, Griffith LE, et al: Elevated cardiac troponin levels in critically ill patients: Prevalence, incidence, and outcomes. Am J Crit Care 15(3):280–289, 2006
MacKenzie JR: Predicting CAD events. C-reactive protein: A marker for atherosclerotic risk. Nurse Pract 29(6):14–27, 2004

Cardiac Diagnostic Tests

Applebaum E, Botnar R, Yeon S, Manning W: Coronary magnetic resonance imaging: current state of the art. Coron Artery Dis 16(6):345–353, 2005
Bosen D, Flemming M: Electrophysiologic testing. Dimens Crit Care Nurs 22(1):10–19, 2003
Di Carli MF, Dorbala S: Cardiac PET-CT. J Thorac Imag 22(1): 101–106, 2007
Heger JW, Niemann JT, Criley JM: Cardiology, 5th ed. Philadelphia: Lippincott Williams & Wilkins, 2004
Kern MJ: The Cardiac Catheterization Handbook, 4th ed. St. Louis: Mosby, 2003
Kuo D, Dilsician V, Prasad R, White C: Emergency cardiac imaging: State of the art. Cardiol Clin 8:1–13, 2005
Murphy JG (ed): Mayo Clinic Cardiology: Concise Textbook, 3rd ed. Rochester, MN: Informa Healthcare, 2006
Raggi P, Taylor A, Fayad Z, et al: Atherosclerotic plaque imaging: Contemporary role in preventive cardiology. Arch Intern Med 165(20):2345–2353, 2005
Reiff PA, Gutierez JD: Use of the insertable loop recorder to detect cardiac arrhythmias during syncopal episodes. Medsurg Nurs 13(2):105–109, 2004
Watkins MW: Recent advances in cardiac computed tomography. Coron Artery Dis 17(2):97–98, 2006
Wilkerson JT, Cohn JN, Wellens HJ, Holmes DR (eds): Cardiovascular Medicine, 3rd ed. New York: Springer, 2007
Zak J: Mapping ventricular tachycardia. Crit Care Nurse 26(5): 13–20, 2006

Electrocardiographic Monitoring

Drew BJ: Pulling it all together: Case studies on ECG monitoring. AACN Adv Crit Care 18(3):305–317, 2007

Erickson BA: Identifying complete heart block in elderly patients. Am Nurse Today 1(2):16–23, 2006

Flanders SA: ST-segment monitoring: Putting standards into practice. AACN Adv Crit Care 18(3):275–284, 2007

Goldich G: Understanding the 12-lead ECG, Part I. Nursing2006 36(11):36–41, 2006

Goldich G: Understanding the 12-lead ECG, Part II. Nursing2006 36(12):36–41, 2006

Jacobson C: Tools for teaching arrhythmias. AACN Adv Crit Care 17(2):230–232, 2006

Jacobson C: Tools for teaching arrhythmias: Wide QRS beats and rhythms. AACN Adv Crit Care 17(3):353–358, 2006

Jacobson C: Tools for teaching arrhythmias. Wide QRS beats and rhythms: Part II. AACN Adv Crit Care 18(1):91–96, 2007

Jacobson C: Atrioventricular dissociation. AACN Adv Crit Care 18(2):221–224, 2007

Jacobson C: Causes of bigeminy. AACN Adv Crit Care 18(3):330–332, 2007

Jacobson C: Narrow QRS tachycardias. AACN Adv Crit Care 18(3):264–274, 2007

Jalırsdoerfer M, Giuliano K, Stephens D: Clinical usefulness of the EASI 12-lead continuous electrocardiographic monitoring system. Crit Care Nurse 25(5):28–37, 2005

Kern LS, McRae ME, Funk M: ECG monitoring after cardiac surgery: Post-operative atrial fibrillation and the atrial electrogram. AACN Adv Crit Care 18(3):294–304, 2007

Leeper B: Saving lives with continuous ST-segment monitoring. Am Nurse Today 2(2):12–14, 2007

Lim W, Qushmaq I, Cook DJ, Devereaux PJ, et al: Reliability of electrocardiogram interpretation in critically ill patients. Crit Care Med 34(5):1–6, 2006

Sommargren CE, Drew BJ: Preventing torsades de pointes by careful cardiac monitoring in hospital settings. AACN Adv Crit Care 18(3):285–293, 2007

Hemodynamic Monitoring

Adams K: Hemodynamic assessment: The physiologic basis for turning data into clinical information. AACN Clin Issues 15(4):534–546, 2004

Ahrens T: Hemodynamics in sepsis. AACN Adv Crit Care 17(4):435–445, 2006

Berton C, Cholley B: Equipment review: New techniques for cardiac output measurement. Oesophageal Doppler, Fick principle using carbon dioxide, and pulse contour analysis. Crit Care 6(3):216–221, 2002

Blissitt P: Hemodynamic monitoring in the care of the critically ill neuroscience patient. AACN Adv Crit Care 17(3):327–340, 2006

Bridges E: Pulmonary artery pressure monitoring: When, how and what else to use. AACN Adv Crit Care 17(3):286–303, 2006

Cottingham CA: Resuscitation of traumatic shock: A hemodynamic review. AACN Adv Crit Care 17(3):317–326, 2006

Dulak SB: What the waveforms reveal [Online]. RN Web 66(9):56–63, 2003. Available at: http://www.rnweb.com

Fawcett JAD: Hemodynamic Monitoring Made Easy. Philadelphia: Elsevier, 2006

Goodrich C: Continuous central venous oximetry monitoring. Crit Care Nurs Clin N Am 18(2):203–209, 2006

Hameed SM, Aird WE, Cohn SM: Oxygen delivery. Crit Care Med 13(Suppl 12):S658–S667, 2003

Johnson K: Diagnostic measures to evaluate oxygenation in critically ill adults: Implications and limitations. AACN Clin Issues 15(4):506–524, 2004

Leeper B: Monitoring right ventricular volumes: A paradigm shift. AACN Clin Issues 14(2):208–219, 2003

Moore K: Critical care hemodynamic parameters and pharmacologic interventions. Crit Care Nurs Clin N Am 14(1):71–76, 2002

Pinsky MR: Hemodynamic evaluation and monitoring in the ICU. Chest 132:2020–2079, 2007

Weigand DL, Carlson KK: AACN Procedure Manual for Critical Care. St Louis: Elsevier Saunders, 2005

Woods SL, Froelicher ES, Motzer SA, Bridges E: Cardiac Nursing. Philadelphia: Lippincott Williams & Wilkins, 2004

18

Patient Management: Cardiovascular System

Marla J. De Jong • Kathryn Escalera •
Vicki Coombs • Kenneth Rempher •
Dulce Obias-Manno • Conrad Gordon

DISCLAIMER STATEMENT

*Opinions or assertions contained herein are the private
views of the authors and are not to be construed as
official or as reflecting the views of the Department of
the Air Force or the Department of Defense.*

Objectives

Based on the content in this chapter, the reader should be able to:

1. Compare and contrast commonly used fibrinolytics, anticoagulants, and platelet inhibitors used to affect the thrombotic process.

2. Describe the four classes of antiarrhythmic drugs.

3. Explain how inotropic drugs improve myocardial function.

4. Discuss the rationale for using phosphodiesterase III inhibitor, angiotensin-converting enzyme inhibitor, and vasodilator drugs for patients with cardiovascular disease.

5. Compare and contrast the four major classes of antihyperlipidemic drugs.

6. Compare and contrast the indications and contraindications for percutaneous coronary interventions (PCI), including percutaneous transluminal coronary angioplasty and intracoronary stenting.

7. Summarize interventions for complications associated with PCI procedures.

8. List potential nursing diagnoses and the interventions for each diagnosis in the patient undergoing an interventional cardiology procedure.

9. Discuss the indications for percutaneous balloon valvuloplasty.

10. Describe the physiological effect of intra-aortic balloon pump (IABP) counterpulsation therapy.

11. Explain indications for and contraindications to IABP therapy.

12. Describe a ventricular assist device and its indications and mechanism of action.

13. Discuss nursing interventions for the patient receiving IABP therapy or ventricular circulatory assistance.

14. Describe the indications, procedure, and nursing management for electrical cardioversion.

15. Explain the indications, procedure and nursing management for radiofrequency catheter ablation.

16. Describe the indications for a permanent pacemaker.

17. Explain the components and functions of a pacemaker.

18. Describe modes of pacing using the pacemaker code.

19. Explain complications of pacing and appropriate interventions.

20. Discuss the nursing management of the patient with a pacemaker.

㉑ Describe the indications for an implantable cardioverter–defibrillator (ICD).

㉒ Describe the ICD components and function.

㉓ Explain the nursing management of a patient with an ICD.

㉔ Describe causes of cardiopulmonary arrest.

㉕ Explain steps of cardiopulmonary resuscitation.

㉖ Discuss roles of members of the resuscitation team.

㉗ Explain indications, procedure, and nursing management for defibrillation.

㉘ Discuss the rationale for using hypothermia as part of cardiopulmonary arrest management.

㉙ Describe pros and cons of having family members present in a cardiopulmonary arrest situation.

● Pharmacological Therapy

Cardiovascular disease continues to be the leading cause of death for men and women in the United States. However, recent and remarkable pharmacological advances have reduced morbidity and mortality related to cardiovascular disease.

Critical care nurses are responsible for preparing and administering potent drugs that affect the patient's cardiovascular function. Furthermore, nurses continuously evaluate the effects of these drugs and use detailed patient assessment data to guide the titration of these drugs.

This section summarizes drugs that are commonly used in critical care settings to treat cardiovascular disease. Recent research data are included to provide a scientific basis for drug therapy. Pharmacotherapy advances continually occur; therefore, changes in drug therapy are common. Critical care nurses frequently use current drug books or guides before administering drugs because nurses must know the drug's indications, effects, contraindications, dosage, method of administration, and adverse effects. Finally, many patients require treatment with numerous cardiovascular drugs; therefore, it is important to consider how drugs interact with other drugs.

• Fibrinolytics, Anticoagulants, and Platelet Inhibitors

Atherosclerotic plaque rupture or vascular endothelium damage initiates a complex platelet reaction, consisting of adhesion, activation, and aggregation. The platelet aggregate accelerates thrombin production through the coagulation cascade. When thrombin, a potent agonist for further platelet activation and coagulation cascade activity, converts fibrinogen to fibrin, a nonsoluble fibrin thrombus forms. For further information about the coagulation process, see Chapter 45. An arterial thrombus may transiently or persistently occlude coronary artery blood flow, causing acute coronary syndrome (ACS). For further information about ACS, see Chapter 21. Fibrinolytic, anticoagulant, and platelet inhibitor drugs affect different phases of the thrombotic process.

FIBRINOLYTICS

Fibrinolytic agents are indicated for patients with acute ST-segment elevation myocardial infarction (STEMI). The drugs are not effective and should not be administered to patients without ST-segment elevation or to patients with nonspecific electrocardiogram (ECG) changes.[1,2] Clinicians may give fibrinolytics to patients with ST depression if a true posterior myocardial infarction is suspected.[1] Fibrinolytic agents either directly or indirectly convert plasminogen to plasmin, which in turn lyses the thrombus. Early fibrinolytic therapy has been shown to dissolve the thrombus, reestablish coronary blood flow, minimize infarct size, preserve left ventricular function, and reduce morbidity and mortality.[1] Table 18-1 summarizes commonly used fibrinolytic agents.

Many researchers continue to evaluate the efficacy of fibrinolytic agents in conjunction with other medications such as glycoprotein (GP) IIb/IIIa inhibitors and low–molecular-weight heparins (LMWHs). Much research focuses on the benefit of fibrinolysis versus a primary percutaneous coronary intervention (PCI).[1] See Percutaneous Coronary Interventions and Percutaneous Balloon Valvuloplasty for further discussion. The Assessment of the Safety and Efficacy of a New Thrombolytic (ASSENT)-2 trial reported nearly identical mortality rates when tissue plasminogen activator (t-PA) and tenecteplase were compared.[3] The Global Utilization of Streptokinase and t-PA for Occluded Coronary Arteries (GUSTO) V trial found that half-dose reteplase plus abciximab did not reduce mortality significantly more than full-dose reteplase[4]; however, combination therapy may be considered to prevent reinfarction in patients with anterior acute myocardial infarction (AMI) who are younger than 75 years of age and who have no risk factors for bleeding.[1] A substudy of the Integrilin and Tenecteplase in Acute Myocardial Infarction (INTEGRITI) trial found that combination therapy with reduced-dose tenecteplase and high-dose eptifibatide was associated with faster ST-segment recovery and less recurrent ischemia than full-dose tenecteplase.[5]

The decision to administer fibrinolytic therapy is based on the patient's cardiovascular physical assessment data and ECG. Unless contraindicated

Table 18-1 • Fibrinolytic Drugs

	Action	Indications	Dose	Half-Life (min)
Alteplase	Binds to fibrin in a thrombus and converts plasminogen to plasmin	AMI Acute ischemic stroke Acute massive PE Cathflo Activase only: to restore function of a central venous access device (for patients ≥ 30 kg, instill 2 mg in 2 mL solution into blocked catheter; dose may be repeated if first dose not effective after 2 h)	Accelerated infusion: 100 mg IV over 90 min (15 mg IV bolus; 50 mg IV over next 30 min; 35 mg IV over next 60 min) 3-h infusion: 100 mg over 3 h (60 mg in the first h with 6–10 mg as a bolus, 20 mg over the second h, and 20 mg over the third h)	<5
Reteplase	Catalyzes the cleavage of plasminogen to generate plasmin	AMI	10 U + 10 U IV bolus (each 10 U given over 2 min; second bolus given 30 min after first bolus)	13–16
Tenecteplase	Binds to fibrin and converts plasminogen to plasmin	AMI	Weight-based dose IV over 5 sec: >60 kg = 30 mg ≥60 to <70 kg = 35 mg ≥70 to <80 kg = 40 mg ≥80 to <90 kg = 45 mg ≥90 kg = 50 mg	20–24
Streptokinase	Binds with plasminogen to produce a complex that converts plasminogen to plasmin	AMI Acute PE Acute, extensive DVT Acute arterial thrombosis or embolism (slowly instill 250,000 IU in 2 mL solution into occluded cannula and clamp for 2 h) Occluded arteriovenous cannulae	1,500,000 IU IV within 60 min	23

AMI, acute myocardial infarction; DVT, deep venous thrombosis; IV, intravenous; PE, pulmonary embolism.

(Box 18-1), fibrinolytics should be given to patients with acute STEMI (1) whose symptoms began within the previous 12 hours and who have ST-segment elevation greater than 0.1 mV in two or more contiguous precordial leads or in two or more adjacent limb leads, or (2) who have a new-onset left bundle branch block.[1] Fibrinolytic therapy produces the greatest mortality reduction when initiated within the first 0 to 4 hours of symptom onset; however, fibrinolytics may be administered up to 12 hours after symptom onset. The goal is to administer a fibrinolytic drug within 30 minutes of presentation. Patients are at risk for recurrent thromboembolism; therefore, aspirin and heparin are given to most patients who receive fibrinolytic therapy.[1,6]

Reperfusion may be manifested by decreased or resolved ST-segment elevation, abrupt cessation of chest pain, early peak of serum cardiac markers, and reperfusion dysrhythmias such as premature ventricular contractions (PVCs), ventricular tachycardia (VT), accelerated idioventricular rhythm, and atrioventricular (AV) blocks. In contrast, reocclusion may be evidenced by recurrent chest pain and ST-segment elevation, further myocardial ischemia or infarction, lethal dysrhythmias, cardiogenic shock, or death. The most common adverse effects of fibrinolytic therapy are bleeding, intracranial hemorrhage, stroke, and reperfusion dysrhythmias. For more details about the use of fibrinolytic therapy for AMI, see Chapter 21.

Box 18-1 • Contraindications for Fibrinolytic Therapy

- Active internal bleeding
- Any history of intracranial hemorrhage
- Ischemic stroke within 3 mo
- Intracranial neoplasm, arteriovenous malformation, or aneurysm
- Recent intracranial or intraspinal surgery
- Recent closed-head or facial trauma within 3 mo
- Suspected aortic dissection
- Severe uncontrolled hypertension
- Bleeding diathesis

ANTICOAGULANTS

Anticoagulants such as unfractionated heparin, LMWHs, direct thrombin inhibitors, and warfarin (Coumadin) limit further fibrin formation and help prevent thromboembolism.[7]

Unfractionated heparin, the most commonly used anticoagulant drug for acute conditions, is indicated for ACS, venous thromboembolism, PCIs, and surgical revascularization and for patients receiving alteplase, reteplase, or tenecteplase. Heparin prevents clot formation by combining with antithrombin III and inhibiting circulating thrombin. However, unfractionated heparin does not lyse thrombi and is not an optimal anticoagulant because of its narrow therapeutic range, low bioavailability, varied anticoagulant response, requirement for parenteral administration and activated partial thromboplastin time (APTT) monitoring, and risk for bleeding, heparin-induced thrombocytopenia (HIT), and hypersensitivity reactions.

The dosage for unfractionated heparin varies according to its indication and route of administration. When used in conjunction with alteplase (Activase), reteplase (Retavase), or tenecteplase (TNKase), the recommended heparin dosage is 60 unit/kg intravenous (IV; maximum 4,000 units) bolus given when the alteplase infusion is started, followed by an infusion of 12 units/kg/hour (maximum 1,000 units/hour) for ST-segment elevation AMI.[1,8] When IV heparin is administered for AMI with non–ST-segment elevation and unstable angina, an initial IV bolus of 60 to 70 units/kg (maximum 5,000 units) followed by a 12 to 15 units/kg/h infusion is recommended.[8] The heparin infusion rate is adjusted to maintain an APTT of 50 to 70 seconds for 48 hours. Protamine sulfate reverses the effects of heparin; however, protamine may cause a life-threatening anaphylactic reaction.

LMWHs, such as enoxaparin (Lovenox) and dalteparin (Fragmin), are small fragments derived from unfractionated heparin and are appealing alternatives to heparin for patients with unstable angina, non–ST-segment elevation AMI (NSTEMI), or deep venous thrombosis. Table 18-2 summarizes these drugs, which inhibit clot formation by blocking factor Xa and thrombin. Investigators have shown that enoxaparin is superior to unfractionated heparin for patients with STEMI, unstable angina, and non–Q-wave myocardial infarction (NQWMI).[9–12] In contrast, the Superior Yield of the New Strategy of Enoxaparin, Revascularization and Glycoprotein IIb/IIIa Inhibitors (SYNERGY) trial found no difference between unfractionated heparin and enoxaparin in the setting of early invasive treatment of ACS.[13] Results from the Thrombolysis in Myocardial Infarction (TIMI) 11B trial and a meta-analysis indicated that enoxaparin and aspirin reduced death, myocardial infarction, and the need for urgent revascularization more effectively than heparin and aspirin for patients with unstable angina or NSTEMI.[14,15]

The advantages of LMWHs are their longer half-life, more predictable anticoagulation effect, greater bioavailability, and cost-effectiveness. In addition, LMWHs are administered subcutaneously twice daily and do not require APTT monitoring.

The most common adverse effects of LMWHs include bleeding, thrombocytopenia, elevated aminotransferase levels, and pain, erythema, ecchymosis, or hematoma at the injection site. Because LMWHs have different molecular weight distribution profiles, activities, and plasma clearance rates, they must not be used interchangeably with each other or unfractionated heparin.

Bivalirudin (Angiomax), a direct thrombin inhibitor, may be administered as an alternative to unfractionated heparin in low-risk patients who undergo PCI or patients with HIT.[16] Data from the Randomized Evaluation of PCI Linking Angiomax to Reduced Clinical Events (REPLACE)-1 and -2 trials showed similar clinical outcomes for patients who were randomized to received either bivalirudin or unfractionated heparin.[17–19] The IV bolus dose for bivalirudin is 0.75 mg/kg, followed by an infusion of 1.75 mg/kg/hour for the duration of the PCI procedure. An additional bolus dose of 0.3 mg/kg may be given in 5 minutes depending on results of the activated clotting time (ACT). The infusion may be continued for 4 hours after the PCI procedure.

Lepirudin (Refludan) is a direct thrombin inhibitor used to prevent thromboembolic complications for patients with HIT and thromboembolic disease. After an IV bolus dose of 0.4 mg/kg (maximum 44 mg), an infusion is initiated at 0.15 mg/kg/hour (maximum 16.5 mg/hour). The infusion rate is adjusted to maintain an APTT ratio of 1.5 to 2.5 times the baseline value. As with other anticoagulants, the major adverse effects of lepirudin are bleeding complications.

Argatroban (Acova) is another direct thrombin inhibitor indicated for prophylaxis or treatment of thrombosis in HIT. The recommended initial dose is 2 µg/kg/minute given as a continuous infusion. Dose adjustments are made to maintain an APTT ratio of 1.5 to 3.0 times the baseline value.

Warfarin, an oral drug used for chronic anticoagulation therapy, interferes with the synthesis of vitamin K–dependent clotting factors such as factors II, VII, IX, and X. The most common cardiovascular indications for warfarin include post-AMI anticoagulation for high-risk patients, dilated cardiomyopathy, atrial fibrillation (AF), heart failure (HF), venous thromboembolism, mobile mural thrombus, and presence of a prosthetic heart valve. The Coumadin Aspirin

Table 18-2 • Low-Molecular-Weight Heparins

	Indications	Absolute Bioavailability	Dose for Patients with USA or Non–Q-wave AMI	Peak Effect	Half-Life
Dalteparin	USA (with aspirin) Non–Q-wave AMI (with aspirin) Prophylaxis of DVT	87%	120 IU/kg (maximum 10,000 IU) SC q12h	4 h	3–5 h
Enoxaparin	USA (with aspirin) Non–Q-wave AMI (with aspirin) Prophylaxis and treatment of DVT	100%	1 mg/kg SC q12h	3–4.5 h	4.5 h

AMI, acute myocardial infarction; DVT, deep venous thrombosis; SC, subcutaneous; USA, unstable angina.

Reinfarction Study (CARS) investigators reported that warfarin and aspirin combination therapy did not provide more benefits than aspirin monotherapy for patients after AMI.[20] Conversely, results of a recent meta-analysis indicated that warfarin plus aspirin combination therapy is associated with decreased recurrent AMI, stroke, and revascularization, but with increased major bleeding.[21] Although high-intensity oral anticoagulation (international normalized ratio [INR]: 3.0 to 4.0) and moderate-intensity anticoagulation (INR: 2.0 to 3.0) plus aspirin lower the risk for untoward outcomes such as AMI, stroke, and death, warfarin treatment regimens are more inconvenient and place patients at greater risk for significant bleeding.[22] Thus, oral anticoagulants are not routinely administered after infarction.

Contraindications for warfarin include uncontrolled hypertension; severe hepatic or renal disease; bleeding diathesis; gastrointestinal (GI) or genitourinary (GU) bleeding; cerebral or dissecting aortic aneurysm; recent central nervous system, eye, or other major surgery; recent trauma; pregnancy (first and third trimesters); pericarditis; pericardial effusion; spinal puncture; and recent diagnostic procedures with the potential for uncontrolled bleeding. Patients must be able and willing to adhere to this somewhat complicated therapy.

Warfarin is usually started at 5 to 10 mg daily but should be decreased for the elderly and patients with liver or renal impairment and HF. The dose is titrated according to the patient's INR. Because warfarin levels do not peak for 3 to 4 days, acute anticoagulant therapy is continued until the INR is at the desired level for the patient's condition, usually 2.5 to 3.5. The INR is evaluated daily until it is therapeutic. Once the INR is therapeutic on a stable warfarin dose, less frequent INR monitoring is appropriate. Elevated INR levels predispose the patient to bleeding, warfarin's most common adverse effect.

Patient education is an important part of warfarin therapy. Warfarin interacts with numerous drugs and foods; safe treatment depends on the patient's knowledge of therapy.

PLATELET INHIBITORS

Aspirin, the most widely used platelet inhibitor, inhibits thromboxane A_2, a platelet agonist, and prevents thrombus formation and arterial vasoconstriction. Aspirin is used to decrease mortality for patients with AMI; to reduce incidence of nonfatal AMI and mortality for patients with stable angina, unstable angina, or previous myocardial infarction; and to prevent graft closure after coronary artery bypass graft (CABG) surgery and coronary artery thrombus after PCI. Aspirin is also indicated to reduce the risk for nonfatal stroke and death in patients with a history of ischemic stroke or transient ischemia due to platelet emboli. Aspirin is not indicated for primary prevention of AMI. Patients with a history of aspirin intolerance, GI or GU bleeding, peptic ulcers, severe renal or hepatic insufficiency, or bleeding disorders should not take aspirin.

Common aspirin dosages range from 75 to 325 mg daily. Depending on the indication, patients may take aspirin for a few weeks or indefinitely. Unless contraindicated, patients with symptoms of ACS should immediately chew 160 to 325 mg of nonenteric coated aspirin. A 325-mg aspirin suppository is recommended for patients unable to take oral drugs or for patients with severe nausea, vomiting, or upper GI disorders. Aspirin may cause stomach pain, nausea, vomiting, GI bleeding, subdural or intracranial hemorrhage, thrombocytopenia, coagulopathy, and a prolonged prothrombin time.

The adenosine diphosphate receptor antagonists clopidogrel (Plavix) and ticlopidine (Ticlid) prevent adenosine diphosphate–induced platelet activation and platelet aggregation, resulting in an irreversible and noncompetitive inhibition of platelet function.

▶ Clopidogrel is indicated to reduce new AMI, new stroke, and vascular death in patients with ACS (both STEMI and NSTEMI) or atherosclerosis as documented by recent stroke, recent AMI, or established peripheral arterial disease.

▶ Ticlopidine is used generally for patients who cannot tolerate aspirin.

If CABG is planned within 1 week, clopidogrel should be withheld. In the Clopidogrel in Unstable Angina to Prevent Recurrent Events (CURE) trial, patients with NSTEMI received either placebo and aspirin or clopidogrel and aspirin. Clopidogrel reduced the composite end point of cardiovascular death, nonfatal AMI, and stroke but was associated with increased bleeding.[23] A CURE substudy showed that clopidogrel reduced the risk for cardiovascular death, AMI, and stroke at 30 days and 12 months in patients with ACS.[24] The Clopidogrel as Adjunctive Reperfusion Therapy (CLARITY)-TIMI 28 trial demonstrated the benefit of adding clopidogrel to aspirin, fibrinolytic, and unfractionated heparin therapy for patients with STEMI. Treatment with a loading dose of 300 mg followed by a daily dose of 75 mg resulted in a 36% reduction in the composite end point of an occluded infarct-related artery, death, or recurrent myocardial infarction before angiography.[25] A recent study was stopped early when findings showed that oral anticoagulation prevented stoke, embolism, AMI, and vascular death better than clopidogrel plus aspirin for patients with AF.[26]

Recent guidelines recommend that patients receive a loading dose of clopidogrel at least 6 hours before PCI.[16] Patients with a drug-eluting stent (DES) should take clopidogrel for a minimum of 3 to 6 months after PCI; however, patients at low risk for bleeding should continue it for 12 months.[16] The dosage for clopidogrel is 75 mg daily with or without food. A loading dose of 300 to 600 mg is often used to achieve a rapid onset of action. Loading doses as high as 900 mg have been given during clinical trials.[27] The effects of clopidogrel begin immediately; steady-state platelet inhibition is achieved after 3 to 7 days of therapy. Once clopidogrel is discontinued, bleeding times and platelet function normalize within 3 to 7 days. Major adverse effects include bleeding disorders, GI upset, thrombotic thrombocytopenic purpura, and neutropenia. Patients receiving clopidogrel have less GI upset, hemorrhage, and abnormal liver function than patients receiving aspirin.

With ticlopidine, a dosage of 250 mg is administered twice daily with food to increase absorption and minimize GI irritation. A loading dose of 500 mg can be given to achieve platelet inhibition more quickly. Maximal platelet aggregation inhibition occurs after 4 to 7 days of therapy. Once ticlopidine is discontinued, bleeding times and platelet function normalize within 2 weeks. Major adverse effects include bleeding, neutropenia, agranulocytosis, thrombotic thrombocytopenic purpura, elevated liver aminotransferases, and GI irritation.

Three GP IIb/IIIa inhibitors include abciximab (ReoPro), tirofiban (Aggrastat), and eptifibatide (Integrilin; Table 18-3). These drugs inhibit the GP IIb/IIIa receptor, the final common pathway for platelet aggregation; inhibit thrombus formation; and prevent platelet aggregation. These three drugs are all administered in conjunction with either enoxaparin or unfractionated heparin. Box 18-2 lists the contraindications to GP IIb/IIIa inhibitors. Adverse effects for this class of drugs include bleeding, thrombocytopenia, stroke, and allergic reactions.

Many clinical trials have been performed to evaluate GP IIb/IIIa inhibitors, and it appears that these drugs are most beneficial for patients with ACS who are to undergo PCI and who are at high risk for AMI. A meta-analysis of ACS and PCI trials indicated that GP IIb/IIIa inhibitors reduced the combined end point of AMI or death at 48 to 96 hours, 30 days, and 6 months.[28] Data show favorable benefits when IIb/IIIa inhibitors are used with coronary stents.[29] In another study, the combination of half-dose tenecteplase plus abciximab reduced in-hospital reinfarction rates and refractory ischemia but not mortality.[30] Practice guidelines for PCI intervention recommend a GP IIb/IIIa inhibitor for patients with ACS or

Table 18-3 • Glycoprotein IIb/IIIa Inhibitors

	Indications	Dose	Concurrent Aspirin and Heparin Therapy	Half-Life
Abciximab	Adjunct to PCI USA that does not respond to conventional therapy and when PCI is planned within 24 h	PCI: IV bolus of 0.25 mg/kg 10–60 min before PCI; then continuous IV infusion of 0.125 µg/kg/min (maximum 10 µg/min) for 12 h USA with planned PCI: IV bolus of 0.25 mg/kg; then 10 µg/min IV infusion for 18–24 h, concluding 1 h after PCI	Yes	First phase, <10 min; second phase, 30 min; remains in circulation up to 10 days in a platelet-bound state
Eptifibatide	ACS: Non-Q-wave AMI or USA, including patients who are managed medically or with PCI PCI	ACS: 180 µg/kg bolus IV, then 2 µg/kg/min infusion up to 72 h, discharge, or CABG; if PCI performed, continue IV infusion up to discharge or for up to 18–24 h post-PCI (whichever comes first), allowing up to 96 h of therapy; for patients with a creatinine between 2 and 4 mg/dL, reduce infusion to 1 µg/kg/min PCI: 180 µg/kg IV bolus immediately before PCI; then 2 µg/kg/min IV infusion and a second 180 µg/kg bolus IV 10 min after the first bolus; continue infusion until discharge or for up to 18–24 h; a minimum of 12 h of infusion is recommended; for patients with a creatinine between 2 and 4 mg/dL, 180 µg/kg IV bolus immediately before PCI, then 1 µg/kg/min IV infusion, and a second 180 µg/kg bolus IV 10 min after the first bolus	Yes	2.5 h; platelet function returns to normal approximately 4 h after stopping the infusion
Tirofiban	ACS: Non-Q-wave AMI or USA, including patients who are managed medically or with PCI	0.4 µg/kg/min IV for 30 min., then 0.1 µg/kg/min IV infusion through angiography or for 12–24 h after PCI; for patients without signs of refractory ischemia who do not proceed to angiography and angioplasty, continue infusion for at least 48 h; for patients with severe renal insufficiency, give half the usual rate of infusion	Yes	1.4–2.2 h; platelet function returns to near baseline 4–8 h after stopping the infusion

ACS, acute coronary syndrome; CABG, coronary artery bypass grafting; IV, intravenous; PCI, percutaneous coronary intervention; USA, unstable angina.

Box 18-2 • Contraindications for Glycoprotein IIb/IIIa Inhibitors

- Internal bleeding
- Bleeding diathesis within 30 days
- Intracranial neoplasm, arteriovenous malformation, or aneurysm
- Stroke within 30 days or any hemorrhagic stroke
- Thrombocytopenia with prior exposure to tirofiban
- Aortic dissection
- Major surgery or severe trauma within the previous month
- Severe hypertension
- Pericarditis (tirofiban)
- Concurrent use of another glycoprotein IIb/IIIa inhibitor
- Dependence on dialysis or serum creatinine ≥4.0 mg/dL (eptifibatide)

NSTEMI who undergo PCI.[16] Guidelines for the management of patients with STEMI recommend abciximab as early as possible before PCI.[1]

• Antiarrhythmics

Antiarrhythmic drugs are used to restore the heart to a regular rhythm. The therapeutic window is small, and these drugs may have a toxic effect. Caution must be used to prevent complications. Antiarrhythmics are classified by their effect on the cardiac action potential—whether they block β-adrenoreceptors; or sodium, potassium, or calcium channels. The action of these drugs is complex; drugs within the same class can work differently, and actions of those in different classes may overlap (Table 18-4). Table 18-5 summarizes antidysrhythmic drugs that are commonly used

in critical care settings. Refer to Chapter 16 for more specific information regarding the cardiac action potential.

CLASS I ANTIARRHYTHMIC DRUGS

Class I antiarrhythmics stabilize the cell membrane by blocking the influx of sodium through fast channels. Class I drugs are further categorized on the basis of the action and effects of the specific medications.

Class IA antiarrhythmics include quinidine (Quinate), procainamide (Pronestyl), and disopyramide (Norpace). These drugs do not improve mortality, may cause life-threatening dysrhythmias, and interact with other drugs commonly used for cardiovascular disease.

Class IB antiarrhythmics are lidocaine and mexiletine (Mexitil). Lidocaine, a less effective but acceptable alternative to procainamide for ventricular dysrhythmias, is no longer use prophylactically for patients with AMI or asymptomatic ventricular dysrhythmias.

Class IC antiarrhythmics are flecainide (Tambocor) and propafenone (Rythmol). Because these drugs are prodysrhythmic and may increase mortality, they are not commonly prescribed.

In general, research data do not support the effectiveness of class I antiarrhythmics. The current trend is to treat ventricular dysrhythmias with class II and class III antiarrhythmics, cardioversion, ablative techniques, and implantable cardioverter–defibrillators (ICDs).[31]

CLASS II ANTIARRHYTHMIC DRUGS

β-Adrenergic blockers are class II drugs that interfere with sympathetic nervous system stimulation, contributing to decreased heart rate, depressed AV node

	Table 18-4 • Classification of Antidysrhythmic Medications	
Class	**Action**	**Medication Examples**
IA	Inhibits fast sodium channel, decreases automaticity, depresses phase 0, and prolongs the action potential duration	Quinidine Procainamide Disopyramide
IB	Inhibits fast sodium channel, depresses phase 0 slightly, and shortens action potential duration	Lidocaine Mexiletine
IC	Inhibits fast sodium channel, depresses phase 0 markedly, slows His-Purkinje conduction profoundly leading to a prolonged QRS duration	Flecainide Moricizine (plus IA and IB effects) Propafenone
II	Depresses phase 4 depolarization, blocks sympathetic stimulation of the conduction system	Esmolol Propranolol Sotalol (plus class III effects) Acebutolol
III	Blocks potassium channel, prolongs phase 3 repolarization, prolongs action potential duration	Amiodarone Sotalol Ibutilide Dofetilide
IV	Inhibits inward calcium channel, depresses phase 4 depolarization, lengthens repolarization in phases 1 and 2	Verapamil Diltiazem

Table 18-5 • Selected Antiarrhythmic Medications

Drug	Antiarrhythmic Indications	Antiarrhythmic Dose	Route	Effect on ECG	Major Adverse Effects
Procainamide	VT, VF; SVTs including WPW syndrome, AF, atrial flutter	IV: 20 mg/min IV infusion (maximum total dose 17 mg/kg). Then infusion of 1–4 mg/min to maintain therapeutic drug level PO: up to 50 mg/kg/d given in divided doses q3h to maintain therapeutic drug level	IV, PO	→ QRS → QTI	Hypotension with IV use, asystole, ventricular fibrillation, positive antinuclear antibody test, lupus syndrome, rash, fever, heart block, torsades de pointes, headache, agranulocytosis
Lidocaine	VT, VF	1.0–1.5 mg/kg IV bolus; may repeat 0.5–0.75 mg/kg IV every 5–10 min for total of 3 mg/kg. Then infusion of 1–4 mg/min	IV; ETT if no patent IV (2–4 mg/kg)	None	Bradycardia, blurred vision, hypotension, tremors, dizziness, tinnitus, convulsions, mental status changes
Flecainide	AF and PSVTs (atrioventricular nodal reentrant tachycardia, atrioventricular reentrant tachycardia) in patients without structural heart disease; life-threatening ventricular dysrhythmias (VT)	100–200 mg PO q12h	PO	→ PRI → QRS 0/→ QTI	Ventricular dysrhythmias, dizziness, dyspnea, headache, fatigue, nausea, palpitations
Esmolol	SVT including AF and atrial flutter; noncompensatory ST	500 μg/kg/min IV loading dose for 1 min. Then 50 μg/kg/min infusion for 4 min. Repeat loading dose every 5 min and increase infusion by 50 μg/kg/min increments until desired therapeutic effect or maximum of 300 μg/kg/min.	IV	↓ HR 0/→ PRI 0/← QTI	Hypotension, nausea, diaphoresis, dizziness, headache, weakness, somnolence, heart block, bronchospasm, thrombophlebitis from extravasation
Propranolol	SVTs, ventricular dysrhythmias, digitalis-induced tachydysrhythmias, premature ventricular contractions	IV: 1–3 mg not exceeding 1 mg/min PO: 10–30 mg t.i.d. to q.i.d.	IV PO	↓ HR 0/→ PRI 0/← QTI	Hypotension, heart block, bradycardia, HF, bronchospasm, fatigue, nausea, vomiting, gastric pain, constipation, diarrhea
Sotalol	Life-threatening ventricular dysrhythmias (VT, VF); maintenance of NSR in patients with symptomatic AF or atrial flutter who are currently in NSR	80 mg PO b.i.d; may be increased to 240–640 mg/d given in 2–3 divided doses	PO	↓ HR → PRI 0/→ QTI	Bradycardia, AV block, dizziness, HF, bronchospasm, gastric pain
Ibutilide	AF, atrial flutter	1 mg IV infusion over 10 min (<60 kg, 0.01 mg/kg). May repeat either dosage in 10 min	IV	→ QTI	Hypotension, torsades de pointes, VT, BBB, bradycardia, nausea
Dofetilide	AF, atrial flutter; maintenance of NSR after conversion	125–500 μg PO b.i.d. depending on creatinine clearance	PO	→ QTI	Torsades de pointes, bradycardia

Drug	Indications	Dose	Route	ECG	Side effects
Amiodarone	Recurrent VF or hemodynamically unstable VT in patients refractory to other drugs; unlabeled uses: AF and maintenance of NSR; SVTs including WPW syndrome; rate control in AF or atrial flutter when other therapies ineffective	IV: Loading infusion of 150 mg over 10 min; 360 mg over next 6 h; 540 mg over next 18 h. May follow with maintenance infusion of 0.5 mg/min. For breakthrough VF or VT, supplemental infusions of 150 mg IV over 10 min. PO: Loading dose of 800–1,600 mg q.d. for 1–3 wk. Then 600–800 mg q.d. for 1 mo. Maintenance dose 100–400 mg/d	IV PO	→ PRI → QTI	Heart block, cardiac arrest, bradycardia, hypotension, VT, pneumonitis, liver disease, hypothyroidism or hyperthyroidism, photosensitivity, solar dermatitis, blue discoloration of skin, malaise, paresthesias, nausea, vomiting, constipation, visual disturbances, anorexia
Verapamil	PSVTs including WPW syndrome; ventricular rate control in AF, atrial flutter	IV: 5–10 mg over 2 min; may give 10 mg 30 min after first dose. PO: 240–480 mg/d in 3–4 divided doses	IV PO	↓ HR → PRI	Hypotension, heart block, HF, bradycardia, headache, dizziness, edema, nausea, constipation
Diltiazem	Ventricular rate control in AF, atrial flutter; PSVT including WPW syndrome	IV: 0.25 mg/kg over 2 min; may give 0.35 mg/kg after 15 min. May follow with an infusion of 5–15 mg/h for up to 24 h	IV for antidysrhythmic indications	↓/O HR → PRI	Bradycardia, heart block, edema, hypotension, nausea, dizziness, flushing, headache, fatigue
Adenosine	PSVT including WPW syndrome; idiopathic VT; used diagnostically to evaluate VT, SVT, latent preexcitation	6 mg IV over 1–2 sec followed by rapid saline flush. After 1–2 min, may give 12 mg. A second 12-mg dose may be given in 1–2 min if needed.	IV	→ PRI	Facial flushing, light-headedness, headache, bradycardia, dyspnea, heart block, asystole, chest pain, nausea
Atropine	Symptomatic sinus bradycardia, AV block, asystole, bradycardic PEA	Asystole or PEA: 1 mg IV push; repeat every 3–5 min to maximum of 0.04 mg/kg; bradycardia: 0.5–1.0 mg IV every 3–5 min to maximum of 0.04 mg/kg	IV; ETT if no patent IV (1–2 mg)	↑ HR	Palpitations, tachycardia, blurred vision, dry mouth, altered taste, nausea, urinary retention
Digoxin	Ventricular rate control in AF	IV: loading dose of 0.4–0.6 mg with additional doses of 0.1–0.3 mg q4–8h. Maintenance dose of 0.125–0.5 mg/d. PO: loading dose of 0.5–0.7 mg with additional doses of 0.125–0.375 mg q6–8h. Maintenance dose of 0.125–0.5 mg/d	IV PO	↓ HR → PRI ← QTI	Heart block, bradycardia, weakness; toxicity: dysrhythmias, anorexia, nausea, vomiting, headache, fatigue, depression, confusion, hallucination

AF, atrial fibrillation; AV, atrioventricular; BBB, bundle branch block; ECG, electrocardiogram; ETT, endotracheal tube; HF, heart failure; HR, heart rate; IV, intravenous; NSR, normal sinus rhythm; PEA, pulseless electrical activity; PO, oral; PSVT, paroxysmal supraventricular tachycardia; ST, sinus tachycardia; SVT, supraventricular tachycardia; VF, ventricular fibrillation; VT, ventricular tachycardia; WPW, Wolff-Parkinson-White; ↑, increased; ↓, decreased; →, prolonged; ←, shortened; O, little or no effect.

conduction, decreased contractility, and decreased myocardial oxygen demand. This class of drugs has a broad spectrum of activity and an established safety record and is currently the best class of antiarrhythmics for *general* use.[32]

β-Blockers are categorized as cardioselective (inhibition of β_1 receptors) or nonselective (inhibition of β_1 and β_2 receptors). Inhibition of β_1 receptors causes decreased heart rate, slowed conduction through the AV node, and depressed cardiac function. Inhibition of β_2 receptors causes bronchoconstriction, vasoconstriction, and decreased glycogenolysis. Table 18-6 indicates the β activity of selected β-blockers.

Unless contraindicated, β-blockers should be given indefinitely to all patients with a history of AMI, ACS, or left ventricular dysfunction with or without symptoms of HF.[33] Other indications include tachydysrhythmias, continuing or recurrent ischemic pain, hypertension, and HF. Acebutolol, esmolol, propranolol, and sotalol and are approved to treat dysrhythmias. All β-blockers, except esmolol and sotalol, are indicated for hypertension.

Numerous trials have demonstrated the effectiveness of β-blockers for dysrhythmias and other cardiovascular disorders such as hypertension and HF. The Carvedilol Post-Infarct Survival Control in Left Ventricular Dysfunction (CAPRICORN) investigators reported that, compared with placebo, carvedilol reduced mortality and recurrent, nonfatal AMIs for patients with AMI and left ventricular dysfunction who were being treated with angiotensin-converting enzyme (ACE) inhibitors.[34] Three studies involving patients with HF were stopped early because β-blockers reduced mortality significantly more than the placebo. The Carvedilol Prospective Randomized Cumulative Survival Trial (COPERNICUS) researchers found that carvedilol significantly reduced hospitalization and mortality rates for patients with severe, chronic HF.[35]

Unless contraindicated, β-blockers should be a part of early treatment for patients with acute coronary syndromes.[36,37] Metoprolol (Lopressor), propranolol (Inderal), atenolol (Tenormin), timolol, and nadolol (Corgard) are approved for angina, whereas metoprolol and atenolol are indicated as first-line drugs for AMI. The first dose is given intravenously, and successive doses are usually given orally. The final end goal is reduction of the patient's resting heart rate to 55 to 60 beats/minute.

β-Blockers are contraindicated in patients with severe asthma or bronchospasm, severe chronic obstructive pulmonary disease, cardiogenic shock, severe left ventricular failure, bradycardia (<60 beats/minute), or second- and third-degree heart block. Cardioselective β-blockers are sometimes used with caution for patients with pulmonary disease. It is important to remember that cardioselective drugs lose their selectivity at higher doses.

Adverse effects of β-blockers include bradycardia, heart block, hypotension, HF, bronchospasm, cold extremities, insomnia, fatigue, and depression. Some patients who experience these adverse effects may respond better to a different β-blocker.

CLASS III ANTIARRHYTHMIC DRUGS

Class III antiarrhythmic drugs include amiodarone (Cordarone), sotalol (Betapace), ibutilide (Corvert), and dofetilide (Tikosyn). It is important to know each drug's unique properties because individual agents contain unique properties not shared by other class III drugs.

Amiodarone is indicated for the treatment of VT as well as AF and flutter. A meta-analysis showed that amiodarone decreased AF, ventricular tachydysrhythmias, stroke, and length of stay after cardiac surgery[38]; in addition, for patients with either AMI or HF, the drug decreased total mortality by 13% and deaths from dysrhythmia by 29%.[39] Current recommendations for patients with STEMI rank amiodarone ahead of other antidysrhythmics.[1] A small study showed that when compared with placebo, prophylactic, short-term oral amiodarone decreased postoperative AF, VT, and cerebrovascular accident (CVA) after open heart surgery for patients 60 years of age or older who were already receiving β-blockers.[40]

The advanced cardiac life support algorithms include amiodarone as a first-line option for treating ventricular fibrillation, pulseless VT, wide-complex tachycardia, and preexcited AF.[41] Limitations of amiodarone include its variable onset of action, intolerable adverse effects, dangerous drug interactions, and life-threatening complications associated with chronic therapy.[31,32]

Ibutilide and dofetilide are class III drugs that are indicated for AF and atrial flutter. Ibutilide inhibits potassium current and enhances sodium current, prolonging repolarization. Dofetilide blocks the rapid potassium current channel, prolonging the action potential duration and refractory period. Although these drugs may cause a prolonged QT interval and torsades de pointes, they have fewer systemic adverse effects than amiodarone and sotalol.

·::::· Table 18-6 • Selected β-Blockers		
Medication	**Cardioselective**	**Nonselective**
Acebutolol	X	
Atenolol	X	
Betaxolol	X	
Bisoprolol	X	
Carvedilol		X
Esmolol	X	
Labetalol		X
Metoprolol	X	
Nadolol		X
Pindolol		X
Propranolol		X
Sotalol		X
Timolol		X

CLASS IV ANTIARRHYTHMIC DRUGS

The class IV calcium channel blocker antiarrhythmics, verapamil and diltiazem, decrease automaticity of the sinoatrial (SA) and AV nodes, slow conduction, and prolong the AV nodal refractory period. These agents have negative inotropic and peripheral vasodilation effects. In addition, they have antiplatelet and anti-ischemic effects. Calcium channel blockers are primarily indicated for angina, hypertension, and supraventricular tachycardia (SVT). Verapamil (Calan) and diltiazem (Cardizem) are contraindicated for usual forms of VT, severe sinus bradycardia, sick sinus syndrome, Wolff-Parkinson-White (WPW) syndrome with AF, digoxin toxicity, hypotension, HF, AV conduction defects, and severe aortic stenosis, and they are not standard therapies for AMI. Adverse effects include hypotension, AV block, bradycardia, headache, dizziness, peripheral edema, nausea, constipation, and flushing.

Calcium channel blockers do not decrease mortality after AMI, and in some cases, these agents may be harmful.[1] Calcium antagonists, in general, should only be used when β-blockers are contraindicated or maximal dosage has been reached without effect.[42]

UNCLASSIFIED ANTIARRHYTHMIC DRUGS

Adenosine is a first-line antiarrhythmic that effectively converts narrow-complex paroxysmal supraventricular tachycardia (PSVT) to normal sinus rhythm by slowing conduction through the AV node. This agent is effective in terminating arrhythmias due to reentry involving the SA and AV nodes; however, it does not convert AF, atrial flutter, or VT to sinus rhythm. It is also used to differentiate between VT and SVT, treat rare forms of idiopathic VT, and reveal latent pre-excitation in patients with suspected WPW syndrome.[32] The dose is 6 mg rapid IV bolus followed by a rapid saline flush. If the 6-mg dose in ineffective, a dose of 12 mg may be administered twice. The half-life of adenosine is less than 10 seconds; therefore, adverse effects are short-lived.

Magnesium sulfate is the drug of choice for treating torsades de pointes. Magnesium is also used for refractory VT and ventricular fibrillation, as well as for life-threatening arrhythmias due to digitalis toxicity. Its mechanism of action is unclear; however, it has calcium channel blocking properties and inhibits sodium and potassium channels. The dose for patients in cardiac arrest is 1 to 2 g diluted in 10 mL of D_5W given by IV push. Adverse effects include hypotension, nausea, depressed reflexes, and flushing.

Atropine, a parasympatholytic agent, is a first-line drug used to treat symptomatic bradycardia and slowed conduction at the AV node. It is also indicated for asystole or bradycardic pulseless electrical activity. Atropine reduces the effects of vagal stimulation, thus increasing heart rate and improving cardiac function. It is important not to increase the heart rate excessively in patients with ischemic heart disease because this may increase myocardial oxygen consumption and worsen ischemia.

Digoxin (Lanoxin) is a mild positive inotrope with antidysrhythmic and bradycardic actions. It inhibits the sodium–potassium pump, causing a rise in intracellular sodium. This rise promotes calcium influx and ultimately enhances myocardial contractility. Digoxin also activates the parasympathetic system, causing a decreased heart rate and increased AV nodal inhibition. Digoxin is primarily indicated for patients with both HF and chronic AF.[43] In addition, digoxin may be used to control a rapid ventricular rate associated with non-preexcitation AF or atrial flutter and in combination with verapamil, diltiazem, or β-blockers for patients without HF.[41,43] Digoxin is not currently used for paroxysmal AF, acute SVTs, or acute left ventricular failure, or as part of inotropic therapy regimens.[43]

The doses and therapeutic blood levels for digoxin are controversial. No longer is it common to administer loading doses.[43] Most patients on digoxin benefit from a low dose that also reduces the incidence of toxicity.[43] Toxicity is a common occurrence and is frequently associated with serious dysrhythmias. Routine doses are individualized based on the patient's diagnosis, symptoms, underlying disease processes, age, response to therapy, and blood levels. Levels of 0.5 to 1.0 ng/mL are recommended for patients with HF, and levels of 0.8 to 2 ng/mL for those with dysrhythmias.

Signs and symptoms of digitalis toxicity include palpitations, syncope, dysrhythmias, elevated digoxin level, anorexia, vomiting, diarrhea, nausea, fatigue, confusion, insomnia, headache, depression, vertigo, facial pain, and colored or blurred vision. Digitalis levels may be increased by the concurrent use of quinidine, verapamil, amiodarone, captopril, diltiazem (Capoten), esmolol (Brevibloc), propafenone (Rythmol), indomethacin (Indocin), quinine, or ibuprofen (Motrin). Finally, hypokalemia, hypomagnesemia, and hypothyroidism may predispose patients to digitalis toxicity. Serum levels are drawn if toxicity is suspected.

• Inotropes

Cardiovascular function is regulated by two divisions of the autonomic nervous system, the sympathetic and parasympathetic systems. Refer to Chapter 32 to review this information. Adrenoreceptor stimulation leads to a variety of effects; therefore, it is important to understand which receptors each drug stimulates (Table 18-7).

Inotropic drugs are used to increase the force of myocardial contraction and cardiac output. Inotropic drugs include sympathomimetics, such as dopamine (Intropin), dobutamine (Dobutrex), epinephrine, isoproterenol (Isuprel), and norepinephrine; and the phosphodiesterase inhibitors inamrinone and milrinone (Primacor). These drugs are commonly given to patients with ventricular dysfunction or cardiogenic shock. Enhanced ventricular contraction increases stroke volume, cardiac output, blood pressure, and coronary artery perfusion. As the ventricles empty more completely, ventricular filling pressures, preload,

Table 18-7 • Adrenergic Receptors Affecting Cardiovascular Function

Receptor	Location	Effects of Stimulation
β_1	Heart	Positive inotropic (increased contractility) and chronotropic action (increases rate)
β_2	Bronchial smooth muscle	Bronchodilation
	Vascular smooth muscle	Vasodilation
	Atrioventricular node	Positive dromotropic action (increased conduction velocity)
α_1	Vascular smooth muscle	Vasoconstriction
	Heart	Weak positive inotropic and chronotropic actions
α_2	Presynaptic sympathetic nerve endings	Inhibition of norepinephrine release
Dopaminergic	Kidney and splanchnic vessels	Renal and splanchnic vessel vasodilation

and pulmonary congestion are decreased. However, as contractility and heart rate increase, myocardial oxygen demand also increases. Myocardial ischemia can occur if a myocardial oxygen supply–demand mismatch develops. The nurse must closely monitor the patient for evidence of ischemia, angina, and dysrhythmias.

DOPAMINE

Dopamine, the most widely used inotropic drug, is administered to patients with conditions that cause hypotension, decreased cardiac output, and oliguria. Dopamine directly stimulates dopaminergic, β-adrenergic, and α-adrenergic receptors and promotes release of norepinephrine from sympathetic nerve terminals. Dopamine is given by continuous IV infusion, and its dose is titrated to achieve the desired effect. Increased myocardial contractility results from dosages of 3 to 10 µg/kg/minute. Higher dosages predominantly cause vasoconstriction and increased blood pressure. Dopamine is usually given through a central line to enhance its distribution and to avoid extravasation, which may cause local vasoconstriction and tissue necrosis. Adverse effects include tachycardia, palpitations, dysrhythmias, angina, headache, nausea, vomiting, and hypertension.

DOBUTAMINE

Dobutamine acts on β_1 receptors and increases myocardial contractility. Dobutamine is used after cardiac surgery; during some cardiac diagnostic stress procedures; and for patients with HF, shock, or other conditions that cause poor cardiac contractility or a low cardiac output. The dosage for dobutamine is 2 to 20 µg/kg/minute by continuous IV infusion. Adverse effects include tachycardia, dysrhythmias, blood pressure fluctuations, headache, and nausea.

EPINEPHRINE

Epinephrine stimulates α_1, β_1, and β_2 receptors and is given for a variety of indications, including cardiac arrest, symptomatic bradycardia, severe hypotension,

anaphylaxis, and shock. In the intensive care unit (ICU), epinephrine is given by continuous IV infusion through a central line, as an IV bolus, or through an endotracheal tube. Continuous IV dosages of 1 to 2 µg/minute stimulate β_1 receptors to increase cardiac output by increasing heart rate and myocardial contractility. At higher dosages, epinephrine stimulates α receptors, causing profound vasoconstriction, increased blood pressure and systemic vascular resistance (SVR), and decreased renal and splanchnic perfusion. Epinephrine may cause dysrhythmias, tachycardia, cerebral hemorrhage, pulmonary edema, headache, dizziness, nervousness, myocardial ischemia, and angina. Vasopressin is now used as an alternative to epinephrine for treatment of shock-refractory ventricular fibrillation, asystole, or pulseless electrical activity.[41] Vasopressin promotes smooth muscle contraction and increases peripheral vascular resistance. The dosage for patients with cardiac arrest is 40 units given by IV push. The drug may also be given as an infusion. Adverse effects include dysrhythmias, myocardial ischemia, angina, myocardial infarction, tremors, vertigo, sweating, and water intoxication.

ISOPROTERENOL

Isoproterenol (Isuprel) stimulates β_1 and β_2 receptors to increase myocardial contractility, cardiac output, heart rate, and blood pressure. Currently, isoproterenol is used mainly to increase heart rate after cardiac transplantation. Other indications include refractory torsades de pointes, β-blocker overdose, and symptomatic bradycardia when an external pacemaker is not available. The IV dosage is 0.5 to 10 µg/minute by continuous infusion. Isoproterenol causes a variety of adverse effects, including dysrhythmias, tachycardia, palpitations, myocardial ischemia, hypotension, pulmonary edema, bronchospasm, headache, nausea, vomiting, and sweating.

NOREPINEPHRINE

Norepinephrine (Levophed) primarily affects α receptors, causing peripheral vasoconstriction, increased blood pressure, and increased SVR. The increased

SVR may actually increase myocardial oxygen demand and work, thus decreasing cardiac output. Norepinephrine is used for patients with cardiogenic shock and significant hypotension accompanied by a low SVR. The dosage is 2 to 12 µg/minute by continuous IV infusion. Adverse effects include tachycardia, bradycardia, dysrhythmias, headache, hypertension, and tissue necrosis from extravasation.

• Phosphodiesterase III Inhibitors

The phosphodiesterase III inhibitors amrinone and milrinone increase contractility, venous vasodilation, and peripheral arterial vasodilation by inhibiting an enzyme that breaks down cyclic adenosine monophosphate. Both drugs reduce ventricular filling pressures and tend to decrease arterial pressure; however, they minimally affect heart rate.

Amrinone is used for severe HF that is refractory to other drugs. An IV bolus dose of 0.75 mg/kg is given over 2 to 3 minutes. A maintenance IV infusion of 5 to 10 µg/kg/minute is titrated to the desired effect. Adverse effects include hypotension, tachycardia, dysrhythmias, and thrombocytopenia.

Milrinone is used for the short-term treatment of acute HF. The IV bolus dose of 50 µg/kg is given over 10 minutes and is followed by a maintenance IV infusion of 0.375 to 0.75 µg/kg/minute. Patients who receive milrinone may experience ventricular dysrhythmias, hypotension, headache, bronchospasm, and thrombocytopenia.

• Vasodilators

Vasodilators decrease preload and afterload. Preload is the distending force that stretches the ventricular muscle at the end of filling. The greater the stretch, the better the contraction. However, if the cells are overstretched, contractile force decreases. Afterload is the force against which the heart has to work to eject its contents. If afterload is too low, blood pressure and tissue perfusion may be low. If afterload is too high, the heart has to work harder.

NITRATES

Patients with myocardial ischemia or infarction may have an increased preload and afterload, which further strains their hearts. Nitrates cause peripheral vasodilation, which in turn decreases venous return to the heart and reduces preload. These drugs promote coronary artery vasodilation, improve collateral blood flow, reduce platelet aggregation, enhance perfusion to ischemic myocardium, and decrease myocardial oxygen demand, thus reducing ischemia, chest pain, and infarct size. Nitrates reduce blood pressure and previously elevated pulmonary vascular resistance, SVR, and central venous and pulmonary capillary wedge pressures. At high doses, nitrates reduce afterload by arterial vasodilator effects.

Nitrates are indicated for acute angina; large anterior AMI; AMI associated with acute and chronic HF, acute pulmonary edema, persistent ischemia, or hypertension; angina unresponsive to other therapies; and prophylaxis of effort angina. However, nitrates have shown little mortality benefit for AMI. Contraindications to IV nitrates include, but are not limited to, hypotension, uncorrected hypovolemia, hypertrophic obstructive cardiomyopathy, and pericardial tamponade. When a right ventricular AMI is suspected, nitrates are used with extreme caution because these patients require an adequate venous return to maintain cardiac output and blood pressure. Patients should not receive nitrates for 24 hours after sildenafil (Viagra), vardenafil (Levitra), or tadalafil (Cialis) use because the resulting drug interactions predispose patients to life-threatening hypotension.

Nitrates are available in a variety of dosage forms. In the ICU, nitrates are often given by the IV, sublingual, or topical routes. An IV nitroglycerin drip is initiated at 5 to 20 µg/minute and increased every 5 to 15 minutes, up to 200 µg/minute, to achieve the desired effects. When used to treat or prevent angina, a 0.3- to 0.6-mg tablet is placed under the patient's tongue and may be repeated twice at 5-minute intervals. The usual dose for nitroglycerin ointment is 1 to 2 inches every 8 hours; however, treatment is often initiated with 0.5 inch and increased gradually to achieve the desired effects.

The adverse effects of nitrates include headache, hypotension, syncope, and tachycardia. Tolerance may develop to the antianginal, hemodynamic, and antiplatelet effects of nitrates, especially with continuous or high-dose therapy; however, dosing regimens that allow for nitrate-free intervals may prevent this occurrence.[44]

NITROPRUSSIDE SODIUM

Nitroprusside (Nitropress) is a potent arterial and venous vasodilator that is used to treat severe left ventricular HF, hypertension after coronary artery bypass grafting, hypertensive crisis, and dissecting aneurysm. Nitroprusside decreases SVR and increases cardiac output. The usual IV infusion dosage is 0.5 to 10 µg/kg/minute; however, to prevent cyanide toxicity, the maximal dose should not be given for longer than 10 minutes. The dose is titrated to effect; if blood pressure does not respond after 10 minutes, the drug is discontinued. Because nitroprusside is sensitive to light, the infusion bag is covered with an opaque material to prevent the drug's degradation. Adverse effects include hypotension, myocardial ischemia, nausea, vomiting, abdominal pain, and cyanide toxicity.

NESIRITIDE

Nesiritide (Natrecor), a recombinant form of human B-type natriuretic peptide, is identical to the hormone produced by the left ventricle in response to volume overload and increased wall stress. A venous and arterial vasodilator, nesiritide reduces preload and afterload and increases cardiac output without increasing heart rate. Nesiritide is indicated for acutely decompensated HF with dyspnea at rest or with minimal activity and is often used in conjunction with IV diuretics. However, clinicians have curtailed use of nesiritide[45] after results of clinical trials raised concerns about renal toxicity[46] and increased mortality.[47] The goal of ongoing prospective clinical trials is to assess nesiritide's efficacy and safety. The bolus dose is 2 µg/kg/minute, followed by an IV infusion of 0.01 to 0.03 µg/kg/minute. Contraindications include cardiogenic or distributive shock, valvular stenosis, constrictive pericarditis, and restrictive or obstructive cardiomyopathy. Adverse effects include hypotension, bradycardia, ventricular dysrhythmias, angina, dizziness, and apnea.

• Angiotensin-Converting Enzyme Inhibitors

ACE inhibitors are indicated to treat HF, hypertension, AMI with or without left ventricular dysfunction or failure, and asymptomatic left ventricular dysfunction. They are also used to decrease morbidity and mortality for patients at high risk for AMI, stroke, or cardiovascular death. Unless contraindicated, patients with a STEMI with anterior infarction, pulmonary congestion, or left ventricular ejection fraction less than 40% should receive an ACE inhibitor within 24 hours.[1]

The ACE inhibitors block the conversion of angiotensin I to the potent vasoconstrictor angiotensin II, reduce aldosterone synthesis, and may promote fibrinolysis.[48] As a result, these agents mitigate left ventricular remodeling, increase cardiac output, and decrease sodium retention, blood pressure, central venous pressure, SVR, pulmonary vascular resistance, and pulmonary capillary wedge pressure.

Numerous research trials conducted in the late 1980s through the early 2000s showed that ACE inhibitors prevent HF, prevent hospitalization due to HF, and decrease mortality.[49-55] Meta-analyses showed that ACE inhibitors decrease mortality after AMI.[56,57] In addition, ACE inhibitors reduce untoward events such as recurrent AMI, rehospitalization, and mortality in patients with HF regardless of whether they had a recent AMI.[58] Results of other trials showed that ACE inhibitors reduced cardiovascular events for patients who had stable coronary artery disease (CAD) or who were at high risk for cardiovascular events but without HF or low ejection fraction.[59,60]

Table 18-8 summarizes selected ACE inhibitors. All ACE inhibitors are contraindicated in pregnancy, angioedema, bilateral renal artery stenosis, and pre-existing hypotension, and they should be used with caution for patients with renal failure or hyperkalemia. Patients with impaired renal function, hypotension, or concurrent diuretic use should receive a lower dosage. Adverse effects of ACE inhibitors include hypotension, dizziness, angioedema, cough, headache, fatigue, nausea, vomiting, diarrhea, hyperkalemia, and renal function impairment.

• Antihyperlipidemics

Cholesterol reduction is an important part of therapy for patients with cardiovascular disease. Patients are encouraged to modify their diet and lifestyle before

Table 18-8 • Selected Angiotensin–Converting Enzyme Inhibitors

Drug	Indications	Usual Initial Dose	Usual Maintenance Dose
Benazepril	HTN	10 mg PO q.d.	20–40 mg/d PO in 1–2 doses
Captopril	HTN	25 mg PO b.i.d. to t.i.d.	25–150 mg PO b.i.d. to t.i.d.
	HF	25 mg PO t.i.d.	50–100 mg PO t.i.d.
	LVD post-AMI	6.25–12.5 mg PO t.i.d.	50 mg PO t.i.d.
Enalapril	HTN	1.25 mg IV q6h	1.25–5 mg IV q6h
		5 mg PO q.d.	10–40 mg/d PO in 1–2 doses
	HF	2.5 mg PO b.i.d.	2.5–20 mg PO b.i.d.
	Asymptomatic LVD	2.5 mg PO b.i.d.	10 mg PO b.i.d.
Fosinopril	HTN	10 mg PO q.d.	20–40 mg PO q.d.
	HF	10 mg PO q.d.	20–40 mg PO q.d.
Lisinopril	HTN	10 mg PO q.d.	20–40 mg PO q.d.
	HF	5 mg PO q.d.	5–20 mg PO q.d.
	AMI	2.5–5 mg PO q.d.	10 mg PO q.d.
Quinapril	HTN	10–20 mg PO q.d.	20–80 mg/d PO in 1–2 doses
	HF	5 mg PO b.i.d.	20–40 mg/d PO in 2 doses
Ramipril	HTN	2.5 mg PO q.d.	2.5–20 mg/d PO in 1–2 doses
	HF post-AMI	2.5 mg PO b.i.d.	5 mg PO b.i.d.
Trandolapril	HTN	1 mg PO q.d.	2–4 mg PO q.d.
	HF post-AMI	1 mg PO q.d.	4 mg PO q.d.
	LVD post-AMI	1 mg PO q.d.	4 mg PO q.d.

AMI, acute myocardial infarction; HF, heart failure; HTN, hypertension; IV, intravenous; LVD, left ventricular dysfunction; PO, oral.

reverting to drug therapy. The pharmacological management of hyperlipidemia decreases morbidity and mortality from coronary heart disease.[61,62] Recent evidence suggests that intensive statin therapy can regress coronary atherosclerosis.[63] The primary target of antihyperlipidemic therapy is low-density lipoprotein (LDL) cholesterol.[62] According to the Adult Treatment Panel III, the goal LDL cholesterol level is (1) less than 160 mg/dL for patients with zero or one risk factor, (2) less than 130 mg/dL for patients with two or more risk factors, and (3) less than 100 mg/dL for patients with documented coronary heart disease (CHD) or CHD risk equivalents (e.g., diabetes, stroke, peripheral arterial disease).[62,64] An LDL cholesterol goal of less than 70 mg/dL may be preferred for patients at highest risk.[64] A total cholesterol level of less than 200 mg/dL is desirable, and a high-density lipoprotein (HDL) cholesterol less than 40 mg/dL is considered low.[64] Drug therapy with LDL cholesterol–lowering drugs is recommended for patients with (1) zero or one risk factor and an LDL cholesterol level greater than or equal to 190 mg/dL, (2) two or more risk factors and an LDL cholesterol level greater than or equal to 130 mg/dL, and (3) documented CHD or CHD risk equivalents and an LDL cholesterol level greater than or equal to 100 mg/dL.[62,64] Drug therapy is also appropriate when triglycerides are 200 mg/dL or greater.[64] Finally, patients with borderline-high triglycerides (150 to 199 mg/dL) and CHD or CHD risk equivalents may receive drugs to raise the HDL cholesterol.[64]

There are four major classes of antihyperlipidemic drugs:

▶ Hydroxymethylglutaryl coenzyme-A (HMG-CoA) reductase inhibitors (statins) decrease total and LDL cholesterol, decrease triglycerides, and increase HDL cholesterol by inhibiting the rate-limiting enzyme that promotes cholesterol biosynthesis.

▶ Nicotinic acid inhibits lipolysis in adipose tissue and inhibits hepatic production of very–low-density lipoprotein (VLDL) cholesterol, thus decreasing cholesterol, triglycerides, VLDL cholesterol, and LDL cholesterol, as well as increasing HDL cholesterol.

▶ The bile acid sequestrants bind bile acids in the intestine and form an insoluble complex that is excreted in the feces. Because bile acids are not absorbed, there is ultimately an increased hepatic synthesis of bile acids from cholesterol that may be evident by a slightly increased triglyceride level. However, plasma total and LDL cholesterol actually decrease owing to an increased clearance rate.

▶ The fibrates inhibit peripheral lipolysis and decrease the hepatic extraction of free fatty acids, which reduces triglyceride production. These agents decrease total cholesterol, triglycerides, and VLDL cholesterol, and they increase HDL-C.

Ezetimibe (Zetia) is a newer cholesterol absorption inhibitor that selectively inhibits the intestinal absorption of cholesterol. It is used more effectively when combined with a statin to further reduce LDL cholesterol.

Table 18-9 summarizes selected drugs used to treat hyperlipidemia. Combination drugs have become increasingly popular; therefore, it is essential that nurses know which drugs may be contained within

Table 18-9 • Selected Lipid-Lowering Drugs

Drug	Usual Initial Dose	Major Adverse Effects
Simvastatin	20–40 mg PO q.d. in the evening	Headache, abdominal pain, constipation, diarrhea, liver damage, myopathy
Pravastatin	40 mg PO q.d. at bedtime	Headache, nausea, vomiting, diarrhea, abdominal pain, flatulence, constipation, dizziness, musculoskeletal pain, liver damage, myopathy
Atorvastatin	10–20 mg PO q.d.	Constipation, diarrhea, flatulence, dyspepsia, heartburn, headache, abdominal pain, nausea, arthralgia, back pain, myopathy, liver damage, asthenia, insomnia
Lovastatin	20 mg PO q.d. with the evening meal	Headache, abdominal pain, diarrhea, nausea, vomiting, constipation, flatulence, liver damage, myopathy, back pain
Rosuvastatin	10 mg PO q.d.	Headache, nausea, vomiting, diarrhea, dyspepsia, abdominal pain, constipation, muscle pain, liver damage, asthenia, depression, dizziness, insomnia, paresthesia
Fenofibrate	130–200 mg PO q.d. with a meal (dose depends on brand name of drug)	Abdominal pain, constipation, diarrhea, nausea, liver damage, headache, back pain, dizziness, insomnia
Nicotinic acid	250 mg PO q.d. following the evening meal	Flushing, sensation of warmth, pruritus, tingling, headache, gastrointestinal upset, dizziness, hepatotoxicity
Gemfibrozil	600 mg PO b.i.d. 30 min before the morning and evening meals	Fatigue, dyspepsia, abdominal pain, diarrhea, nausea, vomiting, cholelithiasis, myopathy, dizziness, tiredness, decreased sexual drive, impotence, depression, blurred vision, impaired hepatic and renal function
Cholestyramine	4 g PO q.d. to b.i.d. at mealtime	Constipation, impaction, abdominal pain, flatulence, gastrointestinal bleeding, bleeding tendencies
Colestipol	Granules: 5 g PO q.d. to b.i.d. before meals. Tablets: 2 g PO q.d. to b.i.d. before meals	Constipation, impaction, abdominal pain, flatulence, gastrointestinal bleeding, bleeding tendencies
Ezetimibe	10 mg PO q.d. with or without food	Diarrhea, abdominal pain, back pain, joint pain, sinusitis

one tablet or capsule. For example, currently available combinations include aspirin and pravastatin (Pravachol), lovastatin (Mevacor) and extended-release niacin, and ezetimibe (Zetia) and simvastatin (Zocor). Future "polypills" may include one pill that contains a statin, an ACE inhibitor, and aspirin.

Percutaneous Coronary Interventions and Percutaneous Balloon Valvuloplasty

• Percutaneous Coronary Interventions

HISTORICAL BACKGROUND

Cardiovascular disease is the number one cause of death in the United States. The American Heart Association estimates that 71,300,000 Americans have one or more types of cardiovascular disease.[1] The estimated treatment cost of cardiovascular disease to Americans is $403.1 billion per year.[1]

The first major advance in the palliative treatment of CAD was the implantation of an aortocoronary saphenous vein bypass graft in 1967. Since that time, CABG has been refined and has been the treatment of choice for many patients with CAD. However, the first percutaneous transluminal coronary angioplasty (PTCA), performed by Andreas Gruentzig in 1977, marked another major innovation in the treatment of CAD.

Since the late 1970s, techniques to treat CAD have expanded beyond PTCA. Today, the term PCI is used to describe less invasive procedures to treat CAD and includes PTCA, laser angioplasty, atherectomy, and stenting. These interventions are described in this chapter.

The path to PCI began in 1964, when Dotter and Judkins introduced the concept of mechanically dilating a stenosis in a blood vessel with a technique of inserting a series of progressively larger catheters to treat peripheral vascular disease. After experimenting with this technique, Gruentzig modified the procedure by placing a polyvinyl balloon on the tip of a catheter; the balloon was passed into a narrowed vessel and then inflated. This revised procedure produced a smoother luminal surface with less trauma than the Dotter-Judkins approach and reduced the risk for complications, including vessel rupture, subintimal tearing, and embolism. Gruentzig performed successful dilation of more than 500 peripheral lesions. He subsequently designed a smaller version of the dilation catheter for use within the coronary arterial tree. Gruentzig performed the first human PTCA in 1977.[2] Improvements in technique and device technology during the past three decades have made PCI the treatment of choice for the management of CAD.

PTCA is a nonsurgical technique used as an alternative to CABG in the treatment of obstructive CAD. When indicated and if successful, PTCA can alleviate myocardial ischemia, relieve angina pectoris, and prevent myocardial necrosis. PTCA is the hallmark procedure and serves as the basis of almost all other percutaneous intracoronary interventions. During PTCA, a coaxial catheter system is introduced into the coronary arterial tree and advanced into an area of coronary artery stenosis. A balloon attached to the catheter is then inflated, increasing the luminal diameter and improving blood flow through the dilated segment. Several inflations ranging from 30 to 300 seconds may be performed.

PHYSIOLOGICAL PRINCIPLES

The process that leads to successful dilation is complex and not clearly defined. Angiographic evaluation and animal and human histological studies indicate that PTCA stretches the vessel wall, leading to fracture of the inelastic atherosclerotic plaque and to tearing or cracking within the intima and media of the vessel. This cracking or slight dissection of the inner lumen of the vessel may be necessary for successful dilation.[2]

COMPARISONS BETWEEN PERCUTANEOUS CORONARY INTERVENTION AND CORONARY ARTERY BYPASS GRAFTING

As an alternative treatment for CAD, PCI compares favorably with CABG in terms of risk, success rate, the patient's physical capacity after the procedure, length of hospital stay, and cost.[3]

Mortality rates associated with first-time PCI and CABG are somewhat similar. The in-hospital death rate for patients undergoing PCI ranges from 0% to 2%; the CABG mortality rate ranges from 1.5% to 4%.[4] In the event that a second surgical procedure becomes necessary to alleviate the symptoms of progressive CAD, the mortality and complication rates for the bypass procedure are significantly greater than for a second PCI. Seven-year survival data in the Bypass Angioplasty Revascularization Investigation (BARI) trial revealed that CABG offers a survival benefit to diabetic patients compared with PTCA (76.4% versus 55.7%). There was no difference in the survival rates of nondiabetic patients with CABG versus PTCA (86.4% versus 86.8%).[5] Three-year outcome data after stenting compared with CABG for the treatment of multivessel disease revealed similar mortality rates.[6,7]

Successful PCI, which is defined as a significant reduction of the luminal diameter stenosis without in-hospital death, myocardial infarction, or CABG, ranges from 80% to 100%, depending on the severity of the patient's angiographic and clinical presentation. In a study by Bentivoglio and colleagues, the cumulative 2-year survival rates were 96% and 95% among patients with stable and unstable angina, respectively, with event-free survival (i.e., no death, myocardial infarction, or CABG) in 79% and 76%, respectively.[8] Among patients with multivessel PCI, the actuarial survival rates were 97% at 1 year and 88% at 5 years in a study by O'Keefe and colleagues.[9] Seven years after PTCA, Dorros and associates reported a survival rate of 90% in patients with simple single-vessel angioplasty and 95% in patients with simple multivessel angioplasty.[10] Long-term survival data in the era of stenting revealed that survival rates remain approximately the same (92% to 97%) [7,11] Data regarding long-term survival in patients who have received DES are being collected at this time.

In the Coronary Artery Surgery Study, graft patency after CABG was 90% at 2 months, 82% at 18 months, and 82% at 5 years. The 10-year survival rate was 82%.[12]

Restenosis or patency data differ greatly between CABG and PCI. Within 6 months after angioplasty, 20% to 30% of lesions recur or restenose. Bare metal intracoronary stenting reduces the incidence of restenosis by an additional 5% to 10%. DES placement further reduces the risk for restenosis to approximately 2%.[13-15] Recently, late loss, defined as late restenosis following DES, has been observed. Stent manufacturers are addressing the concern of late loss through DES platform design and a variety of drug coatings applied directly to the stent. The mean occlusion rate for bypass grafts is approximately 18% during the first 5 years and 4% to 5% in 5 to 10 years.[7]

Psychological advantages of PTCA over surgery may argue favorably for the less invasive procedure. The emotional stress of awaiting dilation is less than that of awaiting surgery. However, this reduction in anxiety is partly offset by the risk for psychological crisis if the angioplasty fails and surgery—especially emergent (immediate) surgery—is needed. The psychological impact of this discouraging situation is significant, but it occurs in a relatively low percentage of cases.

Barring complications with either procedure, PCI requires a hospital stay of 12 to 24 hours, whereas CABG requires a stay of 3 to 7 days. Because the average hospital stay is shorter with PCI and because it is performed in the cardiac catheterization laboratory under local anesthesia, the average cost of PCI may be substantially lower than that of CABG. However, the following factors can increase the cost of PCI:

▶ Complications occurring during the procedure that necessitate emergency surgery (e.g., coronary perforation, acute closure)

▶ Lesions that recur, requiring repeat dilation, or bypass surgery

▶ Surgical standby, which is provided in different levels to correspond to the risk associated with each PCI

▶ Lesions that require multiple devices to alleviate the lesion

▶ Complications associated with the anticoagulation regimen or arterial and venous access

In general, after a PCI, patients can expect a faster return to work (5 to 7 days) as opposed to patients who have had a CABG (6 to 8 weeks). Depression in patients following CABG is common, although reports of quality of life in both groups are similar. [16]

In conclusion, the major advantages of PCI compared with CABG may include reduced mortality and morbidity, shorter convalescence, and lower cost to the patient and third-party payers.

DIAGNOSTIC TESTS FOR PATIENT SELECTION: PERCUTANEOUS CORONARY INTERVENTION AND CORONARY ARTERY BYPASS GRAFTING

Before deciding between PCI and CABG, all objective evidence of coronary insufficiency must be documented. Noninvasive methods of evaluation that may be used before and after PCI include standard treadmill stress testing and thallium stress and redistribution myocardial imaging. These tests allow the physician to discover the areas of ischemia in the myocardium when the patient is subjected to stress (i.e., exercise; see Chapter 17 for a discussion of these tests). It is necessary that nurses familiarize themselves with the results of thallium stress tests because an understanding of the patient's diagnosis, related symptoms, and indications for PCI promotes informed patient care.

Coronary angiography performed by cardiac catheterization, another method of documenting coronary insufficiency, is performed if the previous tests suggest the presence of coronary artery disease. Although this procedure is more invasive than treadmill testing and thallium imaging, it is the gold standard test to pinpoint the location of any stenoses and the degree of involvement of the artery or arteries (see Chapter 17 for a discussion of this test). This procedure yields a 35-mm, VHS tape cineangiogram, or digital image of the coronary artery anatomy. The physician can then analyze the areas of narrowing (stenosis) and gain precise information to decide the appropriate treatment (Figs. 18-1 and 18-2).

EQUIPMENT FEATURES

Since the introduction of the PCI procedure, the device technology has been refined and improved, resulting in fewer contraindications, lower rates of mortality, and fewer incidences of emergent bypass surgery.

The guiding catheters used to direct and support the advancement of the dilation catheter into the appropriate coronary artery ostium have an outer diameter of 6 to 10 French (Fr). The tips of the guiding catheters have curves that are preshaped for selective access to either the right or left coronary artery.

Balloon dilation systems have evolved since Gruentzig's original design, in which the guide wire tip and catheter shaft were integral. In the early days of

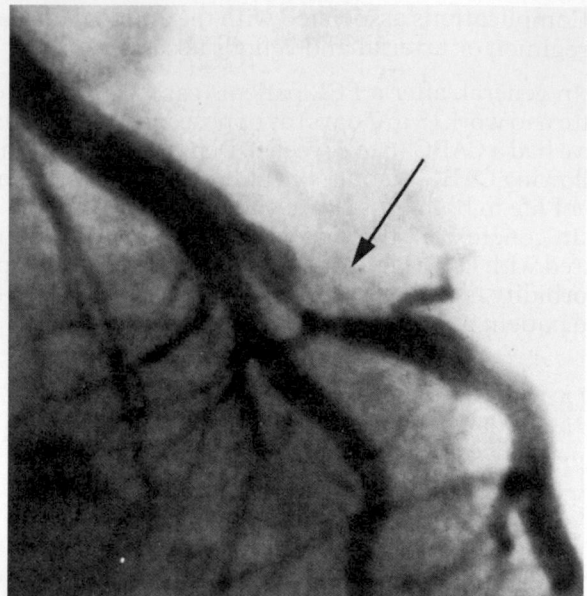

Figure 18-1 • An eccentric stenosis in the left anterior descending artery. The term *eccentric* defines a plaque involving only one side of the intraluminal wall. (Courtesy of John B. Simpson, MD, Palo Alto, CA.)

PTCA, physicians were limited by catheter performance and could address lesions only in the proximal anatomy. In 1982, Simpson introduced a coaxial "over-the-wire" system, an improvement that has become predominant in current catheter designs. The

main innovation is an independently movable guide wire within the balloon dilation catheter. This guide wire can be manipulated to select the correct vessel despite side branches and permits safe advancement of the dilation catheter across the lesion. Currently, the available guide wires measure between 0.010 and 0.018 inch in diameter and thus usually pose little threat of interference with the blood flow through a stenosis.

Coronary balloon dilation catheter shafts range in size from 2.0 to 4.2 Fr, small enough for easy passage through the guiding catheter and for visualization around the catheter during contrast injection. Figure 18-3 shows the contrast injection through the guiding wire to verify position. The balloon dilation catheter has one or more radiopaque markers that can be imaged by fluoroscopy, allowing the interventional cardiologist to position the balloon accurately across the lesion. The inflated balloon size ranges from 1.5 to 5 mm in diameter and from 10 to 40 mm in length. The size (inflated diameter) of the balloon to be used for a particular PCI procedure is usually the same as the smallest-diameter segment of the coronary artery proximal or distal to the stenosis (i.e., 3-mm vessel, 3-mm balloon). Lesion and balloon length also are approximated. Figure 18-4 shows the key components of the PTCA balloon dilation catheter.

The interventional cardiologist manually inflates the balloon with a contrast-filled, disposable inflation device that connects to the side arm or balloon lumen of the coronary dilation catheter. The device incorporates a pressure gauge that indicates the amount of pressure exerted against the balloon wall during inflation. Balloon pressure is measured in pounds per square inch (psi) or atmospheres (atm). The average initial inflation is between 60 and 150 psi or 4 to 10 atm and lasts from 30 to 180 seconds. Longer inflations may promote a smoother, more regular vessel

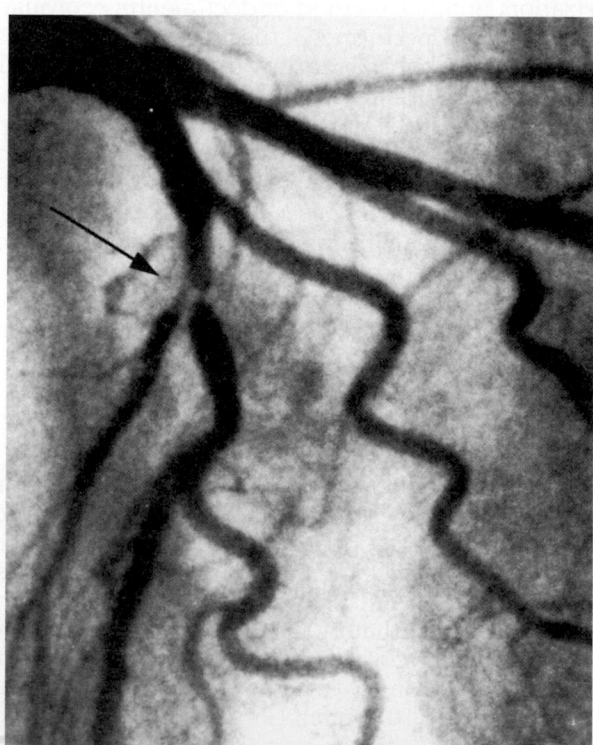

Figure 18-2 • A coronary arteriogram of the circumflex artery illustrating a concentric stenosis. The term *concentric* defines a plaque involving the intraluminal wall circumferentially, giving a dumbbell appearance. (Courtesy of John B. Simpson, MD, Palo Alto, CA.)

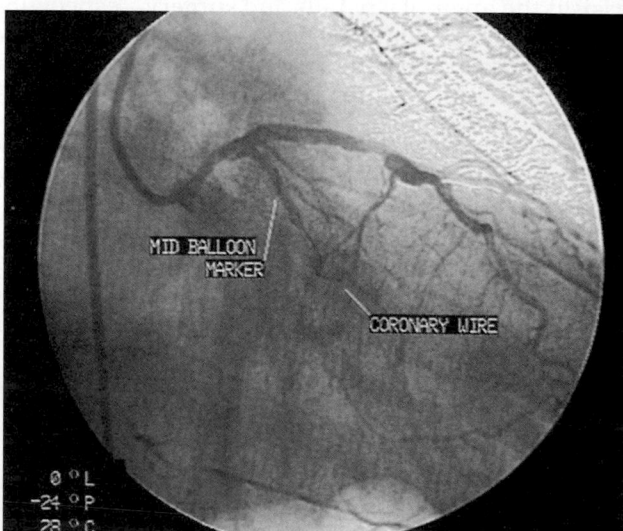

Figure 18-3 • Contrast injection through the guiding catheter to verify position. The coronary guide wire tip is located at the occlusion of the circumflex artery, and the coronary balloon is positioned in the proximal vessel. (Reprinted with permission of Advanced Cardiovascular Systems [ACS] Inc., Santa Clara, CA.)

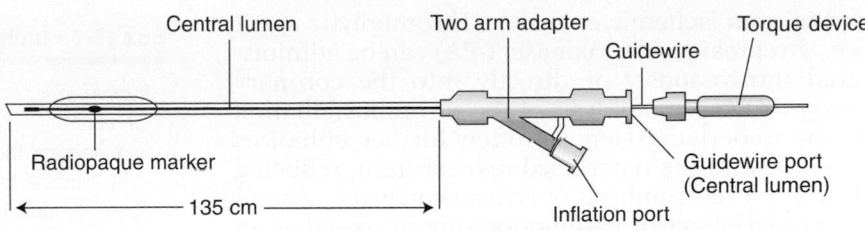

Figure 18-4 • PTCA balloon dilation catheter illustrating the key components of the system. (Reprinted with permission of Advanced Cardiovascular Systems [ACS] Inc., Santa Clara, CA.)

wall as assessed by angiography and are used primarily for the treatment of major dissections and abrupt closure. Extended inflations are performed safely with perfusion catheters that simultaneously dilate and perfuse the coronary artery.

Many factors must be considered when selecting the most appropriate equipment for performing PCI. Technological advances have occurred. Several newly developed balloon dilation catheter systems have improved the success and safety associated with PCI.

Many interventional cardiologists consider the coaxial "over-the-wire" system a workhorse catheter because it can approach any anatomy well. However, the interventional cardiologist might select a rapid-exchange system to accomplish more easily the dilation of a bifurcation lesion. This type of device incorporates a "rail" system that facilitates the exchange process. A fixed-wire catheter is used to reach and dilate lesions in distal, tortuous anatomy, and its small shaft also makes it an option for the use of two coronary dilation catheters in one guiding catheter when the strategy calls for side-by-side balloons; this is also referred to as a "kissing balloon" technique.

Each PCI intervention also encompasses an inflation strategy. The main elements of an inflation strategy are the duration and pressure of balloon inflation required to open a lesion. Today, balloons that can withstand greater pressure for the treatment of calcific lesions are available.

The outcome of any PCI procedure is greatly affected by (1) the selection of a guiding catheter that provides a platform for the advancement of the dilation system while preserving flow to the coronary artery, and (2) the selection of a balloon dilation system and intracoronary DES that best address the vessel's anatomy, the lesion's location, and lesion characteristics.

INDICATIONS FOR AND CONTRAINDICATIONS TO PERCUTANEOUS CORONARY INTERVENTION

Indications

When choosing to treat with PCI, the physician's purpose is to alleviate angina pectoris unrelieved by medical treatment and to reduce the risk for myocardial infarction in symptomatic patients and asymptomatic patients with significant stenosis. Indications for PCI have expanded as device technology, techniques, and operator experience have improved.

PCI is indicated in coronary arteries that have at least a 70% narrowing. Arteries with less narrowing are not considered appropriate for PCI because they are equally at risk for abrupt closure, which can have serious consequences. Patients with surgical risk factors, such as severe underlying noncardiac diseases, advanced age, and poor left ventricular function, are particularly suited for PCI because successful dilation obviates the need for an operation that would be poorly tolerated.

An example of the wide spectrum of candidacy for PCI is the accepted practice of treating patients with multivessel disease. The common technique for dilating multiple lesions is to dilate the most critical stenosis first. With successful dilation of this "culprit" lesion, remaining lesions are dilated in stages (i.e., at different intervals during the procedure or over several days). However, dilation of multiple vessels is technically more demanding and carries a higher risk for complications.

Another expanded indication is the approach to treating the patient with a totally occluded vessel. Early in PCI practice, acute and chronic total occlusions disqualified a patient for the procedure because the stenosis could not be crossed with the guide wire and balloon dilation catheter without causing severe trauma to the artery. Refinement of device technology and greater physician experience have allowed dilation of total occlusions attempts in appropriate candidates. Total occlusions of short duration (i.e., 3 months or less) are easier to cross and dilate successfully than total occlusions of longer duration (chronic total occlusions).

Additional candidates for PCI are those who have undergone CABG in whom symptoms have recurred because of stenosis and graft closure or progression of coronary disease in the native vessels or in vein grafts. For these candidates, successful PCI makes second surgery, with its increased potential for complications, unnecessary. It is thought that the proliferative disease in the graft wall generates fibrous stenosis that is much less dense than most fibrotic tissue in the native vessels, so certain vein graft stenoses respond favorably to percutaneous intervention.

Historically, patients experiencing an AMI as documented by significant ST-segment elevation, increased cardiac enzyme levels, and pain unrelieved by thrombolysis, surgery, or pharmacological treatment, were treated with complete bed rest in a coronary care unit. Today, if thrombus and underlying stenosis are causing the infarction, thrombolytic therapy, PCI, or both offer alternatives. If a blood clot has impeded flow to the distal myocardium and precipitates an ischemic episode, a thrombolytic agent (i.e., streptokinase, urokinase, t-PA) can be administered intravenously or directly into the coronary artery. On successful lysis of the thrombus, dilation of the underlying stenosis often further enhances blood flow to the reperfused myocardium, reducing the risk for rethrombosis or critical narrowing caused by normal or spastic vasomotion superimposed on an organic stenosis.

Primary PCI is a dilation of an infarct-related coronary artery during the acute phase of an AMI without prior administration of a thrombolytic agent. Meyer and associates first used PTCA in the AMI setting in 1982.[17] They reported an 81% success rate in PTCA of the infarct-related artery after intracoronary thrombolytic therapy. In 1999, Grines reported a stand-alone PTCA success rate of 97% with a patency rate of 53% 2 years after PTCA.[18] Parameters routinely assessed in patients selected to receive primary angioplasty are depicted in Box 18-3.

In the setting of AMI, PCI may benefit patients deemed ineligible for traditional medical therapy. Such patients include those in cardiogenic shock, those believed to be at high risk for bleeding complications (CVA, prolonged cardiopulmonary resuscitation [CPR], bleeding diathesis, severe hypertension, or recent surgery), and those of advanced age (>75 years). Primary PCI does not preclude the use of thrombolytics if residual thrombus is observed. Primary PCI may offer distinct advantages in reducing the length of hospital stay and eliminating the need for additional intervention in many cases. Indications for PCI are summarized in Box 18-4.

Complications of primary PCI include retroperitoneal or vascular hemorrhage, other bleeding requiring transfusion, late restenosis, and early acute reocclusion (subacute thrombosis). These complica-

---

Box 18-4 • Indications and Contraindications for PCI

Indications	*Contraindications*
Clinical	
Symptomatic (angina unrelieved by medical therapy)	
Asymptomatic but with severe underlying stenosis	
Stable/unstable angina	
Acute myocardial infarction	
High-risk surgical candidates	
Anatomical	
Severe stenosis (≥70%)	Mild stenosis (<70%)
Proximal and distal lesions	
Single and multivessel disease	
Bifurcation lesions	
Ostial lesions	
Totally occluded vessels	
Bypass graft lesions	
"Protected" and unprotected left main coronary artery (previous LAD or LCX coronary artery bypass graft)	

LAD, left anterior descending artery; LCX, left circumflex artery.

---

tions occur at approximately the same rate as those experienced in routine elective PCI.

Contraindications

There are very few contraindications to PCI. Patients with left main CAD were once not considered candidates for PCI. The obvious drawback of PCI in left main artery disease is the possibility of acute occlusion or spasm of the left main artery during the procedure, which would result in severe left ventricular dysfunction. Patients who have a "protected" left main artery (i.e., have had previous bypass surgery to the left anterior descending or circumflex arteries with patent grafts present) are often candidates for PCI. One-year clinical outcomes of protected and unprotected left main coronary artery stenting revealed that those who had unprotected left main stenting had increased major adverse cardiac events, and their survival was decreased at 1 year. However, left main stenting should be considered in the absence of other options. [19] For high-risk patients (i.e., patients with left main vessel disease, severe left ventricular dysfunction, or dilation of the last remaining patent artery), percutaneous support devices may improve the safety of PCI. These devices include perfusion balloons, intra-aortic balloon counterpulsation, coronary sinus retroperfusion, and cardiopulmonary support.

PROCEDURE

The PCI procedure is carried out in a sterile fashion, with the use of local anesthesia and either the Judkins (percutaneous femoral) approach or, less often, the Sones (brachial cut-down) approach (Fig. 18-5).

Box 18-3 • Parameter Evaluated in Patients Selected to Receive Primary Angioplasty

- Age
- Hemodynamic status
- Angiographic anatomy:
  - Single-, double-, or triple-vessel disease
  - Vessel involvement: LAD, RCA, LCX
  - Lesion location ostial: proximal, mid, or distal disease
  - Percent grade stenosis
  - Thrombolysis in myocardial infarction (TIMI) flow: 0, I, II, III
  - Left ventricular ejection fraction (%)
- Presence of chest pain consistent with acute myocardial infarction
- Electrocardiogram evidence of acute myocardial infarction:
  - 1 mm ST elevation in two contiguous leads
  - or
  - 1 mm ST depression believed to represent reciprocal changes to an area of infarction

LAD, left anterior descending artery; LCX, left circumflex artery; RCA, right coronary artery.

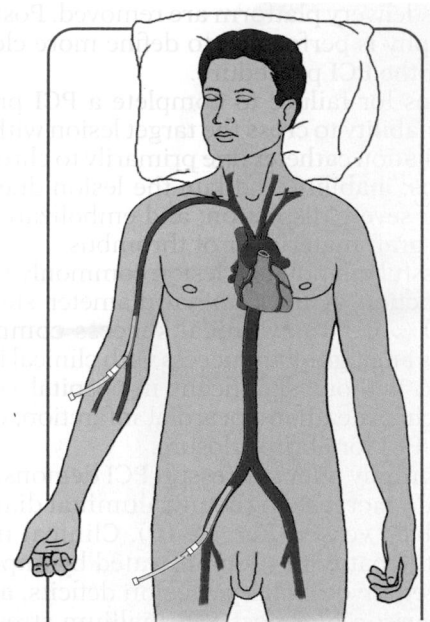

Figure 18-5 • Two approaches to left heart catheterization. The Sones technique uses the brachial artery, and the Judkins technique uses the femoral artery. With either method, the catheter is passed retrograde through the ascending aorta to the left ventricle. (Reprinted with permission of Advanced Cardiovascular Systems [ACS] Inc., Santa Clara, CA.)

With the Judkins approach, the interventional cardiologist cannulates the femoral vein and artery percutaneously by inserting a needle (usually 18-gauge) containing a removable obturator. The obturator is then removed to confirm by the presence of blood flow that the outer needle is within the lumen of the vessel. Once proper placement is established, a guide wire is introduced through the outer cannula into the artery to the level of the diaphragm. The cannula then is removed and replaced by a valved introducer sheath. The sheath provides hemostasis and support at the puncture site in the groin and reduces potential arterial trauma if multiple catheter exchanges are necessary. The guiding catheter is preloaded with a 0.038-inch J-wire and introduced into the sheath. The 0.038-inch J-wire is advanced over the arch, and the guiding catheter is advanced over the wire. The 0.038-inch J-wire is removed, and the guiding catheter is rotated precisely to the appropriate coronary ostium. The procedure also may be accomplished by the Sones approach, in which a brachial cutdown is used to isolate the brachial vein and artery. A small arteriotomy is made, and the catheter is passed to the level of the aortic arch.

Regardless of the mode of access, coronary angiography is then carried out in both the left anterior oblique (30 degrees) and right anterior oblique (60 degrees) views. These views allow for visualization of the heart along its transverse and longitudinal planes. Opposing views provide a thorough assessment of both the lesion and the anatomical approach. A "freeze frame" of each view is obtained as a road map or guide throughout the procedure. A final lesion assessment is made, confirming lesion severity and vessel diameter for appropriate balloon and stent sizing.

If PCI is indicated, the patient may be anticoagulated with 5,000 to 10,000 units of heparin to prevent the formation of clots on or in the catheter system during the procedure. Intracoronary nitroglycerin is kept on the sterile field throughout the procedure and given intermittently as needed for vasospasm and for dilation to facilitate visualization of the culprit coronary artery.

The balloon dilation catheter and intracoronary stent system is introduced into the guiding catheter through a bifurcated adapter that provides access and is a port for contrast injections and aortic pressure measurement. The balloon dilation catheter, stent, and guide wire are advanced to the tip of the guiding catheter while their position is checked by fluoroscopy (Fig. 18-6). The guide wire then is advanced and manipulated to negotiate the branches of the coronary artery. Proper advancement can be confirmed by injecting contrast through the guiding catheter and fluoroscopically visualizing the coronary tree.

Once the guide wire is positioned safely beyond the stenosis, the balloon dilation catheter (with or without a stent) can be advanced slowly over the guide wire into the narrowing without risk for injury to the intima (Fig. 18-7).

Exact placement of the dilation balloon and stent in the stenosis is facilitated under fluoroscopy by the radiopaque marker on the balloon and by contrast injections for visualization. Initially, the balloon is inflated at 1 to 2 atm of pressure to confirm its position. Many PTCA balloon catheters expand at both ends and not in the center, where they are pinched by the stenosis (Figs. 18-8 and 18-9). The central indentation usually disappears as the stenosis is dilated. After each inflation, the interventional cardiologist injects a small bolus of contrast medium to assess any changes in coronary blood flow through the stenosis and to assess any increase in luminal diameter. At this time, the need for additional inflations is

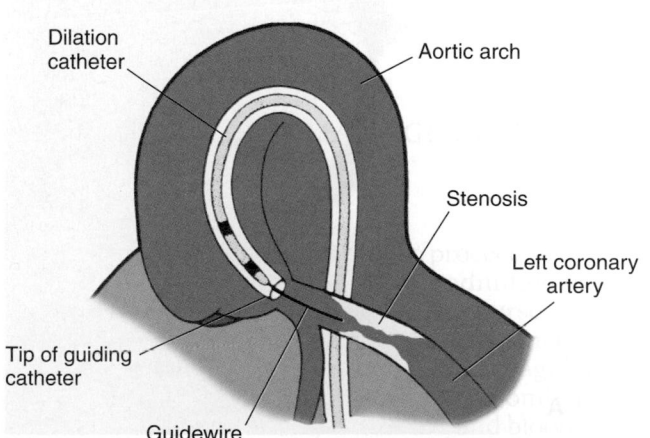

Dilation catheter

Aortic arch

Stenosis

Left coronary artery

Tip of guiding catheter

Guidewire

Figure 18-6 • The advancement of the coronary dilation catheter to the tip of the guiding catheter, which is positioned in the left coronary artery, is facilitated by fluoroscopy. (Reprinted with permission of Advanced Cardiovascular Systems [ACS] Inc., Santa Clara, CA.)

also is sensitive and becomes irritable when the flow of oxygen-rich blood decreases, as it does for a controlled period of time during placement and inflation of the dilation balloon and stent across the lesion. The irritability arising from hypokalemia, ischemia, or both can give rise to life-threatening ventricular dysrhythmias.

Elevation in the levels of serum creatinine, BUN, or both may indicate problems in kidney function. Good kidney function is important because during PCI, radiopaque contrast material (which allows fluoroscopic visualization of the coronary anatomy and of catheter placement) is introduced into the bloodstream.[20] This contrast material is a hyperosmotic solution that the kidneys must filter and excrete from the blood. High levels of creatinine and BUN may reflect decreased renal filtration capability and vulnerability of the kidney in processing the extra load of radiopaque solution. Instances of acute renal failure have resulted from high doses of radiopaque contrast. A study by Rihal and colleagues reported a 3.3% incidence rate of contrast-induced renal failure following PCI. Contrast-induced renal failure occurs more frequently in patients who are diabetic, in patients who are dehydrated, and in patients with higher baseline creatinine levels.[21] The nurse should ensure that the patient is adequately hydrated, either orally or with IV solutions, to avoid falsely high electrolyte levels. Trends in creatinine and BUN levels, in conjunction with measurement of urine output, can be used to monitor kidney function.

Informed Consent

The informed consent for the PCI procedure is obtained from the patient before the procedure after a detailed discussion of the potential complications, anticipated benefit, and alternative therapies. This discussion should be conducted before any preoperative sedation. The nurse plays an important role in answering any questions that the patient and his or her family may have regarding the procedure and follow-up care.

Preoperative Medications

Twenty-four hours before the procedure, the patient's medications should include aspirin, 325 mg once a day, for its antiplatelet effect. Diabetic patients taking metformin should be advised to discontinue this medication before their procedure because it is contraindicated with intravascular contrast agents. Anticoagulants such as warfarin are often withheld for a number of days before the PCI procedure. Studies have shown that administration of clopidogrel before and after a PCI decrease adverse events such as acute closure and subacute thrombosis.[22,23]

Surgical Standby

Surgical standby for PCI is controversial at this time. Surgical availability is required, but the degree to which the operating room is held for availability varies according to the patient's risk factors, patient acuity, and hospital policies. Many smaller community hospitals across the United States are performing PCI procedures without in-house surgical standby.

These patients are typically low risk and reside near larger academic centers that can accept the patient by immediate transfer if complications arise during the PCI. A comparison of patients treated with PCI at hospitals without on-site cardiac surgery with those treated only with thrombolytic therapy reveals that the former group has better clinical outcomes at 1, 3, and 6 months.[24]

Nursing Management During Percutaneous Coronary Intervention

Both before and during the procedure, nurses in the cardiac catheterization laboratory are responsible for understanding all aspects of equipment use and patient care. They should be experienced in advanced cardiac life support and be knowledgeable about the proper administration of emergency medications and the correct application of emergency equipment, including the defibrillator, the intra-aortic balloon pump, the ventilator, and the temporary pacemaker. They observe and communicate with the patient intermittently and report any changes in patient status to the physician. The nurse monitors the ECG and arterial pressure, noting significant changes that may accompany the administration of drugs, symptoms of ischemia, or chest pain. The nurse must recognize signs and symptoms of contrast sensitivity, such as urticaria, blushing, anxiety, nausea, and laryngospasm. The nurse should understand the proper assembly and use of all PCI equipment and should be able to troubleshoot any situation that might arise.

The patient's anticoagulation status during the PCI procedure is of utmost importance. Subtherapeutic levels may result in serious complications, including acute closure or thrombotic events. An ACT should be measured in the catheterization laboratory at baseline (before the PTCA), 5 minutes after the heparin bolus (usually 5,000 to 10,000 units), and every 30 minutes thereafter for the duration of the procedure. ACT levels of 250 to 300 seconds are desirable after the initial heparin bolus. Subsequent boluses of 2,000 to 5,000 units of heparin may be required to achieve and maintain these ACT levels during the PCI procedure.

Patients at high risk for abrupt closure or with unstable lesions, such as in the setting of AMI, may be administered a platelet GP IIb/IIIa antagonist in addition to aspirin and heparin. This is referred to as a "facilitated PCI." These agents are typically initiated just before or during PCI. Eptifibatide or tirofiban should be administered, in addition to aspirin and either unfractionated heparin or LMWH, to patients with continuing ischemia, an elevated troponin, or other high-risk features in whom an invasive management strategy is not planned.[24]

After the PCI is complete, the nurse instructs the patient in the precautions necessary to prevent bleeding from the puncture site. Box 18-5 presents patient teaching.

After the procedure, the patient is transferred to a telemetry unit or catheterization recovery area for observation. Common nursing diagnoses and collaborative problems for patients undergoing PCI are listed in Box 18-6.

Box 18-5 • TEACHING GUIDE:
Precautions Post-PTCA

- Remain on bed rest for 4 to 6 h.
- Maintain the involved leg in a straight position (for Judkins technique).
- Avoid an upright position.
- Avoid vigorous use of the abdominal muscles, as in coughing, sneezing, or moving the bowels.

Nursing Management After Percutaneous Coronary Interventions

The nurse in the coronary care or telemetry unit plays an important role in observing and assessing the patient's recovery. Post-PCI care is designed to monitor the patient closely for signs and symptoms of myocardial ischemia. The most overt symptom of a possible complication, early recurrence of angina pectoris, requires prompt nursing action.

As soon as possible on receiving the patient from the cardiac catheterization laboratory, the nurse attaches the ECG monitor, which allows a quick initial cardiac assessment and establishes a baseline if the patient's condition should change suddenly. The nurse assesses the patient's status from head to toe, noting the overall skin color and temperature and carefully observing the level of consciousness. After the patient is transferred

Box 18-6 **Examples of Nursing Diagnoses and Collaborative Problems for the Patient Having PCI or PBV**

- Risk for Decreased Cardiac Output related to mechanical factors that affect preload, afterload, and left ventricular function
- Risk for Decreased Cardiac Output related to electrical factors affecting rate, rhythm, or conduction
- Risk for Decreased Cardiac Output related to structural changes (dissection, thrombus, or arterial spasm at PCI site), resulting in myocardial ischemia or infarction
- Risk for Decreased Cardiac Output related to increased preload and pulmonary congestion related to temporary mechanical factors (e.g., balloon inflation during PBV)
- Risk for Decreased Cardiac Output related to left-to-right shunt with mitral PBV or late cardiac tamponade
- Risk for Impaired Peripheral Perfusion related to hematoma, thrombus formation, or infection associated with cannulation site
- Risk for Impaired Cerebral Perfusion related to embolism from procedure site, left ventricle, or left atrium
- Risk for Pain related to angina or stretching of the valve during dilation
- Risk for Fluid Volume Deficit related to renal sensitivity to contrast material or diuretic therapy
- Deficient Knowledge related to illness and impact on patient's future
- Anxiety/Fear related to lack of knowledge of PCI/PBV, acute care environment, and potential for surgery

to the bed and attached to the monitor, the nurse listens closely to heart and breath sounds. The nurse evaluates the peripheral circulation by noting peripheral skin color and temperature and the presence and quality of dorsalis pedis and posterior tibial pulses.

Because the Judkins technique is used most often in PCI to access the vasculature, most patients have an entry port in either the right or the left groin through which sheaths have been placed percutaneously in a vein and artery. If the Sones technique is used, there is an arterial catheter in the brachial area (see Fig. 18-5). A variety of mechanical devices and clamps may be used to facilitate hemostasis after sheath removal. The insertion of collagen plugs or the application of a surgical suture around the opening of the blood vessel is also routinely performed to obtain hemostasis. After sheath removal, the nurse pays careful attention to the area distal to the puncture site, checking pulses frequently and reporting immediately to the physician any changes that may indicate bleeding. Bleeding at the sheath site may result in a major hematoma that can require surgical evacuation or compromise distal blood flow to the lower extremity. To prevent excessive bleeding and to aid hemostasis, the physician may order that a 5-lb sandbag be placed over the puncture site after sheath removal.

The nurse instructs the patient on the importance of keeping the involved leg straight and the head of the bed angled at 45 degrees or less. To prevent clotting in the lumens of the introducing sheaths, an IV infusion is attached to the venous sheath, and a pressurized arterial flush is attached to the arterial line. This arrangement also ensures patency should an immediate return to the cardiac catheterization laboratory be necessary because of a complication. The physician chooses both the type of solution to be infused through the venous sheath and the rate of infusion. His or her decision depends on the patient's fluid volume status.

Although initial post-PCI laboratory blood tests vary by institution, they may include coagulation studies, cardiac enzymes, and serum electrolytes. Elevation of the cardiac enzymes can indicate that a silent myocardial infarction has occurred (i.e., infarction unannounced by chest pain). If a cardiac enzyme laboratory value is abnormal, the nurse notifies the physician immediately because the patient's postoperative care might need to be modified to prevent further injury.

The nurse plays a significant role in observing and assessing angina that recurs soon after a PCI procedure. Any chest pain demands immediate and careful attention because it may indicate either the start of vasospasm or impending subacute thrombosis. The patient may describe angina as a burning, squeezing heaviness or as sharp mid-sternal pain. Other signs and symptoms of myocardial ischemia include ischemic ECG changes (elevation of the ST segments or T-wave inversion), dysrhythmias, hypotension, and nausea. The nurse notifies the physician immediately of any such change in the patient's condition because it is impossible to tell merely by observation whether the change indicates a transient vasospastic episode, which can be resolved with vasodilation therapy, or an acute occlusion requiring emergent intervention (repeat PCI or CABG).

If vasodilation therapy is indicated, it may be administered as described subsequently unless the patient is hypotensive; in that case, vasodilation is contraindicated. At the first sign of vasospasm, the nurse gives oxygen by mask or nasal cannula. For fast, temporary (and possibly permanent) relief, 0.4 mg of nitroglycerin, 5 mg of isosorbide, or 10 mg of nifedipine is administered sublingually. In addition, the IV drip of nitroglycerin should be titrated to maintain a blood pressure adequate to ensure coronary artery perfusion and to alleviate chest pain.

In conjunction with the onset of the chest pain, a 12-lead ECG reading is recorded to document any acute changes. If the angina resolves and any acute ECG changes caused by medical therapy disappear, it is safe to assume that a transient vasospastic episode occurred; however, if the angina continues and the ECG changes persist, redilation or emergency bypass surgery should be considered.

If the post-PCI course is uncomplicated, the sheaths are removed after 2 to 4 hours, and a pressure dressing is applied to the site. A variety of mechanical clamps or hemostasis devices may be used to facilitate hemostasis after sheath removal. Many times, the sheaths are removed before the patient leaves the cardiac catheterization laboratory, and a hemostasis device is utilized. The patient must continue complete bed rest for 4 to 6 hours after the sheaths are removed. A normal, low-sodium, or low-cholesterol diet may be resumed, depending on the preference of the physician and the needs of the patient.

During the recovery period, the nurse can introduce the patient to the rehabilitation process, emphasizing lifestyle modifications to combat the advance of CAD. Efforts should be made during this instruction to reinforce the importance of aerobic conditioning with regular, moderate exercise. Risk factor and secondary prevention are also discussed, including stress reduction, weight loss, and smoking cessation. See Box 18-5 for instructions for the patient after PCI. Box 18-7 describes implications for the older patient.

After PCI, the patient is asked to take medications that help prevent thrombus formation and maintain maximal dilation at the culprit lesion site. All patients should be routinely sent home on aspirin for the antiplatelet effect. Aspirin is continued indefinitely. Clopidogrel (Plavix) should be administered to patients who receive one or more DESs. Clopidogrel should be continued for at least 1 to 3 months and may be administered indefinitely.[22,23] However, in patients taking clopidogrel in whom elective CABG is planned, the drug should be withheld for 5 to 7 days. Often, long-acting nitrates, calcium channel blockers, ACE inhibitors, and lipid-lowering agents are added to the medical regimen. The nurse may be responsible for explaining to the patient the indications for the specific medications ordered by the physician, including side effects and signs of overdose. The nurse should also answer any questions that the patient may have regarding his or her follow-up care.

Box 18-7 • CONSIDERATIONS FOR THE OLDER PATIENT: Before and After PCI

- Assess whether the patient will have assistance in the home with meals, cleaning, self-care, and transportation to medical appointments.
- Closely monitor kidney function before and after PCI because elderly patients may be sensitive to small amounts of radiocontrast.
- Monitor vital signs frequently, including temperature, because elderly patients are prone to excessive body heat loss.
- Assess all preexisting comorbidities: arthritis, peripheral vascular disease, diabetes, and so forth.
- Provide clear, precise, written instructions in preparation for discharge.
- Assess ability to purchase/afford required medications.

Box 18-8 summarizes medications currently associated with PCI.

Four to 6 weeks after the patient's discharge, an exercise treadmill stress test and a thallium imaging study may be performed to test the efficacy of the PCI. Compared with the pre-PCI tests, an increase in exercise capacity and a decrease in or disappearance of exercise-induced chest pain (without ST-segment changes) suggest improved blood flow and normalization of cardiac function in the previously hypoperfused muscle. Treadmill stress testing should be repeated at 6 months and then annually after PCI.

COMPLICATIONS

The indications for PCI have expanded to include patients with more severe CAD (i.e., total occlusions, multivessel disease, recent or ongoing myocardial infarction, poor left ventricular function). The rate of complications associated with PCI has not increased. Major complications that can result in ischemia and possible severe left ventricular dysfunction necessitating emergent CABG include angina unrelieved by maximal administration of nitrates and calcium channel blockers (see Box 18-8), myocardial infarction, coronary artery spasm, abrupt closure of a dilated segment, coronary artery dissection leading to occlusion, and restenosis. See Box 18-6 for nursing diagnoses and collaborative problems for the patient having PCI or percutaneous balloon valvuloplasty.

Angina, Myocardial Infarction, and Vasospasm

Some degree of angina is anticipated during the PCI procedure owing to the temporary occlusion of the involved vessel during dilation. This angina is handled with intracoronary nitroglycerin or removal of the balloon dilation catheter while the guide wire is left across the lesion. Evidence of persistent chest pain after PCI, reflected in changes in heart rate and blood pressure and elevated ST segments, indicates ischemia predisposing to an insult to the myocardium

Box 18-8 • Drug Therapy Summary of Medications Most Often Associated With PCI

Anticoagulants/Antiplatelets

Aspirin
Indications: Prophylaxis of coronary and cerebral arterial thrombus formation
Actions: Blocks platelet aggregation
Dosage: 80–325 mg q.d., PO
Adverse effects: Well tolerated; nausea, vomiting, diarrhea, headache, and vertigo occasionally

Heparin (fractionated)
Indications: Prophylaxis of impending coronary occlusion and prophylaxis of peripheral arterial embolism
Actions: Inhibits clotting of blood and formation of fibrin clots; inactivates thrombin, preventing conversion of fibrinogen to fibrin; prevents formation of a stable fibrin clot by inhibiting the activation of fibrin stabilizing factor; inhibits reactions that lead to clotting but does not alter normal components of blood; prolongs clotting time but does not affect bleeding time; does not lyse clots
Dosage: Varies with indications; IV or intra-arterial: 10,000 U at start of PCI
Adverse effects: Uncontrollable bleeding, hypersensitivity

Low–Molecular-Weight Heparin
(Enoxaparin Sodium, Dalteparin Sodium)
Indications: Treatment of unstable angina and myocardial ischemia, complete and non–Q-wave myocardial infarction.
Action: Prevents clotting of blood and formation of thrombin.
Dosage
   Enoxaprin: 1 mg/kg SC q12h for 2–8 days
   Dalteparin sodium: 120 µg/kg SC q12h for 5–8 days
Adverse effects: Thrombocytopenia, hematoma, pain or reaction at the injection site, rash, hemorrhage, fever.

Glycoprotein IIb/IIIa Antagonists
(Abciximab, Eptifibatide, Tirofiban)
Indications: Prevention of clotting and abrupt closure during interventional procedures and to prevent restenosis.
Action: Block the receptor on the platelet membrane that leads to the final common pathway of platelet aggregation.
Dosage
   Abciximab: 0.25 mg/kg IV bolus followed by 0.125 µg/kg/min infusion for 12–24 h after PCI
   Eptifibatide: 135 µg/kg IV administered immediately before PCI followed by 0.5 µg/kg/min for 20–24 h
   Tirofiban: 180 µg/kg IV bolus followed by 1.2–2 µg/kg/min infusion for 72–96 h after PCI
Adverse effects: Thrombocytopenia, hemorrhage, nausea, hematoma

Clopidogrel (Plavix)
Indications: Reduction of atherosclerotic events (acute myocardial infarction [AMI], stroke, and vascular death) in patients with atherosclerosis documented by a recent stroke or AMI or established peripheral arterial disease
Action: Blocks platelet aggregation

Dosage: 75 mg once daily
Adverse effects: Diarrhea, rash, gastrointestinal disturbances, hemorrhage, neutropenia.

Coronary Vasodilators

Isosorbide Dinitrate (Isordil, Sorbitrate)
Indications: Prophylaxis of angina
Actions: A nitrate that acts as a smooth muscle relaxant; causes coronary vasodilation without increasing myocardial oxygen consumption; secondary to general vasodilation, blood pressure decrease
Dosage
   Sublingual: 2.5–10 mg q2–3h PRN angina
   Oral: 5–40 mg q.i.d.
   Sustained-action oral: 40 mg q6–12h
Adverse effects: Cutaneous vasodilation that can cause flushing; headache, transient dizziness, and weakness; excessive hypotension

Nitroglycerin
Indications: Control of blood pressure and angina pectoris
Actions: Potent vasodilator that affects primarily the venous system; selectively dilates large coronary arteries increasing blood flow to ischemic subendocardium
Dosage
   Sublingual: 0.3–0.4 mg PRN chest pain
   Topical (patch): 2.5–10 mg/d; indicated for primary, secondary, or nocturnal angina due to more sustained effect
   IV: 5 µg/min to start—titrate to patient response (no fixed dose due to variable response in different patients)
Adverse effects: Excessive and prolonged hypotension; headache; tachycardia, palpitations; nausea, vomiting, apprehension; retrosternal discomfort

Calcium Channel Blockers

Nifedipine (Procardia), Diltiazem (Cardizem)
Indications: Angina pectoris due to coronary artery spasm and fixed vessel disease; hypertension; dysrhythmias
Actions: Inhibit calcium ion flux across the cell membrane of the cardiac muscle and vascular smooth muscle without changing serum calcium concentration; decrease afterload through peripheral arterial dilation and
1. Reduce systemic and pulmonary vascular resistance
2. Vasodilate coronary circulation
3. Decrease myocardial oxygen demands and increases myocardial oxygen supply
Dosage
   Nifedipine: 10–30 mg t.i.d. to q.i.d., PO
   Diltiazem: 30–90 mg t.i.d. to q.i.d., PO
Adverse effects: Contraindicated in patients with sick sinus syndrome; hypertension after IV use; gastrointestinal distress; headache, vertigo, flushing; peripheral edema, occasional increase in angina, tachycardia
See text for full discussion of antidysrhythmics.

and requiring immediate intervention. Coronary artery spasm sometimes requires emergent surgical intervention (CABG) when the vasoconstriction, occlusion, or ischemia cannot be reversed through the administration of nitrates.

Abrupt Closure of Dilated Segment

Abrupt closure is a serious complication of coronary artery dilation that occurs in approximately 3% of those undergoing angioplasty.[15] An estimated 70% to 80% of abrupt closures occur while the patient is still in the cardiac catheterization laboratory. Approximately one third to one half of those patients whose vessel abruptly closes undergo a successful repeat dilation. Abrupt closure can be caused by coronary artery dissection, coronary artery spasm, and thrombus formation. Treatment options include immediate repeat dilation, emergent CABG surgery, or pharmacological therapy. To maintain blood flow through the occlusion while the patient is being prepared for emergent CABG surgery, the physician can use a perfusion balloon catheter, which has side holes along its shaft to allow blood to flow through the catheter at the site of occlusion and perfuse the distal myocardium.

Coronary Artery Dissection

Coronary artery dissection or an intimal tear in the coronary artery can be visualized in the form of intraluminal filling defects or extraluminal extravasation of contrast material. Mild interruptions in the intraluminal wall are an expected result of the splitting and stretching of the intima on inflation of the balloon dilation catheter at the lesion site. However, a dissection may cause a major luminal obstruction associated with coronary artery occlusion, leading to deterioration in blood flow with resultant severe ischemia or myocardial infarction that requires emergent bypass surgery.

Restenosis

Restenosis of a dilated lesion occurs in approximately 20% to 30% of PCI cases within the first 6 months after a procedure with a bare metal stent. Restenosis occurs less often with PCI procedures utilizing a DES. Over-the-counter remedies such as fish oil derivatives have proved unbeneficial. Pharmacological agents to reduce restenosis are currently being investigated (prostacyclins, new anticoagulants, platelet antibodies, and corticosteroids) but have shown little benefit to date.

The development of devices to remove atherosclerotic plaque (atherectomy catheters) and implantable devices to maintain the opening mechanically (stents) has provided effective adjuncts or alternatives to PTCA for the problem of recurring lesions. Restenosis of de novo lesions after atherectomy is similar in character and prevalence to that in PTCA; however, intracoronary stenting has resulted in a lower restenosis rate in native and vein graft lesions of approximately 10%.

The cause of restenosis still is unclear. It appears to be the result of an excessive healing response to balloon dilation that exposes the subintimal structures of the vessel to circulating blood. These exposed areas are then potential sites for platelet adhesion and aggregation and for thrombus formation. The degree of this "healing" response varies from lesion to lesion and may be influenced by the clinical and angiographic factors associated with restenosis that were discussed previously. Factors associated with increased incidence of restenosis are listed in Box 18-9.

Other Complications

Other major complications of PCI requiring medical intervention are coronary perforation, which may be treated with a sheathed stent to stop the leak of blood into the pericardium; bradycardia, which requires temporary pacing; VT or ventricular fibrillation, which requires immediate defibrillation; and a central nervous system event causing transient or persistent neurological deficit.

Peripheral vascular complications occurring primarily at the catheter site include arterial thrombosis, excessive bleeding that causes a significant hematoma, pseudoaneurysm, femoral arteriovenous fistula, and arterial laceration. If any of these complications persists or compromises distal blood flow to the involved extremity, surgical intervention may be required.

Table 18-10 summarizes the complications that may result from PCI, including general signs of the complications and possible interventional actions.

Box 18-10 provides a Collaborative Care Guide for a complete outline of care for the patient undergoing PCI.

OTHER INTERVENTIONAL CARDIOLOGY TECHNIQUES

The immediate and long-term efficacy of PCI in treating symptomatic patients with single-vessel disease has been well established. In many centers, PTCA

Box 18-9 • Factors Associated With Increased Incidence of Restenosis

Clinical Factors
Severe angina
Noncompliance with antiplatelet regimen
Diabetes
Smoking cigarettes
Substance abuse
Uncontrolled hyperlipidemia

Angiographic Factors
Lesion location
Lesion length
Lesion severity before and after percutaneous coronary intervention
Adjacent arterial diameter
Gaps between overlapping stents

Table 18-10 • Complications of PCI

Complications	General Signs/Symptoms	Possible Interventions
Angina	Chest pain or anginal equivalent	CABG or repeat PCI
Myocardial infarction	Dysrhythmias: tachycardia, bradycardia, ventricular tachycardia/fibrillation, ST elevation	Redo PCI Oxygen
Abrupt reclosure Dissection/intimal tear Hypotension	Marked hypotension Acute electrocardiogram changes (ST segment change) Nausea/vomiting	Medications: vasodilators (nitrates), calcium channel blockers, analgesics, anticoagulants, vasopressors Intra-aortic balloon pump
Coronary branch occlusion	ST elevation	Possible repeat PCI
Restenosis	Angina pectoris Positive exercise test	Redo PIC Coronary artery bypass graft
Marked change in heart rate: bradycardia, ventricular tachycardia, ventricular fibrillation	Rate below 60 beats/min Rate above 250 beats/min No discernible cardiac rhythm Pallor Loss of consciousness Hypotension	Temporary pacemaker Defibrillation Medications: antidysrhythmics, vasopressors
Vascular: excessive blood loss	Hypotension Decreased urine output (from hypovolemia) Decreased hemoglobin/hematocrit Pallor Hematoma at puncture site	Possible surgical repair Fluids Transfusion Oxygen Flat in bed or in Trendelenburg position
Allergic	Hypotension, urticaria, nausea/vomiting, hives, laryngospasm, erythema, shortness of breath	Medications: antihistamines, steroids, antiemetics Clear liquids/NPO Oxygen With anaphylaxis: fluids for volume expansion, epinephrine, vasopressors for hypotension
Central nervous system events	Changes in level of consciousness Hemiparesis Hypoventilation/respiratory depression	Oxygen Discontinue/withhold sedatives Medication: narcotic antagonist as a respiratory stimulant Computed tomography, magnetic resonance imaging

Miscellaneous complications: conduction defects, pulmonary embolism, pulmonary edema, coronary air embolism, respiratory arrest, febrile episode, nausea, minor bleeding.

also is routinely and successfully used in patients with multivessel disease. The safety and efficacy with which angioplasty has been used have fostered research into treating patients with unstable angina, AMI, and cardiogenic shock.

Technologies have been developed to address the challenges associated with complex PCI. These include laser angioplasty, thrombectomy devices, atherectomy devices, DES, brachytherapy, and distal protection devices.

Laser Angioplasty

The acronym LASER stands for "light amplification through stimulated emission of radiation." Through a series of mirrors and lenses, the laser beam is directed into a catheter containing numerous glass fibers. These fibers transmit the light energy through the catheter to the plaque that is to be ablated.[25] The laser is used to ablate plaque or as an adjunct to other PCI procedures to make a pathway in total occlusions to facilitate the passage of a PTCA balloon or stent.

Laser angioplasty is performed much like a standard PCI procedure. The guide catheter is advanced to the ostium of the coronary artery targeted by fluoroscopy. Once the lesion location is ascertained through contrast injection, a guide wire is advanced up and through the lesion. Before the laser is activated, everyone in the room (including the patient) must don protective eyewear. The laser catheter is then advanced through the guide wire and brought into contact with the lesion. Depending on antici-

Box 18-10 • COLLABORATIVE CARE GUIDE for the Patient Undergoing PCI

OUTCOMES	INTERVENTIONS
Oxygenation/Ventilation Patient will maintain normal arterial blood gases, or pulse oximeter reading.	• Provide supplemental oxygen per face mask or nasal cannula per hospital post-PCI protocol. • Monitor blood gases/pulse oximeter per protocol. • Auscultate breath sounds when taking vital signs. • Monitor for signs of pulmonary edema or respiratory distress.

Circulation/Perfusion
The patient will have stable vital signs following PCI.
	• Monitor blood pressure, heart rate, respiration rate, arterial puncture site, distal pulses, and distal motor function and sensation:
	    q15min × 4, q30min × 4
	    q1h × 4, then q4h

There is no evidence of post-PCI myocardial ischemia or infarction due to coronary reocclusion (e.g., no electro-cardiogram changes or angina).	• Monitor cardiac rhythm in leads specific to myocardium most affected by PCI location. • Administer medications to treat coronary artery spasms (e.g., nifedipine and nitroglycerin). • Administer heparin per protocol.
There is no evidence of cardiac dysrhythmias after PCI.	• Report type and frequency of dysrhythmias. • Administer antidysrhythmic medication as indicated and ordered. • Temporary transvenous or external pacemaker and defibrillator are readily available.
There is no evidence of bleeding at the puncture site.	• Monitor site for hematoma as above with vital signs. • Assess for tenderness, ecchymosis, warmth over puncture site. • Apply direct pressure to puncture site for 15 to 30 min after sheath is removed. • Apply sandbag to puncture site if oozing continues, per hospital protocol. • Apply a pressure dressing to puncture site when oozing has stopped. • Monitor activated clotting time, prothrombin time, partial thromboplastin time, and platelets, reporting coagulopathies per protocol.
There is no evidence of arterial occlusion at puncture site.	• Monitor involved extremity with vital signs for mottling, coolness, pallor, diminished pulses, numbness, tingling, pain, and so forth.
Fluids/Electrolytes Patient is euvolemic.	• Monitor intake and output. • Obtain type and cross-match, complete blood count, electrolytes prior to PCI. • Maintain IV patency.
Renal function is maintained after administration of radiographic IV contrast.	• Obtain pre-PCI and post-PCI blood urea nitrogen, creatinine, and electrolytes. • Closely monitor urine output; report if less than 30 mL/h. • Monitor urine specific gravity or osmolarity for clearance of IV contrast. • Administer diuretic agents as ordered.
Mobility/Safety	• The patient is on bed rest for 4 to 6 hours post-PCI per hospital protocol. • While sheath is in place and while on bed rest, keep head of bed less than 45 degrees.

(continued)

Box 18-10 • COLLABORATIVE CARE GUIDE for the Patient Undergoing PCI (Continued)

OUTCOMES	INTERVENTIONS
Skin Integrity Patient's skin will remain intact.	• Assess skin immediately after PCI for pressure areas. • Reposition to relieve pressure from bony prominences, maintaining alignment of extremity involved in procedure. • Consider pressure relief/reduction mattress.
Nutrition Nutritional intake is reestablished. Patient does not experience nausea or vomiting after PCI.	• Resume PO fluids and diet per protocol. • Monitor swallowing and protective airway reflexes while patient is receiving sedatives or narcotics. • Monitor nausea and vomiting. • Administer antiemetic medication as appropriate.
Comfort/Pain Control Patient will not experience anginal pain. Patient will not experience pain from mobility restrictions.	• Instruct patient to verbalize discomfort and pain. • Evaluate severity and location of pain, distinguishing angina from other causes of discomfort. • Administer nitrates or narcotics per order or protocol for angina. • Evaluate patient response to medication. • Reposition patient frequently, keeping involved extremity straight. • Use mattress overlay or egg crate for comfort. • Administer analgesics as appropriate, after distinguishing joint or muscular pain from angina.
Psychosocial Patient and family state risks associated with PCI. Patient uses personal support systems to reduce anxiety.	• Provide information for informed procedural consent. • Encourage verbalization of questions, concerns, and fears. • Encourage significant other to visit in early postprocedural recovery phase. • Validate patient/significant others' understanding of surgery and illness. • Initiate referrals to social services, clergy, and so forth as necessary.
Teaching/Discharge Planning Patient and family are prepared for possibility of emergent repeat PCI or cardiac surgery. Patient cooperates with post-PCI mobility restrictions. Patient states lifestyle changes required to reduce risk for worsening coronary artery disease.	• Preprocedure teaching includes discussion regarding causes for coronary reocclusion or perforation and rationale for surgery or repeat PCI. • Provide preprocedure and postprocedure instruction and rationale for bed rest and limited movement of involved extremity. • Provide verbal and written instruction/information regarding risk factors and pathophysiology, activity, diet, stress reduction, medication administration, and appropriate times/indications to seek medical attention.

pated lesion morphology, energy settings are chosen that will presumably suffice to ablate the plaque. The laser settings include the fluency (millijoules per square millimeter) to be delivered and the repetition rate (pulses per second). The plaque is then vaporized by the laser energy. Several passes down the length of the lesion may be performed. Laser success is determined by fluoroscopy and coronary injections with contrast dye. If there is residual stenosis

after use of the laser, adjunctive PCI procedures, including stenting, can be performed to achieve an optimal final result (Fig. 18-11).

Stenotic lesions best suited for laser angioplasty include those that are long and diffuse (longer than 15 to 20 mm), ostial in location, highly calcified, in vein grafts, and totally occluded. Risks associated with laser angioplasty include perforation of the coronary artery, dissections, and aneurysms. Now

358

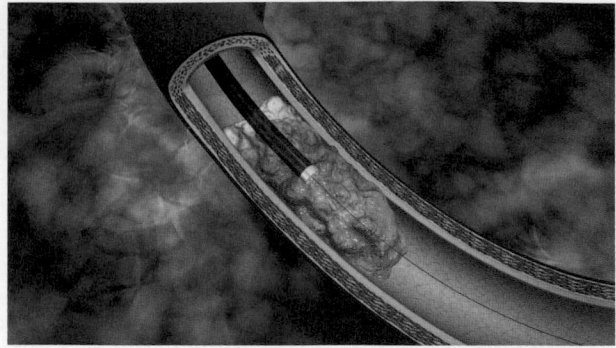

Figure 18-11 • LASER ablation of a coronary artery stenosis.

considered a "niche" procedure, laser angioplasty is performed less frequently in the percutaneous treatment of cardiovascular disease.

Atherectomy

Atherectomy is the process of removing atherosclerotic plaque from the coronary artery by cutting or ablating and thus "debulking" the lesion. Atherectomy devices include directional coronary atherectomy (DCA) and rotational ablation (Rotablator).

Potential complications of all atherectomy devices include perforation of the coronary artery, abrupt closure, embolization distal to the lesion site, and myocardial infarction. The rate of restenosis and other complications is comparable to that with standard balloon angioplasty and less successful than those results achieved with DESs.

Directional Coronary Atherectomy

The DCA device is a cutting catheter that is inserted over a guide wire into the coronary artery across the stenotic lesion (Fig. 18-12). It is positioned so that the opening for the blade faces the lesion. A low-pressure balloon on the opposite side of the catheter is inflated, thus forcing the atherosclerotic plaque into the opening near the cutting blade. The cutting blade turns at approximately 1,200 revolutions per minute (rpm) and is then slowly advanced along the length of the lesion, cutting the plaque and collecting it in the catheter nosecone. The DCA catheter is turned a complete 360 degrees in the artery to shave all sides of the

atherosclerotic plaque with repeated passes. The procedure is repeated until the atherosclerotic plaque is sufficiently removed. The catheter, laden with plaque, is then withdrawn from the patient.

Rotational Ablation Device

The Rotablator device (Boston Scientific, Natick, MA) is a high-speed rotating, abrasive, burr-tipped catheter that ablates the atherosclerotic plaque in the coronary artery. The Rotablator has proved especially effective in complex stenotic lesions that are calcified, tortuous, small in diameter, ostial, or diffuse in character. The device consists of a football-shaped, diamond-studded burr attached to a drive shaft. The Rotablator is advanced over a guide wire to the lesion site. The burr rotates at 160,000 to 190,000 rpm and pulverizes the atherosclerotic plaque into microparticles that are absorbed into the patient's circulatory system. The spinning burr is advanced across the lesion several times to debulk the stenotic lesion. Adjunctive balloon angioplasty may be performed after use of the Rotablator device (Fig. 18-13).

The AngioJet device (Possis) is a thrombectomy system used to extract clot from coronary arteries, saphenous vein grafts, or peripheral arteries. The system consists of three components: (1) the drive unit (Fig. 18-14A); (2) the pump set, which achieves isovolumetric balance between the fluid and thrombus that is removed from the artery and the fluid that is delivered (see Fig. 18-14B); and (3) the catheter, which is disposable and 4- to 6-Fr compatible (see Fig. 18-14C). The AngioJet System has been shown to be safe and effective in removing fresh clot from patients undergoing PCI for AMI[26] and in instances in which there is clot in saphenous vein grafts.[27]

Stents

Intracoronary stents are hollow stainless steel tubes that act as "scaffolding" in the coronary artery. Currently, more than 100 different stents have received U.S. Food and Drug Administration (FDA) approval. After predilation with a PTCA balloon catheter, most stents are premounted on a balloon catheter and

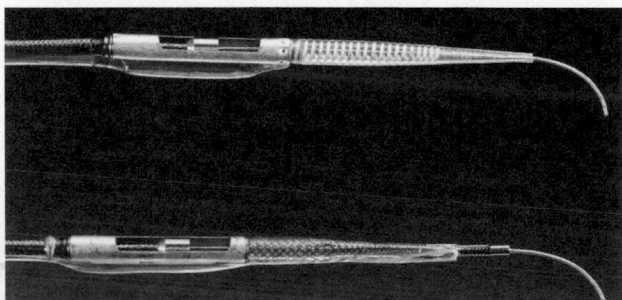

Figure 18-12 • Directional coronary atherectomy catheters: Simpson Coronary AtheroCaths. (Courtesy of Guidant/Advanced Cardiovascular Systems, Santa Clara, CA.)

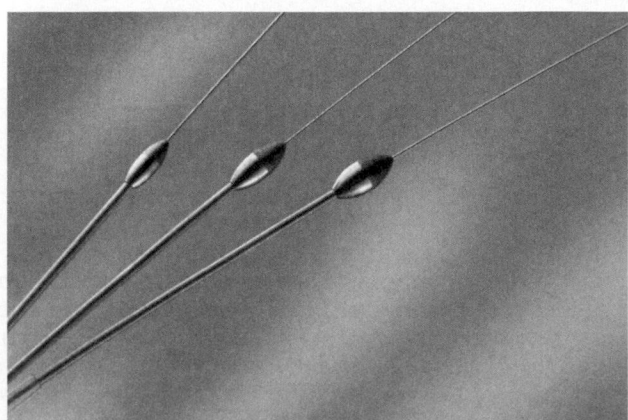

Figure 18-13 • Rotational ablation catheters in different sizes. (Courtesy of SCIMED/Boston Scientific Corporation, Maple Grove, MN.)

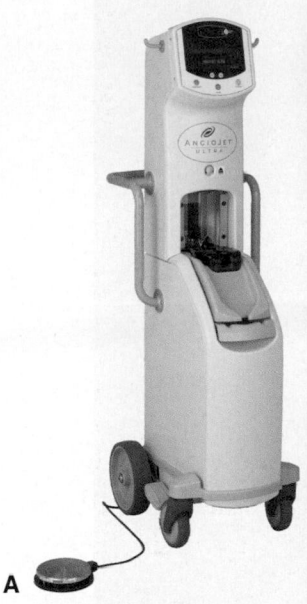
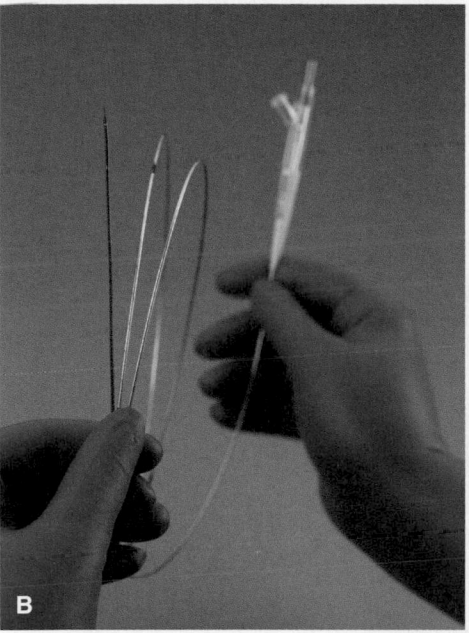
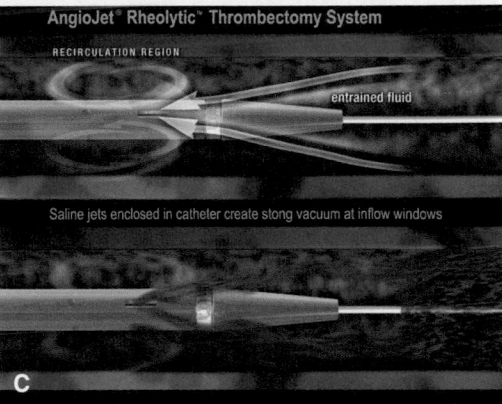

Figure 18-14 • **A:** AngioJet Ultra Console. Power and control console for AngioJet Rheolytic Thrombectomy System. **B:** The AngioJet Spiroflex Thrombectomy Catheter is a 4-French thrombectomy catheter with a spiral-cut shaft for tracking. **C:** The mechanism of action of the AngioJet Thrombectomy Catheter. (Courtesy of Possis Medical Inc., Minneapolis, MN.)

inserted through the guide catheter along a guide wire to the lesion site. Once placed across the stenotic lesion, the balloon is inflated, and the stent is expanded and left in the coronary artery.

Traditional and older stent designs are bare metal. Because many bare metal stent designs are stainless steel, they are potent thrombogenic prostheses. Stent thrombus is a major short- and long-term complication. Success of the stenting procedure depends on endothelialization of the stent to provide a smooth flow of blood in the coronary artery and through the stent, yet controlled to prevent stent thrombosis. Anticoagulation and antiplatelet medication regimens are crucial to successful stenting and long-term prognosis. Stenting has been shown in numerous trials to reduce restenosis rates and improve long-term prognosis. Stents made of newer alloys and compounds are currently undergoing investigation. DESs are coated with drugs such as heparin, paclitaxel, sirolimus, or rapamycin. It is believed that the gradual release of these drugs into the coronary vasculature at the site of the atherosclerotic plaque inhibits restenosis by limiting smooth muscle cell proliferation and inflammation but allowing re-endothelialization to proceed normally. At this time, the FDA-approved DESs include a sirolimus-coated stent called Cypher (Cordis) (Fig. 18-15) and the paclitaxel-coated stent called Taxus (Boston Scientific) (Fig. 18-16). Complications of bare metal stents or DESs may include bleeding at the access site, stent migration, coronary artery dissection, and abrupt closure.

Brachytherapy

Intracoronary radiation (brachytherapy) is potentially a potent antiproliferative therapy that is cur-

rently being investigated for use in conjunction with PCI and might therefore provide a means for effective reduction of restenosis. The radiation therapy is emitted in the form of temporarily implanted or inserted radioactive sources, such as seeds, radioactive stents, or radioactive liquid–filled balloons. Radiation works particularly well in inhibiting new growth by attacking the newer, more aggressive neoplastic cells, while often having little effect on normal tissue.[28] In brachytherapy, endovascular low-dose radiation is applied at the site of balloon dilation or stent implantation by a catheter system. Two types of radiation are used to treat restenosis: γ and β emitters. γ Emitters create a radiation field for a considerable distance away from their source. This requires that the treatment be con-

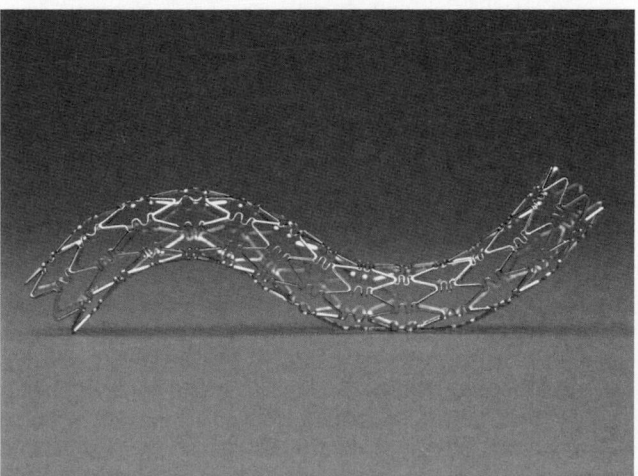

Figure 18-15 • Fully expanded cipher stent. Used with permission of Cordis Corporation.

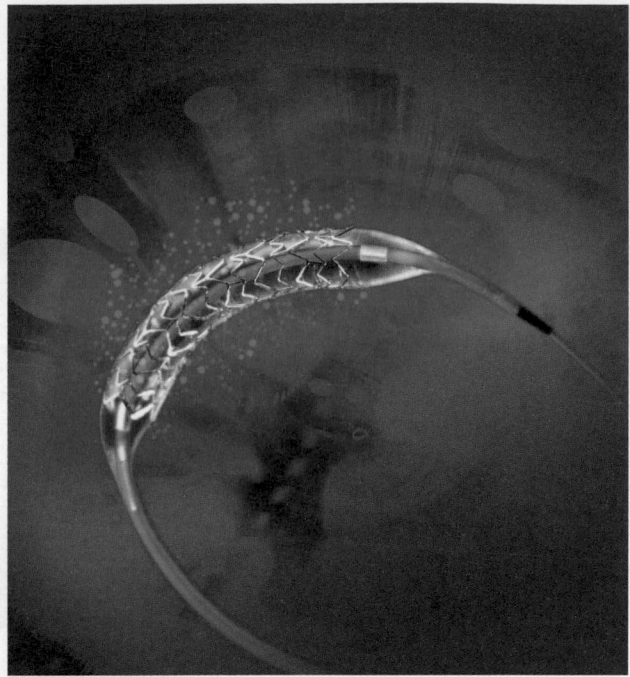

Figure 18-16 • Expanding Taxus stent prior to delivery balloon removal. (Photograph courtesy of Boston Scientific Corporation, 2006.)

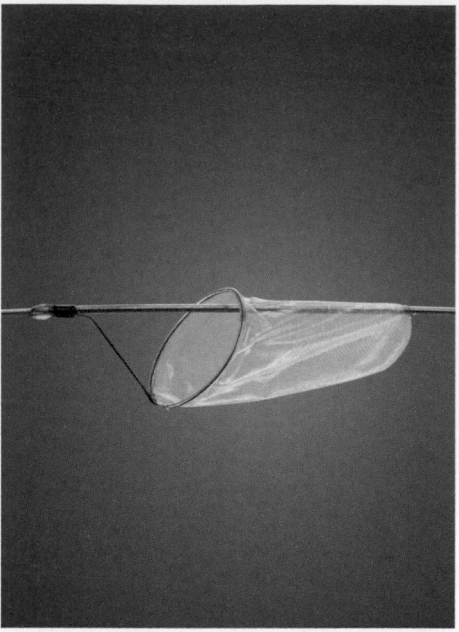

Figure 18-17 • Distal protection devices. Deployed filter wire device. (Photograph courtesy of Boston Scientific Corporation, 2006.)

ducted in a heavily lead-shielded cardiac catheterization laboratory. γ-Emitter intensity is lower than that of β emitters, and γ emitters must be left in place 14 to 45 minutes, depending on the strength of the source used. β Sources, with a higher intensity of radiation near the source, can be more concentrated, enabling the brachytherapy to last only 3 to 10 minutes. The β source can be shielded with only approximately 0.5 inch of Lucite. The FDA currently approves the use of brachytherapy only for in-stent restenosis.

Distal Protection Devices

Distal embolization of particulate matter can complicate PCI and peripheral interventional procedures. Tiny microemboli can be showered distally (downstream of the lesion) during revascularization procedures. This can cause end-organ ischemia, AMI, serum cardiac enzyme elevation, stroke, and left ventricular dysfunction. Distal protection devices are designed to reduce or eliminate distal embolization during PCI and peripheral interventions. Distal protection devices are often used during PCI of saphenous vein grafts and during carotid procedures.

To date, the only distal protection devices approved by the FDA are the PercuSurge GuardWire (Medtronic, Santa Rosa, CA) and the FilterWire (Boston Scientific) (Fig. 18-17). The PercuSurge device consists of a guide wire with a low-pressure occlusive balloon on the distal end. The balloon is inflated to prevent distal embolization, and an aspiration catheter removes the debris from the treated vessel before the balloon is deflated and antegrade flow is restored. The FilterWire device contains a low-profile filter mounted on an angioplasty wire. The filter contains small holes that permit antegrade blood flow while trapping microemboli and thus providing distal protection. Because these distal protection devices are quickly becoming the standard of care for degenerated saphenous veins grafts and carotid stenting, device manufacturers may seek indications for use in ACS interventions and other peripheral procedures in the near future.

• Interventions for Peripheral Arterial Disease

Peripheral arterial disease (PAD) is a condition that affects approximately 12 million Americans.[29] The disease results from the accumulation of plaque in the arteries. It constricts normal blood flow and can result in heart attack, stroke, extremity amputation, and death if left untreated. Patients with PAD have a 5-year mortality rate of 30%.[30] Refer to Chapter 19 for a discussion of aortic aneurysms and peripheral arterial disease and Chapter 22 for surgical management of carotid disease (endarterectomy). Until recent advances in technology made minimally invasive and percutaneous approaches possible, medical or surgical intervention for these cardiovascular diseases was the only option.

Remote endarterectomy is a minimally invasive endovascular procedure for complete superficial femoral artery revascularization. It provides treatment of lower extremity arterial disease and serves as an alternative to bypass surgery. The benefits of the remote endarterectomy approach are (1) preservation of the native vessel, (2) less invasive than surgery (3) no limitation of future surgical options, (4) potentially faster and easier recovery for the patient compared with bypass procedures, and (5) comparable long-term clinical outcomes to surgical endarterectomy.

Percutaneous treatment is an emerging approach in the management of PAD. Angioplasty, atherectomy, and stenting of the carotid arteries, aorta, renal arteries, iliac and femoral arteries, and upper extremities are routinely performed in many medical institutions. Before undergoing a percutaneous intervention, most patients require magnetic resonance angiography, arterial duplex mapping, or angiography. Percutaneous transluminal angioplasty of the peripheral arteries involves placing a balloon in the blood vessel at the site of the blockage and inflating the balloon to open the blood vessel. Stents can also be inserted into the clogged vessel to serve as scaffolding in opening it. Thrombolytic therapy can also be delivered to the site of the blockages before initiating angioplasty or stenting. Atherectomy, or debulking the peripheral blood vessels, has also been shown to be beneficial in some cases before angioplasty or stenting.

Much attention is given to percutaneous intervention for carotid stenoses. As with most percutaneous interventions, the possibility of a small groin incision and same-day discharge is attractive. Today, technology is aimed at preventing cerebral emboli from forming during carotid angioplasty and stenting. Although promising, carotid angioplasty and stenting remain under investigation in comparison to traditional carotid endarterectomy procedures.

Abdominal aortic aneurysms and thoracic aortic aneurysms can also be treated percutaneously. Endovascular stent grafts are metal-lined fabric tubes that reinforce an aneurysm in a blood vessel. It essentially relines the blood vessel and decreases the incidence of aneurysm rupture. The stent graft seals tightly above and below the aneurysm (Fig. 18-18). The graft is stronger than the weakened aorta and permits

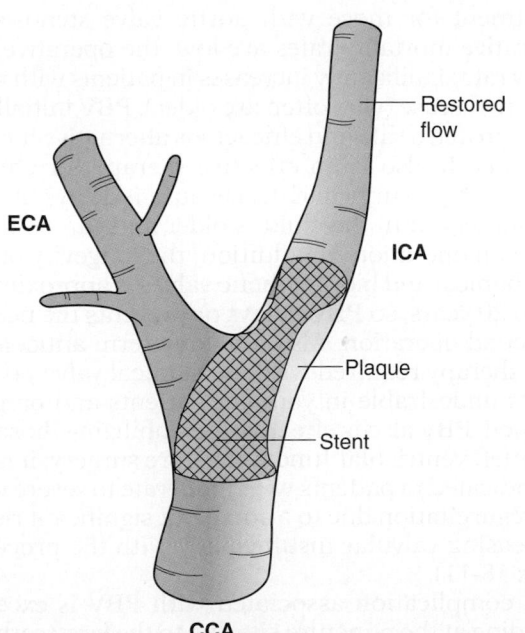

Figure 18-18 • Endovascular stent graft (AAA). CCA, common carotid artery; ECA, external carotid artery; ICA, internal carotid artery.

blood to pass through without exerting pressure on the aneurysm. Patients are candidates for endovascular stent grafting if aneurysms measure 5 cm wide, the aneurysm and aorta contour are conducible to stent grafting, and the blood vessels are large enough to pass guiding catheters, angioplasty balloons, and the stent graft. Potential complications of endovascular stent grafting include endoleaks (leaking of blood around the graft), migration of the stent graft, infection, and restenosis.

Postprocedure care of the patient with PAD is similar to that of patients undergoing PCI of the coronaries. Groin incision observation, extremity assessment, and vital sign measurement are important components of postprocedure care. Patient education and discharge planning should include aggressive management of cardiovascular risk factors such as smoking cessation, reduction of blood glucose, exercise regimens, and lowering blood pressure and cholesterol. Antiplatelet therapy is also indicated for the patient undergoing percutaneous treatment of PAD.

With the various tools and technologies available to the interventional cardiologist, as well as improved pharmacological adjunctive therapy, the future should bring further improvement in the efficacy and predictability of PCI and in the long-term patency of involved atherosclerotic vessels in the coronary system and in the peripheral arterial system.

• Percutaneous Balloon Valvuloplasty

Percutaneous balloon valvuloplasty (PBV) is a non-surgical technique for increasing blood flow through stenotic cardiac valves using dilation catheters. This relatively new procedure is similar to PCI procedures in that a catheter system is inserted percutaneously and advanced to the region of narrowing using fluoroscopic guidance. A dilation catheter then is inflated to increase the valvular opening and improve blood flow.

HISTORICAL BACKGROUND

The first cases of balloon dilation of stenotic cardiac valves were reported in 1979 and 1982, when physicians successfully dilated pulmonary valve stenoses. This technique was considered an effective alternative to open heart surgery, although long-term results could not yet be evaluated. Because surgical commissurotomy was successful in treating mitral valve stenoses and because of the initial success with pulmonary valve dilation, physicians began percutaneous dilation of mitral valves in 1984 to avoid the need for thoracotomy. These procedures improved cardiac function with no serious procedural complications.

The number of PBVs does not approach the volume of PCI procedures. This is due partly to the lesser incidence of valve disease compared with CAD.

Assuming patients have long-term clinical improvement associated with PBV, the advantages compared with surgery are similar to those of PCI versus CABG.

PBV is less traumatic, requires no anesthesia, is associated with lower morbidity and a shorter hospital stay, causes no scarring, and is less expensive. Minimally invasive surgical procedures are also available and include mini-thoracotomy approaches.

PATHOPHYSIOLOGY OF STENOTIC VALVES

Stenotic valves are caused by calcific degeneration, congenital abnormalities, or rheumatic heart disease. Calcific aortic and mitral valve degeneration now appears to be the most frequent causes of valve disease requiring surgical treatment. Refer to Chapter 19 for a discussion of the pathophysiology and clinical manifestations of specific stenotic valves.

DIAGNOSTIC TESTS FOR PERCUTANEOUS BALLOON VALVULOPLASTY AND VALVE REPLACEMENT

Before deciding on the appropriate intervention, the physician evaluates the patient for evidence and severity of valvular stenosis. A variety of noninvasive tests allow the physician to determine the degree of left atrial or left ventricular hypertrophy, pulmonary venous congestion or hypertension, valvular rigidity, and transvalvular gradient. In a 12-lead ECG, the magnitude of the R wave in the precordial leads reflects the presence of left ventricular hypertrophy associated with atrioventricular stenosis. The presence of broad, notched P waves reflects left atrial hypertrophy associated with mitral valve stenosis. A chest radiograph illustrates the presence of calcium in or around the valve, left ventricular or atrial hypertrophy, and pulmonary venous congestion or congestive heart failure (CHF). A two-dimensional echocardiogram is used to scan the cardiac valves and chambers. A Doppler ultrasound study allows measurement of the transvalvular gradient, indirect calculation of valve area, and assessment of valvular regurgitation. With this information, the physician is able to (1) estimate the size of the valve orifice, (2) visualize the degree of valve leaflet movement, and (3) determine the extent of left ventricular or atrial hypertrophy.

Right and left heart catheterization is performed if the previous tests indicate valvular disease. Although this procedure is invasive, it is required to determine the pressures within each of the cardiac chambers and to confirm transvalvular gradients. Once the pressures and gradients are obtained, a series of radiographs may be taken by injecting radiopaque contrast medium, either in the aorta to visualize aortic regurgitation or in the left ventricle to visualize mitral regurgitation. This procedure yields a cineangiogram illustrating the function of the cardiac valves and chamber sizes.

After this series of tests, the physician can analyze the valves closely, gaining precise information with which to decide the mode of treatment. The nurse should be familiar with the results of these tests because a better understanding of the patient's diagnosis and related symptoms, and thus of the reasons for intervention, promotes better care.

EQUIPMENT FEATURES

Although PBV and PCI catheters are based on similar designs, there are important differences, primarily because of the larger diameters of heart valves compared with coronary arteries. One major difference is the outer diameter of the catheters. PBV catheter shafts range from 7 to 9 Fr. PBV balloons range from 15 to 25 mm in diameter when inflated. A 10- to 14-Fr introducing sheath may be used at the arterial or venous puncture site to allow for introduction of the valve dilation catheter.

A large guide wire, 0.035 to 0.038 inch, also is used to provide the added stiffness and support required to introduce the dilatation catheter. PBV dilation catheters have radiopaque markers similar to PCI catheter systems for fluoroscopic imaging.

INDICATIONS FOR AND CONTRAINDICATIONS TO PERCUTANEOUS BALLOON VALVULOPLASTY

The use of PBV initially was limited by the fear of embolization of calcific debris, disruption of the valve ring, acute valvular regurgitation, and valvular restenosis. The incidence of these complications continues to be a concern. Both major and minor complications have been reported in numerous early studies; however, these complications must be assessed in terms of the patient population in which the procedure is performed.

Although surgical valve replacement is an effective treatment for those with aortic valve stenosis and operative mortality rates are low, the operative mortality rate significantly increases in patients with multisystem disease (who often are older). PBV initially has been proved a safe and efficacious alternative for these patients. It also is an effective therapy for children who are high surgical risks because it delays the need for surgery until the child is older and can better tolerate an operation. In addition, the longevity of both mechanical and bioprosthetic valves is approximately 10 to 20 years, so PBV delays or prevents the need for a second operation. Also, the long-term anticoagulation therapy required with mechanical valve prostheses is undesirable in younger patients and pregnant women. PBV also is effective for stabilizing those with poor left ventricular function before surgery; it is contraindicated in patients with moderate to severe valvular regurgitation due to a small but significant risk for increasing valvular insufficiency with the procedure (Box 18-11).

A complication associated with PBV is excessive bleeding at the puncture site due to the large catheters required to perform dilation. The development of smaller catheters may reduce the incidence of bleeding. As with PCI, PBV catheters are being refined

Box 18-11 • Indications and Contraindications for PBV

Clinical Indications
High-risk surgical patients (advanced age, severe
    pulmonary hypertension, renal failure, pulmonary
    dysfunction, left ventricular dysfunction)
Unstable presurgical patients
Patients not candidates for chronic anticoagulation

Anatomical Indications
Moderate to severe valvular narrowing
Moderate to severe valvular calcification
Mild valvular regurgitation

Anatomical Contraindications
Inability to access vasculature
Thrombus
Severe valvular regurgitation
History of embolic events

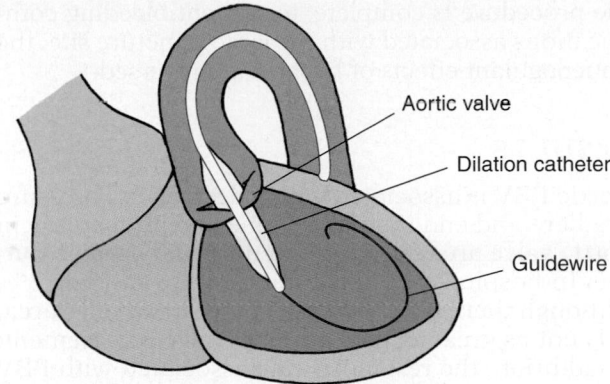

Figure 18-19 • Cross-sectional view of heart illustrating guide wire and dilation catheter positions across the aortic valve. The guide wire is curved to prevent ventricular dysrhythmias or puncture.

continually to increase procedural safety, time, and efficacy.

PROCEDURE

The procedure is performed in the cardiac catheterization laboratory and involves many of the same steps as PCI (see earlier section on PCI procedure). Right and left heart catheterization is repeated to evaluate hemodynamic status and to obtain baseline transvalvular gradients. Coronary angiography, when indicated, is repeated to determine whether the patient still meets the criteria for valvuloplasty. Thorough repeat evaluation is necessary because a patient's status can change, precluding treatment with this intervention.

The angiographic catheter is replaced either by an introducing sheath or a dilation catheter. In mitral PBV, a venous puncture is made in the right femoral vein. During both aortic and mitral PBV, maintaining patent IV and radial or femoral arterial lines is important to administer medications and draw blood samples.

In aortic PBV, once the sheaths are in place, the patient is anticoagulated with 5,000 to 10,000 units of heparin to prevent clot formation in the catheter system. The dilation catheter and guide wire then are advanced to the root of the ascending aorta. The guide wire is advanced across the stenotic aortic valve, and the dilation catheter is advanced over the guide wire (Fig. 18-19). Exact placement of the dilation catheter is facilitated by fluoroscopy and radiopaque markers on the balloon.

In mitral PBV, a pacing catheter may be positioned through a separate venous sheath at the level of the inferior vena cava or right atrium and placed on standby. The mitral valve then is approached either by way of the femoral artery and aortic valve or, in most cases, through the right heart by perforating the atrial septum to enter the left atrium. Once the mitral valve has been accessed, the patient is anticoagulated with 5,000 to 10,000 units of heparin. The dilation

catheter is then advanced over the guide wire through the atrial septal puncture and across the mitral valve (Fig. 18-20). Again, exact placement of the dilation catheter in the valve is facilitated by fluoroscopy and radiopaque markers on the balloon.

Average inflation time of the dilation catheter is 15 to 60 seconds in aortic valvuloplasty and 10 to 30 seconds in mitral valvuloplasty. During dilation of either valve, the nurse monitors blood pressure closely because of the imposed decrease in cardiac output. Once the dilation catheter has been deflated, blood pressure should return to normal. During dilation of the mitral valve, there is a temporary increase in the pulmonary artery wedge pressure (PAWP). Once the dilation catheter has been deflated, the PAWP should return to baseline. Dysrhythmias such as VT, ventricular fibrillation, or sinus bradycardia also may occur during dilation.

Once maximal dilation has been obtained, the catheter is removed. Hemodynamic measurements, including transvalvular gradients, are repeated to determine efficacy of the procedure. Repeat angiography is done to assess for valvular regurgitation. When

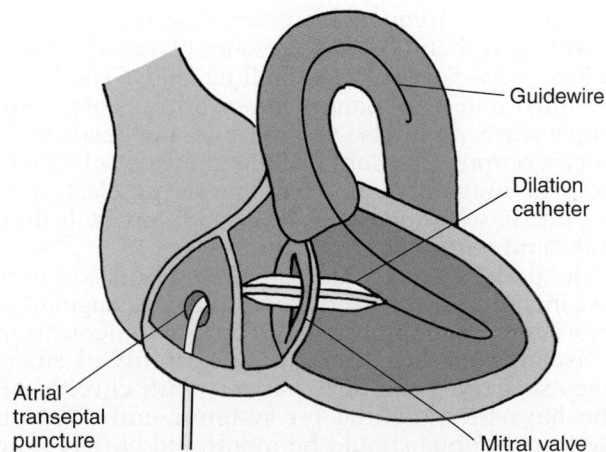

Figure 18-20 • Cross-sectional view of heart illustrating guidewire and dilation catheter placed through an atrial trans-septal puncture and across the mitral valve. The guide wire is extended out the aortic valve into the aorta for catheter support.

the procedure is complete, to prevent bleeding complications associated with the large puncture site, the anticoagulant effects of heparin are reversed.

RESULTS

Aortic PBV is associated with a decrease in pressure gradient and end-systolic volume and an increase in aortic valve area, ejection fraction, and cardiac output. In-hospital mortality rates range from 1% to 3%. Although there is an increase in the aortic valve area, it is not as great as with surgical valve replacement. In addition, the restenosis rate associated with PBV is high. Therefore, aortic valvuloplasty is indicated primarily for older and high-risk surgical patients and generally is considered a palliative, not a curative, procedure.

Results of mitral valvuloplasty are more dramatic. There is a more significant increase in valve area and cardiac output and a decrease in valve gradient, PAWP, and mean pulmonary arterial pressure. The operative mortality rate has been reported as 1.5%, and sustained clinical improvement has been reported in 63% to 90% of cases. Late deaths occur in approximately 5% to 10% of patients.

Three mechanisms have been postulated for the improvement of valvular function due to PBV: (1) fracture of calcific nodules adherent to leaflets (most frequent); (2) separation of fused commissures; and (3) stretching of the anulus and leaflet structure.

ASSESSMENT AND MANAGEMENT
Patient Preparation

The patient is admitted to the hospital the day of the PBV procedure. The goal of nursing care is to reduce the cardiac workload, monitor fluid and electrolyte balance, and reduce psychological stress so that the patient remains hemodynamically stable.

In most cases, the patient does not have invasive pressure monitoring lines in place before the procedure. The nurse therefore carefully monitors signs and symptoms of CHF: narrowing in the arterial pulse pressure, more frequent increases in heart rate during activity, peripheral edema, presence of a cough, complaints of dyspnea, or rales in lung fields. The nurse also must note any changes in sensorium, color, skin temperature, and pulse volume, and any decrease in urinary output. To monitor fluid and electrolyte balance, the nurse obtains a baseline serum electrolyte level and baseline body weight. In addition, daily fluid intake and output are recorded.

The patient's medications before admission may have included diuretics, digoxin, and anticoagulants. Before the procedure, any anticoagulant medication is discontinued because of the possibility of emergency surgery. Therefore, patients with chronic AF who have the potential for systemic embolization due to thrombus should be monitored closely. The nurse also monitors preliminary laboratory tests and notifies the physician of any abnormalities. (See the section on patient preparation for PTCA for further information on these tests.)

After the patient fully understands the procedure, the physician must obtain an informed consent for PBV, anesthesia, and surgery. Surgical standby usually is provided during PBV due to possible complications requiring emergency valve replacement.

Nursing Assessment and Management
During Percutaneous Balloon Valvuloplasty

The nurse continuously monitors pulmonary artery pressure and PAWP and is aware of changes in tracings that may suggest symptoms of CHF or pulmonary edema. In the presence of severe hypotension, the nurse should be prepared to start an IV infusion of dopamine or norepinephrine (Levophed). In the case of ventricular dysrhythmias, a lidocaine drip should be available for infusion.

After Percutaneous Balloon Valvuloplasty

The nurse is important in the patient's recovery. The goal of postvalvuloplasty nursing care is to maintain adequate cardiac output, maintain fluid and electrolyte balance, and verify hemostasis at the puncture site. Alterations in cardiac output can be caused by dysrhythmias secondary to valve manipulation, resulting in edema near the bundle of His; left-to-right atrial shunt through the transseptal puncture created during mitral valvuloplasty; cardiac tamponade; alteration in circulating fluid volume; or blood loss. Alteration in fluid and electrolyte balance results from diuretic therapy and contrast medium used during catheterization. Bleeding at the puncture site is secondary to the combined effect of systemic anticoagulation and the large diameter of catheters used.

Because fluids are important in the hemodynamic balance of the patient with valvular disease, the volume of IV fluids is recorded to establish an accurate intake and output. The decreased circulating volume from diuretic medications given before PBV, combined with improved stroke volume after successful PBV, can be reflected as a decrease in cardiac output. Therefore, careful monitoring of central venous pressure, pulmonary artery pressure, PAWP, and blood pressure, in addition to heart rate, urinary output, and electrolyte balance, is essential in the evaluation and assessment of circulating fluid volume and cardiac pumping status.

In addition, the nurse assesses the patient's status from head to toe, noting overall skin color and temperature and carefully observing the level of consciousness and neurological signs. The nurse also listens closely to heart and breath sounds. Circulation distal to the puncture site is evaluated by noting peripheral skin color and temperature in addition to the presence and quality of the dorsalis pedis and posterior tibial pulses.

Finally, the presence of any drainage on the puncture site dressing or tenderness during palpation should be noted to establish a baseline for the possibility of increased pericatheter bleeding. The nurse reports immediately any changes that may indicate excessive bleeding. Bleeding at the sheath site may result in a hematoma requiring surgical evacuation. To prevent excessive bleeding and to aid hemostasis,

Box 18-12 • DISCHARGE PLANNING GUIDE:
The Cardiac Patient After PCI or PBV

Physiological
- Restrict physical activities first week after PCI/PBV
- No lifting over 10 lb the first 2 wk after PCI
- May resume exercise program after exercise stress test
- Follow prescribed low-fat diet
- Consider cardiac rehabilitation
- Limit alcohol to three drinks per week
- Notify physician of any oozing, bleeding, or pain at puncture site
- Notify physician of fever or other signs of infection
- Notify physician or call 911 for any chest discomfort not relieved with three nitroglycerin tablets taken 5 minutes apart
- Weight loss if indicated

Psychosocial
- No smoking or exposure to second-hand smoke
- May resume sexual activities after exercise stress test
- Stress management
- Recognize signs of depression
- Compliance with medication regimen
- Compliance with medical appointments

Box 18-13 • RED FLAG: Complications
Associated With PBV

- Embolization of calcific debris
- Valve ring disruption
- Valvular regurgitation
- Valvular restenosis
- Bleeding at arterial puncture site
- Left ventricular perforation
- Severe hypotension
- Transient ischemia
- Vascular trauma
- Atrial septal defect (with mitral PBV)
- Aortic dissection
- Aortic rupture
- Cardiac tamponade
- Chordae tendineae rupture

the physician may order a sandbag or clamp placed over the puncture site.

If the patient has documented CAD, the physician also may request a serum cardiac enzyme panel. Particular attention should be paid to creatine kinase (CK) and CK isoenzymes (see Nursing Management After Percutaneous Coronary Interventions). The nurse should be aware of the signs and symptoms of myocardial ischemia in addition to the appropriate interventions.

The nurse instructs the patient about the importance of keeping the involved leg straight for the first few hours after valvuloplasty.

Post-PBV laboratory evaluation may include prothrombin time, hemoglobin and hematocrit, coagu-

lation studies, serum electrolytes, creatine kinase, ECG, and chest radiograph. Box 18-6, under Nursing Management During Percutaneous Coronary Interventions, lists nursing diagnoses and collaborative problems for patients undergoing PBV. Implications for home care for the patient after PCI or PBV are described in Box 18-12.

Complications

A common in-hospital complication associated with PBV is bleeding at the arterial puncture site due to the large diameter of the catheters needed to dilate the valve anulus. In addition, in mitral PBV, a common complication is left-to-right shunting secondary to septal dilation, again due to the large diameter of the dilation catheters. Systemic embolization in both mitral and aortic PBV is a potential and significant complication, although its incidence is low. There have been few reports of significant increases in valvular regurgitation. Complications associated with PBV are listed in Box 18-13.

Intra-Aortic Balloon Pump Counterpulsation and Mechanical Circulatory Support

Intra-Aortic Balloon Pump Counterpulsation

Harken and colleagues of Boston originally described the concept of counterpulsation in 1958 when, in an attempt to increase coronary artery perfusion, they used femoral access to remove blood during systole and replace it during diastole. Intra-aortic balloon pump (IABP) counterpulsation was first introduced clinically by Kantrowitz and associates in 1967. This therapeutic approach was instituted for treatment of two patients with left ventricular failure after AMI.

Since that time, IABP has become a standard treatment for medical and surgical patients with acute left ventricular failure that is unresponsive to pharmacological and volume therapy.

IABP counterpulsation is designed to increase coronary artery perfusion pressure and blood flow during the diastolic phase of the cardiac cycle by inflation of a balloon in the thoracic aorta. Deflation of the balloon, just before systolic ejection, decreases the impedance to ejection (afterload) and thus left ventricular work, with subsequent decreased myocardial oxygen consumption. Inflation and deflation counterpulse each heart beat. With improved blood flow and effective reduction in left ventricular work, the desired results are increased coronary artery perfusion and decreased afterload with subsequent increase in cardiac output. Goals are directed toward increasing oxygen supply to the myocardium, decreasing left ventricular work, and improving cardiac output. Before IABP, no single therapeutic agent was capable of meeting these three goals.

The American College of Cardiology and the American Heart Association (ACC/AHA) guidelines for management of AMI consider IABP counterpulsation therapy a class I recommendation for the following conditions: (1) hypotension, defined as systolic blood pressure less than 90 mm Hg, or 30 mm Hg below baseline mean arterial pressure (MAP), in patients with STEMI who do not respond to other interventions; (2) low output state in patients with STEMI; and (3) cardiogenic shock that has not been quickly reversed with pharmacological agents in patients with STEMI.[1] The ACC/AHA guidelines also regard IABP counterpulsation to be a class I recommendation when used with other medical therapy for patients with STEMI and recurrent ischemic-type chest discomfort with signs of hemodynamic instability, poor left ventricular function, or a large area of myocardium at risk.[1]

PHYSIOLOGICAL PRINCIPLES

Greater work is required to maintain cardiac output in the failing heart. With this added work requirement, oxygen demand increases. These circumstances may occur at a time when the myocardium already is ischemic and coronary artery perfusion is unable to meet the oxygen demands. As a result, left ventricular performance diminishes even further, resulting in decreased cardiac output. A vicious cycle ensues that is difficult to interrupt (Fig. 18-21). Without interruption of the cycle, cardiogenic shock may be imminent. This cycle can be broken with IABP therapy by increasing aortic root pressure during diastole through inflation of the balloon. With increased

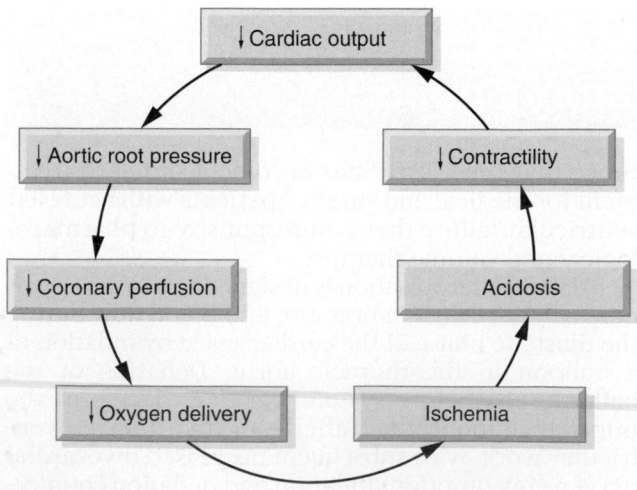

Figure 18-21 • Cycle leading to cardiogenic shock.

aortic root pressure, the perfusion pressure of the coronary arteries is increased.

Effective therapy for the patient in left ventricular failure also involves decreasing myocardial oxygen demand. Four major determinants of myocardial oxygen demand are afterload, preload, contractility, and heart rate. IABP counterpulsation therapy can have an effect on all these factors. It decreases afterload directly and affects the other three determinants indirectly as cardiac function improves. Because IABP therapy assists the left heart, only the left ventricle is discussed here.

Afterload and Preload

The greatest amount of oxygen required during the cardiac cycle is for the development of afterload (see Chapter 16). With greater impedance to ejection, afterload increases, resulting in increased myocardial oxygen demand. Impedance to ejection is caused by the aortic valve, aortic end-diastolic pressure, and vascular resistance. Greater aortic end-diastolic pressures require higher afterload to overcome impedance and ejection. Vascular resistance increases impedance when vessels become vasoconstricted. Vasodilation or lower vascular resistance decreases afterload by decreasing impedance to ejection. Deflation of the balloon in the aorta just before ventricular systole lowers aortic end-diastolic pressure. This decreases impedance to ejection and decreases left ventricular workload. In this way, IABP can effectively decrease the oxygen demand of the heart.

A person in acute left ventricular failure has increased volume in the ventricle at end-diastole (preload; see Chapter 16) as a result of the heart's inability to pump effectively. This excessive increase in preload increases the workload of the heart. IABP therapy helps decrease excessive preload by decreasing impedance to ejection. With decreased impedance, there is more effective forward flow of blood and more efficient emptying of the left ventricle.

Contractility

Contractility refers to the velocity and vigor of contraction during systole. Although vigorous contractility requires more oxygen, it is a benefit to cardiac function because it ensures good, efficient pumping, which increases cardiac output. In the patient with HF, cardiac contractility is depressed. The biochemical status of the myocardium directly affects contractility. Contractility is depressed when calcium levels are low, catecholamine levels are low, and ischemia is present with resultant acidosis.

IABP counterpulsation can increase oxygen supply, thereby decreasing ischemia and acidosis. In this way, IABP therapy contributes to improved contractility and better cardiac function (see Fig. 18-21).

Heart Rate

Heart rate is a major determinant of oxygen demand because the rate determines the number of times per minute the high pressures must be generated during systole. Normally, myocardial perfusion takes place during diastole. Coronary artery perfusion pressure is determined by the gradient between aortic diastolic pressure and myocardial wall tension. PAWP estimates wall tension and resistance to perfusion by approximating left ventricular end-diastolic volume. It can be expressed by the following equation:

Coronary perfusion pressure =

aortic diastolic pressure – myocardial wall tension

Tension in the muscle retards blood flow, which is why approximately 80% of coronary artery perfusion occurs during diastole. With faster heart rates, diastolic time becomes shortened, with very little change occurring in systolic time. A rapid heart rate not only increases oxygen demand but decreases the time available for oxygen delivery. In acute ventricular failure, a person may not be able to maintain cardiac output by increasing the volume of blood pumped with each beat (stroke volume) because contractility is depressed. Cardiac output is a function of both stroke volume and heart rate:

Cardiac output = stroke volume × heart rate

If stroke volume cannot be increased, heart rate must increase to maintain cardiac output. This increase is very costly in terms of oxygen demand.

By improving contractility, IABP therapy helps improve myocardial pumping and the ability to increase stroke volume. Decreasing afterload also increases pumping efficiency. With improved myocardial function and cardiac output, the need for compensatory tachycardia diminishes. IABP counterpulsation increases coronary artery perfusion pressure by increasing aortic diastolic pressure during inflation of the balloon, resulting in improved blood flow and oxygen delivery to the myocardium.

The physiological effects of IABP therapy are summarized in Box 18-14. Proper inflation of the balloon increases oxygen supply, and proper deflation of the balloon decreases oxygen demand. Timing of inflation and deflation is crucial and must coincide with the cardiac cycle.

Box 18-14 • Direct Physiological Effects of IABP Therapy

Inflation
↑ Aortic diastolic pressure
↑ Aortic root pressure
↑ Coronary perfusion pressure
↑ Oxygen supply

Deflation
↓ Aortic end-diastolic pressure
↓ Impedance to ejection
↓ Afterload
↓ Oxygen demand

EQUIPMENT FEATURES

The intra-aortic balloon catheter and the balloon mounted on the end are constructed of a biocompatible polyurethane material. Filling of the balloon is achieved with a pressurized gas that enters through the catheter. Because of its low molecular weight, helium is the pressurized gas of choice. Balloon size should be determined by the patient's physical stature to optimize counterpulsation (Table 18-11). With inflation, the addition of the balloon volume into the aorta acutely increases aortic pressure and retrograde blood flow back toward the aortic valve. With deflation, the sudden evacuation of the balloon volume acutely decreases aortic pressure. Catheters have a central lumen with which aortic pressure can be measured from the tip of the balloon.

INDICATIONS FOR INTRA-AORTIC BALLOON PUMP COUNTERPULSATION

Two major applications of IABP therapy are for treatment of cardiogenic shock after myocardial infarction and for acute left ventricular failure after cardiac surgery. Other applications of IABP therapy for patients with cardiac pathophysiological conditions are noted in Box 18-15.

Cardiogenic Shock

Treatment of cardiogenic shock is complicated, and the mortality rate remains high. Cardiogenic shock develops in approximately 15% of patients with myocardial infarction.

Initially, patients are treated with various inotropic drugs, vasopressors, and volume. A lack of, or minimal response in, cardiac output, arterial pressure, urine output, and mental status after this therapy indicates a need for assisted circulation with IABP therapy. Once hypotension is present, the self-perpetuating process of injury is in effect. Control of further injury and improvement in survival require early reversal of the shock state.

After IABP therapy is instituted, improvement should be observed within 1 to 2 hours. At this time, steady improvement should be seen in cardiac output, peripheral perfusion, urine output, mental status, and pulmonary congestion. With improved cardiac function, a decrease in central venous pressure and PAWP also should be seen. Average peak effect should be achieved within 24 to 48 hours.

Table 18-11 • IABP Balloon Size Guidelines

Patient Height	Balloon Volume	Body Surface Area
<5'4"	30 mL	≤1.8 m^2
5'4"–6'0"	40 mL	>1.8 m^2
>6'0" (or aortic diameter >20 cm)	50 mL	>1.8 m^2

368

> **Box 18-15 • Indications for IABP Therapy**
>
> - Cardiogenic shock after acute infarction
> - Left ventricular failure in the postoperative cardiac surgery patient
> - Severe unstable angina
> - Postinfarction ventricular septal defect or mitral regurgitation
> - Short-term bridge to cardiac transplantation

Postoperative Left Ventricular Failure

Although the best outcomes result when IABP counterpulsation is initiated at least 2 hours before cardiac surgery, a successful reduction in the mortality rate has been achieved by using IABP therapy for patients with acute left ventricular failure after cardiac surgery.[2] Two major conditions might lead to postoperative pump failure: severe preoperative left ventricular dysfunction and intraoperative myocardial injury.

IABP counterpulsation therapy can be used to wean patients from cardiopulmonary bypass (CPB) and to provide postoperative circulatory assistance until left ventricular recovery occurs. In these situations, early recognition of failure is evidenced by the heart's inability to support circulation after CPB. Early recognition and treatment are crucial if left ventricular failure is to be reversed.

Unstable Angina

IABP counterpulsation therapy may be used during PCI for patients with unstable angina or mechanical problems. In this situation, PCI procedures usually are followed by emergency cardiac surgery. Patients in this category include those with unstable angina, postinfarction angina and postinfarction ventricular septal defects, or mitral regurgitation from papillary muscle injury with resultant cardiac failure. IABP counterpulsation therapy has been used successfully to control the severity of angina in patients in whom previous medical therapy has failed. The use of IABP therapy for patients with cardiac failure after ventricular septal rupture or mitral valve incompetence aids in the promotion of forward blood flow, which decreases shunting through the septal defect and decreases the amount of mitral regurgitation.

CONTRAINDICATIONS TO INTRA-AORTIC BALLOON PUMP COUNTERPULSATION

There are few contraindications to the use of IABP therapy. A competent aortic valve is necessary if the patient is to benefit from IABP therapy. With aortic insufficiency, balloon inflation would only increase aortic regurgitation and offer little, if any, augmentation of coronary artery perfusion pressure. In fact, the patient's HF could be expected to become worse.

Severe peripheral vascular occlusive disease also is a relative contraindication to the use of IABP therapy. Occlusive disease would make insertion of the catheter difficult and possibly interrupt blood flow to the distal extremity or cause dislodgment of plaque formation along the vessel wall, resulting in potential emboli. In patients who absolutely require IABP therapy, insertion can be achieved through the thoracic aorta, thus bypassing diseased peripheral vessels. Any previous aortofemoral or aortoiliac bypass graft contraindicates femoral artery insertion.

In addition, the presence of an aortic aneurysm is a contraindication to the use of IABP therapy. A pulsating balloon against an aneurysm may predispose the patient to dislodgment of aneurysmal debris with resultant emboli. A more serious complication is rupture of the aneurysm; it is possible for the catheter to perforate the wall of the aneurysm during insertion.

PROCEDURE

Insertion

Proper positioning of the balloon is in the thoracic aorta just distal to the left subclavian artery and proximal to the renal arteries (Fig. 18-22). The most commonly used method of catheter placement is percutaneous insertion using a Seldinger technique, although other approaches have been described. The most common alternative is direct insertion into the thoracic aorta. Because this requires a median sternotomy incision, it is restricted to cardiac surgical patients whose chests have been opened for the surgery.

Once in place, the catheter is attached to a machine console that has three basic components: a monitoring system, an electronic trigger mechanism, and a drive system that moves gas in and out of the balloon. Monitoring systems have the capability of displaying the patient's ECG and an arterial waveform showing the effect of balloon inflation–deflation. Consoles also are capable of displaying a balloon waveform that illustrates the inflation and deflation of the balloon itself. The standard trigger mechanism for the balloon pump is the R wave that is sensed from the patient's ECG. This trigger signals the beginning of each cardiac cycle for the drive system. Other possible triggers include systolic arterial pressure or pacemaker spikes on the ECG. Adjustment of exact timing is controlled on the machine console. The drive system is the actual mechanism that drives gas into and out of the balloon by alternating pressure and vacuum.

Timing

Two primary methods of timing can be used with IABP therapy: conventional timing and real timing. Conventional timing uses the arterial waveform as the triggering mechanism to determine both inflation and deflation of the balloon. Real timing uses the same point of reference (the dicrotic notch on the arterial waveform) for balloon inflation but uses the ECG signal as the trigger for balloon deflation. Real timing is discussed briefly after conventional timing.

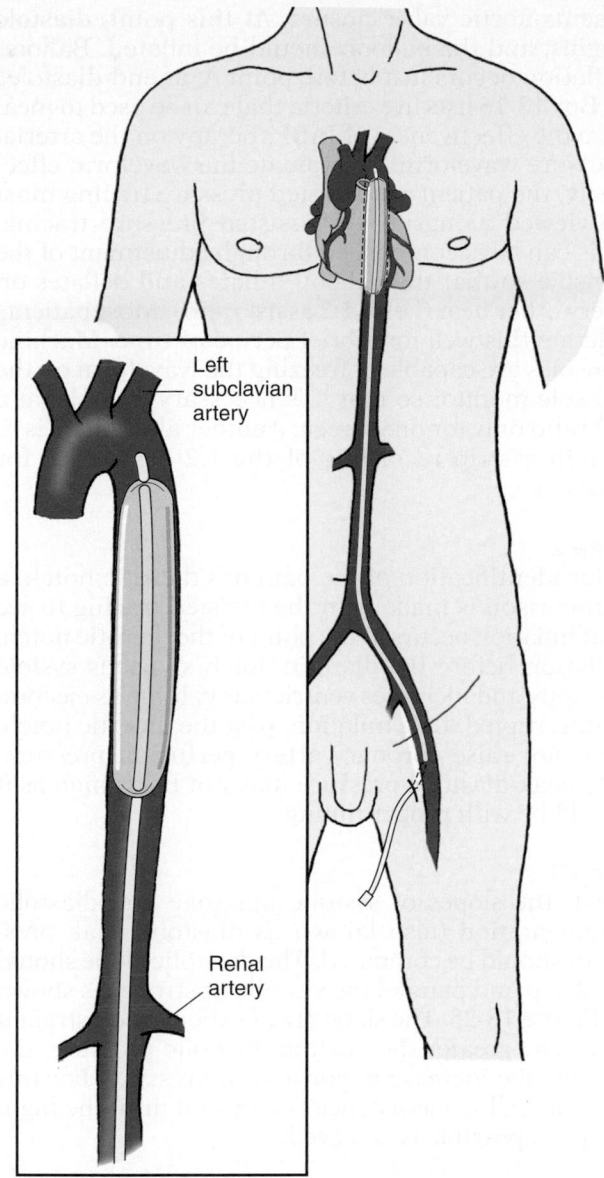

Figure 18-22 • Proper position of the balloon catheter; illustrating percutaneous insertion.

Conventional Timing

The first step to proper timing of the balloon pump using conventional timing is the identification of the beginning of systole and diastole on the arterial waveform. Systole begins when left ventricular pressure exceeds left atrial pressure, forcing the mitral valve closed.

There are two phases of systole: isovolumetric contraction and ejection. Once the mitral valve is closed, isovolumetric contraction begins and continues until enough pressure is generated to overcome impedance to ejection. When ventricular pressure exceeds aortic pressure, the aortic valve is forced open, initiating ejection, or phase two. Ejection continues until pressure in the left ventricle falls below pressure in the aorta. At this point, the aortic valve closes, and diastole begins.

Closing of the aortic valve creates an artifact on the arterial waveform that is called the dicrotic notch.

The dicrotic notch is used as a timing reference to determine when balloon inflation should occur. Inflation should not occur before the notch because systole has not been completed.

After the aortic valve closes, two phases of diastole begin: isovolumic relaxation and ventricular filling. After the aortic valve closes, there is a period in which neither the aortic nor mitral valve is open. The mitral valve remains closed because left ventricular pressure still is higher than left atrial pressure. This phase is isovolumic relaxation. When left ventricular pressure falls below left atrial pressure, the mitral valve is forced open by the higher pressure in the left atrium. This begins the filling phase of diastole. Balloon inflation should continue throughout diastole. Deflation should be timed to occur at end-diastole, just before the next sharp systolic upstroke on the arterial waveform.

Figure 18-23 illustrates the cardiac cycle with left atrial, left ventricular, and aortic pressures superimposed on one another. Figure 18-24 illustrates a radial artery waveform with the beginning of systole and diastole marked.

Real Timing

The main difference between the two timing methods is balloon deflation and the triggering mechanism used. Real timing uses the ECG as the trigger signal for balloon deflation. The QRS complex is recognized as the onset of ventricular systole, and balloon deflation occurs at this time. Triggering off the R wave allows for balloon deflation to occur at the time of systolic ejection and not before (as with conventional timing). This timing mechanism is more effective in patients with irregular heart rhythms because balloon deflation occurs on recognition of the R wave (systolic ejection). It does not need to be approximated by the operator or an algorithm, as in conventional timing. Both a rapid deflation mechanism and a reliable ECG signal are necessary for IABP using real timing to augment blood pressure effectively. Balloon inflation with real timing occurs at the onset of diastole as triggered by the dicrotic notch on an arterial waveform, just as in conventional timing.

Advances in IABP technology have led to the development of automatic timing mechanisms currently

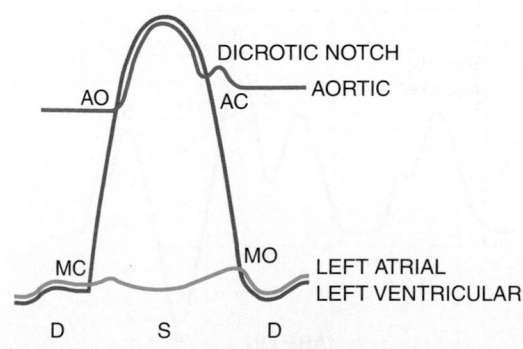

Figure 18-23 • Cardiac cycle of the left heart with aortic, left ventricular, and left atrial pressure waveforms. AC, aortic valve closure; AO, aortic valve opening; D, diastole; MC, mitral valve closure; MO, mitral valve opening; S, systole.

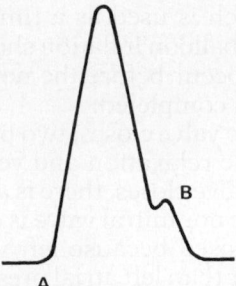

Figure 18-24 • Arterial waveform, with **A** representing the point of balloon deflation before the systolic upstroke, and **B** representing balloon inflation at the dicrotic notch, at diastole.

available in some IABP models. Automatic timing therapy is possible because of special IABP catheters that have fiber optic pressure sensors in the tip.[3] These pressure sensors, capable of transmitting real-time pressure signals at the speed of light, use windkessel model algorithms to calculate real-time aortic flow from aortic pressure.[3] This allows the balloon pump to determine the precise time when the aortic valve closes with each contraction of the heart, regardless of the patient's heart rhythm. The closure of the aortic valve signals the onset of diastole, and balloon inflation occurs.

INTERPRETATION OF RESULTS

Waveform Assessment

Analysis of the arterial pressure waveform and the effectiveness of IABP therapy is an important nursing function. Nurses must be able to recognize and correct problems in balloon pump timing. Figure 18-25 illustrates the five points that are assessed on the waveform.

Step 1

The first step in timing assessment is the ability to recognize the beginnings of systole and diastole on the arterial waveform, as shown in Figure 18-25. Systole begins at point A, where the sharp upstroke begins. Point B marks the dicrotic notch, which rep-

resents aortic valve closure. At this point, diastole begins, and the balloon should be inflated. Balloon deflation occurs just before point A, at end-diastole.

Box 18-16 lists five criteria that can be used to measure the effectiveness of IABP therapy on the arterial pressure waveform. To evaluate the waveform effectively, the patient's unassisted pressure tracing must be viewed alongside the assisted pressure tracing. This can be accomplished through adjustment of the console so that the balloon inflates and deflates on every other beat (i.e., a 1:2 assist ratio). Most patients tolerate this well for a brief period of time. Machine consoles are capable of freezing the waveform on the console monitor so that it is necessary to assist at a 1:2 ratio only for one screen. Another alternative is to obtain a strip recording of the 1:2 assistance for analysis.

Step 2

After identification of the patient's dicrotic notch, a comparison is made with the assisted tracing to see that inflation occurs at the point of the dicrotic notch. Inflation before the dicrotic notch shortens systole abruptly and increases ventricular volume as ejection is interrupted. Late inflation, past the dicrotic notch, does not raise coronary artery perfusion pressure. The peak-diastolic pressure may not be as high as it would be with proper timing.

Step 3

Next, the slopes of systolic upstroke and diastolic augmentation (also known as diastolic peak pressure) should be compared. The diastolic slope should be sharp and parallel the systolic upstroke, as shown in Figure 18-25. The slope always should be a straight line. The greater the peak in diastolic pressure, the greater the increase in aortic root pressure. For this reason, balloon assistance is adjusted until the highest peak possible is achieved.

Step 4

Deflation should occur just before systole, causing an acute drop in aortic end-diastolic pressure. This quick deflation displaces approximately 40 mL of volume. The result is an end-diastolic dip in pressure that reduces the impedance to the next systolic ejection. The end-diastolic pressure without the balloon assistance should be compared with the end-diastolic pressure with the dip created by balloon deflation.

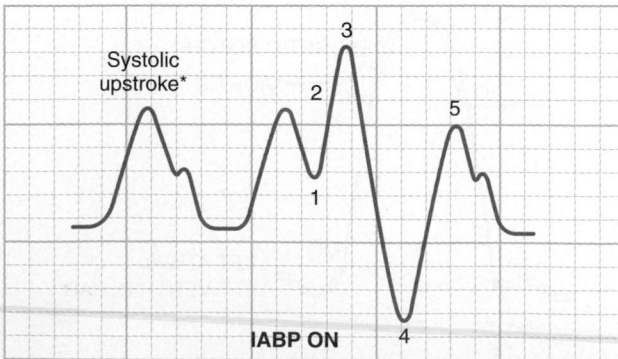

Figure 18-25 • Inspection of the arterial waveform with intra-aortic balloon assistance should include observation of (1) inflation point; (2) inflation slope; (3) diastolic peak pressure/diastolic augmentation; (4) end-diastolic dip; and (5) next systolic peak.

Box 18-16 • Criteria for Assessment of Effective IABP Therapy on the Arterial Pressure Waveform

- Inflation occurs at the dicrotic notch.
- Inflation slope is parallel to the systolic upstroke and is a straight line.
- Diastolic augmentation peak is greater than or equal to the preceding systolic peak.
- An end-diastolic dip in pressure is created with balloon deflation.
- The following systolic peak (assisted systole) is lower than the preceding systole (unassisted systole).

Optimally, a pressure difference of at least 10 mm Hg should be obtained. Better afterload reduction is achieved with the lowest possible end-diastolic dip.

The point of deflation also is crucial. Deflation that is too early allows pressure to rise to normal end-diastolic levels preceding systole. In this situation, there is no decrease in afterload. Deflation that is too late encroaches on the next systole and actually increases afterload because of greater impedance to ejection from the presence of the still-inflated balloon during systolic ejection.

Figure 18-26 demonstrates possible errors in timing.

Step 5

Finally, if afterload has been reduced, the next systolic pressure peak will be lower than the unassisted systolic pressure peak. This implies that the ventricle did not have to generate as great a pressure to overcome impedance to ejection. This may not always be seen because the systolic pressure peak also represents the compliance of the vasculature. If the vasculature is noncompliant due to atherosclerotic disease, the systolic peak may not change very much.

Balloon Fit

The fit of the balloon to any particular patient's aorta determines how well these criteria are met. Ideally, approximately 80% of the aorta is occluded with balloon inflation. In a dilated aorta, in which less than 80% occlusion occurs, the effect of inflation and deflation is not as dramatic on the waveform. When a patient is hypotensive or hypovolemic, the balloon does not have as pronounced an effect on the waveform because there is less volume displacement as the balloon inflates or deflates. See Table 18-11 for a review of balloon size guidelines.

ASSESSMENT AND MANAGEMENT

Patients requiring IABP are managed much like any other critically ill patient in cardiogenic shock or acute left ventricular failure. Nursing assessment and

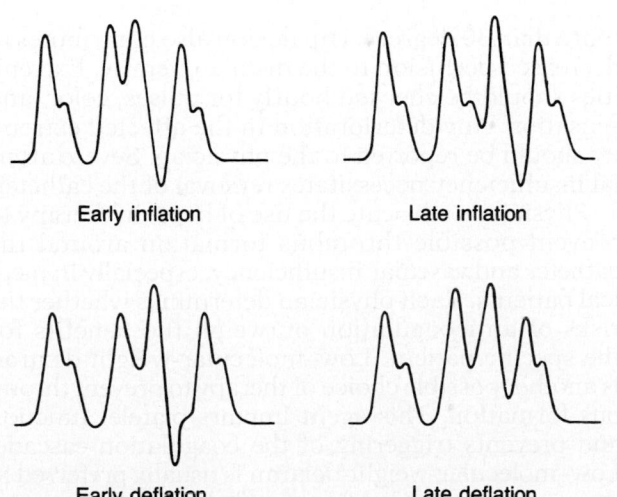

Figure 18-26 • Illustration of possible errors occurring with timing.

Early inflation Late inflation

Early deflation Late deflation

management of these conditions are discussed in Chapter 54. Additional nursing skills and assessment considerations specific to IABP therapy must be included in the care of these patients. These are summarized in Box 18-17. Nursing diagnoses and collaborative care problems for patients with an IABP are listed in Box 18-18.

System Monitoring

Cardiovascular System

Monitoring the cardiovascular system is extremely important in determining the effectiveness of IABP therapy. The basis for this assessment includes vital signs, cardiac output, heart rhythm and regularity, urine output, color, perfusion, and mentation.

Vital Signs Three important vital signs with respect to IABP therapy are heart rate, MAP, and PAWP. Effective IABP therapy causes a decrease in all three parameters. Acute changes in the MAP may indicate volume depletion. Critically ill patients tolerate little change in their volume status. The PAWP is an important parameter for monitoring volume and provides the clinician with an early indication of volume depletion or overload.

Blood pressure readings require special consideration. Because the balloon inflates during diastole, peak-diastolic pressure may be higher than peak-systolic pressure. Most IABP consoles have monitoring systems capable of distinguishing systole from peak diastole; however, some monitoring equipment can distinguish only peak pressures from low-point pressures. For this reason, a monitor's digital display of systolic pressure actually may represent peak-diastolic pressure. It is advisable to record blood pressure as systolic, peak-diastolic, and end-diastolic—that is, 100/110/60. These pressures can be read from a strip recording of the arterial waveform.

Heart Rhythm and Regularity Heart rhythm and regularity are important considerations. Early recognition and treatment of dysrhythmias are crucial for effective IABP support. Irregular dysrhythmias may inhibit efficient IABP therapy with some types of consoles because timing is set by the regular R-R interval on the ECG. A safety feature of all balloon pump consoles is automatic deflation of the balloon for premature QRS complexes. One particular IABP model tracks real time versus any average of beats, so it more effectively tracks dysrhythmias. If the dysrhythmia persists and timing is ineffective, another alternative might be use of the systolic peak on the arterial waveform as the trigger mechanism for balloon inflation. The primary goal in dysrhythmias is to treat the dysrhythmia.

Other Observations Urine output, color, perfusion, and mentation all are important assessment parameters for determining the adequacy of cardiac output. All should improve in patients responsive to IABP therapy. Any deterioration in these signs also might indicate a fall in cardiac output. Cardiac output measurement is indicated when deterioration is

Box 18-17 • NURSING INTERVENTIONS for IABP Counterpulsation and Ventricular Assist Devices (VADs)

IABP Nursing Interventions

- Verify correct timing using assist ratio of 1:2 and document settings hourly.
- Reevaluate timing for any change in the heart rate greater than 10 beats/min.
- Maintain proper balloon volume and refill as needed every 2 to 4 h. Use automatic filling mode if available. Avoid hip flexion, which may impair gas movement in and out of IABP catheter.
- Maintain good arterial waveform and adequate electro-cardiogram (ECG) signal for evaluation of timing.
- Transduce aortic arterial line to the IABP per unit protocol.
- Reduce or eliminate situations that will interfere with the IABP's ability to maintain proper assist ratio. Notify physician of the development of tachycardias or irregular rhythms, and treat dysrhythmias with drug therapy or pacing as ordered. Use appropriate trigger (i.e., ECG, arterial pressure, pacing).
- Use pacer modes only if the patient is 100% paced.
- Notify physician of significant changes in balloon pressure waveform.

VAD Nursing Interventions

- Assess and maintain adequate filling pressures during immediate postoperative phase.
- Monitor and assess heart rate, blood pressure, mean arterial pressure, pump flow, urine output, and neurological status hourly. Treat changes as ordered.
- Assess and change equipment level for devices that require specific placement of equipment for adequate pump flow.
- Evaluate pump flow and rate of VAD in relation to native heart rate and activity level of patient.
- Manage VAD function and volume status as ordered to maintain adequate device output.

General Nursing Interventions

- Monitor and record temperatures every 4 h and PRN.
- Observe all insertion sites and incisions for signs of infection. Maintain sterile technique with dressing changes.
- Change any dressing that is wet or not intact.
- Change all infusion lines and infusion bags per unit protocol.
- Culture any site with suspicious drainage, redness, or swelling.

- Notify physician of elevation in white blood cell count.
- Treat patient with antibiotics as ordered.
- Auscultate and document breath sounds every 2 to 4 h.
- Assist patient with pulmonary toilet (i.e., coughing, deep breathing, frequent turning). Suction intubated patients as needed.
- Use pulse oximeter to monitor patients with abnormal blood gases, excessive secretions, or respiratory difficulty.
- Extubate patient and increase activity level as tolerated—particularly those with VADs.
- Document quality of peripheral pulses and neurological status before AIBP or VAD insertion. Assess and document quality of pulses, skin perfusion, and neurological status per protocol. Evaluate peripheral perfusion with any complaints of leg/foot pain by patient.
- Notify physician of any changes in pulses or neurological status.
- Maintain anticoagulation as ordered.
- Avoid hip flexion, which might obstruct flow to the affected extremity, by keeping the cannulated leg straight and the bed at angle less than 30 degrees.
- Always maintain balloon motion to avoid thrombus formation on the balloon.
- Assess skin integrity, and document any redness and ulcerations over bony prominences.
- Use sheepskin, foam pads, and specialty beds as needed. Turn patient every 2 h.
- Ensure that skin remains clean and dry.
- Maintain adequate nutrition by encouraging oral intake or implementing use of parenteral or enteral nutrition when necessary.
- Maintain alarm volumes, monitor noise at lowest level possible, and minimize unnecessary noise in the room.
- Talk with patient and reorient to date and time frequently.
- Encourage family visits.
- Explain all procedures and activities to the patient.
- Organize care to allow for periods of uninterrupted sleep. Turn the lights off in room at night if possible.
- Sedate patient if necessary and as tolerated per physician orders.

---

evident, when a major change in volume or pharmacological therapy has been instituted, and during weaning from IABP support.

The left radial pulse and the cannulated extremity should be frequently assessed. A decrease, absence, or change in character of the left radial pulse may indicate that the balloon has advanced up the aorta and may be partially obstructing or has advanced into the left subclavian artery.

The presence of the balloon catheter in the femoral or iliac artery predisposes the patient to impaired circulation of the involved extremity. The affected extremity needs to be kept relatively immobile. Because flexion of the hip may kink the catheter and impair balloon pumping, it may be helpful to use a knee immobilizer to remind the patient to avoid hip flexion. The head of the bed also should not be elevated

more than 30 degrees. Hip flexion also contributes to decreased perfusion to the distal extremity. Extremities should be checked hourly for pulses, color, and sensation. Any deterioration in the affected extremity should be reported to the physician. Severe arterial insufficiency necessitates removal of the catheter.

Physicians advocate the use of heparin therapy to prevent possible thrombus formation around the catheter and vascular insufficiency, especially in medical patients. Each physician determines whether the risks of anticoagulation outweigh the benefits for the specific patient. Low–molecular-weight dextran is another possible choice of therapy to prevent thrombus formation. This agent impairs platelet function and prevents triggering of the coagulation cascade. Low–molecular-weight-dextran is usually preferred in the cardiac surgical patient for the first 24 hours.

- Decreased Cardiac Output related to alterations in preload
- Decreased Cardiac Output related to alterations in afterload
- Decreased Cardiac Output related to alterations in heart rate and rhythm
- Ineffective Cardiopulmonary Tissue Perfusion related to left ventricular failure
- Ineffective Cardiopulmonary Tissue Perfusion related to unstable angina
- Ineffective Cardiopulmonary Tissue Perfusion related to improper IABP timing
- Risk for Infection related to invasive procedure
- Impaired Mobility in Bed related to dependency on mechanical device
- Risk for Impaired Skin Integrity related to decreased perfusion
- Disturbed Sleep Pattern related to disruption in circadian rhythm
- Knowledge Deficit with IABP related to lack of history with device

Pulmonary System

Many patients on IABP therapy require intubation and ventilatory assistance. Some of these patients may have respiratory insufficiency secondary to fluid overload associated with HF. The immobile, intubated patient is always at risk for respiratory infections and the development of atelectasis. Turning the patient is appropriate provided modifications are implemented to keep the extremity cannulated by the balloon catheter straight. Daily chest radiographs are needed to follow pulmonary status and to inspect IV catheter placement. The position of the balloon catheter also can be determined in this manner.

Renal System

Patients in cardiogenic shock or severe left ventricular failure are at risk for the development of acute renal failure. In the shock state, the kidneys suffer the consequences of hypoperfusion; therefore, urine output and quality should be monitored closely. Serum BUN, creatinine, and creatinine clearance are monitored daily to assess renal function. Creatinine clearance indicates renal dysfunction and possible failure much earlier than elevated serum creatinine. Any acute, dramatic drop in urine output may be an indication that the catheter has slipped down the aorta and is obstructing the renal arteries.

Weaning

Indications for Weaning

Weaning patients from balloon assistance usually can begin 24 to 72 hours after insertion. Some patients require longer periods of support. Weaning can begin when there is evidence of hemodynamic stability that does not require excessive vasopressor support. Ide-

ally, vasopressor support is minimal when weaning begins. After the balloon is removed, it is much easier to increase vasopressor support than to reinsert a balloon catheter for hemodynamic support.

The patient should exhibit signs of adequate cardiac function, demonstrated by good peripheral pulses, adequate urine output, absence of pulmonary edema, and improved mentation. Good coronary artery perfusion is indicated by an absence of ventricular ectopy and no evidence of ischemia or injury on the ECG.

Complications may require abrupt cessation of IABP. This may or may not result in reinsertion of another balloon catheter. Severe arterial insufficiency evidenced by a loss of pulses in the distal extremity, pain, and pallor is definitely an indication to remove the balloon catheter from that particular insertion site. Any balloon that develops a leak also requires removal. The physician may choose to reinsert the balloon catheter in another extremity or to replace the faulty balloon if the patient is hemodynamically unstable. Depending on the philosophy of the institution and physician, a deteriorating, irreversible situation also might be an indication for weaning or discontinuing balloon pump support. Box 18-19 lists major indications for weaning from IABP therapy.

Approaches to Weaning

Weaning is commonly achieved by decreasing the assist ratio from 1:1 to 1:2 and so on until the minimal assist ratio is achieved on any particular console. A patient may be assisted at the first decrease for up to 4 to 6 hours. The minimal amount of time should be 30 minutes. During this time, the patient must be assessed for any change in hemodynamic status. An increase in heart rate, a decrease in blood pressure, and a decrease in cardiac output indicate a deterioration in hemodynamic status. Weaning should be discontinued temporarily, and therapy should be adjusted before another weaning attempt is made. If the first decrease in assist ratio is tolerated, the assist ratio is decreased to minimum, with 1 to 4 hours allowed for each new assist ratio. The patient must be assessed continually for any indications of intolerance

Box 18-19 • RED FLAG: Indications for Weaning From IABP

- Hemodynamic stability
  - Cardiac index >2 L/min
  - Pulmonary artery wedge pressure <20 mm Hg
  - Systolic blood pressure >100 mm Hg
- Minimal requirements for vasopressor support
- Evidence of adequate cardiac function
  - Good peripheral pulses
  - Adequate urine output
  - Absence of pulmonary edema
  - Improved mentation
- Evidence of good coronary perfusion
  - Absence of ventricular ectopy
  - Absence of ischemia on the electrocardiogram
- Severe vascular insufficiency
- Deteriorating, irreversible condition

to the process. Although less common, weaning can also occur by decreasing balloon volume, which is controlled from the console in many models.

COMPLICATIONS SPECIFIC TO INTRA-AORTIC BALLOON PUMP THERAPY

Patients with IABP counterpulsation need to be monitored for development of poor blood flow to the cannulated extremity, which could lead to compartment syndrome. It may occur within the first 24 hours of support or not until several days after catheter insertion. Compartment syndrome is caused by a rise in the tissue pressure in one of the compartments of the affected lower extremity. Bone, muscle, nerve tissue, and blood vessels all are enclosed by a fibrous membrane called the fascia, and this enclosed space is called a compartment. It is nonyielding, so a rise in volume in the compartment increases the pressure in the compartment. The patient with IABP in whom limb ischemia develops from decreased capillary flow can suffer cellular and capillary damage that leads to increased capillary permeability. The resultant transudation of fluid into the closed compartment space increases tissue pressure to a level that can interfere with capillary blood flow. When this degree of tissue pressure is reached, tissue viability may be threatened. Treatment is directed at improving blood flow. Pressure release by fasciotomy may be needed to prevent tissue death.

Decreased circulating platelets in the first 24 hours of IABP therapy and a minimal decrease in red blood cell count have been reported; however, these problems are not thought to be significant. There is a low incidence of balloon leakage and rupture. These complications may result from balloon inflation against a calcific, atherosclerotic plaque in the aorta. This disruption in the balloon surface may be as small as a pinhole or may be a large tear. The associated danger is gas embolism. In addition, the risk for entrapment is minimal but still exists. Table 18-12 provides additional details about injury secondary to balloons.

Insertion of the catheter in cases of severe atherosclerotic vascular disease may result in arterial perforation or occlusion. Any leak is an indication for immediate balloon removal. Iatrogenic dissection of the aorta is rare but has been reported. Arterial insufficiency is the most common complication of IABP therapy. Arterial insufficiency may be permanent, or it may be relieved by aortofemoral or ileofemoral bypass grafting. Neuropathy in the catheterized extremity is another reported complication.

• Mechanical Circulatory Support

When there is profound myocardial injury, the augmentation of systemic blood pressure by IABP counterpulsation may not be adequate for patient survival. Use of IABP for circulatory support requires that a patient have a functioning left ventricle because IABP augments cardiac output only by 8% to 10%. Patients with severe, acute left ventricular failure after a myocardial infarction, after a surgical procedure, or from end-stage HF may need a mechanism for replacing left ventricular function. Circulatory support with a ventricular assist device (VAD) has become a successful treatment for patients with cardiac failure refractory to pharmacological therapies, revascularization procedures, and IABP counterpulsation. These devices are capable of supporting circulation until the heart recovers or a donor heart is obtained for transplantation. As of 2003, left ventricular devices have been used as a bridge to transplantation in more than 3,500 patients. Nearly 50% of recent implantable device recipients are discharged home.[4]

Interest in the research and development of artificial circulatory support devices has existed since the 1930s. CPB, an early example of these efforts, was successfully implemented in the 1950s. A National Institutes of Health initiative helped organize and support these efforts on a national level. Michael DeBakey became the first clinician to support a postcardiotomy patient with a left ventricular bypass pump successfully in 1966. An impetus for continued research during the 1960s and 1970s was the limited early success with heart transplantation. At that time, the focus of

Table 18-12 • Injuries Secondary to Balloons		
Injury	Assessment Findings	Nursing Intervention
Balloon rupture	Presence of bright red blood or flecks of dried blood in the catheter or helium delivery line Gas alarm sounds Decreased augmentation Signs of embolic event Entrapment (may be the first indication)	Immediate removal of the catheter by the appropriate personnel Before removal: Turn pump off Clamp the line Place the patient on left side in Trendelenburg position
Balloon entrapment	Balloon pressure waveform indicates leaks Small amounts of blood in tubing or flecks of dried blood in tubing	Surgical removal is usually indicated Physician may consider pharmacological dissolution of clot with thrombolytics Physician may consider use of Fogerty embolectomy to remove fresh clot

research was the development of a device that could support the failing heart until sufficient cardiac function had returned. Current research focuses on the use of these devices as a bridge to heart transplantation and as a method of permanent cardiac support for patients with end-stage cardiac disease.

PHYSIOLOGICAL PRINCIPLES

Patients who are candidates for ventricular assistance suffer from HF resulting from ischemic or myopathic heart disease. Both disease processes lead to a reduction in cardiac output and oxygen delivery. The physiological response of the body to this low output state is vasoconstriction and increased systemic vascular resistance. Although these compensatory mechanisms are meant to protect and preserve cardiovascular function in the short term, a vicious cycle develops that is characterized by compromised cardiac contractility and a low ventricular ejection fraction. Hypotension ensues, leading to hemodynamic instability requiring the use of pharmacological agents and possibly IABP therapy for cardiovascular support. Should the patient continue to deteriorate despite drug therapy and IABP, a VAD may be necessary for survival. Hemodynamically, these patients usually demonstrate a cardiac index of less than 2 L/minute/m², a PAWP of greater than 20 mm Hg, and a systolic blood pressure of less than 80 mm Hg despite pharmacological therapies and the use of IABP counterpulsation.

Restoration of adequate blood flow and preservation of end-organ function are the fundamental goals of short- or long-term VAD use. Hemodynamics and perfusion improve as the VAD assumes the workload of the failing ventricle. Ventricular assistance may involve supporting one or both ventricles depending on the extent of myocardial damage and ventricular failure.

Left ventricular support usually requires cannulation of the left ventricle with a conduit that leads to the device. The ascending aorta, which receives the output from the device, is also cannulated with a conduit. In certain situations, the left atrium may be cannulated instead of the left ventricle. Circulation in the patient supported by a left ventricular assist device (LVAD) is similar to the normal circulatory process. Venous blood returns to the right heart, passes through the lungs to be oxygenated, and then returns to the left atrium through the pulmonary veins. Blood then passes from the left atrium through the left ventricle and into the LVAD. The LVAD then ejects blood into the ascending aorta during pump systole.

In situations that necessitate biventricular support, two pump units function in synchrony to assume the roles of the native right and left ventricles. One pump supports right heart circulation while the other supports left heart circulation. The addition of right ventricular assistance requires cannulation of the right atrium for inflow to the pump and the pulmonary artery for outflow from the right ventricular assist device (RVAD). During biventricular assistance, blood is diverted from the right atrium to the lungs through the RVAD, bypassing the right ventricle. Circulation continues to the left heart, where the LVAD undertakes support of systemic circulation. Univentricular or biventricular assistance relieves the ventricles of its workload by acting as the primary pump supporting pulmonary circulation or systemic blood pressure. Reducing ventricular workload decreases cardiac oxygen demand.

DEVICES

Several VADs are available for use. Certain devices are commercially available, whereas others require special exemption for investigational purposes. Although no universal classification system exists, the devices can be categorized according to four general functional characteristics: the intended duration of support (short term versus long term), the type of support provided (univentricular versus biventricular), the actual physical placement of the device (internal versus external), and the type of blood flow produced (pulsatile versus nonpulsatile). Short-term support usually refers to assistance for patients expected to recover from episodes of acute left ventricular failure secondary to myocardial infarction or surgical procedures. Long-term ventricular assistance may be an option for people awaiting heart transplantation, or it may provide an alternative method of permanent cardiac support.

Nonpulsatile Pumps

Centrifugal and roller pumps are examples of nonpulsatile VADs capable of providing univentricular (to either ventricle) or biventricular support. Centrifugal pumps introduce blood near the center of a rapidly spinning disk that accelerates blood toward the periphery of the disk. They are primarily used for short-term ventricular assistance when myocardial recovery is expected. These devices have been used, infrequently, as bridges to transplantation. Both types are approved by the FDA and are commercially available. Centrifugal and roller pumps are extracorporeal devices designed to support circulation of the patient's blood. Because these devices do not generate pulsatile blood flow, IABP is often used in conjunction with them to create a pulse. Blood is transported from the cannulated chamber to an external pump console that circulates the blood back to the corresponding great vessel by a separate cannula. Should right ventricular failure be identified after placement of an LVAD, an RVAD can be added for additional support with these devices.

These devices can be inserted relatively quickly and are adequate methods of deploying short-term circulatory assistance. Methods of cannulation and physical placement of the equipment limit the mobility and activity level of the patient. Patients supported by these VADs are often sedated and paralyzed. A commonly used centrifugal pump is the BioMedicus.

Axial pumps, other types of nonpulsatile pumps, use corkscrew-type impellers that propel blood by rapid rotation. These pumps are much more compact than centrifugal pumps and operate at much higher rotational speeds.[5] In addition, they weigh less than centrifugal pumps, are more compact, and therefore are more comfortable for patients.

Extracorporeal membrane oxygenation (ECMO) or CPB systems are alternative methods of temporary CPR involving circulatory support and oxygenation of the patient's blood. CPB is primarily used for operative situations but has demonstrated effectiveness as a mechanism of support for patients unable to wean from the pump perioperatively or for those requiring cardiopulmonary support refractory to conventional efforts. Circulation of blood between the patient and an external pump is supported by cannulation of the femoral vessels. Venous blood is diverted from central venous circulation; pumped through a membrane oxygenator, where oxygen and carbon dioxide are exchanged; and returned to the arterial circulation through the femoral artery cannula. A heating mechanism in the pump console helps maintain body temperature during circulatory support.

Rapid deployment without the need for surgical intervention and the ability to provide hemodynamic stabilization for a brief period are the major advantages of these resuscitative devices. CPB and ECMO allow time for further assessment and intervention during episodes of acute hemodynamic decompensation. Disadvantages include the need for continuous anticoagulation and the inability to provide extended circulatory support. The presence of occlusive peripheral vascular disease could be a contraindication to use of these devices.

Pulsatile Pumps

Implantable Pulsatile Pumps

Implantable pumps were designed with the intention of providing long-term left ventricular support while allowing the patient a certain amount of physical independence. A few devices have successfully supported a patient for greater than 1 year while awaiting heart transplantation. Many patients with the implantable devices have been physically rehabilitated by participating in regular physical therapy programs and normal activities of daily living while being supported with a VAD. This might better prepare them physically to endure the transplantation process. Examples of the implantable devices are the HeartMate IP and the Novacor left ventricular assist system (LVAS). The Novacor device operates on electricity, whereas the HeartMate IP operates as a pneumatic unit.

Surgical implantation of the VAD necessitates a sternotomy and the use of CPB. Device placement is in an abdominal pocket just below the left diaphragm. Typically, the inflow conduit is tunneled through the diaphragm and anastomosed to the apex of the left ventricle. The outflow conduit is brought around the diaphragm and is anastomosed to the ascending aorta. Drivelines extending from the implanted device are tunneled through the patient's skin and connected to a portable, external power source. This power source may be a portable console or battery pack that is worn by the patient (Fig. 18-27). Either situation allows the

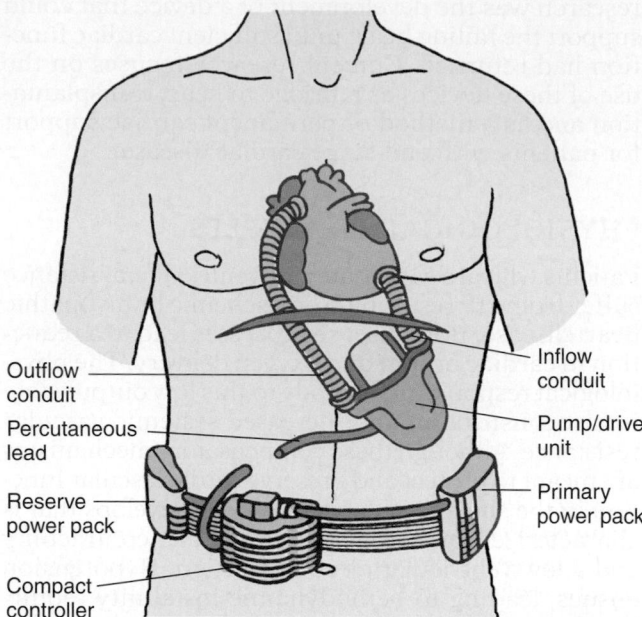

Outflow conduit

Percutaneous lead

Reserve power pack

Compact controller

Inflow conduit

Pump/drive unit

Primary power pack

Figure 18-27 • Portable, implantable left ventricular assist device. (Artwork courtesy of the Novacor Division, Baxter Healthcare Corporation, Oakland, CA.)

patient mobility and independence during the recovery period.

Pump units of the implantable VADs are encapsulated in rigid housing and consist of a blood pump sac and single or dual pusher plates (depending on the particular device). Inflow and outflow conduits have valves that support unidirectional blood flow. These devices work on the principle of converting electrical or pneumatic energy to mechanical energy. This mechanical energy activates the pusher plates, causing them to compress the blood sac at the appropriate time. Blood sac compression causes ejection of the blood out of the pump sac and into the ascending aorta through the outflow conduit. These devices have stroke volumes of 70 to 83 mL and can support pump outputs of greater than 10 L/minute. Depending on the device implanted, long-term anticoagulation may be necessary to prevent thromboembolic events.

External Pulsatile Pumps

Two commonly used external pulsatile devices are the Thoratec VAD and the Abiomed pump. Both devices have successfully supported patients postcardiotomy and patients bridged to heart transplantation.

The Thoratec VAD is a pneumatically driven device that is positioned externally on the recipient's upper abdomen. Placement of this device requires a sternotomy incision and use of CPB. The structure of the pump drive, the inflow and outflow conduits, and the cannulation techniques of the chambers and great vessels are all similar to that of the implantable devices. A major difference is that the cannulas supporting the blood flow pass through the patient's chest wall to the externally positioned pump. One advantage of this device is the ability to provide univentricular or biventricular support, depending on the extent of HF. Figure 18-28 is an example of biventricular support. Another advantage is that due to its external placement, small patient body size is less of a contraindication when considering the need for ventricular assistance.

Another external VAD, the Abiomed pump, is designed for short-term univentricular or biventricular support. It has been used in patients when myocardial recovery is expected and as a bridge to transplantation. Components consist of cannulas for venous and arterial access, blood pumps to support unidirectional blood flow and systemic circulation, and a pneumatically driven console that provides the power source. Cannulation sites for this device are either atria, the pulmonary artery, and the ascending aorta. Filling of the blood pumps occurs passively by gravity; therefore, the blood pumps must be positioned securely below the level of the heart to promote adequate blood flow into their chambers (Fig. 18-29). The internal bladders operate in a fill-to-empty mode. Pumps positioned too high fill insufficiently, and pumps that are too low have a prolonged filling time, each adversely affecting patient hemodynamics. Nursing interventions specific to the Abiomed include monitoring and adjusting the level of the blood pumps and monitoring filling pressures to ensure adequate volumes necessary to support optimal flow through the system. Use of this device significantly impairs patient mobility.

Advances in Mechanical Circulatory Support

In November 2002, the FDA approved the Thoratec HeartMate SNAP-VE LVAS for permanent implantation, also known as "destination therapy," in patients

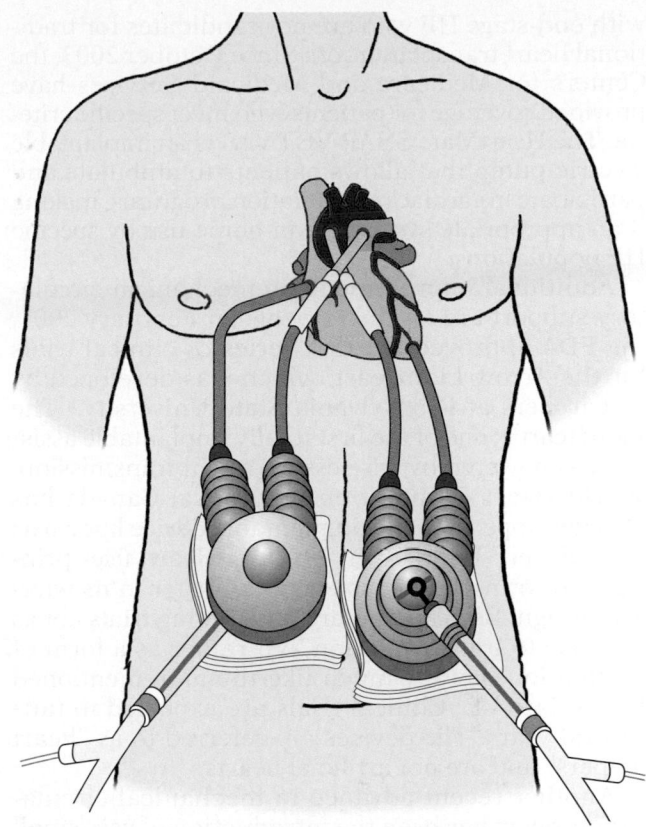

Figure 18-28 • Thoratec pneumatic ventricular assist device. External placement with biventricular assist capabilities. (Courtesy of Kathy J. Vaca, RN, Department of Surgery, St. Louis Health Sciences Center, St. Louis, MO.)

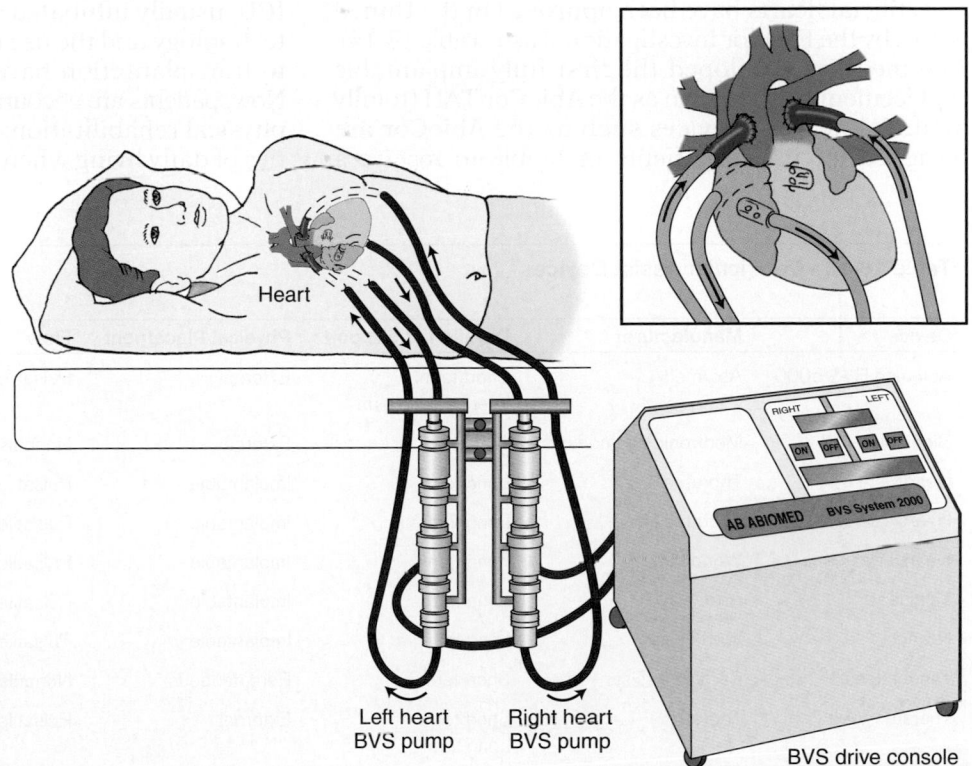

Figure 18-29 • Abiomed biventricular support system. (Artwork courtesy of ABIOMED Cardiovascular, Inc., Danvers, MA.)

with end-stage HF who are not candidates for traditional heart transplantation. Since October 2003, the Centers for Medicare and Medicaid Services have provided coverage for patients who meet specific criteria. The HeartMate SNAP-VE LVAS is an implantable electric pump that allows patients to ambulate and participate in cardiac rehabilitation programs, making it an appropriate system for in-home use by specific HF populations.

Additional improvements in mechanical circulatory support are on the horizon. In February 2001, the FDA approved the first series of clinical trials for the Arrow LionHeart, which was developed by researchers at Pennsylvania State University.[6] The LionHeart is one of the first totally implantable assist devices powered by wireless electrical transmission. World Heart Corporation of Ottawa, Canada has also developed a totally implantable device known as HeartSaver.[7] HeartSaver, like LionHeart, uses principles of transcutaneous energy transfer in its wireless design. Both models are undergoing trials not as a bridge to transplantation, but rather as a form of destination therapy much like the aforementioned HeartMate VE. Clinical trials are expected to take several years. The devices are referred to as "heart helpers" and are not artificial hearts.

Another recent advance in mechanical circulatory support has been the introduction of very small pumps that can be incorporated into a transvascular catheter. Major surgical procedures are required for implantation of all other models of VADs, whereas catheter-based LVADs can be placed percutaneously.[8] Several such devices are in development, including the TandemHeart LVAD, which is an extracorporeal centrifugal LVAD. Table 18-13 provides a comprehensive review of VADs.

Artificial hearts have been approved in the United States by the FDA for investigational use (Table 18-14). Abiomed has developed the first fully implantable replacement heart known as the AbioCor TAH (totally artificial heart).[7] Devices such as the AbioCor are designed for use in patients ineligible to receive a VAD, such as those with both right- and left-sided HF. The AbioCor received Humanitarian Device Exemption from the FDA in September of 2006. In addition, SynCardia Systems has developed the CardioWest device, which is an implantable pneumatic artificial heart. The FDA approved its use as a bridge to transplantation in 2004 (however, destination implants are being performed in Europe).[9] Whereas the AbioCor is a self-contained device, the CardioWest device is designed such that patients are connected to a large console by tubes through their chest wall.

Modes of Operation

With the exception of the Abiomed device, the pulsatile pumps have several modes of operation. Two primary modes depend on the patient's ECG or the rate of blood flow through the pump during each cardiac cycle. In the ECG trigger mode, the pump initiates blood ejection in conjunction with the patient's QRS complex; the R wave acts as the trigger for pump systole. The second mode is a dynamic mode that allows the pump to respond to the changing heart rate, depending on patient activity level. Pump systole and cardiac output depend on the blood flow sensed by the device, which is programmed to respond to changes in pump filling rate as blood passes from the left ventricle into the blood sac of the pump drive. This ability is particularly important as a patient's level of activity increases during the recovery phase after implantation. A third mode of operation, rarely used clinically, is a fixed-rate mode that functions independently of the native heart.

NURSING IMPLICATIONS

Historically, VAD recipients have received care in the ICU, usually intubated and sedated. Evolution of the technology and the use of portable devices as bridges to transplantation have changed the mode of care. Now, patients are encouraged to be independent, pursue physical rehabilitation, and engage in normal activities of daily living when possible (Fig. 18-30). Certain

Table 18-13 • Ventricular Assist Devices

Device	Manufacturer	Duration of Support	Physical Placement	Flow	Drive System
Abiomed BVS 5000	Abiomed	Short term Intermediate term	External	Pulsatile	Pneumatic
Biomedicus	Medtronic-Biomedicus	Short term	External	Nonpulsatile (centrifugal)	Electric
HeartMate IP	Thoratec	Long term	Implantable	Pulsatile	Pneumatic
HeartMate VE	Thoratec	Long term	Implantable	Pulsatile	Electric
HeartSaver	World Heart	Long term	Implantable	Pulsatile	Electric
LionHeart	Arrow	Long term	Implantable	Pulsatile	Electric (wireless)
Novacor	World Heart	Long term	Implantable	Pulsatile	Electric
TandemHeart	Cardiac Assist	Short term	Percutaneous	Nonpulsatile (centrifugal)	Electric
Thoratec VAD	Thoratec	Short term Long term	External	Pulsatile	Pneumatic

Table 18-14 • Total Artificial Heart

Device	Manufacturer	Flow	Drive System
Abiocor	Abiomed	Pulsatile	Hydraulic
CardioWest	SynCardia	Pulsatile	Pneumatic

patients may even be discharged from the hospital. Nurses have an opportunity to be instrumental in the coordination of patient care and outcomes management in this new patient population.

During the immediate postoperative phase, the critical care nurse must be cognizant of the physiological responses expected and the common postoperative complications associated with device implantation. The nurse determines whether the equipment is functioning appropriately by monitoring parameters associated with adequate tissue perfusion and improved end-organ function because these are the primary goals of VAD implantation. Hemodynamic instability and the maintenance of adequate filling pressures are critical issues in the immediate postoperative period. Other issues the critical care nurse encounters include, but are not limited to, dysrhythmias, bleeding complications, infections, thromboembolic events, and possible mechanical problems associated with the devices.

Psychosocial issues and patient education dominate the nursing focus during periods of extended

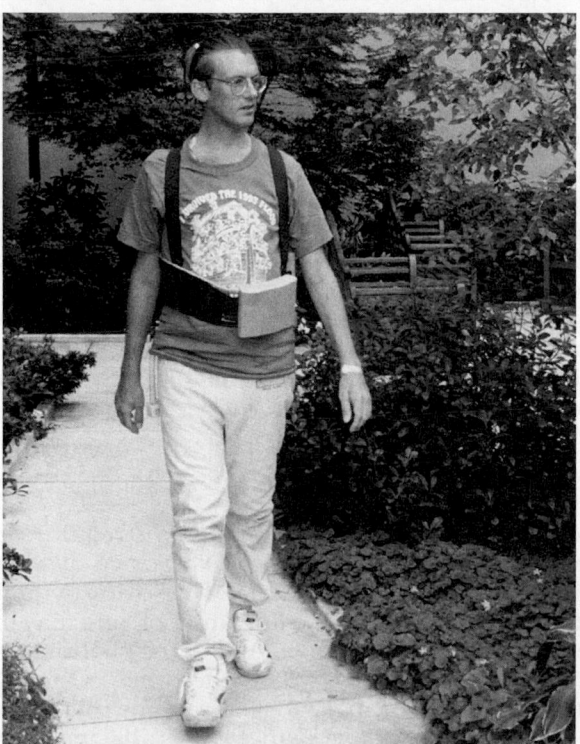

Figure 18-30 • Wearing the portable left ventricular assist system, a patient is able to enjoy the independence of outdoor activities. Some patients may take day trips or be discharged from the hospital. (Photograph courtesy of Stanford Health Services, Stanford, CA.)

support with a VAD; most of these patients require minimal direct nursing care once stabilized and discharged from the ICU. Increased independence in activities of daily living, continued physical rehabilitation, and patient education are emphasized. All aspects of the rehabilitation phase should include the recipient's family members or identified support person. As patients are discharged, they and their primary caregivers need to be educated about the operation of the equipment and how to troubleshoot malfunctions. A person capable of operating the VAD needs to accompany the patient at all times. Nursing must facilitate the integration of the patient's lifestyle with the boundaries created by having a VAD implanted for extended support. Feelings of isolation may unfold because investigational device protocols governed by the FDA may restrict the patients' social activity and geographical mobility.

An advanced-practice nurse is in a pivotal position to assume the role of case manager facilitating the implementation of clinical paths, protocols, and procedures related to patient progress from the acute to chronic phases of rehabilitation. Nursing education facilitated by a clinical nurse specialist is vital to patient care as increasing numbers of nurses on the general floors, and possibly the outpatient setting, are exposed to this patient population. As more patients receive the portable devices and approach the possibility of hospital discharge, case management will be a principal facet of patient care.

• Complications Associated With Intra-Aortic Balloon Pump Therapy and Circulatory Support

BLEEDING

Prolongation of bleeding times is a side effect of exposure to CPB, which is normally reversed in the early postoperative period. With the use of mechanical circulatory support, the continued exposure of blood to an artificial surface causes trauma to platelets. A cascade of events involving the platelets, white blood cells, fibrinolytic system, and complement system occurs. The frequency and severity of bleeding associated with artificial circulatory devices have been reduced by improved surgical techniques and methods of maintaining hemostasis, the reversal of heparin, the infusion of coagulation factors (platelets, fresh frozen plasma), and continued experience with the equipment. Episodes of severe bleeding are usually corrected within the first 24 hours after surgical implantation of a VAD.

Factors associated with increased postoperative bleeding in VAD recipients are preoperative and postoperative use of anticoagulants; coagulopathies secondary to cardiogenic shock, HF, and extended CPB exposure; and the use of multiple cannulation sites. Hemodynamic instability, a reduction in native cardiac output and device output, a risk for ischemia to target organs, and possible cardiac tamponade are all deleterious events associated with uncontrolled bleeding in the patient supported with a VAD. In the patient receiving IABP therapy, bleeding is usually related to use of continuous anticoagulation or the development of coagulopathies. Bleeding commonly occurs at the insertion site of the balloon catheter. In both patient populations, nursing interventions include observing external cannulation sites for oozing, monitoring changes in vital signs (particularly hemodynamic parameters, such as filling pressures for VAD recipients) and laboratory values, and regularly assessing adequate tissue perfusion.

THROMBOEMBOLIC EVENTS

Placement of IABP puts a patient at risk for thromboembolic events. At the time of insertion, plaque may become dislodged from the vessel wall, or emboli may break off a thrombus that has formed on the indwelling catheter or balloon. Both situations can impair circulation to distal extremities and other vital organs or cause a stroke. Continuous anticoagulation with a heparin infusion is required during IABP therapy; dextran infusions may also be used.

The development of a thrombus and the migration of emboli have been reported with the use of mechanical circulatory support. Anticoagulation regimens and the prevention of embolic events are unresolved issues in the clinical management of VAD recipients. Currently, anticoagulation therapy is managed differently depending on the device that is inserted. Devices used for short-term support require prophylactic use of low-dose heparin infusions. Similar to IABP, dextran infusions may be used in conjunction with heparin. Patients supported with the Novacor, HeartMate, and Thoratec devices who require long-term support are at greater risk secondary to extended periods of exposure to the device. These patients are usually managed with heparin infusions in the immediate postoperative phase. During the extended support period, the heparin is weaned, and warfarin (Coumadin) therapy is initiated to maintain the prothrombin time at an INR of 3 to 4.[10] Antiplatelet agents, such as dipyridamole (Persantine), may be used in conjunction with warfarin therapy. Obtaining baseline and postimplantation neurological assessments; monitoring peripheral pulses, especially those distal to cannulation sites; and assessing tissue perfusion are critical to the early recognition and intervention of any embolic event.

RIGHT VENTRICULAR FAILURE

Right ventricular failure continues to be a significant problem associated with LVAD implantation. Right ventricular failure develops in 20% to 25% of LVAD recipients after device implantation secondary to the physiological effects of the LVAD on systemic circulation.[11-12] Because the pumping capabilities of the device exceed those of the impaired left ventricle, systemic circulation and right ventricular preload

increase, subsequently increasing right ventricular workload. Right ventricular output is increased in a patient with a healthy right ventricle. However, a patient with underlying right ventricular failure may not be able to handle this augmentation in circulatory volume. Evidence of primary right ventricular dysfunction may not become apparent until the right heart is challenged by the cardiac output of the LVAD.[12-13] When right ventricular failure develops after LVAD implantation, vasodilators and IV inotropes, such as prostaglandin E$_1$, isoproterenol (Isuprel), and epinephrine, are used to reduce pulmonary pressures and improve right ventricular contractility. It may be possible to add an RVAD for additional support if pharmacological intervention is unsuccessful. Clinical practice has shown that the addition of an RVAD after LVAD placement is a poor prognostic indicator.[6]

INFECTION

People requiring mechanical circulatory assistance and IABP therapy are at increased risk for infection secondary to the surgical procedures and the presence of external cannulas, pumps, drivelines, and so forth. Many of these patients suffer from chronic illness that renders them more immunocompromised. Infection may be related to surgical wounds after device insertion, invasive monitoring lines, drain placement, pulmonary status, or nutritional status. Early recognition of signs and symptoms of infection and early intervention can prevent the development of sepsis. Early detection is particularly important because some of these patients await heart transplantation, and an infection could preclude transplantation. Diligent handwashing, changing or removing invasive lines or drainage tubes when appropriate, adherence to sterile dressing techniques and schedules, and the use of appropriate prophylactic antibiotics are effective barriers to the development of infection. Early extubation and mobilization are goals for patients with the implanted devices. Primary nursing interventions include monitoring invasive sites for signs of infection, encouraging good pulmonary toilet, increasing activity level as tolerated, and promoting adequate nutrition.

DYSRHYTHMIAS

Most patients with cardiomyopathy who require some form of circulatory assistance experience dysrhythmias before insertion of a device. These dysrhythmias often continue after device implantation and may hinder device function, depending on the rhythm. Dysrhythmias should be treated when they occur, and attempts should be made to restore sinus rhythm.

Circulatory assistance with IABP is affected by dysrhythmias. Diastolic augmentation and systolic assistance decrease in the presence of irregular rhythms, such as AF or sinus rhythm with frequent ectopy. These rhythm changes make it difficult to manage the timing of balloon inflation and deflation. Lethal ventricular dysrhythmias need to be treated conventionally because IABP is designed only to augment existing cardiac output.

Right ventricular function and the maintenance of adequate pump output are of primary concern in LVAD recipients with lethal ventricular dysrhythmias. These patients may lack sufficient right ventricular function to support cardiac output during ventricular dysrhythmia even though left ventricular function has been assumed by the LVAD. Although LVAD flow and mean blood pressure have been known to decrease by approximately 20%, it has been demonstrated that patients with LVADs do tolerate sustained lethal ventricular dysrhythmias without the need for RVAD support. Symptoms associated with these rhythms and low-flow states are usually weakness and palpitations.[14] Patients receiving biventricular support should be able to maintain adequate device outputs despite the dysrhythmia because left and right ventricular function has been taken over by the VAD. AF is usually tolerated by these patients even though it may have some effect on right heart function. Severe bradycardia and tachydysrhythmia need to be addressed because they will change pump flow and output. Cardiac rhythms require close monitoring for any acute changes.

NUTRITIONAL DEFICITS

Nutritional status is an important element of any recovery process. Many patients have had end-stage HF and are nutritionally depleted before any surgical intervention, placing them at a higher risk for nutritional deficits during the postoperative phase. Adequate nutrition is necessary for wound healing. Obtaining dietary consultation, encouraging increased oral intake, and providing flexibility with meals will assist these patients in meeting their nutritional goals. Patients supported by IABP and VADs that require intubation and sedation require parenteral or enteral feedings. Those with implanted devices eventually progress to a regular diet but may need smaller, more frequent meals. Experiencing feelings of fullness or early satiety is not uncommon for these patients due to the abdominal placement of the device.

PSYCHOSOCIAL FACTORS

Balloon and VAD insertion are usually unplanned, emergent interventions for a deteriorating condition. Abundant monitoring is frightening for both patient and family; therefore, explanations of procedures and surroundings are very important. Family members need to be prepared before visiting their loved one immediately after device insertion. The goal is to alleviate anxiety and to help the patient and family feel more secure in a foreign environment. Honest communication is important. This helps the family members recognize changes in their loved one's condition and make informed, realistic decisions regarding the patient's care. Putting the family in contact with nonmedical personnel who can objectively provide emotional support is often beneficial. Issues that families and patients struggle with are fear, hopelessness, and death.

Critically ill patients often suffer from disorientation and sleep deprivation. Immobility and unfamiliar noises of the ICU tend to increase stress and anxiety. Mechanisms to help alleviate this stress and anxiety include frequent reorientation by the nursing staff and contact with family members. Better organization of time and procedures also reduces stress because it allows the patient longer periods of uninterrupted rest.

Management of Dysrhythmias

• Electrical Cardioversion

Electrical cardioversion is used to convert sustained supraventricular or ventricular tachydysrhythmias to sinus rhythm, especially when the patient has an unstable rhythm that causes hemodynamic collapse. It may be used electively for recent-onset dysrhythmias that do not respond to antidysrhythmic drugs. As opposed to defibrillation, which delivers an unsynchronized current to the heart, cardioversion delivers a shock that is synchronized with the heart's activity. By setting the automatic external defibrillator (AED) to the synchronized mode, the device detects the patient's R wave and delivers the shock during ventricular depolarization. As a result, there is no danger of causing ventricular fibrillation, which can occur when a shock is delivered during ventricular repolarization (on the T wave). Indications for synchronized, external cardioversion and recommendations for initial joules (J) used are listed in Table 18-15.[1,2] Precautions and relative contraindications for cardioversion are listed in Table 18-16.

The energy needed to convert monomorphic VT with a pulse may be as low as 100 J initially, followed by 200, 300, or 360 J, as necessary for conversion. The energy required for conversion of atrial flutter may start at 5 to 50 J when a biphasic waveform defibrillator is used.[3] The energy required to convert AF is greater, starting at 200 J.[2] After conversion to sinus rhythm, antidysrhythmic therapy may be initiated for rhythm maintenance. Although recommendations are made for the amount of joules needed to convert various rhythms, the actual energy needed may vary depending on the duration of the dysrhythmia, transthoracic impedance, and the waveform morphology of the defibrillator (i.e. monophasic versus biphasic).[3]

Table 18-15 • Indications and Energy Requirements for Cardioversion	
Indications	**Energy in Joules (J) Monophasic Waveform***
Monomorphic ventricular tachycardia with a pulse	100–360
Atrial flutter	50
Atrial fibrillation	200 initially

*The energy requirement when using a biphasic waveform defibrillator varies but is usually less compared with a monophasic waveform automatic external defibrillator.

PROCEDURE

The steps for cardioversion are as follows:

1. Explain the procedure to the patient and obtain informed consent.

2. Restrict the patient's food and water for 6 to 8 hours before cardioversion, unless emergency cardioversion is required.

3. If the patient is on chronic digitalis, confirm that digoxin levels are therapeutic. Patients with digitalis toxicity should not undergo elective cardioversion until levels are normalized.

4. Record a 12-lead ECG and vital signs, establish an IV line, monitor O_2 saturation levels, and ready all necessary resuscitation equipment.

5. Turn on the defibrillator and monitor, and attach the monitoring electrodes to the patient's chest. Avoid placing the electrodes in the area where the defibrillation paddles will be positioned. Some devices permit both monitoring and defibrillation through disposable defibrillation patches.

6. Select a monitoring lead that provides a good ECG pattern with a tall R wave. If monitoring by way of the disposable defibrillator patches, select "paddles" lead.

7. Turn on the synchronizer mode button. The size of the R wave or the monitored lead may need to be adjusted until the synchronization marker appears on each R wave.

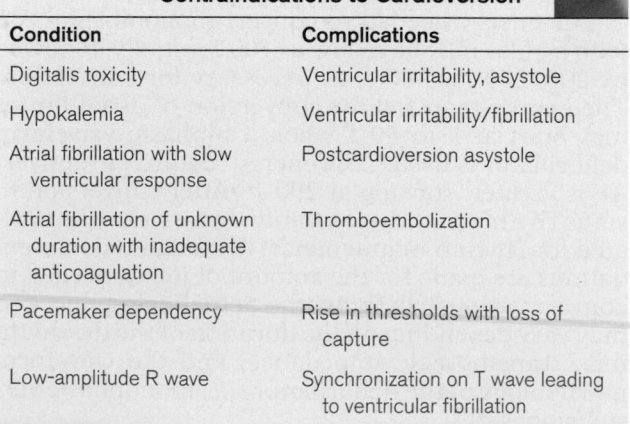

Table 18-16 • Precautions/Relative Contraindications to Cardioversion	
Condition	**Complications**
Digitalis toxicity	Ventricular irritability, asystole
Hypokalemia	Ventricular irritability/fibrillation
Atrial fibrillation with slow ventricular response	Postcardioversion asystole
Atrial fibrillation of unknown duration with inadequate anticoagulation	Thromboembolization
Pacemaker dependency	Rise in thresholds with loss of capture
Low-amplitude R wave	Synchronization on T wave leading to ventricular fibrillation

8. Sedate the patient, and maintain an adequate airway.

9. Remove paddles from the defibrillator and apply a generous amount of electrode gel to the metal surface. Take care not to smear electrode gel between the two paddles on the chest. Disposable pregelled defibrillator patches may be selected rather than standard paddles.

    a. If hands-free gel patches are used, disconnect the paddles from the defibrillator and connect the terminal pin of the patches to the defibrillator using an adaptor. Place the sternum patch to the right of the sternum, just below the clavicle, and the apex patch below the anterior/axillary margin of the left chest. Apply each patch firmly from the center to the periphery, ensuring that there are no air pockets, which can cause electrical arcing and skin burns.

    b. If using paddles, apply firmly, one just below the right clavicle and the other over the apex of the heart. Make sure paddles or patches are away from electrode wires or from an implanted pacemaker or ICD generator.

10. Set the desired energy level.

11. Press the charge button. A light will flash until paddles are fully charged.

12. Reconfirm the synchronization markers on the R waves on the monitor.

13. Call out "clear" and visually check to make sure no one is touching the patient or the bed.

14. While applying 25 pounds of firm pressure on the paddles, push and hold both paddle discharge buttons until the defibrillator discharges. Maintain contact on the chest wall until the machine has delivered the shock. There will be a momentary delay from the pressing of the discharge button to delivery of the shock because of the synchronization with the R wave. Failure to keep the paddles on the chest can result in failure to cardiovert and burns to the chest.

15. Assess the patient's rhythm, airway, and vital signs.

16. Subsequent shocks may need to be delivered. If so, be certain to select the synchronized mode.

17. If the patient's rhythm deteriorates to ventricular fibrillation, turn off the synchronizer and immediately defibrillate the patient, starting with 200 J and increasing to 360 J as needed.

18. After cardioversion, observe the patient for changes in rhythm, blood pressure, and respirations. Patients with AF converting with sinus pauses may have underlying tachy-brady syndrome. Be prepared for transcutaneous pacing if needed, or have atropine sulfate readily available. If a patient has a pacemaker, the pacemaker may need to be interrogated or reprogrammed because a temporary rise in capture thresholds may follow cardioversion. Older pacemaker models may revert to a reset or backup mode.

19. Antidysrhythmic agents may need to be initiated to maintain sinus rhythm.

20. Monitor the patient's respiratory status and level of consciousness because sedation was delivered before the procedure. Inspect the chest wall for any signs of burns and treat appropriately.

21. Clean the paddles thoroughly before storing them.

22. Document the procedure, the outcomes of the procedure, and the patient's status in the medical record.

• Catheter Ablation

Catheter ablation is an invasive procedure used for the treatment of tachydysrhythmias. The technique involves percutaneous catheter insertion through a vein or artery, positioned into the heart to deliver energy (e.g. radiofrequency, microwave frequencies). Delivery of energy to cardiac tissue through a catheter electrode tip limits the tissue damage to targeted areas responsible for the initiation or conduction of the dysrhythmia.

Clinical use of catheter ablation of cardiac tissue started in the early 1980s with direct current shocks delivered through a catheter attached to a defibrillator. Because this technique was associated with significant risk, safer means to ablate tissue were investigated.

Radiofrequency energy, the primary source of energy used to ablate cardiac tissue, is produced by alternating current delivered at 500 kHz through the tip of the catheter in unipolar fashion. The circuit is completed through a grounding pad applied on the patient's skin. Resistive heat is created as the energy dissipates around the active electrode, which results in a small localized lesion in cardiac tissue. Tissue temperatures of 50°C or higher lead to irreversible tissue injury. If properly targeted, this localized area of damage can prevent the initiation of the dysrhythmia (the "focus") or interrupt the conduction (the "accessory pathway") of the dysrhythmia. The size of the resulting lesion depends on the electrode temperature, power delivered, and duration of the alternating current used. When tissue temperature exceeds 100°C, formation of coagulum and char at the electrode tissue interface prevents further energy delivery and adds the risk for steam venting to the endocardial tissue, possibly causing perforation. Electrode cooling (e.g., through saline irrigation) reduces the risk for overheating and allows for larger lesion size delivered by higher power. The size, shape, and electrode material of the ablating catheter also influence the resulting lesion.[4]

INDICATIONS FOR ABLATION

A PSVT can be treated with radiofrequency ablation. Most PSVTs are caused by either atrioventricular nodal reentrant tachycardia (AVNRT) or by atrioventricular reentrant tachycardia (AVRT). PSVT also can be caused by intra-atrial reentrant tachycardia. Recurrent symptomatic or life-threatening ventricular dysrhythmias also may be indications for ablation. Indications for catheter ablation procedures are included in the American Heart Association and Heart Rhythm Society (formerly North American Society of Pacing and Electrophysiology; NASPE) policy statement on catheter ablation.[5]

The most common mechanism for SVT is reentry,[3] which occurs when conduction of an impulse through myocardial tissue is initially blocked (or functionally refractory, unresponsive to stimuli) in one direction. The advancing wavefront proceeds through an alternate slower route. As the previously refractory pathway recovers, the electrical impulses return through that pathway and then find their way back down to the alternate slower route. As a result, a circuitous reentrant pattern of conduction occurs.

Atrioventricular Nodal Reentrant Tachycardia

The compact AV node can utilize two functional pathways for conduction—slow and fast—setting the stage for AVNRT. When this phenomenon is observed in the electrophysiology laboratory, the AV node is described as having dual physiology. AVNRT, the most common type of PSVT, occurs when an AV node with dual physiology is stimulated by a premature atrial contraction. The fast pathway, which is preferentially used in normal sinus rhythm, has not recovered, so the impulse travels down the slow pathway and activates the ventricles. On surface ECG, this initiating rhythm would be viewed as a premature atrial contraction with a long PR interval. The impulse then returns back up to the atria from the ventricles through the fast pathway, which has now recovered excitability, then back down again to the ventricles through the slow pathway, causing the reentrant circuit to perpetuate. Selective ablation of the slow pathway is the preferred method of treating AVNRT. The fast-pathway ablation sites are closer to the compact AV node, and ablation of the fast pathway may be complicated by high-grade AV block.

Atrioventricular Reentrant Tachycardia

In the normal heart, the AV node and the bundle of His serve as the connection between the atria and the ventricles for the conducting system. AVRT rhythms are characterized by the presence of additional accessory pathways that link conduction between the atria and the ventricles. Conduction through accessory pathways may start from the atria to the ventricles (antegrade conduction), from the ventricles to the atria (retrograde conduction), or in both directions. AVRT rhythms result when circular movement of the impulse occurs because of the ability of the accessory pathways to conduct signals in either direction.

In WPW syndrome, an electrocardiographic pattern associated with PSVT and sometimes associated with Ebstein's anomaly of the tricuspid valve, the person has one or more anomalous conduction accessory pathways linking the atria and the ventricles. Because of the presence of these accessory pathways, the person with WPW syndrome is prone to AVRT and AF with rapid ventricular response. When rapidly conducting, these PSVTs may deteriorate into ventricular fibrillation. Ablation of the accessory pathways is used to interrupt the rapid limb of the reentrant circuit and eliminate the offending dysrhythmias.

Atrial Fibrillation or Flutter

Ablation may be indicated for patients with AF or flutter with a rapid ventricular response that has not been controlled by pharmacological therapy. The AV junction may be ablated, completely disrupting communication from the atria to the ventricles. Successful ablation results in complete heart block with a ventricular rate of 40 to 60 beats/minute. A permanent pacemaker is implanted after AV junction ablation to ensure the presence of a reliable rhythm and adequate rate as well as to reduce the risk for bradycardia-dependent torsades de pointes.

In addition, ablation for AF can be performed by creating lines of block around the anatomical triggers (e.g., around the orifice of the pulmonary vein), or when the focus is identified, by electrically isolating the foci. The various techniques require special catheters and mapping equipment. However, not all types of AF are amenable to this procedure, and the etiology and trigger of the dysrhythmia needs to be elucidated before a decision is made to carry out the ablation.

Ablation therapy for primary atrial flutter is indicated in those patients who have reentrant circuits within the right atrium. Ablation lesions are directed at creating a line of block usually along a narrow isthmus between the inferior vena cava and tricuspid annulus to interrupt the circuit. When successful, atrial flutter ablation can provide a permanent cure for atrial flutter. Unlike AV node ablation, atrial flutter ablation does not require permanent pacemaker implantation.

Ventricular Dysrhythmias

The success of ablation for the treatment of VT depends on the cause of the dysrhythmia. Radiofrequency ablation has been shown to be effective in patients with VT in structurally normal hearts and in patients with VT due to bundle branch reentry. The technique also has had some limited success in patients with hemodynamically stable, monomorphic VT associated with a healed myocardial scar. However, it is not unusual to have multiple morphologies (forms) of VT in this population, and some unstable morphologies may not be amenable to ablation.

PROCEDURE

Before an ablation, the patient undergoes an electrophysiological study (EPS) to evaluate the electrical activity of the heart. The EPS is an invasive test in which catheters are placed in the heart to record intracardiac electrograms (IC-EGM). The test provides information about the sequence of electrical activation of the heart in sinus rhythm and any abnormal sequence of activation during an induced dysrhythmia. An electrical map is inferred from the electrical recordings to help identify the focus of a dysrhythmia or locate an accessory pathway. The map guides the placement of the ablating catheter.

After the catheters are positioned, ECG recordings are made from the surface electrodes on the patient's chest and EGMs from the intracardiac electrodes. Programmed electrical stimulation (PES) is then performed to induce the dysrhythmia so that its mechanism and pathway can be evaluated. Once a diagnosis of the dysrhythmia is confirmed, an ablating catheter is positioned in the targeted area of the heart. Additional catheters are positioned to stimulate atrial and ventricular tissue. The ablation catheter contains multiple electrodes designed to localize the site of the dysrhythmia and to deliver the ablation current. The distal tip of the catheter can be flexed to facilitate access to the tissue and to ensure direct contact. Fluoroscopy and the electrogram pattern from the catheter, as well as special mapping equipment and intracardiac ultrasound, help the physician determine the appropriate target area. The clinical ECG of the tachycardia is a useful template of the target dysrhythmia when several morphologies are induced.

When the appropriate site is identified, the radiofrequency current is applied for several seconds until the target tip temperature is achieved. Longer application time is allowed when a cooled or irrigated catheter tip is used. Several lesions may be required to eliminate the abnormal conducting tissue. Successful elimination of the target site is determined by examining the ECG and EGM tracings and confirmed when the dysrhythmia is no longer inducible. When the procedure is finished, the intracardiac catheters and venous or arterial sheaths are removed, and efforts to attain hemostasis at the insertion site are implemented.

NURSING MANAGEMENT

The nurse plays a vital role in the care of the patient undergoing radiofrequency ablation. In consultation with the electrophysiologist, the nurse provides information to the patient and family about what to expect before, during, and after the procedure. The psychosocial support provided by the nurse may be key in helping the patient and family cope with the uncertainties of dysrhythmia management.

Preablation

The nurse participates in educating the patient and family about radiofrequency ablation (Box 18-20). During the preablation period, the nurse records a 12-lead ECG, continuously monitors the patient's cardiac rhythm, and treats any dysrhythmias per the physician's orders. Other baseline data obtained include vital signs, breath sounds, fluid status, serum chemistries, prothrombin time, and complete blood counts. Antidysrhythmic drugs may be discontinued

---

Box 18-20 • Preablation Teaching

- Purpose of the procedure
- The patient's dysrhythmia and how the procedure will help
- Interventions before transport to the electrophysiology laboratory
- The electrophysiology laboratory:
    The appearance of the laboratory
    The equipment in the laboratory
    The personnel in the laboratory
- The use of IV conscious sedation
    The amnesic/analgesic effect of conscious sedation
    Possible side effects such as nausea, vomiting, or hypotension
- Sensations associated with the procedure:
    Cool sensation from cleansing agents
    Pressure sensation from catheter insertion
    Palpitations, dizziness, or other sensations when the patient's dysrhythmia is induced
    Possible mild burning sensation during ablation
    Restlessness or back discomfort from lying immobilized
- Anticipated length of the procedure
- Potential for placement of a permanent pacemaker
- Anticipated after effects:
    Skipped beats or faster than usual resting rate may be felt initially
    Mild chest discomfort or burning may occur for a few days
    "Skin effect," which is a dark outline of the grounding or defibrillation pad, may persist indefinitely

---

2 to 3 days before the procedure to allow provocation of the dysrhythmia during the procedure. The patient receives nothing by mouth for about 8 hours before the procedure. It is important to verify that a female patient is not pregnant because of x-ray exposure during the test. No activity restrictions are imposed before the procedure.

During Ablation

The nurse in the electrophysiology laboratory is responsible for monitoring the patient throughout the procedure and assisting the physician with necessary interventions. The nurse must be competent in advanced cardiac life support so that an emergency situation can be handled appropriately.

In the laboratory, the nurse explains each intervention to the patient and helps put the patient at ease. The nurse connects the patient to a cardiac monitor and physiological recorder and applies a grounding pad for the radiofrequency catheter, AED patches, automatic blood pressure device, and pulse oximeter. Oxygen is provided by nasal cannula. If not already in place, an IV line is inserted. IV conscious sedation is administered to ensure patient comfort. A urinary catheter is inserted if the procedure is anticipated to be lengthy. Both groins and the right subclavian vein sites are shaved and the skin prepared. A sterile field is established and maintained throughout the procedure. A lead apron may be placed under the patient's lower back to block fluoroscopy radiation from penetrating the reproductive system.

Throughout the procedure, the nurse monitors hemodynamic status, ACT if heparin is used, sedation level, and patient comfort. Communication with the patient is essential so that the patient is kept informed about the progress of the procedure, and anxiety and fear are minimized. The nurse also warns the patient that a burning sensation may be felt for a brief time during the actual ablation.

Postablation

Thorough assessment and monitoring of the patient are continued after the ablation procedure. Essential components of the assessment include vital signs, cardiac rhythm, catheter insertion sites, peripheral pulses, and level of consciousness. The patient may remain drowsy for several hours and experience nausea and vomiting as a result of the medications. When an arterial site has been used, leg immobilization and bed rest are maintained for about 6 hours. If only venous sites were used, the patient may begin ambulation in about 4 hours. The nurse assesses the patient for any pain or discomfort and provides comfort measures if indicated. Fluid volume status is checked, and when stable, the urinary catheter is removed.

During the postablation period, the nurse carefully assesses the patient for any evidence of complications. Table 18-17 lists potential complications of radiofrequency ablation and associated signs and symptoms.

• Cardiac Pacemakers

Electrical stimulation of the heart was tried experimentally as early as 1819. In 1930, Hyman noted that he could inject the right atrium with a diversity of

---

Table 18-17 • Potential Complications of Radiofrequency Ablation and Associated Signs and Symptoms

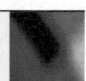

Complications	Signs and Symptoms
Cardiac perforation	Tachycardia, hypotension, dyspnea, pleuritichest pain
Cardiac tamponade	Hypotension, distended neck veins, muffled heart sounds, pulsus paradoxus, change in level of consciousness
Coronary artery spasm	Chest pain, electrocardiogram changes
Pneumothorax	Dyspnea, decreased oxygen saturation decreased breath sounds
Cerebral embolus	Slurred speech, blurred vision, headache, seizures
Pulmonary embolus	Chest pain, dyspnea, tachycardia
Femoral artery dissection	Bruit at site of pulse, hematoma, retroperitoneal bleed
Deep venous thrombosis	Swelling of leg at site of catheter insertion, calf pain

substances and restore a heartbeat. He devised an "ingenious apparatus" that he labeled an artificial pacemaker, which delivered a rhythmic charge to the heart. In 1952, Zoll demonstrated that patients with Stokes-Adams syndrome could be sustained by the administration of current directly to the chest wall. In 1957, Lillehei affixed electrodes directly to the ventricles during open heart surgery.

From 1958 to 1961, implantable pacemakers became accepted treatment for complete heart block. In the 1970s and 1980s, AV synchrony and "physiological" pacing became available. At the start of the first decade of the 21st century, clinical trials on right and left ventricular (biventricular) pacing made tremendous progress. Biventricular pacing is achieved by positioning an additional lead in one of the coronary sinus branches to stimulate the left ventricle, nearly simultaneous with the right ventricle. Commonly referred to as cardiac resynchronization therapy, biventricular pacing is used for symptom improvement and treatment of HF in patients with moderate to severe left ventricular dysfunction and intraventricular delay. Intraventricular delay is not uncommon in dilated cardiomyopathy and is recognized as the prolongation of QRS interval on ECG, as in bundle branch block. Biventricular stimulation improves left ventricular function by synchronizing the activation of the intraventricular septum and the left ventricular free wall.[6]

Currently, technological advances have resulted in smaller pacemakers with longer battery life and numerous programmable options in most models. Furthermore, the goal of individualized, physiological pacing has been achieved with recent advances.

INDICATIONS FOR CARDIAC PACING

Cardiac pacing is most commonly indicated for conditions that result in failure of the heart to initiate or conduct an intrinsic electrical impulse at a rate adequate to maintain perfusion. Pacemakers are necessary when dysrhythmias or conduction defects compromise the electrical system and the hemodynamic response of the heart. The original pacemakers were designed to treat bradydysrhythmias, whereas today's pacemakers may treat bradydysrhythmias and tachydysrhythmias. Further research and advances in technology also have allowed the use of pacemakers in heart conditions such as HF, hypertrophic cardiomyopathy, and neurocardiogenic syncope.[6,7]

Critical care nurses work with members of the health care team to assess potential pacemaker patients who may exhibit dysrhythmias, atherosclerotic heart disease, AMI, or other conditions that alter the conduction of the heart. To assist medical professionals in determining the clinical criteria for pacemaker implantation, a Joint Committee of the American College of Cardiology, American Heart Association, and Heart Rhythm Society (formerly NASPE) was formed to establish uniform criteria for pacemaker implantation.[7] The committee divided its recommendations for implantation into three classes. Class I includes conditions for which there is evidence

or general agreement that a given procedure or treatment is useful and effective. Class II includes conditions for which there is conflicting evidence or a divergence of opinion about the usefulness or efficacy of a procedure or treatment. (In class IIa, usefulness or efficacy is favored by the weight of evidence or opinion, and in class IIb, usefulness or efficacy is less well established by evidence or opinion.) Class III includes conditions for which there is evidence or general agreement that the procedure or treatment is not useful or effective and in some cases may be harmful. The revised 2002 committee recommendations for pacemaker implantation are summarized in Box 18-21.[7]

THE PACEMAKER SYSTEM

The pacemaker system, which consists of a pulse generator and one to three leads with electrodes, performs two main functions: diagnosis and treatment. The diagnostic function is to sense intrinsic cardiac activity; the treatment function is to emit an electrical impulse that excites endocardial cells and produces a wave of depolarization in the myocardium. Clinical terminology related to pacemakers is listed in Box 18-22.

Permanent Pacing Systems

The Pulse Generator

The pulse generator for a permanent pacemaker is composed of a lithium iodide battery source and electronic circuits enclosed in a hermetically sealed metal container. The generator weighs 20 to 30 g and is 5 to 7 mm thick (Fig. 18-31). The longevity of most permanent pacemakers is about 6 to 12 years, depending on the percentage of pacing the heart requires over time. Most permanent pulse generators are inserted in a subcutaneous pocket in the pectoral region below the clavicle (Fig. 18-32).

The Lead System

The lead is a wire that provides the communication network between the pulse generator and the heart muscle. One or more electrodes are at the distal end of the lead and provide sensing and pacing of the heart muscle. In a bipolar lead, the negative electrode (cathode) is at the tip, and the positive electrode (anode) is about 1 to 3 cm proximal to the tip (Fig. 18-33).

The permanent pacemaker lead is typically inserted either through a subclavian vein or a cephalic vein through the chest wall. Alternate insertion sites include the external jugular, internal jugular, and rarely, femoral vein. The lead is then positioned with fluoroscopic guidance and affixed in the right atrial appendage or in the apex of the right ventricle, or in both locations. A third lead may be inserted in a coronary sinus branch to stimulate the left ventricle for biventricular pacing. The leads must provide adequate electrical stimulation, sufficient insulation, and the endurance to withstand pulsatile turbulence.

The permanent pacemaker lead can be affixed to the myocardium with a lead fixation mechanism. Called

Box 18-21 • Indications for Permanent Cardiac Pacing*

Atrioventricular Block

Class I: Third-degree and advanced second-degree atrio-ventricular (AV) block at any anatomical level, associated with any one of the following conditions: (1) symptomatic bradycardia; (2) asystole greater than or equal to 3.0 s or any escape rate less than 40 beats/min in awake, symptom-free patients; (3) dysrhythmias and other medical conditions that require drugs that result in symptomatic bradycardia; (4) post-AV node ablation; (5) postoperative AV block that is not expected to resolve after cardiac surgery; and (6) neuromuscular diseases with AV block

Class IIa: (1) Asymptomatic third-degree AV block at any anatomical site with average awake ventricular rates of 40 beats/min or faster especially if cardiomegaly or left ventricular dysfunction is present; (2) asymptomatic type II second-degree AV block with a narrow QRS; (3) asymptomatic type I second-degree AV block at intra- or infra-His levels found at electrophysiological study (EPS) performed for other indications; and (4) first- or second-degree AV block with symptoms similar to those of pacemaker syndrome.

Class IIb: (1) Marked first-degree AV block (more than 0.30 s) in patients with left ventricular dysfunction and symptoms of congestive heart failure in whom a shorter AV interval results in hemodynamic improvement; and (2) neuromuscular diseases such as myotonic muscular dystrophy, Kearns-Sayre syndrome, Erb's dystrophy (limb-girdle), and muscular atrophy with any degree of AV block (including first-degree AV block) with or without symptoms.

Class III: Asymptomatic first-degree AV block and type I second-degree AV block, transient AV block

Chronic Bifascicular or Trifascicular Block

Class I: (1) Intermittent complete heart block, (2) type II second-degree AV block, and (3) alternating bundle-branch block

Class IIa: (1) Syncope not demonstrated to be due to AV block when other likely causes have been excluded, specifically VT; (2) prolonged His–ventricular (HV) interval on EPS; (3) incidental finding of pacing-induced, nonphysiological infra–His block at EPS

Class IIb: (1) Neuromuscular diseases such as myotonic muscular dystrophy, Kearns-Sayre syndrome, Erb's dystrophy (limb-girdle), and peroneal muscular atrophy with any degree of fascicular block with or without symptoms

Class III: Fascicular block without AV block or symptoms and asymptomatic fascicular block with first-degree AV block

Atrioventricular Block After Acute Myocardial Infarction

Class I: (1) Persistent type II second-degree AV block with bilateral bundle branch block or third-degree AV block after AMI; (2) transient advanced (second- or third-degree) infranodal AV block and associated bundle branch block; (3) persistent and symptomatic second- or third-degree AV block.

Class IIb: (1) Persistent second- or third-degree AV block at the AV node level (the level of AV block may need to be verified with an EPS

Class III: Transient AV block

Sinus Node Dysfunction

Class I: Sinus node dysfunction with documented symptomatic bradycardia and symptomatic chronotropic incompetence

Class IIa: Sinus node dysfunction occurring spontaneously or as a result of necessary drug therapy, with heart rate less than 40 beats/min, asymptomatic, syncope of unexplained origin with provoked sinus node dysfunction during EPS

Class IIb: In minimally symptomatic patients, chronic heart rate less than 40 beats/min while awake.

Class III: Asymptomatic sinus node dysfunction; sinus node dysfunction with symptomatic bradycardia due to nonessential drug therapy

Tachydysrhythmias

Class I: Sustained pause-dependent ventricular tachycardia (VT), with or without prolonged QT, in which the efficacy of pacing is thoroughly documented

Class IIa: (1) High-risk patients with congenital long QT syndrome (overdrive suppression); (2) symptomatic recurrent supraventricular tachycardia (SVT) refractory or intolerant to drugs and failing ablation; (3) AV reentrant or AV node reentrant SVT not responsive to medical or ablative therapy

Class IIb: (1) Recurrent SVT or atrial flutter that is reproducibly terminated by pacing as an alternative to drug therapy or ablation; (2) prevention of symptomatic, drug refractory, recurrent atrial fibrillation (AF) in patients with coexisting sinus node dysfunction.

Class III: (1) Tachydysrhythmias that are accelerated or converted to fibrillation by pacing or in the presence of rapidly conducting AV pathways; (2) torsades de pointes VT due to reversible causes

Hypersensitive Carotid Sinus Syndrome and Neurocardiogenic Syncope

Class I: Recurrent syncope associated with clear, sponta-neous events provoked by carotid sinus stimulation, asys-tole of >3 s induced by minimal carotid sinus pressure in the absence of any medication that depresses sinus and AV node conduction

Class IIa: (1) Recurrent syncope without clear, provocative events and a hypersensitive cardioinhibitory response; (2) recurrent neurocardiogenic syncope associated with bradycardia reproduced by a head-up tilt

Class III: A hyperactive cardioinhibitory response to carotid sinus stimulation in the absence of symptoms or in the presence of vague symptoms such as dizziness, lightheadedness, or both

*Box does not include indications for special population and specific conditions.
Adapted from Gregoratos G, Abrams J, Epstein AE, et al: ACC/AHA/NASPE 2002 guideline update for implantation of cardiac pacemakers and antiarrhythmia devices: Summary article. A report of the American College of Cardiology/American Heart Association Task Force on Practice Guidelines (ACC/AHA/NASPE Committee to Update the 1998 Pacemaker Guidelines). J Cardiovasc Electrophysiol 13(11):1183–1199, 2002.

drugs. To maintain sterility at the connection site and terminal tip of the catheter, a sterile protective sleeve over the catheter can be used before insertion and then connected to the end of the sheath after satisfactory position is confirmed. The sheath entry site should be covered with an antiseptic ointment and a self-adhesive, semipermeable transparent dressing. A small label above the dressing, initialed by the nurse, should indicate time and date of application.

Epicardial Temporary Pacing Systems

Placement of epicardial wires provides another method for temporary pacing. This method can be accomplished by thoracotomy or through a subxiphoid incision with the placement of pacing electrodes directly on the outer surface of the heart. Epicardial wires often are used as a temporary adjunct during and after open heart surgery. The pacing wires are attached to the epicardial surface of the heart, and the proximal end is brought outside through the chest incision and either connected to a temporary pacemaker generator or capped and then connected if the need for pacing arises. The wires are extracted without reopening the incision, even after scar tissue has formed over the tips.

Transcutaneous Temporary Pacing Systems

Another method of temporary pacing is known as external transcutaneous pacing. This method involves placing large gelled electrode patches directly on the chest wall. The cathode or negative electrode is applied anteriorly to the left of the sternum, and the anode or positive electrode is applied straight posteriorly on the patient's back and then connected to an external transcutaneous pacemaker (Fig. 18-35). Transcutaneous pacing can cause significant discomfort, and the patient should be informed and adequately sedated, if necessary. Transcutaneous pacing is used when temporary transvenous pacing is not immediately available. In patients with profound asystolic arrest, the transcutaneous pacemaker should not be relied on indefinitely.

Transthoracic Temporary Pacing Systems

Transthoracic pacing is a temporary pacing method used as a last resort in an emergency situation. This method involves introduction of a pacing needle in the anterior wall of the heart. Transthoracic pacing has limited success rates and a high potential for complications.

The temporary pulse generator is an external device powered by a 9-volt alkaline or lithium replaceable battery (Fig. 18-36). Often called a temporary pacemaker, the device contains several controls that regulate the current output, rate, sensitivity, and the mode of pacing; and for dual-chamber pacing, base and upper rate, AV interval and refractory period settings can be chosen. A dual-chamber pulse generator has separate terminals for the atrial and ventricular inputs. The wires should be labeled appropriately in the proximal portion: atrial or ventricular. Care should be taken not to interchange the electrode positions when attaching leads to the pulse generator. Nursing assessment and intervention guidelines for temporary transvenous pacemaker placement are summarized in Box 18-23.

PACEMAKER FUNCTIONING

When the pacemaker system functions appropriately, it senses and treats the heart rhythm dysfunction. The sensing function is the ability of the pacemaker to detect the heart's intrinsic activity, and the sensing amplitude is the largest intrinsic signal that is consistently detected by the pacemaker electrode (e.g., the R wave is usually the largest signal sensed by the ventricular lead). At the site of the sensing electrode, the amplitude of the intrinsic depolarization wave is measured in millivolts (mV). The smallest number on the sensor control represents the most

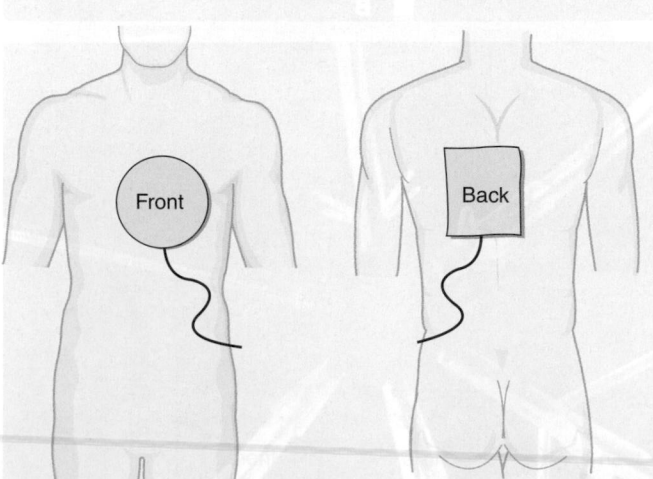

Figure 18-35 • Transcutaneous pacing. Electrodes are placed on anterior and posterior chest walls and attached to the external pacing unit.

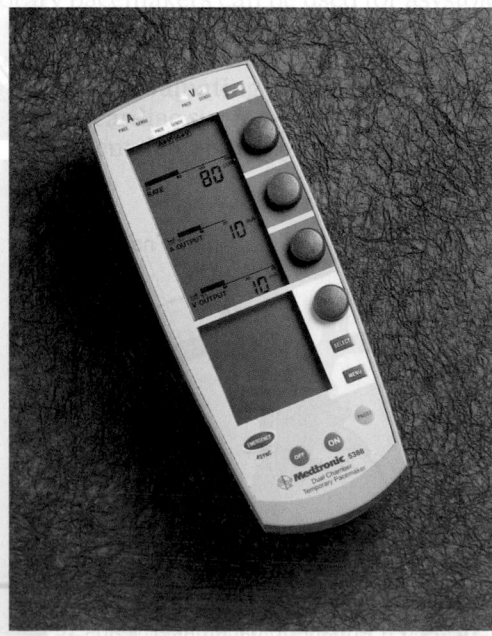

Figure 18-36 • A dual-chamber temporary pacemaker. (Courtesy of Medtronic, Minneapolis, MN.)

Box 18-23 • NURSING INTERVENTIONS for the Patient With a Temporary Transvenous Pacemaker

Assessment
- During insertion:
    Vital signs, O₂ saturation, peripheral pulses
    Level of sedation/sedative agents used
    Continuous cardiac rhythm monitoring
    Date, time, method, and site of insertion
    Location of wire inserted (atrial, ventricular, atrial and
        ventricular)
    Measured values: capture (mA) threshold and intrinsic
        amplitude (mV)
    Patient's tolerance of procedure
    Complications
    12-lead electrocardiogram (ECG)
    Final settings: mode, rate, output, and sensitivity
- After insertion:
    Rate setting, mV setting, mA setting, mode of operation
        (demand, asynchronous) and atrioventricular interval
        (if appropriate)
    Pacemaker turned off or on
    Rhythm strip, capture and intrinsic, if appropriate;
        12-lead ECG
    Status on insertion site and sutures (if present)
    Chest x-ray done, results on chart
- Every change of shift:
    Pacemaker turned off or on
    Pacemaker secured appropriately to patient
    All connections are secure
    Setting for rate, mA, sensitivity, mode of operation,
        atrioventricular interval (if appropriate)
    Rhythm strip (and with any clinical change or intervention)

Sensing and capture thresholds (compare to baseline)
Presence/absence of hiccupping or muscle twitching
Status of insertion site and sutures (if present)
Signs of infection (redness, pain, fever, pus)
Pulse perfusion distal to insertion site (if appropriate)
Connective ends of pacer wires covered (as appropriate)

Intervention
- Continuous cardiac monitoring
- Pacemaker generator:
    Verify replacement 9-volt battery available.
    Verify connections are intact.
- Wear rubber/latex gloves when handling the connective
    ends of pacer wires.
- Cover connective ends of pacer wires to prevent micro-
    shock hazard.
- Label epicardial pacer wires *atrial* or *ventricular*.
- Clean and dress pacer wire insertion site(s) daily with
    gauze dressing or transparent dressing per institutional
    protocol. Label time and date of dressing change
    and initial.

Documentation
- Document in Critical Care Flow Sheet/Nursing Notes:
    Assessments
- Instructions to patient/family
    Pacing wire insertion site care
    Pacing and sensing thresholds (print ECG strips)
    Pacing problems, nursing interventions, and results of
        interventions
    Complications/problems

sensitive setting, in mV, and it indicates the smallest signal the pacemaker will sense. If the heart's intrinsic amplitude is smaller than the sensitivity setting, undersensing occurs. This can occur when the electrode has inadequate contact with the heart tissue. The drawback in setting pacemaker sensitivity at its most sensitive setting is that oversensing may occur, such as when the pacemaker senses extraneous signals (e.g., T waves) or signals from the other chamber. If oversensing occurs, the pacemaker stimulus may be inhibited (Fig. 18-37).

When intrinsic heart rate is adequate, the pacemaker responds by inhibiting a pacing stimulus. When intrinsic heart rate drops to the programmed minimum rate, the pacemaker delivers a stimulus through the lead. When the pacemaker discharges, an artifact known as a pacing spike appears on the ECG, as shown in Figure 18-38. As a result of this stimulus,

the cardiac chamber containing the pacemaker lead is depolarized. *Capture* is the term used to indicate depolarization of the atria or ventricle in response to a pacing stimulus. The minimal amount of voltage required from the pacemaker to initiate consistent capture is known as the pacing threshold. This threshold level is determined by establishing successful pacing at higher energy and then gradually decreasing the energy output of the generator until capture ceases. The pacing threshold is expressed as milliamperage (mA) in the temporary generator and voltage (V) in the permanent pulse generator, within a given pulse width duration. The generator output is then set at 2 or 3 times the threshold level to allow for an adequate safety margin.

Many factors affect the pacing threshold. These include hypoxia, hyperkalemia, antidysrhythmic drugs, catecholamines, digoxin toxicity, and corticosteroids.

Figure 18-37 • Failure to discharge or oversensing with pacing inhibition. In the first half of the strip, the sensing amplifier may have detected electrical noise (oversensing) causing pacemaker inhibition.

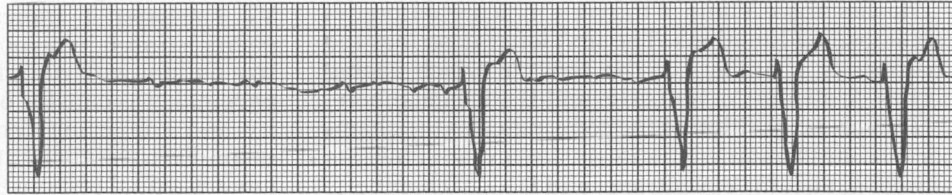

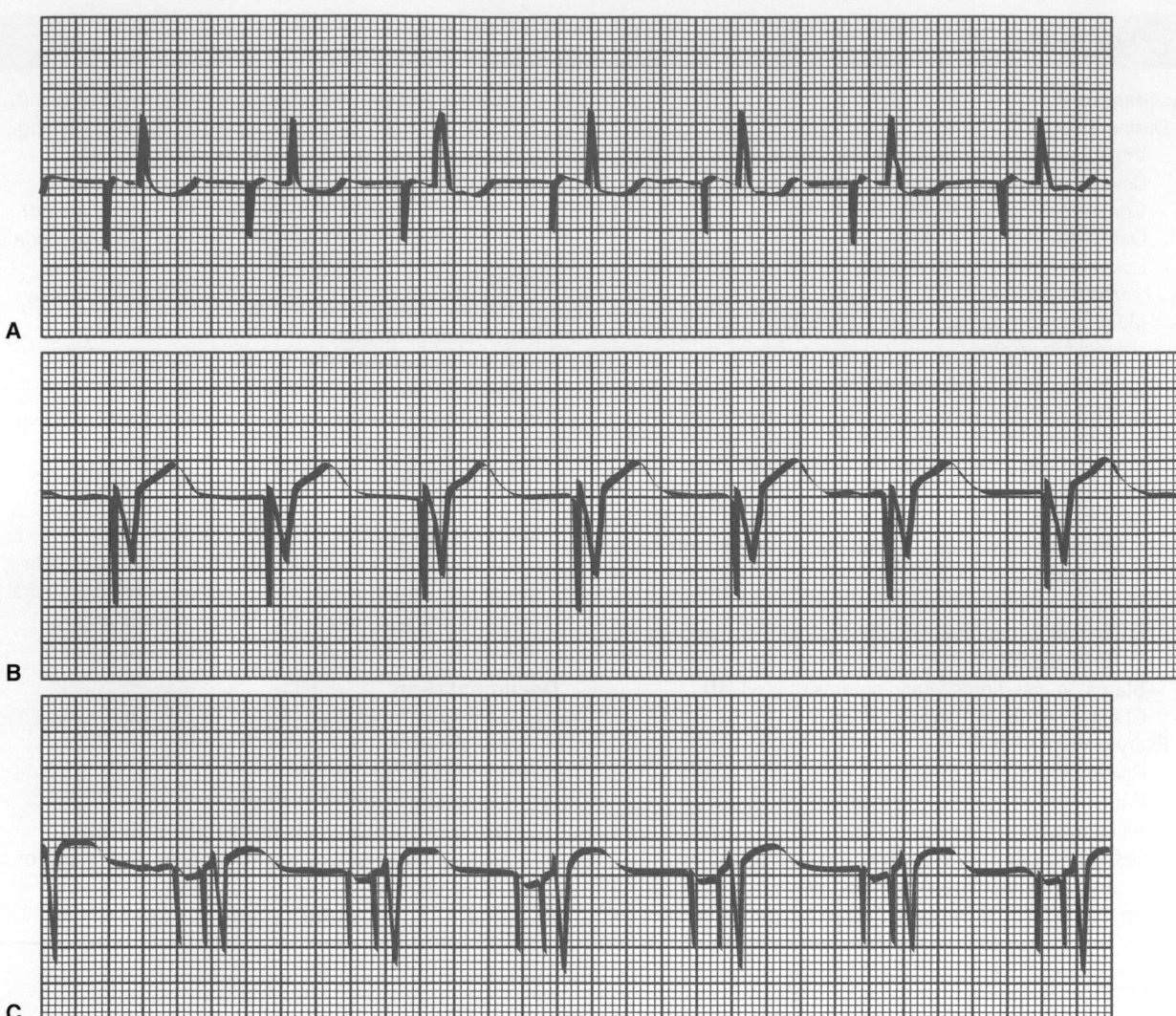

Figure 18-38 • Strip **A** shows an atrial pacemaker. Note that each pacing stimulus is followed by a P wave. Strip **B** shows a ventricular pacemaker. Note that each pacing stimulus is followed by a wide QRS complex. Strip **C** shows a dual-chamber pacemaker. Note that the first spike is followed by a P wave and the second spike is followed by a QRS complex. All strips show 1:1 capture.

THE PACEMAKER CODE

Since the initial use of cardiac pacemakers, the technology has become so complex and diverse that a coding system has been formed to identify the various modes of pacemaker operation. Initially developed in 1974, the pacemaker coding system has undergone several revisions. The most recent version of the code was developed in 2002 through the joint efforts of the American Heart Association and Heart Rhythm Society (formerly NASPE) and the British Pacing and Electrophysiology Group (BPEG).[8] The NASPE/BPEG Generic Pacemaker Code is shown in Table 18-18 and is simply called the NBG pacemaker code.

The first three letters of the code indicate antibradycardia pacing functions. The first letter describes the chamber or chambers of the heart in which pacing occurs: A, atrium; V, ventricle; and D, dual chamber.

The second position of the code indicates the chamber or chambers in which intrinsic cardiac activity is sensed: A, atrium; V, ventricle; and D, dual chamber.

The third position of the code denotes the pacemaker's response to sensed intrinsic cardiac activity. The letter "I" means that the pacemaker is inhibited from firing in response to a sensed intrinsic event. For example, if the pacemaker is set to a rate of 70, and if the patient's intrinsic rate exceeds 70 beats/minutes, the pacemaker will not fire. The pacemaker fires only if the patient's intrinsic rate drops below the paced rate. Thus, the pacemaker functions on demand and is known as a demand pacemaker. Because the pacemaker is inhibited by adequate intrinsic heart activity, there is no danger of the pacemaker firing at an inappropriate time that could initiate a dangerous cardiac dysrhythmia, such as VT. The letter "T" indicates a pacemaker that triggers pacing stimuli in response to a sensed intrinsic beat. In a patient with complete AV block, a dual-chamber pacemaker is capable of sensing intrinsic atrial activity and triggering ventricular pacing stimulus in response to a sensed atrial event. The letter "D" designates a dual response (inhibited pacing output and

Table 18-18 • The NBG Pacemaker

		Position—Category		
I: Chamber(s) Paced	II: Chamber(s) Sensed	III: Response to Sensing	IV: Rate Modulation	V: Multisite Pacing
O = none	O = none	O = none	O = none	O = none
A = atrium	A = atrium	T = triggered	R = rate modulation	A = atrium
V = ventricle	V = ventricle	I = inhibited		V = ventricle
D = dual (A +V)	D = dual (A +V)	D = dual (T + I)		D = dual (A + V)

Adapted from North American Society of Pacing and Electrophysiology/British Pacing and Electrophysiology Group: The revised NASPE/BPEG generic code for antibradycardia, adaptive-rate, and multisite pacing. Pacing Clin Electrophysiol 25(2):260–264, 2002.

triggered pacing after sensed event). The letter "O" in the third position designates a mode in which the pacemaker does not respond to sensed intrinsic activity. Pacemaker insensitivity to intrinsic activity is known as asynchronous pacing. This can be achieved by setting the sensitivity to the highest number or programming to asynchronous mode (i.e., DOO, VOO). Permanent pacemakers also may be switched to an asynchronous mode temporarily by placement of a large magnet over the pulse generator. This maneuver causes the pacemaker to fire in an asynchronous mode, allowing the physician to assess for appropriate firing and capture when the patient's rhythm is overridden by the fixed pacing pulse.

The fourth position of the code describes the presence or absence of rate modulation. The letter "O" denotes no rate modulation, and the letter "R" means that rate modulation is active. This is a feature in which the pacing rate varies in response to a physiological variable. The physiological variables used are mechanical vibration, acceleration, or minute ventilation. When patients increase their activity, the pacer detects the physiological response (e.g., muscle vibration, increased respiratory rate) and increases the pacing rate to meet increased metabolic demands.

The fifth position of the code describes whether multisite pacing is present. The letter "A" means that there are stimulation sites in each atrium, more than one stimulation site in either atrium, or any combination of these two. The letter "V" means that there are stimulation sites in each ventricle, more than one stimulation site in either ventricle, or any combination of these two. The letter "O" means that no multisite pacing is present.

In clinical parlance, the absence of a fourth or fifth letter designation signifies no rate modulation and no multisite pacing. The first three positions are required when describing pacemaker mode, although all positions may be indicated for completeness.[8]

PACING MODES

Knowledge of the five-letter pacemaker code helps the critical care nurse determine the type of implanted device, the intended mode of operation, and the actual mode of operation. Modes of operation can be classified as single- and dual-chamber modes.

Single-Chamber Modes of Operation

A VVIR mode is a commonly used mode of operation for permanent ventricular pacemakers. Devices with this mode of operation are characterized by ventricular pacing, ventricular sensing, inhibited response to sensed intrinsic events, rate modulation, and no multisite pacing. The rate modulation feature offers the benefit of adjusting the paced rate in response to metabolic demand. This rate modulation feature is not used in temporary pacing; therefore, the mode is designated as VVI. A disadvantage of the VVIR and the VVI modes is the lack of hemodynamic benefit from AV synchrony provided by dual-chamber pacing. However, in chronic AF with slow ventricular response rates, VVIR is the appropriate mode to use. A ventricular demand pacemaker with rate modulation and biventricular pacing would have the designated code VVIRV. (The letter "V" in the fifth position indicates the presence of multisite pacing in the ventricles.)

An AAI is a mode of operation for permanent atrial pacemakers. With this mode of operation, there is atrial pacing, atrial sensing, inhibited response to sensed events, and no rate modulation or multisite pacing. Temporary atrial pacemakers most often are set to an AAI mode and are particularly useful in overdrive pacing of atrial dysrhythmias. These modes of pacing can only be used for patients with normal AV node conduction. An advantage of these modes is the presence of AV synchrony.

Dual-Chamber Modes of Operation

DDD mode provides dual-chamber pacing, dual-chamber sensing, dual response to sensed events (inhibited or triggered), and no rate modulation, or multisite pacing. DDDR mode has the additional feature of rate modulation. VDD mode paces only in the ventricle, but this mode senses atrial and ventricular events and has dual response to sensed events. Therefore, an atrial event (P wave) will trigger a ventricular event. If an intrinsic R wave is sensed, ventricular pacing is inhibited. This mode is particularly useful in patients with intact sinus node function but with high-grade AV block.

PACEMAKER MALFUNCTION

Permanent Pacemaker Malfunction

Pacemaker malfunction can be a result of an inappropriate programmed function (pseudomalfunction) or a true component malfunction. Although pacemakers are now manufactured to provide more complex capabilities and are generally considered to be more reliable, unanticipated pacemaker malfunction (e.g., "recall") continues to occur.[9] For this reason, it is important for the patient to know the manufacturer, model, and serial number of his or her pacemaker components (pulse generator and leads) and to ascertain that they have been appropriately registered with the manufacturer. This is usually provided to the patient after the implant procedure, and the patient is given an implanted device identification card.

Safety alerts or recalls are issued when devices of a certain lot or model are associated with component or battery failure. Most manufacturers have toll-free telephone numbers that can provide information on recalls or safety alerts. However, it is important that the patient contact his or her physician, who can provide advice concerning the implications of such recalls or safety alerts. At times, simple programming or monitoring may be all that is needed.

Temporary Pacemaker Malfunction

Temporary pacemaker malfunction should be addressed systematically. First and foremost, immediate action is required to restore pacemaker capture when the patient has no underlying rhythm. These steps are to be followed:

1. Increase pulse generator output (in mA) to the highest setting, asynchronous mode (VOO, DOO).
2. Check patient hemodynamics, simultaneous multiple ECG lead recordings; intervene if appropriate with transcutaneous pacing, atropine sulfate, or isoproterenol.
3. Check all connections.
4. Replace pulse generator or battery; be prepared for transcutaneous pacing backup during change.

Proceed with trouble shooting if the patient is stable. Table 18-19 describes troubleshooting strategies for temporary pacemaker malfunction.

Types of Malfunction

Failure to Discharge

If stimulus discharge from the pacemaker causes an artifact, or "spike," to appear on the ECG, failure to discharge may be manifested in absence of the artifact and unexplained loss of pacing. The cause of this failure may be within the generator itself, either processor or battery failure. Processor failure is not common, but battery failure is more prevalent among patients who are noncompliant with follow-up or unaware of the longevity of their pacemaker battery. This may be evaluated by measuring the output values of the generator through a programmer.

In extreme cases, the generator fails to communicate with the programmer. Replacement of the generator must occur immediately. If the situation is emergent, the physician may insert a temporary transvenous pacemaker to support the patient hemodynamically until the permanent pacemaker problem can be corrected.

Failure to Capture

Failure of the pacing stimulus to capture the ventricles or atria is noted by the absence of the QRS or P wave immediately after the pacemaker artifact on the ECG (Fig. 18-39). Failure to capture may be caused by elevated threshold, a lead impedance problem, or impending battery depletion. These conditions may create insufficient output delivery to meet the capture threshold. If the patient is pacemaker dependent and becomes symptomatic, drug therapy (atropine, isoproterenol), transcutaneous pacing, or CPR may be required until the cause of the problem is found and corrected.

Oversensing

Oversensing occurs when the pacemaker detects events other than those intended. For example, in VVI pacing, if large T waves are sensed in addition to the R wave, the pacemaker is inhibited, and pacing at a slower than programmed rate may be noted. Similarly, electromagnetic interference may result in inappropriate sensing and as a result, incorrectly activate the inhibited or triggered mode of a dual-chamber pacemaker. Oversensing may be caused by electrode displacement, inappropriate sensitivity settings, or impending lead fracture. A partially fractured lead often allows signals to saturate the sensing amplifier, causing oversensing and inhibition of pacing output in demand mode. On the surface ECG, oversensing mimics failure to discharge because oversensing may cause inhibition of the pacing stimuli (see Fig. 18-38). For example, in a DDD pacemaker, a sensed P wave usually triggers a ventricular stimulus after completing the timed P-V interval; however, if the ventricular lead senses an intrinsic signal (e.g., oversensing noise), the ventricular stimulus is inhibited. The only way to confirm oversensing is to examine intracardiac electrograms through a programmer. If noise is recorded on the intracardiac electrogram, then the problem is due to oversensing.

To correct suspected oversensing in a temporary pacemaker system, the nurse should check the connection between the temporary pacemaker and the lead. Electrical noise from an improperly connected lead could cause oversensing. Electromagnetic interference should be investigated, and the grounding wires of all electrical equipment should be checked. The sensitivity may be decreased by turning the dial toward asynchronous, toward a higher mV value. Oversensing due to partial wire fracture in a temporary transvenous bipolar catheter may also be corrected by converting to a unipolar system. To diagnose, an intracavitary ECG is obtained by connecting a single pole to a surface V lead using an alligator clamp connector and obtaining a V1 precordial recording. The recording

Table 18-19 • Troubleshooting a Temporary Pacemaker

Problem	Cause	Intervention
Failure to discharge: No evidence of pacing stimulus, patient's heart rate below programmed rate	Due to battery depletion or pulse generator failure, output or timing circuit failure	Replace battery or generator.
	Due to loose cable connection	Check all connections for tightness.
Failure to capture: Pacing stimulus not followed by electrocardiogram (ECG) evidence of depolarization	Due to lead dislodgment	Review chest film, turn patient to left lateral decubitus position until lead can be replaced.
	Due to broken connector pins or fractured extension connecting cable	Connect wire directly to generator to diagnose cable problem, replace connecting cable.
	Due to incompatibility of wire pins with cable or to generator	Ascertain a secure fit of the exposed pin to the cable or the generator, adjust connection or replace pulse generator.
	Due to output setting (mA) too low	Check capture thresholds and adjust output to a two- to threefold safety margin.
	Due to perforation	Review 12-lead ECG, report signs of perforation, stabilize hemodynamics.
	Due to lead fracture without insulation break	Check intracavitary ECG; if evidence of fracture in one pole, unipolarize lead; if total fracture, replace lead.
	Due to increase in pacing threshold from medication or metabolic changes	Check laboratory test results, correct metabolic alterations, review medications and vital signs, increase output.
Oversensing: Device detects noncardiac electrical events and interprets them as depolarization	Due to oversensitive setting	Reduce sensitivity (value [in millivolts] should be larger to make pacer less sensitive); if patient is pacer dependent (no intrinsic R wave), program to asynchronous mode until problem is corrected.
	Due to device detecting tall T waves and interpreting them as R waves	Increase ventricular refractory period beyond T wave.
In dual-chamber pacing, cross-talk is a form of oversensing: The device detects signals from the other chamber and inhibits; in atrial channel, R waves are detected as P waves.	Caused by atrial lead dislodgment	Recheck atrial capture thresholds; if high, dislodgment is probable.
In ventricular channel, atrial pacing stimulus afterpotential is detected as an R wave, with V pacing inappropriately inhibited	Due to high output from atrial channel	Reduce output from atrial channel, decrease ventricular channel sensitivity (higher millivolt value).
	Due to electrical interference, improperly grounded electrical devices	Remove nongrounded equipment.
Undersensing: Device fails to detect intrinsic cardiac activity and fires inappropriately	Due to asynchronous mode setting (VOO, DOO, AOO)	Reprogram to synchronous mode (VVI, DDD, AAI).
	Due to small intrinsic amplitude	Increase sensitivity (turn sensitivity dial toward lower millivolt value).
	Due to lead dislodgment	Recheck capture thresholds; if high, lead probably dislodged and needs repositioning.
	Due to lead insulation break	Check lead with pacing system analyzer, if impedance too low (<200 ohms), insulation break is likely, and lead needs to be replaced or can be temporarily placed in unipolar configuration.

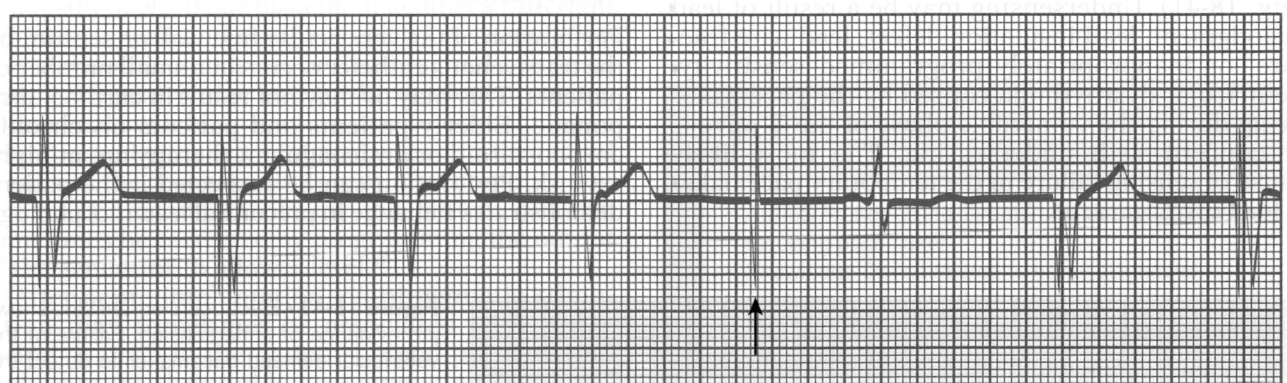

Figure 18-39 • Electrocardiogram strip showing evidence of failure to capture. Note that pacing stimulus is not followed by a QRS complex.

An important aspect of preimplantation of a pacemaker includes an assessment of patient's medical as well as social history. For example, knowledge of a previous fracture to the clavicle may lead to avoidance of implantation on the same side of the fractured clavicle because of potential anatomical distortion. A subclavian approach may be avoided in a person with a history of a collapsed lung or previous lobectomy. A patient with a right arm arterial-venous fistula is best served with a left-sided implant. For social history, avocations such as hunting, professional sport activities, and even just preferential arm dexterity come into consideration. For example, the right pectoral region should not be used in a right-handed tennis player.

To assess patients with pacemakers accurately, the nurse must understand the pacemaker code to know the type of pacer used and the intended mode of the device. The nurse must be aware of the patient's underlying rhythm so that if the pacemaker fails, the nurse is prepared to treat any life-threatening dysrhythmias.

A thorough assessment also helps the nurse determine the patient's physiological response to pacing therapy. Important parameters to assess include pulse rate, underlying cardiac rhythm, blood pressure, activity tolerance, and evidence of dizziness, syncope, dyspnea, palpitations, or edema. The nurse should be attentive to results of chest radiographs, blood tests, and other relevant laboratory tests. If a permanent pacemaker has been implanted, the incision is examined for swelling, redness, drainage, hematoma, and tenderness.

Psychosocial assessment is another essential component of comprehensive care of the patient with a cardiac pacemaker. Patients' psychosocial responses to the need for cardiac pacing may differ. Some may be relieved to have a device that supports the functioning of their heart, whereas others may be anxious about the technology and express fears of dying. If a permanent pacemaker is implanted, patients and families should be encouraged to join support groups where they can share their fears and concerns with others who are dependent on pacing technology.

Patient and Family Education

A planned and systematic approach to teaching the patient and family about cardiac pacing is a vital part of nursing care. Teaching a patient about pacemakers begins at the time the decision for pacemaker insertion is made. The nurse can begin by eliciting the patient's previous knowledge of pacemakers and clarifying any misconceptions. Nothing is assumed about the patient's understanding. If appropriate, the difference between heart block and heart attack is clarified. The patient may confuse cardiac monitoring with pacing and become anxious when the monitoring electrodes are removed.

The patient and family should be told why the pacemaker is necessary. The anatomy of the heart is discussed in general terms when explaining the need

for pacing and how the pacemaker takes the place of or complements spontaneous rhythm. The insertion procedure and the immediate postinsertion care that can be expected are explained.

Many booklets and media presentations are available to aid the nurse in teaching the pacemaker patient. Visual and written guidelines are helpful for the patient and family to review after discharge from the hospital.

The depth of teaching that is appropriate and the teaching tools used may depend on the patient's age, intellect, attention span, vision, and interest in learning. Initial teaching should be confined to the positive aspects of life with a pacemaker. Knowledge of the function and care of the pacemaker are of no interest until the patient is able to accept it as part of life. Box 18-25 provides a guide for teaching patients and families about living with a pacemaker.

Electrocardiogram Monitoring

Careful monitoring of the ECG of the patient with a cardiac pacemaker is an essential component of comprehensive patient assessment. The first step in the analysis involves examining the strip for evidence of pacemaker stimulation. This evidence is noted by the presence of pacing spikes on the strip. Unipolar pacing spikes are usually tall and visible, but bipolar pacing spikes may not be visible in certain leads. Each pacing spike should result in capture. If the pacing lead is in the atria, a pacing spike is followed by a P wave. If the pacing wire is in the ventricle, the spike is followed by a wide QRS complex (Fig. 18-43B). However, a narrower QRS following a pacing spike does not necessarily mean there is pacemaker malfunction. When fusion is present, the patient spike appears right before the intrinsic QRS (see Fig. 18-43A). Biventricular pacing (pacing both ventricles) for cardiac resynchronization in HF also results in a narrower QRS.

The sensing function of the pacemaker is evaluated next. If the pacemaker does not sense intrinsic cardiac activity (undersensing), inappropriate pacemaker spikes may appear throughout the underlying rhythm. An oversensing problem can be detected when the pacemaker senses events other than the intrinsic rhythm and is inappropriately inhibited in that chamber or causes a triggered response in the other chamber.

The third step in evaluating the ECG is to measure various intervals in milliseconds (msec). Each small box on the ECG paper represents 40 msec, and one large box represents 200 msec. The duration of each interval is compared with the programmed setting for that interval.

The first interval, the pacing interval, is the amount of time between two consecutive pacing spikes in the chamber being paced. This interval is used to determine the pacing rate. To calculate the pacing rate, the nurse counts the number of milliseconds between two consecutive atrial spikes or two consecutive ventricular spikes (Fig. 18-44). To convert from milliseconds to beats per minute, the following formula is

Box 18-25 • Living With a Pacemaker

Patient Activity

- Start passive and active range-of-motion exercises on the affected arm 48 h after implantation to avoid "frozen shoulder." For those with new leads implanted, avoid abduction of the affected arm above the shoulder level for 4 to 6 wk to prevent lead dislodgment.
- Avoid activities that may result in high impact or stress at the implantation site.
- Return to work at the discretion of your physician after discussing the type of work you do and what your job entails.
- Return to whatever degree of sexual activity you prefer.
- Your pacemaker will set off the alarm on metal-detector devices in airports, so avoid going through the detector gates. Show your pacemaker identification card. A manual search may be done or a magnetic wand may be used. Do not allow the wand to linger at the pacemaker site for an indefinite amount of time because the magnet in the wand may temporarily put the pacemaker in asynchronous mode. The metal detector or wand will not cause any permanent damage to your pacemaker.

Signs of Pacemaker Malfunction

- Be alert for symptoms of pacemaker malfunction: those associated with decreased perfusion of the brain, heart, or skeletal muscles. Be particularly mindful of return of symptoms you experienced before pacemaker implantation.
- Report any dizziness, fainting, shortness of breath, undue fatigue, or fluid retention. Fluid retention includes sudden weight gain, "puffy ankles," "tightness of rings," and so forth.
- Take pulse once daily upon awakening. Report a pulse rate more than 5 beats/min slower than that at which pacemaker is set.
- Be aware that the pulse may be somewhat irregular if it is a demand pacemaker and has some spontaneous beats and paced beats. This does not signify pacemaker malfunction.

Signs of Infection

- Report any redness, swelling, warmth, drainage, or increase in soreness at the implantation site.
- Report fever of undetermined etiology.

Medications

- Antibiotics are usually given within 24 h of pacemaker implantation. Report any unusual reactions.
- Medications that were withdrawn before pacemaker implantation may need to be restarted. Check with your physician about beta blockers, digitalis, or blood thinners. Know the name of the medication and the dose, frequency of administration, side effects, and use of each medication.
- If warfarin is restarted, levels should be rechecked after reinitiation of the medication.

Considerations for Home Care

- Carry a pacemaker identification card at all times. This card shows the brand and model of pacemaker, the date of insertion, and the implanting physician.
- Wear a medical alert bracelet or necklace stating a pacemaker is worn.
- Adhere to a schedule of follow-up visits with your physician or clinic. The follow-up visit will include an interval history and electrocardiogram recording. Many pacemaker clinics have specialized equipment available to determine pacemaker and lead performance and to predict battery longevity. Some clinics have the capability for obtaining some of this information by telephone, reducing the necessity for travel to the clinic. However, when pacemaker follow-up is done by phone transmission, have the pacemaker checked at least once a year in the pacemaker clinic. Many problems related to the pacemaker pocket or intermittent failure of components cannot be picked up through telephone transmission tests.
- If you have any symptoms similar to those before pacemaker insertion, have the pacemaker checked. Be alert for other symptoms of malfunction such as unexplained dizzy spells, fatigue, or slow pulse.
- Inform any physician or dentist of the pacemaker and of the medications being taken.

Pulse Generator Replacement

- Follow-up is intensified when the pacemaker battery approaches its elective replacement indicator. Avoid extended absences or vacations without consulting your physician at this time.
- Be aware that when the battery depletes, the generator stops working.
- The battery cannot be removed from the generator, so the entire generator is replaced when the battery is low.
- Generator replacement can be done within a 24-h stay, as long as the leads are in good condition. Usually only the generator needs to be replaced.

Considerations for the Older Patient

- Report any changes in skin condition at the pacemaker site. Sudden weight loss or poor nutritional status may predispose elderly patients to pocket erosion.
- Report symptoms such as fatigue, neck pulsations, and lack of energy. Loss of atrioventricular synchrony in patients with single-chamber VVI pacemakers may result in pacemaker syndrome.
- If the pacemaker feels like it is "flipping" inside the pocket, report it to your doctor and do not reposition it. When the skin is loose or when the patient "twiddles" with the pacemaker, the leads can become tangled and coiled and may fracture.

used: 60,000 msec/minute divided by the number of milliseconds between pacing spikes equals the pacing rate.

The next interval to measure is the AV interval, also known as the AV delay. This interval is analogous to the PR interval on the ECG. The AV interval is measured from the beginning of an intrinsic P wave or an atrial pacing spike to the beginning of the intrinsic QRS complex or the ventricular pacing spike (see Fig. 18-44).

The third interval to measure is the ventriculo-atrial (VA) interval, also called the atrial escape inter-

Because of their size and weight, these ICD pulse generators required implantation in the patient's abdomen. Currently used ICD pulse generators are not much larger than the earlier models of pacemakers and can be implanted in the pectoral area. The size of the device is shown in Figure 18-45. Lithium silver vanadium oxide (Li/SVO) batteries provide the power source for ICDs. Improved circuit design has expanded the capabilities and functions of the ICD.

The Lead System

Lead systems sense the life-threatening ventricular dysrhythmia and deliver a shock to convert the dysrhythmia. Initially, the lead system consisted of a pair of epicardial patches for energy delivery and epicardial coils for sensing. The leads were often implanted at the time of CABG surgery, when indicated, or by the subxiphoid approach. The sensing coils were later replaced with a long transvenous lead positioned in the right ventricular endocardium. These leads were tunneled down from the subclavian insertion site to the generator in the abdomen. Improved lead design and smaller generators paved the way for prepectoral implantation. At this time, previously implanted epicardial leads are used only with replacement of ICD generators, when the leads are deemed to be usable. Newer implants use bipolar or tripolar transvenous leads for sensing and defibrillation. The sensing electrodes are bipoles at the tip of the lead. One unipolar coil in the distal portion of the ventricular lead serves as the defibrillation cathode, whereas another coil in the mid-proximal portion or the ICD generator serves as the defibrillation anode, giving rise to the term "active can" or "hot can." With dual-chamber ICDs, an additional bipolar electrode in the right atrium provides atrial sensing and pacing. In biventricular ICDs, a third lead is inserted in the coronary sinus and positioned in the lateral vein for left ventricular stimulation and resynchronization of the ventricles.

Ideally, the ICD generator is implanted in the left pectoral area so that the heart is central to the vector of the defibrillation current (Fig. 18-46). Improvements in lead design have allowed ease of implantation

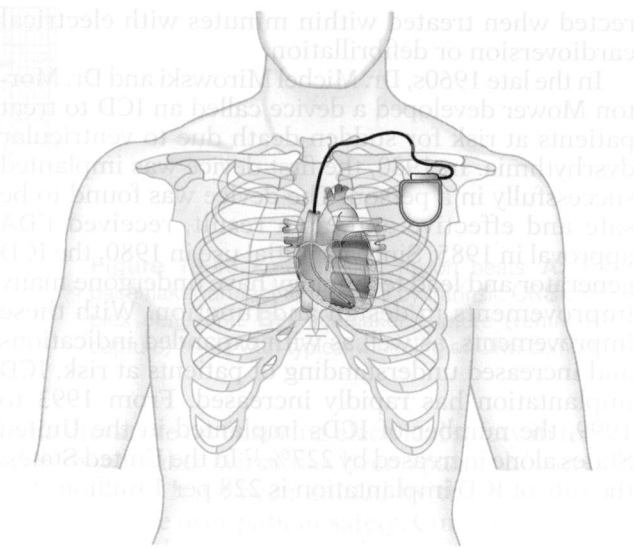

Figure 18-46 • The implantable cardioverter–defibrillator (ICD) mechanical system consists of a generator and a sensing/pacing/defibrillating electrode.

not very dissimilar to that of permanent pacemaker implantation. It is no longer unusual for a patient to be discharged a day after ICD implantation.

IMPLANTABLE CARDIOVERTER–DEFIBRILLATOR FUNCTIONING

ICDs have been categorized into "generations," based on their functionality. The first-generation ICDs were nonprogrammable devices that used a factory-specified rate criterion to detect ventricular dysrhythmias and delivered a shock at a preset energy level. In the mid-1980s, the second generation of the device became available and included programmable features, among them bradycardia and antitachycardia pacing and synchronized cardioversion. These features allowed the use of tiered therapy, the term used to describe different levels of therapy to treat a dysrhythmia. Table 18-20 illustrates the concept of tiered therapy. The first tier of therapy is usually antitachycardia pacing, which involves the carefully timed delivery of pacing stimuli. If antitachycardia pacing is not successful, the second tier of therapy is initiated by a low-energy synchronized cardioversion. The joules for cardioversion can be programmed anywhere from 1 to 36 J, with the highest output dependent on device specifications. Some devices allow multiple attempts at cardioversion. If cardioversion is not successful, the third tier of therapy, defibrillation, is used. The energy delivered for defibrillation can be programmed to a maximum of 36 J, again depending on the model and capacity of a device. The number of defibrillation attempts varies with different devices, but six attempts is usually the maximum. If the patient is successfully converted to a life-compatible rhythm, but the rate is slow, ventricular demand pacemaker is initiated. Bradycardia pacing is usually

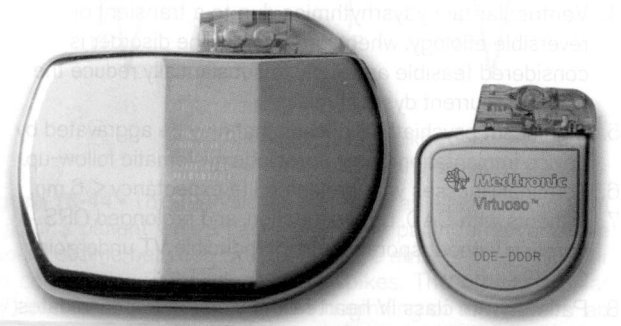

Figure 18-45 • Implantable cardioverter–defibrillators, old and new models. Note the decrease in size and weight that has been achieved with the newer generation, allowing prepectoral implantation. (Courtesy of Medtronic Inc. Minneapolis, MN.)

Table 18-20 • Implantable Cardioverter–Defibrillator: Tiered Therapy

Type of Therapy*	Mode/Energy Level	Condition(s)
Bradycardia pacing	VVI/DDD/VDD	Bradycardia Heart failure
Antitachycardia pacing (ATP)	Burst/ramp ATP	SVT VT (120–180 beast/min)
Low-energy cardioversion	1–8 J	VT (180–210 beats/min)
High-energy cardioversion	15–36 J	VT (>210 beats/min)
Defibrillation†	30–36 J	VF

*Therapy and detection intervals (rate of tachycardia detected) are programmable in most models.
†Maximal energy delivered varies among manufacturers and models.
SVT, supraventricular tachycardia; VF, ventricular fibrillation; VT, ventricular tachycardia.

intended for brief periods of pacing until normal rhythm resumes except in biventricular pacing, in which 100% pacing in the ventricles is desirable.

Today's ICDs have many programmable features that allow the physician to tailor the device to the patient's needs. Bradycardia pacing therapies with biventricular pacing are common features of current ICDs. The availability of an atrial sensing lead allows for a more specific SVT discrimination algorithm. To improve discrimination of tachydysrhythmias, the device allows programming of discrimination algorithms, which withhold VT therapy when PSVT is confirmed. Some devices also have separate tiers of therapy for atrial tachycardia and AF or flutter.

All current ICDs are "noncommitted"; that is, therapy is aborted if the tachycardia terminates even while the ICD is charging. Patients with non-sustained VT need not suffer the discomfort of an inappropriate shock. Third-generation defibrillators have additional features, including memory and event retrieval. Event retrieval may involve successive R-wave analysis or the recording of an electrogram during therapy. These methods document the dysrhythmia before and after the therapy, allowing the physician to analyze the problematic rhythm. These data can be correlated to the patients' symptoms to help further diagnose the dysrhythmia.

Current devices also have the ability to deliver PES using a programmer. PES, a noninvasive method similar to EPS, is used to induce a dysrhythmia to determine the device's ability to successfully terminate it with programmed therapies. It can also be used to ascertain the integrity of the shocking coil, to determine whether a suspected lead problem exists, and to define the defibrillation threshold (DFT) of a patient. The DFT is the lowest amount of energy tested that successfully converts ventricular fibrillation. Certain antidysrhythmic drugs can increase DFTs. For the sake of patient safety, the device should be capable of delivering at least 10 J above the patients' DFT.

PES minimizes the need to test the device in a laboratory situation where catheters are placed in the patient's heart to induce the rhythm disturbance. Testing is done through the device itself, thus reducing the risk associated with the invasive procedure.

THE IMPLANTABLE CARDIOVERTER–DEFIBRILLATOR CODE

The cardiac pacemaker code previously discussed has limited ability to describe modes of ICD function. As a result, in 1993, the American Heart Association and Heart Rhythm Society (formerly NASPE) and BPEG developed the NASPE/BPEG Defibrillator Code.[14] Known as the NBD defibrillator code, it describes ICD capabilities and operation.

The first position of the code indicates the shock chamber—none, atrium, ventricle or dual (O, A, V, or D). The second position indicates the chamber in which antitachycardia pacing is delivered—also coded O, A, V, or D. Position three indicates the means by which tachydysrhythmia is detected, either with the intracardiac electrogram (E) or by hemodynamic means (H). Most current ICDs detect dysrhythmias through intracardiac electrograms. The fourth position of the code is the three- or five-letter code for the pacemaker capability of the device. For example, a ventricular defibrillator with EGM tachydysrhythmia detection and with adaptive rate ventricular antibradycardia pacing would be labeled VOE-VVIR.

NURSING MANAGEMENT

The critical care nurse plays a key role in the pre-implantation and postimplantation management of patients with an ICD. Patient teaching is one of the most important tasks of the critical care nurse. Topics for discussion are included in the Box 18-27. Patients and families need to understand why an ICD is indicated, the purpose of an ICD, the basic parts of the ICD system, and how the ICD functions. Once the physician has determined the type of system to be used, the nurse reinforces the physician's explanation of how the device will be implanted and where the leads and pulse generator will be placed. The patient and family should be informed of the expected length of hospitalization and plans for follow-up care. Many resources for patient education are available from manufacturers of ICDs, including printed materials and videotapes. In addition, the patient and family may find it helpful to meet with a person

Box 18-27 • Implantable Cardioverter-Defibrillator (ICD) Teaching

- Why an ICD is indicated
- Purpose of an ICD
- Components of an ICD
- How the ICD works
- How a shock feels
- How the ICD will be implanted
- Expected length of hospitalization
- Postimplant activities of daily living
- Rate cutoff and therapies programmed in the ICD
- Plans for follow-up care
- When to call the doctor
- Importance of an ICD identification card and medical alert bracelet or necklace
- What the patient and family should do if a shock occurs
- Safety precautions
- Support groups

Box 18-28 • TEACHING GUIDE: ICD

- Carry an ICD identification card.
- Wear a medical alert necklace or bracelet.
- Carry a list of your medications and dosages.
- Keep emergency phone numbers readily available.
- Call your physician after receiving a shock if you do not feel completely recovered.
- Call your physician immediately if you receive more than one shock or several in succession.
- Inform family, significant others, coworkers, and traveling companions about your ICD.
- When traveling by air, inform airline security personnel of your ICD.
- Encourage your family members to take a CPR course.

who has an ICD. This person may be able to alleviate any fears or clarify misconceptions about living with an ICD.

In the postimplantation period, the nurse continuously monitors the patient for the development of any ventricular dysrhythmias and intervenes if necessary. If the patient experiences a sustained VT and no therapy is delivered, it may be that the rate of the tachycardia is below the programmed rate cutoff or that undersensing of the tachydysrhythmias is occurring. Knowledge of the parameters of the ICD and the rate of the patient's dysrhythmia can help the critical care nurse assess this situation correctly. A patient with an ICD who has a sustained, hemodynamically unstable rhythm should not be treated any differently from one without an ICD. External cardioversion can be given in an emergency in the absence of therapy from the patient's ICD. Care should be taken not to apply paddles near or above the ICD generator.

The nurse must be aware of the programmed settings and features of the patient's ICD to provide safe and competent care. Device information should be readily available at the bedside and clearly documented in the patient's chart. If the device fires, the status of the patient and the patient's rhythm is assessed and documented. When a device fires in the absence

of dysrhythmias, there is a high probability of oversensing due to a dislodged lead, loose connection at the header, or an oversensitive setting. Immediate intervention by the EP service is necessary to avoid further discomfort to the patient.

Other immediate postoperative care (wound care, activity instructions) is very similar to that of the patient after pacemaker implantation (see Box 18-25). Furthermore, because the operative approach is almost identical to that of a pacemaker, the complications that one might expect from a pacemaker implant can also be encountered after ICD implantation.

After consulting with the implanting physician, the nurse provides discharge instructions about resuming daily activities. Patients are usually cautioned against swimming or boating alone, climbing ladders, and operating equipment that may produce sparks or cause electromagnetic interference. Patient and family teaching points (Box 18-28) should be reviewed with the patient and family with discharge instructions.

Discussion of psychosocial issues regarding living with an ICD also should be part of the discharge preparation. Although the emotional adjustment varies with each patient, many have fears about receiving their first shock. Other potential patient concerns include alterations in body image, return to work, participation in recreational activities, and reaction of family and friends to the device. If support groups are available, the patient and family should be encouraged to join.

Cardiopulmonary Resuscitation

In any ICU, there is an increased chance that the patient's condition will deteriorate. The cessation of breathing and circulation is known as cardiopulmonary arrest. This condition is also referred to as sudden cardiac arrest, or SCA. When a patient is determined to be in cardiopulmonary arrest, seconds matter. Unless definitive action is taken within 4 to

6 minutes, the patient will suffer irreversible brain injury. Prompt intervention is necessary if the patient is going to have a chance of survival. Immediate and effective CPR often prevents fatal complications. CPR is divided into basic life support (BLS), which is discussed in this chapter, and advanced cardiac life support (ACLS).[1] The ACLS guidelines developed by the

American Heart Association can be found in Appendix 1. This section of the chapter outlines assessment, procedures, interventions, and roles of the nurse in the cardiopulmonary arrest situation. Box 18-29 defines some common terms used during CPR.

• Causes of Cardiopulmonary Arrest

Box 18-30 outlines some of the causes of cardiopulmonary arrest. There are many additional causes of cardiopulmonary arrest. Determination of the cause of the arrest is secondary to rapid intervention. Once intervention to preserve life has been initiated, the cause of the arrest can then be ascertained, and any specific interventions designed to correct the underlying cause can be added to the BLS and ACLS measures.

• Assessment and Management of the Patient in Cardiopulmonary Arrest

Before implementing the resuscitative measures in a code situation, the patient must first be assessed. A myriad of technological monitoring devices are used in the ICU, but it is the everyday physical assessment skills used by nurses that are most accurate in determining a patient's status.

DETERMINE RESPONSIVENESS

The nurse first determines the patient's responsiveness before initiating CPR. The nurse should take no more than 10 seconds to check for breathing and a pulse before initiating CPR. If the patient is unresponsive, the nurse calls for help ("initiate a code") and initiates BLS measures following the acronym ABC (airway–breathing–circulation). Box 18-31 summarizes the ABCs of resuscitation.

POSITION THE PATIENT

The patient should be placed in a supine position on a firm, flat surface. This position enables the rescuer to open the airway and assess for the presence and

---

Box 18-30 • Causes of Cardiopulmonary Arrest

Cardiac Causes
- Myocardial infarction
- Heart failure
- Dysrhythmia
- Coronary artery spasms
- Cardiac tamponade

Pulmonary Causes
- Respiratory failure secondary to respiratory depression
- Airway obstruction
- Impaired gas exchange, such as in acute respiratory distress syndrome
- Impaired ventilation, such as pneumothorax
- Pulmonary embolus
- Electrolyte imbalances
- Hyperkalemia
- Hypomagnesemia
- Hypercalcemia/hypocalcemia

Procedures
- Pulmonary artery catheterization
- Cardiac catheterization
- Surgery

Miscellaneous
- Drug toxicity
- Drug side effects

Box 18-31 • Airway, Breathing, and Circulation

Airway
- Open patient's airway using head tilt–chin lift maneuver (jaw thrust for cervically injured patients).
- Observe for spontaneous breathing.
- If patient is not breathing:
  Place oropharyngeal airway (if possible).
  Suction as necessary.

Breathing
- Connect Ambubag to 100% oxygen.
- Deliver two slow, initial breaths (2 s per breath).
- Maintain seal around patient's mouth and nose.
- Observe for chest rise and fall.
- Monitor pulse oximeter.
- Auscultate for bilateral breath sounds.

Circulation
- Check for carotid pulse and other signs of circulation.
- If no signs of circulation are present:
  Perform chest compressions at rate of 100/min followed by two slow breaths using a 30:2 ratio for compressions to breaths.
  After four cycles, recheck the carotid pulse.
- Continue to assess the effectiveness of CPR by:
  Watching the electrocardiogram monitor to assist with ensuring rate.
  Palpating pulses (radial, femoral, pedal) to determine effectiveness.

Box 18-29 • Common Terms in Cardiopulmonary Resuscitation

Cardiac arrest: Abrupt cessation of effective cardiac pumping activity, resulting in cessation of circulation
Code: Informal term for emergency resuscitation
Crash cart: Emergency cart (see Table 18-21)
Resuscitation: Restoration of vitals signs by mechanical, physiological, and pharmacological means
Clinical death: Absence of vital signs
Biological death: Irreversible cellular changes

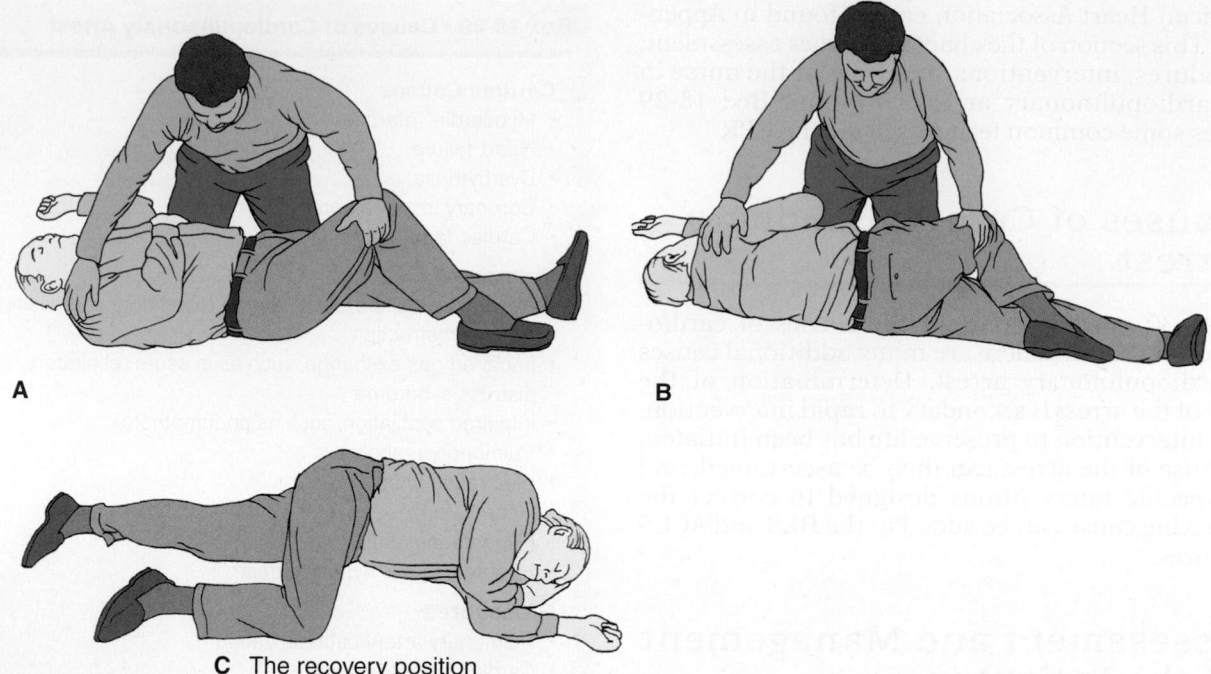

C   The recovery position

Figure 18-47 • BLS—The recovery position. How to place a person in the recovery position if unresponsive but breathing. (From Hazinski MF, Cummins RO, Field JM [eds]: 2000 Handbook of Cardiovascular Care for Healthcare Providers. Dallas: American Heart Association, 2000.)

effectiveness of any spontaneous breathing. If the patient is in a standard hospital bed, a resuscitation board is placed under his or her torso when help arrives. If the patient is in a specialty bed, the CPR setting on the bed is selected.

If the patient is found to be breathing effectively and there is no evidence of trauma, the patient is placed in the recovery position. The recovery position is used to reduce the possibility of airway obstruction by the tongue or by secretions or emesis. To place the patient in the recovery position, the rescuer kneels next to the shoulder of the patient. The rescuer lifts the arm of the patient nearest the rescuer and bends it at the elbow. The arm is then positioned so that the patient's palm of the hand is turned upward and moved toward the patient's face. The rescuer then lifts the leg of the patient furthest from the rescuer and crosses it over the patient's body, moving it toward the rescuer. One hand of the rescuer supports the patient's head during turning and the second hand is used to turn the patient's hips toward the rescuer (Fig. 18-47). Caution must be used when moving patients with suspected or actual spinal cord injuries. One rescuer should ensure that the patient's head remains in a neutral position.

AIRWAY

The nurse assesses for an adequate airway. The patient is positioned to ensure an open, patent airway. The patient is placed in the supine position, and the airway is opened using the head tilt–chin lift method. In this method, the head is tilted back, and the chin is raised to stretch the airway and advance the tongue in preparation for ventilation (Fig. 18-48).

In the case of patients with confirmed or suspected cervical spine injuries, the jaw thrust method is used (Fig. 18-49). The patient's head and neck must not be

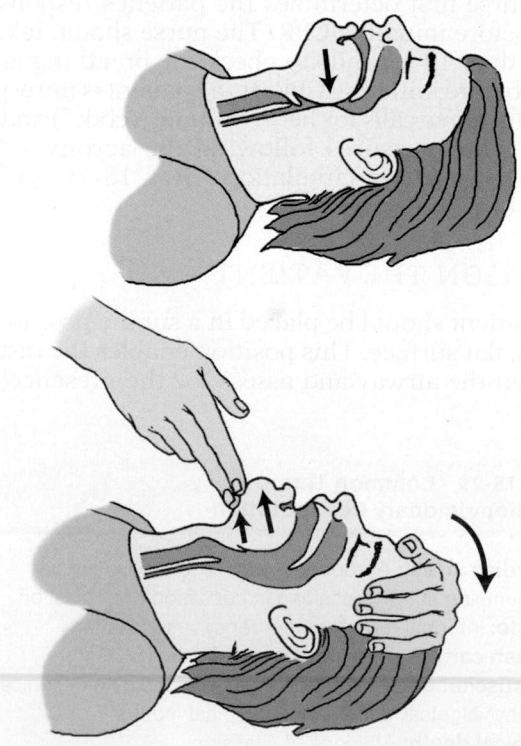

Figure 18-48 • Opening the airway with the back head tilt–chin lift maneuver.

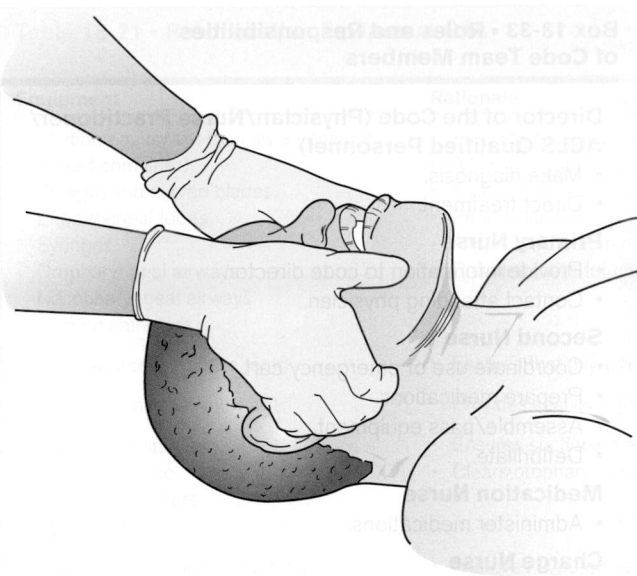

Figure 18-49 • The jaw thrust maneuver without head extension is used if cervical spine trauma is suspected.

moved in an effort to ensure that no damage is done to the cervical spinal cord. Keeping the head in a neutral position, the rescuer places a hand on each side of the patient's head behind the temporomandibular joint and gently pushes the jaw forward. This will open the airway enough to allow for ventilation.

If spontaneous respirations have not returned once a patent airway has been established, then the patient must be assisted with breathing.

BREATHING

Using a bag-valve device (BVD), also known as an Ambu bag, oxygen is delivered as rescue breaths. The BVD is connected to 100% high-flow oxygen, and the mask portion is placed over the patient's mouth and nose. If the patient has an endotracheal tube or tra-

cheostomy tube, there is an adapter that allows for delivery of breaths through an artificial airway. The bag reservoir is then squeezed to deliver the breaths. Observation of the patient's chest is necessary to determine whether the delivered breaths are actually ventilating the lungs. A second person assisting with CPR should auscultate all lung fields to confirm that the delivered breaths are reaching the lungs. Pulse oximetry is used to determine oxygenation.

When one person is performing CPR, two slow breaths are delivered initially. A pulse check should be performed after the delivery of two rescue breaths. If a pulse is detected, rescue breaths are delivered at a rate of 10 to 12 per minute for an adult patient.

CIRCULATION

If no pulse is detected after two initial rescue breaths, then chest compressions must be initiated per BLS protocol. External cardiac compression is a simple technique performed by standing at either side of the patient, placing the heel of one hand 2 to 3 finger-breadths above the xiphoid process, and placing the heel of the other hand over the first. Firm compressions are applied directly downward, and the sternum is depressed between 1.5 and 2 inches and released abruptly. The chest must be allowed to fully recoil between compressions. This rhythm is maintained at the rate of approximately 100 times per minute. A 30:2 compression–ventilation ratio is used, with a pause to provide the ventilation. If the patient is mechanically ventilated, there is no need for an interruption in compressions.[1] To be effective, these techniques must be learned correctly and applied skillfully[1] (Fig. 18-50). A recent study indicates that compressions-only CPR is favorable to conventional CPR in an out-of-hospital arrest situation.[2]

If one person must apply both ventilation and compression, it is best to give two complete ventilations mouth-to-mouth or by other readily available means, followed by 30 external cardiac compressions. This

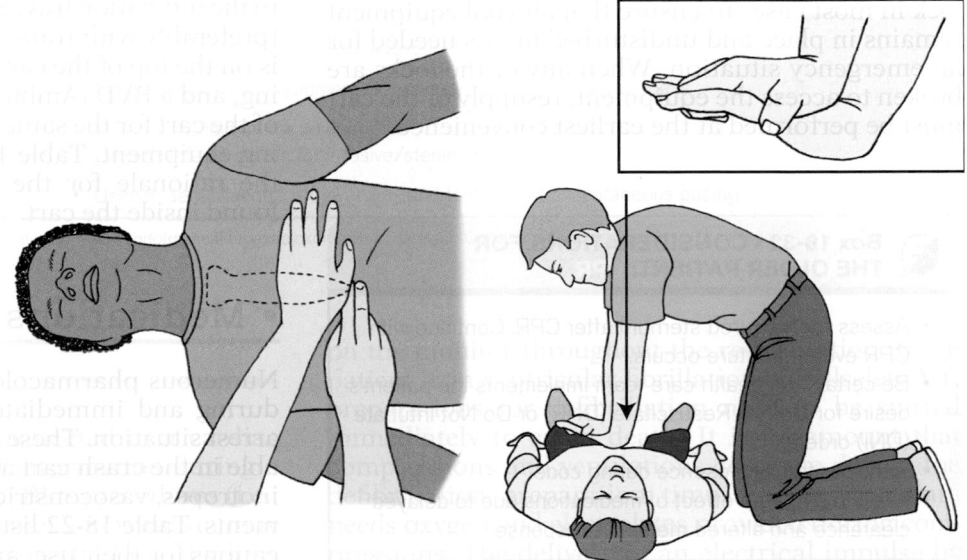

Figure 18-50 • External chest compression. *Left,* proper hand position over lower portion of sternum. *Right,* correct rescuer position.

Table 18-22 • Medications Used to Treat a Patient in Cardiopulmonary Arrest

Drug	Class	Uses	Dosages
Adenosine	Antidysrhythmic	SVT, AF	6 mg rapid IV followed by 10 mL NS flush Repeat twice with 12 mg Max. dose: 30 mg
Amiodarone	Antidysrhythmic	VT, SVT, AF, VF	150–300 mg bolus, 1 mg/min for 6 h, then 0.5 mg/min for 18 h
Atropine	Anticholinergic	Bradycardia, PEA	0.5–1.0 mg IV Max. dose: 3 mg
Bretylium tosylate	Antidysrhythmic	VT, VF	
Calcium chloride	Electrolyte	Hyperkalemia, hypocalcemia, calcium channel blocker toxicity	Syringe 10 mL of 10% solution (100 mg/mL), 2–4 mg/kg
Dobutamine	Inotrope; β₁ agonist	Decreased cardiac output	5–20 µg/kg/min
Dopamine	Inotrope; β₁ agonist	Hypotension	5–20 µg/kg/min
Epinephrine	Catecholamine	VF	Syringe 1:10,000, 1-mg bolus IV Repeat q3–5min
Isoproterenol	Catecholamine; β agonist	VT, VF	Drip 0.5–5 µg/min
Lidocaine	Antidysrhythmic	VT, VF	Bolus 1–1.5 mg/kg Drip 20–50 µg/kg/min
Magnesium sulfate	Electrolyte	Torsades de pointes	Drip 1–2 g/50 mL NS
Nitroglycerin	Coronary vasodilator	Myocardial infarction, angina	5–100 µg/min
Procainamide	Antidysrhythmic	VT, VF	Bolus 5–10 mg/kg over 8–10 min Drip 20–30 mg/min
Sodium bicarbonate	Alkalinizer	Acidosis	50 mEq syringe Normal dose is 1 mEq/kg
Verapamil	Calcium channel blocker	SVT	2.5–5 mg IV over 2 min Repeat 5–10 mg in 15–30 minutes

AF, atrial fibrillation; NS, normal saline; PEA, pulseless electrical activity; SVT, supraventricular tachycardia; VF, ventricular fibrillation; VT, ventricular tachycardia.

an external defibrillator simultaneously depolarizes most of the ventricular cells during ventricular fibrillation and the reentry abnormalities of VT. If the conditions are right, and there has not been too much damage to the heart's intrinsic electrical conduction system, the SA node may resume its function as the pacemaker of the heart.

If indicated, an external countershock should be applied as soon as the instrument is available. The defibrillator paddles are positioned so that the heart is in the current pathway. The anterior apex, also known as the anterolateral or sternum–apex position, is used most often. The anterior paddle is placed firmly on the patient's upper right chest below the clavicle and to the right of the sternum. The apex paddle is positioned firmly on the patient's lower left chest in a mid-axillary line (Fig. 18-51).

A growing body of evidence indicates that early defibrillation can convert a patient's rhythm from ventricular fibrillation more than 90% of the time. In a change to previous defibrillation protocols, defibrillation should be attempted using one shock, with immediate resumption of CPR. If a monophasic defibrillator is used, it should be set at 360 J. If a biphasic device is used, it should be set at either 120 or 200 J;

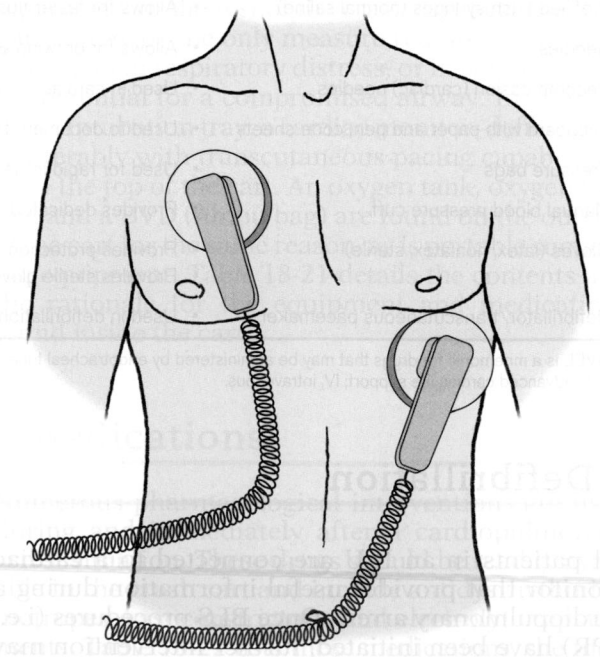

Figure 18-51 • Standard positioning of defibrillator paddles.

this setting is device specific, so familiarity with which defibrillator is on the unit is very important.[1]

Following this first shock, five cycles of CPR should be performed. If the patient remains in a shockable rhythm, then a second shock should be delivered. After each subsequent shock, five more cycles of CPR should be performed before determining whether the patient is in a shockable rhythm.[1] All personnel are advised to avoid touching the patient or bed when the shock is delivered. Immediate resumption of artificial circulation and ventilation (CPR) should occur after each countershock if no pulse returns. Box 18-34 outlines the procedure for defibrillation.

Defibrillators are classified based on the type of waveform used by the defibrillator. Since the early 1970s, monophasic defibrillators have been used. This type of defibrillator provides a shock that flows in one direction from one paddle or electrode pad to the other. In more recent years, newer technology has been developed that changes the way the electrical current flows during defibrillation. Known as a biphasic defibrillator, this newer type delivers the current in two phases. The current initially flows in one direction, then flows in the opposite direction. The biphasic wave uses less peak current, so there is less damage to the heart during defibrillation.[3] ICDs are devices that are designed to shock patients out of potentially fatal dysrhythmias. ICDs have used biphasic technology for more than a decade, but only recently did transthoracic biphasic defibrillation become possible.

• Automatic External Defibrillator

Studies have shown that the sooner a patient in ventricular fibrillation is defibrillated, the greater the chance for survival. The development of the AED has improved the survivability of individuals suffering from potentially life-threatening dysrhythmias. The AED allows for defibrillation to be performed in a variety of settings by personnel trained in the use of the AED but not BLS or ACLS.

The AED consists of a computerized detection system that recognizes the patient's inherent heart rhythm and delivers a defibrillatory countershock when necessary. This cycle of rhythm analysis followed by countershock lasts approximately 30 seconds. AEDs are now found in airports, train stations, sports stadiums, and shopping malls. AEDs are also available in most hospitals in common areas, general floors, and laboratories. The widespread availability of these devices allows for a much quicker response time when a person experiences cardiac arrest.[4]

• Transcutaneous Pacing

A combination defibrillator–transcutaneous pacemaker is usually found on top of the crash cart. The large pacing electrodes ("combination pads") used in defibrillation can also be used to pace a patient transcutaneously. Transcutaneous pacing may be used as a "bridge" (temporary measure) until either a transvenous or permanent pacemaker can be placed.

A nurse, nurse practitioner, or physician quickly and easily initiates transcutaneous pacing. This procedure is noninvasive and therefore is low risk and saves time during an arrest situation. Indications for transcutaneous pacing include new complete (third-degree) heart block or symptomatic bradycardia (unresponsive to drug therapy). The pacing electrodes are also placed when the patient's rhythm changes to a new second-degree, Mobitz II heart block. Transcutaneous pacing also is used when invasive (transvenous) pacing is unsuccessful or contraindicated, such as after the use of thrombolytics and for the patient with sepsis.

The transcutaneous pacemaker is used in a "demand mode" for bradycardia and asystole; it paces the heart only when needed. This mode is safer because the chance of firing on the T wave ("R-on-T phenomenon") is greatly reduced. When the pacemaker is used in an asynchronous mode, the heart is paced at a fixed rate, regardless of the heart's intrinsic rate or rhythm. The pacemaker may fire on the T wave, producing either AF or VT. Box 18-35 outlines the procedures for transcutaneous pacing.

The nurse must ensure that a conscious patient understands what is happening. Much technical jargon and various personnel are involved when a patient is having noninvasive temporary pacing. The nurse is responsible for placing the pacing pads in an anteroposterior configuration, which allows for more effective pacing. Figure 18-52 shows the proper placement of the electrodes. The skin is not shaved, which means that there is no skin irritation. No alcohol or adhesive should be used so that the electrical current is not compromised. The nurse sets the pacing rate and stimulation threshold. Blood pressure should be taken using the right arm to avoid interference from the pacemaker.

Box 18-34 • Indications and Procedure for Defibrillation

Indications
- Pulseless ventricular tachycardia
- Ventricular fibrillation

Procedure
1. Apply defibrillator pads to patient.
2. Turn on defibrillator.
3a. Charge defibrillator to 200 joules for monophasic device.
3b. Change biphasic defibrillation to 120 or 200 J, depending on device.
4. Ensure all personnel are not touching patient or bed.
5. Deliver shock.
6. Determine effectiveness of treatment. Check pulse and observe patient's rhythm.
7. Continue CPR.
8. Be prepared to deliver subsequent shocks per advanced cardiac life support protocol.

Box 18-35 • Indications and Procedure for Transcutaneous Pacing

Indication
- Complete (third-degree) heart block

Procedure
1. Explain procedure to patient.
2. Clip excess hair from chest. Ensure skin is dry.
3. Apply anterior electrode to chest at the fourth intercostal space to the left of the sternum.
4. Apply posterior electrode to patient's back in the area of the left scapula.
5. Connect pacing electrodes to transcutaneous pacemaker.
6. Set pacemaker mode, heart rate, and output.
7. Turn unit on.
8. Assess for effectiveness of pacing:
   - Observe for pacemaker spike with subsequent capture.
   - Assess heart rate and rhythm.
   - Assess blood pressure.
   - Check level of consciousness.
   - Observe for patient anxiety/pain and treat accordingly.

Transcutaneous pacing requires diligent monitoring by the nurse. A loss of capture can occur if the electrodes fail to keep good contact with the skin. Inappropriate pacing may result if the pacemaker cannot detect the heart's intrinsic rhythm. In either case, the nurse must recognize the problem and reposition the patient or the electrodes to ensure efficacious transcutaneous pacing.

• Therapeutic Hypothermia

Unconscious adult patients who suffer out-of-hospital cardiac arrest due to ventricular fibrillation and are resuscitated in the field may benefit from induced

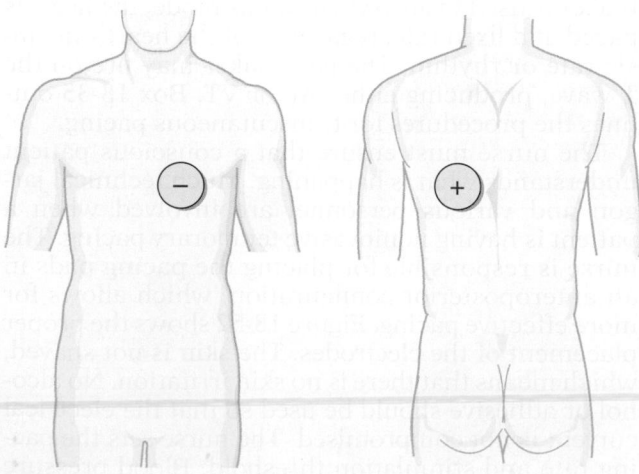

Figure 18-52 • Standard position of transcutaneous pads.

mild hypothermia. During cardiac arrest, blood flow to the brain is compromised, and even prompt interventions may not counteract the deleterious effects of this hemodynamic compromise. The cerebral metabolic rate for oxygen, or $CMRO_2$, is reduced when the body temperature is reduced. Apoptosis (programmed cell death) and the production of free radicals are reduced in a hypothermic state. Studies have shown that the cooling of the patient after cardiac arrest may preserve neurological function. This therapy is currently contraindicated in children of any age, although research continues. There is evidence that supports hypothermic therapy for cardiac arrest caused by dysrhythmias.[5]

• Family Presence in Cardiac Arrest Situations

One aspect of the treatment of cardiopulmonary arrest that has gained attention in recent years is the issue of family presence during a code. Nurses have voiced strong opinions for both sides of the issue. Health care institutions have become more flexible, and they are more accommodating of families and visitors. Some emergency departments and ICUs have protocols in place regarding having loved ones at the bedside while resuscitation efforts are taking place. Every effort must be made to have a knowledgeable person explain to the family what measures are being implemented and the rationale. By involving the family in this manner, they can make more informed decisions about the continuation of resuscitation.[6]

Many family members express a desire to be with the patient during CPR for various reasons. Some want to be reassured that all resuscitative efforts were attempted. There are those who want to have a chance to say goodbye at the moment of death, rather than in the hours or days after death. One of the most often cited reasons for wanting to be with the patient is to make sure that the death is painless.

When discussing advanced directives with patients and their families, the techniques of resuscitation are often described. In the event of a cardiac arrest situation, some family members have seen these measures taking place and make the determination to terminate resuscitation.

The recognition of families after a successful resuscitation must be experienced in order to appreciate it. When the family sees a team of health care professionals working against time to save a patient, they express the realization that nurses, physicians, respiratory therapists, and others combine to provide excellent and compassionate care.

Many nurses and physicians believe that family presence during CPR detracts from their performance and that individuals who have an emotional attachment to the patient hinder their efforts. Rules must be in place to escort family members from the room if the rescuers cannot perform resuscitative measures effectively.

• Clinical Applicability Challenges

Case Study

Mr. K. is a 76-year-old patient who has been admitted to the cardiac surgery intensive care unit just before shift change. He has just come from the operating room, where he had a mitral valve repair and three-vessel coronary artery bypass graft. His prior medical history includes coronary artery disease, myocardial infarction 1 year ago, atrial fibrillation, heart failure, and diabetes mellitus type 2. Medications at home include atorvastatin, lisinopril, metoprolol, nitroglycerin SL, furosemide, metformin, and rosiglitazone.

Initial set postsurgery laboratory results for Mr. K. reveal sodium, 135 mEq/L; potassium, 7.2 mEq/L; chloride, 96 mEq/L; CO_2, 18 mmol/L; blood urea nitrogen, 32 mg/dL; creatinine, 1.6 mg/dL; calcium, 8.8 mg/dL; magnesium, 1.8 mEq/L, and phosphate, 3.2 mg/dL. The patient is on mechanical ventilation. Endotracheal tube placement is confirmed by x-ray. He is still sedated from the surgery. Although his heart rate and blood pressure were within acceptable limits on admission, his heart rate is now 140 beats/minute, and his blood pressure has dropped to 98/50 mm Hg, with a mean arterial pressure of 66 mm Hg. The patient's level of consciousness has declined. Jugular venous distention is now noted to be 3 cm. There is a positive hepatojugular reflex. Heart sounds are muffled, which is contrary to the postoperative report the nurse received.

1. What surgical complication is most likely responsible for Mr. K.'s hemodynamic and neurological status changes?

2. What are some potential complications if this condition remains untreated?

3. What interventions would improve the patient's hemodynamic status?

Review Questions

1. Which of the following fibrinolytic drugs is given as a single bolus over 5 seconds?
   a. Alteplase
   b. Lidocaine
   c. Tenecteplase
   d. Streptokinase

2. Which of the following would amiodarone be used to treat?
   a. Ventricular dysrhythmias only
   b. Atrial dysrhythmias only
   c. Asystole only
   d. Both ventricular and atrial dysrhythmias

3. Which of the following are actions involving inotropic drugs?
   a. Increase myocardial contractility and cardiac output
   b. Decrease myocardial oxygen requirements
   c. Increase risk for pulmonary congestion
   d. Can stop a myocardial infarction

4. Angiotensin-converting enzyme inhibitors are used to treat
   a. hypercholesterolemia.
   b. acute myocardial infarction and heart failure.
   c. peripheral vascular disease.
   d. ventricular tachycardia.

5. The utilization of drug-eluting stents in the management of coronary artery disease maybe advantageous in comparison to bare metal stents and stand-alone percutaneous transluminal coronary angioplasty in terms of
   a. cost.
   b. rate of restenosis.
   c. complications.
   d. length of hospital stay.

6. Facilitated percutaneous coronary intervention (PCI) refers to
   a. Percutaneous transluminal coronary angioplasty within 1 hour after administration of a thrombolytic in acute myocardial infarction (AMI).
   b. Administration of a glycoprotein IIb/IIIa inhibitor as an adjunct to PCI.
   c. PCI without prior administration of a glycoprotein IIb/IIa inhibitor in AMI.
   d. Administration of a glycoprotein IIb/IIIa inhibitor after a thrombolytic has failed to open the vessel in AMI.

7. Restenosis is defined as
   a. a reoccurrence of the blockage in a coronary or peripheral artery.
   b. a stenotic coronary valve.
   c. excision of plaque from the coronary artery.
   d. the dissolution of a thrombus in a coronary or peripheral artery.

8. The signs and symptoms of an acute closure after an interventional cardiology procedure are
   a. ST segment elevation, angina, and dysrhythmias.
   b. fever, headache, and angina.
   c. shortness of breath, angina, and headache.
   d. angina, sudden cardiac death, and oozing from the puncture site.

9. The treatment of coronary artery disease with coronary artery bypass graft and percutaneous coronary intervention are comparable in terms of
   a. degree of invasiveness.
   b. length of hospitalization.
   c. cost.
   d. cardiac risk factor modification requirements after the procedure.

10. Which of the following are Food and Drug Administration–approved treatments for coronary artery disease?
    a. Percutaneous transluminal coronary angioplasty (PTCA), laser, stem cell therapy, and directional coronary atherectomy
    b. PTCA, drug-eluting stents, laser, and directional coronary atherectomy

c. Thrombectomy, PTCA, magnetic resonance angiography, and drug-eluting stents

d. PTCA, stem cell therapy, and percutaneous balloon valvuloplasty

11. A nurse is caring for Mr. E., a 58-year-old man who has had an extensive myocardial infarction and is on day 3 of IABP therapy. During the nursing assessment, the patient complains of chest and back pain, and he is short of breath. He also tells the nurse that he has been spitting up blood. What is the most likely cause of the patient's signs and symptoms?
a. Pneumonia
b. Pulmonary embolism
c. Right ventricular failure
d. Tachycardia

12. A nurse is caring for a patient in the critical care unit who requires intra-aortic balloon pump (IABP) therapy. During rounds, the physician tells her that the patient's IABP catheter has moved down the aorta. She immediately goes to the patient's bedside to conduct an assessment. Which of the following is she most likely to find at this early stage?
a. Low urine output
b. Increased heart rate
c. High blood pressure
d. Severe back pain

13. A nurse is caring for a patient in the critical care unit who is receiving left ventricular assist device therapy. Which of the following is most likely to be included in his plan to ensure proper nutrition?
a. Asking the family to leave at meal time
b. Requesting a soft mechanical diet
c. Obtaining a dietary consult
d. Ensuring a fixed meal schedule

14. Mr. S. is a 63-year-old patient in the critical intensive care unit receiving IABP therapy after cardiac surgery. The attending surgeon is considering weaning Mr. S from the IABP. Which of the following physiological parameters will most likely contribute to the decision to wean?
a. Cardiac index < 2 L/min
b. Pulmonary artery wedge pressure (PAWP) > 20 mm Hg
c. Dobutamine at 15 µg/kg/min
d. Systolic blood pressure of 120 mm Hg

15. A 45-year-old woman presents to the emergency department with 4-day history of palpitations, nausea, and dizziness. She denies history of coronary artery disease or myocardial infarction but reports she is taking a drug once daily to help control her heartbeat and a blood thinner. Her blood pressure is 160/85 mm Hg and pulse 60 to 120 bpm. Bedside rhythm monitoring reveals atrial fibrillation with moderate ventricular response. What laboratory tests should be ordered before considering cardioversion?
a. Quinidine levels, electrolytes, liver function tests
b. Diltiazem level, thyroid function tests, electrolytes

c. Lipid profile, liver function tests, electrolytes
d. Digoxin level, electrolytes, and prothrombin time/international normalized ratio (PT/INR)

16. A 65-year-old woman returns to her room after pacemaker implantation. She is still heavily sedated, but the initial blood pressure reading is 85/50 mm Hg with a pulse of 105 beats/min in sinus tachycardia. Pulse oximetry reading is 88%. Which of the following diagnostic procedures should be performed to correctly rule out cardiac tamponade?
a. Arterial blood gas
b. Two-dimensional echocardiogram
c. Pacemaker interrogation
d. Chest radiograph

17. Ms. G. has just been admitted to your unit after the implantation of a VVIRO pacemaker. A VVIRO pacemaker is one that
a. paces the atria, senses the atria, is inhibited, and is rate modulated.
b. paces the ventricle, senses the ventricle, is inhibited, and is rate modulated.
c. paces both ventricles synchronously, senses both ventricles, and is inhibited.
d. paces both atria synchronously, senses both atria, and is inhibited.

18. The rhythm strip of a patient with an AAIRO pacemaker shows atrial pacing 80 beats/minute. When examining the patient's rhythm, what would you expect to see?
a. A pacing spike followed by a P wave and then a normal QRS
b. No P waves and a pacing spike followed by a wide QRS
c. A pacing spike followed by a P wave and another pacing spike followed by a wide QRS
d. Normal P waves followed by a pacing spike and then a normal QRS

19. A 70-year-old man with an implantable cardioverter–defibrillator (ICD) reports a firing while he is in the shower. Interrogation of the ICD shows ventricular tachycardia that does not respond to antitachycardia pacing and the ICD ramps up to a single cardioversion shock that converts the dysrhythmia. What do you tell the patient?
a. Avoid taking a shower, just use the tub or sponge baths.
b. Be prepared to be admitted to the hospital for drug initiation.
c. Report to his physician if firings occur frequently or in succession.
d. Call his physician daily with reports.

20. A ventilated patient with an endotracheal tube is undergoing cardiopulmonary resuscitation. During a pause in compressions, the cardiac monitor shows narrow QRS complexes and a heart rate of 55 beats/minute with a palpable pulse. Which of the following actions should the nurse take first?
a. Administer amiodarone (Cordarone), 300 mg intravenously over 10 minutes.
b. Check endotracheal tube placement.

c. Obtain an arterial blood gas sample.

d. Administer atropine 1 mg intravenously.

21. Preparation is the key to successful resuscitation. Which of the following responses is most appropriate to prepare for a cardiopulmonary emergency?

a. Have nasal oxygen ready.

b. Place an oropharyngeal airway at the bedside.

c. Keep the medication cart locked up for safety.

d. Do not start an IV line unless necessary.

22. It has been established that a patient is in third-degree heart block, and a transcutaneous pacemaker is attached to the patient. The pacemaker is set in "demand" mode. This setting is used in order to avoid

a. conversion to second-degree heart block.

b. inadvertent defibrillation of the sinoatrial node.

c. having the patient become symptomatic.

d. R-on-T phenomenon

23. Therapeutic hypothermia is used in some cardiac arrest situations because

a. apoptosis is increased in a hypothermic state.

b. cooling of the extremities allows for better perfusion of vital organs.

c. neurologic function may be preserved.

d. Children can tolerate the fluctuation in temperature better.

24. Family presence at the bedside during resuscitative efforts is contraindicated if

a. the patient's safety is at risk.

b. there is obvious bleeding or biohazard conditions.

c. the patient is on contact isolation precautions.

d. the nurse has not had time to explain the situation.

References

Pharmacological Therapy

1. Antman EM, Anbe DT, Armstrong PW, et al: ACC/AHA guidelines for the management of patients with ST-elevation myocardial infarction: A report of the American College of Cardiology/American Heart Association Task Force on Practice Guidelines (Committee to Revise the 1999 Guidelines for the Management of Patients With Acute Myocardial Infarction). Circulation 110:e82–e293, 2004

2. Armstrong PW, Collen D, Antman E: Fibrinolysis for acute myocardial infarction: The future is here and now. Circulation 107:2533–2537, 2003

3. Assessment of the Safety and Efficacy of a New Thrombolytic (ASSENT-2) Investigators: Single-bolus tenecteplase compared with front-loaded alteplase in acute myocardial infarction: The ASSENT-2 double-blind randomised trial. Lancet 354:716–722, 1999

4. The GUSTO V Investigators: Reperfusion therapy for acute myocardial infarction with fibrinolytic therapy or combination reduced fibrinolytic therapy and platelet glycoprotein IIb/IIIa inhibition: The GUSTO V randomised trial. Lancet 357:1905–1914, 2001

5. Roe MT, Green CL, Giugliano RP, et al: Improved speed and stability of ST-segment recovery with reduced-dose tenecteplase and eptifibatide compared with full-dose tenecteplase for acute ST-segment elevation myocardial infarction. J Am Coll Cardiol 43:549–556, 2004

6. White HD, Gersh BJ, Opie LH: Antithrombotic agents: Platelet inhibitors, anticoagulants, and fibrinolytics. In Opie LH Gersh BJ: Drugs for the Heart. Philadelphia: Elsevier Saunders, 2005, pp 275–319

7. Santiago P, Tadros P: Non-ST-segment elevation syndromes: Pharmacologic management, conservative versus early invasive approach. Postgrad Med 112:47–68, 2002

8. Menon V, Berkowitz SD, Antman EM, et al: New heparin dosing recommendations for patients with acute coronary syndromes. Am J Med 110:641–650, 2001

9. Antman EM, Morrow DA, McCabe CH, et al: Enoxaparin versus unfractionated heparin with fibrinolysis for ST-elevation myocardial infarction. N Engl J Med 354:1477–1488, 2006

10. Antman EM, Cohen M, McCabe C, et al: Enoxaparin is superior to unfractionated heparin for preventing clinical events at 1-year follow-up of TIMI 11B and ESSENCE. Eur Heart J 23:308–314, 2002

11. Fox KA, Antman EM, Cohen M, et al: Comparison of enoxaparin versus unfractionated heparin in patients with unstable angina pectoris/non-ST-segment elevation acute myocardial infarction having subsequent percutaneous coronary intervention. Am J Cardiol 90:477–482, 2002

12. Goodman SG, Cohen M, Bigonzi F, et al: Randomized trial of low molecular weight heparin (enoxaparin) versus unfractionated heparin for unstable coronary artery disease: One-year results of the ESSENCE Study. Efficacy and Safety of Subcutaneous Enoxaparin in Non-Q Wave Coronary Events. J Am Coll Cardiol 36:693–698, 2000

13. Ferguson JJ, Califf RM, Antman EM, et al: Enoxaparin vs unfractionated heparin in high-risk patients with non-ST-segment elevation acute coronary syndromes managed with an intended early invasive strategy: Primary results of the SYNERGY randomized trial. JAMA 292:45–54, 2004

14. Antman EM, Cohen M, Radley D, et al: Assessment of the treatment effect of enoxaparin for unstable angina/non-Q-wave myocardial infarction: TIMI 11B ESSENCE meta-analysis. Circulation 100:1602–1608, 1999

15. Antman EM, McCabe CH, Gurfinkel EP, et al: Enoxaparin prevents death and cardiac ischemic events in unstable angina/non-Q-wave myocardial infarction: Results of the thrombolysis in myocardial infarction (TIMI) 11B trial. Circulation 100:1593–1601, 1999

16. Smith SC Jr, Feldman TE, Hirshfeld JW Jr, et al: ACC/AHA/SCAI 2005 Guideline Update for Percutaneous Coronary Intervention—Summary article: A report of the American College of Cardiology/American Heart Association Task Force on Practice Guidelines (ACC/AHA/SCAI Writing Committee to Update the 2001 Guidelines for Percutaneous Coronary Intervention). Circulation 113:156–175, 2006

17. Lincoff AM, Bittl JA, Harrington RA, et al: Bivalirudin and provisional glycoprotein IIb/IIIa blockade compared with heparin and planned glycoprotein IIb/IIIa blockade during percutaneous coronary intervention: REPLACE-2 randomized trial. JAMA 289:853–863, 2003

18. Lincoff AM, Bittl JA, Kleiman NS, et al: Comparison of bivalirudin versus heparin during percutaneous coronary intervention (the Randomized Evaluation of PCI Linking Angiomax to Reduced Clinical Events [REPLACE]-1 trial). Am J Cardiol 93:1092–1096, 2004

19. Lincoff AM, Kleiman NS, Kereiakes DJ, et al: Long-term efficacy of bivalirudin and provisional glycoprotein IIb/IIIa blockade vs heparin and planned glycoprotein IIb/IIIa blockade during percutaneous coronary revascularization: REPLACE-2 randomized trial. JAMA 292:696–703, 2004

20. Coumadin Aspirin Reinfarction Study (CARS) Investigators: Randomised double-blind trial of fixed low-dose warfarin with aspirin after myocardial infarction. Coumadin Aspirin Reinfarction Study (CARS) Investigators. Lancet 350:389–396, 1997

21. Rothberg MB, Celestin C, Fiore LD, et al: Warfarin plus aspirin after myocardial infarction or the acute coronary syndrome: Meta-analysis with estimates of risk and benefit. Ann Intern Med 143:241–250, 2005

22. Hirsh J, Fuster V, Ansell J, et al: American Heart Association/American College of Cardiology Foundation guide to warfarin therapy. J Am Coll Cardiol 41:1633–1652, 2003

23. The Clopidogrel in Unstable Angina to Prevent Recurrent Events Trial Investigators: Effects of clopidogrel in addition to aspirin in patients with acute coronary syndromes without ST-segment elevation. N Engl J Med 345:494–502, 2001

24. Yusuf S, Mehta SR, Zhao F, et al: Early and late effects of clopidogrel in patients with acute coronary syndromes. Circulation 107:966–972, 2003

25. Sabatine MS, Cannon CP, Gibson CM, et al: Addition of clopidogrel to aspirin and fibrinolytic therapy for myocardial infarction with ST-segment elevation. N Engl J Med 352:1179–1189, 2005

26. The ACTIVE Writing Group on behalf of the ACTIVE Investigators: Clopidogrel plus aspirin versus oral anticoagulation for atrial fibrillation in the Atrial Fibrillation Clopidogrel Trial With Irbesartan for Prevention of Vascular Events (ACTIVE W): A randomised controlled trial. Lancet 367:1903–1912, 2006

27. Montalescot G, Sideris G, Meuleman C, et al: A randomized comparison of high clopidogrel loading doses in patients with non-ST-segment elevation acute coronary syndromes: The ALBION (Assessment of the Best Loading Dose of Clopidogrel to Blunt Platelet Activation, Inflammation and Ongoing Necrosis) trial. J Am Coll Cardiol 48:931–938, 2006

28. Kong DF, Califf RM, Miller DP, et al: Clinical outcomes of therapeutic agents that block the platelet glycoprotein IIb/IIIa integrin in ischemic heart disease. Circulation 98:2829–2835, 1998

29. Lincoff AM, Califf RM, Moliterno DJ, et al, for the Evaluation of Platelet IIb/IIIa Inhibition in Stenting Investigators: Complementary clinical benefits of coronary-artery stenting and blockade of platelet glycoprotein IIb/IIIa receptors. N Engl J Med 341:319–327, 1999

30. The Assessment of the Safety and Efficacy of a New Thrombolytic Regimen (ASSENT)-3 Investigators: Efficacy and safety of tenecteplase in combination with enoxaparin, abciximab, or unfractionated heparin: The ASSENT-3 randomised trial in acute myocardial infarction. Lancet 358:605–613, 2001

31. Woosley RL Indik JH: Antiarrhythmic drugs. In Fuster V, Alexander RW, O'Rourke RA (eds): Hurst's The Heart. New York: McGraw-Hill, 2004, pp 949–973

32. DiMarco JP, Gersh BJ, Opie LH: Antiarrhythmic drugs and strategies. In Opie LH, Gersh BJ (eds): Drugs for the Heart. Philadelphia: Elsevier Saunders, 2005, pp 218–274

33. Smith SC Jr, Allen J, Blair SN, et al: AHA/ACC guidelines for secondary prevention for patients with coronary and other atherosclerotic vascular disease: 2006 Update. Circulation 113:2363–2372, 2006

34. The CAPRICORN Investigators: Effect of carvedilol on outcome after myocardial infarction in patients with left-ventricular dysfunction: The CAPRICORN randomised trial. Lancet 357:1385–1390, 2001

35. Packer M, Fowler MB, Roecker EB, et al, for the Carvedilol Prospective Randomized Cumulative Survival (COPERNICUS) Study Group: Effect of carvedilol on the morbidity of patients with severe chronic heart failure: Results of the carvedilol prospective randomized cumulative survival (COPERNICUS) study. Circulation 106:2194–2199, 2002

36. 2005 American Heart Association guidelines for cardiopulmonary resuscitation and emergency cardiovascular care: Part 7.4—monitoring and medications. Circulation 112:IV-78–IV-83, 2005

37. Gibler WB, Cannon CP, Blomkalns AL, et al: Practical implementation of the guidelines for unstable angina/non-ST-segment elevation myocardial infarction in the emergency department: A scientific statement from the American Heart Association Council on Clinical Cardiology (Subcommittee on Acute Cardiac Care), Council on Cardiovascular Nursing, and Quality of Care and Outcomes Research Interdisciplinary Working Group, in Collaboration With the Society of Chest Pain Centers. Circulation 111:2699–2710, 2005

38. Aasbo JD, Lawrence AT, Krishnan K, et al: Amiodarone prophylaxis reduces major cardiovascular morbidity and length of stay after cardiac surgery: A meta-analysis. Ann Intern Med 143:327–336, 2005

39. Amiodarone Trials Meta-Analysis Investigators: Effect of prophylactic amiodarone on mortality after acute myocardial infarction and in congestive heart failure: Meta-analysis of individual data from 6500 patients in randomised trials. Lancet 350:1417–1424, 1997

40. Giri S, White CM, Dunn AB, et al: Oral amiodarone for prevention of atrial fibrillation after open heart surgery, the Atrial Fibrillation Suppression Trial (AFIST): A randomised placebo-controlled trial. Lancet 357:830–836, 2001

41. Field JM, Hazinski MF Gilmore D (eds): Handbook of Emergency Cardiovascular Care for Healthcare Providers. Dallas: American Heart Association, 2006

42. 2005 American Heart Association guidelines for cardiopulmonary resuscitation and emergency cardiovascular care: Part 8—stabilization of the patient with acute coronary syndromes. Circulation 112:IV–89–IV–110, 2005

43. Poole-Wilson PA, Opie LH: Digitalis, acute inotropes, and inotropic dilators: Acute and chronic heart failure. In Opie LH Gersh BJ (eds): Drugs for the Heart. Philadelphia: Elsevier Saunders, 2005, pp 149–183

44. O'Rourke RA: Optimal medical management of patients with chronic ischemic heart disease. Curr Probl Cardiol 26:189–238, 2001

45. Hauptman PJ, Schnitzler MA, Swindle J, et al: Use of nesiritide before and after publications suggesting drug-related risks in patients with acute decompensated heart failure. JAMA 296:1877–1884, 2006

46. Sackner-Bernstein JD, Skopicki HA, Aaronson KD: Risk of worsening renal function with nesiritide in patients with acutely decompensated heart failure. Circulation 111:1487–1491, 2005

47. Sackner-Bernstein JD, Kowalski M, Fox M, et al: Short-term risk of death after treatment with nesiritide for decompensated heart failure: A pooled analysis of randomized controlled trials. JAMA 293:1900–1905, 2005

48. Opie LH, Poole-Wilson PA, Pfeffer MA: Angiotensin-converting enzyme (ACE) inhibitors, angiotensin-II receptor blockers (ARBs), and aldosterone antagonists. In Opie LH Gersh BJ (eds): Drugs for the Heart. Philadelphia: Elsevier Saunders, 2005, pp 104–148

49. Jong P, Yusuf S, Rousseau MF, et al: Effect of enalapril on 12-year survival and life expectancy in patients with left ventricular systolic dysfunction: A follow-up study. Lancet 361:1843–1848, 2003

50. The CONSENSUS Trial Study Group: Effects of enalapril on mortality in severe congestive heart failure. Results of the Cooperative North Scandinavian Enalapril Survival Study (CONSENSUS). N Engl J Med 316:1429–1435, 1987

51. The SOLVD Investigators: Effect of enalapril on survival in patients with reduced left ventricular ejection fractions and congestive heart failure. N Engl J Med 325:293–302, 1991

52. The SOLVD Investigators: Effect of enalapril on mortality and the development of heart failure in asymptomatic patients with reduced left ventricular ejection fractions. N Engl J Med 327:685–691, 1992

53. Pfeffer MA, Braunwald E, Moye LA, et al: Effect of captopril on mortality and morbidity in patients with left ventricular dysfunction after myocardial infarction: Results of the sur-

vival and ventricular enlargement trial. The SAVE Investigators. N Engl J Med 327:669–677, 1992

54. Cleland JG, Erhardt L, Murray G, et al: Effect of ramipril on morbidity and mode of death among survivors of acute myocardial infarction with clinical evidence of heart failure: A report from the AIRE Study Investigators. Eur Heart J 18: 41–51, 1997

55. Cohn JN, Johnson G, Ziesche S, et al: A comparison of enalapril with hydralazine-isosorbide dinitrate in the treatment of chronic congestive heart failure. N Engl J Med 325: 303–310, 1991

56. Domanski MJ, Exner DV, Borkowf CB, et al: Effect of angiotensin converting enzyme inhibition on sudden cardiac death in patients following acute myocardial infarction: A meta-analysis of randomized clinical trials. J Am Coll Cardiol 33:598–604, 1999

57. ACE Inhibitor Myocardial Infarction Collaborative Group: Indications for ACE Inhibitors in the early treatment of acute myocardial infarction: systematic overview of individual data from 100 000 patients in randomized trials. Circulation 97: 2202–2212, 1998

58. Flather MD, Yusuf S, Kober L, et al, for the ACE-Inhibitor Myocardial Infarction Collaborative Group: Long-term ACE-inhibitor therapy in patients with heart failure or left-ventricular dysfunction: A systematic overview of data from individual patients. Lancet 355:1575–1581, 2000

59. Fox KM: Efficacy of perindopril in reduction of cardiovascular events among patients with stable coronary artery disease: Randomised, double-blind, placebo-controlled, multicentre trial (the EUROPA study). Lancet 362:782–788, 2003

60. The Heart Outcomes Prevention Evaluation Study Investigators: Effects of an angiotensin-converting-enzyme inhibitor, ramipril, on cardiovascular events in high-risk patients. N Engl J Med 342:145–153, 2000

61. Part 5: Acute Coronary Syndromes. Circulation 112:III-55–III-72, 2005

62. Grundy SM, Cleeman JI, Merz CN, et al, for the Coordinating Committee of the National Cholesterol Education Program. Implications of recent clinical trials for the National Cholesterol Education Program Adult Treatment Panel III guidelines. Circulation 110:227–239, 2004

63. Nissen SE, Nicholls SJ, Sipahi I, et al, for the ASTEROID Investigators: Effect of very high-intensity statin therapy on regression of coronary atherosclerosis: The ASTEROID trial. JAMA 295:1556–1565, 2006

64. Expert Panel on Detection Evaluation, and Treatment of High Blood Cholesterol in Adults: Executive summary of the third report of the National Cholesterol Education Program (NCEP) Expert Panel on detection, evaluation, and treatment of high blood cholesterol in adults (Adult Treatment Panel III). JAMA 285:2486–2497, 2001

Percutaneous Coronary Interventions and Percutaneous Balloon Valvuloplasty

1. American Heart Association: Heart Disease and Stroke Statistics—2006 Update. Dallas: American Heart Association, 2006

2. Antoniucci D (ed): Primary Angioplasty. Rome: Taylor & Francis Publishing, 2004

3. Serruys PW, Unger F, Sousa JE, et al, for the Arterial Revascularization Therapies Study Group: Comparison of coronary artery bypass grafting and stenting for the treatment of multivessel disease. N Engl J Med 344:1117–1124, 2001

4. Society of Thoracic Surgeons: National Adult Cardiac Surgical Database Report 2000–2001. Chicago: Author, 2004

5. Detre K, et al: New approaches to coronary interventions. J Am Coll Cardiol 35:1122–1129, 2000

6. Legrand VM, Serruys PW, Unger F, et al, for the Arterial Revascularization Therapy Study (ARTS) Investigators: Three-year outcome after coronary stenting versus bypass surgery for the treatment of multivessel disease. Circulation 109: 1114–1120, 2004

7. Serruys PW, Unger F, Sousa JE, et al: Five-year outcomes after coronary stenting versus bypass surgery for the treatment of multivessel disease: The final analysis of the Arterial Revascularization Therapies Study (ARTS) randomized trial. J Am Coll Cardiol 46(4):575–581, 2005

8. Bentivoglio LG, Holubkov R, Kelsey SF, et al: Short and long term outcome of percutaneous transluminal coronary angioplasty in unstable versus stable angina pectoris: A report of the 1985/1986 NHLBI PTCA registry. Cathet Cardiovasc Diagn 23:227–238, 1991

9. O'Keefe JH Jr, Rutherford BD, McConahay DR, et al: Multivessel coronary angioplasty from 1980 to 1989: Procedural results and long-term outcome. J Am Coll Cardiol 16: 1097–1102, 1990

10. Dorros G, Iyer SS, Hall P, et al: Percutaneous coronary angioplasty in 1001 multi-vessel coronary disease patients: An analysis of different patient subsets. J Interv Cardiol 4: 71–80, 1991

11. Hannan EL, Racz MJ, Walford G, et al: Long-term outcomes of coronary artery bypass grafting versus stent implantation. N Engl J Med 352(21):2174–83, 2005

12. Alderman EL, Bourassa MG, Cohen LS, et al, for the CASS Investigators: Ten-year follow-up of survival and myocardial infarction in the randomized coronary artery surgery study. Circulation 82:1629–1646, 1990

13. U.S. Food and Drug Administration and Center for Devices and Radiological Health: Cypher sirolimus-eluting coronary stent on RAPTOR over-the-wire delivery system or RAPTOR-RAIL rapid exchange delivery system. Rockville, MD: Author, 2003

14. Ellis S, Stone GW, Popma JJ, et al: Relationship between angiographic late loss and target lesion revascularization after coronary stent implantation: Analysis from the TAXUS IV Study. J Am Coll Cardiol 45(8):1206–1200, 2005

15. Colombo A, Drzewiecki J, Banning A, et al: Randomized study to assess the effectiveness of slow-and moderate-release polymer-based paclitaxel-eluting stents for coronary artery lesions, Circulation 108:788–794, 2003

16. Mallik S, Krumholz HM, Lin ZQ, et al: Patients with depressive symptoms have lower health status benefits after coronary artery bypass surgery. Circulation 111(3):250–253, 2005

17. Meyer J, Merx W, Schmitz H, et al: Percutaneous transluminal coronary angioplasty immediately after intracoronary streptolysis of transmural myocardial infarction. Circulation 66: 905–913, 1982

18. Grines CL: Primary angioplasty in myocardial infarction. J Am Coll Cardiol 33:640–646, 1999

19. Kelley MP, Klugherz BD, Hashemi SM, et al: One-year clinical outcomes of protected and unprotected left main coronary artery stenting. Eur Heart J 24(17):1554–1559, 2003

20. Gruberg L, Mintz GS, Mehran R, et al: The prognostic implications of further renal function deterioration within 48 hours of interventional coronary procedures in patients with pre-existent chronic renal insufficiency. J Am Coll Cardiol 36(5): 1542–1548, 2000

21. Rihal CS, Textor SC, Grill DE, et al: Incidence and prognostic importance of acute renal failure after percutaneous coronary intervention. Circulation 105:2259, 2002

22. Mahta SR, Yusuf S, Peters RJ, et al: Effects of pretreatment with clopidogrel and aspirin followed by long term therapy in patients undergoing percutaneous coronary intervention: The PCI-CURE Study. Lancet 358:527–533, 2001

23. Steinhubl SR, Berger PB, Mann JT, for the Clopidogrel for Reduction of Events During Observation (CREDO) Investigators: Early and sustained dual oral antiplatelet therapy

following percutaneous coronary intervention: A randomized controlled trial. JAMA 288:2411–2420, 2002

24. Aversano T, Aversano LT, Passamani E, et al: Thrombolytic therapy versus primary percutaneous coronary intervention for myocardial infarction in patients presenting to hospitals without on-site cardiac surgery: A randomized controlled trial. JAMA 287:1943–1951, 2002

25. Braunwald E, Antman EM, Beasley JW, et al: ACC/AHA Guideline Update for the Management of Patients with Unstable Angina and Non-ST Segment Elevation Myocardial Infarction-2002: Summary article. Circulation 106:1893–1900, 2002

26. Goodkind J, Coombs VJ, Golobic RA: Excimer laser angioplasty. Heart Lung 22:26–35, 1993

27. Antoniucci D, Valenti R, Migliorini A, et al: Comparison of rheolytic thrombectomy before direct infarct artery stenting versus direct stenting alone in patients undergoing percutaneous coronary intervention for acute myocardial infarction. Am J Cardiol 93:1033–1035, 2004

28. Ho PC, Leung CY: Rheolytic thrombectomy with distal filter embolic protection as adjunctive therapies to high-risk saphenous vein graft intervention. Cathet Cardiovasc Intervent 61:202–205, 2004

29. Waksman R, Robinson KA, Crocker IR, et al: Intracoronary radiation before stent implantation inhibits neointima formation in stented porcine coronary arteries. Circulation 92:1383–1386, 1995

30. American Diabetes Association: Consensus Statement, 2003.

Intra-Aortic Balloon Pump Counterpulsation and Mechanical Circulatory Support

1. Antman EM, Smith SC, Alpert JS, et al: ACC/AHA guidelines for the management of patients with ST-elevation myocardial infarction—executive summary. A report of the American College of Cardiology/American Heart Association Task Force on Practice Guidelines (Writing Committee to revise the 1999 guidelines for the management of patients with acute myocardial infarction). Circulation 110:588–636, 2004

2. Marra C, DeSanto LS, Amarelli C, et al: Coronary artery by-pass grafting in patients with severe left ventricular dysfunction: A prospective, randomized study. Int J Artif Organs 25:141, 2002

3. Schreuder JJ, Castiglioni A, Donelli A, et al: Automatic intra-aortic balloon pump timing using an intrabeat dicrotic notch prediction algorithm. Ann Thorac Surg 79(3):1017–1022; discussion, 1022, 2005

4. Stevenson LW, Kormos RL: Mechanical Support 2000: Current applications and future trial design. J Am Coll Cardiol 37:340–370, 2001

5. Song X, Throckmorton AL, Untaroiu A, et al: Axial flow blood pumps. Asaio J 49(4):355–364, 2003

6. Heart Assist Pump. The Penn State Heart Devices page. Retrieved November 1, 2003, from http://www/psu/edu/ur/heartdevices/asstpump.htm

7. Delgado DH, Rao V, Ross HJ, et al: Mechanical circulatory assistance: State of the art. Circulation 106:2046–2050, 2002

8. Boehmer JP, Popjes E: Cardiac failure: mechanical support strategies. Crit Care Med 34(9 Suppl):S268–277, 2006

9. Gray NA Jr, Selzman CH: Current status of the total artificial heart. Am Heart J 152(1):4–10, 2006

10. Holman WL, Bourge BC, McGriffin DC, et al: Ventricular assist: Experience with a pulsatile heterotropic device. Semin Thorac Cardiovasc Surg 6(3):147–153, 1994

11. McCarthy PM, Sabik JF: Implanted circulatory support devices as a bridge to heart transplantation. Semin Thorac Cardiovasc Surg 6(3):174–180, 1994

12. Farrar DJ: Ventricular interactions during mechanical circulatory support. Semin Thorac Cardiovasc Surg 6(3):163–168, 1994

13. Dasse KA, Frazier OH, Graham TR: The physiology of left ventricular assistance. In Lewis T, Graham TR (eds): Mechanical Circulatory Support. London: Edward Arnold, 1995, pp 13–25

14. Oz MC, Rose EA, Slater J, et al: Malignant ventricular rhythms are well tolerated in patients receiving long-tern ventricular assist devices. J Am Coll Cardiol 24:1688–1691, 1994

Management of Dysrhythmias

1. Cummins RO: Textbook of Advanced Cardiac Life Support. Dallas: American Heart Association, 2001

2. Fuster V, Ryden LE, Asinger RW, et al: ACC/AHA/ESC Guidelines for the management of patients with atrial fibrillation: A report of the American College of Cardiology/American Heart Association Task Force on Practice Guidelines and the European Society of Cardiology Committee for Practice Guidelines and Policy Conferences (Committee to develop guidelines for the management of patients with atrial fibrillation): J Am Coll Cardiol 38:(4), 2001

3. Blomstrom-Lundqvist C, Scheinman MM, Aliot EM, et al: ACC/AHA/ESC guidelines for the management of patients with supraventricular arrhythmias—executive summary. A report of the American College of Cardiology/American Heart Association Task Force on Practice Guidelines and the European Society of Cardiology Committee for Practice Guidelines (writing committee to develop guidelines for the management of patients with supraventricular arrhythmias) developed in collaboration with NASPE-Heart Rhythm Society: J Am Coll Cardiol 42(8):1493–1531, 2003

4. Haines DE: Biophysics of radiofrequency lesion formation. In Huang SKS, Wood MA (eds): Catheter Ablation of Cardiac Arrhythmias. Philadelphia: Elsevier, 2006, pp 3–48

5. Scheinman M, Calkins H, Gillette P, et al, for the North American Society of Pacing and Electrophysiology. NASPE Policy Statement on Catheter Ablation: Personnel, Policy, and Therapeutic Recommendations. Pacing Clin Electrophysiol 26(3):789–799, 2003

6. Michael R, Bristow MD, Leslie A, et al, for the Comparison of Medical Therapy, Pacing, and Defibrillation in Heart Failure (COMPANION) Investigators: Cardiac-resynchronization therapy with or without an implantable defibrillator in advanced chronic heart failure. N Engl J Med 350(21):2140–2150, 2004

7. Gregoratos G, Abrams J, Epstein AE, et al: ACC/AHA/NASPE 2002 guideline update for implantation of cardiac pacemakers and antiarrhythmia devices: Summary article. A report of the American College of Cardiology/American Heart Association Task Force on Practice Guidelines (ACC/AHA/NASPE Committee to Update the 1998 Pacemaker Guidelines). J Cardiovasc Electrophysiol 13(11):1183–1199, 2002. Available at: http://www.acc.org

8. Bernstein AD, Daubert JC, Fletcher RD, et al: The revised NASPE/BPEG generic code for antibradycardia, adaptive-rate, and multisite pacing. North American Society of Pacing and Electrophysiology/British Pacing and Electrophysiology Group. Pacing Clin Electrophysiol 25(2):260–264, 2002. Available at: http://www.hrsonline.org

9. Maisel WH, Moynahan M, Zuckerman BD, et al: Pacemaker and ICD generator malfunctions: Analysis of Food and Drug Administration annual reports. JAMA 295(16):1901–1906, 2006

10. Obias-Manno D: Clinical considerations for the allied professional: Programming issues in cardiac resynchronization therapy. Heart Rhythm 2(2):216–217, 2005

11. Heart and Stroke Statistical Update (online). American Heart Association, 2006. Available at: http://www.Americanheart.org.

12. Winters S, Packer D, Marchlinski F, et al: Consensus statement on indications, guidelines for use, and recommendations for follow-up of implantable cardioverter defibrillators. Pacing Clin Electrophysiol 24(2):262–269, 2001

13. Seidl K, Senges J: Worldwide utilization of implantable cardioverter/defibrillators now and in the future. Card Electrophysiol Rev 7(1):5–13, 2003

14. Bernstein AD, Camm AJ, Fisher JD, et al: The NASPE/BPEG defibrillator code. PACE 16:1776–1780, 1993

Cardiopulmonary Resuscitation

1. American Heart Association: 2005 American Heart Association guidelines for cardiopulmonary resuscitation and emergency cardiovascular care. Circulation 112(Suppl IV), 2005
2. SOS-KANTO Study Group: Cardiopulmonary resuscitation by bystanders with chest compression only (SOS-KANTO): An observational study. Lancet 369(9565):920–926, 2007
3. Mair M: Monophasic and biphasic defibrillators: The evolving technology of cardiac defibrillation. Am J Nurs 103(8):58–60, 2003
4. Powers C, Martin K: When seconds count, use an AED. Am J Nurs 102(Suppl):8–10, 2002
5. Nolan JP, Morley PT, Vander Hoek TL, et al: Therapeutic hypothermia after cardiac arrest: An advisory statement by the Advanced Life Support Task Force of the International Liaison Committee on Resuscitation. Circulation 108:118–121, 2003
6. Tucker T: Family presence during resuscitation. Crit Care Nurs Clin North Am 14:177–185, 2002

Other Selected Readings

Percutaneous Coronary Interventions and Percutaneous Balloon Valvuloplasty

Astin F, Jones K: Changes in patients' illness representation before and after elective percutaneous transluminal coronary angioplasty. Heart Lung 35(5):293–300, 2006
Dumont CJ, Keeling AW, Bourguignon C, et al: Predictors of vascular complications post diagnostic cardiac catheterization and percutaneous coronary interventions. Dimens Crit Care Nurs 25(3):137–142, 2006
Lins S, Guffey D, Van Riper S, Kline-Rogers E: Decreasing vascular complications after percutaneous coronary interventions: Partnering to improve outcomes. Crit Care Nurse 26(6):38–46, 2006
Reigle J, Molnar HM, Howell C, Dumont C: Evaluation of inpatient interventional cardiology. Crit Care Nurs Clin North Am 18(4):523–530, 2006
Smith PK, Califf RM, Tuttle RH, et al: Selection of surgical or percutaneous coronary intervention provides differential longevity benefit. Am Thorac Surg 82:1420–1429, 2006
Ulvik B, Wentzel-Larsen T, Hanestad BR, et al: Relationship between provider-based measures of physical function and self-reported health-related quality of life in patients admitted for elective coronary angioplasty. Heart Lung 35(2):90–100, 2006

Intra-Aortic Balloon Pump Counterpulsation and Mechanical Circulatory Support

Boehmer JP, Popjes E: Cardiac failure: Mechanical support strategies. Crit Care Med 34(9 Suppl):S268–277, 2006
Golson J: Technology overview: The left ventricular assist device. J Clin Eng 31(1): 31–35, 2006
Portner PM: The state of destination therapy for the treatment of congestive heart failure. Curr Opin Organ Transplant 11:546–552, 2006
Shipgood L: Investigating the suitability of the intra-aortic balloon pump for patients in cardiogenic shock. Br J Cardiac Nurs 1(11):520–526, 2006

Management of Dysrhythmias

Angerstein RL, Thronson F, Rasmussen MJ: Enhancing care of cardiac resynchronization therapy patients: Device diagnostics and clinical application. J Cardiovasc Nurs 21(5):397–404, 2006
Bindra PS, Marchlinski FE: Ablation of ventricular fibrillation and tachycardia. Curr Cardiol Rep 7(5):342–348, 2005
Bleakley JF, Akiyama T, for the Canadian Cardiovascular Society, American Heart Association, North American Society of Pacing and Electrophysiology (NASPE), and European Society of Cardiology: Driving and arrhythmias: Implications of new data. Cardiac Electrophysiol Rev 7(1):77–79, 2003
Bubien RS, Ching EA, Kay GN: Cardiac defibrillation and resynchronization therapies: Principles, therapies, and management implications. AACN Clin Issues 15(3):340–361, 2004

Burkhardt JD, Wilkoff BL: Malfunctions in implantable cardiac devices: Putting the risk in perspective. Cleve Clin J Med 72(9):736, 738, 742, 2005
Chapnick MT: Radiofrequency catheter ablation. RN 68(10): 40–44, 2005
Chiu C, Sequeira IB: Diagnosis and treatment of idiopathic ventricular tachycardia. AACN Clin Issues 15(3):449–461, 2004
Dougherty CM, Pyper GP, Frasz HA: Description of a nursing intervention program after an implantable cardioverter defibrillator. Heart Lung 33(3):183–190, 2004
Fetzer SJ: The patient with an implantable cardioverter defibrillator. J Perianesth Nurs 18(6):398–413, 2003
Finch NJ, Leman RB: Clinical trials update: Sudden cardiac death prevention by implantable device therapy. Crit Care Nurs Clin North Am 17(1):33–38, 2005
Gura MT: Implantable cardioverter defibrillator therapy. J Cardiovasc Nurs 20(4):276–287, 2005
Gura MT, Foreman L: Cardiac resynchronization therapy for heart failure management. AACN Clin Issues 15(3):326–339, 2004
Irwin ME: Cardiac pacing device therapy for atrial dysrhythmias: how does it work? AACN Clin Issues 15(3):377–390, 2004
Jenkins LS, Brodsky M, Schron E, et al: Quality of life in atrial fibrillation: The Atrial Fibrillation Follow-up Investigation of Rhythm Management (AFFIRM) study. Am Heart J 149(1): 112–120, 2005
Leroy SS, Russell M: Long QT syndrome and other repolarization-related dysrhythmias. AACN Clin Issues 15(3):419–431, 2004
Obias-Manno D: Risk stratification and primary prevention of sudden cardiac death: Sudden death prevention. AACN Clin Issues 15(3):404–418, 2004
O'Brien MC, Langberg J, Valderrama AL, et al: Implantable cardioverter defibrillator storm: Nursing care issues for patients and families. Crit Care Nurs Clin North Am 17(1):9–16, 2005
Sealey B, Lui K: Diagnosis and management of vasovagal syncope and dysautonomia. AACN Clin Issues 15(3):462–477, 2004
Shea J: Quality of life issues in patients with implantable cardioverter defibrillators: Driving, occupation, and recreation. AACN Clin Issues 15(3):478–489, 2004
Sweesy MW: Understanding electromagnetic interference. Heart Rhythm 1(4):523–524, 2004
Sweesy MW, Holland JL, Smith KW: Electromagnetic interference in cardiac rhythm management devices. AACN Clin Issues 15(3):391–403, 2004
Thomas S, Friedmann E, Kao CW, et al: Quality of life and psychological status of patients with implantable cardioverter defibrillators. Am J Crit Care 15(4):389–398, 2006
Thompson EJ, Reich DA, Meadows JL: Radiofrequency ablation in the pulmonary veins for paroxysmal, drug-resistant atrial fibrillation. Dimens Crit Care Nurs 23(6):255–263, 2004
Timothy PR, Rodeman BJ: Temporary pacemakers in critically ill patients: Assessment and management strategies. AACN Clin Issues 15(3):305–325, 2004
Trusty JM, Beinborn DS, Jahangir A: Dysrhythmias and the athlete. AACN Clin Issues 15(3):432–448, 2004
Weiss EM, Buescher T: Atrial fibrillation: treatment options and caveats. AACN Clin Issues 15(3):362–376, 2004
Weinstock J, Wang PJ, Homoud MK, et al: Clinical results with catheter ablation: AV junction, atrial fibrillation and ventricular tachycardia. J Interv Card Electrophysiol 9(2):275–288, 2003
Yee R, Connolly S, Noorani H: Clinical review of radiofrequency catheter ablation for cardiac arrhythmias. Can J Cardiol 19(11):1273–1284, 2003

Cardiopulmonary Resuscitation

Benjamin M, Holger J, Carr M: Personal preferences regarding family member presence during resuscitation. Acad Emerg Med 11(7):750–753, 2004
Bourdreaux ED, Francis JL, Loyacano T: Family presence during invasive procedures and resuscitations in the emergency department critical review and suggestions for future research. Am J Emerg Med 40:193–205, 2002
Clark AP, Aldridge MD, Guzzetta CE, et al: Family presence during cardiopulmonary resuscitation. Crit Care Nurs Clin North Am 17(1):23–32, 2005

Cummins RO, Hazinski MF, Kerber RE, et al: Low-energy biphasic waveform defibrillation: Evidence-based review applied to emergency cardiovascular care guidelines. Circulation 97: 1654–1667, 1998

Duran C, Oman K, Abel J, et al: Attitudes toward and beliefs about family presence: A survey of healthcare providers, patients' families, and patients. Am J Crit Care 16(3):270–283, 2007

Ellison S: Nurses' attitudes toward family presence during resuscitative efforts and invasive procedure. J Emerg Nurs 29:515–521, 2003

Halm MA: Family presence during resuscitation: A critical review of the literature. Am J Crit Care 14(6):494–511, 2005

Henderson DP, Knapp JF: Report of the national consensus conference on family presence during pediatric cardiopulmonary resuscitation and procedures. J Emerg Nurs 32(1):23–29, 2006

Holzhauser K, Finucane J, DeVries SM: Family presence during resuscitation: A randomized controlled trial of the impact of family presence. Australas Emerg Nurs 8(4):139–147, 2006

Howard PK: Documentation of resuscitation events. Crit Care Nurs Clin North Am 17(1):39–44, 2005

Keresztes PA, Brick K: Therapeutic hypothermia after cardiac arrest. Dimens Crit Care Nurs 25(2):71–76, 2006

Lasater M: The role of thermoregulation in cardiac resuscitation. Crit Care Nurs Clin North Am 17(1):97–102, 2005

Long RE: Using stimulation to teach resuscitation: an important patient safety tool. Crit Care Nurs Clin North Am 17(1):1–8, 2005

Maclean SL, Guzzette CE, White C, et al: Family presence during cardiopulmonary resuscitation and invasive procedures: Practices of critical care and emergency nurses. Am J Crit Care 12:246–257, 2003

Mangurten J, Scott SH, Guzzetta CE, et al: Effects of family presence during resuscitation and invasive procedures in a pediatric emergency department. J Emerg Nurs 32(3):225–233, 2006

McClenathan BM, Torrington KG, Uyehara CF: Family member presence during cardiopulmonary resuscitation: A survey of US and international critical care professionals. Chest 122: 2204–2211, 2002

Meischke HW, Rea TD, Eisenberg MS, et al: Intentions to use an automated external defibrillator during a cardiac emergency among a group of seniors trained in its operation. Heart Lung 31:25–29, 2002

Mian P, Warchal S, Whitney S, et al: Impact of a multifaceted intervention on nurses' and physicians' attitudes and behaviors toward family presence during resuscitation. Crit Care Nurse 27(1):52–61, 2007

Oddo M, Schaller MD, Feihl F, et al: From evidence to clinical practice: Effective implementation of therapeutic hypothermia to improve patient outcome after cardiac arrest. Crit Care Med 34(7):1865–1873, 2006

Peters R, Boyde M: Improving survival after in-hospital cardiac arrest: The Australian experience. Am J Crit Care 16(3): 240–247, 2007

Peterson R: Teaching cardiopulmonary resuscitation via the web. Crit Care Nurse 26(3):55–59, 2006

Riwitis C, Twibell RS: Family presence during resuscitation: The in's and out's. Am Nurse Today 1(2):12–15, 2006

Rone T, Sauls JL: Recommendations of the international guidelines 2000 conference on cardiopulmonary resuscitation and emergency cardiac care: An overview. Crit Care Nurs Clin North Am 17(1):51–58, 2005

Samson RA, Berg RA, Bingham R, et al: Use of automated external defibrillators for children: An update. Pediatrics 112: 163–168, 2003

Sanford M, Pugh D, Warren NA: Family presence during CPR: New decisions in the twenty-first century. Crit Care Nurs Q 25(2):61–66, 2002

Smith MA: Use of vasopressors in the treatment of cardiac arrest. Crit Care Nurs Clin North Am 17(1):71–76, 2005

Swor R, Compton S, Farr L, et al: Perceived self-sufficiency in performing and willingness to learn cardiopulmonary resuscitation in an elderly population in a suburban community. Am J Crit Care 12:65–70, 2003

Wenzel V, Krismer AC, Arntz R, et al: A comparison of vasopressin and epinephrine for out-of-hospital cardiopulmonary resuscitation. N Engl J Med 350:105–113, 2004

Whitcomb JJ, Blackman VS: Cardiopulmonary resuscitation: How far have we come? Dimens Crit Care Nurs 26(1):1–6, 2007

Williams JM: Family presence during resuscitation: To see or not to see? Nurs Clin North Am 37:211–220, 2002

Common Cardiovascular Disorders

Sue Apple

19

Objectives

Based on the content in this chapter, the reader should be able to:

1 Differentiate between pericarditic and ischemic chest pain.

2 Explain the long-term effect of endocarditis on the heart valves.

3 Discuss key differences in the clinical management of dilated and hypertrophic cardiomyopathy.

4 Describe key differences in clinical presentation between arterial and venous peripheral vascular disease.

5 Compare and contrast the clinical findings of chronic aortic aneurysm with those of acute aortic dissection.

6 Compose a plan of care for the patient in hypertensive crisis covering the first hour of treatment.

The first intensive and coronary care units were developed in the mid-1960s to treat patients with acute myocardial infarction. Since those early days, critical care nurses have expanded their focus to include care of patients with a wide spectrum of cardiovascular diseases. In addition to acute myocardial infarction, these disorders include inflammation and infections of the heart muscle, pericardium, and valves, as well as diseases involving the aorta and peripheral vascular system. This chapter reviews several common cardiovascular disorders, including pericarditis, myocarditis, endocarditis, cardiomyopathies, peripheral vascular disease, aortic diseases, and hypertensive crisis.

• Infection and Inflammation of the Heart

Infectious and inflammatory diseases of the heart have multiple etiologies, making diagnosis and treatment a clinical challenge. Patients may present with acute pain mimicking myocardial infarction, or may seek medical attention because of fatigue and vague flu-like symptoms that fail to resolve over a period of weeks. Because of the permanent damage these diseases can cause to structures of the heart, patients often face serious long-term cardiac disability.

PERICARDITIS

The pericardium surrounds the external surface of heart and the roots of the great vessels. It is composed of two layers: an outer tough fibrous pericardium and an inner serous layer.[1,2] The serous pericardium has two layers: the parietal and the visceral. The parietal layer lines the internal surface of the fibrous membrane. The parietal pericardium extends to the great vessels, where it then folds over on itself to form the inner visceral layer, also known as the epicardium (Fig. 19-1). Between these two layers is 10 to 50 mL of clear serous fluid, which acts as a lubricant. The pericardium helps restrain the

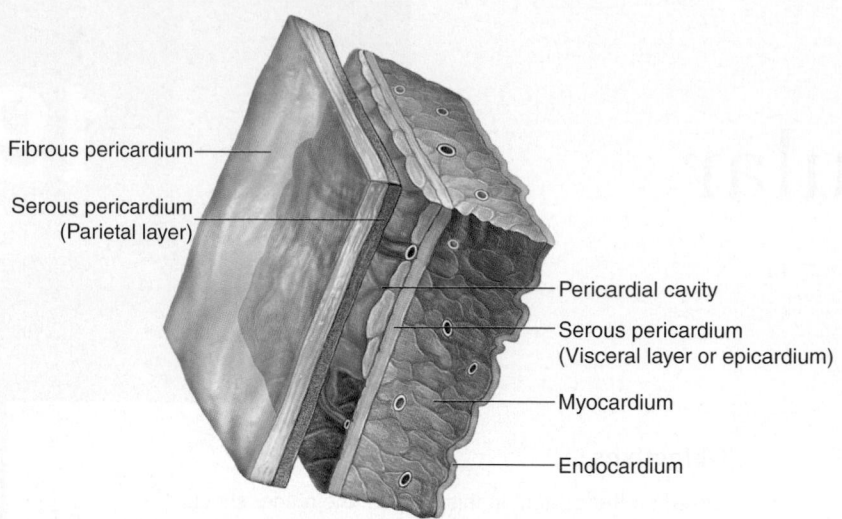

Fibrous pericardium

Serous pericardium
(Parietal layer)

Pericardial cavity

Serous pericardium
(Visceral layer or epicardium)

Myocardium

Endocardium

Figure 19-1 • Section of the heart identifying the pericardium, myocardium, and endocardium. (Reprinted with permission from Holcomb SS: Recognizing and managing different types of carditis. Nursing2005 35(6):6–11, 2005.)

heart and isolate it from infections in the surrounding structures.[3,4]

Pericarditis is inflammation of the pericardium. Acute pericarditis is pericarditis that lasts no longer than 1 or 2 weeks.[4,5] Inflammation often involves the adjoining diaphragm. Pericarditis can be a primary disease or occur secondarily as the result of some other disorder, such as acute myocardial infarction or renal failure.[5,6] The etiology of pericarditis varies. However, in almost 90% of patients diagnosed with acute pericarditis, the exact cause is unknown (idiopathic).[4,5] Causes of pericarditis are listed in Box 19-1. Dressler's syndrome refers to the development of pericarditis, malaise, fever, and elevated white blood cell count appearing weeks to months after a myocardial infarction. This syndrome is believed to be the result of an autoimmune reaction that occurs after the infarct.[3] Infectious pericarditis remains a problem in the immunocompromised patient.[7]

Repeated episodes of pericarditis can lead to the formation of adhesions between the layers of the pericardium or between the pericardium and adjacent structures, resulting in constrictive pericarditis.[8] In constrictive pericarditis, the primary problem is failure of the heart to fill during diastole because of its inability to expand. Unless the diseased pericardium is removed surgically, diastolic filling continues to be impaired, eventually leading to a decrease in cardiac output and systemic signs of heart failure. Even with successful surgical removal of the diseased pericardium, the long-term survival rate is poor.[4,8]

Assessment

Important clues to the diagnosis of pericarditis can be obtained from the history and physical examination. The primary symptom in acute pericarditis is chest pain.[4,6] The pain tends to be pleuritic in nature and classically is made worse by breathing deeply or lying supine. Because of pain from breathing, patients frequently complain of dyspnea. Relief is often obtained by sitting up, leaning forward, and taking shallow breaths. The chest pain of pericarditis may be difficult to distinguish from ischemic chest pain.[5] Differential diagnoses of chest pain are summarized in Table 19-1. One clue in the differentiation is that ischemic chest pain is not relieved by a change in the patient's position.

There may also be general symptoms of an infection, such as a low-grade fever, tachycardia, or malaise. The presence of a pericardial friction rub confirms the diagnosis; however, absence of a rub does not rule out pericarditis. The classic friction rub produces a rasping or scraping high-pitched sound that varies with the cardiac cycle. The rub may wax and wane and may even transiently disappear during the course of the illness. It is best heard with the diaphragm of the stethoscope placed over the lower to middle left sternal edge.[3,6]

There are no specific guidelines for the evaluation or management of acute pericarditis. The electrocardiogram (ECG) is the most important test in establishing the diagnosis.[4] It classically shows diffuse ST-segment elevation with an upward concavity and

Box 19-1 • Causes of Pericarditis

- Idiopathic (usually presumed to be viral)
- Infectious
- Bacterial
- Tuberculosis
- Autoimmune or inflammatory
- Systemic lupus erythematosus
- Drugs
- Vaccinations
- Neoplasms
- Radiation therapy
- Following device implantation, such as an implantable defibrillator
- Acute myocardial infarction
- Trauma to the chest wall or myocardium, including cardiopulmonary surgery
- Chronic renal failure requiring dialysis

Table 19-1 • Differential Diagnosis of Chest Pain

Diagnosis	Onset of Pain	Quality of Pain	Relieved by
Angina pectoris	Sudden, after heavy meal or exertion	Crushing Squeezing Choking	Rest, nitrates
Acute myocardial infarction	Varies, may be associated with feeling of doom	Similar to angina, but more severe	No relief with rest
Pericarditis	Varies, may be preceded by "flu-like" symptoms for several days to weeks	Pleuritic Sharp, stabbing	Sitting up Shallow breathing NSAIDs
Acute aortic dissection	Sudden, may be associated with syncope Intense from the onset	Ripping Tearing Worst pain in patient's life	No relief

NSAIDs, nonsteroidal anti-inflammatory drugs.

PR-segment depression (Fig. 19-2). This contrasts with the ECG seen in acute myocardial injury, which typically shows upward convexity in leads facing the infarct zone (Fig. 19-3).[4-6] The chest radiograph may not be helpful. Although the echocardiogram is usually normal in acute pericarditis, it is indicated in patients with suspected pericardial disease.[9]

Laboratory tests include complete blood count, cardiac enzymes (which may be elevated if the inflammation extends to the myocardium), rheumatoid factors, and antinuclear antibody titers. Blood cultures may be indicated if there is evidence of infection. Viral studies may be obtained if the rest of the diagnostic workup is negative.

Management

Treatment goals for the patient with pericarditis are to relieve symptoms, eliminate any possible causative agents, and monitor for complications such as constrictive pericarditis or pericardial effusions that could lead to cardiac tamponade.[3,6] Symptom relief includes the use of nonsteroidal anti-inflammatory drugs such

as aspirin or ibuprofen. Steroids may be indicated in resistant cases in which infectious causes have been excluded. Anticoagulants should be avoided in the patient recovering from myocardial infarction.

Most episodes of pericarditis abate over 2 to 6 weeks. Rarely do patients experience recurrent episodes. Athletes with acute pericarditis should not participate in competitive sports until the acute phase is over (Box 19-2).[10]

MYOCARDITIS

Myocarditis is an inflammation of the myocardium.[3,11] Primary myocarditis is believed to be related to an acute viral infection or an autoimmune response to the infection. Secondary myocarditis is inflammation related to a specific organism. Potential causes of both types, which can occur in any age group, are listed in Box 19-3. The prevalence is unknown because the clinical presentation is so varied and often subacute.[12] Myocarditis can be a devastating illness that evolves into a chronic, progressive disease with a poor prognosis. The disorder may result in dysrhythmias,

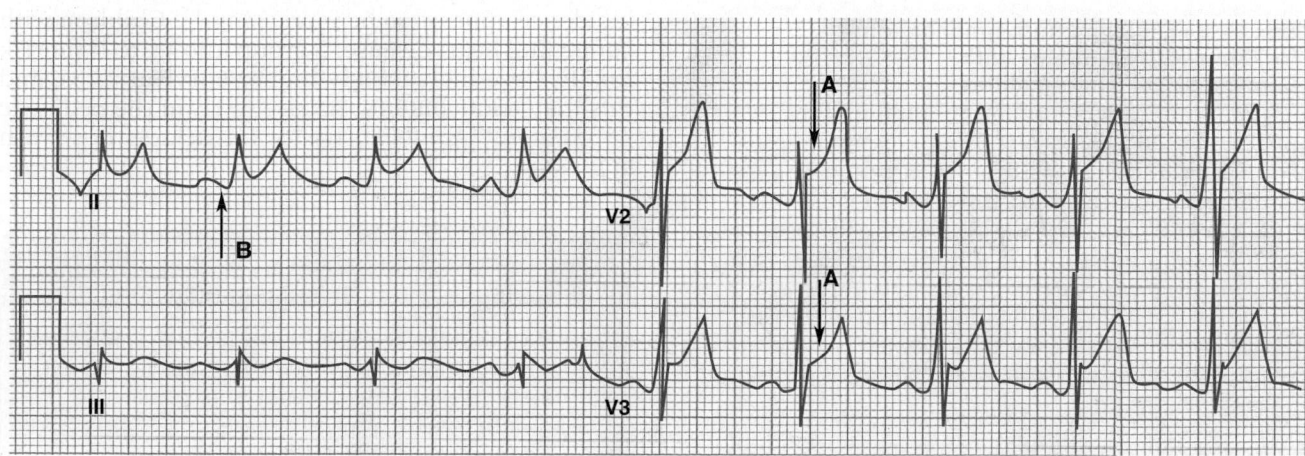

Figure 19-2 • The 12-lead electrocardiogram in acute pericarditis. Note the diffuse upward concavity ST changes (**A**) and the PR-segment depression (**B**).

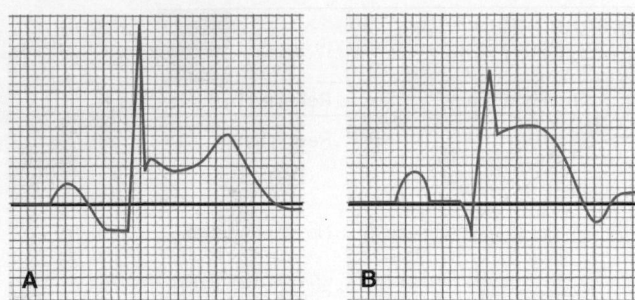

Figure 19-3 • ST-segment changes seen in (**A**) acute pericarditis and (**B**) myocardial infarction.

congestive heart failure, or death.[11] It is also recognized as a cause of sudden death in young athletes.[10]

Assessment

The clinical presentation of myocarditis is variable. With viral myocarditis typically there is a delay before the onset of cardiac symptoms such as congestive heart failure or dysrhythmias.[3,11] The presence of vague symptoms, such as fatigue, dyspnea, palpitations, and precordial discomfort, accompanied by a slight rise in serum enzymes and nonspecific ST-T wave changes on the ECG, may point to the diagnosis of myocarditis. Definitive diagnosis requires a positive endomyocardial biopsy.[11,12] However, lack of a positive biopsy does not rule out myocarditis. Current research is focused on finding a more reliable and safe method of diagnosing this complex disease.[12]

Management

Management of myocarditis depends on the etiology and clinical presentation; however, treatment is largely supportive.[3] Although myocarditis evokes a severe inflammatory response, treatment with corticosteroids or immunosuppressive agents has not been effective in changing the clinical course.[11,12] Some episodes of myocarditis resolve without further sequelae. In other patients, a subacute disease develops with persistent

laboratory findings of inflammation (e.g., an increased white blood cell count or an elevated sedimentation rate). Athletes with myocarditis should withdraw from competitive sports for a period of at least 6 months following the onset of disease (see Box 19-2).[10]

Box 19-4 lists nursing diagnoses for a patient with myocarditis. Many of the skills required by the nurse to care for the patient with myocarditis are similar to those needed in the care of the patient with heart failure. In addition, the nurse must be prepared to help the patient and family deal with the unexpected reality of a potentially lethal disease that often has no cure and may require heart transplantation.[3]

ENDOCARDITIS

Endocarditis is an infection of the endocardial surface of the heart, including the valves, caused by bacterial, viral, or fungal agents.[13,14] Infectious endocarditis (IE) is a serious illness associated with considerable morbidity and mortality. The incidence of IE varies with the specific population under study, but overall the incidence appears to be increasing.[3,13] Children with congenital heart disease, a group known to be at risk for IE, have increasingly higher survival rates, and this may contribute to the rise of IE in the pediatric population.[15] Adults at risk for IE include those with mitral valve prolapse or rheumatic heart disease, those who abuse intravenous drugs, and patients with prosthetic valves or long-term indwelling devices (Box 19-5).[3,13,16,17] Common infectious organisms include streptococci, enterococci, and *Staphylococcus aureus*.

The development of IE is a complex process that requires the occurrence of several critical elements.[3,13,17] First, there must be endothelial damage that exposes the basement membrane of the valve to turbulent blood flow. Next, this exposure, especially in patients in a hypercoagulable state, must lead to the development of a platelet and fibrin clot on the valve leaflet. These clots, or vegetations, must be exposed to bacteria by way of the bloodstream, such as occurs after dental manipulations or urological procedures. Finally, bacterial proliferation must take place. Bacteria proliferate on these vegetations for two reasons: (1) the turbulent blood flow across the valves helps concentrate the numbers of bacteria near the vegetation; and (2) the vegetation itself covers the bacteria with layers of platelets and fibrin, protecting the bacterial colony from the body's natural defense mechanisms. The infected vegetation interferes with normal valve function and eventually damages the valve structure. These incompetent valves eventually lead to severe heart failure. Particles from the infected vegetation or severely damaged valve can break loose and cause peripheral emboli.[3,13,14,17]

Assessment

Symptoms of endocarditis usually occur within 2 weeks of the precipitating bacteremia and are related to four underlying processes: bacteremia or fungemia, valvulitis, immunologic response, and peripheral emboli (Box 19-6).[13,16] Nonspecific complaints, such as general malaise, anorexia, fatigue, weight loss, and night sweats, are common. Because symptoms are nonspecific, a careful history focusing on risk factors for IE and a physical examination are needed to alert the nurse to the potential diagnosis of endocarditis.[3] Fever and a new or changed heart murmur are present

---

Box 19-5 • Risk Factors for Endocarditis

Native Valve Endocarditis
- Mitral valve prolapse
- Congenital heart disease
- Rheumatic heart disease
- Degenerative valve disease (such as aortic stenosis)
- Age greater than 60 years
- Intravenous drug abuse

Prosthetic Valve Endocarditis
Early (Within 60 Days of Surgery)
- Nosocomial infections
- Indwelling catheters
- Endotracheal tubes

Late (After 60 Days)
- Dental, genitourinary, or gastrointestinal manipulations

Box 19-6 • Clinical Features of Endocarditis

- Fever
- Heart murmurs
- Splenomegaly
- Petechiae
  Splinter hemorrhages
  Osler's nodes (small, raised, tender nodules that occur on the fingers or toes)
  Janeway lesions (small erythematous or hemorrhagic lesions on the palms or soles)
- Musculoskeletal complaints
- Systemic or pulmonary emboli
- Neurological manifestations
  Headache
  Mycotic aneurysms

---

in almost all patients.[13] The nurse should suspect IE in any patient with these clinical findings.[3,14]

Definitive diagnosis of IE includes persistent bacteremia caused by typical IE pathogens and evidence of myocardial involvement such as echocardiographic visualization of a vegetation or new or worsening murmur (Duke criteria).[18,19] Three separate sets of blood cultures are usually drawn. Meticulous site preparation is necessary to avoid contamination.[3]

Management

Rapid diagnosis of IE, initiation of appropriate treatment, and early identification of complications are the keys to good patient outcomes.[3,16] Antibiotic therapy is based on the results of the cultures and the clinical setting (i.e., native valve versus prosthetic valve IE). Recommended therapies have been revised to account for a dramatic increase in drug resistance among common IE organisms.[16] Treatment should not be delayed while waiting for identification of the specific organism but should begin as soon as blood cultures are drawn. Immediate surgical intervention is indicated in the presence of severe congestive heart failure secondary to valve dysfunction, uncontrolled infections, and prosthetic valve dysfunction or dehiscence.

Cure of IE is difficult and requires complete eradication of the bacterial colony from the vegetation. This usually involves a prolonged course of antibiotics.[3,16] Box 19-7 outlines considerations for discharge planning for the patient with endocarditis.

• Cardiomyopathies

The cardiomyopathies are diseases of the heart muscle that cause cardiac dysfunction resulting in heart failure, dysrhythmias, or sudden death.[20–22] Since 1995, the cardiomyopathies have been separated into distinct categories: dilated, hypertrophic, restrictive, arrhythmogenic right ventricular cardiomyopathy, and unclassified.[23] However, advances in molecular genetics and improvements in diagnostic imaging

Box 19-8 • Cardiomyopathies and Their Classification

Definition

"Cardiomyopathies are a heterogeneous group of diseases of the myocardium associated with mechanical and/or electrical dysfunction that usually (but not invariably) exhibit inappropriate ventricular hypertrophy or dilatation and are due to a variety of causes that frequently are genetic. Cardiomyopathies either are confined to the heart or are part of generalized systemic disorders, often leading to cardiovascular death or progressive heart failure–related disability." (Maron et al., 2006, p. 1809)

Classification

Primary cardiomyopathies are solely or predominantly confined to heart muscle. Primary cardiomyopathies are classified according to etiology and include genetic (such as hypertrophic cardiomyopathy), mixed genetic and non-genetic (such as dilated cardiomyopathy), and acquired (such as inflammatory or peripartum cardiomyopathy).

   Secondary cardiomyopathies have myocardial involvement as part of systemic disorders (such as amyloidosis or diabetes).

Adapted from Maron BJ, Towbin JA, Thiene G, et al: Contemporary definitions and classification of the cardiomyopathies: An American Heart Association scientific statement from the Council on Clinical Cardiology, Heart Failure and Transplantation Committee; Quality of Care and Outcomes Research and Functional Genomics and Translational Biology Interdisciplinary Working Groups; and Council on Epidemiology and Prevention. Circulation 113:1807–1816, 2006.

have revealed that the cardiomyopathies are more heterogeneous, which has led to proposal of a new definition and classification scheme (Box 19-8).[20] This section focuses on the most common types of primary cardiomyopathies in Western countries: dilated and hypertrophic cardiomyopathies (Table 19-2).

DILATED CARDIOMYOPATHY

Dilated cardiomyopathy (DCM) is characterized by increased myocardial cavity size in the presence of normal or reduced left ventricular wall thickness and impaired systolic function.[20,21] The heart gradually assumes a globular shape accompanied by ventricular chamber dilation.[22] As ventricular dilation progresses, mitral and tricuspid insufficiency develop as the valve leaflets are stretched and separated. Dysrhythmias such as ventricular tachycardia as well as conduction defects commonly occur.

DCM is the third most common cause of heart failure, the most common cause of heart failure in the

Table 19-2 • Primary Cardiomyopathies

Cardiomyopathy	Pathology	Clinical Manifestations	Management
Dilated (DCM)	Systolic dysfunction Chamber dilation with normal left ventricular wall thickness *Increased atrial chamber size* *Increased ventricular chamber size* *Decreased muscle size*	• Congestive heart failure • Fatigue, weakness • Dysrhythmias • Systemic or pulmonary emboli	• Identify and eliminate potential causes such as alcohol • Symptomatic treatment • Manage heart failure, dysrhythmias • Biventricular pacing or implantable cardioverter defibrillator in selected patients • Genetic testing • Family screening to identify asymptomatic members with DCM
Hypertrophic (HCM)	Diastolic dysfunction Marked hypertrophy of left ventricle, occasionally also of right ventricle, and usually (but not always) disproportionate hypertrophy of septum *Thickened interventricular septum* *Left ventricular hypertrophy*	• Dyspnea • Angina • Fatigue • Syncope • Palpitations • Dysrhythmias • Congestive heart failure • Sudden death	• Symptomatic treatment • Medications • Implantable cardioverter defibrillator • Septal wall ablation or surgery in select patients • Volume reduction surgery • Genetic testing • Family screening to identify asymptomatic members with HCM

Images reprinted with permission from the Anatomical Chart Company: Atlas of Pathophysiology. Springhouse, PA, Springhouse, 2001.

young, and the most frequent cause of heart transplantation.[20] It occurs most frequently in middle-aged men, and 20% to 35% of cases are familial.[20,22] In most cases, the specific cause is unknown. The etiology of DCM is various, including familial and genetic factors, viral infections (i.e., past episodes of viral myocarditis), immunological defects, and exposure to toxins.[20,21,24] Many researchers believe that alcohol is the most prevalent toxic cause of DCM.[21]

Assessment

The natural history of DCM is not well defined. Some patients remain asymptomatic or have minimal clinical findings. Symptoms usually develop gradually and are typically related to left ventricular heart failure. The presence of right-sided heart failure is associated with poor prognosis.[3,21] Laboratory tests include screening for potentially reversible causes, including human immunodeficiency virus. The echocardiogram is needed to differentiate the primary abnormality and determine the ejection fraction. Cardiac catheterization may be needed to exclude coronary artery disease.[3,21,24]

Management

Treatment goals include identifying and eliminating potential causes of DCM. Patients and their families should be questioned carefully about alcohol consumption because myocardial damage related to alcohol is reversible if detected early and the patient abstains from further drinking.[3,21,24] Clinical management is focused on control of heart failure and other problems such as dysrhythmias or intracoronary thrombus. Biventricular pacing may be helpful in medically refractory patients with severely symptomatic heart failure and a prolonged QRS on the ECG, dilated left ventricle, and poor ejection fraction.[25] Implantable cardioverter-defibrillators (ICDs) may also be indicated in select patients to prevent sudden death associated with lethal dysrhythmias.[25] Only heart transplantation and some medical therapies have been shown to prolong life.[21]

HYPERTROPHIC CARDIOMYOPATHY

Hypertrophic cardiomyopathy (HCM) is distinguished by a hypertrophied, nondilated left ventricle that is not related to any obvious cause such as hypertension or aortic valve stenosis.[20,21] The most characteristic feature of HCM is diastolic dysfunction. The heart is able to contract but is not able to relax and remains abnormally stiff in diastole. In a few patients, septal wall hypertrophy occurs, leading to a left ventricular outflow tract obstruction during systole.[3,21,26]

HCM is probably the most frequently occurring cardiomyopathy in the United States. It appears to be a common autosomal dominant genetic malformation; indeed, it is probably the most common genetic cardiovascular disorder, affecting approximately 1 in 500 of the population.[20,22,26]

Sudden death is a catastrophic outcome of HCM, usually from a ventricular dysrhythmia, in asymptomatic or mildly symptomatic people of any age group. In the United States, HCM is a leading cause of sudden death in competitive athletes as well as in people participating in recreational sports.[10,27] The risk for sudden death is constant; mortality is higher in younger patients.[3] Early identification of patients at risk for HCM (and therefore, sudden death) is imperative. However, there is no agreement on the best method to identify people at high risk at this time.[21,26]

Assessment

Many patients with HCM are asymptomatic or have only mild complaints.[3,21,24] The condition is often found unexpectedly during investigation of heart murmurs or family screening. The most common symptom is dyspnea, which may be exacerbated with exertion. Presyncope and syncope also frequently occur. Left ventricular hypertrophy (LVH) present on the echocardiogram confirms the diagnosis. Borderline LVH may be a normal finding in competitive athletes.[20]

Management

The goals of management include controlling symptoms, preventing complications, and reducing the risk for sudden death.[3,21] Genetic screening and counseling are also indicated.[26] Most symptomatic patients can be medically managed. ICDs are indicated in patients who have survived an episode of sudden death or have documented potentially lethal ventricular dysrhythmias.[25] In patients with symptoms resulting from septal hypertrophy, percutaneous ablation with ethanol or surgery to remove a portion of the septum may by necessary.[3,21]

Psychosocial concerns are important as patients and families try to cope with this debilitating and potentially fatal illness. They must deal with feelings of uncertainty and loss of control as well as the financial impact of a serious chronic illness.

• Peripheral Vascular Disease

Peripheral vascular disease includes a group of distinct disorders involving the arteries, veins, and lymphatic vessels of the peripheral circulation—the noncardiac diseases that affect the circulation as a whole.[28,29] The next section focuses on peripheral arterial and venous disease.

PERIPHERAL ARTERIAL DISEASE

Peripheral arterial disease (PAD) refers to processes that cause obstruction to the blood supply of the lower or upper extremities.[28,29,30] The incidence of PAD depends on the population studied and the method used to establish the diagnosis. In general, symptomatic PAD is a disease of the elderly found more commonly in men aged 70 years and older.[28,29] Although the incidence of PAD increases steadily with age, the disease is more likely to occur in patients of any age with risk factors for atherosclerosis, such as smoking or diabetes. Other risk factors for PAD include hypertension, lipid disorders, family history, postmenopausal state, and hyperhomocysteinemia.[28,29] With the aging of the population of the United States, management of PAD is a major focus not only of prevention and cure but also of maintenance of quality of life and independence (Box 19-9).

Atherosclerosis is the most common cause of PAD. The disease develops in major bifurcations and areas of acute angulations (Fig. 19-4). In people with diabetes, there is greater involvement of the smaller and more distal vessels. Upper extremity involvement is less common than lower extremity involvement.[28]

Thromboangiitis obliterans, or Buerger's disease, is a severe, chronic inflammatory disease affecting the intermediate and small arteries of the extremities. It may also involve adjacent veins and nerves. The etiology is unknown, but it is associated with heavy smoking, especially in young people. The chronic inflammatory process is often followed by thrombosis, with vascular lesions and fibrous obliteration of the vessel.[29]

Assessment

Clinical signs of PAD reflect the blood's inability to circulate freely to the extremity. Symptoms depend on the extent of the disease and the presence of collateral circulation. The classic symptom of PAD is intermittent claudication, experienced as a cramping, burning, or aching pain in the legs or buttocks that is relieved with rest.[28-31] Symptoms do not correlate with the extent of the disease. If the PAD is extensive and multilevel, the patient may present with "rest pain," that is, a sensation of burning or numbness in the foot or toes. Patients also experience trophic changes, such as hair loss on the extremities, thickening of the nails, and drying of the skin. Acute arterial obstruction, such as occurs with an embolism, results in the sudden onset of extreme pain and other signs of acute arterial obstruction (Box 19-10).[28-30]

Practice guidelines should be incorporated in the evaluation of the patient at risk for PAD.[28] This includes a careful vascular examination of the extremities and assessment of all peripheral pulses, including the measurement of segmental pressures in the legs and the ankle/brachial index (ABI). The ABI is the ratio of ankle to brachial systolic blood pressure. A normal ABI should be 1.0 or greater. Patients with critical limb ischemia may have an ABI of less than 0.518 (Fig. 19-5).[28,29]

Treadmill exercise testing can provide an objective measurement of the patient's walking ability as well as an evaluation of possible coronary artery disease.

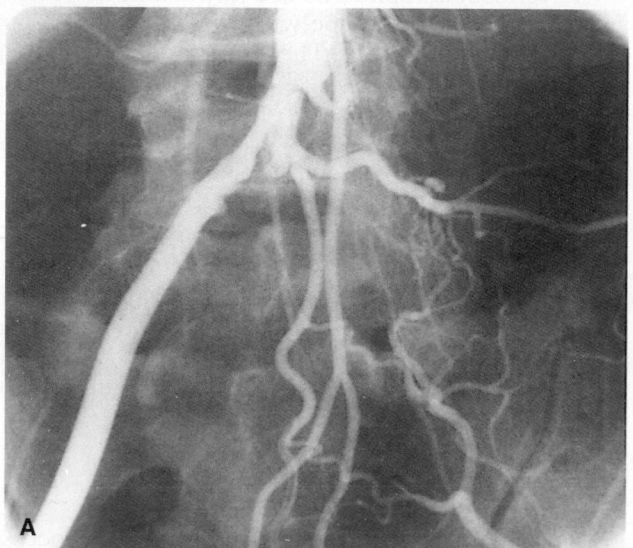

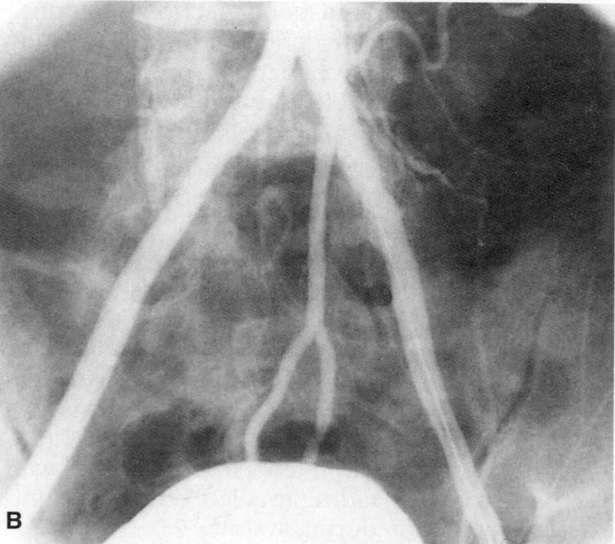

Figure 19-4 • A: A baseline angiogram demonstrating a total occlusion of the left iliac artery. In addition, there is a significant stenosis of the right common iliac artery and occlusion of the internal iliac arteries. **B:** The final result following angioplasty and stenting of the right and left common iliac arteries with Palmaz stents. (Reprinted with permission from Laird JR, Lansky AJ: Percutaneous transluminal angioplasty for the treatment of peripheral vascular disease. In Apple S, Lindsay J Jr [eds]: Principles and Practice of Interventional Cardiology. Philadelphia, Lippincott Williams & Wilkins, 2000, p 196.)

Box 19-10 • Clinical Features of Vascular Obstruction

Acute Arterial Occlusion
- Pain
- Pulselessness
- Pallor
- Paresthesia
- Paralysis

Deep Venous Thrombosis (DVT)
- Pain in calf with dorsiflexion of foot (Homans' sign)
- Pain when standing
- Inflammation
- Swelling
- Tenderness
- Redness, soreness

Noninvasive imaging such as magnetic resonance or computed tomography (CT) may be required to evaluate the extent of disease fully. Angiography is usually limited to revascularization procedures (see Fig. 19-4) or presurgical evaluation.[28,29]

Management

PAD is associated with an increased risk for atherosclerotic adverse events; the mortality rate is high in symptomatic patients.[29,30] Therefore, treatment goals

■ EVIDENCE-BASED PRACTICE HIGHLIGHT: PERIPHERAL ARTERIAL DISEASE

Excerpted from Hirsch AT, Haskal ZJ, Hertzer NR, et al: ACC/AHA 2005 practice guidelines for the management of patients with peripheral arterial disease (lower extremity, renal, mesenteric, and abdominal aortic): A collaborative report from the American Association for Vascular Surgery/Society for Vascular Surgery, Society for Cardiovascular Angiography and Interventions, Society for Vascular Medicine and Biology, Society of Interventional Radiology, and the ACC/AHA Task Force on Practice Guidelines (Writing Committee to Develop Guidelines for the Management of Patients With Peripheral Arterial Disease). Circulation 113:e463–e654, 2006.

Risk factors for lower extremity peripheral arterial disease include:

- Age >50 years and with diabetes or other atherosclerosis risk factors such as smoking or lipid disorder
- Age 50–69 years and with a history of smoking or diabetes
- Age 70 years or older
- Symptoms of claudication or ischemic rest pain
- Abnormal pulses in the lower extremities
- Presence of other vascular disease such as atherosclerotic, coronary, carotid, or renal artery disease

Examination of these patients should include:

- Assessment of walking impairment, claudication, ischemic rest pain, and/or the presence of nonhealing wounds
- Comprehensive pulse evaluation and visual inspection of the feet
- Questions concerning family history of abdominal aortic aneurysms in patients older than 50 years of age

include modifying or eliminating risk factors (especially smoking), improving leg symptoms, and maintaining limb viability. Risk factor modification incorporates national guidelines; these include immediate smoking cessation as well as aggressive treatment of hypertension, diabetes, and lipid disorders, with medication, if necessary. Other pharmacological agents include antiplatelets (aspirin or clopidogrel [Plavix]) to reduce the risk for myocardial infarction and stroke and cilostazol (Pletal) to increase walking distance. In patients with claudication, exercise improves overall walking ability. Peripheral interventional procedures, such as balloon angioplasty, are successful in restoring circulation in many cases. Surgical bypass may be required when severe or diffuse arterial obstruction is present.[28–30] Implications for home care of a patient with peripheral arterial disease are given in Box 19-11.

VENOUS DISEASE

Phlebitis is inflammation of the vessel wall occurring as the result of direct injury to the vein or as a complication of varicose veins. It can lead to the formation of a thrombus, a solid obstruction within the vein that can break loose and form a venous thromboembolism (VTE).[32,33] Factors that predispose a patient to thrombus formation are vessel wall injury, stasis of blood, and increased blood coagulability (Virchow's triad).[32,34] These three conditions have been recognized as causative factors in the development of thrombophlebitis since 1846.

An estimated 100,000 to 300,000 cases of VTE occur in the United States each year.[32,34] This incidence increases with aging.[34,35] More than half of the cases of VTE involve deep vein thrombosis (DVT),[34] and others include pulmonary embolism (PE). Because VTE is associated with significant morbidity and mortality, it is important for the nurse to be familiar with risk factors for VTE as well as current recommendations for treatment. (See Chapter 26 for information concerning pulmonary embolism.[33,36])

Assessment

DVT is characterized by pain, swelling, tenderness, and increased temperature over the affected area (see Box 19-10). The patient also exhibits a positive Homans' sign (pain in the calf with passive dorsiflexion of the foot).[32] However, these clinical findings are not specific for DVT. Accurate diagnosis usually requires diagnostic testing such as compression ultrasonography.[34]

Management

The focus of care for the patient with VTE is to relieve symptoms, increase blood flow and prevent complications. Patients with DVT are at high risk for PE. Treatment strategies include anticoagulant therapy to prevent the formation of emboli, followed by long-term warfarin use to prevent recurrence. Specific

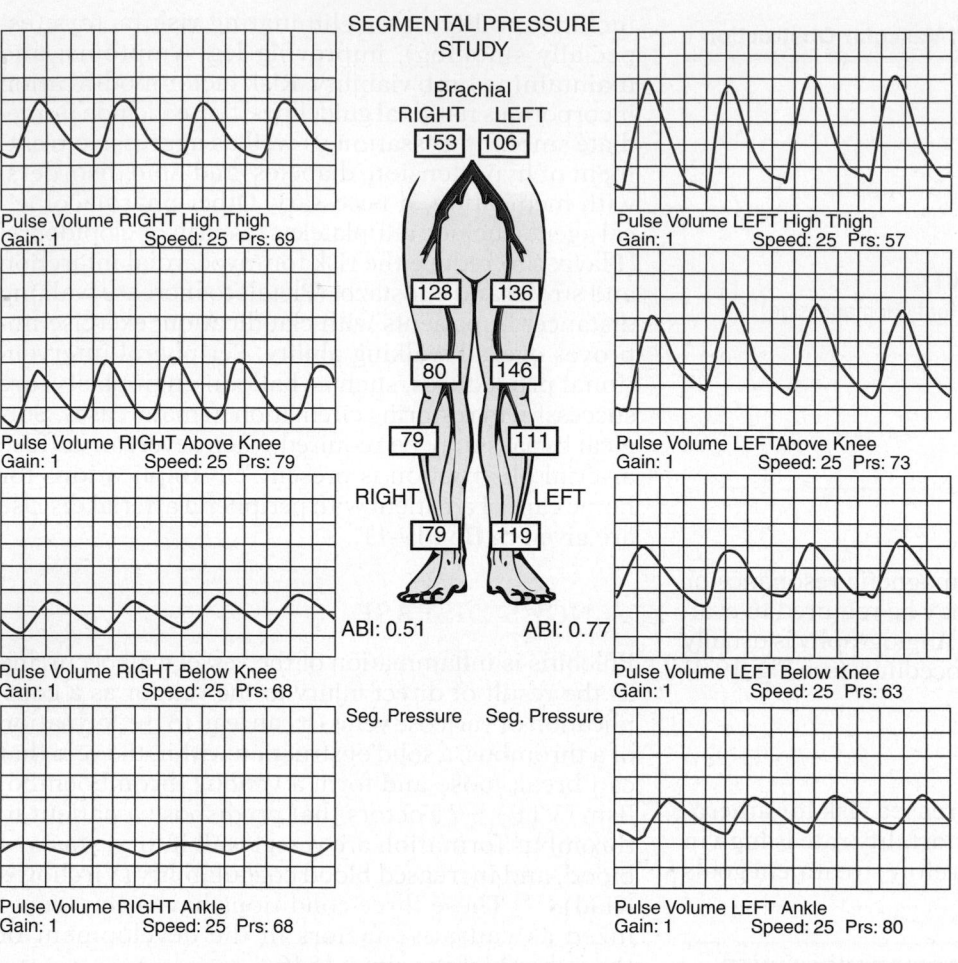

SEGMENTAL PRESSURE STUDY

Brachial
RIGHT   LEFT
153   106

Pulse Volume RIGHT High Thigh
Gain: 1   Speed: 25 Prs: 69

128   136

Pulse Volume RIGHT Above Knee
Gain: 1   Speed: 25 Prs: 79

80   146

Pulse Volume RIGHT Below Knee
Gain: 1   Speed: 25 Prs: 68

79   111

RIGHT   LEFT

79   119

ABI: 0.51   ABI: 0.77

Seg. Pressure   Seg. Pressure

Pulse Volume RIGHT Ankle
Gain: 1   Speed: 25 Prs: 68

Pulse Volume LEFT High Thigh
Gain: 1   Speed: 25 Prs: 57

Pulse Volume LEFTAbove Knee
Gain: 1   Speed: 25 Prs: 73

Pulse Volume LEFT Below Knee
Gain: 1   Speed: 25 Prs: 63

Pulse Volume LEFT Ankle
Gain: 1   Speed: 25 Prs: 80

Figure 19-5 • Segmental pressures and ankle/brachial indices (ABIs) indicating bilateral lower extremity occlusive disease with more severe involvement of the right lower extremity. There is also a probable significant stenosis of the left subclavian artery, which explains the difference between the right and left brachial pressures (Prs, pressures). (Reprinted with permission from Saucedo JF, Laird JR: Peripheral vascular disease. In Apple S, Lindsay J Jr [eds]: Principles and Practice of Interventional Cardiology. Philadelphia, Lippincott Williams & Wilkins, 2000, p 47.)

therapy depends on the patient's history and clinical setting.[33] Bleeding is the most common complication of therapy. Patient teaching includes safe administration of home anticoagulation as well as behaviors to decrease the recurrence of DVT.[32]

• Aortic Disease

The aorta is the longest and strongest artery in the body.[37] However, over time, congenital, degenerative, hemodynamic, and mechanical factors stress this elas-

---

Box 19-11 • DISCHARGE PLANNING GUIDE:
Peripheral Arterial Disease

- Ensure that the patient has a prescription for exercise based on current assessment of the patient's physical ability.
- Develop a smoking cessation plan with the patient based on current assessment of the patient's willingness to quit.
- Target management of critical risk factors (such as diabetes and hypertension) based on current clinical guidelines.
- Arrange for adjunct pharmacotherapy as indicated.
- Follow-up is crucial to success in permanently changing behaviors.

---

tic vessel. The result is dilation of the aortic wall, leaving the patient at risk for aortic dissection or rupture.[38]

AORTIC ANEURYSM

Aortic aneurysms are defined as a localized dilation of the aorta to a size greater than 1.5 times its normal diameter.[37] Aneurysms are classified according to their shape, morphology, and location (Fig. 19-6). Fusiform aneurysms, the more common type, are diffuse dilations of the entire circumference of the artery. Saccular aneurysms are localized balloon-shaped outpouchings. Aneurysms may be thoracic or abdominal; rarely, they are both.

True aneurysms involve the entire vessel wall and are classified as fusiform or saccular. False aneurysms are not actually aneurysms but are formed when blood leaks through the wall of the aorta and is contained by the surrounding tissues (a contained rupture).[37]

Abdominal Aortic Aneurysm

Abdominal aortic aneurysms (AAAs), which are more common than thoracic aortic aneurysms, occur more frequently in men. Smoking is the leading risk factor for AAAs, followed closely by age, hypertension, lipid disorders, and atherosclerosis.[37] Atherosclerosis is probably a major cause of AAAs, but other factors such as genetic and environmental almost certainly

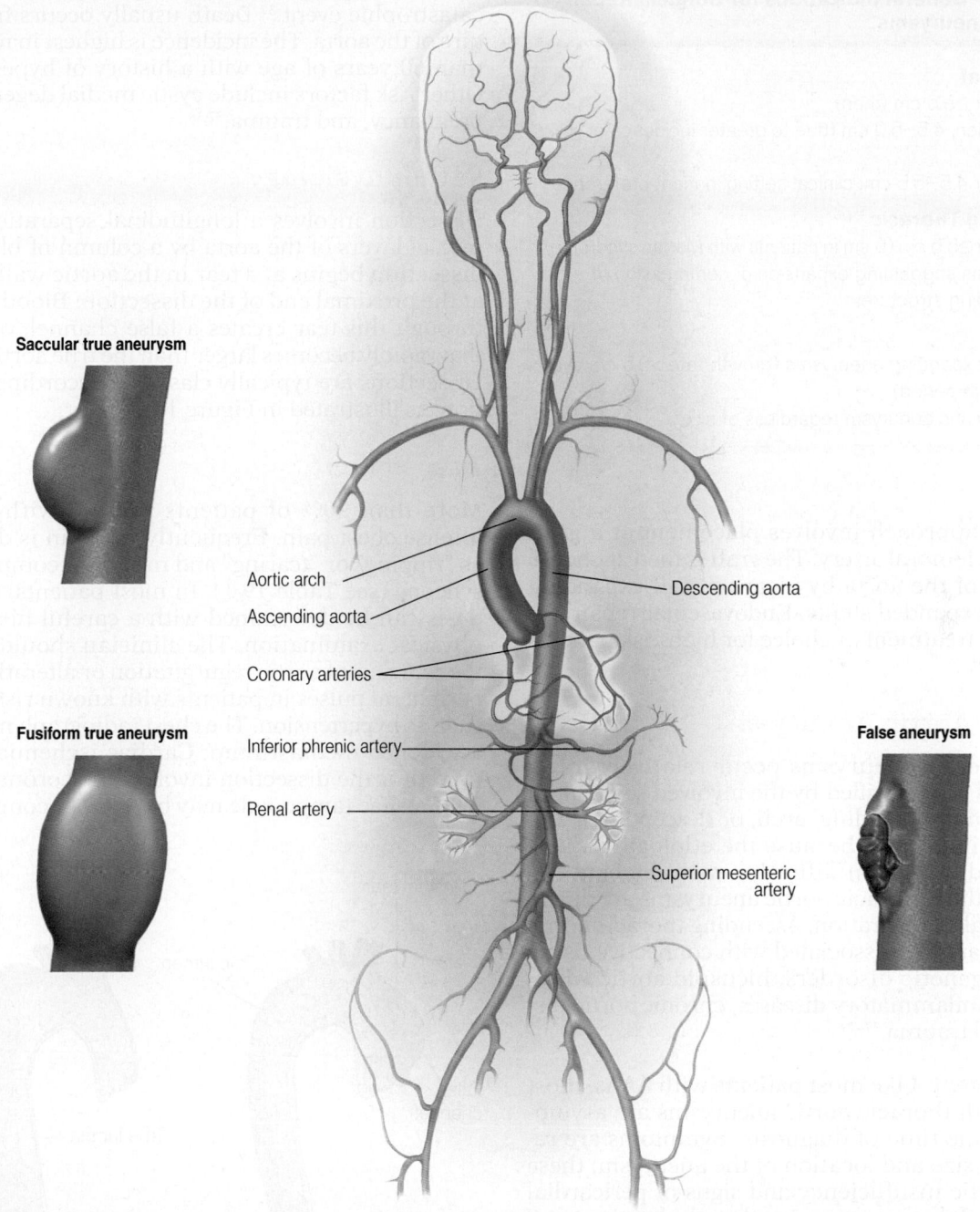

Saccular true aneurysm

Fusiform true aneurysm

False aneurysm

Aortic arch

Ascending aorta

Coronary arteries

Inferior phrenic artery

Renal artery

Descending aorta

Superior mesenteric artery

Figure 19-6 • Types of aortic aneurysms. (Reprinted with permission from the Anatomical Chart Company: Atlas of Pathophysiology. Springhouse, PA, Springhouse, 2001, p 37.)

contribute to their development.[39] The major risk from AAAs is rupture, which is associated with a high rate of mortality.

Assessment Most patients with AAAs are asymptomatic; they are typically identified during health screening for another problem. Abdominal or back pain is the most common complaint. Worsening of symptoms is usually related to expansion or rupture of the aneurysm.

Detection of AAAs by physical examination is difficult, especially in obese patients. The abdomen is examined for the presence of bruits or masses, and peripheral pulses are carefully evaluated. Abdominal ultrasonography is the most practical method of confirming the diagnosis.[37–39]

Management Management of AAAs includes control of hypertension and elimination of risk factors, such as smoking. The patient should be followed with serial noninvasive tests, such as ultrasonography. Treatment of aneurysms involves surgical repair, which is usually indicated for AAAs larger than 5.5 cm (Box 19-12).[40]

In addition to surgery, AAAs may be repaired by a minimally invasive approach using an endovascular

Box 19-12 • General Indications for Surgical Repair of Aortic Aneurysms

Abdominal
- Diameter ≥5.5 cm (men)
- For women, 4.5–5.0 cm (due to greater incidence of rupture)
- Diameter 4.5–5.5 cm; clinical setting, patient preference

Ascending Thoracic
- Diameter ≥5.5 (5 cm in patients with Marfan syndrome)
- Symptoms suggesting expansion or compression of surrounding structures

Other
- Rapidly expanding aneurysms (growth rate >0.5 cm over a 6-month period)
- Symptomatic aneurysm regardless of size

graft. This approach involves placement of a graft through the femoral artery. The graft is then anchored to the wall of the aorta by means of self-expanding or balloon-expanded stents. Endovascular repair has become the treatment of choice for high-risk patients with AAAs.[41]

Thoracic Aortic Aneurysm

Thoracic aortic aneurysms occur relatively infrequently and are classified by the involved segment of the aorta (root, ascending, arch, or descending). The location is important because the etiology, natural history, and treatment differ for each segment.[37,39] Most ascending thoracic aortic aneurysms are due to cystic medial degeneration. Ascending thoracic aortic aneurysms are also associated with connective tissue disorders, genetic disorders, bicuspid aortic valve, infections, inflammatory diseases, chronic aortic dissection, and trauma.[37–39]

Assessment Like most patients with AAAs, most patients with thoracic aortic aneurysms are asymptomatic at the time of diagnosis. Symptoms are related to the size and location of the aneurysm; these include aortic insufficiency and signs of pericardial tamponade if the aneurysm involves the aortic root.[37] Rupture or acute dissection of a thoracic aneurysm can be fatal. Less than half of patients with rupture survive to hospitalization, and by 24 hours, mortality is almost 80%.[37]

Management For most ascending thoracic aortic aneurysms, surgical repair is indicated at a diameter of 5.5 cm or more.[39] These indications vary according to the clinical situation and the existence of comorbidities. Repair of descending thoracic aneurysms is recommended when the diameter is 6 cm or more.[39]

AORTIC DISSECTION

Acute aortic dissection is the most common and the most lethal process involving the aorta. Mortality rates are very high, approaching 1% per hour for this catastrophic event.[37] Death usually occurs from rupture of the aorta. The incidence is highest in men older than 60 years of age with a history of hypertension. Other risk factors include cystic medial degeneration, pregnancy, and trauma.[37,38]

Pathophysiology

Dissection involves a longitudinal separation of the medial layers of the aorta by a column of blood. The dissection begins at a tear in the aortic wall, usually at the proximal end of the dissection. Blood pumped through this tear creates a false channel, or lumen, that rapidly becomes larger than the true aortic lumen. Dissections are typically classified according to location, as illustrated in Figure 19-7.

Assessment

More than 90% of patients present with sudden, intense chest pain. Frequently the pain is described as "ripping" or "tearing" and may be accompanied by syncope (see Table 19-1). In most patients, the diagnosis can be determined with a careful history and physical examination. The clinician should look for the murmur of aortic regurgitation or alteration of the peripheral pulses in patients with known risk factors, such as hypertension. The chest radiograph may show a widened mediastinum. Cardiac ischemia may be present if the dissection involves the coronary arteries. Cardiac tamponade may be another complication

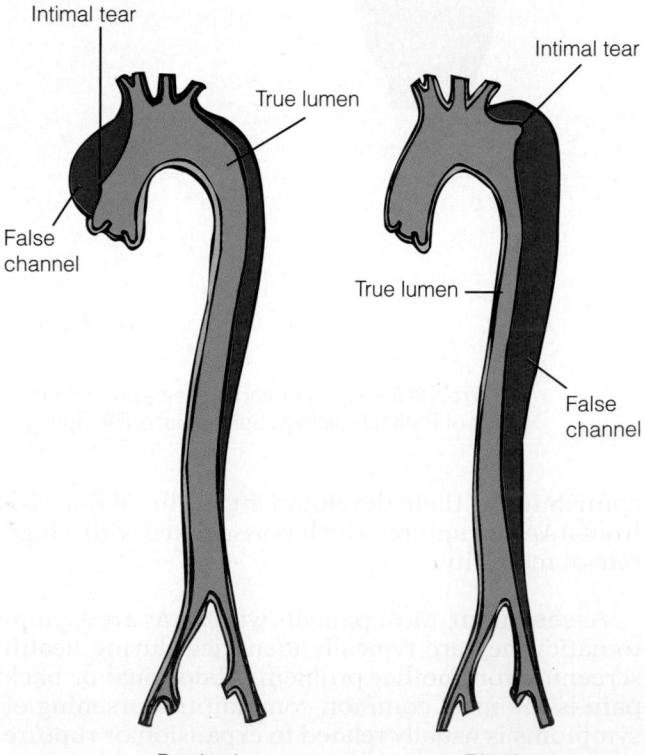

Figure 19-7 • Two major patterns of aortic dissection. Blood pumps through a tear in the wall, creating a false channel or lumen. The false channel rapidly becomes larger than the true lumen.

of dissection involving the aortic root. Neurological deficits may occur if the aortic arch vessels are involved. Dissections involving the renal arteries result in elevated serum creatinine, decreased urine output, and severe hypertension that is difficult to manage.

To confirm the diagnosis of acute aortic dissection, transesophageal echocardiography or contrast medium–enhanced CT may be ordered.[37–39]

Management

Survival of the acute phase depends on the location of the dissection, the severity of the complications, and the rapidity with which the diagnosis is confirmed. Clinical management focuses on controlling the blood pressure and on pain management. Surgery is the treatment of choice when the dissection involves the ascending aorta.[37,38]

• Hypertensive Crisis

Hypertension affects approximately 50 million people in the United States and is a major controllable risk factor for the development of cardiovascular diseases.[42,43] Recognition of the extent of this risk led to the inclusion of a new category in the classification of hypertension, prehypertension, which includes individuals with a systolic blood pressure of 120 to 139 mm Hg or a diastolic blood pressure of 80 to 89 mm Hg (Table 19-3). People with prehypertension should be counseled to adopt healthy lifestyle modifications to reduce their risk for cardiovascular disease.

Patients with high blood pressure are at risk for experiencing a hypertensive crisis. A hypertensive crisis or emergency is defined as an acute elevation of blood pressure (>180/120 mm Hg) that is associated with acute or imminent target organ damage.[42] This rare but potentially fatal condition strikes about 1% to 2% of hypertensive patients, occurring more frequently in African American men and in elderly patients.

PATHOPHYSIOLOGY

A hypertensive crisis is characterized by a marked rapid increase in blood pressure that initially leads to intense vasoconstriction as the body attempts to

protect itself from the elevated pressure. If the blood pressure remains critically high, compensatory vasoconstriction fails, resulting in increased pressure and blood flow throughout the vascular system. In the cerebral circulation, this may quickly lead to hypertensive encephalopathy.[42,43] Hypertensive crisis is associated with a variety of clinical situations (Box 19-13).

ASSESSMENT

Most patients who present with hypertensive crisis are critically ill and in need of immediate treatment. Clinical findings depend on the degree of vascular injury.[43] Signs of encephalopathy include headache, visual disturbances, confusion, nausea, and vomiting. Examination of the eyes may reveal cotton-wool exudates and hemorrhages, indicating damage to retinal nerves and rupture of retinal blood vessels; papilledema is diagnostic of increased intracranial pressure. Chest pain may represent acute coronary syndrome or aortic dissection. Depending on the damage to the kidneys, the patient may present with decreased urine output (oliguria) or azotemia (excess urea in the blood).[43,44]

MANAGEMENT

The goal is to reduce the mean blood pressure within 1 hour of starting treatment, and to prevent or reverse target organ damage.[42,45,46] Several intravenous medications are indicated in the treatment of hypertensive crises; the choice depends on availability and the clinical situation (Table 19-4). Constant monitoring is necessary to avoid lowering the

---

Table 19-3 • Classification of Blood Pressure for Adults

Blood Pressure Classification	Systolic (mm Hg)	Diastolic (mm Hg)
Normal	<120	and <80
Prehypertension	120–139	or 80–89
Stage 1 hypertension	140–159	or 90–99
Stage 2 hypertension	≥160	or ≥100

Adapted from the Seventh Report of the Joint National Committee on Prevention, Detection, Evaluation, and Treatment of High Blood Pressure (JNC 7). May 2003. Available at: http://www.nhlbi.nih.gov/guidelines/hypertension.

Box 19-13 • Summary of Hypertensive Crisis

Causes
- Acute or chronic renal disease
- Exacerbation of chronic hypertension
- Sudden withdrawal of antihypertensive medications

Associated Clinical Situations
- Acute cerebrovascular syndrome
    - Acute stroke
    - Hypertensive encephalopathy
- Acute cardiovascular syndromes
    - Myocardial infarction
    - Unstable angina
    - Pulmonary edema
- Aortic dissection
- Extensive burns
- Postoperative period
- Pheochromocytoma
- Eclampsia

Management
- Intravenous medications with continuous arterial pressure monitoring
- Goal is to reduce mean arterial blood pressure over 1 hour by no more than 25% while avoiding hypoperfusion

Table 19-4 • Intravenous Medications in Hypertensive Emergencies*

Drug	Class	Onset of Action	Adverse Effects
Sodium nitroprusside	Vasodilator	Immediate	Hypotension, nausea, vomiting, muscle twitching, thiocyanate and cyanide toxicity, methemoglobinemia
Nitroglycerin	Vasodilator	1–2 min	Hypotension, reflex tachycardia, headache, tolerance with prolonged use
Labetalol	Adrenergic blocker	<5 min	Nausea, vomiting, bronchospasm, heart block
Fenoldopam	Vasodilator	<5 min	Reflex tachycardia, headache, nausea
Esmolol	Adrenergic blocker	Immediate	Hypotension, heart block
Nicardipine	Calcium channel blocker	5–6 min	Reflex tachycardia, headache, nausea, vomiting, flushing
Enalaprilat	Angiotensin-converting enzyme inhibitor	10–15 min	Hypotension, renal failure
Hydralazine	Vasodilator	15–30 min	Reflex tachycardia, headache, exacerbation of angina pectoris

*Choice of agent depends on the etiology of the hypertensive emergency and the clinical setting.
Adapted from Mansoor GA, Frishman WH: Comprehensive management of hypertensive emergencies and urgencies. Heart Dis 4:358, 2002; and Tuncel M, Ram VCS: Hypertensive emergencies: Etiology and management. Am J Cardiovasc Drugs 3(1):21–31, 2003.

blood pressure too quickly. This is best accomplished with an intra-arterial catheter.

Once the blood pressure has been stabilized, treatment goals depend on the etiology of the crisis. All patients require careful long-term management to control their blood pressure and prevent future episodes.

• Clinical Applicability Challenges

Case Study

Ms. V. is a 19-year-old Hispanic woman who has been admitted to the intensive care unit (ICU) from the delivery room for an episode of acute pulmonary edema that developed during the birth of her first child. She has recently entered the United States from Central America; she arrives at the hospital alone and speaks very little English. Through an interpreter, it is determined that she has received no prenatal care and is taking no medications. She denies any past medical problems, but she has never seen a physician before. She denies using tobacco, alcohol, or drugs.

Physical examination reveals an enlarged heart, presence of an S$_3$ and S$_4$, and a murmur of mitral regurgitation. A chest radiograph demonstrates marked cardiac enlargement. A transthoracic echocardiogram reveals severe left ventricular enlargement and dysfunction; ejection fraction is estimated at 35% (normal is 50%–70%). Based on the results of these tests, Ms. V. is diagnosed with peripartum cardiomyopathy.

Ms. V. is currently on the cardiac stepdown unit receiving the following medications: enalapril, 5 mg twice a day; carvedilol, 25 mg twice a day; digoxin, 0.25 mg daily; amlodipine, 5 mg daily; furosemide, 40 mg daily; milrinone, 0.50 µg/kg/min.

She is also on a low-sodium diet and fluid restriction. This morning her vital signs are as follows: temperature, 98.2°F (36.8°C); blood pressure, 90/52 mm Hg; heart rate, 120 beats/minute; respiratory rate, 28 breaths/minute; and pulse oximetry, 92% on 2 L by nasal cannula. Telemetry (electrocardiographic) reveals sinus tachycardia with frequent premature ventricular contractions. Crackles are present in both lung bases. Laboratory results are as follows: potassium, 2.9 mEq/L; blood urea nitrogen, 45 mg/dL; creatinine, 2.0 mg/dL; brain natriuretic peptide, 50 pg/mL; troponin, 0.02 ng/mL; white blood cells, 9.0 × 10^3 mL; hemoglobin, 10.0 g/dL; and hematocrit, 30.3%.

During morning report, you learn that Ms. V. is refusing medications, stating that they are making her "feel bad." She has minimal contact with the health care team, largely because of the language barrier. Ms. V. also complains bitterly about her diet, and she now obtains high-calorie, high-sodium food from an outside source. Although she is frequently on the telephone, she has no visitors.

1. What are the priority medical problems for Ms. V.?
2. What are the priority nursing actions for Ms. V.?
3. What are some potential long-term problems facing Ms. V.?

Review Questions

1. A nurse is evaluating a 16-year-old athlete who collapsed on a football field and required emergency resuscitation. Which statement by the mother has the greatest implication for the entire family?
   a. She states that her other three sons once fainted during football practice but never required hospitalization.

b. She states that her son would not have fainted if he had eaten breakfast.

c. She states that her son probably just over-exerted himself trying to perform better than his brothers.

d. She states that her father and uncle have diabetes and high blood pressure.

2. A nurse is evaluating a patient who presents to the emergency department with a severe headache for the past 3 days. Which findings should alert the nurse to prepare for immediate reduction of the blood pressure (BP)?

a. BP, 150/90 mm Hg; complaints of headache, weakness, and fatigue; normal neurological examination; urine output 90 mL/hour

b. BP, 190/130 mm Hg; complaints of headache, weakness, and fatigue; nausea, vomiting; urine output 15 mL/hour

c. BP, 160/100 mm Hg; complaints of headache, weakness, and fatigue; loss of appetite; has not voided for several hours

d. BP, 160/90 mm Hg; complaints of headache, weakness, and fatigue; normal neurological examination; temperature 102.2°F (39°C)

3. A 54-year-old man with a history of poorly controlled hypertension has been admitted to evaluate new-onset chest pain. While assessing the patient, the nurse also asks him about his pain. Which of the following findings leads the nurse to suspect dissecting aortic aneurysm?

a. The pain occurred suddenly in the patient's back and was so intense that he fainted.

b. The patient is leaning forward while sitting in a chair; he states that this relieves the pain.

c. The pain increases with exercise but goes away with rest.

d. The pain is present everywhere in the chest but is worse with coughing.

4. A nurse is preparing discharge instructions for a 42-year-old man with endocarditis who will be receiving home intravenous antibiotic therapy. Information about which of the following should be included?

a. Signs and symptoms of infection, management of chest pain, care of the access site

b. Recording daily temperature, care of the access site, avoiding crowds until therapy is complete

c. Signs and symptoms of infection, care of the access site, procedures requiring antibiotic prophylaxis

d. Care of the access site, screening of family members and genetic counseling, signs and symptoms of infection

5. A nurse is assessing a 70-year-old man with claudication. Which finding has the greatest implication for the patient's care?

a. The patient is a widower who lives in a retirement community.

b. The patient has gout.

c. The patient drives himself to appointments to his health care provider.

d. The patient smokes.

References

1. Bond EF: Cardiac anatomy and physiology. In Woods SL, Sivarajan Froelicher ES, Motzer SA, Bridges EJ (eds): Cardiac Nursing, 5th ed. Philadelphia, Lippincott Williams & Wilkins, 2005, pp 3–48

2. Porth CM: Pathophysiology: Concepts of Altered Health States, 7th ed. Philadelphia, Lippincott Williams & Wilkins, 2005, pp 536–539

3. McNeill MM: Pericardial, myocardial, and endocardial disease. In Woods SL, Sivarajan Froelicher ES, Motzer SA, Bridges EJ (eds): Cardiac Nursing, 5th ed. Philadelphia, Lippincott Williams & Wilkins, 2005, pp 776–793

4. LeWinter MM, Kabbani S: Pericardial diseases. In Zipes DP, Libby P, Bonow RO, Braunwald E (eds): Braunwald's Heart Disease, 7th ed. Philadelphia, Elsevier Saunders, 2005, pp 1757–1780

5. Lange RA, Hillis LD: Acute pericarditis. N Engl J Med 351(21):2195–2202, 2004

6. Carter T, Brooks CA: Pericarditis: Inflammation or infarction? J Cardiovasc Nurs 20(4):239–244, 2005

7. Maisch B, Ristic AD: Practical aspects of the management of pericardial disease. Heart 89:1096–1103, 2003

8. Wang A, Bashore TM: Undercover and overlooked. N Engl J Med 351(10):1014–1019, 2004

9. American College of Cardiology/American Heart Association/American Society of Echocardiography: 2003 Guideline Update for the Clinical Application of Echocardiography. Retrieved July 14, 2006, from http://www.americanheart.org

10. Maron BJ, Ackerman MJ, Nishimura RA, et al: Task Force 4: HCM and other cardiomyopathies, mitral valve prolapse, myocarditis, and Marfan syndrome. J Am Coll Cardiol 45: 1340–1345, 2005. Retrieved July 18, 2006, from http://content.onlinejacc.org/cgi/content/full/45/8/1318

11. Baughman KL, Wynne J: Myocarditis. In Zipes DP, Libby P, Bonow RO, Braunwald E (eds): Braunwald's Heart Disease, 7th ed. Philadelphia, Elsevier Saunders, 2005, pp 1697–1717

12. Baughman KL: Diagnosis of myocarditis: Death of Dallas criteria. Circulation 113:593–595, 2006

13. Karchmer AW: Infective endocarditis. In Zipes DP, Libby P, Bonow RO, Braunwald E (eds): Braunwald's Heart Disease, 7th ed. Philadelphia, Elsevier Saunders, 2005, pp 1633–1658

14. Fink AM: Endocarditis after valve replacement surgery. Am J Nurs 106:40–51, 2006

15. Ferrieri P, Gewitz MH, Gerber MA, et al: Unique features of infective endocarditis in childhood. Circulation 105:2115–2126, 2002

16. Baddour LM, Wilson WR, Bayer AS, et al: Infective endocarditis: Diagnosis, antimicrobial therapy, and management of complications. A statement for healthcare professionals from the Committee on Rheumatic Fever, Endocarditis, and Kawasaki Disease, Council on Cardiovascular Disease in the Young, and the Councils on Clinical Cardiology, Stroke, and Cardiovascular Surgery and Anesthesia, American Heart Association: Endorsed by the Infectious Diseases Society of America. Circulation 111:e394–e434, 2005

17. Moreillon P, Que Y: Infective endocarditis. Lancet 363:139–149, 2004

18. Durak DT, Lukes AS, Bright DK, for the Duke Endocarditis Service: New criteria for diagnosis of infective endocarditis: Utilization of specific echocardiographic findings. Am J Med 96:200–209, 1994

19. Li JS, Sexton DJ, Mick N, et al: Proposed modifications to the Duke criteria for the diagnosis of infective endocarditis. Clin Infect Dis 30:633–638, 2000

20. Maron BJ, Towbin JA, Thiene G, et al: Contemporary definitions and classification of the cardiomyopathies: An American Heart Association scientific statement from the Council on Clinical Cardiology, Heart Failure and Transplantation

Management of patients with heart failure requires a collaborative effort on the part of physicians, nurses, pharmacologists, and dietitians as well as other allied health professionals. The care of patients with heart failure extends across all parts of the medical system. Patients with heart failure may be located in ambulatory care, acute care, critical care, and rehabilitation care facilities. As patients take charge of their own disease prevention, the home serves as another location.

• Definition

Heart failure is a clinical syndrome characterized by shortness of breath, dyspnea on exertion, paroxysmal nocturnal dyspnea, orthopnea, and peripheral or pulmonary edema. Not all patients have all these clinical indicators. Heart failure is a general term used to describe the general clinical syndrome regardless of the kind of heart failure or the etiology that produces the symptoms. Congestive heart failure is so named because the interruption in circulation related to failure of the heart to function normally leads to congestion in the vascular beds of the lungs and peripheral tissues, resulting in respiratory symptoms and peripheral edema. The revised guidelines recently published by a joint American College of Cardiology (ACC) and American Heart Association (AHA) task force use the preferred term *heart failure* rather than congestive heart failure because patients with chronic heart failure rarely demonstrate the rales and alveolar edema associated with congestion.[2] For this reason, it is important to look at the way heart failure is classified because the pathophysiology and etiology are keys to appropriate management.

• Classification

Heart failure is more difficult to understand when signs and symptoms are common to more than one type of failure and when types of heart failure are used interchangeably. Several categories are used to describe and classify heart failure. Using these categories to organize information about heart failure and for discussion of any individual patient case makes diagnosis, management, and outcome evaluation clearer.

ACUTE VERSUS CHRONIC

The terms *acute* and *chronic* are used to describe both the onset of symptoms of heart failure and the intensity of symptoms. Heart failure of acute onset refers to the sudden appearance of symptoms, usually over days or hours. Acute symptoms have progressed to a point at which immediate or emergency intervention is necessary to save the patient's life. Heart failure of chronic onset refers to the develop-

ment of symptoms over months to years. Chronic symptoms represent the baseline condition, the limitations the patient lives with on a daily basis. If the cause of the acute onset or the acute symptoms is not reversible, then the heart failure may become chronic. For example, a patient who has an acute MI with severe damage to the left ventricle has acute heart failure with pulmonary edema, causing lasting damage to the left ventricle. As a result, the patient has poor contractility (and, therefore, dyspnea on exertion) after the MI has resolved. The patient's acute onset of heart failure has left him or her with chronic symptoms.

LEFT-SIDED HEART FAILURE VERSUS RIGHT-SIDED HEART FAILURE

Left-Sided Heart Failure   WATCH & LEARN

Left-sided heart failure refers to failure of the left ventricle to fill or empty properly. This leads to increased pressures inside the ventricle and congestion in the pulmonary vascular system. Left-sided heart failure may be further classified into systolic and diastolic dysfunction (Fig. 20-1).

Systolic Dysfunction Systolic dysfunction is usually estimated by ejection fraction, or the percentage of the left ventricular end-diastolic volume (LVEDV) that is ejected from the ventricle in one cycle. If the LVEDV is 100 mL and the stroke volume is 60 mL, the ejection fraction is 60%. Normal ejection fraction is 50% to 70%. Systolic dysfunction is defined as an ejection fraction of less than 40% and is caused by a decrease in contractility. The ventricle is not emptied adequately because of poor pumping, and the end result is decreased cardiac output.

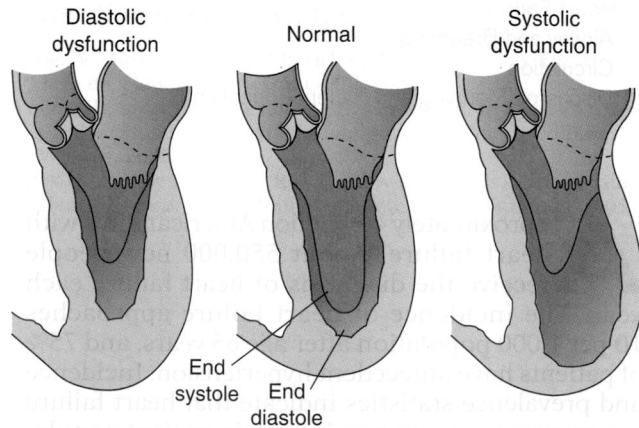

Figure 20-1 • Heart failure due to systolic and diastolic dysfunction. The ejection fraction corresponds to the difference between the end-diastolic and end-systolic volumes. Normal systolic and diastolic function with normal ejection fraction (*middle*); diastolic dysfunction with decreased ejection fraction due to decreased diastolic filling (*left*); systolic dysfunction with decreased ejection fraction due to impaired systolic function (*right*). (From Porth CM: Pathophysiology: Concepts of Altered Health States, 7th ed. Philadelphia, Lippincott Williams & Wilkins, 2005, p 608.)

Diastolic Dysfunction Diastolic dysfunction is less well defined and more difficult to measure, and it is often referred to as heart failure with preserved left ventricular function. Pumping is normal or even increased, with an ejection fraction as high as 80% at times. Diastolic dysfunction is caused by impaired relaxation and filling. Left ventricular filling, a complex process that takes place during diastole, is a combination of passive filling and atrial contraction. If the ventricle is stiff and poorly compliant (due to aging, uncontrolled hypertension, or volume overload), relaxation is slow or incomplete. If the heart rate is fast, diastole is short, or if the patient has atrial fibrillation, there is no organized atrial contraction. These mechanisms all reduce filling of the ventricle and contribute to diastolic dysfunction, therefore decreasing cardiac output.

Right-Sided Heart Failure

Right-sided heart failure refers to failure of the right ventricle to pump adequately. The most common cause of right-sided heart failure is left-sided heart failure, but right-sided heart failure can exist in the presence of a perfectly normal left ventricle and does not lead to left-sided heart failure. Right-sided heart failure can also result from pulmonary disease and primary pulmonary artery hypertension (where it is referred to as cor pulmonale). Acute onset of right-sided heart failure is often caused by pulmonary embolus.

CLASSIFICATION SYSTEMS

New York Heart Association Functional Classification

The New York Heart Association (NYHA) Functional Classification is a measure of how much the symptoms of heart failure limit the activities of patients (Box 20-1). Although ejection fraction is used to define left ventricular function, ejection fraction is poorly correlated with the patient's functional capacity or prognosis.[3]

Box 20-1 • New York Heart Association (NYHA) Functional Classification of Heart Failure

Class I: No limitation of physical activity. Ordinary physical activity does not cause undue fatigue or dyspnea.

Class II: Slight limitation of physical activity. Comfortable at rest, but ordinary physical activity results in fatigue or dyspnea.

Class III: Marked limitation of physical activity without symptoms. Symptoms are present even at rest. If any physical activity is undertaken, symptoms are increased.

Class IV: Unable to carry on any physical activity without symptoms. Symptoms are present even at rest. If any physical activity is undertaken, symptoms are increased.

Box 20-2 • American College of Cardiology (ACC)/ American Heart Association (AHA) Guidelines for Stages of Heart Failure*

A Patients at high risk for heart failure because of the presence of conditions that are strongly associated with the development of heart failure. Such patients have no identified structural or functional abnormalities of the pericardium, myocardium, or cardiac valves and have never shown signs or symptoms of heart failure.

B Patients who have structural heart disease that is strongly associated with the development of heart failure but who have never shown signs or symptoms of heart failure.

C Patients who have current or prior symptoms of heart failure associated with underlying structural heart disease

D Patients with advanced structural heart disease and marked symptoms of heart failure at rest despite maximal medical therapy and who require specialized interventions.

New York Heart Association classification is applicable only to stages C and D.

American College of Cardiology/ American Heart Association Guidelines

The ACC/AHA Guidelines outline four stages of heart failure that are useful for organizing the prevention, diagnosis, management, and prognosis for patients with heart failure[2] (Box 20-2). These stages are not meant to replace the NYHA functional classification but rather to augment it. Only stages C and D are applicable to the NYHA functional classification system.

• Factors That Determine Cardiac Output

The underlying result of all types of heart failure is insufficient cardiac output. That is, the volume of blood pumped by the heart in 1 minute is inadequate. Some patients may have a normal cardiac output at rest, but they do not have the reserve function to increase cardiac output to meet the increased demands of exercise, hypoxemia, or anemia. Therefore, it is important to understand the physiological basis of cardiac output and review the mechanisms of compensation of decreased cardiac output. (See Chapter 16 for a review of cardiovascular physiology.)

OXYGEN DEMAND

The required cardiac output is determined by the body's metabolic demand for oxygen. At rest, the body needs sufficient oxygen to burn calories to support cellular function, as measured by basal metabolic rate. Oxygen delivery to the tissues depends on arterial

440

oxygen content (CaO_2) and cardiac output. CaO_2, a combination of arterial oxygen saturation (SaO_2) and hemoglobin, is constant in healthy people. Any factor that increases metabolic demand for oxygen, such as exercise, fever, hyperthyroidism, or trauma, increases cardiac output. If CaO_2 is decreased, as it is in hypoxemia or anemia, then cardiac output increases to ensure sufficient oxygen to meet the metabolic demand. Exercise or fever in a patient with anemia puts a tremendous burden on the heart to supply sufficient oxygen to meet the metabolic demands.

A person with a healthy heart has sufficient reserve to meet this increased metabolic demand and increase cardiac output. At best, a patient with myocardial ischemia, cardiomyopathy, valvular disease, dysrhythmia, or lung disease may not be able to meet the metabolic demand for oxygen associated with exercise. At worst, the patient with one or more of these problems may not be able to meet the basal metabolic demand for oxygen and becomes symptomatic, even at rest.

MECHANICAL FACTORS

Cardiac output equals stroke volume multiplied by heart rate.

Stroke Volume

Stroke volume results from the complex interaction of preload, afterload, and contractility. Preload stretches the ventricle, and as the ventricle begins to contract, the volume of blood pumped is equally dependent on both the loading and the efficiency and force of the contraction. Approximately 60% of resting blood volume is located in the venous reservoir. This stored volume can be recruited to increase preload and therefore contractility and stroke volume.

To optimize stroke volume, these factors must be balanced; they must increase and decrease in relation to each other. Resting stroke volume can be increased by increasing preload, increasing contractility, and decreasing afterload. This happens with exercise, as does an increase in blood pressure and a neurohormonally regulated decrease in afterload. All these processes produce an increase in stroke volume. However, increased heart rate raises cardiac output much more than increased stroke volume because the ability to increase stroke volume is limited, even in a healthy heart.

Preload Preload is the volume of blood in the ventricle at the end of diastole.[4] Because of the curvilinear relationship of volume and pressure in the heart, volumes are often estimated using pressure. Volume in the heart is difficult to measure, and left ventricular end-diastolic pressure is used to estimate LVEDV and therefore preload. However, it is impossible to measure left ventricular end-diastolic pressure on a regular basis outside the catheterization laboratory; pulmonary artery wedge pressure (PAWP) is used to estimate left ventricular end-diastolic pressure. Central venous pressure and right atrial pressure are used to estimate right ventricular end-diastolic

pressure. In a person with a healthy heart, central venous pressure is an adequate estimate of left ventricular end-diastolic pressure because variation is most often related to total-body volume that affects the right and left ventricles equally. In a patient with heart or lung disease, central venous pressure does not reliably reflect left ventricular end-diastolic pressure; in these patients, many factors in addition to total-body volume may affect left ventricular end-diastolic pressure.

Afterload Afterload is the resistance to the flow of blood from the heart. Afterload depends on the competency of the heart valves, especially the aortic valve, and vascular resistance. Vascular resistance is a major contributor to blood pressure, which equals resistance multiplied by the volume or flow through the artery. Resistance is a function of both the compliance and the diameter of the artery. The ventricle must overcome resistance to open the aortic valve before any blood is pumped. A high resistance may decrease stroke volume; there is less energy to pump blood after the aortic valve is opened. Similarly, a stenotic aortic valve reduces stroke volume because stenosis restricts the opening and therefore increases the resistance to blood flow.

Contractility Contractility is the force and velocity with which the ventricle contracts. Contractility involves the alignment of actin and myosin fibers in the cardiac muscle fibers. Starling described the relationship between stretch of the muscle fibers and the velocity with which they contract. The filling of the ventricular cavity with blood stretches the muscle fibers, and the fuller the ventricle, the more stretch it has, and the more energy it has to overcome resistance and pump blood. This relationship is referred to as the Frank-Starling curve or the Frank-Starling law. Compensatory mechanisms in heart failure that attempt to maintain the cardiac output are shown in Figure 20-2.

An increase in muscle mass increases the number of fibers available for contraction and therefore increases contractility. Sufficient oxygen is also necessary for normal contraction. Calcium plays a critical role in the alignment of actin and myosin. The alignment of the fibers and the connective tissues contributes to the elliptical shape of the ventricle that makes the contraction more efficient.

Heart Rate

As stated earlier, cardiac output equals stroke volume multiplied by heart rate. Therefore, just doubling the heart rate doubles cardiac output without changing stroke volume. The immediate response to a decrease in stroke volume, a decrease in arterial oxygen content, or an increase in metabolic demand is an increase in heart rate. However, at a certain point, increasing the heart rate can actually decrease the stroke volume and therefore cardiac output as well. Because the ventricle fills during diastole, preload becomes compromised at higher heart rates

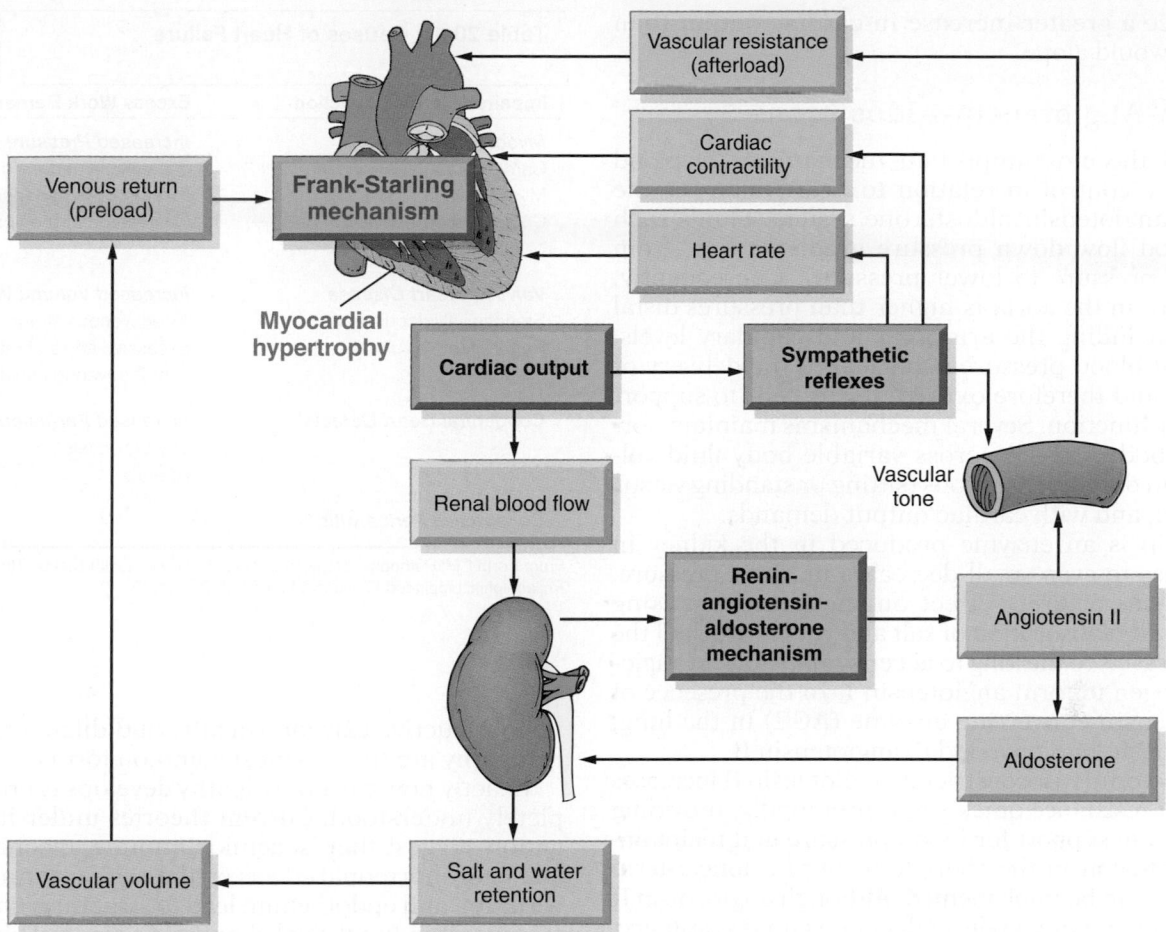

Figure 20-2 • Compensatory mechanisms in heart failure. The Frank-Starling mechanism, sympathetic reflexes, renin–angiotensin–aldosterone mechanism, and myocardial hypertrophy work to maintain cardiac output in the failing heart. (From Porth CM: Pathophysiology: Concepts of Altered Health States, 7th ed. Philadelphia, Lippincott Williams & Wilkins, 2005, p 605.)

because of the shortened diastolic filling time. A decrease in preload compromises contractility.

The physiological role of heart rate in the regulation of cardiac output involves more than just the absolute rate. Cardiac rhythm is important. As previously stated, rapid tachycardia can compromise stroke volume. Any rhythm that does not include a rhythmic atrial contraction, such as atrial fibrillation and flutter, junctional rhythms, ventricular rhythms, and ventricular pacing, can compromise filling and therefore stroke volume and cardiac output. A heart rate that is too slow, such as that which occurs in third-degree atrioventricular (AV) block or sick sinus syndrome, may compromise cardiac output, not by decreasing stroke volume, but by decreasing overall cardiac output.

NEUROHORMONAL MECHANISMS

Metabolic demand for oxygen is the primary factor in the regulation of cardiac output, and the mechanical relationships between loading and contractility provide a means to regulate it. Neurohormones are the messengers that initiate, coordinate, and mediate the complex processes that meet the dynamic need for cardiac output.

Catecholamines

Catecholamines are released from the adrenal medulla as part of the primitive "fight or flight" response to any stressor. Stressors can be physiological or psychological. Epinephrine and norepinephrine as well as cortical hormones, such as cortisol and aldosterone, are released.

Epinephrine and norepinephrine are the key catecholamines involved in the regulation of the cardiovascular system. The heart and blood vessels contain α- and β-adrenergic receptors that bind with these hormones to support cardiac output and blood pressure. Norepinephrine has almost exclusively α-adrenergic properties that increase vascular resistance and therefore blood pressure. Epinephrine has both α- and β-adrenergic properties. β-Agonist effects include increased heart rate, increased contractility, and vasodilation. The net effect of epinephrine is increased cardiac output; it increases stroke volume by increasing contractility and decreasing afterload. The increases in heart rate and stroke volume together produce a greater increase in cardiac output than either would alone.

Renin-Angiotensin-Aldosterone System

One of the most important mechanisms of blood pressure control in relation to heart failure is the renin–angiotensin–aldosterone system. Fluids such as blood flow down pressure gradients (i.e., from higher pressure to lower pressure). Consequently, pressure in the aorta is higher than pressures distal to it, including the arteriolar and capillary levels. Arterial blood pressure is critical to the delivery of blood (and therefore oxygen) to the cells to support cellular function. Several mechanisms maintain normal blood pressure across variable body fluid volumes, in different positions (sitting or standing versus supine), and with cardiac output demands.

Renin is an enzyme produced in the kidney in response to even small decreases in blood pressure. Renin has a direct effect on the kidney, causing increased reabsorption of salt and water. Much of the renin travels to the lung to act enzymatically on angiotensinogen to form angiotensin I. In the presence of angiotensin-converting enzyme (ACE) in the lung, angiotensin I is converted to angiotensin II.

A powerful vasoconstrictor, angiotensin II increases arterial resistance quickly and profoundly, providing immediate support for blood pressure and maintaining perfusion in the short term until a longer-term strategy can be implemented. Although angiotensin II has a much more modest effect on venous resistance, it does increase venous resistance and therefore venous return. Angiotensin II also stimulates the adrenal cortex to release aldosterone. Aldosterone then acts on the kidney to increase salt reabsorption in the distal tubule, and this salt increases water reabsorption in the kidney, resulting in increased circulating volume. Increased circulating volume is the longer-term strategy. The renin–angiotensin–aldosterone system initiates a process that assumes any decrease in blood pressure is a volume loss (e.g., hemorrhage), and the long-term strategy is to replace that loss.

• Pathophysiology

The physiological principles discussed in the previous section form the basis for understanding the patient's signs, symptoms, responses, and compensation for the disease process as well as the basis for management strategies. Heart failure has many causes (Table 20-1).

CARDIOMYOPATHY

The distinguishing pathophysiological factor in heart failure is the presence of a cardiomyopathy, but cardiomyopathy is not synonymous with heart failure.[2] Literally, cardiomyopathy is a progressive pathological process in the heart muscle. Cardiomyopathy may be congenital or acquired; this discussion is limited to acquired cardiomyopathy. Hypertrophic,

Table 20-1 • Causes of Heart Failure

Impaired Cardiac Function	Excess Work Demands
Myocardial Disease	**Increased Pressure Work**
Cardiomyopathies	Systemic hypertension
Myocarditis	Pulmonary hypertension
Coronary insufficiency	Coarctation of the aorta
Myocardial infarction	
Valvular Heart Disease	**Increased Volume Work**
Stenotic valvular disease	Arteriovenous shunt
Regurgitant valvular disease	Excessive administration
	of intravenous fluids
Congenital Heart Defects	**Increased Perfusion Work**
	Thyrotoxicosis
	Anemia
Constrictive Pericarditis	

From Porth CM: Pathophysiology: Concepts of Altered Health States, 7th ed. Philadelphia, Lippincott Williams & Wilkins, 2005, p. 608.

nonobstructive cardiomyopathy and dilated cardiomyopathy are the two most common forms.

Exactly how cardiomyopathy develops is not completely understood. Current theories under investigation suggest that ischemic, immune, mechanical, and neurohormonal effects on the pericardium, myocardium, and endothelium lead to structural changes that result in functional changes. Structural changes at the cellular level include replacement of contractile and elastic muscle cells with fibrotic elements, which leads to stiffness of the ventricles and smooth muscle layers in the arteries. In hypertrophic cardiomyopathy, the heart muscle becomes thickened, with increased mass and poor relaxation. In dilated cardiomyopathy, the ventricular chamber dilates, thins, and changes from a normally elliptical shape to a less efficient spherical shape, reducing contractility and impairing emptying. Both stiffness and spherical remodeling may occur in the same heart, leading to a compromised cardiac output from impaired relaxation and impaired emptying. Stiffening of arteries seen in aging, atherosclerosis, and arteriosclerosis decreases stroke volume and exacerbates the ventricular wall stress by overfilling the ventricle. The heart attempts to maintain cardiac output in the face of a decreased stroke volume by increasing heart rate, which decreases relaxation time and impairs filling. This endless spiral of dysfunction is manifested by the progressive nature of heart failure.

The resulting decrease in cardiac output leads to activation of the renin–angiotensin–aldosterone system and the release of catecholamines. As previously described, these neurohormones were meant to respond to temporary decreases in blood pressure such as hemorrhage, but in cardiomyopathy, the problem is chronic. Consequently, the neurohormonal effects, which were intended to be temporary, become permanent and become part of the problem instead of the solution to a decreased cardiac output.

The persistence of these neurohormones is hypothesized to be the mechanism by which the ventricle remodels from an elliptical shape to spherical, further decreasing its pumping efficiency. The realignment of the muscle fibers has been attributed to long-term exposure to aldosterone. Furthermore, long-term exposure to catecholamines leads to down-regulation of β-adrenergic receptors and contributes to decreased contractility.[5,6]

Hypertrophic Cardiomyopathy

Hypertrophic cardiomyopathy is an increase in muscle mass in the ventricle. The result is a measurable increase in the thickness of the ventricular wall. Hypertrophy is the response to a prolonged increase in resistance (afterload). Hypertrophy may result from prolonged or uncontrolled hypertension; it may also occur in patients with aortic stenosis, mitral stenosis, or primary pulmonary artery hypertension. Increased muscle mass results in increased energy and therefore increased contraction. However, the increase in mass decreases compliance of the ventricle and slows relaxation. The decreased compliance and slower relaxation make ventricular filling more difficult, resulting in a decrease in cardiac output even though contractility may be normal or actually increased.

Dilated Cardiomyopathy

Dilated cardiomyopathy is an increase in the size of the ventricular chamber without an increase in wall size and is a response to decreased contractility. A decrease in contractility may occur for many reasons, including ischemia, alcohol abuse, endocrine disorders, pregnancy, viral infections, and valvular disease. The result of the decrease in contractility (ejection fraction <40%) is an increase in end-systolic volume. Over time, the ventricle dilates to accommodate the increased intraventricular volumes (preload). The increased preload in a normal heart would lead to an increase in stroke volume, but in the dilated heart, the increased volume leads to a decreasing stroke volume. Dilated cardiomyopathy can be further divided into two types: ischemic and nonischemic.

Ischemic Cardiomyopathy Ischemic cardiomyopathy is the result of oxygen levels that are inadequate to meet the metabolic demands of the myocardial cells. It occurs when there is obstruction in the coronary arteries and may be acute or chronic. Oxygen is essential to the function of cells. It is necessary for the metabolism of nutritional substrates and the formation of adenosine triphosphate (ATP), which powers all intracellular processes. When oxygen is inadequate, ATP becomes insufficient, and the calcium, sodium, and potassium pumps fail, leading to interruptions in both the mechanical and electrical function of the cells. The net result is a decrease in contractility and dysrhythmia. If oxygen is restored to the muscle cells, function returns and the dysrhythmia disappears.

If the ischemia is severe or persists, the muscle tissue dies, causing an MI. Dead muscle cannot regenerate and is replaced with scar tissue. The larger the scar, the larger the dysfunction. The decrease in muscle mass leads to decreased energy for pumping blood and therefore decreased cardiac output. The goal in treatment of unstable angina and acute MI is preservation of muscle mass to prevent systolic dysfunction.

If an MI is small, the damage may be insufficient to cause heart failure because there is still enough muscle to meet the body's demands for oxygen at rest and with exercise. The ejection fraction may still be within the normal range, although it may be decreased somewhat owing to the myocardial damage. However, repeated damage from subsequent infarctions or persistent ischemia in other areas of the heart muscle may exhaust the reserve function. "Hibernating" myocardium is an area of myocardial cells that are not dead (MI) but lack sufficient oxygen and nutrient substrates to contract. Once a patient is stable after an MI, it is important to identify any viable myocardium that may be hibernating because of reversible ischemia. If perfusion can be restored to this viable but underperforming myocardium, ventricular function can be improved.

If an MI is very large, or critical structures such as the chordae tendineae are involved, then the consequences may be life-threatening. Damage or rupture of the chordae may lead to acute, severe mitral regurgitation and profound heart failure. The loss of ventricular pumping function that results from a massive MI or smaller repeated MIs may produce such an acute loss of pump function that all the body's compensatory mechanisms are not effectively able to overcome the deficit in cardiac output.

This condition represents cardiogenic shock, in which cardiac output is severely inadequate and the left ventricle empties poorly (see Chapter 54). Consequently, left ventricular end-diastolic pressure increases, pulmonary artery pressures increase, and pulmonary edema results. End-organ damage due to inadequate oxygen begins to occur depending on the function of the organ. The skin becomes cool, perhaps clammy and pale. The respiratory rate increases to supply as much oxygen as possible to the blood being pumped because the pulmonary edema severely decreases the effective area for gas transport. The pulmonary edema makes the lungs heavy and less compliant and reduces the effective tidal volume. Increases in respiratory rate are necessary to maintain minute volume. In addition, the tissues that are not adequately supplied with oxygen begin to produce lactic acid, leading to metabolic acidosis. The short-term compensation for metabolic acidosis is an increase in minute volume, or hyperpnea. The patient complains of feeling short of breath even at rest and may not be able to breathe in any recumbent position.

The hierarchy of protection in times of inadequate perfusion preserves most of the cardiac output for the brain, heart, and kidneys. Autoregulation mechanisms are present in all these organs to preserve pressure gradients and blood flow even when blood pressure and flow are compromised in other areas such as the skin, muscle, and gut. Indications that the brain is inadequately perfused are confusion, disorientation, somnolence, and agitation. Early indications of inadequate renal flow are an increase in blood urea nitrogen (BUN) and creatinine. Early on, the normal 10:1 to 20:1 ratio of BUN to creatinine increases to greater than 20:1; this signals the onset of prerenal azotemia. If perfusion is restored to the kidney at this time, the BUN and creatinine levels return to normal, as does kidney function. If the poor perfusion is profound or prolonged, the kidneys become damaged, and the BUN and creatinine continue to increase, although the ratio returns to normal. This ischemic damage to the kidneys is known as acute tubular necrosis and may be reversible.

If cardiogenic shock persists uncorrected for an extended period, the damage cannot be reversed, and the patient will die. Even if the patient is treated appropriately, further damage may occur in areas where the oxygen demand is lower than that of the brain and kidneys. Prolonged episodes of low cardiac output may lead to ileus, bowel infarction, liver failure, and increased risk for pneumonia and skin breakdown.

Patients who survive the initial episode of acute heart failure may recover completely if an intervention such as angioplasty or coronary artery bypass restores perfusion to the heart muscle and the damage to the remaining muscle is not severe. Chronic heart failure eventually develops in many patients and is characterized by the same symptoms as acute heart failure, but usually at a lower intensity; the body has had time to compensate for the decreased cardiac output. Usually, chronic heart failure does not have the intense limitations associated with acute heart failure. Patients often modify their activity to match the limited reserve of cardiac output available.

Nonischemic Cardiomyopathy Nonischemic cardiomyopathy results from several causes. A large number of people have idiopathic dilated cardiomyopathy. For some as yet unknown reason, their hearts dilate, remodel, and become ineffective pumps. Others have myocarditis, often due to viral infection of the myocardium, hypothyroidism or hyperthyroidism, valvular disease, human immunodeficiency virus (HIV), or hemochromatosis. In addition, myocarditis may be bacterial or idiopathic. Nonischemic cardiomyopathy may also result from pregnancy, heavy alcohol use, hypertension, and tachycardia. Heart failure that results from hypothyroidism or hyperthyroidism, hemochromatosis, valvular disease, and tachycardia is reversible and disappears when these problems are corrected.

Nonischemic cardiomyopathy, like ischemic cardiomyopathy, may be acute or chronic. Patients with chronic disease are often quite limited in their ability to carry out everyday activities. The mechanism by which the dilation is triggered and progresses is not well understood. Dilated cardiomyopathy, whether ischemic or nonischemic, produces symptoms after all the compensatory mechanisms have been exhausted.

Consequently, unless the onset of symptoms is acute, pathological changes may be quite advanced before activity is sufficiently limited and the patient seeks medical care. However, myocarditis frequently has an acute onset. The patient feels fine and is free of symptoms before fatigue and dyspnea on exertion, or, occasionally, pulmonary edema, suddenly develop. Dysfunction results from inflammation of the heart muscle. Metabolic function of inflamed muscle cells is impaired; the cells do not contract properly, leading to decreased cardiac output. Severity of the condition ranges from cardiogenic shock to mild limitation of activity. Once the initial acute phase passes, the patient has a low ejection fraction, with varying levels of physical limitation of activity and shortness of breath, or chronic heart failure.

Alcoholism, hypertension, and idiopathic etiologic factors are nonischemic conditions that may lead to dilated cardiomyopathy over longer periods—months to years as opposed to days to weeks with acute onset. As the ventricle begins to dilate, compensatory mechanisms, including the previously described catecholamines and other neurohormonal factors, begin to work. The proposed mechanism by which the ventricle remodels from the normal, efficient elliptical dimensions to a thin-walled, inefficient spherical shape involves constant exposure of the myocardium to these neurohormones. The natural progression is from dilation without symptoms, to compensated heart failure, to uncompensated heart failure, to refractory heart failure. Patients most often present when their heart failure is no longer compensated and symptoms interfere with normal daily activities. At this point, medication may relieve all or most symptoms. However, the structural changes that occur are progressive, and, even with medication, symptoms worsen over time. Medication can be adjusted to treat the worsening symptoms, but eventually, the medications will not be enough, and the patient dies. Mortality is usually due to worsening of the cardiac output, leading to system failure or sudden death from ventricular dysrhythmia. Before the stage of refractory heart failure is reached, much can be done to control the patient's symptoms, improve activity tolerance, control the progression of the disease, and improve quality of life.

DYSRHYTHMIA

Heart failure is commonly associated with dysrhythmias, both atrial and ventricular. The structural and metabolic changes that occur in heart failure frequently lead to dysrhythmia, and the dysrhythmia itself may lead to heart failure.

Atrial Dysrhythmias

Atrial tachycardias may cause heart failure in two ways. First, the shortened diastole leads to decreased filling and may cause or aggravate diastolic dysfunction, resulting in decreased cardiac output and the symptoms of heart failure. When the tachycardia is caused by atrial fibrillation, the loss of atrial kick increases the impact of the atrial dysrhythmia on left ventricular dysfunction. In one study, systolic dysfunction developed in 11% of patients with atrial fibrillation, and 6% of the patients died.[7]

Atrial fibrillation is a significant problem in patients with heart failure. The most common sustained dysrhythmia, atrial fibrillation, affects 2.2 million Americans. The median age for atrial fibrillation is 75 years; it affects 8.8% of Americans older than 80 years. The risk for stroke is increased 5 times in patients who have this dysrhythmia.[8] The incidence of both atrial fibrillation and heart failure increases with age, increasing the likelihood that patients with heart failure will also have atrial fibrillation at some time.

Ventricular Dysrhythmias

Ventricular dysrhythmias, in particular premature ventricular beats and nonsustained ventricular tachycardia (NSVT), are common in patients with dilated cardiomyopathy, whether ischemic or nonischemic. Sudden death from ventricular dysrhythmia or bradycardia accounts for 30% to 40% of deaths associated with heart failure.[9] The presence of premature ventricular beats or even NSVT has not been shown to be reliably predictive of risk for sudden death for any particular patient. However, the presence of these dysrhythmias does appear to reliably reflect a globally impaired myocardium.

Several mechanisms play a role in the development of ventricular dysrhythmias. The low ejection fraction leads to stretch of the myocardial fibers, thus increasing excitability. Excitability is also affected by the presence of increased catecholamines; increased sympathetic tone; and, on occasion, antiarrhythmic drugs. Activation of the renin–angiotensin–aldosterone system contributes to the overall environment that generates dysrhythmia. Ischemia leads to failure of the sodium–potassium pump, and the loss of potassium from the cell increases the risk for premature ventricular beats. Scar tissue from previous infarctions and surgery can stimulate dysrhythmia. Electrolyte shifts involving potassium, calcium, and magnesium are often associated with prolonged or aggressive diuretic use. Lung disease such as emphysema or chronic bronchitis is often comorbid with heart failure, and the lung disease may lead to hypoxemia, which contributes to the genesis of ventricular dysrhythmias. The traditional sources of ventricular dysrhythmia that occur in patients without heart failure, such as reentry, enhanced automaticity, and delayed after-potentials, may also be involved.

ACUTE EXACERBATION OF CHRONIC HEART FAILURE

Patients with chronic heart failure may live from day to day with no symptoms of heart failure or well-controlled symptoms. However, chronic heart failure may become acutely worse, resulting in an increase in symptoms and limitations associated with left ventricular dysfunction. Several factors may lead to an exacerbation.

Alcohol, anemia, hypoxemia, hypertension, ischemia, and worsening left ventricular function may trigger an acute exacerbation. Any factor that increases oxygen demand, and therefore demand for increased cardiac output beyond the ability of the ventricle to function (e.g., hypertension, tachycardia, anemia, exercise), causes an exacerbation. Similarly, any factor that depresses the function of the already compromised ventricle leads to exacerbation (e.g., alcohol, drugs that exert a negative inotropic effect such as calcium channel blockers and β-blockers). As the ventricle is called on to work harder, it works less efficiently, and the left ventricular end-diastolic pressure increases, leading to increased pulmonary artery pressures. The increased pulmonary artery pressures, in turn, lead to orthopnea, possibly pulmonary edema, elevated venous pressures, liver congestion, lower extremity edema, and paroxysmal nocturnal dyspnea. Patients may also present with lower blood pressures, more rapid heart rates, and prerenal azotemia. Potentially, the acute decompensation is reversible if treated quickly and aggressively.

• Assessment

Heart failure has long been defined by the presence of pulmonary edema characterized by bibasilar rales or crackles. Once, the absence of crackles ruled out heart failure. However, chronic heart failure is a persistent, not episodic, condition, and it rarely includes pulmonary edema and crackles. History, physical examination, diagnostic procedures, and hemodynamic evaluation all contribute to diagnosing heart failure, perhaps determining its cause, and evaluating the success of therapy.

HISTORY

The symptoms of heart failure are nonspecific (i.e., they are common to many disease processes). The history is used to put the symptoms into a context that may lead to their interpretation as heart failure and not pulmonary disease, deconditioning, or other conditions that produce shortness of breath, dyspnea on exertion, fatigue, and swelling of the lower extremities. History alone does not confirm the diagnosis, but it helps determine what follow-up examination and diagnostic tests may be appropriate.

Onset

The basic question is, "When did the symptoms start?" The answer to this question helps categorize the condition as acute or chronic. Most patients indicate an acute onset of 2 weeks or less if this is their first visit for their symptoms. If they are asked additional questions about their activity tolerance for the past year or so, patients with chronic heart failure note a gradual slowing of activity to match the amount of energy available or to control symptoms. The recent identification of symptoms indicates that the patient is now aware of them or they have become unbearable. Acuity is important because reversible ischemia is a potentially life-threatening etiology that may present acutely. When identified and treated, chronic heart failure can be avoided, and perhaps a patient's life may be saved.

Duration

It is important to know whether the symptoms are persistent and independent of activity or come and go with activity, change of position, food ingestion, or other events. This helps differentiate between heart failure and other conditions that can cause the same symptoms. Heart failure symptoms typically worsen with activity and improve with rest. Cough and shortness of breath may increase when lying down and improve with sitting up. Hiatal hernia and gastric reflux may produce shortness of breath, chest pain, and cough but typically occur after eating and more often in the evening. Lung disease or sleep apnea may also cause the shortness of breath that occurs at rest or awakens the patient at night, characteristic of heart failure. History alone does not establish the diagnosis, but it does help determine what follow-up examination and diagnostic tests may be appropriate.

Severity

Severity of symptoms is important to determine because it is the basis for establishing functional class (see Box 20-1). Severity of symptoms is also an important standard for the evaluation of the success of therapy. A major goal of therapy is symptomatic improvement or, if possible, elimination of symptoms. The evaluation of severity requires that patients be asked certain questions about their symptoms (Table 20-2).

Comorbid Diseases

Many patients with heart failure have comorbid disorders that contribute to or aggravate their heart failure. The most common of these diseases are coronary artery disease (CAD), hypertension, diabetes mellitus, chronic obstructive pulmonary disease (COPD), and chronic renal insufficiency. Worsening of one or more comorbid diseases may lead to an exacerbation of stable chronic heart failure. In the case of CAD, hypertension, and diabetes, heart failure may be the long-term result of complications of these disease processes. Identification and tight control of these comorbid diseases contribute to the control and treatment of the symptoms of heart failure.

Medications

It is very important to obtain a complete list of medications taken by the patient, with dosages. The list should include both prescription and nonprescription medications. In cases of new-onset heart failure, even old medications may contribute to the severity of symptoms. For example, patients who have been treated with a calcium channel blocker for hyper-

Table 20-2 • Assessment of Severity of Heart Failure

Symptom	Measure(s)	Questions
Orthopnea	Number of pillows patient sleeps on regularly	How many pillows do you sleep on at night? If more than one, is it for comfort or because you cannot breathe with one or two?
Dyspnea on exertion	Number of blocks patient can walk without stopping to rest or catch breath Number of flights of stairs patient can climb without stopping to rest or catch breath Number of times patient must rest while doing activities of daily living such as toileting or minor housework	How many blocks and flights of stairs can you walk without stopping to rest or catch your breath? Do you stop because you cannot go further or because you want to avoid getting short of breath? For patients who are limited by peripheral vascular disease or orthopedic problems: Do you stop because you cannot breathe or because of pain? Which comes first?
Paroxysmal nocturnal dyspnea	Average number of times per night or week	After you go to bed, do you ever have to sit up suddenly to catch your breath? How much time passes before you can breathe normally? Do you need to do anything besides sit up to relieve the shortness of breath?
Dizziness or lightheadedness	Presence or absence (of real concern when symptom occurs when the patient is standing and persists or occurs with activity)	Do you ever become dizzy or lightheaded? What are you doing when this occurs?
Chest pain or pressure*	Presence or absence	Do you have chest pain or pressure? Do you become short of breath with the chest pain or pressure? Which comes first, the pain or the shortness of breath?†

*Chest pain should be fully investigated to determine whether active ischemia is present. This is especially true in patients who are presenting for the first time for evaluation of symptoms of heart failure. Once ischemia has been ruled out, patients may still have chest pain, and it should be evaluated by using these assessment questions.
†Chest pain that comes after shortness of breath is often caused by the heart failure.

tension and now present with a decreased ejection fraction and heart failure may improve when the medication is changed and does not depress myocardial function. Other medications may contribute to heart failure. Patients taking over-the-counter medications such as nonsteroidal anti-inflammatory drugs (NSAIDs) may present with worsening heart failure and renal function because of the effect of the NSAIDs on renal blood flow. NSAIDs block the effect of prostaglandins, which the body secretes to maintain renal blood flow in the context of decreased cardiac output. Cold medicines with systemic decongestants can lead to increased blood pressure that precipitates worsening symptoms of heart failure.

Psychosocial Factors

Noncardiac factors may also affect patients with heart failure. Because many affected patients are elderly, they may have problems remembering to fill prescriptions or take medications. Financial hardships may force them to choose between buying medication and buying food. Transportation may depend on friends or family who may be unreliable. Housekeeping may be difficult or impossible because of fatigue and shortness of breath. Patients living on the second or third floor of buildings without elevators may become isolated and lonely. Depression is not uncommon; the exact incidence is not known. Ongoing family dysfunction and family members who depend on the patient for care and financial support (e.g., grandchildren, dependent adult children) add a burden to the patient's management. Illiteracy is still prevalent; even patients who can read may not read medication instructions correctly. Some patients may skip diuretic doses when visiting places where they are uncertain about access to bathroom facilities; they may not take the diuretic when they return home.

Although many of these factors are significant, they may not be obvious until the patient has visited the same health care facility many times. Early case management and skillful discharge planning depend on recognizing these problems before they lead to repeated hospitalizations and increased mortality.

Substance Abuse

Alcohol and drug (e.g., cocaine) use is also important because it may contribute to the development and progression of heart failure. If alcohol use is the cause of cardiomyopathy, abstinence may lead to complete reversal. Patients who have substance abuse problems often forget to buy or take medication. They may be homeless, which increases the likelihood that they will not return to the health care facility for regular follow-up.

PHYSICAL EXAMINATION

The physical findings in heart failure differ depending on whether the patient has (1) acute or chronic heart failure or (2) systolic or diastolic dysfunction.

When the physiological changes of left ventricular dysfunction occur over a long period, the body adapts and compensates. Consequently, many of the findings on physical examination are normal, despite moderate to severe disease. However, when the problem occurs acutely, there is no time for compensation or adaptation, and the symptoms and consequences are severe. Patients with chronic heart failure due to systolic dysfunction who do have abnormal findings have them persistently. Patients with diastolic dysfunction may have abnormal findings only during an exacerbation.

One or more of the following findings characterizes acute exacerbation. The patient may be volume overloaded by 5 to 50 pounds over dry weight; dry weight is the patient's weight when he or she is euvolemic. Patient self-monitoring is often geared to maintenance of dry weight; maintaining dry weight within 1 to 2 pounds can frequently prevent exacerbation. A second finding is often renal insufficiency characterized by an increase in both BUN and creatinine, with a ratio of BUN to creatinine of greater than 20:1. The third finding is decreased cardiac output manifested by increased dyspnea on exertion and decreased exercise tolerance in general, often described as "fatigue." Patients may also complain of increased orthopnea, paroxysmal nocturnal dyspnea, or both. Some patients have all of the findings, and it is not unusual for patients to be short of breath at rest (NYHA class IV) or demonstrate Cheyne-Stokes respirations.

General Findings

Patients with acute heart failure or acute exacerbation of chronic heart failure appear ill; they are often breathing rapidly, looking anxious, and either sitting up straight or leaning forward and resting their arms on a table or their knees. Patients with stable, chronic heart failure may be quite comfortable but may have evidence of cachexia, muscle wasting, and thin skin.

Vital Signs

Patients with systolic dysfunction may have quite low, but asymptomatic, blood pressures (systolic, 80 to 99 mm Hg; diastolic, 40 to 49 mm Hg). Heart rates may be rapid (90 beats/minute or more), or lower at rest. Patients with diastolic dysfunction may or may not be hypertensive.

Serial weights are very important in following fluid status. Daily weights, when performed properly on a calibrated scale, are more accurate estimates of fluid status than intake and output. Daily weights can be used to evaluate fluid status because 1 L of water weighs 1 kg. Overnight fluctuations in weight are always related to water retention or diuresis.

Neck

Jugular venous pressure is an estimate of right heart filling pressures. When either the total-body fluid volume or right atrial pressure increases, the jugular venous pressure increases, and the vein dilates.

Jugular venous pressure is estimated by identifying the internal jugular vein and measuring the height of the pulse from the level of the clavicle in centimeters. The patient's head is elevated to 45 degrees. It is important not to use the external jugular vein, which often appears distended and prominent in patients with normal volume and pressure.

Lungs

It is necessary to determine the respiratory rate and observe the depth of respiration as well as the respiratory rhythm. It is not unusual for patients with severe NYHA class IV heart failure to have a Cheyne-Stokes respiratory pattern. The heart failure may be chronic and persistently class IV or may represent an acute exacerbation.

Results of auscultation of the chest may be completely normal. Because patients with increased pulmonary artery pressures have increased lymph drainage over time, fluid does not collect in the alveoli. Rales or crackles are sounds made by air bubbling through water in the alveoli, and if no water is present, the sounds are not audible. When pressures increase suddenly, water is forced into the alveoli by increased hydrostatic pressure. Consequently, in acute heart failure and acute exacerbation, in which pulmonary edema is common, bibasilar crackles occur. The presence of unilateral crackles or nondependent crackles is indicative of a pulmonary process, not heart failure. Pulmonary edema can cause wheezing that may be difficult to distinguish from reactive airway disease, such as asthma.

Heart

Progression from left-sided heart failure to left-sided and right-sided heart failure or chronic elevations of pulmonary artery pressure often results in a visible, palpable right ventricular or pulmonary artery pulsation at the left sternal border. The point of maximal impulse may be extremely displaced. In advanced heart failure, it may be at the posterior axillary line and at the fifth or sixth intercostal space.

Figure 20-3 shows the areas of cardiac auscultation that are examined in a patient with heart failure. The first (S_1) and second (S_2) heart sounds are expected. The sudden appearance of a third heart sound (S_3) is a warning of impending or worsening heart failure. In chronic heart failure, S_3 is a common and chronic finding. A fourth heart sound (S_4) is common in patients with long-standing hypertension and is not considered ominous. However, in severe heart failure, all four heart sounds may be heard; this is known as a summation gallop.

When valvular disease is the cause of heart failure, a heart murmur associated with the diseased valve is heard. In patients with dilated cardiomyopathy, a mitral regurgitation murmur is commonly heard. This holosystolic murmur is best heard at the left sternal border or, in patients with very large hearts, at the apex. The mitral valve is usually structurally intact. The dilation of the left ventricle in chronic heart fail-

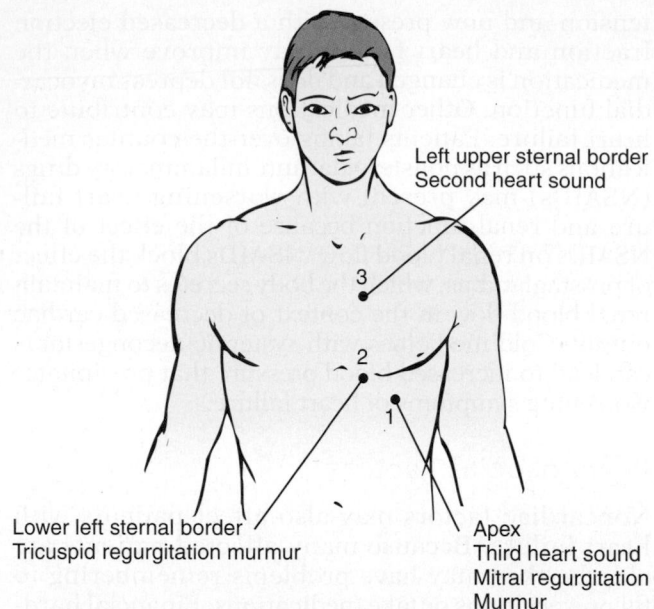

Left upper sternal border
Second heart sound

Lower left sternal border
Tricuspid regurgitation murmur

Apex
Third heart sound
Mitral regurgitation
Murmur

Figure 20-3 • Cardiac auscultation in the patient with heart failure.

ure dilates the mitral annulus and prevents the close approximation of the valve leaflets. Consequently, blood regurgitates back across the mitral valve into the left atrium with each systole.

When a mitral regurgitation murmur develops acutely, as when there is damage to the papillary muscles that open and close the mitral valve, severe, acute heart failure results. The sudden appearance of a mitral regurgitation murmur in a patient with MI is a warning of impending heart failure. The disappearance of this murmur in a patient with severe systolic dysfunction suggests a worsening of the heart failure; the ventricle cannot pump enough to generate the turbulence necessary to make the sound of the murmur.

Tricuspid regurgitation develops in patients with right-sided heart failure alone or from left-sided heart failure for the same reasons as mitral regurgitation. This murmur is also a holosystolic murmur and is heard at the right sternal border. It may be increased with inspiration. When both mitral regurgitation and tricuspid regurgitation murmurs are present, it may be impossible to distinguish between them.

Abdomen

It is necessary to palpate and percuss the abdomen to identify any ascites and the lower liver edge. High right atrial pressures that are translated into high venous pressures characterize right-sided heart failure, and the liver becomes a reservoir for the increased venous volume and increases in size (hepatomegaly) when congested. Once the liver becomes engorged, pressure increases in the portal vein and in the capillaries of the intestines. When the lymph system is no longer able to drain off sufficient fluid to relieve the pressure, ascites develops. Ascites is the transudation or third spacing of fluid and sometimes protein into the abdominal cavity. In the absence of hepatomegaly and ascites, a congested liver may conceal significant fluid. Eliciting hepatojugular reflux may identify this concealed fluid. To assess hepatojugular reflux, it is necessary to observe the internal jugular vein while pressing on the liver. When the height of the pulse increases or the vein engorges, hepatojugular reflux is positive.

Extremities

The lower extremities are inspected for the presence of edema. The edema associated with heart failure is bilateral, dependent, and pitting. Unilateral or non-pitting edema is not related specifically to heart failure, and other causes such as arterial insufficiency, myxedema, or lymphedema should be suspected.

In the ambulatory patient, the edema can be assessed by pressing the skin over the tibia. Pitting here is referred to as pretibial edema. The edema is usually graduated and worse in the ankles than at the calf, and is greater than at the thigh if the edema is present that high. In patients who are confined to bed, the edema is dependent posteriorly, and pretibial edema may be absent even in frank fluid overload. The patient must be assessed for pitting edema on the backs of the legs, the buttocks, and back. Occasionally, an ambulatory patient is so volume overloaded that presacral edema develops. To assess presacral edema and the presence of pitting, press the skin over the sacrum against the bone.

There are several schemes for describing the severity of pitting edema. None is superior to another; consistency is the most important factor. It is less important whether a series of pluses on a scale from 0 for no edema to 4+ for severe edema is based on the depth of the pit or the height of the edema on the lower extremity. When in doubt about the scale, a clear description of the depth of the pit and the level of the edema communicates the condition more effectively than a subjective number. A clear description allows for better continuity between clinicians and a better estimate of improvement.

Long-standing venous stasis and the consequent edema produce skin color and texture changes. The skin becomes leathery and discolored and may be hard to assess. These changes always indicate that the edema is chronic and not acute. Acute increases in the chronic edema may also be hard to assess. Pressing the skin firmly to the side of the tibia instead of directly over it may be of some help. Figure 20-4 shows the physical assessment findings of a patient with ACC/AHA class D chronic heart failure.

LABORATORY STUDIES

Laboratory studies are used to rule out some reversible causes of systolic dysfunction and to monitor the effects of management strategies. On initial evaluation of a patient presenting with new-onset heart failure, a battery of baseline laboratory studies is ordered (Table 20-3).

In addition to the studies listed in Table 20-3, patients who take digoxin are monitored periodically to determine whether the dose should be adjusted. The initial digoxin level is drawn 2 weeks after initia-

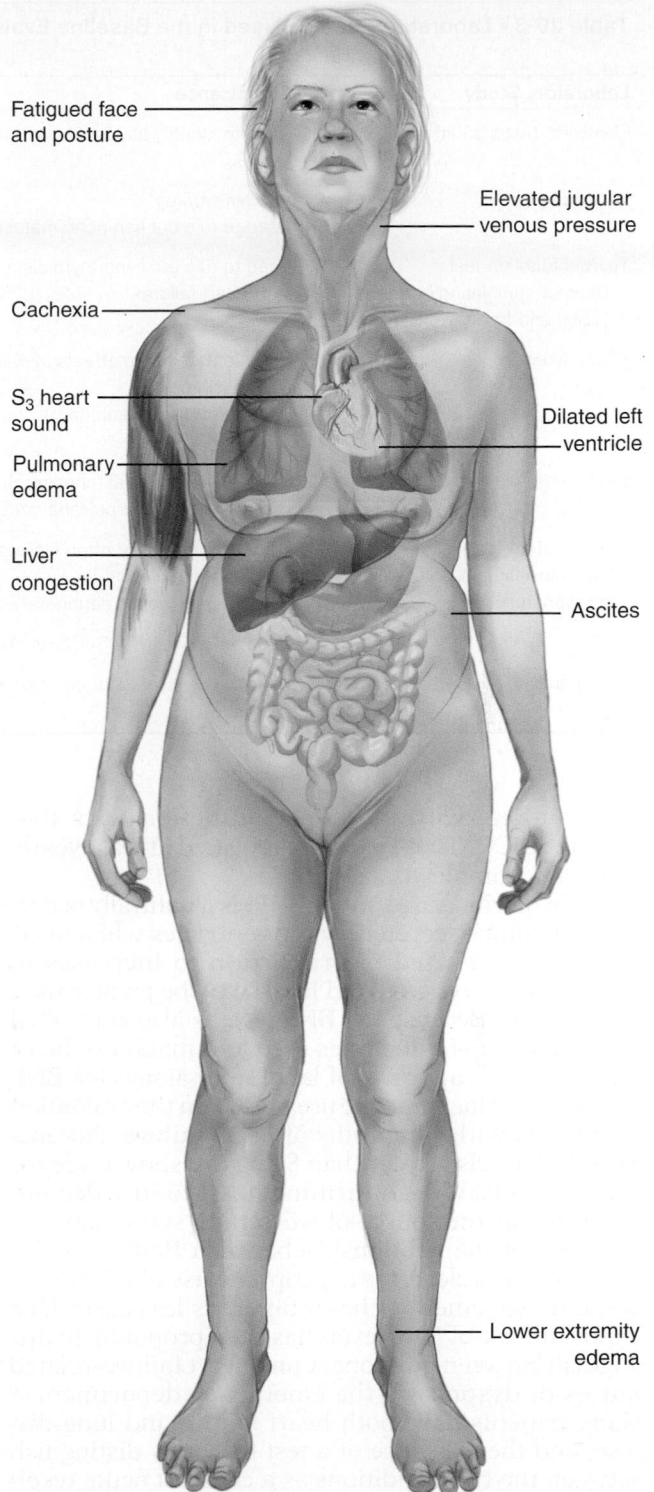

Figure 20-4 • Physical examination findings for the person with ACC/AHA class D chronic heart failure.

tion of the therapy and then as indicated by signs and symptoms or suspicion of toxic levels. Patients receiving anticoagulation therapy with warfarin are also monitored regularly, using the international normalized ratio (INR) to adjust the dose. Before the initiation of amiodarone, patients have thyroid function and liver function tests performed to obtain baseline

Table 20-3 • Laboratory Studies Used in the Baseline Evaluation of New-Onset Heart Failure

Laboratory Study	Significance	When Performed
Complete blood count	Used to identify any anemia or infection	Yearly if no specific indication With any exacerbation
Iron studies	Anemia workup Used to rule out hemochromatosis	As needed to evaluate any treatment for iron-deficiency anemia
Thyroid function tests (thyroid-stimulating hormone [TSH] and free thyroxine [T4])	Used to rule out hyperthyroidism or hypothyroidism as a cause of heart failure	No follow-up unless indicated before initiation of amiodarone
Electrolytes	Used to assess the effects of diuresis, in particular on potassium Hyponatremia is common	With changes in diuretic dose, aggressive diuresis, and titration of drugs that affect potassium (ACE inhibitors, angiotensin receptor blockers, spironolactone)
Blood urea nitrogen and creatinine	Used to assess renal function; BUN:creatinine ratio distinguishes between prerenal azotemia and kidney disease	With increased edema or an exacerbation With titration of ACE inhibitors
Liver function tests, especially albumin, bilirubin, and alkaline phosphatase (AP)	Bilirubin and AP are often elevated in liver congestion caused by heart failure Low albumin makes peripheral edema more difficult to reduce	With any exacerbation Before initiation of lipid-lowering drugs or amiodarone
HIV	Used to rule out HIV/AIDS as etiologic factor	As indicated by history or change in status
Lipid panel	Used to assess risk for coronary artery disease and nutritional status	Yearly or more often as indicated to evaluate treatment

values, along with pulmonary function tests that include DLCO. These tests are repeated at least yearly and if any complications occur.

Brain natriuretic peptide (BNP) is a naturally occurring substance secreted by the ventricles when overfilled. It is elevated in proportion to increases in end-diastolic pressure, and levels may be greater than 1000 pg/mL. Because the BNP level is also correlated with PAWP, it is sometimes used as a marker of heart failure. Recent approval of laboratory assays for BNP and pro-BNP facilitate the use of BNP in the evaluation of patients with symptoms of heart failure. Patients with BNP levels greater than 80 pg/mL show evidence of elevated PAWP, confirming heart failure decompensation as the source of worsening symptoms.

Although the relationship between BNP level and heart failure is clear, the appropriate use of BNP levels in the management of heart failure is less clear. One important use of BNP levels has been proposed: to distinguish between pulmonary and heart failure–related causes of dyspnea in the emergency department.[10] Many patients have both heart failure and lung disease, and the existence of a test that may distinguish between the two conditions as a cause of acute respiratory problems is a real advantage for individualizing and targeting treatment. In addition, BNP has been proposed as a marker for adequacy of treatment and for acute progression of heart failure, but the reliability of BNP for this use has not been established.[11]

DIAGNOSTIC STUDIES

Diagnostic studies are used to establish baseline values, identify potentially reversible etiologies, evaluate the effectiveness of treatment, and assess changes in condition. Several invasive and noninvasive tests are performed routinely when heart failure is suspected. Some tests are performed initially, when the symptoms of heart failure are first identified; some on a regular basis; and others only if indicated.

Electrocardiography

The electrocardiogram (ECG) is used to assess rate and rhythm, and it is also useful in the diagnosis of dysrhythmias, conduction defects, and MI. In addition, an ECG is often used to identify atrial enlargement and ventricular hypertrophy. However, in such cases, an echocardiogram is more helpful because it can quantify these structural changes.

ECGs are useful in the identification of the atrial fibrillation and ventricular dysrhythmias common in patients with heart failure. Sudden exacerbation of symptoms of heart failure often results from new-onset atrial fibrillation, especially when it is associated with a rapid ventricular response. An ECG can also distinguish frequent premature ventricular beats, which are common in acute and chronic heart failure. Episodes of asymptomatic NSVT often occur in patients who are monitored in ICUs, in telemetry units, or with Holter monitors. These asymptomatic dysrhythmias are usually not treated, and their prognostic importance is unclear. In contrast, symptomatic ventricular tachycardia, even if it is nonsustained, requires evaluation and usually results in placement of an implantable cardioverter–defibrillator.

Conduction defects are also common in patients with heart failure. A left bundle branch block is the most common conduction defect in patients with systolic dysfunction and may make interpretation of the ECG very difficult. New anterior ischemia or infarct may be impossible to identify because of this block. Bundle branch blocks and AV blocks require a 12-lead ECG for diagnosis.

ECGs are also useful in diagnosing ischemia, MI, and prior MI that may explain new-onset heart failure. For patients who do not present with typical chest pain (such as those with diabetes mellitus and women), the ECG may show a prior MI that was never diagnosed. New-onset heart failure may be the first indication of MI. An ECG is completed as part of the workup for new-onset heart failure and then repeated as necessary for any new symptoms that may reflect new ischemia or a rhythm change. In addition, ECGs are performed on inpatients who experience chest pain to rule out ischemia as the source of the pain.

Echocardiography

Echocardiography uses the reflection of sound waves off cardiac structures to recreate a two-dimensional representation of the heart chambers, walls, valves, and large vessels such as the aorta, pulmonary artery, and vena cava. This technique provides information about both the structure and function of the heart and is used to measure ejection fraction, evaluate valve structure and competence, and describe wall motion abnormalities. The addition of Doppler to the traditional echocardiogram allows for the evaluation of volume and direction of blood flow through the vessels and the heart. The reliability of echocardiography is greatly influenced by the competence of the echocardiographic technician and the cardiologist who interprets the echocardiograph. Echocardiography is of limited use in patients who are obese, have very large breasts, or have an increased anteroposterior chest diameter and air trapping (e.g., patients with COPD).

Transesophageal echocardiography may be performed in addition to the transthoracic echocardiography previously described. The limitations of the transthoracic procedure can be remedied by the use of the transesophageal procedure; however, the risks are increased because the transponder must be passed down the esophagus, and conscious sedation is often required. The ability to assess the mitral valve and to identify transmural clots is greatly improved when transesophageal echocardiography is used.

Radionuclide Ventriculography

A radionuclide ventriculogram or multigated acquisition (MUGA) scan is a precise means of calculating ejection fraction using a radioactive isotope. A MUGA scan is currently the gold standard for calculation of ejection fraction because it is not based on the subjective analysis of the person who "reads" it. A MUGA scan can describe abnormal wall motion, dilation, and wall thickness, in addition to ejection fraction. Valve function and flow direction cannot be evaluated by MUGA scan.

Chest Radiography

Chest radiography is useful in screening the patient with shortness of breath or dyspnea on exertion. It allows the clinician to rule out infection or pneumonia, COPD, or a mass as the cause of the patient's symptoms. Chest radiography may also help identify pulmonary edema and chronic congestion. However, because changes in the patient's condition and fluid status may not be apparent on a chest radiograph for several days, this procedure is not helpful in evaluating therapy.

Exercise Testing

When ischemia is suspected as the primary cause of the heart failure, stress testing may be used to confirm or rule out this diagnosis. When the body is physically stressed (i.e., when oxygen demand is increased, such as in exercise), heart rate and cardiac output increase. This increase requires an increased oxygen supply to the heart muscle. If the supply of oxygen is not sufficient, portions of the heart muscle become ischemic and function is decreased. For patients who can exercise, a treadmill or bike is used to provide stress, and function is measured by radioisotope uptake or echocardiography; areas of the heart that are inadequately perfused are indicated. For patients who are unable to exercise, pharmacological agents such as adenosine, dipyridamole, or dobutamine are used to simulate the increased demand for oxygen caused by exercise.

Exercise (or the pharmacological surrogate), combined with radionuclide scanning, is more sensitive and specific for the diagnosis of stress-induced myocardial ischemia than exercise testing alone. With a stress thallium test, uptake of a radioactive isotope of thallium is measured with a gamma camera at the time of peak stress or symptom development. Areas of the heart that are underperfused either do not absorb the thallium or absorb it incompletely or more slowly than the well-perfused areas. In some cases, sestamibi is used instead of thallium, and a picture is taken 12 or 24 hours later to determine whether more of the marker has been absorbed, suggesting that the heart muscle that appeared nonfunctional at first is still viable and would benefit from revascularization.

A stress echocardiogram may be used instead of a stress thallium test. Instead of the injection of an isotope such as thallium, the patient is stressed with exercise or pharmacological alternatives, and an echocardiogram is performed. The patient with ischemic myocardium may have changes in dilation, ejection fraction, or segmental wall motion that indicate that the dysfunction is related to inadequate perfusion.

In most cases, a positive stress test (i.e., one that shows stress-induced, reversible ischemia) leads to a cardiac catheterization. This procedure involves injecting radiopaque dye into the coronary arteries to evaluate the patency of the coronary arteries. Depending on the size, location, and number of lesions found in the coronary arteries, the patient undergoes balloon angioplasty and possibly receives a stent, or is referred for coronary artery bypass surgery. In many cases, correction of the perfusion abnormality completely reverses the heart failure and systolic dysfunction.

Cardiopulmonary exercise testing is used to determine whether dyspnea on exertion is more related to cardiovascular causes (ventricular dysfunction), pulmonary causes (COPD, restrictive lung disease), or deconditioning. Such testing is performed when a precise measure of activity limitation is needed or when a patient is being evaluated for heart transplantation. The patient is exercised on a treadmill or exercise bicycle while a 12-lead ECG is obtained and blood pressure is measured in response to graded exercise. In addition, all the patient's expired gases are collected and carbon dioxide is measured. This allows for the measurement of oxygen consumption, cardiac index, and anaerobic threshold.

HEMODYNAMICS

The basics of hemodynamic monitoring are discussed in Chapter 17. The application of hemodynamic monitoring in the assessment and management of acute heart failure and acute exacerbation of chronic heart failure is discussed here. It may be necessary to obtain more sensitive information about fluid status, cardiac function, and symptom causation to guide evaluation and therapy. For most patients with acute heart failure or acute exacerbation of chronic heart failure, the problem is obvious based on history and physical examination. The problem is a combination of decreased cardiac output and increased left ventricular end-diastolic pressure related to volume overload, added to poor contractility. Precise quantification of the low cardiac output or the estimation of left ventricular end-diastolic pressure by PAWP does not change the basic assessments made on physical examination and does not affect management.

Indications for Hemodynamic Monitoring

The decision to use aggressive diuresis or inotropes is not based on any specific numerical values for PAWP or cardiac output. Pulmonary artery catheters are common in critical care units today, but they are expensive and not without risk. The potential benefit of more specific, guided management must be weighed against the risk associated with pulmonary artery catheter placement.

Three types of patients with heart failure have clear indications for hemodynamic monitoring in the management of their condition. In the first type, the patient has been empirically started on inotropes and intravenous (IV) diuretics but has not responded appropriately by diuresis and improved symptoms. The second type of patient has both COPD and heart failure. At times, only pulmonary artery pressure measurements can differentiate the source of the current decompensation. However, BNP testing may be as effective in this setting. The third type of patient continues to have peripheral edema or ascites and has renal function parameters indicating worsening prerenal azotemia. This patient may benefit from a clearer definition of fluid balance; without the aid of a pulmonary artery catheter, it may be impossible to determine fluid status.

In summary, a pulmonary artery catheter is indicated in the following situations:

► The patient does not respond to empirical therapy for heart failure.
► Differentiation between pulmonary and cardiac causes of respiratory distress is necessary.
► Complex fluid status needs to be evaluated.

These categories are not mutually exclusive, and there is much overlap. They are discussed separately here, for clarity.

Inadequate Response to Empirical Therapy Respiratory distress, volume overload, and renal insufficiency are common indicators of acute heart failure or acute exacerbation of chronic heart failure. Typically, the patient needs inotropic support and IV diuresis to resolve the problem. These therapies are usually started empirically, and the patient's improvement is monitored as a basis for titration of dose. In most patients, improvement follows rapidly, and after 2 to 3 days of therapy, the inotrope is gradually discontinued, and the patient is restarted on oral therapy in preparation for discharge.

Cardiac Versus Pulmonary Cause of Symptoms In the minority of patients who do not respond to empiric therapy, a pulmonary artery catheter may be helpful in identifying any additional factors that have contributed to the persistence of symptoms, especially cardiac and pulmonary causes. It may be particularly difficult to differentiate the cause of worsening dyspnea on exertion, orthopnea, and paroxysmal nocturnal dyspnea in patients with both pulmonary disease and known heart failure. In COPD and in exacerbations of heart failure, results of history and physical examination are often identical. Pulmonary artery pressures, PAWP, and cardiac output or cardiac index can be very useful in distinguishing COPD from acute heart failure and therefore targeting therapy decisions based on the correct diagnosis. In patients with a predominantly pulmonary cause of their respiratory symptoms, pulmonary artery systolic and diastolic pressures are elevated, but PAWP, cardiac output, and cardiac index are normal. In patients with a primarily cardiac cause, pulmonary artery systolic and diastolic pressures are also elevated, but the PAWP is elevated and the cardiac output or cardiac index is decreased.

As with all PAWP readings, the measurement should be recorded on a paper printout and read at end-expiration. Most patients with dilated cardiomyopathy have some degree of mitral regurgitation. Mitral regurgitation causes V waves on the waveform; the greater the mitral regurgitation, the higher the V waves. This makes it even more important to read the PAWP from a tracing because most monitors average the highs and lows and return a falsely elevated PAWP if the value is read from the digital readout of the monitoring system.

Patients with long-standing heart failure due to dilated cardiomyopathy also tend to have higher-than-normal PAWP values even at baseline, and values of 18 to 22 mm Hg are not uncommon, even in patients who are euvolemic. Reducing their volume status to the point of normal PAWPs usually results in a decrease in cardiac output and an increase in renal insufficiency because the higher pressures are necessary for ventricular filling. Readings of PAWP must be evaluated in conjunction with cardiac output and physical findings to determine the optimum PAWP for any individual patient.

Fluid Status Patients may respond initially to IV diuresis with or without inotropes. After this initial diuresis, they begin to have a decreased urine output associated with increasing BUN and creatinine in the presence of persistent peripheral edema. They are frequently referred to as intravascularly dry.

The strategy for dealing with this problem is unclear. Insertion of a pulmonary artery catheter may determine whether high pulmonary artery pressures are the cause and whether those pulmonary artery pressures are elevated because of an elevated left ventricular end-diastolic pressure. The readings can then be evaluated in light of the patient's serum albu-min and any comorbid diseases such as primary liver failure, sepsis, or vascular insufficiency.

PULSE OXIMETRY

Pulse oximetry is frequently monitored in patients with heart failure. Unfortunately, routine intermittent monitoring is of little value. At best, it gives irrelevant information, and at worst, it enables a false sense of security over the patient's oxygen delivery status (Box 20-3). The results of pulse oximetry should be normal. Decreased estimates of oxygen saturation are usually not the result of heart failure unless the patient has severe pulmonary edema.

A low pulse oximetry reading in patients with heart failure and no pulmonary edema suggests that pulmonary disease is complicating the heart failure. Hypoxemia rarely occurs in the absence of comorbid pulmonary disease. Even patients with Cheyne-Stokes respirations associated with an acute exacerbation may have oxygen saturations greater than 95%. The pulse oximetry reading is only half of the information needed to assess oxygenation accurately. The oxygen saturation is meaningless unless the hemoglobin level

---

Box 20-3 • Pulse Oximetry

Pulse oximetry (SpO_2) estimates arterial oxygen saturation (SaO_2) or the percentage of hemoglobin (Hgb) saturated with oxygen. Oxygen saturation and hemoglobin are the two major components of arterial oxygen content (CaO_2). The dissolved oxygen in the arterial blood (PaO_2) contributes only a tiny portion of the arterial oxygen content. Arterial oxygen content multiplied by cardiac output (CO) equals tissue oxygen delivery (DO_2). If arterial oxygen content is decreased for any reason, cardiac output (mostly heart rate) increases to compensate. This is why patients with anemia or hypoxemia are tachycardic. As long as cardiac output can increase to compensate for a decreased CaO_2, tissues have sufficient oxygen to carry out their functions and the patient is asymptomatic. When a patient cannot increase cardiac output, as in heart failure, then even modest decreases in CaO_2 produce symptoms and increase the likelihood of an exacerbation or death.

$$(SaO_2 \times Hgb \times 1.34) + (PaO_2 \times 0.0031) = CaO_2$$

$$CaO_2 \times CO \times 10 = DO_2$$

Most nurses would be concerned about a patient with a pulse oximetry reading of 85%, but not one with 98%. The following examples demonstrate that the patient with normal hemoglobin and a pulse oximetry reading of 85% has more oxygen in the blood and a better oxygen delivery than a person with a 98% saturation and a hemoglobin of 10. The patients in all these examples have a normal cardiac output at rest but cannot increase cardiac output in response to decreasing arterial oxygen content.

A patient with normal blood gases and a 5-L cardiac output would have a calculated oxygen delivery of 1,000 mL O_2/minute:

$$(SaO_2 \times Hgb \times 1.34) + (PaO_2 \times 0.0031) = CaO_2$$

$$(0.98 \times 15 \times 1.34) + (90 \times 0.0031) =$$
$$19.7 + 0.3 = 20 \text{ mL } O_2/\text{min}$$

$$CaO_2 \times CO \times 10 = DO_2$$

$$20 \text{ mL } O_2/\text{min} \times 5000 \text{ mL} \times 10 = 1000 \text{ mL } O_2/\text{min}$$

Suppose a patient has a low SaO_2 and normal hemoglobin:

$$(SaO_2 \times Hgb \times 1.34) + (PaO_2 \times 0.0031) = CaO_2$$

$$(0.85 \times 15 \times 1.34) + (60 \times 0.0031) =$$
$$17.085 + 0.186 = 17.271 \text{ mL } O_2/\text{min}$$

$$CaO_2 \times CO \times 10 = DO_2$$

$$17.271 \text{ mL } O_2/\text{min} \times 5,000 \text{ mL} \times 10 = 863.55 \text{ mL } O_2/\text{min}$$

Suppose a patient has a normal SaO_2 and low hemoglobin:

$$(SaO_2 \times Hgb \times 1.34) + (PaO_2 \times 0.0031) = CaO_2$$

$$(0.98 \times 10 \times 1.34) + (98 \times 0.0031) =$$
$$13.132 + 0.3 = 13.44 \text{ mL } O_2/\text{min}$$

$$CaO_2 \times CO \times 10 = DO_2$$

$$13.44 \text{ mL } O_2/\text{min} \times 5,000 \text{ mL} \times 10 = 672 \text{ mL } O_2/\text{min}$$

Suppose a patient has low SaO_2 and low hemoglobin:

$$(SaO_2 \times Hgb \times 1.34) + (PaO_2 \times 0.0031) = CaO_2$$

$$(0.85 \times 10 \times 1.34) + (60 \times 0.0031) =$$
$$11.39 + 0.186 = 11.58 \text{ mL } O_2/\text{min}$$

$$CaO_2 \times CO \times 10 = DO_2$$

$$11.58 \text{ mL } O_2/\text{min} \times 5,000 \text{ mL} \times 10 = 579 \text{ mL } O_2/\text{min}$$

is known as well. Even normal arterial oxygen content in a patient with decreased cardiac output and no reserve may lead to tissue hypoxia. If the arterial oxygen content is decreased, as it is in patients with low hemoglobin (patients are rarely transfused unless the hemoglobin is less than 10 g/dL), the patient with heart failure may not be able to increase cardiac output enough to compensate.

Pulse oximetry may be of some value when used continuously in an ICU for patients with acute pulmonary edema. Particularly in patients with ischemic cardiomyopathy and MI, continuous monitoring may alert the nursing staff to impending ischemia or adverse effects of analgesia or conscious sedation.

• Management of Chronic Heart Failure

Heart failure is not a true disease but rather a manifestation of disease. Management is based on the same therapeutic principles that apply to any disease. The cause of disease should be identified and then treated. If an etiologic factor cannot be identified or cannot be treated, then its manifestations should be treated. Often, the cause of heart failure is not identified, and even when it is, it may not be reversible. Reversible causes of heart failure have been discussed previously and are not addressed here. Isolated right-sided heart failure (cor pulmonale) also is not addressed here.

Heart failure due to diastolic dysfunction is a complex and poorly defined entity. Few studies of investigational medications or therapies have included patients with diastolic dysfunction, and consequently there is little in the way of evidence-based therapy. In general, treatment strategies are directed toward controlling blood pressure, fluid volume, and heart rate and rhythm. There is no consensus as to how this control should be established and maintained.

Chronic heart failure secondary to dilated cardiomyopathy and systolic dysfunction is better defined. This section discusses the current evidence-based guidelines for the management of chronic heart failure and acute exacerbation. When appropriate, management of acute heart failure is distinguished from acute exacerbation; the use of IV inotropes, diuresis, and afterload reduction is similar in both conditions.

PHARMACOLOGICAL TREATMENT

The ACC and the AHA have published a consensus of evidence-based guidelines for the pharmacological management of heart failure[2] (Table 20-4). These guidelines present the most current recommendations based on available clinical trials for the medical management of heart failure. For example, heart failure in older patients has particular management implications (Box 20-4).

Angiotensin-Converting Enzyme Inhibitors

ACE inhibitors are the mainstay of standard therapy for heart failure today; they represent one third of the classic three-drug combination used. The Studies of Left Ventricular Dysfunction (SOLVD) and Cooperative North Scandinavian Enalapril Survival Study (CONSENSUS) trials demonstrated improvement in mortality as well as symptom management and exercise tolerance in even the sickest of patients with heart failure.[12,13] ACE inhibitors are typically started at low doses and titrated to target doses established in clinical trials. Studies have shown that ACE inhibitors were being underprescribed for appropriate patients, and the Assessment of Treatment With Lisinopril and Survival (ATLAS) trial found that being on the medication alone was not sufficient and that target doses used in the clinical trials were necessary to achieve the optimum results.[14]

ACE inhibitors work by blocking the renin–angiotensin–aldosterone system, resulting in vasodilation and antagonism of aldosterone and decreasing afterload and sodium reabsorption. Blockage of the long-term effects of myocardial cell exposure to the renin–angiotensin–aldosterone system is hypothesized to be the mechanism by which ACE inhibitors decrease mortality and limit the progression of remodeling.[15]

ACE inhibitors do have some side effects. Some patients are allergic to ACE inhibitors and experience angioedema, a potentially fatal reaction that involves edema of the mouth, pharynx, and larynx. There is no way to predict which patients will have this reaction, but when it presents, it is critical that the medication be stopped and a notation be made in the patient record so that it is not prescribed again. Patients should also be educated about the names of potential ACE inhibitors and why they should not be taken.

A troubling but not dangerous cough develops in some patients who take ACE inhibitors. Typically, after starting ACE inhibitors, patients may complain of a persistent, dry, nonproductive cough. The cough is not related to patient position or time of day, and it disappears when the ACE inhibitor is discontinued.

Hyperkalemia develops in some patients who take ACE inhibitors. Like the cough, the hyperkalemia resolves when the drug is discontinued. Serum potassium levels greater than 6.0 mEq/L are potentially dysrhythmogenic and should be treated with exchange resin. Patients with serum creatinine levels greater than 1.5 µg/dL are often denied ACE inhibitors in the mistaken belief that they will develop renal failure if they are given ACE inhibitors. In fact, patients with elevated creatinine levels are no more likely to develop an increased creatinine than patients with a normal creatinine when the ACE inhibitors were started.[16] The two types of patients most likely to show increased creatinine when started on ACE inhibitors are patients with renal artery stenosis and those with hypovolemia.

Patients receiving ACE inhibitors also have decreased blood pressure. It is not uncommon to see asymptomatic systolic pressures of 80 to 99 mm Hg, and diastolic pressures may be 40 to 59 mm Hg. These low pressures are not symptomatic because perfusion of the brain and kidneys is not compromised as it might be in a patient with normal systolic function.

Table 20-4 • Medications Used in the Treatment of Heart Failure

Agent	Action	Starting Dose	Target Dose	Indications, Contraindications, Adverse Effects
Chronic Heart Failure				
ACE inhibitors Lisinopril Enalapril Captopril	Block renin–angiotensin –aldosterone system, decrease symptoms and mortality Block conversion of angiotensin I to angiotensin II for afterload reduction	Lisinopril: 2.5–5 mg qd Enalapril: 2.5–5 mg bid Captopril: 6.25–12.5 tid	Lisinopril: 20–40 mg qd Enalapril: 10–20 mg bid Captopril: 50 mg tid	May cause angioedema, hyper- kalemia, increased creatinine, symptomatic hypotension
Hydralazine	Pure vasodilator Used to decrease afterload	10–25 mg PO q6–8h	75 mg PO q6h or 100 mg PO q8h	May cause tachycardia Used for intolerance of ACE inhibitors, for additional blood pressure control, or for afterload reduction in severe mitral regurgi- tation or atrial insufficiency
Nitrates Isosorbide dinitrate Isosorbide mononitrate	Decrease preload, relieve angina, decrease orthopnea	Isosorbide dinitrate: 10 mg q6h (hold midnight dose) Isosorbide mononitrate: 30 mg qd	Isosorbide dinitrate: up to 40 mg q6h (hold midnight dose) Isosorbide mononitrate: up to 120 mg qd	Dose limited by symptoms such as headache or hypotension Use least dose that relieves symptoms
Digoxin	Oral inotrope Blocks neurohormonal bombardment of heart	0.125–0.25 mg PO qd	Same	Limited by renal excretion; smaller doses used when creatinine is >1.3 mg/dL Dose should be decreased in patients receiving amiodarone
Diuretics Furosemide Metolazone	Control fluid volume	Furosemide: 20–40 mg (in patient who has never been on diuretics) Metolazone: 2.5–5 mg qd	Up to 320 mg bid if nec- essary to control fluid Metolazone 10 mg qd if necessary in addition to furosemide	Diuretic dosage requirements are higher during aggressive diuresis than during maintenance Combination of furosemide and metolazone is very powerful, and loss of potassium, magnesium, and calcium can be dramatic, increas- ing risk for dysrhythmia
Spironolactone	Blocks effects of aldos- terone and protects potassium	25 mg qd	25 mg qd	May cause hyperkalemia, so potas- sium should be monitored regularly May cause gynecomastia in men
β-blockers Metoprolol SR Carvedilol Bisoprolol	Improve symptoms, increase exercise tolerance, decrease hospitalizations and mortality	Metoprolol SR: 12.5 mg qd Carvedilol: 3.125 mg bid Bisoprolol: 1.25 mg qd	Metoprolol SR: 100–200 mg qd Carvedilol: 25–50 mg bid Bisoprolol: 10 mg qd	May precipitate exacerbation during initiation and titration Monitor weight and heart rate care- fully; do not stop drugs suddenly Benefit is long term and may not be evident for up to 3 months
Acute Heart Failure and Acute Exacerbation of Chronic Heart Failure				
Inodilators Dobutamine Milrinone	Increase contractility, decrease afterload and therefore increase cardiac output Increased forward flow decreases left ventricular end-diastolic pressure	Dobutamine: 2–5 µg/kg/min Milrinone: 0.2–0.3 µg/kg/min (with or without loading dose)	Dobutamine: 5–15 µg/kg/min Milrinone: 0.375–0.7 µg/kg/min	Use smallest dose that produces desired hemodynamic effect May cause tachycardia and ventricu- lar dysrhythmias Can be given effectively to patients who are receiving β-blockers
Dopamine	Increases renal perfusion and improves diuresis	1–3 µg/kg/min	1–3 µg/kg/min	The higher the dose, the more likely dopamine is to increase afterload Do *not* give through a peripheral line
Nitroprusside	Used for afterload reduction and blood pressure control	0.5 µg/kg/min	Up to 1.5 µg/kg/min	High doses or prolonged administra- tion is associated with increased cyanide levels and should be avoided

(continued)

Table 20-4 • Medications Used in the Treatment of Heart Failure (Continued)

Agent	Action	Starting Dose	Target Dose	Indications, Contraindications, Adverse Effects
Nesiritide	Used for afterload reduction	2 µg/kg/min bolus with 0.01 µg/kg/min infusion	Increase by 0.005 µg/kg/min to maximum of 0.3 µg/kg/min	Use caution if systolic blood pressure <90 mm Hg
Hydralazine	Used for afterload reduction and blood pressure control	5–10 mg IV q4h PRN	5–10 mg IV q4h PRN	May cause tachycardia

The increased flow or stroke volume more than compensates for the decrease in resistance, and the tissues actually receive more blood and therefore oxygen than they would at a higher resistance and pressure. It is unnecessary to hold or decrease ACE inhibitors for asymptomatic hypotension.

For patients who truly cannot tolerate ACE inhibitors, other options are available. The use of hydralazine and nitrates preceded the studies on ACE inhibitors, and these drugs have similar mortality benefits. Hydralazine must be taken 3 or 4 times a day, and many patients have trouble complying with a multidose medication regimen. Long-acting nitrates are used in conjunction with the hydralazine. Once-a-day preparations such as isosorbide mononitrate or a nitroglycerin patch may be used if compliance is a problem. Isosorbide dinitrate can be used if a rest period of at least 6 to 8 hours is taken.

Another option for patients who cannot take ACE inhibitors because of cough is an angiotensin II receptor blocker. Losartan, valsartan, and candesartan were studied in the treatment of heart failure. Early results suggest that these agents are effective in patients who are not taking ACE inhibitors. Valsartan and candesartan have FDA indications for heart failure.

Digoxin

Cardiac glycosides have been used for centuries in the empirical management of heart failure. However, until recently, no objective evidence indicated that digitalis preparations made any actual difference in the management of heart failure. Beginning in 1993, the Prospective Randomized Study of Ventricular Failure and the Efficacy of Digoxin (PROVED) trial and, more recently, the Randomized Assessment of Digoxin on Inhibitors of Angiotensin-Converting Enzyme (RADIANCE) and Digitalis Investigation Group (DIG) trials provided evidence that digoxin is of value in the treatment of heart failure.[17] Although none of the studies has shown that digoxin affects mortality, they all have consistently shown that digoxin leads to improvement in symptom management and exercise tolerance as well as decreased hospitalizations for heart failure.

The benefit of digoxin has long been thought to be due to its inotropic effects. However, it is a very weak inotrope. The long-term benefit of digoxin may be in its proven blockade of neurohormones such as norepinephrine. As discussed previously, long-term exposure of the myocardium to catecholamines is hypothesized to cause progression of heart failure.

Digoxin should be given in daily doses of 0.125 mg. Lower doses are used in patients who have renal insufficiency or also take amiodarone. Digoxin is safe and has few, if any, adverse effects as long as the blood levels remain less than 2.0 ng/mL. No studies have identified a therapeutic level for digoxin in heart failure or guidelines for interpreting drug levels.[2] The traditional therapeutic levels given in studies of atrial fibrillation may be excessively high; lower levels (i.e., 1.0 ng/mL) may be equally beneficial and safer.

Diuretics

Since furosemide became available in the 1960s, diuretics have become a mainstay of heart failure management. Edema, a common finding in patients with heart failure, is the result of volume expansion in response to neurohormonally mediated salt and

---

Box 20-4 • CONSIDERATIONS FOR THE OLDER PATIENT: HEART FAILURE

Most patients with heart failure are elderly, and many fit the category of "old old." They have a variety of limitations and comorbid diseases that may or may not relate to heart failure, as well as a remarkable resiliency and adaptability not found in younger patients. Therefore, it is critical to evaluate their limitations and strengths on an individual basis. It is important to treat the comorbid diseases aggressively according to patients' wishes and to include them in the planning and treatment decisions at all levels.

It is also critical to assess fall risk, activity level, visual acuity, manual dexterity, cognitive ability, and memory when administering, evaluating, or teaching about any medication. For some older patients, the assistance of a family member or friend is critical to successful medication adherence. Financial considerations are also important because many older patients are on Medicare and have a limited drug plan to pay for expensive medications. Having to choose between medication and food is no choice.

water retention. In certain conditions (e.g., ascites, pleural effusions), "third spacing" of fluids is a common result of excess volume and increased hydrostatic pressure. Edema worsens when patients are unwilling or unable to reduce sodium in their diets. Patients who have advanced heart failure are frequently malnourished and may have low serum albumin levels with a consequent decrease in osmotic gradients to pull fluids back into the circulation. Patients who are symptomatic from volume overload feel dramatically better when they are diuresed to their dry weight. Drugs such as ACE inhibitors and β-blockers work best in euvolemic patients.

Loop diuretics such as furosemide are standard therapy for diuresis in patients with heart failure.[18] More expensive loop diuretics are available but have not been shown to be superior to furosemide. Loop diuretics are threshold drugs, and the threshold varies from patient to patient. This means that the appropriate dosage must be determined by the patient's response. In a patient who requires oral doses of 200 mg of furosemide to maintain dry weight, 100 mg twice daily is not sufficient. Doses in excess of 200 mg daily may be necessary. When patients are receiving oral doses of 240 mg or more, yet continue to have edema or have increased edema, diuretic resistance must be considered. Loop diuretics should not be abandoned; however, a brief course of IV diuretic or the addition of a thiazide such as metolazone until the edema is controlled may be required.

The combination of loop and thiazide diuretics works more efficiently than either type of diuretic alone. However, this drug combination should be reserved for refractory edema, and when the edema resolves, an appropriate dose of loop diuretic should be determined and continued.

As heart failure progresses or when exacerbations occur, dose adjustments are necessary. Patients should be taught to weigh themselves daily and record their weights. Increases of 2 pounds or more overnight or of 5 pounds or more in a week are water weight, which can be controlled with additional doses of diuretic (1 L [1.06 quarts] of water weighs 1 kg [2.2 pounds]). Some patients can manage their fluid balance with a sliding-scale diuretic, much like patients with diabetes mellitus manage their blood glucose with sliding-scale insulin.

Spironolactone

Spironolactone is a weak diuretic with potassium-sparing properties. It is not used specifically for its diuretic activity. The Randomized Aldactone Evaluation Study (RALES) trial[19] studied mortality in patients with NYHA class III or IV heart failure who took spironolactone as well as ACE inhibitors, digoxin, and diuretics. The results were a 30% reduction in mortality in patients who received only 25 mg/day of spironolactone. The reasons for the decreased mortality are unclear, but the hypothetical mechanism is that spironolactone blocks aldosterone and its damaging effects on heart muscle. Of theoretical concern is the addition of another potassium-sparing drug to the regimen of patients who are already taking an ACE inhibitor, which also spares potassium. However, few patients had serum potassium levels high enough to discontinue the spironolactone. Many of those patients tolerated every-other-day administration of spironolactone well, with excellent results.

β-Blockers

Intuitively, β-blockers, with their negative inotropic properties, ought to be the least likely intervention to benefit patients with systolic dysfunction. For many years, the prevailing standard of care specifically excluded β-blockers for patients with ineffective heart pumps. During the past 30 years, both small studies and large, multicenter, international, randomized, placebo-controlled studies challenged this idea. Meta-analysis of the smaller studies and primary analysis of the recent studies documented a 34% improvement in mortality in NYHA class II and III heart failure. Other long-term benefits of β-blockers include improved exercise tolerance, better symptom control, fewer hospitalizations, and improved ejection fraction.

Short-term use of β-blockers makes heart failure worse. Consequently, β-blockers should be used as a long-term strategy that is begun only when patients are stable using optimum background therapy with ACE inhibitors, digoxin, and diuretics. β-Blockers should not be started when a patient is in the midst of an exacerbation. The specific drug used should be started at a very small dose and gradually increased to the target range. The initiation and titration of β-blockers are beyond the scope of this text but are outlined in detail elsewhere.[20]

Under no circumstances should β-blockers be stopped suddenly. The rebound tachycardia can be fatal, especially in patients with coronary insufficiency. Patients who come into the hospital because of an exacerbation of heart failure who are on β-blockers should continue taking the β-blocker. If a temporal relationship exists between titration of the β-blocker dose and the onset of the exacerbation, the dose should be reduced to the last well-tolerated dose. Patients who are taking β-blockers may receive inotropes without discontinuing the β-blocker and may respond well because of the up-regulation of β-adrenergic receptors.

Calcium Channel Blockers

First-generation calcium channel blockers such as diltiazem, verapamil, and nifedipine should be avoided in patients with systolic dysfunction. These drugs exert a strong negative inotropic effect without the long-term benefits of β-blockers. Second-generation calcium channel blockers such as amlodipine or felodipine have been used in patients with heart failure because they are vasodilators with minimal negative inotropic effects. They are most commonly used to control blood pressure in patients who are on target doses of ACE inhibitors but continue to have blood pressure levels that exceed the recommendations of the Seventh Report of the Joint National Committee on Detection, Evaluation and Treatment of High

Blood Pressure (JNC-7).[21] (The JNC-7 recommends that blood pressure in patients with heart failure be less than 130/80 mm Hg.)

Nitrates

Nitrates are venodilators, and their primary effect is to decrease preload. As coronary vasodilators, they are used to treat angina. In very high doses, they may lower blood pressure, but they are not first-line drugs for the treatment of hypertension. When given to patients who are volume depleted or have right ventricular infarctions, nitrates may lead to abrupt hypotension, which is the result of inadequate preload to maintain stroke volume and cardiac output.

Nitrates are used in heart failure to help alleviate the symptoms of orthopnea and dyspnea on exertion.[22] Often, when patients lie down, the increased venous return (preload) leads to increased pulmonary artery pressure because the volume is too great for the weakened left ventricle. This sudden increase in preload and pulmonary artery pressure causes the sensation of dyspnea. Sitting up reduces the preload and relieves the symptoms. Nitrates decrease preload and mediate the volume of blood presented to the left ventricle, thus helping to control dyspnea. For this reason, nitrates may be used for patients who do not have angina specifically for the management of orthopnea and dyspnea on exertion.

NONPHARMACOLOGICAL TREATMENT

Role of the Patient

Several strategies can be used to manage symptoms and prevent hospitalization of patients with heart failure.[23,24] The participation and commitment of the patient is necessary for success.

Sodium restriction is critical. Patients often believe that if they no longer use a salt shaker, they have eliminated all excess salt from their diet, and they may be surprised to learn that canned soup and canned vegetables are extremely high in salt. Education about the natural salt content of foods and the salt that is added as part of food processing is essential. Patients must be taught to read labels and shop for foods that provide optimum nutrition with minimal salt.

Alcohol use should be stopped. As noted previously, alcohol is a powerful cardiac depressant. Many patients have read that a glass of wine or a drink each day decreases the risk for coronary artery disease. Although this may be true, the studies were performed in patients who did not have systolic dysfunction. It is important to clarify this fact and explain to the patient the adverse effects of alcohol.

Exercise should be encouraged. Patients with heart failure have limited stamina, and the goal is to increase stamina with low-level exercise over a longer period of time instead of intense exercise for short periods of time. Obviously, some patients with heart failure start at a higher level of functioning and have a better exercise tolerance than patients with advanced heart failure. Exercise for patients with heart failure is not the same as that for development of cardiovascular fitness, and heart rate is not a good indicator of exercise efficacy.

Patients with heart failure should be encouraged to maintain their level of activity. Walking is by far the best recommended exercise. Neither speed nor distance is important. Patients should aim for 15 to 20 minutes each day without stopping to rest or "catch their breath" at whatever pace they are able to manage. Some patients need to take many rests before they begin to exercise, and it may be quite a while before they can exercise for this length of time even at low levels. Weight-lifting is not recommended because this activity increases afterload and may worsen symptoms.

The most important thing patients can do to stay out of the hospital and control symptoms is to take their medication. The second most important activity is to measure their weight every day. An overnight weight change of more than 3 pounds is due to water weight. If patients take and record their weight every day, modest fluid accumulations of 1 quart or less can be identified. Patients can be diuresed before they become so fluid overloaded that hospitalization for IV diuresis is necessary.

Fluid restrictions are punishing, and there is no evidence that water restriction has any value in the absence of significant hyponatremia. Likewise, there is no physiological basis for decreasing or controlling edema by fluid restriction, or any evidence that restricting fluids is effective.[25] The problem for patients with heart failure is the retention of sodium, which "holds on" to water. Restricting sodium does decrease or control edema, as discussed in the section on diuretics.

Implantable Cardioverter–Defibrillator

In dilated cardiomyopathy, the incidence of sudden death from ventricular tachycardia or ventricular fibrillation is very high. Asymptomatic ventricular tachycardia is common, but its prognostic impact is unknown. For patients who have syncopal episodes or survive sudden death, an implantable cardioverter–defibrillator is usually indicated. An implantable cardioverter–defibrillator interrupts life-threatening dysrhythmias. If this device fires frequently or symptomatic NSVT occurs, amiodarone may be added to the regimen for rhythm control. See Chapter 18 for more information about the implantable cardioverter–defibrillator.

Biventricular Pacing

In a select group of patients with heart failure and intraventricular conduction delays (QRS duration >130 milliseconds), biventricular pacing or cardiac resynchronization may improve cardiac output and therefore symptoms and exercise tolerance.[26] Pacing both ventricles of the spherically dilated heart reproduces the bottom-to-top contraction of a normal ventricle that is lost with myocardial remodeling and bundle branch block.

EVIDENCE-BASED PRACTICE HIGHLIGHT: MANAGEMENT OF HEART FAILURE

Excerpted from: Heart Failure Society of America. Disease management in heart failure. J Card Fail 12(1):e58–e69, 2006.

It is recommended that heart failure disease management programs include the following components, based on patient characteristics and needs (strength of evidence = B):

- Comprehensive education and counseling individualized to patient needs
- Promotion of self-care, including self-adjustment of diuretic therapy in appropriate patients (or with family member or caregiver assistance)
- Emphasis on behavioral strategies to increase adherence
- Vigilant follow-up after hospital discharge or after periods of instability
- Optimization of medical therapy
- Increased access to providers
- Early attention to signs and symptoms of fluid overload
- Assistance with social and financial concerns

It is recommended that heart failure disease management include integration and coordination of care between the physician and heart failure care specialists and with other agencies, such as home health and cardiac rehabilitation (strength of evidence = C).

It is recommended that patients in a heart failure disease management program be followed until they or a family member or caregiver demonstrates independence in following the prescribed treatment plan, adequate or improved adherence to treatment guidelines, improved functional capacity, and symptom stability. Higher-risk patients with more advanced heart failure may need to be followed permanently. Patients who experience increasing episodes of exacerbation or who demonstrate instability after discharge from a program should be referred again to the service (strength of evidence = B).

Rating scheme for the strength of the evidence: A, randomized, controlled, clinical trials (may be assigned based on results of a single trial); B, cohort and case-control studies (post hoc, subgroup analysis, and meta-analysis; prospective observational studies or registries); C, expert opinion (observational studies—epidemiological findings; safety reporting from large-scale use in practice).

• Management of Acute Exacerbations of Heart Failure

Acute exacerbations of heart failure are an acute worsening of chronic heart failure and may occur for many reasons. Left ventricular function may deteriorate; heart failure is a progressive disease. If function deteriorates beyond the patient's ability to compensate, then symptoms worsen. Although heart function may be stable, the development of other problems such as pneumonia, anemia, dysrhythmia, hypertension, or trauma may tax the ability of the compromised heart to increase cardiac output to meet the increased metabolic demand. Dietary lapses, medication disruption, or lack of vigilance on the part of the patient regarding progressive water weight gain may all contribute to exacerbation. If possible, it is important to identify the cause of an exacerbation so that a long-term strategy to control the underlying problem can be implemented. However, in the intervening period, an acute exacerbation must be treated aggressively, often to save the life of a patient.

The main concerns for the care of patients with acute exacerbations of chronic heart failure are the same as in any patient with a life-threatening condition. They start with the basic priorities: airway, breathing, and circulation. Once these issues are addressed, etiologic factors and long-term strategies can become the focus of care.

AIRWAY AND BREATHING

For most patients with acute symptoms of heart failure, airway patency is not a problem. Likewise, oxygenation is not usually compromised unless pulmonary edema is severe or a comorbid pulmonary disease is present. However, when the acute onset of heart failure or the acute exacerbation is accompanied by profound pulmonary edema, such as in MI or flash pulmonary edema, the airway may become compromised. With severe pulmonary edema, surfactant may be washed out of the alveoli, decreasing lung compliance and making ventilation difficult. In patients who also have COPD or restrictive lung disease, the compromise in compliance may make normal minute ventilation difficult if not impossible. An indication that normal minute ventilation is not being maintained is increased partial pressure of arterial carbon dioxide ($PaCO_2$) associated with increased work of breathing and respiratory acidosis. For example, a patient may initially do well but tire as the increased work of ventilating wet lungs is prolonged.

Intubation

The usual indications for endotracheal intubation in patients with heart failure are the same as for patients in respiratory distress. Intubation and assisted ventilation are indicated if patients are unable to maintain oxygenation or ventilation. Patients who have pulmonary edema and a persistent oxygen saturation of less than 90% on 100% oxygen should be intubated and supported until they can obtain oxygen on their own. If the increased work of breathing is leading to fatigue of the respiratory muscles and the $PaCO_2$ is rising in association with a falling pH, intubation is indicated even if the patient is able to breathe unaided. The intubation may not be required for more than 12 to 24 hours, but it may be better to protect the airway than to try to intubate a patient after respiratory arrest. See Chapter 25 for more information about the care of the patient on a mechanical ventilator.

Diuresis

Once the airway is protected, attention is directed toward reducing the pulmonary edema. In most cases, aggressive IV diuresis is indicated. The presence of bilateral crackles on physical examination is not always an indication of total-body volume excess. Evaluation of crackles, along with peripheral edema, liver congestion or ascites, and renal function, allows for a better assessment of fluid status than crackles alone. If the patient is determined to be volume overloaded, then IV diuretics facilitate the excretion of excess fluid rapidly and quickly make the patient feel better.

Aggressive diuresis usually starts with the patient's oral dose of loop diuretic in IV form. An adequate diuretic response is about 1 L of urine within 2 hours of the IV dose. If urine output is less than 1 L, the dose is doubled until a maximum dose is reached (for furosemide, a 400-mg single dose) or until the 1 L urine output goal is met. If the IV loop diuretic is not sufficient to produce this level of diuresis, a thiazide such as metolazone may be given orally along with the loop diuretic.[18] The desired weight loss is 1 to 2 kg/day until the patient's dry weight is reached. Initial weight loss may be greater. Careful monitoring of potassium and magnesium is indicated. If the creatinine begins to rise in response to the diuresis, then the ACE inhibitor should be held until after the diuresis is complete.

CIRCULATION

Once the airway is protected and breathing is adequate to maintain oxygen and carbon dioxide levels, the circulation of blood to perfuse cells and supply oxygen for cellular function becomes the priority. Two indicators are used to determine the adequacy of perfusion. The first indicator is function of organ systems. Inadequate perfusion affects the brain, leading to confusion and change in level of consciousness; the kidneys, leading to increased BUN and creatinine; and the gastrointestinal system, leading to ileus and liver failure. The second indicator is metabolic acidosis. If perfusion is severely inadequate or prolonged past the capacity of the body to buffer the lactic acid produced, the level of sodium bicarbonate decreases, as does the pH, producing metabolic acidosis. Metabolic acidosis is a system-wide measure of inadequate oxygen to meet the metabolic demands of tissues.

Hypotension alone is not sufficient to diagnose hypoperfusion in patients with heart failure because many such patients are chronically hypotensive. Hypotension associated with hypoperfusion should be treated in a way that increases flow without increasing afterload. The problem is decreased cardiac output caused by decreased contractility. Whether the patient has acute heart failure associated with cardiogenic shock or acute exacerbation of chronic heart failure, the goal of treatment should be to increase cardiac output. Several interventions increase cardiac output.

The normal physiological response to decreased cardiac output is vasoconstriction and increased afterload. In patients with heart failure, afterload may be increased without a dramatic increase in blood pressure, and it is not safe to assume that a low blood pressure means a decreased afterload. Decreasing afterload increases stroke volume, and even in patients with low blood pressures, the increase in stroke volume and perfusion more than compensates for the low blood pressure.

Optimize Hemodynamics

One way to increase cardiac output is to optimize preload. If a patient is dehydrated or fluid overloaded, contractility is compromised.

Decreased preload is usually related to iatrogenic overdiuresis. However, patients who are on stable doses of diuretics may become dehydrated if they become hyperglycemic or experience vomiting and diarrhea while continuing to take the prescribed diuretic dose. Careful fluid repletion usually corrects this problem and improves cardiac output. The symptomatic hypotension and increased BUN and creatinine that are the hallmarks of decreased preload should quickly return to baseline levels.

More commonly, increased preload is a problem; patients are total-body volume overloaded. The combination of fluid overload and decreased contractility leads to cardiopulmonary congestion with increased pulmonary artery pressures and overfilling of the heart. When the heart is overfilled, it becomes stiff and does not empty or fill well. The result is compromised stroke volume and sometimes localized ischemia. The ischemia further worsens contractility. Patients may present with classic angina even if they have no documented CAD. Diuresis with IV loop diuretics often restores the pressure–volume dynamics that optimize stroke volume. For patients who do not respond to diuresis, increasing contractility may decrease preload.

Increase Contractility

To increase cardiac output, it is necessary to increase contractility and decrease afterload. Drugs that directly increase contractility are called inotropes. All inotropes increase myocardial oxygen consumption. To be useful in patients with heart failure, there must be greater improvement in oxygen delivery than in oxygen consumption. For this reason, inotropes such as epinephrine and isoproterenol are not used.

The following are indications for the use of inotropes:

▶ Low cardiac output and high PAWP, especially with symptomatic hypotension
▶ High PAWP with poor response to diuretics in volume-overloaded patients
▶ Severe right-sided heart failure that is the direct result of left ventricular failure

► Symptoms of heart failure at rest despite excellent maintenance therapy

Dopamine is also an excellent inotrope at mid-level doses. However, because dopamine is also a vasoconstrictor, especially at higher doses, it increases afterload in patients with heart failure and decreases stroke volume or, at the very least, does not increase it. Although there are no data to support its use, so-called renal-dose dopamine has been used frequently in patients with heart failure.[27] The use of renal-dose dopamine has been based on the knowledge that the effects of dopamine are dose related. At low doses of 1 to 3 μg/kg/min, the hypothesized main effect of dopamine is stimulation of dopaminergic receptors that dilate renal and splanchnic circulations. Higher doses have inotropic and vasoconstrictor activity. Even low-dose dopamine should not be used routinely.

Drugs called inodilators are used to stimulate β-adrenergic receptors located in the heart and blood vessels to increase contractility and cause vasodilation.[27] The two inodilators most commonly used in ICUs are dobutamine and milrinone. Although these drugs have different pharmacological mechanisms, they both increase stimulation of β-adrenergic receptors. Because they stimulate β-adrenergic receptors, they are also chronotropic (i.e., they increase heart rate), and they must be used carefully and titrated slowly in patients with tachycardia or ventricular dysrhythmia.

The effect of inotropes and inodilators can be measured when a pulmonary artery catheter is in place. As the drugs are titrated to optimum doses, cardiac output increases, and the PAWP decreases. Urine output should increase, and BUN and creatinine should return to baseline levels. Any organ function that was compromised because of inadequate perfusion should improve.

Vasodilation

Sometimes an inodilator alone is not sufficient to decrease afterload adequately. In patients with cardiogenic shock or patients who have an exacerbation related to hypertensive emergency, the afterload is the primary limiting factor. Decreasing and controlling the blood pressure or decreasing the workload of the damaged myocardium requires immediate treatment, and vasodilation with parenteral medications is necessary to maintain life or limit end-organ damage. Nitroprusside has the most rapid onset with the shortest half-life of any of these medications. It provides for rapid, efficient decrease in blood pressure, and the effect is limited to minutes if the medication is stopped because of an exaggerated response. Nitroprusside must be given as a continuous drip and requires reliable monitoring of blood pressure in a setting where emergency resuscitation is available.

Nesiritide, a BNP, has been approved as a vasodilator for treatment of acute decompensation of chronic heart failure.[28,29] It is unclear whether this vasodilator has any advantages over nitroprusside or nitroglycerin. Studies are underway to answer remaining questions about nesiritide, such as whether it is more effective than less expensive inodilators or more effective in patients with renal dysfunction.

For intermittent blood pressure control, IV or oral hydralazine provides vasodilation with a decrease in afterload, without any negative inotropic effects. Sublingual nifedipine should never be used to control blood pressure.[2] IV nitroglycerin is valuable in decreasing preload and in treating angina associated with hypertensive emergency, but it is not a good afterload reducer or antihypertensive.

Intra-aortic balloon counterpulsation has proved very successful in reducing afterload in cardiogenic shock by augmenting perfusion pressure and decreasing the workload of the left ventricle. Intra-aortic balloon counterpulsation is often critical to survival in patients with acute MI who suffer acute left ventricular failure. Intra-aortic balloon counterpulsation is used for a limited time for support of the patient until a revascularization procedure can restore oxygenation and function or until the stunned myocardium has recovered somewhat (in a patient who cannot be revascularized). For a more detailed discussion of intra-aortic balloon counterpulsation, see Chapter 18.

Heart Rate

Heart rate and rhythm must be optimized for adequate cardiac output. If the heart rate is too slow, such as in sick sinus syndrome, second- or third-degree AV block, or sinus bradycardia, stroke volume cannot be increased adequately to compensate, resulting in an exacerbation. A heart rate that is too slow or too fast can compromise filling and, in patients with ischemia, can contribute directly to decreased contractility. A fast rate may be a compensation for a decreased stroke volume and usually responds to increasing stroke volume.

The administration of β-adrenergic inotropes may improve heart rate along with the inotropic effect and greatly improve cardiac output. However, the reason for the bradycardia must be identified and treated if the improvement is to be sustained. In many cases, problems with bradycardia result from ischemic damage to the conduction system. In this situation, a permanent pacemaker resolves the problem. If the bradycardia is the result of active ongoing ischemia, a temporary pacemaker along with treatment of the ischemia is indicated. (For a more detailed discussion of cardiac pacemakers, see Chapter 18.) If the bradycardia is the result of medication, the medication should be held or discontinued until the indication for the medication can be reevaluated. In this situation, β-blockers may be held for 24 to 36 hours but should not be discontinued suddenly. If the bradycardia is the result of β-blockers, temporary pacing may be required while the drug is titrated down.

Sinus tachycardia is usually the result of decreased stroke volume and therefore cardiac output. Treatment of the tachycardia without increasing stroke volume leads to worsening end-organ perfusion. Sinus tachycardia usually resolves if the underlying decrease in stroke volume is corrected.

When the tachycardia is caused by atrial flutter or atrial fibrillation with rapid ventricular response, the heart rate is the cause of the problem, and it is necessary to control this directly. If the patient is unconscious secondary to the heart rhythm, direct-current countershock cardioversion is indicated. Otherwise, mechanical methods such as the Valsalva maneuver or carotid massage may be helpful. If medication is required to slow the rhythm, amiodarone is the least dangerous medication to use in systolic dysfunction. Calcium channel blockers such as verapamil and diltiazem are powerful negative inotropes and may aggravate the low–cardiac-output state. In many cases, the tachycardia is associated with ischemia or hypertensive crisis, and treatment of the underlying problem also treats the tachycardia.

After the patient is stabilized and cardiac output has been supported by inodilators or vasodilators, any uncontrolled comorbid diseases that may have triggered or worsened the exacerbation must be treated. Anemia with a hemoglobin level of less than 10 g/dL should usually be treated with transfusion. Pneumonia or other infection should be diagnosed and treated with the appropriate antibiotics. Blood glucose should be controlled using insulin if necessary. Examples of nursing diagnoses for heart failure are shown in Box 20-5.

DISCHARGE PLANNING AND PATIENT EDUCATION

Many times, severe exacerbations requiring hospitalization can be avoided. If a weight gain of 2 to 3 pounds can be treated with intermittent extra doses of diuretic, then 15- and 20-pound weight gains that require hospitalization will not occur. Helping patients control both their heart failure and their comorbid diseases empowers them instead of victimizing them and gives them a sense of control that also helps to limit hospitalization. There have been many reports of improved quality of life, decreased hospitalizations, and decreased cost of care for patients in disease management programs.[30–32]

Home care provides many opportunities for disease management. As the home care nurse enters the patient's environment, the opportunities for teaching become evident. Even in situations in which the number of visits after a hospital stay is limited, such as with patients covered by Medicare, there are many opportunities for the home care nurse not only to assess but also to intervene (Box 20-6).

Discharge planning begins with the first day of hospitalization. A program of education, referral, and follow-up is initiated with the goal of preventing further hospitalization. Patient teaching is necessary (Box 20-7). Clearly, patients must be on target levels of standard medications to reap the benefits of the clinical studies that have been done in heart failure. However, patients must work in collaboration with health care providers to maximize this benefit (Box 20-8).

• Clinical Applicability Challenges

Case Study

Mrs. K., a 68-year-old Caucasian woman, has been admitted to the ICU with shortness of breath at rest. Vital signs are as follows: blood pressure, 218/100 mm Hg; heart rate, 110 beats/min; and respiratory rate, 38 breaths/min. She has run out of her antihypertensive medication for the fourth time this year and only came to the hospital because of her breathing difficulties.

On examination, Mrs. K. is pale and clammy sitting upright in a chair. She has bibasilar crackles to her scapulae, and her heart rhythm is irregularly irregular. She has pitting edema bilaterally to her thighs, jugular venous pulsation to the earlobe, and hepatojugular reflux. A chest radiograph shows bilateral infiltrates. An echocardiogram shows a left ventricular ejection fraction of 78% with estimated pulmonary artery pressures of 50 to 55 mm Hg. Laboratory values are unremarkable.

Box 20-7 • TEACHING GUIDE:
Living With Heart Failure

Medications
- Take all medications as instructed. If you cannot afford them, please let your provider know so that you can be put in touch with someone to help.
- Do not stop taking medication because you feel better. These are lifetime medications in most instances. Some of the medications will need to be adjusted over time, but your health care provider will discuss the changes with you.
- You may be taking several drugs. These medications do not interfere with each other, and they are given together so that they can work together to do more than any one or two of them can do alone.
- Do not let your medication supply run out because stopping some medications suddenly can cause serious problems.
- Take your medications about the same time every day.
- If you are going out for a few hours and will not have easy access to a bathroom when you need it, hold off on your diuretic until you return home. Do not skip a day's dose of diuretic because this could lead to serious water accumulations and worsening of your heart failure.

Diet
- Restrict your salt intake by removing the salt shaker from the table and the food preparation area. Do not add salt to any food you are cooking or any food on your plate.
- Avoid foods that have a high salt content naturally or because of the way they are preserved. Foods such as canned soup, canned vegetables, canned meats, foods frozen in sauces, cold cuts, sauerkraut, dill pickles, cheese, and processed foods of any kind are loaded with salt. Seasonings such as garlic and onion salt, Old Bay, and monosodium glutamate are the same as salt. Avoid salt substitutes because they are made with potassium; in combination with the medications you are taking, they can lead to potassium excesses. Avoid fast food such as hamburgers, french fries, fried chicken, and tacos.
- Seasonings such as pepper, Mrs. Dash, onion and garlic powder, herbs, seeds, and spices are acceptable.
- Fresh or frozen vegetables (frozen without sauces), fresh lean meats and poultry, and fish (not fried) are all good choices.

Daily Weights
- Weigh yourself every day at about the same time and record the value.
- The best time to weigh yourself is in the morning when you first get up and after you go to the bathroom.

- Weigh yourself without clothes if possible.
- Record your weight and the date in a daily diary. Bring this diary with you to the office when you visit your health care provider.
- Call if your weight goes up more than 2 lb overnight and does not go back to baseline the next day, or if you gain more than 3 lb in a week.

Activity
- Stay as active as possible.
- The stronger your skeletal muscles are, the easier it is for your heart.
- Do not use heart rate as a measure of adequacy of exercise effort.
- If you get tired or short of breath, stop and rest and then try again. The goal is 15 to 20 minutes of continuous activity each day.
- There are no speed or distance goals, and walking at whatever pace you can accomplish is a good choice. Home-making and gardening are good choices as well. Choose an activity that you enjoy.
- Shortness of breath is uncomfortable but not dangerous. It is an indication that you are nearing the end of your exercise tolerance for this period, but once your breathing normalizes, you can go again. If you stop before you get short of breath out of fear, you will not be able to increase your activity tolerance.
- If you have any questions about how much exercise you can tolerate, discuss it with your health care provider. That person is the best advisor for you because you are well known.
- Do not lift weights unless your health care provider has specifically said it is an acceptable activity for you.

Call Your Health Care Provider if:
- Your weight increases or decreases suddenly.
- You begin waking up at night short of breath and need to sit up to breathe.
- You start needing more pillows at night to breathe when you lie down or you are unable to lie down.
- You become short of breath at rest.
- You cannot walk up stairs that you used to climb regularly because now it makes you too short of breath or tired.
- Your feet and legs start to swell.
- You faint or feel as though you are going to faint.
- You become dizzy and weak when you stand.

On admission, Mrs. K. is started on lisinopril, 5 mg orally once per day, and given 20 mg of IV furosemide. She is also given 5 mg of IV metoprolol × 3 over the first 24 hours, which results in worsened shortness of breath and frothy sputum. Blood gases show hypoxemia and hypercarbia. She is intubated and placed on a ventilator. Because of her worsening condition, a pulmonary catheter is put in place. Readings are as follows: right atrial pressure, 26 mm Hg; pulmonary artery pressure, 68/54 mm Hg; pulmonary artery wedge pressure, 36 mm Hg, and cardiac index, 1.1 L/min/m². Shortly after the readings are taken, she has a cardiac arrest, from which she cannot be resuscitated.

1. Mrs. K. experienced fluid overload and hypertension. The level of symptoms associated with her blood pressure constituted a hypertensive

Box 20-8 • COLLABORATIVE CARE GUIDE for the Patient With Acute Decompensation of Chronic Heart Failure

OUTCOMES	INTERVENTIONS

Oxygenation/Ventilation

There will be adequate oxygen to meet the metabolic demands of the tissue.

Minimum arterial oxygen content evidenced by:
1. Hemoglobin (Hgb) ≥ 10 g/dL
2. SpO_2 ≥ 90%

- Consider the transfusion of RBCs if Hgb ≤9.0 g/dL.
- Supplemental oxygen to maintain SpO_2 >90%.
- Consider intubation and mechanical ventilation if patient develops respiratory acidosis or cannot maintain oxygen saturation on 100% oxygen by mask
- Consider primary pulmonary problem as cause of hypoxemia and check brain natriuretic peptide (BNP) level.

The patient's symptom of dyspnea will be managed.
1. Patient denies dyspnea at rest
2. Patient reports increased activity before feeling sufficient dyspnea to limit activity
3. NYHA class equal to or better than baseline before decompensation

- Elevate head of bed or allow patient to select upright position that best relieves dyspnea.
- Apply damp washcloth to patient's face.
- Use a fan or other means to create air movement across the patient's face.
- Encourage the patient to ambulate as soon and as much as possible once dyspnea at rest is relieved.

Circulation/Perfusion

Cardiac output will be maximized.
Optimum cardiac output evidenced by:
1. Cardiac index > 2.0
2. SvO_2 > 50%
3. Urine output > 30 mL/h
4. Baseline level of consciousness and orientation

- Optimize preload with diuresis, fluid administration, or vasodilation with agent such as nitroglycerin, nitroprusside, or nesiritide.
- Increase contractility with inotrope such as milrinone or dobutamine.
- Decrease afterload with diuresis and vasodilation.

Hypotension will be asymptomatic, and the patient's blood pressure is at baseline.

- Determine the patient's baseline blood pressure; systolic pressure may be <90 mm Hg.
- If blood pressure is less than baseline, assess for orthostatic decreases in blood pressure and increases in heart rate that would suggest dehydration.
- Continue to give angiotensin-converting enzyme inhibitors and other afterload reducers if hypotension is asymptomatic.
- If patient is symptomatic on standing keep on bed rest until orthostasis resolves.
- If patient is orthostatic, symptomatic, and blood urea nitrogen and creatinine levels are elevated, hold diuretics and consider giving intravenous normal saline.

Fluids/Electrolytes

Euvolemia will be achieved. Euvolemia evidenced by:
1. Absence of peripheral edema
2. Absence of ascites
3. Documented dry weight
4. Baseline blood urea nitrogen and creatinine
5. Moist mucous membranes

- Administer loop diuretic sufficient to produce 1 L of urine output within 2 h of administration.
- Obtain daily weights.
- Strive for a weight loss of 1–2 kg/day until dry weight is achieved.
- Monitor electrolytes at least daily.
- Replenish potassium, magnesium, and calcium as needed.
- Measure serum albumin.
- If inadequate response to loop diuretics add metolazone or inotropes as above
- Report new or worsened rales to physician.

Teaching/Discharge Planning

Rehospitalization will be prevented.

- Assess the patient's understanding of medication regimen.
- Assess the patient's reading ability before giving written instructions.
- Include a family member in the discussions if the patient has trouble reading, seeing, or remembering.
- Consider a means of preparing medications so that the patient has to open only one container each day.

Box 20-8 • COLLABORATIVE CARE GUIDE for the Patient With Acute Decompensation of Chronic Heart Failure (Continued)

OUTCOMES	INTERVENTIONS
	• Teach the patient the importance of daily weights to follow fluid balance. • Have the patient weigh himself each day and record. Call physician if weight is 3–5 lb over baseline. • Have the patient or family member repeat early signs and symptoms of worsening heart failure and when to call physician for them. • Teach the patient about foods that have a high sodium content. • Encourage the patient to abstain from alcohol. • Encourage the patient to walk and stay as active as possible. • Consider case management referral or social work referral if the patient has multiple admissions or problems obtaining medications.

emergency. Why was Mrs. K.'s hypertensive emergency not recognized? What should the health care team have done differently?

2. What role did atrial fibrillation play in Mrs. K.'s heart failure?

3. What might have been done to address Mrs. K.'s frequent problems with taking her medications?

Review Questions

1. Which of the following statements best describes heart failure?
   a. It is episodic.
   b. It is present even when symptoms are controlled.
   c. It is the result of poor eating habits and obesity.
   d. It is not preventable.

2. Which of the following classes of drugs should be avoided in patients with heart failure?
   a. β-Blockers
   b. Diuretics
   c. Nonsteroidal anti-inflammatory drugs
   d. Nitrates

3. Standard medications used in the treatment of heart failure may cause dangerous increases in what electrolyte?
   a. Potassium
   b. Sodium
   c. Chloride
   d. Magnesium

4. The recommended standard medication regimen for patients with heart failure includes which five drugs?
   a. Angiotensin-converting enzyme (ACE) inhibitors, β-blockers, diuretics, aldosterone inhibitors, and digoxin
   b. Angiotensin II receptor blockers, β-blockers, digoxin, calcium channel blockers, and diuretics

   c. ACE inhibitors, diuretics, digoxin, nitrates, and calcium channel blockers
   d. Hydralazine, digoxin, nitrates, β-blockers, and amiodarone

5. Elevation in which biomarker is associated with heart failure exacerbation in the patient who presents to the emergency department with shortness of breath?
   a. Troponin I
   b. Norepinephrine
   c. Brain natriuretic peptide
   d. Creatinine kinase

6. Which of the following statements best describes appropriate instruction about exercise for patients with heart failure?
   a. Choose a vigorous activity and exercise until you are short of breath.
   b. Walk at your own pace until you need to rest and then walk more while building up your time.
   c. Exercise until your heart rate is 65% of predicted maximum.
   d. Use graduated weights to build muscle for improved endurance.

References

1. Heart Disease and Stroke Statistics—2006 Update: A report from the American Heart Association Statistics Committee and Stroke Statistics Subcommittee. Circulation 113:85–151, 2006

2. American College of Cardiology and American Heart Association: 2005 Guideline update for the diagnosis and management of chronic heart failure in the adult. J Am Coll Cardiol 46:1116–1143, 2005

3. New York Heart Association: Diseases of the Heart and Blood Vessels: Nomenclature and Criteria for Diagnosis, 6th ed. Boston, Little, Brown, 1964

4. Harding SE: The failing cardiomyocyte. Heart Fail Clin 1(2): 171–181, 2005

5. Packer M: Evolution of the neurohormonal hypothesis to explain the progression of chronic heart failure. Eur Heart J 16(Suppl f):4–6, 1995

6. Tang WHW, Francis GS: Neurohormonal upregulation in heart failure. Heart Fail Clin 1(1):1–9, 2005

7. Miyasaka Y, Barnes Me, Gersh BJ, et al: Incidence and mortality risk of congestive heart failure in atrial fibrillation patients: A community-based study over two decades. Eur Heart J 27(8): 936–941, 2006

8. Boriani G, Diemberger I, Martignani C, et al: The epidemiological burden of atrial fibrillation: A challenge for clinicians and health care systems. Eur Heart J 27(8):893–894, 2006

9. Daniel MB, Nelson CL, Anstrom KJ, et al, for the SCD-HeFT Investigators: Cost-effectiveness of defibrillator therapy or amiodarone in chronic stable heart failure: Results from the sudden cardiac death in heart failure trial (SCD-HeFT). Circulation 114(2):135–142, 2006

10. Maisel A: B-type natriuretic peptide levels: A potential "white count" for congestive heart failure. J Card Fail 7:183–193, 2001

11. Wright GA, Struthers AD: Natriuretic peptides as a prognostic marker and therapeutic target in heart failure. Heart 92(2): 149–151, 2006

12. Garg R, Yusuf S: Overview of randomized trials of angiotensin-converting enzyme inhibitors on mortality and morbidity in patients with heart failure. Collaborative Group on ACE Inhibitor Trials. JAMA 273(18):1450–1456, 1995

13. Milfred-LaForest SK: Pharmacotherapy of systolic heart failure: A review of recent literature and practical applications. J Cardiovasc Nurs 14(4):57–75, 2000

14. Nicklas JM, Cohn JN, Pitt B: What does ATLAS really tell us about "high" dose angiotensin-converting enzyme inhibition in heart failure? J Card Fail 6(2):165–168, 2000

15. Arnlov J, Ramachandran SV: Neurohormonal activation in populations susceptible to heart failure. Heart Fail Clin 1(1): 11–23, 2005

16. Solomon SD, Rice MM, Jablonski KA, et al, for the Prevention of Events With ACE Inhibition (PEACE) Investigators: Renal function and effectiveness of angiotensin-converting enzyme inhibitor therapy in patients with stable coronary disease in the prevention of events with ACE inhibition (PEACE) trial. Circulation 114(1):16–31, 2006

17. The Digitalis Investigation Group: The effect of digoxin on mortality and morbidity in patients with heart failure. N Engl J Med 336(8):525–533, 1977

18. Gupta S, Neyses L: Diuretic usage in heart failure: A continuing conundrum in 2005. Eur Heart J 26(7):644–649, 2005

19. Pitt B, Zannad F, Remme WJ, et al, for the Randomized Aldactone Evaluation Study Investigators: The effect of spironolactone on morbidity and mortality inpatients with severe heart failure. N Engl J Med 341(10):709–717, 1999

20. Clelend JGF, Huan L, Windram J: Are there clinically important differences between beta-blockers in heart failure? Heart Fail Clin 1(1):57–66, 2005

21. Chobanian AV, Bakris GL, Black HR, et al: National High Blood Pressure Education Coordinating Committee: The seventh report of the joint national committee for prevention, detection, evaluation, and treatment of high blood pressure. The JNC-7 Report. JAMA 289(19):2560–2571, 2003

22. Elkayam U: Nitrates in heart failure. Cardiol Clin 12(1):73–85, 1994

23. Krumholz HM, Butler J, Miller J, et al: Prognostic importance of emotional support for elderly patients hospitalized with heart failure. Circulation 97(10):958–964, 1998

24. Carlson B, Riegel B, Moser DK: Self care abilities of patients with heart failure. Heart Lung 30(5):351–359, 2001

25. Heart Failure Society of America: 2006 Comprehensive heart failure practice guideline. J Cardiac Fail 12:e1–e122, 2006

26. Tarcho JA: Biventricular pacing. N Engl J Med 355(3):288–294, 2006

27. Mehra MR: Optimizing outcomes in the patient with acute decompensated heart failure. Am Heart J 151(3):571–579, 2006

28. Moe GW: B-type natriuretic peptide in heart failure. Curr Opin Intern Med 5(4):385–391, 2006

29. Kayser SR: The use of nesiritide in the management of acute decompensated heart failure. Prog Cardiovasc Nurs 17(2): 89–95, 2002

30. Rich MW: Heart failure disease management: A critical review. J Card Fail 5(1):64–75, 1999

31. Atkinson RC, Branum K: Home-based disease management in congestive heart failure. Home Health Care Manage Pract 13(2):106–113, 2001

32. Stewart S, Horowitz JD: Home-based intervention in congestive heart failure: Long-term implications on readmission and survival. Circulation 105:2861–2866, 2002

Other Selected Readings

Albert N: Evidence-based nursing care for patients with heart failure. AACN Adv Crit Care 17(2):170–185, 2006

Ammar H, Malani AK, Gupta C, Dobyan D: Brain natriuretic peptide, clinical reasoning, and congestive heart failure. Am J Crit Care 15(6):614–616, 2006

Ancheta I: B-type natriuretic peptide rapid assay: A diagnostic test for heart failure. Dimens Crit Care Nurs 25(4):149–154, 2006

Ancheta I: A retrospective pilot study: Management of patients with heart failure. Dimens Crit Care Nurs 25(5):228–243, 2006

Clark A, McDougall G: Cognitive impairment in heart failure. Dimens Crit Care Nurs 25(3):93–100, 2006

Gary R: Self-care practices in women with diastolic heart failure. Heart Lung 35(1):9–19, 2006

Hou N, Chui M, Eckert G, et al: Relationship of age and sex to health-related quality of life in patients with heart failure. Am J Crit Care 13(2):153–161, 2004

Luttik ML, Jaarsma T, Veeger N, van Veldhuisen DJ: Marital status, quality of life, and clinical outcomes in patients with heart failure. Heart Lung 35(1):3–8, 2006

Miller-Davis C, Marden S, Leidy NK: The New York Heart Association classes and functional status: What are we really measuring? Heart Lung 35(4):217–224, 2006

Quinn C: Low-technology heart failure care in home health: Improving patient outcomes. Home Healthcare Nurse 24(8): 533–540, 2006

Redeker N, Stein S: Characteristics of sleep in patients with stable heart failure versus a comparison group. Heart Lung 35(4): 252–261, 2006

Sneed NV, Paul SC: Readiness for behavioral change in patients with heart failure. Am J Crit Care 12(6):444–453, 2003

Stoltzfus S: The role of noninvasive ventilation: CPAP and BiPAP in the treatment of congestive heart failure. Dimens Crit Care Nurs 25(2):66–70, 2006

Tsao L, Gibson CM: Heart failure: An epidemic of the 21st century. Critical Pathways in Cardiology: A Journal of Evidence-Based Medicine 3(4):194–204, 2004

Acute Myocardial Infarction

Patricia Gonce Morton

21

Atherosclerosis
    Pathophysiological Principles
    Risk Factors
Acute Coronary Syndrome
Angina Pectoris
    Pathophysiological Principles
    Classification of Angina
    Assessment
    Management
Myocardial Infarction
    Pathophysiological Principles
    Assessment
    Management
    Complications
    Cardiac Rehabilitation

Objectives

Based on the content in this chapter, the reader should be able to:

❶ Explain the pathophysiology and risk factors for atherosclerosis.

❷ Describe the classification, assessment, and management of patients with angina pectoris.

❸ Compare and contrast the pathophysiological principles and assessment findings of a patient with angina pectoris versus a patient with a myocardial infarction.

❹ Discuss the diagnostic tests used for a patient with a myocardial infarction.

❺ Summarize principles of managing the patient with a myocardial infarction in the early phase, intensive care phase, and intermediate care phase of management.

❻ Describe the complications for a patient with a myocardial infarction.

❼ Explain the principles of cardiac rehabilitation and patient education.

Cardiovascular disease is a significant global health problem, accounting for the death of about one third of people in the world. About 80% of these deaths occur in developing countries.[1] A total of 80.7 million American adults (one in three) have one or more types of cardiovascular disease. In the United States, cardiovascular disease continues to be the leading cause of death, accounting for 36.3% of all deaths in 2004.[2] About 2,400 Americans die each day from cardiovascular disease; this represents an average of 1 death every 37 seconds.[2]

Cardiovascular disease claims about as many lives each year as cancer, chronic lower respiratory disease, accidents, and diabetes mellitus combined. Of those who die from cardiovascular disease, the majority die as a result of coronary heart disease (myocardial infarction [MI] and angina pectoris), which is the largest killer of American men and women.[2] About every 26 seconds, an American has a coronary event, and about every minute, a person dies from one. About 38% of the people who have a coronary event in a given year die as a result. The death rate for coronary heart disease is 150.2 per 100,000. The death rate from coronary heart disease for black men (223.9 per 100,000) exceeds that for white men (194.2 per 100,000), and the death rate for black women (148.7 per 100,000) exceeds that for white women (114.7 per 100,000). About 50% of men and 64% of women who die suddenly of coronary heart disease have no previous symptoms of the disease. In the United States, the estimated direct (health care expenditures) and indirect (lost productivity) costs for 2008 for coronary heart disease total $156.4 billion.[2]

About 770,000 Americans have a new MI each year, and about 430,000 have a recurrent MI annually. An additional 190,000 silent first MIs occur each year. The average age at the time of the first MI is 64.5 years for men and 70.4 years for women.[2] For adults between 40 and 69 years of age, 8% of white men, 12% of white women, 14% of black men, and 11% of black women die within 1 year following a first MI. The estimated average number of years of life lost due to an MI is 15.[2]

As overwhelming as the mortality and morbidity statistics appear, much progress has been made in the prevention, diagnosis, and management of cardiovascular disease. Since the Framingham Study of risk factors in 1951 and the development of coronary care units in the 1960s, the critical care nurse has played a major role in helping to reduce the mortality associated with heart disease. The critical care nurse uses advanced assessment skills, rapid decision making, and therapeutic interventions to treat the patient in the acute phase of cardiovascular disease. Patient education and psychological support provided by the nurse have enabled patients and their families to return home and maximize their health status.

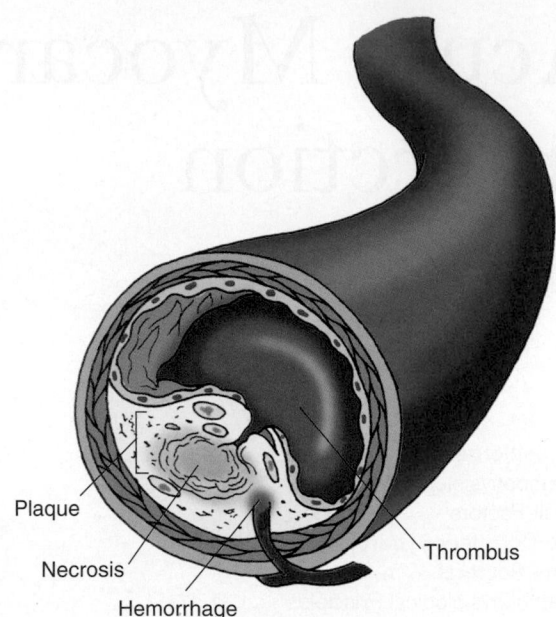

Figure 21-1 • Thrombosis of an atherosclerotic plaque. It may partially or completely occlude the lumen of the vessel. (From Bullock BL: Pathophysiology: Adaptations and Alterations in Function, 4th ed. Philadelphia: Lippincott-Raven, 1996.)

• Atherosclerosis

Atherosclerosis is a major cause of cardiovascular disease. The term atherosclerosis comes from the Greek words *athere*, meaning "gruel" or "paste," and *sclerosis*, meaning "hardness."

PATHOPHYSIOLOGICAL PRINCIPLES

Atherosclerosis is a complex, insidious process, beginning long before symptoms occur. Although the process is not completely understood, scientific evidence suggests that it begins when the inner, protective layer of the artery (endothelium) is damaged. Three known causes of the damage include elevated levels of cholesterol and triglycerides in the blood, hypertension, and cigarette smoking.[3]

Gradually, as fatty substances, cholesterol, cellular waste products, calcium, and fibrin pass through the vessel, they are deposited in the inner lining of an artery. As a result of the deposition of these materials, a lipid plaque with a fibrous covering, also known as an atheroma, builds up, and blood flow in the artery becomes partially or completely blocked.

The injury to the vessel and the resulting accumulation of these substances in the inner lining of the artery cause white blood cells, smooth muscle cells, and platelets to aggregate at the site. As a result, a matrix of collagen and elastic fibers form, and the endothelium becomes much thicker. The core of the fibrous plaque can become necrotic, and hemorrhage and calcification may result. A thrombosis may also form, thus contributing even more to the blockage of the vessel lumen (Fig. 21-1). These fibrous plaques are most often found in the coronary, popliteal, and internal carotid arteries and in the abdominal aorta.

Because of the fibrous plaque, the amount of blood flow through the artery is reduced, resulting in decreased supply of oxygen to tissues. However, symptoms often do not occur until 75% or more of the blood supply to the area is occluded. The occurrence of symptoms may depend to an extent on the development of collateral circulation. Collateral vessels are small arteries that connect two larger arteries or different segments of the same artery. Under normal conditions, these collateral arteries carry very little of the blood flow. As the larger artery gradually occludes, pressure builds on the proximal side of the occlusion. As a result, flow is redirected through the collateral vessels, which enlarge and dilate over time (Fig. 21-2). Blood is then allowed to flow around an area of blockage through these alternate routes.

Scientific advances have highlighted the role of inflammation in the pathophysiological process of atherosclerosis. The classic signs and symptoms of inflammation include redness, pain, heat, and swelling. They indicate that the injured tissue is in the process of restoring homeostasis, which includes three phases: vasodilation and increased permeability of the blood vessels; emigration of phagocytes from the blood into the tissue; and tissue repair. This process of restoring homeostasis is meant to be protective, but in the setting of atherosclerosis, the process has been found to be destructive. The atherosclerotic plaque continues to develop, aided by inflammatory molecules, and a fibrous cap forms over the lipid core. As the cap matures, inflammatory substances weaken the cap and cause it to rupture. Once the cap is ruptured, the coagulation cascade is initiated, and a clot is formed, resulting in obstruction of blood flow in the vessel.

Markers of inflammation are now being used to assess the risk for atherosclerosis. C-reactive protein

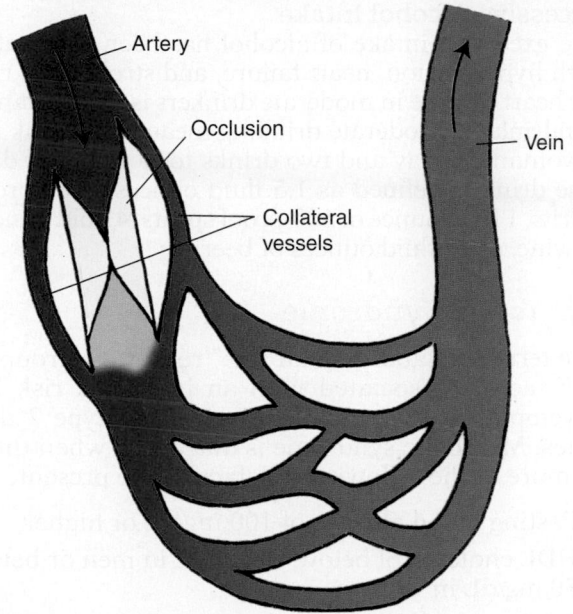

Figure 21-2 • Collateral circulation can develop for slowly developing lesions to provide myocardial blood flow until the atherosclerosis progresses beyond the limits of collateral supply. (From Bullock BL: Pathophysiology: Adaptations and Alterations in Function, 4th ed. Philadelphia: Lippincott-Raven, 1996.)

(CRP) is an acute-phase protein that increases during systemic inflammation. A newer, more sensitive CRP blood test called a highly sensitive C-reactive protein (hs-CRP) can be used to determine the risk for heart disease. High levels of hs-CRP have consistently predicted recurrent coronary events in patients with unstable angina and MI. An hs-CRP less than 1.0 mg/dL is associated with a low risk for developing cardiovascular disease, a value between 1.0 and 3.0 mg/dL with a moderate risk, and a value greater than 3.0 mg/dL with a high risk.[4]

RISK FACTORS

The cause of atherosclerosis is not clearly known. Through epidemiological studies, risk factors for the development of atherosclerosis have been identified. These risk factors are usually classified into two groups: major risk factors and contributing risk factors. Major risk factors are those that have been shown through research to increase significantly the risk of cardiovascular disease. Contributing risk factors are known to be associated with an increased risk for cardiovascular disease, but their significance and prevalence are still under investigation. Major risk factors are further divided into those that are uncontrollable and those that can be lowered by modification, treatment, or control.

Major Uncontrollable Risk Factors

Age
There is an increased incidence of all types of atherosclerotic disease with aging. More than 83% of people who die from coronary heart disease are 65 years of age and older. At older ages, women who have an MI are more likely than men to die from it within a few weeks.[5]

Heredity
The tendency to develop atherosclerosis seems to run in families, although the risk is presumed to be a combination of environmental and genetic influences. Even when other risk factors are controlled, the chance for developing coronary artery disease increases when there is a familial tendency. Most people with a strong family history of cardiovascular disease also have one or more additional risk factors.

Race
Rates of cardiovascular disease are higher in African Americans, Mexican Americans, Native Americans, Native Hawaiians, and some Asian Americans. High blood pressure, which is more severe in African Americans than Caucasians, contributes to a higher rate of heart disease. Higher rates of obesity and diabetes in Mexican Americans, American Indians, and Native Hawaiians help account for their higher rates of cardiovascular disease.[3]

Gender
Men have a greater risk for coronary artery disease than woman, and men have MIs at a younger age. However, after menopause, the death rate from coronary disease rises in women, but it never reaches the risk level of men.[3]

Major Risk Factors That Can Be Modified, Treated, or Controlled

Cigarette Smoking
A smoker's risk for an MI is double that of a nonsmoker. Smoking is the biggest risk factor for sudden cardiac death. A smoker's risk for an MI is more than twice that of a nonsmoker's risk. Smokers are more likely to die from the infarction and to die within 1 hour than nonsmokers. Exposure to environmental smoke also increases the risk for heart disease in nonsmokers.[3]

High Blood Cholesterol
High cholesterol levels increase the risk for coronary artery disease. Middle-aged adults with a total blood cholesterol level below 200 mg/dL have a relatively low risk for coronary artery disease. A total blood cholesterol level in the range of 200 to 239 mg/dL represents a moderate but increasing risk. When the level rises above 240 mg/dL, the risk for coronary artery disease is about double.[3]

Most cholesterol in the blood is carried in low-density lipoprotein (LDL), often called "bad" cholesterol. This type of cholesterol is deposited in the artery walls, and high blood levels of LDL increase the risk for coronary heart disease. An LDL level of less than 100 mg/dL is optimal.[3]

High-density cholesterol (HDL) removes cholesterol from tissues and transports the excess cholesterol back to the liver, where it is metabolized. For this reason, HDL is often called "good" cholesterol. A low level of HDL (<40 mg/dL) is associated with a higher risk for coronary artery disease.[3]

Triglyceride is the most common type of fat in the body, and the normal levels vary by age and sex. The rate of atherosclerotic development seems to be accelerated by a combination of high triglycerides with either high amounts of LDL or low amounts of HDL.[3]

Hypertension   CONCEPTS in action ANIMATION

Hypertension is a major risk factor that is termed the silent killer because it has no specific symptoms and no early warning signs. A higher percentage of men than women have hypertension until 45 years of age. The percentage of men and women with hypertension is similar between the ages of 45 and 54 years. After age 54 years, a much higher percentage of women have hypertension.

In the United States, the prevalence of hypertension in blacks is among the highest in the world, and this value is increasing. Compared with whites, hypertension develops in blacks earlier in life, with average blood pressures that are significantly higher.[2]

Physical Inactivity

A lack of physical activity plays a significant role in the development of heart disease. When lack of regular exercise is combined with overeating and obesity, high cholesterol can result and further increase the risk for heart disease. Even moderate levels of regular, low-intensity exercise have been shown to be beneficial in the prevention of heart disease.[3]

Obesity and Overweight

Approximately 66% of the U.S. adult population is overweight, and about 31.4% is considered obese.[2] Obesity and excess weight are associated with an increased mortality rate from coronary artery disease and stroke. Excess weight is also linked with an increased incidence of hypertension, insulin resistance, diabetes, and dyslipidemia. Central obesity (intra-abdominal fat) appears to be a stronger predictor of cardiovascular disease than peripheral or subcutaneous obesity. The waist measurement and the body mass index (a measure of weight relative to height) are the recommended means to estimate a person's body fat. A higher risk for cardiovascular disease is found for women with a waist greater than 35 inches and for men with a waist greater than 40 inches.[3]

Diabetes Mellitus

Diabetes mellitus is associated with a markedly increased risk for cardiovascular disease. This increased risk occurs even if the person maintains control of blood glucose levels. About 75% of people with diabetes die of some form of heart or blood vessel disease.[3,5]

Contributing Risk Factors

Stress

A person's response to stress may be a contributing factor to cardiovascular disease. The behaviors that a person engages in when under stress (such as smoking and overeating) may contribute to the risk for cardiovascular disease.[3,5]

Excessive Alcohol Intake

The excessive intake of alcohol has been associated with hypertension, heart failure, and stroke. The risk for heart disease in moderate drinkers is lower than in nondrinkers. Moderate drinking means one drink for a woman per day and two drinks for a man per day. One drink is defined as 1.5 fluid ounces of 80-proof spirits, 1 fluid ounce of 100-proof spirits, 4 fluid ounces of wine, or 12 fluid ounces of beer.[5]

Metabolic Syndrome

The term "metabolic syndrome" refers to a group of risk factors associated with an increased risk for developing cardiovascular disease and type 2 diabetes. Metabolic syndrome is diagnosed when three or more of the following risk factors are present:

▶ Fasting blood glucose of 100 mg/dL or higher
▶ HDL cholesterol below 40 mg/dL in men or below 50 mg/dL in women
▶ Triglycerides of 150 mg/dL or higher
▶ Waist circumference of 102 cm or higher in men or 88 cm or higher in women
▶ Systolic blood pressure of 130 mm Hg or higher, or diastolic pressure of 85 mm Hg or higher, or drug treatment for hypertension[2]

About 47 million people have metabolic syndrome in the United States. These people are at increased risk for developing diabetes and cardiovascular disease. They also have increased mortality from cardiovascular disease of all causes.[2]

• Acute Coronary Syndrome

The term acute coronary syndrome is used to describe patients with clinical symptoms compatible with acute myocardial ischemia. This term includes unstable angina and acute MI. Unstable angina refers to unexpected chest pain or discomfort that usually occurs while at rest. Patients with MI are further classified into one of two groups: those with ST-segment elevation MI and those with non–ST-segment elevation MI.[2,6]

• Angina Pectoris

The term angina comes from the Latin word meaning "to choke." Angina pectoris is the term used to describe chest pain or discomfort that results from coronary artery disease. The patient may describe the sensation as pressure, fullness, squeezing, heaviness, or pain.

PATHOPHYSIOLOGICAL PRINCIPLES

Angina pectoris is caused by transient, reversible myocardial ischemia precipitated by an imbalance between myocardial oxygen demand and myocardial oxygen supply. In most cases, angina pectoris is the result of a reduced oxygen supply. The most common cause of a reduced supply of oxygen is atherosclerotic narrowing of the coronary arteries. A nonocclusive thrombus develops on a disrupted atherosclerotic plaque, resulting in a reduction in myocardial perfusion. As blood flow to the myocardium decreases, autoregulation of coronary blood flow occurs as a compensatory mechanism. The smooth muscles of the arterioles relax, thus decreasing resistance to blood flow in the arteriolar bed. When this compensatory mechanism can no longer meet the metabolic demands, myocardial ischemia occurs, and the person feels pain.

A less common cause of unstable angina is dynamic obstruction resulting from intense focal spasm of a coronary artery. The spasm is caused by hypercontractility of vascular smooth muscle, endothelial dysfunction, or abnormal constriction of small resistance vessels. As a result of the spasm, perfusion to the myocardium is interrupted, thus reducing the supply of oxygen.[6]

Arterial inflammation may be another cause of decreased oxygen supply that results in unstable angina. The inflammatory process may cause arterial narrowing, plaque destabilization, rupture, and thrombogenesis. More recent research has contributed to a better understanding of the role of inflammation in acute coronary syndromes. The role of an infection in the inflammatory process is under investigation.[4,6]

A marked increase in oxygen demand is another cause of unstable angina. Conditions such as fever, tachycardia, and thyrotoxicosis may result in an increased oxygen demand that is unable to be met, especially if the patient has underlying coronary artery disease.[6]

When the balance between oxygen supply and demand is not met, the myocardial tissue's need for oxygen and nutrients continues. The same work of pumping blood must be accomplished with less available energy and oxygen. The tissue that depends on the blood supply becomes ischemic as it functions with less oxygenated blood. Anaerobic metabolism can provide only 6% of the total energy needed. Glucose uptake by the cells is markedly increased as glycogen and adenosine triphosphate stores are depleted. Potassium rapidly moves out of the myocardial cells during ischemia. An acidotic cellular bath develops, further compromising cellular metabolism.

CLASSIFICATION OF ANGINA

Many terms are used clinically to describe angina. Stable angina (also known as chronic stable angina, classic angina, or exertional angina) is a term used to describe paroxysmal substernal pain that is usually predictable. The pain occurs with physical exertion or emotional stress and is relieved by rest or nitroglycerin.[3]

Unstable angina, also called preinfarction angina or crescendo angina, refers to cardiac chest pain that usually occurs while at rest. The patient with unstable angina has more prolonged and severe chest discomfort than the person with stable angina. Unstable angina is a type of acute coronary syndrome and requires immediate treatment because the patient is at increased risk for acute MI, cardiac dysrhythmias, or cardiac sudden death.[3]

Variant angina, also known as Prinzmetal's angina or vasospastic angina, is a form of unstable angina. Variant angina usually occurs at rest, most often between midnight and 8:00 a.m. It does not usually occur after exertion or emotional stress. Variant angina is the result of coronary artery spasm. Most people who experience variant angina have severe coronary atherosclerosis of at least one major coronary artery, and the spasm occurs very near the area of blockage.[3]

The Canadian Cardiovascular Society also has proposed a classification system for grading for angina. Each stage of the four-class system is described in Box 21-1.

ASSESSMENT

History

The five most important factors that indicate a likelihood of ischemia due to coronary artery disease are obtained rapidly during the history. These factors include a description of the symptoms, information about a prior history of coronary artery disease, the patient's sex and age, and the number of risk factors present.[6]

The nurse uses the N, O, P, Q, R, S, T method of pain assessment when taking the patient's history. For a review of the assessment questions, see Box 17-1. After determining the patient's normal baseline, the

---

Box 21-1 • Grading of Angina Pectoris by the Canadian Cardiovascular Society Classification System

Class I: Ordinary physical activity does not cause angina, such as walking, climbing stairs. Angina occurs with strenuous, rapid, or prolonged exertion at work or recreation.

Class II: Slight limitation of ordinary activity occurs. Angina occurs when walking or climbing stairs rapidly, walking uphill, walking or climbing stairs after meals, in cold, in wind, under emotional stress, or during the few hours after awakening. Angina occurs when walking more than two level blocks and climbing more than one flight of ordinary stairs at a normal pace and in normal conditions.

Class III: Ordinary physical activity is markedly limited. Angina occurs when walking one to two level blocks and climbing one flight of stairs in normal conditions and at a normal pace.

Class IV: Physical activity without discomfort is impossible; anginal symptoms may be present at rest.

From Campeau L: Grading of angina pectoris [letter]. Circulation 54:522–523, 1976; copyright 1976, American Heart Association, Inc; used with permission.

nurse asks about the time of onset of the pain. The nurse determines causes (provocative) of the pain and any measures the patient has used to relieve the pain (palliative). The pain of angina is often brought on by exertion or emotion. It may also occur after meals, exposure to cold, and at rest. Patients with angina often obtain relief from the pain with rest or by taking sublingual nitroglycerin. As the angina becomes more severe (unstable angina), the pain may occur at rest or be caused by less exertion and is no longer relieved with rest or sublingual nitroglycerin. The quality of anginal pain is frequently described as deep, poorly localized chest or arm discomfort. Patients often describe heaviness, squeezing, choking, or smothering sensations. When asked about region and radiation of the pain, patients report substernal, left-sided chest, or epigastric pain that may radiate to the left arm, neck, back, or jaw. The severity of the pain is evaluated by asking the patient to rate the pain on a scale of 0 to 10, with 10 being the worst pain they have experienced. Additional information is obtained related to time. The nurse asks how long the pain lasts, how frequently it occurs, and the time of day it occurs. Finally, the nurse asks about associated symptoms such as dyspnea, nausea, vomiting, and diaphoresis. Box 21-2 summarizes the assessment findings for a patient with myocardial ischemia. Based on the information obtained, the angina may be classified as one of three principal presentations: rest angina; new onset (<2 months) severe angina; and increasing angina (in intensity, duration, or frequency).[6]

The older patient, especially women, who experiences angina may have a different presentation because of changes in neuroreceptors. Considerations for the older patient are described in Box 21-3.

Physical Examination

The physical examination helps determine the cause of the pain, detect comorbid conditions, and assess any hemodynamic consequences of the pain. When the vital signs are taken, the nurse should measure the blood pressure in both arms of the patient. If the physical examination is performed during an anginal episode, the patient may present with tachycardia and pulsus alternans. During the initial phase of an anginal episode, the patient may be hypertensive. The patient may exhibit pallor with cold, clammy skin. On further examination of the skin, the nurse may detect xanthomas, which are yellow nodules or plaques, especially on the skin. Xanthomas may be indications of hypercholesterolemia. Carotid or femoral bruits may be auscultated, indicating the possible presence of obstructive cardiovascular disease. The nurse may hear a paradoxical split of S_2 or auscultate an S_3 heart sound. Both sounds are indicators of left ventricular failure. An S_4 may be heard, which is suggestive of decreased left ventricular compliance. Deficits in peripheral pulses may indicate peripheral vascular disease.

Diagnostic Tests

A 12-lead electrocardiogram (ECG) is a standard diagnostic test for patients with angina and should be obtained immediately in patients with chest discomfort. During the anginal episode, the ECG may show T-wave inversions and ST-segment depressions in the ECG leads associated with the anatomical region of myocardial ischemia (Fig. 21-3). Transient ST-segment changes (≥0.05 mV) that occur during a symptomatic episode while at rest and that resolve

---

Box 21-2 • The N, O, P, Q, R, S, T Characteristics of Chest Pain Due to Myocardial Ischemia

N–Normal
- The patient's baseline before the onset of the pain

O–Onset
- The time when the pain/discomfort started

P–Precipitating and Palliative Factors

Precipitating
- Exercise
- Exercise after a large meal
- Exertion
- Walking on a cold or windy day
- Cold weather
- Stress or anxiety
- Anger
- Fear

Palliative
- Stop exercise.
- Sit down and rest.
- Use sublingual nitroglycerin; pain of myocardial infarction is often not relieved by sublingual nitroglycerin.

Q–Quality
- Heaviness
- Tightness
- Squeezing
- Choking
- Suffocating
- Viselike

R–Region and Radiation
- Substernal with radiation to the back, left arm, neck, or jaw
- Upper chest
- Epigastric
- Left shoulder
- Intrascapular

S–Severity
- Pain rated on a scale of 0 to 10, with 10 being the worst pain ever experienced, often rated as 5 or above

T–Time
- Pain lasts from 30 seconds to 30 minutes.
- Pain can last longer than 30 minutes for unstable angina or myocardial infarction.

Box 21-3 • CONSIDERATIONS FOR THE OLDER PATIENT: Acute Coronary Syndrome

Coronary artery disease is more common and more severe in the older patient. Older patients often present with special problems because of their numerous comorbidities, such as diminished β-sympathetic response, increased cardiac afterload due to decreased arterial compliance and arterial hypertension, cardiac hypertrophy, and ventricular diastolic dysfunction.[11]

The older patient is more likely to present with atypical symptoms such as dyspnea, confusion, weakness, or fainting rather than with typical substernal chest pain. Because of differences in amount and distribution of subcutaneous fat, the older person may develop anginal symptoms more quickly when exposed to cold. The older person should be taught to dress in warm clothing and to recognize feelings of weakness, shortness of breath, or fainting as possible indicators of angina.

when the patient is asymptomatic are highly suggestive of severe coronary artery disease.[6] Ectopic beats may also be present during an anginal episode. The ECG should be compared with previous ECGs. Between anginal episodes, the ECG may appear normal. Ambulatory ECG monitoring may be used to assist in the diagnosis of angina, especially for patients with angina at rest.

Biochemical cardiac markers are useful in determining both the diagnosis and the prognosis of acute coronary syndromes. For a more detailed discussion of cardiac markers, see Chapter 17. A cardiac-specific troponin (troponin T or troponin I) is the preferred marker to obtain in all patients who present with chest discomfort consistent with acute coronary syndrome. For patients who present to the hospital within 6 hours of the onset of symptoms consistent with acute coronary syndrome, an early marker of cardiac injury such as myoglobin, in conjunction with a late marker such as troponin, may be obtained. If the patient has a negative cardiac marker within 6 hours of the onset of chest discomfort, another sample should be drawn in the 6- to 12-hour period after onset of chest discomfort.[6] Additional blood tests include chemistry, complete blood count, and coagulation studies.

Other diagnostic tests include exercise stress testing in which the ECG and blood pressure are monitored before, during, and after exercise. The exercise stress test is especially useful in risk stratification of patients. For patients who are unable to exercise, pharmacological stress testing may be done in which the medication increases myocardial oxygen demand while the patient remains inactive. Intravenous (IV) medications used for pharmacological stress testing include adenosine, dobutamine, and dipyridamole.

Cardiac imaging studies usually start with chest radiographs, although they have limited value in diagnosing coronary heart disease. Thallium-201 or technetium-99m sestamibi perfusion imaging can be used with exercise or pharmacological stress testing to detect perfusion defects. Positron emission tomography (PET) may be helpful in differentiating ischemic from infarcted myocardium. Echocardiography is performed to evaluate wall motion abnormalities and thickness, valvular function, and ejection fraction. Magnetic resonance imaging (MRI) and coronary computed tomographic angiography may be used to view structural cardiovascular abnormalities when other diagnostic techniques (e.g., the echocardiogram) are inconclusive or ambiguous.

Coronary angiography is an invasive diagnostic test that provides a definitive diagnosis of coronary artery disease. Results from coronary angiography are used to guide the decision whether to manage the patient medically or surgically. For further discussion of cardiovascular diagnostic tests, see Chapter 17.

MANAGEMENT

The goal of therapy for the patient with angina pectoris is to restore the balance between oxygen supply and oxygen demand. The nurse assesses the patient's vital signs and mental status frequently. The patient is placed on a cardiac monitor for ischemia and dysrhythmia detection. The patient is placed on bed rest until stabilized to minimize oxygen demands. Supplemental oxygen may be given to unstable patients to increase oxygen supply. A pulse oximeter and arterial blood gases are used to evaluate oxygenation status.

Pharmacological Therapy

Pharmacological therapy is an important component in the management of patients with angina pectoris. The severity of symptoms, hemodynamic status of the patient, and medication history guide the drug regimen.

Nitroglycerin is a mainstay of therapy and is used sublingually or as a spray for acute anginal attacks. If three sublingual tablets (0.4 mg) or spray taken 5 minutes apart (no more than 3 sprays in 15 minutes) does not relieve the pain of angina, IV nitroglycerin may be useful. IV nitroglycerin should be started at a rate of 10 μg/minute by continuous infusion and titrated up by 10 μg/minute every 3 to 5 minutes until some symptom or blood pressure response is noted. If signs and symptoms are relieved, there is no need to continue to increase the dose. However, if relief is not obtained, the dose can be increased until a blood pressure response is noted. A ceiling dose of 200 μg/minute is

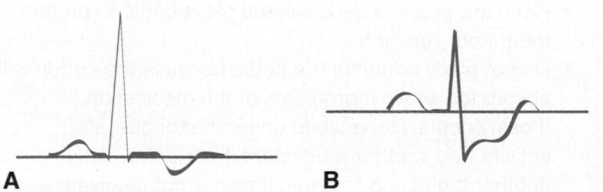

Figure 21-3 • Inversion of T wave (**A**) and depression of ST segment (**B**). (From Bullock BL: Pathophysiology: Adaptations and Alterations in Function, 4th ed. Philadelphia: Lippincott-Raven, 1996.)

recommended. Once patients have been pain free and have no other indications of ischemia for 12 to 24 hours, the IV nitroglycerin should be discontinued and replaced with oral or topical nitrates.[6]

Morphine sulfate is indicated for patients whose symptoms are not relieved after three serial sublingual nitroglycerin tablets or whose symptoms recur with adequate anti-ischemic therapy. A dose of 1 to 5 mg IV is recommended to relieve symptoms and maintain comfort. The nurse carefully monitors the patient's respiratory rate and blood pressure, especially if the patient continues to receive IV nitroglycerin.[6]

β-Blockers may be used to decrease myocardial oxygen consumption by reducing myocardial contractility, sinus node rate, and atrioventricular (AV) node conduction velocity. The reduction in myocardial contractility reduces the work of the heart and decreases myocardial oxygen demand. The slowing of the heart rate helps increase the time for diastolic filling, thus improving blood flow to the coronary arteries. β-Blockers are started orally within the first 24 hours for patients with unstable angina and non–ST-segment elevation MI.[6]

Calcium channel blockers may be beneficial for the patient with unstable angina and non–ST-segment elevation MI. Calcium channel blockers decrease myocardial oxygen demand by decreasing afterload, contractility, and heart rate. Verapamil and diltiazem have been shown to have the greatest benefit. The nurse carefully monitors the patient for side effects such as hypotension, worsening heart failure, bradycardia, and AV block. Calcium channel blockers can be administered to treat ischemia-related symptoms in patients unresponsive to or intolerant of nitrates and β blockers.[6]

The combination of aspirin, an anticoagulant, and an additional antiplatelet drug is recommended for the patient with unstable angina or non–ST-segment elevation MI. Aspirin should be administered as soon as the diagnosis of unstable angina or non–ST-segment elevation MI is made or suspected, unless contraindicated. For additional antiplatelet therapy, two drugs are approved: ticlopidine and clopidogrel. Anticoagulant therapy also is recommended to modify the disease process and its consequences for the patient with unstable angina and non–ST-segment elevation MI. Several drugs are available, and it is difficult to determine which is preferred based on the current research. Anticoagulant drugs that may be used include unfractionated heparin and low-molecular-weight heparin, as well as two new anticoagulants: fondaparinux (a factor XA inhibitor) and bivalirudin (direct thrombin inhibitor).[6]

Invasive Therapy

Invasive therapy may be indicated for the management of patients with unstable angina. Intra-aortic balloon pump (IABP) support may be used in the critically ill patient to provide increased coronary artery perfusion and to decrease afterload. Percutaneous transluminal coronary angioplasty (PTCA) and stent placement may be used for treating patients with unstable angina. See Chapter 18 for a more detailed discussion of the IABP, PTCA, and stent placement. Coronary artery bypass grafting (CABG) is another invasive option for treatment. See Chapter 22 for a more detailed discussion of cardiac surgery.

Risk Factor Modification

Risk factor modification may help prevent an anginal episode or delay the worsening of existing angina. Patients should be encouraged to stop smoking, achieve or maintain optimal weight, and exercise daily. Diet and medications may be prescribed to control hypertension, diabetes, and hyperlipidemia. Patient education, including home care considerations, is essential for patients with angina pectoris. Patient education guidelines and home care considerations are described in Box 21-4.

Box 21-4 • TEACHING GUIDE:
Angina Pectoris

Activity and Exercise
- Participate in a daily program of exercise that does not precipitate pain.
- Alternate activity with periods of rest and moderate activity level as needed.

Diet
- Eat a well-balanced diet with an appropriate caloric intake.
- If obese, participate in a supervised weight-reduction program.
- Avoid activity immediately after meals.
- Restrict intake of caffeine because it can increase heart rate.
- Maintain a diet low in fat.

Smoking
- Participate in a smoking cessation program. Smoking can increase heart rate, blood pressure, and blood carbon monoxide levels.
- Avoid smoke-filled environments.

Cold Weather
- Avoid exposure to cold and windy weather. Exercise indoors when necessary.
- When outdoors, dress in warm clothing, and cover mouth and nose with a scarf.
- Use a moderate pace of walking in cold weather.

Medications
- Carry sublingual nitroglycerin at all times.
- Keep the pills in a dark-colored glass bottle to protect them from sunlight.
- Do not place cotton in the bottle because the cotton will absorb the active ingredients of the medication.
- If pain occurs, place tablet under the tongue, stop activity, and wait for medication to dissolve. Take another tablet in 3 to 5 min if pain is not resolved.
- If pain continues, seek immediate care.
- Be aware of side effects of nitroglycerin, including headache, flushing, and dizziness.

• Myocardial Infarction

Prolonged ischemia caused by an imbalance between oxygen supply and oxygen demand causes MI. The prolonged ischemia causes irreversible cell damage and muscle death. Although multiple factors can contribute to the imbalance between oxygen supply and oxygen demand, the presence of a coronary artery thrombosis characterizes most MIs. In a classic investigation, DeWood and colleagues demonstrated that 87% of patients studied in the first 4 hours after onset of MI symptoms had a thrombotic occlusion.[7] The incidence of thrombotic occlusion decreases to 65% at 12 to 24 hours.

MI can be determined from several different perspectives, including clinical, electrocardiographic, biochemical, imaging, and pathological. The European Society of Cardiology, the American College of Cardiology Foundation, the American Heart Association, and the World Heart Federation developed a joint consensus document for the redefinition of MI.[1] Their clinical classification of an acute MI is shown in Box 21-5.

PATHOPHYSIOLOGICAL PRINCIPLES

Most patients who sustain an MI have coronary atherosclerosis. The thrombus formation occurs most often at the site of an atherosclerotic lesion, thus obstructing blood flow to the myocardial tissues. Plaque rupture is believed to be the triggering mechanism for the development of the thrombus in most patients with an MI. As mentioned previously, the role of inflammatory processes in the development of atherosclerotic plaque is an area of intense scientific investigation. Cardiovascular risk factors play a role in endothelial damage, resulting in endothelial dysfunction. The dysfunctioning endothelium contributes to the activation of the inflammatory response and the formation of atherosclerotic plaques. When the plaques rupture, a thrombus is formed at the site that can occlude blood flow, thus resulting in an MI. Figure 21-4 shows the atherosclerotic plaque in stable angina and in acute coronary syndromes.

Irreversible damage to the myocardium can begin as early as 20 to 40 minutes after interruption of blood flow. However, the dynamic process of infarction may not be completed for several hours. Necrosis of tissue appears to occur in a sequential fashion. Reimer and associates demonstrated that cellular death occurs first in the subendocardial layer and spreads like a "wave front" throughout the thickness of the wall of the heart.[8] Using dogs, they showed that the shorter the time between coronary occlusion and coronary reperfusion, the greater the amount of myocardial tissue that could be salvaged. Their classic work indicates that a substantial amount of myocardial tissue can be salvaged if flow is restored within 6 hours after the onset of coronary occlusion. For the clinician, this means time is muscle.

The cellular changes associated with an MI can be followed by the development of infarct extension (new myocardial necrosis), infarct expansion (a disproportionate thinning and dilation of the infarct zone), or ventricular remodeling (a disproportionate thinning and dilation of the ventricle).

Size of the Infarction

Several factors determine the size of the resulting MI. These factors include the extent, severity, and duration of the ischemic episode; the size of the vessel; the amount of collateral circulation; the status of the intrinsic fibrinolytic system; vascular tone; and the metabolic demands of the myocardium at the time of the event. MIs most often result in damage to the left ventricle, leading to an alteration in left ventricular function. Infarctions can also occur in the right ventricle or in both ventricles.

The term transmural infarction is used to imply an infarction process that has resulted in necrosis of the

---

Box 21-5 • Clinical Classification of Different Types of Myocardial Infarction

Type 1
Spontaneous myocardial infarction related to ischemia due to a primary coronary event such as plaque erosion and/or rupture, fissuring, or dissection

Type 2
Myocardial infarction secondary to ischemia due to either increased oxygen demand or decreased supply (e.g., coronary artery spasm, coronary embolism, anemia, arrhythmias, hypertension, hypotension)

Type 3
Sudden unexpected cardiac death, including cardiac arrest, often with symptoms suggestive of myocardial ischemia, accompanied by presumably new ST elevation, or new left bundle branch block, or evidence of fresh thrombus in a coronary artery by angiography and/or at autopsy, but death occurring before blood samples could be obtained, or at a time before the appearance of cardiac biomarkers in the blood

Type 4a
Myocardial infarction associated with percutaneous coronary intervention

Type 4b
Myocardial infarction associated with stent thrombosis as documented by angiography or at autopsy

Type 5
Myocardial infarction associated with coronary artery bypass grafting

From Thygesen K, Alpert JS., White, HD, on behalf of the Joint ESC/ACCF/AHA/WHF Task Force for the Redefinition of Myocardial Infarction: Universal definition of myocardial infarction. Circulation 116:2637, 2007.

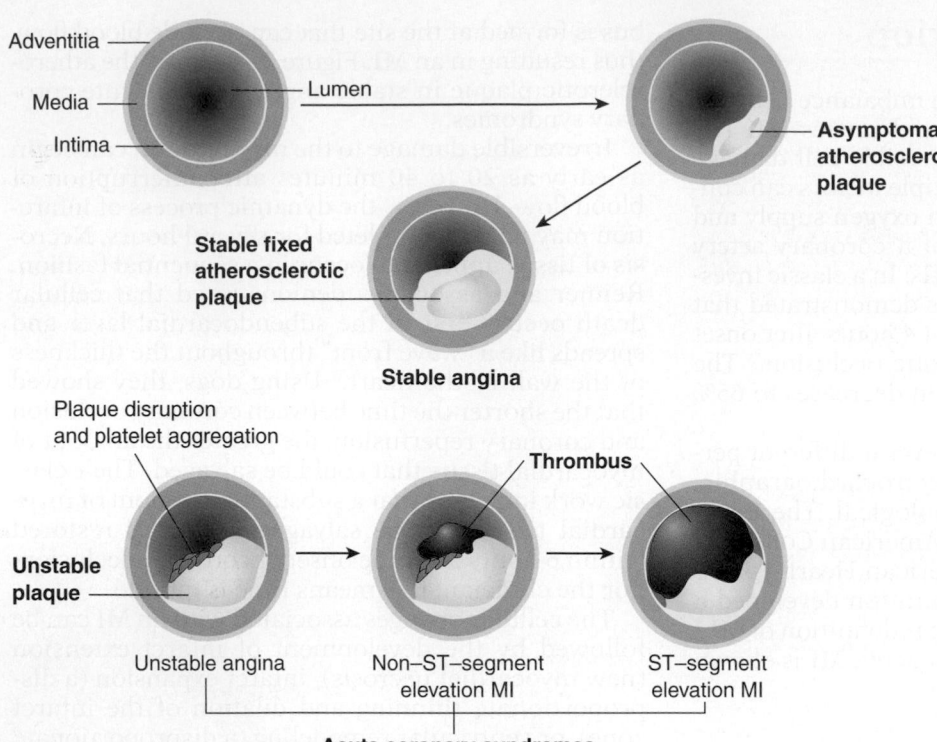

Figure 21-4 • Atherosclerotic plaque. Stable fixed atherosclerotic plaque in stable angina and the unstable plaque with plaque disruption and platelet aggregation in the acute coronary syndromes. (From Porth CM: Pathophysiology: Concepts of Altered Health States, 6th ed. Philadelphia: Lippincott Williams & Wilkins, 2002, p 495.)

tissue in all the layers of the myocardium. Because the heart functions as a squeezing pump, systolic and diastolic efforts can be significantly altered when a segment of the heart muscle is necrotic and nonfunctional. If the area of the transmural infarction is small, the necrotic wall may be dyskinetic, a term meaning "difficulty in moving." If the damage to the myocardial tissue is more extensive, the myocardial muscle may become akinetic, meaning "without motion."

The normal myocardial muscle contracts with systole and relaxes with diastole. When normal motion is not possible because of infarction, diastolic filling and systolic pumping are altered. As a result, cardiac output is compromised. The larger the area of infarction, the greater is the impact on ventricular function.

Location of the Infarction

In addition to size, location of the infarction is an important determinant of ventricular function. MIs can be located in the anterior, septal, lateral, posterior, or inferior walls of the left ventricle. In more recent years, clinicians have acknowledged the presence and clinical significance of MIs occurring in the right ventricle.

Anterior Left Ventricle

Infarctions of the anterior wall of the left ventricle and the interventricular septum result from occlusion of the left anterior descending (LAD) coronary artery. The LAD coronary artery supplies oxygenated blood to the anterior wall of the left ventricle, the interventricular septum, and the ventricular conducting tissue. (See Chapter 16 for a more detailed discussion of coronary artery anatomy and physiology.) Anterosep-

tal wall MIs are the most frequent type of infarction and have the potential for causing a significant amount of left ventricular dysfunction. Patients with an anteroseptal MI are at high risk for heart failure, pulmonary edema, cardiogenic shock, and death because of an inadequate pump. Anteroseptal wall MIs are also associated with increased risk for intraventricular conduction disturbances, such as bundle branch blocks and fascicular blocks, which are also known as hemi-blocks.

Lateral and Posterior Left Ventricle

Infarctions of the lateral and posterior walls of the left ventricle result from occlusion of the left circumflex vessel. In addition to supplying oxygenated blood to the lateral and posterior walls, the left circumflex vessel is the source of blood supply to the sinoatrial (SA) node in about 50% of the population and to the AV node in about 10% of the population. Infarctions of the lateral and posterior walls are less common than infarctions of the anteroseptal wall. Although muscle necrosis occurs with lateral and posterior wall MIs, the impact on left ventricular function is usually less than for patients with anteroseptal MI. Patients with a lateral or posterior wall MI are also at risk for dysrhythmias associated with dysfunction of the SA or AV nodes. Examples include sinus arrest, wandering atrial pacemaker, sinus pause, or junction rhythm.

Inferior Left Ventricle

Infarctions of the inferior wall result from occlusion of the right coronary artery. The right coronary artery supplies oxygenated blood to the inferior wall and the right ventricle. In addition, it is the source of blood supply to the SA node in about 50% of the population and the AV node in about 90% of the population.

Infarctions of the inferior wall are less common than anteroseptal MIs but occur more frequently than MIs of the lateral or posterior walls. The potential impact on left ventricular function usually is less for a patient with an inferior wall MI than for a patient with an anteroseptal wall infarct. Because the right coronary artery supplies oxygenated blood to much of the conducting tissue, patients are at frequent risk for dysrhythmias related to altered function of the SA and AV nodes.

Right Ventricle

The right coronary artery provides the blood supply to the inferior wall and the right ventricle. Consequently, right coronary artery disease causing an inferior wall MI is likely to be associated with concomitant right ventricular infarction. Approximately 33% to 50% of patients with an inferior wall MI have associated right ventricular involvement.[9,10] Patients may experience significant hemodynamic compromise due to biventricular dysfunction. As a result, patients with a right ventricular infarction and hemodynamic abnormalities with a concurrent inferior wall MI have a significantly higher mortality rate (25% to 30%).[11] Dysrhythmias associated with right ventricular infarction involve dysfunction of the SA and AV nodes.

Type of Infarction

Patients with chest pain may present with or without ST-segment elevations on their ECG. In most patients with ST-segment elevation, a Q wave ultimately develops on the ECG, and the term Q-wave MI is used to describe the type of MI they experience. In a much smaller number of patients who present with ST-segment elevation, a Q wave does not develop, and the term non–Q-wave MI is used to classify these patients. Patients who present without ST-segment elevations are diagnosed with either unstable angina or a non–ST-segment elevation MI[11] (Fig. 21-5).

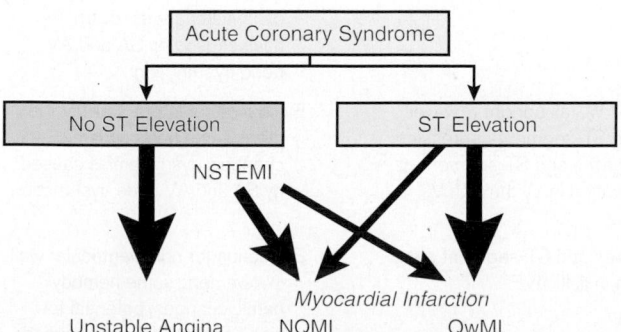

Figure 21-5 • Acute coronary syndrome. Patients may present with or without ST-segment elevation on electrocardiography. Most patients with ST-segment elevation (*large arrows*) ultimately develop a Q-wave AMI (QwMI), whereas a minority (*small arrow*) develop a non–Q-wave AMI (NQMI). Patients who present without ST-segment elevation are experiencing either unstable angina or NSTEMI (non–ST segment elevation MI). (Redrawn with permission from Braunwald E, et al: ACC/AHA Practice Guidelines. American College of Cardiology, 2002.)

The ST segment is the portion of the ECG tracing from the end of the QRS complex to the beginning of the T wave. Normally, the ST segment is isoelectric, meaning it joins the QRS complex at the baseline. When the ST segment is elevated, the amount of elevation is measured in millimeters on the ECG paper.

A Q wave is a portion of the QRS complex on the ECG. Specifically, the Q wave is the initial downward deflection of the QRS complex. A Q wave is not present on the normal ECG. The presence of significant Q waves indicates an MI. For a review of ECG waveforms, see Chapter 17.

ASSESSMENT

The nursing assessment of a patient with a probable MI must be organized and thorough. It is best to start with the history because this establishes rapport and provides valuable data. The history is followed by the physical examination and evaluation of diagnostic tests. Based on the data, a management plan is developed initially for the acute phase. Once the patient is stabilized, plans for cardiac rehabilitation are initiated.

History

The most common presenting complaint of a patient with an MI is the presence of chest discomfort or pain. Other assessment findings are similar to those described in Box 21-2. Like patients with angina, patients with MI describe a heaviness, squeezing, choking, or smothering sensation. Patients often describe the sensation as "someone sitting on my chest." The substernal pain can radiate to the neck, left arm, back, or jaw. Unlike the pain of angina, the pain of an MI is often more prolonged and unrelieved by rest or sublingual nitroglycerin. For a review of the assessment questions, see Box 17-1.

Associated findings on history include nausea and vomiting, especially for the patient with an inferior wall MI. These gastrointestinal complaints are believed to be related to the severity of the pain and the resulting vagal stimulation. Patients may initially seek relief of the gastrointestinal symptoms through antacids and other home remedies, thus delaying their decision to go the hospital. Additional complaints described during the history include diaphoresis, dyspnea, weakness, fatigue, anxiety, restlessness, confusion, shortness of breath, or a sense of impending death.

After the patient is stabilized, a more comprehensive history is obtained. Information about risk factors, previous cardiac illnesses and surgeries, and family history is important to acquire. This information will be useful in guiding patient education, cardiac rehabilitation, and care at home.

Physical Examination

On physical examination, patients usually appear restless, agitated, and in distress. They often assume a position to promote breathing and alleviate pain.

The skin is cool and moist. Vital signs may reveal a low-grade fever, hypertension, and tachycardia from increased sympathetic tone or hypotension and bradycardia from increased vagal tone. The pulse may be irregular and faint.

The cardiovascular examination may reveal additional abnormalities. When the patient is placed in the left lateral decubitus position, abnormalities of the precordial pulsations can be felt. These abnormalities include a lack of a point of maximal impulse or the presence of diffuse contraction. On auscultation, the first heart sound may be diminished as a result of decreased contractility. A fourth heart sound is heard in almost all patients with MI as a result of decreased left ventricular compliance. A third heart sound may be detected due to left ventricular systolic dysfunction. Transient systolic murmurs may be heard because of papillary muscle dysfunction. After about 48 to 72 hours, many patients acquire a pericardial friction rub.[12] Additional findings on physical examination, such as jugular venous distention, may be related to the development of complications such as heart failure or pulmonary edema. Breathing may be labored and rapid, and fine crackles, coarse crackles, or rhonchi may be heard when auscultating the lungs. These sounds may indicate the presence of heart failure or pulmonary edema.

Patients with right ventricular infarcts may present with jugular venous distention as well as peripheral edema and elevated central venous pressure. Their lungs may be clear because the failing right ventricle has not provided adequate forward flow.

Diagnostic Tests

The Electrocardiogram

When a coronary artery becomes about 70% occluded and oxygen demand exceeds oxygen supply, myocardial ischemia may result. If the ischemic state is not corrected, injury to the myocardium may occur. Eventually, if adequate blood flow to the myocardium is not restored, an MI may result. Ischemia and injury are reversible processes; however, infarction is not.

An ECG can be used to detect patterns of ischemia, injury, and infarction. When the heart muscle becomes ischemic, injured, or infarcted, depolarization and repolarization of the cardiac cells are altered, causing changes in the QRS complex, ST segment, and T wave in the ECG leads overlying the affected area of the heart. Table 21-1 shows location of the MI, the artery affected, findings from the ECG, and clinical implications.

Ischemia Myocardial ischemia may be a transient finding on ECG, or ischemic patterns may be more prolonged due to the presence of ischemic tissue surrounding a region of infarcted tissue. On the ECG, myocardial ischemia results in T-wave inversion

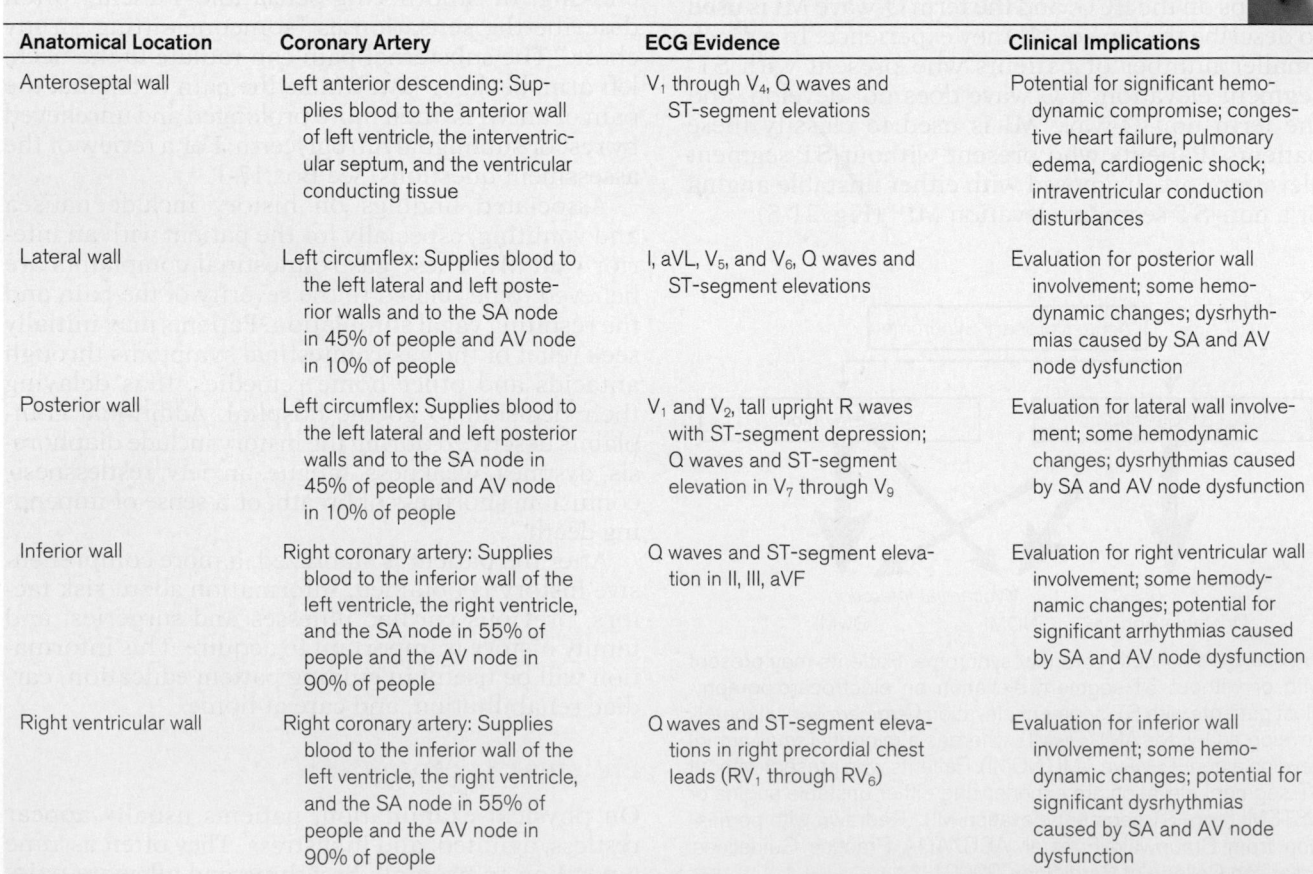

Table 21-1 • Location of Myocardial Infarction, Electrocardiographic (ECG) Findings, and Clinical Implications

Anatomical Location	Coronary Artery	ECG Evidence	Clinical Implications
Anteroseptal wall	Left anterior descending: Supplies blood to the anterior wall of left ventricle, the interventricular septum, and the ventricular conducting tissue	V_1 through V_4, Q waves and ST-segment elevations	Potential for significant hemodynamic compromise; congestive heart failure, pulmonary edema, cardiogenic shock; intraventricular conduction disturbances
Lateral wall	Left circumflex: Supplies blood to the left lateral and left posterior walls and to the SA node in 45% of people and AV node in 10% of people	I, aVL, V_5, and V_6, Q waves and ST-segment elevations	Evaluation for posterior wall involvement; some hemodynamic changes; dysrhythmias caused by SA and AV node dysfunction
Posterior wall	Left circumflex: Supplies blood to the left lateral and left posterior walls and to the SA node in 45% of people and AV node in 10% of people	V_1 and V_2, tall upright R waves with ST-segment depression; Q waves and ST-segment elevation in V_7 through V_9	Evaluation for lateral wall involvement; some hemodynamic changes; dysrhythmias caused by SA and AV node dysfunction
Inferior wall	Right coronary artery: Supplies blood to the inferior wall of the left ventricle, the right ventricle, and the SA node in 55% of people and the AV node in 90% of people	Q waves and ST-segment elevation in II, III, aVF	Evaluation for right ventricular wall involvement; some hemodynamic changes; potential for significant arrhythmias caused by SA and AV node dysfunction
Right ventricular wall	Right coronary artery: Supplies blood to the inferior wall of the left ventricle, the right ventricle, and the SA node in 55% of people and the AV node in 90% of people	Q waves and ST-segment elevations in right precordial chest leads (RV_1 through RV_6)	Evaluation for inferior wall involvement; some hemodynamic changes; potential for significant dysrhythmias caused by SA and AV node dysfunction

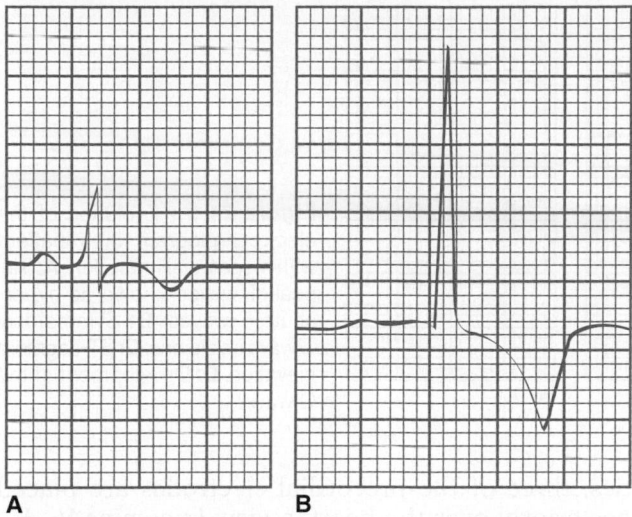

Figure 21-6 • T-wave inversion seen with ischemia (**A**) versus T-wave inversion seen with left ventricular hypertrophy (**B**).

or ST-segment depression in the leads facing the ischemic area. The inverted T wave representative of ischemia is symmetrical, relatively narrow, and somewhat pointed. In contrast, asymmetrical inversion of the T wave usually does not indicate ischemia. Instead, it may signify ventricular hypertrophy or bundle branch block (Fig. 21-6). ST-segment depressions of 1 to 2 mm or more for a duration of 0.08 second may indicate myocardial ischemia. Ischemia also should be suspected when a flat or depressed ST segment makes a sharp angle when joining an upright T wave rather than merging smoothly and imperceptibly with the T wave (Fig. 21-7).

Injury ECG patterns of myocardial injury indicate a state of cellular damage beyond ischemia. Like ischemia, myocardial injury is a reversible process if interventions are instituted rapidly. As described previously, the injury process begins in the subendocardial layer and moves throughout the thickness of the wall of the heart like a wave. If the injury process is not interrupted, it eventually results in a transmural MI.

On ECG, the hallmark of acute myocardial injury is the presence of ST segment elevations. In the normal ECG, the ST segment should not be elevated more

than 1 mm in the standard leads or more than 2 mm in the precordial leads. With an acute injury, the ST segments in the leads facing the injured area are elevated. The elevated ST segments also have a downward concave or coved shape and merge unnoticed with the T wave (Fig. 21-8).

Infarction When myocardial injury persists, MI is the result. The pattern of the ECG indicative of an MI is seen on the ECG in stages and involves changes in the T wave, the ST segment, and the Q wave in the leads overlying the infarcted area. Figure 21-9 shows the evolution of the ECG in an MI. During the earliest stage of MI, known as the hyperacute phase, the T waves become tall and narrow. This configuration is referred to as hyperacute or peaked T waves. Within a few hours, these hyperacute T waves invert.

Next, the ST segments elevate, a pattern that usually lasts from several hours to several days. In addition to the ST-segment elevations in the leads of the ECG facing the injured heart, the leads facing away from the injured area may show ST-segment depression. This finding is known as reciprocal ST-segment changes. Reciprocal changes are most likely to be seen at the onset of infarction, but their presence on the ECG does not last long. Reciprocal ST-segment depressions may simply be a mirror image of the ST-segment elevations. However, others have suggested that reciprocal changes may reflect ischemia due to narrowing of another coronary artery in other areas of the heart.[13]

The last stage in the ECG evolution of an MI is the development of Q waves, the initial downward deflection of the QRS complex. Q waves represent the flow of electrical forces toward the septum. Small, narrow Q waves may be seen in the normal ECG in leads I, II,

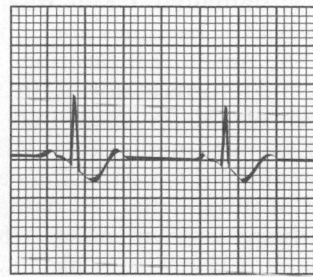

Figure 21-7 • An ST-segment pattern consistent with myocardial ischemia. Notice how the ST segment forms a sharp angle when joining an upright T wave rather than merging smoothly and imperceptibly with the T wave.

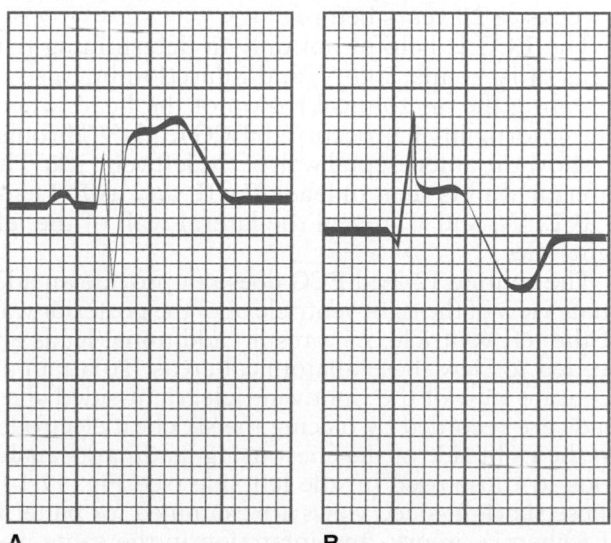

Figure 21-8 • ST-segment pattern consistent with acute myocardial injury. **A:** ST-segment elevation without T-wave inversion. **B:** ST-segment elevation with T-wave inversion. The elevated ST segments have a downward concave or coved shape and merge unnoticed with the T wave.

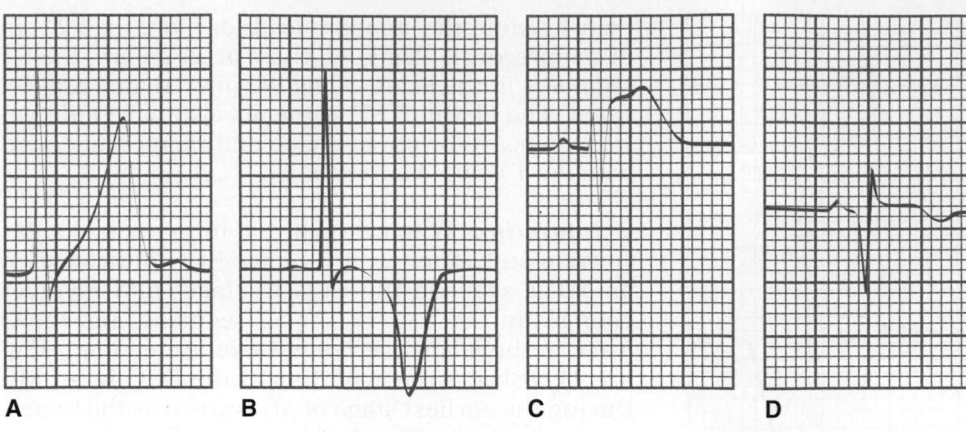

Figure 21-9 • Evolution of the electrocardiogram in a patient with myocardial infarction. **A:** Tall peak T waves known as hyperacute T waves. **B:** Symmetrical T-wave inversions. **C:** ST-segment elevation. **D:** Development of the Q wave.

III, aVR, aVL, V_5, and V_6. Q waves compatible with an MI are usually 0.04 second or more in width or one fourth to one third the height of the R wave. Q waves indicative of infarction usually develop within several hours of the onset of the infarction, but in some patients, they may not appear until 24 to 48 hours after the infarction.

Within a few days after the MI, the elevated ST segments return to baseline. Persistent elevation of the ST segment may indicate the presence of a ventricular aneurysm. The T waves may remain inverted for several weeks, indicating areas of ischemia near the infarct region. Eventually, the T waves should return to their upright configuration. The Q waves do not disappear and therefore always provide ECG evidence of a previous MI.

The ECG pattern can be used to distinguish acute MIs from "old" MIs. Abnormal Q waves accompanied by ST-segment elevations indicate an acute MI. Abnormal Q waves accompanied by a normal ST segment indicate a previous MI. How long ago the infarction occurred cannot be determined by the ECG. The pattern could signify an infarction that occurred 2 weeks or 20 years before.

The ECG is helpful not only in determining patterns of ischemia, injury, and infarction but also in revealing the anatomical region of the heart where the abnormality has occurred. ECG leads V_1 through V_4 show the anteroseptal wall of the left ventricle. The inferior wall is seen in leads II, III, and aVF. Leads I, aVL, V_5, and V_6 reveal the lateral wall of the left ventricle.

The routine 12-lead ECG does not provide an adequate view of the right ventricle or of the posterior wall of the left ventricle. As a result, additional leads are needed to view these anatomical areas. To attain an accurate view of the right ventricle, right-sided chest leads are recorded by placing the six chest electrodes on the right side of the chest using landmarks analogous to those used on the left side (see Fig. 17-14). These six right-sided views are examined for patterns of ischemia, injury, and infarction in the same way left-sided chest leads are evaluated.

Detection of posterior wall abnormalities is also difficult on the standard 12-lead ECG because none of the 6 chest leads provides an adequate view of the posterior wall. To detect posterior wall abnormali-

ties, three of the precordial electrodes are placed posteriorly over the heart, a view known as V_7, V_8, and V_9. V_7 is positioned at the posterior axillary line; V_8 at the posterior scapular line; and V_9 at the left border of the spine. All three posterior leads are positioned along the same horizontal line established by V_6. The recording is examined for evidence of ischemia, injury, or infarction using the same criteria as described previously. If posterior leads were not recorded, it may still be possible to detect posterior wall abnormalities. To do so, the principle of reciprocal change is used. When an infarction in the posterior wall is suspected, the leads anatomically opposite the posterior wall are examined. These include V_1 and V_2 because the anterior wall is anatomically opposite the posterior wall. If tall R waves with ST-segment depressions are noted in V_1 and V_2, the pattern is consistent with a posterior wall MI. Figures 21-10 through 21-13 show the 12-lead ECGs of patients with MIs.

Laboratory Tests

When myocardial cells are damaged by an infarction, biochemical markers are released into the bloodstream and can be detected by laboratory tests. The presence of abnormally high levels of biochemical markers, their distribution, and the time pattern for their appearance and disappearance make them very useful in the diagnosis of acute MI. For a more detailed discussion of laboratory tests, see Chapter 17.

Creatine Kinase Creatine kinase (CK) is an enzyme found mainly in heart and skeletal muscles. When heart muscle is damaged, CK is released into the blood. The level of CK becomes abnormal within 6 to 8 hours after the onset of infarction, peaks within 12 to 28 hours, and returns to normal in 24 to 36 hours. The isoenzymes of CK are measured to determine whether the CK came from the heart (MB) or the skeletal muscle. Elevation of CK-MB offers a more definitive indication of myocardial cell damage than total CK alone. For the patient with an MI, CK-MB appears in the serum in 3 to 12 hours, peaks in 24 hours, and returns to normal levels in about 48 to 72 hours.[11]

New assay techniques to measure CK-MB based on monoclonal antibodies offer greater sensitivity and specificity than conventional means. In addition,

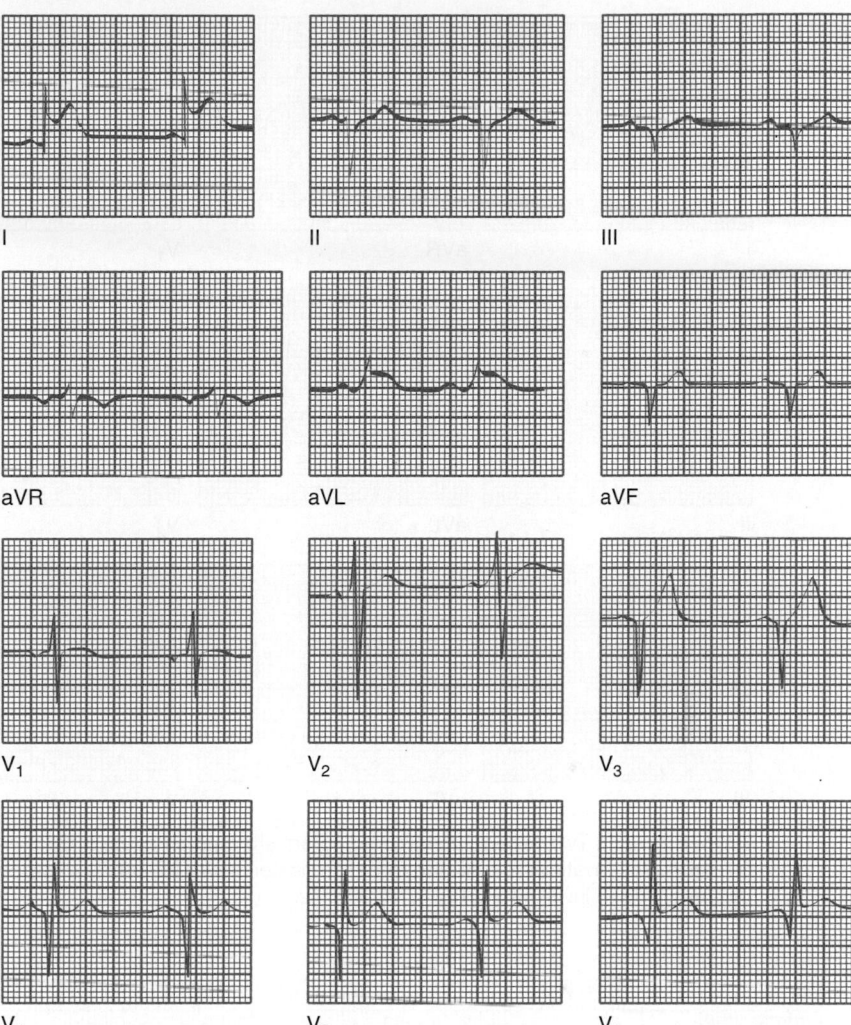

Figure 21-10 • Twelve-lead electrocardiogram showing an acute lateral wall myocardial infarction. ST-segment elevations can be seen in leads I, aVL, V5, and V6. Note also the deep Q waves in II, III, and aVF and normal ST segments, indicating a previous inferior wall myocardial infarction.

the results can be available in 30 minutes, which provides a distinct advantage in the diagnosis of an MI, especially in the emergency department.

Creatine Kinase Isoforms When the myocardial cells release CK-MB, it is quickly transformed into two isoforms, also known as subforms. $CK\text{-}MB_1$ is the isoform found in the plasma, and $CK\text{-}MB_2$ is found in the tissues. In the normal person, these two isoforms are found in about equal amounts, resulting in a ratio of approximately 1. In the patient with an MI, the $CK\text{-}MB_2$ level rises, resulting in a $CK\text{-}MB_2/CK\text{-}MB_1$ ratio greater than 1. This ratio can be rapidly measured in the laboratory and provides an excellent diagnostic marker for acute MI. The $CK\text{-}MB_2$ to $CK\text{-}MB_1$ ratio has improved sensitivity and specificity for diagnosis of MI within the first 6 hours compared with conventional assays for CK-MB. Isoform $CK\text{-}MB_2$ is also a sensitive test for detecting an early extension of an MI during the first 24 hours.[11]

Myoglobin Myoglobin is an oxygen-binding protein found in skeletal and cardiac muscle. Myoglobin's release from ischemic muscle occurs earlier than the release of CK. As a result, elevation of serum levels of myoglobin can be detected soon after the onset of symptoms. The myoglobin level can elevate within 1 to 4 hours of acute MI and peaks within 6 to 7 hours. Because myoglobin is also present in skeletal muscle, an elevated myoglobin level is not specific for the diagnosis of MI. Consequently, its diagnostic value in detecting an MI is limited. However, the early release of myoglobin makes it valuable in helping to detect MI.[11]

Troponin Troponin is a contractile protein with two subforms (troponin T and troponin I) that are highly specific for cardiac muscle. Troponin levels are not detected in the healthy person, and skeletal muscle injury does not affect the level. Troponin has been found to be a sensitive marker during the early hours after an MI. Troponin I levels rise in 3 to 12 hours, peak at 24 hours, and remain elevated for 5 to 10 days. Troponin T levels rise in 3 to 12 hours, peak in 12 hours to 2 days, and remain elevated for 5 to 14 days.[11] Because the cardiac troponins are highly sensitive and specific for MI, they are the preferred biomarker for diagnosing this coronary event.[11]

Other Diagnostic Tests

Patients with an MI should have a chest radiograph. An echocardiogram may be done to detect struc-

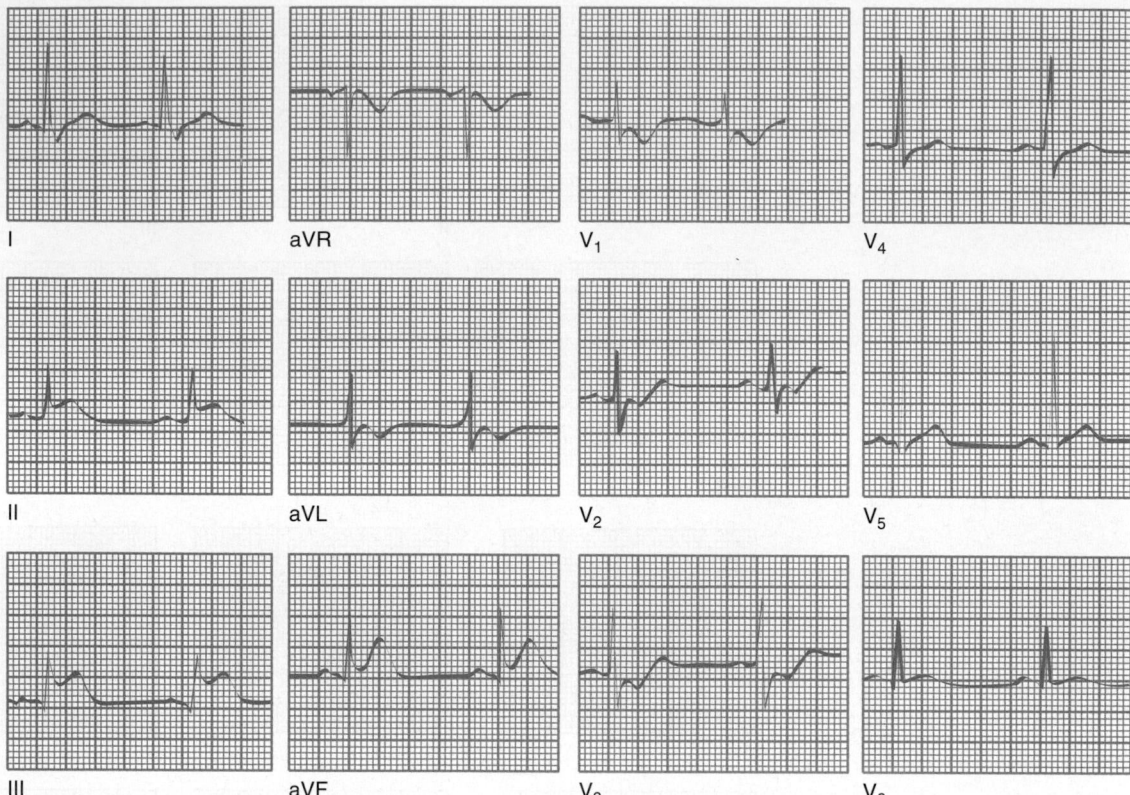

Figure 21-11 • Twelve-lead electrocardiogram showing an acute inferior wall myocardial infarction. Note the ST-segment elevations in II, III, and aVF. The posterior wall infarction is evidenced by a tall R wave, ST-segment depression, and inverted T wave in V1 and V2.

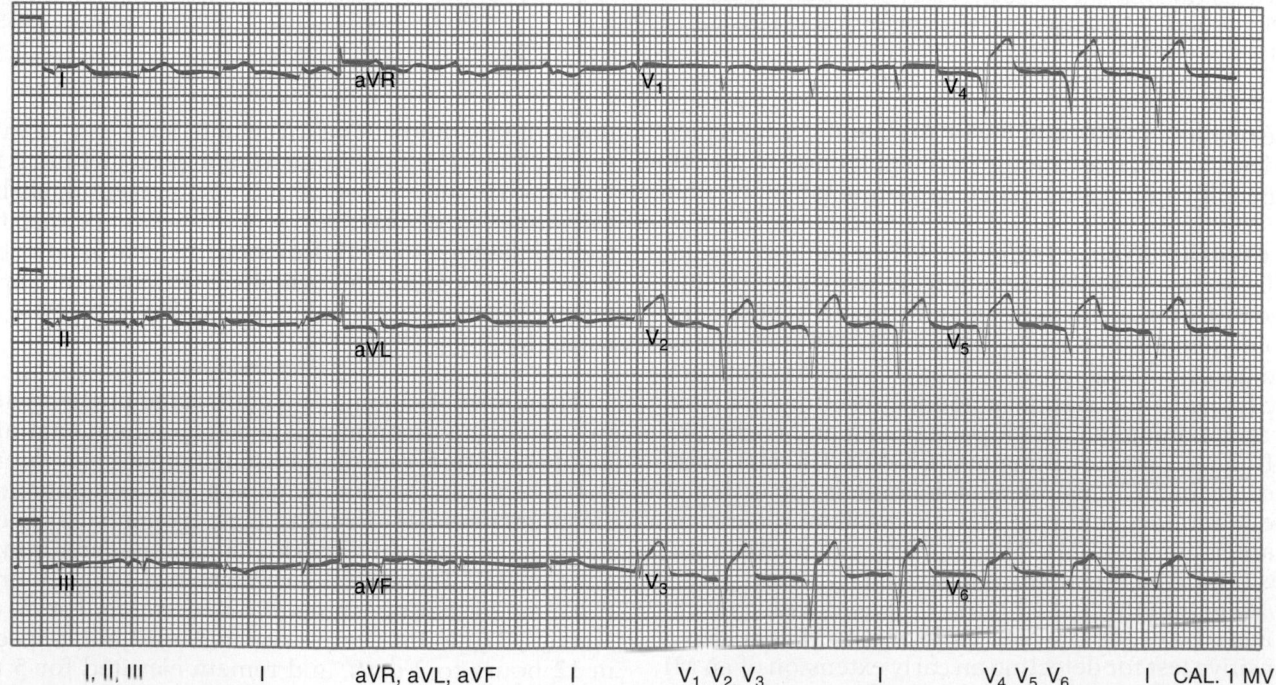

Figure 21-12 • Twelve-lead electrocardiogram showing an acute anterior and lateral wall myocardial infarction. Note the ST segment elevations and Q waves in I, aVL, V5, and V6 (lateral), and V2, V3, and V4 (anterior).

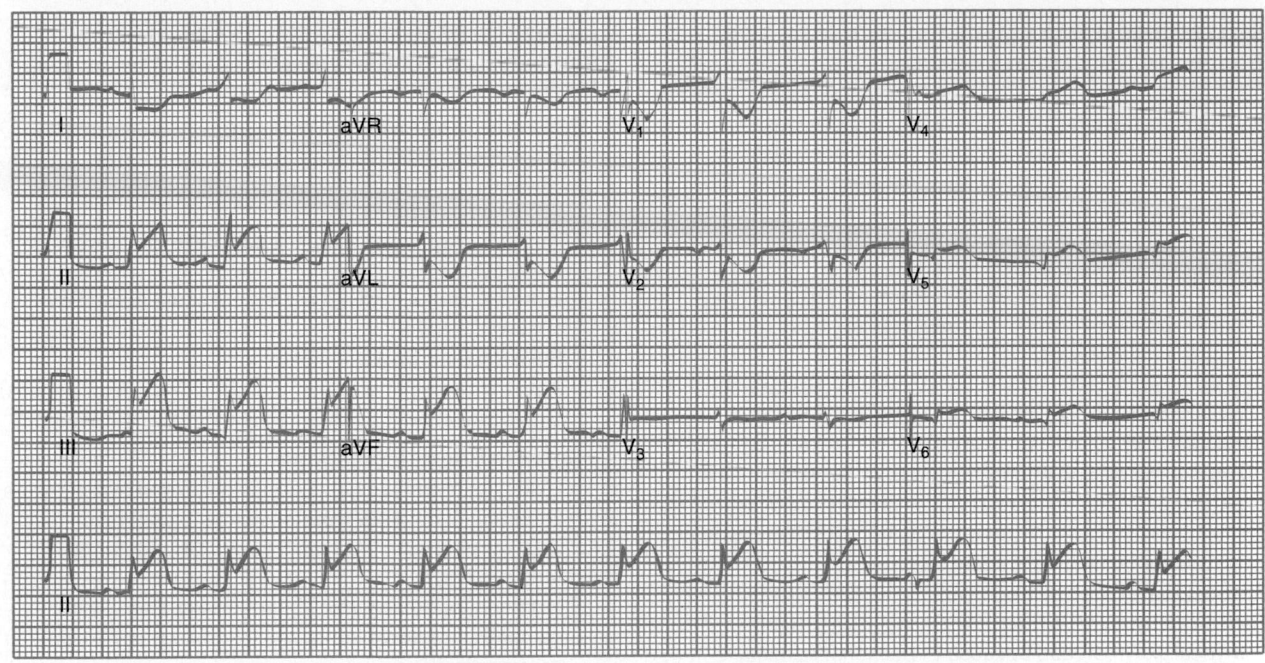

Figure 21-13 • Twelve-lead electrocardiogram showing right ventricular infarction. The six chest leads have been positioned on the right side of the chest. Note the ST segment elevation in RV4, RV5, and RV6. The ECG also shows elevated ST segments in the inferior leads (II, III, aVF). Patients with an inferior wall MI often also have an infarction in the right ventricle.

tural abnormalities such as valvular problems. Other tests may include radionuclide angiography, MRI, magnetic perfusion imaging, digital subtraction angiography, and single-photon emission computed tomography (SPECT) radionuclide imaging. For a more detailed discussion of these diagnostic tests, see Chapter 17.

MANAGEMENT

Early Management

When a patient with a possible MI arrives in the emergency department, the diagnosis and initial management of the patient must be rapid because the benefit of reperfusion therapy is greatest if therapy is initiated quickly. An initial evaluation of the patient should occur ideally within the first 10 minutes after arrival.[11] The patient's history and 12-lead ECG are the primary methods used to determine initially the diagnosis of MI. The ECG is examined for the presence of ST-segment elevations of 1 mm or greater in contiguous leads. This pattern provides evidence of thrombotic coronary arterial occlusion. The patient is placed on a continuous cardiac monitor with ST-segment monitoring capabilities.

If the initial screening suggests an MI, the interventions listed in Box 21-6 are initiated. The nurse checks the vital signs frequently, establishes IV access, and continuously assesses the patient's cardiac rhythm. Blood is drawn for serum cardiac markers, hematology, chemistry, and lipid profile. A chest radiograph and echocardiogram, obtained as soon as possible, are useful in ruling out an aortic dissection and acute pericarditis. During the initial evaluation, the patient

and family may be anxious, necessitating brief and clear explanations of the interventions. Reassurance and support are essential components of the nurse's responsibilities.

Fibrinolytic Therapy

If the patient is diagnosed with an MI, fibrinolytic therapy may be used to establish reperfusion if there are no contraindications to its use. Fibrinolytic drugs lyse coronary thrombi by converting plasminogen to plasmin. This conversion causes the degradation of fibrin and fibrinogen, resulting in clot lysis. Box 21-7 lists contraindications to fibrinolytic therapy.[11]

The goal is to complete the assessment of the patient and the administration of the fibrinolytic drug (if indicated) within 30 minutes of the patient's arrival to the emergency department. Fibrinolytic therapy provides maximal benefit if given within the first 3 hours after the onset of symptoms. There is a time-dependent decrease in efficacy of fibrinolytic therapy.[11]

For the patient receiving fibrinolytic therapy, two to three 18-gauge peripheral IV lines are usually started. One line is for the fibrinolytic agent, and one to two lines are for the administration of other drugs. Subclavian and jugular sites are avoided because they are noncompressible, and blood could be lost into the chest or neck. Some type of blood sampling device is also inserted so that peripheral venous punctures can be avoided.

The patient is closely monitored during and after the infusion of a fibrinolytic agent. The nurse assesses the patient for resolution of chest pain, normalization of elevated ST segments, development of reperfusion dysrhythmias, any allergic reactions, evidence of

Box 21-6 • Initial Management of the Patient With a Suspected Myocardial Infarction

Action: Administer aspirin, 160 to 325 mg chewed.

Rationale: Aspirin is used because it diminishes platelet aggregation. This effect is important because platelets are one of the main components in thrombus formation when a coronary plaque is disrupted. Aspirin has been shown to reduce mortality rates independently in patients with acute myocardial infarction. Patients diagnosed with a myocardial infarction should be continued on aspirin indefinitely.

Action: After recording the initial 12-lead ECG, place the patient on a cardiac monitor and obtain serial ECGs.

Rationale: The 12-lead ECG is central in the decision pathway for the diagnosis and treatment of the patient. The patient is placed on a continuous cardiac monitor after the 12-lead ECG is recorded to detect dysrhythmias and to monitor ST-segment changes.

Action: Give oxygen by nasal cannula.

Rationale: Hypoxemia often occurs in patients with a myocardial infarction because of pulmonary edema. If severe pulmonary edema is present and the patient is in respiratory distress, intubation may be necessary. A pulse oximeter is often applied, and, when time permits, an arterial blood gas may be drawn.

Action: Administer sublingual nitroglycerin (unless the systolic blood pressure is less than 90 mm Hg or the heart rate is less than 50 or greater than 100 beats/minute). Give 0.4 mg every 5 minutes for a total of 3 doses.

Rationale: Nitroglycerin helps to promote vasodilation but is relatively ineffective in relieving pain in the early stages of a myocardial infarction. Intravenous nitroglycerin is recommended for patients with acute myocardial infarction with persistent pain, for control of hypertension, or for management of pulmonary congestion.

Action: Provide adequate analgesia with morphine sulfate.

Rationale: Morphine is the drug of choice to relieve the pain of a myocardial infarction. The drug is given intravenously in small doses (2–4 mg) and can be repeated every 5 min until the pain is relieved. Close respiratory and blood pressure monitoring are indicated because morphine can depress respirations and cause hypotension.

Action: Administer β-blocker.

Rationale: During the first few hours after the onset of ST-segment elevation, myocardial infarction, β-blocking agents may diminish myocardial oxygen demand by reducing heart rate, systemic arterial pressure, and myocardial contractility.

From Antman, EM, Anbe DT, AR, Armstrong PW, et al: ACC/AHA guidelines for the management of patients with ST-elevation myocardial infarction. A report of the American College of Cardiology/American Heart Association Task Force on Practice Guidelines (Committee to revise the 1999 guidelines for the management of patients with acute myocardial infarction). Circulation 110:e82–e293, 2004.

Box 21-7 • Contraindications and Cautions for Fibrinolysis in ST-Elevation Myocardial Infarction*

Absolute Contraindications
- Any prior intracranial hemorrhage
- Known structural cerebral vascular lesion (e.g., arteriovenous malformation)
- Known malignant intracranial neoplasm (primary or metastatic)
- Ischemic stroke within 3 mo *except* acute ischemic stroke within 3 h
- Suspected aortic dissection
- Active bleeding or bleeding diathesis (excluding menses)
- Significant closed-head or facial trauma within 3 mo

Relative Contraindications
- History of chronic, severe, poorly controlled hypertension
- Severe uncontrolled hypertension on presentation (SBP greater than 180 mm Hg or DBP greater than 110 mm Hg)†
- History of prior ischemic stroke greater than 3 mo, dementia, or known intracranial pathology not covered in contraindications
- Traumatic or prolonged (greater than 10 min) CPR or major surgery (<3 wks)
- Recent (within 2–4 wks) internal bleeding
- Noncompressible vascular punctures
- For streptokinase/anistreplase: prior exposure (more than 5 d ago) or prior allergic reaction to these agents
- Pregnancy
- Active peptic ulcer
- Current use of anticoagulants: the higher the INR, the higher the risk of bleeding

SBP, systolic blood pressure; DBP, diastolic blood pressure; CPR, cardiopulmonary resuscitation; INR, international normalized ratio; MI, myocardial infarction.
*Viewed as advisory for clinical decision making and may not be all inclusive or definitive.
†Could be an absolute contraindication in low-risk patients with MI.
Used with permission from Antman EM, Anbe DT, Armstrong PW, et al: ACC/AHA guidelines for the management of patients with ST-elevation myocardial infarction. A report of the American College of Cardiology/American Heart Association Task Force on Practice Guidelines (Committee to revise the 1999 guidelines for the management of patients with acute myocardial infarction). Circulation 110:e127, 2004.

bleeding, and the onset of hypotension. Commonly seen reperfusion dysrhythmias include an accelerated idioventricular rhythm, ventricular tachycardia, and AV heart block.

Evaluation of complications remains a key nursing intervention. The patient is closely monitored for evidence of reocclusion of the coronary artery. Indicators of reocclusion include chest pain, ST-segment elevation, and hemodynamic instability. Close observation for evidence of bleeding also is essential. The patient is carefully assessed for indications of subcutaneous or mucous membrane bleeding. The nurse also monitors the patient for signs of internal bleeding, including positive results of urine and stool for blood or altered levels of consciousness due to intracranial bleeding.

Percutaneous Coronary Intervention

Early reperfusion of myocardial tissue is essential to preserve myocardial function. In addition to pharmacological therapy, percutaneous coronary intervention (PCI) is an effective alternative to reestablish blood flow to ischemic myocardium. PTCA, an invasive procedure in which the infarct-related coronary artery is dilated with a balloon catheter, is the type of PCI used. Once the artery is opened by the balloon, a stent may be placed in the artery. PTCA is used for patients who present within 12 hours of the onset of symptoms, and it also can be performed in patients whose ischemic symptoms persist. This therapeutic intervention necessitates the availability of a cardiac catheterization laboratory and skilled personnel at all times.[11] (See Chapter 18 for a more detailed discussion of the PTCA procedure.)

Evaluation of patients for PTCA is similar to that of fibrinolytic therapy. The accessibility of the lesion in the coronary artery is an additional factor that must be considered. PTCA may be an excellent reperfusion alternative for patients ineligible for fibrinolytic therapy. The nurse must carefully monitor the patient after a PTCA for evidence of complications. These complications can include retroperitoneal or vascular hemorrhage, other evidence of bleeding, early acute reocclusion, and late restenosis. If the PCI is not successful, the patient may be evaluated for an emergent coronary artery bypass grafting procedure.

Intensive and Intermediate Care Management

The management goal for the patient in the intensive care unit and intermediate care unit continues to be maximizing cardiac output while carefully minimizing cardiac workload. To achieve this goal, the patient frequently has vital signs taken and continues on a cardiac monitor with ST-segment monitoring. The lead selected for monitoring should be based on the infarct location and underlying rhythm. Serial ECGs and serial evaluations of serum cardiac markers of infarction are recorded. Serum hematology and chemistry are monitored.

For the first 12 hours of hospitalization, patients who are hemodynamically stable and free of ischemic-type chest discomfort remain on bed rest with bedside commode privileges. Activity level increases gradually in hemodynamically stable patients. Careful attention is paid to maximal pain relief. Nitroglycerin is not an appropriate substitute for analgesics. A pulse oximeter is used to monitor oxygen saturation continuously and is a good indicator of early hypoxemia. When the oxygen saturation level is stable for more than 6 hours, the need for continuous oxygen therapy should be reassessed.[11]

The patient is often not given anything by mouth until pain free. When pain free, the patient is given clear liquids and progressed to a heart-healthy diet as tolerated. Daily weights are recorded, and intake and output are measured to detect fluid retention. Stool softeners are administered so that the patient avoids a Valsalva maneuver. During a Valsalva maneuver, forced expiration against a closed glottis causes sudden and significant changes in systolic blood pressure and heart rate. These changes may influence regional endocardial repolarization and place the patient at risk for ventricular dysrhythmias. Nursing diagnoses and collaborative care problems for patients with acute MI are listed in Box 21-8.

Pharmacological Therapy
Prophylactic antidysrhythmics during the first 24 hours of hospitalization are not recommended. However, easy access to atropine, lidocaine, amiodarone, transcutaneous pacing patches, transvenous

> **Box 21-8** Examples of Nursing Diagnoses and Collaborative Problems for the Patient With Acute Myocardial Infarction
>
> - Chest Pain related to myocardial infarction, angina
> - Decreased Cardiac Output: Electrical factors affecting rate, rhythm, or conduction
> - Decreased Cardiac Output: Mechanical factors related to preload, afterload, or left ventricular failure
> - Knowledge Deficit related to illness and impact on patient's future
> - Anxiety, Stress related to fear of illness, death, and critical care environment
> - Activity Intolerance related to decreased cardiac output or alterations in myocardial tissue perfusion
> - Risk for Ineffective Tissue Perfusion related to thrombolytic therapy impact

pacing wires, a defibrillator, and epinephrine are essential for management of dysrhythmias. Daily aspirin is continued on an indefinite basis. Clopidogrel may be used for patients who are intolerant of aspirin.[11]

Angiotensin-converting enzyme (ACE) inhibitors are administered orally within the first 24 hours to patients with anterior wall MI, pulmonary congestion, or left ventricular ejection fraction less than 40%, in the absence of hypotension. ACE inhibitors help prevent ventricular remodeling (dilation) and preserve ejection fraction.[11]

During the first several days after ST-segment elevation MI, it is important to normalize the patient's blood glucose levels. An insulin infusion may be required to achieve this goal.[11]

Patients with a documented magnesium deficit should receive magnesium. Patients with torsades de pointes ventricular tachycardia with prolonged QT intervals also should be treated with magnesium.[11]

IV β-blocker therapy should be administered within the initial hours of the evolving infarction, followed by oral therapy provided there are no contraindications. β-Blockers are one of the few pharmacological agents that have been shown to reduce morbidity and mortality in the patient with an MI. They reduce oxygen demand by decreasing the heart rate and contractility. They also increase coronary artery filling by prolonging diastole. Calcium channel blockers may be given to patients in whom β-blocker therapy is ineffective or contraindicated.[11] The continuation of nitrate therapy beyond the first 24 to 48 hours may be useful for patients with recurrent angina or persistent heart failure.[11]

IV unfractionated heparin or low-molecular-weight heparin is used in patients after ST-segment elevation MI who are at high risk for systemic emboli. The risk is highest in patients with an anterior MI, atrial fibrillation, cardiogenic shock, or a previous embolus.[11]

Hemodynamic Monitoring
Use of a pulmonary artery catheter for hemodynamic monitoring is indicated in the patient with MI who has severe or progressive congestive heart failure or

pulmonary edema, cardiogenic shock, progressive hypotension, or suspected mechanical complications, such as ventricular septal defect, papillary muscle rupture, or pericardial tamponade.[11] The pulmonary artery wedge pressure (PAWP) is closely followed for assessment of left ventricular filling pressures. A PAWP below 18 mm Hg may indicate volume depletion, whereas a PAWP greater than 18 mm Hg indicates pulmonary congestion or cardiogenic shock. Using the thermodilution technique, frequent measurements of cardiac output and cardiac index can be made to evaluate hemodynamic status further. In some situations, monitoring venous oxygen saturation may also be useful. For a more detailed discussion of hemodynamic monitoring, see Chapter 17.

Invasive arterial monitoring is indicated for patients with MI who have severe hypotension or for those receiving vasopressor or vasodilator drugs. The collaborative care guide for the patient with an MI (Box 21-9) provides further information about the care of these patients.

Additional Diagnostic Tests

Computer Imaging Tests One category of computer imaging test is radionuclide imaging and radionuclide angiography. Radionuclide studies provide information about the presence of coronary artery disease as well as the location and quantity of ischemic and infracted myocardium. A radioactive tracer is injected into the patient, and computer generated images are created. Radionuclide tests include thallium tests, multiple gated acquisition (MUGA) scans, and infarct scintigraphy.

Another type of computer imaging test is MRI. This diagnostic test uses strong magnets and low-energy radio frequency signals to reveal structural and functional abnormalities of the heart and aorta. Coronary magnetic resonance angiography uses the principles of MRI in combination with a contrast medium to create images of vessel walls and the presence of any plaques.

Computed tomography (CT) is a type of computer imaging study that provides cross-sectional images of the chest, including the heart and aorta. CT angiography involves a CT scan of the heart after injection of a contrast medium. In addition to providing information about the structure of the heart, CT angiography offers information about the circulation of blood in the heart and coronary arteries. Electron-beam CT is a type of ultrafast CT and is considered the gold standard for detecting and quantifying the amount of calcium in coronary plaques. Electron beam CT can note the formation of an atherosclerotic plaque before the development of significant stenotic lesions.[3,14]

Cardiac positron tomography (PET) is another type of computed imaging test. PET combines CT imaging with radionuclide agents to detect coronary artery disease and injured but viable myocardial muscle. PET is a helpful test to determine myocardial muscle viability.

SPECT is a computed imaging test that involves the injection of a radionuclide agent followed by a series of computed graphics of the chest. SPECT is used to determine the extent and severity of blood flow abnormalities and coronary artery disease.[3,14]

A more detailed discussion of computed imaging tests can be found in Chapter 17.

Echocardiogram An echocardiogram is a non-invasive ultrasonographic test involving the transmission of high-frequency sound waves into the heart. This commonly used diagnostic test helps determine ejection fraction, segmental wall motion, systolic and diastolic ventricular volumes, valve function, mural thrombi, pericardial fluid, intracardiac tumors, and aortic dissection.[14] Two-dimensional, Doppler, and transesophageal echocardiograms are the most frequently used types of echocardiograms for patients with an MI. (See Chapter 17 for further discussion of echocardiograms.)

Stress Test Stress testing, also known as exercise electrocardiography, may be performed before discharge or within the first 3 weeks after discharge. The test is intended to assess the patient's functional capacity and ability to perform activities of daily living, to evaluate the efficacy of the patient's medical therapy, and to risk-stratify the patient based on the likelihood of a subsequent cardiac event. Stress testing may be combined with perfusion imaging to determine better the size of the infarction. (See Chapter 17 for further discussion of stress testing.)

Coronary Angiography During the course of hospitalization, patients may be further evaluated by coronary angiography. Results of the angiography help the physician determine whether a PTCA or placement of a stent is indicated, or if the patient is a candidate for CABG. (A more detailed discussion of PTCA can be found in Chapter 18, and a more detailed discussion of CABG can be found in Chapter 22.)

COMPLICATIONS

The nurse closely monitors the patient with MI for evidence of complications. Numerous complications can occur, and a list of possible complications is provided in Box 21-10. Prompt recognition and management of complications are essential in reducing mortality and morbidity.

Vascular Complications

Recurrent myocardial ischemia can occur in patients and is often transient. A recurrent MI is another possible complication. If the reinfarction occurs within the first 24 hours, it may be hard to diagnose because the cardiac serum markers have not yet returned to baseline. Early recognition and management are essential for both of these vascular complications. Efforts are made to lower myocardial oxygen demand and to relieve pain. Emergent PTCA or surgical revascularization may be considered.

Myocardial Complications

Cardiogenic shock is the most serious myocardial complication of MI. It occurs because of the loss of

Box 21-9 • COLLABORATIVE CARE GUIDE for the Patient With Myocardial Infarction

OUTCOMES	INTERVENTIONS
Oxygenation/Ventilation	
Patient has arterial blood gases within normal limits and pulse oximeter value >90%.	• Assess respiratory rate, effort, and breath sounds q2–4h. • Obtain arterial blood gases per order or signs of respiratory distress. • Monitor arterial saturation by pulse oximeter. • Provide supplemental oxygen by nasal cannula or face mask for the first 6 h, then as needed. • Provide intubation and mechanical ventilation as necessary. (Refer to Chapter 25, Mechanical Ventilation Care Guide.)
There is no evidence of pulmonary edema on chest x-ray and by clear breath sounds. There is no evidence of atelectasis.	• Obtain chest x-ray daily. • Administer diuretics per order. • Monitor signs of fluid overload as described below. • Encourage nonintubated patients to use incentive spirometer, cough, and deep breath q4h and PRN. • While on bed rest, turn side to side q2h.
Circulation/Perfusion	
Vital signs are within normal limits, including MAP >70 mm Hg and cardiac index >2.2 L/min/m2.	• Monitor HR and BP q1–2h and PRN during acute failure phase. • Assist with pulmonary artery catheter insertion. • Monitor PAP and PAWP, CVP, or right atrial pressure (RAP) q1h and cardiac output, SVR, and PVR q6–12h if pulmonary artery catheter is in place. • Maintain patent IV access. • Administer positive inotropic agents, and reduce afterload with vasodilating agents guided by hemodynamic parameters and physician orders. • Evaluate effect of medications on BP, HR, and hemodynamic parameters. • Prepare patient for intra-aortic balloon pump assist if necessary.
Patient has no evidence of congestive heart failure due to decreased cardiac output.	• Restrict volume administration as indicated by PAWP or CVP values. • Assess for neck vein distention, pulmonary crackles, S_3 or S_4, peripheral edema, increased preload parameters, elevated a wave of CVP, RAP, or PAWP waveform. • Monitor 12-lead ECG qd and PRN.
Patient has no evidence of further myocardial dysfunction, such as altered ECG or cardiac enzymes.	• Monitor cardiac markers, magnesium, phosphorus, calcium, and potassium as ordered. • Monitor ECG for changes consistent with evolving MI. • Consider obtaining right precordial chest leads, 12-lead ECG, if inferior wall/right ventricle is involved. • Report and treat abnormalities per protocols or orders.
Dysrhythmias are controlled.	• Provide continuous ECG monitoring in the appropriate lead. • Document rhythm strips every shift. • Anticipate need for/administer pharmacological agents to control dysrhythmias.
After fibrinolytic therapy, patient will have relief of pain; no evidence of bleeding; no evidence of allergic reaction.	• Assess, monitor, and treat pain as described below. • Monitor signs of reperfusion, such as dysrhythmias, ST-segment return to baseline, early rise and peak in CK.

(continued)

Box 21-9 • COLLABORATIVE CARE GUIDE for the Patient With Myocardial Infarction (Continued)

OUTCOMES	INTERVENTIONS
	• Monitor for signs of bleeding, including neurological, GI, and GU assessment.
	• Monitor PT, aPTT, ACT per protocol.
	• Have anticoagulant antidotes available.
	• Assess for itching, hives, sudden onset of hypotension or tachycardia.
	• Administer hydrocortisone or diphenhydramine (Benadryl) per protocol.
There is no evidence of cardiogenic shock, cardiac valve dysfunction, or ventricular septal defect.	• Monitor ECG, heart sounds, hemodynamic parameters, level of consciousness, and breath sounds for changes.
	• Report and treat deleterious changes as indicated.
Fluids/Electrolytes	
Renal function is maintained as evidenced by urine output >30 mL/h, normal laboratory values.	• Monitor intake and output q1–2h.
	• Monitor BUN, creatinine, electrolytes qd and PRN. Take daily weights.
	• Administer fluid volume and diuretics as ordered.
Mobility/Safety	
Patient will comply with ADL limitations.	• Provide clear explanation of limitations.
	• Provide bed rest with bed side commode privileges first 6 h.
	• Progress to chair for meals, bathing self, bathroom privileges. Continually assess patient response to all activities.
Patient will not fall or accidentally harm self.	• Provide environment to prevent falls, bruising, or injury.
	• Use self-protective devices as indicated and per hospital policy.
Skin Integrity	
Patient has no evidence of skin breakdown.	• Turn side to side q2h while patient is on bed rest.
	• Evaluate skin for signs of pressure areas when turning.
	• Consider pressure relief/reduction mattress for high-risk patients.
	• Use Braden scale (see Chap. 51) to monitor risk for skin breakdown.
Nutrition	
Caloric and nutrient intake meet metabolic requirements per calculation (e.g., basal energy expenditure).	• Provide appropriate diet: oral, parenteral, or enteral feeding.
	• Provide clear or full liquids the first 24 h.
	• Restrict sodium, fat, cholesterol, fluid, and calories if indicated.
	• Consult dietitian or nutritional support services.
Patient has normal laboratory values reflective of nutritional status.	• Monitor albumin, prealbumin, transferrin, cholesterol, triglycerides, total protein.
Comfort/Pain Control	
Patient has relief of chest pain.	• Use visual analog scale to assess pain quantity.
There is no evidence of pain, such as increased HR, BP, RR, or agitation during activity or procedures.	• Assess quality, duration, location of pain.
	• Administer IV morphine sulfate, and monitor pain and hemodynamic response.
	• Administer analgesics appropriately for chest pain and assess response.
	• Monitor physiological response to pain during procedures or after administration of pain medication.
	• Provide a calm, quiet environment.
Psychosocial	
Patient demonstrates decreased anxiety by calm demeanor and vital signs during, for example, procedures, discussions.	• Assess vital signs during treatments, discussions, and so forth.

(continued)

Box 21-9 • COLLABORATIVE CARE GUIDE for the Patient With Myocardial Infarction (Continued)

OUTCOMES	INTERVENTIONS
	• Provide explanations and stable reassurance in calm and caring manner. • Cautiously administer sedatives and monitor response.
Patient/family demonstrate understanding of MI and treatment plan by asking questions and participating in care.	• Consult social services and clergy as appropriate. • Assess coping mechanism history. • Allow free expression of feelings. • Encourage patient/family participation in care as soon as feasible. • Provide blocks of time for adequate rest and sleep.
Teaching/Discharge Planning Patient reports occurrence of chest pain or discomfort. Family demonstrates appropriate coping during the critical phase of an acute MI. In preparation for discharge to home, patient understands activity levels, dietary restrictions, medication regimen, what to do if pain recurs.	• Explain importance of reporting all episodes of chest pain. • Provide frequent explanations and information to family. • Encourage family to ask questions regarding treatment plan, patient response to therapy, prognosis, and so forth. • Make appropriate referrals and consults early during hospitalization. • Initiate family education regarding heart-healthy diet, cardiac rehabilitation program, stress-reduction strategies, management of chest pain, after crisis phase has passed.

contractile forces in the heart resulting in left ventricular dysfunction. Cardiogenic shock is the most common cause of in-hospital death for patients with MI, with a mortality rate of nearly 80%.[15] (For a more detailed discussion of cardiogenic shock, see Chapter 54.)

Clinical manifestations of cardiogenic shock include a rapid, thready pulse; a narrow pulse pressure; dyspnea; tachypnea; inspiratory crackles; distended neck veins; chest pain; cool, moist skin; oliguria; and decreased mentation. Arterial blood gas analysis reveals a decreased PaO_2 and respiratory alkalosis. Hemodynamic findings include a systolic blood pressure less than 85 mm Hg, a mean arterial blood pressure less than 65 mm Hg, a cardiac index less than 2.2 L/minute/m², and a PAWP greater than 18 mm Hg. Cardiac enzymes may show an additional rise or a delay in reaching peak values.

The goal of treatment for cardiogenic shock is to minimize myocardial workload and maximize myocardial oxygen delivery. Immediate actions must be taken to improve tissue perfusion and preserve viable myocardium. To improve oxygenation, supplemental oxygen is given to the patient and, if necessary, the patient may be intubated and placed on a mechanical ventilator. Efforts are aimed toward restoring blood

Box 21-10 • Complications of Acute Myocardial Infarction

Vascular Complications
• Recurrent ischemia
• Recurrent infarction

Myocardial Complications
• Diastolic dysfunction
• Systolic dysfunction
• Congestive heart failure
• Hypotension/cardiogenic shock
• Right ventricular infarction
• Ventricular cavity dilation
• Aneurysm formation (true, false)

Mechanical Complications
• Left ventricular free wall rupture
• Ventricular septal rupture
• Papillary muscle rupture with acute mitral regurgitation

Pericardial Complications
• Pericarditis
• Dressler's syndrome
• Pericardial effusion

Thromboembolic Complications
• Mural thrombosis
• Systemic thromboembolism
• Deep venous thrombosis
• Pulmonary embolism

Electrical Complications
• Ventricular tachycardia
• Ventricular fibrillation
• Supraventricular tachydysrhythmias
• Bradydysrhythmias
• Atrioventricular block (first, second, or third degree)

From Becker RC: Complicated myocardial infarction. Crit Pathways Cardiol 2(2):125–152, 2003.

pressure. This may require discontinuation of vaso-dilator drugs and drugs with negative inotropic effects. An IV dopamine drip may be initiated to improve the patient's blood pressure and improve myocardial contractility. Dobutamine may be used to improve contractility, especially in low cardiac output states. Nitroprusside, a vasodilator, may be used with a vasopressor to improve cardiac output by decreasing peripheral vascular resistance and reducing left ventricular preload. Treatment may also require the use of an IABP. This invasive device helps improve coronary artery perfusion and decrease left ventricular afterload. (For a more detailed discussion of IABP therapy, see Chapter 18.)

Mechanical Complications

The most catastrophic mechanical complications of MI are intraventricular septal rupture and left ventricular free wall rupture. These clinical situations develop rapidly and result in almost immediate physiological deterioration.

Ventricular Septal Wall Rupture

Ventricular septal rupture occurs in about 2% to 4% of patients with an MI and accounts for approximately 15% of all in-hospital deaths.[15] The greatest risk for ventricular septal wall rupture is within the first 24 hours and continues for up to 5 days.[15] The patient presents with a new, loud, holosystolic murmur associated with a thrill felt in the parasternal area. In addition, the patient has progressive dyspnea, tachycardia, and pulmonary congestion. Oxygen samples taken from the right atrium, right ventricle, and pulmonary artery show a higher PaO_2 in the right ventricle than in the right atrium because the oxygenated left ventricular blood is shunted to the right ventricle. This testing can be accomplished during pulmonary artery catheterization. Urgent cardiac catheterization and surgical correction are needed. The patient can be supported with fluid administration, inotropic support (dopamine and dobutamine), afterload reduction (nitroprusside), and IABP counterpulsation until emergency surgery is possible. Some fibrosis of the tissue is needed for suturing. Often it is impossible to maintain the patient medically until this occurs.

Left Ventricular Free Wall Rupture

Left ventricular free wall rupture occurs in about 1% to 2% of patients with MI and accounts for approximately 10% to 15% of in-hospital deaths.[15] It occurs more frequently than rupture of the intraventricular septum or the papillary muscle. Left ventricular free wall rupture is more likely to occur either within the first 24 hours after MI or 3 to 5 days after MI.[11] Left ventricular free wall rupture is more likely to occur in patients older than 70 years of age, women, hypertensive patients, and patients with their first MI. The patient experiences prolonged chest pain, dyspnea, sudden hypotension, jugular venous distention, tamponade, and ECG evidence of electrical–mechanical dissociation. This event occurs so suddenly and with such severity that lifesaving efforts are often futile.

Pericardial Complication

Pericarditis is common after MI and can occur as soon as the first 3 days after infarction or as late as several weeks after infarction. The patient reports chest pain that may be confused with ischemic pain. The precordial pain of pericarditis intensifies with deep breathing, coughing, swallowing, and lying flat. The pain is lessened when the patient sits up and leans forward. The patient may have a fever, with a temperature usually less than 38.6°C, that lasts for several days. On auscultation, a friction rub often can be heard along the left sternal border. Some friction rubs are transient; therefore, the absence of such a rub is not conclusive. The ECG often shows concave upward ST-segment elevation on five or more leads. Anti-inflammatory agents, such as aspirin, indomethacin, and corticosteroids, are given in usual doses for 7 to 14 days.[15,16]

Thromboembolic Complications

Thromboembolisms occur in about 5% to 10% of patients with MI. These patients are often predisposed to deep venous thrombosis (DVT) because of the systemic inflammatory response associated with infarction, immobility, venous stasis, and reduced cardiac output. Pulmonary embolism develops in about 10% to 15% of patients with DVT. After MI, patients are also at risk for systemic emboli that usually originate in the wall of the left ventricle. These emboli can occlude the cerebral, renal, mesenteric, or iliofemoral artery. Patients are systemically anticoagulated with unfractionated or low–molecular-weight heparin followed by warfarin (Coumadin) for 6 to 12 months.[15]

Electrical Complications

Cardiac dysrhythmias and conduction disturbances often accompany acute MIs and can be life-threatening. The causes of electrical complications are many and include myocardial ischemia, myocardial necrosis, altered autonomic tone, electrolyte imbalances, acid–base disturbances, and adverse drug effects.[15,16]

Cardiac Dysrhythmias

Ventricular dysrhythmias that occur in the prehospital phase cause the majority of sudden cardiac deaths. Ischemic myocardium has a lower fibrillatory threshold, and few ventricular dysrhythmias are considered benign after an infarct. Patients may experience tachydysrhythmias or bradydysrhythmias during the hospital phase of treatment. Supraventricular rhythms may be the result of high left atrial pressures caused by left ventricular failure.

Conduction Disturbances

Conduction disturbances after MI can include those caused by SA node, AV node, or ventricular conducting tissue abnormalities. The right coronary artery supplies the SA node in about half of all patients, and the left circumflex coronary artery supplies the SA node in the other half. Because the right coronary artery is also the source of oxygenated blood for the inferior, right posterior, and right ventricular walls, patients with inferior, right posterior, or right ventricular wall MIs are at risk for conduction disturbances resulting from poor SA node functioning. Patients with lateral wall MIs also are at risk for SA nodal conduction disturbances because the left circumflex vessel supplies the lateral wall of the heart.

The right coronary artery also is the source of oxygenated blood for the AV node in about 90% of people. Therefore, patients with inferior, right posterior, or right ventricular wall infarctions due to right coronary artery occlusion are at risk for AV nodal conduction disturbances. First-degree heart block and Mobitz type I (Wenckebach) block may appear, but often are transient. These rhythm disturbances may progress to complete heart block and require pacing therapy.

The LAD coronary artery is the primary source of blood supply to the bundle of His and bundle branches. Therefore, patients with an anterior wall MI caused by an LAD occlusion are at risk for ventricular conduction defects. Conduction defects, such as right bundle branch block, left bundle branch block, anterior fascicular block, posterior fascicular block, bifascicular block, or trifascicular block, may occur.

For patients with MI, the nurse continuously monitors the cardiac rate and rhythm, assesses the apical and peripheral pulses, auscultates the heart, and monitors blood pressure and other indicators of hemodynamics such as urine output and level of consciousness. The goals of therapy for cardiac dysrhythmias and conduction disturbances are to restore normal rate, rhythm, and AV synchrony and to maintain adequate cardiac output. To achieve these goals, pharmacological therapy may be indicated. Cardio-version may be used to treat patients with supraventricular dysrhythmias such as atrial fibrillation or atrial flutter. Transcutaneous pacing may be indicated in an emergent situation for heart block dysrhythmias until a transvenous temporary pacemaker can be initiated. The patient may require permanent pacemaker implantation to maintain an adequate rate and rhythm. Some patients may require an implantable cardioverter–defibrillator to manage ventricular dysrhythmias. (For a more detailed discussion of pacemakers and implanted cardioverter–defibrillators, see Chapter 18.)

CARDIAC REHABILITATION

Preparation for discharge must begin early in the patient's course of hospitalization. Patient and family education is an essential component of the process. A severely compromised, critically ill patient may lack the ability to process and retain new information but usually is motivated to learn after the life-threatening event. Guidelines for patient and family education after an acute MI are described in Table 21-2.

Cardiac rehabilitation is recommended for most patients after MI. Cardiac rehabilitation involves a combination of prescribed exercise, education, and counseling. The goals of cardiac rehabilitation are to limit the adverse physiological and psychological effects of heart disease, modify risk factors, reduce the risk for sudden death or reinfarction, control cardiac symptoms, stabilize or reverse the atherosclerotic process, and enhance the patient's psychosocial and vocational status.[11] Components of cardiac rehabilitation programs include exercise, smoking cessation, lipid management, weight control, blood pressure

Table 21-2 • Patient Teaching: Goals After Acute Myocardial Infarction

Content	When Mastery of Content Is To Be Expected:		
	Acute Phase	Before ICU Discharge	At Hospital Discharge
Pathophysiology of heart disease	Can identify angina, using 0–10 pain scale for reference	Can initiate treatment of angina (rest, nitroglycerin, O_2 use)	Knowledgeable about medications, when to seek medical assistance
Environment of hospital	Understands procedures	Asks appropriate questions	Knowledgeable about disease process and therapy
Lifestyle modifications	Complies with activity limitations	Can state relationship between activity and cardiac workload	Can progress activity as tolerated
	Complies with dietary limitations	Begins light activity	Placement in cardiac rehabilitation program
		States risk factors	Can state dietary restrictions
		Selects appropriate meals	
Treatment of disease	Accepts medications as ordered	Can identify medications	Knowledgeable about medications, dose, timing, action, and side effects
		Can identify risk factors	Plans for risk factor reduction
			Begins cardiac rehabilitation program
Emotional adaptation	Able to define support system	Begins to communicate about lifestyle changes	Involves self and loved ones in plans for lifestyle changes
		Becomes involved with resolving emotions related to surviving a critical illness	Expresses feelings
			Participates in group recovery program

control, psychological interventions, and guidance for return to work. Cardiac rehabilitation programs have been shown to improve the patient's functional capacity and quality of life and to decrease emotional distress, risk for subsequent coronary events, and cardiovascular mortality. Although the benefits of cardiac rehabilitation are well known, fewer than one third of patients receive information or counseling about cardiac rehabilitation before being discharged from the hospital.[11]

Family members of patients with MI should be included in the educational process so that they can learn about heart disease and help the patient achieve the goals of rehabilitation. Family members also should be given the opportunity to learn cardiopulmonary resuscitation because most episodes of cardiac arrest in patients with MI occur within the first 18 months after discharge from the hospital.[11]

• Clinical Applicability Challenges

Case Study

Mrs. K., a 78-year-old black female, was brought to the emergency department (ED) by an ambulance at 8:30 a.m. She described substernal chest pain with radiation to her back that began 2 hours ago. The pain is not relieved by rest or sublingual nitroglycerin. She describes the pain as dull and rates it a 9 on a scale of 10. She feels nauseated and vomited once before coming to the hospital. Mrs. K. has a history of hypertension, obesity, diabetes, and elevated cholesterol. She is allergic to penicillin and developed hives and a rash when she previously took penicillin.

On physical examination, she was awake, alert, oriented, and cooperative. Her skin was cool and diaphoretic. Blood pressure was 94/48 mm Hg; heart rate, 112 beats/minute and irregular; respiratory rate, 24 breaths/minute on 2 L O_2 per nasal cannula; temperature, 98°F (36.7°C). Her cardiac examination revealed S_1, S_2, and an S_3. She had no jugular venous distention. Peripheral pulses were present but thready, and there was 1+ pedal edema bilaterally. Auscultation of her lungs revealed bilateral basilar crackles. She had no evidence of cyanosis or clubbing. Her abdominal examination showed positive bowel sounds in all four quadrants. Her abdomen was soft and nontender with no palpable masses.

The nurse immediately recorded a 12-lead ECG that showed 4-mm ST-segment elevation in leads II, III, and aVF. Blood samples were drawn that revealed an elevated CK level positive for MB. Her troponin level was also abnormal. Mrs. K. was given an aspirin, and an intravenous (IV) line was started. Her pain was treated with IV morphine sulfate. Mrs. K. was diagnosed with an acute inferior wall MI and was treated in the coronary care unit.

1. On physical examination, you noted that Mrs. K. had pedal edema and bilateral basilar crackles, and you heard an S_3 heart sound. What may these findings indicate?

2. Mrs. K. was diagnosed with an inferior wall myocardial infarction. What coronary artery is most likely occluded and what potential complications are priorities for you to monitor?

3. You are caring for Mrs. K. during her second day in the coronary care unit. She complains of chest pain that is made worse by taking a deep breath. The pain is relieved when she sits up and leans forward. She has developed a fever of 38°C. What is the most likely cause of these findings? What else should the nurse assess?

Review Questions

1. You are providing discharge education to Mr. J. after his hospitalization for unstable angina. You know that he is 72 years of age and had a father who died of heart disease. Mr. J. has hypertension, sleeps only about 6 hours per night, and admits to including few fruits in his diet. Which of the following should be your priority in educating him about risk factors for heart disease?
   a. Diet
   b. Hypertension
   c. Sleep
   d. Family history

2. You are caring for Ms. L. who was recently admitted to your unit with a diagnosis of unstable angina. Ms. L. now describes the onset of chest pain and rates the pain 8 on a scale of 10. The pain is substernal and dull. When you record her 12-lead electrocardiogram, you notice ST-segment elevations of 4 mm in leads V_1 through V_4. This abnormal finding in leads V_1 through V_4 indicates which of the following:
   a. A pattern of acute myocardial injury in the anteroseptal wall
   b. A pattern of acute myocardial injury in the lateral wall
   c. A pattern of ischemia in the anteroseptal wall
   d. A pattern of ischemia in the lateral wall

3. Mr. S. is a patient in the coronary care 2 days after myocardial infarction. His vital signs are: temperature, 37°C; pulse, 118 beats/minute and thready; respirations, 28 breaths/minute; and blood pressure, 82/58 mm Hg. On physical exam, you note the following: cool moist skin, distended neck veins, inspiratory crackles, and decreased urine output (from 100 mL;/hour in the night to 40 mL/hour). What complication from myocardial infarction is Mr. S. most likely experiencing?
   a. Left ventricular free wall rupture
   b. Ventricular septal wall rupture
   c. Cardiogenic shock
   d. Frequent premature ventricular contractions

4. Ms. G. has been diagnosed with an anteroseptal myocardial infarction. Disease in which of the fol-

lowing coronary arteries most likely caused her myocardial infarction?

a. Right coronary artery
b. Posterior descending coronary artery
c. Left circumflex coronary artery
d. Left anterior descending coronary artery

5. When administering sublingual nitroglycerin, what is the most important parameter to assess?

a. Pulse
b. Blood pressure
c. Temperature
d. Cardiac rhythm

References

1. Thygesen K, Alpert JS., White, HD, on behalf of the Joint ESC/ACCF/AHA/WHF Task Force for the Redefinition of Myocardial Infarction: Universal definition of myocardial infarction. Circulation 116:2634–2653, 2007

2. American Heart Association: Heart Disease and Stoke Statistics: 2008 update. Dallas, American Heart Association, 2008

3. American Heart Association: Heart and Stoke Facts. Dallas, American Heart Association, 2003

4. American Heart Association: Inflammation, Heart Disease, and Stroke: The Role of C-reactive Protein.

5. American Heart Association: Risk Factors and Coronary Heart Disease.

6. Anderson JL, Adams CD, Antman EM, et al: ACC/AHA 2007 guidelines for the management of patients with unstable angina/non-ST-segment elevation myocardial infarction: Executive summary. A Report of the American College of Cardiology/American Heart Association Task Force on Practice Guidelines (Writing Committee to Revise the 2002 Guidelines for the Management of Patients With Unstable Angina/Non-ST-Elevation Myocardial Infarction). Circulation 116:803–877, 2007

7. DeWood MA, Spores J, Notske R, et al: Prevalence of total coronary occlusion during the early hours of transmural myocardial infarction. N Engl J Med 303:897–902, 1980

8. Reimer KA, Lower JE, Rasmussen MM, et al: The wave front phenomenon of ischemic cell death. 1. Myocardial infarct size versus duration of coronary occlusion in dogs. Circulation 56:786–794, 1977

9. Bueno H, Lopez-Palop R, Bermejo J, et al: In hospital outcome if elderly patients with acute inferior myocardial infarction and right ventricular involvement. Circulation 96(2):436–441, 1997

10. Kinch J, Ryan T: Right ventricular infarction. N Engl J Med 330(17):1211–1216, 1994

11. Antman EM, Anbe DT, Armstrong PW, et al: ACC/AHA guidelines for the management of patients with ST-elevation myocardial infarction. A report of the American College of Cardiology/American Heart Association Task Force on Practice Guidelines (Committee to revise the 1999 guidelines for the management of patients with acute myocardial infarction). Circulation 110:e82–e293, 2004

12. Becker RC: Complicated myocardial infarction. Crit Pathways Cardiol 2(2):125–152, 2003

13. Grauer K: A Practical Guide to ECG Interpretation, 2nd ed. St. Louis: Mosby-Year Book, 1998

14. Soine L, Hanrahan M: Nuclear and other imaging studies. In Woods SL, Froelicher ES, Motzer SA, Bridges EJ: Cardiac Nursing, 5th ed. Philadelphia: Lippincott Williams & Wilkins, 2005, pp 319–325

15. Becker RC: Complicated myocardial infarction. Crit Pathways Cardiol 2(2):125–152, 2003

16. Del Bene S, Vaughan A: Acute coronary syndromes. In Woods SL, Froelicher ES, Motzer SA, Bridges EJ: Cardiac Nursing, 5th ed. Philadelphia: Lippincott Williams & Wilkins, 2005, pp 550–584

Other Selected Readings

Albert NM: Switching to once-daily evidence-based beta-blockers in patients with systolic heart failure or left ventricular dysfunction after myocardial infarction. Crit Care Nurse 27(6):62–72, 2007

Alonzo A: The effect of health care provider consultation on acute coronary syndrome care-seeking delay. Heart Lung 36(5):307–318, 2007

Andersson SI, Pesonen E, Ohlin H: Perspectives that lay persons with and without health problems show toward coronary heart disease: An integrated biopsychosocial approach. Heart Lung 36(5):330–338, 2007

Coughlin RM: Attacking anterior-wall myocardial infarction in time. Am Nurse Today 3(1):26–31, 2008

DeVon HA, Ryan CJ, Ochs AL, Shapiro M: Symptoms across the continuum of acute coronary syndromes: Differences between women and men. Am J Crit Care 17(1):14–24, 2008

Gelfand EV, Cannon CP: Myocardial infarction: Contemporary management strategies. J Intern Med 262:59–77, 2007

Goldich G: Understanding 12-lead ECG: Part I. Nursing 2006 36(11):36–41, 2006

Goldich G: Understanding 12-lead ECG: Part II. Nursing 2006 36(12):36–41, 2006

Hildingh C, Fridlund B, Lidell E: Women's experiences of recovery after myocardial infarction: A meta-synthesis. Heart Lung 36(6):410–417, 2007

King KB, McGuire MA: Symptom presentation and time to seek care in women and men with acute myocardial infarction. Heart Lung 36(4):235–243, 2007

Miracle VA: Coronary artery disease in women: The myth still exists. Dimens Crit Care Nurs 25(5):209–215, 2006

Noureddine S, Arevian M, Adra M, Puzantian H: Response to signs and symptoms of acute coronary syndrome: differences between Lebanese men and women. Am J Crit Care 17(1):26–35, 2008

Purgason K: Broken hearts: Differentiating stress-induced cardiomyopathy from acute myocardial infarction in the patient presenting with acute coronary syndrome. Dimens Crit Care Nurs 25(6):247–253, 2006

Rosenfeld AG: State of the heart: Building science to improve women's cardiovascular health. Am J Crit Care 15(6):556–567, 2006

Thuresson M, Jarlov MB, Lindahl B, et al: Thoughts, actions, and factors associated with prehospital delay in patients with acute coronary syndrome. Heart Lung 36(6):398–409, 2007

22

Cardiac Surgery

Nancy Munro

Objectives

Based on the content in this chapter, the reader should be able to:

❶ Discuss advantages and disadvantages of off-bypass coronary artery surgery.

❷ Discuss the indications for transmyocardial laser revascularization.

❸ Compare and contrast the pathophysiological impacts of stenosis and insufficiency in the mitral and aortic valves.

❹ Explain the cardiopulmonary bypass process.

❺ Describe five key assessment areas in the early postoperative period.

❻ Discuss the impact of the inflammatory response in patients after coronary artery surgery.

❼ Discuss causes of postoperative hypotension in a cardiac surgery patient, as well as assessments and interventions for same.

Despite emphasis on modifying and eliminating risk factors, cardiovascular disease remains a leading cause of disability and death in the United States. Development of new treatments, such as thrombolytic and anticoagulation therapy, balloon and laser angioplasty, and coronary artery stenting, has improved medical management of cardiac disease. These nonsurgical approaches are discussed in Chapter 18. However, surgical intervention remains the treatment of choice in some patients. In particular, cardiac surgery is sometimes necessary in two common conditions, coronary artery disease (CAD) and valvular disease.

• Indications for Cardiac Surgery

CORONARY ARTERY DISEASE

Pathophysiology

A detailed discussion of the pathophysiology of CAD is found in Chapter 21.

Surgical Treatment

Coronary Artery Bypass Graft Surgery

In coronary artery bypass graft (CABG) surgery, native vessels or conduits are "harvested" during the initial phase of surgery to reroute or bypass blood flow past diseased areas of the coronary arteries. The first saphenous vein aortocoronary bypass graft was performed in 1964. Since then, the use of CABG surgery has become an acceptable treatment for CAD. Compared with medical treatment, CABG surgery has proved effective in relieving angina and improving exercise tolerance, and it prolongs life in patients with left main CAD and three-vessel disease with poor left ventricular function.[1]

Increased use of percutaneous transluminal coronary angioplasty and stenting has decreased the need for CABG surgery in many cases. Patients selected for such surgery today are older; have more advanced coronary disease; have more impaired left ventricular function; and, in many cases, have had previous CABG surgery. To decrease the mortality associated with bypass surgery, it is necessary to consider several factors: urgency of operation, age, previous heart surgery, sex, left ventricular ejection fraction, percentage stenosis of the left main coronary artery, and number of major coronary arteries with greater than 70% stenosis.[1]

Desired characteristics for a graft or conduit are (1) diameter similar to the coronary arteries, (2) no disease or wall abnormalities, and (3) adequate length. Commonly used grafts include saphenous vein grafts and internal mammary artery grafts, although other potential grafts are being explored.

Saphenous Vein Grafts Saphenous vein grafts are used to bypass the obstruction in the coronary artery by anastomosing one end of the vein to the aorta (proximal anastomosis) and the other end to the coronary artery just past the obstruction (distal anastomosis). Saphenous vein grafts may be simple, with an end-to-side anastomosis to the aorta and the coronary artery, or sequential (also called skip), with an end-to-side anastomosis to the aorta, a side-to-side anastomosis to one coronary artery, and an end-to-side anastomosis to another coronary artery (Fig. 22-1).

Although the saphenous vein can be taken from above or below the knee, a vein from below the knee is generally preferred because it is close in diameter to the size of the coronary artery. To remove the vein, an incision is made along the inner aspect of the leg. Alternatively, small incisions can be made in the area of the vein, and a flexible fiberoptic scope is inserted to visualize the vessel and remove it. The fiberoptic method of vein removal is associated with improved wound healing and reduced complications involving the incision site.[2]

Fifty percent of saphenous vein grafts are occluded after 10 years. Three main processes account for saphenous vein failure: thrombosis, fibrointimal hyperplasia, and atherosclerosis. Thrombosis is most common in the first month but may occur as long as 1 year after surgery. Fibrointimal hyperplasia occurs predominantly between 1 month and 5 years and may result in a 25% decrease in luminal vessel diameter. Atherosclerosis begins as early as 1 year after surgery and is fully developed after 5 years. Aspirin is the drug recommended for use postoperatively to prevent early saphenous vein graft closure and should be continued indefinitely.[1] To decrease the incidence of occlusion of grafts from the saphenous vein, grafts from other vessels are being used.[3]

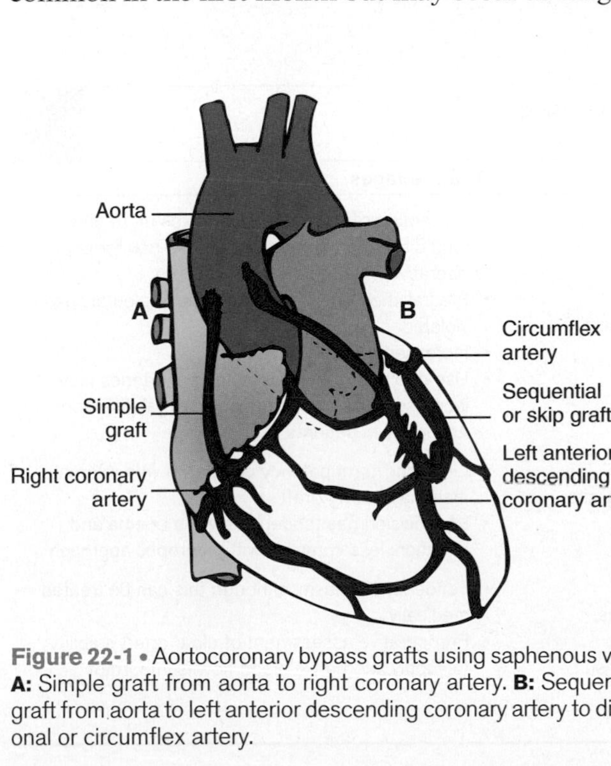

Internal Mammary Artery Grafts The internal mammary artery is a preferred alternative to the saphenous vein for surgical revascularization. The internal mammary artery is used as a pedicle graft (i.e., the proximal end remains attached to the subclavian artery) to bypass diseased coronary arteries. Both the left and the right internal mammary artery can be used. Because the left internal mammary artery is longer and larger than the right, it is usually used to bypass the left anterior descending coronary artery. The right internal mammary artery is anastomosed to the right coronary artery or the circumflex coronary artery.

The internal mammary artery, the second branch of the subclavian artery, descends the anterior chest wall just lateral to the sternum behind the costal cartilage. To isolate the internal mammary artery, the pleural space is entered, the internal mammary artery is dissected free from the chest wall, and the intercostal artery branches are cauterized.

Compared with saphenous vein grafts, internal mammary artery grafts have superior graft patency rates; 90% were patent 10 years after surgery. In addition, internal mammary artery grafts exhibit less atherosclerosis over time, and they have been associated with lower long-term morbidity and improved long-term survival.[1]

Other Grafts The search for other native vessels to serve as conduits continues as patients return for reoperation. The use of the radial artery has gained popularity; occlusion rates have lowered as harvesting techniques have improved. The radial artery, a thick, muscular artery, is prone to spasm with mechanical stimulation, and to prevent spasm, the artery is perfused with a calcium channel blocker solution during surgery and minimally stimulated. After the radial artery has been implanted, spasm has not been a major factor, and patency rates of 84% for 5 years have been reported.[4] Initiation of nitroglycerin followed by oral nitrates (isosorbide mononitrate) postoperatively has helped decrease the occurrence of spasm; results have been better than with calcium channel blockers.[5]

Acceptable alternative conduits must have short- and long-term acceptable patency rates. The right gastroepiploic artery, which is harvested by extending the sternotomy incision toward the umbilicus and dissecting the artery off the greater curvature of the stomach, is used for coronary grafting. Patency rates have been acceptable, but long-term data are not available.[1] Homologous (non-native) conduits using the saphenous vein, umbilical vein, or bovine internal

Figure 22-1 • Aortocoronary bypass grafts using saphenous vein. **A:** Simple graft from aorta to right coronary artery. **B:** Sequential graft from aorta to left anterior descending coronary artery to diagonal or circumflex artery.

mammary artery have resulted in poor patency rates and therefore are not recommended.[1] A comparison of common conduits used for revascularization is presented in Table 22-1.

Off-Pump Coronary Artery Bypass Graft Surgery

CABG surgery actually began as a surgical procedure performed on a beating heart because the cardiopulmonary bypass machine was not yet available. Once the cardiopulmonary bypass machine was perfected, "beating heart" surgery was used less often. This machine, also called a pump oxygenator, assumes the job of oxygenating the patient's blood and circulating it throughout the body. However, complications associated with cardiopulmonary bypass have led surgeons to reconsider performing CABG surgery "off pump" (OPCABG)—in other words, on beating hearts—in the hope of improving patient outcome.

Initially, surgeons wanted to avoid using the midline sternotomy incision and use the less invasive "mini" left and right thoracotomy approaches while performing CABG surgery, on or off bypass. This approach, which is known as minimally invasive direct coronary artery bypass grafting (MIDCABG), restricts the number of grafts that can be performed because the small incision does not allow access to the entire heart surface. Grafts to the left anterior descending artery are most frequent. Depending on where the "mini" incision is placed, grafts to the right coronary artery and the posterior descending artery can also be made.[6] Experience with MIDCABG has not been as successful as anticipated, but the technique is still used depending on the patient situation. The trend is toward using the median sternotomy incision but performing the grafting process off bypass.

In the 1990s, as neurological complications associated with the cardiopulmonary bypass machine, especially cognitive dysfunction, became more prominent, OPCABG surgery was reinstituted.[7] The initial results of OPCABG surgery have been promising but sometimes difficult to compare with the large data pool for on-pump CABG surgery. Length of stay in patients after OPCABG surgery has decreased compared with length of stay in patients who have had on-pump CABG surgery.[8] In addition, neurological dysfunction seems less after OPCABG surgery. However, Peel and colleagues have demonstrated that the stroke rate is similar in patients who undergo OPCABG compared with those who undergo on-pump CABG; after OPCABG, the symptoms of the stroke appear 48 to 72 hours after surgery, and after on-pump CABG, the symptoms of stroke occur immediately after surgery.[9] The explanation for this finding is that systemic inflammatory response syndrome (SIRS; discussed in detail in Chapter 54) causes diffuse microembolic events that take time to develop. The microembolization is the result of the inflammation of the endothelium, which activates the coagulation cascade.

The significance of these differences for patient care after OPCABG surgery is not well documented in the nursing literature because OPCABG surgery is a new procedure. Data from institutions with larger numbers of patients who have had this surgery seem to suggest that emphasis should be placed on anticoagulation interventions.[9] Traditional agents such as heparin (weight-based protocols), aspirin, clopidogrel (Plavix), and low–molecular-weight heparin are aggressively implemented to prevent platelet activation and suppress activation of the coagulation cascade. Nursing assessment focuses on the detection of embolic events in any body system and monitors for side effects of anticoagulation such as gastrointestinal

Table 22-1 • Common Conduits Used for Coronary Artery Bypass Grafting

Type of Graft	Advantages	Disadvantages
Internal mammary artery	• Vascular endothelium adapted to arterial pressure and high flow, resulting in decreased intimal hyperplasia and atherosclerosis • Improved long-term patency • Retains nerve innervation and therefore its ability to adapt diameter to blood flow • No leg incision • Diameter closer to coronary artery	• Dissection off the chest wall takes more time; long dissection time may increase risk for postoperative bleeding • Pleural chest tube needed because pleural space violated • Increased postoperative pain • Use of bilateral internal mammary arteries may increase risk for infection and sternal infection, especially in patients with diabetes
Saphenous vein	• Technically easier to harvest • Longer length (if able) may allow for several grafts	• Less long-term patency compared with internal mammary artery graft • Leg incision has tendency toward edema and infection; less common with fiberoptic approach
Radial artery	• Technically easier to harvest • Better patency rate compared with saphenous vein graft • Vascular endothelium adapted to arterial pressure and high flow, resulting in decreased intimal hyperplasia and atherosclerosis	• Tendency to spasm, although this can be treated medically • Preoperative assessment of ulnar artery's ability to supply alternative blood flow is important

bleeding and heparin-induced thrombocytopenia. Because SIRS can develop in 48 to 72 hours, the critical care nurse must continually reassess the patient who has undergone OPCABG surgery and report any changes that may occur, especially with regard to neurological changes or electrocardiographic (ECG) ST-segment monitoring. If the thoracotomy approach is used, the increased need for pain medication may decrease patient compliance to cough and deep-breathe postoperatively. A high index of suspicion is the key nursing intervention after OPCABG surgery and may improve patient outcome.

Transmyocardial Laser Revascularization

Transmyocardial laser revascularization (TMR; TMLR) may be an option for patients who continue to have unstable angina that is refractory to interventions. Eligible patients usually have had prior CABG surgery, multiple cardiac interventions with maximal medication manipulation, or both. A laser probe is inserted into the wall of the left ventricle to create channels that encourage revascularization. The location and number of channels created depend on the patient's preoperative cardiac performance. Revascularization theoretically occurs through two mechanisms: (1) angiogenesis, and (2) direct channel patency and endothelialization.[10] With angiogenesis, the formation of new blood vessels or the modeling of existing blood vessels increases collateral flow to the dysfunctional areas. Direct channel patency with endothelialization may result in direct perfusion to impaired walls of the left ventricle. Although the actual mechanisms are not clearly understood, the clinical outcomes are promising. In TMR, revascularization takes months to develop, which should be emphasized to the patient and family. In TMR, three types of lasers of different wavelengths are used: holmium:YAG, excimer, and carbon dioxide. All produce clean channels with minimal tissue trauma.[10]

Care of patients after TMR is similar to care after cardiovascular surgery, with some special concerns. The life of patients who have had TMR can become relatively normal, but careful observation is required. In TMR, patients have sustained direct myocardial insult that can result in a decrease in left ventricular function 48 to 72 hours after the surgery. Inotropic support using dobutamine or milrinone may be required for several days. Vigilant monitoring of fluid status is necessary because congestive failure tends to occur, although patients have higher filling pressures because the desired effects of TMR develop over time. Antiarrhythmic therapy may also be necessary because there may be irritable foci in the ventricle; amiodarone is frequently used. Angina may occur, but because the channel areas are denervated in TMR, the patient may not be able to perceive anginal pain. Continuous ST-segment monitoring is needed to detect any changes that occur. Nitrates are started as part of the medication regimen. Anticoagulation is initiated to prevent myocardial infarction and also to maintain the patency of the channels.[11]

VALVULAR DISEASE

Cardiac valves maintain the unidirectional flow of blood. If structural changes occur as a result of disease, this function is disrupted. Disease causes either valvular stenosis or insufficiency (regurgitation; Fig. 22-2). The stenotic valve has a narrowed orifice that creates a partial obstruction to blood flow, resulting in increasing pressure behind the valve and decreasing forward blood flow. The insufficient valve is incompetent or leaky; blood flows backward, increasing the pressure and volume behind the valve. Stenosis and insufficiency can occur alone or in combination, in the same valve, or in more than one valve. Abnormalities can affect the tricuspid, pulmonic, mitral, and aortic valves. This discussion focuses on mitral and aortic abnormalities, which are more common and produce profound hemodynamic changes.

The diagnosis of valvular disease is suggested by the history, clinical signs and symptoms, physical examination, and auscultation of the characteristic murmur (see Chapter 17). Diagnosis is confirmed by echocardiography and catheterization of both sides of the heart, at which time valvular gradients are measured. To determine the gradient across the mitral valve, left atrial and left ventricular pressures are measured during diastole. A gradient of more than 15 to 20 mm Hg (i.e., left atrial diastolic pressure is 15 to 20 mm Hg higher than left ventricular diastolic pressure) means that severe mitral stenosis exists. Valve area is also calculated during cardiac catheterization. The normal mitral valve area is 4 to 6 cm². An area less than 1.5 cm² signifies critical mitral stenosis, and surgery is indicated.

To determine the gradient across the aortic valve, the left ventricular and aortic root pressures are measured during systole. A gradient of more than 50 mm Hg is associated with clinically significant aortic stenosis. Normal aortic valve area is 2.6 to 3.5 cm². Hemodynamically significant aortic stenosis occurs if the valve area is less than 1 cm². Valvular insufficiency is diagnosed by regurgitation of the contrast medium backward through the incompetent valve.

Pathophysiology

Mitral Stenosis
Mitral stenosis (Fig. 22-3A) occurs most frequently as a result of rheumatic heart disease. The disease process causes fusion of the commissures and fibrotic contraction of valve leaflets, commissures, and chordae tendineae. As forward flow from the left atrium to the left ventricle decreases, cardiac output falls, creating a decrease in systemic perfusion. Blood backed up behind the stenotic valve causes left atrial dilation and increased left atrial pressure. This pressure is reflected backward into the pulmonary circulation, and with prolonged high pressures, fluid moves from the pulmonary capillaries into the interstitial space and eventually the alveoli. Pulmonary hypertension develops, which can eventually lead to right-sided heart failure. As a result of this pathophysiology, patients with mitral stenosis present with fatigue, exertional dyspnea, orthopnea, and even pulmonary

Mitral valve

Atrioventricular (AV) valve

Normal

Stenotic

Insufficient

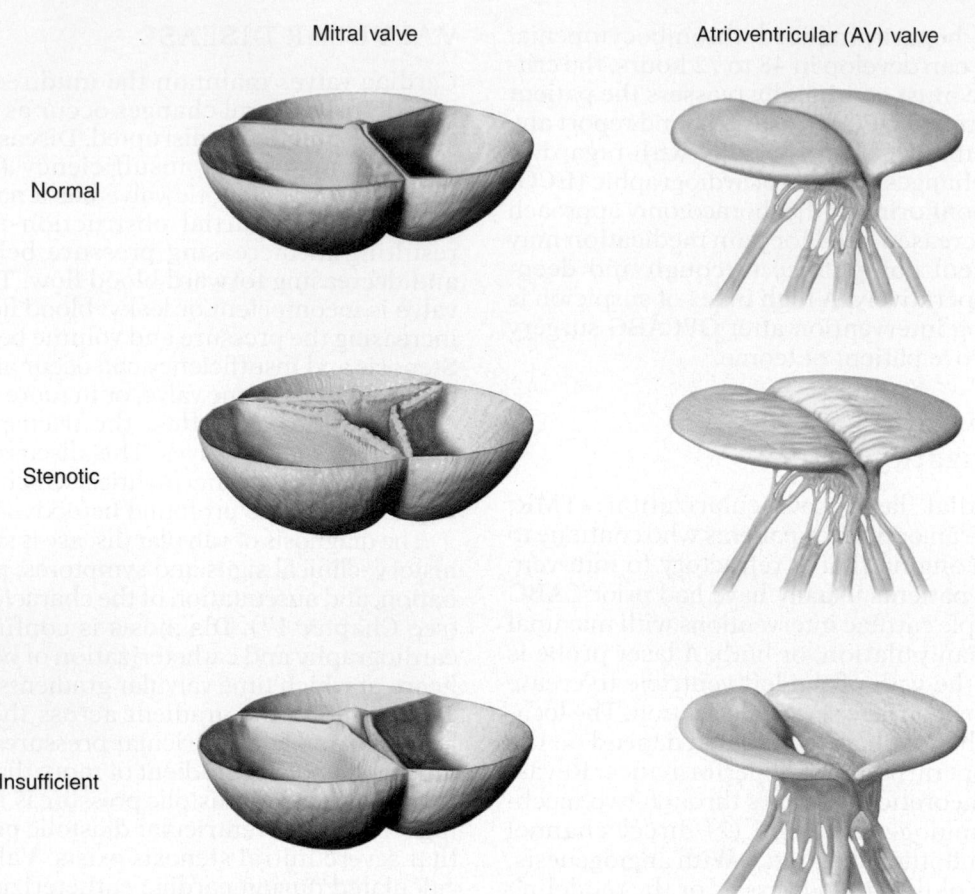

Figure 22-2 • Normal and diseased heart valves. (From Anatomical Chart Company: Atlas of Pathophysiology. Springhouse, PA, Springhouse, 2002, pp 74–75.)

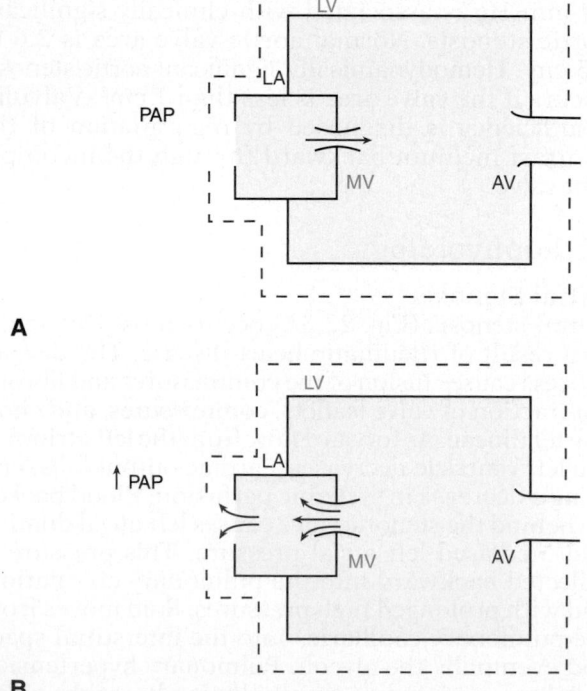

A

B

Figure 22-3 • Mitral valve dysfunction. **A:** Mitral stenosis. **B:** Mitral insufficiency. AV, aortic valve; LA, left atrium; LV, left ventricle; MV, mitral valve; PAP, pulmonary artery pressure.

edema. Left atrial dilation causes atrial fibrillation in 40% to 50% of affected patients.

Mitral Insufficiency

Mitral insufficiency (see Fig. 22-3B) can occur acutely or develop over a period of time. Chronic mitral insufficiency may result from rheumatic heart disease, myxomatous degeneration of the mitral valve, degenerative changes associated with aging, or left ventricular dilation. The basic valve dysfunction is caused by thickening or stretching of the leaflets, resulting in backward blood flow. During ventricular systole, some of the left ventricular blood regurgitates into the atrium rather than being ejected through the aortic valve. This regurgitation decreases the forward cardiac output. Left ventricular hypertrophy occurs in an attempt to improve the cardiac output, but the hypertrophy can actually worsen the regurgitation. Left ventricular volume overload causes left ventricular dilation. Regurgitant flow into the left atrium causes increased left atrial pressure and dilation. This volume overload can be reflected backward to the pulmonary circulation; however, pulmonary and right-sided heart symptoms usually do not develop until late in the disease process. As a result of this pathophysiology, patients with chronic mitral insufficiency commonly present with fatigue, palpitations, and sometimes shortness of breath.

Acute mitral insufficiency may result from endocarditis, chest trauma, or myocardial infarction. Endocarditis erodes or perforates the valve leaflets or chordae. Trauma may rupture the chordae. Myocardial infarction may cause papillary muscle rupture, allowing blood to flow backward into the left atrium during ventricular systole. Because of the acute nature of the valve dysfunction, there is inadequate time for dilation or hypertrophy to compensate. In acute mitral insufficiency, cardiac output decreases dramatically, cascading into pulmonary edema and shock. The treatment of choice for acute mitral regurgitation with hemodynamic compromise is emergent mitral valve replacement.

Aortic Stenosis

Aortic stenosis may develop as a result of rheumatic fever, calcification of a congenital bicuspid valve, or calcific degeneration, especially in elderly patients. The resultant fusion of the commissures and fibrous contractures of the cusps leads to obstruction of left ventricular outflow. Forward cardiac output is diminished, and the left ventricle hypertrophies to maintain the cardiac output. As the stenosis worsens, compensation fails, and volume and pressure overload in the left ventricle causes left ventricular dilation. Increased left ventricular pressures are reflected backward through the left atrium and pulmonary vasculature (Fig. 22-4A).

Diminished cardiac output in the person with aortic stenosis may lead to two major problems—angina and syncope. Extreme left ventricular hypertrophy increases myocardial oxygen demand at the same time that cardiac output and coronary artery perfusion are decreased. Ischemic myocardium develops, which may lead to angina. Syncope occurs in the late stages of aortic stenosis, when the forward cardiac output cannot increase to meet the body's demands. As a person with severe aortic stenosis exercises, the blood vessels to the skeletal muscles dilate to increase the blood supply. The normal response to this increased demand is increased cardiac output. However, the person with aortic stenosis is unable to respond in such a way. The vasodilation without a concomitant increase in cardiac output results in insufficient cerebral perfusion and syncope. Patients with aortic stenosis also experience exertional dyspnea, orthopnea, and paroxysmal nocturnal dyspnea.

Aortic Insufficiency

Aortic insufficiency, like mitral insufficiency, can occur acutely or develop over a period of time. Chronic aortic insufficiency is commonly caused by rheumatic fever and aneurysm of the ascending aorta. Rheumatic disease results in thickened and retracted valve cusps, whereas aortic aneurysm causes annular dilation. Both conditions prevent the edges of the valve leaflets from approximating, allowing blood to regurgitate backward from the aorta into the left ventricle during ventricular diastole. Forward cardiac output decreases, and left ventricular volume and pressure increase. Left ventricular hypertrophy ensues. Eventually, the increase in left ventricular pressure is reflected backward into the left atrium and pulmonary circulation (see Fig. 22-4B). Patients with chronic aortic insufficiency present with fatigue, and they have a low diastolic blood pressure and a widened pulse pressure. The pulse may rise rapidly and collapse suddenly (water-hammer or Corrigan's pulse) because of the forceful ventricular contraction and subsequent diastolic regurgitation from the aortic root into the left ventricle. Angina may occur because aortic insufficiency creates an imbalance between left ventricular myocardial oxygen supply and demand. As left ventricular hypertrophy worsens, the oxygen demand increases, but regurgitant flow from the aortic root during diastole decreases coronary artery perfusion.

Acute aortic insufficiency may be caused by blunt chest trauma, ruptured ascending aortic aneurysm, or infective endocarditis. Left-sided heart failure and pulmonary edema develop rapidly in the patient with acute aortic insufficiency because compensatory left ventricular hypertrophy does not have time to develop. In response to the diminished cardiac output, systemic vascular resistance (SVR) increases to maintain the blood pressure. The elevated SVR increases the degree of regurgitation and worsens the situation.

Surgical Treatment

The goals of valvular surgery are to relieve symptoms and restore normal hemodynamics. Surgery is indicated before left ventricular function deteriorates significantly and the patient's activity becomes severely

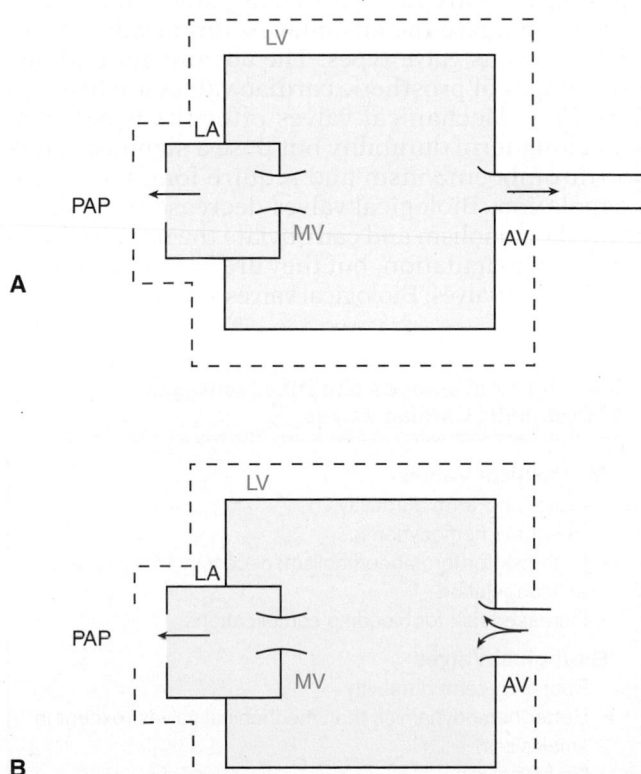

Figure 22-4 • Aortic valve dysfunction. **A:** Aortic stenosis. **B:** Aortic insufficiency. AV, aortic valve; LA, left atrium; LV, left ventricle; MV, mitral valve; PAP, pulmonary artery pressure.

limited, or before severe signs and symptoms, such as angina or syncope from aortic stenosis or pulmonary hypertension from mitral stenosis, develop. Percutaneous balloon valvuloplasty, a procedure that is indicated primarily for patients considered too high risk for surgery, is discussed in Chapter 18. Surgical intervention consists of either valve reconstruction or valve replacement. Because valve reconstruction is associated with decreased operative mortality and fewer thromboembolic and anticoagulation-related complications than valve replacement, valve reconstruction is gaining popularity.

Valve Reconstruction

With the development of transesophageal echocardiography to assess the effectiveness of repair during surgery, the use of valve reconstruction is increasing. Most valve reconstruction procedures are performed on the mitral valve. Compared with mitral valve replacement, reconstruction eliminates the need for long-term anticoagulation, decreases the risks for thromboembolism and endocarditis, decreases the need for reoperation, and increases survival. However, for aortic valve disorders, most attempts at reconstruction have not been successful because of late insufficiency and restenosis.

A common reconstruction technique for mitral stenosis is commissurotomy. Although not indicated for patients with severe mitral stenosis, commissurotomy may be effective for patients with moderate stenosis with minimal calcification and regurgitation. During commissurotomy, the fused commissures are surgically divided. Calcified tissue is débrided and fused, and shortened chordae are incised. This procedure improves leaflet mobility and increases the mitral valve area, decreasing the degree of stenosis.

Another technique for treatment of mitral insufficiency is reconstruction. If annular dilation causes the regurgitation, annuloplasty can be performed using sutures or a prosthetic ring (e.g., Carpentier-Edwards annuloplasty ring). The ring is sewn around the mitral annulus so that excess annular tissue is drawn up. Suturing and the ring reduce the circumference of the enlarged annulus so that the edges of the leaflets coapt, diminishing regurgitation. If the chordae tendineae are stretched or ruptured, surgical shortening or transposition of chordae to substitute for ruptured chordae can be effective. Redundant mitral leaflets are repaired by resecting a portion of the leaflet, and perforated valve leaflets can be reconstructed by patching. Such repairs are usually supported by an annuloplasty ring.

Reconstruction procedures are more likely to be successful if performed early in the course of the disease, before left ventricular function deteriorates and irreparable damage occurs. Anticoagulation is not usually needed after valve repair unless an annuloplasty ring is used. In such cases, anticoagulants are given for only 3 months until the ring is endothelialized. If reconstruction cannot be accomplished, valves are replaced.

Valve Replacement

The first valve replacement was performed by Harken and Starr in 1960 with a caged ball prosthesis. Since then, many new valve designs have evolved. Valve replacement surgery is done through a median sternotomy incision, and cardiopulmonary bypass and myocardial preservation techniques (discussed in detail later in this chapter) are used. The mitral valve is approached through the left atrium. Rather than excising the native valve, the chordae and papillary muscles are preserved when the prosthetic valve is sutured in place. This technique helps maintain left ventricular function and ejection fraction. The aortic valve is approached through the ascending aorta. The native aortic valve is excised, the annulus is sized, and the prosthetic valve of correct size is sutured to the annulus. Once the surgery is completed, the patient is transferred to the intensive care unit (ICU).

Ideally, a prosthetic valve would be durable, last for a patient's life, and perform exactly like a normal human valve. The valve would have normal hemodynamics with unimpeded, nonturbulent blood flow through a central opening, no transvalvular gradient, and no regurgitation when closed. It would be nonthrombogenic and not damaging to blood components, and acceptable to the patient in terms of noise and the need for anticoagulation. Unfortunately, no artificial valve currently meets these criteria, so research continues.

Two major types of prosthetic valves are available—mechanical and biological. Mechanical valves are made entirely of synthetic materials, whereas biological valves combine synthetic materials with chemically treated biological tissues. When choosing an appropriate valve for a particular patient, it is necessary to compare the advantages and disadvantages of the various valve types. The advantages and disadvantages of prosthetic cardiac valves are listed in Box 22-1. Mechanical valves offer the benefits of good long-term durability but pose a significant risk for thromboembolism and require long-term anticoagulation. Biological valves decrease the risk for thromboembolism and can obviate the need for long-term anticoagulation, but they are not as durable as mechanical valves. Biological valves studied at autopsy

---

Box 22-1 • Advantages and Disadvantages of Prosthetic Cardiac Valves

Mechanical Valves
- Good long-term durability
- Adequate hemodynamics
- High risk for thromboembolism; necessity for long-term anticoagulation
- Increased risk for bleeding complications

Biological Valves
- Poor long-term durability
- Better hemodynamics than mechanical valves (except in small sizes)
- No hemolysis
- Low incidence of thromboembolism; possibly no necessity for anticoagulation
- Fewer bleeding complications

have shown structural deterioration beginning as early as 6 years after implantation, and their total useful lifetime is usually considered to be less than 10 years.

Patients with a long life expectancy may receive mechanical valves because they are particularly durable. Older patients may receive biological valves because less calcification and deterioration occur in older people, long-term durability is less important, and the risk for anticoagulation may increase with advancing age. Biological valves are indicated for patients who are unable to comply with an anticoagulation regimen, for those in whom a long-term anticoagulation regimen is contraindicated, and for women of childbearing age who plan to become pregnant (the anticoagulant warfarin crosses the placental barrier).

Mechanical Valves Mechanical valves include the caged ball, tilting disk, and bileaflet designs (Fig. 22-5). The caged ball valve consists of a plastic or metal ball inside of a metal cage attached to a sewing ring. When pressure behind the valve increases, the ball is forced down into the cage, and blood flows around it. When pressure in front of the valve increases, the ball is forced upward against the sewing ring, preventing regurgitant flow. An example of the caged ball valve is the Starr-Edwards valve (see Fig. 22-5C, D).

Hemodynamically, the ball in the cage produces a central obstruction to blood flow, which can result in a small stenotic pressure gradient, and ventricular outflow may be partially obstructed because of the cage's size and high profile. Because of the thrombogenicity of the plastic and metal and the turbulent

flow around the ball and through the cage, blood clots can form on or around the valve. Thromboembolism is a common problem, and chronic anticoagulant therapy is essential. Caged ball valves have good long-term durability.

The tilting disk valve is constructed of a disk held in place by struts attached to a sewing ring. When the pressure behind the valve increases, the disk tilts open approximately 60 to 80 degrees, allowing blood to flow around it. When the pressure in front of the valve increases, the disk tilts back flush with the sewing ring to close. Because of its semicentralized flow and lower profile, the tilting disk valve produces less obstruction to blood flow and has better hemodynamic characteristics than the caged ball valve. The tilting disk valve has good long-term durability, but the risk for thromboembolism requires long-term anticoagulant therapy. Examples of the tilting disk valve are the Medtronic-Hall and the Omniscience valves.

The bileaflet tilting disk valve, which consists of two pyrolytic carbon semicircular disks or leaflets hinged to a sewing ring, is the newest type of mechanical valve (see Fig. 22-5A, B). When the pressure behind the valve increases, the leaflets open perpendicular to the sewing ring, and blood flows through the central opening with minimal obstruction. When pressure in front of the valve increases, the leaflets return to their flat position against the sewing ring, preventing insufficiency. The bileaflet tilting disk valve has good hemodynamic characteristics and durability, but it is thrombogenic and requires long-term anticoagulation. An example of the bileaflet tilting disk valve is the St. Jude Medical valve.

Biological Valves Biological prostheses, or tissue valves, offer another alternative for valve replacement. The porcine heterograft is constructed of an excised pig aortic valve preserved in glutaraldehyde and mounted on a frame attached to a sewing ring. Examples of porcine valves are the Hancock and the Carpentier-Edwards valves. Biological prostheses provide good hemodynamics, except in smaller sizes, where obstruction to flow can occur and a gradient can develop. Their main advantage is the lower risk for thromboembolism compared with mechanical valves. Because most thromboembolic events occur during the first 3 months after implantation before the sewing ring is endothelialized, most patients with biological valves receive anticoagulants during that time only. However, the decision regarding anticoagulation must be based on the patient's condition. Patients in chronic atrial fibrillation undergoing mitral valve replacement frequently receive long-term anticoagulation therapy even with a biological prosthesis because of stagnant blood flow in the atria, which predisposes to clot formation.

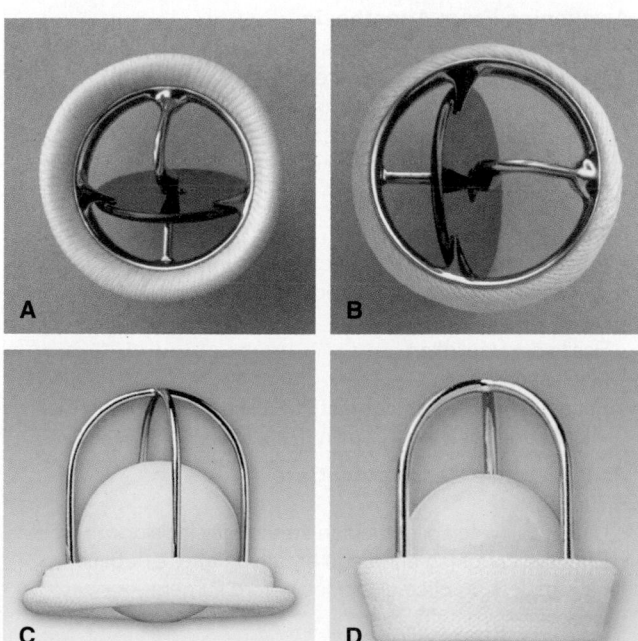

Figure 22-5 • A: Medtronic Hall Easy-Fit, aortic model. **B:** Medtronic Hall Easy-Fit, mitral model. **C:** Starr-Edwards Silastic ball valve, aortic model. **D:** Starr-Edwards Silastic ball valve, mitral model. (A and B courtesy of Medtronic Heart Valves, Minneapolis, MN; C and D courtesy of Edwards Life Sciences, Irvine, CA.)

• Cardiac Surgery

With managed care, rising costs, and the demand for high-quality care, cardiac surgery has come under increased scrutiny. The unique challenge for the critical care nurse is to integrate theoretical knowledge, assessment skills, and problem-solving ability to provide optimal nursing care and maintain high-quality outcomes while decreasing resource consumption, yet always keeping the patient as the focus.

PREOPERATIVE PHASE

Preoperative preparation for cardiac surgery includes physiological and psychological components. The physiological preparation is similar to that for any preoperative patient and includes history, physical examination, chest radiography, and an ECG. The history and physical examination are extremely important; they can provide information about previous neurological status, current medications, and any other coexisting conditions (e.g., diabetes mellitus, pulmonary disease, renal disease). The chest radiograph can give the surgeon general information about aortic calcification, and the ECG provides baseline information about the patient's heart rhythm. Laboratory tests include complete blood count (CBC), electrolytes, prothrombin time (PT), partial thromboplastin time (PTT), blood urea nitrogen (BUN), and creatinine. Pulmonary function tests and arterial blood gases (ABGs) may be performed if a patient has underlying pulmonary problems. Cost is always a consideration; only necessary tests should be ordered.

Effective preoperative teaching, which reduces anxiety and physiological responses to stress before and after surgery, is an important aspect of psychological preparation. The surgical procedure and the intraoperative and postoperative experiences are explained. The patient usually is not in the ICU before surgery, and a tour of the ICU helps familiarize the patient and family with the specialized equipment and environment. The sight of a patient who is successfully recovering from cardiac surgery helps instill confidence and allay anxiety. Incorporating family members or significant others in the education process is pivotal in patient care. Specific teaching topics related to the patient's stay in the ICU are listed in Box 22-2.

Numerous invasive lines are placed in the patient before surgery and are used for monitoring during and after surgery. These include a thermodilution pulmonary artery catheter, arterial line, and Foley catheter. Use of the pulmonary artery catheter has become controversial recently, and whether it is used is determined primarily by the patient's preoperative left ventricular function. The patient is intubated, and a nasogastric tube and additional intravenous (IV) lines may also be inserted.

INTRAOPERATIVE PHASE
Surgical Approach

The surgical approach most commonly used for myocardial revascularization and valve surgery is median

---

Box 22-2 • Preoperative Teaching About the Intensive Care Unit Experience for the Patient Undergoing Cardiac Surgery

Equipment to Point Out
- Cardiac monitor
- Arterial line
- Thermodilution catheter
- IV lines and IV infusion pumps
- Endotracheal tube and ventilator
  Suctioning
  Explain how to communicate when intubated; unable to talk
  Explain when extubation can be anticipated
- Foley catheter (increased sensation to urinate)
- Chest tubes (anticipated removal)
- Pacing wires
- Nasogastric tube
- Soft hand restraints

Incisions and Dressings to Expect
- Median sternotomy or other incision
- Leg incision (if saphenous vein is used)

Patient's Immediate Postoperative Appearance
- Skin yellow owing to use of Betadine solution in operating room
- Skin pale and cool to touch because of hypothermia during surgery
- Generalized "puffiness," especially noticeable in neck, face, and hands, because of third spacing of fluid given during cardiopulmonary bypass

Awakening From Anesthesia
- Patient recovers in the intensive care unit (ICU); does not go to the postanesthesia care unit
- Each patient recovers from anesthesia differently
- Patient may feel certain sensations
- Patient may hear certain noises
- Patient may be aware or able to hear but unable to respond

Discomfort
- Amount of discomfort to be expected
- When pain might be expected
- Relief mechanisms
  Positioning/splinting
  Medications
  Patient-controlled analgesia (PCA) and the importance of early administration of pain medication

Postoperative Respiratory Care
- Turning
- Use of pillow to splint median sternotomy incision
- Effective coughing and deep breathing after extubation; have patient practice exercises before surgery
- Incentive spirometry
- Early mobilization

Miscellaneous
- Postoperative activity progression
- Hospital visiting policy in intensive care area
- Avoiding use of arms to protect stability of sternotomy

sternotomy. The sternum is split with a sternal saw from the manubrium to below the xiphoid process, and the ribs are spread to expose the anterior mediastinum and pericardium. After the pericardium is opened and the heart and aorta are exposed, the patient is placed on cardiopulmonary bypass.

As myocardial revascularization has become increasingly sophisticated, new interventions to minimize the invasive nature of the surgery have been developed. The number of patients undergoing reoperations using CABG surgery has increased, and if the mediastinal approach is used in a reoperation, injury to old bypass grafts or embolization of debris due to manipulation of diseased grafts may cause problems.[12] A smaller lateral thoracotomy incision is often used to decrease the risks associated with reentry into the mediastinum. The choice of incision is based on the specific needs of each patient and the experience of the surgeon.

Cardiopulmonary Bypass

Cardiac surgery as it is known today was made possible by the development and practical application of cardiopulmonary bypass by Gibbon in 1953.[1] Because the heart must be still (not beating) and empty during the surgery, a cardiopulmonary bypass machine is used, unless OPCABG surgery is to be performed. Before the bypass is implemented, the tubing of the machine is primed with a balanced electrolyte solution. Blood can be used if indicated. The patient's deoxygenated venous blood is brought to the pump either through one cannula placed in the right atrial appendage or by two cannulas, one of which is placed directly in the inferior vena cava and the other directly in the superior vena cava. Another cannula is placed in the ascending aorta to return oxygenated blood to the patient's systemic circulation (Fig. 22-6). Heparin is administered throughout cardiopulmonary bypass to prevent massive extravascular coagulation as the blood circulates through the mechanical parts of the bypass system. After bypass is established, the blood is pumped through the circuit by a series of roller-type pumps that, unlike normal heart function, produce a nonpulsatile flow. Venous blood from the patient flows through the venous cannula to the cardiotomy reservoir and then into the oxygenator, where exchange of oxygen and carbon dioxide occurs. The blood then travels through the heat exchanger, where it is cooled initially and later rewarmed.

During bypass, the patient's core body temperature is lowered to 28° to 32°C (82.4° to 89.6°F) to decrease metabolism. For each 1°C drop of body temperature, the metabolic demands of the body decrease by 7%. This reduction in metabolic demands helps protect the major organ systems from possible ischemic injury and adverse effects of nonpulsatile perfusion during cardiopulmonary bypass.

Oxygenated blood is filtered and returned to the patient's ascending aorta through the arterial cannula (see Fig. 22-6). Once extracorporeal circulation is established and systemic hypothermia is achieved, the aorta is cross-clamped just above the coronary

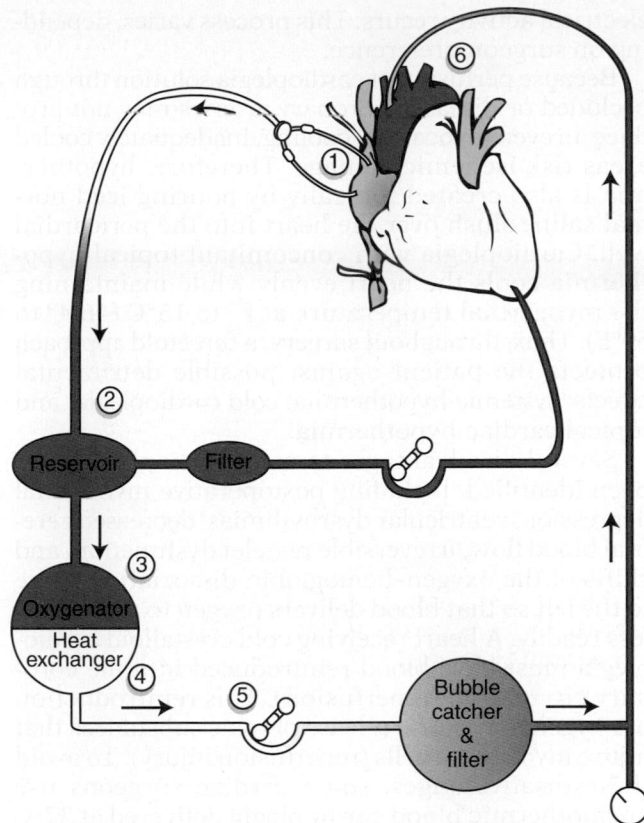

Figure 22-6 • Blood flow through the circuit of the cardiopulmonary bypass machine: (1) Patient's deoxygenated blood enters the bypass circuit from the venous cannulas in the superior and inferior vena cavae. (2) The reservoir holds the blood temporarily. (3) The oxygenator removes carbon dioxide from and adds oxygen to the patient's blood. (4) The heat exchanger initially cools the blood and then rewarms the blood. (5) Roller pumps pump the blood through the circuit and back to the patient. (6) Oxygenated blood is returned to the ascending aorta by way of the aortic cannula.

arteries, and either crystalloid or blood cardioplegia solution is infused into the aortic root. The formula varies, but cardioplegia solution is a balanced electrolyte solution high in potassium. Oxygenated blood from the bypass circuit or oxygenated crystalloid can be added to the cardioplegia solution.

After the aorta is cross-clamped, no blood circulates through the coronary arteries, so the myocardium becomes ischemic. Cold cardioplegia solution at 4°C (39.2°F) is infused into the aortic root under pressure. As it circulates through the coronary arteries, the high potassium concentration causes immediate asystole and relaxation, and the cold produces myocardial hypothermia. Asystole and hypothermia protect against myocardial ischemia by decreasing the metabolic needs of myocardial tissue. The cardioplegia solution provides a substrate for ongoing cellular metabolism and ensures appropriate pH and calcium ion levels for myocardial preservation.[13] The inclusion of blood or oxygenated crystalloid in the cardioplegia solution lessens myocardial ischemia by supplying oxygen. Cardioplegia solution may be infused into the aortic root continuously or intermittently every 15 to 30 minutes and whenever cardiac electrical activity recurs. This process varies, depending on surgeon preference.

Because perfusion of cardioplegia solution through occluded or diseased coronary arteries may not produce an even myocardial cooling, inadequately cooled areas risk ischemic damage. Therefore, hypothermia is also created topically by pouring iced normal saline slush over the heart into the pericardial well. Cardioplegia with concomitant topical hypothermia cools the heart evenly while maintaining the myocardial temperature at 8° to 15°C (46.4° to 59°F). Thus, throughout surgery, a threefold approach protects the patient against possible detrimental effects: systemic hypothermia, cold cardioplegia, and topical cardiac hypothermia.

Several disadvantages to cold cardioplegia have been identified, including postoperative myocardial depression, ventricular dysrhythmias, decreased cerebral blood flow, irreversible platelet dysfunction, and shifts of the oxygen–hemoglobin dissociation curve to the left so that blood delivers oxygen to the tissues less readily. A heart receiving cold crystalloid cardioplegia must have blood reintroduced into the coronary circulation (reperfusion). This reintroduction of oxygen may cause release of toxic substances that injure myocardial cells (reperfusion injury). To avoid these disadvantages, some cardiac surgeons use normothermic blood cardioplegia delivered at 37°C (98.6°F), which keeps the heart at a normal temperature. This intervention is now recommended with the urgent/emergent CABG surgery for acute myocardial infarction to protect myocardium that may be acutely depressed.[1] With the warm technique, topical cardiac hypothermia is not used, and systemic hypothermia may or may not be used. Advantages of warm cardioplegia include more frequent spontaneous return of normal sinus rhythm after surgery, better postoperative left ventricular function and cardiac index, less use of inotropic agents, and less postoperative bleeding. Patients who have undergone warm cardioplegia require less time on the ventilator and almost no rewarming technology in the ICU.

After surgery is completed, the heat exchanger rewarms the blood to return the patient's core temperature to 37°C (98.6°F) if hypothermic techniques were used. After air is vented from the heart chambers and the aortic root, the aortic cross-clamp is removed so that blood again perfuses the coronary arteries, warming the myocardium. As perfusion and rewarming continue, a spontaneous cardiac rhythm may resume, ventricular fibrillation may develop (necessitating internal defibrillation), or pacing may be used to initiate a rhythm. After a reliable rhythm with a rate adequate to maintain the cardiac output and blood pressure is established, total cardiopulmonary bypass is reduced to partial bypass. During partial bypass, some of the patient's blood circulates through the heart and lungs, while some continues to circulate through the pump. If adequate arterial pressures are maintained, the patient's heart then assumes total responsibility for the cardiac output, and bypass is discontinued.

After the heart can maintain an adequate cardiac output, the cannulas are removed from the right atrium and aorta. Heparinization is reversed by the administration of protamine sulfate. If adequate cardiac output cannot be maintained during the weaning process, positive inotropic agents or intra-aortic balloon counterpulsation can be instituted (see Chapter 18).

Completion of Surgery

If the need for postoperative cardiac pacing is anticipated, temporary pacing electrodes are placed on the epicardial surface of the heart and brought out through the chest wall on either side of the median sternotomy incision. Ventricular pacing electrodes are typically located to the left and atrial wires to the right of the sternum (Fig. 22-7).

Chest tubes placed in the mediastinum and pericardial space for drainage are brought out through stab wounds just below the median sternotomy. If the pleural space has been entered, pleural tubes are also placed. Smaller, more flexible chest drains are being used instead of the stiff, larger-bore tubes to enhance drainage of the pleural and mediastinal space.[14] After adequate hemostasis is obtained, the edges of the sternum are approximated with stainless steel wires, the incision is closed, and dressings are applied.

POSTOPERATIVE PHASE

Patients are transported directly to the ICU, where they recover from anesthesia and usually remain for 24 hours after surgery. Patients arrive in the ICU with numerous lines and tubes (e.g., endotracheal tube, hemodynamic monitoring lines). Immediate postoperative care involves cardiac monitoring and

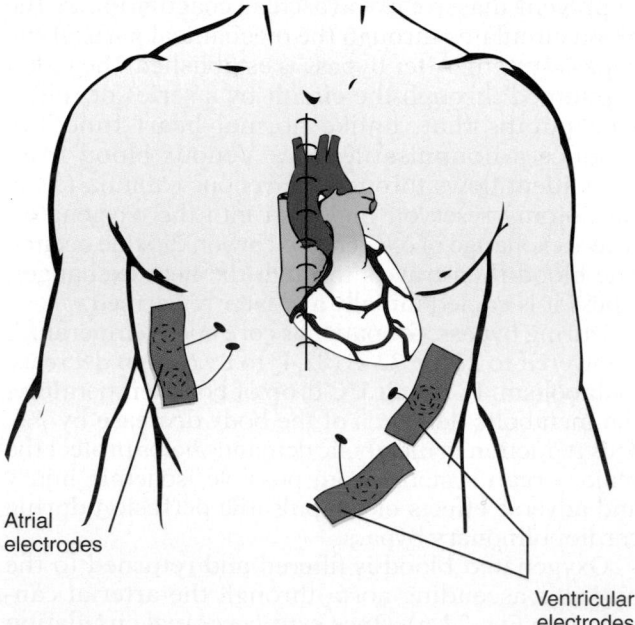

Atrial electrodes

Ventricular electrodes

Figure 22-7 • Temporary epicardial pacing wires: position of atrial and ventricular wires on chest wall.

maintenance of oxygenation and hemodynamic stability, as described in Box 22-3. Because cardiopulmonary bypass produces abnormal blood interface and altered blood flow patterns, it has profound physiological effects (Table 22-2).

The postoperative course depends on the patient's preoperative condition. Factors that may increase mortality include age; sex; previous similar surgery (resurgery); preoperative occurrence of acute myocardial infarction; and concomitant conditions such as diabetes mellitus, peripheral vascular disease, renal insufficiency, and chronic obstructive pulmonary disease (COPD).[1] Whether the surgery is elective or emergent may also influence outcome. Awareness of these conditions helps the critical care nurse anticipate problems. Accurate assessments, vigilant monitoring, and proper interventions are critical in stabilizing patients who have just undergone cardiac surgery. Box 22-4 lists some nursing diagnoses and collaborative problems in cardiac surgery. Box 22-5 presents a collaborative care guide for the patient after such surgery. Certain patient populations present special problems. Box 22-6 lists factors to consider in management of the older cardiac patient.

Box 22-3 • Nursing Responsibilities in Caring for the Cardiac Surgery Patient in the Immediate Postoperative Period

Priority Interventions Performed by the Critical Care Team on Arrival

- Attach patient to bedside cardiac monitor and note rhythm.
- Attach pressure lines to bedside monitor (arterial and pulmonary artery); level and zero transducers and note pressure values and waveforms.
- Obtain cardiac output/index and note existing inotropic or vasoactive drips.
- After ventilator is connected to endotracheal tube, auscultate breath sounds bilaterally.
- Apply end-tidal carbon dioxide ($ETCO_2$) device to ventilator circuit and note waveform and value (best indicator of endotracheal tube placement).
- Apply pulse oximetry device to patient and note SpO_2 value and waveform.
- Check peripheral pulses and perfusion signs.
- Monitor chest tubes and character of drainage: amount, color, flow. Check for air leaks.
- Measure body temperature and initiate rewarming if temperature < 96.8°F (36°C).

Once the Patient Is Determined to Be Hemodynamically Stable

- Measure urine output and note characteristics.
- Obtain clinical data (within 30 minutes of arrival).
- Obtain chest radiograph.
- Obtain 12-lead electrocardiogram (ECG).
- Obtain routine blood work within 15 minutes of arrival; tests may include ABGs, potassium, glucose, PTT, hemoglobin (varies with institution).
- Assess neurological status.
- Test pacemaker function by assessing capture and sensing.

Prevention of Hypothermia

Whether the cardiac procedure is performed on or off bypass, hypothermia is a common side effect. During rewarming on cardiopulmonary bypass, the patient's core temperature is returned to 98.6°F (37°C). However, as this warmed blood begins to circulate to the periphery, heat transfer to the surrounding tissues again causes the core temperature to decline. Patients frequently enter the ICU with a temperature in the 95° to 96.8°F (35° to 36°C) range. OPCABG surgery causes hypothermia because of heat loss secondary to prolonged exposure to cool operating room temperatures. Hypothermia causes peripheral vasoconstriction and a shift of the oxygen–hemoglobin dissociation curve to the left, which means that less oxygen is released from the hemoglobin to the tissues. Hypothermia can also impair coagulation because all enzyme systems in the body depend on a tight temperature range for optimal performance.[15]

The nurse assesses the patient's temperature on ICU admission using pulmonary artery or tympanic membrane temperature; if performed properly, both are considered accurate indicators of core temperature. Rectal temperature does not correlate with core temperature measurements until 8 hours after surgery, and bladder temperature differs significantly from core temperature with rapid cooling and rewarming. Increasing the room temperature and using radiant heat, blankets, or a warming blanket are effective techniques for increasing core temperature. Rewarming should occur slowly to prevent hemodynamic instability due to rapid vasodilation.

It is important to prevent shivering, which occurs most often from 90 to 180 minutes after ICU admission, because it increases metabolic rate, oxygen consumption, carbon dioxide production, and myocardial workload. If left ventricular function is compromised, shivering should be managed with a neuromuscular blocker in combination with simultaneous sedation to avoid further cardiac compromise. In unusual situations, the patient may experience discomfort with shivering, which can be treated with meperidine (Demerol).

After rewarming, many patients experience an overshoot in body temperature. One etiological theory is that narcotics and anesthetics administered during surgery reset the hypothalamic regulatory center, altering peripheral blood flow and feedback.[16] A cold, constricted peripheral vascular bed may also be a factor in preventing heat dissipation. If the patient is bleeding after surgery, correction of temperature is imperative to aid in the return of normal coagulation enzyme function and clotting ability.

Monitoring for Systemic Inflammatory Response Syndrome

Any process, including surgery, initiates the inflammatory process called SIRS. In recent years, research in critical care medicine has focused on SIRS because it may be the cause of many patient problems. An

Table 22-2 • Effects of Cardiopulmonary Bypass

Effects	Clinical Implications
Increased Capillary Permeability Interface between blood and nonphysiological surfaces or bypass circuit leads to • Complement activation that increases capillary permeability • Platelet activation—platelets secrete vasoactive substances that increase capillary permeability • Release of other vasoactive substances that increase capillary permeability	Large amounts of fluid move from the intravascular to the interstitial space during and up to 6 h after cardiopulmonary bypass. Patient becomes edematous.
Hemodilution Solution used to prime extracorporeal circuit dilutes patient's blood. Secretion of vasopressin (ADH) is increased. Levels of renin–angiotensin–aldosterone are increased because of nonpulsatile renal perfusion. Total body water is increased.	Decreased blood viscosity improves capillary perfusion during nonpulsatile flow and hypothermia. Hgb and Hct decrease. Levels of coagulation factors are decreased because of dilution. Intravascular colloid osmotic pressure is decreased, contributing to movement of fluid from intravascular to interstitial spaces. Water is retained at collecting tubule of kidney. Aldosterone causes retention of sodium and water at renal tubule. Weight gain occurs.
Altered Coagulation Procoagulant effects: • Interface between blood and nonendothelial surfaces of bypass circuit activates intrinsic coagulation cascade. • Platelet damage activates intrinsic pathway. Anticoagulant effects: • Interface between blood and nonendothelial surfaces of bypass circuit causes platelets to adhere to tubing and to clump; abnormal platelet function; activation of coagulation cascade, which depletes clotting factors; denaturization of plasma proteins, including coagulation factors. • Coagulation factors are decreased as a result of hemodilution.	Risk for microemboli is increased. Platelet count decreases by 50% to 70% of baseline. Abnormal postoperative bleeding occurs. Possibility of bleeding diathesis exists.
Damage to Blood Cells Exposure of blood to nonendothelial surfaces causes mechanical trauma and shear stress. • Platelet damage occurs. • Red blood cell hemolysis occurs. • Leukocytes are damaged.	Platelet count is decreased. Free hemoglobin and hemoglobinuria are increased. Hct is decreased. Immune response is diminished.
Microembolization Emboli form from tissue debris, air bubbles, platelet aggregation.	Microemboli to body organs (brain, lungs, kidney) are possible.
Increased Systemic Vascular Resistance (SVR) Catecholamine secretion is increased when cardiopulmonary bypass is initiated. Renin secretion is due to nonpulsatile flow to kidney. Hypothermia develops.	Hypertension is possible. Increased SVR may decrease cardiac output.

entire "body" inflammatory response may occur after CABG surgery that appears to be an infection. Symptoms and signs include fever, tachycardia, tachypnea, and an increased white blood cell count. To attempt to differentiate between SIRS and infection or sepsis, the American College of Chest Physicians convened a consensus conference in 1997.[17] The conference developed definitions differentiating the two conditions (Box 22-7), which are now used frequently by critical care experts.

SIRS is a natural defense mechanism that is initiated when tissue or vessels are injured. A vascular injury, the inflammatory response, and the coagulation cascade are interrelated. An event that dis-

rupts the integrity of the endothelium, such as trauma from cutting the vessel or hypoxia in a few endothelial cells, triggers the process. Once the injury occurs, a local inflammatory reaction begins with the release of mediators called cytokines from "protector" cells (e.g., lymphocytes, macrophages). These mediators signal other cells (e.g., neutrophils, monocytes) to the injured area, which release other mediators. The endothelium then releases vasodilating mediators (e.g., nitric oxide), which increase blood flow to the area, thereby increasing oxygen delivery. Counter-regulatory mediators cause vasoconstriction to balance vasodilatory actions. Platelets are attracted to the area to start the coagulation process. As a

---

Box 22-4 | **Examples of Nursing Diagnoses and Collaborative Problems for Cardiac Surgery Patients**

- Decreased Cardiac Output related to changes in ventricular preload, afterload, and contractility
- Decreased Cardiac Output related to cardiac dysrhythmias
- Impaired Tissue Perfusion related to cardiopulmonary bypass, decreased cardiac output, hypotension
- Impaired Tissue Perfusion related to microembolization secondary to the systemic inflammatory response syndrome (SIRS) process
- Impaired Gas Exchange related to cardiopulmonary bypass, anesthesia, poor chest expansion, atelectasis, retained secretions
- Impaired Comfort related to endotracheal tube, surgical incision, chest tubes, rib spreading
- Anxiety related to fear of death, intensive care unit environment
- Risk for Fluid Volume Deficit related to abnormal bleeding
- Risk for Infection related to surgical procedure, invasive lines, drainage tubes, hypoventilation, retained secretions

---

result of the endothelial damage, increased capillary permeability inevitably occurs.[18] This highly complex process is discussed in more detail in Chapter 54.

It was once believed that the cardiopulmonary bypass machine was the major trigger of SIRS; this prompted experts to reconsider the use of this machine. However, Vallely and colleagues have demonstrated that OPCABG surgery also initiates a SIRS response involving the release of different mediators from the on-pump procedure.[7] Few interventions limit SIRS; the inflammatory process is so complex that it has been difficult to develop medications to counter all the numerous reactions. Steroids have been shown to decrease SIRS somewhat if given before surgery, but they should be used with caution, especially in patients with diabetes mellitus.[1] Nursing responsibilities focus on refining assessment skills to increase early detection of embolic events in any system, especially the nervous, cardiovascular, pulmonary, and renal systems. It is important to have a high degree of suspicion when assessing patients and providing postoperative care.

Controlling Pain

After cardiac surgery, the patient may experience pain resulting from the chest or leg incision, the chest tubes, rib spreading during surgery, and care activities. The ICU environment may accentuate the pain physiologically because of light and noise, as well as psychologically because of separation and fear. Pain often stimulates the sympathetic nervous system, increasing heart rate and blood pressure, which can be detrimental to the patient's hemodynamics. Discomfort can also result in diminished chest expansion, increased atelectasis, and retention of secretions.

Although pain perception varies from person to person, a median sternotomy incision is usually less painful than a thoracotomy incision, and most people report that the pain is most severe the first 3 to 4 days after surgery. Discomfort from the leg incision often worsens after the patient is ambulatory, especially if leg swelling occurs. Stretching of back and neck muscles as the ribs are spread and immobilization for several hours during surgery can cause back and neck discomfort. Patients who have internal mammary artery grafts may have increased pain because of increased stretching of the intercostal muscles and the incision into the parietal pleura, which is richly innervated.

Angina after CABG surgery may indicate graft failure; therefore, the nurse must be able to differentiate angina from incisional pain. Typical median sternotomy pain is localized; does not radiate; and can be sharp, dull, aching, or burning. It is often worse with deep breathing, coughing, or movement. Angina is usually precordial or substernal; not well localized; and frequently radiates to arms, neck, or jaw. It is often described as a pressure sensation and is not affected by respiration or movement.

One of the goals of nursing management is a thorough assessment of the patient's pain using a pain scale; administration of analgesics based on the reported pain intensity; provision of adequate pain relief as reported by the patient; and alleviation of factors that enhance pain perception, such as anxiety and fear. The common analgesic agents used are morphine sulfate, fentanyl, and hydromorphone (Dilaudid), as needed. These drugs can be supplemented with nonsteroidal anti-inflammatory drugs (NSAIDs), such as ketorolac (Toradol), which decrease pain through a different mechanism. Caution should be used in administering NSAIDs to patients with compromised renal function. Patient-controlled analgesia pumps are frequently used to allow the patient to control administration of pain medication. Interventions such as intercostal nerve blocks and spinal analgesia are less common. Regardless of the mechanism used, pain control is aggressively pursued to ensure comfort and rapid mobilization, which in turn can lessen complications. Alternative therapies such as music therapy and guided imagery may also be useful in controlling pain.

Preventing Cardiovascular Complications

Volume Resuscitation

Adequate intravascular volume to provide preload is a primary concern. Increased capillary permeability due to SIRS causes intravascular volume to shift into the interstitial spaces. To maintain optimal cardiac performance and blood pressure, proper volume resuscitation is imperative. A variety of fluids may be used, including normal saline, hetastarch, and

Box 22-5 • COLLABORATIVE CARE GUIDE for the Patient After Cardiac Surgery

OUTCOMES	INTERVENTIONS
Oxygenation/Ventilation Patient will have arterial blood gases within normal limits and pulse oximeter value > 92%. Pulmonary edema will be minimized on chest x-ray and demonstrated by improved breath sounds. Atelectasis will be improved. Chest tubes will remain patent.	• Obtain arterial blood gases per protocol. • Correlate pulse oximeter and end-tidal CO_2 with arterial blood gas results. • Adjust ventilator settings after consulting with the respiratory therapist and physician. • Wean from mechanical ventilation per protocol using the expertise of respiratory therapy. • Extubate when patient is hemodynamically stable; able to protect airway. • Provide supplemental oxygen after extubation. • Encourage use of incentive spirometer, cough and deep breath q 2 to 4 h after extubation. • Milk chest tubes if necessary to facilitate forward drainage movement.
Circulation/Perfusion Patient will maintain adequate clinical perfusion. Vital signs will be within normal limits, including MAP > 70 mm Hg; cardiac index will be in a suitable range for the patient's left ventricular function. Patient will be euthermic.	• Monitor PA and PAWP, CVP or RAP, cardiac output, SVR, and PVR per protocol if pulmonary artery catheter is in place. • Monitor ECG, ST segments, and arterial blood pressure continuously. • Administer positive inotropic agents and reduce afterload with vasodilating agents guided by hemodynamic parameters and physician orders. • Regulate volume administration as indicated by PAWP or CVP values. • Evaluate effect of medications on BP, HR, and hemodynamic parameters. • Monitor and treat dysrhythmias per protocol and physician orders. • Anticipate need for temporary cardiac pacing; wires will be properly isolated for electrical safety. • Prepare patient for intra-aortic balloon pump assist if necessary. • Congestive heart failure due to decreased cardiac output or perioperative MI will be minimized by collaborating with a physician. • Assess for neck vein distention, pulmonary crackles, S_3 or S_4, peripheral edema, increased preload parameters, elevated "a" wave of CVP, RAP, or PAWP waveform. • Monitor 12-lead ECG if ECG changes observed. • Assess temperature q 1 h. • Warm patient 1°C per hour by using warming blankets, lights, and fluid warmer.
Hematological Issues Patient will have minimal bleeding and avoid cardiac tamponade.	• Chest tube drainage will be < 200 mL/h. • Monitor for signs of cardiac tamponade (hypotension, pulsus paradoxus, tachycardia, PA pressure equalization). • Evaluate chest x-ray for widened mediastinum, consulting with a physician as needed. • Monitor PT, PTT, ACT, CBC per protocol. • Administer protamine, blood products, and other procoagulants per order or protocol. • Monitor vasoactive drug need and report marked increase of drugs to physician immediately because this change may indicate possible tamponade.

(continued)

Box 22-5 • COLLABORATIVE CARE GUIDE for the Patient After Cardiac Surgery (Continued)

OUTCOMES	INTERVENTIONS
Fluids/Electrolytes Patient will maintain or improve preoperative renal function.	• Renal function will be maintained as evidenced by urine output of approximately 0.5 mL/kg/h. • Potassium will be replaced to maintain K^+ > 4.0 mEq/L. • Monitor intake and output q 1–2 h. • Monitor BUN, creatinine, electrolytes, Mg, PO_4. • Record daily weights. • Administer fluid volume or diuretics as ordered.
Mobility/Skin Integrity Patient will maintain range of motion and muscle strength and will have intact skin integrity	• Turn patient side to side every 2 h while on bed rest and evaluate skin closely. • Mobilize out of bed after extubation. • Progress activity to chair for meals, bathroom privileges, increased distance walking, delegating to assistive personnel as indicated. • Monitor vital signs, respiratory effort during activity.
Incisions will heal without evidence of infection.	• Check stability of sternotomy incision daily, especially with diabetic patients. • Assess sternotomy and leg incision for redness, swelling, drainage. • Apply compression hose and elevate legs to reduce edema. • Caloric and nutrient intake meet metabolic requirements per calculation for long-term patients. • Monitor prealbumin for trends on long-term patients.
Comfort and Pain Control Patient will have relief of surgical pain. Patient will demonstrate no evidence of pain or anxiety such as increased HR, BP, RR, or agitation during activity or procedures. Timely administration of pain medication will be a priority.	• Assess quality, duration, location of pain. Use visual analog scale to assess pain quantity. • Provide a calm environment. Provide for adequate periods of rest and sleep.
Teaching/Discharge Planning Patient and family will understand need for: Tests, procedures, treatments. Self-protective devices as indicated and per hospital policy. In preparation for discharge to home, patient will understand activity levels, dietary restrictions, medication regimen, incision care.	• Consult nutritional support services. • Make appropriate social work referrals early during hospitalization. • Initiate family education regarding heart-healthy diet, physical activity limitations (e.g., lifting over 10–15 lb, driving restrictions), stress reduction strategies, management of pain, incision care.

hyperosmolar fluids (e.g., 3% saline).[19] No fluid is definitively recommended. If the patient is bleeding, blood products should be the fluid of choice. If the patient's blood pressure is unresponsive to moderate infusion rates, usually 500 mL is infused using a pressure bag and a large-bore catheter. Hemodynamic parameters, including a low central venous pressure (CVP) (<8 to 10 mm Hg), low pulmonary artery diastolic pressure, and low pulmonary artery wedge pressure (PAWP) (<14 to 18 mm Hg), in combination with a low cardiac index (<2.5 L/minute/m²), help guide interventions.[15] Caution should be exercised in using these numerical values as absolute goals.

The preoperative condition of the heart is important to consider. If the patient has had a recent myocardial infarction or poor left ventricular performance, higher pressures may be required to maintain optimal cardiac work. The patient with a hypertrophied left ventricle, especially with valvular disease, is heavily dependent on volume resuscitation.

The effectiveness of all interventions must be assessed against the patient's response. Mottling of the extremities, especially the knees, and the character of the peripheral pulses (especially dorsalis pedis) are clinical indications of perfusion.[20] The combination of weak pulses and mottled knees may indicate hypoperfusion. Resolution of these clinical findings, as well as improved pressure values, signals the return of adequate perfusion. The astute critical care nurse continually monitors the appearance of the extremities and the pulses.

Monitoring for Dysrhythmias

Dysrhythmias are a major issue after CABG surgery. The hemodynamic response to a change in cardiac rhythm dictates the speed of the intervention in

Box 22-6 • CONSIDERATIONS FOR THE OLDER PATIENT: After Cardiac Surgery

Physiological Changes

Cardiovascular System
- Increased stiffness of myocardial muscle
- Increased stiffness of peripheral vasculature and decreased ability to adjust to changes in blood volume
- Replacement of cells in conduction system with collagen and elastin
- Decreasing number of pacemaker cells in the sinoatrial (SA) and atrioventricular (AV) nodes
- Decreased cardiac responsiveness to β-adrenergic stimulation

Pulmonary System
- Breakdown of elastin and collagen, which impairs elastic recoil of lung
- Thoracic cage less compliant
- Decreased expiratory muscle strength and mucociliary clearance

Renal System
- Progressive loss of cortical nephrons and decrease in corticomedullary concentration gradient
- Impaired renal concentrating ability
- Decreased clearance of medications excreted by the kidneys (may be reduced by up to 40% by 80 years of age)

Gastrointestinal System
- Decreased and more variable gastrointestinal absorption of medications
- Decline in liver function, resulting in decreased hepatic breakdown of medications

Musculoskeletal System
- Skeletal osteoporosis

Immune System
- Immune response may be decreased, especially if concomitant malnutrition and decrease in serum proteins

Neurological System
- Decline in neurotransmitters
- Increased risk for acute confusion

Response to Medications
- Decreased percentage of lean body tissue
- Increased percentage of body fat
- Decrease in body water

Clinical Effect
- Higher filling pressures (pulmonary artery diastolic [PAD] pressure and pulmonary artery wedge pressure [PAWP])
- Decreased ability for vasoconstriction with position change, leading to orthostatic hypotension
- SA and AV node impairment
- Cardiac output maintained by increase in stroke volume
- Slowing of renal response to dehydration
- Decreased effectiveness of fluid conservation
- Toxic medication levels or abnormally prolonged duration of action
- Sensitive to drugs with narrow therapeutic range, such as digoxin
- More intense medication effect and longer duration of action for medications broken down in liver (e.g., benzodiazepines)
- As a result of decreased body water, water-soluble medications concentrated in the bloodstream, resulting in higher serum drug levels
- Fat-soluble medications stored in fat; increase in fat tissue may result in slower therapeutic response and longer duration of action as drug is released slowly from fat

Patient Teaching
- Accommodate sensory deficits.
  - Ensure hearing aids are in and functional.
  - Speak loudly and face patient.
  - Use large print, easy-to-read materials.
- Teach one thing at a time, and ensure patient understands before moving on.
- Start with simple and progress to more complex information.
- Teach both patient and caregiver.

Adapted from Dixon V: Effects of vascular surgery on the elderly vascular patient. J Vasc Nurs 17:86–88, 1999.

---

patients who have undergone CABG surgery, as in all critical care patients. In emergent situations, advanced cardiac life support (ACLS) algorithms are used. Knowledge of the patient's baseline rhythm is important. The types of dysrhythmias that may occur range from premature atrial contractions to ventricular fibrillation and asystole.

Sinus tachycardia is very common and may result from many factors. Some of the more common causes are sympathomimetic drugs, SIRS, hypovolemia, fever, and pain. Prolonged periods of tachycardia may be harmful due to decreased coronary artery filling time. Sinus bradycardia may occur, but it is not anticipated because patients are in a sympathetically responsive state. In many cases, preoperative β-blockade may be the cause.

Causes of premature atrial contractions are usually electrolyte disturbances, ischemia or infarction, or hypoperfusion. Frequent premature atrial contractions may be a precursor to atrial fibrillation and occur very commonly, especially in patients with a previous history of pulmonary or valve disease in which the atria can be distended. The simple treatment for premature atrial contractions is repletion of potassium and magnesium. Maintenance of adequate potassium

Box 22-7 • Definition of Systemic Inflammatory Response Syndrome (SIRS)

SIRS is defined by the presence of two or more of the following conditions:

Temperature	>100.4°F (38°C) or <96.8°F (36°C)
Heart rate	>90 beats/min
Respiratory rate	>20 breaths/min or $Paco_2$ <32 mm Hg
White blood cell count	>12,000 cells/m³, <4000 cells/m³, or >10% immature (bands) cells

Sepsis is a systemic response to documented infection and is determined by the same criteria as SIRS.

(range, 4 to 4.5 mEq/L) and IV infusion of 2 g magnesium may minimize premature atrial contractions.

Atrial fibrillation may occur after CABG surgery, and prevention is a high priority. Cardiac decompensation or cerebrovascular accidents are the major risks associated with atrial fibrillation. For new-onset atrial fibrillation, the goal is conversion to sinus rhythm using antiarrhythmics, especially amiodarone. The loading dose is 150 mg IV over 10 minutes followed by a 1 mg/minute drip for 6 hours, then a 0.5 mg/minute drip for 18 hours. Additional loading may be necessary. Procainamide, an older drug, can be used if amiodarone is contraindicated. The loading dose is up to 1 g IV at a rate of 20 mg/minute, followed by a 2 mg/minute drip until the dysrhythmia is corrected. Control of the ventricular response is a goal and can be achieved using diltiazem, starting with a loading dose up to 0.75 mg/kg IV followed by a drip, which is usually started at 5 mg/hour. Combination of antiarrhythmics may be used but should be monitored carefully. If atrial fibrillation persists or reoccurs for more than 24 hours, warfarin anticoagulation for 4 weeks may be needed.[1] For chronic atrial fibrillation, conversion is not a goal unless the patient has been anticoagulated because of the risk for atrial thrombus and possible embolization. If emergent cardioversion is required in the immediate postoperative period and anticoagulation is not an option, echocardiography, either Doppler or transesophageal, may be performed to check for thrombus formation in the left atrium.

Heart block arrhythmias occur in patients with valve surgery secondary to the edema at the surgical site, near the conduction system. Resolution of this rhythm is usually attained 48 to 72 hours after surgery once the edema has decreased. Myocardial ischemia and infarction also cause the heart block. Patients who have had cardiac surgery have an advantage with the placement of epicardial pacing wires. Use of these wires allows better control of ventricular response compared with the use of drugs such as atropine and isoproterenol. Atrial pacing is preferred if the atrioventricular (AV) node is intact because it allows optimal hemodynamics with an atrial contraction. If the AV node is not functioning properly, AV sequential pacing may be required. Ventricular pacing is the last choice. If pacing is required for more than 72 hours, permanent pacemaker placement should be considered, especially in patients who have had valve surgery. An in-depth discussion of pacing can be found in Chapter 18.

The occurrence of tachyarrhythmias may lead to emergent situations. If the patient is hemodynamically unstable in a fast rhythm, the first intervention is cardioversion, following ACLS guidelines. If ventricular dysrhythmias develop, electrical or pharmacological interventions are necessary. If premature ventricular contractions appear after surgery, 2 to 4 g IV of magnesium may help resolve this problem. The new ACLS guidelines de-emphasize the use of lidocaine and recommend amiodarone as the drug of choice, especially in patients with poor left ventricular function. If ventricular tachycardia deteriorates

into ventricular fibrillation or other rhythms with no pulse, cardiopulmonary resuscitation should be started immediately; medical personnel should be prepared to open the chest at the bedside to determine and correct the cause of arrest.

Improving Cardiac Contractility

Contractility may be depressed because of the exposure of the heart muscle to manipulation, temperature change, and possible hypoperfusion. The first step taken to improve performance is to ensure optimal volume resuscitation; it will quickly become clear if volume does not increase the cardiac output and index. The addition and titration of sympathomimetic drugs is a common part of the care of patients with decreased contractility. Various drugs, including epinephrine, dobutamine, and milrinone, may be used. Dopamine is another drug that can increase contractility but may cause unwanted tachycardia. The choice of drug varies with institution and health care provider.

As the drug of choice is added, the cause of the ventricular dysfunction should be pursued. Myocardial ischemia and infarction typically cause decreased cardiac function, but other factors may be sources of the problem. Stunned myocardium, the transient depression of left ventricular function due to a temporary reduction of myocardial blood flow, may cause transient dysfunction; it is usually associated with normally functioning myocardium.[21] Hibernating myocardium is chronically impaired yet viable myocardial tissue, which results in left ventricular dysfunction at rest because of persistently hypoperfused myocardium or repeated stunning.[21] This state can lead to more chronic dysfunction. The state of the right ventricle should also be considered. If a patient had a right ventricular infarct preoperatively, surgery should be delayed up to 4 weeks to allow recovery of function.[1] If right ventricular dysfunction develops after CABG surgery, use of nitric oxide is one of the more effective interventions. Evaluation of cardiac work is not limited to cardiac output and cardiac index. Cardiac biomarkers can be used in the first 24 hours after CABG surgery. Creatine kinase muscle band (MB) is one parameter that can be monitored, and if it is greater than 5 times the upper limit of normal, the patient may have sustained myocardial damage.[1] In the more complicated cases, sampling of mixed venous blood gases/mixed venous saturation (SvO_2) and the arterial–venous difference in oxygen may be useful. These values are indicators of oxygen transport and consumption and can help direct therapy. Although continuous SvO_2 monitoring may be used in patients with severe myocardial dysfunction, it is not a standard intervention; it is costly and has not been shown to make a difference in outcomes.

The intra-aortic balloon pump (IABP) is a mechanical method used to improve coronary perfusion in any of the previously mentioned situations.[1] For a complete discussion of IABP, see Chapter 18. Mechanical factors may lead to depressed cardiac function. Cardiac tamponade, the most common such factor, may require surgical correction. This topic is discussed later in the chapter. Whatever the cause, time and support of function are usually the major factors that improve cardiac performance. However, protracted periods of time with mechanical or pharmacological support may be the signal to start to consider the placement of a ventricular assist device, usually as a bridge to heart transplantation.

Controlling Blood Pressure

A reduction in SVR is another clinical maneuver that can increase cardiac performance. If the patient has an adequate blood pressure (mean arterial pressure [MAP] > 70 mm Hg or systolic blood pressure > 120 mm Hg) without pharmacological support (α-agonist agents to increase blood pressure), afterload reduction should be started even if the patient is on inotropic support. Various agents, including nitroprusside, nitroglycerin, hydralazine, labetalol, and angiotensin-converting enzyme (ACE) inhibitors such as captopril, can be used. The necessary speed of response dictates the choice of drug. For example, IV drugs, especially nitroprusside, rapidly cause a reduction in afterload. Other agents, such as hydralazine and ACE inhibitors, can then be used to augment this effect. ACE inhibitors should be used with caution in patients with impaired renal function because this drug category can exacerbate renal dysfunction. The previously named drugs also reduce blood pressure; in the immediate postoperative period, this is very important in maintaining the integrity of the grafts.

Preventing Pulmonary Complications

Postoperative pulmonary function depends on preoperative function. The degree of preoperative evaluation in preparation for surgery has changed in the current era of cost containment. If the patient has a significant pulmonary history (e.g., COPD, pulmonary hypertension), baseline pulmonary function tests and ABGs can be very helpful in setting goals in the postoperative period. These tests may help predict how the patient will respond to mechanical ventilation.

The causes of pulmonary dysfunction after cardiac surgery can be attributed to changes that occur with the inflammatory response. Various triggers, such as surgical trauma and regional myocardial ischemia, activate the complement system and release cytokines, leading to an egress of neutrophils and fluid across endothelium. These triggers can also cause end-organ dysfunction, including organs such as the lungs.[7] Such changes in the lungs can lead to alterations in microcirculation and gas exchange that ultimately result in ventilation–perfusion mismatching, shunting, and atelectasis.[15]

Mechanical ventilation is required to achieve adequate oxygenation and ventilation. Adequate oxygenation is achieved by adjusting the level of oxygen delivered by the ventilator; the usual starting point is 40% to 50% oxygen. Effective oxygenation is monitored using pulse oximetry with intermittent ABG sampling. Positive end-expiratory pressure (PEEP) is a standard intervention used to help keep the alveoli open and improve oxygenation. PEEP usually starts at 5 cm H_2O but can be increased to 10 cm H_2O or more if hypoxemia is present. Care must be taken when increasing PEEP because it can decrease preload, thereby decreasing cardiac output and blood pressure. The initial mode for the ventilator is usually assist-control ventilation and is changed to continuous positive airway pressure (CPAP) when the patient is awake, stable, and ready to be weaned for extubation.

Adequate ventilation is maintained by selecting tidal volumes that are appropriate for body size as well as setting a sufficient rate for the ventilator tidal volumes. Monitoring of ventilation should include end-tidal CO_2 monitoring, which should be correlated with the partial pressure of carbon dioxide ($PaCO_2$) on an ABG. End-tidal carbon dioxide monitoring is also used to confirm proper endotracheal tube placement.

The recent implementation of newer techniques in cardiac anesthesia, which allows for faster recovery times, has led to shorter times on mechanical ventilation. Weaning from mechanical ventilation is a quick process in patients who have undergone CABG surgery. Once the patient has displayed the ability to follow commands and the strength to protect the airway, a short CPAP trial is instituted. The patient can be extubated if (1) cardiac performance is good (cardiac index > 2.2 L/minute/m²), (2) adequate oxygenation and ventilation are achieved without acidosis, and (3) chest tube bleeding is minimal. Aggressive use of incentive spirometry and physical mobility ensures proper pulmonary function. Continual assessment by the critical care nurse is very important. Auscultation of breath sounds should be performed at frequent intervals and as the patient's condition dictates. Diminished breath sounds, especially in the left lower lobe, are common because left lower lobe atelectasis is an expected postoperative outcome. Observation of the work of breathing is also important, and signs such as tachypnea, use of accessory muscles, and prolonged expiratory time can indicate compromised pulmonary function. Bronchodilator therapy may be indicated and should be continued if the patient was using bronchodilators at home.

Prolonged mechanical ventilation may be a complication of cardiac surgery. Protracted poor cardiac function requires continued mechanical ventilation. Phrenic nerve damage due to cold preservation techniques for myocardial protection or physical transection is another cause of ventilatory failure due to diaphragm dysfunction. Acute respiratory distress syndrome associated with SIRS, a hypoperfusion state, or both, can also be a reason for prolonged ventilator days. A tracheostomy should be considered in patients with compromised pulmonary function because it can enhance the ventilator weaning process and promote patient comfort. Expert nursing and multidisciplinary care of the patient in ventilatory failure using weaning protocols may make a difference in patient outcome.[22,23]

Preventing Neurological Complications

Neurological recovery of the cardiac surgery patient depends on several factors, such as preoperative neurological state; age (>70 years); presence of conditions such as aortic atherosclerosis, hypertension, and diabetes mellitus; and use of the IABP.[1] The usual course of neurological recovery is much faster since anesthetic agents have changed. Narcotics and benzodiazepines, with neuromuscular blockade, are used now, and gases are used less.[15] There is little need for sedation when the patient is transported from the operating room unless hemodynamic instability is present. The patient is allowed to wake up and recover from the anesthesia as soon as possible. There may be some barriers to this process, including age and renal failure. The elderly patient is not able to metabolize narcotics and paralytics as quickly as a younger patient and may require a longer recovery time. If the patient is difficult to arouse and has pinpoint pupils, reversal of narcotics with naloxone (Narcan) may be indicated. Naloxone diluted 0.4 mg in 10 mL normal saline and given 1 to 2 mL IV every 5 minutes is a delicate method of regaining level of consciousness that does not reverse pain control. If the patient does not have good muscle strength, reversal of neuromuscular blockade is indicated. Glycopyrrolate, 0.6 mg IV, and neostigmine, 3 mg IV (or more), are used. The patient in renal failure is not able to clear these drugs and probably needs reversal of both narcotics and neuromuscular blockade agents to expedite extubation.

Once the patient is awake, continual evaluation using the standard neurological examination that assesses the level of consciousness and motor and sensory ability is mandatory. Postoperative neurological deficits are divided into two categories: (1) major focal deficits (stroke), stupor, or coma; and (2) deterioration in intellectual function.[1] The best predictor of stroke is proximal aortic atherosclerosis, which is the source of emboli that are released with the manipulation of the aorta, especially during cannulation or cross-clamping. Hypoxia, hypoperfusion, hemorrhage, or metabolic abnormalities may also cause strokes.[1] Cognitive changes are more difficult to detect because there may be deficits in memory, language, and psychomotor function. The family of the patient may be helpful in detecting any subtle changes. These changes are most noticeable immediately after surgery but may still be present 12 to 36 months after the procedure.[24] Confirmation of a stroke can be performed with computed tomography or magnetic resonance imaging of the head, but these studies may need to be repeated; embolic events do not immediately appear on scans. Prevention of such a catastrophic event is difficult, but the risk can be reduced by patient selection and procedure selection.[24] If a patient has known carotid disease, maintaining higher blood pressure may help increase perfusion of the cerebral tissues. Thrombolytic therapy, which is used successfully in other patients with emboli, cannot be used after surgery in the patient who has just had CABG surgery because of bleeding concerns.

Monitoring Postoperative Bleeding

Postoperative bleeding is expected; the challenge is to know when and how to intervene. Anticoagulation interventions that have improved outcomes for the cardiac patient in general confound bleeding problems in the patient who has had CABG surgery. Timely correction of bleeding problems can decrease both the occurrence of complications and the cost of patient care. Preoperative anticoagulation such as thrombolytics and antiplatelet therapy (aspirin and clopidogrel) hamper coagulation, and their effects are difficult to reverse; reversal may not even be an option, and postoperative bleeding may increase. It is recommended that that if the patient is receiving clopidogrel, it should be stopped 5 days before surgery.[1]

Drainage and decompression of the pericardial and pleural spaces are required after cardiac surgery. Traditionally, chest tubes were large, rigid tubes, which were very uncomfortable for patients. Recently, smaller, more flexible chest tubes with bulb suction have been introduced to decrease discomfort, increase early ambulation, and decrease the accumulation of pleural effusions. Large postoperative pleural effusions may require increased hospital days or rehospitalization. These tubes are longer and more flexible to enhance pleural drainage; they have been found to decrease clinically significant pleural effusions at 6-week follow-up.[14]

Vigilant monitoring of chest tube drainage is imperative to anticipate impending problems. Chest tube drainage is monitored hourly. The usual chest tube output can range from 100 to 200 mL/hour, with periods of increased drainage due to a change in position or temperature. Measurement of drainage may be required at more frequent intervals (every 15 or 30 minutes) if drainage is high.

If the chest tube output continues to be greater than 200 mL/hour, then intervention is necessary. Protamine, the first level of intervention, is given at 1 mg for every 100 units of heparin to reverse the effects of heparin, which is used in the surgical process (both on and off bypass).[25] PTT is commonly used to monitor the intrinsic pathway of the coagulation cascade, which heparin affects. Additional protamine may be necessary, especially if the patient is hypothermic, because a "rebound" phenomenon may occur. Aggressive rewarming is very important in a patient who has increased bleeding because the coagulation cascade, with its enzymatic reactions, cannot function properly at hypothermic temperatures. However, as the patient's temperature rises, heparin is reactivated, causing increased bleeding. Platelet infusion (usually 6 units per infusion) is used next to help decrease bleeding. It is important to remember that a platelet infusion can cause a blood product reaction because each infusion may be from multiple donors. Before surgery, patients require therapy to make platelets dysfunctional, thus preventing thrombus formation in the coronary arteries. Causes of platelet dysfunction and postoperative bleeding include medications such as aspirin; the bypass machine itself; the IABP, which mechanically destroys platelets; and heparin-induced thrombocytopenia, a recent phenomenon in which heparin exposure disables platelet function.

Follow-up coagulation studies act as a guide to the need for further infusions as well as monitoring blood loss, but they are not absolute parameters. If bleeding is increasing, a PT can be ordered to monitor the extrinsic pathway of the coagulation cascade and determine whether other factors need to be replaced. An elevated PT (>15 seconds) may indicate that bleeding is due to a lack of factors such as fibrinogen that can be replaced using fresh frozen plasma, usually 4 to 6 units/infusion. The overall goal is to determine whether bleeding is due to a coagulopathy or surgical bleeding. Chest tube bleeding that exceeds 500 mL/hour is considered surgical bleeding and mandates surgical reexploration.

Other therapeutic interventions may also be used to decrease bleeding. Coagulation factors such as cryoprecipitate (factors I and VIII) and factor VII are indicated in severe bleeding. Various drugs such as aminocaproic acid (Amicar), a potent inhibitor of fibrinolysis; aprotinin, a serine-protease inhibitor that blocks kallikrein at the beginning of the coagulation cascade; and desmopressin acetate (DDAVP), which influences factor VIII and enhances platelet adhesion, can be administered to promote coagulation.[25] Autotransfusion of mediastinal chest tube drainage using special drainage systems has been used to decrease blood transfusion requirements. However, the possibility that reinfusion can stimulate fibrinolysis and exacerbate bleeding is a concern, and therefore this treatment method is not recommended for routine use (especially in low-risk patients).[1]

Intraoperative measures to prevent bleeding include minimizing hemodilution, minimizing autologous losses, and optimizing coagulation status with full rewarming and antifibrinolytics.[26] Blood loss requires replacement, which should be considered carefully. Transfusion of red blood cells not only can increase exposure to infectious diseases, especially hepatitis and human immunodeficiency virus (HIV), but also is associated with increased immunosuppressive and microcirculatory complications.[27] The hemoglobin level indicated for transfusion is a controversial issue. Recent research has indicated that a restrictive transfusion strategy (hemoglobin <7 g/dL) has demonstrated a lower mortality rate in patients who are less critically ill. Autotransfusion of chest drainage also has been used, but there are no clear data that support improved outcomes with this intervention.

Cardiac tamponade is a serious complication of increased postoperative bleeding that occurs when excessive fluid or blood accumulates in the pericardial space, resulting in increasing pressure on the right atrium and ventricle that can lead to collapse of those structures. Tamponade may develop rapidly or slowly, depending on how fast blood accumulates in the pericardial sac. When a patient is treated for excessive bleeding, it is important to monitor the chest tube drainage closely and maintain patency. Decreasing cardiac output and blood pressure and significant increases in pharmacological support

(especially norepinephrine [Levophed]) are important warning signs. The mechanism of cardiac tamponade is the collapse of the lower pressure chambers of the right heart as a result of the increasing and equalizing of the CVP, pulmonary artery diastolic pressure, and the PAWP. This increase and equalization of the three values is classic evidence of cardiac tamponade. However, the clinical situation can be a late finding, and decreasing cardiac performance and blood pressure, despite volume resuscitation, is an earlier indicator. An arterial line waveform with significant respiratory variation (best illustration of an increased pulsus paradoxus) is another warning sign that cardiac tamponade is pending.[28] Definitive diagnosis is made with an echocardiogram (two-dimensional or transesophageal).

Interventions to prevent tamponade include stripping and milking chest tubes when the blood begins to clot, although stripping the tubes can generate increased negative pressure. Because the chambers (atria and ventricles) are being compressed, cardiac pressures, especially CVP, may be elevated. Another useful intervention involves the infusion of volume even with increased pressure to keep the structures from collapsing. Performing a pericardial window is the best surgical intervention.

Preventing Renal Complications

The postoperative course of renal function is influenced by preoperative function. Preoperative risk factors are age; history of moderate to severe congestive heart failure; prior CABG surgery; and preexisting conditions, including type 1 diabetes mellitus and renal disease (serum creatinine 1.4 to 2.0 mg/dL).[1] The usual postoperative course also depends on whether the surgery was performed on or off bypass. After on-bypass CABG surgery, brisk initial urine output is expected because of the priming of the bypass circuit with mannitol and the possible use of diuretics. The output diminishes as these effects decrease with time. After OPCABG surgery, there is a smaller urine volume because patients are not exposed to these interventions. Some patients are able to autodiurese excess volume, but as the inflammatory response diminishes within 24 to 48 hours, the leaky capillary membranes seal and extra interstitial fluid shifts into the intravascular space, increasing the need for pharmacological diuresis with agents such as furosemide. Electrolyte repletion with potassium and magnesium after diuresis is also important to maintaining a regular cardiac rhythm. A slight metabolic acidosis may be present in the patient with existing renal failure and may persist after surgery. If acidosis is present, the source (respiratory, metabolic, or combined) should be determined to intervene appropriately. The focus of interventions is to remove excess fluid while protecting metabolic and cardiac function.

Oliguria
Decreasing urine output (<0.5 mL/kg/hour) is usually caused by decreased renal perfusion. Obvious causes such as Foley catheter obstruction or malposition

may often be overlooked and should be considered initially, so that mechanical problems may be ruled out. Decreased cardiac function may also cause a decrease in urine output. Hypovolemia is a very common problem that can be addressed with fluid boluses, and monitoring pulmonary artery pressures and the cardiac output/cardiac index shortly after fluid infusions indicates whether the intervention was therapeutic. Caution must be exercised when adding volume because excess fluid can cause decreased function in compromised myocardial muscle. In that situation, inotropic agents or vasoactive drugs may be required. Determining the patient's baseline blood pressure is important so that control of vasoactive drugs can be titrated according to a perfusion pressure (MAP or systolic blood pressure) that the patient's kidneys require.

If none of these interventions is successful, diuresis may be necessary. Loop diuretics (e.g., furosemide) are the usual first-line drugs. If urine output does not increase, larger doses may be indicated, or other diuretics that act on other areas of the renal tubular system, such as thiazides, may be added. Creatinine and BUN are closely monitored.

Renal Failure

If acute renal failure develops, dialysis is necessary. The method used depends on patient condition and practitioner preference. Continuous venovenous hemofiltration (CVVH) and hemodialysis are among the several methods that may be used. CVVH is preferred in the patient who is severely hemodynamically compromised because it is more gradual and minimizes preload compromise, which could decrease cardiac performance. Patients who undergo dialysis require fluid restriction, nutrition modification for prolonged renal dysfunction, and other standard interventions, such as dietary modifications to decrease protein and potassium intake. Chapter 31 provides a further discussion of renal failure. Unfortunately, the mortality rate due to acute renal failure in postoperative cardiac surgery patients is greater than 60%.[1]

Preventing Endocrine Complications

Diabetes mellitus is one of the major risk factors for the development of cardiovascular disease. This disease affects almost all systems in the body and requires that the vigilant clinician continually monitor blood sugar and maintain strict glucose control. In the initial postoperative period, a blood glucose level less than 200 mg/dL is particularly important in managing wound healing. Aggressive intervention using an insulin drip initially has reduced the incidence of deep sternal wound infections by 50%.[1] Once good glucose control has been achieved, insulin is given subcutaneously, and glucose levels are followed closely. Such insulin therapy also decreases the incidence of diabetic ketoacidosis or hyperosmolar coma. It is important to remember that whereas hyperglycemia is detrimental, severe hypoglycemia can be fatal. The need for vigilant blood glucose monitoring cannot be overemphasized.

Adrenal insufficiency may occur, especially in patients who were receiving steroids at regular intervals before surgery. The administration of steroids can suppress adrenal function. To prevent suppression, postoperative stress doses of hydrocortisone (100 mg every 8 hours) should be given, and the patient's regular dose should be restarted. If the patient is taking vasoactive drugs and is not weaning off the drips, adrenal insufficiency is considered; this condition may be the result of hypoperfusion of the adrenal gland. Cortisol levels are low and confirm adrenal insufficiency.

Thyroid dysfunction, especially hypothyroidism, is common in elderly persons and women. Although perioperative effects do not result in dysfunction, preoperative function is an important consideration, and undiagnosed dysfunction may become apparent in the postoperative period because the thyroid hormones, especially triiodothyronine (T_3), can have cardiovascular effects.

Preventing Gastrointestinal Complications

Fortunately, the gastrointestinal aspects of the postoperative course are uneventful and similar to those of general surgery. After extubation, the patient remains NPO for up to the first 8 hours, with a nasogastric tube in place to decompress the stomach. The patient is then allowed to have small amounts of ice or water. This relatively simple aspect of nursing care is very important for the postoperative patient, who may experience significant thirst because of the anticholinergic drugs that were given before surgery. The use of ice pops and ginger ale can help with compliance and decrease the possibility of nausea, vomiting, and aspiration.

Complications such as cholecystitis, pancreatitis, and bowel infarction rarely occur. Their pathogenesis is not always clear but is attributed to splanchnic hypoperfusion and general gastrointestinal ischemia. Thorough assessment of the abdomen looking for pain, distention, or tympany may help discover subtle abnormalities. Lactate levels greater than 2.5 mmol/L may indicate splanchnic hypoperfusion. However, they may also be the result of nonpulsatile flow of the bypass machine, which may cause a release of angiotensin II, exacerbating splanchnic ischemia.[15] The need for further evaluation is dictated by the clinical presentation.

Monitoring for Infection

In the early postoperative period, hypothalamic resetting is the cause of temperature derangement. Febrile reactions are usually attributed to SIRS and to overshoot from rewarming. If the fever (temperature >100.4°F [38°C]) persists for more than 48 to 72 hours, infection should be considered. Prevention of infection is the major goal of all programs. This goal is achieved through the prudent use of antibiotics, vancomycin, and a cephalosporin (e.g., cefazolin, ceftazidime). Timing of antibiotic administration is pivotal. For optimal results, preoperative doses should be completely infused before the skin is cut. Antibiotic dosing depends on preoperative renal function. A short postoperative course should also be anticipated.

Mediastinitis is the major infection in patients who have undergone CABG surgery and may be a devastating complication that increases the length of hospital stay and mortality. Risk factors associated with mediastinitis are obesity; prior cardiac surgery; preexisting type 1 diabetes mellitus; and perioperative factors such as excessive electrocautery use and use of both internal mammary arteries, resulting in compromised blood flow to the chest wall. Therapy is an extended antibiotic course and plastic surgery. The aggressive regulation of blood sugar using insulin drips initially instead of subcutaneous administration has been shown to decrease the occurrence of mediastinitis.[1] This intervention is also used in cases that do not involve CABG; a decrease in mortality has been demonstrated.[29] It is very important to instruct the patient not to use the arms excessively when moving and to use a "cough pillow" with coughing (a small pillow that is placed on the sternal incision and squeezed when coughing). Other interventions, such as having the patient sleep on his or her back, are also important. Following these instructions may help maintain the stability of the sternum.

Patient Teaching and Discharge Planning

With managed care, capitation, rising costs, and limited resources, the usual length of hospitalization after cardiac surgery is 4 to 7 days. Discharge planning that begins at admission is imperative because of the short length of hospital stays. Box 22-8 summarizes patient teaching about cardiac postoperative care, and Box 22-9 contains a discharge planning guide for the post–cardiac surgery patient.

Box 22-8 • TEACHING GUIDE: Recovering From Cardiac Surgery

General Instructions
- Avoid lifting heavy objects (10–15 lb or more) for first 3 mo.
- Avoid strenuous arm movement such as golf or tennis. When getting in and out of chair or bed, use legs. Arms should not bear weight and should be used only for balance.
- Do not drive for 6 wk after surgery. (May ride in automobile.)
- Follow physician's instructions for activity progression.
- Resume sexual activity when you can climb two flights of stairs without stopping (with physician's recommendations).
- Use alternative positions for 3 to 4 mo to decrease stress on sternum; avoid side-lying and prone positions.
- Inspect and cleanse surgical incisions daily with soap and water.
- Understand medications, including reason for taking, dosage, frequency, and side effects.
- Follow dietary restrictions.
- Understand how much pain to expect and how to manage it.

Risk Factors
- Follow instructions on individual risk factors, their impact on health after cardiac surgery, and how to modify them.
- Seek referrals as appropriate (e.g., for a weight loss program or a smoking cessation program).

Follow-Up With Physician
- Know how and when to schedule follow-up appointments.
- Be alert for signs and symptoms of infection, such as fever, increased redness, tenderness, drainage, or swelling of incisions.
- Report palpitations, tachycardia, or an irregular pulse (if normally regular) to the physician immediately.
- Seek follow-up care if you experience dizziness or increased fatigue, sudden weight gain or peripheral edema, shortness of breath, or chest pain.

• Carotid Endarterectomy

Stenosis or occlusion of the carotid arteries is usually due to atherosclerotic disease and may cause stroke, a leading cause of morbidity and mortality in the United States. Carotid endarterectomy is the most common noncardiac vascular procedure performed to restore flow to the carotid arteries and is designed to decrease the risk for stroke and stroke-related death.[30]

The right carotid artery is a branch of the innominate artery that arises from the right side of the aortic arch. The left common carotid artery arises directly from the aortic arch. At the level of the thyroid, the common carotids bifurcate into the external and internal carotids. Located near this bifurcation, in the carotid sinus, are the carotid chemoreceptors, which are sensitive to blood carbon dioxide and oxygen levels, and the baroreceptors, which help regulate blood pressure. The external carotid arteries supply blood to the structures in the head and neck, excluding the eyes

and brain. The internal carotid arteries give rise to the ophthalmic arteries and the posterior communicating, anterior cerebral, and middle cerebral arteries, which help supply blood to the brain (Fig. 22-8).

Patients with carotid artery occlusive disease may have sudden dysphagia, unilateral motor weakness, expressive aphasia, dizziness, memory deficits, or monocular blindness.[31] They often exhibit signs of vascular disease in other parts of the body, such as the heart (CAD) or the legs (peripheral arterial disease). Risk factors for carotid artery occlusive disease are associated with stroke and should guide patient care. Hypertension is the most important risk factor for stroke, and blood pressure regulation is essential in the postoperative period. Issues such as cigarette smoking, hyperlipidemia, alcohol consumption, and postmenopausal use of estrogen may also affect patient care.[30]

Patients with risk factors for carotid artery occlusive disease must be examined carefully. A carotid bruit can usually be auscultated over the artery due to turbulent flow through the narrowed artery. Carotid Doppler ultrasonography is usually performed to estimate the presence and amount of stenosis, but angiography is the most reliable method to determine the exact amount of stenosis. Magnetic resonance angiography, which is less invasive, may also be used.

INDICATIONS FOR CAROTID ENDARTERECTOMY

Carotid artery occlusive disease is part of the systemic atherosclerotic process, which is reviewed in Chapter 21. Carotid endarterectomy is indicated for recently symptomatic patients with 70% to 99% carotid artery stenosis.[31] This surgery should not be considered for symptomatic patients with less than 50% stenosis; these patients have better outcomes if treated medically.[31] To be considered for carotid endarterectomy, patients should be between 40 and 75 years of age, with a 5-year life expectancy.[31]

SURGICAL PROCEDURE

A skin incision is made along the lower anterior border of the sternocleidomastoid muscle just below the angle of the jaw, and the common, internal, and external carotid arteries are isolated. The carotid arteries on the operative side must be clamped. Clamping puts the ipsilateral cerebral hemisphere and eye at risk for ischemia and infarct because the only perfusion to these areas occurs through the circle of Willis and collaterals, which may be inadequate. To prevent thromboembolus formation while the arteries are clamped, a heparin bolus may be given before clamping. Adequacy of circulation is determined by continuous electroencephalographic monitoring in the operating room. If circulation is determined to be inadequate, a temporary bypass or shunt may be placed from the common carotid artery to the distal portion of the internal carotid to provide continued intraoperative perfusion. Patients treated with shunts often include those with contralateral carotid stenosis, neurological deficits, history of cerebrovascular accidents, and stroke in evolution.

Endarterectomy or removal of the ulcerated or stenotic atheromatous plaque is then performed, and the artery is closed. If primary closure will cause a narrowing, a patch may be used.

POSTOPERATIVE CARE

After extubation in the recovery room, patients are transferred to the ICU with ECG monitoring, an arterial line, CVP monitoring, and oxygen. Traditionally, patients stay in the ICU for 24 hours. However, cost concerns have led to monitoring patients in an intermediate care unit and reducing the hospital stay to 1 day.[32]

Controlling Blood Pressure

Blood pressure is commonly labile up to 24 hours after surgery because of surgically induced abnormalities of the carotid baroreceptor sensitivity. This is characterized as baroreflex failure syndrome and is usually associated with bilateral surgical procedures.[30] Preoperative hypertension is thought to be the most important determinant of postoperative hypertension, which means that the critical care nurse must be aware of the patient's preoperative blood pressure range. Increased blood pressure may also increase the risk for wound bleeding and possible hematoma formation. The goal of blood pressure regulation is a systolic blood pressure between 120 and 170 mm Hg. A systolic blood pressure greater than 170 mm Hg should be treated with nitroprusside or other IV agents, whereas one less than 120 mm Hg should be treated with IV fluid or with a phenylephrine drip if the patient is unresponsive to volume.

Wound Care

To minimize stress on the operative site, the patient's head and neck are kept in alignment. The dressing and the area behind the patient's neck and shoulders

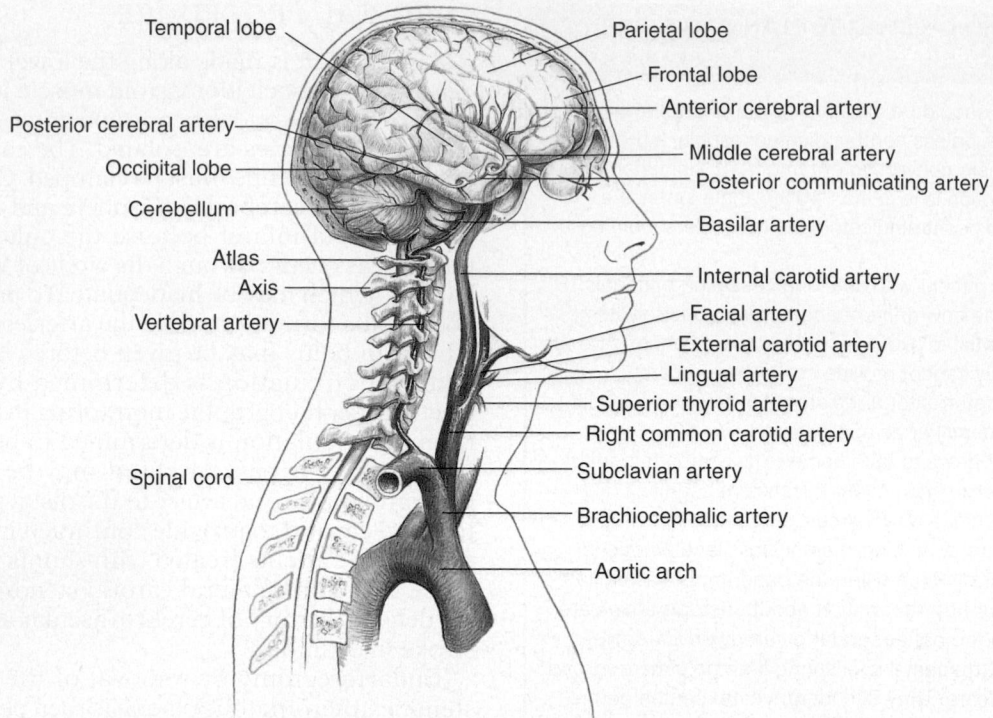

Figure 22-8 • Branches of the right external carotid artery. (From Anatomical Chart Company: Atlas of Pathophysiology. Springhouse, PA, Springhouse, 2001, p 39.)

are assessed for the presence of blood. Persistent oozing from deep tissue, coughing, straining during extubation, and disruption of suture lines may all lead to bleeding into the operative site. The risk for bleeding can be further aggravated by anticoagulation with heparin, aspirin, or antiplatelet therapy. The nurse assesses the neck size, comparing the operative side with the nonoperative side. Swelling could indicate hematoma formation. Any patient complaints of difficulty talking, swallowing, or breathing should be reported to the physician immediately. If a hematoma is suspected because of tracheal compression by a hematoma, surgical evacuation may be indicated. Wound hematomas occur in about 5.5% of patients.[30]

Preventing Neurological Complications

Brain injury, local nerve injury, or both may occur. Perioperative stroke occurs in approximately 3% of patients and may be due to embolization of atheromatous debris, air from the operative site, or low flow during carotid artery clamping.[31] Neurological assessment includes monitoring level of consciousness, pupil reactivity, eye movement, orientation, appropriateness of response, and motor function (flexion, extension, and hand grips) for the first 24 hours. Abnormalities should be reported to the physician immediately.

Hyperperfusion syndrome occurs in patients with high-grade stenosis. Theoretically, the hemisphere distal to the stenotic area has suffered hypoperfusion that causes the small blood vessels to remain maximally dilated with a loss of autoregulation. Once the stenosis is repaired, autoregulation is still par-

alyzed, but a marked increase in blood flow occurs that cannot be controlled with vasoconstriction to protect the capillaries. Edema or hemorrhage to the area results.[31] Strict blood pressure control is imperative.

Several cranial nerves (CN) traverse the surgical area and can be exposed to trauma. The most commonly affected are CN VII (the facial nerve), CN X (the vagus nerve), CN XII (the hypoglossal nerve), and CN XI (the spinal accessory nerve). Specific functional assessment for each nerve should be performed after surgery, including those listed in Table 22-3. If a deficit is present, the nurse should notify the physician and explain to the patient how it occurred and that the deficit is usually temporary.

HOME CARE CONSIDERATIONS

Patients are usually discharged on the first or second postoperative day. Aspirin (81 or 325 mg/day) should be prescribed postoperatively for at least 3 months to reduce the possibility of stroke, myocardial infarction, or death.[31] The critical care nurse plays an essential role in the care of the patient who has had a carotid endarterectomy. Although considered a vascular surgical procedure, postoperative complications usually manifest as neurological symptoms, and the nurse must assess the patient for subtle neurological changes. Patient education is also a key component of care. Patients and their families should understand that the patient has an underlying cardiovascular disease and that risk factor modification is necessary. Education should include the items listed in Box 22-10.

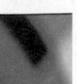

Table 22-3 • Postoperative Functional Assessment of Cranial Nerves Following Carotid Endarterectomy

Nerve	Nerve Intervention	Functional Assessment	Functional Damage
Facial nerve (VII)	Motor function of facial muscles	Ability to smile and frown	Asymmetrical contraction of the mouth
Vagus nerve (X)	Motor and sensory function of larynx and throat	Quality and tone of voice and ability to swallow	Difficult swallowing, hoarseness, speech problems, loss of gag reflex
Hypoglossal nerve (XII)	Muscles to tongue	Movement of tongue	Difficult swallowing, speech problems, deviation of tongue, sometimes airway damage
Spinal accessory nerve (XI)	Trapezius and sternocleidomastoid muscles	Ability to shrug shoulders and raise arm to horizontal position	Shoulder may sag, difficulty raising shoulder against resistance, difficulty raising arm to horizontal position

Box 22-10 • TEACHING GUIDE:
Recovering From Carotid Endarterectomy

Risk Factor Reduction
• Stop smoking.
• Eat a low-fat diet.
• Control hypertension if present.

Activity
• There are usually no restrictions on activity. It is all right to move your neck in a normal manner.

Incision Care
• Bruising and discoloration are common.
• Wash the incision site with soap and water.

General
• Be familiar with signs and symptoms of incisional infection.
• Notify your physician of visual defects, changes in memory or sensation, or an inability to swallow or speak.
• Be knowledgeable about medication indications, including reason for taking, dosage, frequency, and side effects.
• Keep physician appointments.

• Clinical Applicability Challenges

Case Study

Mr. M., a 63-year-old man who has had coronary artery bypass graft surgery with three grafts and moderate left ventricular dysfunction preoperatively (ejection fraction ~ 35%), has arrived in the intensive care unit from the operating room after 8 hours in surgery. He is receiving dobutamine at 5 µg/kg/minute to improve cardiac performance. An internal mammary artery graft to the left anterior descending coronary artery and saphenous vein graft to the right coronary artery and diagonal artery were performed using bypass. Past medical history is significant for diabetes mellitus that is not well controlled because of patient noncompliance. He was treated for tuberculosis 20 years ago, and he also has renal insufficiency. To maintain a cardiac index greater than 2.2 L/minute/m², he continues to require dobutamine and cannot wean off the medication. On postoperative day 2, he is still intubated, on dobutamine at 7 µg/kg/minute, with a cardiac index of 2.0 L/minute/m² and a pulmonary artery occlusion pressure of 22 mm Hg. His urine output is marginal at 25 mL/hour (preoperative weight is 80 kg).

1. What do you think was occurring in this patient situation?
2. What would be your immediate intervention?
3. What interventions would be the most important to make the physician aware of?

Review Questions

1. One advantage of the saphenous vein graft compared with the internal mammary artery graft is that
   a. the saphenous vein graft remains patent longer.
   b. the saphenous vein graft is easier to perform.
   c. fibrointimal hyperplasia does not occur with the saphenous vein graft.
   d. postoperative pain is less with the internal mammary artery graft.

2. Off-pump coronary artery bypass graft (CABG) surgery was reinstituted in the 1990s because on-pump CABG surgery became associated with an increase in what type of complications?
   a. Vascular
   b. Renal
   c. Gastrointestinal
   d. Neurologic

3. With mitral insufficiency, the pathophysiology includes thickening or stretching of the valve leaflets, which leads to
   a. myocardial ischemia.
   b. stroke.
   c. left ventricular hypertrophy.
   d. increased forward cardiac output.

4. A patient who has a long life expectancy and needs a valve replacement should receive
   a. a mechanical valve.
   b. a tissue valve.
   c. either a mechanical or tissue valve.
   d. a porcine valve.

5. During bypass, the patient's core body temperature is lowered to decrease oxygen consumption. This intervention can increase postoperative coagulopathy due to
   a. optimizing the chemical environment for the coagulation cascade.
   b. increased production of coagulation factors.
   c. alteration in platelet function.
   d. minimal endothelial damage and activation.

6. Pain control in the postoperative period is important in order to improve outcomes. Which one of the following is NOT a result of good pain control?
   a. increased mobility.
   b. improved pulmonary parameters.
   c. improved gastric motility.
   d. decreased level of consciousness.

7. One of the major nursing interventions in this patient population is volume resuscitation. Which step is most helpful in volume resuscitation?
   a. Infusing volume through a large-bore access
   b. Using "999" rate on the IV pump
   c. Always using a central line
   d. Infusing the volume through a peripheral line

8. Cardiac tamponade is a complication of cardiac surgery that needs to be recognized early. Which of the following is a less sensitive finding when trying to recognize tamponade?
   a. Equalization of the pulmonary artery pressures
   b. Elevated central venous/right atrial pressure
   c. Decreased cardiac output
   d. Drop in blood pressure

9. After a carotid endarterectomy, you assess that the patient has the tongue deviating to one side. The most likely cause is
   a. surgical damage to the hypoglossal nerve (cranial nerve [CN] XII).
   b. stroke affecting the right side of the brain.
   c. stroke affecting the left side of the brain.
   d. surgical damage to the vagus nerve (CN X).

10. Improving glycemic control in the coronary artery bypass graft patient population can
   a. improve gastric motility.
   b. decrease wound infections.
   c. improve mobility.
   d. decrease cardiac performance.

References

1. Eagle K, Guyton R, Davidoff R, et al: ACC/AHA 2004 guideline update for coronary bypass graft surgery. J Am Coll Cardiol 110:e340–431, 2004
2. Felisky C, Paull D, Hill M, et al: Endoscopic greater saphenous vein harvesting reduces the morbidity of coronary artery bypass surgery. Am J Surg 183:576–579, 2002
3. Nwasokwa O: Coronary artery bypass graft disease. Ann Intern Med 123:528–545, 1995
4. Acar C, Ramshey A, Pagny JY: The radial artery for coronary artery bypass grafting: Clinical and angiographic results at five years. J Thorac Cardiovasc Surg 116:981–989, 1998
5. Shapira O, Xu A, Vita J, et al: Nitroglycerin is superior to diltiazem as a coronary bypass conduit vasodilator. J Thorac Cardiovasc Surg 117:906–911, 1999
6. Emery RW, Arom KV, Holter AR, et al: Advances in coronary artery surgery. In Franco KL, Verrier E (eds): Advanced Therapy in Cardiac Surgery, 2nd ed. Hamilton, Ontario: BC Decker, 2003, pp 124–130
7. Vallely M, Bannon P, Kritharides L: The systemic inflammatory response syndrome and off-pump cardiac surgery. Heart Surg Forum 4(Suppl):S7–S13, 2001
8. Magee M, Jablouski K, Stamou S, et al: Elimination of cardiopulmonary bypass improves early survival for multivessel coronary artery bypass patients. Ann Thorac Surg 73:1196–1202, 2002
9. Peel GK, Stamou SC, Dullum MK, et al: Chronological distribution of stroke after minimally invasive versus conventional coronary artery bypass. J Am Coll Cardiol 43(5):752–756, 2004
10. Horvath KA: Transmyocardial laser revascularization. In Franco KL, Verrier E (eds): Advanced Therapy in Cardiac Surgery, 2nd ed. Hamilton, Ontario: BC Decker, 2003, pp 131–137
11. Lynn-McHale D, Hambach C, Carter T, et al: Transmyocardial laser revascularization. J Cardiovasc Nurs 12:17–28, 1998
12. Lytle BW: Coronary artery reoperations. In Cohn LH, Edmunds LH (eds): Cardiac Surgery in the Adult, 2nd ed. New York: McGraw-Hill Medical Publishing Division, 2003, pp 659–679
13. Kaiser L, Kron I, Spray T: Mastery of Cardiothoracic Surgery. Philadelphia: Lippincott-Raven, 1998
14. Lancey R, Gaca C, Vander Salm T: The use of smaller, more flexible chest drains following open heart surgery. Chest 119:19–24, 2001
15. Corso P, Hockstein M: New techniques in management of the cardiac surgery patient. In Shoemaker W, Ayres S, Grenvik A, et al (eds): Textbook of Critical Care. Philadelphia, WB Saunders, 2002, pp 1130–1155
16. Sladen R, Berend J, Fassero J, et al: Comparison of vecuronium and meperidine on the clinical and metabolic effects of shivering after hypothermic cardiopulmonary bypass. J Cardiothorac Vasc Anesth 9:147–153, 1995
17. Muckart D, Bhagwanjee S: American College of Chest Physicians/Society of Critical Care Medicine Consensus Conference: Definitions of the systemic inflammatory response syndrome and allied disorders in relation to critically injured patients. Crit Care Med 25:1789–1795, 1997
18. Harvey M: Systemic inflammatory response syndrome and multiorgan dysfunction syndrome. In Kinney M, Dunbar S, Brooks-Braun J, et al (eds): AACN Clinical Reference for Critical Care Nursing. St. Louis: Mosby, 1998
19. Sirieix D, Hongnat M, Delayaance M, et al: Comparison of the acute hemodynamic effects of hypertonic or colloid infusions immediately after mitral valve repair. Crit Care Med 27:2159–2165, 1999
20. Le Conte P, Coutaut V, N'Guyeu J, et al: Prognostic factors in acute cardiogenic pulmonary edema. Am J Emerg Med 17:329–332, 1999
21. Brown T: Hibernating myocardium. Am J Crit Care 10:84–90, 2001
22. Ely E, Meade M, Haponik E, et al: Mechanical ventilator weaning protocols driven by non-physician health-care professionals: Evidence-based clinical practice guidelines. Chest 120(6 Suppl):454S–463S, 2001
23. Burns S, Dempsey E: Long-term ventilator management strategies: Experiences in two hospitals. AACN Clin Issues 11:424–441, 2000
24. Jarcia JP, Venkataramana V, Gold JP: Prevention of neurologic injury during cardiac and great vessel surgery. In Franco KL, Verrier E (eds): Advanced Therapy in Cardiac Surgery, 2nd ed. Hamilton, Ontario: BC Decker, 2003, pp 74–82
25. Limbird L, Hardin J (eds): Goodman & Gilman's the Pharmacological Basis of Therapeutics. New York: McGraw-Hill, 2001

26. Rosengart TK: Blood conservation for open heart surgery. In Franco KL, Verrier E (eds): Advanced Therapy in Cardiac Surgery, 2nd ed. Hamilton, Ontario: BC Decker, 2003, pp 37–45

27. Hebert P, Wells G, Blajchman M, et al, and the Transfusion Requirements in Critical Care Investigators for the Canadian Critical Care Trials Group: A multicenter, randomized, controlled clinical trial of transfusion requirements in critical care. N Engl J Med 340:409–417, 1999

28. Shoemaker WC: Pericardial tamponade. In Shoemaker W, Ayres S, Grenvik A, et al (eds): Textbook of Critical Care. Philadelphia: WB Saunders, 2002, pp 1097–1101

29. Van den Berghe G, Vounters P, Weekers F, et al: Intensive insulin therapy in the critically ill patients. N Engl J Med 345: 1359–1367, 2001

30. Bettmann M, Katzen B, Whisnant J, et al: A statement for healthcare professionals from a special writing group of the Stroke Council, American Heart Association. Circulation 97: 121–123, 1998

31. Chaturvedi S, Bruno A, Feasby, T et al: Carotid endarterectomy: An evidence-based review. Report of the Therapeutics and Technology Assessment Subcommittee of the American Academy of Neurology. Neurology 65:794–801, 2005

32. Brown M, Fitzgerald C, Morse K, et al: Cardiovascular surgery. In Kinney M, Dunbar S, Brooks-Brunn J, et al (eds): AACN Clinical Reference for Critical Care Nursing. St. Louis: Mosby, 1998, pp 383–428

Other Selected Readings

Barnason S, Zimmerman L, Nieveen J, Hertzog M: Impact of a telehealth intervention to augment home health care on functional and recovery outcomes of elderly patients undergoing coronary artery bypass grafting. Heart Lung 35(4):225–233, 2006

Brantman L, Howie J: Use of amiodarone to prevent atrial fibrillation after cardiac surgery. Critical Care Nurse 26(1):48–59, 2006

Doering L, Cross R, Magsarili M, et al: Utility of observer-rated and self-report instruments for detecting major depression in women after cardiac surgery: A pilot study. Am J Crit Care 16(3):260–269, 2007

Dupuis G, Kennedy E, Lindquist R, et al. Coronary artery bypass graft surgery and cognitive performance. Am J Crit Care 15(5): 471–479, 2006

Eastwood G: Evaluating the reliability of recorded fluid balance to approximate body weight change in patients undergoing cardiac surgery. Heart Lung 35(1):34–44, 2006

Elliott D, Lazarus R, Leeder S: Health outcomes of patients undergoing cardiac surgery: Repeated measures using short form–36 and 15 dimensions of quality of life questionnaire. Heart Lung 35(4):245–251, 2006

Gallagher R, McKinley S: Stressors and anxiety in patients undergoing coronary artery bypass surgery. Am J Crit Care 16(3): 248–259, 2007

Godfrey B, Parten C, Buckner E: Identification of special care needs: The comparison of the cardiothoracic intensive care unit patient and nurse. Dimens Crit Care Nurs 25(6):275–282, 2006

Marwitz Kallenbach A, Rosenblum J: Carotid endarterectomy: Creating the 1-day stay. Crit Care Nurse 20:23–36, 2000

McCormick K, Naimarc B, Tate R: Uncertainty, symptom distress, anxiety, and functional status in patients awaiting coronary artery bypass surgery. Heart Lung 35(1):34–45, 2006

Okkonen E, Vanhanen H: Family support, living alone, and subjective health of a patient in connection with a coronary artery bypass surgery. Heart Lung 35(4):234–244, 2006

Rosborough D: Cardiac surgery in elderly patients: Strategies to optimize outcomes. Crit Care Nurse 26(5):24–33, 2006

Scherr K, Urquhart G, Eichorst C, Bulbuc C: Paraplegia after coronary artery bypass graft surgery: Case report of a rare event. Crit Care Nurse 26(5):34–45, 2006

Sendelbach S, Lindquist R, Watanuki S, Savik K: Correlates of neurocognitive function of patients after off-pump coronary artery bypass surgery. Am J Crit Care 15(3):290–298, 2006

Wynne R, Botti M, Copley D, Bailey M: The normative distribution of chest tube drainage volume after coronary artery bypass grafting. Heart Lung 36(1):35–42, 2007

Respiratory System

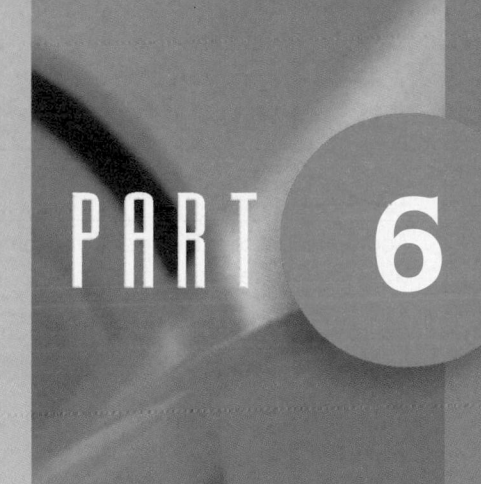

PART 6

INTERNET RESOURCES

Topic	Web Page Address
Acute Respiratory Distress Syndrome Support Group	www.ards.org
Allergy and Asthma Network Mothers of Asthmatics	www.aanma.org
American Association for Respiratory Care (AARC)	www.aarc.org
American College of Chest Physicians	www.chestnet.org
American Lung Association	www.lungusa.org
American Thoracic Society	www.thoracic.org
Auscultation Assistant	www.wilkes.med.ucla.edu/inex.htm
British Thoracic Society	www.brit-thoracic.org.uk
Canadian Thoracic Society	www.lung.ca/cts
Club for Kids with Asthma	www.asthmabusters.org
Educational Website Dedicated to Patient Safety	www.capnography.com
Emphysema Foundation for Our Right to Survive	www.emphysema.net
European Federation of Allergy and Airways Diseases Patients' Association	www.efanet.org
Global Initiative for Chronic Obstructive Lung Disease	www.goldcopd.com
Grafxsman's Pulmonary Monitoring with Graphics	www.hometown.aol.com/grafxsman/index.html
National Heart, Lung, and Blood Institute	www.nhlbi.nih.gov/index.htm
National Institute of Allergy and Infectious Diseases	www.niaid.nih.gov
National Lung Health Education Program	www.nlhep.org
Network ARDS in Children	www.meb.uni-bonn.de/ards
Respiratory Nursing Society	www.respiratorynursingsociety.org
Second Wind Lung Transplant Association, Inc.	www.2ndwind.org
Society of Thoracic Surgeons	www.sts.org
Ventworld Website	www.ventworld.com
Virtual Hospital Website	www.vh.org
World Health Organization	www.who.int

Anatomy and Physiology of the Respiratory System

23

Karen L. Johnson

Anatomy of the Respiratory System
   The Thorax
   The Conducting Airways
   The Respiratory Airways
   The Lung Circulation
   The Pulmonary Lymphatics
Physiology of the Respiratory System
   Ventilation
   Diffusion
   Perfusion
   Relationship of Ventilation to Perfusion
   Gas Transport
   Regulation of Respiration

Objectives

Based on the content in this chapter, the reader should be able to:

❶ Identify the major structures of the respiratory system that are located in the thorax.

❷ Describe the movement of air through the airways from the nose to the alveoli.

❸ Discuss the function of surfactant in maintaining alveolar inflation.

❹ Differentiate the function of bronchial and pulmonary circulations.

❺ Describe the mechanics of ventilation in terms of air movement into and out of the lungs, lung compliance, and airway resistance.

❻ Explain four factors that affect the diffusion of gases across the alveolar–capillary membrane.

❼ Identify physiological and pathophysiological conditions that produce a ventilation–perfusion mismatch.

❽ Discuss conditions that affect the relationship described in the oxyhemoglobin dissociation curve and how these conditions affect oxygen exchange.

❾ Describe the function of the chemoreceptors and lung receptors.

The structures of the respiratory system allow gases to move between the external environment and the internal environment. The cardinal function of the respiratory system is gas exchange, a process by which oxygen moves from the air into the blood and carbon dioxide moves out of the blood and is exhaled to the external environment. The respiratory system also has several other functions, including regulation of acid–base balance, metabolism of some compounds, and filtration of inhaled unwanted materials. Intact respiratory structures and proper functioning of the respiratory system are necessary for transport of gases in and out of the body. Knowledge of respiratory anatomy and physiology helps the nurse understand respiratory assessment techniques, principles of respiratory system management, and common disorders of the respiratory system.

• Anatomy of the Respiratory System

THE THORAX

The thorax contains the major structures of the respiratory system. These structures include the bony thoracic cage, the muscles of ventilation, the lungs, the pleural space, and the mediastinum (Fig. 23-1). The thoracic cage is a rigid, yet flexible, structure. Its bony structure protects the major organs in the thoracic cavity. Flexibility allows for inhalation/inflation and exhalation/deflation of the lungs. The thoracic cage consists of 12 vertebrae, each with a pair of ribs. Posteriorly, each rib is attached to a vertebra (Fig. 23-2). Anteriorly, the first seven ribs are attached to the sternum (Fig. 23-3). The 8th, 9th, and 10th ribs

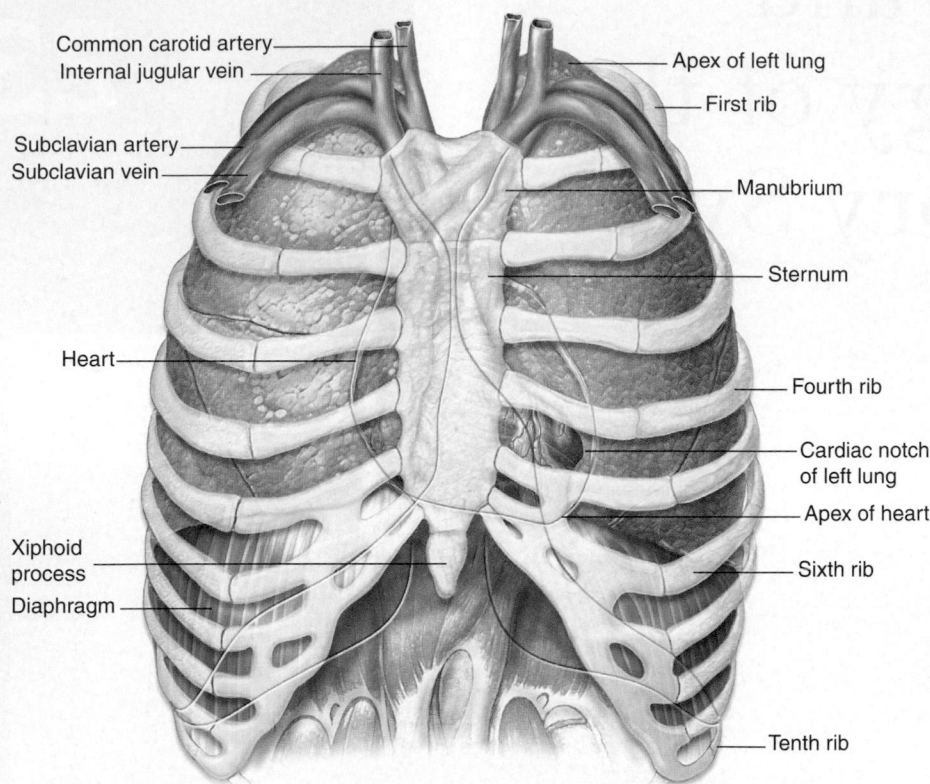

Common carotid artery
Internal jugular vein
Subclavian artery
Subclavian vein
Heart
Xiphoid process
Diaphragm

Apex of left lung
First rib
Manubrium
Sternum
Fourth rib
Cardiac notch of left lung
Apex of heart
Sixth rib
Tenth rib

Figure 23-1 • Thoracic contents. (From Anatomical Chart Company: Atlas of Human Anatomy. Springhouse, Springhouse, PA, 2001, p 149.)

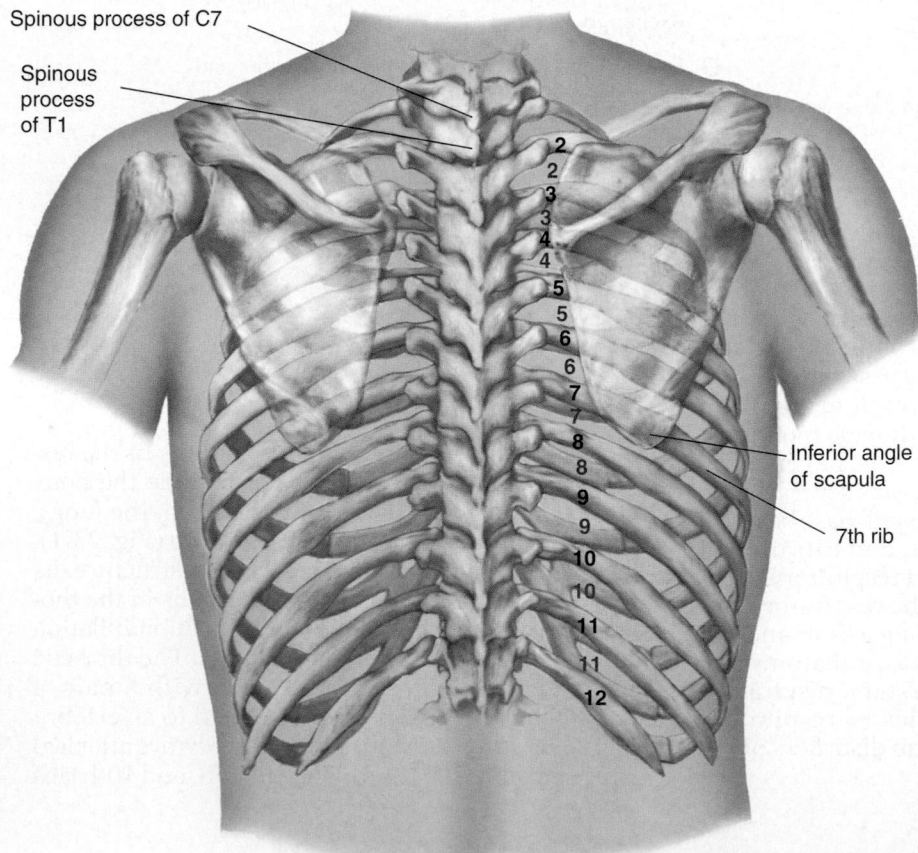

Spinous process of C7
Spinous process of T1

Inferior angle of scapula
7th rib

Figure 23-2 • Posterior thoracic cage. (From Bickley LS: Bates' Guide to Physical Examination and History Taking, 9th ed. Philadelphia, Lippincott Williams & Wilkins, 2006, p 243.)

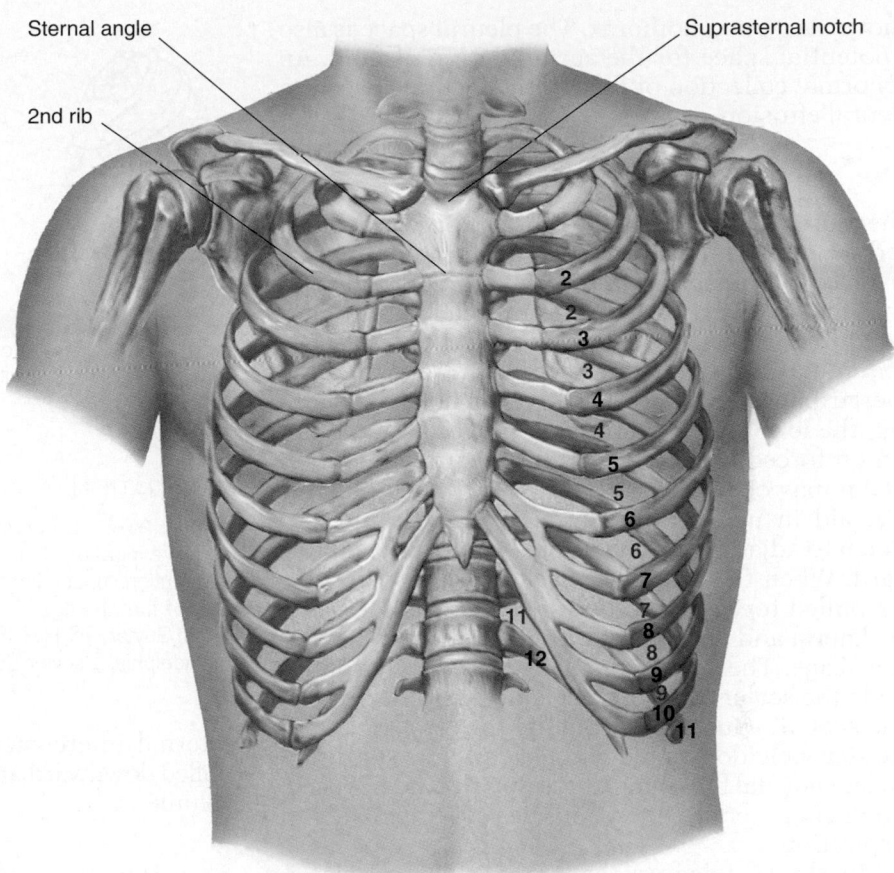

Sternal angle

2nd rib

Suprasternal notch

Figure 23-3 • Anterior thoracic cage. (From Bickley LS: Bates' Guide to Physical Examination and History Taking, 8th ed. Philadelphia, Lippincott Williams & Wilkins, 2003, p 210.)

are attached by cartilage to the ribs above them. The 11th and 12th ribs are called "floating ribs" because they are not attached anteriorly to another structure.

The Lungs, Mediastinum, and Pleural Space

Positioned within, and protected by, the thoracic cage, the lungs are located on either side of the chest. These air-filled, spongy structures are attached to the body only at the pulmonary ligament at the mediastinum. The right lung contains three lobes, and the left lung contains only two lobes because of the space limitation imposed by the heart. The base of each lung rests anteriorly at the level of the sixth rib at the midclavicular line and at the eighth rib at the mid-axillary line. The apices extend 2 to 4 cm above the inner aspects of the clavicles.

The space between the two lungs is the mediastinum. The mediastinum contains the heart, blood vessels, lymph nodes, thymus gland, nerve fibers, and esophagus.

Pleural membranes surround the lungs and line the thoracic wall. The parietal pleura is the membrane lining the chest wall, and the visceral pleura overlays the lung parenchyma (Fig. 23-4). A thin layer of serous fluid in the small space between these two pleurae allows the parietal and visceral pleurae to slide over each other during inspiration and expiration. The pressure within the pleural space is called the intrapleural pressure. The intrapleural pressure

is normally less than the pressures within the lung. It is this negative pressure that keeps the lungs inflated. If the intrapleural space loses its negative pressure (by exposure to atmospheric pressure; for example, as a result of chest trauma), the lung collapses, a condition

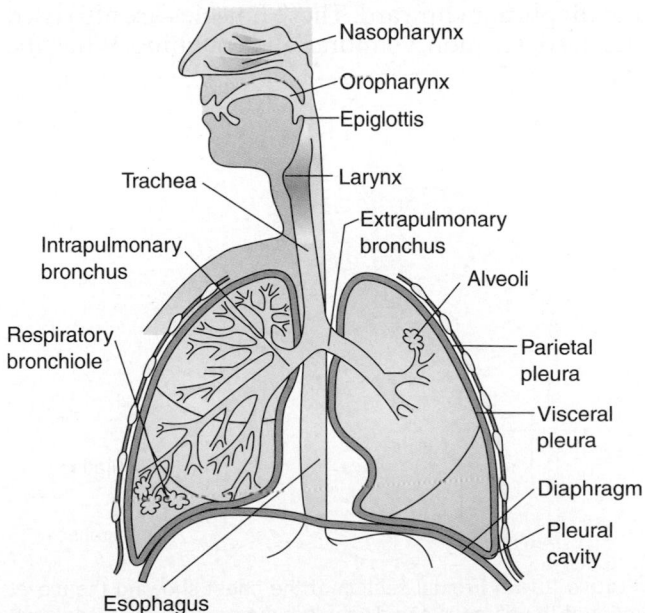

Nasopharynx

Oropharynx

Epiglottis

Trachea

Larynx

Extrapulmonary bronchus

Intrapulmonary bronchus

Alveoli

Respiratory bronchiole

Parietal pleura

Visceral pleura

Diaphragm

Pleural cavity

Esophagus

Figure 23-4 • Structures of the respiratory system. (From Porth CM: Pathophysiology: Concepts of Altered Health States, 7th ed. Philadelphia, Lippincott Williams & Wilkins, 2005, p 634.)

known as a pneumothorax. The pleural space is also a potential space for the accumulation of fluid. An abnormal collection of fluid in the pleural space is a pleural effusion.

The Respiratory Muscles

The muscles that elevate the thoracic cage are classified as *muscles of inspiration*.[1] The major muscle involved with inspiration is the diaphragm. The diaphragm is a thin, dome-shaped muscle that is innervated by the phrenic nerves. When it contracts, the abdominal contents are forced downward, and the chest expands vertically (Fig. 23-5). In normal breathing, the level of the diaphragm moves about 1 cm, but on forced inspiration, a total excursion of up to 10 cm may occur.[2] The external intercostal muscles also aid in inspiration (Fig. 23-6). These muscles attach to adjacent ribs and slope downward and forward. When the external muscles contract, the ribs are pulled forward and upward, and this increases the lateral and anteroposterior diameters of the thoracic cage. The accessory muscles of inspiration include the scalene and sternocleidomastoid muscles. The scalene muscles elevate the first two ribs, and the sternocleidomastoid muscles raise the sternum.[2] During normal breathing, these muscles are not used, but during exercise, these muscles contract to aid in inspiration.

Muscles that depress the thoracic cage are classified as *muscles of expiration*.[1] Expiration is a largely passive process during normal breathing. During expiration, the diaphragm relaxes, and the elastic recoil of the lungs, chest wall, and abdominal structures compresses the lungs. Expiration can become an active process during exercise. The abdominal and intercostal muscles can increase expiratory effort (see Fig. 23-5). When the abdominal muscles contract, the intra-abdominal pressure increases and pushes the diaphragm upward. These muscles are also used during defecation, vomiting, and coughing. When the

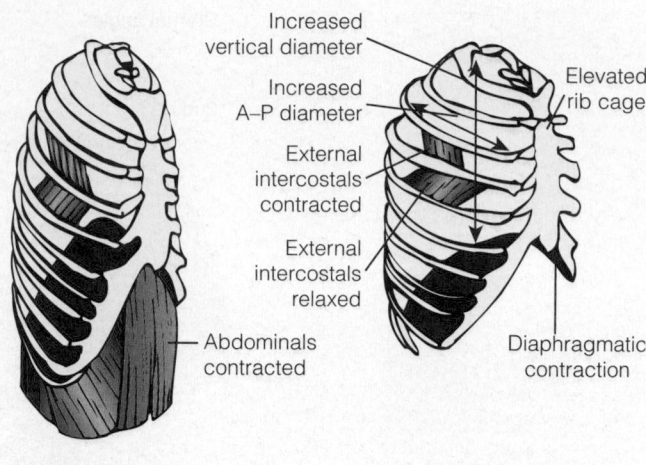

EXPIRATION   INSPIRATION

Figure 23-6 • Contraction and expansion of the thoracic cage during expiration and inspiration, demonstrating diaphragmatic contraction, function of the intercostals, and elevation and depression of the rib cage. A–P diameter, anterior–posterior diameter. (From Guyton AC, Hall JE: Textbook of Medical Physiology, 11th ed. Philadelphia, Elsevier Science, 2006, p 472.)

internal intercostal muscles contract, the ribs are pulled downward and inward, decreasing the thoracic volume.

THE CONDUCTING AIRWAYS

The conducting airways include the nasopharynx, oropharynx, trachea, bronchi, bronchioles, and the terminal bronchioles (see Fig. 23-4). These airways— a series of tubes that become more numerous and narrow as they penetrate deeper into the lungs (Fig. 23-7)—warm, humidify, and filter air that is inhaled as it is channeled to the gas exchange region. Because the conducting airways contain no alveoli and do not participate in gas exchange, they constitute the *anatomic dead space*. The volume in the anatomic dead space is approximately 150 mL.[3]

The Nasopharynx and Oropharynx

The nasopharynx is the preferred route for entrance of air into the respiratory tract during normal breathing because it filters and warms inspired air.[4] The outer passages are lined with coarse hairs that filter large particles. The upper portion of the nasal cavity supplies warmth and moisture to the air inhaled. If nasal passages are plugged or when larger volumes of gases need to be exchanged (e.g., during exercise), the oropharynx provides an alternate route. Obstruction of the oropharynx leads to immediate cessation of ventilation ("choking"). Foreign bodies and swelling of the pharyngeal airways due to infection, injury, or allergic reaction can also cause airway obstruction.

The Epiglottis

The epiglottis is located posterior to the root of the tongue (see Fig. 23-4). It is a leaf-shaped piece of car-

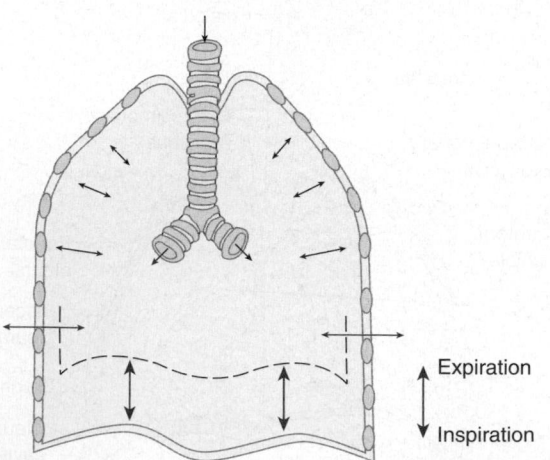

Figure 23-5 • Frontal section of the chest showing the movement of the rib cage and diaphragm during inspiration and expiration. (From Porth CM: Pathophysiology: Concepts of Altered Health States, 7th ed. Philadelphia, Lippincott Williams & Wilkins, 2005, p 641.)

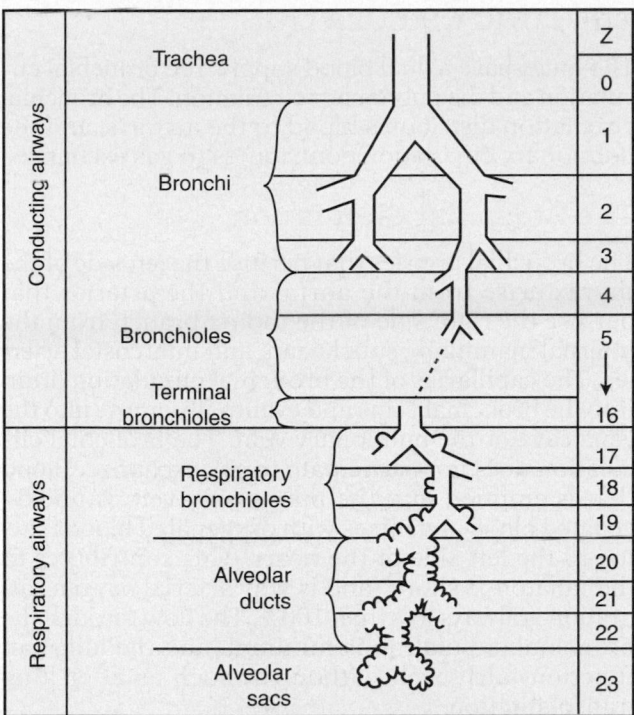

Figure 23-7 • Idealization of the human airways. Note that the first 16 generations (Z) make up the conducting airways, and generations 17 to 23 make up the respiratory airways. Throughout childhood, the airways increase in diameter and length, and the number and size of the alveoli increase until adolescence, when respiratory development matures to that of an adult. (From West JB: Respiratory Physiology: The Essentials, 7th ed. Philadelphia, Lippincott Williams & Wilkins, 2005, p 6.)

tilage that moves up and down. During inhalation, the epiglottis moves upward to allow air to move through the trachea. During swallowing, it moves downward to cover the larynx and allow food and liquid to pass into the esophagus. During defecation, especially during defecation associated with straining and constipation, inhaled air is temporarily held in the lungs by closure of the glottis. Contraction of the intra-abdominal muscles causes an increase in the intra-abdominal and intrathoracic pressures. These collective processes are called the *Valsalva maneuver*. The Valsalva maneuver can be dangerous because the abrupt increase in intrathoracic pressure can significantly reduce venous return and therefore cardiac output.

The Tracheobronchial Tree

The tracheobronchial tree consists of the trachea, bronchi, and bronchioles. The trachea is a hollow tube, or "windpipe," that connects the larynx and the major bronchi of the lungs (see Fig. 23-4). The trachea is primarily smooth muscle and is supported by horseshoe-shaped rings of cartilage that prevent the trachea from collapsing during coughing or bronchoconstriction of the smooth muscle.

The end of the trachea divides, forming the two large mainstem bronchi. The point at which the trachea divides is called the *carina*. The carina is innervated with sensory neurons. When the carina

is stimulated (e.g., during tracheal suctioning), the cough reflex and bronchoconstriction are elicited. The right mainstem bronchus is wider and shorter than the left bronchus. Thus, the right mainstem bronchus is the most common site of aspiration of foreign bodies. The right and left mainstem bronchi divide into branches that become smaller and more numerous as they divide (Fig. 23-8). The right and left mainstem bronchi divide into lobar and segmental bronchi, which divide into bronchioles, which become terminal bronchioles. The terminal bronchioles are the smallest airways without alveoli. The mainstem bronchi are similar in structure to the trachea, in that they are airways supported by cartilage rings. However, as the bronchi extend into the lungs, the cartilage rings become irregular and smaller until they disappear at about the level of the respiratory bronchioles. Here, smooth muscle wraps around the bronchioles. Contraction of these muscles (bronchospasm) causes narrowing of the bronchioles and impairs gas flow.[4]

THE RESPIRATORY AIRWAYS

The terminal bronchioles branch into the respiratory airways. These airways include the respiratory bronchioles, the alveolar ducts, and the alveolar sacs (see Fig. 23-7). The respiratory zone makes up most of the lung, its volume being about 2.5 to 3 L.[5]

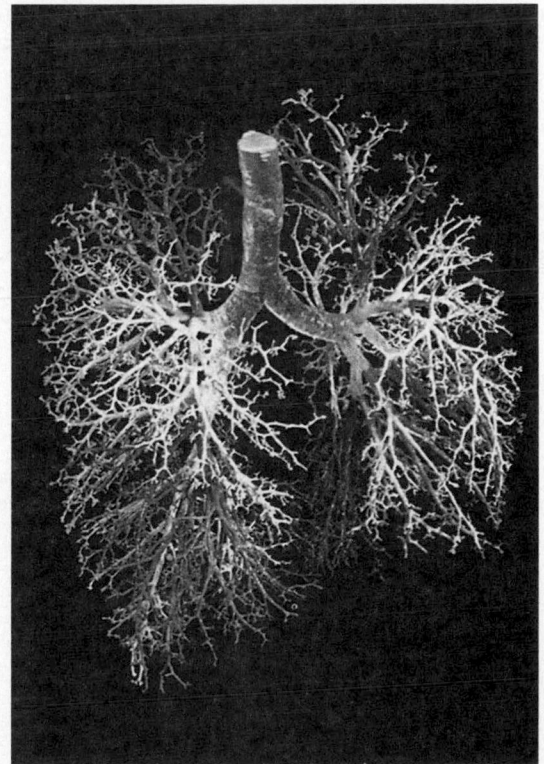

Figure 23-8 • Cast of the airways of a human lung. The alveoli have been pruned away, allowing the conducting airways from the trachea to the terminal bronchioles to be seen. (From West JB: Respiratory Physiology: The Essentials, 7th ed. Philadelphia, Lippincott Williams & Wilkins, 2005, p 5.)

The Respiratory Bronchioles

Each respiratory bronchiole forms a lobule. The lobule is the smallest functional unit of the lung and is where gas exchange takes place. A lobule consists of an arteriole, the pulmonary capillaries, and a venule (Fig. 23-9). Blood enters through a pulmonary artery and exits through a pulmonary vein. This is the only place in the body where highly oxygenated blood flows through a vein.

The Alveoli

Each respiratory bronchiole gives rise to several alveolar ducts that terminate in a cluster of alveoli, as shown in Figure 23-9. The alveolus is the end point of the respiratory tract, and it is here where gas exchange takes place. The alveoli are thin-walled, cup-shaped structures. There are approximately 300 million alveoli in the adult lung, with a total surface area of 85 square meters.[5] The alveoli also contain macrophages that perform a phagocytic role. These cells move from alveolus to alveolus, removing foreign substances and keeping the alveoli sterile.

Alveolar structures are composed of two types of cells: type I alveolar cells and type II alveolar cells. *Type I alveolar cells* are flat squamous epithelial cells and comprise approximately 90% of the total alveolar surface area. Gas exchange takes place along these cells. *Type II alveolar cells* secrete pulmonary surfactant. Surfactant is a lipoprotein that decreases surface tension in the alveoli. This prevents collapse of the smaller airways during expiration and makes it easier to inflate the alveoli during inspiration. Therefore, injury to type II alveolar cells leads to alveolar collapse and impaired pulmonary gas exchange.

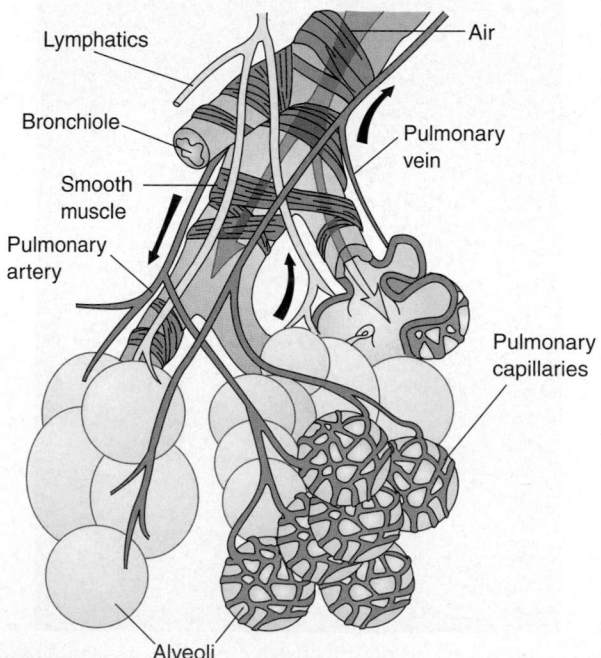

Figure 23-9 • Lobule of the lung, showing the bronchial smooth muscle fibers, pulmonary blood vessels, and lymphatics. (From Porth CM: Pathophysiology: Concepts of Altered Health States, 7th ed. Philadelphia, Lippincott Williams & Wilkins, 2005, p 637.)

THE LUNG CIRCULATION

The lungs have a dual blood supply: the bronchial circulation and the pulmonary circulation. The bronchial circulation distributes blood to the airways, and the pulmonary circulation contributes to gas exchange.

The Bronchial Circulation

The bronchial arteries that perfuse the left side of the thorax arise from the aorta, and the arteries that perfuse the right side of the thorax branch from the internal mammary, subclavian, and intercostal arteries. The capillaries of the bronchial circulation drain into the bronchial veins and eventually empty into the vena cava or the pulmonary vein. The bronchial circulation does not participate in gas exchange. Blood that is emptied into the pulmonary vein is unoxygenated blood and mixes with oxygenated blood flowing to the left side of the heart. This contributes to the "anatomic shunt" and is why arterial oxygen saturation is always less than 100%. The flow through the bronchial circulation is minimal, and the lung can function fairly well without it, such as after lung transplantation.[5]

The Pulmonary Circulation

The pulmonary circulation arises from the pulmonary artery and provides for the gas exchange function of the lung (Fig. 23-10). As shown in Figure 23-10, deoxygenated blood leaves the right ventricle and enters the pulmonary artery. The blood passes from the pulmonary artery through a series of branching arteries to the capillaries, and then back through a series of venules to the pulmonary vein.

In the walls of the alveoli, the capillaries form a dense network (see Fig. 23-9). The diameter of a capillary segment is about 10 μm, just large enough for one red blood cell.[5] The extreme thinness of the blood–gas barrier is extremely efficient for gas exchange but also means these capillaries are easily damaged. Increasing pressure in the alveoli (such as occurs with high levels of positive end-expiratory pressure) or increasing volume in the alveoli (such as occurs with mechanical ventilation with large tidal volumes) can damage capillaries, causing them to leak plasma into the alveolar spaces. Each red blood cell spends about 0.75 second in the capillary network and during this time probably transverses two or three alveoli.[5] Almost complete equilibrium of oxygen and carbon dioxide between alveolar gas and capillary blood can occur during this very brief time.

The pulmonary artery receives the whole output from the right ventricle. However, the resistance of the pulmonary circuit is extremely low, compared with the systemic vascular resistance, because the pulmonary vascular structures do not have vascular smooth muscle like the systemic vascular structures do. Thus, systolic and diastolic pressures in the pulmonary circulatory system are much lower. Normal pulmonary artery pressures are 20 to 30/8 to 15 mm Hg. Just as hypertension can develop in the systemic circulatory system, hypertension can occur within the pul-

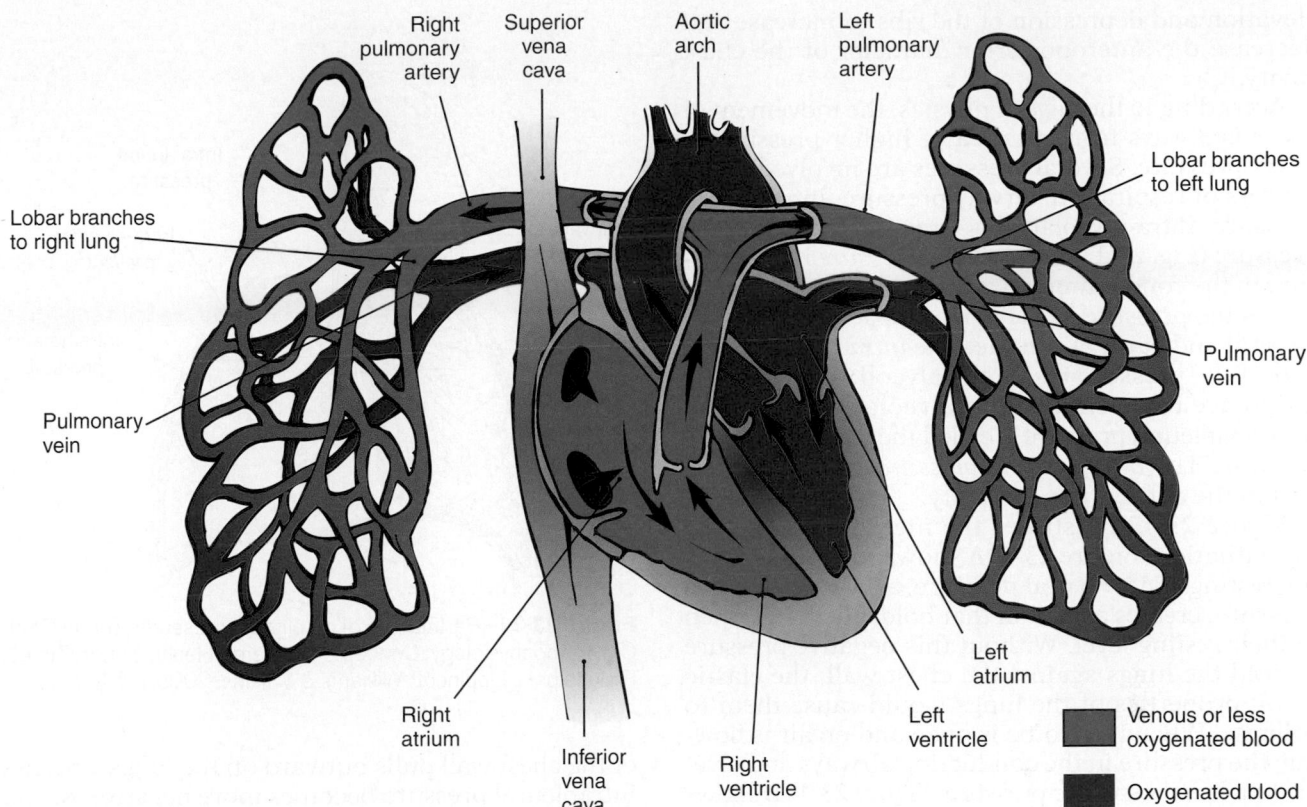

Right pulmonary artery

Superior vena cava

Aortic arch

Left pulmonary artery

Lobar branches to left lung

Lobar branches to right lung

Pulmonary vein

Pulmonary vein

Left atrium

Right atrium

Left ventricle

Inferior vena cava

Right ventricle

Venous or less oxygenated blood

Oxygenated blood

Figure 23-10 • Circulation from the right heart to the lungs and left heart.

monary circulatory system and is called pulmonary hypertension.

THE PULMONARY LYMPHATICS

The lungs represent the largest surface area of the body that is exposed to an increasingly hostile environment.[5] Fortunately, the lungs have multiple mechanisms to handle inhaled particles. The nose filters large particles. Particles that deposit in the conducting airways are removed by cilia that line the airways. The cilia brush the particles up toward the epiglottis, where they are then swallowed. Particles in the alveoli are phagocytosed by macrophages or leukocytes. Foreign materials that reach the alveoli are then removed by lymphatic tissue. The lungs have a vast supply of lymphatic tissue. The lymphatic vessels parallel the pulmonary vasculature (see Fig. 23-9). They surround the lobule and aid in the removal of particles and protein from the interstitial spaces. These vessels eventually drain into lymph nodes located at the hila of the lungs.

• Physiology of the Respiratory System

The goals of respiration are to provide oxygen to tissues and to remove carbon dioxide. The physiology of respiration involves the following three processes: (1) *ventilation*, or the movement of air between the atmosphere and the alveoli; (2) *diffusion* of oxygen and carbon dioxide between the pulmonary capillaries and the alveoli; and (3) *transport* of oxygen and carbon dioxide in the blood to and from the cells.[6]

VENTILATION

During ventilation, the movement of air into the lungs is known as *inhalation,* and the movement of air out of the lungs is known as *exhalation.* Air flows from a region of higher pressure to a region of lower pressure. To initiate a breath, a drop in pressure in the alveoli must precipitate airflow into the lungs.

The Mechanics of Ventilation

Ventilation is a complex process with multiple variables, including the change in pressures and the integrity of the muscles responsible for moving air in and out of the lungs, the compliance of the lungs, and the resistance afforded by the airways. Collectively, these variables are referred to as the *mechanics of ventilation.*

Movement of Air Into and Out of the Lungs The movement of air in and out of the lungs requires muscles to expand and contract the chest cavity and a change in gas pressures to facilitate movement of air from one compartment to another. The lungs can be expanded and contracted in two ways: (1) by downward and upward movement of the diaphragm to lengthen and shorten the chest cavity, and (2) by elevation and depression of the ribs to increase and decrease the anteroposterior diameter of the chest cavity.[1]

According to the laws of physics, the movement of gases is always from an area of higher pressure to lower pressure. Several pressures are involved in the process of respiration: airway pressure, intrapleural pressure, intra-alveolar pressure, and intrathoracic pressure (Fig. 23-11). The *airway pressure* is the pressure in the conducting airways. The *intrapleural pressure* is the pressure in the narrow space between the visceral and parietal pleurae. The *intra-alveolar pressure* is the pressure inside the alveoli. The pressure difference between the intra-alveolar pressure and the intrapleural pressure is called the *transpulmonary pressure*. The *intrathoracic pressure* is the pressure within the entire thoracic cavity.

Figure 23-12 illustrates the mechanics involved in ventilation. Figure 23-12A shows the pressures in the resting state. Pleural pressure, a slightly negative pressure, creates a suction that holds the lungs open to their resting level. Without this negative pressure to hold the lungs against the chest wall, the elastic recoil properties of the lungs would cause them to collapse. When the glottis is open and no air is flowing, the pressure in the conducting airways and alveoli equals atmospheric pressure. Figure 23-11B shows the pressures during inspiration. During inspiration, as the diaphragm and intercostal muscles contract, the volume of the chest cavity increases. Expansion

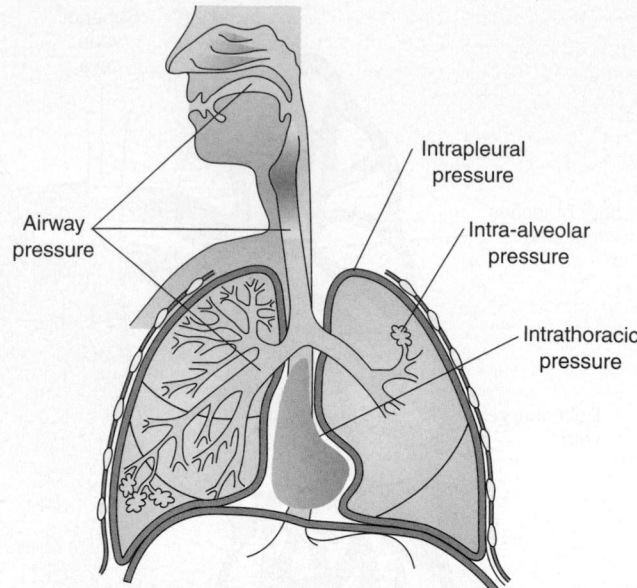

Figure 23-11 • Partitioning of respiratory pressures. (From Porth CM: Pathophysiology: Concepts of Altered Health States, 7th ed. Philadelphia, Lippincott Williams & Wilkins, 2005, p 640.)

of the chest wall pulls outward on the lungs, and the intrapleural pressure becomes more negative. As the alveolar pressure becomes more negative, air flows in from the atmosphere through the conducting airways to the alveoli. After inspiration, the muscles relax,

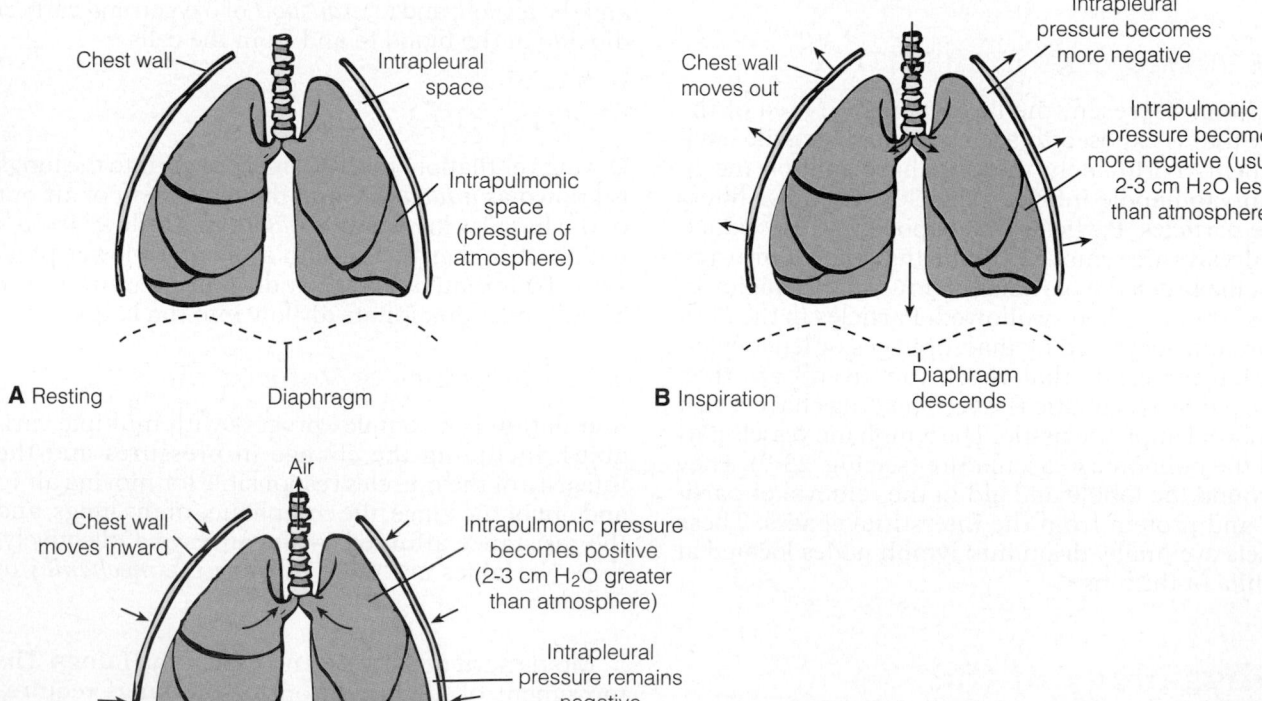

Figure 23-12 • Phases of ventilation. **A:** No air movement (resting). **B:** Air moves from the environment to the intrapulmonic space (inspiration). **C:** Air moves from the intrapulmonic space to the environment (expiration).

and the chest cavity returns to its resting position. With this decrease in chest size and resultant compression of the lungs, the intra-alveolar pressure builds and forces air out of the lungs during expiration. One respiratory cycle consists of one inhalation and one exhalation. At rest, inhalation requires 1 second and exhalation lasts 2 seconds.

Lung Compliance The extent to which the lungs expand is called *compliance*. Compliance is a measurement of distensibility, or how easily a tissue is stretched. If compliance is reduced, it is more difficult to expand the lungs for inspiration. And conversely, if compliance is increased, it is easier to expand lung tissue. Compliance is expressed as the ratio of the change in lung volume to the change in lung pressure.

$$Compliance = \frac{Change\ in\ lung\ volume\ (L)}{Change\ in\ lung\ pressure\ (cm\ H_2O)}$$

Compliance can be appreciated by comparing the ease of blowing up a new balloon that is stiff and resistant with one that has been previously blown up and is more compliant. Lung compliance is determined by the elastin and collagen fibers of the lung and the surface tension in the alveoli.

Lung tissue is made up of elastin and collagen fibers. Collagen fibers resist stretching and make lung inflation difficult, whereas elastin fibers are easily stretched and increase the ease of lung inflation. When elastin fibers are replaced with scar tissue, such as that which occurs with pulmonary fibrosis or interstitial lung disease, the lungs become stiff and noncompliant.

The fluid lining the alveoli has a high surface tension. When the surface tension is high, the moist interior surfaces of an alveolus are difficult to separate from one another, and more energy is required to open and fill the alveolus with air during inspiration. When the surface tension is low, the alveoli walls separate more easily, requiring less effort for alveolar filling during inspiration. Recall that a lipoprotein substance called *surfactant*, which is secreted by type II alveolar cells, decreases the surface tension of these fluids in the alveoli.

Surfactant has four important effects on lung inflation: it lowers the surface tension; increases lung compliance and ease of inflation; provides for stability and more even inflation of the alveoli; and assists in preventing pulmonary edema by keeping the alveoli dry.[4] Without surfactant, lung inflation is extremely difficult. The type II alveolar cells that produce surfactant do not mature until the 26th to 28th weeks of gestation.[4] Premature infants do not have sufficient amounts of surfactant, which leads to alveolar collapse and severe respiratory distress, a condition known as *infant respiratory distress syndrome*. Lack of surfactant or inefficient surfactant production may also play a role in the development of *acute respiratory distress syndrome* (ARDS) in adults.

Airway Resistance Airflow in the conducting airways is affected not only by pressure differences between the atmosphere and alveoli but also by the resistance that air encounters as it moves through the airways. According to Poiseuille's law, the resistance to flow is inversely proportional to the fourth power of the radius ($R = 1/r^4$). If the radius of the tube that gas is flowing through is cut in half, the resistance is increased 16-fold ($2 \times 2 \times 2 \times 2 = 16$). In the respiratory airways, this means that small changes in airway diameter can have enormous effects on airflow resistance. Normally, airway resistance is so small that only small changes in pressure are needed to move large volumes of air into the lungs. But in conditions that decrease airway diameter, such as those caused by pulmonary secretions or bronchospasm, marked increases in airway resistance occur. To maintain the same rate of airflow as before the onset of increased airway resistance, people with these conditions must increase the driving pressure (or respiratory effort) to move air.

Assessment of Ventilation

Minute ventilation is the volume of air inhaled and exhaled per minute. It is calculated by multiplying tidal volume (V_T) and respiratory rate. At rest, minute ventilation is approximately 7,500 mL/minute.

Not all the air that enters the airways reaches the alveoli where gas exchange takes place. The part of V_T that does not participate in alveolar gas exchange is called *dead space ventilation*. Dead space ventilation includes anatomical dead space volume and physiological dead space volume. Anatomical dead space is the amount of air in the conducting airways and is normally about 2 mL/kg, or about 150 mL.[7] Anatomical dead space depends on body posture and disease states. In certain disease states, such as chronic obstructive pulmonary disease (COPD), anatomical dead space is larger than normal. Physiological dead space occurs when ventilation is normal but perfusion to the alveoli is reduced or absent. This can occur with certain disease states, such as reduced cardiac output or pulmonary embolism. Dead space increases the partial pressure of arterial carbon dioxide ($PaCO_2$) because blood that is carrying carbon dioxide back from the tissues cannot reach the alveoli.

The *alveolar ventilation* is the volume of fresh gas entering the respiratory zone each minute. Alveolar ventilation is of key importance because it represents the amount of fresh inspired air available for gas exchange.[3] Alveolar ventilation is the minute ventilation minus dead space. It is inversely proportional to $PaCO_2$ levels. If one breathes excessively, alveolar ventilation is increased, and $PaCO_2$ decreases. If alveolar ventilation is decreased, $PaCO_2$ levels increase.

Pulmonary Volumes and Capacities

The flow of air in and out of the lungs provides tangible measures of lung volumes. Although referred to as "pulmonary function" measures, in reality these volumes represent "pulmonary anatomy" measures. In the evaluation of ventilation, structure or anatomy often determines function.

Ventilatory or pulmonary function tests measure the ability of the chest and lungs to move air into and out of the alveoli. Pulmonary function tests include

Table 23-2 • Factors Affecting Alveolar–Capillary Gas Exchange

Factors Affecting Gas Exchange	Examples
Surface area available for diffusion	Removal of a lung or diseases such as emphysema and chronic bronchitis, which destroy lung tissue or cause mismatching of ventilation and perfusion
Thickness of the alveolar–capillary membrane	Conditions such as pneumonia, interstitial lung disease, and pulmonary edema, which increase membrane thickness
Partial pressure of alveolar gas	Decreasing the partial pressure of a gas in the inspired air (e.g., ascent to high altitudes) decreases the gradient for diffusion; increasing the partial pressure of a gas in the inspired air (e.g., oxygen therapy) increases the gradient for diffusion
Solubility and molecular weight of the gas	Carbon dioxide, which is more soluble in the cell membranes, diffuses across the alveolar–capillary membrane more rapidly than oxygen

From Porth CM: Pathophysiology: Concepts of Altered Health States, 6th ed. Philadelphia, Lippincott Williams & Wilkins, 2002, p 594.

mechanism of this response, called *hypoxic vasoconstriction*, is not known.[9] Hypoxic vasoconstriction has the effect of directing blood flow away from hypoxic areas of the lung. By diverting blood flow from these areas, the deleterious effects on gas exchange are reduced.

RELATIONSHIP OF VENTILATION TO PERFUSION

Distribution of Ventilation

Not all areas of the lung have the same ventilation. Body position affects distribution of ventilation. In a seated or standing position, lower regions of the lung ventilate better than upper zones. In a supine position, the apex and base of the lung ventilate about the same; however, ventilation in the lowermost (posterior) lung is greater than that of the uppermost (anterior) lung. In a lateral position, the dependent lung is best ventilated.[3]

Distribution of Perfusion

As with ventilation, the distribution of pulmonary blood flow is affected by body position and gravity. In the upright position, blood flow is better at the base of the lungs than the apex of the lungs. In the supine position, the blood flow from apex to base is almost uniform, but blood flow in the posterior (dependent) regions of the lung exceeds that of the anterior regions. In the prone position, the same holds true: blood flow in the dependent region (now the anterior chest) exceeds that of the posterior chest.

Considerable inequality of blood flow exists within the human lung (Fig. 23-15). The uneven distribution of blood flow can be explained by the hydrostatic pressure differences in the blood vessels. In zone 1, alveolar pressures exceed pulmonary arterial and pulmonary venous pressures. The capillaries are basically squashed flat by the pressure in the alveoli, and there is no blood flow. In zone 2, pulmonary arterial pressures are greater than alveolar pressures, so some blood flow occurs. Blood flow here is determined by the differences in arterial and alveolar pressures. In zone 3, there is minimal alveolar pressure influence on the pulmonary vasculature, and blood flow is determined in the usual way by the arteriovenous pressure difference.

Matching of Ventilation to Perfusion

Effective pulmonary gas exchange depends on a balance, or matching of ventilation to perfusion (Fig. 23-16A). Two factors may interfere with the matching of ventilation to perfusion: dead space and shunt. As previously described in this chapter, dead

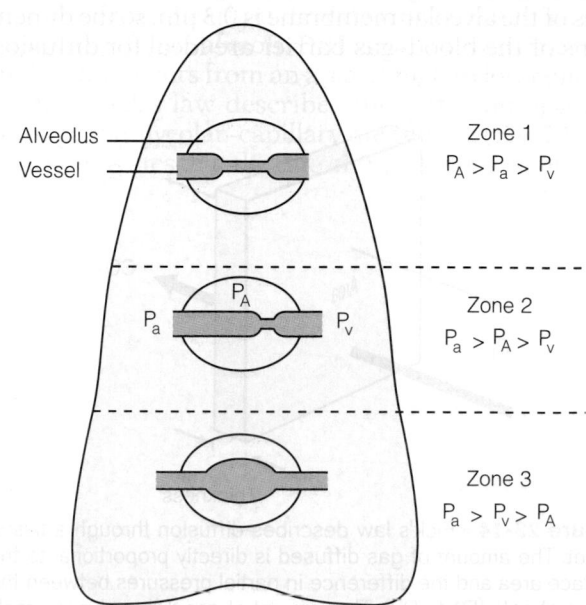

Figure 23-15 • Explanation of the uneven distribution of blood flow in the lung, based on the pressures affecting the capillaries. P_A, alveolar pressure; Pa, arterial pressure; Pv, venous pressure. (From West JB: Respiratory Physiology: The Essentials, 7th ed. Philadelphia, Lippincott Williams & Wilkins, 2005, p 44.)

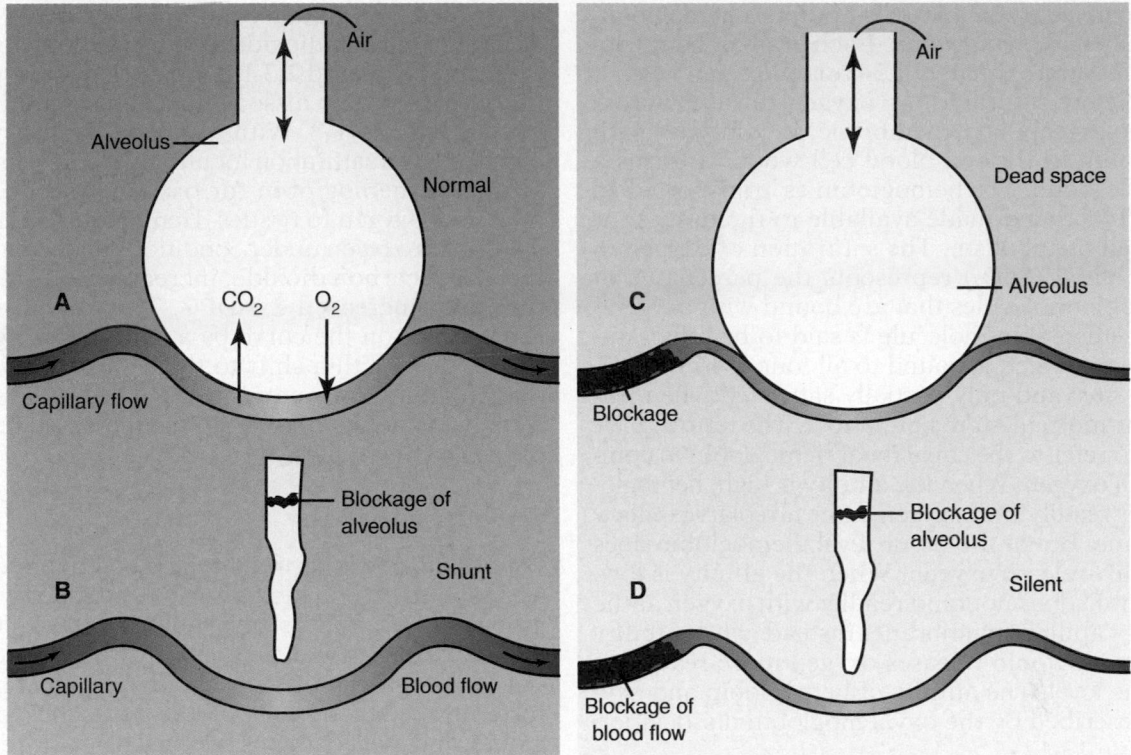

Figure 23-16 • A schematic representation of various ventilation–perfusion situations. **A:** Normal unit with normal ventilation and normal perfusion. **B:** Low ventilation/perfusion ratio—alveoli with no ventilation but normal perfusion. **C:** High ventilation/perfusion ratio—alveoli with normal ventilation but no perfusion. **D:** Silent unit—alveoli with no ventilation and no perfusion. CO_2, carbon dioxide; O_2, oxygen. (From Smeltzer SC, Bare BG: Brunner and Suddarth's Textbook of Medical Surgical Nursing, 11th ed. Philadelphia, Lippincott Williams & Wilkins, 2008, p 559.)

space refers to areas in the respiratory system that do not participate in gas exchange. The air in the conducting airways (about 150 mL) does not participate in gas exchange and is referred to as *anatomical dead space*. Anatomical dead space increases with intubation. In zone 1 of the lung, the region is ventilated but not perfused, and this is referred to as *alveolar dead space*. Other areas of the lung may also contain alveolar dead space, such as that which occurs with collapsed alveoli from atelectasis or pneumonia. Shunt refers to blood that bypasses, or shunts by, alveoli without picking up oxygen. There are two types of shunts: anatomical and physiological. With an anatomical shunt, blood moves from the right side to the left side of the heart without passing through the lungs. Anatomical shunts occur with congenital heart diseases. With a physiological shunt, blood is shunted past alveoli without picking up sufficient amounts of oxygen.

A ventilation–perfusion imbalance, known as a ventilation–perfusion mismatch, occurs when there is inadequate ventilation, inadequate perfusion, or both. Three types of ventilation–perfusion imbalances may occur:

▶ *Physiological shunt* (low ventilation–perfusion ratio). When perfusion exceeds ventilation, the ratio is low, and a shunt is present. A shunt means that blood passes by alveoli without gas exchange occur-

ring. A low ventilation–perfusion ratio is seen with pneumonia, atelectasis, tumor, or a mucous plug (see Fig. 23-16B).

▶ *Alveolar dead space* (high ventilation/perfusion ratio). When ventilation exceeds perfusion, the ratio is high and an alveolar dead space develops. The alveolus has inadequate perfusion available, and gas exchange cannot occur. A high ventilation/perfusion ratio is seen with a pulmonary embolus, pulmonary infarction, cardiogenic shock, and mechanical ventilation associated with high tidal volumes (see Fig. 23-16C).

▶ *Silent unit.* When both ventilation and perfusion are decreased, a silent unit occurs. A silent unit is seen with pneumothorax and severe ARDS (see Fig. 23-16D).

GAS TRANSPORT

Oxygen

CONCEPTS in action **ANIMATION**

Oxygen is carried in the blood in two forms: dissolved and attached to hemoglobin. The partial pressure of oxygen in arterial blood (PaO_2) represents the level of dissolved oxygen in plasma. Less than 3% of all oxygen is carried in this form. Ninety-seven percent of oxygen carried in the blood is bound to hemoglobin and is called *oxyhemoglobin*. Each gram of hemoglobin carries approximately 1.34 mL of oxygen when it is completely saturated. As oxygen diffuses across the alveolar–capillary membrane, it combines with hemoglobin in the red blood cell where it forms a reversible bond. Oxyhemoglobin is transported in arterial blood and made available to the tissues for use in cell metabolism. The saturation of oxygen in arterial blood (SaO_2) represents the percentage of hemoglobin molecules that are bound with oxygen.

The hemoglobin molecule is said to be fully saturated when oxygen is bound to all four of its oxygen-binding sites and only partially saturated when less than four molecules are bound to it. The term *affinity* is used to refer to the capacity of hemoglobin to combine with oxygen. When the affinity is high, hemoglobin binds readily with oxygen at the alveolar–capillary membrane. But at the tissue level, hemoglobin does not readily release oxygen. When the affinity is low, hemoglobin does not bind readily with oxygen at the alveolar–capillary membrane. Instead, when affinity is low, hemoglobin releases oxygen more readily at the tissue level. The affinity of hemoglobin and oxygen is described by the oxyhemoglobin dissociation curve (Fig. 23-17).

The oxyhemoglobin dissociation curve is a graphic depiction of the relationship between oxyhemoglobin saturation (the percentage of hemoglobin combined with oxygen, or the SaO_2) and the arterial oxygen tension (PaO_2) to which it is exposed. The initial part of the curve is very steep and then flattens at the top. The flat portion represents the binding of oxygen to hemoglobin in the lungs. The steep portion of the curve (between 40 and 60 mm Hg) represents the release of oxygen from the hemoglobin that occurs in the capillaries. At an arterial oxygen tension (PaO_2) of 40 mm Hg, hemoglobin molecules are still about 70% to 75% saturated with oxygen. This provides a reserve supply of oxygen that can be given to the tissues in cases of emergency or strenuous exercise.

Hemoglobin's affinity for oxygen is influenced by pH, carbon dioxide concentration, temperature, and 2,3-diphosphoglycerate (2,3-DPG). 2,3-DPG is a metabolically important phosphate compound found in the blood in different combinations under different metabolic conditions.[10] Hemoglobin binds more readily with oxygen under conditions of increased pH, decreased carbon dioxide, decreased body temperature, and decreased 2,3-DPG. This is represented on the oxyhemoglobin dissociation curve as a shift to the left (see Fig. 23-17). With a shift to the left, there is higher oxygen saturation for any given PaO_2, increased affinity of hemoglobin for oxygen, and decreased release of oxygen to tissues. Hemoglobin more readily releases oxygen under conditions of decreased pH, increased carbon dioxide, increased body temperature, and increased 2,3-DPG. This relationship is represented on the curve by a shift to the right (see Fig. 23-17). With a shift to the right, there is lower oxygen saturation for any given PaO_2, decreased affinity of hemoglobin for oxygen, and increased release of oxygen to the tissues.

Carbon Dioxide

Carbon dioxide is carried in the blood in three forms: as dissolved carbon dioxide (10%), attached to hemoglobin (30%), and as bicarbonate (60%).[4] Carbon dioxide is formed as a metabolic byproduct. It diffuses out of the cell and into the capillaries. Most of it diffuses into red blood cells, where it attaches to hemoglobin, and most of that is released from the red blood cell as bicarbonate. In the pulmonary capillaries, the concentration of carbon dioxide is greater in the capillaries than in the alveoli, so the carbon dioxide moves down this concentration gradient and diffuses into the alveoli and is exhaled. An increased rate of exhalation leads to greater elimination of carbon dioxide. The transport of carbon dioxide has a profound effect on the acid–base status of the blood and the body as a whole. The lung excretes more than 10,000 mEq of carbonic acid per day, compared with the kidney, which excretes less than 100 mEq of fixed acids per day.[11] Therefore, by altering alveolar ventilation (and subsequently, the elimination of carbon dioxide), the body is able to exert precise control over its acid–base balance.

REGULATION OF RESPIRATION

Breathing is controlled by both the nervous system and chemical regulation. Nervous system regulation is achieved by the respiratory centers, which are located in the medulla and pons (i.e., the brainstem). Chemi-

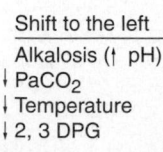

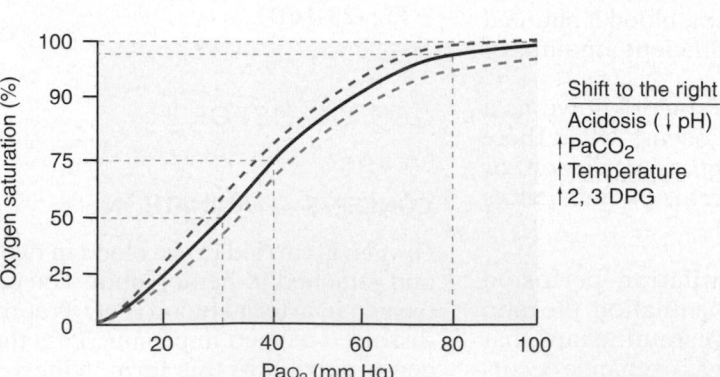

Shift to the left

Alkalosis (↑ pH)
↓ PaCO₂
↓ Temperature
↓ 2, 3 DPG

Shift to the right

Acidosis (↓ pH)
↑ PaCO₂
↑ Temperature
↑ 2, 3 DPG

Figure 23-17 • Oxyhemoglobin dissociation curve. The shift to the left indicates a higher oxygen saturation at any given arterial oxygen tension (PaO_2), an increased affinity of hemoglobin for oxygen, and a decreased release of oxygen to the tissues. A shift to the right indicates a lower oxygen saturation at any given PaO_2, a decreased affinity of hemoglobin for oxygen, and an increased release of oxygen to the tissues.

cal regulation of breathing occurs through chemoreceptors, which respond to blood pH and the levels of oxygen and carbon dioxide in the blood. Chemoreceptors are located near the respiratory center in the medulla, in the carotid arteries, and in the aortic arch.

Brainstem Centers and the Respiratory Cycle

Unlike the heart, the lungs have no spontaneous rhythm. Ventilation depends on rhythmic operation of brainstem centers and intact pathways to the respiratory muscles. There are two centers in the medulla: a center that stimulates inspiration by diaphragmatic contraction (by way of phrenic nerves) and another center that innervates both inspiratory and expiratory intercostal and accessory muscles (Fig. 23-18). The pons also contains two centers involved in controlling respiration: the pneumotaxic center and the apneustic center. The apneustic center produces sustained inspiration if stimulated. Voluntary control and involuntary control are further established by descending fibers from other brain centers. Neural control of ventilation is illustrated in Figure 23-18. In breathing at rest, the following sequence is thought to occur. The neurons innervating the inspiratory muscles fire bursts of impulses to these muscles, leading to inspiration. These neurons also stimulate the pneumotaxic center.

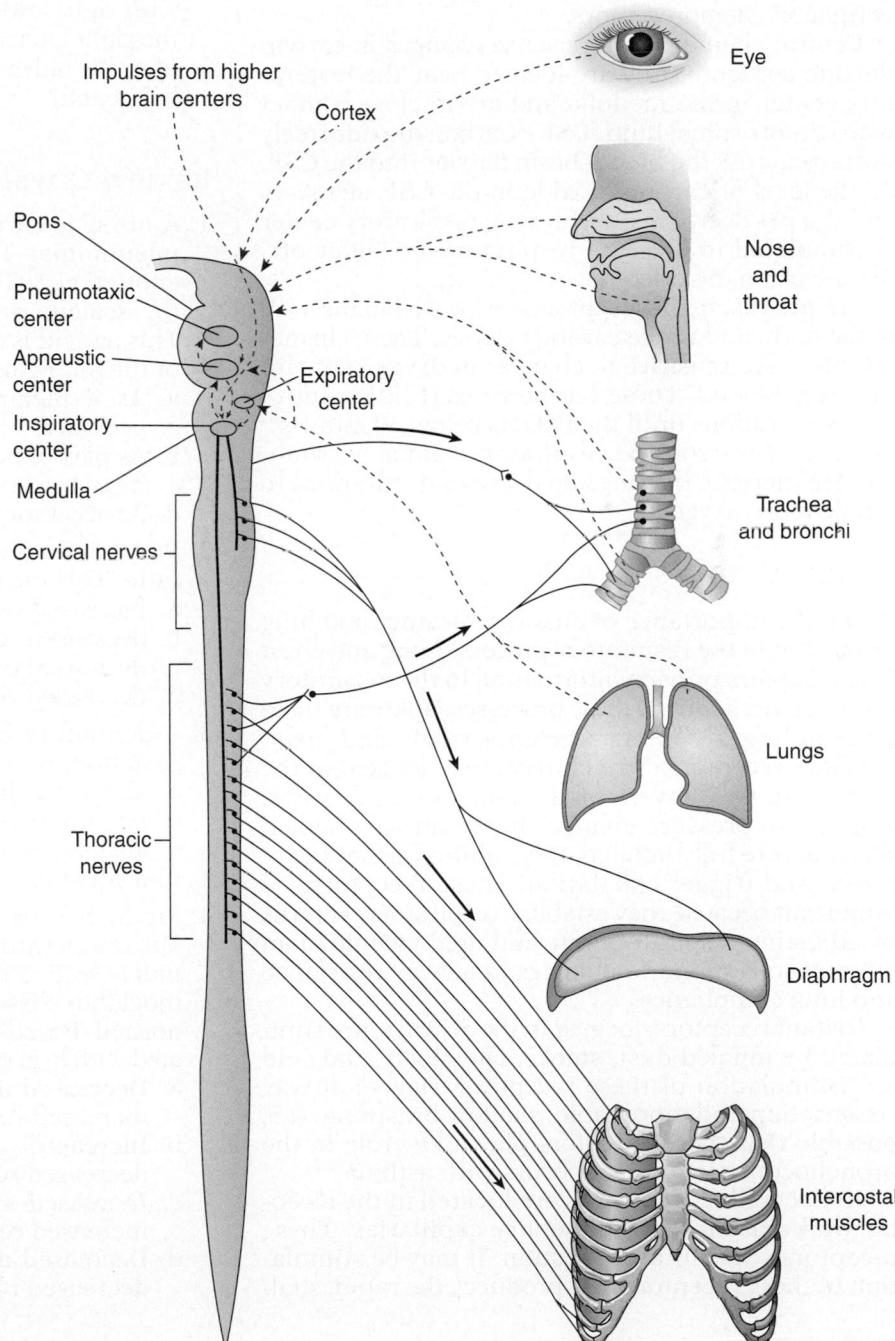

Figure 23-18 • Schematic representation of activity in the respiratory center. Impulses traveling over afferent neurons activate central neurons, which activate efferent neurons that supply the muscles of respiration. Respiratory movements can be altered by a variety of stimuli.

This center, in turn, fires inhibitory impulses back to the inspiratory neurons, causing a halt in inspiration. Expiration follows passively. After expiration, the inspiratory neurons are again stimulated to fire automatically. During exercise or other occasions when more vigorous ventilation occurs, the expiratory neurons of the medulla are postulated to participate in this sequence, causing active exhalation.

Chemoreceptors

Chemoreceptors are like radar screens planted in the body to monitor blood levels of carbon dioxide and oxygen. Signals from these receptors are transmitted to the respiratory center, and ventilation is adjusted to maintain these gases in a normal range. There are two types of chemoreceptors: central chemoreceptors and peripheral chemoreceptors.

Central chemoreceptors sense changes in carbon dioxide content. They are located near the respiratory center in the medulla and are in close contact with cerebrospinal fluid (CSF). Carbon dioxide freely diffuses across the blood–brain barrier into the CSF. As the level of carbon dioxide in the CSF increases and the pH decreases, the nearby respiratory center is stimulated to increase respirations to "blow off" more carbon dioxide.

Peripheral chemoreceptors are located in the arch of the aorta and in the carotid arteries. These chemoreceptors are sensitive to changes in oxygen content in arterial blood. These receptors exert little control over respirations until the PaO_2 is below 60 mm Hg.[4] When this occurs, the respiratory center is stimulated to increase the rate and depth of respirations to inhale more oxygen.

Lung Receptors

Recall the importance of airway resistance and lung expansion in the respiratory process. Lung and chest wall receptors provide information to the respiratory center on the status of these processes. There are three types of lung receptors: stretch, irritant, and juxtacapillary receptors. Stretch receptors, located in the smooth muscle layers of the conducting airways, respond to pressure changes in the airways. When the lungs are fully inflated, they inhibit further inspiration and trigger exhalation. These receptors are important because they establish respiratory patterns by adjusting respiratory rate and tidal volume in an attempt to respond to changes in airway resistance and lung compliance.

Irritant receptors, located in the airways, are stimulated by inhaled dust, smoke, chemicals, and cold air. Stimulation of these receptors triggers airway constriction and more rapid, shallow breathing. It is possible that these receptors play a key role in the bronchoconstriction that occurs with asthma.[4]

Juxtacapillary receptors are located in the alveolar wall close to the pulmonary capillaries. These receptors sense lung congestion. It may be stimulation of these receptors that produces the rapid, shallow breathing that is characteristic in patients with pneumonia and pulmonary edema.

• Clinical Applicability Challenges

Short-Answer Questions

1. Describe the muscles involved in inspiration and expiration.
2. The nurse notes that a patient has increased work of breathing. Discuss three factors that may cause an increase in work of breathing. Identify a pathological condition that affects each factor.
3. Analyze the following situation: Mr. P. is admitted with right lower lobe pneumonia. He is placed in the right lateral decubitus position. Within 5 minutes, his pulse oximeter reading is 80%. What has happened?

Review Questions

1. A nurse is caring for a 92-year-old patient with pneumonia. The patient states, "I cannot get enough air!" The nurse notes the patient is using the scalene and sternocleiodomastoid muscles. This patient is using these muscle groups in which of the following ways?
   a. As a means of increasing intra-abdominal pressure
   b. As part of normal inspiration
   c. As accessory muscles of inspiration
   d. As accessory muscles of expiration
2. Pneumonia results in a low ventilation/perfusion ratio. This mean that there is
   a. increased ventilation with decreased perfusion.
   b. decreased ventilation with increased perfusion.
   c. decreased perfusion in relation to ventilation.
   d. decreased ventilation in relation to perfusion.
3. A premature infant, who was born at 25 weeks' gestation, is at high risk for developing
   a. alveolar collapse.
   b. pneumothorax.
   c. alveolar dead space.
   d. a silent unit.
4. Mr. M. has just returned from the operating room. His temperature on arrival in the intensive care unit is 95°F (35°C). Hypothermia causes the oxyhemoglobin dissociation curve to shift away from normal. Based on the direction of this shift associated with hypothermia, which statement is correct?
   a. Decreased affinity of hemoglobin for oxygen; increased release of oxygen to tissues
   b. Increased affinity of hemoglobin for oxygen; decreased release of oxygen to tissues
   c. Increased affinity of hemoglobin for oxygen; increased release of oxygen to tissues
   d. Decreased affinity of hemoglobin for oxygen; decreased release of oxygen to tissues

5. A nurse notes a high $PaCO_2$ value on arterial blood gas results. A compensatory mechanism for this hypercapnia is an increase in respiratory rate through stimulation of
   a. central chemoreceptors.
   b. peripheral receptors.
   c. irritant chemoreceptors.
   d. juxtacapillary receptors.

References

1. Guyton AC, Hall JE: Pulmonary ventilation. In Guyton AC, Hall JE (eds): Textbook of Medical Physiology, 11th ed. Philadelphia, Lippincott Williams & Wilkins, 2006, pp 471–482
2. West JB: Mechanics of breathing. In West JB (ed): Respiratory Physiology: The Essentials, 7th ed. Philadelphia, Lippincott Williams & Wilkins, 2005, pp 93–120
3. West JB: Ventilation. In West JB (ed): Respiratory Physiology: The Essentials, 7th ed. Philadelphia, Lippincott Williams & Wilkins, 2005, pp 13–23
4. Porth CB: Control of respiratory function. In Porth CB (ed): Pathophysiology: Concepts of Altered Health States, 7th ed. Philadelphia, Lippincott Williams & Wilkins, 2005
5. West JB: Structure and function. In West JB (ed): Respiratory Physiology: The Essentials, 7th ed. Philadelphia, Lippincott Williams & Wilkins, 2005, pp 1–11
6. Johnson KL: Diagnostic measures to evaluate oxygenation in critically ill adults. AACN Clin Issues 15:506–524, 2004
7. Pierce NLP: Practical physiology of the pulmonary system. In Pierce LNB (ed): Management of the Mechanically Ventilated Patient. Philadelphia, Lippincott Williams & Wilkins, 2007, pp 26–60
8. West JB: Diffusion. In West JB (ed): Respiratory Physiology: The Essentials, 7th ed. Philadelphia, Lippincott Williams & Wilkins, 2005, pp 25–34
9. West JB: Blood flow and metabolism. In West JB (ed): Respiratory Physiology: The Essentials, 7th ed. Philadelphia, Lippincott Williams & Wilkins, 2005, pp 35–53
10. Guyton AC, Hall JE: Transport of oxygen and carbon dioxide in blood and tissue fluids. In Guyton AC, Hall JE (eds): Textbook of Medical Physiology, 11th ed. Philadelphia, Lippincott Williams & Wilkins, 2006, pp 502–513
11. West JB: Gas transport by the blood. In West JB (ed): Respiratory Physiology: The Essentials, 7th ed. Philadelphia, Lippincott Williams & Wilkins, 2005, pp 75–92

Other Selected Readings

Berry BE, Pinard AE: Assessing tissue oxygenation. Crit Care Nurse 22(3):22–42, 2002
Bickley LS, Hoekelman RA: Bates' Guide to Physical Examination, 8th ed. Philadelphia, Lippincott Williams & Wilkins, 2003
Pierce LNP: Management of the Mechanically Ventilated Patient, 2nd ed. Philadelphia: Lippincott Williams & Wilkins, 2007
Smeltzer SC, Bare BG: Brunner & Suddarth's Textbook of Medical-Surgical Nursing, 11th ed. Philadelphia, Lippincott Williams & Wilkins, 2008
Wilkins RL, Stoller JK, Scanlan CL (eds): Egan's Fundamentals of Respiratory Care, 8th ed. St Louis: Mosby, 2003

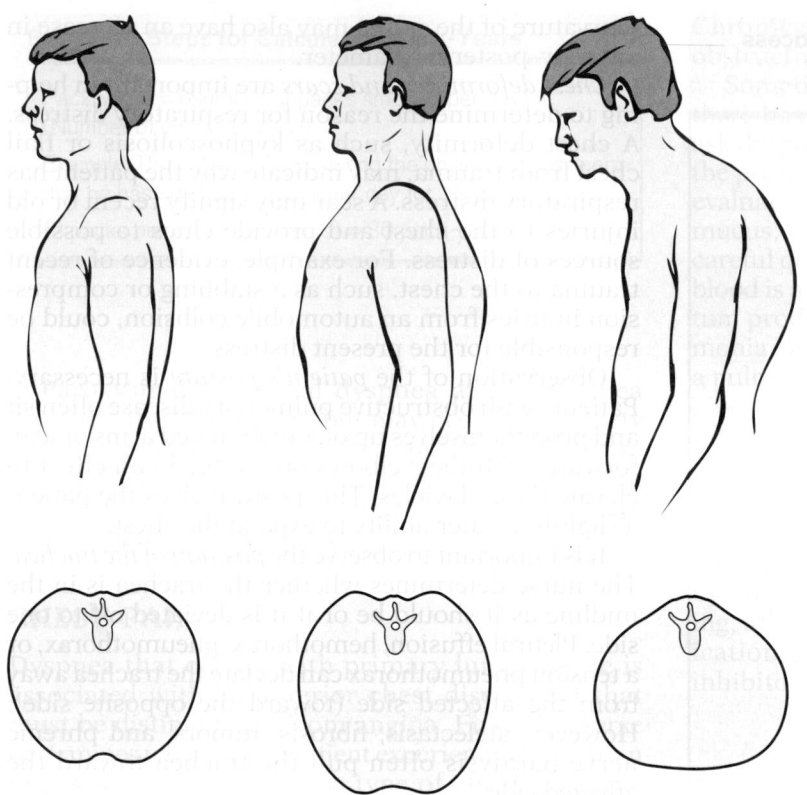

Figure 24-1 • Deformities and configurations of the human thorax. **A:** Normal chest. **B:** "Barrel chest," a chest deformity that typically results from emphysema. **C:** Kyphosis, a chest deformity that is most common in older adults.

A. Normal   **B.** "Barrel chest"   **C.** Kyphosis

sive inflammatory arthritis that typically affects the spine and sacroiliac joints, may be present. General chest expansion is limited in this condition. During the inspection, the nurse compares the expansion of the upper chest with that of the lower chest. The nurse also observes the movement of the diaphragm to determine whether the patient with obstructive pulmonary disease is concentrating on expanding the lower chest and using the diaphragm properly. Expansion of one side of the chest versus the other side is important to note because atelectasis, especially that caused by a mucus plug, may cause unilaterally diminished chest expansion because the air is unable to move equally through the pulmonary bed. Abnormal chest expansion may also occur with flail chest, in which the chest collapses instead of expanding during inspiration. Flail chest may result from broken or fractured ribs that are unable to maintain the integrity of the chest wall during respiration. The nurse also notes whether the abdomen and chest rise and fall together as they should or if the effort is not coordinated; is there symmetry of respiratory effort? Asynchronous respiratory effort decreases the quality of respiration at the cost of increased work of breathing and often precedes the need for ventilatory support.

A pulmonary embolus, pneumonia, pleural effusion, pneumothorax, or any problem associated with chest pain, such as fractured ribs, may lead to diminished chest expansion. An endotracheal or nasotracheal tube positioned beyond the trachea into one of the mainstem bronchi (usually the right) is a serious cause of diminished expansion of one side of the chest. If the tube slips into the right mainstem bronchus, the left lung is not expanded, and the patient may experience atelectasis on the left side and hypoxemia.

Examination of the *patient's extremities* may provide additional information about the patient's respiratory status. Clubbing of the fingers is an enlargement of the distal portion of the finger and is seen in many patients with respiratory and cardiovascular diseases (Fig. 24-2). Although the exact cause is not known, chronic hypoxia is a contributing factor. It is also important to assess the extremities for edema and peripheral cyanosis.

PALPATION

Chest palpation may indicate lung or chest abnormalities. To palpate the chest, the nurse places his or her hand flat against the patient's chest. When the patient speaks, sounds are generated by the larynx, and these sounds travel along the bronchial tree, resulting in a resonant motion of the chest wall. *Tactile fremitus* is the ability to feel the sound on the chest wall. Tactile fremitus is more easily palpated over the large bronchi and is more difficult to palpate over the distant lung fields.

To assess tactile fremitus, the nurse asks the patient to say "ninety-nine" while moving his or her hands over the posterior surfaces of the chest wall (Fig. 24-3). Tactile fremitus should be symmetrical. Tactile fremitus may be diminished or absent if there is an increase

Table 24-1 • Respiration Patterns

Type	Description	Pattern	Clinical Indication
Normal	12 to 20 breaths/min and regular		Normal breathing pattern
Tachypnea	>24 breaths/min and shallow		May be a normal response to fever, anxiety, or exercise. Can occur with respiratory insufficiency, alkalosis, pneumonia, or pleurisy
Bradypnea	<10 breaths/min and regular		May be normal in well-conditioned athletes. Can occur with medication-induced depression of the respiratory center, diabetic coma, neurologic damage
Hyperventilation	Increased rate and increased depth		Usually occurs with extreme exercise, fear, or anxiety. Causes of hyperventilation include disorders of the central nervous system, an overdose of the drug salicylate, or severe anxiety.
Kussmaul	Rapid, deep, labored		A type of hyperventilation associated with diabetic ketoacidosis
Hypoventilation	Decreased rate, decreased depth, irregular pattern		Usually associated with overdose of narcotics or anesthetics
Cheyne-Stokes respiration	Regular pattern characterized by alternating periods of deep, rapid breathing followed by periods of apnea		May result from severe congestive heart failure, drug overdose, increased intracranial pressure, or renal failure. May be noted in elderly persons during sleep, not related to any disease process
Biot's respiration	Irregular pattern characterized by varying depth and rate of respirations followed by periods of apnea		May be seen with meningitis or severe brain damage
Ataxic	Significant disorganization with irregular and varying depths of respiration		A more extreme expression of Biot's respirations indicating respiratory compromise
Air trapping	Increasing difficulty in getting breath out		In chronic obstructive pulmonary disease, air is trapped in the lungs during forced expiration

Figure 24-2 • In clubbing, the angle between the nail plate and the proximal nail fold increases to 180 degrees or more. Clubbing of the fingers is seen in patients with respiratory and cardiovascular disease. (Photo from Bickley LS: Bates' Guide to Physical Examination and History Taking, 9th ed. Philadelphia: Lippincott Williams & Wilkins, 2007, p 150. Line art from Weber J, Kelley J: Health Assessment in Nursing, 3rd ed. Philadelphia: Lippincott Williams & Wilkins, 2007, p 185.)

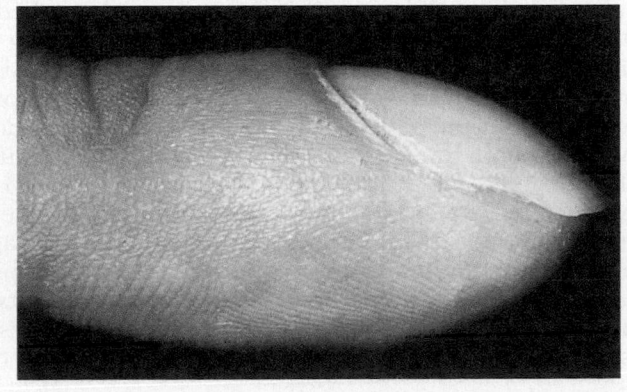

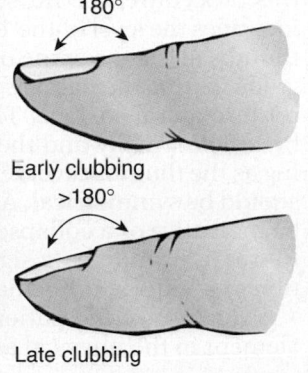

180°

Early clubbing

>180°

Late clubbing

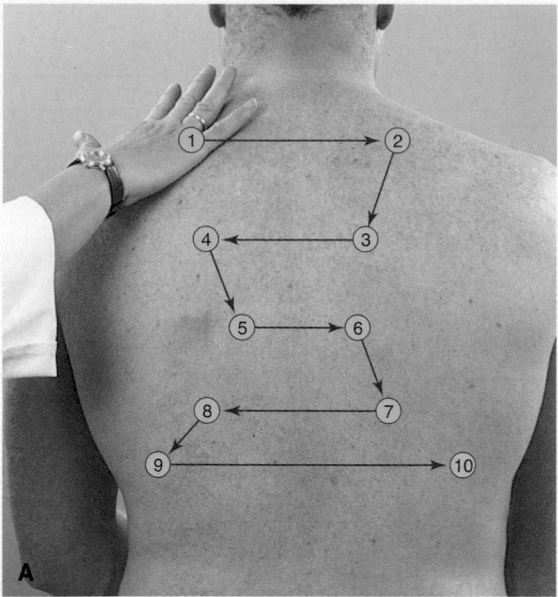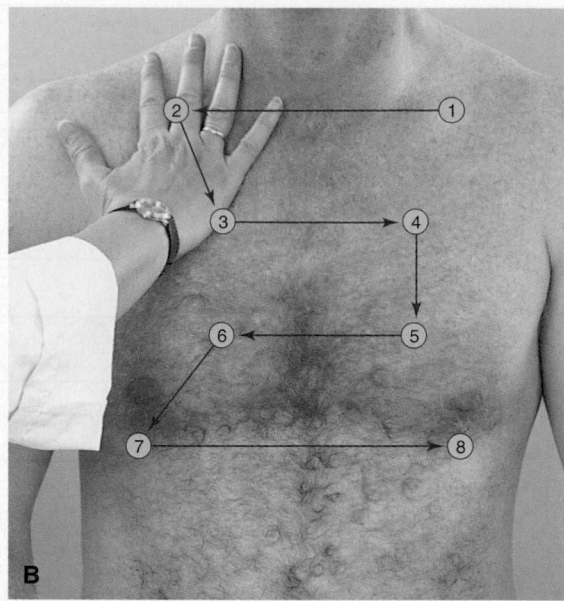

Figure 24-3 • Palpating the thorax is performed in a sequential fashion, starting near the neck and moving systematically downward. **A:** Posterior thorax. **B:** Anterior thorax. (From Weber J, Kelley J: Health Assessment in Nursing, 3rd ed. Philadelphia: Lippincott Williams & Wilkins, 2007, pp 311, 320.)

in air per unit volume of lung because air impedes the transmission of sound. For example, patients with emphysema have little or no tactile fremitus on physical examination. Tactile fremitus is slightly increased by the presence of solid substances, such as the consolidation of a lung due to pneumonia. Other respiratory conditions causing an alteration in tactile fremitus are listed in Table 24-2.

Palpation is also used to assess for subcutaneous emphysema, a condition in which air "leaks" out of the alveolus and moves through the subcutaneous tissue. By moving the fingers in a gentle rolling motion across the chest and neck, it is possible to feel the pockets of air underneath the skin. Feeling subcutaneous emphysema is often likened to the "crunch" of Rice Krispies under the skin. Subcutaneous emphysema may result from a pneumothorax, small pockets of alveoli that have burst with increased pulmonary pressure, or the use of positive end-expiratory pressure. In severe cases, the subcutaneous emphysema may spread into the lower thorax, arms, and face.

Evaluation of thoracic expansion during respiration also requires palpation (Fig. 24-4). To perform this procedure, the nurse stands behind the patient, identifies the level of the 10th rib, and places his or her thumbs along the spine using the bony processes as a guide, letting the palms come in light contact with the posterolateral surface. The nurse asks the patient to breathe normally and then deeply, both times watching as the thumbs diverge. Expansion of the chest wall should be symmetrical. Asymmetrical expansion may be indicative of a collapsed lung or unilateral disease. Retractions may be a sign of obstruction to inspiration and require immediate attention.

Palpation of the patient's trachea is an important element in the physical assessment of the respiratory system. To palpate the trachea to evaluate the midline position, the nurse positions his or her index finger in the suprasternal notch, feeling each side of the notch and palpating the tracheal rings (Fig. 24-5). The trachea should be in the midline position directly above the suprasternal notch.

PERCUSSION

Percussion of the chest results in slight motion of the chest wall and underlying structures, causing audible and tactile vibrations. To percuss a patient's chest, the nurse presses one finger from the nondominant hand flat against the chest and uses a fingertip from the dominant hand to strike the knuckle pressed against the chest (Fig. 24-6). Normally, the chest has a resonant or hollow percussion note. In diseases in which there is increased air in the chest or lungs, such as pneumothorax and emphysema, there can be hyperresonant percussion notes. However, these loud, low-pitched sounds are sometimes difficult to detect.

More important is a flat percussion note (e.g., the sound that is heard when percussing over a part of the body that contains no air). A flat percussion note is a soft, high-pitched sound that is more easily distinguished by noting the change in sound when one moves from percussing an area with air to an area with no air. It is more likely to be heard if a large pleural effusion is present in the lung beneath the examining hand. A dull percussion note is medium in intensity and pitch. It is heard if atelectasis or consolidation due to pneumonia, pulmonary edema, or pulmonary hemorrhage is present. A tympanic drumlike sound is a high-pitched noise heard if asthma or a large pneumothorax is present. See Table 24-2 for a description of percussion sounds associated with various respiratory pathologies.

AUSCULTATION

In chest auscultation, the diaphragm of the stethoscope is pressed firmly against the chest wall. The sequence for auscultating the posterior and anterior thorax is given in Figure 24-7. The nurse listens to the intensity or loudness of breath sounds. Normally, there is a fourfold increase in loudness of breath sounds when a patient takes a maximal deep breath as opposed to quiet breathing. Sounds are louder in the upper and central chest when listening to the larger bronchus and become quieter as the smaller airways are auscultated. The intensity of the breath sounds may be diminished because of decreased flow through the airways or the presence of substances between the lungs and the stethoscope. In pleural thickening, pleural effusion, pneumothorax, and obesity, an abnormal substance (fibrous tissue, fluid, air, or fat) lies between the stethoscope and the underlying lung; this substance insulates the breath sounds from the stethoscope, making the breath sounds seem less loud. In airway obstruction, such as COPD or atelectasis, the intensity of breath sounds is diminished. With shallow breathing, there is diminished air movement through the airways, and the breath sounds are not as loud. With restricted movement of the thorax or diaphragm, there are diminished breath sounds in the restricted areas.

In general, four types of sounds are heard in the normal chest (Table 24-3). *Vesicular breath sounds* are quiet, low-pitched sounds, and the inspiratory phase is longer than the expiratory phase. *Bronchovesicular breath sounds* are medium in pitch, and the inspiratory and expiratory phases are of equal length. *Bronchial breath sounds* are higher pitched and louder compared with vesicular sounds, and the expiratory phase is longer than the inspiratory phase. *Tracheal breath sounds* are loud, high-pitched sounds, and the inspiratory and expiratory phases are about equal in length.

Bronchial breath sounds are heard over the manubrium not only in the normal state but when consolidation is present, as in pneumonia. Bronchial breath sounds are also heard above a pleural effusion in which the normal lung is compressed and sounds are transmitted through the tissue, which is not participating in airflow. Wherever there is bronchial breathing, there also may be two associated changes: E to A changes and whispered pectoriloquy.

An *E to A change* occurs when the patient says "E" and the nurse listening with a stethoscope actually hears an "A" sound rather than an "E" sound. This occurs if consolidation is present. *Egophony* is the term used to describe voice sounds that are distorted.

Whispered pectoriloquy is the presence of loud, clear sounds heard through the stethoscope when the patient whispers. Normally, the whispered voice is heard faintly and indistinctly through the stethoscope. The increased transmission of voice sounds indicates that air in the lungs has been replaced by fluid as a result of pneumonia, pulmonary edema, or hemorrhage.

Adventitious sounds are additional breath sounds heard with auscultation and include discontinuous sounds, continuous sounds, and rubs. Discontinuous sounds are brief, nonmusical, intermittent sounds and include fine and coarse *crackles*. (Crackles were formerly known as *rales*.) Fine crackles are soft, high-pitched, very brief popping sounds that occur most commonly during inspiration. Crackles result from fluid in the airways or alveoli, or from the opening of collapsed alveoli. Restrictive pulmonary disease results in crackles during late inspiration, whereas obstructive pulmonary disease results in crackles during early inspiration. Crackles become coarser as the air moves through larger fluid accumulations, such as in bronchitis or pneumonia. Crackles that clear with coughing are not associated with significant pulmonary disease. When assessing crackles, the nurse also notes their loudness, pitch, duration, amount, location, and timing in the respiratory cycle.[1]

Continuous adventitious breath sounds are longer in duration than crackles and include wheezes and rhonchi. *Wheezes* are continuous musical sounds that are longer than crackles in duration and persist throughout the respiratory cycle. Wheezes (also known as sibilant wheezes) are continuous, high-pitched adventitious sounds that have a shrill quality. They are caused by the movement of air through a narrowed or partially obstructed airway, such as in asthma, COPD, or bronchitis.

Rhonchi, another type of continuous adventitious breath sound, are deep, low-pitched rumbling noises that are sometimes referred to as sonorous wheezes or gurgles. The presence of rhonchi indicates the presence of secretions in the large airways.[1] Conditions such as bronchitis cause sonorous wheezing. These sounds may clear somewhat with coughing.

A *friction rub* is a crackling, grating sound heard more often with inspiration than expiration. The sound of friction results from the visceral and parietal pleurae rubbing against each other. A friction rub can be heard with pleural effusion, pneumothorax, or pleurisy. It is important to distinguish a pleural friction rub from a pericardial friction rub. To determine the origin of the rub, the nurse asks the patient to hold his or her breath while the lungs are auscultated. If the sounds continue while the patient is holding his or her breath, it is most likely a pericardial friction rub; a pleural friction rub stops when breathing stops.

In elderly people, unique anatomical and physiological characteristics manifest in different assessment findings. Box 24-4 shows specific respiratory assessment findings in older patients.

• Respiratory Monitoring

PULSE OXIMETRY

Approximately 3% of oxygen is dissolved in the plasma (Box 24-5). The partial pressure of oxygen dissolved in the arterial blood is measured by the PaO_2. The normal

(text continues on page 554)

Table 24-2 • Physical Examination Signs in Selected Respiratory Disorders

Condition	Trachea	Percussion Note
Normal	Midline	Resonant
Bronchitis	Midline	Resonant
Consolidation	Midline	Dull over the airless area
Atelectasis	May be shifted toward the involved side	Dull over the airless area

Bronchial inflammation and constriction with mucus

Consolidation

Collapsed portion of lung

Breath Sounds	Tactile Fremitus and Transmitted Voice Sounds	Adventitious Sounds
Vesicular,* except perhaps bronchovesicular and bronchial sounds over the large bronchi and trachea, respectively	Normal	None, except perhaps a few transient inspiratory crackles at the bases of the lungs
Normal	Normal	None or scattered coarse crackles in early inspiration and perhaps expiration; or wheezes or rhonchi
Bronchial over the involved area	Increased over the involved area with bronchophony, egophony, and whispered pectoriloquy	Late inspiratory crackles over the involved area
Usually absent when the bronchial plug persists; exceptions—right upper lobe atelectasis, where adjacent tracheal sounds may be transmitted	Usually absent when the bronchial plug persists; exceptions (e.g., right upper lobe atelectasis), may be increased	None

Crackles

Crackles   Unaffected

Tracheal sounds adjacent to right upper lobe atelectasis

(continued)

Table 24-2 • Physical Examination Signs in Selected Respiratory Disorders (Continued)

Condition	Trachea	Percussion Note
Pleural effusion	Toward the opposite side in a large effusion	Dull to flat over the fluid

Fluid in the pleural space

Pneumothorax	Toward the opposite side if much air	Hyperresonant or tympanitic over the pleural air

Air in the pleural space

Emphysema	Midline	Diffusely hyperresonant

Abnormally distended alveoli

Asthma	Midline	Normal to diffusely hyperresonant

Bronchospasm

* The thickness of the bars indicates intensity; the steeper the incline, the higher the pitch.
Adapted from Bickley LS: Bates' Guide to Physical Examination and History Taking (8th Ed), pp 242–243.
Philadelphia, Lippincott Williams & Wilkins, 2003.

Breath Sounds	Tactile Fremitus and Transmitted Voice Sounds	Adventitious Sounds
Decreased to absent, but bronchial breath sounds possibly heard near the top of a large effusion	Decreased to absent, but may be increased toward the top of a large effusion	None, except a possible pleural rub

May hear rub

Near top of effusion

| Decreased to absent over the pleural air | Decreased to absent over the pleural air | None, except a possible pleural rub |

Unaffected side

Over pleural air

| Decreased to absent | Decreased | None, or the crackles, wheezes, and rhonchi of associated chronic bronchitis |

Crackles

Wheeze

| Often obscured by wheezes | Decreased | Wheezes, possibly crackles |

Wheeze

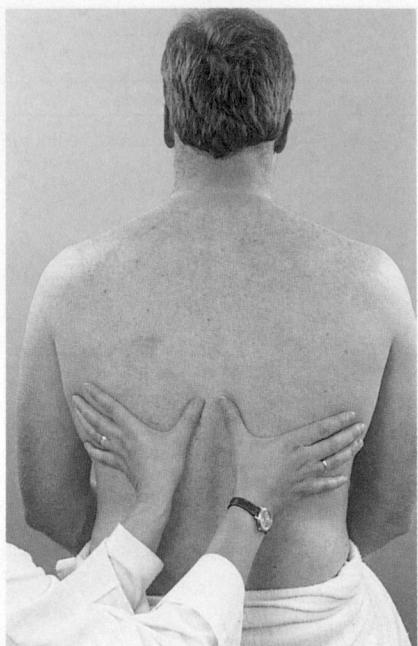

Figure 24-4 • Palpating chest expansion. The thumbs are positioned at the level of the 10th rib. (From Weber J, Kelley J: Health Assessment in Nursing, 3rd ed. Philadelphia, Lippincott Williams & Wilkins, 2007, p 312.)

PaO_2 is 80 to 100 mm Hg at sea level. The remaining 97% of oxygen is attached to hemoglobin molecules in red blood cells. Each gram of hemoglobin can carry a maximum of 1.34 mL of oxygen. The percentage of saturation of hemoglobin is defined as the amount of oxygen that hemoglobin is carrying compared with the

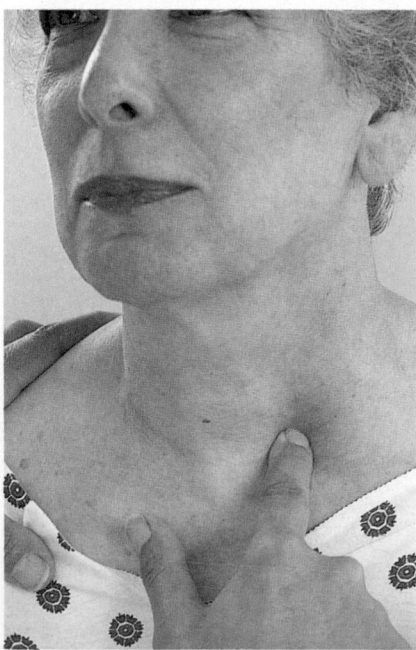

Figure 24-5 • Palpating the trachea. The trachea should be midline, above the suprasternal notch. (Photograph © B. Proud. From Weber J, Kelley J: Health Assessment in Nursing, 3rd ed. Philadelphia: Lippincott Williams & Wilkins, 2007, p 203.)

amount of oxygen that hemoglobin (Hgb) can carry, expressed as a percentage:

$$\text{Percent O}_2 \text{ saturation of Hgb} =$$

$$\frac{\text{Amount of O}_2 \text{ Hemoglobin is carrying}}{\text{Amount O}_2 \text{ Hemoglobin can carry}} \times 100$$

Because the amount of oxygen that hemoglobin can carry is a constant 1.34 mL/g,

$$1.34 \text{ mL/g} \times \text{g Hgb} \times \% \text{ saturation Hgb} =$$

$$\text{mL of O}_2 \text{ that Hgb is carrying}$$

The arterial oxygen saturation of hemoglobin is known as the SaO_2. The normal SaO_2 ranges from 93% to 99%.

The relationship between PaO_2 and SaO_2 is depicted by the oxyhemoglobin dissociation curve (Fig. 24-8). The initial part of the curve is very steep and flattens at the top. The flattened part means that large changes in the PaO_2 result in only small changes in SaO_2. A critical point of the curve occurs when the PaO_2 drops below 60 mm Hg. At this point, the curve drops sharply, signifying that a small decrease in PaO_2 is associated with a large decrease in SaO_2.

When the curve shifts to the right, there is a reduced capacity for hemoglobin to combine with oxygen, resulting in more oxygen released to the tissues. When the curve shifts to the left, there is an increased capacity for hemoglobin to combine with oxygen, resulting in less oxygen released to the tissues. See Chapter 23 for a more detailed discussion of the oxyhemoglobin dissociation curve.

A pulse oximeter, illustrated in Figure 24-9, is a device used to measure a value known as SpO_2 (oxygen saturation as measured by pulse oximetry). The SpO_2 reflects the arterial oxygen saturation of hemoglobin. Through oximetry, light-emitting and light-receiving sensors quantify the amount of light absorbed by oxygenated/deoxygenated hemoglobin in arterial blood. The value displayed on the pulse oximeter is an average of numerous readings taken in a 3- to 10-second period. This reduces the effects of pressure waveform variation caused by patient activity. Usually, the sensors are in a clip placed on a finger or ear lobe and allow for evaluation of the quality of the pulsatile waveform. Improvements in technology have resulted in a decrease in artifact caused by motion.[2] A newer device has been developed in which the oximeter sensor is placed on the forehead.[3] For assessment of pulse oximetry in infants, flexible probes can measure saturation when placed on the palm, arm, penis, or foot.

Oximetry should not be used in place of arterial blood gas (ABG) monitoring. Instead, pulse oximetry may be used to assess trends in oxygen saturation when the correlation between arterial blood and pulse oximetry readings has been established. Values obtained by pulse oximetry are unreliable when vasoconstricting medications or intravenous dyes are used and when shock, cardiac arrest, or severe anemia is present. Pulse oximetry has limited usefulness in

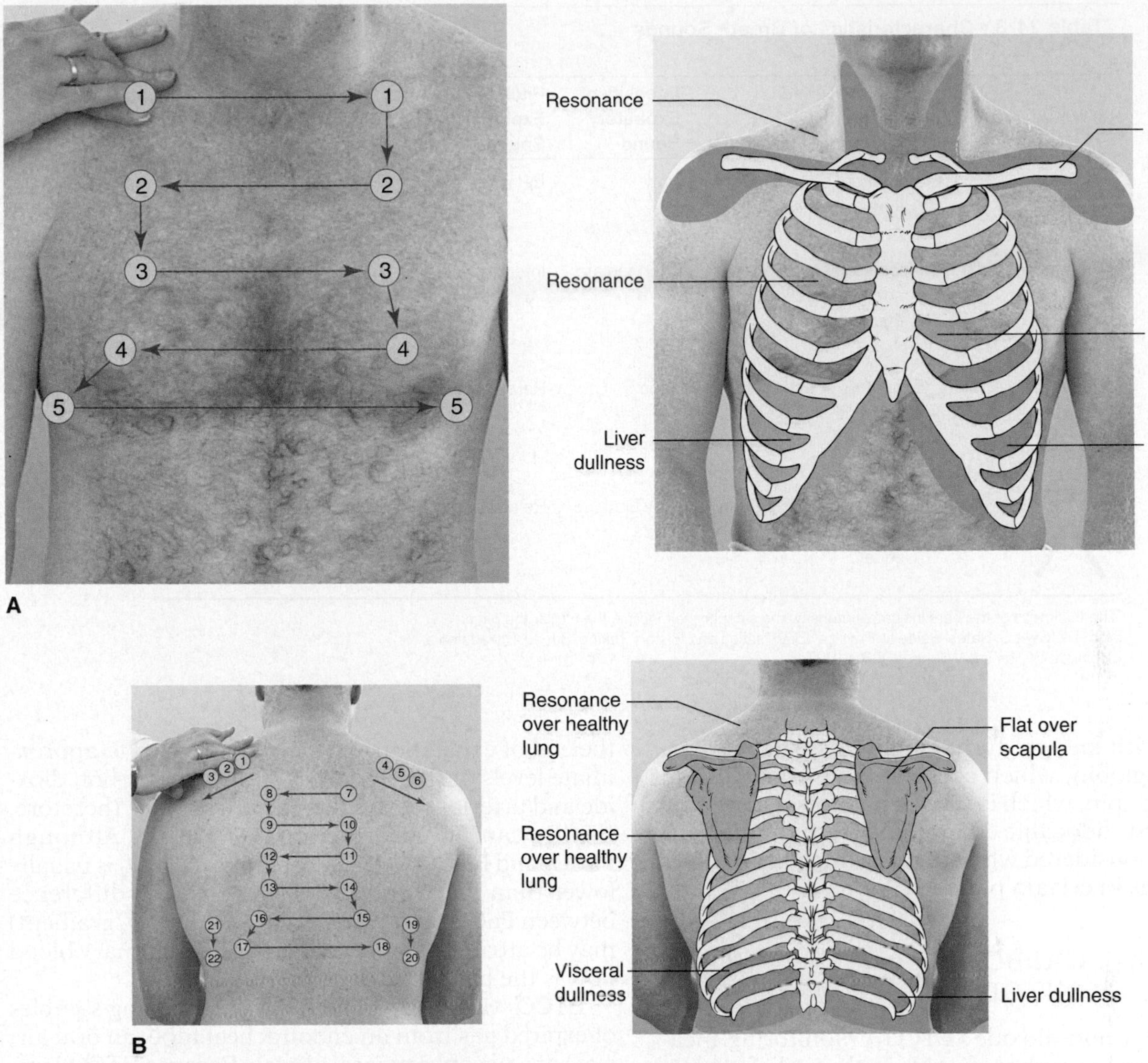

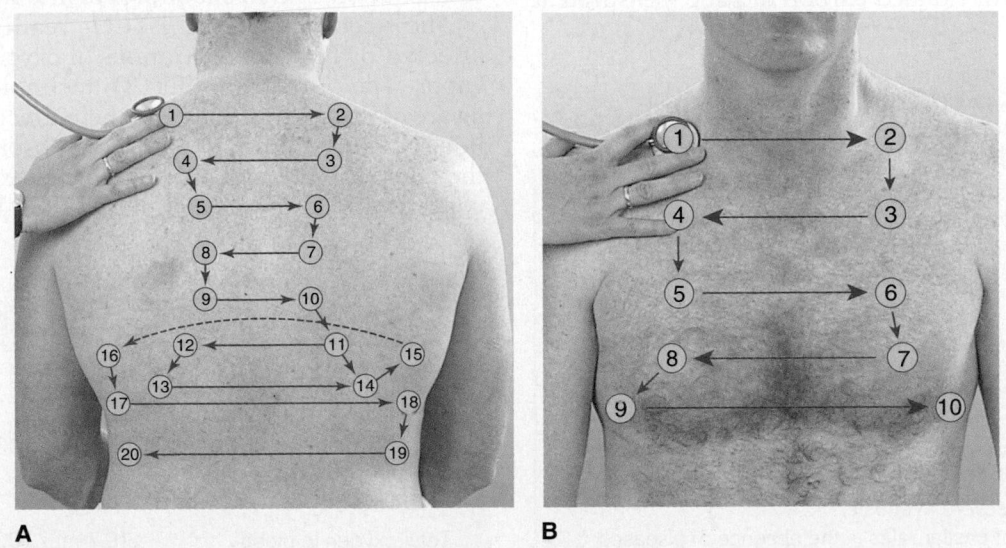

Figure 24-6 • Percussing the thorax is performed in a sequential fashion, starting near the neck and moving systematically downward. **A:** Anterior thorax. **B:** Posterior thorax. (From Weber J, Kelley J: Health Assessment in Nursing, 3rd ed. Philadelphia: Lippincott Williams & Wilkins, 2007, pp 313, 321.)

Figure 24-7 • Auscultating the chest is performed in a sequential fashion, starting near the neck and moving systematically downward. **A:** Posterior thorax. **B:** Anterior thorax. (From Weber J, Kelley J: Health Assessment in Nursing, 3rd ed. Philadelphia: Lippincott Williams & Wilkins, 2007, pp 316, 322.)

Table 24-3 • Characteristics of Breath Sounds

	Duration of Sounds	Intensity of Expiratory Sound	Pitch of Expiratory Sound	Locations Where Heard Normally
Vesicular*	Inspiratory sounds last longer than expiratory ones.	Soft	Relatively low	Over most of both lungs
Bronchovesicular	Inspiratory and expiratory sounds are about equal.	Intermediate	Intermediate	Often in the first and second interspaces anteriorly and between the scapulae
Bronchial	Expiratory sounds last longer than inspiratory ones.	Loud	Relatively high	Over the manubrium, if heard at all
Tracheal	Inspiratory and expiratory sounds are about equal.	Very loud	Relatively high	Over the trachea in the neck

*The thickness of the bars indicates intensity; the steeper their incline, the higher the pitch.
From Bickley LS: Bates' Guide to Physical Examination and History Taking, 8th ed. Philadelphia, Lippincott Williams & Wilkins, 2003, p. 227.

patients with known dyshemoglobins, such as carboxyhemoglobin, which is elevated in smokers, and methemoglobin, which is seen in patients undergoing nitrate and lidocaine therapy. These limitations should be considered when interpreting pulse oximetry readings in certain patients.

END-TIDAL CARBON DIOXIDE MONITORING

End-tidal carbon dioxide ($ETCO_2$) monitoring measures the level of carbon dioxide at the end of exhalation, when the percentage of carbon dioxide dissolved in the arterial blood ($PaCO_2$) approximates the percentage of alveolar carbon dioxide ($PACO_2$). Therefore, samples of exhaled carbon dioxide measured at the end of exhalation ($ETCO_2$) can be used to approximate levels of $PACO_2$. Levels of alveolar carbon dioxide and arterial carbon dioxide are similar; therefore, $ETCO_2$ can be used to estimate $PaCO_2$. Although $PaCO_2$ and $ETCO_2$ values are similar, $ETCO_2$ is usually lower than $PaCO_2$ by 2 to 5 mm Hg. The difference between $PaCO_2$ and $ETCO_2$ ($PaCO_2 - ETCO_2$ gradient) may be attributed to several factors; pulmonary blood flow is the primary determinant.

$ETCO_2$ values are obtained by monitoring samples of expired gas from an endotracheal tube, an oral airway, or a nasopharyngeal airway. Because $ETCO_2$ provides continuous estimates of alveolar ventilation, its measurement is useful for monitoring the patient during weaning from a ventilator, in cardiopulmonary resuscitation, and in endotracheal intubation.

The accuracy of the $ETCO_2$ readings may be affected by high concentrations of oxygen and water vapor. The nurse using $ETCO_2$ technology must be aware of these conditions and their effect on the monitor being used. Impaired infrared absorption due to the interaction of carbon dioxide and oxygen in high concentrations may cause falsely low $ETCO_2$ mea-

Box 24-4 • CONSIDERATIONS FOR THE OLDER PATIENT: Respiratory Assessment

- Decreased ability to hold breath during examination
- Increased hyperresonance (caused by increased distensibility of the lungs)
- Decreased chest wall expansion
- Decreased use of respiratory muscles
- Increased use of accessory muscles secondary to calcification of rib articulations
- Less subcutaneous tissue
- Possible pronounced dorsal curvature
    Kyphosis (abnormal convexity of the spine—see Fig. 24-1C)
    Gibbus (severe kyphosis)
- Presence of basilar rales in the absence of disease (should clear after a few coughs)

Box 24-5 • How Oxygen Is Carried in the Blood

Oxygen dissolved in the plasma measured as PaO_2	0.3 mL/100 mL of blood
Oxygen combined with hemoglobin measured as SaO_2	19.4 mL/100 mL of blood
Total oxygen in blood	19.7 mL/100 mL of blood

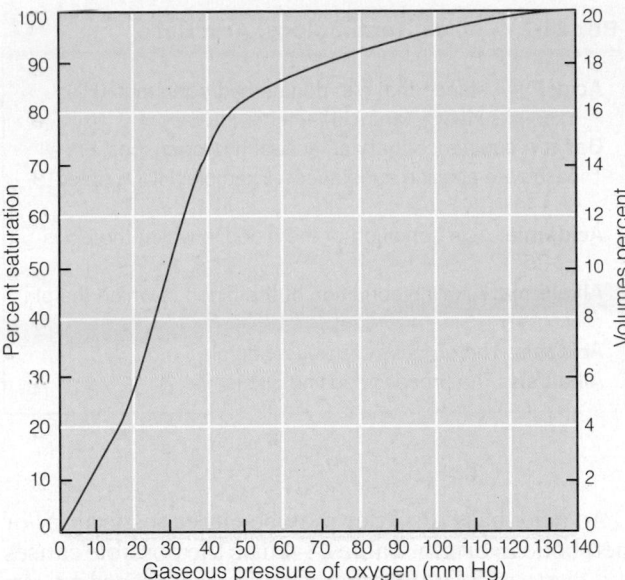

Figure 24-8 • Oxyhemoglobin dissociation curve.

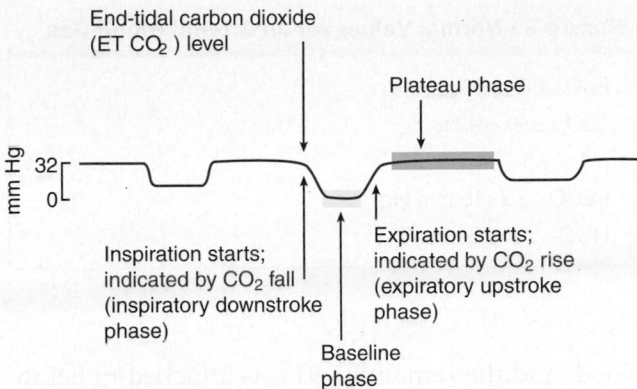

Figure 24-10 • Capnogram tracing, with four phases labeled. CO_2, carbon dioxide.

beginning of the expiratory phase, when carbon dioxide–free air in the anatomical dead space is exhaled. This value should be zero in a healthy adult.

2. The second phase is the expiratory upstroke, which represents the exhalation of carbon dioxide from the lungs. Any process that delays the delivery of carbon dioxide from the patient's lungs to the detector prolongs the expiratory upstroke. Conditions such as COPD and bronchospasm are known physiological causes of prolonged expiratory upstroke. Mechanical obstructions such as kinked ventilator tubing may also cause prolonged expiratory upstroke.

3. The third phase begins as carbon dioxide elimination rapidly continues; a plateau on the capnogram indicates the exhalation of alveolar gases. The ETCO2 is the value generated at the very end of exhalation, indicating the amount of carbon dioxide exhaled from the least ventilated alveoli.

4. The fourth phase is known as the inspiratory downstroke. The downward deflection of the waveform is caused by the washout of carbon dioxide that occurs in the presence of the oxygen influx during inspiration.

ARTERIAL BLOOD GASES

In an ABG test, a sample of arterial blood is drawn and analyzed to help determine the quality and extent of pulmonary gas exchange and acid–base status. The ABG test measures PaO_2, SaO_2, $PaCO_2$, pH, and the bicarbonate (HCO_3) level. The procedure involves obtaining arterial blood from a direct arterial puncture or from an arterial line often placed in the radial artery. More recent technology allows the continuous monitoring of ABGs using a fiberoptic sensor placed in the artery. Normal ABG values are given in Box 24-6.

Measuring Oxygen in the Blood

Oxygenation may be measured using an ABG by evaluating the PaO_2 and the SaO_2. As mentioned previously, only 3% of oxygen is dissolved in the arterial

surements, and the interference of water vapor with the absorption of infrared light may cause falsely elevated measurements. The nurse must combine ETCO2 readings with a variety of other clinical data.

The exhaled carbon dioxide waveform is displayed on the monitor as a plot of ETCO2 versus time called a capnogram, which provides the nurse with a continuous graphic reading of the patient's ETCO2 level with each exhaled breath. Changes in the waveform indicate clinical abnormalities, mechanical abnormalities, or both, and require immediate assessment by the nurse or other trained professional.

On a capnogram, the waveform is composed of four phases, each one representing a specific part of the respiratory cycle (Fig. 24-10):

1. The first phase is the baseline phase, which represents both the inspiratory phase and the very

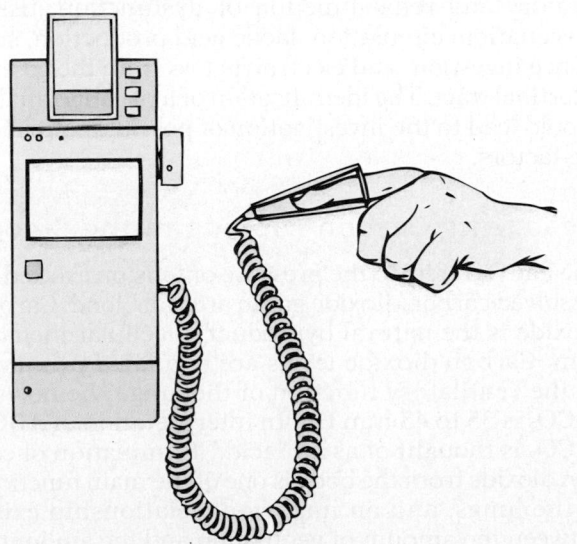

Figure 24-9 • Pulse oximetry monitor.

blood, and the remaining 97% is attached to hemoglobin in the red blood cells.

The normal PaO_2 is 80 to 100 mm Hg at sea level (barometric pressure of 760 mm Hg). For people living at higher altitudes, the normal PaO_2 is lower because of the lower barometric pressure. PaO_2 tends to decrease with age. For patients who are 60 to 80 years of age, a PaO_2 of 60 to 80 mm Hg is normal. An abnormally low PaO_2 is referred to as hypoxemia. Hypoxemia may result from many conditions, which are most commonly grouped according to their origin: intrapulmonary (disturbances in the lung), intracardiac (disturbance of flow to or from the heart, which impedes pulmonary flow or function), or perfusion (inadequate perfusion of the lung tissues, which causes decreased oxygen uptake from the alveoli) deficits.

The normal SaO_2 ranges between 93% and 97%. SaO_2 is an important oxygenation value to assess because most oxygen supplied to tissues is carried by hemoglobin.

Measuring pH in the Blood

The pH is a measure of the hydrogen ion concentration in the blood and provides information about the acidity or alkalinity of the blood. A normal pH is 7.35 to 7.45. As hydrogen ions accumulate, the pH drops, resulting in acidemia. Acidemia refers to a condition in which the blood is too acidic. Acidosis refers to the process that caused the acidemia.

A decrease in hydrogen ions results in an elevation of the pH and alkalemia. Alkalemia refers to a condition in which the blood is too alkaline. Alkalosis refers to the process that causes the alkalemia. Box 24-7 reviews the terms used in acid–base balance.

Acids An acid is a substance that can donate a hydrogen ion (H^+) to a solution. There are two different types of acids: volatile acids and nonvolatile acids.

Volatile acids are those that can move between the liquid and gaseous states. Once in the gaseous state, these acids can be removed by the lungs. The major acid in the blood serum is carbonic acid (H_2CO_3). This acid is broken down into carbon dioxide and water by an enzyme produced in the kidneys.

Nonvolatile ("fixed") acids are those that cannot change into a gaseous form and therefore cannot be excreted by the lungs. They can only be excreted by the kidneys (a metabolic process). Examples of nonvolatile acids are lactic acid and ketoacids.

An acid–base disorder may be either respiratory or metabolic in origin. Table 24-4 lists the possible causes and signs and symptoms of acid–base disorders. An excess of either kind of acid results in acidemia. If carbon dioxide from volatile acids accumulates, then respiratory acidosis exists. If nonvolatile acids accumulate, then metabolic acidosis exists.

Alkalemia may be the result of losing too many acids from the serum. If too much carbon dioxide is lost, the result is respiratory alkalosis. If there are less than normal amounts of nonvolatile acids, the result is metabolic alkalosis.

Bases A base is a substance that can accept a hydrogen ion (H^+), thereby removing it from the circulating serum. The main base found in the serum is bicarbonate (HCO_3). The amount of bicarbonate that is available in the serum is regulated by the kidney (a metabolic process). If there is too little bicarbonate in the serum, the result is metabolic acidosis. If there is too much bicarbonate in the serum, the result is metabolic alkalosis.

Conditions leading to acidemia or alkalemia are influenced by a multitude of physiological processes (see Table 24-4). Some of these processes include respiratory and renal function or dysfunction, tissue oxygenation, circulation, lactic acid production, substance ingestion, and electrolyte loss from the gastrointestinal tract. The identification of a pH abnormality should lead to the investigation of possible contributing factors.

Measuring Carbon Dioxide in the Blood

The $PaCO_2$ refers to the pressure or tension exerted by dissolved carbon dioxide gas in arterial blood. Carbon dioxide is the natural byproduct of cellular metabolism. Carbon dioxide levels are regulated primarily by the ventilatory function of the lung. The normal $PaCO_2$ is 35 to 45 mm Hg. In interpretation of ABGs, $PaCO_2$ is thought of as an "acid." Elimination of carbon dioxide from the body is one of the main functions of the lungs, and an important relationship exists between the amount of ventilation and the amount of carbon dioxide in blood.

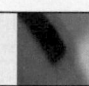

Table 24-4 • Possible Causes and Signs and Symptoms of Acid–Base Disorders

Condition	Possible Causes	Signs and Symptoms

Respiratory Acidosis
PaCO$_2$ > 45 mm Hg
pH < 7.35
	Central nervous system depression
	  Head trauma
	  Oversedation
	  Anesthesia
	  High cord injury
	Pneumothorax
	Hypoventilation
	Bronchial obstruction and atelectasis
	Severe pulmonary infections
	Heart failure and pulmonary edema
	Massive pulmonary embolus
	Myasthenia gravis
	Multiple sclerosis
		Dyspnea
		Restlessness
		Headache
		Tachycardia
		Confusion
		Lethargy
		Dysrhythmias
		Respiratory distress
		Drowsiness
		Decreased responsiveness

Respiratory Alkalosis PaCO$_2$ < 35 mm Hg pH > 7.45	Anxiety and nervousness Fear Pain Hyperventilation Fever Thyrotoxicosis Central nervous system lesions Salicylates Gram-negative septicemia Pregnancy	Light-headedness Confusion Decreased concentration Paresthesias Tetanic spasms in the arms and legs Cardiac dysrhythmias Palpitations Sweating Dry mouth Blurred vision

Metabolic Acidosis
HCO$_3$ < 22 mEq/L
pH < 7.35
	Increased acids
	  Renal failure
	  Ketoacidosis
	  Anaerobic metabolism
	  Starvation
	  Salicylate intoxication
	Loss of base
	  Diarrhea
	  Intestinal fistulas
		Headache
		Confusion
		Restlessness
		Lethargy
		Weakness
		Stupor/coma
		Kussmaul respiration
		Nausea and vomiting
		Dysrhythmias
		Warm, flushed skin

Metabolic Alkalosis
HCO$_3$ > 26 mEq/L
pH > 7.45
	Gain of base
	  Excess use of bicarbonate
	  Lactate administration in dialysis
	  Excess ingestion of antacids
	Loss of acids
	  Vomiting
	  Nasogastric suctioning
	  Hypokalemia
	  Hypochloremia
	  Administration of diuretics
	  Increased levels of aldosterone
		Muscle twitching and cramps
		Tetany
		Dizziness
		Lethargy
		Weakness
		Disorientation
		Convulsions
		Coma
		Nausea and vomiting
		Depressed respiration

If a patient hypoventilates, carbon dioxide accumulates, and the PaCO$_2$ value increases above the upper limit of 45 mm Hg. The retention of carbon dioxide results in respiratory acidosis. Respiratory acidosis may occur even with normal lungs if the respiratory center is depressed and the respiratory rate or quality is insufficient to maintain normal carbon dioxide concentrations.

If a patient hyperventilates, carbon dioxide is eliminated from the body, and the PaCO$_2$ value decreases below the lower limit of 35 mm Hg. The loss of carbon dioxide results in respiratory alkalosis.

Measuring Bicarbonate in the Blood

Bicarbonate (HCO$_3$), the main base found in the serum, helps the body regulate pH because of its ability to accept a hydrogen ion (H$^+$). The concentration of bicarbonate is regulated by the kidneys and is referred to as a metabolic process of regulation. The normal bicarbonate level is 22 to 26 mEq/L. Bicarbonate may be thought of as a "base" (alkaline). When the bicarbonate level increases above 26 mEq/L, a metabolic alkalosis exists. Metabolic alkalosis results from a gain of base (alkaline) substances or a loss of metabolic acids. When the bicarbonate level decreases below 22 mEq/L, a metabolic acidosis exists. Metabolic acidosis results from a loss of base (alkaline) substances or a gain of metabolic acids.

Alterations in Acid–Base Balance

Disturbances in acid–base balance result from an abnormality of the metabolic or respiratory system. If the respiratory system is responsible, it is detected by the carbon dioxide in the serum. If the metabolic system is responsible, it is detected by the bicarbonate in the serum.

Respiratory Acidosis Respiratory acidosis is defined as a $PaCO_2$ greater than 45 mm Hg and a pH of less than 7.35. Respiratory acidosis is characterized by inadequate elimination of carbon dioxide by the lungs and may be the result of inefficient pulmonary function or excessive production of carbon dioxide.

Respiratory Alkalosis Respiratory alkalosis is defined as a $PaCO_2$ less than 35 mm Hg and a pH of greater than 7.45. Respiratory alkalosis is characterized by excessive elimination of carbon dioxide from the serum.

Metabolic Acidosis Metabolic acidosis is defined as a bicarbonate level of less than 22 mEq/L and a pH of less than 7.35. Metabolic acidosis is characterized by an excessive production of nonvolatile acids or an inadequate concentration of bicarbonate for the concentration of acid within the serum.

Metabolic Alkalosis Metabolic alkalosis is defined as a bicarbonate level of greater than 26 mEq/L and a pH of greater than 7.45. Metabolic alkalosis is characterized by excessive loss of nonvolatile acids or excessive production of bicarbonate.

Interpreting Arterial Blood Gas Results

When interpreting ABG results, three factors must be considered: (1) oxygenation status, (2) acid–base status, and (3) degree of compensation. A suggested approach for interpreting ABG results is presented in Box 24-8, along with sample values for interpretation.

Evaluating Oxygenation It is necessary to examine the patient's oxygenation status by evaluating the PaO_2 and the SaO_2. If the PaO_2 value is less than the patient's norm, hypoxemia exists. If the SaO_2 is less than 93%, inadequate amounts of oxygen are bound to hemoglobin.

Evaluating Acid–Base Status The first step in evaluating acid–base status is the examination of the arterial pH. If the pH is less than 7.35, acidemia exists. If the pH is greater than 7.45, alkalemia exists.

The second step in evaluating acid–base status is examination of the $PaCO_2$. A $PaCO_2$ of less than 35 mm Hg indicates a respiratory alkalosis, whereas a $PaCO_2$ of greater than 45 mm Hg signifies a respiratory acidosis.

Box 24-8 • Interpretation of Arterial Blood Gas (ABG) Results

Approach

1. Evaluate oxygenation by examining the PaO_2 and the SaO_2.
2. Evaluate the pH. Is it acidotic, alkalotic, or normal?
3. Evaluate the $PaCO_2$. Is it high, low, or normal?
4. Evaluate the HCO_3. Is it high, low, or normal?
5. Determine whether compensation is occurring. Is it complete, partial, or uncompensated?

Examples

Sample blood gas: Case 1

PaO_2	80 mm Hg	Normal
SaO_2	95%	Normal
pH	7.30	Acidemia
$PaCO_2$	55 mm Hg	Increased (respiratory cause)
HCO_3	25 mEq/L	Normal

Conclusion: Respiratory acidosis (uncompensated)

Sample blood gas: Case 2

PaO_2	85 mm Hg	Normal
SaO_2	90%	Low saturation
pH	7.49	Alkalemia
$PaCO_2$	40	Normal
HCO_3	29 mEq/L	Increased (metabolic cause)

Conclusion: Metabolic alkalosis with a low saturation (uncompensated)

The third step in evaluating acid–base status is examination of the bicarbonate level. If the bicarbonate value is less than 22 mEq/L, metabolic acidosis is present. If the bicarbonate value is greater than 26 mEq/L, metabolic alkalosis exists.

Occasionally, patients present with both respiratory and metabolic disorders that together cause an acidemia or alkalemia. For example, alkalosis could result from an increase in bicarbonate and a decrease in carbon dioxide, or an acidosis could result from a decrease in bicarbonate and an increase in carbon dioxide. A patient with metabolic acidosis from acute renal failure could also have a very slow respiratory rate that causes the patient to retain carbon dioxide, creating a respiratory acidosis. Therefore, the ABG reflects a mixed respiratory and metabolic acidosis. Box 24-9 lists examples of mixed gases.

Box 24-9 • Arterial Blood Gases in Mixed Respiratory and Metabolic Disorders

MIXED ACIDOSIS	MIXED ALKALOSIS
pH: 7.25	pH: 7.55
$PaCO_2$: 56 mm Hg	$PaCO_2$: 26 mm Hg
PaO_2: 80 mm Hg	PaO_2: 80 mm Hg
HCO_3: 15 mEq/L	HCO_3: 28 mEq/L

Determining Compensation If the patient presents with an alkalemia or acidemia, it is important to determine whether the body has tried to compensate for the abnormality. If the buffer systems in the body are unable to maintain normal pH, then the renal or respiratory systems attempt to compensate. If the problem is respiratory in origin, the kidneys work to correct it. If the problem is renal in origin, the lungs try to correct it. It may take as little as 5 to 15 minutes for the lungs to recognize a metabolic presentation and start to correct it. It may take up to 1 day for the kidneys to correct the respiratory-induced problem. One system will not overcompensate; that is, a compensatory mechanism will never make an acidotic patient alkalotic or an alkalotic patient acidotic.

The respiratory system responds to metabolic-based pH imbalances in the following manner:

▶ Metabolic acidosis: increase in respiratory rate and depth
▶ Metabolic alkalosis: decrease in respiratory rate and depth

The renal system responds to respiratory-based pH imbalances in the following manner:

▶ Respiratory acidosis: increase in hydrogen secretion and bicarbonate reabsorption
▶ Respiratory alkalosis: decrease in hydrogen secretion and bicarbonate reabsorption

ABGs are defined by their degree of compensation: uncompensated, partially compensated, or completely compensated. To determine the level of compensation, the pH, carbon dioxide, and bicarbonate are examined. First, it is determined whether the pH is acidotic or alkalotic. In some cases, the pH is not within the normal range, indicating an acidosis or alkalosis. If it is within the normal range, it is important to determine on which side of 7.40 (midpoint of the normal pH range) the pH lies. For example, a pH of 7.38 is tending toward acidosis, whereas a pH of 7.41 is tending toward alkalosis. Next, an evaluation is made to see whether carbon dioxide or bicarbonate has changed to account for the acidosis or alkalosis. Finally, it is determined whether the opposite system (metabolic or respiratory) has worked to try to shift back toward a normal pH. The primary abnormality (metabolic or respiratory) is correlated with the abnormal pH (acidotic or alkalotic). The secondary abnormality is an attempt to correct the primary disorder. By using the rules for defining compensation in Box 24-10, it is possible to determine the compensatory status of the patient's ABGs.

MIXED VENOUS OXYGEN SATURATION

Mixed venous oxygen saturation ($S\overline{v}O_2$) is a parameter that can be measured to evaluate the balance between oxygen supply and oxygen demand. Blood obtained from a vein in an extremity gives information mostly about that extremity; it can be quite misleading if the metabolism in the extremity differs from the metabolism of the body as a whole. This difference is accen-

---

Box 24-10 • Compensatory Status of Arterial Blood Gases

Uncompensated: pH is *abnormal*, and *either* the CO_2 or HCO_3 is also abnormal. There is no indication that the opposite system has tried to correct for the other.

In the example below, the patient's pH is alkalotic as a result of the low (below the normal range of 35–45 mm Hg) CO_2 concentration. The renal system value (HCO_3) has not moved out its normal range (22–26 mEq/L) to compensate for the primary respiratory disorder.

PaO_2:	94 mm Hg	Normal
pH:	7.52	Alkalotic
$PaCO_2$:	25 mm Hg	Decreased
HCO_3:	24 mEq/L	Normal

Partially compensated: pH is *abnormal*, and *both* the CO_2 and HCO_3 are also abnormal; this indicates that one system has attempted to correct for the other but has not been completely successful.

In the example below, the patient's pH remains alkalotic as a result of the low CO_2 concentration. The renal system value (HCO_3) has moved out its normal range (22–26 mEq/L) to compensate for the primary respiratory disorder but has not been able to bring the pH back within the normal range.

PaO_2:	94 mm Hg	Normal
pH:	7.48	Alkalotic
$PaCO_2$:	25 mm Hg	Decreased
HCO_3:	20 mEq/L	Decreased

Completely compensated: pH is *normal* and *both* the CO_2 and HCO_3 are abnormal; the normal pH indicates that one system has been able to compensate for the other.

In the example below, the patient's pH is normal but is tending toward alkalosis (>7.40). The primary abnormality is respiratory because the $PaCO_2$ is low (decreased acid concentration). The bicarbonate value of 18 mEq/L reflects decreased concentration of base and is associated with acidosis, not alkalosis. In this case, the decreased bicarbonate has completely compensated for the respiratory alkalosis.

PaO_2:	94 mm Hg	Normal
pH:	7.44	Normal, tending toward alkalosis
$PaCO_2$:	25 mm Hg	Decreased, primary problem
HcO_3:	18 mEq/L	Decreased, compensatory response

---

tuated if the extremity is cold or underperfused (e.g., in shock), if the patient has performed local exercises with the extremity (e.g., opening and closing the fist), or if there is local infection in the extremity.

Sometimes blood is sampled through a central venous pressure (CVP) catheter in the hope of obtaining mixed venous blood, but even in the superior vena cava or right atrium where a CVP catheter ends, there is usually incomplete mixing of venous return from various parts of the body. For complete mixing of the blood, it is necessary to obtain a blood sample from a pulmonary artery catheter. Use of the pulmonary artery catheter provides a sample of blood that has returned from the extremities and has been mixed in the right ventricle.

Oxygen measurements of mixed venous blood indicate whether the tissues are being oxygenated, but $S\bar{v}O_2$ does not distinguish the independent contributions of the heart and the lungs. $S\bar{v}O_2$ indicates the adequacy of the supply of oxygen relative to the demand for oxygen at the tissue levels. Normal $S\bar{v}O_2$ is 60% to 80%; this means that supply of oxygen to the tissues is adequate to meet the tissue's demand. However, a normal value does not indicate whether compensatory mechanisms were needed to maintain the perfusion. For example, in some patients, an increase in cardiac output is needed to compensate for a low supply of oxygen.

A low $S\bar{v}O_2$ may be caused by a decrease in oxygen supply to the tissues or an increase in oxygen use due to a high demand. A decrease in oxygen supply results from low hemoglobin, hemorrhage, or low cardiac output. An increase in oxygen demand results from hyperthermia, pain, stress, shivering, or seizures. An $S\bar{v}O_2$ of 40% to 60% may occur in heart failure, and values less than 40% may indicate profound shock. A decrease in $S\bar{v}O_2$ often occurs before other hemodynamic changes and, therefore, is an excellent clinical tool in the assessment and management of critically ill patients. The goals of interventions for a low $S\bar{v}O_2$ include increasing the oxygen supply by blood transfusions or by increasing cardiac output. Treatment may also be aimed at eliminating the cause of the high demand.

A high $S\bar{v}O_2$ value indicates that oxygen supply exceeds demand or a decrease in the demand. Elevated $S\bar{v}O_2$ values are associated with increased delivery of oxygen (high fraction of inspired oxygen [FiO_2]) or with decreased demand from hypothermia, hypothyroidism, or anesthesia. An elevated $S\bar{v}O_2$ also is seen in the early stages of septic shock when the tissues are unable to use the oxygen. Table 24-5 summarizes possible causes of abnormalities in $S\bar{v}O_2$.

A pulmonary artery catheter with an oximeter built into its tip that allows continuous monitoring of $S\bar{v}O_2$ provides ongoing assessment of oxygen supply and demand imbalances. If a catheter with a built-in oximeter is not available, the nurse can draw blood from the pulmonary artery through a regular pulmonary artery catheter, send the sample to the laboratory for blood gas and $S\bar{v}O_2$ analysis, and use the information in the same manner.

• Respiratory Diagnostic Studies

CHEST RADIOGRAPHY

Chest radiography is a valuable diagnostic tool that clinicians frequently use to assess anatomical and physiological features of the chest and to detect pathological processes. X-rays pass through the chest wall

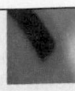

Table 24-5 • Possible Causes of Abnormalities in Mixed Venous Oxygen Saturation ($S\bar{v}O_2$)	
Abnormality	**Possible Cause**
Low $S\bar{v}O_2$ < 60%	***Decreased oxygen supply***
	Low hematocrit from anemia or hemorrhage
	Low arterial saturation and hypoxemia from lung disease, ventilation–perfusion mismatches
	Low cardiac output from hypovolemia, heart failure, cardiogenic shock, myocardial infarction
	Increased oxygen demand
	Increased metabolic demand, such as hyperthermia, seizures, shivering, pain, anxiety, stress, strenuous exercise
High $S\bar{v}O_2$ > 80%	***Increased oxygen supply***
	Supplemental oxygen
	Decreased oxygen demand
	Anesthesia, hypothermia, early stages of sepsis
	Technical problems
	False high reading because of wedged pulmonary artery catheter
	Fibrin clot at end of catheter

and make it is possible to visualize various structures. Dense tissues, such as bones, absorb the x-ray beam and appear as opaque or white on the radiograph. Blood vessels and blood-filled organs, such as the heart, are moderately dense structures and appear as gray areas on the radiograph. During inspiration, normal lungs fill with air and appear black on the radiograph. When parts of the lungs fill with fluid, which is a more dense material, the lungs appear white.

The nurse uses the radiograph as an assessment parameter to validate clinical findings and suspected abnormalities. Using a systematic approach, the nurse examines the radiograph by comparing the film with previous films. The approach can be to examine the film starting in the periphery and then to move toward the center of the chest, or to start centrally and move outward toward the soft tissue. Whatever the method, the objects of scrutiny are the soft tissue areas, the bony structures, the inner layers just under the bone, and the internal structures.

The nurse examines the soft tissues on the radiograph by looking for homogeneity, beginning with lateral areas and moving medially. Air visualized in the lateral soft tissue may indicate the presence of a pneumothorax.

Bony structures inspected on the chest film include the ribs, clavicles, sternum, manubrium, spine, and vertebrae. Approximately eight to nine ribs should overlie lung tissue on the normal chest film. The nurse examines the ribs for the presence of fractures by following the curve of each rib, beginning anteriorly and moving around posteriorly. Like the ribs, the other bony structures are examined for correct position and intactness.

The contour of the diaphragm is also visible on the radiograph. Normally, the diaphragm is rounded with sharp, pointed costophrenic angles. Pleural effusions may cause the angles to become blunted. The top of the diaphragm is apparent at about the sixth rib. A lowered diaphragm may indicate hyperinflation caused by emphysema.

The nurse assesses lung parenchyma by comparing right and left sides, moving top to bottom. Normal air-filled lungs should appear black or very dark compared with the bones and heart. It is important in the evaluation to look for symmetry. Abnormally high density on one side of the chest may indicate edema, a mass, pleural effusion, or pneumonia.

Interlobar fissures separate the lobes of the lungs. The minor fissure in the right lung is usually visible in the frontal film. Displacement of the normal fissures seen on the film may indicate the presence of atelectasis or lobar collapse.

The trachea should appear midline over the thoracic vertebrae. The trachea can shift toward areas of atelectasis and away from areas of pneumothorax, pleural effusion, or tumors.

VENTILATION–PERFUSION SCANNING

Ventilation–perfusion scanning is a nuclear imaging test used to evaluate a suspected alteration in the ventilation–perfusion relationship. (See Chapter 23 for a discussion of ventilation–perfusion relationships.) A ventilation–perfusion scan is helpful in detecting the percentage of each lung that is functioning normally, diagnosing and locating pulmonary emboli, and assessing the pulmonary vascular supply.

The ventilation–perfusion scan consists of two parts: a ventilation scan and a perfusion scan. In the ventilation scan, the patient inhales radioactive gas, which follows the same pathway as air in normal breathing. In pathological conditions, the diminished areas of ventilation are visible on the scan. In the perfusion scan, a radioisotope is injected intravenously, enabling visualization of the blood supply to the lungs. When a pulmonary embolus is present, the blood supply beyond the embolus is restricted, revealing poor or no visualization of the affected area.

Ventilation–perfusion scans are often not useful in patients dependent on mechanical ventilation because the ventilation component of the scan is difficult to perform. Ventilation–perfusion mismatches may make interpretation of ventilation–perfusion scans difficult in patients with lung diseases, such as pneumonia. Because of these limitations, pulmonary angiography may be appropriate in the critically ill patient, especially if a pulmonary embolus is suspected.

PULMONARY ANGIOGRAPHY

Pulmonary angiography involves the rapid injection of a radiopaque substance for radiographic studies of the pulmonary vasculature. Suspected pulmonary embolus is the most common indication for pulmonary angiography. A radiopaque substance is injected into one or both arms, the femoral vein, or a catheter that has been placed in the pulmonary artery. A positive test result is indicated by the impaired flow of the radiopaque substance through a narrowed vessel or by the abrupt cessation of flow of the substance in a vessel.

BRONCHOSCOPY

Bronchoscopy involves the direct visualization of the larynx, trachea, and bronchi through a flexible fiberoptic bronchoscope. Bronchoscopy is used diagnostically to examine tissues, collect secretions, determine the extent and location of a pathologic process, and obtain a biopsy. In addition, bronchoscopy is used therapeutically as a means to remove foreign bodies or secretions from the tracheobronchial tree, treat postoperative atelectasis, and excise lesions.

In preparation for a bronchoscopy, a history and physical examination should be performed. A chest radiograph, clotting studies, and ABGs also are obtained. The patient often receives intravenous sedation or analgesia before the procedure. If the purpose of the bronchoscopy is therapeutic, medications that suppress a cough or diminish secretions are avoided (e.g., intratracheal topical anesthetics, atropine, and codeine).

Careful monitoring of the patient is indicated after a bronchoscopy. The nurse assesses for any evidence of complications, which may include laryngospasm, fever, hemodynamic changes, cardiac dysrhythmias, pneumothorax, hemorrhage, or cardiopulmonary arrest.

THORACENTESIS

In thoracentesis, a needle is inserted into the pleural space to remove air, fluid, or both; obtain specimens for diagnostic evaluation; or instill medications. A chest radiograph, coagulation studies, and patient education are essential before a thoracentesis. Some patients may require medication to reduce anxiety. Unlike bronchoscopy, thoracentesis requires the cooperation of the patient; therefore, a local anesthetic, rather than moderate sedation, is used to minimize the pain and discomfort that accompanies the procedure. During the procedure, the patient is placed either in a chair or on the edge of the bed in an upright position with arms and shoulders raised so that the ribs lift and separate, allowing easier needle insertion. If a patient is unable to lift his or her arms, sitting on the bed with the arms placed above the head on a table is an alternative position.

During thoracentesis, the nurse's primary function is to provide comfort for the patient, perform ongoing assessment of the patient's respiratory system, dress the wound with sterile dressings on completion of the procedure, and send labeled laboratory specimens as ordered. Post-thoracentesis nursing care includes assessment for complications, including pneumothorax, pain, hypotension, and pulmonary edema.

SPUTUM CULTURE

Sputum specimens are often part of the respiratory assessment. Because healthy patients do not produce sputum, obtaining a specimen requires the patient to cough to bring up sputum from the lungs. It is essential that the nurse distinguish sputum from saliva before sending the specimen to the laboratory.

In most cases, sputum specimens are obtained to examine for culture and sensitivity. The specimen is examined for specific microorganisms and their corresponding drug sensitivities. In addition, sputum specimens are also required for studies of cytology and acid-fast bacilli. Culture of acid-fast bacilli requires serial collection (usually over 3 days) and is used to identify the presence of tuberculosis and mycobacteria.

PULMONARY FUNCTION TESTS

The flow of air in and out of the lungs provides tangible measures of lung volumes. Although these volumes are referred to as measures of "pulmonary function," in reality they are measures of pulmonary anatomy. In the evaluation of ventilation, structure or anatomy often determines function. Ventilatory or pulmonary function tests measure the ability of the chest and lungs to move air into and out of the alveoli.

Pulmonary function tests include volume measurements, capacity measurements, and dynamic measurements. These measurements are influenced by exercise and disease. Age, sex, body size, and posture are other variables that are taken into consideration when the test results are interpreted. Figure 23-13 in Chapter 23 illustrates pulmonary function tests showing normal lung volumes and capacity.

Volume Measurements

Volume measurements show the amount of air contained in the lungs during various parts of the respiratory cycle. Measures of lung volume include tidal volume (V_T), inspiratory reserve volume (IRV), expiratory reserve volume (ERV), and residual volume (RV; see Chapter 23, Table 23-1).

Capacity Measurements

Capacity measurements quantify part of the pulmonary cycle. They are a combination of the previous volumes and include inspiratory capacity (IC), functional residual capacity (FRC), vital capacity (VC), and total lung capacity (TLC; see Chapter 23, Table 23-1).

Dynamic Measurements

The following measurements, called dynamic measurements, provide data about airway resistance and the energy expended in breathing (work of breathing).

▶ Respiratory rate or frequency is the number of breaths per minute. At rest, the respiratory rate is about 15 breaths/minute.
▶ Minute volume, sometimes called minute ventilation, is the volume of air inhaled and exhaled per minute. It is calculated by multiplying tidal volume by respiratory rate. At rest, the minute volume is approximately 7,500 mL/minute.

▶ Dead space is the part of the tidal volume that does not participate in alveolar gas exchange. The dead space (measured in milliliters) is the air contained in the airways (anatomical dead space) plus the volume of alveolar air that is not involved in gas exchange (physiological dead space; e.g., air in an unperfused alveolus due to pulmonary embolism or, more commonly, air in underperfused alveoli). Adult anatomical dead space is usually equal to the body weight in pounds (e.g., 140 mL in a 140-lb person). In a healthy person, dead space is composed only of anatomical dead space. Physiological dead space occurs in certain disease states. Dead space is calculated by subtracting the partial pressure of arterial carbon dioxide ($PaCO_2$) from the partial pressure of alveolar carbon dioxide ($PACO_2$). The normal value of dead space in healthy adults is typically less than 40% of the tidal volume. The dead space/tidal volume ratio is used to follow the effectiveness of mechanical ventilation.

▶ Alveolar ventilation, the complement of dead space, is expressed as the volume of tidal air that is involved in alveolar gas exchange. This volume is represented as volume per minute by the symbol $\dot{V}_A$. $\dot{V}_A$ is a measure of ventilatory effectiveness. It is more relevant to the blood gas values than either the dead space or tidal volume because these last two measures include physiological dead space. $\dot{V}_A$ is calculated by subtracting the dead space (V_D) from the tidal volume (V_T) and multiplying the result by the respiratory rate (f):

$$\dot{V}_A = (V_T - V_D) \times f$$

About 2,300 mL of air (FRC) remains in the lung at the end of expiration. Each new breath introduces about 350 mL of air into the alveoli. The ratio of new alveoli air to total volume of air remaining in the lungs is:

$$\frac{350 \text{ mL}}{2,300 \text{ mL}}$$

Therefore, new air is only about one seventh of the total volume contained in the lungs. The normal is 5,250 mL/minute (350 mL/breath × 15 breaths/minute = 5,250 mL/minute). A normal breath (V_T) can replace 7,500 mL of air per minute (500 mL/breath × 15 breaths/minute = 7,500 mL/minute), requiring 0.008 second/mL:

$$\frac{1 \text{ minute}}{7,500 \text{ mL}} \times \frac{60 \text{ seconds}}{1 \text{ minute}} = 0.008 \text{ seconds/mL}$$

Therefore, the FRC of the lungs can be completely replaced in 18.4 seconds (2,300 mL × 0.008 second/mL = 18.4 seconds) if air diffusion is uniform. This slow turnover rate prevents rapid fluctuations of gas concentrations in the alveoli with each breath.

• Clinical Applicability Challenges

Case Study

Mr. J. is a 75-year-old man who has been admitted to the cardiac care unit with a diagnosis of exacerbated congestive heart failure. He has a history of two myocardial infarctions and is status post–triple coronary artery bypass graft (CABG × 3) 4 years ago.

On admission to the unit, Mr. J. is profoundly short of breath, restless, and tachycardic. His daughter who accompanied him to the hospital tells you that Mr. J. is uncharacteristically confused. On physical examination, his respiratory rate is 32 breaths/minute, and he is using accessory muscles for breathing. His heart rate is 126 beats/minute, and his blood pressure is 100/64 mm Hg. His mucous membranes are pale, and he has a Glasgow Coma Scale score of 14. On auscultation, you hear coarse crackles in both bases with some audible expiratory wheezing. During assessment of breath sounds, when you ask the patient to whisper, you are able to clearly hear the sounds he makes through the stethoscope. In addition, his jugular veins are visibly distended at 45 degrees. arterial bloods gases (ABGs) are PaO_2, 68 mm Hg; $PaCO_2$, 49 mm Hg; HCO_3, 29 mEq/L; and pH, 7.31.

1. What three findings from Mr. J.'s assessment are consistent with a diagnosis of heart failure?

2. Describe some of the differences in respiratory assessment of the older patient.

3. What are some immediate signs of respiratory distress that you recognize in Mr. J. even before you begin to auscultate his lungs or draw the ABG?

4. Why is Mr. J. tachypneic?

5. Why were you able to hear Mr. J. so clearly with the stethoscope when he whispered? What is this condition called?

6. How would you interpret the ABG results? Is Mr. J. compensating?

Review Questions

1. A nurse in the progressive care unit is caring for a patient admitted with a diagnosis of heart failure. During her shift, she notices that the patient's respiratory status progressively worsens. Her assessment yields significant dyspnea with adventitious breath sounds bilaterally in the bases. In addition, she notices that the patient is lethargic. When explaining the patient's condition to the attending physician, she receives an order for an arterial blood gas. The values returned include the following: PaO_2, 82%; SaO_2, 94%; pH, 7.30; $PaCO_2$, 53 mm Hg; and HCO_3, 24 mEq/L. The patient's condition is described by which of the following:
   a. Respiratory acidosis
   b. Metabolic acidosis
   c. Metabolic alkalosis
   d. Respiratory alkalosis

2. A critical care unit nurse is caring for a 78-year-old female patient admitted with a primary diagnosis of acute coronary syndrome. During his assessment, the nurse hears basilar crackles bilaterally that clear with a cough. In addition, he notices that the patient's chest wall expansion is decreased and that the patient has some rather pronounced dorsal curvature of the spine. The nurse is not alarmed because he understands that these are typical findings in older adult patients. Which of the following is another physical assessment finding often present in the older adult?
   a. Kussmaul respirations
   b. Clubbing of the fingers
   c. Decreased use of respiratory muscles
   d. Diffuse hyperresonance

3. A nurse in the intensive care unit is completing an assessment on a 30-year-old male patient who presents status post–open reduction and internal fixation of the left femur. During her assessment of the otherwise healthy male, the nurse auscultates breath sounds over the trachea. What are the characteristics of the breath sounds is she likely to hear?
   a. Soft, low-pitched sounds where inspiration is longer than expiration
   b. Loud, high-pitched sounds where expiration is longer than inspiration
   c. Very loud, high-pitched sounds where inspiration and expiration are equal
   d. Moderately loud sounds, with an intermediate pitch where inspiration and expiration are equal

4. A cardiothoracic critical care nurse is preparing for the return of a patient from the cardiac operating room where the patient just underwent a triple bypass. Because of the general impact of anesthesia and surgery on the respiratory process, the critical care nurse understands the importance of continuous monitoring to assess the patient's gas exchange. Which of the following methods of assessment is most appropriate in this case?
   a. End-tidal monitoring
   b. Pulse oximetry
   c. Arterial blood gas
   d. Physical assessment

5. A patient in the cardiac care unit is status post–myocardial infarction, and based on his assessment, the nurse believes that the patient is experiencing cardiogenic shock. During morning rounds, the nurse shares his assessment of the patient's condition with the medical team. To better understand the patient's perfusion status, the attending physician orders $S\overline{v}O_2$ monitoring. The patient's initial $S\overline{v}O_2$ reading is 56%. Which of the following items is a likely contributor to the patient's low $S\overline{v}O_2$?
   a. Wedged pulmonary artery catheter
   b. Low cardiac output state
   c. Fibrin clot at the end of the $S\overline{v}O_2$ catheter
   d. Hypothermia

References

1. Bickley LS, Szilagyi PG: Bates' Guide to Physical Examination and History Taking, 9th ed. Philadelphia: Lippincott Williams & Wilkins, 2007
2. Giuliano KK, Higgins TL: New-generation pulse oximetry in the care of critically ill patients. Am J Crit Care 14(1):26–37, 2005
3. Fernandez M, Burns K, Calhoun B, et al: Evaluation of a new pulse oximeter sensor. Am J Crit Care 16(2):146–152, 2007

Other Selected Readings

Ahrens T, Sona C: Capnography applications in acute and critical care. AACN Clin Issues 14(2):123–132, 2003

Attin M, Cardin S, Doering L, et al: An educational project to improve knowledge related to pulse oximetry. Am J Crit Care 11(6):529–534, 2002

Berry BE, Pinard AE: Assessing tissue oxygenation. Crit Care Nurse 22(3):22–42, 2002

Branson RD, Mannheimer PD: Forehead oximetry in critically ill patients: The case for a new monitoring site. Respir Care Clin North Am 10:359–367, 2004

Ruffolo DC, Headley JM: Regional carbon dioxide monitoring: A different look at tissue perfusion. AACN Clin Issues 14(2):168–175, 2003

St. John RE: End-tidal carbon dioxide monitoring. Crit Care Nurse 23(4): 83–88, 2003

Weber J, Kelley J: Health Assessment in Nursing, 3rd ed. Philadelphia: Lippincott Williams & Wilkins, 2007

Patient Management: Respiratory System

25

Charles A. Fisher • Donna L. Charlebois •
Sidenia S. Tribble • Paul K. Merrel

Objectives

Based on the content in this chapter, the reader should
be able to:

❶ Summarize the desired outcomes of the various
    bronchial hygiene therapies.

❷ Compare and contrast situations in which chest
    physiotherapy (including postural drainage) is
    useful versus contraindicated situations.

❸ Discuss two goals of oxygen delivery.

❹ Describe the nursing assessment of patients on
    oxygen therapy.

❺ Explain three complications of oxygen therapy.

❻ Compare and contrast indications for, and
    complications of, orotracheal intubation versus
    nasotracheal intubation.

❼ Identify four iatrogenic procedures or therapies that
    can lead to pneumothorax.

❽ Compare and contrast the principles governing
    chest tube drainage systems.

❾ Discuss nursing interventions necessary to prevent
    complications in a patient with a chest tube
    drainage system.

❿ Discuss the pharmacology for the treatment of
    bronchospasm in asthma and chronic obstructive
    pulmonary disease.

⓫ Explain causes of agitation in critically ill patients.

⓬ Define respiratory failure, and list three causes.

⓭ Differentiate between the principles of negative-
    pressure ventilation and positive-pressure ventilation.

⓮ Differentiate between pressure-cycled and volume-
    cycled ventilators in positive-pressure ventilation.

⓯ Compare and contrast the following ventilator
    modes: assist-control, synchronized intermittent
    mandatory, pressure-support, and pressure-
    controlled ventilation.

⓰ Summarize strategies to maximize oxygen delivery
    with the goal of achieving a nontoxic FiO_2 setting.

⓱ Summarize adverse effects of positive end-
    expiratory pressure, how they are identified, and
    the appropriate treatment.

⓲ Compare and contrast the advantages and
    disadvantages of tracheostomy versus
    endotracheal intubation.

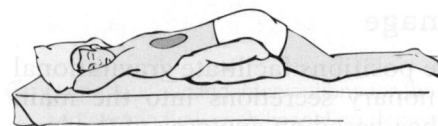

A. Face-lying—hips elevated 16–18 inches on pillows, making a 30°–45° angle.
Purpose: to drain the posterior lower lobes.

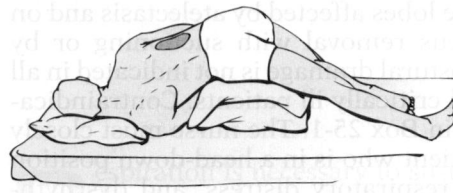

B. Lying on the left side—hips elevated 16–18 inches on pillows.
Purpose: to drain the right lateral lower lung segments.

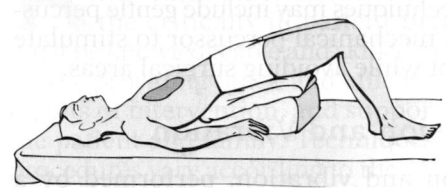

C. Back lying—hips elevated 16–18 inches on pillows.
Purpose: to drain the anterior lower lung segments.

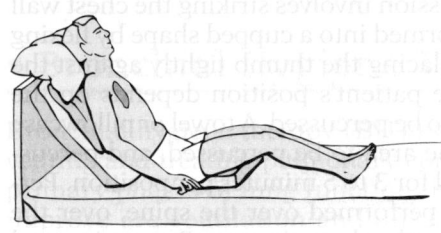

D. Sitting upright or semireclining.
Purpose: to drain the upper lung field and allow more forceful coughing.

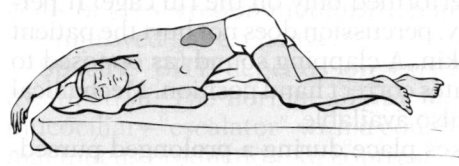

E. Lying on the right side—hips elevated on pillows forming a 30°–45° angle.
Purpose: to drain the left lower lobes.

Figure 25-2 • Positions used in lung drainage.

Box 25-1 • RED FLAG: Contraindications to Chest Physiotherapy

Contraindications to Postural Drainage
• Increased intracranial pressure
• After meals/during tube feeding
• Inability to cough
• Hypoxia/respiratory instability
• Hemodynamic instability
• Decreased mental status
• Recent eye surgery
• Hiatal hernia
• Obesity

Contraindications to Percussion/Vibration
• Fractured ribs/osteoporosis
• Chest/abdominal trauma or surgery
• Pulmonary hemorrhage or embolus
• Chest malignancy/mastectomy
• Pneumothorax/subcutaneous emphysema
• Cervical cord trauma
• Tuberculosis
• Pleural effusions/empyema
• Asthma

atelectasis caused by mucus obstruction and diseases that result in increased sputum production (at least 30 mL/day) such as cystic fibrosis and bronchiectasis.[6] Bronchoscopy is an alternative treatment to remove mucus plugs that result in atelectasis. CPT may produce bronchospasm in asthmatics and spread infected material to uninfected lung tissue in patients with unilateral pneumonia.

The inclusion of CPT in the plan of care should be individualized and evaluated in terms of derived benefit versus potential risks. In addition, CPT should be discontinued when it fails to promote treatment goals. In patients who cannot tolerate CPT, turning the patient laterally every 2 hours aids in mobilizing secretions for removal with cough or suctioning. Progressive mobility from sitting up in a chair, to weight bearing, and to ambulation is used in all ventilated patients as part of pulmonary hygiene as well as increasing patient strength and endurance. Patients with an artificial airway or an ineffective cough may require suctioning after CPT.

To be effective, CPT must be accompanied by the postural drainage position specific to the affected area of the lung. Patients with unilateral disease are positioned with the healthy lung down for better ventilation and perfusion.[7] Positioning the patient with the diseased lung down is likely to cause hypoxemia with ventilation-perfusion mismatching and shunting. Positioning is altered if the patient has a lung abscess. In such cases, the preferred position is with the diseased lung down because the abscessed lung in a gravity-dependent position can drain its purulent contents into the opposite lung. The abscessed lung would then contaminate the healthy lung.

Patient Positioning

Studies have demonstrated improved oxygenation in patients with acute respiratory failure who were placed in the prone position although this maneuver may not ultimately improve survival.[8] Prone positioning is an advanced technique used with critically ill ventilated patients who have acute lung injury (ALI) or acute respiratory distress syndrome (ARDS) with a low PaO_2/FiO_2 ratio. The enhanced oxygenation is attributed to recruitment of collapsed lung areas related to body position change allowing dependent lung regions to have improved perfusion and ventilation.[9] Prone positioning involves multiple personnel and specialized beds or equipment, and it should be performed only by specially trained staff to prevent the many complications related to prone positioning.

Patients who are ventilated benefit from having the head of the bed elevated 30 degrees at all times.[10] The rationale is to promote lung expansion, prevent the aspiration that can occur in the recumbent position in intubated patients, and prevent ventilator-associated pneumonia (VAP). Keeping the head of the bed elevated 30 degrees, with the associated reduction in VAP, is included in the ventilator bundle to prevent VAP and is part of the Institute for Healthcare Improvement's 5 Million Lives Campaign.[11,12] Mobilization of the patient contributes to improved oxygenation, secretion removal, and airway patency. Using lateral rotational therapy beds is more effective than the inconsistent nursing care of turning every two hours at minimum.[13] (See the *American Association of Critical-Care Nurses [AACN] Protocols for Practice, Care of Mechanically Ventilated Patients, 2nd edition*, for a complete explanation of prone therapy.)

Mobilization of the patient using continuous lateral rotation therapy (CLRT) improves oxygenation and blood flow to the lung tissue in affected regions.[5,8–10] CLRT is defined as continuous lateral positioning of less than 40 degrees for 18 of 24 hours daily. The lateral positioning improves blood flow and ventilation in the superior lung regions. CLRT may help reduce pneumonia, although it may not reduce days on the ventilator or the length of hospital stay. The results do not show improved mortality for ventilated patients using either prone positioning or rotational therapy. However, with CLRT, the improved oxygenation and recruitment lead to a reduction in VAP and in the cost associated with VAP, and with prone positioning, there is improved oxygenation. The rotation should be at the maximum to each side, and rotation should be continuous for 18 of 24 hours to obtain best outcomes.

Rotation therapy with Kinetic Therapy refers to beds that rotate greater than or equal to 40 degrees and to CLRT beds that rotate to less than 40 degrees. Note that the best evidence-based research involves Kinetic Therapy. Both types of beds may include percussion and vibration modules that allow frequent use of those functions to further improve secretion mobilization.

Positioning of critically ill patients remains a nursing intervention not only for ventilated patients to improve oxygenation but to prevent pressure ulcers. The additional benefit from CLRT over conventional nurse turning is skin ulcer prevention.[14–17] Turning by nurses has become more significant, with the Joint Commission (formerly Joint Commission on Accreditation of Healthcare Organizations) mandated safety goal of requiring the risk assessment and reassessment for pressure ulcers followed by implementing actions to prevent them.[18] Turning every 2 hours allows the nurse to assess pressure points on the torso and extremities, including the back of the head, and this is even more important in patients with low perfusion. Guidelines should be in place for the use of a scale such as the Braden scale to assess for pressure ulcer risk.[19,20] The Braden scale is a tool to reassess for increased risk factors daily; its use should be followed by consulting the wound care team and providing additional actions to treat pressure ulcers. Repositioning manually, using CLRT or prone positioning, requires care to avoid causing tissue injury when positioning for extended periods. Prolonged positioning in any one position leaves a patient at risk for developing a pressure ulcer, and turning can result in the pulling out of various tubes or lines. The critical care staff should be well trained in prone positioning, monitoring tubes and lines during rotation therapy, and preventing prolonged pressure in lateral positions. Low-pressure airflow mattresses may help reduce skin ulcer occurrence but should not be relied on as a primary prevention method. Mobilization of ventilated patients using rotation therapy specialty beds is one method for nurses to improve patient outcomes of improved oxygenation; this technique also helps prevent VAP and skin ulcers. Ultimately, the critically ill patient should progress to weight-bearing positions, sitting up in a chair, and, with physical therapy, to ambulation that improves overall physical reconditioning toward return to independent functioning.

• Oxygen Therapy

The administration of oxygen therapy to a patient is designed to correct hypoxemia (low oxygen blood levels). When tissue oxygen availability is decreased, it is referred to as hypoxemia. If external or internal respiration is impaired, supplemental oxygen is vital to maintain the patient's cellular function. Oxygen therapy corrects hypoxemia, decreases the work of breathing, and decreases myocardial work. Any disease process that alters the gas exchange can cause hypoxemia.

Asthma, bronchitis, pneumonia, ALI and ARDS, COPD, and emphysema are disease processes that alter oxygen supply. Traumatic events that lead to pneumothorax or hemothorax, as well as surgical events such as pneumonectomy and lobectomy, or events causing large pleural effusions can significantly alter gas exchange. Oxygen delivery by nasal cannula may provide sufficient additional oxygen to reduce air hunger and shortness of breath. A patient with COPD may also need continuous oxygen because of permanent alterations in the lungs, which result in lowered oxygen delivery, especially with stress, illness, infection, and exercise. Patients with COPD and emphysema require close monitoring for carbon dioxide retention and narcosis associated with the delivery of too high a concentration of oxygen. These patients normally tolerate higher levels of carbon dioxide because their chemoreceptors no longer respond to the normally accepted partial pressure of carbon dioxide (PCO_2) levels and serum pH. These patients' primary drive to breathe comes from their oxygen, rather than carbon dioxide, levels. The desired goals for all patients on oxygen therapy are stable arterial oxygen saturation (SaO_2) level, eupneic respirations, and a decrease in anxiety and shortness of breath. These goals should be accomplished through delivery of the least amount of supplemental oxygen needed, so the nurse continuously monitors the patient on oxygen for the desired result and complications (Box 25-2). Appropriate physician or advanced practice nurse orders are necessary to initiate this therapy.

PATIENT ASSESSMENT

Assessment of the patient's oxygen need is based on the disease process and the severity of the hypoxemia. The nursing assessment considers the patient's level of consciousness, vital signs (including the rate and depth of breathing), nail bed color, airway patency or presence of an artificial airway, SaO_2, and ABGs. The use of accessory muscles or abdominal breathing may indicate severe distress, and the inability to speak (or the tendency to respond using only one-syllable words) is ominous. A patient with asthma who comes in with bilateral wheezes but who can communicate in complete sentences is less likely to have increased dyspnea and require intubation than the patient with asthma who sits bolt upright, only nods the head to questions, and is using the shoulder and neck accessory muscles to breathe. Accessory muscle use in any patient is usually a sign of respiratory fatigue. Laboratory data, including hemoglobin, hematocrit, ABGs, and chest radiographs, may be obtained to assist in correcting electrolyte and pH imbalances. A full assessment, which may include collection of a blood gas, takes time, whereas assessment of the person's vital signs, SaO_2, and respiratory effort and symptoms is possible to do quickly and repeatedly. To establish baseline activity tolerance and respiratory function, it may be necessary to involve the family if the patient is not able to communicate in complete sentences. Clinicians need to compare the usual symptoms exhibited by a patient with asthma or COPD with the presenting symptoms to establish the severity of the patient's illness. They should initiate oxygen therapy for distress and hypoxemia. After a thorough assessment including laboratory data, it is necessary to adjust the oxygen delivery method to meet the therapeutic goal.

The patient's acuity and underlying disease process dictate the level of oxygen delivery required. The choice of oxygen delivery method is based on the assessment and presentation of the patient, the SaO_2 on room air, and the desired outcome. The desired oxygen level for a patient with COPD may be much lower than that for a patient with pneumonia who does not have COPD. The patient with pneumonia tolerates higher levels of oxygenation for longer periods than the patient with COPD, who is susceptible to carbon dioxide narcosis.

After giving oxygen, it is necessary to reassess the patient. Signs of improvement include reduction of respiratory rate, a more comfortable breathing pattern, an increased SaO_2, and the patient's own subjective statement of improved breathing with decreased anxiety or distress. Altered mental status may indicate hypoxemia but may also be due to pH, electrolyte, or carbon dioxide changes. The nurse assesses the patient's respiratory status as often as needed until the desired results are achieved. ABGs guide therapy, especially in patients known to have carbon dioxide retention or continued lethargy or sedation and in those unable to clear secretions. Ultimately, the ABGs indicate success or failure of efforts to correct the underlying hypoxemia.

OXYGEN DELIVERY SYSTEMS

Several methods of oxygen delivery are available. The choice of a delivery method depends on the patient's condition. Oxygen delivery systems are traditionally divided into high-flow and low-flow systems (Box 25-3).

Low-flow oxygen devices work by supplying oxygen at flow rates less than the patient's inspiratory volume, usually 1 to 10 L/minute. The rest of the volume is pulled from room air (entrained). Because of this oxygen and room air mixing (entrainment), the actual fraction of inspired oxygen (FiO_2) delivered to

Box 25-2 • RED FLAG: Complications of Oxygen Therapy

- Respiratory arrest
- Discomfort with skin breakdown from straps and masks
- Dry mucous membranes, epistaxis, or infection in the nares
- Oxygen toxicity (prolonged high levels seen in acute lung injury or acute respiratory distress syndrome)
- Absorptive atelectasis
- Carbon dioxide narcosis (manifested by altered mental status, confusion, headache, somnolence)

Box 25-3 • Oxygen Delivery Methods With Delivered Fraction of Inspired Oxygen (FiO$_2$)

Nasal Cannula–Low-Flow Device

FLOW (L/MIN)	FiO$_2$
1	21%–25%
2	25%–28%
3	28%–32%
4	32%–36%
5	36%–40%
6	40%–44%

High-Flow Nasal Cannula

FLOW (L/MIN)	FiO$_2$
1–35	21%–100%

High-Flow Nasal Cannula

The high-flow nasal cannula (e.g., AquinOx system) is adjusted for the desired clinical effect depending on the arterial blood gas, SaO$_2$, and breaths per minute. These high-flow systems allow for humidification at 100% with high levels of oxygen delivery maintaining nasal mucosa moisture not possible with a low-flow nasal cannula. The nurse should monitor the SaO$_2$ closely when switching from another oxygen delivery device for at least 30 to 60 minutes, evaluate arterial blood gas as needed, and assess patient tolerance. Be aware of clinical contraindications with increased oxygen delivery.

Facemask–Low-Flow Device

FLOW (L/MIN)	FiO$_2$
5–6	40%
6–7	50%
7–10	60%

Face Tent–Low-Flow Device

Variable oxygen delivery of 21%–50%; depends on patient breathing (21% delivered with compressed air and up to 50% delivered with 10 L/min oxygen flow attached). Air is mixed with the oxygen flow in the mask, resulting in variable delivery with humidification. Often used for humidification as well as oxygen delivery in patients who do not like the claustrophobic feeling associated with more traditional masks.

Venturi Mask–Low-Flow Device

OXYGEN FLOW (MINIMAL RATE)	FiO$_2$ SETTING*
4 L/min	25%
4 L/min	28%
6 L/min	31%
8 L/min	35%
8 L/min	40%
10 L/min	50%

*FiO$_2$ setting is based on Venturi setting/adapter used and oxygen flow.

NON-REBREATHER MASK–LOW-FLOW DEVICE

The non-rebreather mask is used in severe hypoxemia to deliver the highest oxygen concentration. The one-way valve on one side allows for the exhalation of carbon dioxide. The mask delivers 80%–95% FiO$_2$ at a flow rate of 10 L/min depending on the patient's rate and depth of breathing, with some room air entrained through the open port on the mask. However, the mask should fit snugly to prevent additional entrainment of room air.

Tracheostomy Collar and T-Piece–Low-Flow Device

The T-piece is a T-shaped adapter used to provide oxygen to either an endotracheal or tracheostomy tube. The flow rate should be at least 10 L/min with humidification. Flow can also be provided by a ventilator. The tracheostomy collar may also be used and is generally the preferred method because it is more comfortable than the T-piece. The strap on the tracheostomy collar is adjusted to keep the collar on top of the tracheostomy. With both the T-piece and tracheostomy collar, the goal is to provide a high enough flow rate to ensure that there is a minimal amount of entrained room air.

---

the patient is difficult to specify. Low-flow oxygen devices are suitable for patients with normal respiratory patterns, rates, and ventilation volumes. High-flow oxygen devices supply flow rates high enough to accommodate 2 to 3 times the patient's inspiratory volume, at 1 to 35 L/minute. These devices are suitable for patients with high oxygen requirements because high-flow devices deliver 100% O$_2$ and maintain 100% humidification essential to prevent drying of the nasal mucosa.

Oxygen delivery devices all deliver different levels of oxygen. Device selection is based on the desired FiO$_2$.[13] For example, a patient admitted with pneumonia who has an SaO$_2$ of 88% might improve to the desired level with a nasal cannula at 2 L/minute. In contrast, a patient who has an SaO$_2$ of 88% but who also has a PaO$_2$ of 52 mm Hg and is using accessory muscles may require a higher liter flow or a non-rebreather oxygen mask. Both patients are monitored for improved SaO$_2$, respiratory rate and pattern, and ABG improvement. If increased distress, desaturation, or both are noted, more extreme interventions (such as intubation) may be necessary.

If lower concentrations of oxygen are needed, the system selected is usually nasal cannula. The cannula can be used even with mouth breathers because oxygen fills the nasopharynx and, with inspiration, oxygen is entrained. A patient who is primarily a mouth breather with sinusitis needs to be monitored closely for nasal cannula effectiveness or placed on mask oxygen delivery. The exact concentration of oxygen depends on the patient's inspired tidal volume (V$_T$). If the patient hypoventilates, the oxygen concentration increases in the upper airway. In contrast, if hyperventilation occurs, the concentration of oxygen decreases because of large amounts of room air diluting the oxygen delivered. A simple calculation for nasal cannula delivery is to add another 4% for each liter FiO$_2$ delivered to the room air value of 21% (see Box 25-3). Each of the other oxygen delivery devices delivers a variable FiO_2, based on breathing pattern and what device is used, as well as the oxygen flow in liters per minute.

If the oxygen concentration must be constant, as is the case for patients with COPD, Venturi systems (e.g., the Venturi mask) are used. The Venturi mask delivers an exact percentage of oxygen regardless of the patient's tidal volume. Patients with COPD may require oxygen delivery by the Venturi system. These patients are "sensitive" to oxygen, and a small increase in the percentage of FiO_2 delivered may result in an elevated $PaCO_2$ and respiratory depression. The patient with COPD may have a respiratory drive based on his or her PaO_2, and with this disease process, ventilation decreases with an increased FiO_2, resulting in hypercapnia. The carbon dioxide level can be detected through serial ABG monitoring, which may reveal large increases in $PaCO_2$ with small increases in oxygen flow.

As higher concentrations of oxygen are required, the nasal cannula is replaced by a mask system. A simple mask delivers the lowest concentrations of oxygen, and a non-rebreather mask delivers the highest concentration. The alternative to a non-rebreather for high FiO_2 delivery is the high-flow nasal cannula system. The high-flow nasal cannula is used on a variety of patients with higher oxygen requirements. For example, patients may be those just off the ventilator with low oxygen saturation, for prevention of dry secretions with the increased humidity (100%); those in pulmonary rehabilitation with decreased exercise tolerance; and those with COPD and asthma, for whom high-flow nasal cannula systems improve breathing rate and dyspnea. The AquinOx system allows high liter oxygen flow through a nasal cannula with humidification at flows of 35 L/minute.[21,22] The high-flow nasal cannula can be more comfortable and allow improved tolerance by providing a constant temperature and high humidity without condensation and moisture buildup in the tubing, which would enter the nose in a low-flow nasal cannula. The other advantage of the high-flow nasal cannula is the ability to deliver a range of FiO_2, up to 100%, to meet patient oxygen demand. If a patient's PaO_2 and SaO_2 cannot be maintained using the non-rebreather mask or high-flow nasal cannula, respiratory failure, with the need for intubation and mechanical ventilation, is imminent.

COMPLICATIONS OF OXYGEN DELIVERY

The delivery of oxygen can cause discomfort, skin breakdown, and other complications. Long-term oxygen by nasal cannula, even with humidification, can cause dry mucous membranes, epistaxis, or infection in the sinuses. Nasal cannula tubing, facemasks (including the straps), and tracheostomy collars can cause skin breakdown along the face, bridge of the nose, back of the neck, or behind the ears. Oxygen delivery can fail if the tubing is disconnected from the wall, leading to hypoxemia with dysrhythmias or increased dyspnea. The edematous or malnourished patient is at higher risk for alteration in skin integrity,

and contaminated oxygen delivery devices should be replaced. Contamination can occur with copious secretions coughed onto a tracheostomy collar or with mucus on any other device used. A "no smoking" rule must be enforced for all patients while on oxygen therapy to prevent fires.

The nurse routinely inspects the skin and mucous membranes of the mouth and nares for signs of breakdown. Should skin injury occur, further breakdown can be prevented by providing skin barriers or cushions, and possibly changing to another type of device. For example, if the bridge of the nose is irritated by a facemask, then switching to a nasal cannula may relieve the discomfort to the nose, as long as the patient receives the same oxygen level. The mask may cause some patients anxiety, with feelings of suffocation, and, as with all devices, the nurse should ensure the patients' comfort. The nasal cannula can cause breakdown behind the ears or on the upper lip, and even in the nares. Because oxygen delivered by nasal cannula is not highly humidified, except from high-flow devices, it may cause drying of mucous membranes in the nose. Finally, it is necessary to change disposable humidification systems according to manufacturer specifications to prevent infections from the systems. Oxygen humidification sets for any device need routine changing at least every 72 hours. The key to preventing any complication, including hypoxemia, is accurate and timely assessment of oxygenation parameters and monitoring for complications of the therapies by the nurse.

Oxygen toxicity starts to occur in patients breathing a concentration of more than 50% for longer than 24 hours. Patients who are ventilated with high oxygen concentration for prolonged periods are at risk for oxygen toxicity. To prevent the pathological cellular changes of oxygen toxicity, the patient's FiO_2 should be decreased as tolerated to the lowest possible setting as long as the PaO_2 remains greater than 60 mm Hg. The pathophysiological changes that occur with oxygen toxicity occur at the alveolar level and may progress from capillary leaking to pulmonary edema and possibly to ALI if the high FiO_2 continues for several days. Once the oxygen concentration is decreased to safer levels, the pathophysiological cellular changes may reverse, but if high FiO_2 levels continue, there may be permanent cellular changes and pulmonary function impairment.

Carbon dioxide narcosis is a risk in patients with COPD who are "sensitive" to oxygen, and an increased FiO_2 may result in an elevated $PaCO_2$, hypoventilation, and respiratory depression or respiratory arrest. Oxygen must therefore be administered with caution to patients with COPD and often at low levels to prevent respiratory depression. Patients on high FiO_2 may develop absorptive atelectasis. Absorptive atelectasis is a result of less nitrogen in the delivered gas mixture. Because nitrogen is not absorbed, it normally exerts a pressure within the alveoli, keeping the alveoli open. When nitrogen is "washed out," the oxygen replacing it is absorbed, resulting in alveolar collapse (atelectasis).

Respiratory arrest is a complication that can occur even in patients on oxygen therapy. Nurses prevent this complication by monitoring the patient's overall respiratory status, neurological assessment, vital signs with SaO_2, and ABGs to evaluate for signs of impending respiratory failure. Respiratory arrest can also occur for reasons such as mucus plugging within the tracheobronchial airways or plugging of a tracheostomy or endotracheal tube. Respiratory failure from fatigue due to increased work of breathing can occur quickly in a patient with pulmonary compromise, such as a patient with COPD and new-onset pneumonia. Aspiration of food or gastric contents can also lead to respiratory arrest, and this occurs regularly in hospitalized patients with dysphagia (e.g., as from a stroke or secondary to prolonged intubation with vocal cord paralysis). The nurse must monitor the vulnerable patient more frequently when there is a clear comorbidity that may result in respiratory failure or arrest.

• Artificial Airways

Rigorous BHT and carefully monitored oxygen therapy may eliminate the need for an artificial airway or ventilatory support. An artificial airway and ventilatory support become mandatory if these measures fail to provide adequate oxygenation and removal of carbon dioxide. Artificial airways have a fourfold purpose:

▶ Establishment of an airway
▶ Protection of the airway, with the cuff inflated
▶ Provision of continuous ventilatory assistance
▶ Facilitation of airway clearance

Knowledgeable, aggressive nursing care is required to maintain airway patency, maximize therapeutic effects, and minimize damage to the patient's natural airway.

The selection of the appropriate artificial airway is important. Because all artificial airways increase airway resistance, it is essential that the largest tube possible be used for intubation. The cuff on the endotracheal or tracheostomy tube must be very compliant (soft) so that trauma to the trachea, vocal cords, and subglottic area is minimized. The competency of the cuff must be established before intubation. Approximately 10 mL of air is injected into the cuff before use, and the clinician checks for leaks.

NASOPHARYNGEAL AND OROPHARYNGEAL AIRWAYS

If a patient is sedated and lying supine or becomes unconscious, tongue and airway muscle tone is decreased, causing the tongue to occlude the airway. Although an oropharyngeal or nasopharyngeal airway will maintain the air passage, it will not eliminate the potential for aspiration. Figure 25-3 illustrates some frequently used artificial airways. The nasopharyngeal airway (nasal trumpet) is a flexible tube that is

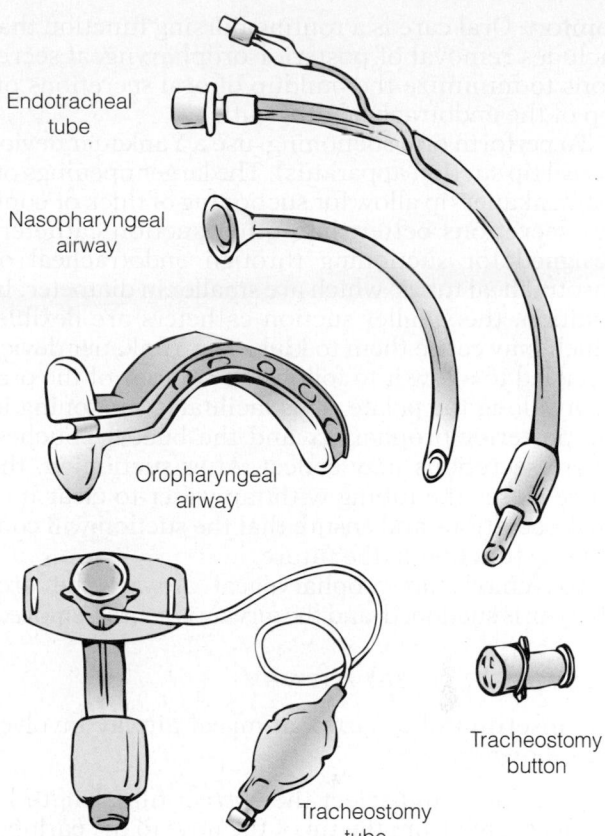

Figure 25-3 • Five frequently used artificial airways.

inserted nasally past the base of the tongue to maintain airway patency. This airway may be better tolerated than the oropharyngeal airway in patients with an intact gag reflex.[23,24]

Oropharyngeal Airway

An oropharyngeal airway is never placed in a conscious patient because it stimulates the gag reflex and can cause vomiting and aspiration. Before placing an artificial airway, the nurse makes sure any possible obstruction is cleared. Insertion of an oropharyngeal airway follows three steps:

1. Gently open the patient's mouth using a crossed finger technique or a modified jaw thrust.
2. Hold down the tongue with a depressor and guide the airway over the back of the tongue. (An optional method is to position the tip of the airway toward the roof of the mouth, with the curved end toward the roof, and gently advance the airway by rotating it 180 degrees.)
3. Monitor the patient frequently for airway patency by listening to breath sounds. Provide oropharyngeal suction as needed for emesis or oral secretions.

Oral suctioning is important to maintain oral hygiene when the patient is intubated because the patient's ability to swallow can be limited. The nurse performs oral suctioning as needed for copious oral secretions and after suctioning the endotracheal or tracheostomy tubes to maintain oral hygiene and comfort. Oral care is a routine nursing function that includes removal of posterior oropharyngeal secretions to minimize the buildup of oral secretions on top of the endotracheal tube cuff.

To perform oral suctioning, use a Yankauer device (tonsil tip suction apparatus). The larger openings on the Yankauer tip allow for suctioning of thick or copious secretions better than other suction catheters designed for suctioning through endotracheal or nasotracheal tubes, which are smaller in diameter. In addition, the smaller suction catheters are flexible, which may cause them to kink. The Yankauer device is angled to allow it to follow the contour of the oral cavity along the palate. This facilitates suctioning in the posterior oropharynx and the buccal pouches, where secretions may collect. After suctioning, the nurse rinses the tubing with tap water to clear it of thick secretions and ensure that the suction will continue to function in the future.

To remove an oropharyngeal airway, the oropharynx is suctioned, and the airway is gently removed.

Nasopharyngeal Airway

The insertion of a nasopharyngeal airway involves the following steps:

1. Determine and select the correct tube length by measuring from the tip of the nose to the earlobe. Use a tube with the largest outer diameter that fits the patient's nostril.
2. Lubricate the tube with water, water-soluble jelly, or lidocaine jelly, which alleviates discomfort.
3. Reassure the patient and familiarize him or her with the procedure.
4. Insert the airway into the nostril up to the end of the nasal trumpet.
5. Have the patient exhale with the mouth closed. (If the tube is in the correct position, air can be felt exiting from the tube opening.)
6. Open the patient's mouth, depress the tongue, and look for the tube's tip just behind the uvula.

In patients who require frequent nasotracheal suctioning, nasopharyngeal airways are frequently used to prevent patient discomfort and airway trauma from repeated suction catheter introduction through the nares. Nasotracheal suctioning is best done using a red rubber suction catheter, which is more flexible and better tolerated than standard plastic catheters. Nasotracheal suctioning is done as a sterile procedure. The catheter is lubricated with water-soluble jelly and passed to the back of the nasopharynx initially. Supplemental oxygen is given before suctioning and in between each suction attempt. The oxygen can be given using a manual resuscitation bag (MRB) with mask and gently bagging with each inspiration to provide a high FiO_2. Other high-flow devices, such as a Venturi mask, may also be used. The nurse or respiratory therapist then asks the patient to cough, which opens the epiglottis and allows the catheter to be advanced. A change in the sound of the cough and the return of sputum with suctioning indicates passage into the tracheal tree. The technique of nasotracheal suctioning is difficult and should only be attempted by experienced practitioners. The novice intensive care unit nurse should seek the help of experienced clinicians to learn this skill.

The nasopharyngeal airway may have to be gently rotated to withdraw it from the nares. Be prepared for the potential for epistaxis with nasopharyngeal airway removal. Prior history of epistaxis or known coagulopathy should be carefully reviewed before placing a nasopharyngeal airway or performing nasotracheal suctioning that may lead to bleeding.

ENDOTRACHEAL TUBES

An endotracheal tube is inserted if the patient needs ventilation or protection of the airway from aspiration. Equipment listed in Box 25-4 is assembled before intubation. The endotracheal tube can be inserted nasally or orally. The advantages and disadvantages of each placement are listed in Table 25-1.

To reduce the incidence of complications, personnel with rigorous credentials must perform tracheal intubation. The nurse explains the procedure to the patient and family. The patient is positioned on his or her back with a small blanket under the shoulder blades to hyperextend the neck and open the airway.[25] Air is injected (10 mL) into the endotracheal cuff before insertion to ensure an intact cuff, and then the cuff is deflated. The stylet is a malleable thick wire with a blunt end used to stiffen the flexible endotracheal tube for insertion. The end of the stylet must be kept at least 1 inch from the end of the endotracheal tube to prevent perforation of the trachea. The stylet is inserted to the correct position, and the remaining stylet is bent over the distal end of the endotracheal tube to maintain endotracheal tube stiffness. The physician or other qualified health care professional shapes the endotracheal tube with the stylet to facilitate placement through the vocal cords prior to insertion.

Box 25-4 • Equipment for Endotracheal Intubation

- Laryngoscope with blades and intact bulb
- Suction setup with Yankauer suction
- Correct size endotracheal tube with stylet*
- 10-mL syringe for cuff inflation
- Adhesive tape, twill tape, or commercial endotracheal tube holder
- Magill forceps (may be used with nasal intubation)
- Pulse oximetry
- Oxygen source
- Manual resuscitation bag with mask
- End-tidal CO_2 monitor or disposable detector
- Sedation and paralytic medication

*In adults, tube size is usually 8.0 initially unless the procedure is difficult, the patient is small, or a difficult intubation is anticipated, in which case smaller sizes are used. An endotracheal tube larger than 7.0 mm facilitates bronchoscopy.

Table 25-1 • Airway Placement

Type	Advantages	Disadvantages
Nasal endotracheal	Patient comfort Prevents tube obstruction from biting Easily anchored and reduced risk for extubation Oral hygiene more effective Used in patients with maxillofacial trauma or cervical spine injuries	Can kink and obstruct airway Predisposes to acute sinusitis, which may result in bacteremia Epistaxis a frequent complication Pressure necrosis of the nares Tube and cuff can cause tracheoesophageal fistula, erosion, and vocal cord paralysis High risk for shearing off nasal polyps in patients with asthma Limited usually to 6.0–6.5 tube size that prevents bronchoscopy later*
Oral endotracheal	Less trauma during intubation than nasal route Permits use of a larger endotracheal tube* Avoids nasal/sinus complications	Predisposes to mouth sores Uncomfortable for patient Pressure sores develop on lips, gums, and tongue Easily obstructed by biting, necessitates a bite block Tube and cuff can cause tracheal damage, tracheoesophageal fistula, and vocal cord paralysis Tube, bite block, and tube-securing tape complicate oral hygiene Self-extubation easier (from patient pushing on endotracheal tube with tongue) Difficult to secure (beards, failure of tape to adhere to skin) Makes communication difficult

*Facilitates work of breathing because the larger endotracheal tube allows improved flow, and bronchoscopy is done only with an endotracheal tube of at least 7.5 mm.

Before the procedure, the nurse confirms that the suction is working properly. Using an MRB and mask, the nurse preoxygenates the patient. The physician may use topical anesthetics, sedatives, or a short-acting neuromuscular blocking agent to facilitate rapid and nontraumatic intubation. Newer short-acting intravenous (IV) anesthetics facilitate rapid intubation, and a lidocaine bolus reduces the reflex to cough.

The nurse assists during intubation by providing suction as necessary and monitoring the patient's SaO_2 by pulse oximetry as well as the patient's heart rate and blood pressure. Intubation attempts should be held and the patient oxygenated with the MRB if the SaO_2 falls below 90%. Hypoxemia during intubation may cause bradycardia, hypotension, dysrhythmias, and other complications.

After placement of the endotracheal tube, the cuff is inflated. It is necessary to auscultate the chest bilaterally for equal breath sounds and the abdomen for evidence of esophageal intubation. Waterproof tape is used to secure the endotracheal tube, and the centimeter mark is noted at the lips, teeth, or nostril for the nasotracheal tube. The level of the endotracheal tube must be noted to prevent changing of position, which could result in either right mainstem bronchus placement with left lung collapse or self-extubation. A portable chest radiograph is obtained immediately after the insertion to confirm proper tube placement, which is about 2 to 3 cm above the carina (but below the clavicular heads as appropriate).

Complications of endotracheal tube placement are noted in Box 25-5. Initially during intubation, complications of hypoxemia, gastric intubation, mainstem intubation, and oral or tracheal tissue damage can

occur. Vomiting during the procedure can lead to aspiration with resultant lung injury. If the patient has prolonged hypoxemia and hypercapnia (as might result with a difficult intubation), dysrhythmias such as bradycardia or tachycardia can occur, possibly leading to hypotension or hypertension.

Once the patient is intubated, potential complications include disconnection, failure of the ventilator, tube obstruction, sinusitis, and tracheoesophageal fistula. Vocal cord paralysis or laryngeal or tracheal stenosis may present after extubation. Accidental extubation in a critically ill patient is a preventable complication. The most challenging cases involve confused patients who attempt to self-extubate. Orienting the

Box 25-5 • RED FLAG: Complications of Intubation

- Laryngospasm/bronchospasm
- Hypoxemia/hypercapnia during intubation
- Laryngeal edema resulting in stridor with extubation
- Trauma/bleeding to nasal, oral, esophageal, tracheal, or laryngeal sites
- Fractured teeth
- Nosocomial infection (pneumonia, sinusitis, abscess)
- Displacement of tube (right mainstem intubation, gastric intubation)
- Aspiration of oral or gastric contents
- Tracheal stenosis/tracheomalacia
- Laryngeal damage, paralysis, and necrosis
- Dysrhythmias, hypertension, hypotension

patient to the need for the endotracheal tube and assuring the patient that you will help make him or her more comfortable are the first interventions. Occasionally, physical or pharmacological restraints are necessary.

Many of the complications can be avoided by ensuring adequate fixation of the endotracheal tube, securing ventilator tubing properly, suctioning only as needed, and following other care maintenance protocols. These include providing oral care to remove secretions and maintaining the head of the bed elevated at 30 degrees to help prevent aspiration. Following aseptic policies decreases nosocomial infections, and maintaining proper cuff pressure helps prevent tracheal erosion. Ultimately, the long-term ventilated patient, intubated longer than 72 hours, may require a tracheostomy to continue ventilatory support and weaning.

Suctioning

The presence of an artificial tube prevents glottic closure. As a result, the patient is unable to use the normal clearing mechanism (i.e., effective coughing). Additionally, the foreign object increases production of secretions. Suctioning, therefore, becomes paramount to removing secretions and maintaining airway patency. Suctioning is not without risks and should be done only when needed.[26] Complications of suctioning are listed in Box 25-6. Indications for suctioning include visual observation of secretions in the airway, determination of the presence of secretions or mucus plugs by chest auscultation, coughing, an increase in peak airway pressure, a decrease in tidal volume during pressure ventilation, or deterioration of the patient's oxygenation as noted by decreased SaO_2.

The procedure for suctioning is presented in Box 25-7. The nurse performs suctioning as a sterile procedure, using practices recommended by the Centers for Disease Control and Prevention (CDC). In-line suction catheters are available for use in patients on high levels of positive end-expiratory pressure (PEEP) who do not tolerate disconnection of the ventilator tubing for suctioning. Additionally, in-line suction catheters are used for patients with copious secretions requiring frequent suctioning and for those with grossly bloody secretions. Patients who

are identified as having the potential for long-term mechanical ventilation and patients who have been reintubated following a failed extubation are candidates for the use of the continuous aspiration of subglottic secretions (CASS) endotracheal tube. This device is used to prevent the subglottic accumulation of secretions that may lead to aspiration and is discussed as part of the VAP section.[27]

Hyperoxygenation and Saline Instillation

The patient must be hyperoxygenated using the ventilator set to 100% if an in-line system is used. Patients not on ventilators also need to be hyperoxygenated before suctioning. The patient should be instructed to take deep breaths while connected to a 100% oxygen source. Patients incapable of taking a deep breath should be assisted using an MRB with mask, timing a squeeze on the MRB with the patient's own breath.[28] The presence of epiglottitis or croup is an absolute contraindication to any kind of suctioning of patients without an artificial airway.

The routine instillation of normal saline has become increasingly questionable. In a test tube, saline and sputum act as oil and water, and they do not form a mixture. Therefore, it is unlikely that saline instillation liquefies or increases the amount of sputum obtained during suction. In addition, saline instillation causes oxygenation to decrease and may predispose patients to nosocomial infection by transporting bacteria to lower airways.[29–31]

Endotracheal tube care and cuff pressure monitoring are discussed in more detail later in this chapter, under Ventilatory Support, Assessment and Management. After the patient is intubated, the patient loses the ability to communicate easily. This inability to communicate can become a major stressor during the ventilated period.

• Chest Tubes

The chest tube is a drain. Its purposes are to remove air, fluid, or blood from the pleural space; restore negative pressure to the pleural space; re-expand a collapsed or partially collapsed lung; and prevent reflux of drainage back into the chest. Chapter 23 provides a review of the anatomical and physiological principles of the lungs and chest that helps explain how chest tube systems work.

EQUIPMENT

Equipment needed for chest tube insertion is listed in Box 25-8.

Chest Tube

Most chest tubes are multifenestrated transparent tubes with distance and radiopaque markers. This enables the physician or other qualified health care professional to visualize the tube on chest radio-

---

Box 25-6 • RED FLAG: Complications of Suctioning

- Hypoxemia
- Dysrhythmias
- Vagal stimulation (bradycardia, hypotension)
- Bronchospasm
- Elevated intracranial pressure
- Atelectasis
- Tracheal mucosal trauma
- Bleeding
- Nosocomial infection

Box 25-7 • Procedure for Suctioning

Equipment

Sterile suction catheter*
Sterile gloves
Sterile normal saline for irrigation, only when indicated
Sterile disposable container

Technique

1. Perform routine procedures before suctioning: Administer medication, assemble equipment, explain the procedure to the patient, adjust bed to comfortable working position, prepare suction pressure, wash hands, prepare and open equipment and supplies, and don gloves.
2. Hyperoxygenate the patient with 100% oxygen, using a manual resuscitation bag (MRB) or the ventilator. If the ventilator method is used, preoxygenation must last at least 2 minutes. Return to the previous oxygen setting after suctioning is completed. (Clinical research shows that the use of the patient's ventilator for preoxygenation delivers higher oxygen concentrations and lower peak pressures than those generated with an MRB.)[9] In patients who do not tolerate suctioning with hyperoxygenation, a positive end-expiratory pressure (PEEP) attachment should be on the MRB at the appropriate setting, or in-line suctioning should be used to avoid loss of PEEP and desaturation.
3. Quickly but gently, insert the catheter as far as possible into the artificial airway without application of suction.

For tracheostomy patients, limit the distance to just beyond the end of the tracheostomy device.

4. Withdraw the catheter 1 to 2 cm, and apply intermittent suction while rotating and removing the catheter. Limit suction pressure to 80 to 120 mm Hg. Aspiration should not exceed 10 to 15 seconds. (Prolonged aspiration can lead to severe hypoxemia, hemodynamic instability, and ultimately cardiac arrest.) Tracheostomy patients are usually suctioned for a briefer period of 3–5 seconds because of the very short device.
5. Do not instill sterile normal saline unless the patient has thick secretions and trial use has shown that it improves secretion removal. Routine saline instillation has been shown to decrease oxygenation and have other negative effects.[28–31]
6. Hyperoxygenate the patient before and after each subsequent pass of the catheter for at least 30 seconds, and before reconnection to the ventilator.
7. Monitor heart rate and rhythm and pulse oximetry during and after suctioning.
8. Discontinue the procedure if the patient does not tolerate it, as evidenced by dysrhythmias, bradycardia, or a drop in SaO_2.
9. Remove equipment.
10. Perform oral hygiene. Cleanse suction tubing with a water rinse to remove secretions into the suction container.
11. Wash your hands.
12. Document procedure.

Suction catheter sized for either endotracheal tube or tracheostomy; with tracheostomy, the red rubber or more flexible suction catheter brand is used to prevent tracheal bleeding.

---

graph and position it correctly in the pleural space. All openings in the tube must be placed within the rib cage to ensure that air leaks do not develop either in subcutaneous tissue or outside the chest wall. Chest tubes are categorized as pleural or mediastinal, depending on the location of the tube's tip. Patients can have more than one tube in different locations, depending on the purposes of the tubes.

Box 25-8 • Equipment for Chest Tube Insertion

- Chest tube tray or thoracotomy tray (with scalpel)
- Chest tube
- 1% Lidocaine
- Syringe for lidocaine infiltration
- Topical antiseptic
- Sterile gloves
- Large hemostats
- Suture material (0-0 or 2-0 silk) on a cutting needle
- Bacteriostatic ointment or petroleum gauze
- Sterile gauze with a slit
- Tape—both wide and narrow, or an occlusive dressing
- Chest tube drainage system and suction
- Sterile water for water-seal systems
- Medication for pain and sedation

Larger tubes (20 to 36 French) are used to drain blood or thick pleural drainage. Smaller tubes (16 to 20 French) are used to remove air.

Drainage System

To reestablish intrapleural negative pressure, a seal for the chest tube that prevents outside air from entering the system is required. The simplest way to accomplish this is to use an underwater system of drainage. A review of multichamber systems can provide a basis for understanding all the commonly used disposable drainage units. Knowledge of these systems enables the nurse to safely manage the most complex chest tube drainage setup. Modern chest drainage systems are composed of disposable materials and may be configured in either two- or three-chamber systems. The two-chamber system has a water seal and a collection chamber, whereas the three-chamber system adds a suction control chamber.

Two-Chamber System

In a two-chamber system, the first chamber is the collection receptacle, and the second chamber is the water seal. In a disposable system that requires water, sterile water is added to the second chamber to the 2-cm level to achieve the seal. This level represents the negative pressure that is exerted on the pleural space as the water closes the chest drain to outside air, acting as a one-way valve. The water seal allows air to escape while preventing outside air from entering the pleural space. A fluid level higher than 2 cm H_2O exerts a greater negative pressure on the pleural space and may prevent resolution of the air leak. In addition, a higher column of water in the water seal chamber can make breathing more difficult because the patient has a longer column of fluid to move during respiration. Figure 25-4 depicts disposable chest drainage systems.

The patient's chest tube is connected to a 6-foot length of latex tubing that is attached to an outlet on the top of the drainage collection chamber. The second chamber (the water seal) has a vent that remains open, allowing air from the pleural space to escape as it bubbles through the water seal to the atmosphere. Except for the vented cap, the drainage system from the chest tube insertion site to the bottle is airtight.

The fluid level in the water seal fluctuates ("tidals") during respiration. During inspiration, pleural pressures become more negative, causing the fluid level in the water seal chamber to rise. During expiration, pleural pressures become more positive, causing the fluid level to descend. If the patient is being mechanically ventilated, this process is reversed. Bubbling should be seen only in the underwater seal chamber during expiration (or during inspiration with positive-pressure ventilation) as air and fluid drain from the pleural cavity. Constant bubbling indicates an air leak in either the system or a bronchopleural fistula; this is discussed further under Assessment and Management.

Three-Chamber System

In the three-chamber system, a suction control chamber is added to the two-chamber system. This is the safest way to regulate the amount of suction. In a disposable system that requires water, suction is achieved by adding water to the prescribed level in the suction chamber, usually –20 cm H_2O, and newer waterless suction systems adjust with a dial to the desired suction in centimeters of water.

In this system, it is the height of the water column in the third chamber, not the amount of wall suction, that determines the suction amount applied to the chest tube, most commonly –20 cm H_2O. Once the wall suction exceeds the force necessary to "lift" this column of fluid, any additional suction simply pulls air from a vented cap atop the chamber up through the water. The amount of wall suction applied to the third chamber should be sufficient to create a "gently rolling" bubble in the suction control chamber. Vigorous bubbling results in water loss through evaporation, changing suction pressure and increasing the noise level in the patient's room. It is important to assess for water loss and to add sterile water as necessary to maintain the prescribed level of suction. The bubbling should be assessed for gentle action, and the water level (–20 cm H_2O) is assessed every 8 hours and when the patient's clinical status changes.

Suction

Dry suction (waterless) systems use a spring mechanism to control the suction level and can provide higher levels of suction with easier setup.[32] The dry suction systems can be easily adjusted for any setting between –10 and –40 cm H_2O, and allow for safer use if the device is accidentally tipped over. If this happens, the drainage can be returned to the correct collection chamber without replacing the unit, resulting in cost savings. This system affords the patient a quieter environment. Dry suction systems that can deliver higher levels of suction may be necessary in patients with large bronchopleural fistulas, hemorrhage, or obesity.

The Emerson pleural suction pump may be used instead of wall suction. It can be set up using a two- or three-bottle system as well as a disposable chest drainage system. In contrast to the wall unit, the pressure control knob on the front of the pump controls the suction generated. The amount of pressure is registered on the suction dial.

Heimlich valves are reserved for the treatment of pneumothoraces (usually spontaneous or traumatic, or in the field by paramedics) on an outpatient basis. The valve is composed of a small-bore chest tube attached to a one-way valve, which is enclosed in a plastic case. The one-way valve allows air to escape but not reenter the pleural space. The Heimlich valve is not appropriate for fluid removal.[33]

CHEST TUBE PLACEMENT

If injury, surgery, or any disruption in the integrity of the lungs and chest cavity occurs, placement of a chest tube is warranted. In addition, iatrogenic pneumothorax can occur in the intensive care unit during thoracic central line placement, thoracentesis, high mechanical ventilation pressures, or cardiopulmonary resuscitation (CPR), or after transbronchial lung biopsy. Indications for chest tube placement are listed in Table 25-2.

Chest tube insertion can be accomplished in the operating room, in the emergency department, or at the bedside. Placement is based on the principle that, because of their different densities and weights, air rises, and liquid sinks. The insertion site for air removal is near the second intercostal space along the mid-clavicular line. The insertion site for liquid drainage is near the fifth or sixth intercostal space on the mid-axillary line. Fluid may occasionally become loculated (walled off), requiring ultrasound or computed tomography (CT) guidance for drainage tube placement. After heart surgery, placement can be in the mediastinum to drain blood from around the heart.

The nurse prepares the patient and family for the procedure, answering any questions they may have. The nurse also prepares the patient physically. Because parietal pleurae are innervated from the intercostal and phrenic nerves, this is a painful procedure, and administration of analgesics is indicated. The patient is placed in Fowler's or semi-Fowler's

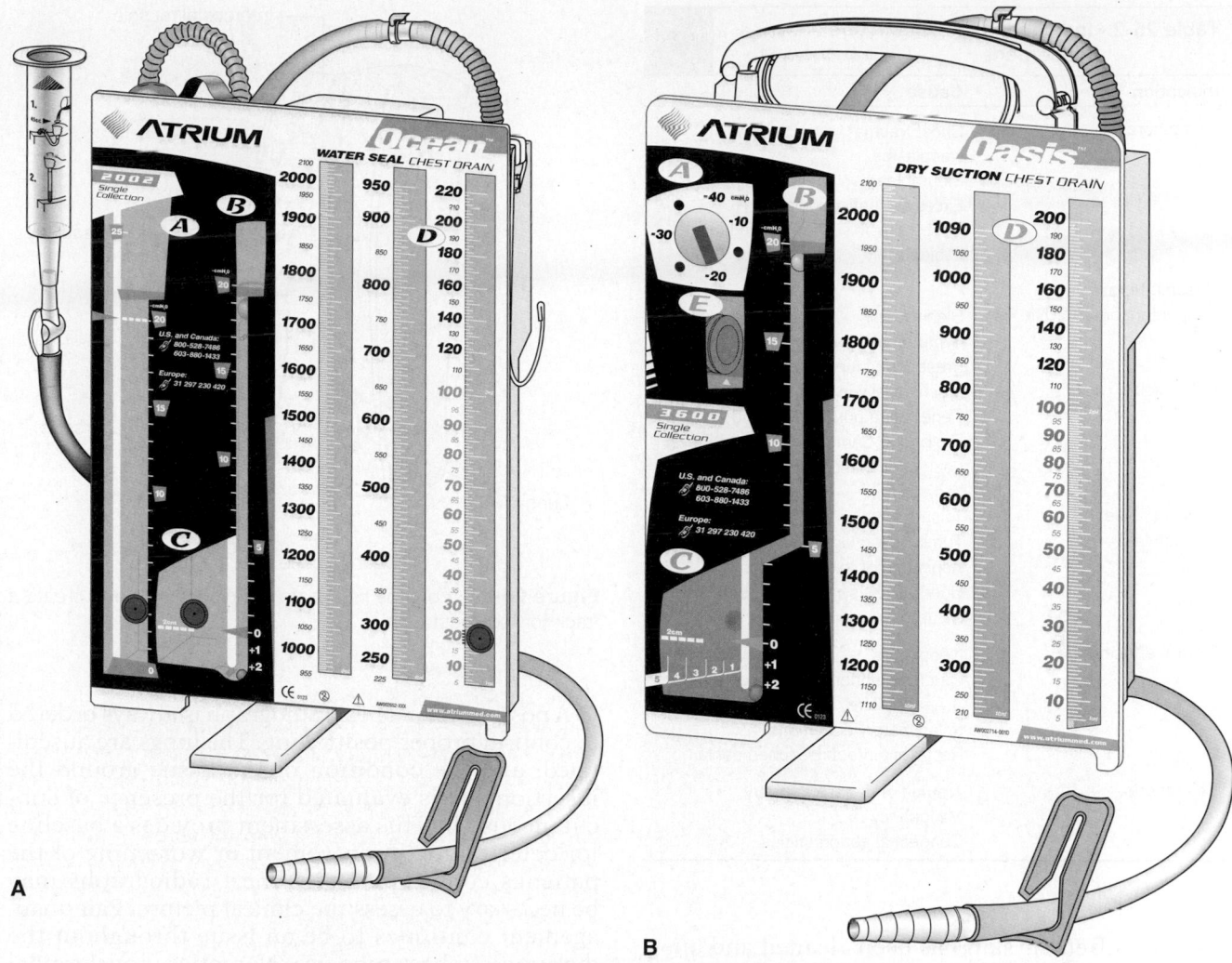

Figure 25-4 • Chest tube drainage systems. **A:** The Atrium Ocean is an example of a water seal chest drain system composed of a drainage chamber and water seal chamber. The suction control is determined by the height of the water column in that chamber (usually 20 cm). (A, suction control chamber; B, water seal chamber; C, air leak zone; D, collection chamber). **B:** The Atrium Oasis is an example of a dry suction water seal system that uses a mechanical regulator for vacuum control, a water seal chamber, and a drainage chamber. (A, dry suction regulator; B, water seal chamber; C, air leak monitor; D, collection chamber; E, suction monitor bellows.) Courtesy of Atrium Medical Corporation, Hudson, New Hampshire.

Chest drainage units (CDUs) work with the same three chambers shown in the examples above. The collection chamber collects fluid with air passing through, the water seal prevents air going back into the patient, and a suction control chamber allows suction level settings depending on the medical condition. A collection chamber allows fluid totals up to 2,000 mL. This allows for assessment of type of drainage, amount of drainage, and rate changes, with some models having a sampling port. The water seal chamber is the one-way valve action that prevents air from returning to the chest while allowing air removal as in pneumothorax. The water seal chamber is filled to the −2 cm H_2O level that maintains a slight negative pleural pressure and prevents air entering the pleural space when the CDU is off suction and on water seal. The suction control chamber is either the dry suction or a water-filled chamber. Water-filled suction is set by adjusting the water level that, with continuous high suction, evaporates, changing the suction level. Nursing care includes assessing the water level daily with suction off to refill the chamber to the desired level. Dry suction uses a mechanical system that allows the set suction level to be maintained regardless of the external suction level applied. The bellow window on dry suction systems allows a visual check that correct suction is applied; the colored indicator rises when sufficient suction is applied to maintain the set suction level from −10 to −40 cm H_2O. The wall suction regulator should be adjusted to −80 mm Hg with a continuous gentle bubbling in the water seal chamber. All CDUs follow these same functions of collection, water seal, and suction regulation chambers, and the nurse adheres to manufacturer instructions concerning proper setup and monitoring of the system.

Table 25-2 • Indications for Chest Tube Placement	
Indication	**Cause**
Hemothorax	Chest trauma
	Neoplasms
	Pleural tears
	Excessive anticoagulation
	Post-thoracic surgery/open lung biopsy
Pneumothorax	
Spontaneous: >20%	Bleb rupture
	Symptomatic patient
	Presence of lung disease
Tension	Mechanical ventilation
	Penetrating puncture wound
	Prolonged clamping of chest tubes
	Lack of seal in chest tube drainage system
Bronchopleural fistula	Tissue damage
	Tumor (esophageal cancer)
	Aspiration of toxic chemicals
	Boerhaave's syndrome (spontaneous rupture)
Pleural effusion	Neoplasms
	Cardiopulmonary disease, congestive heart failure
	Inflammatory conditions
	Recurrent infections/pneumonia
Chylothorax	Trauma or thoracic surgery
	Malignancy
	Congenital abnormalities

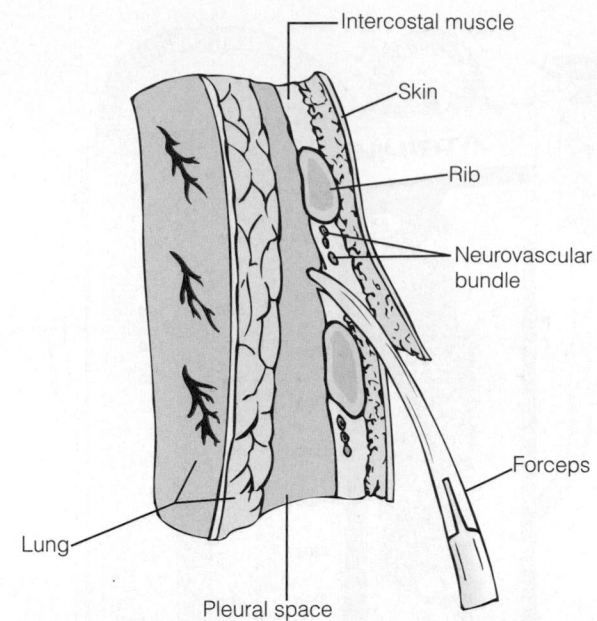

Figure 25-5 • Forceps penetrate the pleural space to create a track for the chest tube.

position. After the skin has been cleaned and anesthetized, the physician or other qualified health care professional makes a small skin incision. A hemostat is used to penetrate the pleural space (Fig. 25-5). The tract made by the hemostat is then dilated with a sterile, gloved finger. The proximal end of the tube is clamped with the hemostat and then inserted into the pleural space. If the placement is difficult, a metal trocar can be used to penetrate the chest wall, leaving the tube in place and removing the trocar.

After insertion, the external end of the tube is connected to a chest drainage unit (CDU). It is important to remember that the ends of both the chest tube and the drainage system tubing must remain sterile as they are connected. To prevent the tube from dislodging, the tube is sutured to the skin around the insertion site. The ends of the suture are wrapped around the tube and tied off. Bacteriostatic ointment or petroleum gauze can be applied to the incision site. Petroleum gauze has been preferred because it is thought to prevent air leaks; however, it also has the potential to macerate the skin and predispose the site to infection. A 4 × 4 gauze pad with a split is positioned over the tube and taped occlusively to the chest. All connections from the insertion site to the drainage collection system are securely taped to prevent air leaks as well as inadvertent disconnection. The proximal tube is taped to the chest to prevent traction on the tube and sutures if the patient moves.

A postinsertion chest radiograph is always ordered to confirm proper positioning. The lungs are auscultated, and the condition of the tissue around the insertion site is evaluated for the presence of subcutaneous air. This assessment provides a baseline for determining improvement or worsening of the patient's condition. Daily chest radiographs may be necessary to assess the clinical picture. Pain management continues to be an issue throughout the duration of chest tube use. Narcotics, nonsteroidal anti-inflammatory drugs, and the lidocaine patch (Lidoderm) may help reduce pain. The application of a lidocaine-infused patch proximal to the incision or at the chest tube incision site, which slowly releases medication over 12 to 24 hours, is an additional pain relief tool.[34] Dressings are changed per institutional protocol, or as needed if soiled or loose. It is necessary to assess chest tube output every 2 hours, looking for sudden cessation or increase to greater than 200 mL/hour or a sudden change in the character of the drainage.[35]

Chest tubes are removed after drainage is minimal and 12 to 24 hours after the chest tube is on water seal. Placement to water seal only (without suction) identifies persistent air leaks or reaccumulation of fluid with a repeat chest radiograph. Other indications for removal of the chest tube are listed in Box 25-9. When the tube is connected to water seal, disconnect the suction tube to facilitate atmospheric venting. Premature clamping or removal of the tube may cause reaccumulation of the pneumothorax.

Before removing the chest tube, the patient is placed in a Fowler's or semi-Fowler's position (head of bed elevated 45 to 90 degrees). Premedication is recommended to alleviate pain and discomfort. The dressing over the insertion site is removed, and the area is cleaned. The suture is clipped. The tube is removed in one quick movement at peak inspiration or during expiration to prevent entraining air back into the pleural cavity through the chest tube eyelets. Immediately after tube removal, the lung fields are auscultated for any change in breath sounds, and an occlusive sterile dressing is applied over the site. A chest radiograph is usually obtained several hours later to look for the presence of residual air or fluid.

ASSESSMENT AND MANAGEMENT

Nursing care is directed at maintaining patency and proper functioning of the chest tube drainage system. Vigilant and expert nursing care can prevent serious complications in the patient with a chest tube and drainage system. The latex tubing is frequently drained into the collection container. Coiling the latex tubing loosely on the bed prevents kinks and pooling of blood in a dependent loop hanging on the floor. Ensure that the patient does not inadvertently lie on the tubing. The chest tube drainage system is never raised above the chest or the drainage will back up into the chest. At frequent intervals, check the chest tube drainage system for drainage, suction level, and water seal integrity. The system should be secured to the foot of the patient's bed or taped to the floor to avoid accidental overturning and possible reaccumulation of the pneumothorax. Inspect all tubing connections for leaks, and secure them with tape to prevent accidental disconnection.

To check for chest tube patency and respiratory cycle fluctuations, it is necessary to momentarily disconnect the suction (system placed only to water seal—not clamped). Use a step-by-step system to evaluate and troubleshoot the system:

1. Assess cardiopulmonary status and vital signs every 2 hours and as needed.
2. Check and maintain tube patency every 2 hours and as needed.
3. Monitor type and amount of drainage.
4. Mark amount of drainage on collection chamber in hourly or shift increments and document in output record.
5. Prevent dependent loops from forming in tubing; ensure that the patient does not inadvertently lie on the tubing.
6. Refill water systems with sterile water to the water seal level and prescribed suction level (secondary to evaporation).
7. Assess for "tidaling" in the water seal chamber with respiration or mechanical ventilation breaths.
8. Assess for the location of air leaks (constant bubbling in the water seal chamber). Turn off the suction. Begin at the insertion site; occlude the chest tube or drainage tube (briefly) below each connection point until the drainage unit is reached.
9. Check that all tubing connections are securely sealed and taped. Another technique for sealing the connections is to use a banding gun that secures a plastic loop around the connections to prevent air leakage.[35]
10. Assess the patient for pain, intervene as needed, and reassess appropriately. Pain management may include narcotics, analgesics, lidocaine patch, and the use of nonsteroidal anti-inflammatory medications.
11. Assess the actual chest tube insertion site for signs of infection and subcutaneous emphysema with dressing changes.
12. Change the dressing twice daily or per unit guideline, when soiled, and when ordered.[32]

Drainage Monitoring

The nurse assesses and documents the color, consistency, and amount of drainage, while remaining alert to significant changes. A sudden increase indicates hemorrhage or sudden patency of a previously obstructed tube. A sudden decrease indicates chest tube obstruction or failure of the chest tube or drainage system. The following nursing actions are recommended to reestablish chest tube patency:

▶ Attempt to alleviate the obstruction by repositioning the patient.
▶ If the clot is visible, straighten the tubing between the chest and drainage unit and raise the tube to enhance the effect of gravity.

Studies have suggested that milking and stripping techniques may not be beneficial for maintenance of chest tube patency.[35] These techniques may excessively increase intrapleural and intrapulmonary pressures, affecting ventricular function, or causing trauma from aspiration of lung tissue into chest tube eyelets. However, this procedure may be necessary in cases of active bleeding to prevent blood clotting in the tubing that could lead to cardiac or pleural tamponade.[32]

Water Seal Monitoring

Monitoring the water seal of the chest tube drainage system is as important as observing the drainage. Visual checks are made to ensure water seal chambers are filled to the 2-cm water line. If suction is applied, the nurse ensures that the water line in a water-controlled suction chamber is at the ordered level (usually –20 cm H_2O) because water evaporates over time, decreasing the amount of suction being applied. It is important to add only sterile water to the system. If an Emerson pleural suction pump is used, the nurse checks the suction gauge for the desired suction level. It is essential that the air vent opening is never occluded. Disconnect the suction tubing briefly to accurately assess the water level in the chamber (water suction control) only after clamping the tubing. Then reattach the tubing and open the clamp. Never leave the tubing clamped because this can result in pneumothorax or buildup of fluid in the chest, leading to respiratory distress.

Respiratory fluctuations are observed in the water seal chamber. The absence of fluctuations can indicate that the lung is re-expanded or that there is an obstruction in the system. Continuous vigorous bubbling in the water seal chamber, without suction, indicates continued pneumothorax, or it can indicate the tube has been displaced or disconnected, or the drainage system is damaged. It is necessary to check the entire system for disconnections and to inspect the chest tube to see if it is displaced outside the chest. In the setting of mechanical ventilation at high volumes and pressures, bubbling in a chest tube system that persists may indicate a bronchopleural fistula when there is no pneumothorax or other known cause.

Positioning

The ideal position for a patient with a chest tube is semi-Fowler's. Turning the patient every 2 hours enhances air and fluid evacuation. The nurse teaches patients how to support or "splint" the chest wall near the tube insertion site using a pillow, bath blanket, or their arms. The nurse also encourages coughing, deep breathing, and ambulation. Administration of pain medication before these exercises decreases pain and enhances lung expansion.

COMPLICATIONS

The most serious complication resulting from chest tube placement is tension pneumothorax, which can develop if there is any obstruction in the chest tube drainage system. Clamping chest tubes as a routine practice predisposes patients to this complication. Clamping of chest tubes is recommended in only two situations:

▶ To locate the source of an air leak if bubbling occurs in the water seal chamber (*clamping is only momentary*)
▶ To replace the chest tube drainage unit (*clamping is only momentary*)

If the tube must be clamped, padded hemostats are used to avoid cutting the vinyl chest tube.

Occasionally, the chest tube may fall out or be accidentally pulled out. In such a circumstance, the insertion site is quickly sealed off using petroleum gauze covered with dry gauze and occlusive tape dressing to prevent air from entering the pleural cavity.

TRANSPORTING THE PATIENT WITH CHEST TUBES

As in any transport situation for critically ill patients, constant assessment is necessary to prevent inadvertent chest tube removal, resulting in recurrent pneumothorax. Maintain chest drainage system integrity by positioning the drainage system below the level of the chest. Secure the system to the foot of the bed, and ensure that the tubing does not become crushed or kinked. If the system requires suction to evacuate the pleural space, then portable suction must be implemented. The nurse performs frequent assessment of the patient and the drainage system per unit guidelines as needed, to check for air leaks, dressing integrity, water seal integrity, water level, and drainage.

• Pharmacological Agents

BRONCHODILATOR THERAPY

Asthma is characterized by recurrent airway inflammation and increased hypersensitivity to a wide range of stimuli (noxious fumes and gases, air pollutants, animal dander, extreme cold, and exercise). The hypersensitivity leads to hyperreactivity of the airways with obstruction, with widely variable symptoms even in the same person. Asthma is an episodic disease with recurrent exacerbations and periods without symptoms. Management goals include symptom control to maintain normal activities, prevention of exacerbations, and minimization of pharmacological side effects and toxicity. Pharmacological therapy is designed around multiple classes of drugs and is aimed at reducing inflammation, treating acute symptoms, and maintaining a plan for the short- and long-term therapy. The agents discussed in Table 25-3 include short- and long-acting bronchodilators, corticosteroids, anti-inflammatory agents, and other agents. Bronchospasm may also be present in COPD and can be treated with the same pharmacological agents.

Delivery of agents typically has been by propellant inhalers, with dosage dependent on the number of puffs per treatment using a metered dose inhaler (MDI). The breath, depth, inspiratory flow rate, and use of a spacer (versus administering just into the mouth) create variable medication delivery. Cleaning and proper fitting together of the actuator to the valve stem, and onto a spacer (if used), are necessary. The preferred MDI method involves using a spacer—a tube attached to the inhaler to hold the medication until it is breathed in by the patient. In many patients, this makes MDIs easier to use and deposits medications into the lungs better. Dry powder inhalers (DPIs) allow some asthma medications to be taken in a dry powder form. The difference between DPIs and MDIs is that DPIs do not use a propellant, only a medication. Patient inhalation ensures delivery into the lungs. Patients must practice the proper use of these devices, maintain consistent inspiratory flow, and consistently use a spacer or aim the device directly

Table 25-3 • Action, Dosage, and Side Effects of Pulmonary Drugs

Agent	Usual Dose	Common Adverse Effects	Comments
Advair Diskus (salmeterol and fluticasone combination)	Comes as dry powder inhaler in three dose combinations (fluticasone and salmeterol): 100/50, 250/50, and 500/50 µg of each drug. Taken twice daily for long-term maintenance treatment of asthma in patients 4 years of age and older and for chronic obstructive pulmonary disease (COPD) associated with bronchitis.	Serious allergic reactions: rash; hives; swelling of the face, mouth, and tongue; breathing problems; increased blood pressure; fast and irregular heartbeat; chest pain; headache; tremor; nervousness; throat irritation	Advair is not indicated for relief of acute bronchospasm. Contraindicated in status asthmaticus or acute episodes of asthma or COPD. Patient should call health care provider immediately if any of the following occur: breathing problems worsen; use of short-acting β_2-agonist medicine frequently, increased daily doses, or the short-acting β_2-agonist is not helping; peak flow meter results decrease; asthma symptoms do not improve after using Advair regularly for 1 week
Albuterol (Proventil, Ventolin)	Aerosol inhaler: 1–2 inhalations every 4–6 h Solution for inhalation: 2.5 mg three to four times a day	Palpitations, tachycardia, anxiety, irritability, tremor, gastrointestinal (GI) upset, cough, dry mouth, hoarseness, flushing, headache	Shake well before using; allow 1 full minute between inhalations; use as a continuous nebulizer for severe asthma or inline on a ventilator
Metaproterenol (Alupent, Metaprel)	Aerosol inhaler: 2–3 inhalations every 3–4 h Maximal dose: 12 inhalations daily Solution for nebulizer inhalation: one treatment every 4–6 h	Palpitations, tachycardia, anxiety, irritability, tremor, GI upset, cough, dry mouth, hoarseness, flushing, headache	Shake well before using; allow 1 full minute between inhalations
Salmeterol (Serevent)	Asthma/bronchospasm: 1–2 inhalations every 12 h Maximal dose: 4 inhalations daily	Palpitations, tachycardia, anxiety, irritability, tremor, GI upset, cough, dry mouth, hoarseness, flushing, headache	Shake well before using; allow 1 full minute between inhalations; should not be used for relief of acute asthmatic symptoms
Terbutaline (Brethine, Bricanyl)	Asthma/bronchospasm: Aerosol: 1–2 inhalations every 4–6 h	Palpitations, tachycardia, anxiety, irritability, tremor, GI upset, cough, dry mouth, hoarseness, flushing, headache	Shake well before using; allow 1 full minute between inhalations
Beclomethasone (Beclovent, Vanceril)	Aerosol: 2 inhalations three to four times a day or 4 inhalations twice daily Maximal dose: 20 inhalations daily	Throat irritation, hoarseness, coughing, dry mouth, oral thrush, adrenal suppression with large doses over prolonged period; rare cases of immediate and delayed hypersensitivity reactions	Use bronchodilator therapy several minutes before using inhaled steroid therapy to enhance penetration
Methylprednisolone (Solu-Medrol)	125 mg IV every 6 h initially; taper dose according to patient response; may switch to oral prednisone when tapering	Hyperglycemia, impaired immune response, hypertension, fluid retention, psychosis, steroid myopathy, fragile skin	Avoid long-term use because of adverse effects
Prednisone (Deltasone)	40–60 mg four times a day initially, then taper based on patient response	Hyperglycemia, impaired immune response, hypertension, fluid retention, osteoporosis, hyperkalemia	Avoid long-term oral therapy if possible; inhaled therapy is preferred for chronic use if necessary
Triamcinolone (Azmacort)	Initial dose: 2 inhalations three to four times a day Maximal dose: 16 inhalations daily	Throat irritation, hoarseness, coughing, dry mouth, oral thrush; adrenal suppression with large doses over prolonged period	Use bronchodilator therapy several minutes before using inhaled steroid therapy to enhance penetration
Ipratropium (Atrovent)	Aerosol inhalation Initial dose: 2 inhalations four times a day Maximal dose: 12 inhalations daily	Cough, dry mouth, nervousness, agitation, dizziness, headache, GI upset, palpitations, urinary retention, constipation, worsening narrow angle glaucoma	Must be used regularly to achieve benefit in patients with COPD
Cromolyn (Intal, Gastrocrom, NasalCrom)	20 mg inhaled, capsule or nebulizer solution, or 2 sprays of aerosol four times a day	Lacrimation, urinary frequency, dizziness, headache, rash, cough, wheezing, nasal irritation, sneezing, epistaxis, unpleasant taste	Must be used regularly to achieve benefit
Nedocromil (Tilade)	2 inhalations four times a day	Cough, pharyngitis, rhinitis, bronchospasm, dry mouth, unpleasant taste, GI upset, dizziness, headache	Must be used regularly to achieve benefit

(continued)

Table 25-3 • Action, Dosage, and Side Effects of Pulmonary Drugs (Continued)

Agent	Usual Dose	Common Adverse Effects	Comments
Theophylline (Aerolate, Bronkodyl, Elixophyllin, Quibron-T, Slo-bid, Slo-Phyllin, Theo-Dur, Theolair, Uniphyl)	Asthma/bronchospasm Regular release preparations: Initial dose: 16 mg/kg (up to 400 mg) in three to four divided doses Time-release preparations: Initial dose: 12 mg/kg (up to 400 mg) in two to three divided doses Maximal dose: 13 mg/kg daily Therapeutic range: 10–20 mg/L (some references list 5–15 mg/L)	GI irritation, diarrhea, increased gastrointestinal reflux, palpitations, tachycardia, potentiation of diuresis Toxic levels: possible cardiac dysrhythmias, convulsions, and death	Do not chew or crush enteric-coated or sustained-release capsules or tablets; take at the same time, with or without food each day; do not change from one brand to another without consulting a physician (different therapeutic response to formulations). Drug–drug interactions: agents that may decrease theophylline concentrations include phenobarbital, phenytoin, ketoconazole, rifampin, and smoking. Agents that may increase theophylline concentrations include allopurinol, cimetidine, corticosteroids, erythromycin, and ciprofloxacin.
Montelukast (Singulair) and other agents such as zafirlukast (Accolate) and zileuton (Zyflo)	Montelukast: 10 mg PO once a day before bed Zafirlukast: 20 mg twice daily in adults, 1 h before or 2 h after meals Zileuton: 600 mg 4 times a day (adults)	Montelukast: dizziness, fatigue, abdominal pain, rash, asthenia, influenza, cough, nasal congestion. Accolate: pharyngitis, headache, rhinitis, gastritis Zafirlukast: dyspepsia, abdominal pain, nausea	Drug–drug interactions: Montelukast: rifampin and phenobarbital may increase montelukast concentrations; adjust dosage for hepatic disease. Zafirlukast: monitor liver isoenzymes every 2 to 3 mo; not to be used in patients with hepatic dysfunction. Zileuton: may alter effects of warfarin, theophylline, and propranolol; liver enzymes are checked once a month for 3 mo and once every 2 to 3 mo afterward.
DNase (Pulmozyme)	2.5 mg inhaled daily	Laryngitis, hoarseness, hemoptysis	Evaluate for thick, tenacious secretions
Budesonide (Pulmicort)	1–4 puffs twice daily Maximal dose: 4 puffs twice daily (for asthma)	Hypercortisolism, diarrhea, indigestion, nausea, arthralgia, dizziness, headache, epistaxis, dry nasal mucosa, nasal stinging or burning, respiratory tract infection, sinusitis, throat irritation	Drug interactions with bupropion, erythromycin, itraconazole, and ketoconazole Do not break or chew capsules; take capsule in the morning. After inhalation, rinse mouth and spit.
Fluticasone propionate (Flonase)	Oral aerosol inhalation: Starting doses with prior therapy of: Inhaled bronchodilators alone, dose 88 µg twice daily; maximal dose, 440 µg twice daily Inhaled corticosteroids, dose 88 to 220 µg twice daily; maximal dose, 440 µg twice daily Oral corticosteroids, initial dose, 440 µg twice daily may increase to 880 µg twice daily; maximal dose, 880 µg twice daily Oral powder inhalation: starting dose with previous therapy of: Bronchodilators only, starting dose 100 µg twice daily; maximal dose, 500 µg twice daily Inhaled corticosteroids, starting dose 100 to 250 µg twice daily; maximal dose, 500 µg twice daily Oral corticosteroids, 500 to 1,000 µg twice daily; maximal dose, 1,000 µg twice daily	Pharyngeal candidiasis, epistaxis, pharyngitis	Contraindicated with bupropion and interacts with darunavir, ritonavir, and tipranavir Contraindicated with hypersensitivity to fluticasone or other ingredients; severe allergy to milk proteins (inhalation powder); status asthmaticus or other acute episodes of asthma

into the mouth to achieve consistent medication dosage. Patients may range in age from 5 years to elderly, although they must be able to inhale forcefully enough to breathe in the medication. As with MDIs, patients need training to follow the directions and process for each form of DPI inhaler.

The Diskus inhaler is a version of the DPI. Usually it contains a set number of metered doses such as a long-acting β_2-agonist (e.g., Serevent) or the newer combination of Flovent and Serevent called Advair. The Diskus type of medication is used for asthma control and not for an acute asthma attack because the medication is long acting for daily use. A spacer is not used with the Diskus inhaler. The patient has to breathe in deeply and steadily, hold the breath for up to 10 seconds, and then slowly exhale. With the Diskus inhaler, it is important to point out that the mouthpiece should never be washed in water and that the inhaler should not be placed in water. In addition, the patient does not breathe into the Diskus before inhaling.

Bronchodilators

Bronchodilators act principally to dilate the airways by relaxing bronchial smooth muscles. The goals of bronchodilator therapy are to relax the airways, mobilize secretions, and reduce mucosal edema. Bronchodilator therapy can be delivered through MDIs, preferably with a spacer attachment, or nebulization. Regardless of the mode of delivery, assessment before, during, and after the therapy is essential.

Assessment before and after treatment includes breath sounds, pulse, and respiratory rate. The last two commonly increase during bronchodilator therapy and can remain elevated for as long as 1 to 1.5 hours after treatment. ABGs may be indicated. (In people with asthma, measurement of peak expiratory flow rate with a peak flow meter before and after a treatment measures the improvement in severity of airway obstruction.) Objective evaluation is crucial, but subjective information is also valuable. How does the patient feel? Is breathing better than before the treatment? How long does the effectiveness of the treatments last? What, if any, are the side effects (jitteriness, palpitations, inability to concentrate, increased heart rate) and how long do these symptoms last?

Bronchodilators may be divided into three categories based on their mechanism and site of action. These are β_2-adrenergic agonists, anticholinergic agents, and methylxanthines.

β_2-Adrenergic Agonists

The bronchodilator effects of β-adrenergic agonists result from the stimulation of β_2-adrenergic receptors in the lung bronchial smooth muscle. In addition, these agents may decrease the release of mediators from mast cells and basophils. β_1-Adrenergic receptors in the heart may also be stimulated and lead to undesired cardiac effects. Newer β-agonists are more specific for the β_2-receptor, although they retain some β_1 activity.

β-Agonists may be administered orally or inhaled. Aerosolized or inhaled therapy is preferred and has been shown to produce comparable bronchodilation and fewer systemic adverse effects.

β-Agonists are the bronchodilators of choice for the treatment of acute exacerbation of asthma because of their rapid onset of action. They produce less bronchodilation in patients with COPD than in those with asthma. Albuterol (2.5 to 5 mg diluted in 3 mL normal saline) is the bronchodilator of choice in the acute setting and may be administered by continuous or intermittent frequent nebulization (every 15 to 20 minutes), then scheduled on a PRN basis depending on patient response.[36] Until recently, all available inhaled β-agonists, such as albuterol, had short durations of action (4 to 6 hours). Salmeterol is the first long-acting β-agonist, with a duration of action of 12 hours. Salmeterol cannot be used for acute exacerbations of asthma because of its slow onset of action. The medication DuoNeb combines albuterol and ipratropium, allowing for a synergistic effect of both a bronchodilator and an anticholinergic agent, as discussed later. In addition, Advair Diskus combines a long-acting β_2-adrenergic agonist, salmeterol, with fluticasone propionate, an inhaled corticosteroid, to provide twice-daily dosing for patients who do not achieve adequate control using other asthma medications.

Anticholinergic Agents

Anticholinergic agents produce bronchodilation by reducing intrinsic vagal tone to the airways. They also block reflex bronchoconstriction caused by inhaled irritants.

Atropine is the prototype anticholinergic agent but is used infrequently. It is readily absorbed from the respiratory tract but produces unwanted systemic effects (e.g., blurred vision, drying of respiratory secretions, tachycardia, and anxiety). Ipratropium, a quaternary amine that is not well absorbed from the respiratory tract, produces fewer systemic adverse effects and has taken the place of atropine. It is most effective in patients with COPD when used on a regular basis. It decreases submucosal gland secretion and relaxes bronchial smooth muscle. Ipratropium should not be used alone in acute exacerbations because of its slower onset of effect compared with β-agonists. It has been shown to be effective during status asthmaticus when administered through a nebulizer in combination with β-agonists as in DuoNeb.

Methylxanthines

The use of methylxanthines in the treatment of bronchospastic airway disease is controversial. The mechanism of action of these agents is poorly understood. They inhibit phosphodiesterase, an enzyme that catalyzes the breakdown of cyclic adenosine monophosphate. They may also possess some degree of anti-inflammatory activity and may augment respiratory muscle contractility.

Theophylline, the prototype methylxanthine, may be used chronically in the treatment of bronchospastic disease but is usually considered third- or fourth-line therapy. Some patients with severe disease that is not controlled with β-agonists, anticholinergics, or anti-inflammatory agents may benefit from theophylline. Aminophylline, the IV form of theophylline, is rarely used in acute exacerbations because of the lack of evidence that it is beneficial in this situation.

Theophylline has a narrow therapeutic index. Depending on the clinical situation, serum drug concentration should be monitored to ensure efficacy and prevent toxicity. The accepted therapeutic range is 10 to 20 µg/mL, although some references use 5 to 15 µg/mL.[36] Theophylline interacts with a variety of other medications that may alter its serum concentration. These include erythromycin, ciprofloxacin, and cimetidine. Patients with liver disease or congestive heart failure eliminate theophylline more slowly and may be at an increased risk for toxicity. The level should be monitored 12 to 24 hours after the loading dose is administered and frequently as clinical condition and liver and renal function dictate.

Anti-inflammatory Agents

Anti-inflammatory agents interrupt the development of bronchial inflammation and have a prophylactic or preventive action. They may also reduce or terminate ongoing inflammation in the airway. Anti-inflammatory agents include corticosteroids, mast cell stabilizers, and leukotriene receptor antagonists.

Corticosteroids
Corticosteroids are the most effective anti-inflammatory agents for the treatment of reversible airflow obstruction. Corticosteroid therapy should be initiated simultaneously with bronchodilator therapy because the onset of action may be 6 to 12 hours. They may be administered parenterally, orally, or as aerosols. In acute exacerbations, high-dose parenteral steroids (e.g., intravenous methylprednisolone) are used and then tapered as the patient tolerates. Short courses of oral therapy may be used to prevent the progression of acute attacks. Long-term oral therapy is associated with systemic adverse effects and should be avoided if possible. If necessary, the chronic use of inhaled corticosteroids, such as fluticasone (Flovent) or budesonide (Pulmicort), is preferred because of the decreased risk for systemic adverse effects.

Mast Cell Stabilizers
The two available mast cell stabilizers are cromolyn and nedocromil. They are thought to stabilize the membrane and prevent the release of mediators from mast cells. These agents are not indicated for acute exacerbations of asthma because they are used *prophylactically* to prevent acute airway narrowing after exposure to allergens (e.g., exercise, cold air). A 4- to 6-week trial may be required to determine the efficacy in individual patients. The desired end point is to reduce the frequency and severity of asthma attacks and enhance the effects of concomitantly administered bronchodilator and steroid therapy. As a result, it may be possible to decrease the dose of bronchodilators or corticosteroids in patients who respond to mast cell stabilizers.

Leukotriene Receptor Antagonists
Leukotriene receptor antagonists, such as montelukast, may be used in the management of exercise-induced bronchospasm, asthma, allergic rhinitis, and urticaria. These agents block the activity of endogenous inflammatory mediators, particularly leukotrienes. These mediators cause increased vascular permeability, mucus secretion, airway edema, bronchoconstriction, and other inflammatory cell process activities. Leukotriene receptor antagonists are administered once daily and are usually well tolerated. They are not to be administered for acute conditions but as a part of an ongoing program of therapy.[37]

Cystic Fibrosis Agent (DNase)

DNase is used in cystic fibrosis patients to break down molecules in tenacious secretions to facilitate expectoration as well as decrease the amount of medium for bacterial growth. This also improves gas flow through airways. It is administered in an inhaled form either daily or twice daily.[37]

ANTIBIOTICS

Pneumonia is often treated empirically until the results of cultures and sensitivities are available. Then, the antibiotic regimen is tailored to eradicate the specific pathogenic organism (Table 25-4). Commonly, broad-spectrum antibiotics or combination therapy is used. The critically ill patient is at increased risk for developing pneumonia due to mechanical ventilation, decreased immune responses, use of corticosteroids, debilitated general health, and cross-infection by health care workers. Antibiotic therapy should be driven by institutional protocols to prevent antibiotic overuse and following guidelines for antimicrobial selection to limit resistance.

Empiric therapy for community-acquired pneumonia includes therapy directed toward the most common organisms associated with this type of pneumonia. These organisms include *Streptococcus pneumoniae* and *Haemophilus influenzae*. Methicillin-resistant *Staphylococcus aureus* (MRSA) should be suspected in patients admitted to the hospital from a nursing home. *Legionella* species should be suspected in patients with severe multilobar pneumonia. Patients infected with the human immunodeficiency virus should be empirically treated for *Pneumocystis carinii* pneumonia.

Hospital-acquired pneumonia (HAP) is often associated with gram-negative bacilli, such as *Pseudomonas aeruginosa*, or it may be polymicrobial. HAP is the new term for pneumonia that develops at least 48 hours after hospitalization; formerly, it was known as nosocomial pneumonia, and it includes VAP. Aspiration is a concern in mechanically ventilated patients or patients unable to protect their airway. Aspiration pneumonia is associated with anaerobic organisms (e.g., *Actinomyces* species). Atypical organisms (*Mycoplasma pneumoniae*, *Chlamydia pneumoniae*, and *Legionella* species) should also be considered, as should viral infection. Patients should have a quantitative sputum culture to identify species on admission, and they may require bronchoscopy for specimen collection.

Table 25-4 • Antibiotic Therapy in Pulmonary Disease

Pulmonary Infection	Empiric Therapy
Community-acquired pneumonia (CAP)	
Outpatient	Clarithromycin, 500 mg twice daily PO for 10 days; or azithromycin, 500 mg PO once, then 250 mg/d for 4 days
Hospitalized with CAP	Cefuroxime, 750 mg q8h IV, or ceftriaxone 1–2 g daily, or cefotaxime 2 g q6h IV; or ampicillin/sulbactam 1.5–3 g q6h IV; adjust dose for renal function
Methicillin-resistant *Staphylococcus aureus* (MRSA) pneumonia	Vancomycin, 750–1500 mg q12h IV; adjust dose for weight and renal function
Legionella pneumonia	Cefuroxime, 750 mg q8h IV, or ceftriaxone 1 g/d IV, or piperacillin-tazobactam, 3.375 g q6h IV; plus azithromycin 500 mg/d IV, or levofloxacin 500 mg/d IV
Pneumocystis carinii pneumonia	Trimethoprim-sulfamethoxazole, 15 mg/kg (as trimethoprim) every 6–8 h; adjust dose for renal function
Hospital-acquired (nosocomial) pneumonia (HAP)	Cefuroxime, 750 mg q8h IV, or ceftriaxone, 1 g/d IV, or piperacillin-tazobactam, 3.375 g q6h IV, or clindamycin plus aztreonam; adjust for renal function; if *Pseudomonas* species infection is suspected, double coverage with the addition of aminoglycoside or ciprofloxacin, 500 mg q12h IV plus one of the following: piperacillin, 4 g q6h IV, or piperacillin-tazobactam, 4.5 g q6h IV, or cefepime 1–2 g q12h IV, or imipenem, 500 mg q8h IV; adjust dose for renal function
Aspiration pneumonia	Use the HAP treatment above and include clindamycin, 450–900 mg q8h IV, or piperacillin-tazobactam, 3.375 g q6h IV; adjust dose for renal function
Mycoplasma pneumoniae	Erythromycin, 500 mg four times a day for 7–10 days; azithromycin, 500 mg day, 1,250 mg over 4 days; or clarithromycin, 250 mg PO twice daily for 7 to 14 days
Chlamydia pneumoniae	Azithromycin, 500 mg day, 1,250 mg over 4 days; or clarithromycin, 250 mg PO twice daily for 7–14 days Doxycycline, 100 mg twice daily for 7–10 days

SEDATIVE AGENTS

Critically ill patients frequently require pharmacological intervention for analgesia, sedation, control of anxiety, and facilitation of mechanical ventilation. The selection of appropriate pharmacological agents is based on the cause of the agitation (Box 25-10), underlying illness, possible adverse effects, history of previous drug use, and cost. Agents most commonly used in the intensive care unit include opiates, benzodiazepines, haloperidol (Haldol), and propofol

---

Box 25-10 • Etiologies of Agitation in Critically Ill Patients

Pain
Mechanical ventilation
Dyspnea
Hypoxemia
Metabolic disarray
Withdrawal from alcohol or drugs
Anxiety
Sleep deprivation
Immobility
Sepsis
Age
Steroid administration
Alzheimer's disease
Hearing or vision deficit (severe)

(Diprivan) (Table 25-5). Specifically, haloperidol is recommended for patients with delirium, and opiates are used synergistically to treat pain.

Several agents can be given as bolus doses, by continuous infusion, or by using a combination of the two approaches, although some drugs, such as haloperidol, are limited to bolus dosing. When administering these agents by continuous infusion, it is important to monitor the patient's response closely and adjust the dose to meet his or her individual needs. This is best accomplished by using an objective sedation rating scale for consistent assessment and documentation of the medication's efficacy. Such a protocol can help prevent the prolonged use of these agents and can lower the cumulative amount required for the control of pain or agitation. This can contribute to a decreased length of hospital stay and decreased length of mechanical ventilation.[38–41]

When using a continuous infusion, if an increase in dosage is necessary, an additional small bolus dose should be given to facilitate rapid increase to the new desired blood level. To prevent withdrawal symptoms, dosages given to patients who have received large amounts of opiates or benzodiazepines for 2 or more weeks must be tapered gradually. For example, the dose may be decreased by 25% a day. Some protocols promote the conversion of benzodiazepine infusions to the enteral route before stopping the infusion. Enteral administration is performed to maintain an appropriate level of sedation and to wean patients who have required prolonged sedation, usually over

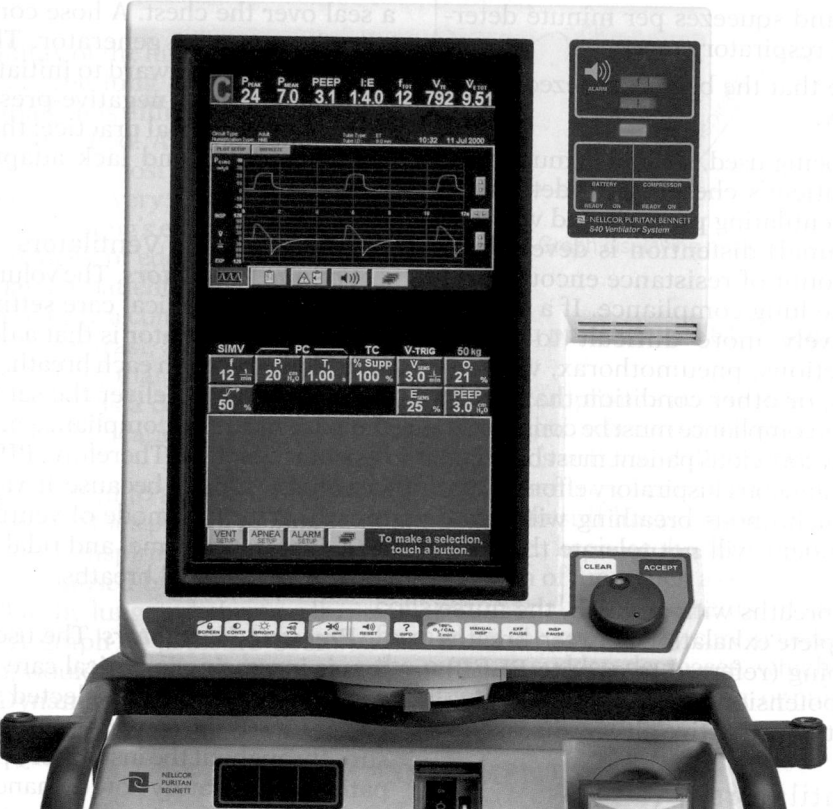

Figure 25-8 • The Puritan-Bennett 840 (PB 840) Ventilator System. The close-up photos of the screens and controls are an example of the type of controls used with computer-controlled ventilators.

The controls on the PB 840 are simple to use. This ventilator has a battery system allowing for transport with bottled oxygen. Dual screens display monitoring and alarm data in the upper screen and ventilator settings in the lower screen. On the top of the upper screen are the patient's ventilator parameters, indicating respiratory rate, tidal volume, minute volume, positive end-expiratory pressure, inspiratory pressure limit, and other values. Primary ventilator controls are accessed by screen touch boxes, and then a value or mode is selected by turning the select knob on the right followed by touching the "Accept" button for changes made. There is also a cancel button to remove changes before entering them. The nurse should be familiar with each ventilator system; each uses similar controls, but configurations of screens and touch buttons differ. The PB 840 also has additional quick action buttons along the bottom of the controls for 100% FiO_2 setting that lasts 2 minutes. This function allows preoxygenation before suctioning, or if the SaO_2 drops, it can improve oxygenation until troubleshooting of the patient and ventilator identifies the problem. An alarm pause button along the bottom controls only stops alarms for 2 minutes during therapy such as suctioning. Current alarms are viewed on the upper display screen, with the two most urgent alarms visible for review. There is a three-tiered system of warning lights on the right upper corner with red (three lights blink rapidly) for high-urgency situations that require immediate attention, yellow (two lights blink slowly) for medium-urgency situations that require prompt attention, and yellow (one light is steadily lit) for low-urgency situations that indicate a change in the ventilator system. Alarm sounds also increase to the highest level continuous with reduced intensity or duration sounds for the other alarm levels. There is an alarm reset button that resets the alarms, but if the condition persists, the alarm reactivates until the problem is corrected with the patient or the ventilator. Only registered respiratory therapists should enter the ventilator setting controls for adjustments. The nurse should be familiar with the alarm pause and 100% FiO_2 setting. He or she should know the alarm levels to respond immediately for high-urgency situations and be able to know the meaning of the alarm problem displayed in the upper screen for this ventilator. Familiarity with this and other ventilator manufacturers' alarm systems and controls is essential for every nurse who cares for ventilated patients.

and necrotizing tracheobronchitis, when used in the absence of adequate humidification.[49]

VENTILATOR MODES

Several different modes of ventilatory control are available on ventilators. Figure 25-9 and Table 25-7 compare these modes. Volume modes include assist-control (A/C) mode and synchronized intermittent mandatory ventilation (SIMV) mode. Pressure modes include pressure support ventilation (PSV) mode, pressure-controlled ventilation (PCV) mode, airway pressure release ventilation (APRV) mode, volume-guaranteed pressure options (VGPO) mode, continuous positive airway pressure (CPAP)/PEEP mode, and noninvasive BiPAP mode. There is no one best mode

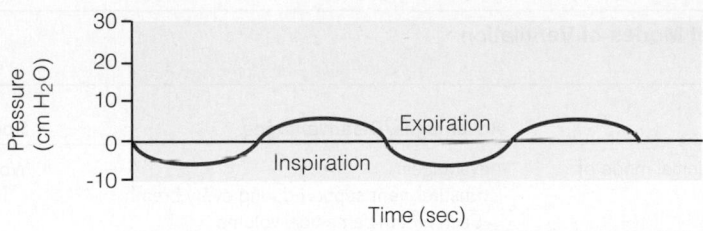

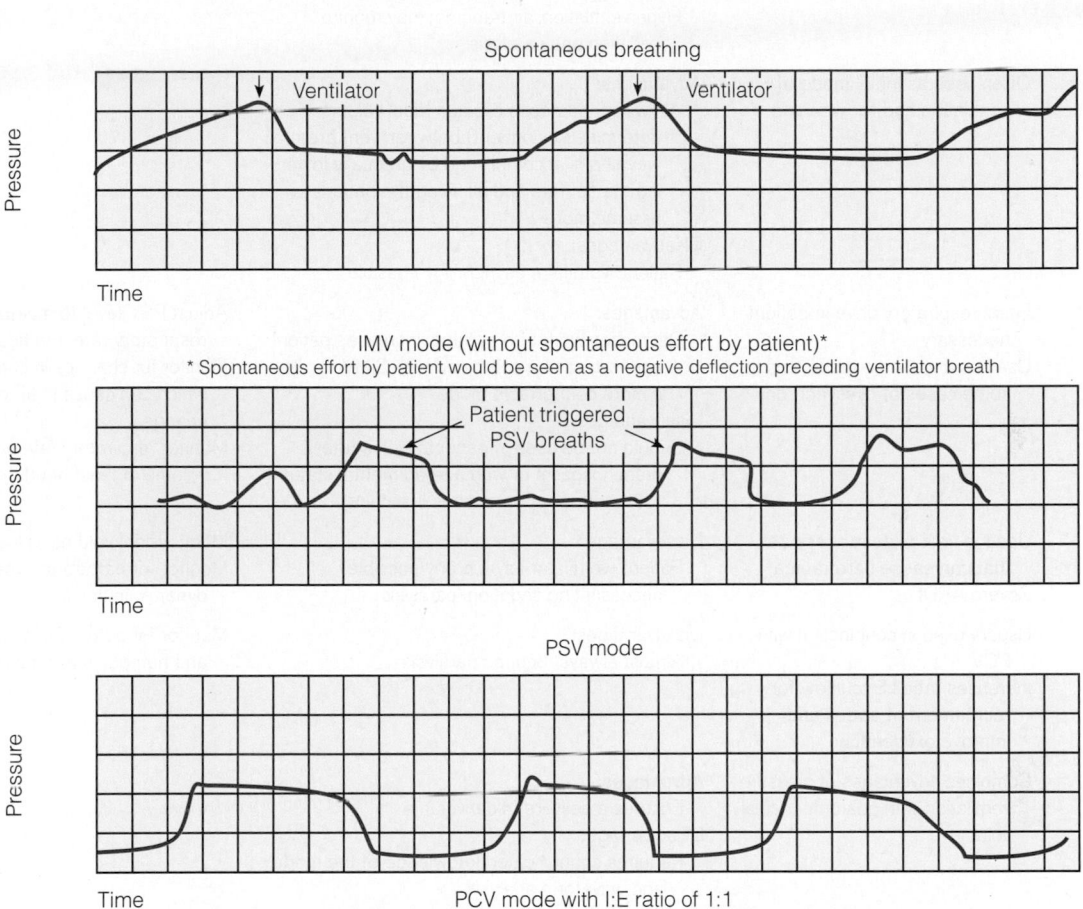

Figure 25-9 • Comparison of ventilatory modes using continuous airway pressure monitoring.

for managing patients in respiratory failure, although each mode has its advantages and disadvantages.

Volume Modes

Assist-Control Mode
In A/C mode, a mandatory (or "control") rate is selected. If the patient wishes to breathe faster, he or she can trigger the ventilator and receive a full-volume breath. This mode of ventilation is often used to fully support a patient, such as when the patient is first intubated or when the patient is too weak to perform the work of breathing (e.g., when emerging from anesthesia).

Synchronized Intermittent Mandatory Ventilation Mode
In SIMV mode, the rate and tidal volume are preset. If the patient wants to breathe above this rate, he or she may. However, unlike the A/C mode, any breaths

taken above the set rate are spontaneous breaths taken through the ventilator circuit. The tidal volume of these breaths can vary drastically from the tidal volume set on the ventilator because the tidal volume is determined solely by the patient's spontaneous effort. Adding pressure support (discussed in the next section) during spontaneous breaths can minimize the risk for increased work of breathing. In the past, SIMV was used as a popular weaning mode. To wean the patient, the mandatory breaths were gradually decreased, thereby allowing the patient to assume more and more of the work of breathing.

Pressure Modes

Pressure Support Ventilation Mode
PSV mode augments or assists spontaneous breathing efforts by delivering a high flow of gas to a selected pressure level early in inspiration and maintaining that level throughout the inspiratory phase. The

Table 25-7 • Comparison of Modes of Ventilation

Ventilatory Mode	Indications	Advantages/Disadvantages	Special Monitoring

A/C	Often used as initial mode of ventilation	Advantages:
		  Ensures vent support during every breath
		  Each breath same tidal volume
		Disadvantages:
		  Hyperventilation, air trapping; may require sedation and paralysis
			Work of breathing may be increased if sensitivity or flow rate is too low.

SIMV	Often used as initial mode of ventilation and for weaning	Advantages:
		  Allows spontaneous breaths (tidal volume determined by patient) between vent breaths; weaning is accomplished by gradually lowering the set rate and allowing the patient to assume more work
		Disadvantages:
		  Patient–ventilator asynchrony possible	

PSV	Intact respiratory drive in patient necessary
	Used as a weaning mode, and in some cases of dyssynchrony
		Advantages:
		  Decreases work of breathing; increases patient comfort; can be combined with SIMV to allow a more comfortable mode
		Disadvantages:
		  Should not be used in patients with acute bronchospasm or with altered mental status with reduced spontaneous breathing
			Adjust PSV level to maintain desired respiratory rate and tidal volume.
			Monitor for changes in compliance, which can cause tidal volume to change.
			Monitor respiratory rate and tidal volume at least hourly.

PCV	Used to limit plateau pressures that can cause barotrauma Severe ARDS	Disadvantages: Patient–ventilator asynchrony possible, necessitating sedation/paralysis	Monitor tidal volume at least hourly. Monitor for barotrauma, hemodynamic instability.
IRV	Usually used in conjunction with PCV Increases ratio I:E to allow for recruitment of alveoli and improve oxygenation	Disadvantages: Almost always requires paralysis	Monitor for auto-PEEP, barotrauma, and hemodynamic instability.

VGPO	Combines advantages of pressure ventilation with guaranteed tidal volume	Advantages:
		  Ensures a delivered tidal volume
		Disadvantages:
		  Requires sophisticated knowledge of the mode and waveform analysis	

CPAP	Constant positive airway pressure for patients who breathe spontaneously	Advantages:
		  Used in intubated or non-intubated patients
		Disadvantages:
		  On some systems, no alarm if respiratory rate falls
			Monitor for increased work of breathing.

Noninvasive (BiPap)	Nocturnal hypoventilation in patients with neuromuscular disease, chest wall deformity, obstructive sleep apnea, and COPD; to prevent intubation; to prevent reintubation initially after extubation	Advantages:
		  Decreased cost when patients can be cared for at home; no need for artificial airway
		Disadvantages:
		  Patient discomfort or claustrophobia
			Monitor for gastric distention, air leaks from mouth, aspiration risk.

patient's effort determines the rate, inspiratory flow, and tidal volume. When PSV mode is used as a stand-alone mode of ventilation, the pressure support level is adjusted to achieve the approximate targeted tidal volume and respiratory rate. At high pressure levels, PSV mode provides nearly total ventilatory support.

Specific uses of PSV are to promote patient comfort and synchrony with the ventilator, to decrease the work of breathing necessary to overcome the resistance of the endotracheal tube, and for weaning.

As a weaning tool, PSV is thought to increase the endurance of the respiratory muscles by decreasing the physical work and oxygen demands during spontaneous breathing. Because the level of pressure support can be gradually decreased, endurance conditioning is enhanced.

In PSV mode, the inspired tidal volume and respiratory rate must be monitored closely in order to detect changes in lung compliance. Generally, if compliance decreases or resistance increases, tidal volume decreases and respiratory rate increases. PSV mode should be used with caution in patients with bronchospasm or other reactive airway conditions.

Pressure-Controlled Ventilation Mode

The PCV mode is used to control plateau pressures in conditions such as ARDS in which compliance is decreased and the risk for barotrauma is high. It is used when the patient has persistent oxygenation problems despite a high FiO_2 and high levels of PEEP. The inspiratory pressure level, respiratory rate, and inspiratory/expiratory (I:E) ratio must be selected. Tidal volume varies with compliance, and airway resistance must be closely monitored. Sedation and the use of NMB agents are frequently indicated because any patient-ventilator asynchrony usually results in profound drops in the SaO_2. This is especially true when inverse ratios are used. The "unnatural" feeling of this mode often requires muscle relaxants in order to ensure patient-ventilator synchrony.

Most ventilators operate with a short inspiratory time and a long expiratory time (1:2 or 1:3 ratio). This promotes venous return and allows time for air to passively exit the lungs. Inverse ratio ventilation (IRV) mode reverses this ratio so that inspiratory time is equal to, or longer than, expiratory time (1:1 to 4:1). Inverse I:E ratios are used in conjunction with pressure control to improve oxygenation in patients with ARDS by expanding stiff alveoli using longer distending times, thereby providing more opportunity for gas exchange and preventing alveolar collapse.

As expiratory time is decreased, the nurse must monitor for the development of hyperinflation or auto-PEEP. Regional alveolar overdistention and barotrauma may result from excessive total PEEP.[50] When the PCV mode is used, the mean airway and intrathoracic pressure rise, potentially resulting in a decrease in cardiac output and oxygen delivery. Therefore, it is necessary to monitor the patient's hemodynamic status closely.

Airway Pressure Release Ventilation Mode

APRV has been used in trauma and ARDS patients to reduce airway pressure and lower minute volume while allowing spontaneous breathing throughout the ventilator cycle, all with decreased sedation and NMB agent use. APRV mode allows lung protective strategies to be followed with limitation of plateau and peak pressures. The mode functions by having a time-triggered, pressure-limited, time-cycled mode of ventilation. It consists of a high-pressure setting and a low-pressure setting, with recruitment and oxygenation occurring during the high-pressure setting at a long set time interval (5.4 seconds) followed by a brief controlled release (0.6 second) to the low-pressure setting. What this means is that the patient spontaneously breathes both at a set high pressure with preset brief times and at low pressure, which is synchronized during exhalation. Because the patient is breathing spontaneously throughout both high- and low-pressure phases, sedation may be limited. Weaning from APRV is done by decreasing the high-

pressure limit while increasing the time at high pressure. At the same time, the low-pressure limit may be dropped, allowing for reduced mean airway pressure. Usually, the low-pressure limit is reduced to 5 cm H_2O, and as the high pressure is lowered, this allows release to a PEEP level that prevents de-recruitment. When the patient tolerates an FiO_2 of 50% or less, the patient can be switched to PSV and further weaning. This mode may improve oxygenation and prevent VALI and VILI in patients with ARDS or ALI.[51]

Volume-Guaranteed Pressure Options Mode

VGPO mode ensures delivery of a prescribed tidal volume while using a decelerating flow pattern by means of a "pressure" breath. The options include both spontaneous and control rate parameters, and the volume guarantee is provided differently, depending on the ventilator.[52] VGPO can be used in acutely ill patients as well as more stable, weaning patients. Some examples include the volume support and pressure-regulated volume control options (Siemens Medical) as well as pressure augmentation (Bear Medical Systems).

In the acutely ill, unstable patient, this option may provide pressure ventilation while guaranteeing tidal volume and minute ventilation at a set rate. In the spontaneously breathing patient, the option is used as a "safety" when pressure ventilation is desired. The use of a volume guarantee in the spontaneously breathing patient may be especially important at night (when respiratory rates and volumes normally decrease) and in patients for whom secretions are a problem (because secretions increase resistance and result in decreased spontaneous volumes).

Continuous Positive Airway Pressure/Positive End-Expiratory Pressure Mode

CPAP is the term used when PEEP is supplied during spontaneous breathing. PEEP is the term used to describe positive end-expiratory pressure with positive-pressure (machine) breaths. CPAP assists spontaneously breathing patients to improve their oxygenation by elevating the end-expiratory pressure in the lungs throughout the respiratory cycle. CPAP can be used for intubated and nonintubated patients. It may be used as a weaning mode and for nocturnal ventilation (nasal or mask CPAP) to splint open the upper airway, preventing upper airway obstruction in patients with obstructive sleep apnea.

PEEP is positive pressure exerted at the end of exhalation. It is common practice to use low levels of PEEP (2 to 5 cm H_2O) in the intubated patient. PEEP is increased in 2- to 5-cm H_2O increments when FiO_2 levels are greater than 50% to attain an acceptable SaO_2 (greater than 90%) or PaO_2 (greater than 60 to 70 mm Hg). PEEP is most often necessary in patients with refractory hypoxemia (such as those with ARDS) in whom the PaO_2 deteriorates rapidly, despite greater concentrations of oxygen administration.

PEEP is used to keep alveoli stented open, and it may recruit alveolar units that are totally or partially collapsed during any mode of ventilation. This end-expiratory pressure increases the functional residual capacity (FRC) by reinflating collapsed alveoli, maintains the alveoli in an open position, and improves lung compliance. This decreases shunt and improves oxygenation. In addition, there is some evidence that keeping the alveoli open enhances surfactant regeneration. High levels of PEEP should rarely be interrupted because it may take several hours to recruit alveoli again and restore the FRC; until this occurs, oxygenation may suffer.[53]

In the patient who does not have adequate circulating blood volume, institution of PEEP decreases venous return to the heart, decreases cardiac output, and decreases oxygen delivery to the tissues. If hypotension or decreased cardiac output results from PEEP application, restoring circulating intravascular volume with administration of intravenous fluids may correct the hypotension. Another serious complication of PEEP is barotrauma. It can occur in any mechanically ventilated patient but is most common when high levels of PEEP are used ($\geq$10 to 20 cm H_2O) in lungs with high ventilating pressures and low compliance and in patients with obstructive airway disease. The development of barotrauma is an emergency and usually requires placement of a chest tube.

Noninvasive Bilateral Positive-Pressure Ventilation Mode

BiPAP is a noninvasive form of mechanical ventilation provided by means of a nasal mask, nasal prongs, or a full facemask. It is used in the treatment of patients with chronic respiratory insufficiency to manage acute or chronic respiratory failure without intubation and conventional mechanical ventilation. It is also used as a bridge to weaning patients from mechanical ventilation and as an alternative to conventional mechanical ventilation in patients who are ventilated in their homes.[50] The system allows the clinician to select two levels of positive-pressure support: an inspiratory pressure support level (referred to as IPAP) and an expiratory pressure called EPAP (PEEP/CPAP level).[36] Because BiPAP allows for the provision of assisted inspiration with ventilator rate set, application of this mode to those patients who hypoventilate as well as obstruct during sleep is possible.

BiPAP is beneficial in patients with worsening hypoventilation, obstructive apneic episodes, or both. It is also useful to prevent intubation in patients with respiratory failure and hypercarbia as well as to prevent reintubation following extubation in borderline cases. Use of a full facemask may increase the risk for aspiration and risk for rebreathing carbon dioxide; therefore, ventilation with a full facemask should be used cautiously. Thick or copious secretions and poor cough may be relative contraindications for BiPAP.[54]

USE OF MECHANICAL VENTILATORS

Setting Ventilator Controls

The nurse must know how to monitor the various ventilators, modes, and controls before giving mechanical ventilatory support to a patient. The following section discusses these various controls and settings and their implications for nursing care. In some institutions, the respiratory therapists share or have complete responsibility for managing the ventilator, but the nurse still needs to be fully aware of the implications for the patient of the mode and level of mechanical support.[45]

Ventilator settings must be frequently evaluated against patient response. Iatrogenically induced complications include overventilation (which causes respiratory alkalosis) and underventilation (which causes respiratory acidosis or hypoxemia). ABG studies determine the effectiveness of mechanical ventilation. Patients with chronic pulmonary disease, however, should be ventilated to stay relatively close to their normal ABG values. This usually means accepting relatively high carbon dioxide levels, lower-than-average oxygenation, or both.

Fraction of Inspired Oxygen

Ventilators allow for adjustment of oxygen percentage (FiO_2) with in-circuit or external oxygen analyzers, thus allowing the nurse to ascertain the FiO_2 being delivered. Initially, a patient is placed on a high level of FiO_2 (60% or higher). Subsequent changes in FiO_2 are based on ABGs and the SaO_2. Usually, the FiO_2 is adjusted to maintain an SaO_2 of greater than 90% (roughly equivalent to a PaO_2 greater than 60 mm Hg). Oxygen toxicity is a concern when an FiO_2 of greater than 60% is required for more than 24 hours; therefore, most clinicians attempt to use strategies to allow for maintenance of an FiO_2 of 60% or less.

Respiratory Rate

The number of breaths per minute delivered to the patient can be directly dialed on most ventilator models. The nurse double-checks the functioning of the ventilator by observing the patient's respiratory rate. In the pressure ventilator, the inspiratory time determines the duration of inspiration by regulating the gas flow rate. The higher the flow rate, the faster peak airway pressure is reached, and the shorter the inspiration; conversely, the lower the flow rate, the longer the inspiration. A very high flow rate may produce turbulence, shallow inspirations, and uneven distribution of volume.

Respiratory rate times tidal volume equals minute ventilation ($RR \times V_T = MV$). In turn, minute volume determines alveolar ventilation. These two parameters are adjusted according to the $PaCO_2$. Increasing the minute volume decreases the $PaCO_2$; conversely, decreasing the minute volume increases the $PaCO_2$. In special cases, hypoventilation or hyperventilation is desired. For example, in a patient with a head injury, respiratory alkalosis may be required to promote cerebral vasoconstriction, with a resultant decrease in ICP. In this case, the tidal volume and respiratory rate are increased to achieve the desired alkalotic pH by manipulating the $PaCO_2$. In contrast, a patient with COPD whose baseline ABGs reflect an elevated $PaCO_2$ should not be hyperventilated. Instead, the goal should be restoration of the baseline $PaCO_2$. These patients usually have a large carbonic acid load, and lowering their carbon dioxide levels rapidly may result in seizures. Rate adjustments may also be necessary to enhance patient comfort or when rapid rates cause air trapping that results in auto-PEEP.

Tidal Volume

In the volume ventilator, the number of milliliters of air to be delivered with each breath is set by the clinician. Traditionally, tidal volumes of 10 to 15 mL/kg of body weight were used. Research has identified a phenomenon of iatrogenic lung injury (VILI or VALI), in which forces produced in the lungs by the large tidal volumes may aggravate the damage inflicted on the lungs by the pathological process that necessitated mechanical ventilation.[47] For this reason, lower tidal volume targets (5 to 8 mL/kg) are now recommended.

Peak Flow

Peak flow is the velocity of gas flow per unit of time and is expressed as liters per minute. On many volume ventilators, this is a separate dial. If auto-PEEP (due to inadequate expiratory time) is present, peak flow is increased to shorten inspiratory time so that the patient may exhale completely. However, increasing peak flow increases turbulence, which is reflected in increasing airway pressures.

Inspiratory Pressure Limit

On volume-cycled ventilators, the inspiratory pressure limit (IPL) control limits the highest pressure allowed in the ventilator circuit. Once the high pressure limit is reached, inspiration is terminated. Therefore, if the IPL is being constantly reached, the designated tidal volume is not being delivered to the patient. The cause of this can be coughing, accumulation of secretions, kinked ventilator tubing, pneumothorax, decreasing compliance, or a pressure limit alarm set too low. IPL is used with pressure support ventilation to adjust the pressure during spontaneous breathing, providing reduced work of breathing. Weaning can be accomplished in the pressure support ventilation mode by reduction of IPL to low levels as the patient increases work of breathing.

Positive End-Expiratory Pressure

The PEEP control adjusts the pressure that is maintained in the lungs at the end of expiration. PEEP and CPAP can be visualized on the respiratory pressure gauge or display. Instead of returning to zero (atmospheric pressure) at the end of expiration, the pressure value drops to the PEEP/CPAP level. Reduction of PEEP is considered if the patient has a PaO_2 of 80 to 100 mm Hg or an FiO_2 of 50% or less, is hemodynamically stable, and has stabilization or improvement of the underlying illness. To evaluate whether the effects of PEEP are beneficial, monitoring of ABGs, SaO_2, compliance, and hemodynamic pressures (including cardiac output and blood pressure) is necessary. Baseline values are obtained before changes in PEEP are made. PEEP is usually increased in increments of 2 to 5 cm H_2O. The patient is monitored for adverse effects, such as hypotension and dysrhythmias. If these occur, the PEEP is reduced. If higher PEEP is tolerated, the patient is stabilized on the new PEEP settings for approximately 15 minutes. The monitored parameters are then repeated.

Hemodynamic measurements (cardiac output, pulmonary artery pressure [PAP], CVP, and pulmonary artery wedge pressure [PAWP]) are taken at end expiration with the patient on PEEP. Accuracy in selecting the point of end expiration on the waveform tracing is facilitated by using continuous airway monitoring (Fig. 25-10).[55] PEEP does not need to be discontinued before obtaining hemodynamic measurements. Hemodynamic measurements can be inaccurate (as an indicator of volume status) if a patient is on high PEEP or the position of the transducer is not leveled at the phlebostatic axis. The position of the catheter within the pulmonary circulation should also be verified on a chest radiograph.

Attempts are made to minimize removing the patient from the ventilator when using high levels of PEEP. Oxygenation can deteriorate and be slow to rebound because it takes a significant amount of time for the effects of PEEP to be reestablished. Therefore, if the patient is being oxygenated using an MRB, it must be equipped with a valve that allows levels of PEEP to be dialed in. An in-line suction apparatus may be helpful to prevent breaking the PEEP circuit to suction the patient.

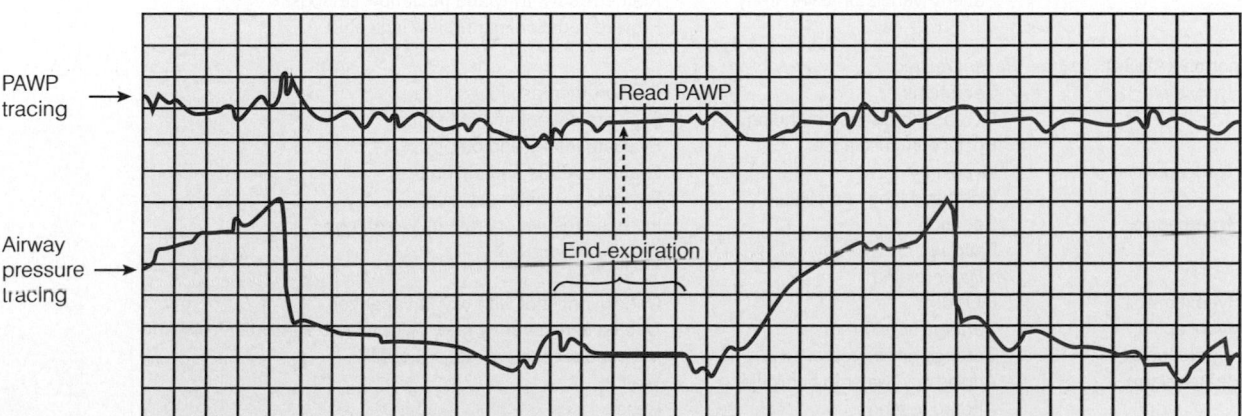

Figure 25-10 • Use of continuous airway pressure monitoring to assist in identifying point of end-expiration.

Sensitivity

The sensitivity function controls the amount of patient effort needed to initiate an inspiration, as measured by negative inspiratory effort. Increasing the sensitivity (requiring less negative force) decreases the amount of work the patient must do to initiate a ventilator breath. Likewise, decreasing the sensitivity increases the amount of negative pressure that the patient needs to initiate inspiration and increases the work of breathing.

Responding to Alarms

Mechanical ventilators are used to support life. Alarm systems are necessary to warn the nurse of developing problems. Alarm systems can be categorized according to volume and pressure, high and low. Low-pressure alarms warn of disconnection of the patient from the ventilator or circuit leaks. High-pressure alarms warn of rising pressures. Electrical failure alarms are necessary for all ventilators. A nurse or respiratory therapist must respond to every ventilator alarm. Alarms must never be ignored or disarmed. Some clinical troubleshooting guidelines are presented in Table 25-8.

Ventilator malfunction is a potentially serious problem. Nursing or respiratory therapists perform ventilator checks every 2 to 4 hours, and recurrent alarms may alert the clinician to the possibility of an equipment-related issue. When device malfunction is suspected, a second person manually ventilates the patient while the nurse or therapist looks for the

Table 25-8 • Troubleshooting the Ventilator

Problem	Possible Causes	Action
Volume or pressure alarm	*Patient related*	
	Patient disconnected from ventilator	Reconnect STAT.
		Auscultate neck for possible leak around endotracheal tube (ETT) cuff.
	Loss of delivered V_T	Review chest film for endotracheal tube placement—may be too high.
		Check for loss of V_T through chest tube.
	Decrease in patient-initiated breaths	Evaluate patient for cause: check respiratory rate, arterial blood gases (ABGs), last sedation.
	Increased compliance	May be due to clearing of secretions or relief of bronchospasms.
	Ventilator related	
	Leaks	Check all tubing for loss of connection, starting at patient and moving toward humidifier.
		Check for change in ventilator settings.
		(*Note:* If problem is not corrected STAT, use mandatory resuscitation bag until ventilator problem is corrected.)
High-pressure or peak-pressure alarm	*Patient related*	
	Decreased compliance	
	Increased dynamic pressures	Suction patient.
		Administer inhaled β-agonists.
		If sudden, evaluate for pneumothorax.
		Evaluate chest film for ETT placement in right mainstem bronchus.
		Sedate if patient is bucking the ventilator or biting the ETT.
	Increased static pressure	Evaluate ABGs for hypoxia, fluids for overload, chest film for atelectasis.
		Auscultate breath sounds.
	Ventilator related	
	Tubing kinked	Check tubing.
	Tubing filled with water	Empty water into a receptacle: Do not drain back into the humidifier.
	Patient–ventilator asynchrony	Recheck sensitivity and peak flow settings.
		Provide sedation/paralysis if indicated.
Abnormal (ABGs)	*Patient related*	
Hypoxemia	Secretions	Suction. Increase FiO_2
	Increase in disease pathology	Evaluate patient and chest film.
	Positive fluid balance	Evaluate Intake and output.
Hypocapnia	Hypoxia	Evaluate ABGs and patient.
	Increased lung compliance	Evaluate for wean potential.
Hypercapnia	Sedation	Increase respiratory rate or V_T settings.
	Fatigue	
	Ventilator related	
Hypoxemia	FiO_2 drift	Check ventilator with oxygen analyzer.
Hypocapnia	Settings not correct	Decrease respiratory rate, V_T, or minute ventilation (MV).
Hypercapnia	Settings not correct	Increase respiratory rate, V_T, or MV.
Heater alarm	Adding cold water to humidifier	Wait.
	Altered setting	Reset.
	Cold air blowing on humidifier	Redirect air flow.

cause. If a problem cannot be promptly corrected by ventilator adjustment, a different machine is procured so that the ventilator in question can be taken out of service for analysis and repaired by technical staff.

Ensuring Humidification and Thermoregulation

Mechanical ventilation bypasses the upper airway, thereby negating the body's protective mechanism for humidifying and warming inspired air. These two processes must be added to the ventilator circuit in the form of a humidifier with a temperature control. All air delivered by the ventilator passes through the water in the humidifier, where it is warmed and saturated. Because of this, insensible water loss is decreased. In most instances, the temperature of the air is about body temperature. In some rare instances (severe hypothermia), the air temperatures can be increased. Caution is advised because prolonged inhalation of gas at high temperatures can cause tracheal burns. An empty humidifier contributes to drying the airway, often with resultant mucus plugging and less ability to suction out secretions.

As air passes through the ventilator to the patient, water condenses in the corrugated tubing. This moisture is considered contaminated and must be drained into a receptacle and not back into the sterile humidifier. If the water is allowed to build up, resistance is developed in the circuit, and PEEP is generated. In addition, if moisture accumulates near the endotracheal tube, the patient can aspirate the water. The nurse and respiratory therapist jointly are responsible for preventing this condensation buildup. The humidifier is an ideal medium for bacterial growth. Institutional policies should describe the frequency of ventilator circuit changes.

COMPLICATIONS OF MECHANICAL VENTILATION

Complications that can occur with mechanical ventilation are listed in Box 25-12. Although all these adverse consequences occur over time in some ventilated patients, the incidence of these complications can be minimized by good preventive care practices.

Aspiration

Aspiration can occur before, during, or after intubation. The potential for developing nosocomial pneumonia or ARDS is increased if aspiration occurs. The risk for aspiration after intubation can be minimized by maintaining appropriate cuff inflation, evacuation of gastric distention with suction, suctioning of the oropharynx (especially before cuff deflations), and elevation of the head of the patient's bed 30 degrees or more at all times.[27] Elevation of the head of the bed is limited when the patient has femoral site IV lines; however, the bed can be raised up to 15 to 20 degrees and then placed in slight reverse Trendelenburg to approximate 30 degrees of elevation.

Box 25-12 • Complications of Mechanical Ventilation

Airway
- Aspiration
- Decreased clearance of secretions
- Ventilator-acquired pneumonia

Endotracheal Tube
- Tube kinked or plugged
- Rupture of piriform sinus
- Tracheal stenosis or tracheomalacia
- Mainstem intubation with contralateral lung atelectasis
- Cuff failure
- Sinusitis
- Otitis media
- Laryngeal edema

Mechanical
- Hypoventilation with atelectasis
- Hyperventilation with hypocapnia and respiratory alkalosis
- Barotrauma (pneumothorax or tension pneumothorax, pneumomediastinum, subcutaneous emphysema)
- Alarm "turned off"
- Failure of alarms or ventilator
- Inadequate nebulization or humidification
- Overheated inspired air, resulting in hyperthermia

Physiological
- Fluid overload with humidified air and sodium chloride (NaCl) retention
- Depressed cardiac function and hypotension
- Stress ulcers
- Paralytic ileus
- Gastric distention
- Starvation
- Dyssynchronous breathing pattern

Barotrauma and Pneumothorax

Mechanical ventilation involves "pumping" air into the chest, creating positive pressures during inspiration that may lead to barotrauma. If PEEP is added, the pressures are increased and continued throughout expiration. These positive pressures, especially with PEEP greater than 10 to 15 cm H_2O, can spontaneously rupture an alveolus or emphysematous bleb in the patient with COPD. Air then escapes into, and is trapped in, the pleural space, accumulating until it begins to collapse the lung. Eventually the collapsing lung impinges on the mediastinal structures, compressing the trachea and eventually the heart; this is called tension pneumothorax. Signs and symptoms of tension pneumothorax are listed in Box 25-13. Signs of pneumothorax include extreme dyspnea, hypoxemia (indicated by a decrease in SaO_2), and an abrupt increase in PIP. Breath sounds may be decreased or absent on the affected side; however, this sign may not be reliable in the patient on positive-pressure ventilation. Observation of the patient may reveal a tracheal deviation (to the opposite side) or the sudden development of subcutaneous emphysema. The most ominous signs of tension pneumothorax are hypotension and bradycardia that can deteriorate into a cardiac arrest without timely medical intervention. The physician or other qualified health care professional may decompress the chest by inserting a needle to evacuate the trapped air until a chest tube can be inserted.

Ventilator-Associated Pneumonia

VAP is the second most common HAP and the leading cause of death from nosocomial infections.[27,56–60] The incidence of nosocomial pneumonia is increased 10-fold in intubated patients, and the risk for developing VAP is especially great in critically ill patients who are mechanically ventilated. Factors that lead to nosocomial pneumonia are oropharyngeal colonization, gastric colonization, aspiration, and compromised lung defenses. Mechanical ventilation, reintubation, self-extubation, presence of a nasogastric tube, and supine position are a few of the associated risk factors for VAP. Maintenance of the natural gastric acid barrier in the stomach plays a major role in decreasing incidence and mortality from nosocomial pneumonia. The widespread use of antacids or histamine (H$_2$) blockers can predispose the patient to nosocomial infections because they decrease gastric acidity (increase alkalinity). These medications are used to guard against stress bleeding and may increase colonization of the upper gastrointestinal tract by bacteria that thrive in a more alkaline environment.

VAP is defined as nosocomial pneumonia in a patient who has been mechanically ventilated (by endotracheal tube or tracheostomy) for at least 48 hours at the time of diagnosis. A patient should be suspected of having a diagnosis of VAP if the chest radiograph shows new or progressive and persistent infiltrates. Other signs and symptoms can include a temperature higher than 100.4°F (38°C), leukocytosis, new-onset purulent sputum or cough, and worsening gas exchange.

There are numerous strategies for the prevention of VAP. The first step is to prevent colonization by pathogens of the oropharynx and gastrointestinal tract. Basic nursing care principles, such as meticulous handwashing and the use of gloves when suctioning patients orally or through the endotracheal tube, are essential. Gloves should also be worn when suctioning through closed-suction devices. In addition, critically ill patients have an increased risk for colonization by the microorganisms contributed by poor oral hygiene. Oral care for a mechanically ventilated patient involves brushing the patient's teeth (at least every 8 hours), using antimicrobial solutions and alcohol-free mouthwash to cleanse the mouth, applying a water-based mouth moisturizer to maintain the integrity of the oral mucosa, and thoroughly suctioning oral and subglottic secretions. Chlorhexidine oral rinse is one agent that provides antimicrobial action and is used in many institutions. An oral care protocol should be in place for every adult critical care unit using the current evidence-based research and practice.[56,61]

In patients receiving enteral feedings, the head of the bed should be elevated 30 to 45 degrees (unless contraindicated) to decrease the risk for aspiration.[27] Long-term nasally placed endotracheal and gastric tubes (i.e., longer than 3 days) should be placed orally unless contraindicated or not tolerated by the patient. This intervention reduces the risk for the patient developing sinusitis, which is associated with the development of VAP. Sinusitis is relatively common in nasally intubated patients and can cause bacteremia and sepsis. Signs of sinusitis (fever, purulent nasal drainage) must be reported immediately. Lastly, the use of an endotracheal tube that provides a port for the CASS appears to prevent the development of VAP in the first week of intubation, and it may decrease the overall incidence of VAP but does not affect mortality or length of stay.[27] The use of the CASS endotracheal tube is typically reserved for those patients who can be identified as potentially requiring long-term ventilation.

The advent of the ventilator bundle, which incorporates gastrointestinal and deep venous thrombosis prophylaxis, along with getting the patient out of bed, oral care, and keeping the head of the bed elevated 30 to 45 degrees, has reduced the incidence of VAP in many institutions. These procedures should be included as an integral part of the care of ventilated patients.[61]

Decreased Cardiac Output

Decreased cardiac output, as reflected by hypotension, may be observed at the initiation of mechanical ventilation. Although this is often attributed to the drugs used for intubation (narcotics, sedatives, and NMB agents all reduce blood pressure), the most important contribution to this phenomenon is lack of sympathetic tone and decreased venous return due to the effects of positive pressure within the chest. In addition to hypotension, other signs and symptoms can include unexplained restlessness, decreased levels of consciousness, decreased urine output, weak peripheral pulses, slow capillary refill, pallor, fatigue, and chest pain. Increasing fluids to correct

⧉ EVIDENCE-BASED PRACTICE HIGHLIGHT: VENTILATOR-ASSOCIATED PNEUMONIA*

Expected Practice:

- All patients receiving mechanical ventilation, as well as those at high risk for aspiration (e.g., decreased level of consciousness; with enteral tube in place), should have the head of the bed (HOB) elevated at an angle of 30 to 45 degrees unless medically contraindicated.
- Use an endotracheal (ET) tube with a dorsal lumen above the endotracheal cuff to allow drainage by continuous suctioning of tracheal secretions that accumulate in the subglottic area.
- Do not routinely change, on the basis of duration of use, the patient's ventilator circuit.

Supporting Evidence:

- Critically ill patients who are intubated for >24 hours are at 6 to 21 times the risk of developing ventilator-associated pneumonia (VAP)[1–3] and those intubated for <24 hours are at 3 times the risk of VAP.[4] Other risk factors for VAP include decreased level of consciousness, gastric distention, presence of gastric or small intestine tubes, and a trauma or COPD diagnosis. VAP is reported to occur at rates of 10 to 35 cases /1,000 ventilator days, depending on the clinical situation.[3]

- Aspiration of oral and/or gastric fluids is presumed to be an essential step in the development of VAP. Pulmonary aspiration is increased by supine positioning and pooling of secretions above the ET tube cuff.[1,5,6]
- Morbidity and mortality associated with the development of VAP are high, with mortality rates ranging from 20% to 41%.[4,7–8] Development of VAP increases ventilator days, critical care and hospital lengths of stay (LOS) by 4, 4 and 9 days, respectively,[2,7] and results in >$40,000 additional costs / VAP case.[2,6]
- Compared to supine positioning, studies have shown that simple positioning of the HOB to 30 degrees or higher significantly reduces gastric reflux and VAP (8% versus 34%, respectively),[4,9–12] yet national surveys and reports in the literature describe poor compliance rates with HOB elevation in critical care units.[4,13–15]
- Studies on the use of special ET tubes which remove secretions pooled above the cuff with continuous suction decrease VAP by 45% to 50%.[16–19]
- Studies on the frequency of ventilator circuit changes have found no increase in VAP with prolonged use.[20–22]
- National regulatory and expert consensus groups include these interventions as critical to decrease VAP.[1,23–25]

References

1. Weinstein R, Chinn R, Larson E, et al: Guidelines for prevention of healthcare-associated pneumonia. MMWR Morb Mort Wkly Rep (in press)

2. Rello J, Ollendorf D, Oster G, et al: Epidemiology and outcomes of ventilator-associated pneumonia in a large US database. Chest 122:2115–2121, 2002

3. Craven D: Epidemiology of ventilator-associated pneumonia. Chest 117:186S–187S, 2000

4. Kollef M: Ventilator-associated pneumonia: A multivariate analysis. JAMA 270:1965–1970, 1993

5. Torres A, Serra-Batiles J, Ros E, et al: Pulmonary aspiration of gastric contents in patients receiving mechanical ventilation: The effect of body position. Ann Intern Med 116:540–542, 1992

6. Craven D, Rosa F, Thornton D, et al: Nosocomial pneumonia: Emerging concepts in diagnosis, management and prophylaxis. Curr Opin Crit Care 8:421–429, 2002

7. Bercault N, Boulain T: Mortality rate attributable to ventilator-associated nosocomial pneumonia in an adult intensive care unit: A prospective case-control study. Crit Care Med 29:2303–2309, 2001

8. Heyland D, Cook D, Griffith L, et al: The attributable morbidity and mortality of ventilator-associated pneumonia in the critically ill patient. Am J Resp Crit Care Med 159:1249–1256, 1999

9. Ibanez J, Penafiel A, Raurich J, et al: Gastroesophageal reflux in intubated patients receiving enteral nutrition: Effect of supine and semi recumbent positions. J Parente Enter Nutr 16:419–422, 1992

10. Orozco-Levi M, Torres A, Ferrer M, et al: Semi-recumbent position protects from pulmonary aspiration but not completely from gastroesophageal reflux in mechanically ventilated patients. Am J Respir Crit Care Med 152:1387–1390, 1995

11. Drakulovic M, Torres A, Bauer T, et al: Supine body position as a risk factor for nosocomial pneumonia in mechanically ventilated patients: A randomized trial. Lancet 354:1851–1854, 1999

12. Dotson R, Robinson R, Pingleton S: Gastroesophageal reflux with nasogastric tubes: Effect of nasogastric tube size. Am J Respir Crit Care Med 149:1659–1662, 1994

13. Zack J, Garrison T, Trouillion E, et al: Effect of an educational program aimed at reducing the occurrence of ventilator-associated pneumonia. Crit Care Med 30:2407–2412, 2002

14. Berenholtz S, Pronovost P: Barriers to translating evidence into practice. Curr Opin Crit Care 9:321–325, 2003

15. Grap M, Cantly M, Munro C, et al: Use of backrest elevation in critical care: Pilot study. Am J Crit Care 8:475–480, 1999

16. Valles J, Artigas A, Rello J, et al: Continuous aspiration of subglottic secretions in preventing ventilator-associated pneumonia. Int Care Med 122:179–186, 1995

17. Mahul P, Auboyer C, Jospe R, et al: Prevention of nosocomial pneumonia in intubated patients: respective role of mechanical subglottic secretion drainage and stress ulcer prophylaxis. Int Care Med 18:20–25, 1992

18. Kollef M, Skubas N, Sundt T: A randomized clinical trial of continuous aspiration of subglottic secretions in cardiac surgery patients. Chest 116:1339–1346, 1999

(continued)

╬ **EVIDENCE-BASED PRACTICE HIGHLIGHTS: VENTILATOR-ASSOCIATED PNEUMONIA* (Continued)**

19. Cook D, KeJonge B, Brochard L, Brun-Buisson C: Influence of airway management on ventilator-associated pneumonia: Evidence from randomized trials. JAMA 279:761–787, 1998

20. Dreyfuss D, Djedaini K, Weber P, et al: Prospective study of nosocomial pneumonia and of patient circuit colonization during mechanical ventilation with circuit changes every 48 hours versus no change. Am Rev Respir Dis 143:738–743, 1991

21. Kotilainen H, Keroack M: Cost analysis and clinical impact of weekly ventilator circuit changes in patients in intensive care unit. Am J Infect Control 25:117–120, 1997

22. Kollef M, Shapiro S, Fraser V, et al: Mechanical ventilation with or without 7-day circuit changes: A randomized controlled trial. Ann Intern Med 123:168–174, 1995

23. Joint Commission on Accreditation of Healthcare Organizations: ICU Core Measures–draft statement. Retrieved September 26, 2003, from http://www.jcaho.org/pms/core+measures/candidate+core+measure+set.htm

24. Parrish C, Krenitsky J, McCray C. Nutritional support for the mechanically ventilated patient. In AACN's Protocols for Practice, Care of the Mechanically Ventilated Patient Series. AACN:Aliso Viejo, 1998.

25. Collard H, Saint S: Prevention of ventilator-associated pneumonia. Agency for Health Care Policy and Research (AHCPR) website: http://www.ahcpr.gov/clinic/ptsafety/chap17a.htm

*Excepted from American Association of Critical-Care Nurses Practice Alert.

the relative hypovolemia usually treats hypotension. However, in this setting, vasopressors may be needed.

Water Imbalance

The decreased venous return to the heart is sensed by the vagal stretch receptors located in the right atrium. This sensed hypovolemia stimulates the release of antidiuretic hormone from the posterior pituitary. The decreased cardiac output, leading to decreased urine output, compounds the problem by stimulating the renin-angiotensin-aldosterone response. The patient who is mechanically ventilated, is hemodynamically unstable, and requires large amounts of fluid resuscitation can experience extensive edema, including scleral and facial edema.

Complications Associated With Immobility

Many complications that contribute to the morbidity and mortality of mechanically ventilated patients are the result of immobility. These complications include muscle wasting and weakness, contractures, loss of skin integrity, pneumonia, and deep venous thrombosis that can result in pulmonary embolus, constipation, and ileus.

Gastrointestinal Problems

Gastrointestinal complications associated with mechanical ventilation include distention (due to air swallowing), hypomotility and ileus (due to immobility and the use of narcotic analgesics), vomiting, and breakdown of the intestinal mucosa due to the lack of normal nutritional intake. This breakdown allows translocation of bacteria from the gut into the bloodstream, leading to increased risk for bacteremia in patients who are unable to be fed enterally. Maintenance of an adequate bowel elimination pattern is necessary to prevent abdominal distention with resulting impingement on diaphragmatic excursion.

Many mechanically ventilated patients are already malnourished because of underlying chronic disease. Research verifies that the many side effects of clinical starvation can lead to pulmonary complications and death, as listed in Box 25-14. Early enteral nutrition is advocated for trauma and critically ill patients with either small-bore or Salem-sump tubes that end in the stomach or small intestine.[62] The advantage of small-bore feeding tubes is comfort, and with postpyloric placement, enteral feeding goal rates can be achieved sooner.[63,64]

Muscle Weakness

The muscles used in respiration, like other muscles, become deconditioned and may even atrophy with prolonged disuse. The ventilated patient's respiratory muscles may not be used (other than passive movement) while on the ventilator, especially if muscle relaxants, heavy sedation, or both have been part of the care plan. A retraining period to exercise and strengthen the respiratory muscles may be neces-

---

Box 25-14 • Side Effects of Clinical Starvation

- Atrophy of respiratory muscles
- Decreased protein
- Decreased albumin
- Decreased cell-mediated immunity
- Decreased surfactant production
- Decreased replication of respiratory epithelium
- Intracellular depletion of adenosine triphosphate
- Impaired cellular oxygenation
- Central respiratory depression

sary before ventilatory support can be discontinued. Especially at risk for "critical illness myopathies" are patients who have been on corticosteroids in combination with NMB agents as well as those with multiorgan failure, sepsis, and ARDS.[65–67]

Muscle weakness also occurs as a result of muscle fatigue. Those patients requiring mechanical ventilation typically have one or more reasons for an increase in the work of breathing. These include an increase in carbon dioxide production, physiological dead space (non–gas-exchanging air passages), or both; decreased lung compliance; and increased airway resistance, as with bronchospasm or thick secretions. When the work of breathing exceeds the capacity of weakened muscles, the patient begins to display abnormal respiratory mechanics with inefficient use of these muscles. This often occurs during a weaning trial after prolonged ventilation. The accepted intervention for fatigue in this setting is returning to muscle rest on the ventilator. However, this carries the risk for contributing further to muscle atrophy.[68] The diaphragm muscle also requires sufficient electrolytes of calcium, magnesium, and phosphorus to optimize function during weaning. The nurse should review electrolyte values daily to ensure these diaphragm-essential electrolytes are kept normalized.[69]

ASSESSMENT AND MANAGEMENT

The patient who needs ventilatory support also needs primary nursing care. One of the greatest contributions the nurse can make to decreasing costs, length of stay, and mortality in patients with respiratory problems is to implement interventions that will prevent or minimize complications. Because mechanical ventilation is supportive rather than curative, focus of care for the mechanically ventilated patient is holistic. The nurse must interact effectively with each member of the health care team to achieve desired patient outcomes. Box 25-15 gives examples of nursing diagnoses and collaborative problems for the patient who needs ventilatory support. Box 25-16 summarizes care of the patient on a ventilator. The mechanical ventilator, the artificial airway, and the care necessary to maintain mechanical ventilation require specialized nursing knowledge and skills, which are discussed in the following sections.

Endotracheal Tube Care

To prevent tube movement, tube migration, or inadvertent extubation, endotracheal tubes must be anchored securely. Anchoring can be accomplished with adhesive tape or with commercially manufactured tube immobilization appliances. Usual practice is to retape the endotracheal tube every 1 to 2 days or when it is soiled or insecure. In orally intubated patients, the position of the endotracheal tube should be changed from side to side to facilitate oral care and to prevent areas of pressure necrosis on the lips, mouth, and tongue.[70] The disadvantage of frequent retaping is that patients with fragile skin or prolonged intubation may incur skin breakdown. Twill tape can be substituted for adhesive tape in these sit-

---

Box 25-15 Examples of Nursing Diagnoses and Collaborative Problems for the Patient Who Needs Ventilatory Support

- Coping, Ineffective
- Fluid Volume, Excess
- Gas Exchange, Impaired
- Breathing Pattern, Ineffective
- Airway Clearance, Ineffective
- Tissue Perfusion, Ineffective (Peripheral, Cardiopulmonary)
- Body Image, Disturbed, related to intubation or tracheostomy
- Thought Processes, Disturbed
- Infection, Risk for
- Activity Intolerance, Risk for
- Airway Clearance, Ineffective
- Anxiety
- Aspiration, Risk for
- Breathing Pattern, Ineffective
- Mobility, Impaired Bed
- Sleep Deprivation
- Ventilatory Weaning Response, Dysfunctional

---

uations and for patients with heavy beards. Retaping by two people is desirable to prevent accidental tube displacement. The final step in retaping is to check tube placement in comparison to placement before retaping. Endotracheal tube placement is verified by radiography following initial intubation. The position in centimeters at the lips/teeth or nostril is recorded; this placement is verified every shift to detect inadvertent position changes. Tube placement is checked, following retaping, by comparing the centimeter markings at the lips/teeth or nostril with the last radiological documentation of position. Placement of an oral bite block can prevent biting on the tube, which can cause airway narrowing (the high-pressure alarm on the ventilator will sound) or tube displacement. Oral inspection and hygiene are of paramount importance when a bite block is used. The use of a swivel connector (connecting the tube to the ventilator circuit), along with anchoring a large loop of tubing to the bed, facilitates patient movement without endotracheal tube movement.

Persistent coughing may suggest that the endotracheal tube has migrated to touch the carina, requiring the tube to be withdrawn to an appropriate level. The pilot cuff balloon is protected from inadvertent disruption; cuff rupture or endotracheal tube occlusion with a mucus plug usually requires reintubation. If a patient is prematurely extubated for any reason, the airway must be kept patent. Oxygenation and ventilation may be provided with an MRB and mask until reintubation can be accomplished.

Tracheostomy Care

In patients requiring long-term mechanical ventilation, the airway is converted to a tracheostomy at some point to prevent the complications of endotracheal

Box 25-16 • COLLABORATIVE CARE GUIDE for the Patient on Mechanical Ventilation

OUTCOMES	INTERVENTIONS
Oxygenation/Ventilation A patent airway is maintained. Lungs are clear to auscultation. Patient is without evidence of atelectasis. Peak, mean, and plateau pressures are within normal limits. Arterial blood gases (ABGs) are within normal limits.	• Auscultate breath sounds q2–4h and PRN. • Suction as needed for rhonchi, coughing, or oxygen desaturation. • Hyperoxygenate and hyperventilate before and after each suction pass. • Monitor airway pressures q1–2h. • Monitor airway pressures after suctioning. • Administer bronchodilators and mucolytics as ordered. • Perform chest physiotherapy if indicated by clinical examination or chest x-ray. • Turn side to side q2h. • Consider kinetic therapy or prone positioning as indicated by clinical scenario. • Get patient out of bed to chair or standing position when stable. • Monitor pulse oximetry and end-tidal CO_2. • Monitor ABGs as indicated by changes in noninvasive parameters, patient status, or weaning protocol.
Circulation/Perfusion Blood pressure, heart rate, cardiac output, central venous pressure (CVP), and pulmonary artery pressure remain stable on mechanical ventilation.	• Assess hemodynamic effects of initiating positive-pressure ventilation (e.g., potential for decreased venous return and cardiac output). • Monitor electrocardiogram (ECG) for dysrhythmias related to hypoxemia. • Assess effects of ventilator setting changes (inspiratory pressures, tidal volume, positive end-expiratory pressure [PEEP], and fraction of inspired oxygen [FIO_2]) on hemodynamic and oxygenation parameters. • Administer intravascular volume as ordered to maintain preload.
Fluids/Electrolytes Intake and output (I & O) measurements are balanced. Electrolyte values are within normal limits.	• Monitor hydration status in relation to clinical examination, auscultation, amount and viscosity of lung secretions. • Assess patient weight, I & O totals, urine specific gravity, or serum osmolality to evaluate fluid balance. • Administer electrolyte replacements (IV or enteral) per physician's order.
Mobility Patients will maintain/regain baseline functional status related to mobility and self-care. Joint range of motion is maintained.	• Collaborate with physical/occupational therapy staff to encourage patient effort/participation to increase mobility. • Progress activity to sitting up in chair, standing at bedside, ambulating with assistance as soon as possible. • Assist patient with active or passive range-of-motion exercises of all extremities at least every shift. • Keep extremities in physiologically neutral position using pillows or appropriate splint/support devices as indicated.
Safety Endotracheal tube will remain in proper position. Proper inflation of endotracheal tube cuff is maintained. Ventilator alarm system remains activated.	• Securely stabilize endotracheal tube in position; use respiratory therapy expertise for best method. • Note and record the "cm" line on endotracheal tube position at lip or teeth. • Use patient self-protective devices or sedation per hospital protocol. • Evaluate endotracheal tube position on chest x-ray daily (by viewing film or by report).

(continued)

Box 25-16 • COLLABORATIVE CARE GUIDE for the Patient on Mechanical Ventilation (Continued)

OUTCOMES	INTERVENTIONS
	• Keep emergency airway equipment and manual resuscitation bag readily available, and check each shift. • Inflate cuff using minimal leak technique, or pressure less than 25 mm Hg by manometer. • Monitor cuff inflation/leak every shift and PRN. • Protect pilot balloon from damage. • Perform ventilator setting and alarm checks q4h (minimum) or per hospital protocol.
Skin Integrity Patient is without evidence of skin breakdown.	• Assess and document skin integrity at least every shift. • Turn side to side q2h; reassess bony prominences for evidence of pressure injury. • When patient is out of bed to chair, provide pressure relief to sitting surfaces at least q1h. • Remove self-protective devices from wrists, and monitor skin per hospital policy.
Nutrition Nutritional intake meets calculated metabolic need (e.g., basal energy expenditure equation). Patient will establish regular bowel elimination pattern.	• Consult dietitian for metabolic needs assessment and recommendations. • Provide early nutritional support by enteral or parenteral feeding, start within 48 hours of intubation. • Monitor actual delivery of nutrition daily with I & O calculations. • Weigh patient daily. • Administer bowel regimen medications as ordered, along with adequate hydration.
Comfort/Pain Control Patients will indicate/exhibit adequate relief of discomfort/pain while on mechanical ventilation.	• Document pain assessment, using numerical pain rating or similar scale when possible. • Provide analgesia as appropriate, document efficacy after each dose. • Prevent pulling and jarring of the ventilator tubing and endotracheal or tracheostomy tube. • Provide meticulous oral care q1–2h with oropharynx suctioning and mouth moisturizer as needed; teeth brushing scheduled at least t.i.d. antimicrobial b.i.d. oral assessment at least daily. • Administer sedation as indicated.
Psychosocial Patient participates in self-care and decision making related to own activities of daily living (ADLs) (e.g., turning, bathing). Patient communicates with health care providers and visitors.	• Encourage patient to move in bed and attempt to meet own basic comfort/hygiene needs independently. • Establish a daily schedule for bathing, time out of bed, treatments, and so forth with patient input. • Provide a means for patient to write notes and use visual tools to facilitate communication. • Encourage visitor conversations with patient in normal tone of voice and subject matter. • Teach visitors to assist with range-of-motion and other simple care delivery tasks, to facilitate normal patterns of interaction.

Teaching/Discharge Planning
Patient cooperates with and indicates understanding of need for mechanical ventilation.
Potential discharge needs are assessed.
	• Provide explanations to patient/significant others regarding:
	    Rationale for use of mechanical ventilation
	    Procedures such as suctioning, airway care, chest physiotherapy
	    Plan for and progress toward weaning and extubation
	• Initiate early social work to screen for needs, resources, and support systems.

intubation, such as tracheal stenosis and vocal cord paralysis. The preferred method of airway management is the tracheostomy tube for long-term ventilation. Past practice involved tracheostomy after 11 and up to 21 days on the ventilator. Current practice promotes earlier tracheostomy at 72 hours after intubation. Studies have been small, although larger ones still show an advantage from defining patients who will benefit from early tracheostomy. At some institutions, practice has been for earlier tracheostomy (e.g., after 3 to 7 days on the ventilator) to facilitate earlier weaning, particularly if the patient has multiple comorbidities and demonstrates difficulty weaning or has trauma or neurological diagnoses associated with prolonged need for an artificial airway.[71–73] Tracheostomy is also performed for patient comfort and safety when mobilizing the patient and may lead to decreased ventilator weaning time. In addition to long-term ventilation, indications for tracheostomy include upper airway obstruction, airway edema from anaphylaxis, failed intubation, multiple intubations (high risk for complications), complications of endotracheal tube intubation, absence of protective reflexes, home care, conditions in which endotracheal tube intubation is not possible (e.g., facial trauma, cervical fractures), and the desire for improved patient comfort.

The advantages of tracheostomy over endotracheal intubation include faster weaning (at least in part because of decreased dead space), enhanced patient comfort, enhanced communication, and the possibility of oral feeding. The tracheostomy is inserted into the trachea, thereby avoiding the mouth, upper airway, and glottis, and this decreases problems of airway resistance and occlusion. Box 25-17 lists the equipment necessary for performing a tracheostomy.

Tracheostomy is not without disadvantages. These include hemorrhage, infection, pneumothorax, and the need for an operative procedure that is itself a risk. Box 25-18 presents complications of tracheostomy. The most serious complication is erosion into the innominate artery, which can result in exsanguination. If bleeding occurs, the cuff can be hyperinflated in an attempt to control bleeding until emergency surgery can be performed. Recently, the practice of bedside percutaneous tracheostomy using a progressive dilation technique has been touted to decrease the morbidity and cost incurred with an operative procedure. Less infection and bleeding have also been given as advantages over the standard procedure performed in the operating room.[72]

The nurse can prevent complications by assessing for them with each patient interaction and during tracheostomy care. Proper fixation of the tracheostomy tube reduces the movement of the tube in the airway and limits friction injury to the tracheal wall or larynx. Maintaining the cuff pressure at the minimum required to prevent air leak on the ventilator reduces the risk for tissue breakdown due to excessive pressure on the trachea wall. The tracheostomy tube must be firmly secured. The ventilator tubing should have enough length to allow movement without pulling on the tracheostomy and to allow for procedures. A tracheostomy swivel connector, with or without flex tubing, reduces the tension on the tracheostomy while the patient is on the ventilator. A confused or very mobile patient can easily self-decannulate; patient restraints may be needed to prevent accidental decannulation. Orienting the patient to the need for an artificial airway and providing pain control and sedation (if needed to improve patient tolerance of the tracheostomy) are measures that are taken before resorting to restraint application. If restraints are needed, it is necessary to obtain a physician's order, with regular review of continued need. The nurse must monitor the patient closely for potential injury and

---

Box 25-17 • Equipment for Tracheostomy

- Percutaneous tracheostomy kit, either percutaneous or surgical*
- Surgical drapes, towels, gowns, gloves and sutures, prep equipment, and antiseptic application or solution
- Suction setup
- Correct size tracheostomy tube*
- 10-mL syringe for cuff inflation
- Twill tape, or Velcro tracheostomy holder†
- Pulse oximetry
- Oxygen source
- Manual resuscitation bag with mask
- End-tidal CO_2 monitor or disposable detector
- Sedation analgesic and paralytic medication
- Bronchoscopy cart (visualize correct placement for percutaneous approach)

---

*In adults, tube size is usually 8.0 mm initially unless the procedure is difficult. Percutaneous tracheostomy kits come with special tracheostomy tubes designed for that use. Smaller sizes can be used, and there are pediatric tracheostomy tubes.
†Initially the tracheostomy tube is sutured to the neck in both surgical and percutaneous procedures. Sutures are removed after 48 to 72 h. Tracheostomy is secured at all times with twill tape or a Velcro tracheostomy holder, even with the sutures in place, to prevent accidental dislodgment.

Box 25-18 • RED FLAG: Complications of Tracheostomy

- Acute hemorrhage at the site
- Air embolism
- Aspiration
- Tracheal stenosis
- Erosion into the innominate artery with exsanguination
- Failure of the tracheostomy cuff
- Laryngeal nerve damage
- Obstruction of tracheostomy tube
- Pneumothorax
- Subcutaneous and mediastinal emphysema
- Swallowing dysfunction
- Tracheoesophageal fistula
- Infection
- Accidental decannulation with loss of airway
- False placement of cannula (not in trachea)
- Weak voice/hoarseness

must perform circulatory checks with removal of restraints frequently.

Tracheostomy care includes frequent changing of tracheal ties and dressing, although initial ties are not changed until at least 24 to 48 hours after placement to allow for hemostasis of the site. The sutures from either a percutaneous or surgical tracheostomy are left in place for 48 to 72 hours or even up to a week (per hospital protocol) to prevent decannulation. As with retaping of the endotracheal tube, changing of tracheostomy ties should be a two-person procedure. The ties should be tied so that one to two fingers can be inserted between the ties and the skin, allowing minimal movement of the tracheostomy tube but maintaining comfort. It is mandatory to maintain a midline position for the tracheostomy to prevent pressure on surrounding tissue. The stoma is cleansed with half-strength hydrogen peroxide, followed by rinse with sterile saline, and observed for wound healing, bleeding, and signs of infection The routine practice of inner cannula cleaning or changes may not be necessary with a disposable inner cannula that can be changed daily. The routine care for tracheostomy is cleaning the tracheostomy site at least every 8 to 12 hours and as needed, changing the inner cannula daily (or according to facility policy), and changing soiled tracheostomy ties as needed, progressing to daily and as-needed care. This longer care interval usually occurs after 7 to 10 days or when secretion and tracheostomy drainage are minimal. The routine care of tracheostomies is always performed as a sterile procedure while in the hospital.[74,75]

If decannulation occurs within the first 7 days of tracheostomy insertion, the patient may be reintubated with an endotracheal tube if emergent tracheostomy tube replacement cannot be done safely. An obturator and a new, appropriately sized tracheostomy tube are kept at the bedside. If inadvertent decannulation occurs after a tract has developed, the tube is carefully replaced using the obturator.

Tube Cuff Pressure Monitoring

Tube cuff pressures are monitored every shift to prevent overdistention and excess pressure on the tracheal wall mucosa, which can cause complications such as tracheal stenosis. If a patient is on the ventilator, the best pressure is the lowest possible pressure without having a loss of inspiratory volume. Physiologically, pressures of about 20 to 30 mm Hg obliterate capillary circulation to the tracheal mucosa. If a cuff leak is suspected, auscultation at the neck for the sound of air escaping above the cuff can determine whether the seal is adequate.

One method used to inflate a cuff is called the minimal occluding volume. Air is injected slowly during ventilator inspiration while auscultation is performed over the trachea. When the harsh "squeak" of air escaping is no longer audible, the minimal occluding volume has been reached, and the tube cuff is occluding the airway without excessive pressure on the trachea. Extra air should not be added. In the intensive care unit, the best practice is actual measurement of cuff pressure using a manometer. This device is

attached to the endotracheal tube pilot balloon to obtain a reading, which should ideally be 20 to 25 mm Hg.[25] If a leak is still present above this level of inflation, slight repositioning of the endotracheal tube within the patient's airway may correct the problem. Changing to a larger or longer endotracheal tube may be necessary with increasing pressures to seal the airway. The cuff pressure is assessed with the manometer every 6 to 8 hours and, when a leak is noted, to help prevent aspiration of subglottic secretions. Whenever a cuff leak is found, the medical team and respiratory care practitioner should be notified. Recurrent cuff leaks may indicate the need for an extra long tube or a larger size to provide for ventilation.

Discharge Planning and Patient Teaching

Discharge planning is necessary for patients who will be discharged to home with tracheostomies. Rationales for tracheostomy care include promotion of ostomy healing, prevention of infection, maintenance of a patent airway, and increased patient comfort. Box 25-19 provides a discharge planning guide for the patient with a tracheostomy.

Box 25-19 • DISCHARGE PLANNING GUIDE: The Patient With a Tracheostomy

- Explain the rationale and procedure for home tracheostomy care to the patient and the caregiver.
- Arrange for home care supplies, oxygen, and suction equipment to be set up at the home before discharge.
- Arrange for home health care for review of care on ongoing monitoring. Aid is necessary if an additional caregiver is needed to hold the tracheostomy in place while changing the tracheal ties if the patient cannot assist.
- Provide a contact number where questions about tracheostomy care can be answered 24 hours per day, 7 days per week.
- Review the tracheostomy care procedure with the caregiver and monitor the caregiver performing this care.
- Ensure that the caregiver can perform the care, following the steps completely, and is able to recite indications for calling the physician or 911.
- If prepackaged tracheostomy kits are not being used, supply the following for home tracheostomy care:
  - Bottles of hydrogen peroxide (H_2O_2) and sterile normal saline (NS) (or sterile water)
  - Twill tape or premade Velcro tracheal ties
  - Disposable sterile cotton swabs, a sterile basin, and a sterile brush or pipe cleaners for inner cannula cleansing
  - Scissors, procedure gloves (nonsterile)
  - Suction equipment, catheters, and self-inflating resuscitation bag and mask, oxygen supply (suctioning with bagging is taught as a separate procedure for home care)
  - Sterile 4 × 4 gauze pads and sterile precut drain sponges to fit the tracheostomy
  - Sterile, packaged disposable inner cannulas
  - Protective eyewear and masks

Teaching the patient and family caregiver tracheostomy care allows for independence and self-care. This is an essential component of discharge teaching. Communication about the procedure and reassurance during the training process reduce anxiety and improve cooperation. The procedure in Box 25-20 is designed for the tracheostomy patient who is going home and who tolerates periods of time off the tracheostomy collar without experiencing a decrease in SaO_2.

Nutritional Support

Respiratory muscles, like all other body muscles, need energy to work. If energy needs are not met, muscle fatigue occurs, leading to discoordination of respiratory muscles and a decrease in tidal volume. Hypomagnesemia and hypophosphatemia have been implicated in muscle fatigue caused by depleted levels of adenosine triphosphate (ATP). Electrolyte imbalances must be corrected and monitored daily for optimal muscle functioning during ventilator weaning. In prolonged starvation, the body cannibalizes the intercostal and diaphragmatic muscles for energy.[68,76]

Metabolic needs in critically ill patients are much higher than in normal subjects. Basic caloric requirements are usually increased by 25% for hospital activity and stress associated with treatment. Adequate nutrition is a prerequisite for weaning from mechanical ventilation; nutritional support should be instituted early. If the gastrointestinal tract is intact, enteral nutrition is preferred and can be provided through a small-bore feeding tube.

Many chronically ill patients, such as those with COPD, have long-standing protein and calorie malnutrition. Initial tube feeding is started slowly, with close monitoring of blood glucose and electrolyte levels. The nurse observes the patient for signs of intolerance, such as diarrhea and hyperosmolar dehydration. If the patient tolerates feedings, the rate is gradually increased until the goal rate is achieved. If tube feedings cannot be tolerated, parenteral hyperalimentation should be considered (see Chapter 40).

Patients who require long-term mechanical ventilation typically need additional calories per day. When available, metabolic cart testing (also called indirect calorimetry) or a 24-hour urine nitrogen test can assess individual nutritional requirements. Nutritionists are invaluable in determining the caloric needs of critically ill patients.[62,63]

Eye Care

Eye care of the ventilator patient is important. Many intensive care unit patients are comatose, sedated, or chemically paralyzed and therefore have lost the blink reflex or ability to close their eyelids completely. This can lead to corneal dryness and ulceration.

Few studies have established the efficacy of one eye care measure over another. Current practices include instillation of lubricating drops or ointment, taping the eyes, applying eye shields, or applying a moisture chamber.[77] Eye care should be scheduled and not on an as-needed basis to ensure 24-hour application. Scleral edema is common in the ventilated patient. Raising the head of the bed may reduce scleral edema.

Oral Care

Frequent oral care must be performed on all mechanically ventilated patients. Oral care not only increases comfort but also preserves the integrity of the oropharyngeal mucosa. An intact mucosa helps prevent infection and colonization of organisms that has been shown to lead to VAP. As noted in the VAP discussion, evidence-based studies note the use of oral care protocols for ventilated adult patients in preventing VAP. Nursing skill manuals do present guidelines for oral care in patients with and without teeth as well as in those who are incapacitated.[26] However, these general oral care guidelines are not suitable for patients with an endotracheal tube and do not promote the prevention of VAP. Oral care in critical care varies with unit guidelines and usually is based on the nurse's experience, knowledge, and product availability.[61] The current literature includes oral care guidelines using every 2-, 4-, and 8-hour interventions with specific interventions of tooth brushing, oral and subglottic suctioning, moisturizer, and oral rinses.[78–82] The CDC recommends that every intensive care unit implement a complete oral care program to prevent oral colonization with use of an antimicrobial rinse.[56] What is still needed is a definitive research study regarding the optimal frequency, products, type of oral rinse, and materials to provide oral care for adult ventilated patients.[58,61,80,81] Including the oral care guideline as part of VAP prevention reduces VAP owing to education of nurses and implementation of practice changes, along with continued quality improvement monitoring of the effectiveness of oral care and VAP protocols.[56,80] Every intensive care unit should either review their oral care guideline or create one with the current evidence-based research and available protocols; they should follow the AACN Practice Alert on Oral Care in the critically ill.[82,83] Suggested guidelines may include the following:

1. Systematic assessment of the oral mucosa performed daily and with each cleaning
2. Handwashing before and after every nursing intervention
3. Routine brushing of teeth to remove dental plaque every 8 hours
4. Cleansing of the mouth every 2 hours and as needed
5. Use of an alcohol-free or antimicrobial (chlorhexidine) oral rinse every 8 or 12 hours to reduce oropharyngeal colonization
6. Suctioning the mouth and subglottic pharynx to minimize aspiration risk and provide a cover for the suction set with replacement every 8 or 24 hours
7. Applying a water-based mouth moisturizer to prevent mucosal drying and maintain oral mucosa integrity

Box 25-20 • Caring for a Tracheostomy at Home

ELEMENT	RATIONALE	PRECAUTIONS AND CONSIDERATIONS
1. Wash hands.	Reduces microorganisms on hands, standard precautions	Protective eyewear or facemask should be worn with copious secretions, especially in patients with forceful coughs
2. Bag and suction trachea as needed to remove secretions.	Preoxygenates to reduce risk for hypoxemia and cough during the tracheostomy care procedure Removes secretions from contaminating the stoma during tracheostomy care and keeps tracheostomy area clean	
3. Don procedure gloves and remove soiled dressing.	Reduces microorganisms	
4. Remove soiled gloves and prepare prepackaged kit or supplies; prepare supplies and place approximately 100 mL in two bowls, one with hydrogen peroxide (H_2O_2) and the other with normal saline (NS).		
5. Don new procedure gloves.	Reduces microorganisms, standard precautions	
6. Moisten cotton swabs and 4 × 4 gauze pads with NS, then cleanse and wipe stoma site, outer cannula, and neck plate. Half-strength H_2O_2 diluted with NS can be used for cleansing; NS alone can be used for this purpose when the tracheostomy wound is well healed. Rinsing with NS is done after using H_2O_2. Wipe under the neck plate. Performed as needed for secretions and 2 to 3 times daily to keep stoma clean.	Cleanses around the outer stoma and tracheostomy plate of secretions. H_2O_2 half-strength diluted with NS is appropriate for cleansing with an NS rinse using 4 × 4 pads or cotton-tipped applicators. Use NS alone to cleanse delicate skin around stoma when H_2O_2 leads to skin irritation. Draw only once from the bowel direction to prevent contamination, using new 4 ×4 or cotton swab each time. Discard each 4 × 4 or cotton swab after one use to prevent contamination.	Cleansing around the stoma before doing the inner cannula prevents contamination of the NS.
7. Remove tracheostomy collar and oxygen supply; remove inner cannula and place into H_2O_2 bowl. (See Precautions and Considerations for use of disposable inner cannulas and single-lumen tracheostomy tubes.)	Inner cannula can now be cleaned. Put on new clean gloves for the inner cannula care.	When using disposable inner cannulas, omit steps 6, 7, 8, and 10. Remove disposable inner cannula and replace with new inner cannula. With single-lumen tracheostomy tubes, skip steps 6, 7, 8, and 10. Periodic cleaning or changing of the inner cannula tube is thought necessary to identify narrowing of the inner cannula from encrusted or tenacious secretions. Tracheostomy care should be done q8h with increased stoma secretions; daily care may be necessary in the very long-term patient. The disposable inner cannula should be changed daily, and the reusable inner cannula cleansed daily as per protocols.[74,75]

(continued)

Box 25-20 • Caring for a Tracheostomy at Home (Continued)

ELEMENT	RATIONALE	PRECAUTIONS AND CONSIDERATIONS
8. Cleanse inner cannula with a small brush or pipe cleaners daily.	Removes debris and thick secretions	
9. Rinse inner cannula with NS poured over the cannula and let soak in the NS; remove and dry inner cannula.	Removes H_2O_2 and debris	Dry inner cannula before replacing to remove NS.
10. Insert and lock dry inner cannula in place. Reinsert at 90 degrees and turn into correct position; make sure the locking tab secures the inner cannula in place.	Secures inner cannula	Insert and lock dry inner cannula in place.
11. Pat dry the skin around the stoma with a dry 4 × 4 pad.	Dry skin reduces likelihood of micro-organism growth and skin breakdown.	
12. Prepare new tracheostomy ties or use premade tie; cut twill tape long enough to wrap around the neck twice.	Length appropriate for wrapping around the neck and tying on the side of the neck	Premade Velcro tracheostomy ties are available and easy to use; review manufacturer's guideline.
13. Have the patient or an assistant hold the tracheostomy securely during tracheostomy tie replacement.	Prevents accidental decannulation	
14. Remove old twill tape or premade tracheostomy tie.	Allows for clean tracheostomy tie application	Patient or assistant holds tracheostomy in place until new tie is secured; if patient unable to assist, tie the new twill tape into place first and then remove the old twill tape or have person stabilize the tracheostomy when replacing ties to prevent decannulation.
15. Apply twill tape and secure through eyes on neck plate; insert both ends into eyes, bring one end back around the neck and tie on one side of the neck; apply Velcro tracheostomy tie through both eyes, adjusting with Velcro to correct tightness.	Resecures the tracheostomy with the knot on the side of the neck; allows knot to be observed when using twill tape. Excessive tightness of the tracheostomy ties decreases circulation under the ties and can be uncomfortable for the patient.	Tighten tracheostomy tie to allow one finger to be inserted between tie and neck to keep tracheostomy in place with comfort. Twill tape loosens when wet, which may lead to an increased risk for tube dislodgment.
16. Tuck the precut drain sponge under the neck plate; change drain sponge as needed. Precut drain sponge is for secretions and may not be needed with a dry stoma.	Absorbs stoma secretions	Use only precut tracheostomy drain gauze; cutting a 4 × 4 pad causes frayed edges that may be a possible source for infection or irritation.
17. Replace tracheostomy collar for humidification and oxygen.	Returns humidified oxygen to tracheal airway	Humidified air or oxygen prevents drying of secretions that can lead to obstruction.
18. Remove all soiled supplies and wash hands after procedure.	Reduces microorganisms and is standard procedure	

Call the Physician or 911

- Indications for calling the physician include elevated temperature, oozing or frank bleeding at the stoma, foul odor from the stoma or secretions, and a change in or increased secretions around the tracheostomy opening. Report any change to the stoma appearance.
- Reasons for calling 911 include obstruction, loss of tracheostomy from the stoma, respiratory distress from other causes, severe bleeding, severe distress from febrile condition, and other potential medical emergencies.

Commercial kits are available that provide the suction catheters, covered tonsil tip suction, toothbrushes with suction, and toothpaste for brushing in individually wrapped sets to prevent contamination.

Psychological Care

The ventilated patient is subjected to extreme physical and emotional stress in the intensive care unit environment. Psychological distress can be caused by sleep deprivation, sensory overstimulation, sensory deprivation for familiar cues, pain, fear, inability to communicate, and commonly used pharmacological agents. Treatments can often seem dehumanizing. In many cases, the prognosis is poor, and the possibility of death is ever present.

Feelings of helplessness and lack of control can be overwhelming. The patient may attempt to gain some element of control through constant demanding or exhibition of other "inappropriate" behavior. If the patient is incapable of dealing with stress through coping mechanisms, he or she may exhibit depression, apathy, and lack of emotional involvement. These reactions may be exacerbated in patients with

---

▦ EVIDENCE-BASED PRACTICE HIGHLIGHT: ORAL CARE IN THE CRITICALLY ILL*

Expected Practice:

- Develop and implement a comprehensive oral hygiene program for patients in critical care and acute care settings who are at high risk for healthcare-associated pneumonia.
  - Brush teeth, gums and tongue at least twice a day using a soft pediatric or adult toothbrush.
  - In addition to brushing, provide oral moisturizing to oral mucosa and lips every 2 to 4 hours.
  - Use an oral chlorhexidine gluconate (0.12%) rinse twice a day during the perioperative period for adult patients who undergo cardiac surgery. Routine use in other populations is not recommended at this time.

Supporting Evidence:

- Colonization of the oropharynx is a critical factor in the development of nosocomial pneumonia.[1-3] Growth of potentially pathogenic bacteria in dental plaque provides a nidus of infection for microorganisms that have been shown to be responsible for the development of ventilator-associated pneumonia (VAP).[2-4] Dental plaque provides a microhabitat for organisms and provides opportunity for adherence either to the tooth surface or to other microorganisms. These microorganisms in the mouth translocate and colonize the lung, which can result in VAP.[3,5] Dental plaque can be removed by brushing. (Level VI)
  - Whereas there are no data associated with critically ill patients, the American Dental Association recommends that healthy people brush teeth twice daily to remove plaque from all tooth surfaces.[6] (Level II)
  - The use of an oral care protocol (brushing with a pediatric toothbrush, mouthwash, and moisturizing gel) reduced oral inflammation and improved oral health.[7] (Level IV)
- Chlorhexidine oral rinse reduced respiratory infections in cardiac surgery patients who received chlorhexidine before intubation as well as postoperatively[8] and reduced nosocomial pneumonia in patients who were intubated for more than 24 hours.[9] However, when chlorhexidine was tested in a more varied ICU population, no difference was observed

in VAP, mortality, or length of stay. Although oropharyngeal colonization by VAP pathogens was reduced with chlorhexidine, its efficacy was insufficient to reduce the incidence of respiratory infections.[10] A recent meta-analysis of chlorhexidine trials found that use of chlorhexidine did not result in significant reduction in the incidence of nosocomial pneumonia, nor in alteration of the mortality rate.[11] The CDC [Centers for Disease Control and Prevention] guidelines recommend use of chlorhexidine only during the perioperative period for adult patients undergoing cardiac surgery; routine use in other critically ill populations is not recommended.[12] (Level V)

- Several studies have tested intervention bundles that included oral care as one of the interventions.[13-14] Whereas these studies demonstrated that bundled interventions decreased nosocomial respiratory infections, the contribution of oral care to the results could not be determined. (Level IV)
- To date, no data have been published from large, well-controlled clinical trials of oral care interventions in critical care patients other than chlorhexidine studies. There are limited clinical reports of infection rates before and after changes in oral care procedures, but these reports have not been published in refereed journals. Whereas some reports have shown a positive effect, the role of oral care in reducing nosocomial pneumonia is not clearly established by such projects, and it is possible that other changes in care occurred in the units and affected the results.

AACN Grading Level of Evidence

Level I: Manufacturer's recommendations only

Level II: Theory based, no research data to support recommendations; recommendations from expert consensus group may exist

Level III: Laboratory data, no clinical data to support recommendations

Level IV: Limited clinical studies to support recommendations

Level V: Clinical studies in more than 1 or 2 patient populations and situations to support recommendations

Level VI: Clinical studies in a variety of patient populations and situations to support recommendations

References

1. *Munro CL, Grap MJ: Oral health and care in the intensive care unit: state of the science. Am J Crit Care 13:25–33, 2004*

2. *Fourrier F, Duvivier B, Boutigny H, et al: Colonization of dental plaque: A source of nosocomial infections in intensive care unit patients. Crit Care Med. 1998;26:301–308.*

(continued)

EVIDENCE-BASED PRACTICE HIGHLIGHTS: ORAL CARE IN THE CRITICALLY ILL* (Continued)

3. Garrouste OM, Chevret S, Arlet G, et al: Oropharyngeal or gastric colonization and nosocomial pneumonia in adult intensive care unit patients: A prospective study based on genomic DNA analysis. Am J Respir Crit Care Med 156:1647–1655, 1997

4. Scannapieco FA, Stewart EM, Mylotte JM: Colonization of dental plaque by respiratory pathogens in medical intensive care patients. Crit Care Med 20:740–745, 1992

5. El-Solh AA, Pietrantoni C, Bhat A, et al: Colonization of dental plaque: A reservoir of respiratory pathogens for hospital-acquired pneumonia in institutionalized elders. Am J Respir Crit Care Med 126:1575–1582, 2004

6. American Dental Association: Oral Health Topics: Cleaning your teeth and gums (oral hygiene). Retrieved September 19, 2006 from http://www.ada.org/public/topics/cleaning.asp

7. Fitch JA, Munro CL, Glass CA, Pellegrini JM: Oral care in the adult intensive care unit. Am J Crit Care 8:314–318, 1999

8. DeRiso AJ, Ladowski JS, Dillon TA, et al: Chlorhexidine gluconate 0.12% oral rinse reduces the incidence of total nosocomial respiratory infection and nonprophylactic systemic antibiotic use in patients undergoing heart surgery. Am J Respir Crit Care Med 109:1556–1561, 1996

9. Houston S, Hougland P, Anderson JJ, et al: Effectiveness of 0.12% chlorhexidine gluconate oral rinse in reducing prevalence of nosocomial pneumonia in patients undergoing heart surgery. Am J Crit Care 11:567–570, 2002

10. Fourrier F, Dubois D, Pronnier P, et al: Effect of gingival and dental plaque antiseptic decontamination on nosocomial infections acquired in the intensive care unit: A double-blind placebo-controlled multicenter study. Crit Care Med 33:1728–1735, 2005

11. Pineda LA, Saliba RG, El Solh AA: Effect of oral decontamination with chlorhexidine on the incidence of nosocomial pneumonia: A meta-analysis. Crit Care 10:R35, 2006

12. Tablan OC, Anderson LJ, Besser R, et al, and the CDC Healthcare Infection Control Practices Advisory Committee: Guidelines for preventing healthcare-associated pneumonia, 2003: Recommendations of CDC and the Healthcare Infection Control Practices Advisory Committee. MMWR Recomm Rep 53(RR-3):1–36, 2004

13. Zack JE, Garrison T, Trovillion E, et al: Effect of an education program aimed at reducing the occurrence of ventilator-associated pneumonia. Crit Care Med 30:2407–2412, 2002

14. Simmons-Trau D, Cenek P, Counterman J, et al: Reducing VAP with 6 Sigma. Nurs Manage 35:41–45, 2004

*Excerpted from American Association of Critical-Care Nurses Practice Alert.

a history of psychiatric problems or drug or alcohol abuse.

Assisted ventilation can precipitate a psychological dependence in those with primary respiratory disorders. If for the first time in years, a patient is receiving enough oxygen to meet metabolic needs and does not have to struggle for air, he or she may be reluctant to give up the ventilator. Weaning can become even more stressful for this patient. Nursing interventions to improve sleep with quiet time, psychiatric consultation, and alternative therapy such as music or massage, in addition to encouraging family support, will benefit the stressed patient. Taking the patient outside on the ventilator (weather permitting), sitting up in a chair, and ambulating on an MRB improve the patient's mental health.[84] Pet therapy, visiting with family and friends, and using a calendar for long-term patients helps keep them oriented. Resumption of home psychotropic medications, especially for depression or other disorders, is essential when compatible with the ongoing medical plan.[85]

Facilitating Communication

A number of interventions can facilitate communication with the patient who has an endotracheal or tracheostomy tube. Before assessing the patient's ability to communicate, provide the patient with his or her eyeglasses or hearing aid (if applicable). Complete explanations from staff members regarding any procedures may help decrease the patient's stress. The caregiver can use verbal and nonverbal communication skills. Nonverbal communication may include sign language, gestures, or lip reading. If the patient is unable to use these forms of nonverbal communication, helpful devices include pencil and paper, "grease" boards, picture or alphabet boards, electronic communication boards, and even a computer.

Once the patient is off the ventilator and tolerating the tracheostomy collar, the tracheostomy patient can communicate by using a cap or speaking valves that occlude the tracheostomy tube. These allow for the passage of air around the tracheostomy to the vocal chords as long as the cuff is deflated. The tracheostomy may be capped for 24 to 48 hours before decannulation, and the patient breathes and speaks around the tracheostomy. The cap is the final test to ensure airway protection by the patient. Two other options to the cap are the Passy-Muir valve and the Shiley speaking valve. The Passy-Muir and Shiley speaking valves are one-way valves that allow air to enter during inspiration and then close to allow the air to flow over the vocal chords with exhalation. These valves each have a side port for oxygen tubing to be attached, providing oxygen support in addition to the humidified air from a tracheostomy collar. The tracheostomy collar should be used nearly continuously to prevent the accumulation of secretions and the drying of the airway mucosa, and neither speaking valve should be used during sleep to prevent aspiration with a deflated cuff. Patients with copious secretions are at risk for obstruction of these valves. They must be monitored very closely. In addition, patients at high risk for aspiration, especially those with laryngeal or pharyngeal dysfunction, should be carefully assessed before one of these devices is used. The nurse should store these valves in a container clearly identified with the patient's name for safekeeping because each type of valve is relatively costly. The patient should be taught to remove the valve with excessive sputum during cough and call for assistance to clean the valve before reuse. The tracheostomy patient with a speaking valve is at increased risk for aspiration because the cuff must be deflated for the patient to communicate.

Caring for the Family

Family members must deal with a strange environment, a critically ill loved one, and the financial strain imposed by the illness. Nursing support is given by familiarizing the family with the physical surroundings, supplying information about visitation policies, and providing frequent progress reports on the patient's condition.[86,87]

Studies show improvement in patient outcomes from increased presence of loved ones during hospitalization. Based on these findings and on increased patient and family satisfaction, many intensive care units have instituted open visitation policies and increased involvement of family members in patient care. Critical care patients and especially the elderly benefit from increased visitation, and the families benefit from improved communication when they are the decision maker.[88,89] Nurses increasingly recognize the importance of family visitation for the patient. The presence of family during invasive procedures or during a code has been associated with positive outcomes, and studies show family and caregivers reported the benefit of being at the bedside.[87]

Often nurses do not consider family needs a priority. Ideally, the nurse establishes open communication with the patient and family, proactively arranges for visits, and provides the family with information. By promoting spiritual and cultural support, scheduled family communication conferences, nursing education on visitation, and open communication, the family has better coping and less stress.[87] A system that includes liberal visitation policies and flexibility for individual patient and family needs promotes a healing environment and supports the family as partners in the care plan.

WEANING FROM MECHANICAL VENTILATION

As soon as mechanical ventilation is started, plans begin for weaning the patient from mechanical support. The process to achieve this goal includes correcting the cause of respiratory failure, preventing complications, and restoring or maintaining physiological and psychological functional status. Patients can be categorized into two groups: those requiring short-term ventilation (3 days or less) and those requiring long-term ventilation (more than 3 days).[85]

Each patient is evaluated daily for readiness to wean. Boxes 25-21 and 25-22 present guidelines for weaning from short-term ventilation and long-term ventilation, respectively. It is important to perform this assessment and address weaning impediments before initiating weaning trials. Many weaning indices have been advocated for use in predicting weaning readiness. Some look exclusively at respiratory factors such as muscle strength and endurance (e.g., negative inspiratory pressure [NIP], PEP weaning index, or rapid shallow breathing index as the ratio of frequency to tidal volume). Others are integrated indices that look at a broad range of physiological factors that influence weaning readiness. Many of these factors individually lack predictability, and often several factors are assessed for weaning readiness.[69,90]

In addition to controversy concerning weaning indices, there is disagreement and lack of evidence regarding which approach to weaning is best. Some clinicians maintain total ventilatory support up until the time of weaning trials; others use intermittent trials of increasing frequency and duration. The theoretical advantages of a gradual approach to weaning support include the following: (1) over time, the patient on partial rather than full ventilation is exposed to lower levels of pressure and volume, therefore reducing the risk for complications; and (2) a weaning approach that requires the patient to perform some level of work to breathe imposes an "exercise" regimen that should reduce deconditioning and atrophy of the muscles used in respiration.[69]

The performance of the diaphragm, as well as accessory muscles of respiration, depends on both the endurance and strength of the muscles. The effectiveness of diaphragmatic contraction is a function of both the resting length of muscle fibers and the speed with which they contract. Both of these factors are affected by physiological changes that change the resting position of the diaphragm. With COPD, the resting length is shorter (weakening force of contraction), and with diaphragmatic distention, ascites, or morbid obesity, the diaphragm must push down abdominal contents as it contracts. Reactive airway disease increases the resistance to airflow, with increased workload for muscles of respiration. Any of these abnormalities can lead to significant fatigue of these muscles and respiratory distress.[76,91]

Respiratory muscle fatigue impedes weaning. It may take as long as 24 hours of complete rest (the mechanical ventilator assumes all of the work of breathing for the patient) for recovery of fatigued respiratory muscles. Therefore, it is common practice to increase ventilatory support at night to ensure rest. This can be accomplished with any of the "resting" modes, so long as the patient's respiratory rate is less than 20 breaths/minute. The intent here is to promote and simulate the normal decrease in rate and work of breathing that occurs during each person's sleep-rest cycle. Newer ventilator modes such as APRV may be useful to allow gradual reduction of support and increased patient work of breathing.[69]

Box 25-21 • Guidelines for Weaning From Short-Term Ventilation

Patients are often intubated electively for surgical or other procedures, or more urgently owing to respiratory distress related to underlying pulmonary disease or traumatic injury. The other common reason for intubation is the need for airway protection because of airway swelling (e.g., as a result of acute inhalation injury) or significant change in mental status (e.g., as with cerebrovascular accident or head injury). Once the procedure is completed or the patient is stabilized, the goal should be extubation as soon as the patient is able to protect the airway. The weaning process in this setting may proceed rapidly, based on individual patient response to reducing ventilatory support.

Readiness Criteria

- Hemodynamically stable, adequately resuscitated, and not requiring vasoactive support
- SaO_2 >90% on FiO_2 ≤40%, positive end-expiratory pressure ≤5 cm H_2O
- Chest x-ray reviewed for correctable factors; treated as indicated
- Metabolic indicators (serum pH, major electrolytes) within normal range
- Hematocrit >25%
- Core temperature >36°C and <39°C
- Adequate management of pain/anxiety/agitation
- No residual neuromuscular blockade
- Arterial blood gases normalized or at patient's baseline

Weaning Intervention

- Reduce ventilator rate, then convert to pressure-support ventilation (PSV) only.

- Wean PSV as tolerated to ≤10 cm H_2O.
- If patient meets tolerance criteria for at least 2 h on this level of support *and* meets extubation criteria (see later), may extubate.
- If patient fails tolerance criteria, increase PSV or add ventilator rate as needed to achieve "rest" settings (consistent respiratory rate <20 breaths/min) and review weaning criteria for correctable factors.
- Repeat wean attempt on PSV 10 cm after rest period (minimum, 2 h). If patient fails second wean trial, return to rest settings and use "long-term" ventilation weaning approach.

Tolerance Criteria

If the patient displays any of the following, the weaning trial should be stopped and the patient returned to "rest" settings.
- Sustained respiratory rate greater than 35 breaths/min
- SaO_2 <90%
- Tidal volume ≤5 mL/kg
- Sustained minute ventilation >200 mL/kg/min
- Evidence of respiratory or hemodynamic distress:
  Labored respiratory pattern
  Increased anxiety, diaphoresis, or both
  Sustained heart rate >20% higher or lower than baseline
  Systolic blood pressure >180 mm Hg or <90 mm Hg

Extubation Criteria

- Mental status: alert and able to respond to commands
- Good cough and gag reflex, able to protect airway and clear secretions
- Able to move air around endotracheal tube with cuff deflated and end of tube occluded

Adapted from evidence-based practice guidelines used in the Surgical/Trauma Intensive Care Unit, University of Virginia Health System, Charlottesville, Virginia.

Weaning trials are discontinued if signs of fatigue or respiratory distress develop. The weaning tolerance criteria and observations are summarized in Boxes 25-21 and 25-22. During physical therapy and activities, it is necessary to monitor the patient for fatigue with use of accessory muscles, increased respiratory rate, and decreased oxygen saturation that indicates respiratory muscle fatigue. The approach to prolonged mechanical ventilation includes aggressive physical therapy and activity to promote muscle conditioning and strength.[69,92,93] The use of sedatives and narcotics during weaning should be limited to only the level of medication clearly needed to control pain or anxiety. Special considerations for weaning an older patient from a ventilator are given in Box 25-23.

Regardless of the mode or approach, certain factors have been found to influence weaning success positively. These include the use of collaborative, multidisciplinary teams to formulate comprehensive plans of care based on assessment of individual patients, the use of standardized weaning protocols that are assigned to each patient based on individual assessment, and the use of critical pathways.[94] The interplay of these strategies, all designed to promote consistency of and rationale for practice, truly leads to outcomes showing that the whole (process) is greater than the sum of its parts.

Short-Term Ventilation Weaning

Patients typically intubated for a short time include those who are intubated for surgical procedures, for an acute exacerbation of an underlying lung disease that can be easily reversed, and for airway protection during an acute neurological event (e.g., drug overdose). Weaning within a short period of time is desirable because physiological changes caused by the mechanical ventilation begin within 72 hours (see Box 25-21).

Frequently used predictive criteria for short-term weaning success are an NIP of less than or equal to −20 cm H_2O (more negative as −30 cm H_2O), PEP of greater than or equal to +30 cm H_2O (more positive as +45 cm H_2O), and spontaneous minute volume of less than 12 L/minute. NIP and PEP give an indication of respiratory muscle strength. The choice of weaning method does not appear to be important.

Weaning procedures may vary slightly from hospital to hospital, but general guidelines remain the same. For instance, weaning is generally initiated in the morning when the patient is rested. The patient is made comfortable, and the nurse elevates the head of

Box 25-22 • Guidelines for Weaning From Long-Term Ventilation

Patients on mechanical ventilation for longer than 72 h or those having failed short-term weaning often display significant deconditioning as a result of acute or chronic complex illness, or both. These patients usually require a period of "exercising" respiratory muscles to regain the strength and endurance needed for successful return to spontaneous breathing. Goals for this process are:

- To have the patient tolerate two to three daily weaning trials of reduction in ventilatory support without exercising to the point of exhaustion
- To rest the patient between weaning trials and overnight on ventilator settings that provide diaphragmatic rest, with minimal or no work of breathing for the patient

Readiness Criteria

- Same as for short-term ventilation (see Box 25-21), with emphasis on hemodynamic stability, adequate analgesia/sedation (record scores on flow sheet), and normalizing volume status

Weaning Intervention

- Transfer to pressure-support ventilation (PSV) mode, adjust support level to maintain patient's respiratory rate at less than 35 breaths/min.
- Observe for 30 min for signs of early failure (same tolerance criteria as with short-term ventilation; see Box 25-21).
- If tolerated, continue trial for 2 h, then return patient to "rest" settings by adding ventilator breaths or increasing PSV to achieve a total respiratory rate of less than 20 breaths/min.
- After at least 2 h of rest, repeat trial for 2 to 4 h at same PSV level as previous trial. If the patient exceeds the tolerance criteria (listed in Box 25-21), stop the trial and return to "rest" settings. In this case, the next trial should be performed at a higher support level than the "failed" trial.
- Record the results of each weaning episode, including specific parameters and the time frame if "failure" observed, on the bedside flow sheet.

- The goal is to increase the length of the trials and reduce the PSV level needed on an incremental basis. With each successive trial, the PSV level may be decreased by 2 to 4 cm H_2O, the time interval may be increased by 1 to 2 h, or both, while keeping the patient within tolerance parameters. The pace of weaning is patient-specific, and tolerance may vary from day to day. Review readiness criteria for correctable factors daily *and* each time the patient "fails" a weaning trial.
- Ensure nocturnal ventilation at "rest" settings (with a respiratory rate of <20 breaths/min) for at least 6 h each night until the patient's weaning trials demonstrate readiness to discontinue ventilatory support.

Discontinuing Mechanical Ventilation

The patient should be weaned until ventilator settings are FiO_2 ≤40%, PSV ≤10 cm H_2O, and positive end-expiratory pressure ≤8 cm H_2O. Once these settings are well tolerated, the patient should be placed on continuous positive airway pressure 5 cm H_2O or (if tracheostomy in place) on tracheostomy collar. If the patient meets tolerance criteria over the first 5 min, the trial should be continued for 1 to 2 h. If clinical observation and arterial blood gases indicate that the patient is maintaining adequate ventilation and oxygenation on this "minimal" support, the following options should be considered:

- If the patient meets extubation criteria (see Box 25-21), this step should be attempted.
- If the patient is on tracheostomy collar, the trials should be continued 2 to 3 times per day with daily increases in time on tracheostomy collar by 1 to 2 h per trial until total time off the ventilator reaches 18 h per day. At this point, the patient may be ready to remain on tracheostomy collar for longer than 24 h unless the tolerance criteria are exceeded.
- Ventilator weaning is considered successful once the patient achieves spontaneous ventilation (extubated or on tracheostomy collar) for at least 24 h.

Adapted from evidence-based practice guidelines used in the Surgical/Trauma Intensive Care Unit, University of Virginia Health System, Charlottesville, Virginia.

the bed. Pharmacological agents for comfort, such as bronchodilators or sedatives, are administered as indicated. By explaining the procedure, the nurse helps the patient through some of the discomfort and apprehension. Before a weaning trial, the nurse ensures a patent airway and provides suction if necessary.

Support and reassurance help the patient through the discomfort and apprehension as the nurse remains with the patient following initiation of the weaning process. The nurse also evaluates and documents the patient's response to weaning.

Long-Term Ventilation Weaning

The process of long-term weaning often takes weeks. It incorporates gradual and progressive conditioning for respiratory and body muscles using a multidisciplinary team approach. Success with whole body conditioning with emphasis on upper body strength and

respiratory muscle function has improved ventilator liberation, and aggressive physiotherapy is necessary.[92] Usually the entire process is complicated, and it involves multiple delays and setbacks. During long-term weaning, the patient may fail a weaning trial and should then be rested on the ventilator up to 24 hours before another trial is attempted.[69] The rest period allows for the recovery of the respiratory muscles. Patients who fail a weaning trial often exhibit rapid, shallow breathing patterns consistent with their respiratory muscle weakness. Regular re-evaluation of the weaning plan by the multidisciplinary team, coupled with continuous communication with the patient and family, is necessary (see Box 25-22).

Methods of Ventilator Weaning

Various methods have been studied for weaning from the ventilator. Controversies exist about which

> **Box 25-23 • CONSIDERATIONS FOR THE OLDER PATIENT: Overcoming Barriers to Ventilator Weaning**
>
> An elderly patient on mechanical ventilation poses a unique challenge to caregivers. Successful weaning requires effective nursing interventions to address the patient's basic care needs.
>
> • **Sleep Deprivation:** Learn the patient's normal sleep habits, establish a restful environment, and minimize interruptions for at least 6 h each night and 2 h of midday rest. Consult the pharmacist or doctor for sleep medication as needed at bedtime.
>
> • **Nutrition, Imbalanced: Less than body requirements; and Fluid Volume, Risk for imbalance:** Consult the registered dietitian and begin delivery of recommended nutrition as soon as possible. Assess patient tolerance and increase to goal rate per order. Evaluate fluid balance each shift (input and output, weight, clinical examination) and discuss changes in intake and the possible need for diuretics with the physician.
>
> • **Pain, Acute; Anxiety; and Confusion, Acute:** Administer analgesia per order, assessing need and effect of intervention by pain scale or physiological parameters. Carefully evaluate possible etiology of anxiety or agitation; when pharmacological intervention is indicated, titrate to achieve desired response using standardized sedation scale to limit sedation. Nonpharmacological interventions are essential in the elderly patient (e.g., orientation to place, date, and time; spiritual; massage). Adjust care for hearing impairment or for other sensory limitations that may contribute to confusion or anxiety.
>
> • **Constipation, Risk for; and Diarrhea:** Learn the patient's "usual" elimination pattern if possible; start with similar intervention and add more aggressive bowel regimen as needed to establish regular bowel movements. Evaluate factors (e.g., medications or narcotics) that may alter bowel function, and ensure adequate hydration by enteral route if possible.
>
> • **Activity Intolerance, Risk for; and Mobility, Impaired bed or physical:** Consult the physical or occupational therapist to evaluate functional capacity and initiate appropriate therapy. Begin getting patient out of bed as soon as possible, and encourage active range-of-motion exercises and participation in activities of daily living.

methods are best. Some of the most common weaning methods include T-piece, CPAP trials, and gradual PSV reduction to minimal settings.[69] Comprehensive assessment of the patient's needs and progress toward weaning, monitoring of the weaning parameters, and following established goals promote successful weaning. Multidisciplinary and comprehensive approaches to weaning based on a health care professional (nurse) monitoring and promoting a weaning plan with continuity have demonstrated positive outcomes.[94]

T-Piece Trial
The T-piece is connected to the patient at the desired FiO_2 (usually slightly higher than the previous venti-

lator setting). The patient's response and tolerance to the trial are continuously observed. The duration of T-piece trials is not standardized, and some clinicians extubate if an initial trial of 30 minutes ends with acceptable ABGs and patient response. Increasing frequency and duration of T-piece trials builds the patient's endurance, with periods of rest on the ventilator between extended trials. When the latter method is used, the patient is generally deemed ready to be extubated after 24 successive hours on a T-piece.

Synchronized Intermittent Mandatory Ventilation Method
The SIMV mode was initially heralded as the optimal weaning mode, allowing some spontaneous breathing (to prevent respiratory muscle atrophy) while providing a backup rate. Weaning with the SIMV method entails a gradual reduction in the number of delivered breaths until a low rate is reached (usually 4 breaths/minute). The patient is then extubated if all other weaning criteria are met. However, low levels of SIMV (fewer than 4 breaths/minute) may result in a high level of work and fatigue. SIMV plus PSV, called synchronized pressure support ventilation (SPSV), may be used to decrease the work of breathing associated with spontaneous breaths. It has been suggested that using SIMV mode may result in prolonged weaning duration.[90] Use of the SPSV mode can easily progress to PSV alone when the patient initiates all breaths by dialing down the ventilator breaths. As a result, PSV "stand alone" mode is often preferred for weaning trials.

Continuous Positive Airway Pressure Method
CPAP entails breathing through the ventilator circuit with a small amount of (or zero) positive pressure. The use of CPAP instead of the use of a T-piece for weaning is controversial. Often the decision to use one over the other is determined by observing the patient's response or is simply based on the clinician's preference.

Pressure-Support Ventilation Method
Low levels of PSV decrease the work of breathing associated with endotracheal tubes and ventilator circuits. Weaning using the PSV mode entails a progressive decrease in IPL to 5 to 10 cm H_2O based on the patient maintaining an adequate tidal volume (6 to 12 mL/kg) and a respiratory rate of less than 25 breaths/minute. PSV is associated with less work of breathing than with volume modes, so longer weaning trials may be tolerated. The 5-cm H_2O IPL is thought to overcome the work of breathing through the endotracheal tube and ventilator tubing. Typically, the IPL is reduced by 2 cm H_2O daily or twice daily following the patient's response to the ventilator change. Tolerance of PSV weaning is assessed as any weaning mode by assessing the patient's response to changes in respiratory rate, SaO_2, and heart rate, along with observing for fatigue (see Boxes 25-21 and 25-22). There is support for use of CPAP, T-piece, or even PSV during a spontaneous breathing trial before extubation because each is an effective method for the weaning readiness trial.[69,90]

Adjuncts to Weaning

Several adjuncts to long-term weaning are used to improve weaning tolerance and patient comfort. The mode on newer ventilators that allows for the regulation of pressure support for the size and type of tube, endotracheal or tracheostomy, adjusts for the type of tube resistance to allow less work of breathing. Called automatic tube compensation on some ventilators, this is another tool to consider during weaning. The fenestrated tracheostomy tube provides for communication during weaning periods, improving patient interaction. The fenestrated tracheostomy tube has an opening in the outer cannula but not the inner cannula. With the inner cannula in place and the cuff inflated, mechanical ventilation is easy. During the weaning process, the inner cannula is removed, the cuff deflated, the outer cannula capped, and supplemental oxygen supplied by nasal cannula. This system permits air to pass the vocal cords, allowing verbal communication by the patient. The cuff should never be inflated while the inner cannula is capped because the patient will be unable to breathe. The speaking valves provide communication during weaning periods for patients with non-fenestrated tracheostomy tubes, which are generally used more frequently. These valves provide less resistance than the fenestrated tracheostomy tube, and each type of speaking valve allows for supplemental oxygen through a side port. Humidified air with a tracheostomy collar is required to keep the airway moist and prevent secretions from drying, especially at night when speaking valves should be removed for sleep. Use of a large endotracheal tube (greater than 7.0 mm) decreases resistance to breathing and decreases the work of breathing. A larger endotracheal tube also supports bronchoscopy to remove secretions when needed. Tracheostomy in many instances is more comfortable for patients and allows for improved oral care, better communication, and tracheostomy collar trials for weaning.

Extubation Criteria

Whichever mode or combination of modes is used for weaning, extubation cannot occur until several criteria are met based on short-term or long-term ventilation (see Boxes 25-21 and 25-22). Before extubation, the patient must be able to maintain his or her own airway, as evidenced by an appropriate level of consciousness and the presence of cough and gag reflexes. In all patients, but especially in those with a history of difficult intubation or reactive airway disease, the cuff-leak test should be performed before extubation. This entails deflation of the tube cuff (after suctioning of the oropharynx) and a brief period of occluding the endotracheal tube in order to demonstrate an air leak with patient inspiration. Absence of a leak can indicate edema and may predict laryngeal stridor after extubation. If the cuff-leak test fails, the patient may be given corticosteroids to reduce edema for 24 to 48 hours and then be reassessed for cuff leak. A direct visualization of the trachea with a bronchoscope may be performed before extubation to determine whether the edema has resolved.

Extubation should never occur unless a qualified person is available to reintubate emergently if the patient does not tolerate extubation. After explaining the procedure and preparing the patient, the nurse suctions the patient's tube and posterior oropharynx. Equipment includes an MRB and mask at bedside. After the nurse loosens the endotracheal tube securing device or tape, the cuff is deflated. The endotracheal tube is removed quickly while having the patient cough. The patient's mouth is suctioned, and humidified oxygen is applied immediately. The patient is evaluated for immediate signs of distress: stridor, dyspnea, and decrease in SaO_2. Treatment of stridor includes inhaled racemic epinephrine and sometimes administration of IV steroids (because steroids do not work immediately, they are given before extubation in those at risk). If these interventions fail, immediate reintubation may be necessary.

HOME CARE AND MECHANICAL VENTILATION

Certain patients requiring invasive mechanical ventilation may be candidates for home care. These patients may require full or partial invasive mechanical ventilation because of neuromuscular weakness, neurogenic hypoventilation, or cardiopulmonary diseases that result in ineffective gas exchange.[95] Conditions that may warrant home care ventilator management include:

▶ Neurological disorders (e.g., ALS, Guillain-Barré syndrome, multiple sclerosis, muscular dystrophy, myasthenia gravis, poliomyelitis, polymyositis, spinal cord injury)
▶ Restrictive disorders (e.g., interstitial pulmonary fibrosis, kyphoscoliosis, obesity, sarcoidosis)
▶ Obstructive disorders (e.g., bronchiectasis, bronchiolitis obliterans, bronchopulmonary dysplasia, chronic bronchitis and emphysema, cystic fibrosis, obesity, sleep apnea syndromes)

A discharge planning guide for a patient who is a candidate for home care management of a ventilator is given in Box 25-24.

NEW FRONTIERS AND CHALLENGES FOR VENTILATED PATIENTS

Ventilated patients present major challenges to nurses because they are prone to iatrogenic complications with higher mortality and morbidity. It is important that nurses apply current evidence-based research and practice to patient care so that clinical and financial outcomes may improve. Research on the use of low-volume ventilation, high-frequency ventilation, and the appropriate fluid management in ARDS presents new challenges for nurses responsible for implementing the changes in clinical practice.

Box 25-24 • DISCHARGE PLANNING GUIDE:
Home Care for Ventilator-Assisted Patients

- The caregivers, patient, nurse, and physician meet to discuss the patient's and caregivers' desire for home care. The team presents a realistic overview, including the need for extensive caregiver teaching before discharge, and the need for a high level of caregiver commitment owing to the extensive daily care needs of the patient.
- This initial meeting is followed by a multidisciplinary meeting with representatives from Nursing, Medicine, Social Work, Physical and Occupational Therapy, Respiratory Therapy, Speech Therapy, Nutrition, and Pharmacy, to discuss the patient's and caregivers' resources and formulate a teaching plan.
- Funding for home care management must be in place before discharge.
- Extensive assessment of the patient's physical status as well as an assessment of home and caregiver resources is imperative before initiating the process of preparing patients and caregivers for home care of a ventilator-assisted patient.

Patient's Physical Status
- Are acute diseases resolved, chronic conditions under control, all infectious processes cured or under definitive treatment?
- Does the patient have stable pulmonary function, minimal ventilator settings (low FIO_2 and simplest ventilatory mode), and pulmonary secretion control with adequate cough or tracheal suction?
- Does the patient have a stable metabolic and nutritional status, and simplified medication and nutrition regimen?

Caregiver Resources
- Are multiple caregivers available (minimum one more for backup)?
- Is the caregiver motivated, realistic, flexible, committed, and in good health?

Home
- Are adequate electrical circuits available for ventilator equipment?
- Is there adequate heating and cooling, a phone, a safe water supply, and storage space?
- Is there adequate room for safe patient evacuation in the case of an emergency?
- Caregiver and patient goals must be identified, and a teaching plan formulated with an approximate timeline toward discharge:
  - Ventilator, tracheostomy, suctioning teaching
  - Nutrition, hydration, medication teaching
  - Patient personal care, hygiene, percutaneous endoscopic gastrostomy care, bowel and bladder care teaching

- Techniques for maintenance of patient's strength and flexibility
- Communication techniques, recreational activities for patient
- Safe patient positioning and transferring techniques
- Troubleshooting tracheostomy and ventilator
- Troubleshooting signs of acute illness, exacerbation of chronic illnesses, or progression of underlying illness
- Emergency plans, caregiver cardiopulmonary resuscitation training
- Conference with patient and caregivers regarding end-of-life issues and wishes, with specific scenarios reviewed
- Conference with patient and caregivers regarding alternatives, if home care does not work out
- Conference regarding ways to meet the psychological needs of the patient and caregivers
- The team performs ongoing evaluation of the patient's and caregivers' readiness and progress toward discharge and adjusts the teaching plan and discharge date accordingly.
- Predischarge and discharge:
  - Caregivers gradually take over the patient's total care while in the hospital, with staff supervising and assisting in troubleshooting.
  - The respiratory therapy home care coordinator assesses the home and arranges for delivery of equipment.
  - The respiratory therapy home care coordinator notifies the local electrical company, fire department, and rescue squad of patient on ventilator before discharge.
  - The respiratory therapy home care coordinator completes home ventilator management teaching.
  - A physician is identified to follow the patient on discharge.
  - A contact person is identified from the hospital unit (case manager, primary nurse).
  - A referral for home health care (e.g., Physical or Occupational Therapy, Speech, Counseling, Nursing, Social Work, Nutrition) is provided.
  - Arrangements are made for ventilation on ventilator to be used at home at least 3 days before discharge.
  - The caregiver changes the tracheostomy before discharge.
  - When the discharge date is established by the team, caregiver, and patient, Social Work arranges for transportation.
  - Equipment needed for transportation home (e.g., suction machine, ventilator) is secured and established to be in good working order.
  - Discharge orders are in place at least 2 days before discharge.
  - Discharge medications are obtained before discharge.

Ventilator weaning by use of weaning teams, outcomes managers, and weaning protocols show promise for future improvement in outcomes, lowering hospital costs, and effective weaning from ventilators with decreased mortality.[94,96–98] These system approaches continue to demonstrate reduction of ven-

tilator days, length of stay, and complications. They will continue to be popular initiatives for hospitals that are attempting to find the best outcomes, quality, and cost-effective solutions for complex patients.

Nurses can use current journals and the Internet to search for information about the most up-to-date information and research. The new nurse should seek access to a health science library database to obtain the most current research for his or her area of practice as well as subscribe to nursing journals. Four excellent sources for the new nurse for advanced topics are (1) the *AACN Procedure Manual for Critical Care*, (2) the AACN Protocols for Practice: Care of the Mechanically Ventilated Patient, (3) the journal titled *AACN Advanced Critical Care*, and (4) *Essentials of Respiratory Care* by Kacmarek and Dimas. These resources provide more in-depth coverage of topics related to ventilators, pathophysiology, and patient care.

The new frontiers of nursing and health care will continue to require that nurses keep abreast of rapidly changing practice by continually updating their knowledge. The key to excellent nursing care is evidence-based practice. The goal for new nurses is to integrate the best evidence-based practice, knowledge, therapies, and clinical skills of ventilator care into all aspects of clinical practice. The ever-changing technology and research of the 21st century will provide nurses with continued challenges to update their clinical practice with the latest evidence-based practice and research to provide the respiratory patient with the highest quality care.

• Clinical Applicability Challenges

Case Study

Mrs. Q, a 74-year-old woman, is admitted with a diagnosis of esophageal cancer. She had an esophagectomy 1 week ago. Following initial extubation, she was reintubated the day of surgery (failed extubation) for respiratory distress, hypercarbia, and inability to clear her secretions. Her history includes a 13-kg weight loss and limited activities of daily living while living at home, limited by her dependence on supplemental oxygen and nasojejunal nutrition. (Her nutrition status was improved by 6 weeks of home therapy before admission.) Her current medications include albuterol, fluticasone, lisinopril, insulin, thyroxine, prednisone, and paroxetine, as well as alprazolam and zolpidem as needed. The current ventilator settings on day 7 of ventilation are: fraction inspired oxygen of 0.40, no rate, positive end-expiratory pressure of 5 cm H_2O, and inspiratory pressure limit (IPL) of 14 cm H_2O with a respiratory rate of 20, tidal volume of 550 mL (current weight 68 kg, a gain of 6 kg from 2 months ago), and minute volume of 10.9 L/minute. Her vital signs are stable, she is afebrile, and her pain is well controlled with scheduled oral and as-needed IV narcotics. She is generally weak and able to turn in bed on her own, for 2 days, she has tolerated 3 times daily sitting up in a chair, and she took her first walk today with physical therapy. She is able to cough out secretions from her endotracheal tube. Nutrition and medications are delivered through a percutaneous endoscopic gastrostomy tube inserted during surgery. She tolerates ventilation with resumption of her as-needed alprazolam and is sleeping better with nocturnal zolpidem.

1. What weaning from the ventilator would you want to do today, and on which settings?
2. When would you consider Mrs. Q. ready for extubation, and what weaning assessment and laboratory tests, including arterial blood gases and chemistry, should be obtained before a second trial extubation?
3. This is day 7 of ventilation following a failed extubation trial the day of surgery, and she has progressed physically. What respiratory assessments do you want to follow while she is working with physical therapy?
4. You observe Mrs. Q. on continuous positive airway pressure (CPAP) for 1 hour, and she remains stable without changes to her respiratory rate, tidal volume, or minute volume, and her arterial blood gases are within normal limits. Would you extubate her after this 1-hour CPAP trial if she complained of feeling exhausted (in a written note)? Indicate what further weaning assessment you would want to obtain.
5. The medical team decides to wait 1 day longer to allow Mrs. Q. to continue on the ventilator with reduced inspiratory pressure limit at 10 cm H_2O. What does reducing the IPL do for work of breathing and the strength and endurance of respiratory muscles?
6. If Mrs. Q. were not on her home medications, which ones would you want to discuss with the medical team?

Review Questions

1. The nurse is caring for an independent and ambulatory patient after thoracic surgery who is experiencing moderate levels of pain when using the incentive spirometer. He also has a productive cough with small amounts of sputum, and his chest radiograph is clear without atelectasis. What other bronchial hygiene therapy will assist this patient in clearing secretions?
   a. EzPAP
   b. Nasotracheal suctioning
   c. Acapella valve
   d. Nebulizer bronchodilator therapy
2. You start your shift by taking report on a newly intubated patient with bilateral upper lobe pneumonia and minimal secretions. The previous shift noted the ventilator settings of FiO_2 0.75, rate 14, mode is assist control with a tidal volume of 450 mL/breath, and positive end-expiratory pressure of 8 cm H_2O. The current arterial blood gas is pH 7.32, PaO_2 82 mmHg, and $PaCO_2$ 42 mmHg,

53. Acosta P, Santisbon E, Varon J: The use of positive end-expiratory pressure in mechanical ventilation. Crit Care Clin 23(2):251–261, 2007

54. Hill NS: Noninvasive positive-pressure ventilation. In Tobin MJ (ed): Principles and Practice of Mechanical Ventilation, 2nd ed. New York: McGraw-Hill, 2006, pp 433–472

55. Albert NM: Procedure 63, cardiac output measurement techniques (invasive). In Lynn-McHale Wiegand DJ, Carlson KK (eds): AACN Procedure Manual for Critical Care, 5th ed. Philadelphia: Elsevier, 2005, pp 482–497

56. Cason CL, Tyner T, Saunders S, Broome L: Nurses' implementation of guidelines for ventilator-associated pneumonia from the Centers for Disease Control and Prevention. Am J Crit Care 16(1):28–38, 2007

57. AACN practice alert: Ventilator-associated pneumonia. AACN Clin Issues 16(1):105–109, 2005

58. Chlebicki MP, Safdar N: Topical chlorhexidine for prevention of ventilator-associated pneumonia: A meta-analysis. Crit Care Med 35(2):595–602, 2007

59. Minei JP, Nathens AB, West M, et al: Guidelines for prevention, diagnosis and treatment of ventilator-associated pneumonia (VAP) in the trauma patient. J Trauma 60(5):1106–1113, 2006

60. Ricart M, Lorente C, Diaz E, et al: Nursing adherence with evidence-based guidelines for preventing ventilator-associated pneumonia. Crit Care Med 31(11):2693–2696, 2003

61. Munro CL, Grap MJ: Oral health and care in the intensive care unit: State of the science. Am J Crit Care 13(1):25–33, 2004

62. Parrish CR, Falls McCray S: Nutrition support for the mechanically ventilated patient. Crit Care Nurs 23(1):77–80, 2003

63. Parrish CR, Krenitsky J, Willcutts K: Nutritional support for mechanically ventilated patients. In Burns SM (ed): AACN Protocols for Practice: Care of the Mechanically Ventilated Patient, 2nd ed. Sudbury, Mass: Jones & Bartlett, 2007, pp 191–252

64. Hildebrandt LA, Fracchia J, Driscoll J, Giroux P: Comparison of post-pyloric vs. gastric enteral formula administration. Top Clin Nutr 17(3):44–51, 2002

65. Luer J: Sedation and neuromuscular blockade in mechanically ventilated patients. In Burns SM (ed): AACN Protocols for Practice: Care of the Mechanically Ventilated Patient, 2nd ed. Sudbury, MA: Jones & Bartlett, 2007, pp 253–284

66. Foster JGW, Clark AP: Functional recovery after neuromuscular blockade in mechanically ventilated critically ill patients. Heart Lung 35(3):178–189, 2006

67. Bercker S, WeberCarstens S, Deja M, et al: Critical illness polyneuropathy and myopathy in patients with acute respiratory distress syndrome. Crit Care Med 33(4):711–715, 2005

68. Pruitt B: Weaning patients from mechanical ventilation. Nursing 36(9):36–42, 2006

69. MacIntyre NR: Evidence-based ventilator weaning and discontinuation. Respir Care 49(7):830–836, 2004

70. St. John RE, Seckel MA: Airway management. In Burns SM (ed): AACN Protocols for Practice: Care of the Mechanically Ventilated Patient, 2nd ed. Sudbury, MA: Jones & Bartlett, 2007, pp 1–57

71. Goettler CE, Fugo JR, Bard MR, et al: Predicting the need for early tracheostomy: A multifactorial analysis of 992 intubated trauma patients. J Trauma 60(5):991–996, 2006

72. Rana S, Pendem S, Pogodzinski MS, et al: Tracheostomy in critically ill patients. Mayo Clin Proc 80(12):1632–1638, 2005

73. Rumbak MJ, Newton M, Truncale T, et al: A prospective, randomized study comparing early percutaneous dilational tracheotomy to prolonged translaryngeal intubation (delayed tracheotomy) in critically ill medical patients [corrected] [published erratum appears in Crit Care Med 32(12):2566, 2004]. Crit Care Med 32(8):1689–1694, 2004

74. Skillings KN, Curtis BL: Procedure 12, tube care. In Lynn-McHale Wiegand DJ, Carlson KK (eds): AACN Procedure Manual for Critical Care, 5th ed. Philadelphia: Elsevier, 2005, pp 79–86

75. Nettina SM: Tracheostomy care (routine). In Mill EJ (ed): Lippincott Manual of Nursing Practice, 8th ed. Philadelphia: Lippincott Williams & Wilkins, 2006

76. Markou NK, Myrianthefs PM, Baltopoulos GJ: Respiratory failure: An overview. Crit Care Nurs Q 27(4):353–379, 2004

77. Joyce N, Evans D: Best practice: Eye care for patients in the ICU. Am J Nurs 106(1):72AA–BB, 2006

78. Murray T, Goodyear Bruch C: Ventilator-associated pneumonia improvement program. AACN Clin Issues 18(2):190–199, 2007

79. Oral care update from prevention to treatment. Nurs Manag 34(5 Suppl 3):1–13, 2003

80. Berry AM, Davidson PM, Masters J, Rolls K: Systematic literature review of oral hygiene practices for intensive care patients receiving mechanical ventilation. Am J Crit Care 16(6):552–562, 2007

81. Tolentino-Delosreyes AF, Ruppert SD, Shiao SPK: Evidence-based practice: Use of the ventilator bundle to prevent ventilator-associated pneumonia. Am J Crit Care 16(1):20–27, 2007

82. Laux L, Herbert C: Decreasing ventilator-associated pneumonia: Getting on board. Crit Care Nurs Q 29(3):253–258, 2006

83. Practice alert. Oral care in the critically ill. AACN News 23(8):4, 2006

84. Bailey P, Thomsen GE, Spuhler VJ, et al: Early activity is feasible and safe in respiratory failure patients. Crit Care Med 35(1):139–145, 2007

85. Pruitt B: Weaning patients from mechanical ventilation. Nursing 36(9):36–42, 2006

86. Damboise C, Cardin S: Family-centered critical care: How one unit implemented a plan. Am J Nurs 103(6):56AA–56EE, 2003

87. Davidson JE, Powers K, Hedayat KM, et al: Clinical practice guidelines for support of the family in the patient-centered intensive care unit: American College of Critical Care Medicine Task Force 2004–2005. Crit Care Med 35(2):605–622, 2007

88. Auerbach SM, Kiesler DJ, Wartella J, et al: Optimism, satisfaction with needs met, interpersonal perceptions of the healthcare team, and emotional distress in patients' family members during critical care hospitalization. Am J Crit Care 14(3):202–210, 2005

89. MacLean SL, Guzzetta CE, White C, et al: Family presence during cardiopulmonary resuscitation and invasive procedures: Practices of critical care and emergency nurses. Am J Crit Care 12(3):246–257, 2003

90. Fenstermacher D, Hong D: Mechanical ventilation: What have we learned? Critical Care Nurs Q 27(3):258–294, 2004

91. Smith-Blair N: Mechanisms of diaphragm fatigue. AACN Clin Issues 13(2):307–319, 2002

92. Martin UJ, Hincapie L, Nimchuk M, et al: Impact of whole-body rehabilitation in patients receiving chronic mechanical ventilation. Crit Care Med 33(10):2259–2265, 2005

93. O'Bryan L, Von Rueden K, Malila F: Evaluating ventilator weaning best practice: A long-term acute care hospital system-wide quality initiative. AACN Clin Issues 13(4):567–576, 2002

94. Burns SM, Earven S, Fisher C, et al: Implementation of an institutional program to improve clinical and financial outcomes of mechanically ventilated patients: One-year outcomes and lessons learned. Crit Care Med 31(12):2752–2763, 2003

95. Eklund MM: Beyond the ICU: Home care management of patients receiving mechanical ventilation. In Burns SM (ed): AACN Protocols for Practice: Care of the Mechanically Ventilated Patient, 2nd ed. Sudbury, MA: Jones & Bartlett, 2007, pp 161–190

96. Burns SM: Weaning from mechanical ventilation. In Burns SM (ed): AACN Protocols for Practice: Care of the Mechanically Ventilated Patient, 2nd ed. Sudbury, MA: Jones & Bartlett, 2007, pp 97–156

97. Dries DJ, McGonigal MD, Malian MS, et al: Protocol-driven ventilator weaning reduces use of mechanical ventilation, rate

of early reintubation, and ventilator-associated pneumonia . . . includes discussion. J Trauma, 56(5):943–952, 2004

98. Henneman E, Dracup K, Ganz T, et al: Using a collaborative weaning plan to decrease duration of mechanical ventilation and length of stay in the intensive care unit for patients receiving long-term ventilation. Am J Crit Care 11(2):132–140, 2002

Other Selected Readings

Andrews PL, Habashi NM: Airway pressure release ventilation: A boost for spontaneous breathing. Am Nurse Today 1(1):10–12, 2006

Burns SM (ed): AACN Protocols for Practice: Care of Mechanically Ventilated Patients, 2nd ed. Sudbury, MA: Jones & Bartlett, 2007

Celik SA, Kanan N: A current conflict: Use of isotonic sodium chloride solution on endotracheal suctioning in critically ill patients. Dimens Critical Care Nurs 25(1):11–14, 2006

Chlan LL, Engeland WC, Anthony A, Guttormson J: Influence of music on the stress response in patients receiving mechanical ventilatory support: A pilot study. Am J Crit Care 16(2): 141–145, 2007

Crimlisk JT, O'Donnell C, Grillone GA: Standardizing adult tracheostomy tube styles: What is the clinical and cost-effective impact? Dimens Crit Care Nurs 25(1):35–43, 2006

Epstein CD, Peerless JR: Weaning readiness and fluid balance in older critically ill surgical patients. Am J Crit Care 15(1):54–64, 2006

Foster JGW, Clark AP: Functional recovery after neuromuscular blockade in mechanically ventilated critically ill patients. Heart Lung 35(3):178–189, 2006

Frazier SK, Stone KS, Moser DK, et al: Hemodynamic changes during discontinuation of mechanical ventilation in medical intensive care unit patients. Am J Crit Care 15(6):580–594, 2006

Frazier SK, Brom H, Widener J, et al: Prevalence of myocardial ischemia during mechanical ventilation and weaning and its effects on weaning success. Heart Lung, 35(6):363–373, 2006

Giuliano KK, Liu LM: Knowledge of pulse oximetry among critical care nurses. Dimens Crit Care Nurs 25(1):44–49, 2006

Guentner K, Hoffman LA, Happ MB, et al: Preferences for mechanical ventilation among survivors of prolonged ventilation and tracheostomy. Am J Crit Care 15(1):65–67, 2006

Happ MB, Swigart VA, Tate JA, et al: Family presence and surveillance during weaning from prolonged mechanical ventilation. Heart Lung 36(1):47–57, 2007

Hsieh HY, Tuite PK: Prevention of ventilator-associated pneumonia: What nurses can do. Dimens Crit Care Nurs 25(5):205–208, 2006

Kacmarek RM, Dimas S: Essentials of Respiratory Care, 4th ed. Philadelphia: Elsevier, 2005

Labeau S, Vandijck DM, Claes B, et al, for the executive board of the Flemish Society for Critical Care Nurses: Critical care nurses' knowledge of evidence-based guidelines for preventing ventilator-associated pneumonia: An evaluation questionnaire. Am J Crit Care 16(4):371–377, 2007

McLean SE, Jensen LA, Schroeder DG, et al: Improving adherence to a mechanical ventilation weaning protocol for critically ill adults: Outcomes after an implementation program. Am J Crit Care 15(3):299–309, 2006

Munro CL, Grap MJ, Elswick RK, et al: Oral health status and development of ventilator-associated pneumonia: A descriptive study. Am J Crit Care 15(5):453–461, 2006

Murray T, Goodyear-Bruch C: Ventilator-associated pneumonia improvement program. AACN Clin Issues 18(2):190–199, 2007

Pruitt B: Weaning patients from mechanical ventilation. Nursing 36(9):36–41, 2006

Rose L: Advanced modes of mechanical ventilation: Implications for practice. AACN Clin Issues 17(2):145–160, 2006

Savian C, Paratz J, Davies A: Comparison of the effectiveness of manual and ventilator hyperinflation at different levels of positive end-expiratory pressure in artificially ventilated and intubated intensive care patients. Heart Lung 35(5):334–341, 2006

Shaffer C: Diagnostic blood loss in mechanically ventilated patients. Heart Lung 36(3):217–222, 2007

Winters AC, Munro N: Assessment of the mechanically ventilated patient: An advanced practice approach. AACN Clin Issues 15(4):525–533, 2004

26

Common Respiratory Disorders

Susan E. Anderson • Debbi Spencer*

Objectives

Based on the content in this chapter, the reader should be able to:

❶ Compare the etiology, pathophysiology, assessment, management, and prevention of community acquired, hospital acquired, and health care associated pneumonia.

❷ Describe the etiology, pathophysiology, assessment, and management of a patient with severe acute respiratory syndrome (SARS).

❸ Discuss the pathophysiology, assessment, and management of pleural effusion.

❹ Describe the pathophysiology, assessment, and management associated with pneumothorax.

❺ Discuss the pathophysiology, assessment, management, and prevention of pulmonary embolism.

❻ Explain the pathophysiology, assessment, management and prevention of chronic obstructive pulmonary disease.

❼ Compare the pathological processes, signs and symptoms, and management of chronic bronchitis and emphysema.

❽ Describe the pathology, assessment, and management of a patient at various points on the asthma continuum, from mild attack to status asthmaticus.

❾ Identify the key characteristics of hypoxemic acute respiratory failure and hypercapnic acute respiratory failure in terms of pathophysiology, assessment, and management.

*The views of the authors are their own and do not reflect the official policy or position of the Department of the Army, the Department of Defense, or the United States Government.

• Pneumonia

Pneumonia remains a common infection found in both the community and hospital, even though there have been advances in identifying people at risk and implementing preventive measures. Critical care nurses encounter pneumonia when it complicates the course of a serious illness or leads to acute respiratory distress. In the United States, pneumonia is the leading cause of death from infectious disease, the second most common nosocomial (hospital-acquired) infection, and the seventh leading cause of death.[1] About 2 to 3 million cases of pneumonia occur every year, leading to more than 10 million outpatient visits and 500,000 hospitalizations.[1,2] In 2003, 63,241 people died of pneumonia at a rate of 21.7 per 100,000 population.[1] The incidence of community-acquired pneumonia (CAP) requiring hospitalization is 4 times higher in elderly patients (>65 years of age) than it is in those 45 to 64 years of age.[3]

CAP is defined by the Infectious Diseases Society of America (IDSA) as an acute infection of the pulmonary parenchyma that is usually associated with at least two symptoms of acute infection. It occurs in a person who has not been hospitalized or has not resided in a long-term care facility for more than 14 days before the onset of symptoms.[2] In the outpatient setting, CAP has a low mortality rate (1% to 5%). However, the mortality rate climbs to 12% in patients requiring hospitalization and to 40% in those requiring admission to the intensive care unit (ICU).[2,4]

Two sets of guidelines regarding treatment of patients with pneumonia have been issued. In the first set, issued by the Pneumonia Patient Outcomes Research Team (PORT), the initial site of treatment should be selected based on three criteria, which include (1) assessment of any preexisting conditions that compromise the safety of the patient being cared for at home, (2) calculation of the Pneumonia Severity Index (PSI), and (3) clinical judgment.[4] The PSI stratifies patients into five risk categories. The higher the score, the higher the risk for death, admission to the ICU, or readmission, and the longer the length of stay.[5] Patients in risk classes I, II, and III are at low risk for death and can most likely be treated safely in the outpatient setting. Patients in risk classes IV and V should be hospitalized, with those in class V being admitted to the ICU[5] (Box 26-1). In the second set of guidelines developed by the American Thoracic Society (ATS), patients with severe CAP require admission to the ICU. Severe CAP is defined as the presence of one of two major criteria or the presence of two of three minor criteria[6] (Box 26-2).

Hospital-acquired pneumonia (HAP), ventilator-associated pneumonia (VAP), and health care–associated pneumonia (HCAP) continue to be important causes of morbidity and mortality despite advances in antimicrobial therapy and advanced supportive measures.[7,8] HAP is defined as pneumonia occurring more than 48 hours after admission to a hospital, which excludes infection that is incubating at the time of admission.[7] HAP occurs at a rate of 5 to 10 cases per 1,000 hospital admissions, and the incidence increases by 6- to 20-fold in patients receiving mechanical ventilation.[9] VAP is defined as the occurrence of pneumonia more than 48 to 72 hours after intubation. If a person experiences a severe episode of HAP requiring intubation and mechanical ventilation, that person should then be managed like a patient with VAP.[7] HCAP is defined as pneumonia in any patient who has been hospitalized in an acute care hospital for 2 or more days within 90 days of infection; has lived in a nursing home or long-term care facility; has received recent intravenous antibiotic therapy, chemotherapy, or wound care within the past 30 days of the current infection; or has received treatment at a hospital or hemodialysis clinic.[8]

The ATS HAP guidelines state that the criteria defining severe CAP can also be used to define severe HAP.[5] Severe HAP may occur in the ICU, with patients receiving mechanical ventilation being at the greatest risk, or it may precipitate admission to the ICU.[6] HAP independently contributes to mortality in critically ill patients; the attributable mortality rate is 33% to 50%.[7]

ETIOLOGY

Bacteria, viruses, mycoplasmas, other infectious agents such as fungi, and foreign material can all cause pneumonia. The specific etiology varies greatly depending on the type of pneumonia (CAP or HAP).[10] *Streptococcus pneumoniae* (pneumococcus) is the predominant pathogen associated with CAP, accounting for 30% to 60% of all occurrences of CAP. It is the most common cause of CAP identified in patients requiring hospitalization. Other organisms considered to be causative agents in CAP include *Haemophilus influenzae, Staphylococcus aureus,* and other gram-negative bacilli.[2] Even in the approximately 50% of cases of CAP in which the causative organism is not identified, *S. pneumoniae* is believed to predominate.[2] Drug-resistant *S. pneumoniae* is frequently seen in individuals older than 65 years of age.[2] Pathogens that should be considered in severe CAP requiring admission to the ICU include *S. pneumoniae, Chlamydia pneumoniae, S. aureus, Mycobacterium tuberculosis, Legionella* species, respiratory viruses, and endemic fungi.[11]

Etiologic factors may be used to classify pneumonia as typical or atypical. Typical pneumonia, caused by pathogens such as *S. pneumoniae, Streptococcus pyrogenes,* and *S. aureus,* is the result of the bacteria multiplying in the alveoli, causing inflammation and accumulation of fluid within the alveoli.[3] Atypical pneumonia is caused by pathogens such as *Mycoplasma pneumoniae, C. pneumoniae,* influenza virus, adenovirus, and *Legionella* species that give rise to inflammatory changes in the alveolar septa and lung interstitium.[3,10]

Time of onset of pneumonia is an important factor in determining the specific pathogens and outcomes in patients with HAP and VAP.[7] HAP and VAP occurring within 4 days of admission are more likely to be caused by bacteria sensitive to antibiotics. HAP and VAP occurring later on are more likely to be caused

Box 26-1 • Patient Outcomes Research Team (PORT) Pneumonia Severity Index

Step 1: Answer questions 1, 2, and 3. If the response is "no" to all three questions, assign patient to Risk Class I and institute outpatient treatment. If the response is "yes" to any one of the three questions, proceed to Step 2 to determine the patient's Risk Class (II-V).

1. **Is the patient older than 50 years of age?**
2. **Does the patient have a history of any of the following coexisting conditions*?**
   Neoplastic disease; Congestive heart failure (CHF); Cerebrovascular disease; Renal disease; Liver disease
3. **Does the patient have any of the following abnormalities on physical examination?**
   Altered mental status**; Pulse ≥ 125/minute; Respiratory rate ≥ 30 breaths/minute; Systolic blood pressure < 90 mmHg; Temperature < 35°C or ≥ 40°C

Step 2: Assess the Following Characteristics

Characteristic	Points assigned	Score
Demographic factor		
Age		
Men	Age (yrs)	
Women	Age (yrs) − 10	
Nursing home resident	+10	
Coexisting illnesses*		
Neoplastic disease	+30	
Liver disease	+20	
Congestive heart failure	+10	
Cerebrovascular disease	+10	
Renal disease	+10	
Physical examination findings		
Altered mental status **	+20	
Respiratory rate ≥ 30 breaths/min	+20	
Systolic blood pressure < 90 mmHg	+20	
Temperature < 35°C (95°F) or ≥ 40°C (104°F)	+15	
Pulse ≥ 125 beat/min	+10	
Laboratory and radiographic findings (if study performed)		
Arterial blood pH < 7.35	+30	
Blood urea nitrogen level > 30 mg/dl	+20	
Sodium level < 130 mmol/L	+20	
Glucose level ≥ 250 mg/dL	+10	
Hematocrit < 30%	+10	
Partial pressure of arterial O_2 < 60 mmHg Or Sat < 90% ***	+10	
Pleural effusion	+10	

Total score is the sum of points to identify the severity score and determine the patient's risk class.

*Neoplastic disease is defined as any cancer—except basal- or squamous-cell cancer of the skin—active at time of presentation or diagnosed within 1 year of presentation. Liver disease is defined as a clinical or histologic diagnosis of cirrhosis or another form of chronic liver disease, such as chronic active hepatitis. Congestive heart failure is defined as systolic or diastolic ventricular dysfunction documented by history, physical examination, and chest x-ray, echocardiogram, multiple gated acquisition scan, or left ventriculogram. Cerebrovascular disease is defined as a clinical diagnosis of stroke or transient ischemic attack or stroke documented by magnetic resonance imaging or computed tomography. Renal disease is defined as a history of chronic renal disease or abnormal blood urea nitrogen or creatinine.
**Altered mental status is defined as disorientation with respect to person, place, or time that is not known to be chronic, stupor, or coma.
***In the Pneumonia PORT cohort study, an oxygen saturation < 90% on pulse oximetry or intubation prior to admission was also considered abnormal.

Step 3: Determine the Patient's Risk Class

Total Score	Risk Class	Mortality*	Recommended Site of Treatment
None (see Step 1)	I	0.1%	Outpatient
< 70	II	0.6%	Outpatient
71 to 90	III	0.9%	Outpatient
91 to 130	IV	9.3%	Inpatient
> 130	V	27%	Inpatient

Adapted with permission.

From Miskovich-Riddle L, Keresztes P: CAP management guidelines. Nurse Practitioner 31(1):43–53, 2006.

Box 26-2 • American Thoracic Society Criteria for Diagnosis of Severe Community-Acquired Pneumonia

Major Criteria

- Need for mechanical ventilation
- Requirement for vasopressors for >4 hours (septic shock)
- Acute renal failure (urine output <80 mL in 4 hours or serum creatinine >2 mg/dL in the absence of chronic renal failure)
- Increase in size of infiltrates by >50% in presence of clinical nonresponse to treatment or deterioration

Minor Criteria

- Respiratory rate >30 breaths/minute
- Systolic BP ≤90 mm Hg
- Diastolic BP <60 mm Hg, multilobar disease
- PaO_2/FiO_2 ratio <250

From American Thoracic Society: Guidelines for the management of adults with community-acquired pneumonia. Am J Respir Crit Care Med 163:1730–1754, 2001, with permission.

by resistant organisms.[7] HAP may be polymicrobial, and common causative pathogens include aerobic gram negative bacilli such as *Escherichia coli*, *Klebsiella pneumoniae*, and *Pseudomonas aeruginosa*, as well as gram-positive cocci such as *S. aureus*.[7] Polymicrobial HAP is particularly common (>50%) in patients receiving mechanical ventilation (VAP). Highly resistant gram-negative organisms (e.g., *P. aeruginosa*, *Acinetobacter* species) and methicillin-resistant *S. aureus* are frequently seen in late-onset HAP but may occur in early-onset HAP in patients with risk factors for these pathogens.[7,9] The spectrum of potential pathogens can be defined by assessment of a variety of factors, including the severity of the pneumonia, presence of comorbidities, prior therapy (including antibiotics), and length of hospitalization.[7]

PATHOPHYSIOLOGY

Pneumonia is an inflammatory response to inhaled or aspirated foreign material or the uncontrolled multiplication of microorganisms invading the lower respiratory tract. This response results in the accumulation of neutrophils and other proinflammatory cytokines in the peripheral bronchi and alveolar spaces.[9] The body's defense system, which includes anatomical, mechanical, humoral, and cellular defenses, is designed to repel and remove organisms entering the respiratory tract. Many systemic diseases increase the patient's risk for pneumonia by altering the respiratory defense mechanism. Pneumonia develops when normal pulmonary defense mechanisms are either impaired or overwhelmed, allowing microorganisms to multiply rapidly. The severity of pneumonia is dependent on the amount of material aspirated, the virulence of the organism, the amount of bacteria in the aspirate, and the host defenses.[9]

The means by which pathogens enter the lower respiratory tract include aspiration, inhalation, hematogenous spread from a distant site, and translocation.

Risk factors that predispose an individual to one of these mechanisms may be categorized as (1) conditions that enhance colonization of the oropharynx, (2) conditions favoring aspiration, (3) conditions requiring prolonged intubation, and (4) host factors.[2,4] Colonization of the oropharynx (colonization is the presence of microorganisms other than the normal flora in the absence of clinical evidence of infection) has been identified as an independent factor in the development of HAP. Gram-positive bacteria and anaerobic bacteria normally live in the oropharynx, and they occupy bacterial binding sites in the oropharyngeal mucosa. When normal oropharyngeal flora are destroyed, these binding sites are susceptible to colonization by pathogenic bacteria. Risk factors associated with oropharyngeal colonization include previous antibiotic therapy, increased age, dental plaque, smoking, and chronic diseases, such as chronic obstructive pulmonary disease (COPD), gastroesophageal reflux disease, alcoholism, diabetes mellitus, and malnutrition.[9,11] The exact role the stomach plays in the development of pneumonia is controversial. In healthy individuals, the stomach is normally sterile because of the bactericidal activity of hydrochloric acid. However, when gastric pH increases above normal (pH > 4), as occurs with the use of histamine type 2 antagonists and antacids for stress ulcer prophylaxis, microorganisms are able to multiply.[7] Gastric colonization increases retrograde colonization of the oropharynx and increases the risk for pneumonia. Individuals at risk for gastric colonization include the elderly; those with achlorhydria, ileus, or upper gastrointestinal disease; and those receiving antacids, histamine-2 antagonists, or enteral feedings.[2,4] The gram-negative or pathogenic gram-positive organisms that have colonized the oropharynx are readily available for aspiration into the tracheobronchial tree.

Aspiration occurs frequently in healthy individuals while they sleep. The risk for clinically significant aspiration is increased in individuals who are unable to protect their airways (e.g., in patients with alcohol abuse, a depressed level of consciousness, or dysphagia; in those who have endotracheal or enteral tubes; or in those receiving enteral feedings). Aspiration of bacteria found in dental plaques is receiving increased attention as a significant source of pneumonia.

Inhalation of bacteria-laden aerosols from contaminated respiratory equipment is another potential source of pneumonia-causing bacteria. Condensate collection in the ventilator tubing can become contaminated with secretions and serve as a reservoir for bacterial growth.[11] Inhalation is an effective entry mechanism for *Legionella* species, *M. tuberculosis*, certain viruses, and fungi. Organisms are carried through small inhaled droplets from the tracheobronchial tree into the lower respiratory tract.[11]

Hematogenous spread serves as a mechanism for the development of pneumonia; the pulmonary circulation provides a potential portal of entry for microbes. The pulmonary capillaries form a dense network in the walls of the alveoli that is ideal for gas exchange. Hematogenous microbes from distant sites of infection can migrate through this network and cause pneumonia. (Pneumonia can also cause bacteremia. Secondary bacteremia after pneumonia has been reported in 6% to 20% of pneumonia cases.) Finally, translocation of bacterial toxins from the gut lumen to the mesenteric lymph nodes and eventually to the lungs may possibly cause bacterial pneumonia. However, translocation has not yet been confirmed as a pathophysiological mechanism.[7]

ASSESSMENT

History

Knowledge of risk factors and symptoms can assist in the identification of potential pathogens causing CAP and HAP. Hemoptysis implies tissue necrosis and is more common with pyogenic streptococcal pneumonia, anaerobic lung abscesses, *S. aureus,* necrotizing gram-negative organisms, and invasive *Aspergillus* species.[9] Extrapulmonary symptoms may indicate specific pathogens; diarrhea and abdominal discomfort are present with *Legionella* species, and otitis media and pharyngitis are present with *M. pneumoniae.*[11] The clinical presentation in the older adult may vary somewhat from what is "typical" in a younger person (Box 26-3).

Historical information may also be extremely helpful in diagnosis of CAP and HAP. It is important to include information about contact with animals, especially birds, bats, rats, and rabbits, which can assist with the diagnosis of histoplasmosis, psittacosis, tularemia, and plague. In addition, a complete history that includes dental hygiene history and place of residence may assist in the differential diagnosis.[9] Diseases that may mimic pneumonia include heart failure, atelectasis, pulmonary thromboembolism, drug reactions, pulmonary hemorrhage, and acute respiratory distress syndrome.

Physical Findings

A comprehensive cardiovascular and pulmonary assessment should be completed, with a focus on the ATS major and minor criteria (see Box 26-1). The nurse assesses for signs of hypoxemia (duskiness or cyanosis) and dyspnea. Patients presenting with new-onset respiratory symptoms (e.g., cough, sputum production, dyspnea, pleuritic chest pain) usually have an accompanying fever and chills. Inspection of the chest includes assessing respiratory pattern and respiratory rate, observing the patient's posture and work of breathing, and inspecting for the presence of intercostal retractions. Percussion of the chest frequently reveals dullness with lobar pneumonia. Decreased breath sounds are heard on auscultation. Crackles or bronchial breath sounds are heard over the area of consolidation.

Extrapulmonary symptoms may include myalgia and gastrointestinal symptoms. Confusion may be a subtle symptom in elderly patients.[11,12]

Diagnostic Studies

The workup for severe CAP and HAP is similar. Diagnostic tests are ordered for two reasons: to determine whether the pneumonia is the cause of the patient's symptoms and to determine the pathogen when pneumonia is present.[7] Table 26-1 summarizes the current ATS recommendations. The diagnostic evaluation must be performed rapidly to prevent delays in initiation of antibiotic therapy.

All patients should have a chest radiograph (posteroanterior and lateral views) to identify both the presence and location of infiltrates. The chest radiograph is helpful in differentiating pneumonia from other conditions and identifying severe pneumonia, which is indicated by the presence of multilobular, rapidly spreading, or cavitary infiltrates.

The value of examining lower respiratory secretions with Gram stain and culturing sputum is controversial. The ATS does not recommend routine use of Gram's stain and sputum culture and advises that results must be interpreted cautiously.[6,7] However, the IDSA recommends routine Gram stain and culture of deep-cough specimens.[2,4] Lower respiratory secretions can be easily obtained in intubated patients using endotracheal aspiration. Nonquantitative endotracheal aspiration cultures may assist in excluding certain pathogens and may be helpful in modifying initial empirical treatment.[2] Routine use of quantitative invasive diagnostic techniques (bronchoscopy with protected specimen brush [PSB] or bronchoalveolar lavage [BAL]) in severe pneumonia is not recommended by the ATS, the Centers for Disease Control and Prevention (CDC), or the IDSA.[2,4,6,7] Current guidelines suggest that BAL or PSB be used only in selected circumstances, such as in nonresponse to antimicrobial therapy, immunosuppression, suspected tuberculosis in the absence of a productive cough, pneumonia with suspected neoplasm or foreign body, or conditions that require lung biopsy.[2,4,6,7] The IDSA recommends HIV testing for people age 15 to 54 years as well.[4] Pneumococcal urinary antigen assay is being recommended as an addition to blood culture testing. The advantage of this test is the rapidity with which results are obtained (within 15 minutes).[4]

Box 26-3 • CONSIDERATIONS FOR THE OLDER PATIENT: PNEUMONIA

- **Presentation.** The usual symptoms (fever, chills, increased white blood count) may be absent. Confusion and tachypnea are common presenting symptoms in older patients with pneumonia. Other symptoms in the older patient include weakness, lethargy, failure to thrive, anorexia, abdominal pain, episodes of falling, incontinence, headache, delirium, and nonspecific deterioration.

- **Prevention.** People 65 years of age and older should receive both the pneumococcal vaccine (a one-time vaccination) and yearly influenza vaccines. The Health Care Financing Agency has approved the use of standing orders to give the vaccines to Medicare patients.

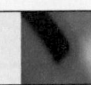

Table 26-1 • Diagnostic Studies in Patients With Severe Community-Acquired Pneumonia or Severe Hospital-Acquired Pneumonia

Study	Rationale
Chest radiograph (anterior–posterior and lateral)	Identify presence and severity of infiltrates. Assess for pleural effusions. Determine severity of pneumonia by identifying the presence of multilobar, rapidly spreading, or cavitary infiltrates.
Two sets of blood cultures from separate sites	Can isolate the etiologic pathogen in 8%–20% of cases.
Complete blood count Serum electrolytes Renal and liver function	Document the presence of multiple-organ dysfunction. Help define severity of illness.
Arterial blood gases	Define severity of illness. Determine need for supplemental oxygen and mechanical ventilation.
Thoracentesis (if pleural effusion >10 mm identified on lateral decubitus film) Pleural fluid studies, including: White blood count with differential Protein Glucose Lactate dehydrogenase (LDH) pH Gram stain and acid-fast stain Culture for bacteria, fungi, and mycobacteria	Rule out empyema.

From data in American Thoracic Society: Guidelines for the management of adults with community-acquired pneumonia. Am J Respir Crit Care Med 163:1730–1754, 2001.

MANAGEMENT

Antibiotic Therapy

Antibiotic therapy is the cornerstone of treatment for both CAP and HAP. Patients should initially be treated empirically, based on the severity of disease and the likely pathogens.[7] Table 26-2 presents ATS guidelines for treatment of severe CAP, and Table 26-3 presents guidelines for treatment of HAP and VAP. Initial therapy should be instituted rapidly. Data show that hospitalized patients with CAP who receive their first dose of antibiotic therapy within 8 hours of arrival at the hospital have reduced mortality at 30 days.[6] Double antibiotic coverage is necessary for people with severe CAP.[9] Initial therapy should not be changed within the first 48 to 72 hours unless progressive deterioration is evident or initial microbiological (blood or respiratory) cultures indicate a need to modify therapy.[6,7]

Factors to consider when determining the duration of therapy include concurrent illness, bacteremia, severity of pneumonia at the onset of antibiotic therapy, infecting pathogens, risk for multidrug resistance, and rapidity of clinical response.[6,7] Recommended duration of therapy is 7 to 10 days for S. aureus or H. influenzae; 10 to 14 days for M. pneumoniae or C. pneumoniae; and 8 to 14 days for P. aeruginosa, Acinetobacter species, multilobar involvement, malnutrition, or a necrotizing gram-negative bacillus.[9]

Supportive Therapy

Common nursing diagnoses and collaborative problems for a patient with a respiratory disorder (such as pneumonia) are given in Box 26-4. Oxygen therapy may be required to maintain adequate gas exchange. Mechanical ventilation to correct hypoxemia is frequently required in both severe CAP and HAP. Humidified oxygen should be administered by mask or endotracheal tube to promote adequate ventilation. Aggressive pulmonary toilet is indicated to mobilize secretions, open closed alveoli, and promote oxygenation. Adequate nutritional support is critical. In addition, a nutritional consult should be initiated with implementation of appropriate enteral or parenteral therapy.

PREVENTION

Pneumonia is the seventh leading cause of death in the United States; therefore, prevention of both CAP and HAP is essential. Primary measures to prevent CAP include the use of influenza and pneumococcal vaccines.[6,7] All immunocompetent patients 50 years of age or older should receive the injected form of the inactivated influenza vaccine. The live attenuated intranasal influenza vaccine is an alternative for people 5 to 49 years of age without chronic disease. The pneumococcal vaccine is recommended for people older than 65 years of age and those with chronic illnesses such as cardiovascular disease, COPD (but not asthma), diabetes mellitus, alcoholism, chronic liver disease, cerebrospinal fluid leaks, and functional or anatomic asplenia; those who belong to special populations, such as Alaska natives or other Native Americans; or those who live in special social settings, such as long-term care facilities.[6,7] The ATS recommends influenza

·⠿· Table 26-2 • Antibiotic Therapy for Severe Community-Acquired Pneumonia*†

Organisms	Therapy‡§
No Risk for Pseudomonas aeruginosa	
Streptococcus pneumoniae (including DRSP)	Intravenous ß-lactam (cefotaxime, ceftriaxone)‖ plus either
Legionella species	Intravenous macrolide (azithromycin)
Haemophilus influenzae	or
Enteric gram-negative bacilli	Intravenous fluoroquinolone
Staphylococcus aureus	
Mycoplasma pneumoniae	
Respiratory viruses	
Miscellaneous	
Chlamydia pneumoniae	
Mycobacterium tuberculosis	
Endemic fungi	
Risk for Pseudomonas aeruginosa	
All of the above pathogens plus *P. aeruginosa*	Selected intravenous antipseudomonal ß-lactam (cefepime, imipenem, meropenem, piperacillin/tazobactam)¶ plus intravenous antipseudomonal quinolone (ciprofloxacin)
	or
	Selected intravenous antipseudomonal ß-lactam (cefepime, imipenem, meropenem, piperacillin/tazobactam)
	plus either
	Intravenous macrolide (azithromycin)
	or
	Intravenous nonpseudomonal fluoroquinolone

* Excludes patients at risk for HIV.
† In roughly one third to one half of the cases no etiology was identified.
‡ Combination therapy required.
§ In no particular order.
‖ Antipseudomonal agents such as cefepime, piperacillin/tazobactam, imipenem, and meropenem are generally active against drug-resistant *S. pneumoniae* (DRSP) and other likely pathogens in this population, but are not recommended for routine use unless the patient has risk factors for *P. aeruginosa*.
¶ If ß-lactam allergic, replace the listed ß-lactam with aztreonam and combine with an aminoglycoside and an antipneumococcal fluoroquinolone as listed.
Reprinted with permission from the American Thoracic Society: Guidelines for the management of adults with community-acquired pneumonia. Am J Respir Crit Care Med 163:1730–1754, 2001.

vaccine for three target groups: persons at a high risk for influenza complications, persons who may transmit influenza to high-risk patients (e.g., health care workers), and any person who wishes to decrease the chance of becoming infected with influenza.[7] High-risk patients include people older than 65 years of age, residents of long-term care facilities, patients with chronic cardiovascular or pulmonary disease, patients who required regular medical care or hospitalization during the preceding year, and pregnant women in the second or third trimester during influenza season. Because cigarette smoking is a risk factor for both HAP and CAP pneumonia, smoking cessation, particularly in patients who have previously had pneumonia, is an important preventive strategy.[7]

A complete understanding of the pathogenesis of HAP enables the critical care nurse to develop strategies about interventions that prevent the onset of pneumonia. The CDC, IDSA, and ATS consider education the cornerstone of an effective infection control program and the prevention of HAP.[4,7] Targets of opportunity in the prevention of HAP include strict infection control, handwashing using an alcohol-based disinfectant, surveillance for pathogens, and early removal of invasive lines.[7] The American Association of Critical-Care Nurses (AACN) has published guidelines for the prevention of VAP as part of their

AACN Practice Alerts (see Chapter 25). According to the evidence-based directive from AACN, in all patients receiving mechanical ventilation as well as those at high risk for aspiration (1) the head of the bed should be elevated at 30 to 45 degrees unless medically contraindicated, (2) endotracheal tubes should have dorsal lumens above the cuff to allow drainage and continuous tracheal secretions, and (3) patient ventilator circuits should be changed based on need because of contamination rather than by routine.[13] The CDC has published comprehensive guidelines on the prevention of HAP.[7] Internet access to the CDC guidelines is available at http://www.cdc.gov.

• Severe Acute Respiratory Syndrome

SARS, a viral illness of the lower respiratory tract, is caused by the SARS-associated coronavirus (SARS-CoV).[14] First reported in Guandong Province, China in February 2003,[15] cases of SARS were subsequently identified in Hong Kong, Viet Nam, Thailand, and Taiwan.[16] More than 8,000 suspected cases of SARS, resulting in 774 deaths, were reported to the World Health Organization (WHO) between December 2002

Table 26-3 • Antibiotic Therapy for Patients With Hospital-Acquired or Ventilator-Associated Pneumonia

Initial Empiric Antibiotic Therapy for Hospital-Acquired Pneumonia or Ventilator-Associated Pneumonia in Patients with No Known Risk Factors for Multidrug-Resistant Pathogens, Early Onset, and Any Disease Severity

Potential Pathogen	Recommended Antibiotic
Streptococcus pneumoniae[†] *Haemophilus influenzae* Methicillin-sensitive *Staphylococcus aureus* Antibiotic-sensitive enteric gram-negative bacilli *Escherichia coli* *Klebsiella pneumoniae* *Enterobacter* species *Proteus* species *Serratia marcescens*	Ceftriaxone *or* Levofloxacin, moxifloxacin, or ciprofloxacin *or* Ampicillin/sulbactam *or* Ertapenem

[†]The frequency of penicillin-resistant *S. pneumoniae* and multidrug-resistant *S. pneumoniae* is increasing; levofloxacin and moxifloxacin are preferred to ciprofloxacin, and the role of other new quinolones, such as gatifloxacin, has not been established.

Initial Empiric Therapy for Hospital-Acquired Pneumonia, Ventilator-Associated Pneumonia, and Health Care–Associated Pneumonia in Patients with Late-Onset Disease or Risk Factors for Multidrug-Resistant Pathogens and All Disease Severity

Potential Pathogens	Combination Antibiotic Therapy*
Pathogens listed in above table and MDR pathogens *Pseudomonas aeruginosa* *Klebsiella pneumoniae* (ESBL+)[‡] *Acinetobacter* species[†]	Antipseudomonal cephalosporin (cefepime, ceftazidime) *or* Antipseudomonal carbepenem (imipenem or meropenem) *or* β-Lactam/β-lactamase inhibitor (piperacillin-tazobactam) *plus* Antipseudomonal fluoroquinolone[‡] (ciprofloxacin or levofloxacin) *or* Aminoglycoside (amikacin, gentamicin, or tobramycin) *plus*
Methicillin-resistant *Staphylococcus aureus* (MRSA) *Legionella pneumophilia*[‡]	Linezolid or vancomycin[†]

*Initial antibiotic therapy should be adjusted or streamlined on the basis of microbiologic data and clinical response to therapy.
[†]If an ESBL+ strain, such as *K. pneumoniae*, or an *Acinetobacter* species is suspected, a carbepenem is a reliable choice. If *L. pneumophila* is suspected, the combination antibiotic regimen should include a macrolide (e.g., azithromycin) or a fluoroquinolone (e.g., ciprofloxacin or levofloxacin) should be used rather than an aminoglycoside.
[‡]If MRSA risk factors are present or there is a high incidence locally.

Initial Intravenous, Adult Doses of Antibiotics for Empiric Therapy of Hospital-Acquired Pneumonia, Including Ventilator-Associated Pneumonia, and Health Care–Associated Pneumonia in Patients with Late-Onset Disease or Risk Factors for Multidrug-Resistant Pathogens

Antibiotic	Dosage*
Antipseudomonal cephalosporin	
Cefepime	1–2 g every 8–12 h
Ceftazidime	2 g every 8 h
Carbepenems	
Imipenem	500 mg every 6 h or 1 g every 8 h
Meropenem	1 g every 8 h
β-Lactam/β-lactamase inhibitor	
Piperacillin-tazobactam	4.5 g every 6 h
Aminoglycosides	
Gentamycin	7 mg/kg per d[†]
Tobramycin	7 mg/kg per d[†]
Amikacin	20 mg/kg per d[†]
Antipseudomonal quinolones	
Levofloxacin	750 mg every d
Ciprofloxacin	400 mg every 8 h
Vancomycin	15 mg/kg every 12 h[‡]
Linezolid	600 mg every 12 h

*Dosages are based on normal renal and hepatic function.
[†]Trough levels for gentamicin and tobramycin should be less than 1 μg/mL, and for amikacin they should be less 4–5 μg/mL.
[‡]Trough levels for vancomycin should be 15–20 μg/mL.

From American Thoracic Society Antibiotic Therapy for Patients With Hospital-Acquired or Ventilator-Associated Pneumonia from American Thoracic Society: Guidelines for the management of adults with hospital-acquired, ventilator-associated, and health care-associated pneumonia. Am J Respir Crit Care Med 171:388–416, 2005.

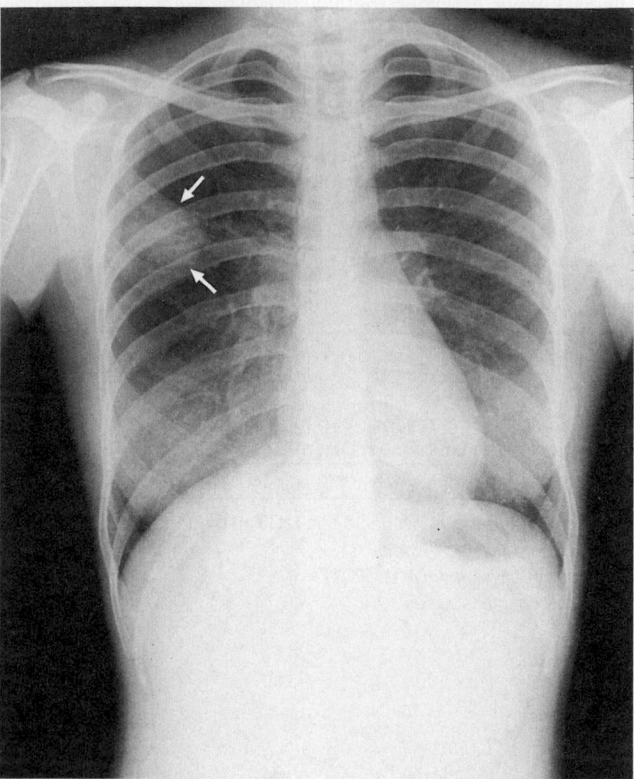

Figure 26-1 • Frontal chest radiograph in a 25-year-old woman showing ill-defined air-space shadowing. (From Lee N, Hui D, Wu A, et al: A major outbreak of severe acute respiratory syndrome in Hong Kong. N Engl J Med 348[20]:1986–1994, 2003. Copyright © 2003. Massachusetts Medical Society. All rights reserved.)

and April 2003.[14] The illness has not been as prevalent in the United States, with only eight people having been hospitalized with evidence of the SARS-CoV.[17] What these people had in common was international travel to a SARS-affected region within 10 days of hospital admission.

The SARS virus is transmitted from person to person by droplets, direct or indirect contact, or viral shedding in feces and urine.[18] Droplets spread when an infected person coughs or sneezes and droplets land on the mucous membranes of the mouth, nose, or eyes of a person who is usually located within a distance of three feet. Direct or indirect contact results when a person touches a surface contaminated with droplets and then touches his or her eyes, nose, or mouth.[17] The virus spreads quickly, and medical personnel are among those commonly infected.[18]

The period from exposure to the onset of symptoms or prodromal phase of SARS is usually 2 to 7 days, although it may be as long as 10 to 14 days. The first symptoms are fever (>38°C), chills, and rigor.[19] Other symptoms include headache, malaise, and myalgias. Mild respiratory symptoms may be present. Inspiratory crackles may be heard at the bases of the lungs. Chest radiographs may be normal, or focal airspace infiltrates may be present in the peripheral lung zones (Fig. 26-1). Initial blood counts indicate lymphopenia, although the neutrophil count and monocyte count are often normal.[19] Sputum and blood cultures are obtained to rule out the other causes of atypical pneumonia to include *M. pneumoniae, C. pneumoniae,* human cytomegalovirus, adenoviruses, respiratory syncytial virus, and influenza viruses.[20]

After 3 to 7 days, the lower respiratory phase begins, as evidenced by a dry, nonproductive cough and dyspnea that may be accompanied by progressive hypoxemia.[21] In up to 20% of the cases, the respiratory illness is severe enough to require intubation and mechanical ventilation.[21] The focal infiltrates progress to more generalized, interstitial infiltrates, and significant consolidation is evident.[19] Findings of ground-glass opacification in the periphery are typical on thoracic computed tomography (CT) scan.[19] Laboratory findings include leukopenia, lymphopenia, and thrombocytopenia on the complete blood count. Serum alanine aminotransferase, creatine kinase (CK), and lactate dehydrogenase (LDH) may be elevated, indicating extensive lung injury.[19] Advanced age, male gender, high peak CK, high LDH, high neutrophil count, and low serum sodium have been found to be predictive of significant illness, ICU admission, and death.[19]

Until SARS is specifically identified, the treatment plan for a patient with a suspected diagnosis of SARS includes empiric therapy using antibiotics effective against typical and atypical pathogens.[20] Antiviral agents such as ribavirin and corticosteroids may be administered as well.[22] In vitro studies suggest that ribavirin may not be effective and possibly may cause serious side effects when used to treat SARS.[23] In an analysis of 110 patients with SARS, 61% had an incident of hemolytic anemia, 57% hypocalcemia, and

46% hypomagnesemia.[24] Ventilatory support may be provided either through noninvasive positive-pressure ventilation or, as patient condition dictates, intubation with mechanical ventilation.

Because SARS is a virulent pathogen, a key part of the care of the patient is the institution of strict infection control measures. Droplet and contact precautions are a necessity. Personal protective equipment, including a gown, gloves, surgical mask or N95 disposable particulate respirator, and face shield, should be worn by those in contact with the patient.[25] A private room with negative flow is recommended.[25] Strict handwashing and decontamination of any equipment used in patient care are a must (Fig. 26-2).[25] When

patients are discharged, they should be instructed to limit their interactions outside the home and not go to any public places until 10 days after resolution of fever and respiratory symptoms.[20]

• Pleural Effusion

The pleural space is a potential space between the visceral and parietal pleurae that lines the lungs and interior chest wall. There is a continuous flow of fluid from the parietal pleura of the chest wall to the visceral pleura, and the fluid is eventually absorbed by the pulmonary lymphatics.

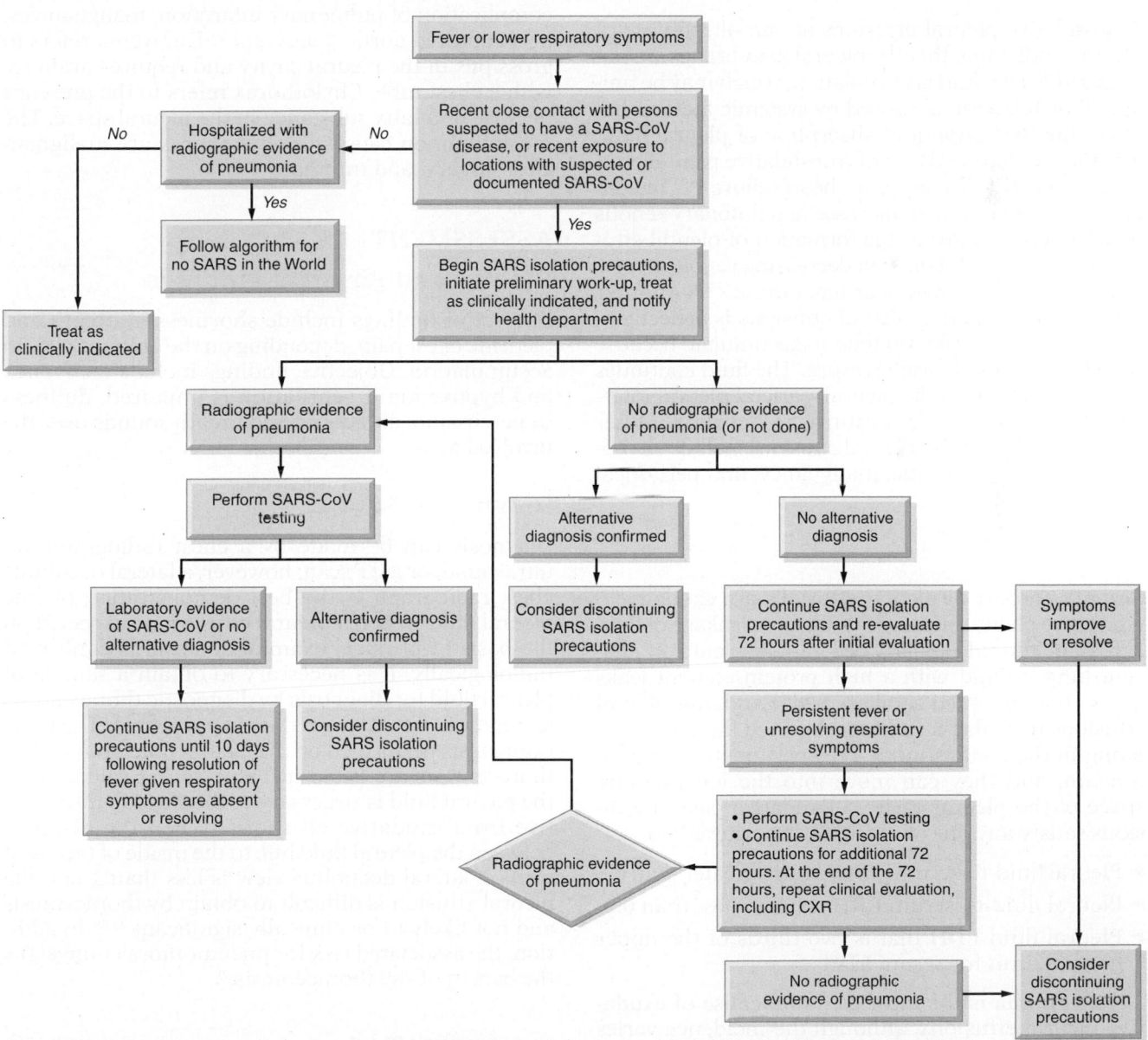

Figure 26-2 • Algorithm for management of patients with fever or lower respiratory symptoms when person-to-person transmission of SARS-CoV is occurring in the world. (From Centers for Disease Control and Prevention: Clinical guidance on the identification and evaluation of possible SARS-CoV disease among persons presenting with community-acquired illness, Version 2, Supplement I: Infection control in healthcare, home, and community settings. Washington, DC, Department of Health and Human Services Centers for Disease Control and Prevention, 2004, pp 1–28.)

PATHOPHYSIOLOGY

Pleural effusion is the accumulation of pleural fluid due to an increased rate of fluid formation, a decreased rate of fluid removal, or both.[26,27] This is caused by at least one of the five following mechanisms:

▶ Increased pressure in subpleural capillaries or lymphatics

▶ Increased capillary permeability

▶ Decreased colloid osmotic pressure of the blood

▶ Increased intrapleural negative pressure

▶ Impaired lymphatic drainage of the pleural space

Transudates

Transudative pleural effusions are an ultrafiltrate of plasma, indicating that the pleural membranes are not diseased.[26] The fluid accumulation, which may be unilateral or bilateral, is caused by systemic factors that affect the formation and absorption of pleural fluid. The most common cause of transudative pleural effusions in the ICU is congestive heart failure.[26,27] In congestive heart failure, an increase in pulmonary venous pressure contributes to the formation of pleural effusions. Treatment focuses on decreasing venous hypertension and improving cardiac output.[28,29] Another cause of transudative pleural effusions is atelectasis, which may cause pleural fluid to accumulate because of a decrease in pleural pressure. The fluid continues to accumulate until the pleural–parietal pleural interstitial pressure gradient returns to normal.[28] Other causes of transudative pleural effusions include cirrhosis, nephrotic syndrome, malignancy, and peritoneal dialysis.

Exudates

Seventy percent of pleural effusions are exudative.[30] Exudative pleural effusions result from leakage of fluid across an injured capillary bed into the pleura or adjacent lung.[26] Fluid with a high protein content leaks across the disrupted capillary bed. Exudative pleural effusions may also result from infected fluid accumulating in the mediastinum, retroperitoneum, or peritoneum, and they can move into the low-pressure space of the pleural cavity.[28] Exudative pleural effusions satisfy any one of the following criteria[26,27]

▶ Pleural fluid-to-serum protein ratio greater than 0.5

▶ Pleural fluid-to-serum LDH ratio greater than 0.6

▶ Pleural fluid LDH that is two thirds of the upper normal limit for serum LDH

Pneumonia is the most common cause of exudative pleural effusions, although the incidence varies with the infective agent. Malignancies are the second most common cause of exudative pleural effusions. Approximately one third of exudative pleural effusions caused by malignancies are bloody. If a massive effusion opacifies an entire hemithorax, metastatic disease should be suspected.

Exudative pleural effusions occur in approximately 30% to 50% of patients with pulmonary embolism.[29,30] The presence of a pleural effusion on chest radiology in a patient with chest pain and dyspnea is suggestive of pulmonary effusion. Mechanisms that produce these effusions include ischemia-induced increased pleural capillary permeability, imbalance in vascular and pleural space hydrostatic pressures, and pleuropulmonary hemorrhage.[29]

A hemothorax is a bloody exudative pleural effusion and is diagnosed by a pleural fluid/blood hematocrit ratio greater than 50%.[26,29,30] Trauma is the most common cause of a hemothorax (see Chapter 55). Hemothorax can result from invasive procedures (placement of central venous catheter, thoracentesis) and anticoagulation therapy. Hemothorax is a rare complication of pulmonary infarction, malignancies, or a ruptured aortic aneurysm.[29] Empyema refers to gross pus in the pleural cavity and requires drainage with a chest tube. Chylothorax refers to the presence of chyle or a fatty substance in the pleural space. The most common causes of chylothorax are malignancies, surgery, and trauma.[31]

ASSESSMENT

History and Physical Findings

Subjective findings include shortness of breath and pleuritic chest pain, depending on the amount of fluid accumulation. Objective findings include tachypnea and hypoxemia if ventilation is impaired, dullness to percussion, and decreased breath sounds over the involved area.

Diagnostic Studies

Diagnosis can be made by a chest radiograph, an ultrasound, or a CT scan; however, a lateral decubitus chest radiograph is the best demonstration of free pleural fluid. When a pleural effusion is suspected on the basis of physical examination and is confirmed radiologically, it is necessary to obtain a sample of pleural fluid for diagnosis by diagnostic thoracentesis (aspiration of fluid from the pleural space). The laboratory tests performed on the pleural fluid obtained by thoracentesis are listed in Table 26-4. Evaluation of the pleural fluid is necessary to distinguish transudative from exudative effusions. When the distance between the pleural fluid line to the inside of the chest wall on lateral decubitus view is less than 1 cm, the pleural effusion is difficult to obtain by thoracentesis and not likely to be clinically significant.[26,29] In addition, the associated risk for pneumothorax outweighs the benefit of the thoracentesis.[29]

MANAGEMENT

Treatment of the underlying cause is necessary. Removal of the pleural effusion by thoracentesis or chest tube placement may be indicated depending on the etiology and size of effusion. The primary indication for therapeutic thoracentesis is relief of dyspnea.

Table 26-4 • Assessment of Pleural Fluid

Test	Comment
Red blood cell count >100,000/mm³	Trauma, malignancy, pulmonary embolism
Hematocrit >50% of peripheral blood	Hemothorax
White blood cell count (WBC)	
>50,000–100,000/mm³	Grossly visible pus, otherwise total WBC less useful than WBC differential
>50% Neutrophils	Acute inflammation or infection
>50% Lymphocytes	Tuberculosis, malignancy
>10% Eosinophils	Most common: hemothorax, pneumothorax; also benign
>5% Mesothelial cells	Asbestos effusions, drug reaction, paragonimiasis; tuberculosis *less likely*
Glucose <60 mg/dL	Infection, malignancy, tuberculosis, rheumatoid
Amylase >200 units/dL	Pleuritis, esophageal perforation, pancreatic disease, malignancy, ruptured ectopic pregnancy
	Isoenzyme profile: salivary–esophageal disease, malignancy (especially lung)
pH <7.2	Isoenzyme profile: pancreatic–pancreatic disease
	Infection (complicated parapneumonic effusion and empyema), malignancy, esophageal rupture, rheumatoid or lupus pleuritis, tuberculosis, systemic acidosis, urinothorax
Triglyceride >110 mg/dL	Chylothorax
Microbiological studies	Etiology of infection
Cytology	Diagnostic of malignancy

Adapted from Sahn SA: State of the art: The pleura. Am Rev Respir Dis 138:184–234, 1988. From Zimmerman LH: Pleural effusions. In Goldstein RH, et al (eds): A Practical Approach to Pulmonary Medicine. Philadelphia, Lippincott-Raven, 1997, p 199.

• Pneumothorax

A pneumothorax occurs if air enters the pleural space between the visceral and parietal pleurae, producing partial or complete lung collapse.

PATHOPHYSIOLOGY

During spontaneous breathing, two opposing forces generate negative pleural pressures. Pressure in the airways is positive during expiration and negative during inspiration.[29] However, pleural pressure remains subatmospheric on both inspiration and expiration.[29] Therefore, airway pressure remains higher than pleural pressure throughout the respiratory cycle. Sudden communication of the pleural space with either alveolar or external air allows gas to enter (Fig. 26-3). When the pleural pressure rises, the elasticity of the lung causes it to collapse. The lung continues to collapse until either the pressure gradient no longer exists or the pleural defect closes.[29,31] Lung collapse produces a decrease in vital capacity, an increase in the alveolar–arterial partial pressure of oxygen ($P_{A}O_2$–PaO_2) gradient, a ventilation–perfusion mismatch, and an intrapulmonary shunt resulting in hypoxemia.[29,31] In the patient without underlying lung disease, hypercapnia does not occur because the uninvolved lung functions to maintain adequate alveolar ventilation. In the patient with underlying pulmonary disease (COPD), hypercapnia is common because the abnormal gas exchange produced by the pneumothorax is superimposed on preexisting abnormal gas exchange.[29]

There are two types of pneumothorax: spontaneous and traumatic. Spontaneous pneumothorax is any pneumothorax that results from the rupture of air into the pleural space without obvious cause. Primary spontaneous pneumothorax occurs in the absence of underlying lung disease, and secondary spontaneous pneumothorax occurs as a complication of underlying lung disease.[29,31] Primary spontaneous pneumothorax occurs primarily in young (adolescence to 30 years of age), tall men. Family history and cigarette smoking are important risk factors.[31–33] Secondary spontaneous pneumothorax largely occurs in patients who have COPD.[30] Other causes of secondary spontaneous pneumothorax include asthma, cystic fibrosis, *Pneumocystis carinii* pneumonia, sarcoidosis, necrotizing pneumonia, and histiocytosis X.[29,31]

The most common causes of a traumatic pneumothorax in critically ill patients are invasive procedures and barotrauma.[29] (See Chapter 55 for a discussion of blunt and penetrating trauma as causes of pneumothorax.) Accidental entry of air into the pleural space during an invasive procedure causes iatrogenic pneumothorax. Central line catheter insertions cause approximately 36,000 pneumothoraces per year, which affect 1% of the patients receiving central line catheters.[29] Pulmonary barotrauma occurs in approximately 1% to 15% of patients receiving positive-pressure mechanical ventilation and in 25% to 78% of patients with acute respiratory distress syndrome.[29] Barotrauma includes parenchymal inter-

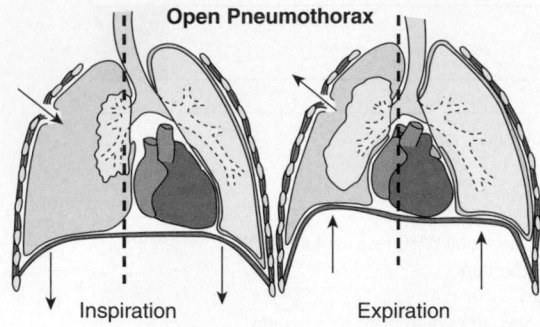

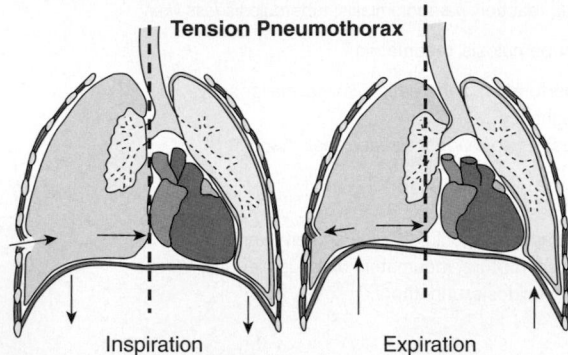

Figure 26-3 • Open or communicating pneumothorax (*top*) and tension pneumothorax (*bottom*). In an open pneumothorax, air enters the chest during inspiration and exits during expiration. There may be slight inflation of the affected lung due to a decrease in pressure as air moves out of the chest. In tension pneumothorax, air can enter but not leave the chest. As the pressure in the chest increases, the heart and great vessels are compressed, and the mediastinal structures are shifted toward the opposite side of the chest. The trachea is pushed from its normal midline position toward the opposite side of the chest, and the unaffected lung is compressed. (From Porth C: Pathophysiology: Concepts of Altered Health States, 7th ed. Philadelphia, Lippincott Williams & Wilkins, 2005, p 692.)

stitial gas, pneumomediastinum, subcutaneous emphysema, pneumoperitoneum, and pneumothorax.[29] Pulmonary interstitial gas or emphysema is the initial radiographic indication of barotrauma. The mechanically ventilated patient is at risk for development of a tension pneumothorax. A tension pneumothorax occurs when the pressure of air in the pleural space exceeds atmospheric pressure. As pressures in the thorax increase, the mediastinum shifts to the contralateral side, placing torsion on the inferior vena cava and decreasing venous return to the right side of the heart[31] (see Fig. 26-3).

ASSESSMENT
History and Physical Findings

The patient complains of sudden onset of acute pleuritic chest pain localized to the affected lung. The pleuritic chest pain is usually accompanied by shortness of breath, increased work of breathing, and dyspnea. Chest wall movement may be uneven because the affected side does not expand as much of the healthy side. Breath sounds are distant or absent. Chest percussion produces a hyperresonant sound. Tachy-

Box 26-5 • RED FLAG: Symptoms of Tension Pneumothorax

- Hypoxemia (early sign)
- Apprehension
- Respiratory distress (severe tachypnea)
- Increasing peak and mean airway pressures, decreasing compliance, and auto–positive end-expiratory pressure (auto-PEEP) in patients receiving mechanical ventilation
- Cardiovascular collapse (heart rate >140 beats/minute with any of the following: peripheral cyanosis, hypotension, pulseless electrical activity)

cardia occurs frequently in all types of pneumothorax. Tension pneumothorax is a life-threatening condition manifested by respiratory distress (Box 26-5).

Diagnostic Studies

To assess for the presence of a pneumothorax, a chest radiograph should be obtained with the patient in the upright or decubitus position. The chest film shows contralateral (opposite side) mediastinal shift, ipsilateral (same side) diaphragmatic depression, and ipsilateral chest wall expansion in the patient with tension pneumothorax.[29] To confirm the size of the pneumothorax, a chest CT maybe obtained.[31] When clinical symptoms of tension pneumothorax are present in a patient on mechanical ventilation, treatment should not be delayed to obtain radiographic confirmation. Arterial blood gases (ABGs) are used to assess for hypoxemia and hypercapnia.

MANAGEMENT

Supplemental oxygen should be administered to all patients with pneumothorax because oxygen accelerates the rate of air resorption from the pleural space.[27,30] If the pneumothorax is 15% to 20%, no medical intervention is required, and the patient is placed on bed rest or limited activity.[34] If the pneumothorax is greater than 20%, then a chest tube is placed in the apical and anterior aspect of the pleural space to assist air removal. Connecting the chest tube to underwater seal drainage alone is usually adequate to resolve the pneumothorax. Initially placing the chest tube to suction risks re-expansion pulmonary edema due to rapid reinflation of the collapsed lung.[29] If the pneumothorax persists after 12 to 24 hours of underwater seal drainage, 15 to 20 cm H_2O suction should be applied to facilitate closure.[30] In approximately one third of patients with COPD, persistent air leaks require multiple chest tubes to evacuate the pneumothorax.[30]

A tension pneumothorax is a life-threatening condition requiring immediate treatment; if untreated, it leads to cardiovascular collapse. If a chest tube is not immediately available, a large-bore (16- or 18-gauge) needle should be placed into the anterior second intercostal space. After needle insertion, a chest tube is placed and connected to underwater seal drainage.

When the tension pneumothorax is relieved, the effect is rapid and occurs as an improvement in oxygenation, a decrease in heart rate, and an increase in blood pressure.

• Pulmonary Embolism

Most incidents of pulmonary embolism occur when a thrombus, which has broken loose and migrated to the pulmonary arteries, causes an obstruction of part of the pulmonary vascular tree (Fig. 26-4).[35] A pulmonary embolism usually results from a deep vein thrombosis (DVT) that has formed in the lower extremities. Other sites of clot formation include the right sight of the heart (as in untreated atrial fibrillation) and other deep vessels of the pelvic region.[36] In North America, venous thromboembolism occurs for the first time in approximately 100 of every 100,000 people.[37] Of these, approximately one third have a symptomatic pulmonary embolus. Major risk factors include age, recent surgery, cancer, and thrombophilia.[36] Risk factors that increase the incidence of venous thromboembolism are listed in Box 26-6. Nonthrombotic causes of pulmonary embolism include fat, air, and amniotic fluid but are much less common than thromboembolism.[36]

PATHOPHYSIOLOGY

A cascade of events begins the process of thromboembolus development. Virchow's triad (venous stasis, hypercoagulability, vein wall damage) has long been acknowledged in the pathophysiology of venous thromboembolism. Venous return from the lower extremities is usually facilitated by contraction of the muscles of the lower extremities during activity. Conditions such as immobility, congestive heart failure, dehydration, and varicose veins contribute to decreased venous return, increased retrograde pressure in the venous system, and stasis of blood with resultant thrombus formation.[38]

Normally there is a balance between activation of clotting factors and the fibrinolytic system that prevents thrombus formation. Hypercoagulability may occur in the presence of trauma, surgery, malignancy, or use of oral contraceptives. In these instances, coagulation may be initiated by contact of factor XII with collagen on exposed subendothelium of damaged vessels, by exposure of blood to tissue factor available as a result of vascular wall damage, by activated monocytes migrating to areas of vascular injury, and by release of activated platelets in response to injury. Factor X may be activated by substances from malignant cells and by substances released from hypoxic endothelial cells.[38] Damage to the vessel wall causes adhesion and aggregation of platelets and contributes to the activation of clotting factors.

Thrombus formation is frequently bilateral and often asymptomatic. Although most thrombi form in the calf, most pulmonary emboli (80% to 90%) arise from venous thrombi that extend into the proximal veins (popliteal and iliofemoral) of the lower extremities.[37] Proximal venous thrombi pose an approximate 50% risk for embolism.[37]

Occlusion of a pulmonary artery by an embolus produces both pulmonary and hemodynamic changes. Alveoli are ventilated but not perfused, producing areas of mismatched ventilation and perfusion. As a result, well-ventilated alveoli are underperfused, and gas exchange is compromised (increased respiratory

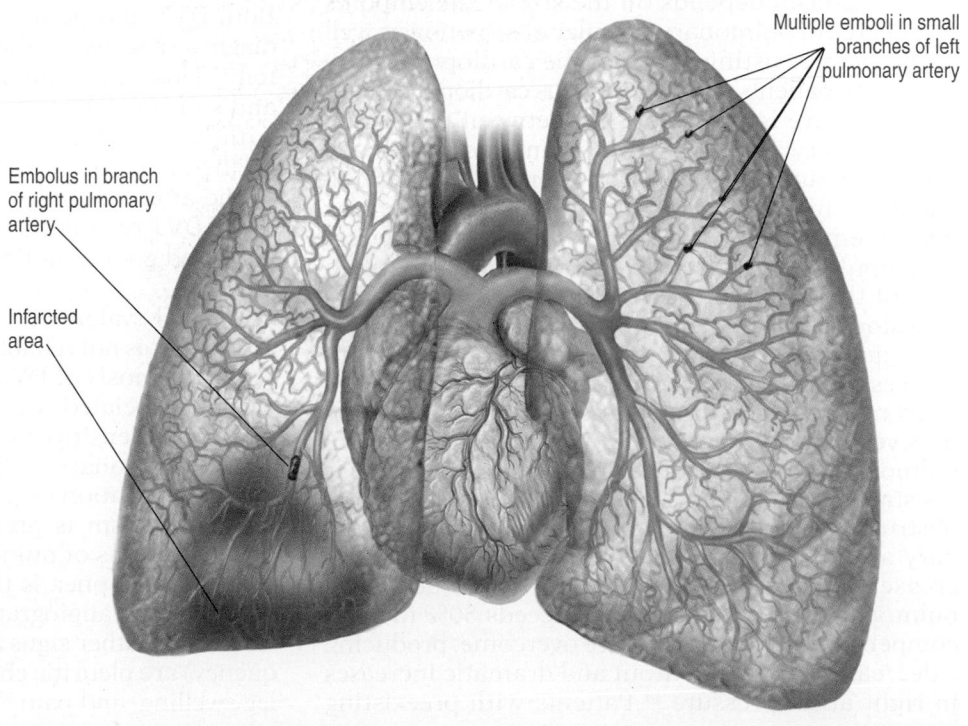

Figure 26-4 • Sites of pulmonary emboli. (From Anatomical Chart Company: Atlas of Pathophysiology. Springhouse, PA, Springhouse, 2002.)

Embolus in branch of right pulmonary artery

Infarcted area

Multiple emboli in small branches of left pulmonary artery

Box 26-6 • Risk Factors for Thromboembolism

Risk Factors for Venous Thromboembolism
Strong Risk Factors
Fracture of the hip, pelvis, or leg
Hip or knee replacement
Major general surgery, major trauma
Spinal cord injury

Moderate Risk Factors
Arthroscopic knee surgery
Central venous lines
Malignancy
Congestive heart or respiratory failure
Hormone replacement therapy, oral contraceptives
Paralytic stroke
Postpartum period
Previous venous thromboembolism
Thrombophilia

Weak Risk Factors
Bed rest for more than 3 days
Immobility due to sitting
Increasing age
Laparoscopic surgery
Obesity
Antepartum period
Varicose veins

Risk Stratification of Thromboemboli for Patients Undergoing Surgery
Low Risk
Uncomplicated surgery in patients aged less than 40 years with minimal immobility postoperatively and no risk factors

Moderate Risk
Any surgery in patients aged 40–60 years
Major surgery in patients aged less than 40 years and no other risk factors
Minor surgery in patients with one or more risk factors

High Risk
Major surgery in patients aged more than 60 years
Major surgery in patients aged 40–60 years with one or more risk factors

Very High Risk
Major surgery in patients aged more than 40 years with previous venous thromboembolism, cancer, or known hypercoagulable state
Major orthopaedic surgery
Elective neurosurgery
Multiple trauma or acute spinal cord injury

From Blann AD, Lip GYH: Venous thromboembolism. BMJ 332(7535):215–219, 2006.

dead space). Pulmonary vascular constriction resulting from a lack of carbon dioxide, which is normally present in pulmonary arterial blood, shifts ventilation from the underperfused alveoli. Accompanying physiological changes include increased minute ventilation, decreased vital capacity, increased airway resistance, and decreased diffusing capacity.[11,36]

The severity of hemodynamic change in pulmonary embolism depends on the size of the embolus and degree of pulmonary vascular obstruction as well as on the preexisting status of the cardiopulmonary system. In patients with no previous cardiopulmonary disease, there is a relationship between the degree of pulmonary artery obstruction and the pulmonary artery pressure. Increased right ventricular afterload results from obstruction of the pulmonary vascular bed by embolism. In patients with no preexisting cardiopulmonary disease, obstruction of less than 20% of the pulmonary vascular bed produces compensatory events that minimize adverse hemodynamic consequences.[36] Cardiac output is maintained by increases in both right ventricular stroke volume and heart rate, and recruitment and distention of pulmonary vessels occur, producing normal or near-normal pulmonary artery pressure and pulmonary vascular resistance.[36] When the degree of pulmonary vascular obstruction exceeds 30% to 40%, increases in pulmonary artery pressure occur, followed by modest increases in right atrial pressure.[24] As the degree of pulmonary artery obstruction exceeds 50% to 60%, compensatory mechanisms are overcome, producing a decrease in cardiac output and dramatic increases in right atrial pressure.[36] Patients with preexisting cardiopulmonary disease have degrees of pulmonary hypertension that are disproportionate to the degree of embolic obstruction.[36] Severe pulmonary hypertension may develop from a relatively small reduction of pulmonary blood flow.

ASSESSMENT

Both DVT and pulmonary embolism are difficult to diagnose because of their nonspecific signs and symptoms. This may result in significant therapeutic delays and substantial morbidity and mortality.[39] Patients with lower extremity DVT may present with pain, erythema, tenderness, swelling, and a palpable cord in the affected limb.[37] However, it is also common that a DVT or embolus produces no significant symptoms and goes unnoticed by patient and practitioner alike.[39]

Clinical evaluation may indicate a need for further studies but is not reliable for confirmation or exclusion of the diagnosis of DVT.[11] Similarly, clinical manifestations associated with pulmonary embolism are not adequately sensitive or specific for diagnosis or exclusion of pulmonary embolism. A diagnostic algorithm for the evaluation of patients with suspected pulmonary embolism is presented in Figure 26-5. Signs and symptoms of pulmonary embolism are listed in Box 26-7. Dyspnea is the most frequent symptom in patients with angiographically confirmed pulmonary embolism. Other signs and symptoms (in order of frequency) are pleuritic chest pain, cough, apprehension, leg swelling, and pain.[35]

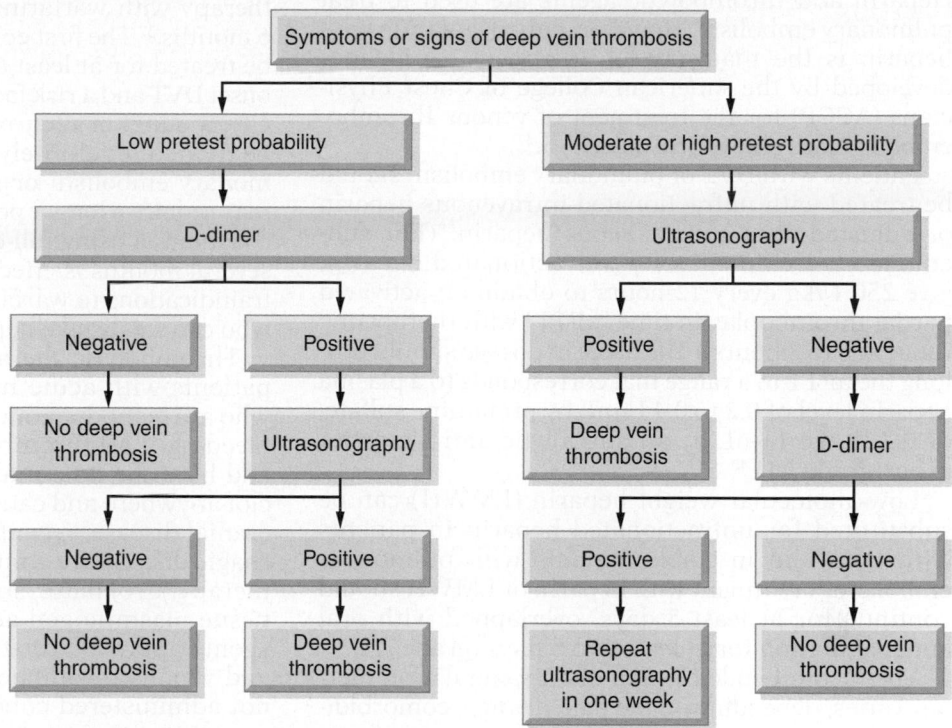

For assessment of pretest probability of suspected deep vein thrombosis:
• Score 1 point each for following: tenderness along entire deep vein system; swelling of entire leg, >3 cm difference in calf circumference; pitting edema; collateral superficial veins; risk factors present (active cancer, prolonged immobility or paralysis, recent surgery, or major medical illness)

• Subtract 2 points for alternative diagnosis likely (for example, ruptured Baker's cyst in rheumatoid arthritis, superficial thrombophlebitis, or infective cellulitis)

Result >3 = high probability; 1-2 = moderate probability; ≤0 = low probability

Figure 26-5 • Diagnostic algorithm for evaluation of patients with symptoms suggestive of acute pulmonary embolism. (From Blann AD, Lip GYH: Venous thromboembolism. BMJ 332[7535]:215–219, 2006.)

 Box 26-7 • RED FLAG: Signs and Symptoms of Pulmonary Embolism

Small to Moderate Embolus
• Dyspnea
• Tachypnea
• Tachycardia
• Chest pain
• Mild fever
• Hypoxemia
• Apprehension
• Cough
• Diaphoresis
• Decreased breath sounds over affected area
• Rales
• Wheezing

Massive Embolus
A more pronounced manifestation of the above signs and symptoms, plus the following:
• Cyanosis
• Restlessness
• Anxiety

• Confusion
• Hypotension
• Cool, clammy skin
• Decreased urinary output
• Pleuritic chest pain: associated with pulmonary infarction
• Hemoptysis: associated with pulmonary infarction

Signs of Pulmonary Embolism in Intensive Care Patients
• Worsening hypoxemia or hypocapnia in a patient on spontaneous ventilation
• Worsening hypoxemia and hypercapnia in a sedate patient on controlled mechanical ventilation
• Worsening dyspnea, hypoxemia, and a reduction in $PaCO_2$ in a patient with chronic lung disease and known carbon dioxide retention
• Unexplained fever
• Sudden elevation in pulmonary artery pressure or central venous pressure in a hemodynamically monitored patient

MANAGEMENT

Heparin and thrombolytic agents are used to treat pulmonary embolism. However, anticoagulation with heparin is the mainstay for treatment. Guidelines developed by the American College of Chest Physicians (ACCP) for the treatment of venous thromboembolism are shown in Table 26-5.[37]

Patients with DVT or pulmonary embolism should be treated with unfractionated intravenous heparin or adjusted-dose subcutaneous heparin. (For subcutaneous treatment with unfractionated heparin, give 250 U/kg every 12 hours to obtain an activated partial thromboplastin time [aPTT] with therapeutic range at 6 to 8 hours.) The heparin dosage should prolong the aPTT to a range that corresponds to a plasma heparin level of 0.2 to 0.4 U/mL by protamine sulfate, or 0.3 to 0.6 U/mL by an amidolytic anti-factor Xa assay (grade A1).[40]

Low–molecular-weight heparin (LMWH) can be substituted for unfractionated heparin in patients with DVT and in stable patients with pulmonary embolism. Treatment with heparin or LMWH should continue for at least 5 days, overlapped with oral anticoagulation for at least 4 to 5 days (grade A1).[40]

The recommended length of anticoagulation therapy varies, depending on the patient's age, comorbidities, and the likelihood of recurrence of pulmonary embolism or DVT. In most patients, anticoagulation therapy with warfarin should be continued for 3 to 6 months.[37] The first episode of idiopathic DVT should be treated for at least 6 months.[11] Patients with new-onset DVT and a risk factor (e.g., cancer, inhibitor deficiency state) or recurrent venous thrombosis should be treated indefinitely.[37] Patients with massive pulmonary embolism or severe iliofemoral thrombosis may require a longer period of heparin therapy.[37] Anticoagulation using full-dose subcutaneous heparin for several months is effective in patients who have contraindications to warfarin (e.g., pregnant women) but who can safely take heparin.[37]

Thrombolytic therapy is only recommended for patients with acute massive pulmonary embolism who are hemodynamically unstable and not prone to bleeding.[39] All thrombolytic agents act systemically and have the potential to lyse a fresh platelet-fibrin clot anywhere and cause bleeding at that site.[37] Intracranial disease, recent surgery, trauma, and hemorrhagic disease are contraindications to thrombolytic therapy. Urokinase, streptokinase, and recombinant tissue plasminogen activator are the thrombolytic agents approved for treating pulmonary embolism and venous thromboembolism. Heparin therapy is not administered concurrently with thrombolytics;

Table 26-5 • American College of Chest Physicians Recommendations for Treatment of Venous Thromboembolism	
Anticoagulation Guidelines for	Recommended Therapy
Unfractionated Heparin	
Suspected VTE	• Obtain baseline aPTT, PT, CBC. • Check for contraindications to heparin therapy. • Give heparin 5,000 U IV. • Order imaging study.
Confirmed VTE	• Re-bolus with heparin 80 U/kg IV, and start maintenance infusion at 18 U/kg/h. • Check aPTT at 6 h; maintain a range corresponding to a therapeutic heparin level. • Start warfarin therapy on day 1 at 5 mg; adjust subsequent daily dose according to INR. • Stop heparin after 4 to 5 days of combined therapy, when INR is >2.0 (2.0–3.0). • Anticoagulate with warfarin for at least 3 mo (target INR 2.5; 2.0–3.0).
Low–Molecular Weight Heparin (LMWH)	
Suspected VTE	• Obtain baseline aPTT, PT, CBC. • Check for contraindication to heparin therapy. • Give unfractionated heparin, 5,000 U IV. • Order imaging study.
Confirmed VTE	• Give LMWH (enoxaparin), 1 mg/kg subcutaneously q12h. • Start warfarin therapy on day 1 at 5 mg; adjust subsequent daily dose according to the INR. • Consider checking platelet count between days 3 and 5. • Stop LMWH after at least 4–5 days of combined therapy, when INR is >2.0 on 2 consecutive days. • Anticoagulate with warfarin for at least 3 mo (goal INR 2.5; 2.0–3.0).

VTE, venous thromboembolism; aPTT, activated partial thromboplastin time; PT, prothrombin time; INR, international normalized ratio; CBC, complete blood count.
From American College of Chest Physicians: Seventh ACCP consensus conference on Antithrombotic and Thrombolytic Therapy. Chest 126(3 Suppl):401S, 428S, 2004.

however, thrombolytic therapy is followed by administration of heparin, then warfarin.

An inferior vena cava filter is recommended to prevent pulmonary embolism in patients with contraindications to heparin therapy (risk for major bleed or drug sensitivity).[39] Placement of an inferior vena cava filter is also recommended in patients with recurring thromboembolism despite adequate anticoagulation, chronic recurrent embolism and pulmonary hypertension, and concurrent surgical pulmonary embolectomy or pulmonary endarterectomy procedures.

PREVENTION

Prevention of venous thromboembolism is essential to decreasing the morbidity and mortality associated with pulmonary embolism. Prophylactic measures are based on the patient's specific risk factors.[41] Preventive measures recommended by the ACCP are listed in Table 26-6.

Chronic Obstructive Pulmonary Disease

COPD is a disease state characterized by airflow limitation that is not fully reversible. The airflow limitation is usually both progressive and associated with an abnormal inflammatory response of the lungs to noxious particles or gases (primarily cigarette smoke) or an inherited deficiency of α_1-antitrypsin.[42] COPD includes two diseases: emphysema and chronic bronchitis.[42] COPD is a major cause of chronic morbidity and mortality, ranking as the fourth leading cause of death in the United States and Europe, with 126,128 deaths in 2003.[42] In 2004, it was estimated that 11.4 million American adults had COPD.[43]

The WHO estimates that COPD shares fourth and fifth place with HIV/AIDS as a single cause of death (behind heart disease, cerebrovascular disease, and acute respiratory infection), and unlike

Table 26-6 • American College of Chest Physicians Recommendations for Prevention of Venous Thromboembolism (VTE)

Patient Population	Recommended Therapy	Grade*
Low-risk general surgery	Early ambulation	C1
Moderate-risk general surgery	LDUH, LMWH, intermittent pneumatic compression, or elastic stockings	A1
Higher-risk general surgery	LDUH, or higher-dose LMWH	A1
Very–high-risk general surgery with multiple risk factors	LDUH, or LMWH combined with intermittent pneumatic compression	B1
Total hip replacement surgery	LMWH, started 12–24 h after surgery Warfarin, started before or immediately after surgery, or Adjusted-dose heparin, started before surgery; Adjuvant use of elastic stockings or intermittent pneumatic compression	A1
Total knee replacement surgery	LMWH, warfarin, or intermittent pneumatic compression	A1
Acute spinal cord injury	LMWH	B1
	Elastic stockings and intermittent pneumatic compression may have benefit when used with LMWH; however, they appear ineffective when used alone	C1
Trauma patients with identifiable risk factor for thromboembolism	LMWH, as soon as safe	A1
	Intermittent pneumatic compression if LMWH will be delayed or is contraindicated	C1
	For high-risk patients with suboptimal prophylaxis, consider screening with duplex ultrasonography or filter placement in the inferior vena cava	C2
Myocardial infarction	LDUH or full-dose anticoagulation	A1
	Intermittent pneumatic compression or elastic stockings when heparin is contraindicated	C1
Ischemic stroke and lower extremity paralysis	LDUH or LMWH	A1
	Intermittent pneumatic compression with elastic stockings	B1
Medical patients with risk factors for VTE (including congestive heart failure and chest infections)	LDUH or LMWH	A1
Patients with long-term indwelling central vein catheters	Warfarin (1 mg/day), or LMWH qd, to prevent axillary–subclavian venous thrombosis	A1
Patients receiving a spinal puncture or epidural catheter placement	LMWH should be used with caution	C1

LDUH, low-dose unfractionated heparin; LMWH, low–molecular-weight heparin.
*A1: Methods strong, results consistent—randomized clinical trials (RCTs), no heterogeneity, effect clear that benefits do (or do not) outweigh risks.
A2: Methods strong, results consistent—RCTs, no heterogeneity, effect equivocal—uncertain whether benefits outweigh risks.
B1: Methods strong, results inconsistent—RCTs, heterogeneity present, effect clear that benefits do (or do not) outweigh risks.
B2: Methods strong, results inconsistent—RCTs, heterogeneity present, effect equivocal—uncertain whether benefits outweigh risks.
C1: Methods weak—observational studies, effect clear that benefits do (or do not) outweigh risks.
C2: Methods weak—observational studies, effect equivocal—uncertain whether benefits outweigh risks.
From American College of Chest Physicians: Seventh ACCP Conference on Antithrombotic and Thrombolytic Therapy. Chest 126(3 Suppl):401S–428S, 2004.

some of the other diseases, the death rates from COPD have increased. The WHO estimates that COPD will be the fifth highest cause of morbidity and mortality by 2020.[44,45]

PATHOPHYSIOLOGY

In COPD, pathologic changes occur in the central airways, peripheral airways, lung parenchyma, and pulmonary vasculature.[42] As the disease progresses, pathophysiological changes usually occur in the following order: mucus hypersecretion, ciliary dysfunction, airflow limitation, pulmonary hyperinflation, gas exchange abnormalities, pulmonary hypertension, and cor pulmonale.[41] The peripheral airways become the major site of obstruction in patients with COPD. The structural changes in the airway wall are the most important cause of the increase in peripheral airway resistance. Inflammatory changes such as airway edema and mucus hypersecretion also contribute to narrowing of the peripheral airways.[11] Mucus hypersecretion is caused by the stimulation of the enlarged mucus-secreting glands and the increased number of goblet cells by inflammatory mediators such as leukotrienes, interleukins, and tumor necrosis factor.[11] Ciliated epithelial cells undergo squamous metaplasia, leading to impaired mucociliary clearance, which is

usually the first physiological abnormality to occur in COPD.[11] This abnormality may be evident for many years before any other abnormalities develop.[11]

Expiratory airflow limitation is an essential finding in COPD. As the disease process progresses, forced expiratory volume in 1 second (FEV_1) and forced vital capacity (FVC) decrease; this is related to the increased thickness of the airway wall, loss of alveolar attachments, and loss of lung elastic recoil. Frequently, the first sign of developing airflow limitation is a decrease in the FEV_1/FVC ratio.[42,44] According to the 2001 Global Initiative for Chronic Obstructive Lung Disease (GOLD), the presence of a postbronchodilator FEV_1 less than 80% of the predicted value, in combination with an FEV_1/FVC ratio less than 70%, confirms the presence of airflow limitation that is not fully reversible (Table 26-7). In severe COPD, air is trapped in the lungs during forced expiration, leading to an abnormally high functional residual capacity (FRC). As FRC increases, this leads to pulmonary hyperinflation.[45]

In advanced COPD, peripheral airway obstruction, parenchymal destruction, and pulmonary vascular irregularities reduce the lung's capacity for gas exchange, resulting in hypoxemia (low blood oxygen) and hypercapnia (high blood carbon dioxide).[42] A ventilation/perfusion ratio mismatch is the driving

Table 26-7 • Stages of Chronic Obstructive Pulmonary Disease (COPD) and Their Treatment

Stage	Characteristics	Recommended Treatment
ALL		• Avoidance of risk factor(s) • Influenza vaccination
0: At Risk	• Chronic symptoms (cough, sputum) • Exposure to risk factor(s) • Normal spirometry	
I: Mild COPD	• FEV_1/FVC <70% • FEV_1 ≥80% predicted • With or without symptoms	• Short-acting bronchodilator when needed
II: Moderate COPD	IIA: • FEV_1/FVC <70% • 50% ≤ FEV_1 <80% predicted • With or without symptoms	• Regular treatment with one or more bronchodilators • Rehabilitation • Inhaled glucocorticosteroids if significant symptoms and lung function response
	IIB: • FEV_1/FVC <70% • 30% ≤ FEV_1 <50% predicted • With or without symptoms	• Regular treatment with one or more bronchodilators • Rehabilitation • Inhaled glucocorticosteroids if significant symptoms and lung function response or if repeated exacerbations
III: Severe COPD	• FEV_1/FVC <70% • FEV_1 <30% predicted or presence of respiratory failure or right heart failure	• Regular treatment with one or more bronchodilators • Inhaled glucocorticosteroids if significant symptoms and lung function response or if repeated exacerbations • Treatment of complications • Rehabilitation • Long-term oxygen therapy if respiratory failure • Consider surgical treatments

FEV_1, forced expiratory volume in 1 second; FVC, forced vital capacity.
Patients must be taught how and when to use their treatment, and treatments being prescribed for other conditions should be reviewed.
β-Blocking agents (including eye drop formulations) should be avoided.
From Pauwels RA, et al: Global strategy for the diagnosis, management, and prevention of chronic obstructive pulmonary disease: National Heart, Lung, and Blood Institute and World Health Organization global initiative for chronic obstructive lung disease (GOLD). Am J Respir Crit Care Med 163:1256–1276, 2001.

force behind hypoxemia in patients with COPD, regardless of the stage of the disease. Chronic hypercapnia usually indicates inspiratory muscle dysfunction and alveolar hypoventilation.[11] As hypoxemia and hypercapnia progress late in COPD, pulmonary hypertension often develops, which causes hypertrophy of the right ventricle, better known as cor pulmonale.[45] Right-sided heart failure leads to further venous stasis and thrombosis that may potentially result in pulmonary embolism and further compromise the pulmonary circulation. Lastly, COPD is associated with systemic inflammation and skeletal muscle dysfunction that may result in limitation of exercise capacity and decline of health status.[11]

ASSESSMENT

History

A detailed medical history of a new patient with known or suspected COPD should include the following:

▶ Exposure to risk factors, such as smoking, and occupational or environmental exposures.

▶ Past medical history, including asthma, allergy, sinusitis or nasal polyps, respiratory infections in childhood, and other respiratory diseases.

▶ Family history of COPD or other chronic respiratory disease.

▶ Pattern of symptom development. COPD typically develops in adults, and most patients are aware of the occurrence of increased breathlessness, increased frequency of winter "colds," and some social restriction for a number of years before seeking medical attention.

▶ History of exacerbations or previous hospitalizations for respiratory disorder. Patients may be conscious of periodic worsening of symptoms even if these episodes have not been identified as acute exacerbations of COPD. Indications for hospital assessment or admission for acute exacerbation of COPD are listed in Box 26-8.

▶ Comorbidities such as heart disease and rheumatic disease, which may also contribute to restriction of activity.

▶ Appropriateness of current medical treatments, such as β-blockers, commonly prescribed for heart disease. β-Blockers are usually contraindicated in COPD.

▶ Impact of disease on patient's life, including limitation of activity, missed work and economic consequences, effect on family routines, or feelings of depression or anxiety.

▶ Social and family support.

▶ Possibilities for reducing risk factors, especially smoking cessation.[44]

Physical Findings

Two patterns of disease are evident in advanced COPD (Table 26-8). These patterns may become increasingly

---

Box 26-8 • Indications for Hospital Assessment or Admission for Acute Exacerbation of Chronic Obstructive Pulmonary Disease

Marked increase in intensity of symptoms, such as sudden development of resting dyspnea
Severe background COPD
Onset of new physical signs (e.g., cyanosis, peripheral edema)
Failure of exacerbation to respond to initial medical management
Significant comorbidities
Newly occurring arrhythmias
Diagnostic uncertainty
Older age
Insufficient home support

Local resources need to be considered.
From Pauwels, RA, et al: Global strategy for the diagnosis, management, and prevention of chronic obstructive pulmonary disease: National Heart, Lung, and Blood Institute and World Health Organization global initiative for chronic obstructive lung disease (GOLD). Am J Respir Crit Care Med 163:1256–1276, 2001.

---

apparent as the disease progresses.[11] A physical examination is rarely diagnostic in COPD, although it remains an important aspect of patient care.[42] The physical examination should include the following:

Inspection

▶ Central cyanosis or bluish discoloration of the mucosal membranes. This feature may be present but is difficult to detect in artificial light and in many racial groups.

▶ Common chest wall abnormalities, which reflect the pulmonary hyperinflation seen in COPD, including relatively horizontal ribs, barrel-shaped chest, and protruding abdomen

▶ Flattening of the hemidiaphragms, which may be associated with paradoxical in-drawing of the lower

---

Table 26-8 • Patterns of Disease in Advanced Chronic Obstructive Pulmonary Disease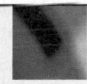

Feature	Type A	Type B
Commonly used name	Pink puffer	Blue bloater
Disease association	Predominant emphysema	Predominant bronchitis
Major symptom	Dyspnea	Cough and sputum
Appearance	Thin, wasted, not cyanotic	Obese, cyanotic
PO_2	↓	↓↓
PCO_2	Normal or ↓	Normal or ↑
Elastic recoil of lung	↓	Normal
Diffusing capacity	↓	Normal
Hematocrit	Normal	Often ↑
Cor pulmonale	Infrequent	Common

From Weinberger SE: Principles of Pulmonary Medicine, 4th ed. Philadelphia, Elsevier Saunders, 2004.

rib cage on inspiration, reduced cardiac dullness, and widening xiphisternal angle

▶ Resting respiratory rate, which is often increased to more than 20 breaths/minute; breathing may be shallow

▶ Pursed-lip breathing, which may serve to slow expiratory flow and permit more efficient lung emptying

▶ Resting muscle activation, which may be indicative of respiratory distress. While lying supine, patients with COPD often use the scalene and sterno-cleidomastoid muscles.

▶ Ankle or lower leg edema, which may be an indication of right heart failure

Palpation and Percussion

▶ Palpation and percussion, which are often unhelpful in COPD

▶ Heart apex beat, which may be difficult to detect due to pulmonary hyperinflation

▶ Pulmonary hyperinflation, which also leads to downward displacement of the liver and an increase in the ability to palpate this organ without its actually being enlarged

Auscultation

▶ Reduced breath sounds. Patients with COPD often have reduced breath sounds.

▶ Wheezing. Occurrence during quiet breathing is a useful indicator of airflow limitation. However, wheezing heard only after forced expiration is of no diagnostic significance.

▶ Inspiratory crackles, which occur in some COPD patients but are of little assistance diagnostically

▶ Heart sounds, which are best heard over the xiphoid area

Symptoms of COPD include cough, sputum production, and shortness of breath on exertion. Indications for ICU admission for patients with acute exacerbation of COPD are listed in Box 26-9.[43]

Box 26-9 • Indications for ICU Admission for Patients with Acute Exacerbation of Chronic Obstructive Pulmonary Disease

Severe dyspnea that responds inadequately to initial emergency therapy
Confusion, lethargy, coma
Persistent of worsening hypoxemia (PaO_2 < 6.7 kPa, 50 mm Hg), or severe/worsening hypercapnia ($PaCO_2$ > 9.3 kPa, 70 mm Hg), or severe/worsening respiratory acidosis (pH < 7.30) despite supplemental oxygen and NIPPV

Local resources need to be considered.
From Pauwels, RA, et al: Global strategy for the diagnosis, management, and prevention of chronic obstructive pulmonary disease: National Heart, Lung, and Blood Institute and World Health Organization global initiative for chronic obstructive lung disease (GOLD). Am J Respir Crit Care Med 163:1256–1276, 2001.

Diagnostic Studies

Laboratory and diagnostic tests in COPD are summarized in Table 26-9.

Spirometry Expiratory airflow limitation is the hallmark diagnostic sign of COPD. Because spirometry is the most reproducible and objective measure of airflow limitation, it remains the gold standard for diagnosing COPD and monitoring its progression.[46] Spirometry is performed in patients with chronic cough and sputum production even without dyspnea. Spirometry measures the maximal volume of air forcibly exhaled from the point of maximal inspiration (FVC) and the volume of air exhaled during the first second of this exercise (FEV_1). The ratio of these two measurements (FEV_1/FVC ratio) is then calculated.[42] Spirometry measurements are evaluated by comparison of the results with appropriate reference values based on age, height, sex, and race.

Figure 26-6 demonstrates a normal spirogram and a spirogram characteristic of a patient with COPD with mild to moderate airflow limitation. Patients with COPD have decreased FEV_1 and FVC, and the degree of spirometric abnormality generally reflects the severity of the disease[45,46] (see Table 26-8). By itself, the FEV_1/FVC ratio is the most sensitive measure of airflow limitation, and an FEV_1/FVC ratio less than 70% is considered an early sign of airflow limitation in patients whose FEV_1 remains normal (≥80% of the predicted value).

Arterial Blood Gases ABG measurements should be performed in all patients in moderate and severe stages of the disease (FEV_1 < 40% predicted) or when clinical signs of respiratory failure or right-sided heart failure are present (i.e., central cyanosis, ankle swelling, increase in the jugular venous pressure).[42] Respiratory failure is indicated by a partial pressure of arterial oxygen (PaO_2) of 60 mm Hg with or without a partial pressure of arterial carbon dioxide ($PaCO_2$) of 45 mm Hg while breathing air at sea level.[46] Several precautions must be taken to ensure accurate results. First, it should be noted if the patient is currently receiving an oxygen source and the amount of oxygen delivered to the patient during the blood gas sample time. Second, if the fraction of inspired oxygen (FiO_2) has been changed, a period of 20 to 30 minutes should elapse before gas tensions are rechecked.[45]

MANAGEMENT

Several different treatment modalities, ranging from exercise training, nutrition counseling, and education, to drug therapy, oxygen use, and surgery, may be effective in the treatment of COPD. See Table 26-7 for therapeutic guidelines for the various stages of COPD. Box 26-10 provides a collaborative care guide for the patient with COPD.

Nonpharmacological Therapy

The main goals of pulmonary rehabilitation are to decrease symptoms, improve quality of life, and increase

Table 26-9 • Laboratory and Diagnostic Tests for Patients With Chronic Obstructive Pulmonary Disease (COPD)

Test	Rationale
Spirometry	Measures FVC and FEV_1
Bronchodilator reversibility	Performed once during diagnosis stage and useful for the following reasons: • To rule out an asthma diagnosis (If FEV_1 returns to predicted normal range after administration of bronchodilator, airflow limitation is likely due to asthma.) • To establish a patient's best attainable lung function at that point in time • To gauge a patient's prognosis (Postbronchodilator FEV_1 is a more reliable prognostic indicator than prebronchodilator FEV_1.) • To assess potential response to treatment (An increase in FEV_1 >200 mL and 12% above prebronchodilator FEV_1 is considered significant.)
Glucocorticosteroid reversibility	Measures significant FEV_1 response (i.e., FEV_1 increase of 200 mL and 15% above baseline)
Chest radiography	Bullous disease may be evident Radiological changes seen include: • Flattened diaphragm on lateral chest film • Increased volume of retrosternal air space (signs of hyperinflation) • Hyperlucency of the lungs • Rapid tapering of vascular markings
Computed tomography and ventilation–perfusion scanning	Assessment of surgical patient to visualize airway and parenchymal disease May assist with differential diagnosis
Arterial blood gases	Performed if FEV_1 <40% predicted or if signs of respiratory failure or right heart failure are present
α_1-Antitrypsin deficiency screening	Indicated for patients in whom COPD develops at <45 years of age or who have a strong family predisposition (α_1-antitrypsin serum level below 15%–20% of normal value is highly suggestive of homozygous α_1-antitrypsin deficiency)
Hematocrit	Smokers can develop polycythemia in the presence of arterial hypoxemia. (Hematocrit >55% is defined as polycythemia.)

FEV_1, forced expiratory volume in 1 second; FVC, forced vital capacity.
From Pauwels RA, et al: Global strategies for the diagnosis, management, and prevention of chronic obstructive pulmonary disease: National Heart, Lung, and Blood Institute and World Health Organization global initiative for chronic obstructive lung disease (GOLD). Respir Care 46:798–825, 2001, with permission.

physical and emotional participation in day-to-day activities.[44] The 2001 GOLD guidelines for the diagnosis, management, and prevention of COPD recommend a comprehensive pulmonary rehabilitation program.

Exercise Training An exercise training program for COPD may consist of bicycle ergometry, treadmill exercise, or timed walking. The exercise may range in frequency from daily to weekly, in duration from 10 to 45 minutes per session and in intensity from 50% peak oxygen consumption to maximum tolerated.[46] Many physicians advise patients to exercise on their own (e.g., walking 20 minutes daily) if they are unable to participate in a structured exercise program. The benefits of pulmonary rehabilitation in COPD patients include the following:[45]

▶ Improved exercise capacity
▶ Reduced (perceived) intensity of breathlessness
▶ Improved health-related quality of life
▶ Reduced number of hospitalizations and days in the hospital
▶ Reduced COPD-associated anxiety and depression
▶ Improved arm function due to strength and endurance training of the upper limbs
▶ Benefits that extend well beyond the immediate period of training
▶ Improved survival

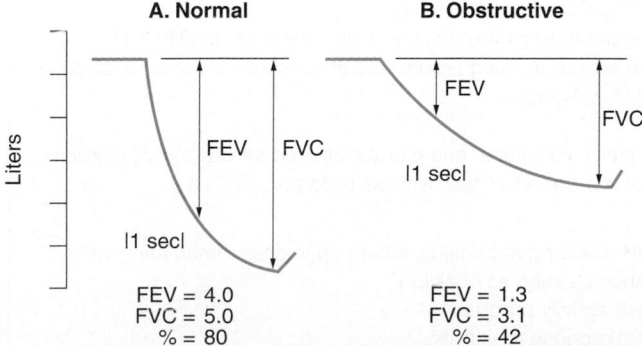

Figure 26-6 • Normal obstructive, obstructive, and restrictive patterns of a forced expiration. FVC, forced vital capacity; FEV, forced expiratory volume. (From West JB: Pulmonary Pathophysiology: The Essentials, 6th ed. Philadelphia, Lippincott Williams & Wilkins, 2003.)

Nutritional Counseling Malnutrition is a common problem in patients with COPD and is present in

Box 26-10 • COLLABORATIVE CARE GUIDE for the Patient With Chronic Obstructive Pulmonary Disease

OUTCOMES	INTERVENTIONS
Oxygenation/Ventilation Patient has arterial blood gases within normal limits and pulse oximeter value >90%.	• Assess respiratory rate, effort, and breath sounds q2–4h. • Obtain arterial blood gases per order or signs of respiratory distress. • Monitor arterial saturation by pulse oximeter. • Provide supplemental oxygen by nasal cannula or face mask using lowest possible FiO_2 and flow rate. • Provide humidification with oxygen. • Provide intubation and mechanical ventilation as necessary (refer to Collaborative Care Guide for the Patient on Mechanical Ventilation, Chapter 25).
Patient maintains normal rate and depth of respiration.	• Monitor respiratory rate, pattern, and effort (e.g., use of accessory muscles). • Assess respirations during sleep; note sleep apnea or Cheyne-Stokes patterns.
Patient has clear chest x-ray.	• Obtain chest x-ray qd.
Patient has clear breath sounds.	• Monitor breath sounds for crackles, wheezes, or rhonchi q2–4h. • Administer diuretics per order. • Administer bronchodilators and mucolytics as indicated.
There is no evidence of atelectasis or pneumonia.	• Encourage nonintubated patients to use incentive spirometer, cough, and deep breathe q2–4h and PRN. • Assess quantity, color, and consistency of secretions. • Turn side to side q2h. • Mobilize out of bed to chair.
Circulation/Perfusion Blood pressure, heart rate, and hemodynamic parameters are within normal limits.	• Monitor vital signs q1–2h. • Monitor pulmonary artery pressures and right atrial pressure q1h and cardiac output, systemic venous resistance, and peripheral venous resistance q6–12h if pulmonary artery catheter is in place. • Assess for signs of right ventricular dysfunction (e.g., increased central venous pressure, neck vein distension, peripheral edema).
Patient is free of dysrhythmias.	• Maintain patent IV access. • Monitor for atrial dysrhythmias due to right atrial dilation and ventricular dysrhythmias due to hypoxemia and hypoxia.
Serum lactate will be within normal limits.	• Monitor lactate qd until it is within normal limits. • Administer red blood cells, positive inotropic agents, colloid infusion as ordered to increase oxygen delivery.
Fluids/Electrolytes Renal function is maintained as evidenced by urine output >30 mL/h, normal laboratory values.	• Monitor intake and output q1–2h. • Monitor blood urea nitrogen, creatinine, electrolytes, Mg, PO_4. • Replace potassium, magnesium, and phosphorus per order or protocol. • Take daily weights.
Patient is euvolemic.	• Administer fluid volume and diuretics based on vital signs, physical assessment, secretion viscosity, as ordered.
Mobility/Safety There is no evidence of loss of muscle tone or strength.	• Promote standing at bedside, sitting up in chair, ambulating with assistance as soon as possible. • Establish activity program. • Monitor response to activity.

(continued)

Box 26-10 • COLLABORATIVE CARE GUIDE for the Patient With Chronic Obstructive Pulmonary Disease (Continued)

OUTCOMES	INTERVENTIONS
Patient maintains joint flexibility.	• Consult with physical therapist. • Use passive and active range of motion q4h while awake.
There is no evidence of infection. White blood cells (WBCs) are within normal limits.	• Monitor systemic inflammatory response syndrome criteria: increased WBC count, increased temperature, tachypnea, tachycardia. • Use strict aseptic technique during procedures and monitor others. • Maintain invasive catheter tube sterility. • Per hospital protocol, change invasive catheters, culture blood, line tips, or fluids.
There is no evidence of DVT.	• Initiate DVT prophylaxis within 24 hours of admission. • Monitor for leg pain, redness, or swelling.
Skin Integrity There is no evidence of skin breakdown.	• Turn side to side q2h. • Remove self-protective devices from wrists, and monitor skin per hospital policy. • Assess risk for skin breakdown using objective tool (e.g., Braden scale). Consider pressure relief/reduction mattress.
Nutrition Caloric and nutrient intake meet metabolic requirements per calculation (e.g., Basal Energy Expenditure).	• Provide parenteral, enteral, or oral nutrition within 48 hours. • Consult dietitian or nutritional support service. • Avoid high-carbohydrate load if patient retains CO_2. • Monitor albumin, prealbumin, transferrin, cholesterol, triglycerides, glucose.
Comfort/Pain Control Patient is comfortable and evaluates pain as <4 on the pain scale.	• Assess pain/comfort q4h. • Administer analgesics and sedatives cautiously, closely monitoring respiratory rate, depth, and pattern. • Differentiate between agitation caused by discomfort or caused by hypoxia before medication administration. • Elevate head of bed to improve breathing comfort.
Psychosocial Patient demonstrates decreased anxiety.	• Assess vital signs during treatments, discussions, and so forth. • Cautiously administer sedatives. • Consult social services, clergy as appropriate. • Provide for adequate rest and sleep. • Provide support during periods of dyspnea.
Teaching/Discharge Planning Patient/significant others understand procedures and tests needed for treatment.	• Prepare patient/significant others for procedures such as chest physical therapy, bronchoscopy, pulmonary artery catheter insertion, or laboratory studies.
Significant others understand the severity of the illness, ask appropriate questions, anticipate potential complications.	• Explain the causes and effects of COPD and the potential for complications, such as pneumonia or cardiac dysfunction. • Encourage significant others to ask questions related to the ventilator, pathophysiology, monitoring, treatments, and so forth.
In preparation for discharge to home, patient understands activity levels, dietary restrictions, medication regimen, metered inhaler.	• Make appropriate referrals and consults early during hospitalization. • Initiate family education regarding proper use of metered inhaler, signs and symptoms of respiratory failure, and appropriate actions.

in the remaining pulmonary parenchyma, which decreases hyperinflation and improves diaphragmatic function.[47] The mean improvement in FEV_1 and FVC is in the range of 5% to 96%, with a decrease in total lung capacity from 1% to 23% after LVRS.[42] Usually, a subsequent mean of 7% to 103% improvement of airflow and exercise capacity occurs.[42] The etiology of this physiological improvement is unclear, but it may be related to increases in elastic recoil properties of the remaining lung.[47] The baseline patient characteristics and lobe involvement have been found to affect long-term mortality rates.[42]

Bilateral LVRS patients show greater improvement than unilateral LVRS. Because of inherent subjectivity in selection of patients and the selection of lung areas to be resected, candidate selection remains controversial.[42] Reports have shown that patients with bilateral upper lobe–dominant disease do somewhat better after LVRS than patients with non–upper lobe disease. Factors associated with good outcome following LVRS include:

▶ Age younger than 75 years
▶ FEV_1 at least >2% predicted
▶ $PaCO_2$ less than 45 mm Hg
▶ PaO_2 more than 60 mm Hg
▶ Predominant upper lobe emphysema on CT scan
▶ Residual volume greater than 150%
▶ Demonstration of severe dyspnea despite optimal medical therapy
▶ Excellent cardiac performance, with left ventricular ejection fraction greater than 45%
▶ No other comorbidities
▶ Demonstrable preoperative motivation to have the surgery with agreement to participate in 4 to 6 weeks of pulmonary rehabilitation[31,45,47]

Contraindications to LVRS include active smoking, marked obesity or cachexia, and inability to undertake pulmonary rehabilitation successfully.[42,47] Depending on the volume of tissue to be removed, LVRS is performed through a median sternotomy or thoracotomy, or using video-assisted thoracoscopic surgery. The target for LVRS, as predetermined by CT and ventilation–perfusion scanning, is the hyperinflated portion of the diseased lung with well-demarcated areas of trapped air or dead space.[47] Usually, tissue from the upper lobe or the least functional lung is removed first.[47] The National Emphysema Treatment Trial is designed to compare LVRS with the best available medical therapy, and the results indicate the following:[42]

▶ Physiological benefits from LVRS may begin to dissipate as early as 1 year after surgery.
▶ Accelerated declines of FEV_1 averaging 100 mL per year may occur and are particularly marked in those patients with the greatest postoperative gains in airflow.
▶ Improvements in dyspnea and exercise tolerance may be sustained for as long as 3 years but may then begin to decline.

Morbidity in LVRS is related to persistent postoperative air leaks, difficulty with postoperative weaning from the ventilator, and postoperative nosocomial pulmonary infections.[47] In addition, a recent study confirmed that older patients and those undergoing cardiac surgery in combination with LVRS are at increased risk for postoperative respiratory failure.[42] Until the results of this and similar controlled studies are known and the risk/benefit ratio is satisfactorily resolved, LVRS will remain an experimental palliative surgical procedure.[45]

Other Surgical Procedures Patients with severe COPD (stage III) may also consider bullectomy and lung transplantation.[42,47] Bullectomy is a surgical procedure for bullous emphysema, which is effective in alleviating dyspnea and improving overall lung function.[42,47] Patients with very advanced COPD are candidates for lung transplantation. Lung transplantation has been shown to improve quality of life and functional capacity.[42,47]

PREVENTION

Influenza vaccines reduce serious illness and death by about 50% in patients with COPD.[44] Vaccines containing killed or live, inactivated viruses are recommended because they are more efficacious in elderly patients with COPD. Vaccines are administered either once (autumn) or twice (autumn and winter) each year. Some experts do recommend pneumococcal vaccine administration once each year for patients with COPD and chronic bronchitis and every other year for asplenic patients or patients at risk for decreased antibody levels (e.g., in transplantation or in chronic renal failure).[42,45]

CHRONIC BRONCHITIS

Chronic bronchitis is defined as the presence of a productive cough for at least 3 months per year over 2 consecutive years, in the absence of other medical causes.[42] During an exacerbation or episode of acute infection, a patient with chronic bronchitis may present with airflow obstruction similar to that of a patient with asthma. However, the difference lies in the fact that, with chronic bronchitis, the primary cause of airflow obstruction is not due to airway hyperreactivity, and there are residual clinical symptoms even when the patient returns to baseline function.[11]

Pathophysiology

Airway obstruction is caused by inflammation of the major and small airways in chronic bronchitis (Fig. 26-7). Subsequently, edema and hyperplasia of submucosal glands and excess mucus excretion into the bronchial tree occur, resulting in a chronic productive cough.[11] Cigarette smoking is the major causal factor in the development of chronic bronchitis.[11] Other causes of chronic airway irritation include air pollutants and occupational exposure to nitrogen,

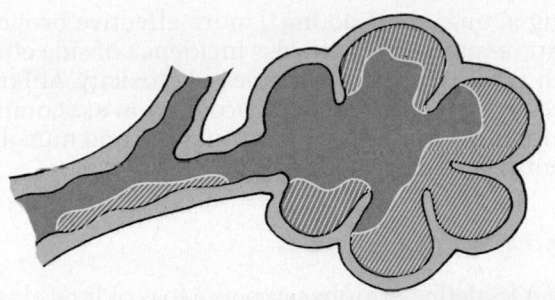

Figure 26-7 • Bronchitis: inflammation and thickening produce narrowing of airways. Lined areas indicate secretions.

sulfur oxides, or endotoxin.[11] Nonspecific pathological changes in the lung, including infiltration of airway mucosa and submucosa with neutrophils and mononuclear cells, smooth muscle hypertrophy, and enlargement of the submucosal secretory glands, may also contribute to the development of chronic bronchitis.[9,11]

Once the airway lumen is occluded by secretions and narrowed by a thickened wall, patients develop airflow obstruction and COPD. Acute bacterial or viral infection in patients with existing chronic bronchitis can increase airway and parenchymal damage, impair mucociliary clearance, obstruct bronchioles, and contribute to chronic epithelial damage and bacterial colonization that further exacerbate symptoms and airway obstruction.[11] Common bacteria isolated from the secretions of patients with chronic bronchitis include *H. influenzae, Haemophilus parainfluenzae, S. pneumoniae,* and *Moraxella catarrhalis.*[11] Even in nonsmoking patients, acute viral infection may lead to the chronic airway inflammation and chronic sputum production characteristic of chronic bronchitis.[9] In contrast to emphysema, chronic bronchitis may have a reversible component if the source of chronic infection or irritation is treated. These patients normally do not have hyperinflation or abnormal diffusion test results.

Assessment

Excessive bronchial secretions and subsequent airway obstruction and vasoconstriction lead to ventilation–perfusion mismatching. Patients do not compensate by increasing their ventilation and, therefore, develop hypoxemia, cyanosis, and eventually cor pulmonale with peripheral edema.[42] Common physical signs and symptoms may include[11]:

▶ Copious sputum expectoration arising from sleep
▶ Sputum that is usually mucoid, often with brownish discoloration
▶ Increased sputum volume or changes in color from whitish to yellow or green (signs of an endobronchial infection)
▶ Hemoptysis occurring during acute exacerbations
▶ Decreased breath sounds, wheezes, or rhonchi
▶ Resting respiratory rate greater than 16 breaths/ minute

▶ Prolonged forced expiratory time (greater than the normal 4 seconds)

Often patients wait to seek medical treatment until they are in severe distress. Manifestations of severe exacerbations of chronic bronchitis are listed in Box 26-12.

Management

Patients with chronic bronchitis without airflow obstruction require no specific pharmacological treatment. An essential prophylactic measure involves rigorous bronchial hygiene to promote the clearance of secretions, which provide an ideal medium for bacterial growth in peripheral airways. It is important to prevent the development of an acute inflammatory process to avoid exacerbations. Other preventive measures include smoking cessation, immunization against influenza virus and *S. pneumoniae,* and prompt antibiotic treatment for acute exacerbations caused by bacterial tracheobronchitis.[11]

Chronic bronchitis with airflow obstruction does require pharmacological treatment. The major goals of drug therapy in chronic bronchitis with COPD are to reverse or slow the progression of airway obstruction and mucosal edema, decrease secretion volume, alleviate bronchial smooth muscle spasm, and decrease airway inflammation.[42] Primary agents include inhaled bronchodilators (β_2-adrenergic agents, anticholinergic agents, corticosteroids) and theophylline.[42] An effective treatment regimen may include using a combination of drugs. By combining drugs with different mechanisms of action and duration of effect

---

Box 26-12 • Manifestations of Severe Exacerbations of Chronic Bronchitis

Constitutional Signs
Temperature frequently subnormal
White blood cell count varies—may be slightly ↑, normal, or ↓

Central Nervous System Disturbances
Headache
Confusion
Hallucinations
Depression
Drowsiness
Somnolence
Coma
Papilledema

Cardiovascular Signs
Diaphoresis
Tachycardia
Blood pressure varies: normal, ↑, or ↓
Vasoconstriction initially followed by vasodilation

Neuromuscular Signs
Fine tremors
Asterixis
Flaccidity
Convulsions

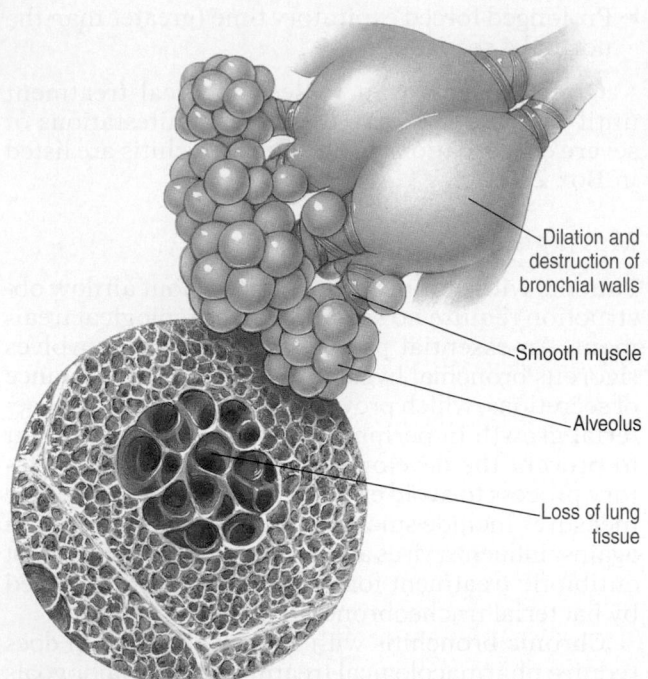

Figure 26-8 • Lung changes in emphysema. Airspaces are enlarged in the emphysematous lung. (From Anatomical Chart Company: Atlas of Pathophysiology. Springhouse, PA: Springhouse, 2002, p 89.)

(long acting, short acting), more effective broncho-dilation may occur with less incidence of side effects such as tachycardia, restlessness, or toxicity. Although excessive cough and mucus production are common symptoms, regular use of antitussives and mucolytic agents is not indicated.[45]

EMPHYSEMA

The ATS defines emphysema as a loss of lung elasticity and abnormal, permanent enlargement of the airspaces distal to the terminal bronchioles with destruction of the alveolar walls and capillary beds without obvious fibrosis (Fig. 26-8).[42] Most patients with COPD have a combination of chronic bronchitis (mucus hypersecretion) and emphysema rather than "pure" bronchitis or emphysema.[41]

There are three types of emphysema: centrilobular emphysema, panacinar emphysema, and paraseptal emphysema (Fig. 26-9). Centrilobular emphysema is most common in smokers and often localizes in the upper lung zones. Panacinar emphysema is most frequently found in patients with α_1-protease inhibitor deficiency and is often localized in the lower lobes. Paraseptal emphysema is also most common in smokers and is localized peripherally, with possible formation of large bullae.[11]

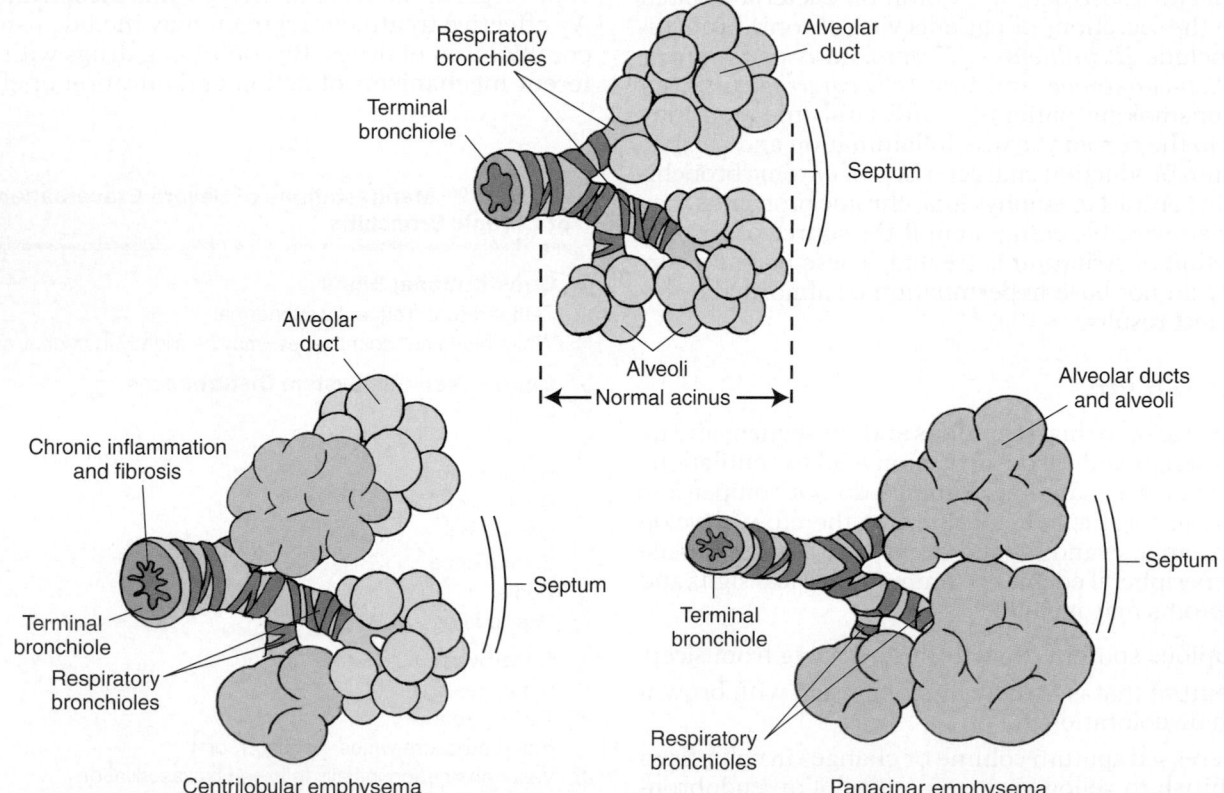

Figure 26-9 • Types of emphysema. The acinus, the gas-exchanging structure of the lung distal to the terminal bronchiole, consists of the terminal bronchiole, respiratory bronchioles, alveolar ducts, alveolar sacs, and alveoli. In centrilobular (proximal acinar) emphysema, the respiratory bronchioles are mainly involved. In paraseptal (distal acinar) emphysema, the alveolar ducts are mainly affected. In panacinar (panlobular) emphysema, the acinus is uniformly damaged. (From Porth CM: Pathophysiology: Concepts of Altered States, 5th ed. Philadelphia, Lippincott-Raven, 1998, p 541. Courtesy of Dmitri Kavetnikov, artist.)

Pathophysiology

The enlargement of the airspaces in emphysema results in hyperinflation of the lungs and increased total lung capacity.[11] Emphysema is believed to result from the breakdown of elastin by enzymes, called proteases, which digest proteins. These proteases, especially elastase, are released from neutrophils, alveolar macrophages, and other inflammatory cells.[42] Two recognized conditions that cause emphysema are smoking and inherited α_1-antitrypsin deficiency. Smoking contributes to increased inflammatory cells in the alveoli, enhanced release of elastase from neutrophils, increased elastase activity in macrophages, and activation of mast cells that release mast cell elastases.[42] α_1-Antitrypsin usually protects the lung from the destructive inflammatory cells; however, the elastic tissue destructive process continues unabated in patients with an inherited α_1-antitrypsin deficiency.[42]

Almost all people who develop emphysema before 40 years of age have an α_1-antitrypsin deficiency. Evidence has shown that cigarette smoking decreases levels of α_1-antitrypsin and increases the number of macrophages in the alveolar walls. This vicious cycle promotes increased numbers of neutrophils. A hereditary deficiency in α_1-antitrypsin is responsible for about 1% of all cases of COPD.[42] Smoking and repeated respiratory tract infections further decrease α_1-antitrypsin levels, adding to the risk for emphysema in people with low α_1-antitrypsin levels.[42]

A common phenomenon in emphysema is spontaneous pneumothorax related to rupture of thinned parenchyma.[11] Patients may experience acute severe dyspnea and respiratory failure depending on the amount of pulmonary reserve (see the discussion of barotrauma in the section on Pneumothorax).

Assessment

Patients with pulmonary emphysema are referred to as "pink puffers" because their oxygen levels are usually satisfactory, and their skin remains pink.[11] There is a proportionate loss of ventilation and perfusion area in the lung. In severe COPD, air is trapped in the lungs during forced expiration, leading to abnormally high residual volume.[11] These patients develop a puffing style of breathing. Common physical examination findings in emphysema include increased basal respiratory rate; barrel-shaped chest; decreased breath sounds; soft, dry crackles in lung bases; right-sided S_3 gallop auscultated substernally; supraclavicular wasting and nasal flaring; and evidence of pulmonary hypertension, including an increased second heart sound, jugular venous distention, and right ventricular heave.[11] Cyanosis may be present in advanced cases of emphysema.

Management

The medical and surgical therapies described for COPD also pertain to patients with emphysema (see section on COPD, Management). Preventive measures include an annual influenza vaccine and a pneumococcal vaccine every 5 to 10 years. Medical therapy involves smoking cessation, pulmonary rehabilitation, and oxygen therapy in all patients who are hypoxemic ($PaO_2 < 55$ mm Hg or $SaO_2 < 88\%$).[42] Pharmacological therapy includes bronchodilators (β_2-agonists, anticholinergics, and theophylline), possibly mucolytics, and α_1-protease inhibitor replacement in young patients with homozygous disease. In addition, adequate nutrition is important. Patients with advanced emphysema ($FEV_1 < 750$ mL) may experience significant weight loss related to a variety of factors, including increased energy expended during breathing secondary to the use of accessory muscles; performing activities of daily living; and reduced caloric intake.[47] Patients who are overweight and hypercapnic should strive to lose weight to diminish the respiratory workload.[42]

Three surgical treatments available for patients with emphysema are LVRS, bullectomy, and lung transplantation. Currently, LVRS is the only recognized therapy that can increase respiratory function (FEV_1, FVC, ABGs, and exercise capacity) in moderate to severe emphysema.[42] For end-stage emphysema, the only definitive surgical treatment is single-lung transplantation. Because of the short supply of donor lungs, lung transplantation is usually reserved for younger patients (<60 years of age) with α_1-protease inhibitor deficiency.[42] Studies have indicated improvements in exercise performance and ABGs after lung transplantation.

• Thoracic Surgery

Thoracic surgery is indicated as part of the management plan for a variety of diseases involving the lungs and the associated structures. Specific surgeries involving removal of part of the lung include wedge resection, lobectomy, pneumonectomy, lung volume reduction, and lung transplantation. Wedge resection or segmentectomy is performed for the removal of benign or malignant lesions; segmentectomy is the preferred method when patients are a poor risk with limited pulmonary reserve.[47] Bleeding may be extensive following the surgery, and two chest drains are usually in place to drain air or blood. Lobectomy may be performed as a treatment for malignant or benign tumors, infections such as bronchiectasis, tuberculosis, or fungal infection.[47] Pneumonectomy is performed to remove one lung, usually because of primary carcinoma or significant infection. LVRS involves the excision of 20% to 30% of the volume of each lung to improve elastic recoil and diaphragmatic function in the patient with moderate to severe emphysema.[47] Lung transplantation may involve one lung or both lungs, or it may be inclusive as part of a heart–lung transplantation. To be considered a viable candidate for lung transplantation, a patient should have advanced lung disease that is unresponsive to other medical therapy and minimal comorbidities. Significant areas of concern involved in this surgery include primary graft failure, lifelong immunosuppressive therapy, and organ rejection.[47]

• Acute Asthma

CONCEPTS in action **ANIMATI◯N**

Asthma is defined as a chronic inflammatory disease of the airways characterized by airway hyperresponsiveness to a variety of stimuli, reversible airflow limitation, and chronic inflammation of the airway submucosa.[48] It is manifested as variable airway obstruction that resolves either spontaneously or after bronchodilator administration.[48] Based on symptoms and lung function, the National Asthma Education and Prevention Program (NAEPP) has classified asthma as mild intermittent, mild persistent, moderate persistent, or severe persistent (Table 26-11).

According to the CDC, asthma is a worldwide epidemic. Asthma affects 7% of the population, or 17 million adults and children in the United States.[49] Asthma accounts for 2 million emergency department visits, 500,000 hospital admissions, and 5,000 deaths annually in the United States, and most cases are believed to be preventable.[48]

PATHOPHYSIOLOGY

Inflammation may be present throughout the bronchial tree, from large airways to the alveoli. This inflammation is characterized by mast cell activation, inflammatory cell infiltration, edema, denudation and disruption of the bronchial epithelium, collagen deposition beneath the basement membrane, goblet cell hyperplasia (which contributes to mucus hypersecretion), and smooth muscle thickening (Fig. 26-10).

This inflammatory process contributes to airway hyperresponsiveness, airflow limitation, pathological damage, and associated respiratory symptoms (i.e., wheezing, shortness of breath, and chest tightness).[11]

Factors contributing to the airflow limitation in asthma include acute bronchoconstriction, airway mucosal edema, chronic formation of mucus plugs, and airway remodeling.[11]

The T lymphocytes (helper T [Th] cells) are believed to play a crucial role in the inflammation process.[49] Th1 cells serve a protective role against airway inflammation, and Th2 cells promote development of chronic airway inflammation. Recent studies suggest that possible early childhood viral and bacterial infections may contribute to Th2 cell stimulation and result in asthma pathogenesis.[49]

The etiology and pathogenesis of asthma are not fully understood. Inhaled irritants such as cigarette smoke, inorganic dusts, and environmental pollutants are common precipitants. These irritants stimulate the irritant receptors in the walls of the larynx and large bronchi, which initiate a reflex arc that travels to the central nervous system and back through the vagus nerve. This in turn induces bronchoconstriction.[11] The most common precipitant of an acute asthmatic exacerbation is an upper respiratory tract viral infection. The proposed mechanism of action is through epithelial damage and airway inflammation.[11] Other potential infectious causal factors include infection with C. pneumoniae, tracheobronchitis related to herpes simplex, and exposure to aspirin or other nonsteroidal anti-inflammatory cyclooxygenase-1 inhibitors, which can lead to life-threatening asthmatic reactions in selected patients.[49] The mechanism of

Table 26-11 • Classification of Asthma Severity

	Symptoms	Nighttime Symptoms	Lung Function
Mild intermittent	Symptoms ≤2 times a week Asymptomatic and normal PEF between exacerbations Exacerbations brief (few hours to few days); intensity may vary	≤2 times a month	FEV_1 or PEF ≥80% predicted PEF variability ≤20%.
Mild persistent	Symptoms >2 times a week but <1 time a day Exacerbations may affect activity	>2 times a month	FEV_1 or PEF >80% predicted PEF variability 20%–30%
Moderate persistent	Daily symptoms Daily use of inhaled short-acting β$_2$-agonist Exacerbations affect activity Exacerbations ≥2 times a week; may last days	>1 time a week	FEV_1 or PEF >60% to <80% predicted PEF variability >30%
Severe persistent	Continual symptoms Limited physical activity Frequent exacerbations	Frequent	FEV_1 or PEF ≤60% predicted PEF variability >30%

FEV_1, forced expiratory volume in 1 second; PEF, peak expiratory flow.
Adapted from National Asthma Education and Prevention Program, Expert Panel Report 2: Guidelines for the Diagnosis and Management of Asthma. National Institutes of Health publication no. 97-4051. Bethesda, MD, National Institutes of Health, 1997.

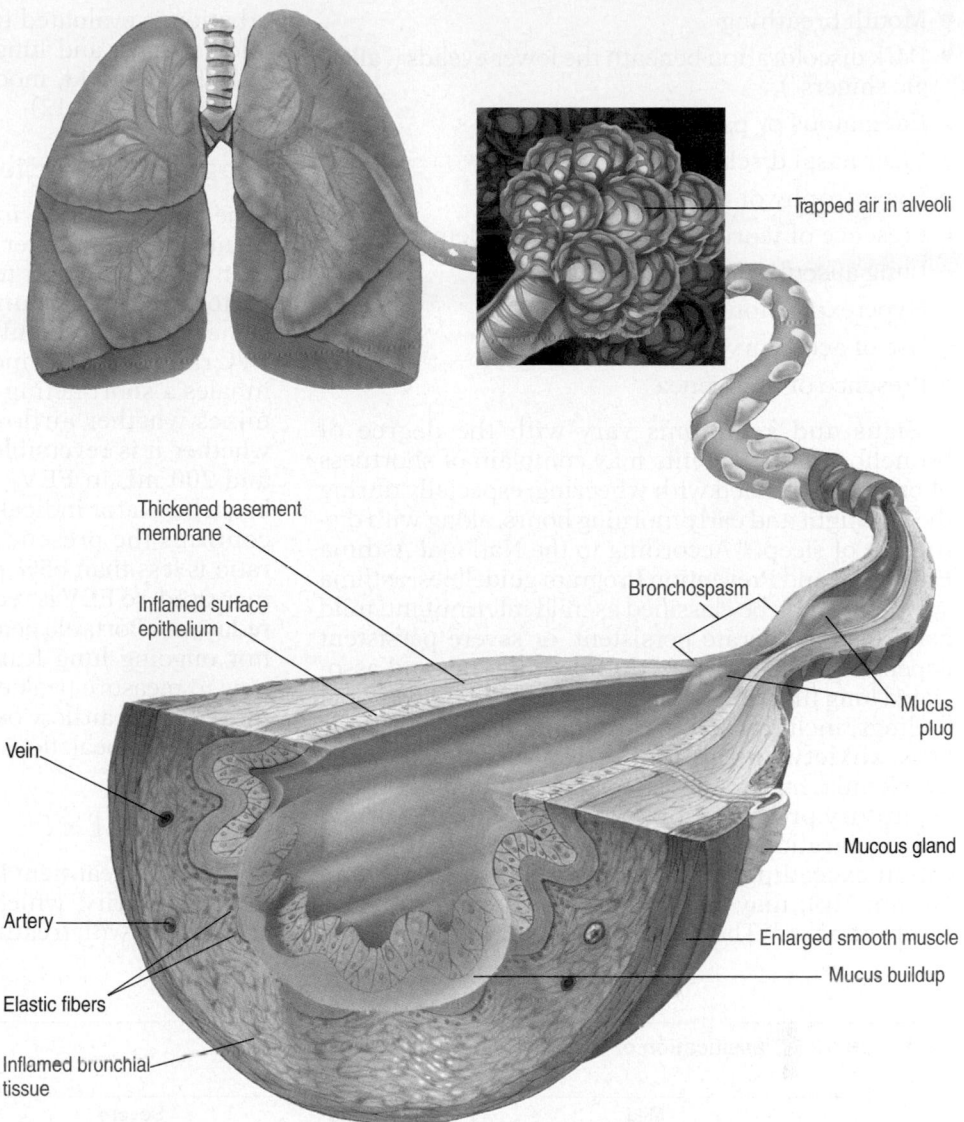

Trapped air in alveoli

Thickened basement membrane

Inflamed surface epithelium

Bronchospasm

Mucus plug

Vein

Mucous gland

Artery

Enlarged smooth muscle

Mucus buildup

Elastic fibers

Inflamed bronchial tissue

Figure 26-10 • Asthmatic bronchus. (From Anatomical Chart Company: Atlas of Pathophysiology. Springhouse, PA: Springhouse, 2002, p 83.)

action in exercise-induced asthma is less clear but thought to be related to hyperemia and stimulation of irritant receptors following the rewarming of cooled airways. Common triggers of asthma exacerbations are given in Box 26-13.

Box 26-13 • Common Triggers of Asthma

- Viral respiratory infections
- Environmental allergens (domestic dust mite, tobacco smoke, animals with fur, cockroach, outdoor and indoor pollens and mold, perfume, wood-burning stoves)
- Exercise, temperature, humidity
- Occupational and recreational allergens or irritants
- Medications (aspirin, nonsteroidal anti-inflammatory drugs, and β-blockers)
- Food (sulfites)
- Emotions

From National Heart, Lung, and Blood Institute, National Institutes of Health: Global Initiative for Asthma. Bethesda, MD, National Heart, Lung, and Blood Institute, 2003, p 249. Also available at: http://www.ICSI.org.

ASSESSMENT

History and Physical Findings

The medical history should address the following areas[50]

► Symptoms and symptom patterns
► Precipitating and aggravating factors
► Development of disease
► Current treatment
► Effect of symptoms on activities of daily living
► Impact of asthma on the patient and family
► Perceptions of the disease by the patient and family (parent, if appropriate)

The physical examination should focus on the following areas[50]:

► Vital signs
► Height, weight, and a comparison of normal values for age
► Inspection of skin for evidence of atopic dermatitis or eczema

► Mouth breathing
► Dark discoloration beneath the lower eyelids ("allergic shiners")
► Edematous or pale nasal mucosa
► Clear nasal discharge
► Hypertrophy of tonsils and adenoids
► Presence of tearing and periorbital edema
► Lung auscultation for wheezing
► Hyperexpansion of the thorax
► Use of accessory muscles
► Presence of tachypnea

Signs and symptoms vary with the degree of bronchospasm. Patients may complain of shortness of breath associated with wheezing, especially during the late night and early morning hours, along with disruption of sleep.[50] According to the National Asthma Education and Prevention Program guidelines, asthma symptoms may be classified as mild intermittent, mild persistent, moderate persistent, or severe persistent depending on frequency, duration, timing, and associated lung function level (see Table 26-11). Additional findings, including tachycardia, retractions, restlessness, anxiety, inspiratory or expiratory wheezing, hypoxemia, hypercapnia, cough, sputum production, expiratory prolongation, cyanosis, and an elevated pulsus paradoxus (systolic blood pressure in expiration exceeding that in inspiration by more than 10 mm Hg), may be observed in patients who have severe attacks.[48] The severity of an acute asthma exacerbation is evaluated using patient symptoms, physiologic signs, and lung function results and can be classified as mild, moderate, severe, and impending failure (Table 26-12).

Diagnostic Studies

Objective measures in the diagnosis and measurement of asthma severity consist of spirometry and pulmonary function testing. Allergy testing may be performed to ascertain precipitating allergens.[50] Spirometry measurements of the FVC, FEV_1, and FEV_1/FVC ratio are performed before and after the patient inhales a short-acting bronchodilator, which determines whether airflow obstruction is present and whether it is reversible. An increase of at least 12% and 200 mL in FEV_1 after inhaling a short-acting bronchodilator indicates significant reversibility and confirms the presence of asthma.[50] The FEV_1/FVC ratio is less than 65% predicted. Airway resistance is increased, so FEV is reduced out of proportion to FVC reduction. Portable peak flow meters are used to monitor ongoing lung function. Patients are instructed how to measure peak expiratory flow, an indicator of the degree of airflow obstruction in the large airways, by using the peak flow meter on a regular basis.[50]

MANAGEMENT

The level of treatment is based on the patient's level of asthma severity, which changes with time, age, and compliance with treatment.[50] Frequent reassessments

Table 26-12 • Classification of Severity of Asthma Exacerbations

	Mild	Moderate	Severe	Impending Respiratory Failure
Symptoms				
Breathlessness	With activity	With talking	At rest	At rest
Speech	Sentences	Phrases	Words	Mute
Signs				
Body position	Able to recline	Prefers sitting	Unable to recline	Unable to recline
Respiratory rate	Increased	Increased	Often >30/min	>30 breaths/min
Use of accessory respiratory muscles	Usually not	Commonly	Usually	Paradoxical thoracoabdominal movement
Breath sounds	Moderate wheezing at mid- to end-expiration	Loud wheezes throughout expiration	Loud inspiratory and expiratory wheezes	Little air movement without wheezes
Heart rate (beats/min)	<100	100–120	>120	Relative bradycardia
Pulsus paradoxus (mm Hg)	<10	10–25	Often >25	Often absent
Mental status	May be agitated	Usually agitated	Usually agitated	Confused or drowsy
Functional Assessment				
PEF (% predicted or personal best)	>80	50–80	<50 or response to therapy lasts <2 h	<50
SaO_2 (%, room air)	>95	91–95	<91	<91
PaO_2 (mm Hg, room air)	Normal	>60	<60	<60
$PaCO_2$ (mm Hg)	<42	<42	≥42	≥42

Adapted from National Asthma Education and Prevention Program, Expert Panel Report 2: Guidelines for the Diagnosis and Management of Asthma. National Institutes of Health publication no. 97-4051. Bethesda, MD, National Institutes of Health, 1997.

of the level of severity are necessary to provide adequate therapy. The overall goals of therapy are to prevent chronic and troublesome symptoms; prevent exacerbations of symptoms; maintain normal activity levels; maintain normal pulmonary function; optimize pharmacotherapy and minimize side effects; and satisfy the patient's and the family's expectations and goals for asthma care.[50] A stepwise pharmacological approach is recommended in treating patients with asthma. The main goal is to gain control quickly and to "step down" to the lowest medication level required to maintain asthma control.[49] A list of quick-relief asthma medications is presented in Table 26-13. A flow chart outlining the stepwise approach is shown in Figure 26-11.

Asthma education and self-management training are critical to helping the asthmatic patient control airway inflammation. The 1997 NAEPP guidelines describe the critical components of asthmatic patient education. An important aspect of asthmatic patient education programs is training in the necessary management skills. These skills include proper medication administration, understanding the need for maintenance medications, knowing the early warning signs of an asthma attack, making decisions on the basis of self-monitoring of symptoms and peak flow results, and maintaining control of environmental asthma triggers (i.e., dust mites, fur-bearing animals).[50] Recent studies have confirmed that appropriate therapy, coupled with structured asthma education, significantly improves short-term compliance with therapy and decreases asthma morbidity.[50] Long-term asthma management requires regular follow-up care with a clinician experienced in long-term asthma to maintain optimal asthma control and avoid preventable complications.[50]

STATUS ASTHMATICUS

Status asthmaticus is a medical emergency. It is an acute refractory asthma attack that has not responded to rigorous therapy with β_2-adrenergic compounds or intravenous theophylline. Patients present with a dramatic picture of acute anxiety, markedly labored breathing, tachycardia, and diaphoresis. Deterioration of pulmonary function results in alveolar hypoventilation with subsequent hypoxemia, hypercapnia, and acidemia. A rising $PaCO_2$ in a patient with an acute asthmatic attack is often the first objective indication of status asthmaticus.[48]

The treatment of status asthmaticus involves the institution of multiple therapeutic modalities. All patients with status asthmaticus demonstrate hypoxemia and require oxygen therapy. Patients are also usually dehydrated and require fluid resuscitation. Pharmacological agents include methylxanthines,

Table 26-13 • Drug Therapy in Asthma

	Examples	Possible Routes of Administration	Mechanism of Action
Bronchodilators			
Sympathomimetics	Epinephrine Metaproterenol Terbutaline Albuterol Salmeterol Formoterol	Inhaled, oral, parenteral (depending on particular drug)	↑ cAMP via stimulation of adenylate cyclase
Xanthines	Theophylline Aminophylline	Oral Oral, parenteral	?↑ cAMP via inhibition of phosphodiesterase; ? anti-inflammatory
Anticholinergics	Ipratropium	Inhaled	Blockade of cholinergic (bronchoconstrictor) effect on airways
Anti-inflammatory drugs			
Corticosteroids	Prednisone Methylprednisolone Beclomethasone Triamcinolone Flunisolide Fluticasone Budesonide	Systemic (oral or parenteral, depending on particular drug) Inhaled	Decreased inflammatory response in airways; ? additional mechanisms
Cromolyn		Inhaled	Inhibition of mediator release from mast cells: ? additional mechanisms
Nedocromil		Inhaled	? Similar to cromolyn
Drugs directed at specific targets			
5-Lipoxygenase inhibitors	Zileuton	Oral	Decreased production of leukotrienes
Leukotriene antagonists	Zafirlukast	Oral	Leukotriene D_4 receptor antagonism
Anti-IgE antibody (approval pending)	Omalizumab	Parenteral	Binds circulating IgE

cAMP, cyclic adenosine monophosphate.
From Weinberger SE: Principles of Pulmonary Medicine, 4th ed. Philadelphia, Elsevier Saunders, 2004.

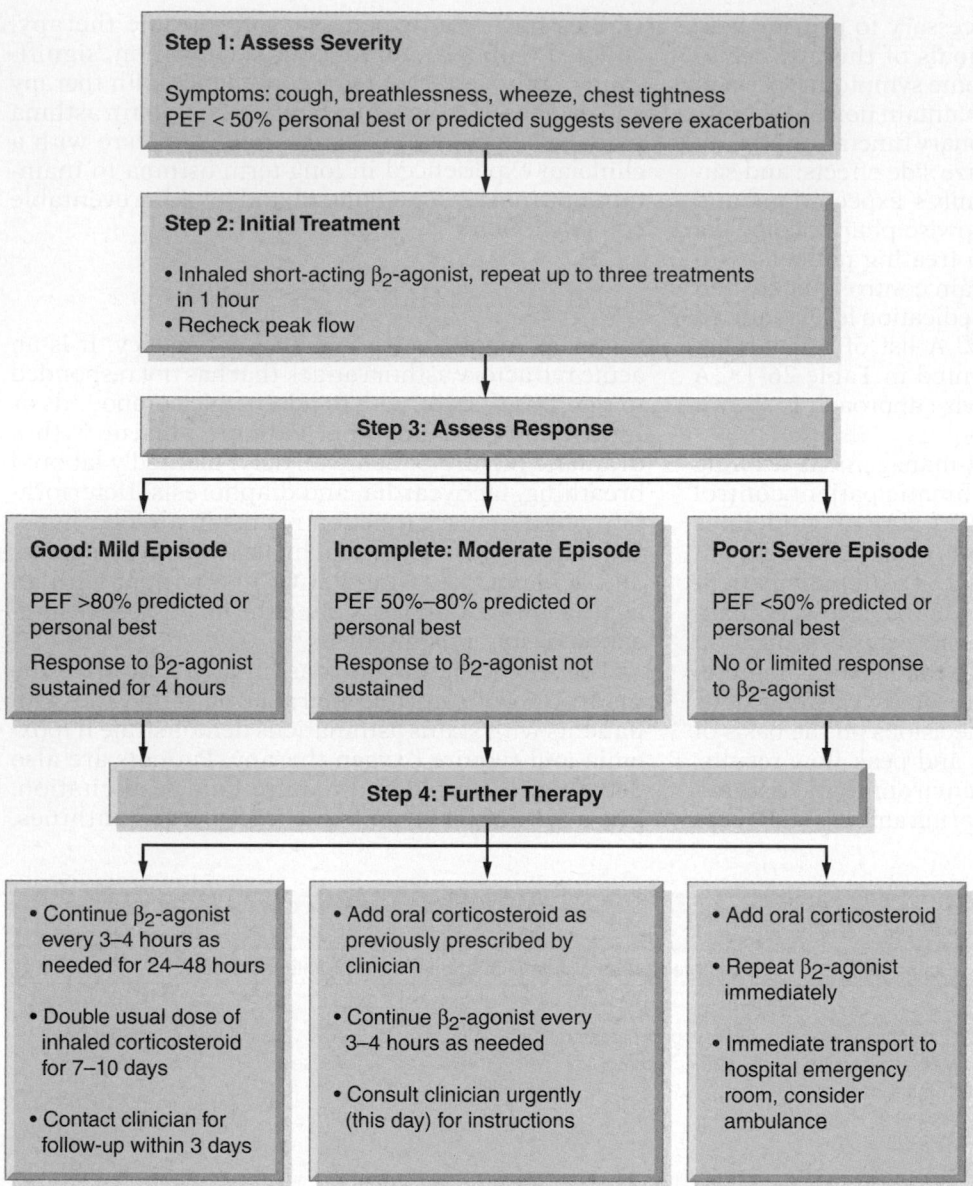

Step 1: Assess Severity

Symptoms: cough, breathlessness, wheeze, chest tightness
PEF < 50% personal best or predicted suggests severe exacerbation

Step 2: Initial Treatment

• Inhaled short-acting β2-agonist, repeat up to three treatments
  in 1 hour
• Recheck peak flow

Step 3: Assess Response

Good: Mild Episode

PEF >80% predicted or
personal best

Response to β2-agonist
sustained for 4 hours

Incomplete: Moderate Episode

PEF 50%–80% predicted or
personal best

Response to β2-agonist not
sustained

Poor: Severe Episode

PEF <50% predicted or
personal best

No or limited response
to β2-agonist

Step 4: Further Therapy

• Continue β2-agonist
  every 3–4 hours as
  needed for 24–48 hours

• Double usual dose of
  inhaled corticosteroid
  for 7–10 days

• Contact clinician for
  follow-up within 3 days

• Add oral corticosteroid as
  previously prescribed by
  clinician

• Continue β2-agonist every
  3–4 hours as needed

• Consult clinician urgently
  (this day) for instructions

• Add oral corticosteroid

• Repeat β2-agonist
  immediately

• Immediate transport to
  hospital emergency
  room, consider
  ambulance

Figure 26-11 • Peak expiratory flow rate–based plan for management of asthma exacerbations. PEF, peak expiratory flow. (Modified from National Asthma Education Program: Expert Panel Report II. Guidelines for the diagnosis and management of asthma. Washington, DC, U.S. Department of Health and Human Services, 1997. NIH Publ. No. 97-4051. From Givelber RJ, O'Connor GT: Asthma. In Goldstein RH, Connell JJ, Karlinsky JB, et al [eds]: A Practical Approach to Pulmonary Medicine. Philadelphia, Lippincott-Raven, 1997, pp 68–84.)

sympathomimetic amines, and corticosteroids.[48] If pulmonary function cannot be improved and respiratory failure ensues, patients may require intubation and assisted ventilation (see Chapter 25). A spontaneous pneumothorax may occur during severe acute asthmatic attacks, as well as during positive-pressure mechanical ventilation (see section on Pneumothorax, Management).

• Acute Respiratory Failure

Acute respiratory failure is a sudden and life-threatening deterioration in pulmonary gas exchange, resulting in carbon dioxide retention and inadequate oxygenation.[51] Acute respiratory failure remains a major cause of morbidity and mortality in the intensive care setting, despite the technological advances in diagnosis, monitoring, and management that have been made in the past four decades.[52] A study of more than 1,400 patients found that 44% of patients diag-

nosed with acute respiratory failure who required admission to the ICU died in the hospital; in the past 20 years, this statistic has not changed significantly.[53,54] Acute respiratory failure may be responsible for as much as 10% to 15% of admissions to medical ICUs and for as many as 50% to 75% of those patients who require ICU hospital stays longer than 7 days.[52]

PATHOPHYSIOLOGY

Acute respiratory failure is defined as a PaO_2 of 50 mm Hg or less, a $PaCO_2$ greater than 50 mm Hg, and an arterial pH less than 7.35.[54,55] This definition is valid only in cases in which baseline ABGs are assumed to be normal.[56] In patients with established chronic hypoxemia or hypercapnia, acute respiratory failure is indicated by the acute deterioration of blood gases relative to their previous levels rather than their absolute values.[56] In patients with chronic lung disease, ABGs associated with classic acute respiratory failure may not be present because these patients have

Box 26-14 • Causes of Acute Respiratory Failure

Intrinsic Lung/Airway Diseases

Large Airway Obstruction
- Congenital deformities
- Acute laryngitis, epiglottitis
- Foreign bodies
- Intrinsic tumors
- Extrinsic pressure
- Traumatic injury
- Enlarged tonsils and adenoids
- Obstructive sleep apnea

Bronchial Diseases
- Chronic bronchitis
- Asthma
- Acute bronchiolitis

Parenchymal Diseases
- Pulmonary emphysema
- Pulmonary fibrosis and other chronic diffuse infiltrative diseases
- Severe pneumonia
- Acute lung injury from various causes (acute respiratory distress syndrome)

Cardiovascular Disease
- Cardiac pulmonary edema
- Massive or recurrent pulmonary embolism
- Pulmonary vasculitis

Extrapulmonary Disorders

Diseases of the Pleura and the Chest Wall
- Pneumothorax
- Pleural effusion
- Fibrothorax
- Thoracic wall deformity
- Traumatic injury to the chest wall: flail chest
- Obesity

Disorders of the Respiratory Muscles and the Neuromuscular Junction
- Myasthenia gravis and myasthenia-like disorders
- Muscular dystrophies
- Polymyositis
- Botulism
- Muscle-paralyzing drugs
- Severe hypokalemia and hypophosphatemia

Disorders of the Peripheral Nerves and Spinal Cord
- Poliomyelitis
- Guillain-Barré syndrome
- Spinal cord trauma (quadriplegia)
- Amyotrophic lateral sclerosis
- Tetanus
- Multiple sclerosis

Disorders of the Central Nervous System
- Sedative and narcotic drug overdose
- Head trauma
- Cerebral hypoxia
- Cerebrovascular accident
- Central nervous system infection
- Epileptic seizure: status epilepticus
- Metabolic and endocrine disorders
- Bulbar poliomyelitis
- Primary alveolar hypoventilation
- Sleep apnea syndrome

---

adapted to blood gas levels outside this range, consistent with their disease process.[27]

Acute respiratory failure may be caused by a variety of pulmonary and nonpulmonary diseases (Box 26-14). Respiratory failure may result from malfunction of the respiratory center, abnormal respiratory neuromuscular system, chest wall diseases, airway obstruction, or parenchymal lung disorders.[56] Many factors may precipitate or exacerbate acute respiratory failure (Box 26-15).

A vicious positive feedback mechanism characterizes the deleterious effects of continued hypoxemia and hypercapnia. Hypoxemia affects every organ and tissue, and hypercapnia impairs cellular functions.[56] Hypoxemia in respiratory failure may be caused by any of these conditions, separately or in various combinations; Table 26-14 lists the causes of hypoxemia.[54,56] Hypercapnia results from alveolar hypoventilation and ventilation–perfusion mismatching when there is no compensation by increased ventilation of well-perfused regions.[57] In acute hypercapnia, arterial blood pH is decreased, indicating acute respiratory acidosis. Patients with advanced COPD and chronic hypercapnia may exhibit an acute rise of $PaCO_2$ to a high level, a decrease of blood pH, and a significant increase in serum bicarbonate during the onset of acute respiratory failure.[57]

Hypoxemia and hypercapnia may have precipitous effects, which include the following[53]:

▶ Increased pulmonary vascular resistance
▶ Cor pulmonale

Box 26-15 • RED FLAG: Precipitating Factors Leading to Acute Respiratory Failure

- Changes of tracheobronchial secretions
- Infection: viral or bacterial
- Disturbance of tracheobronchial clearance
- Drugs: sedatives, narcotics, anesthesia, oxygen
- Inhalation or aspiration of irritants, vomitus, foreign body
- Cardiovascular disorders: heart failure, pulmonary embolism, shock
- Mechanical factors: pneumothorax, pleural effusion, abdominal distension
- Trauma, including surgery
- Neuromuscular abnormalities
- Allergic disorders: bronchospasm
- Increased oxygen demand: fever, infection
- Inspiratory muscle fatigue

From Farzan S: Respiratory failure. In Farzan S (ed): A Concise Handbook of Respiratory Diseases, 4th ed. Stamford, CT, Appleton & Lange, 1997, pp 371–386, with permission.

Table 26-14 • Causes of Hypoxemia in Acute Respiratory Failure

Mechanism	Effect
Inhalation of a hypoxic gas mixture or severe reduction of barometric pressure—occurs in toxic fume inhalation, in fires that consume oxygen in combustion, and at high altitudes because of reduced barometric pressure.	Decrease in the partial pressure of inhaled oxygen
Alveolar hypoventilation—commonly seen in ventilatory failure hypoxemic patients.	Increased alveolar PCO_2 Decreased alveolar PO_2 Arterial hypoxemia
Impairment of diffusion—prevents complete equilibration of alveolar gas with pulmonary capillary blood.	Usually small effect and easily compensated by a small increase in inspired oxygen (FiO_2); present in emphysema and diffuse lung injury
Ventilation–perfusion mismatching—uneven ventilation of various lung regions and units whose perfusion frequently fails to match the changes in ventilation.	Most common cause of oxygen desaturation High ventilation–perfusion units contribute to dead space Supplemental oxygen reverses hypoxemia
Right-to-left shunt—the result of continuous perfusion of nonventilated lung regions.	Indicates closure of air passages, especially the distal airways and alveoli. Classic sign—changes in FiO_2 have little effect on PaO_2 when the true shunt fraction exceeds 30%.
Reduced oxygen in mixed venous blood—may occur from abnormal pulmonary gas exchange, too high or too low cardiac output, or high metabolic rate (fever).	Increased oxygen extraction from arterial blood results in decreased PaO_2.

From Farzan S: Respiratory failure. In Farzan S (ed): A Concise Handbook of Respiratory Diseases, 4th ed. Stamford, CT, Appleton & Lange, 1997, pp 371–386, with permission.

▶ Right-sided heart failure
▶ Impaired left ventricular function
▶ Reduced cardiac output
▶ Cardiogenic pulmonary edema
▶ Diaphragmatic fatigue from increased workload of respiratory muscles

CLASSIFICATION

Acute respiratory failure is classified as acute hypoxemic respiratory failure (type I), acute hypercapnic respiratory failure (type II), or combined hypoxemic and hypercapnic respiratory failure (type I and type II).[57] Type I failure is a direct defect in oxygenation. Type II failure is a direct defect in ventilation. However, in many instances, the distinction is not clear; many patients exhibit signs and symptoms of a combined type I and type II respiratory failure.[57]

Acute Hypoxemic Respiratory Failure (Type I)

Type I acute respiratory failure is the result of abnormal oxygen transport secondary to pulmonary parenchymal disease, with increased alveolar ventilation resulting in a low $PaCO_2$.[56] The principal problem in type I acute respiratory failure is the inability to achieve adequate oxygenation, as evidenced by a PaO_2 of 50 mm Hg or less and a $PaCO_2$ of 40 mm Hg or less. The most common cause of hypoxemia is ventilation–perfusion mismatch.[57] However, right-to-left shunt and alveolar hypoventilation are the most clinically significant causes of type I failure.[52] The major causes of type I respiratory failure are listed in Table 26-15.

Acute Hypercapnic Respiratory Failure (Type II)

Type II acute respiratory failure, or ventilatory failure, is the result of inadequate alveolar ventilation[56] and is characterized by marked elevation of carbon dioxide with relative preservation of oxygenation.[52] Hypoxemia results from reduced alveolar pressure of oxygen (PaO_2) and is proportionate to hypercapnia.[56] Three factors contribute to type II failure: decreased ventilatory drive, respiratory muscle fatigue or failure, and increased work of breathing.[57] Various factors may influence a decreased ventilatory drive, such as medications or drugs (narcotics, benzodiazepines, barbiturates, alcohol), brainstem lesions, hypothyroidism, morbid obesity, and sleep apnea.[52,57] Respiratory muscle fatigue or failure is caused by neuromuscular dysfunction due to the following diseases: amyotrophic lateral sclerosis, Guillain-Barré syndrome, myasthenia gravis, muscular dystrophy, and polymyositis.[57] Increased work of breathing most commonly occurs in COPD (increased dead space) or asthma (elevated airway resistance), and it may also result from thoracic abnormalities (restriction on lungs) such as pneumothorax, rib fractures, or pleural effusions.[57]

Table 26-15 • Evaluation and Management of Common Causes of Acute Respiratory Failure

Etiology	Key Clinical Findings	Key Diagnostic Tests	Specific Therapy
Normal Alveolar–Arterial Gradient: Acute Hypercapnic Respiratory Failure			
Reduced FiO_2	Geographic location (altitude)	Ambient FiO_2	Change location
CNS depression	History of drug overdose, head trauma, or anoxic encephalopathy Comatose	Response to naloxone Toxicology screen Electrolytes (glucose, calcium, sodium) CT head, EEG	Naloxone, charcoal Correct electrolytes Neurological evaluation
Neuromuscular dysfunction	Neck trauma or neuro-muscular disease Received paralytic medications (2)	Cervical spine films Review medications CXR: elevated hemidiaphragms Upright/supine PFTs (reduced VC, NIF, PEF in supine position)	Stabilize cervical spine Discontinue paralytics Noninvasive ventilation
Increased Alveolar–Arterial Gradient: Acute Hypoxemic Respiratory Failure			
Alveoli/interstitium			
Cardiogenic pulmonary edema	Rales, diaphoresis	CXR: pulmonary edema; PA line: elevated PCWP; ECG; echocardiogram	Diuresis Reduce LVEDP
Adult respiratory distress syndrome	Rales PaO_2 <55 mm Hg with FiO_2 >60%	CXR: pulmonary edema; PA line; normal or low PCWP	Treat underlying cause
Pneumonia	Fever Lung sounds: rales and/or egophony	CXR: diffuse or lobar infiltrate CBC: leukocytosis Sputum Gram stain, blood culture	Antibiotics: empirical therapy tailored to likely pathogens
Pleural effusion	Lung sounds: egophony	CXR: pleural effusion; contralateral mediastinal shift Thoracentesis	Drainage Treat underlying cause Consider pleurodesis
Atelectasis	Diminished breath sounds Postoperative	CXR: volume loss, ipsilateral mediastinal shift	Reduce sedation Pulmonary toilet Consider bronchoscopy
Pneumothorax	Diminished breath sounds Chest wall asymmetry Tracheal deviation	CXR: pneumothorax; contralateral mediastinal shift	Decompression: chest tube
Alveolar hemorrhage	Hemoptysis	CXR: localized or diffuse infiltrate; air bronchograms Sputum: hemosiderin-laden macrophages ANCA, antiGBM, sputum AFB, cytology, Gram stain, urinalysis	Protect uninvolved lung Identify bleeding site and etiology If localized, consider resection, embolization
Pulmonary infarct	Tachypnea, tachycardia Pleuritic CP, hemoptysis Risk for DVT; hypercoagulable	CXR: wedge-shaped peripheral infiltrate Abnormal $\dot{V}/\dot{Q}$ scan or PA gram	Heparin anticoagulation Consider thrombolysis and IVC filter
Airways			
Asthma	Wheezing (may be absent if severe airflow obstruction)	Reduced PEF	β-Agonists Corticosteroid Theophylline Consider HELIOX
Chronic obstructive pulmonary disease	Wheezing: infrequent		Titrate oxygen carefully to SaO_2 > 89% β-Agonists Ipratropium bromide Corticosteroid Theophylline Antibiotics: if clinical evidence of infection

(continued)

Table 26-15 • Evaluation and Management of Common Causes of Acute Respiratory Failure (Continued)

Etiology	Key Clinical Findings	Key Diagnostic Tests	Specific Therapy
Acute airway obstruction			
Foreign body	Witnessed aspiration	CXR	Localize and remove foreign body using bronchoscope
Epiglottitis	Odynophagia, drooling	Lateral neck films	Racemic epinephrine, antibiotics, HELIOX
Vascular disease			
Pulmonary embolus	See pulmonary infarct	CXR: nonspecific Abnormal $\dot{V}/\dot{Q}$ scan or PA gram	Heparin anticoagulation Consider thrombolysis and IVC filter
Lymphatic disease			
Lymphangitic carcinomatosis	History of neoplasm	CXR: reticular infiltrates Cytology from PA line	Treat underlying disease

AFB, acid fast bacilli; ANCA, antineutrophilic cytoplasmic antibody; antiGBM, anti–glomerular basement membrane antibody; CBC, complete blood cell count; CNS, central nervous system; CP, chest pain; CT, computed tomography; CXR, chest x-ray; DVT, deep venous thrombosis; ECG, electrocardiogram; EEG, electroencephalogram; HELIOX, helium and oxygen mixture; IVC, inferior vena cava; LVEDP, left ventricular end-diastolic pressure; NIF, negative inspiratory force; PA, pulmonary artery; PA gram, pulmonary arteriogram; PCWP, pulmonary capillary wedge pressure; PEF, peak expiratory flow; PEFR, peak expiratory flow rate; PFTs, pulmonary function tests; VC, vital capacity; $\dot{V}/\dot{Q}$, ventilation–perfusion.

From Powell CA, Joyce-Brady MF: Acute and chronic respiratory failure. In Goldstein RH, et al (eds): A Practical Approach to Pulmonary Medicine. Philadelphia, Lippincott-Raven, 1997, pp 300–302 with permission.

Extensive burns may produce increased carbon dioxide production from the hypermetabolic state, requiring increased minute ventilation.[57] The major causes of type II respiratory failure are listed in Table 26-15, including hypercapnic respiratory failure.[55]

Combined Hypoxemic and Hypercapnic Respiratory Failure (Type I and Type II)

The combined type of acute respiratory failure develops as a consequence of a combined inadequate alveolar ventilation and abnormal gas transport.[56] This condition is commonly seen in asthmatic exacerbations, emphysema complicated by a lower respiratory tract infection, severe pneumonia, pulmonary edema, and pulmonary embolism.[52] Any potential cause of type I failure may lead to combined failure, especially if increased work of breathing and hypercapnia are involved. Situations producing respiratory muscle fatigue or neuromuscular weakness may be compounded by pneumothorax or pleural effusion, which would result in hypoxemia superimposed on the primary hypercapnia.[52]

ASSESSMENT

History

A complete medical and social history should be obtained from the patient or a family member to determine the patient's baseline respiratory status on admission. The ATS has provided specific standards for assessment of adult patients with actual or potential pulmonary dysfunction, which address process and outcome variables.[58] Box 26-16 presents the nursing assessment guide based on these standards. These comprehensive standards are used in assess-

ment, goal setting, intervention, and evaluation to ensure that patients receive high-quality health care.[59] Self-management categories address the patient's capacity for self-care (physical, cognitive, psychosocial, socioeconomic, and environmental). The health care professional will find this a valuable tool in the continual assessment process of patients with pulmonary disorders.

Physical Findings

Presentation of acute respiratory failure may vary, depending on the underlying disease, precipitating factors, and degree of hypoxemia, hypercapnia, or acidosis.[56] It is essential to determine whether intubation and positive-pressure ventilation are required as emergency measures; this is the most critical assessment objective.[52] Typically, intubation and ventilation are necessary in patients with depressed mental status or coma, severe respiratory distress, extremely low or agonal respiratory rate, obvious respiratory muscle fatigue, peripheral cyanosis, or impending cardiopulmonary arrest.[52] Patients with altered mental status are at risk for aspiration of gastric contents. In any of these situations, immediate intervention is vital and should not be postponed pending the results of ABG studies or chest radiography.[52]

The classic symptom of hypoxemia is dyspnea,[33] although this may be completely absent in ventilatory failure resulting from depression of the respiratory center.[56] Other presenting symptoms of hypoxemia include cyanosis, restlessness, confusion, anxiety, delirium, tachypnea, tachycardia, hypertension, cardiac dysrhythmias, and tremor.[33] Peripheral cyanosis of the skin, lips, or nail beds suggests the presence of profound arterial hypoxemia, usually with a PaO_2 less than 50 mm Hg.[52]

Box 26-16 • Nursing Assessment Guide for Adult Patients With Pulmonary Dysfunction

History and Symptoms Profile

Pulmonary Symptoms*
- Dyspnea
- Cough
- Sputum
- Hemoptysis
- Wheeze
- Chest pain (e.g., pleuritic)

Extrapulmonary Symptoms*
- Night sweats
- Headaches on awakening
- Weight changes
- Fluid retention
- Nasal stuffiness, discharge
- Fatigue
- Orthopnea, paroxysmal nocturnal apnea
- Snoring, sleep disturbances, daytime drowsiness
- Sinus problems

Pulmonary Risk Factors
- Smoking history: type (cigarettes, cigar, pipe); amount per day; duration (years)
- Childhood respiratory diseases/symptoms
- Family history of respiratory disease
- Alcohol and chemical substance abuse (e.g., heroin, marijuana, cocaine)
- Environmental exposures: location (e.g., home, work, region); type (e.g., asbestos, silica, gases, aerosols); duration
- Obesity or nutritional depletion
- Compromised immune system function (e.g., IgG deficiency, HIV infection, α_1-antitrypsin deficiency)

Previous History
- Pulmonary problems
- Treatments
- Number of hospitalizations
- Medical diagnosis(es)
- Immunizations

Self-Management Capacity

Physical Ability (0 to 4 scale, 0 = independent, 4 = dependent)
- Lower extremity (e.g., walking, stair climbing)
- Upper extremity (e.g., shampooing, meal preparation)
- Activities of daily living: toileting, hygiene, feeding, dressing
- Activity pattern during a typical day

- Patient statement re: management of problems
- Sensory-perceptual factors (e.g., vision, hearing)

Cognitive Ability
- Mental age
- Memory
- Knowledge about diagnosis and treatment of pulmonary problems, or risk factors of pulmonary disease
- Judgment

Psychosocial-Cultural Factors
- Self-concept: self-esteem, body image, role(s), changes
- Value system (e.g., spiritual and health beliefs)
- Coping mechanisms
  Displaced anger
  Anxiety
  Hostility
  Dependency
  Withdrawal
  Isolation
  Avoidance
  Denial
  Noncompliance
  Acceptance

Socioeconomic Factors
- Social support system
  Family
  Significant others
  Friends
  Community resources
  Government resources
- Financial situation/health insurance
- Employment/disability

Environmental Factors
- Home
- Community
- Worksite
- Health care setting (e.g., hospital, nursing home)

---

*Consider onset, duration, character, and precipitating, aggravating, and relieving factors of symptoms.
IgG, immunoglobulin G.
Modified from American Thoracic Society Medical Section of the American Lung Association: Standards of nursing care for adult patients with pulmonary dysfunction, Am Rev Respir Dis 144:231, 1991. From Krider SJ: Interview and respiratory history. In Wilkins RL, et al (eds): Clinical Assessment in Respiratory Care, 4th ed. St. Louis, Mosby, 2000, p 26, with permission.

The cardinal symptoms of hypercapnia are dyspnea and headache.[33] Other clinical manifestations of hypercapnia include peripheral and conjunctival hyperemia, hypertension, tachycardia, tachypnea, impaired consciousness, papilledema, and asterixis.[33] Uncorrected carbon dioxide narcosis leads to diminished alertness, disorientation, increased intracranial pressure, and ultimately unconsciousness.[52] Other physical findings on examination may include use of accessory muscles of respiration, intercostal or supraclavicular retraction, and paradoxical abdomi-

nal movement if diaphragmatic weakness or fatigue is present.[56] See Box 26-16 for more details concerning assessment findings; see Table 26-15 for more details concerning clinical findings.

Diagnostic Studies

Because the signs and symptoms of acute respiratory failure are nonspecific and insensitive, the physician must request an ABG analysis to determine the exact level of PaO_2, $PaCO_2$, and blood pH in cases of suspected acute respiratory failure. Only determination of the blood gases and pH can confirm the diagnosis.[56] Other diagnostic tests necessary to determine the etiology of acute hypoxemic respiratory failure include chest radiography, sputum examination, pulmonary function testing, angiography, ventilation–perfusion scanning, CT, toxicology screen, complete blood count, serum electrolytes, cytology, urinalysis, bronchogram, bronchoscopy, electrocardiography, echocardiography, and thoracentesis.[55] See Table 26-15 for more details about the use of these diagnostic tests in acute respiratory failure.

MANAGEMENT

Treatment of acute respiratory failure warrants immediate intervention to correct or compensate for the gas exchange abnormality and identify the cause.[55] Therapy is directed toward correcting the cause and alleviating the hypoxia and hypercapnia.[27] Although the recommended therapeutic intervention may vary according to the specific disease's pathological process, general management principles are applicable to every patient with acute respiratory failure. See Table 26-16 for specific therapies for the management of common causes of acute respiratory failure.[55]

If alveolar ventilation is inadequate to maintain PaO_2 or $PaCO_2$ levels related to respiratory or neurological failure, endotracheal intubation and mechanical ventilation may be lifesaving.[17] The initial assessment and the decision to initiate mechanical ventilation should be performed rapidly to minimize the life-threatening complications associated with extended hypoxemia (e.g., cardiac dysrhythmias, anoxic encephalopathy).[55] Controlled oxygen therapy and mechanical ventilation are used to increase PaO_2 by increasing FiO_2 and to normalize pH by increasing minute ventilation.[55] See Chapter 25 for further information on airway management and care of the patient on a ventilator.

Patients with acute hypoxemic respiratory failure should receive immediate treatment with rapidly increased FiO_2 and continuous pulse oximetry monitoring until an SaO_2 of 90% or higher is obtained.[52] Correction of hypoxemia in the acute setting takes precedence over possible attenuation of hypoxic respiratory drive.[52] Therefore, once hypoxemia is reversed, oxygen is titrated to the minimum level necessary for correction of hypoxemia and prevention of significant carbon dioxide retention.[52]

Patients with acute hypercapnic respiratory failure should be immediately assessed for either an impaired central respiratory drive associated with sedative or narcotic therapy or for underlying bronchospasm secondary to an asthma exacerbation or COPD.[52] Reversal agents (opiate antagonists, e.g., naloxone) are used in the case of impaired central respiratory drive, and inhaled bronchodilators and systemic corticosteroids are used in the case of underlying bronchospasm.[52]

• Clinical Applicability Challenges

Case Study

Ms. S. presents to the urgent care clinic with her 75-year-old father, stating that her father just doesn't seem right. On speaking to Mr. S., you discover that he is oriented to self but has difficulty with place and time. He thinks that he has "felt a little under the weather for a couple of days." His daughter states that he has complained of shortness of breath, chills, and lack of appetite for the past 2 or 3 days. In attempting to obtain his medical history, you find out from Ms. S. that her father had an inferior wall myocardial infarction 5 years ago. He smoked two packs of cigarettes per day for 45 years but quit smoking 5 years ago. His daughter is unsure of any medications her father is currently taking.

Mr. S. is a tall, thin, frail elderly man who appears chronically ill and mildly distressed. He rests leaning over the bedside table. Physical examination shows the patient breathing using pursed lips and accessory respiratory muscles; bilateral breath sounds are diminished in the lung bases. He has a productive cough, with thick yellow sputum with green streaks. He has 1+ pitting edema in his lower extremities. A chest radiograph reveals blunted costophrenic angles and diffuse infiltrates in the left lower lobes. The patient's vital signs are as follows: temperature, 101.2°F; pulse, 130 beats/minute; blood pressure, 142/86 mm Hg; and respiratory rate, 28 breaths/minute.

1. What respiratory disorders would you include in your differential diagnosis?
2. What additional diagnostic studies would be useful?
3. What potential infectious organisms would you consider?
4. What treatment modalities would be involved in the plan of care for Mr. S.?
5. Using the Pneumonia Severity Index, what is the recommended site of care for this patient?

Review Questions

1. A tall, 27-year-old construction worker presents with complaints of shortness of breath, acute pleuritic pain, and no breath sounds auscultated on the right. He has no significant medical history except a 25 pack-year history of cigarette smoking. This individual is most likely experiencing
   a. spontaneous pneumothorax.
   b. community-acquired pneumonia.
   c. acute asthma attack.
   d. exacerbation of chronic bronchitis.
2. You are caring for a mechanically ventilated patient in the ICU. A subclavian central line was inserted a few hours ago, and you are waiting for x-ray con-

Table 26-16 • Management in Respiratory Failure

Management Principle	Therapeutic Intervention
Establishment and maintenance of an adequate airway	• Use oropharyngeal or nasopharyngeal tubes for upper airway obstruction during transient loss of consciousness. • Tracheal intubation may be necessary to prevent aspiration, maintain airway patency, and provide effective suctioning. • Strictly adhere to adequate tracheobronchial toilet (i.e., deep breathing, coughing, tracheobronchial suctioning).
Oxygenation	• Increase the inspired oxygen (FiO_2) concentration by administration of oxygen via a Venturi mask or nasal cannula. • Improve cardiac output, correct anemia, and reduce metabolic rates (fever) to improve tissue oxygenation. • Consider continuous positive airway pressure or expiratory positive airway pressure via a nasal or facial mask for alert and cooperative patients. • Mechanical ventilatory support may be needed in more severe cases with refractory and progressive hypoxemia.
Correction of acid–base disturbance	• Correct pH disturbances: In acute hypercapnia with acidosis, improve alveolar ventilation by providing mechanical ventilatory support, establishing and maintaining an adequate airway, treating broncho-spasm, and controlling heart failure, fever, and sepsis. • Consider bicarbonate administration in acute respiratory acidosis or metabolic acidosis.
Restoration of fluid and electrolyte balance	• Prevent excessive intravenous fluid administration and, conversely, poor fluid intake. • Monitor fluid intake and output closely. • Perform daily body weight measurement. • Prevent and treat promptly hypokalemia and hypophosphatemia.
Optimization of cardiac function	• Maintain adequate cardiac output. • Consider use of pulmonary artery catheter for accurate hemodynamic monitoring.
Identification and treatment of underlying correctable conditions and precipitating causes	• Prevent or treat respiratory tract infections (viral, bacterial, or fungal). • Prevent potential airway obstruction by maintenance of proper tracheobronchial hygiene, recognize increased tracheobronchial secretions, changes in their characteristics, or difficulty in their elimination due to various factors. • Identify and treat congestive heart failure appropriately. • Recognize and treat bronchospasm with bronchodilators and corticosteroids. • Assess for organic or metabolic disorder affecting the central nervous system or neuromuscular function. • Assess tolerance to sedative, hypnotic, and narcotic drugs in patients with chronic ventilatory insufficiency. In case of a narcotic drug overdose, a proper antidote may be administered. • Avoid indiscriminate use of oxygen; it may potentiate carbon dioxide retention or result in carbon dioxide narcosis. • Remove air or fluid in the pleural cavity. • Prevent and treat abdominal distention by insertion of a nasogastric tube. • For trauma and surgical patients, assess limitation of the thoracic wall movement, ineffective cough, immobility, and lack of deep breathing. • Control fever and other causes of increased metabolism. • Assess diaphragmatic fatigue; if present, mechanical ventilatory support is indicated to rest these muscles and restore their contractility. • Promptly identify and adequately treat hypophosphatemia, hypokalemia, and hypocalcemia.
Prevention and early detection of potential complications	• Most of these complications occur in mechanically ventilated patients (see Chapter 25).
Nutritional support	• Enteral alimentation is preferred over parenteral feeding because bowel wall integrity is maintained. • Recommend high-lipid formulas over high carbohydrates to limit carbon dioxide production.
Periodic assessment of the course, progress, and response to therapy	• Perform frequent arterial blood gas measurements. • Monitor arterial oxygen saturation by pulse oximetry.
Determination of a need for mechanical ventilatory support	• Continuously assess the patient's respiratory status and need for ventilator support (see Chapter 25).

From Farzan S: Respiratory failure. In Farzan S (ed): A Concise Handbook of Respiratory Diseases, 4th ed. Stamford, CT, Appleton & Lange, 1997, pp 371–386, with permission.

firmation of placement. You notice that the ventilator high-pressure alarms keep going off despite the fact that you have suctioned the patient, and she appears to be resting. You suspect the patient is having a traumatic pneumothorax because the most common cause of traumatic pneumothorax is

a. pneumonia and chronic obstructive pulmonary disease.
b. patients "bucking" the ventilator.
c. invasive procedures and barotraumas.
d. suctioning and chest physiotherapy.

3. The physician has diagnosed your patient as having an empyema and inserts a chest tube. The type of drainage you would most likely see coming from the chest tube would be

a. blood.
b. pus.
c. chyle.
d. serum.

4. The patient who is most likely to have community-acquired pneumonia is an

a. individual who has been hospitalized for 2 weeks with fever, chills, and cough.
b. elderly person who was just transferred to the emergency department from the nursing home complaining of chills, cough, and fever.
c. individual who has not lived in a long-term care facility for 14 days and comes to the clinic with fever, chills, and a cough.
d. elderly person discharged from the hospital to the assisted care facility with a recurrence of chills, cough, and fever.

5. The pathogens that cause pneumonia may enter the lower respiratory tract in the following four ways:

a. Aspiration, inhalation, hematogenous spread, and translocation
b. Aspiration, homologous transfer, translocation, and fomentation
c. Inoculation, translocation, hematemesis spread, and inhalation
d. Ventilation, transmigration, hematogenous spread, and aspiration

6. The three components of Virchow's triad in the pathophysiology of pulmonary embolism include

a. venous stasis, hypocoagulability, and vein wall damage.
b. venous stasis, hypercoagulability, and vein wall damage.
c. venous malformation, hypercoagulability, and arterial wall rupture.
d. venous turbulence, normocoagulability, and vein wall aneurysm.

7. Mr. L is reporting to your surgery clinic for his preoperative evaluation. In reviewing his medications, which of the following would you expect him to be taking if he has COPD?

a. Bronchodilators
b. Antitussives
c. Narcotics
d. Vasodilators

References

1. Hoyert DL, Kung H, Smith BL: Death: Preliminary data for 2003. Natl Vital Stat Rep 53(15):1–48, 2005
2. Bartlett JG, Dowell, SF, Mandell, LA, et al: Practice guidelines for the management of community acquired pneumonia in adults. Clin Infect Dis 31(2):347–382, 2000
3. Miskovich-Riddle L, Keresztes P: CAP management guidelines. Nurse Practitioner 31(1):43–53, 2006
4. Mandell LA, Bartlett JG, Dowell SF, et al: Update of practice guideline for the management of community acquired pneumonia in immunocompetent adults. Clin Infect Dis 37(11):1405–1433, 2003
5. Halm EA, Teirstein AS: Management of community-acquired pneumonia. N Engl J Med 347(25):2039–2045, 2002
6. American Thoracic Society: Guidelines for the management of adults with community-acquired pneumonia. Am J Respir Crit Care Med 163(7):1730–1745, 2001
7. American Thoracic Society: Guidelines for the management of adults with hospital-acquired, ventilator-associated, and healthcare-associated pneumonia. Am J Respir Crit Care Med 171(4):388–416, 2005
8. Leeper KV, Moss M: Bacterial pneumonia. In Hanley ME, Walsh CH (eds): Current Diagnosis and Treatment in Pulmonary Medicine. New York, McGraw-Hill, 2003, pp 361–371
9. Tablan OC, Anderson LJ, Besser R, et al: Guidelines for preventing health-care–associated pneumonia, 2003. MMWR Morb Mortal Wkly Rep 53(RR03):1–36, 2004
10. Lutfiyya MN, Henley E, Chang LF, et al: Diagnosis and treatment of community-acquired pneumonia. Am Fam Physician 73(3):442–450, 2006
11. Weinberger SE: Principles of Pulmonary Medicine, 4th ed. Philadelphia, Elsevier Saunders, 2004
12. Ramsdell J, Narsavage GL, Fink JB, for the American College of Chest Physicians' Home Care Network Working Group: Management of community-acquired pneumonia in the home: An American College of Chest Physicians clinical position statement. Chest 127(5):1752–1763, 2005
13. McKay CA, Speers M: Watch for AACN practice alerts. AACN News 21(2):1–4, 2004. Available at: http://www.aacn.org
14. Centers for Disease Control and Prevention: Clinical guidance on the identification and evaluation of possible SARS-CoV disease among persons presenting with community-acquired illness, Version 2. Washington, DC, Department of Health and Human Services, 2004, pp 1–12. Available at: http://www.cdc.gov/sars
15. Ksiazek TG, Erdman D, Goldsmith CS, et al: A novel coronavirus associated with severe acute respiratory syndrome. N Engl J Med 348(20):1953–1966, 2003
16. Centers for Disease Control and Prevention: Update: Outbreak of severe acute respiratory syndrome—worldwide, 2003. MMWR Morb Mortal Wkly Rep 52(12):241–248, 2003
17. Centers for Disease Control and Prevention: Severe acute respiratory syndrome (SARS) fact sheet, 2005. Available at: http://www.cdc.gov/ncidod/sars/factsheet
18. Kamps BS, Hoffman C (eds): SARS reference, October 2003, pp 14–17. Available from Flying Publisher at: httpp://www.SARSReference.com
19. Lee N, Hui D, Wu A, et al: A major outbreak of severe acute respiratory syndrome in Hong Kong. N Engl J Med 348(20):1986–1994, 2003
20. Centers for Disease Control and Prevention: Update: Outbreak of severe acute respiratory syndrome—worldwide, 2003. MMWR Morb Mortal Wkly Rep 52(13):269–272, 2003
21. World Health Organization: Preliminary clinical description of severe acute respiratory syndrome: Epidemic and pandemic alert and response, 2006. Available at: http://www.who.int/csr/sars/clinical/en

22. Drosten C, Gunther S, Preiser W, et al: Identification of a novel coronavirus in patients with severe acute respiratory syndrome. N Engl J Med 348(20):1967–1976, 2003

23. Booth CM, Stewart TE: Severe acute respiratory syndrome and critical care medicine: The Toronto experience. Crit Care Med 33(1):S53–S60, 2003

24. El-Masri MM, Williamson KM, Fox-Wasylyshyn SM: Severe acute respiratory syndrome: Another challenge for critical care nurses. AACN Clin Issues 15(1):150–159, 2004

25. Centers for Disease Control and Prevention: Clinical guidance on the identification and evaluation of possible SARS-CoV disease among persons presenting with community-acquired illness, Version 2, Supplement I: Infection control in healthcare, home, and community settings. Washington, DC, Department of Health and Human Services Centers for Disease Control and Prevention, 2004, pp 1–28. Available at: http://www.cdc.gov/sars

26. Broaddus VC, Light RW: Pleural effusion. In Mason RJ, et al (eds): Murray & Nadel's Textbook of Respiratory Care (4th Ed), pp 1913–1960. Philadelphia, Elsevier Saunders, 2005

27. Porth C: Disorders of ventilations and gas exchange. In Pathophysiology: Concepts of Altered Health States, 7th ed. Philadelphia, Lippincott Williams & Wilkins, 2005, pp 689–724

28. Zimmerman LH: Pleural effusions. In Goldstein RH, O'Connell JJ, Karlinsky JB, et al (eds): A Practical Approach to Pulmonary Medicine. Philadelphia, Lippincott-Raven, 1997, pp 195–205

29. Huggins JT, Weissberg D, Sahn SA: Pleural diseases in the intensive care unit. In Fink MP, Abraham E, Vincent JL, et al (eds): Textbook of Critical Care, 5th ed. Philadelphia, Elsevier Saunders, 2005, pp 633–646

30. Des Jardin T, Burton GG: Pleural diseases. In Clinical Manifestations and Assessments of Respiratory Diseases, 5th ed. Philadelphia, Elsevier Mosby, 2006, pp 318–327

31. Berk JL: Pneumothothorax. In Goldstein RH, O'Connell JJ, Karlinsky JB, et al (eds): A Practical Approach to Pulmonary Medicine. Philadelphia, Lippincott-Raven, 1997, pp 206–223

32. Strange C: Pleural diseases. In Wilkins RL, Stoller JK, Scanlan CL, et al (eds): Egan's Fundamentals of Respiratory Care, 8th ed. St. Louis, Mosby, 2003, pp 503–519

33. Chesnutt MS, Prendergast TJ: Lung. In Tierney L, McPhee SJ, Papadakis MA (eds): Current Medical Diagnosis and Medical Treatment, 46th ed. New York, McGraw-Hill, 2007, pp 222–315

34. Des Jardin T, Burton GG: Pneumothorax. In Clinical Manifestations and Assessments of Respiratory Diseases, 5th ed. Philadelphia, Elsevier Mosby, 2006, pp 306–316

35. Robinson GV: Pulmonary embolism in hospital practice. BMJ 332(7534):156–160, 2006

36. West JB: Pulmonary Pathophysiology: The Essentials, 6th ed. Philadelphia, Lippincott Williams & Wilkins, 2003

37. Blann AD, Lip GYH: Venous thromboembolism. BMJ 332(7535):215–219, 2006

38. Merli GJ: Pathophysiology of venous thrombosis, thrombophilia, and the diagnosis of deep vein thrombosis–pulmonary embolism in the elderly. Clin Geriatr Med 22:75–92, 2006

39. Nana-Sinkam P: Pulmonary thromboembolism. In Hanley ME, Walsh CH (eds): Current Diagnosis and Treatment in Pulmonary Medicine. New York, McGraw-Hill, 2003, pp 195–203

40. Hirsh J, Raschke R: Heparin and low-molecular-weight heparin: The seventh ACCP conference on antithrombotic and thrombolytic therapy. Chest 126(3):188S–203S, 2004

41. Geerts WH, Pineo GF, Heit JA, et al: Prevention of venous thromboembolism: The seventh ACCP conference on antithrombotic and thrombolytic therapy. Chest 126(3):338S–400S, 2004

42. American Thoracic Society: Standards for the Diagnosis and Management of Patients with COPD. New York, Author, 2004.

43. American Lung Association: Chronic obstructive pulmonary disease (COPD) fact sheet (chronic bronchitis and emphysema), 2006. Available at: http://www.lungusa.org/

44. Petty TL: Chronic obstructive pulmonary disease. In Hanley ME, Walsh CH (eds): Current Diagnosis and Treatment in Pulmonary Medicine. New York, McGraw-Hill, 2003, pp 82–91

45. Pauwels RA, Buist AS, Calverley PM, et al: Global strategy for the diagnosis, management, and prevention of chronic obstructive pulmonary disease: NHLBI/WHO global initiative for chronic obstructive lung disease (GOLD) workshop summary. Am J Respir Crit Care Med 163:1256–1276, 2001.

46. Gerald LB, Bailey WC: Global initiative for chronic obstructive lung disease. J Cardiopulm Rehabil 22(2):234–244, 2002

47. Margereson C, Riley J: Cardiothoracic Surgical Nursing: Current Trends in Adult Care. Maden, MA, Blackwell Publishing, 2003

48. John J, Idell S: Managing severe exacerbations of asthma. Emerg Med 38(4):20–32, 2006

49. Kaminshy DA: Asthma. In Hanley ME, Walsh CH (eds): Current Diagnosis and Treatment in Pulmonary Medicine. New York, McGraw-Hill, 2003, pp 67–81

50. U.S. Department of Health and Human Services: Practical Guide for the Diagnosis and Management of Asthma based on the Expert Panel Report 2: Guidelines for the Diagnosis and Management of Asthma. NIH Publ. No. 97-4053, October 1997, pp 1–52

51. Markou NK, Myrianthefs PM, Baltopoulos GJ, et al: Respiratory failure: An overview. Crit Care Nurs Q 27(4):353–379, 2004

52. Van Hoozen B, Albertson TE: Acute respiratory failure. In Burton GG, Hodgkin JE, Ward JJ: Respiratory Care: A Guide to Clinical Practice, 4th ed. Philadelphia, JB Lippincott, 1997, pp 1107–1132

53. Vasileyev S, Schaap RN, Mortensen JD: Hospital survival rates of patients with acute respiratory failure in modern respiratory intensive care units. Chest 107(4):1083–1088, 1995.

54. Reardon C, et al: Acute respiratory failure. In Crapo JD, Glassroth J, Karlinsky J, et al (eds): Baum's Textbook of Pulmonary Diseases, 7th ed. Philadelphia, Lippincott Williams & Wilkins, 2004, pp 1049–1071

55. Powell CA, Joyce-Brady MF: Acute and chronic respiratory failure. In Goldstein RH, O'Connell JJ, Karlinsky JB, et al (eds): A Practical Approach to Pulmonary Medicine. Philadelphia, Lippincott-Raven, 1997, pp 296–308

56. Farzan S: Respiratory failure. In Farzan S (ed): A Concise Handbook of Respiratory Diseases, 4th ed. Stamford, CT, Appleton & Lange, 1997, pp 371–386

57. Christie HA, Goldstein LS: Respiratory failure and the need for ventilatory support. In Wilkins RL, Stoller JK, Scanlan CL, et al (eds): Egan's Fundamentals of Respiratory Care, 8th ed. St. Louis, Mosby, 2003, pp 913–927

58. American Thoracic Society: Standards of nursing care for adult patients with pulmonary dysfunction. Am Rev Respir Dis 144:231, 1991

59. Krider SJ: Interview and respiratory history. In Wilkins RL, Sheldon RL, Kidder SJ (eds): Clinical Assessment in Respiratory Care, 4th ed. St. Louis, Mosby, 2000, pp 11–50

Other Selected Readings

Allibone L: Assessment and management of patients with pleural effusions. Nursing Stand 20(22):55–64, 2006

Badesch DB, Abman SH, Simonneau G, et al: Medical therapy for pulmonary arterial hypertension: Updated ACCP evidence-based clinical practice guidelines. Chest 131(6):1917–1928, 2007

Behnia M, Cummings O: Desquamative interstitial pneumonia masquerading as acute life-threatening pulmonary embolism. Am J Crit Care 13(3):199–201, 2004

Brozek J, McDonald E, Clarke F, et al: Pneumonia observational incidents and treatments: A multidisciplinary process improvement study. Am J Crit Care 16(3):214–221, 2007

Burns SM: Ventilating patients with acute severe asthma: What do we really know? AACN Adv Crit Care 17(2):186–193, 2006

Caroci A, Lareau S: Descriptors of dyspnea by patients with chronic obstructive pulmonary disease versus congestive heart failure. Heart Lung 33(2):102–110, 2004

Cason C, Tyner T, Saunders S, Broome L: Nurses' implementation of guidelines for ventilator-associated pneumonia from the Centers for Disease Control and Prevention. Am J Crit Care 16(1): 28–38, 2007

Cicutto L, Downey G: Biological markers in diagnosing, monitoring, and treating asthma: A focus on non-invasive measurements. AACN Clin Issues 15(1):97–111, 2004

DeMello D, Kierol-Andrews L, Scalise P: Severe sepsis and respiratory distress syndrome from community-acquired legionella pneumonia: Case report. Am J Crit Care 16(3):317–320, 2007

El-Masri M, Williamson K, Fox-Wasylyshyn S: Severe acute respiratory syndrome: Another challenge for critical care nurses. AACN Clin Issues 15(1):150–159, 2004

Gelinas C, Fortier M, Viens C, et al: Pain assessment and management in critically ill intubated patients: A retrospective study. Am J Crit Care 13(2):126–135, 2004

Goldhill D, Imhoff M, McLean B, Waldmann C: Rotation bed therapy to prevent and treat respiratory complications: A review and meta-analysis. Am J Crit Care 16(1):50–62, 2007

Holcomb S: Asthma update. Dimens Crit Care Nurs 23(3):101–110, 2004

Jeng C, Chang W, Wai P, et al: Comparison of oxygen consumption in performing daily activities between patients with chronic obstructive pulmonary disease and a healthy population. Heart Lung 32(2):121–130, 2003

Kanervisto M, Paavilainen E, Astedt-Kurki P: Impact of chronic obstructive pulmonary disease on family functioning. Heart Lung 32(6):360–367, 2003

Kehl-Pruett W: Deep vein thrombosis in hospitalized patients: A review of evidence-based guidelines for prevention. Dimens Crit Care Nurs 25(2):53–59, 2006

Koschel M: Pulmonary embolism. Am J Nurs 104(6):46–50, 2004

Meek P, Lareau S, Hu J: Are self-reports of breathing efforts and breathing distress stable and valid measures among persons with asthma, persons with COPD, and healthy persons? Heart Lung 32(5):335–346, 2003

Montgomery SS, Burke EM, Wissman SA, et al: Natural course of large spontaneous pneumothorax. Heart Lung 34(5):332–334, 2005

Rabe KF, Beghe B, Luppi F, Fabbri LM: Update in chronic obstructive pulmonary disease 2002. Am J Respir Crit Care 175: 1222–1232, 2007

Ryan B: Pneumothorax: Assessment and diagnostic testing. J Cardiovasc Nurs 20(4):251–253, 2005

Shaughnessy K: Massive pulmonary embolism. Crit Care Nurse 27(1):39–50, 2007

Sims J: An overview of asthma. Dimens Crit Care Nurs 25(6): 264–268, 2006

Smyth M: Acute respiratory failure: Part 1. Failure in oxygenation: When a patient loses the ability to oxygenate the blood. Am J Nurs 105(5):72GG–72OO, 2005

Smyth M: Acute respiratory failure: Part 2. Failure in ventilation: Exploring the other cause of acute respiratory failure. Am J Nurs 105(6):72AA–72DD, 2005

Spector N, Connoly MA, Carlson KK: Dyspnea: Applying research to bedside practice. AACN Adv Crit Care 18(1):45–60, 2007

Tolentino-DelosReyes A, Ruppert S, Yun S, Shiao P: Evidence-based practice: Use of the ventilator bundle to prevent ventilator-associated pneumonia. Am J Crit Care 16(1):20–27, 2007

Tovey C, Wyatt S: Diagnosis, investigation, and management of deep vein thrombosis. BMJ 326:1180–1184, 2003

Vollman KM: Ventilator-associated pneumonia and pressure ulcer prevention as targets for quality improvement in the ICU. Crit Care Nurs Clin North Am 18(4):453–468, 2006

White KA, Ruth-Sahd LA: Bronchiolitis obliterans organizing pneumonia. Crit Care Nurse 27(3):53–66, 2007

Acute Respiratory Distress Syndrome

27

Mary van Soeren • Christina Hurlock-Chorostecki

Objectives

Based on the content in this chapter, the reader should be able to:

❶ Compare and contrast the causes, definition, assessment findings, and outcomes between acute lung injury (ALI) and acute respiratory distress syndrome (ARDS).

❷ Relate the assessment and diagnostic findings of ARDS to the pathophysiological processes.

❸ Describe mechanical ventilation strategies used to prevent ventilator-associated lung injury (VALI).

❹ Explain the management of patients with ARDS and rationales for the interventions.

❺ Review the use of critical care "bundles" as they relate to the care and treatment of patients with ARDS.

❻ Discuss potential complications of ARDS and the related interventions.

A cute respiratory distress syndrome (ARDS) represents a complex clinical syndrome (rather than a single disease process) and carries a high risk for mortality. The severity of the clinical course, the uncertainty of the outcome, and the reliance on the full spectrum of critical care resources for treatment means that the entire health care team is challenged. Since the 1960s, researchers and clinicians have investigated the nature of the pathological process and explored treatment options with the goal of improving outcome. Through this application of research to practice we know that some previous strategies have been ineffective, and innovations in mechanical ventilation, sedation, nutrition and pharmacological intervention remain important research initiatives. A key role for the critical care nurse is early detection and prevention of ARDS. Therefore, with respect to ARDS, it is essential that critical care nurses be knowledgeable about risk factors, assessment tools and protocols, and prevention strategies.

ARDS was first described in 1967 and was termed *adult* (rather than *acute*) respiratory distress syndrome because of a misconception that the syndrome occurred only in adults. Recognition of the prevalence of this syndrome in younger patients led to the current terminology. ARDS is at the extreme end of a continuum of hypoxic acute lung injury (ALI) that results in respiratory failure. In 1994, the American-European Consensus Conference members issued definitions of ALI and ARDS that are widely used by researchers today[1] (Table 27-1).

• Etiology, Diagnostic Criteria, and Incidence

The causes of ARDS are many and diverse.[2] The syndrome may be precipitated by either direct or indirect pulmonary injury, possibly in previously healthy people who are exposed to an insult (Box 27-1). ARDS is acute in onset, and symptoms typically develop over 4 to 48 hours after the inciting insult, making a cause-and-effect association somewhat

**Table 27-1 • Comparison of Acute Lung Injury (ALI)
and Acute Respiratory Distress Syndrome (ARDS)**

Criterion	ALI	ARDS
PaO_2/FiO_2 ratio,* regardless of PEEP level	Less than 300	Less than 200
Chest x-ray	Bilateral infiltrates	Bilateral infiltrates
Pulmonary artery wedge pressure	Less than 18 mm Hg or no indication of left atrial hypertension	Less than 18 mm Hg or no indication of left atrial hypertension

*Ratio of arterial oxygen to inspired oxygen.
PEEP, positive end-expiratory pressure.
Adapted from Bernard GR, Artigas A, Brigham KL, et al: The American-European Consensus conference on ARDS: Definitions, mechanisms, relevant outcomes, and clinical trials co-ordination. Am J Respir Crit Care Med 149:818–824, 1994.

difficult. Recently, several related respiratory disorders have been found presenting with clinical signs of ALI. These disorders may ultimately lead to development of ARDS and include severe acute respiratory syndrome (SARS), discussed in Chapter 26, and transfusion-related acute lung injury (TRALI).

TRALI is the leading cause of transfusion-related mortality in the United States.[3,4] It is theorized that an interaction occurs between the recipient's blood and the donor's, among the bioactive compounds produced during blood storage, or a combination of both.[3,5,6] Clinical presentation is the sudden onset of respiratory distress within 1 to 2 hours after a transfusion of red blood cells or fresh frozen plasma.[3,7] Peak airway pressures are elevated, airway secretions may be frothy, and the chest radiograph shows patchy infiltrates. Management of the patient is supportive and involves the same principles of mechanical ventilation used in ARDS and avoidance of aggressive diuresis. Mechanical ventilation is required in about 70% of cases.[7] The blood bank should be notified of a TRALI case, and the patient should not receive further blood products from that donor.

Diagnostic criteria for ARDS have been difficult to define because ARDS closely resembles several conditions, such as hemodynamic pulmonary edema due to heart failure, diffuse alveolar hemorrhage, acute interstitial pneumonia, idiopathic acute eosinophilic pneumonia, and lung cancer.[8] Diagnostic testing is used to "rule out" these conditions, yet the final diagnosis of ARDS is largely based on clinical presentation. No one test, including radiographic evidence, a plasma brain natriuretic peptide (BNP) less than 500 pg/mL, or a pulmonary artery wedge pressure (PAWP) less than 18 cm H_2O, is truly indicative of ARDS.[9] However, an early feature of ARDS is diffuse alveolar damage (DAD), and recent research findings have shown promise in diagnosing DAD with cytology of bronchoalveolar fluid.[10]

Approximately 190,600 cases of ARDS occur each year in the United States, of which 74,500 result in death.[11] In critical care units, up to 20% of mechanically ventilated patients meet the criteria for ARDS.[12] The patients most at risk for development of ARDS are older than 65 years, with a severe acute illness on presentation such as sepsis or a preexisting chronic

---

Box 27-1 • Causes and Predisposing Conditions for Acute Respiratory Distress Syndrome (ARDS)

Genetic predisposition
Direct injury
- Aspiration (gastric fluids, near-drowning)
- Infectious pneumonia
- Lung contusions with trauma
- Toxic inhalation
- Upper airway obstruction (relieved)
- Severe acute respiratory syndrome (SARS) coronavirus
- Neurogenic pulmonary edema
- Acute eosinophilic pneumonia*
- Bronchiolitis obliterans with organizing pneumonia (BOOP)*
- Miliary tuberculosis*
Indirect pulmonary injury
- Sepsis
- Burns
- Trauma
- Blood transfusion (TRALI)
- Lung or bone marrow transplantation
- Drug or alcohol overdose
- Drug reaction

- Cardiopulmonary bypass
- Acute pancreatitis
- Multiple fractures
- Venous air embolism
- Amniotic fluid embolism
- Pancreatitis

Systemic Inflammatory Response Syndrome (SIRS) Criteria

SIRS is manifested by two or more of the following:
- Temperature greater than 100.4°F (38°C) or less than 96.8°F (36°C)
- Heart rate greater than 90 beats/minute
- Respiratory rate greater than 20 breaths/minute or an arterial carbon dioxide tension ($PaCO_2$) less than 32 mm Hg
- White blood cell count greater than 12,000 cells/mm³ or less than 4,000 cells/mm³ OR more than 10% immature (band) forms

*Specific treatment required.
TRALI, transfusion-related acute lung injury.

disorder,[9,13] those who smoke cigarettes,[14] and those with a history of alcohol abuse.[15] Although sepsis is the most common cause of ARDS,[16] approximately one third of patients who aspirate (e.g., gastric fluids) will develop ARDS.[17] However, any person with one of the potential precipitating causes of ARDS is susceptible, and nurses need to be vigilant for early warning signs. Most patients with ARDS require a period of mechanical ventilation support of days to weeks. Mortality from ARDS varies based on the cause, with current mortality rates estimated to be 25% to 58%.[18,19] Because of improvements in critical care techniques, the cause of death appears to have changed in the past 5 years.[20] Infections such as ventilator-acquired pneumonia (VAP) and multiorgan system failure, not respiratory failure, are now the leading causes of death.[21]

• Pathophysiology

In 1967, Ashbaugh and others described ARDS in case reports of 12 patients presenting with acute tachypnea, decreased lung compliance, diffuse pulmonary infiltrates on chest radiograph, and hypoxemia.[1] Later researchers used histological examination of lungs of patients with ARDS to show lung fibrosis that was unlike other diseases. This led to new understanding that the pathological process was not limited to the lung endothelium but was a result of alterations of lung epithelium and vascular tissue as well as the development of hyaline membranes. Pathological changes in lung vascular tissue, increased lung edema, and impaired gas exchange are hallmarks of the pathophysiology. The pathological pulmonary alterations of ARDS are directly related to a cascade of events resulting from release of cellular and biochemical mediators. The activation, interactions, and multisystem actions of biological mediators are extremely complex.

PATHOLOGICAL CHANGES IN ACUTE RESPIRATORY DISTRESS SYNDROME

Mediators released as a result of either direct or indirect injury can precipitate ARDS, including lipopolysaccharide (LPS) in gram-negative bacterial sepsis.[22] There is a relationship between clinical presentation (severe acute hypoxia resistant to improvement with supplemental oxygen, tachypnea, and dyspnea), mediator release (interleukins, tumor necrosis factor-α [TNF-α], and platelet-activating factor [PAF]), and pathological changes (microvascular permeability, pulmonary hypertension, and pulmonary endothelial damage). Some primary mediators responsible for lung damage in ARDS and their major actions as they relate to ARDS are listed in Table 27-2.[22,23]

Adequate pulmonary gas exchange depends on open, air-filled alveoli, intact alveolar–capillary membranes, and normal blood flow through the pulmonary vasculature. The pathogenesis of ARDS is illustrated in Figure 27-1. Diffuse alveolar–capillary membrane damage occurs and increases membrane permeability, thus allowing fluids to move from the vascular space into the interstitial and alveolar space. Air spaces fill with bloody proteinaceous fluid and debris from degenerating cells, causing interstitial and alveolar edema. As a result, oxygenation is impaired. Inflammatory mediators cause the pulmonary vascular bed to vasoconstrict. Pulmonary hypertension and reduced blood flow to portions of the lung result. Because of the reduction in blood flow and decreased hemoglobin in capillaries, there is a decrease in oxygen available for diffusion and transport, further impairing oxygenation.

The pathological changes affect pulmonary blood vessels, gas exchange, and lung and bronchial mechanics (Fig. 27-2). Ventilation is impaired because of a decrease in lung compliance and an increase in airway resistance. Lung compliance is reduced as a result of the stiffness of fluid-filled, nonaerated lung. The presence of these fluid-filled alveoli alongside collapsed alveoli gives the chest radiograph the classic "patchy" appearance. Surfactant, a substance that normally decreases the surface tension of alveoli, is lost, resulting in alveolar collapse. Mediator-induced bronchoconstriction causes airway narrowing and increased airway resistance, restricting the flow of air into the lungs.

SYSTEMIC INFLAMMATORY RESPONSE SYNDROME

Systemic inflammatory response syndrome (SIRS) describes the inflammatory response occurring throughout the body as a result of some systemic

Table 27-2 • Examples of Pathological Responses to Biological Mediators

Response	Biological Mediators
Persistent inflammatory response	Cytokines: interleukins (IL-1, IL-6), interferon-γ (INF-γ), tumor necrosis factor-α (TNF-α), complement, thromboxane
Endothelial membrane disruption	Complement, thromboxane, kinins, TNF-α, toxic oxygen metabolites, leukotrienes, prostaglandins (PGE_1 and PGE_2)
Selective vasoconstriction	Thromboxane, TNF-α, platelet-activating factor (PAF), toxic oxygen metabolites
Systemic vasodilation	Complement, prostaglandins, TNF-α, IL-1, IL-6
Myocardial depression	Complement, leukotrienes, TNF-α, myocardial depressant factor
Bronchoconstriction	Complement, thromboxane, leukotrienes, PAF

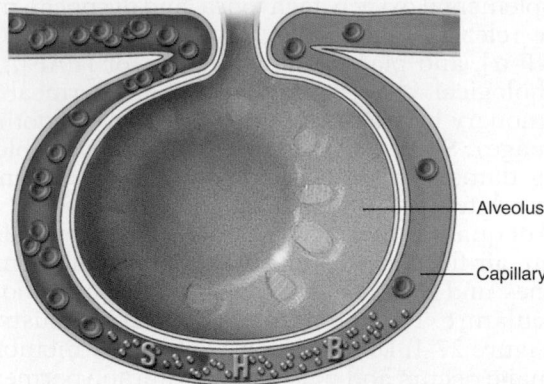

Phase 1. Injury reduces normal blood flow to the lungs. Platelets aggregate and release histamine (H), serotonin (S), and bradykinin (B).

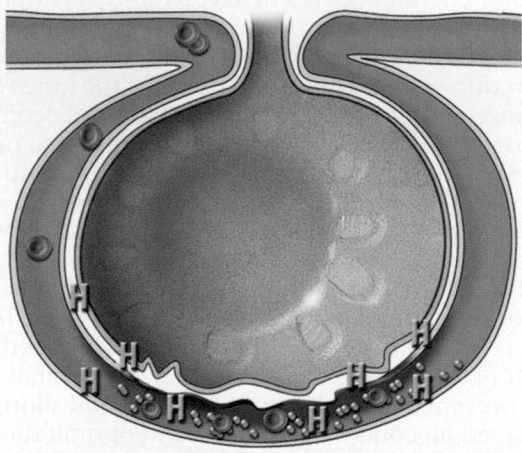

Phase 2. Those substances, especially histamine, inflame and damage the alveolar–capillary membrane, increasing capillary permeability. Fluids then shift into the interstitial space.

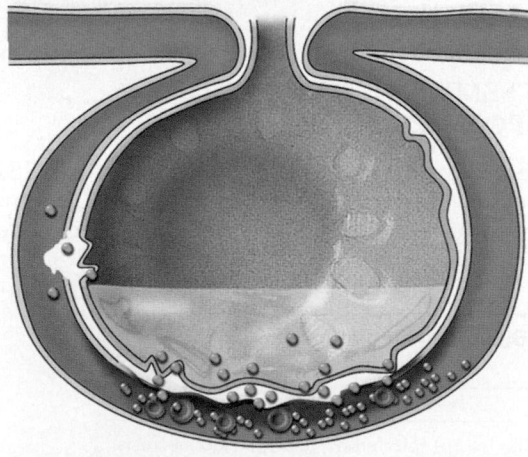

Phase 3. As capillary permeability increases, proteins and fluids leak out, increasing interstitial osmotic pressure and causing pulmonary edema.

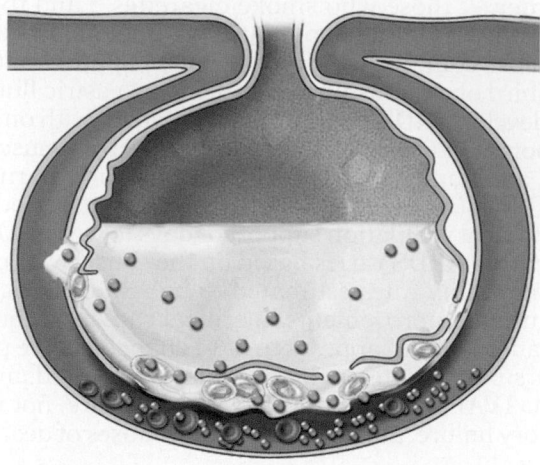

Phase 4. Decreased blood flow and fluids in the alveoli damage surfactant and impair the cell's ability to produce more. As a result, alveoli collapse, impeding gas exchange and decreasing lung compliance.

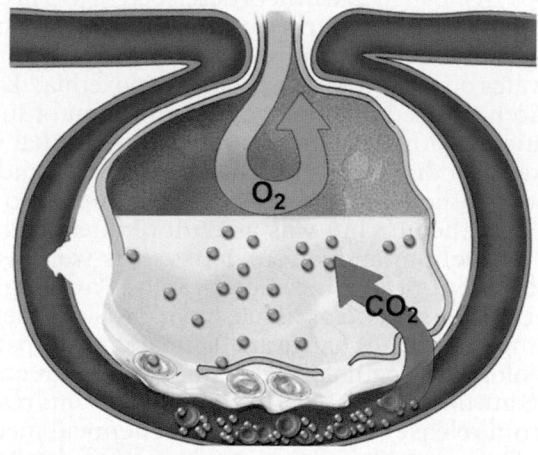

Phase 5. Sufficient oxygen cannot cross the alveolar–capillary membrane, but carbon dioxide (CO_2) can and is lost with every exhalation. Oxygen (O_2) and CO_2 levels decrease in the blood.

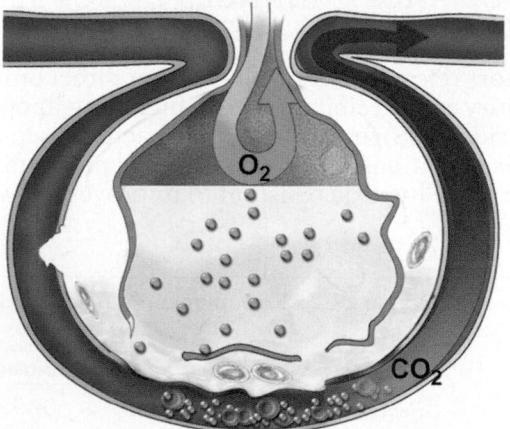

Phase 6. Pulmonary edema worsens, inflammation leads to fibrosis, and gas exchange is further impeded.

Figure 27-1 • Pathogenesis of acute respiratory distress syndrome (ARDS). Changes in lung epithelium and vascular endothelium result in fluid and protein movement, changes in lung compliance, and disruption of the alveoli with accompanying hypoxia. (From Anatomical Chart Company: Atlas of Pathophysiology, 2nd ed. Ambler, PA: Lippincott Williams & Wilkins, 2006, pp 81, 83.)

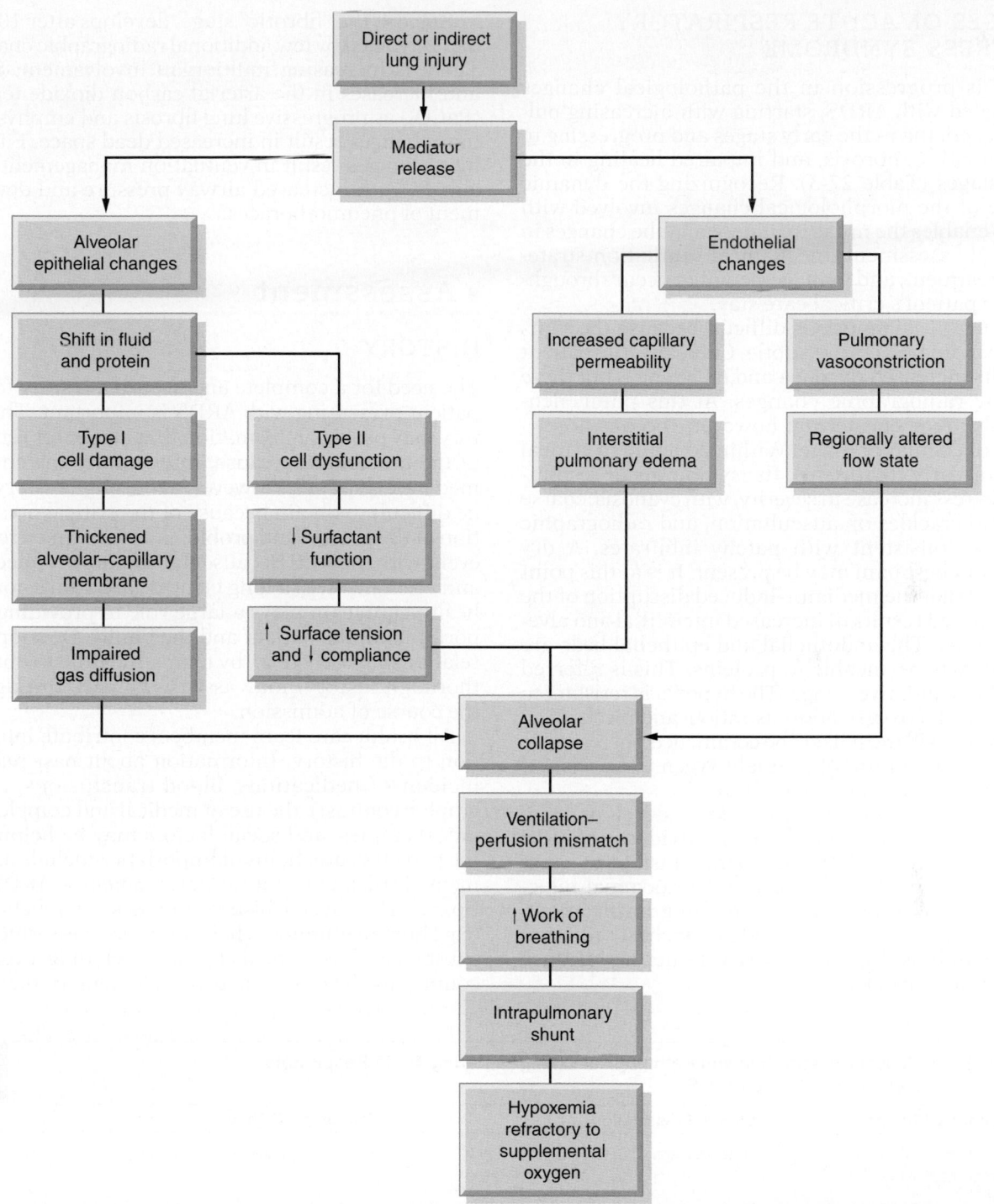

Figure 27-2 • Pathophysiological cascade is initiated by injury resulting in mediator release. The multiple effects result in changes to the alveoli, vascular tissue, and bronchi. The ultimate effect is ventilation–perfusion mismatching and refractory hypoxemia.

insult.[22] Most patients with ARDS manifest the symptoms that define SIRS (see Box 27-1), and the respiratory system may be the earliest and most common organ system to be involved in the systemic response. Thus, an understanding of the pathophysiology of SIRS and knowledge of the interventions used for SIRS are important in relation to ARDS. Often, patients with SIRS develop multisystem organ dysfunction (MODS), primarily in the liver and kidney. As endothelial damage progresses and tissue hypoxia

ensues from the severely impaired gas exchange, the inflammatory response is perpetuated and the SIRS cascade intensifies (up-regulates) with the release of more mediators. ARDS and MODS are therefore part of a vicious cycle and the continuum of SIRS.[22] Determination of the triggers for SIRS and ARDS that are present in some individuals but not others and investigations of how to stop the cascade pathways are the subjects of ongoing research. For a more detailed discussion of SIRS and MODS, see Chapter 54.

STAGES OF ACUTE RESPIRATORY DISTRESS SYNDROME

There is progression in the pathological changes associated with ARDS, starting with increasing pulmonary edema in the early stages and progressing to inflammation, fibrosis, and impaired healing in the later stages (Table 27-3). Recognizing the dynamic nature of the morphological changes involved with ARDS enables the nurse to understand the changes in physical assessment, mechanical ventilation strategies, treatment, and management that occur throughout the patient's critical care stay.

In stage 1, diagnosis is difficult because the signs of impending ARDS are subtle. Clinically, the patient exhibits increased dyspnea and tachypnea, but there are few radiographic changes. At this point, neutrophils are sequestering; however, there is no evidence of cellular damage. Within 24 hours (a critical time for early treatment), the symptoms of respiratory distress increase in severity, with cyanosis, coarse bilateral crackles on auscultation, and radiographic changes consistent with patchy infiltrates. A dry cough or chest pain may be present. It is at this point (stage 2) that the mediator-induced disruption of the vascular bed results in increased interstitial and alveolar edema. The endothelial and epithelial beds are increasingly permeable to proteins. This is referred to as the "exudative" stage. The hypoxia is resistant to supplemental oxygen administration, and mechanical ventilation will most likely be commenced in response to a worsening ratio of arterial oxygen to fraction of inspired oxygen (PaO_2/FiO_2 ratio).

Stage 3, the "proliferative" stage, develops from the 2nd to the 10th day after injury. Evidence of SIRS is now present, with hemodynamic instability, generalized edema, possible onset of nosocomial infections, increased hypoxemia, and lung involvement. Air bronchograms may be evident on chest radiography, as well as decreased lung volumes and diffuse interstitial markings.

Stage 4, the "fibrotic" stage, develops after 10 days and is typified by few additional radiographic changes. There is increasing multiorgan involvement, SIRS, and increases in the arterial carbon dioxide tension ($PaCO_2$) as progressive lung fibrosis and emphysematous changes result in increased dead space. Fibrotic lung changes result in ventilation management difficulties, with increased airway pressure and development of pneumothoraces.

• Assessment

HISTORY

The need for a complete and accurate history for the patient presenting with ARDS is important. The history may provide information that allows for removal of the precipitating cause, interrupting the ensuing mediator response. However, a thorough history may be difficult to obtain because of the critical presentation of the patient and problems associating a remote event with the ALI. Because the outcome is uncertain and often involves a long critical care admission, the health care team plays a large role in providing support to both the patient and the family. Developing a relationship early (e.g., by taking the time to obtain a thorough history) may assist with care throughout the course of admission.

All health care team members contribute information to the history. Information about past relevant incidents (medications, blood transfusions, radiographic contrast), the use of medical and complementary therapies, and social factors may be helpful for the person's care. Items of importance include assessment of risk factors for the development of ARDS (see Box 27-1), a social history to assess risk behaviors (e.g., human immunodeficiency virus status, smoking, substance abuse), medications (including over-the-counter medications), and complementary therapies

---

Table 27-3 • Clinical Presentation and Pathological Changes During Acute Respiratory Distress Syndrome (ARDS)

Radiographic Change	Clinical Presentation	Pathological Change
Stage 1 (first 12 h): Normal chest x-ray	Dyspnea, tachypnea	Neutrophil sequestration, no evidence of cellular damage
Stage 2—Exudative (24 h): Patchy alveolar infiltrate, primarily in dependent lung areas; normal heart size	Dyspnea, tachypnea, cyanosis, tachycardia, coarse crackles, hypoxemia	Neutrophil infiltration, vascular congestion, fibrin strands, increased interstitial and alveolar edema
Stage 3—Proliferative (2–10 days): Diffuse alveolar infiltrates, possibly air bronchograms, decreased lung volume, normal heart size	Hyperdynamic hemodynamic parameters, systemic inflammatory response syndrome (SIRS) presentation	Type II cell proliferation, microemboli formation, increased interstitial and alveolar inflammatory exudate, early deposition of collagen
Stage 4—Fibrotic (>10 days): Persistent infiltrates, new pneumonic infiltrates, recurrent pneumothorax	Multiple organ involvement, difficulty maintaining adequate oxygenation, sepsis, pneumonia	Type II cell hyperplasia, thickening of interstitial wall with fibrosis, macrophages, fibroblasts, remodeling of arterioles, cyst formation

Adapted from van Soeren MH, Diehl-Jones WL, Maykut RJ, et al: Pathophysiology and implications for treatment of acute respiratory distress syndrome. AACN Clin Issues 11(2):179–197, 2000.

(all exogenous substances, including inhalations). This information is obtained in addition to the history of the present illness and presenting signs and symptoms.

PHYSICAL EXAMINATION

Acute respiratory failure initially may present within a few hours to several days, depending on the initial insult, and does not always progress to ARDS.[11] Monitoring patients who meet the SIRS criteria (see Box 27-1) may aid identification of those who are at risk for development of ARDS. No unexplained change in respiratory rate should be taken lightly because there are few reliable early indicators of impending ALI or ARDS. Vital signs throughout the progression of ARDS vary, but the general trend is hypotension, tachycardia, and hyperthermia or hypothermia. Respiration, initially rapid and labored, varies once mechanical ventilation is instituted.

Early signs and symptoms of respiratory failure include tachypnea, dyspnea, and tachycardia. Breath sounds often are clear in this phase (Table 27-4). Patients with acute respiratory failure may exhibit neurological changes, such as restlessness and agitation associated with impaired oxygenation and decreased perfusion to the brain. Use of accessory respiratory muscles is evident. The cardiovascular response is tachycardia to improve cardiac output as compensation for poor tissue oxygenation. These attempts to reduce hypoxia represent an adaptive sympathetic nervous system response. In both ALI and ARDS, these attempts to reduce hypoxia are likely to be ineffective because mediators are already circulating and triggering a cascade of systemic responses.

As the pathological changes progress, lung auscultation may reveal crackles secondary to an increase in secretions and narrowed airways; however, the bubbling crackles of cardiogenic pulmonary edema may be minimal. Assessment must be considered in the context of the presenting or initiating disease. For example, pneumonia, one risk factor for ARDS, may confound the ability to diagnose early-stage lung sound changes. The patient may be increasingly restless and confused secondary to hypoxia. Decreases in arterial oxygen saturation (SaO_2) are early signs of impending decompensation.

The ability to compensate decreases with increasing pathological changes to the lung, pulmonary vasculature, and bronchi. Dependent lung fields have decreased breath sounds as fluid accumulation and alveoli collapse occur. Agitation may give way to lethargy, an ominous sign in which interventions to support ventilation and oxygenation are required quickly. Other later stages of progression result from tissue hypoxia and include dysrhythmias, chest pain, decreased renal function, and decreased bowel sounds. These are indications of multisystem involvement as highly perfused organ systems respond to decreased oxygen delivery with diminished function.

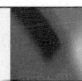

Stage	Physical Examination	Diagnostic Test Results
Stage 1 (first 12 h)	• Restlessness, dyspnea, tachypnea • Moderate to extensive use of accessory respiratory muscles	• *ABG:* Respiratory alkalosis • *CXR:* No radiographic changes • *Chemistry:* Blood results may vary depending on precipitating cause (e.g., elevated white blood cell count, changes in hemoglobin) • *Hemodynamics:* Elevated PAP, normal or low PAWP
Stage 2 (24 h)	• Severe dyspnea, tachypnea, cyanosis, tachycardia • Coarse bilateral crackles • Decreased air entry to dependent lung fields • Increased agitation and restlessness	• *ABG:* Decreased SaO_2 despite supplemental oxygen administration • *CXR:* Patchy bilateral infiltrates • *Chemistry:* Increasing acidosis (metabolic) depending on severity of onset • *Hemodynamics:* Increasingly elevated PAP, normal or low PAWP
Stage 3 (2–10 days)	• Decreased air entry bilaterally • Impaired responsiveness (may be related to sedation necessary to maintain mechanical ventilation) • Decreased gut motility • Generalized edema • Poor skin integrity and breakdown	• *ABG:* Worsening hypoxemia • *CXR:* Air bronchograms, decreased lung volumes • *Chemistry:* Signs of other organ involvement: decreased platelets and hemoglobin, increased white blood cell count, abnormal clotting factors • *Hemodynamics:* Unchanged or becoming increasingly worse
Stage 4 (>10 days)	• Symptoms of MODS, including decreased urine output, poor gastric motility, symptoms of impaired coagulation **OR** • Single-system involvement of the respiratory system with gradual improvement over time	• *ABG:* Worsening hypoxemia and hypercapnia • *CXR:* Air bronchograms, pneumothoraces • *Chemistry:* Persistent signs of other organ involvement: decreased platelets and hemoglobin, increased white blood cell count, abnormal clotting factors • *Hemodynamics:* Unchanged or becoming increasingly worse

ABG, arterial blood gas; CXR, chest radiograph; MODS, multisystem organ dysfunction syndrome; PAP, pulmonary artery pressure; PAWP, pulmonary artery wedge pressure.

In the later stages of ARDS, mechanical ventilation support is required. Consolidation of the lungs with fluid reduces breath sounds. Lung compliance is decreased, and increasing difficulties maintaining ventilation in the face of increasing resistance ensue. Unexplained changes in ventilation (such as a decreased PaO_2 or increased peak inspiratory pressure) cannot be minimized because development of spontaneous pneumothoraces is a frequent complication of ARDS in the later stages. Transmitted sounds, poor air entry throughout all lung fields, and diffuse crackles coupled with ventilation make breath sounds difficult to assess. A further complicating event is myocardial depression, a mediated response. Therefore, despite persistent tachycardia, cardiac output decreases, and hypotension results.

DIAGNOSTIC STUDIES

Throughout the stages of ARDS, the reliance on diagnostic tests is important (see Table 27-4). In the early stages, the need to establish cause may require specific tests, such as blood cultures, bronchoalveolar lavage cultures, and computed tomography (CT) examinations for abscess (e.g., abdominal abscesses). In later stages, further vigilance is required to intervene for early management of any nosocomial infections. Ongoing monitoring of routine blood gases, chemistry, and hematology is performed to ensure stability in metabolic parameters and optimization of existing function. Other laboratory studies are generally nonspecific and may include leukocytosis and lactic acidosis.

The use of bronchoalveolar lavage samples for detection of mediators, particularly elevated amounts of interleukin-1 (IL-1) and TNF-α, as early markers for diagnosis of ARDS remains experimental.[24] Persistence of neutrophils in bronchoalveolar lavage, proinflammatory cytokines (IL-1, TNF-α, IL-8), and elevated plasma surfactant protein D (SP-D) may be indicators of a poor prognosis.[10,25]

Blood Gas Analysis

Deterioration of arterial blood gases (ABGs), despite interventions, is a hallmark of ARDS. Initially, hypoxemia (an arterial oxygen tension, or PaO_2, of <60 mm Hg) may improve with supplemental oxygen; however, refractory hypoxemia (no improvement of PaO_2 with supplemental oxygen) and a persistently low SaO_2 eventually develop. Early in acute respiratory failure, dyspnea and tachypnea are associated with a decreased $PaCO_2$. Hypercarbia develops as gas exchange and ventilation become increasingly impaired. Arterial pH in the early phase may be high (>7.45), a finding that is consistent with respiratory alkalosis secondary to rapid respirations and a low $PaCO_2$. The arterial pH measurements in ARDS are typically lower because of respiratory and ventilatory failure and tissue hypoxia, anaerobic metabolism, and subsequent metabolic acidosis. Base excess and deficit follow a similar trend, depending on the degree of tissue and organ hypoxia.

Measurement of arterial lactate is commonly ordered as an indication of tissue hypoxia and anaerobic metabolism. An elevated blood lactate concentration is common in early ARDS and resolves as oxygenation improves. Lactate measurement is not performed routinely once adequate, although perhaps not optimal, oxygenation has been achieved.

Radiographic Studies

In the early phase of ARDS, the chest radiographic changes are usually negligible. Within a few days, the chest radiographic findings show patchy bilateral alveolar infiltrates, usually in the dependent lung fields. This may be mistaken for cardiogenic pulmonary edema. Over time, these patchy infiltrates progress to diffuse infiltrates, consolidation, and air bronchograms. CT of the chest also shows areas of infiltrates and consolidation of lung tissue. Daily chest radiographs are important in the continuing evaluation of the progression and resolution of ARDS and for ongoing assessment of potential complications, especially pneumothoraces.

Intrapulmonary Shunt Measurement

An intrapulmonary shunt is a type of ventilation–perfusion mismatch. It may be defined as the percentage of cardiac output that is not oxygenated owing to pulmonary blood flowing past collapsed or fluid-filled and nonventilated alveoli (a physiological shunt), absence of blood flow to ventilated alveoli (alveolar dead space), or a combination of both of these conditions (silent unit; see Chapter 23, Fig. 23-16). Normally, an intrapulmonary shunt of 3% to 5% is present in all people. Advanced respiratory failure and ARDS are associated with a shunt of 15% or more because of the pathological changes in blood flow, endothelial disruption, and alveolar collapse. As the intrapulmonary shunt increases to 15% and greater, more aggressive interventions, including mechanical ventilation, are required because this level of shunt is associated with profound hypoxemia and may be life-threatening.

The intrapulmonary shunt fraction (Qs/Qt) is calculated using the arterial oxygen content (CaO_2), the mixed venous oxygen content ($C\bar{v}O_2$), and the capillary oxygen content (CcO_2). Oxygen content is determined by hemoglobin (Hgb), oxygen saturation (SO_2), and partial pressure of oxygen (PO_2), measured by calculating the oxygen content in the pulmonary capillary bed, in the systemic arterial system, and in the mixed venous blood from the pulmonary artery. The intrapulmonary shunt fraction may be estimated using a simple calculation, the ratio of arterial oxygen to inspired oxygen (i.e., the PaO_2/FiO_2 ratio). In general, a PaO_2/FiO_2 ratio greater than 300 is normal, a value of 200 is associated with an intrapulmonary shunt of 15% to 20%, and a value of 100 is associated with an intrapulmonary shunt of more than 20%.

Lung Compliance, Airway Resistance, and Pressures

Lung mechanics are altered in ARDS, resulting in reduced alveolar ventilation and pulmonary gas

Box 27-2 • Examples of Nursing Diagnoses and Collaborative Problems for the Patient With Acute Respiratory Distress Syndrome

- Gas Exchange, Impaired, related to refractory hypoxemia and pulmonary interstitial/alveolar leaks found in alveolar capillary injury states
- Airway Clearance, Ineffective, related to increased secretion production and decreased ciliary motion
- Breathing Patterns, Ineffective, related to inadequate gas exchange, increased secretions, decreased ability to oxygenate adequately, fear, or exhaustion
- Anxiety related to critical illness, fear of death, role changes, or permanent disability
- Infection, Risk for, related to invasive monitoring devices and endotracheal tube

exchange. Lung compliance, or distensibility, is decreased as the alveoli become fluid filled or collapsed. More effort and greater pressure are required to move air into the lungs as they become increasingly "stiff." In addition, the resistance to airflow into and out of the lungs increases with the accumulation of secretions and mediator-induced bronchoconstriction. Because the patient with ARDS requires mechanical ventilation to support oxygenation and ventilation, lung compliance and airway resistance can be evaluated by assessing ventilator pressures and tidal volume changes.

Close monitoring of airway pressures, including the mean airway pressure, the peak inspiratory pressure, and the plateau pressure, is an important component of patient assessment in ARDS. Increases in these pressures as tidal volumes are maintained to achieve a normal $PaCO_2$ indicate reduced compliance and increased resistance to airflow. As airway pressures rise, the lung epithelium is traumatized, resulting in further lung tissue damage. Volutrauma (lung epithelial damage) or barotrauma from persistently elevated airway pressures thus has additional deleterious effects on ventilation and oxygenation.[26]

Possible nursing diagnoses for a patient with ARDS are given in Box 27-2.

• Management

Therapeutic modalities to actually treat ARDS have remained elusive. Although there are multiple potential causes of ARDS, management principles are similar. Treatment is supportive; that is, contributing factors are corrected or reversed, and while the lungs heal, care is taken so that treatment does no further damage. Figure 27-3 describes the current status of the management of ARDS.

In addition, extensive work has gone into creating "bundles," which are elements of care considered core to the management and treatment of specific critical illnesses in intensive care units (ICUs). Recent

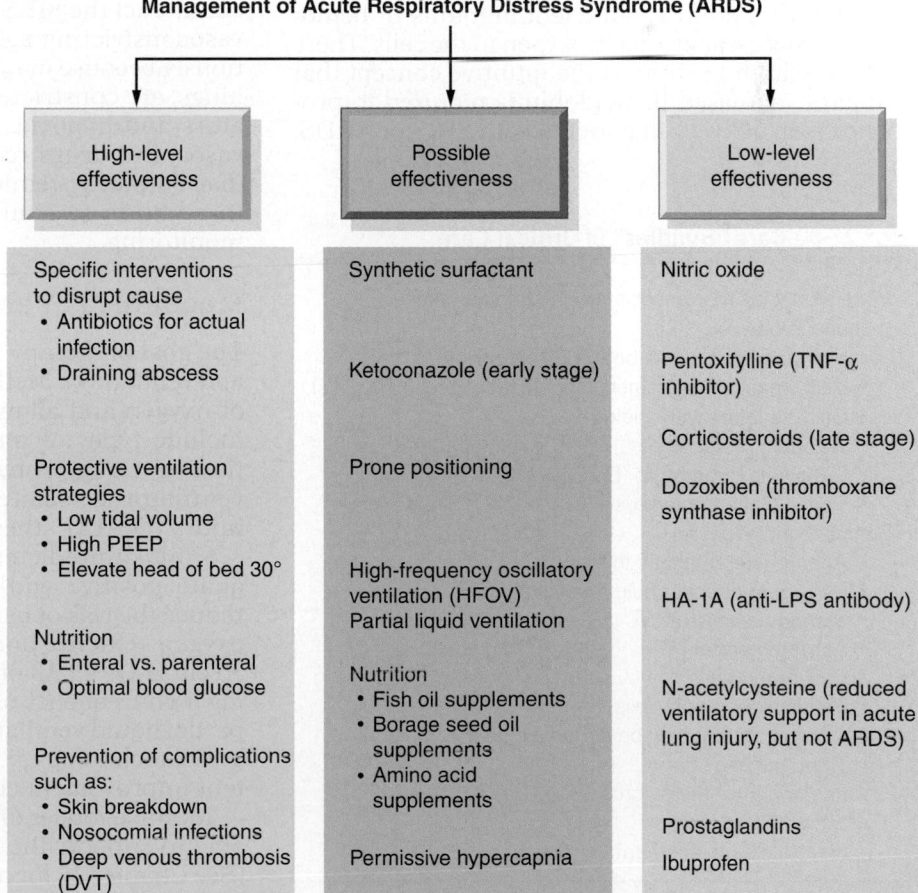

Figure 27-3 • Management of acute respiratory distress syndrome (ARDS). Treatment involves interventions of proven, possible, or minimal to low effectiveness. Therapies supported by multicentered trials are included in the proven list. No items in this list, except specific interventions to disrupt cause, have been shown to treat ARDS; rather, they provide adjunct therapy to reduce complications or length of ventilator days. Items that appear in the possible effectiveness category have support through limited individual studies with promising results. One of the primary issues in obtaining proof of efficacy includes a lack of randomized controlled trials for many treatments currently in use. PEEP, positive end-expiratory pressure; TNF-α, tumor necrosis factor-α.

Management of Acute Respiratory Distress Syndrome (ARDS)

High-level effectiveness	Possible effectiveness	Low-level effectiveness
Specific interventions to disrupt cause • Antibiotics for actual infection • Draining abscess	Synthetic surfactant Ketoconazole (early stage)	Nitric oxide Pentoxifylline (TNF-α inhibitor) Corticosteroids (late stage)
Protective ventilation strategies • Low tidal volume • High PEEP • Elevate head of bed 30°	Prone positioning	Dozoxiben (thromboxane synthase inhibitor)
Nutrition • Enteral vs. parenteral • Optimal blood glucose	High-frequency oscillatory ventilation (HFOV) Partial liquid ventilation	HA-1A (anti-LPS antibody)
Prevention of complications such as: • Skin breakdown • Nosocomial infections • Deep venous thrombosis (DVT)	Nutrition • Fish oil supplements • Borage seed oil supplements • Amino acid supplements Permissive hypercapnia	N-acetylcysteine (reduced ventilatory support in acute lung injury, but not ARDS) Prostaglandins Ibuprofen

reviews of sepsis bundles are used to illustrate many of the core management principles considered for ARDS.[26–28] Box 27-3 lists essential critical care bundles that apply to the management of ARDS. These treatments span prevention at early stages of onset of disease, such as early goal-directed fluid resuscitation and longer-term prevention of complications such as sedation protocols. Regardless, one of the most important roles for critical care nurses is ensuring attention to all these elements to prevent mortality and to aid recovery.

OXYGENATION AND VENTILATION

Oxygen Delivery

Refractory hypoxemia is one of the hallmarks of ARDS; therefore, attention to improving oxygen delivery is paramount. Strategies have attempted to optimize normal oxygen delivery parameters, including hemoglobin, cardiac output, and oxygen saturation. Oxygen delivery (DaO_2) is the amount of oxygen delivered to the tissues and organs every minute and depends on the flow of oxygenated blood through the tissue beds. Parameters that determine DaO_2 are hemoglobin, arterial oxygenation, and cardiac output.

Adequate DaO_2 (>800 mL O_2/minute) is essential to meet tissue requirements for oxygen, thereby preventing anaerobic metabolism and hypoxia, which can trigger and perpetuate SIRS. Critically ill patients with ARDS have high demands for oxygen to maintain organ function.

Hemoglobin combines with oxygen to form oxyhemoglobin; therefore, sufficient amounts of hemoglobin are necessary to carry oxygen to the cells. There is little research to support the intuitive concept that normal or increased hemoglobin is required to promote oxygen delivery in patients with SIRS or ARDS.

Studies on transfusion requirements indicate that values of approximately 8.0 g/dL are sufficient for critically ill patients, except for those with cardiac disease. In addition, there are linkages between blood transfusions and development of ALI.[29] Therefore, transfusion to maintain normal hemoglobin is no longer accepted therapy and should be discouraged.[30]

Cardiac output is typically altered in ARDS because of the SIRS, the effect of hypoxemia on the myocardium, and the decrease in venous return induced by mechanical ventilation.[31] Evaluation of the cardiac output is important to assess oxygen delivery and initiate appropriate interventions. Therapies to optimize cardiac output are directed toward enhancing preload and contractility and normalizing afterload. Use of a thermodilution pulmonary artery catheter to assess oxygen delivery and consumption is routine for patients with ARDS to ensure that the appropriate interventions are instituted.

Fluid management has been used for many years in an effort to balance the type of fluid needed to manage the hallmark edema and decompensation associated with ARDS; however, it is now under review. At the onset of the disease, early goal-directed fluid resuscitation is recommended.[28] Diuretics and reduced fluid administration have been studied to reduce lung edema. Although these strategies result in fewer ventilator days and shorter time spent in the ICU, actual mortality is unchanged.[32]

Positive inotropic agents, such as dopamine or dobutamine, are used to enhance contractility and increase cardiac output. Vasoconstrictors, such as norepinephrine, may be added to the therapies to counteract the SIRS-induced vasodilation. However, vasoconstricting agents must be administered cautiously because many vascular beds, especially in the lungs, are constricted, also as a result of SIRS mediators and hypoxia. Patients receiving inotropic or vasoactive drugs require regular evaluation of cardiac output, systemic vascular resistance, and PAWP, in addition to continuous arterial blood pressure monitoring.

Mechanical Ventilation

The goal of therapy is to improve tissue oxygenation and ventilation. Methods to deliver appropriate levels of oxygen and allow for removal of carbon dioxide include types of mechanical ventilation and positioning. Lung-protective ventilation strategies limit ventilator-associated (or ventilator-induced) lung injury (VALI); these include low tidal volumes (<6 mL/kg predicted body weight), the use of adequate positive end-expiratory pressure (PEEP) to reduce the risk of using a high FiO_2 and precipitating oxygen toxicity, and limiting plateau pressures to 30 cm H_2O.[33–35] All other ventilation therapies, including high-frequency oscillation ventilation (HFOV),[36–38] partial liquid ventilation,[39,40] and extracorporeal lung-assist technology,[41] have not demonstrated consistent improvements in patient outcomes in ARDS.

Multiple modes of mechanical ventilation are available to support the patient with respiratory failure. (See Chapter 25 for a complete discussion of mechan-

---

Box 27-3 • Care "Bundles" in Critical Care

Ventilator: ventilator-associated pneumonia (VAP) "bundle" basics
- Elevated head of the bed 30–45 degrees
- Daily weaning assessment (spontaneous breathing trials)
- Daily sedation withholding
- Weaning protocol
- Deep vein thrombosis (DVT) prophylaxis
- Peptic ulcer prophylaxis

Sepsis "bundle" basics
- Appropriate antibiotic therapy
- Early goal-directed fluid resuscitation
- Steroid administration
- Activated protein C
- DVT prophylaxis
- Peptic ulcer prophylaxis

Other protocols that may be added include:
- Tight glucose control
- Feeding after the pylorus
- Subglottic suctioning
- Electrolyte replacement

ical ventilation.) In general, the principle of "do no harm" includes use of the lowest FiO_2 to achieve adequate oxygenation and use of small tidal volumes to minimize airway pressures, thus preventing or reducing lung damage (barotrauma and volutrauma). Permissive hypercapnia may be necessary to prevent an increased respiratory rate in the face of lower tidal volumes.[42] PEEP prevents collapse and opens alveolar sacs, allowing diffusion of gases across the alveolar–capillary membrane. Recommended values for PEEP are 10 to 15 cm H_2O, but values in excess of 20 cm H_2O are acceptable to reduce inspired oxygen requirements or maintain adequate oxygenation.

Permissive hypercapnia is a strategy that allows the $PaCO_2$ to rise slowly above normal through reduction of tidal volume, therefore limiting the plateau and peak airway pressures. A $PaCO_2$ between 55 and 60 mm Hg and a pH of 7.25 to 7.35 are tolerated when achieved gradually.[42] It is necessary to monitor the increase in $PaCO_2$ to prevent too rapid a rise, and overall values should be no greater than 80 to 100 mg Hg because of the potential effects on cardiopulmonary function. These techniques are not used for patients with cardiac or neurological involvement.

Several modes of mechanical ventilation are directed toward minimizing airway pressures and iatrogenic lung injury, associated with conventional volume-controlled mechanical ventilation.[41] Pressure-controlled ventilation limits the peak inspiratory pressure to a set level (as opposed to volume-controlled ventilation, which delivers a set tidal volume despite the pressure required to move the set volume into the lungs). Pressure-controlled ventilation also uses a decelerating inspiratory airflow pattern to minimize the peak pressure while delivering the necessary tidal volume. Patients on pressure-controlled ventilation mode typically require significant amounts of sedation and pharmacological paralysis to prevent attempts at breathing and dyssynchrony with the ventilator. Airway pressure release ventilation is similar to pressure-controlled ventilation but with the advantage of allowing the patient to initiate breaths; therefore, these patients do not require the same level of sedation or paralysis to achieve pressure-limited ventilation.

Inverse-ratio ventilation is another strategy thought to improve alveolar recruitment. Reversal of the normal inspiratory/expiratory ratio (I/E ratio) to 2:1 or 3:1 prolongs inspiration time, preventing complete exhalation. An inverse I/E ratio is achieved through manipulation of the mechanical ventilator. This increased end-expiratory volume creates auto-PEEP (intrinsic PEEP) that is added to the applied extrinsic PEEP. The theoretical advantages include reduced alveolar pressures and overall PEEP levels. This therapy requires patients to be sedated or given paralytics to improve tolerance.

Novel Ventilation Strategies

HFOV uses very low tidal volumes delivered at rates between 60 and 100 breaths/minute, resulting in lower airway pressures and reduced barotrauma. Deleteri-

ous effects of HFOV include increased trapping of air in the alveoli (auto-PEEP) and increased mean airway pressures to high levels in some patients. Research is ongoing as to the possible effectiveness of this ventilation technique.[36–38]

The use of liquid breathing with perfluorocarbons as the medium for gas exchange is perhaps one of the most exciting of the novel ventilation strategies currently being tested.[39] This technique is thought to provide decreased surface tension, assist with distention of collapsed alveoli, and remove inflammatory debris. In one trial, this therapy led to more ventilator-free days, but further study is needed.[40] This technique requires resources that are not readily available in nonacademic medical centers, which may limit proliferation of its use for some time, even if its efficacy is established.

Extracorporeal lung-assist technology involves the use of large vascular cannulas to remove blood from the patient. A pumping device and circuit circulate the blood, and one or two "artificial lungs" remove carbon dioxide and oxygenate the blood. Extracorporeal membrane oxygenation (ECMO) and extracorporeal carbon dioxide removal (ECCO$_2$R) may potentially be effective in the management of ARDS, but at present their use is controversial.[41] These highly invasive, high-risk technologies allow the lungs to "rest" because near-apneic ventilation or ventilation with small tidal volumes and slow respiratory rates greatly reduces airway pressures while gas exchange takes place in the artificial membrane lungs. The need for intensive resources and personnel with a high degree of expertise, coupled with the potential for devastating complications (particularly intracranial hemorrhage) and a lack of conclusive benefits for patients with ARDS, make extracorporeal lung-assist technology of limited use.

Positioning

Frequent position change is well established as a means to prevent and reverse atelectasis and facilitate removal of secretions from the airways. Although not a treatment for ARDS, elevating the head of the bed greater than 30 degrees is considered necessary care for preventing VAP.

Prone positioning, in the patient's bed or using a Stryker frame, improves pulmonary gas exchange, facilitates pulmonary drainage in the dorsal lung regions, and aids resolution of consolidated dependent alveoli (in the supine position), particularly in the dorsal lung regions. The evidence for the effectiveness of prone positioning, now a common intervention with ARDS, is variable.[43,44] Randomized, controlled trials are underway, and these results will be necessary before support for prone positioning becomes clear.[45] There are alternative explanations for the improved oxygenation associated with prone positioning, and the question of whether the improvement in oxygenation persists beyond a short time remains controversial. The associated risks include loss of airway control through accidental extubation, loss of vascular access, facial edema and development of pressure areas, and difficulties with cardiopulmonary resuscitation. Recommendations on the steps involved in prone positioning appear in Box 27-4.[46]

PHARMACOLOGICAL THERAPY

Most of the pharmacological agents used in the ARDS population are supportive. Researchers developed many agents as treatments directed at specific mediators, with the goal of disrupting or interfering with the development of SIRS. However, most of these promising pharmacological interventions ultimately proved ineffective in humans, notably anti-TNF drugs, most anti-inflammatory mediators, and inhaled gases such as nitric oxide.[47,48] Of the treatments now available, the ones that have some therapeutic promise are surfactant,[49–51] corticosteroids,[52–54] and β-adrenergic agonists,[55] but these remain experimental.

Antibiotic therapy is appropriate in the presence of a known microorganism but should not be used prophylactically. The signs of SIRS are similar to those of infection (i.e., tachycardia, fever, increased white blood cell count), thus creating the temptation to treat the patient with SIRS with antimicrobial therapy. It is essential to identify a source of infection (isolation of specific bacteria through blood, wound, pulmonary, and other cultures) before initiating antibiotics. Prophylactic antibiotic therapy has not been shown to improve outcome. Emphasis is on prevention of infection, especially nosocomial infection related to the use of invasive vascular catheters and ventilators (e.g., VAP).

Bronchodilators and mucolytics are useful in ARDS to assist in maintaining airway patency and reducing the inflammatory reaction and accumulation of secretions in the airways. The response to therapy is evaluated by monitoring airway resistance and pressures and lung compliance.

Exogenous surfactant replacement therapy has been used for several years in neonates with hyaline membrane disease to decrease alveolar surface tension and facilitate the maintenance of open alveoli.[50] Administration of surfactant to adults with ARDS has shown some usefulness but requires further investigation. Clinical trials using synthetic surfactant continue to refine the drug delivery system and synthetic surfactant; however, improvements in the need for ventilation or mortality have not been demonstrated.[51] Administration of corticosteroids to decrease the inflammatory response in late stages of ARDS has been used. However, a large randomized controlled clinical trial did not show improvement in 60-day mortality, and therefore the routine use of corticosteroids is not recommended.[52] Researchers are investigating specific conditions in which these agents may be effective, and therefore their use may be continued on a case-by-case basis until further research is completed.[53,54]

Newer pharmacological agents directed toward blocking mediators and the SIRS inflammatory cascade are under investigation, but none has proved effective in treating ARDS. Nitric oxide is an inhaled gas that causes selective pulmonary vasodilation and therefore reduces the deleterious effects of pulmonary hypertension. Despite widespread use, to date, nitric oxide has not been shown to improve mortality or oxygenation beyond the first 24 hours of therapy.[47,48] Other agents that have demonstrated limited effects on the outcomes of ARDS include[56]:

▶ Antioxidants, such as N-acetylcysteine, a glutathione analogue. This drug replenishes glutathione, a natural antioxidant, possibly decreasing endothelial damage caused by oxygen radicals and limiting the duration of lung injury.

▶ Antilipid mediators, such as prostacyclin (prostaglandin E_1 [PGI_2]),[57] and nonsteroidal anti-inflammatory drugs, such as ibuprofen or indomethacin. These agents theoretically interact with the arachidonic acid cascade metabolites, which produce lung endothelial injury and inflammation. However, a multicenter trial showed that this treatment has no benefit.

▶ Neutrophil elastase inhibitors (e.g., sivelestat sodium hydrate [Sivelestat]). These agents inhibit neutrophil elastase, which is thought to increase vascular permeability, part of the pathological process of ALI and ARDS.[58]

▶ Ketoconazole. This drug inhibits thromboxane A_2 and leukotriene. Prophylactic doses of this drug

---

Box 27-4 • Summary of Key Steps to Consider for Prone Positioning

1. Evaluate with the interdisciplinary team the patient's condition and determine whether a trial of prone positioning is warranted.
2. Organize the team to ensure familiarity with the procedure and patient care while prone.
   - Use your hospital's evidence-based procedure
   - Equipment on site
   - Assign and clarify team roles during proning
3. Prepare the patient for the procedure.
   - Provide explanation to patient and family
   - Consider insertion of feeding tube, nasogastric tube, or both as necessary
4. Assess and document the patient's pre-proning status.
   - Hemodynamic and ventilatory parameters, skin or wound condition, and so forth
5. Protect and maintain the patient's airway.
   - Secure endotracheal tube
   - Apply in-line suction if not already in place
6. Use safety precautions to ensure body position will be maintained during the proning procedure.
7. Administer adequate sedation, analgesic, and anxiolytic medication.
8. Complete the procedure as per protocol. Note: Risks for inadvertent extubation or line displacement are high during the procedure.
9. Assess, evaluate, and monitor the patient's condition.
10. Implement preventive care for pressure areas, eyes, and skin.

are thought to decrease incidence of ARDS. However, once ALI has been diagnosed, no difference has been reported with treatment using this drug.[56]

▶ Pentoxifylline and lisofylline (its derivative). These drugs diminish proinflammatory cytokine expression through different mechanisms; however, human research has indicated no therapeutic benefit.

▶ β_2-Agonists are of more recent interest. These drugs are thought to improve alveolar fluid clearance by restoring fluid transport and ion exchange across the lung.[56] Small studies indicate improved survival, and a larger trial is needed to further understand the impact of this therapy.[55]

Sedation

Effective use of sedation to promote comfort and reduce respiratory effort, thus decreasing oxygen demand, is an important consideration for nurses dealing with patients with ARDS. Neuromuscular blocking agents and general anesthetics such as propofol, although not sedatives, are all used to decrease the work of breathing and facilitate ventilation for patients with ARDS. These have long- and short-term side effects. The risks include polyneuropathy of critical illness, overfeeding with lipids, and prolongation of days requiring ventilation.[59] In addition, neuromuscular blocking agents require concurrent use of sedation to prevent patients who are chemically paralyzed from being alert but unable to move. Frequent assessment of adequacy of both neuromuscular blockade and sedation is an important nursing intervention.

Pain, anxiety, and delirium are all possible reasons for needing pharmacological treatment, and it is important to distinguish between them because each requires a different pharmacological intervention. It is vital to understand why each is being given, what the goals of therapy are, and what the long-term implications of overuse can be. These considerations are balanced with the need to decrease oxygen demand and provide comfort for patients requiring intensive ventilation management and undergoing potentially uncomfortable procedures.

NUTRITIONAL SUPPORT

Early initiation of nutritional support is essential for patients with ARDS because we now realize that nutrition plays an active therapeutic role in recovery from critical illness.[60] There are two major theoretical reasons to use early enteral feeding as a therapeutic intervention in SIRS and ARDS. Mediators (TNF-α and IL-1 in particular) stimulate release of proteolytic enzymes that stimulate protein catabolism from skeletal muscle. Persistent protein loss is compounded by interstitial loss through capillary leak and down-regulation of messenger RNA production of intravascular proteins such as albumin.[61] Earlier in this chapter, reference was made to changes in circulatory patterns due to hypoxic sympathetic nervous system reactions. In this way, there is decreased perfusion to the gut. After resuscitation, increases in neutrophil release further damage the injured, reperfused colon through increased vascular endothelial permeability, thus releasing normal gut bacteria into the systemic circulation and leading to increases in the incidence of peritonitis, pneumonia, and sepsis. The mechanism through which enteral feeding improves outcome remains unproved, but the reduction in mortality in the critically ill who are enterally fed indicates that this practice is of general benefit.

A diet with a balanced caloric, protein, carbohydrate, and fat intake is calculated based on metabolic needs, with particular attention paid to specific amino acids, lipid, and carbohydrate intake. Patients with SIRS or ARDS usually require 35 to 45 kcal/kg/day. High-carbohydrate solutions are avoided to prevent excess carbon dioxide production. Intralipids are judiciously administered to prevent further up-regulation of the lipid mediators of SIRS, which contributes to inflammation and lung injury. Recent innovations in amino acid supplementation are being reviewed because of the role of amino acids in the immune response.[61]

The problem facing the practitioner is the ability to deliver enteral nutrition in the face of decreased gut motility. Insertion of small bowel feeding tubes may be considered. The role of total parenteral nutrition is controversial, and some clinicians rarely use it, either alone or in combination with enteral nutrition.[60] The risk for aspiration associated with enteral feeding needs to be appreciated, and careful monitoring of absorption and gut function is essential.

A collaborative care guide for the patient with ARDS is given in Box 27-5.

• Prevention of Complications

Complications of ARDS are primarily related to SIRS, VALI, and immobility imposed by critical illness. The most serious of these is the development of MODS due to hypoxemia, hypoxia, and the persistent inflammatory response. An entire spectrum of potential complications exists for the critically ill patient. Critical care forums have compiled evidence-based protocols into bundles for two major critical care situations: VAP and sepsis (see Box 27-3). The introduction of care bundles into critical care supports application of evidence to reduce major complications. The implementation of care bundles has been shown effective in reducing length of stay and reducing ventilator days, but consistent application requires teamwork and monitoring.[27,28,62]

Mechanical ventilation with high levels of PEEP, high tidal volumes, and volume-controlled modes predisposes the patient with ARDS to volutrauma and barotraumas, as previously described. Barotrauma may present as a pneumothorax, pneumomediastinum, or subcutaneous or interstitial emphysema. Prompt chest tube insertion is required for the presence of a pneumothorax. Prevention of volutrauma

(text continues on page 686)

Box 27-5 • COLLABORATIVE CARE GUIDE for the Patient With Acute Respiratory Distress Syndrome (ARDS)

OUTCOMES	INTERVENTIONS
Oxygenation/Ventilation Patent airway will be maintained. A PaO_2:FIO_2 ratio of 200 to 300 or more will be maintained, if possible.	• Auscultate breath sounds every 2 to 4 h and as required. • Intubate to maintain oxygenation and ventilation and decrease work of breathing. • Suction endotracheal airway when appropriate (see Chapter 25, Box 25-16, Collaborative Care Guide for the Patient on Mechanical Ventilation). • Hyperoxygenate and hyperventilate before and after each suction pass.
Lung-protective ventilation strategies will be used. Maintain a low tidal volume (<6 mL/kg), a plateau pressure less than or equal to 30 cm H_2O, and positive end-expiratory pressure (PEEP) levels titrated to pressure–volume curve.	• Monitor airway pressures every 1 to 2 h. • Monitor airway pressures after suctioning. • Administer bronchodilators and mucolytics. • Obtain a PEEP study to determine optimal oxygen delivery. • Consider a change in ventilator mode to prevent barotrauma and volutrauma.
The risk for atelectasis, ventilator-associated pneumonia (VAP), and barotrauma will be reduced and oxygenation will be improved.	• Turn side-to-side every 2 h. • Perform chest physiotherapy every 4 h, if tolerated. • Head of bed elevated 30 degrees. • Take chest x-ray daily.
Oxygenation will be maximized (a PaO_2 of 55 to 80 mm Hg or an SaO_2 of 88% to 95%).	• Monitor pulse oximetry and end-tidal carbon dioxide. • Monitor arterial blood gases as indicated by changes in noninvasive parameters. • Monitor intrapulmonary shunt (Qs/Qt and PaO_2/FIO_2 ratio). • Increase PEEP and FIO_2 to decrease intrapulmonary shunting, using lowest possible FIO_2. • Consider permissive hypercapnia to maximize oxygenation. • Monitor for signs of barotrauma, especially pneumothorax. • Consider risk for prolonged hyperoxia and decrease FIO_2 to less than 65% as soon as able.
Circulation/Perfusion Blood pressure, cardiac output, central venous pressure (CVP), and pulmonary artery pressures remain stable related to mechanical ventilation.	• Assess hemodynamic effects of initiation of mechanical ventilation (e.g., decreased venous return and cardiac output). • Monitor electrocardiogram (ECG) for dysrhythmias related to hypoxemia. • Assess hemodynamic effects of changes in inspiratory pressure settings, tidal volume, PEEP, and ventilatory modes. • Assess effects of ventilator setting changes on cardiac output and oxygen delivery. • Administer intravascular volume to maintain preload.
Blood pressure, heart rate, and hemodynamic parameters are optimized to therapeutic goals (e.g., DaO_2 greater than 600 mL O_2/m²).	• Monitor vital signs every 1 to 2 h. • Monitor pulmonary artery pressures and right atrial pressure every hour and cardiac output, systemic vascular resistance, peripheral vascular resistance, DaO_2, and oxygen consumption ($\dot{V}O_2$) every 6 to 12 h, if pulmonary artery catheter is in place. • Administer intravascular volume as indicated by real or relative hypovolemia, and evaluate response. • Consider monitoring gastric mucosal pH as a guide to systemic perfusion.
Serum lactate will be within normal limits.	• Monitor lactate as required until it is within normal limits. • Administer red blood cells, positive inotropic agents, and colloid infusion as ordered to increase oxygen delivery.

(continued)

Box 27-5 • COLLABORATIVE CARE GUIDE for the Patient With Acute Respiratory Distress Syndrome (ARDS) (Continued)

OUTCOMES	INTERVENTIONS
Fluids/Electrolytes Patient is euvolemic. Urine output is greater than 30 mL/h (or >0.5 mL/kg/h).	• Monitor hydration status to reduce viscosity of lung secretions. • Monitor intake and output. • Avoid use of nephrotoxic substances and overuse of diuretics. • Administer fluids and diuretics to maintain intravascular volume and renal function.
There is no evidence of electrolyte imbalance or renal dysfunction.	• Replace electrolytes as ordered. • Monitor blood urea nitrogen (BUN), creatinine, serum osmolarity, and urine electrolytes as required.
Mobility/Safety There is no evidence of complications related to bed rest and immobility.	• Initiate deep venous thrombosis (DVT) prophylaxis. • Reposition frequently. • Mobilize to chair when acute phase is past, hemodynamic stability and hemostasis achieved. • Consult physiotherapist. • Conduct range-of-motion and strengthening exercises when able.
Physiological changes are detected and treated without delay.	• Monitor mechanical ventilator alarms and settings and patient parameters (e.g., tidal volume) every 1 to 2 h. • Ensure appropriate settings and narrow limits for hemodynamic, heart rate, and pulse oximetry alarms.
There is no evidence of infection; white blood cell count is within normal limits.	• Monitor for systemic inflammatory response syndrome (SIRS) criteria (increased white blood cell count, increased temperature, tachypnea, tachycardia). • Use strict aseptic technique during procedures, and monitor others. • Maintain sterility of invasive catheters and tubes. • Change chest tube and other dressings and invasive catheters. • Culture blood and other fluids and line tips when they are changed.
Skin Integrity Skin will remain intact.	• Assess skin every 4 h and each time patient is repositioned. • Turn every 2 h. • Consider pressure relief/reduction mattress, kinetic therapy bed, or prone positioning. • Use Braden Scale to assess risk for skin breakdown.
Nutrition Caloric and nutrient intake will meet metabolic requirements per calculation (e.g., basal energy expenditure).	• Provide enteral nutrition within 24 h. • Consult dietitian or nutritional support service. • Consider small bowel feeding tube if gastrointestinal motility is an issue for enteral feeding. • Monitor lipid intake. • Monitor albumin, prealbumin, transferrin, cholesterol, triglycerides, and glucose.

Comfort/Pain Control
Patient will be as comfortable as possible as evidenced by stable vital signs or cooperation with treatments or procedures.
	• Objectively assess comfort/pain using a pain scale.
	• Provide analgesia and sedation as indicated by assessment.
	• Monitor patient cardiopulmonary and pain response to medication.
	• If patient is receiving neuromuscular blockade for ventilatory control:
	  • Use peripheral nerve stimulator to assess pharmacological paralysis.
	  • Provide continuous or routine (every 1 to 2 h) intravenous sedation and analgesia.

(continued)

Box 27-5 • COLLABORATIVE CARE GUIDE for the Patient With Acute Respiratory Distress Syndrome (ARDS) (Continued)

OUTCOMES	INTERVENTIONS
Psychosocial Patient demonstrates decreased anxiety.	• Assess vital signs during treatments, discussions, and the like. • Cautiously administer sedatives. • Consult social services, clergy, as appropriate. • Provide for adequate rest and sleep.
Teaching/Discharge Planning Patient/significant others understand procedures and tests needed for treatment.	• Prepare patient/significant others for procedures, such as bronchoscopy, pulmonary artery catheter insertion, or laboratory studies. • Explain the causes and effects of ARDS and the potential for complications, such as sepsis, barotrauma, or renal failure.
Significant others understand the severity of the illness, ask appropriate questions, and anticipate potential complications.	• Encourage significant others to ask questions related to the ventilator, the pathophysiology of ARDS, monitoring, and treatments.

and barotrauma by maintaining the lowest possible airway pressures, PEEP, and tidal volumes may be achieved through the use of pressure-limiting modes of mechanical ventilation.

Prevention or reduction in the incidence of VAP can be accomplished through the use of in-line suction catheters. A newer suctioning practice is the use of Hi-Lo Evac tubes that allow continuous or intermittent subglottic suctioning. The Hi-Lo tube has a separate dorsal lumen that opens into the subglottic region, allowing removal of pooled secretions above the cuff. This technique has been shown to reduce aspiration of secretions associated with VAP.[63,64] Sinusitis is associated with VAP. The critical care nurse needs to monitor for nasal secretions and ensure that devices such as nasotracheal or feeding tubes are removed from the nose when these occur. Elevating the head of the bed 30 degrees and feeding the critically ill patient with a feeding tube after the pylorus have been shown to reduce microaspiration and VAP.

Immobility due to bed rest, sedation, or pharmacological paralysis has multisystem effects. Nosocomial pneumonia not infrequently is acquired from accumulation of secretions in the airways and atelectasis secondary to immobilization, with bacterial access through and around the endotracheal tube. Using techniques to reduce the incidence of VAP are important. As discussed, frequent repositioning accompanied by chest physiotherapy will help to reduce stasis of secretions and facilitate removal.

Deep venous thrombosis (DVT) and subsequent pulmonary embolus may be life-threatening complications of immobility. Initiation of DVT prophylaxis within 48 hours of admission minimizes the risk for development of DVT. Low-dose heparin, graded elastic stockings, external pneumatic compression devices, frequent mobilization, and ambulation have shown utility in reducing DVT formation.

The physiological aging process compounds the severity of the metabolic insults and complications of ARDS (Box 27-6).

• Clinical Applicability Challenges

Case Study

Mr. H., a 61-year-old man, is admitted to the hospital for elective cardiac surgery that is not straightforward. He has a cardiac arrest after coming off the bypass machine and has to be rapidly placed back on bypass. An intraaortic balloon pump is placed to support his heart, and he is sent to the intensive care unit for recovery.

Three days after surgery, Mr. H. remains intubated and on inotropic support of vasopressin, 4 units/hour, and epinephrine, 2 µg/minute, with a reduction of milrinone to 0.25 µg/kg/minute. He has a sudden desaturation to 50%, and his FiO_2 is raised to 100% FiO_2. He is placed on assist-control ventilation of 21 breaths/minute, with positive end-expiratory pressure (PEEP) of 8 cm H_2O. His chest sounds clear with no crackles or wheezes. His temperature is 101.1°F (38.4°C). A bronchial lavage is performed, and no pus, fluid, or blood is seen in the airways. As the day progresses, he becomes difficult to ventilate, and he is paralyzed with cisatracurium (Nimbex). He is also sedated with a fentanyl infusion and midazolam (Versed) infusion. His cardiac index is 2.3, heart rate is 76 beats/minute, central venous pressure is 14 mm Hg, pulmonary artery wedge pressure is 15 mm Hg, and systemic vascular resistance index is 1,676 dynes.sec.m²/cm⁵. Arterial gases show PaO_2 of 68 mm Hg, $PaCO_2$ of 39 mm Hg, pH of 7.45, HCO_3 of 26 mEq/L, and O_2 saturation of 95.5%.

The following day, Mr. H. continues to decline on 100% FiO_2. He has developed a mild to moderate bilateral wheeze in his chest. Chest radiography shows small bilateral effusions but is otherwise clear. PaO_2 remains low at 65 mm Hg. Cultures are sent, and empiric broad-spectrum

Box 27-6 • CONSIDERATIONS FOR THE OLDER PATIENT: Acute Respiratory Distress Syndrome (ARDS)

- People who are 65 years of age or older are at increased risk for multisystem organ involvement with less chance of recovering from ARDS; therefore, the mortality rate is increased in this population.
- Because of increased immunosuppression with aging, the elderly are at greater risk for infection; therefore, nosocomial infections, such as urinary tract infections and ventilator-associated pneumonia, are more common.
- Hemodynamic instability adds metabolic insults to already-decreased renal function, thus predisposing this group to renal failure.
- Decreased stroke volume; possible coronary artery disease (CAD), atherosclerosis, or both; and increased systolic blood pressure and peripheral vascular resistance alter hemodynamic recovery.
- Decreased maximal oxygen uptake associated with decreased lung volumes puts elderly patients at greater risk for ventilator-associated lung injury.
- Decreased muscle mass associated with aging makes recovery from prolonged immobility more difficult. Therefore, an elderly person with ARDS may require prolonged rehabilitation.
- Generalized peripheral edema, multiple invasive tests, and prolonged bed rest, combined with the decreased skin integrity associated with old age, increase the elderly patient's potential for development of pressure ulcers and skin tears.
- Elderly patients with ARDS are at risk for not receiving the same quality and quantity of treatment and care as younger patients, due to the effects of ageism. The patient's age is one factor to consider in outcome and prognosis, but not the only one.
- The incidence of comorbid conditions, especially non–insulin-dependent diabetes mellitus and CAD, increases with age. Research findings indicate that the presence of comorbidity increases the risk for death in patients with ARDS.
- The patient and family may request no initiation of, or early removal from, life support based on previously expressed wishes. A person's life experience or vision of risk related to prolonged illness with high possibility of mortality may influence this decision, and these wishes should be respected.

antibiotics are started. With no improvement in the arterial blood gases and the rising pulmonary arterial pressures (47/16 mm Hg), nitric oxide is started at 10 ppm.

Computed tomography (CT) of the thorax is performed the following day to rule out pulmonary embolus and shows bilateral airspace opacity. This is visible on a chest radiograph the following day. A feeding tube is inserted after the pylorus, and enteral feeds are started.

Seven days after surgery, FiO$_2$ remains at 100%, and nitric oxide continues at 10 ppm with no improvement in oxygenation. Temperature remains elevated at 102°F (39.1°C) with a white blood cell count of 8,000/mm^3. All cultures remain negative. Chest radiography shows fluffy white opacities bilaterally and a collapsed right upper lobe. A bronchoscopy is performed to examine the right upper lobe, and copious secretions are removed. Several short attempts at lung recruitment are done, and because there is still no improvement, Mr. H. is placed in the prone position. Once in the prone position, his blood pressure plummets (despite vasopressors), so he is returned to the supine position.

Over the next week, Mr. H. makes small steps forward with his oxygenation yet continues to require high levels of oxygen. A transbronchial biopsy is performed and demonstrates diffuse alveolar damage and organizing pneumonia without evidence of infection. At this time, high-dose corticosteroids are started intravenously and continued for 3 weeks. The dose is tapered off over a 3-month period.

Mr. H. does well after corticosteroids are initiated. However, he has several episodes of ventilator-associated pneumonia before becoming free of the ventilator. He also develops mediastinitis from methicillin-resistant *Staphylococcus aureus,* requiring a 6-week course of vancomycin.

After almost 4 months in hospital, Mr. H. is discharged home. On a follow-up examination, he has recovered to about 60% of his presurgical exercise tolerance. His pulmonary function test shows only mild impairment. CT of his thorax shows scarring and fibrosis in nondependent lung zones and some bronchiectasis in dependent lung zones. This is interpreted as ventilator-acquired (induced) lung injury with stretch injury in the nondependent areas and airway trauma in the dependent airways.

1. What symptoms were presented early in this case that indicated the onset of ARDS?

2. Early enteral feeding was used to support Mr. H. What other care should the nurse advocate for to reduce complications in Mr. H.?

3. What is the evidence that corticosteroids have a positive benefit in treatment of a patient with late-stage acute respiratory distress syndrome?

Review Questions

1. The diagnosis of acute respiratory distress syndrome is made by
   a. careful assessment of radiographic changes.
   b. restlessness and tachypnea.
   c. tachycardia.
   d. none of the above.

2. Strategies to prevent ventilator-associated lung injury include
   a. low tidal volume, low external positive end-expiratory pressure (PEEP), and limiting plateau pressures.
   b. low tidal volume, high external PEEP, and limiting plateau pressures.

c. permissive hypercapnia and variable oxygen delivery.
d. volume-controlled ventilation.

3. Pharmacological treatment for acute respiratory distress syndrome includes
   a. antibiotics for cultured infections.
   b. corticosteroids for late phase anti-inflammatory treatment.
   c. surfactant for reduction in ventilator days.
   d. nitric oxide for reduced mortality

4. Complications associated with acute respiratory distress syndrome may be limited by the following nursing interventions:
   a. Raising the head of the bed at least 30 degrees
   b. Continuous administration of sedation protocols
   c. Bed rest throughout the ventilatory period
   d. Administration of total parental nutrition

5. Acute respiratory distress syndrome may be prevented through
   a. lung-protective ventilation.
   b. prone positioning.
   c. removal of the inciting cause.
   d. use of multiple ventilation strategies.

References

1. Bernard GR, Artigas A, Brigham KL, et al: The American-European Consensus Conference on ARDS: Definitions, mechanisms, relevant outcomes, and clinical trials coordination. Am J Respir Crit Care Med 149:818–824, 1994
2. Dechert RE: The pathophysiology of acute respiratory distress syndrome. Respir Care Clin North Am 9:283–296, 2003
3. Holness L, Knippen MA, Simmons L, Lachenbruch PA: Fatalities caused by TRALI. Trans Med Rev 18:184–188, 2004
4. Toy P, Popovsky MA, Abraham E, et al: Transfusion-related acute lung injury: Definition and review. Crit Care Med 33:721–726, 2005
5. Boshkov LK: Transfusion-related acute lung injury and the ICU. Crit Care Clin 21:479–495, 2005
6. Silliman CC, Boshkov LK, Mehdizadehkashi Z, Elzi DJ: Transfusion-related acute lung injury: Epidemiology and a prospective analysis of etiologic factors. Blood 101:454–462, 2003
7. Kleinman S, Caulfield T, Chan P, et al: Toward an understanding of transfusion-related acute lung injury: Statement of a consensus panel. Transfusion 44:1774–1789, 2004
8. Schwartz MI, Albert RK: "Imitators" of the ARDS: Implications for diagnosis and treatment. Chest 125:1530–1535, 2004
9. Ware LB, Matthay MA: Clinical practice. Acute pulmonary edema. N Engl J Med 353:2788–2796, 2005
10. Esteban A, Fernadez-Segoviano P, Frutos-Vivar F, et al: Comparison of clinical criteria for the acute respiratory distress syndrome with autopsy findings. Ann Intern Med 141:440–445, 2004
11. Rubenfeld GD, Caldwell E, Peabody E, et al: Incidence and outcomes of acute lung injury. N Engl J Med 353:1685–1693, 2005
12. Frutos-Vivar F, Nin N, Esteban A: Epidemiology of acute lung injury and acute respiratory distress syndrome. Curr Opin Crit Care 10:1–6, 2004
13. Luhr OR, Karlsson M, Thorsteinsson A, et al: The impact of respiratory variables on mortality in non-ARDS and ARDS patients requiring mechanical ventilation. Intensive Care Med 26:508–517, 2000
14. Iribarren C, Jacobs DR Jr, Sideny S, et al: Cigarette smoking, alcohol consumption, and risk of ARDS: A 15-year cohort study in a managed care setting. Chest 117:163–168, 2000
15. Moss M, Parsons PE, Steinberg KP, et al: Chronic alcohol abuse is associated with an increased incidence of acute respiratory distress syndrome and severity of multiple organ dysfunction in patients with septic shock. Crit Care Med 31:869–877, 2003
16. Hudson LD, Milberg JA, Anardi, D, Maunder RJ: Clinical risks for development of the acute respiratory distress syndrome. Am J Resp Crit Care Med 151:293–301, 1995
17. Vidar L, Gualis B, Rodriquez A: Clinical resolution in patients with suspicion of ventilator-associated pneumonia: A cohort study comparing patients with and without acute respiratory distress syndrome. Crit Care Med 33:1429–1430, 2005
18. MacCallum NS, Evans TW: Epidemiology of acute lung injury. Curr Opin Crit Care 11:43–49, 2005
19. Brower RG, Lanken PN, MacIntyre N, et al: Higher versus lower positive end-expiratory pressures in patients with the acute respiratory distress syndrome. N Engl J Med 351:327–336, 2004
20. Martin M, Salim A, Murray J, Demetriades D: The decreasing incidence and mortality of acute respiratory distress syndrome after injury: A 5-year observational study. J Trauma. 59:1107–1113, 2005
21. Esteban A, Anzueto A, Frutos F, et al: Characteristics and outcomes in adult patients receiving mechanical ventilation: A 28-day international study. JAMA 287:345–355, 2002
22. Cunneen J, Cartwright M: The puzzle of sepsis: Fitting the pieces of the inflammatory response with treatment. AACN Clin Issues 15:18–44, 2004
23. van Soeren MH, Diehl-Jones WL, Maykut RJ, et al: Pathophysiology and implications for treatment of acute respiratory distress syndrome. AACN Clin Issues 11:179–197, 2000
24. Pittet JF, Mackersie RC, Martin TR, et al: Biological markers of acute lung injury: Prognostic and pathogenic significance. Am J Respir Crit Care Med 155:1187–1205, 1997
25. Eisner MD, Parsons P, Matthay MA, et al: Plasma surfactant levels and clinical outcomes in patients with acute lung injury. Thorax 58:983–988, 2003
26. Winters B, Dorman T: Patient-safety and quality initiatives in the intensive-care unit. Curr Opin Anaesthesiol 19:140–145, 2006
27. Crunden E, Boyce C, Woodman H., Bray B: An evaluation of the impact of the ventilator care bundle. Nurs Crit Care 10:242–246, 2005
28. Resar R, Pronovost P, Haraden C, et al: Using a bundle approach to improve ventilator care processes and reduce ventilator-associated pneumonia. Jt Comm J Qual Saf 31:243–248, 2005
29. Gong MN, Thompson BT, Williams P, et al: Clinical predictors of and mortality in acute respiratory distress syndrome: potential role of red cell transfusion. Crit Care Med 33:1191–1198, 2005
30. Hebert PC, Wells G, Blanjchman MA, et al: A multi-center, randomised, controlled clinical trial of transfusion requirements in critical care. N Engl J Med 340:409–417, 1999
31. National Heart, Lung, and Blood Institute Acute Respiratory Distress Syndrome (ARDS) Clinical Trials Network; Wheeler AP, Bernard GR, Thompson BT, et al: Pulmonary-artery versus central venous catheter to guide treatment of acute lung injury. N Engl J Med 354:2213–2224, 2006
32. National Heart, Lung, and Blood Institute Acute Respiratory Distress Syndrome (ARDS) Clinical Trials Network; Wiedemann HP, Wheeler AP, Bernard GR, et al: Comparison of two fluid-management strategies in acute lung injury N Engl J Med 354:2564–2575, 2006
33. Petrucci N, Iacovelli W: Ventilation with lower tidal volumes versus traditional tidal volumes in adults for acute lung injury and acute respiratory distress syndrome. Cochrane Database Syst Rev 2:CD003844, 2004
34. Villar J, Kacmarek RM, Perez-Mendez L, Aguirre-Jaime A: A high positive end-expiratory pressure, low tidal volume venti-

latory strategy improves outcome in persistent acute respiratory distress syndrome: A randomized, controlled trial. Crit Care Med 34:1311–1318, 2006

35. Kallet RH, Jasmer RM, Pittet JF, et al: Clinical implementation of the ARDS network protocol is associated with reduced hospital mortality compared with historical controls Crit Care Med 33:925–929, 2005

36. Fan E, Mehta S: High-frequency oscillatory ventilation and adjunctive therapies: Inhaled nitric oxide and prone positioning. Crit Care Med 33(Suppl):S182–187, 2005

37. Imai Y, Slutsky AS: High-frequency oscillatory ventilation and ventilator-induced lung injury. Crit Care Med 33(Suppl): S129–134, 2005

38. Wunsch H, Mapstone J: High frequency ventilation versus conventional ventilation for treatment of acute lung injury and acute respiratory distress syndrome. Cochrane Database Syst Rev 1:CD004085, 2004

39. Kacmarek RM, Wiedemann HP, Lavin PT, et al: Partial liquid ventilation in adult patients with acute respiratory distress syndrome. Am J Respir Crit Care Med 173:882–889, 2005

40. Hirchl RB, Pranikoff T, Wise C, et al: Prospective, randomized, controlled pilot study of partial liquid ventilation in adult acute respiratory distress syndrome. Am J Respir Crit Care Med 165:781–787, 2002

41. Bein T, Weber F, Philipp A, et al: A new pumpless extracorporeal interventional lung assist in critical hypoxemia/hypercapnia. Crit Care Med 34:1372–1377, 2006

42. Ni Chonghaile M, Higgins B, Laffey JG: Permissive hypercapnia: Role in protective lung ventilatory strategies. Curr Opin Crit Care 11:56–62, 2005

43. Pelosi P, Brazzi L, Gattinoni L: Prone position in acute respiratory distress syndrome. Eur Respir J 20:1017–1028, 2002

44. Ward NS: Effects of prone position ventilation in ARDS: An evidence-based review of the literature. Crit Care Clin 18:35–44, 2002

45. Mancebo J, Fernandez R, Blanch L, et al: A multicenter trial of prolonged prone ventilation in severe acute respiratory distress syndrome. Am J Respir Crit Care Med 173:1233–1239, 2006

46. Rowe C: Development of clinical guidelines for prone positioning in critically ill adults. Nurs Crit Care 9:50–57, 2004

47. Taylor RW, Zimmerman JL, Dellinger RP, et al: Low dose inhaled nitric oxide in patients with acute lung injury: A randomized controlled trial. JAMA 291:1603–1609, 2004

48. Adhikari N, Granton JT: Inhaled nitric oxide for acute lung injury: No place for NO? JAMA 291:1629–1631, 2004

49. Eisner MD, Parsons P, Matthay MA, et al; Acute Respiratory Distress Syndrome Network: Plasma surfactant protein levels and clinical outcomes in patients with acute lung injury. Thorax 58:983–988, 2003

50. Spragg RG, Lewis JF, Walmrath HD, et al: Effect of recombinant surfactant protein C-based surfactant on the acute respiratory distress syndrome. N Eng J Med 351:884–892, 2004

51. Baudouin SV: Exogenous surfactant replacement in ARDS: One day, some day, or never? N Engl J Med 351:853–858, 2004

52. Steinberg KP, Hudson LD, Goodman RB, et al; National Heart, Lung, and Blood Institute Acute Respiratory Distress Syndrome (ARDS) Clinical Trials Network. Efficacy and safety of corticosteroids for persistent acute respiratory distress syndrome. N Engl J Med 354:1671–1684, 2006

53. Lee HS, Lee JM, Kim MS, et al: Low-dose steroid therapy at an early phase of postoperative acute respiratory distress syndrome. Ann Thorac Surg 79:405–410, 2005

54. Annane D, Sebille V, Bellissant E: Effect of low doses of corticosteroids in septic shock patients with or without early acute respiratory distress syndrome. Crit Care Med 34:22–30, 2006.

55. Perkins GD, McAuley DF, Thickett DR, et al: The Beta-Agonist Lung Injury Trial (BALIT): A randomized placebo-controlled clinical trial. Am J Respir Crit Care Med 173:281–287, 2006

56. Cepkova M, Matthay MA: Pharmacology of acute lung injury and the acute respiratory distress syndrome. J Intensive Care Med 21:119–143, 2006

57. Domenighetti G, Stricker H, Waldispuehl B: Nebulized prostacyclin (PGI2) in acute respiratory distress syndrome: Impact of primary (pulmonary injury) and secondary (extrapulmonary injury) disease on gas exchange. Crit Care Med 29:57–62, 2001

58. Zeiher BG, Artigas A, Vincent JL, et al: Neutrophil elastase inhibition in acute lung injury: Results of the STRIVE study. Crit Care Med 32:1695–1702, 2004

59. Bercker S, Weber-Carstens S, Deja M, et al: Critical illness polyneuropathy and myopathy in patients with acute respiratory distress syndrome. Crit Care Med 33:711–715, 2005

60. Parrish CR, McCray SF: Nutrition support for the mechanically ventilated patient. Crit Care Nurse 23:77–80, 2003

61. Biolo G, Grimble G, Preiser JC, et al: European Society of Intensive Care Medicine Working Group on Nutrition and Metabolism. Metabolic basis of nutrition in intensive care unit patients: ten critical questions. Intensive Care Med 28:1512–1520, 2002

62. Cocanour CS, Peninger M, Domonoske BD, et al: Decreasing ventilator-associated pneumonia in a trauma ICU. J Trauma 61:122–130, 2006

63. Subramanya S: A low-volume, low-pressure tracheal tube cuff reduces pulmonary aspiration. Crit Care Med 34:632–639, 2006

64. Girou E, Buu-Hoi A, Stephan F, et al: Airway colonisation in long-term mechanically ventilated patients: Effect of semi-recumbent position and continuous subglottic suctioning. Intensive Care Med 30:225–233, 2004

Other Selected Readings

ARDS Network Authors: Ketoconazole for early treatment of acute lung injury and acute respiratory distress syndrome: A randomized controlled trial. JAMA 283:1995–2002, 2000

Gattinoni L, Caironi P, Carlesso E: How to ventilate patients with acute lung injury and acute respiratory distress syndrome. Curr Opin Crit Care 11:69–76, 2005

Griffiths MJ, Evans TW: Inhaled nitric oxide therapy in adults. N Engl J Med 353:2683–2695, 2005

Haitsma J, Papadakos P, Lachmann B: Surfactant therapy for acute lung injury/acute respiratory distress syndrome. Curr Opin Crit Care 10:18–22, 2004

Inoue Y, Tanaka H, Ogura H, et al: A neutrophil elastase inhibitor, sivelestat, improves leukocyte deformability in patients with acute lung injury. J Trauma 60:936–943, 2006

Kalhan R, Mikkelsen M, Dedhiya P: Underuse of lung protective ventilation: Analysis of potential factors to explain physician behavior. Crit Care Med 34:300–306, 2006

Lapinsky S, Granton J: Critical care lessons from severe acute respiratory syndrome. Curr Opin Crit Care 10:53–58, 2004

Spragg RG, Lewis JF: Pathology of the surfactant system of the mature lung. Am J Respir Crit Care 163:280–282, 2001

Suter PM: Lung inflammation in ARDS—friend or foe? N Engl J Med 354:1739–1742, 2006

Young P, Pakeerathan S, Blunt M, et al: Comparison of prone positioning and high-frequency oscillatory ventilation in patients with acute respiratory distress syndrome. Crit Care Med 33:2162–2171, 2005

Zeiher BG, Matsuoka S, Kawabata K, et al: Neutrophil elastase and acute lung injury: Prospects for sivelestat and other neutrophil elastase inhibitors as therapeutics. Crit Care Med 30:S281–S287, 2002

Renal System

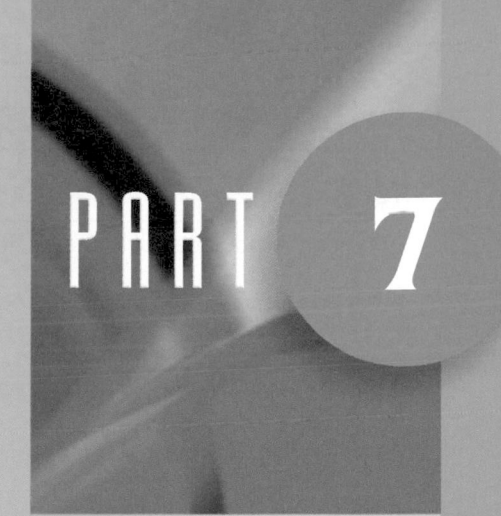

PART 7

INTERNET RESOURCES

Topic	Web Page Address
American Association of Kidney Patients	www.aakp.org
American Nephrology Nurses' Association	www.annanurse.org
American Society for Artificial Internal Organs	www.asaio.com
American Society of Nephrology	www.asn-online.org
Atlas of Diseases of the Kidney	www.kidneyatlas.org
Canadian Association of Nephrology Nurses and Associates	www.cannt.ca
European Renal Association	www.era-edta.org
Forum of End Stage Renal Disease Networks	www.esrdnetworks.org
International Society for Hemodialysis	www.ishd.net
International Society for Peritoneal Dialysis	www.ispd.org
International Society of Nephrology	www.isn-online.org
Kidney and Urologic Foundation of America, Inc.	www.kidneyurology.org
The Kidney Foundation of Canada	www.kidney.ca
Kidney Transplant and Dialysis Association	www.ktda.org
National Institute of Diabetes, Digestive, And Kidney Diseases	www.niddk.nih.gov/
National Kidney and Urologic Diseases Information Clearinghouse	www.kidney.niddk.nih.gov/
National Kidney Foundation	www.kidney.org
Nephron Information Center	www.nephron.com
NephroWorld	www.nephroworld.com
Polycystic Kidney Disease Foundation	www.pkdcure.org/home.htm
Renalnet	www.renalnet.org
TransWeb (Information about Transplantation and Donation)	www.transweb.org
United Network for Organ Sharing	www.unos.org
U.S. Renal Data Systems	www.usrds.org
World Foundation for Renal Care	www.worldrenal.org

Anatomy and Physiology of the Renal System

Kara Adams Snyder

28

Macroscopic Anatomy of the Renal System
Microscopic Anatomy of the Renal System
and Normal Renal Physiology
    Juxtaglomerular Apparatus
    Glomerulus
    Tubules
Hormonal Influences
    Antidiuretic Hormone
    Renin
    Aldosterone
Functions of the Renal System
    Renal Clearance
    Regulation
    Fluid Balance
    Other Renal Functions

Objectives

Based on the content in this chapter, the reader should be able to:

❶ Describe the impact of afferent and efferent blood supply on renal function.

❷ Discuss the structures comprising the nephron: glomerulus, proximal tubule, loop of Henle, and distal and collecting tubules.

❸ Differentiate the functions of the nephron, including glomerular filtration, active and passive transport, and tubular secretion.

❹ Compare normal fluid pressures in the nephron and how they affect glomerular filtration rate.

❺ Explain the relationship of antidiuretic hormone, renin, and aldosterone to fluid regulation by the kidneys.

❻ Explain the mechanisms used by the kidneys to help achieve clearance of substances and maintain homeostasis.

❼ Describe the physiological roles of the predominant electrolytes.

With each contraction of the heart, the kidneys receive 21% of the cardiac output. This means that approximately 1.2 L of blood pass through the kidneys each minute, and the body's entire blood volume is filtered through the kidneys 340 times per day.[1] With this large volume of blood, the kidneys have a dominant role in filtration and a minor role in metabolism. Therefore, the kidneys have a large requirement for pressure and a relatively smaller requirement for oxygen. The regulation and maintenance of the concentration of solutes in the extracellular fluid (ECF) of the body are the primary functions of the kidney. The kidneys remove metabolic waste products and excess concentrations of constituents and conserve substances present in normal or low quantities.

• Macroscopic Anatomy of the Renal System

The kidneys are bean-shaped organs that lie in a retroperitoneal position in the abdomen, one on each side of the vertebral column (Fig. 28-1). The kidneys are partially protected by the last pair of ribs, with the right kidney slightly lower than the left because of the location of the liver. A tough, fibrous coat, known as the renal capsule, surrounds each kidney. The adrenal glands, which are discussed in more detail in Chapter 42, cap the kidneys.

The adult kidneys are approximately 12 cm long, 6 cm wide, and 2.5 cm thick. The kidney weighs about 150 gm, the size of a clenched fist. The size

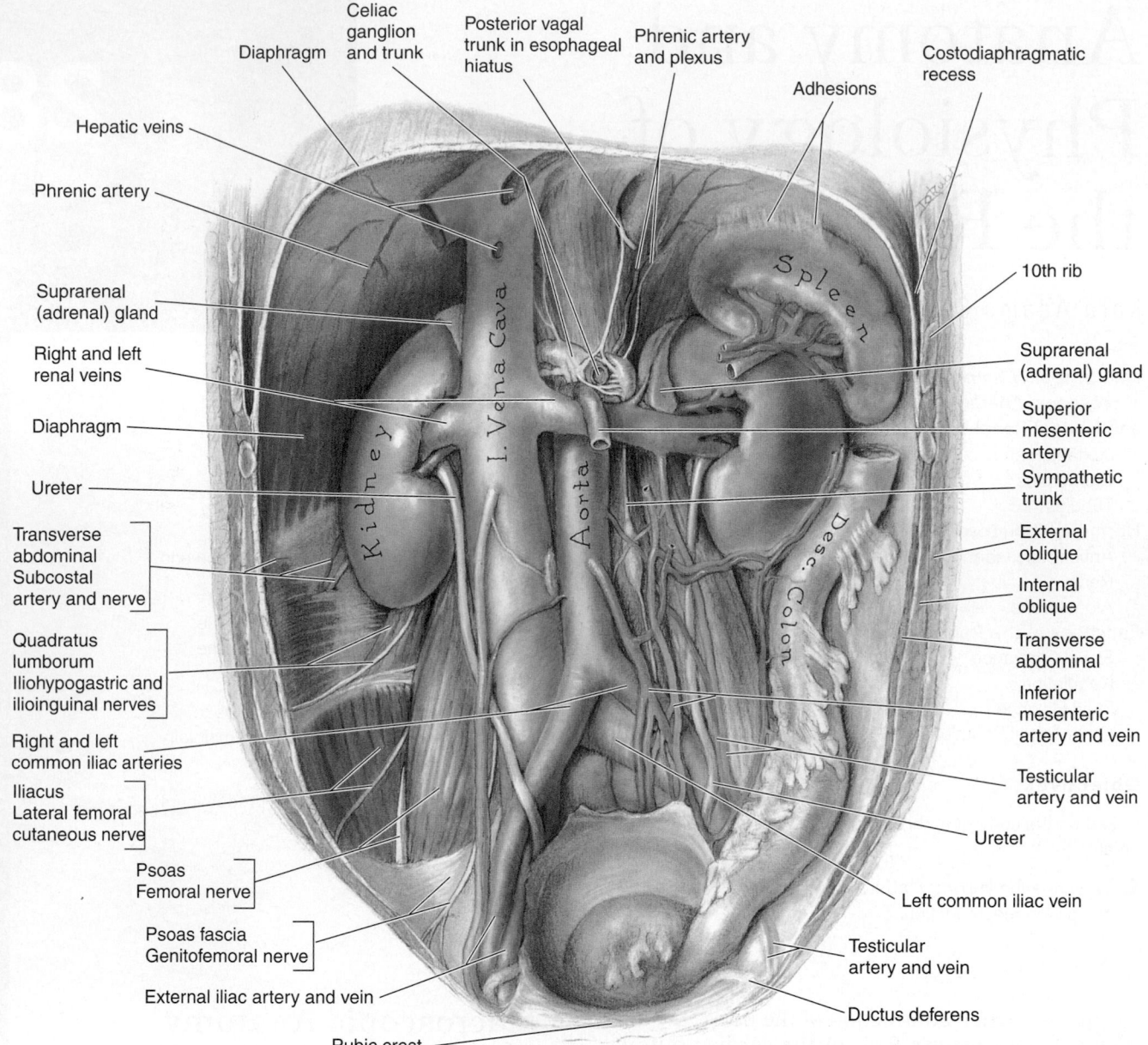

Figure 28-1 • Anatomy of the kidneys and urinary system. (From Moore KL, Dalley AF: Clinically Oriented Anatomy, 4th ed. Philadelphia, Lippincott Williams & Wilkins, 1999, p 281.)

and weight of the kidneys are clinically valuable indicators in ultrasound-guided differential diagnosis of renal failure (see Chapter 29).

There are two distinct layers of the kidney: the renal cortex and the renal medulla (Fig. 28-2). The renal cortex is the outer portion of the kidney and has two regions: the cortical region and the juxtamedullary ("next to the medulla") region. The cortex contains the glomeruli, the proximal tubules, the cortical loops of Henle, the distal tubules, and the cortical collecting ducts. The inner layer, the medulla, in addition to the cortical structures, contains the renal pyramids. The pyramids contain the medullary loops of Henle and the medullary portions of the collecting ducts, which join together to form a minor calyx. Minor calyces come together to form a major calyx. The renal calyces

further join to become the conduit for directing the flow of urine into the ureter.

Urine exits the kidney at an oblique angle through a fibromuscular structure, the ureter. Peristalsis helps maintain the flow of urine through the ureter. The ureter enters the bladder in the trigone region. The trigone region of the bladder is so called for the three structures that form the shape of a triangle: the two ureters and the urethra. The peristaltic actions in the ureter and the angle of entry at the bladder help prevent the reflux of urine. Urine exits the bladder through the urethral orifice via the urethra. The male urethra is about 20 cm long; the female urethra is about 3 to 5 cm long.[1]

On the medial aspect of each kidney there is an indentation known as the hilum. It is through this

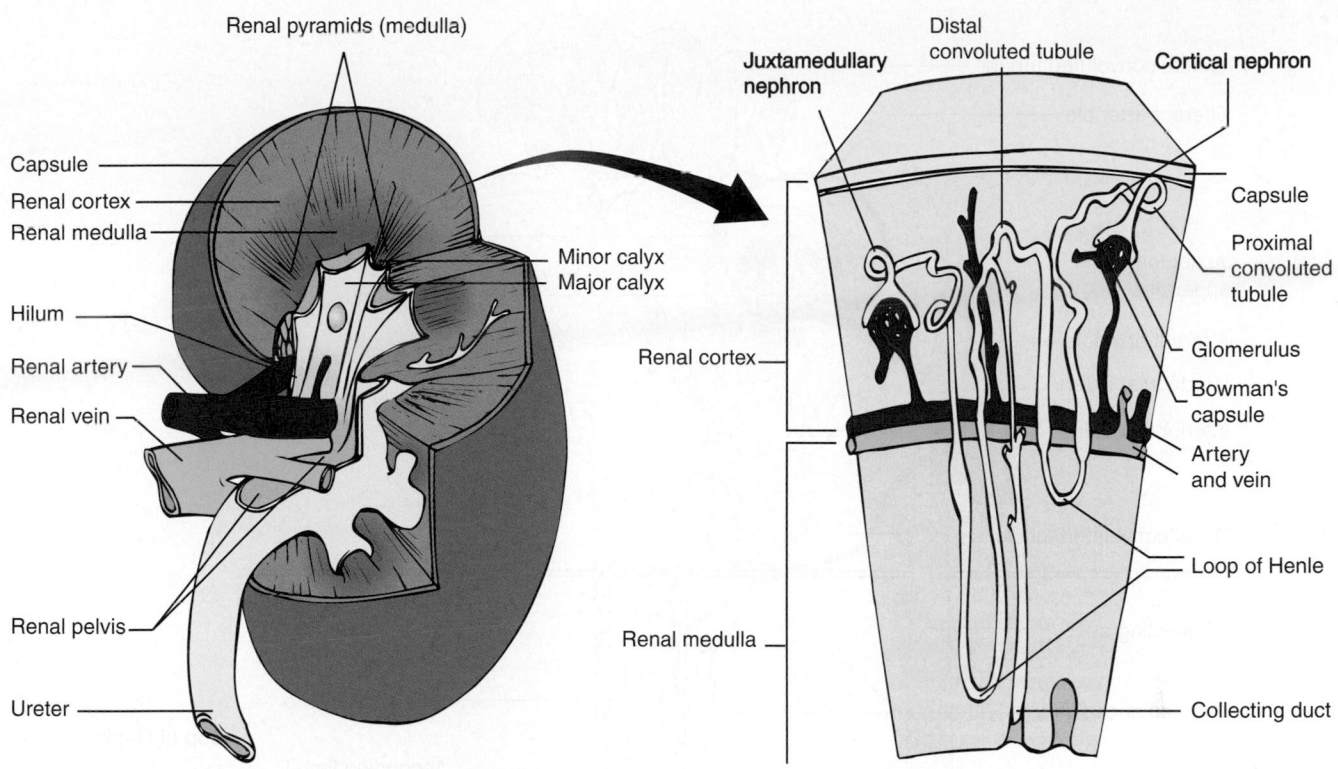

Figure 28-2 • Macroscopic anatomy of the kidney.

indentation that the renal arteries and nerves enter and the renal veins, lymphatics, and ureters exit (see Fig. 28-2).

The kidneys receive their blood supply from the renal artery, a branch of the descending aorta. The renal artery divides into several smaller branches known as the interlobular arteries (Fig. 28-3). Further branching produces numerous afferent arterioles. Each afferent arteriole forms a tuft of capillaries, known as the glomerulus, where blood is filtered. Leaving the glomerulus is the efferent arteriole. The efferent arteriole branches to form a second capillary bed, known as the peritubular capillaries (see Fig. 28-3). The peritubular capillaries surround the loop of Henle to reabsorb more water and solutes as needed for homeostasis. Reconnecting, this vast network of vessels eventually returns to the central circulation through the renal veins.

The kidneys were once thought to function in the normal homeostasis of systemic blood pressure because of the effect of hydrostatic pressure on filtration. It is now known that the glomerular filtration rate (GFR) is relatively stable over a wide range of arterial blood pressures. The reason for this stability is that the afferent arterioles adjust their diameter in response to the pressure of blood coming to them. If the blood pressure decreases, the smooth muscles of the afferent arterioles relax. This causes dilation of these arterioles, which increases the perfusion of the glomeruli and maintains the GFR at its normal rate. Conversely, with an increase in blood pressure, these vessels constrict. However, there is a limit to this autoregulatory mechanism. Below a mean arterial

pressure of 90 mm Hg and above a mean of 250 mm Hg, the GFR is proportional to perfusion pressure.[1] For example, if the systemic blood pressure falls greatly, such as in shock, the GFR falls to near zero, thereby producing near anuria.

• Microscopic Anatomy of the Renal System and Normal Renal Physiology

CONCEPTS in action ANIMATION

Urine, the end product of kidney function, is formed from the blood by the smallest unit of the kidney, the nephron (see Fig. 28-3). Each human kidney consists of about 1 million nephrons, all of which function identically; therefore, kidney function can be explained by describing the function of one nephron (Table 28-1). A nephron is composed of a glomerulus, a proximal tubule, a loop of Henle, and a distal tubule. Several distal tubules drain into a collecting duct.

Approximately 80% of the filtrate is returned to the bloodstream by reabsorption in the proximal tubule.[1] In a healthy person, all the filtered glucose and amino acids; much sodium, chloride, hydrogen, and other electrolytes; and uric acid and urea are reabsorbed here. The proximal tubule cells also secrete substances (e.g., some drugs, organic acids, and organic bases) into the filtrate.

In the loop of Henle, the filtrate (urine) becomes highly concentrated. This part of the nephron is composed of a thin-walled descending portion and

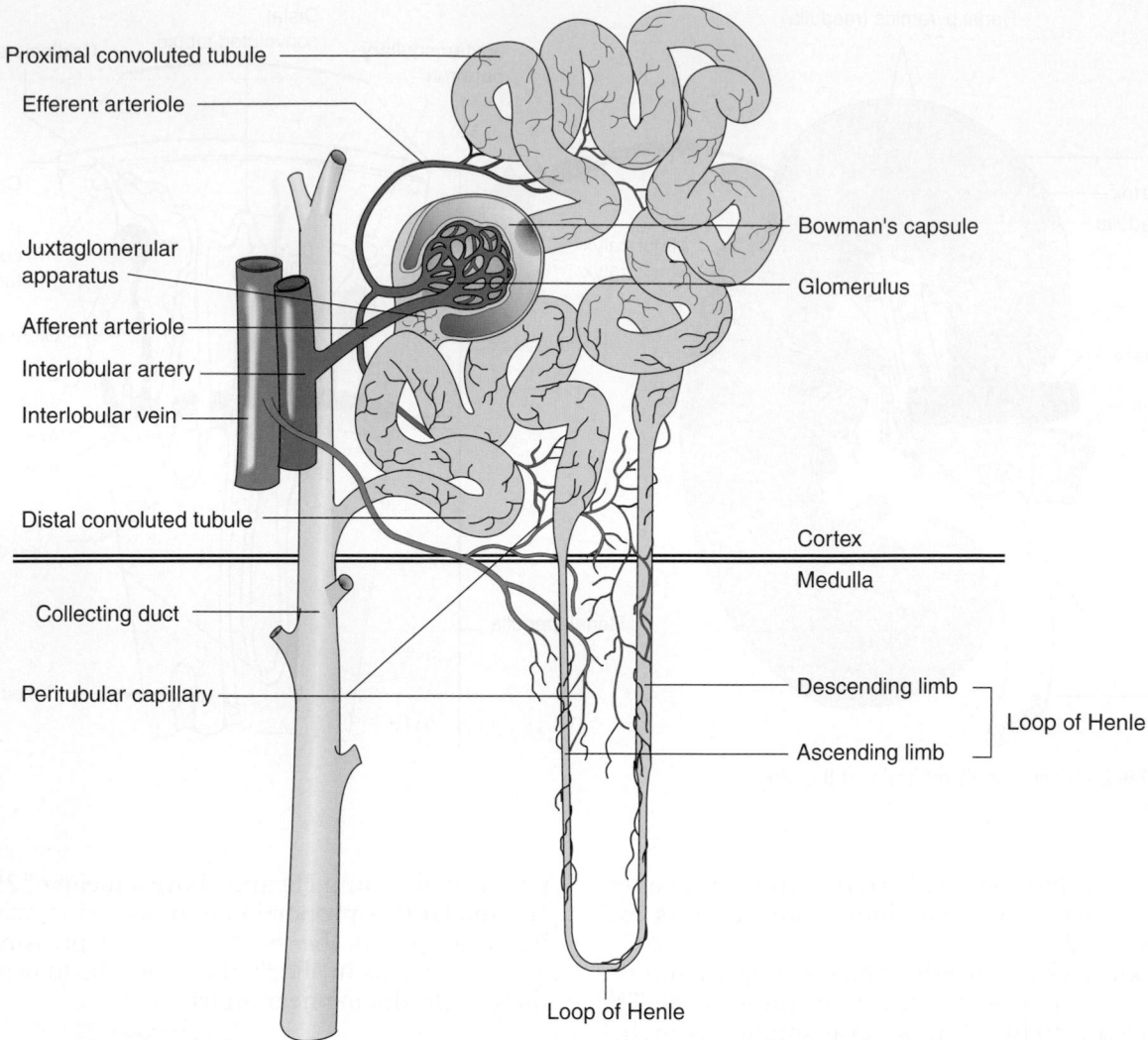

Proximal convoluted tubule

Efferent arteriole

Juxtaglomerular apparatus

Afferent arteriole

Interlobular artery

Interlobular vein

Distal convoluted tubule

Collecting duct

Peritubular capillary

Bowman's capsule

Glomerulus

Cortex

Medulla

Descending limb

Ascending limb

Loop of Henle

Loop of Henle

Figure 28-3 • Renal blood supply. The afferent arteriole feeds the glomerulus. Exiting the glomerulus is the efferent arteriole, which divides into a second capillary network, the peritubular capillaries. (From Porth CM: Pathophysiology: Concepts of Altered Health States, 7th ed. Philadelphia: Lippincott Williams & Wilkins, 2005, p 730.)

a thick-walled ascending portion. Loops of Henle belonging to juxtamedullary nephrons dip into the medulla of the kidney, which contains a highly concentrated interstitial fluid. The thin walls of the descending portion are quite permeable, and this permeability, together with the high concentration of the interstitial fluid at this point, causes water to move by osmosis from the filtrate into the interstitial fluid. This makes the filtrate quite concentrated by the time it reaches the ascending limb of the loop.

The thicker-walled ascending limb is relatively impermeable to water, but it contains ion carriers that actively transport chloride ions out of the filtrate. This creates an electrochemical gradient that "pulls" the positively charged sodium ions out of the filtrate as well. This exit of electrolytes without water now makes the filtrate more dilute than before.

In the distal tubule, sodium again is reabsorbed by active transport, and hydrogen, potassium, and uric acid can be added to the urine by tubular secretion.

The collecting ducts receive the contents from many distal tubules. There is no further electrolyte

reabsorption or secretion, and in the well-hydrated person, no further water reabsorption as well. Water reabsorption without electrolyte reabsorption can occur in the collecting ducts under the stimulus of antidiuretic hormone (ADH).

JUXTAGLOMERULAR APPARATUS

The nephron is arranged so that the initial portion of the distal tubule lies at the juncture of the afferent and efferent arterioles, which is very near the glomerulus. Here, macula densa cells of the distal tubule lie in approximation to the juxtaglomerular cells of the wall of the afferent arteriole. Both these cell types (juxtaglomerular and macula densa cells) plus some connective tissue cells constitute the juxtaglomerular apparatus (Fig. 28-4). A major function of the juxtaglomerular cells is to secrete renin, which thereby initiates the renin–angiotensin–aldosterone system.[2] When a decrease in sodium chloride concentration is sensed, the macula densa cells initiate two signals: one signal to reduce afferent arteriole

Table 28-1 • Nephron Functions

Nephron Structure	Function	Concentration of Filtrate Along the Nephron
Glomerulus	Free filtration of blood through Bowman's capsule to produce filtrate Hydrostatic and osmotic pressure forces create net filtration pressure	Isosmotic
Proximal convoluted tubule	Reabsorbs sodium, potassium, calcium, glucose, ketone bodies, and amino acids by active transport Reabsorbs chloride and bicarbonate by electromechanical gradient Reabsorbs water by osmosis Reabsorbs urea by diffusion	Isosmotic
Loop of Henle		
Thin descending limb	Reabsorbs sodium by active transport Further reabsorption of chloride by electromechanical gradient Reabsorbs water by osmosis Reabsorbs urea by diffusion	Isosmotic
Thick ascending limb	Reabsorbs sodium and chloride by active transport Blocks water reabsorption at thick ascending limb Reabsorbs bicarbonate by electromechanical gradient	Hypo-osmotic
Distal tubule	Reabsorbs sodium by active transport and aldosterone Reabsorbs water by osmosis Reabsorbs phosphorus, chloride, and bicarbonate by electromechanical gradient	Hypo-osmotic
Collecting tubule	Antidiuretic hormone promotes selective water reabsorption Secretes or reabsorbs bicarbonate and hydrogen ions to maintain pH Secretes potassium and hydrogen ions depending on body requirements or effects of drugs Secretes some creatinine Actively reabsorbs potassium	Depends on body requirements for fluid

tone (increasing afferent arteriole hydrostatic pressure) and a second to increase renin release from the juxtaglomerular cells.[2,3] In this manner, the juxtaglomerular apparatus helps maintain and promote glomerular filtration.

GLOMERULUS

The glomerulus consists of a tuft of capillaries fed by the afferent arteriole and drained by the efferent arteriole. The glomerulus is surrounded by Bowman's

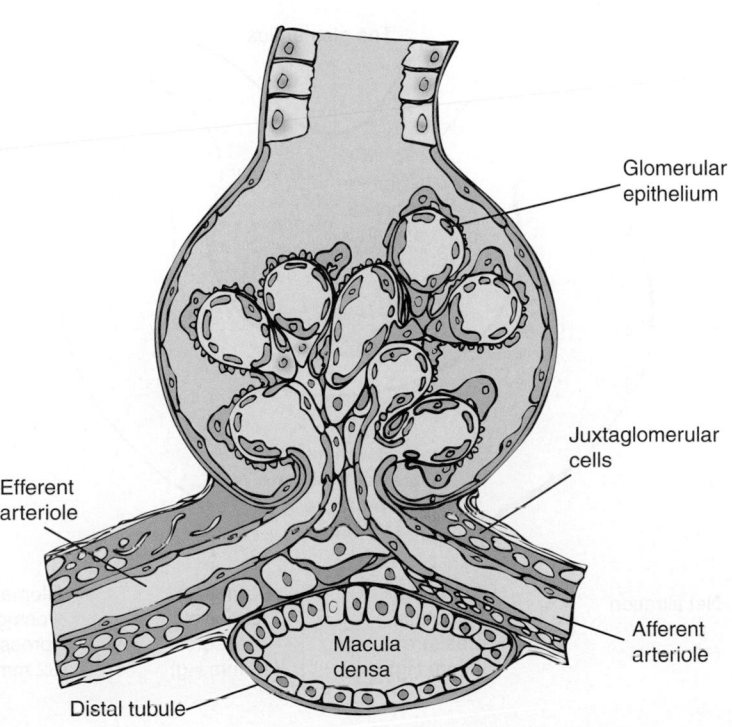

Figure 28-4 • The juxtaglomerular apparatus. The macula densa cells lie in close proximity to the afferent and efferent arterioles, which help to regulate nephron functions.

capsule. High hydrostatic pressure in the afferent arteriole causes rapid filtration. Fluid that is filtered from the capillaries into this capsule then flows into the tubular system, which is divided into four sections: the proximal tubule, the loop of Henle, the distal tubule, and the collecting duct (see Fig. 28-3). Lower hydrostatic pressure in the efferent circulation allows reabsorption. Most of the water and electrolytes are reabsorbed into the blood in the peritubular capillaries that surround the tubular structures. The end products of metabolism remaining in the tubules pass into the urine.

Glomerular filtration is determined by net filtration pressure.[3] Hydrostatic pressure and osmotic pressure forces are major factors. Hydrostatic pressure is driving or "pushing" pressure. Osmotic pressure is defined as the pressure exerted by water (or any solvent) on a semipermeable membrane as it attempts to cross the membrane into an area containing more molecules that cannot cross the semipermeable membrane. The pores in the glomerular capillary make it a semipermeable membrane that permits smaller molecules and water to cross, but prevents larger molecules (e.g., plasma proteins) from crossing. Protein concentrations are the greatest factors in determining an osmotic pressure, and therefore osmotic pressure is often referred to as colloid osmotic pressure.

Four forces are considered when determining net filtration of fluid. These forces are:

1. Glomerular hydrostatic pressure, which promotes filtration
2. Bowman's capsule hydrostatic pressure, which opposes filtration
3. Glomerular colloid osmotic pressure, which opposes filtration
4. Bowman's capsule colloid osmotic pressure, which promotes filtration

Under normal conditions, the concentration of proteins in Bowman's capsule is thought to be negligible and therefore is not considered as part of the net filtration pressure equation (Fig. 28-5). Glomerular hydrostatic pressure is about 60 mm Hg and is autoregulated under most circumstances.[3] Filtrate hydrostatic pressure in Bowman's capsule, about 18 mm Hg, results from the presence of filtrate in the capsule and opposes blood hydrostatic pressure. Glomerular osmotic pressure, derived from protein concentrations in the blood, is about 32 mm Hg. As mentioned, the filtrate also exerts a negligible osmotic pressure. The sum of these pressures is the net gradient that favors movement of filtrate from the bloodstream into Bowman's capsule.

The rate at which the filtrate is formed is the GFR. In the typical healthy person, this amounts to the formation of 125 mL of filtrate per minute.[3] Major clinical factors that influence the GFR are the blood hydrostatic pressure and the filtrate osmotic pressure. Hypoproteinemia, as in starvation, lowers filtrate osmotic pressure and increases the GFR.[3] The GFR decreases with severe hypotension because of a drop in blood hydrostatic pressure, when autoregulatory control may be lost. Other factors that decrease the hydrostatic pressure (and therefore the GFR) are afferent arteriole constriction and renal artery stenosis.

From the 20% to 25% of the cardiac output that goes to the kidneys in a resting adult, about 125 mL of filtrate is produced each minute. This totals 180 L/day and is about 4.5 times the total amount of fluid in the body. Obviously, not all this filtrate could be excreted as urine. As this filtrate passes from Bowman's capsule through the remainder of the nephrons, all but about

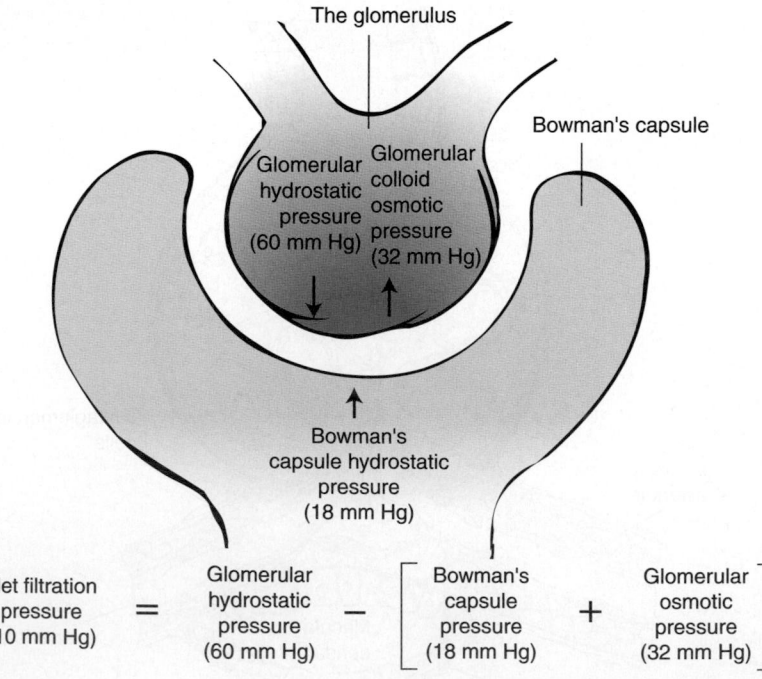

$$\begin{array}{c} \text{Net filtration} \\ \text{pressure} \\ (10 \text{ mm Hg}) \end{array} = \begin{array}{c} \text{Glomerular} \\ \text{hydrostatic} \\ \text{pressure} \\ (60 \text{ mm Hg}) \end{array} - \left[\begin{array}{c} \text{Bowman's} \\ \text{capsule} \\ \text{pressure} \\ (18 \text{ mm Hg}) \end{array} + \begin{array}{c} \text{Glomerular} \\ \text{osmotic} \\ \text{pressure} \\ (32 \text{ mm Hg}) \end{array} \right]$$

Figure 28-5 • Interaction of hydrostatic and osmotic forces for glomerular filtration at Bowman's capsule.

1.5 L/day is returned to the bloodstream. Similarly, at plasma glucose levels of less than 200 mg/dL, none of the filtered glucose is found in the urine when it enters the collecting tubules. The volume and content of the urine are the result of tubular reabsorption and tubular secretion.

TUBULES

Tubular Reabsorption

Reabsorption is accomplished by active transport, osmosis, and diffusion. It occurs in all parts of the nephron as substances moving from the lumen into the peritubular capillaries.

Active Transport Active transport involves the binding of a molecule of a substance to a carrier, which then moves the molecule from one side of the membrane to the other against the concentration gradient of that substance. Because it helps molecules to move in a direction opposite the one they would move by simple diffusion, the carrier acts like a pump. Many processes for active transport use the sodium–potassium pump. Therefore, the small oxygen requirements of the kidneys are closely linked to the active transport processes that occur in the nephron.

In tubular cells, the carrier is located in the cell membrane nearest the peritubular capillaries, and it transports material out of the tubular cell into the peritubular fluid. This lowers the intracellular concentration of the type of molecule being transported. The decreased concentration enables more of those molecules to diffuse from the urine (filtrate) into the tubule cell. These molecules, in turn, exit the cell and enter the peritubular fluid by active transport. The movement of molecules increases the peritubular fluid concentration of the molecule, and this increase stimulates the diffusion of the molecule into the peritubular capillaries. In the nephrons, reabsorption by active transport removes molecules from the filtrate (urine) back to the bloodstream.

Because active transport involves carrier molecules and energy exchanges, there is an upper limit to the number of molecules of a substance that can be transported at one time. This maximal limit for reabsorption rates is called T_{max}. Glucose is an example of a molecule that appears in the same concentrations that it appears in the blood. As serum glucose rises, filtrate glucose also rises. The renal tubules reabsorb the filtered glucose at faster and faster rates, until all of this molecule's active transport mechanisms are being used. At this T_{max}, more glucose is appearing in the filtrate than can be reabsorbed, and glucose is excreted in the urine. This "spilling" of glucose into the urine indicates serum levels higher than T_{max}.

Osmosis The active transport of sodium is responsible for the osmotic reabsorption of water from the filtrate in the proximal (and later, in the distal) tubule. As sodium ions are actively transported out of the cell

and into the peritubular fluid, they make the osmotic pressure of this peritubular fluid higher than that of the cellular or tubular fluid. Water is thereby osmotically "pulled out" of the tubular fluid. Both water and sodium then diffuse into peritubular capillaries and are returned to the bloodstream. This movement of positively charged sodium ions also creates an electrochemical gradient that draws negatively charged ions (especially chloride) out of the tubular fluid and back into the bloodstream.

Diffusion Urea is an example of a molecule that is reabsorbed by diffusion. Under the high pressures in the glomerular capillaries, urea is filtered. In the tubules, as water is reabsorbed into the bloodstream, urea follows by simple diffusion. No selective permeability prevents its return to the bloodstream, and no transport mechanism is required. The reabsorption rates of urea range from 40% to 60% of what is filtered and depend entirely on water reabsorption rates.

Tubular Secretion

Secretion involves active transport and is performed only by distal tubule cells. Substances move from the peritubular capillaries through tubule cells into the filtrate. Many substances that are secreted do not occur naturally in the body (e.g., penicillin). Naturally occurring bodily substances that are secreted include uric acid, potassium, and hydrogen ions.

In the distal tubule, the active transport of sodium uses a carrier system that is also involved in the tubular secretion of hydrogen and potassium ions. In this relationship, every time the carrier transports sodium out of the tubular fluid, it also carries either a hydrogen ion or a potassium ion into the tubular fluid on its "return trip." Thus, for every sodium ion reabsorbed, a hydrogen or potassium ion must be secreted, and vice versa. The choice of cation to be secreted depends on the ECF concentration of these ions (hydrogen and potassium).

Knowledge of this cation exchange system in the distal tubule helps explain some of the relationships that these electrolytes have with one another. For example, it is clear why an aldosterone blocker (such as spironolactone) may cause hyperkalemia. The aldosterone blocker reduces sodium reabsorption. Such reduced reabsorption of sodium also reduces the tubular secretion of either hydrogen or potassium. The hydrogen excess can be buffered by bicarbonate, but the potassium simply rises to above-normal levels, leading to hyperkalemia. Similarly, the cation exchange system helps explain why there can be an initial decrease in plasma potassium in alkalosis or as severe acidosis is corrected therapeutically. In severe acidosis, the nephrons attempt to compensate by increasing hydrogen ion secretion. But as acidosis is therapeutically corrected (e.g., by sodium bicarbonate administration), potassium ions are secreted. As hydrogen ions no longer need to be secreted, potassium ions become the sole exchange for sodium ions, leading, it is thought, to a reduction in plasma potassium.

• Hormonal Influences

Through the reabsorption of sodium and the passive "following" of water and chloride, it is possible to make urine of the same osmolality as blood. However, under conditions of dehydration, urine is very concentrated, whereas if a great deal of water is consumed, urine is more dilute than blood. This final regulation of urine (and, therefore, serum osmolality and volume) is under the influence of three hormones: ADH, renin, and aldosterone.

ANTIDIURETIC HORMONE

Osmoreceptors in the hypothalamus are sensitive to serum osmolality. During dehydration, when serum osmolality rises, osmoreceptors in the hypothalamus respond by stimulating the hypothalamus to secrete ADH, which increases the permeability of collecting tubule cells to water. This permits the reabsorption of water alone (without electrolytes), which in turn decreases the concentration of the ECF. Negative feedback loops regulate ADH secretion. This means that as the concentration of the ECF returns to normal, the stimulus for ADH secretion disappears, and ADH secretion stops.

RENIN

Another hormone that influences urine concentration is renin. When the GFR falls because of dehydration or blood loss, the juxtaglomerular apparatus secretes renin.[2] Subnormal sodium levels in the filtrate also stimulate renin secretion. Renin converts angiotensin, which is secreted by the liver, into angiotensin I. Pulmonary capillary cells in turn convert angiotensin I into angiotensin II (see Chapter 42, Fig. 42-9).

ALDOSTERONE

Angiotensin II constricts the smooth muscle surrounding the arterioles. This increases blood pressure, which increases the GFR. Angiotensin II also triggers the secretion of aldosterone by the adrenal cortex (see Chapter 42, Fig. 42-9). Aldosterone is the third hormone that influences urine osmolality. By increasing sodium reabsorption in distal tubule cells, aldosterone causes an increase in renal water reabsorption. This increases blood pressure and decreases serum osmolality. Simultaneously, potassium is excreted in the urine in exchange for the sodium reabsorption. Therefore, aldosterone also is secreted in response to subnormal serum sodium and elevated potassium levels.

• Functions of the Renal System

RENAL CLEARANCE

From the previous discussion, an important concept in renal function emerges: clearance. As the filtrate moves along the nephron, it contains a large proportion of metabolic end products. These products are removed (cleared) from the blood and exit the body in the urine. Indeed, of each 125 mL of glomerular filtrate formed per minute, about one half, or 60 mL, returns to the blood without urea, and about one half is excreted with urea. Stated another way, 60 mL of plasma is "cleared" of urea each minute in normally functioning kidneys. In the same way, the 125 mL of plasma is also cleared of creatinine, uric acid, potassium, sulfate, phosphate, and so forth each minute. It is possible to calculate renal clearance by simultaneously sampling urine and plasma. By dividing the quantity of substance found in each milliliter of plasma into the quantity found in the urine, the milliliters cleared per minute can be calculated. This method is used as one means of testing kidney function.

Other methods of assessing renal function involve chemicals that are known to be filtered only, or both filtered and secreted. The polysaccharide, inulin, for example, is filtered only and neither absorbed nor secreted. Therefore, the clearance of inulin provides a measure of glomerular filtration. Mannitol can be used similarly. Para-aminohippurate sodium and iodopyracet (Diodrast) are drugs that are secreted in addition to being filtered. As such, their clearance provides an index of plasma flow through the kidneys. They also can be used together with a filtered-only drug in assessing tubular secretion and therefore the health of tubular cells.

The sodium concentration in the urine can also serve as an index of tubular health in certain situations. For example, in acute renal failure, an increased clearance of sodium can indicate acute tubular necrosis. Accordingly, supernormal blood levels of filtered substances (creatinine and other nitrogenous wastes) indicate a decrease in glomerular filtration and therefore in nephron health.

REGULATION

In addition to excreting nitrogenous wastes as urea and other byproducts of metabolism, the kidneys help regulate the electrolyte concentration and the pH of the ECF (i.e., the blood and interstitial fluid of the body).

Electrolyte Concentration

Electrolytes are substances that, when in water, disassociate and become charged. When charged, the solution is capable of carrying an electrical current. Positively charged electrolytes are cations; negatively charged electrolytes are anions. Most electrolytes are dissolved in body fluids, although some are bound to proteins or deposited as solids to form bones and teeth.

Despite the complex physiology associated with electrolytes, they have four main functions in homeostasis:

1. Cell metabolism and contribution to body structures
2. Facilitation of water movement between body compartments
3. Help in the maintenance of acid–base balance
4. Maintenance and production of membrane potentials in nerve and muscle cells

The functions of individual electrolytes are given in Table 28-2. For normal functions to occur, the concentration of electrolytes must be carefully maintained. Energy, usually in the form of adenosine triphosphate (ATP), is often required to maintain this balance. As described earlier in this chapter, the kidneys play a crucial role in electrolyte balance. In addition to being lost in the urine, electrolytes are lost from the gastrointestinal tract in the stool and through the skin in sweat.

Sodium The sodium content of a normal adult is approximately 142 mEq/L of ECF. As the most abundant extracellular electrolyte, sodium exerts an extracellular osmolality, thereby regulating movement of body fluids. Sodium plays a role in nerve impulses through active transport and the sodium–potassium pump. The balance of sodium is carefully regulated by the kidneys, with hormonal influences of aldosterone and ADH. Regulation occurs primarily through reabsorption (or excretion) in the proximal tubule under the influence of aldosterone.

Potassium In contrast to sodium, potassium is the most abundant intracellular electrolyte, with an approximate plasma concentration of only 4.5 mEq/L. Potassium, among other substances and factors, is critical in the maintenance of nervous and impulse conduction in the heart. Because of the small plasma concentration, potassium plays little role in osmotic regulation. Although some potassium may be lost in sweat and feces, the kidneys excrete approximately 80% to 90% of the potassium lost by the body. In cases of hyperkalemia, aldosterone release facilitates increased potassium excretion. Potassium also assists with acid–base regulation through the cellular exchange with hydrogen ions.

Table 28-2 • Electrolyte Functions

Electrolyte	Normal Range	Functions
Sodium (Na$^+$)	135–145 mEq/L	Exerts an extracellular osmolality, thereby regulating movement of body fluids Facilitates nerve impulses through active transport and the sodium–potassium pump
Potassium (K$^+$)	3.5–5 mEq/L	Maintains nervous impulse conduction in the heart Promotes skeletal muscle function Plays small role in osmotic regulation Assists with acid–base regulation
Chloride (Cl$^-$)	100–110 mEq/L	Maintains electroneutrality by passively following the positively charged ions Helps regulate osmotic pressure differences between intracellular and extracellular fluid compartments Regulates body water balance with sodium Combines with H$^+$ in gastric mucosal cells to make hydrochloric acid
Calcium (Ca^{2+})	8.5–10.0 mg/dL (total) 4.4–5.4 mg/dL (ionized)	Major structural component of bones and teeth Plays role in blood coagulation Promotes muscle contraction and nervous impulse transmission Decreases neuromuscular irritability
Phosphorus (PO$_4^-$)	2.5–4.5 mg/dL	A structural component of bones and teeth Helps maintain acid–base balance Energy production (adenosine triphosphate) Delivery of oxygen to tissues as a component of 2,3-DPG
Magnesium (Mg^{2+})	1.8–2.5 mEq/L	Ensures the cross-membrane transport of sodium and potassium in the sodium–potassium pump Promotes neuromuscular excitability Plays role in heart contraction Facilitates transmission of central nervous system impulses Part of many enzymatic reactions for carbohydrate and protein metabolism

Chloride Chloride is the most abundant extracellular anion. Negatively charged, chloride passively follows the positively charged sodium to maintain electroneutrality. Chloride plays an important role in electroneutrality because all positive charges and negative charges must be in equilibrium. Therefore, chloride passively follows the secretion or reabsorption of the predominant cations, sodium and potassium. A large amount of chloride is also found in the gastric mucosal cells in the form of hydrochloric acid.

Calcium Calcium has both structural and functional roles in homeostasis. In the form of calcium phosphate, it is the major structural component of bones and teeth. In the free, plasma form, calcium has a function in clotting, muscle contraction, and nervous impulse transmission. In the ionized form, about half is bound to plasma proteins, such as albumin.

Unlike the other electrolytes, calcium is absorbed from the small intestine under the influence of vitamin D, with the remaining ingested calcium lost in the feces. Excretion also occurs in the proximal convoluted tubule of the kidneys.

Parathyroid hormone (PTH) is produced and released by the parathyroid glands. A low calcium concentration stimulates its release. PTH facilitates the shift of calcium in its solid form (calcium phosphate, found in the bones) to its ionized form. PTH also increases the calcium absorbed from the intestine by signaling the kidneys to activate vitamin D. Reabsorption of calcium at the renal tubules is also increased under the influence of PTH. Calcitonin, secreted by the thyroid gland, is another hormone that plays a comparatively small role in calcium regulation. Calcitonin acts in opposition to PTH in an effort to reduce plasma calcium levels.

Phosphorus Like calcium, phosphorus has both structural and functional roles. Approximately 85% is found in the organic form in bones and teeth. The remaining phosphorus is in the inorganic, ionized forms, HPO_4^{2-} and $H_2PO_4^{-}$. Carried in two forms, phosphate is able to accept or donate an ion, thereby assisting with acid–base balance. The intracellular ionized form plays a role in many critical metabolic processes, with its primary function being the formation of ATP. Phosphorus is required for the delivery of oxygen to tissues because it is the primary substrate for 2,3-diphosphoglycerate.

PTH regulates phosphorus, with effects directly opposite those of calcium. PTH causes an increase in calcium plasma concentration and promotes excretion of phosphorus. PTH also causes release of phosphorus in the bones and shifts it to the ECF. Presumably, this would cause an increase in phosphorus; however, PTH also decreases the transport of phosphate ions by the kidney tubules, so more phosphate ions are lost in the urine.

Magnesium Magnesium is a predominantly intracellular ion. Magnesium ensures the cross-membrane transport of sodium and potassium in the sodium–potassium pump. In addition, magnesium functions in the maintenance of neuromuscular excitability and in the transmission of central nervous system impulses. It also plays a role in enzymatic reactions for carbohydrate and protein metabolism. Often, reactions requiring calcium require magnesium as well.

pH If respiratory buffers for pH regulation are insufficient, the kidneys begin to take part, although much more slowly than the lungs. Although respiratory control of carbon dioxide, and therefore hydrogen ion levels, can take only seconds to achieve, 48 to 72 hours may pass before the renal system can change the serum acid–base balance significantly.

Alkalosis occurs as a result of too few hydrogen ions or too many bicarbonate ions. To compensate, the body must conserve hydrogen ions. In renal compensation for alkalosis, tubular reabsorption of hydrogen ions is increased and secretion is decreased. This increases the hydrogen ion concentration of the ECF and thereby decreases the alkalosis.

Acidosis occurs as a result of too many hydrogen ions or too few bicarbonate ions. To compensate, the body must secrete hydrogen ions. Renal compensation for acidosis involves increasing the hydrogen ion secretion of the tubule cells, especially in the distal tubule cells. In this case, bicarbonate and sodium ions are continually being filtered from the glomerulus. Also, hydrogen ion secretion by distal tubule cells causes an increase in sodium reabsorption. Such sodium reabsorption can increase bicarbonate reabsorption electrochemically. Therefore, as hydrogen ions are being eliminated from the ECF, sodium and bicarbonate ions are being added to it. Both serve to decrease the acidosis (Fig. 28-6).

Urine can be acidified (by hydrogen ion secretion) only to a pH level of 4.0 to 4.5. If the tubular secretion of hydrogen ions was the only mechanism operating, only a few hydrogen ions could be secreted before the critical shut-off level of 4.0 was reached. This would occur because hydrogen would combine with urinary chloride to make hydrochloric acid. Not many of these strong hydrochloric acid molecules are needed to make the urine pH 4.0. The formation of hydrochloric acid would then stop tubular hydrogen ion secretion before sufficient compensation for acidosis could be obtained. This does not occur because tubule cells deaminate certain amino acids and secrete the nitrogenous component as ammonia. This ammonia combines with hydrogen in the urine to form ammonium. Because tubule membranes are not permeable to ammonium, much of it is secreted in this form. Some ammonia combines with chloride to form ammonium chloride.

FLUID BALANCE

The body contains about 60% water in most individuals.[4] This percentage may vary between 50% and 70%, depending on a person's fat content. Adipose tissue has very low water, and therefore people with more fat have a lower percentage of body weight as water. Women have a tendency to have higher body

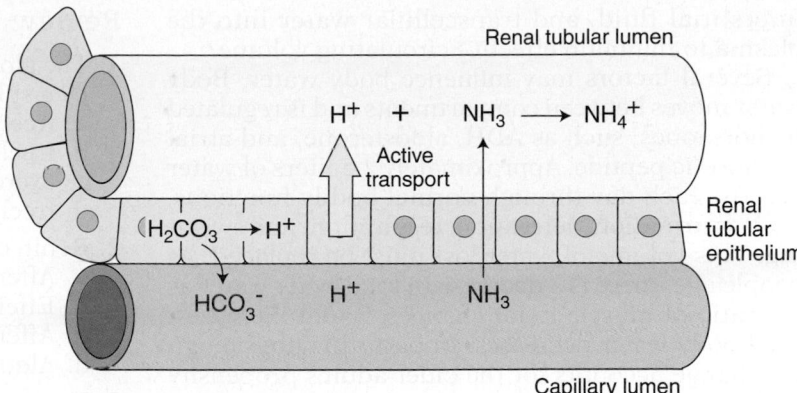

Figure 28-6 • Renal compensation for acidosis. Hydrogen (H^+) is moved from blood into the filtrate by active transport and exits in the urine as ammonium (NH_4^+). HCO_3^-, bicarbonate; NH_3, ammonia.

fat percentages than men and therefore have a lower total-body water (usually around 50%).[4]

Water is distributed among the two main compartments in the body: intracellular fluid (ICF) and ECF. The ICF is the amount of volume within the cell and makes up about two thirds of the total-body water, or about 40% of the body weight. Primarily, the ICF is a solution of ions, including potassium, proteins, and organic ions. The ECF represents the remaining one third of the body water, or about 20% of the body weight. The solution primarily contains sodium chloride and bicarbonate. Figure 28-7 illustrates the different body water compartments.

There are three subcompartments to the ECF: the interstitial fluid (ISF), the plasma, and the transcellular fluid. ISF surrounds the cells but does not circulate. This subcompartment makes up about three fourths of the ECF. The second subcompartment of the ECF is the plasma, which circulates as the extracellular component of blood. Plasma makes up about one fourth of the ECF.

The third subcompartment of ECF is called transcellular fluid. This fluid is neither in the plasma nor in the interstitium; instead, it is the fluid that makes up the digestive juices, cerebrospinal fluid, synovial fluid, pericardial fluid, and mucus. Although the transcellular fluid is only about 1 to 2 liters in total (<1 lb), it plays a very important role in homeostasis. Transcellular fluid helps cushion the heart with each beat, make joint movement smooth, carry critical oxygen and glucose to the brain, and remove bacteria and antigens from the respiratory tract.

There is a constant movement of water between body compartments. For example, in diseases in which there is a lack of plasma oncotic pressure (e.g., liver disease), there may be excessive movement of fluid from the plasma to the interstitium. This additional ISF is reabsorbed by the lymph for recirculation; however, the volume that the lymph system is capable of holding becomes overwhelmed. This then causes edema formation. During times of dehydration, hormonal influences are recruited to pull additional ICF,

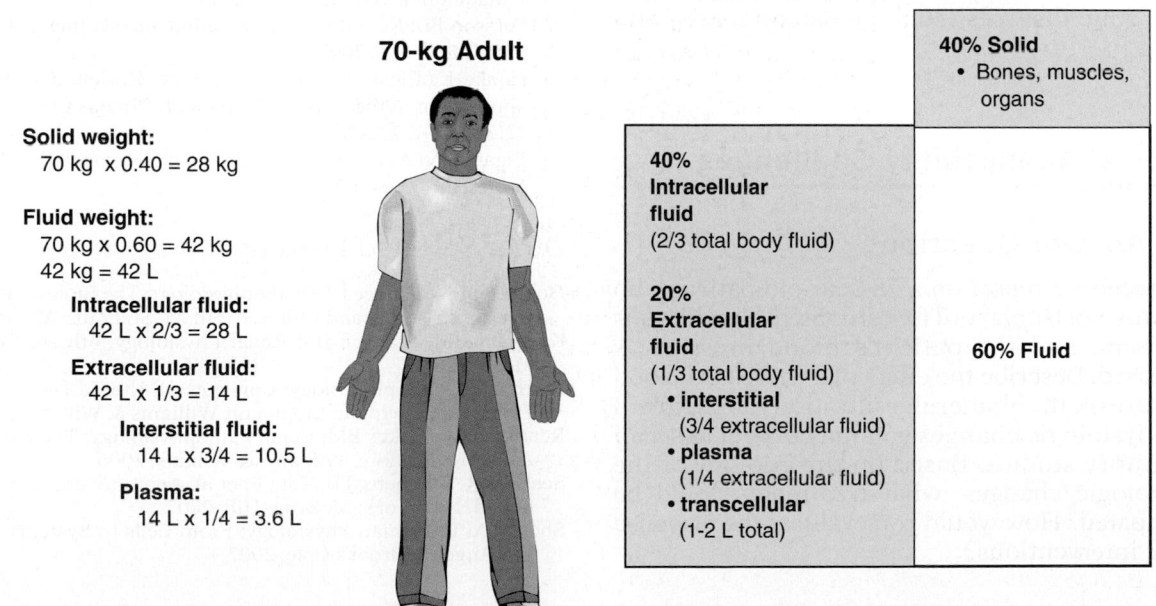

Figure 28-7 • Body water compartments.

interstitial fluid, and transcellular water into the plasma to maintain effective circulating volume.

Several factors may influence body water. Body water moves between compartments and is regulated by hormones, such as ADH, aldosterone, and atrial natriuretic peptide. Approximately 2.5 liters of water are lost each day through normal bodily functions, such as urination, defecation, respiration, and sweating. This volume of water lost must be replaced. As people age, there is a decrease in total-body water as the ratio of muscle to fat changes. As fat increases, total-body water decreases. In part, this physiological change accounts for the older adult's propensity to dehydration.

OTHER RENAL FUNCTIONS

Renal interstitial (not nephron) cells manufacture and secrete two hormones, calcitriol (vitamin D) and erythropoietin, the actions of which are unrelated to urine formation. Calcitriol is a hormone that increases plasma calcium concentration by increasing intestinal absorption of calcium, promoting bone resorption, and stimulating the renal tubular reabsorption of calcium. Erythropoietin is a glycoprotein hormone that stimulates the bone marrow to produce red blood cells. Any process that decreases the oxygen content in the blood, such as bleeding or hypoxemia, is sensed by the kidney and initiates the release of erythropoietin. This increases the arterial oxygen content required to maintain cell integrity.

The kidneys also activate vitamin D. Ingested with food, vitamin D is absorbed in an inert form. The kidneys make vitamin active so that it may assist in the absorption of calcium, which occurs in the intestines. Calcium has many functions as discussed earlier in this chapter. If renal failure occurs, there is a marked reduction in vitamin D and subsequently bioavailable calcium, thereby putting the patient at risk for bone diseases (such as osteoporosis) and bleeding.

• Clinical Applicability Challenges

Short-Answer Questions

1. You receive a report on a 78-year-old patient who is status postsurgery. The estimated blood loss is 3.4 liters, and the patient's blood pressure is decreased. Describe the effect of a decreased blood pressure on the glomerular filtration rate. Explain the physiologic changes you may expect to see in laboratory studies. Based on the etiology of the physiologic changes, what treatments could be anticipated? How would you evaluate the response to the interventions?

Review Questions

1. The glomerular filtration rate is ideally calculated by a substance that is
   a. freely filtered, without secretion or reabsorption.
   b. freely filtered with secretion into the tubule.
   c. excreted in the urine.
   d. freely filtered, with maximal reabsorption.

2. Renin causes which of the following?
   a. Afferent arteriolar dilation
   b. Efferent arteriolar dilation
   c. Afferent arteriolar constriction
   d. Aldosterone inhibition

3. Hyperglycemia increases the osmotic pressure of the filtered urine in the nephron. This would cause which of the following?
   a. Increased sodium and water reabsorption, leading to oliguria.
   b. Decreased sodium and water reabsorption, leading to diuresis.
   c. Decreased glomerular filtration, leading to prerenal azotemia.
   d. Increased glomerular secretion of proteins into the filtrate.

4. Which of the following is caused by calcitonin?
   a. Decreased phosphorus concentration
   b. Potassium secretion
   c. Decreased calcium concentration
   d. Sodium reabsorption

5. Calculate the estimated intracellular body water of a 75-kg man:
   a. 45 liters
   b. 30 liters
   c. 15 liters
   d. 3 liters

References

1. Guyton AC, Hall JE: Textbook of Medical Physiology, 11th ed. Philadelphia: WB Saunders, 2005
2. Persson PB: Renin: Origin, secretion and synthesis. J Physiol 552(3):667–671, 2003
3. Henke K, Eigsti J: Renal physiology: Review and practical application in the critically ill patient. Dimens Crit Care Nurs 22(3):125–132, 2003.
4. Elgart HN: Assessment of fluids and electrolytes. AACN Clin Issues 15(4):607–621, 2005

Other Selected Readings

Huether SE, McCance KL: Pathophysiology: The Biologic Basis for Disease in Adults and Children, 5th ed. St. Louis: Mosby, 2005
Koeppen BM, Stanton BA: Renal Physiology, 4th ed. St Louis: Mosby, 2006
Porth CM: Pathophysiology: Concepts of Altered Health States, 7th ed. Philadelphia: Lippincott Williams & Wilkins, 2005
Rennke HG, Denker BM: Renal Pathophysiology: The Essentials, 2nd ed. Baltimore: Williams & Wilkins, 2006
Seeley RR, Stephens TD, Tate P, et al: Anatomy and Physiology, 8th ed. New York: McGraw-Hill, 2007
Sherwood L: Human Physiology: From Cells to Systems, 6th ed. Los Angeles: Brooks-Cole, 2007

Patient Assessment: Renal System

Kara Adams Snyder

Objectives

Based on the content in this chapter, the reader should be able to:

1 Formulate a plan for collecting history and physical examination data for patients with renal disorders and fluid and electrolyte imbalance.

2 Describe diagnostic and laboratory blood tests used to evaluate renal status.

3 Discuss methods to evaluate fluid balance.

Assessment of the renal system involves determining how well the kidneys perform their many functions. It also includes gathering information about other systems. A careful assessment of the history and physical findings, with interpretation of laboratory and diagnostic test results, provides early clues to the diagnosis of disorders of water and volume imbalance and other complications of renal dysfunction in the critically ill patient.

• History

The patient history provides important information that helps determine the cause, severity, treatment, and management of renal dysfunction. It involves gathering information about the present illness, past health history, family history, personal history, and social history. In addition, relevant information about the status of other body systems is gathered through a review of systems. A guide for renal assessment is summarized in Box 29-1.

To begin, the nurse asks the patient about his or her perception of the chief complaint. The nurse uses the NOPQRST format described in Box 17-1 to learn more about each symptom the patient describes. The significance of the complaint to the patient and its impact on the patient's life should be ascertained. The patient is asked about previous occurrences of the complaint.

Once the patient has described the presenting problem, the nurse inquires about the patient's past health history and family history. This information may offer clues to the underlying cause of the problem. Next the nurse asks about the patient's personal and social history because this information helps the nurse develop an individualized plan of care. The health history concludes with a review of systems. Renal function has an impact on all other body systems, so it is important to ask the patient about each body system.

• Physical Examination

The physical examination provides objective data that are used to substantiate and clarify the history. The history guides the physical examination and helps determine areas of the examination that require more depth. If time permits, the nurse

Box 29-1 • Health History for Renal Assessment

Chief Complaint
- Patient's description of the problem

History of the Present Illness
- Complete analysis of the following signs and symptoms (using the NOPQRST format, see Chapter 17, Box 17-1)
- Frequency
- Urgency
- Hesitancy
- Burning
- Dysuria
- Hematuria
- Incontinence
- Lower back pain
- Pain with urination
- Change in color, odor, or amount of urine
- Thirst
- Change in weight
- Edema

Past Health History
- Relevant antenatal history and immunizations: prematurity; antenatal use of angiotensin-converting enzyme inhibitors, angiotensin-receptor blockers, or nonsteroidal anti-inflammatory drugs (NSAIDs; e.g., ibuprofen); ensuring antenatal vaccination against rubella; screening for cytomegalovirus or toxoplasmosis
- Past acute and chronic medical problems, including treatments and hospitalizations: renal failure; renal calculi; renal cancer; glomerulonephritis; Wegener's granulomatosis; polycystic kidney disease; dialysis, including type, frequency, and duration; urinary tract infections; systemic lupus erythematosus; sickle cell anemia; cancer; AIDS; hepatitis C; heart failure; diabetes; hypertension
- Risk factors: age; trauma; heavy use of ibuprofen, naproxen, or acetaminophen; use of heroin or cocaine
- Past surgeries: kidney transplantation, placement of dialysis fistula
- Past diagnostic tests and interventions: urinalysis, cystoscopy, intravenous pyelography, ultrasound of kidneys, renal biopsy, magnetic resonance imaging, diagnostic tests that have used contrast dyes
- Medications: diuretics, aminoglycosides, antibiotics, NSAIDs
- Allergies and reactions: radiographic contrast media
- Transfusions

Family History
- Health status or cause of death of parents and siblings: hereditary nephritis, polycystic kidney disease, diabetes, high blood pressure

Personal and Social History
- Tobacco, alcohol, and substance use
- Family composition
- Occupation and work environment: exposure to nephrotoxic substances such as organic acids, pesticides, lead, mercury
- Living environment: exposure to nephrotoxic substances such as organic acids, pesticides, lead, mercury
- Diet
- Sleep patterns
- Exercise
- Cultural beliefs
- Spiritual and religious beliefs
- Coping patterns and social support systems
- Leisure activities
- Sexual activity
- Recent travel

Review of Systems
- Skin: dryness, itching
- HEENT: periorbital edema
- Cardiovascular: hypertension, heart failure, vascular disease
- Respiratory: Goodpasture's syndrome
- Gastrointestinal: hepatitis, cirrhosis
- Endocrine: diabetes mellitus
- Neurological: numbness, tingling, burning, tremors, memory loss
- Hematological: sickle cell anemia
- Immune: systemic lupus erythematosus
- Musculoskeletal: rhabdomyolysis, muscle weakness

reviews the chart, including laboratory results, before beginning the physical examination. This can help identify data that require follow-up during the physical examination.

The nurse begins the physical examination by observing the patient's overall appearance, including facial expression, height and weight, position in bed, grooming, personal hygiene, and signs of distress. The nurse observes the patient's level of responsiveness, cognition, and interaction with people, including positive, negative, or unusual responses.

Because patients with renal problems usually have significant problems with fluid and electrolyte balance, the nurse evaluates the patient's volume status throughout the examination. The nurse begins by taking the vital signs. Particular attention is paid to the blood pressure, noting pulse pressure and presence of a positive pulse paradoxus. An elevated temperature may indicate an infection. Patients with chronic kidney disease (CKD) tend to have low temperatures because they are often immunocompromised.

Throughout the physical examination, the nurse inspects the skin on the extremities and trunk for color and evidence of excoriation, bruising, or bleeding; palpates for moistness, dryness, temperature (using the back of the fingers), and edema; and checks mobility and turgor by lifting a fold of skin and noting the ease (mobility) and speed with which it returns into place (turgor). To assess hydration further, the nurse inspects the tongue and mucous membranes in the mouth and looks for a saliva pool under the tongue. Additional volume status assessment is done when examining the neck, as the nurse observes for jugular vein distention and determines the need to measure jugular venous pressure.

The anterior and posterior chest is inspected for respiratory rate, rhythm, depth, and effort. Deformities of the thorax, shape of chest, or bulging of interspaces during expiration are noted. The precordial area is observed and palpated for heaves, pulsations, and thrills. The nurse listens for heart rate and rhythm, extra heart sounds, murmurs, clicks, and pericardial friction rub. Fluid overload often results in the presence of a third or fourth heart sound.

Anterior and posterior lung fields are auscultated. The nurse notes the quality of vesicular breath sounds and the presence of adventitious breath sounds (crackles, wheezes, rubs), which may indicate volume overload.

After auscultating the posterior chest, the nurse can assess kidney tenderness. To do this, the nurse places one hand over the posterior costovertebral angle (CVA). Then, using the fist of the second hand, the nurse gently percusses the CVA and notes whether the patient has discomfort (Fig. 29-1), which is known as CVA tenderness (CVAT).

The nurse inspects the abdomen and then listens for bowel sounds. In addition to auscultating bowel sounds, the nurse auscultates the renal arteries for the presence of bruits by placing the stethoscope above and to the left and right of the umbilicus (Fig. 29-2). A bruit is an abnormal sound that resembles a blowing or swishing noise, similar to the sound of a cardiac murmur. The presence of a renal bruit may indicate renal artery stenosis, which means there may be diminished blood flow to the kidney. This diminished blood flow may result in acute or chronic renal dysfunction.

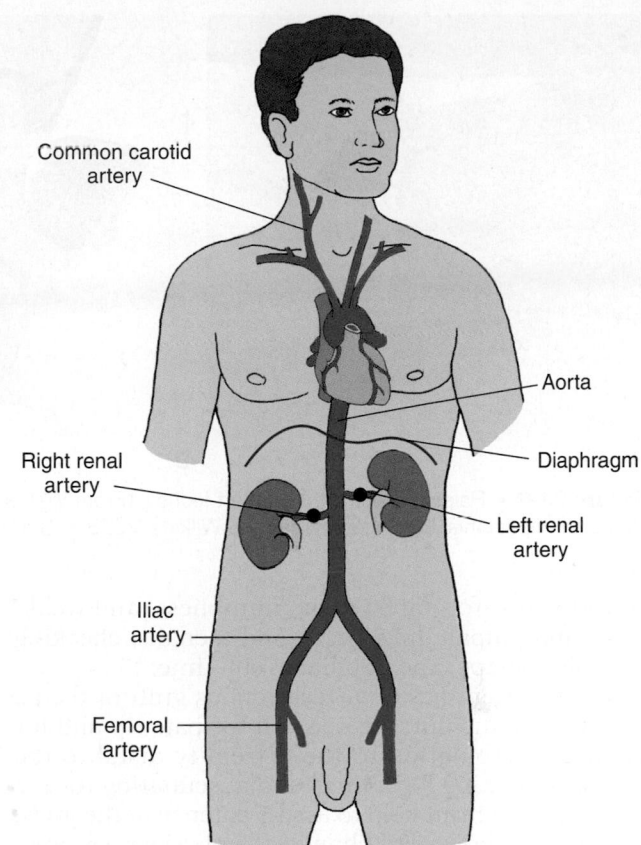

Figure 29-2 • Sites for auscultation of renal bruits.

Next, the nurse percusses and palpates the abdomen, and then palpates the liver border to determine enlargement. If ascites is suspected, the nurse measures abdominal girth and may check for a fluid wave or shifting dullness. During the abdominal examination, the right and left kidneys are palpated by placing one hand under the patient's flank and placing the other examining hand in the quadrant just below the costal margin at the mid-clavicular line. The kidneys are normally not palpable. An enlarged kidney may be palpable, and the enlargement may be due to a cyst, tumor, or hydronephrosis (Fig. 29-3). If indicated by history, the nurse may palpate and percuss the bladder. The bladder cannot be palpated unless it is distended above the symphysis pubis. When palpated, the dome of the distended bladder feels smooth and round. For palpation and percussion of the bladder, the nurse begins at the symphysis pubis and moves upward and outward to estimate the bladder size. A full bladder is dull to percussion (Fig. 29-4).

If the patient is at risk for excess vascular volume, the nurse looks for hypertension; pulmonary edema; crackles; engorged, elevated neck veins; liver congestion and enlargement; heart failure; and shortness of breath. Signs and symptoms related to excess extravascular volume include pitting edema of feet, ankles, hands, and fingers; periorbital edema; sacral edema; and ascites. Table 29-1 presents a scale used to document levels of pitting edema.

While examining the extremities, the nurse can check the quality of the peripheral pulses; observe for

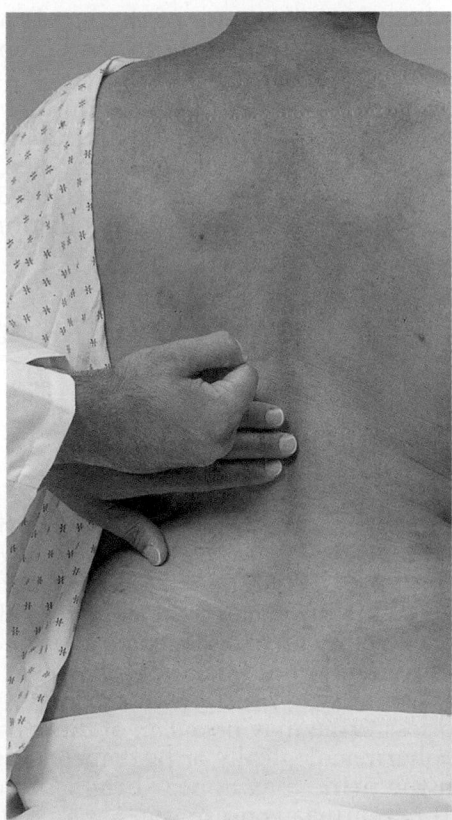

Figure 29-1 • Assessing costovertebral angle (CVA) tenderness. (From Bickley LS: Bates' Guide to Physical Examination, 9th ed. Philadelphia: Lippincott Williams & Wilkins, 2007, p 386.)

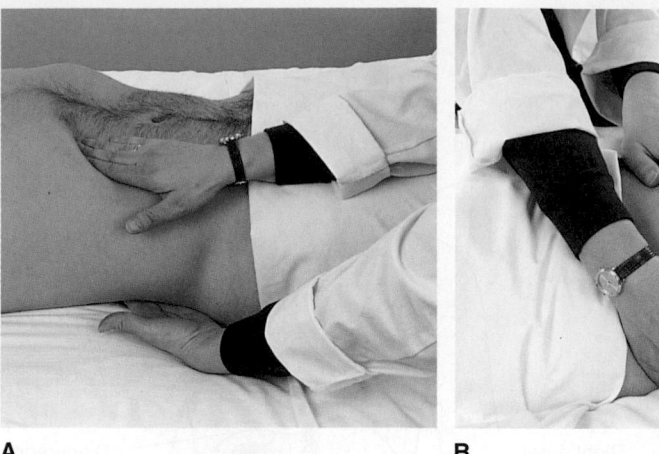
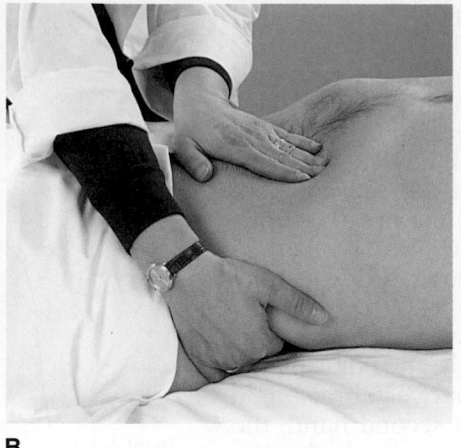
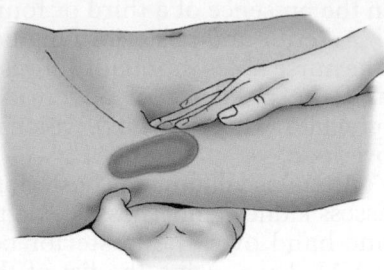

A   **B**   **C**

Figure 29-3 • Palpating the right and left kidney. (From Weber J, Kelley J: Health Assessment in Nursing, 2nd ed. Philadelphia: Lippincott Williams & Wilkins, 2003, p. 390.)

tremors; test for paresthesia, numbness, and weakness; and palpate fingernails and toenails, checking for color, shape, and capillary refill time.

If the patient has an arteriovenous graft or fistula for dialysis, the nurse assesses it for patency and for adequate circulation to the extremity distal to the access. Palpating for a thrill and auscultating for the presence of a bruit help to assess patency of the graft. If assessment reveals a change, the physician or practitioner must be notified urgently because the graft may be saved through radiological or surgical intervention. If the patient has temporary dialysis access, the exit site is inspected for signs of inflammation or infection. Often the lumens of the temporary access have high doses of heparin to maintain patency, so flushing or use of the device is clarified with the physician or practitioner before any manipulation or use of the catheter.

Patients with renal impairment may be at risk for hypocalcemia, hypomagnesemia, or both. Physical assessment of these electrolyte changes can be achieved by checking for Chvostek's and Trousseau's signs. Chvostek's sign occurs when there is facial irritability after tapping the facial nerve in front of the auditory meatus with the finger. Trousseau's sign occurs when there is spasm of the hands and feet (carpopedal spasm) in response to arm compression (e.g., as with a blood pressure cuff).

During the history and examination, the critical care nurse continuously observes the patient's level of consciousness and mental status. If more data are needed, the nurse may use tools such as the Glasgow Coma Scale and Folstein Mini-Mental Examination.

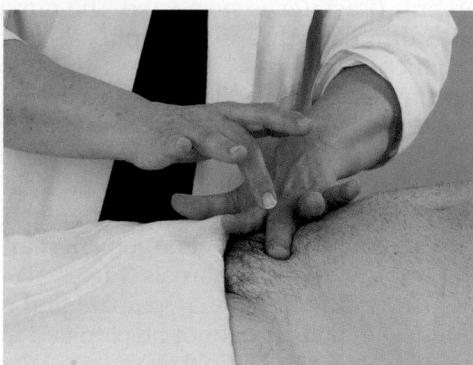

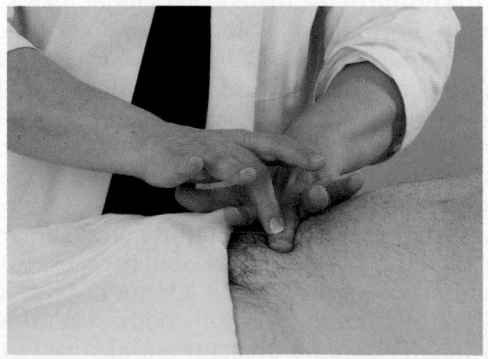

Figure 29-4 • Percussing the bladder. (From Rhoads J: Advanced Health Assessment and Diagnostic Reasoning. Philadelphia: Lippincott Williams & Wilkins, 2006, p. 305.)

• Assessment of Renal Function

LABORATORY STUDIES

Urine Studies

Urinalysis

The nurse inspects the urine for color, clarity, and odor. Normally, the urine is clear and yellow to straw-colored and smells of ammonia. Changes in the characteristics of the urine can indicate kidney damage, infection, excretion of drugs, or the kidney's compensation for systemic homeostatic imbalance. Cloudy urine may indicate infection, whereas very clear and colorless urine may be a sign of diuresis, either induced pharmacologically or by diabetes insipidus. Blood in the urine may appear bright red or dark brown. If hematuria is present in a man older than 50 years of age, additional radiological evaluation (such as cystoscopy) is considered to rule out a malignancy.[1] Urinalysis is used to identify more specifically

Table 29-1 • Assessing Pitting Edema

Scale	Description	Depth of Indentation	Return to Baseline
4+	Severe	8 mm	2–5 minutes
3+	Moderate	6 mm	1–2 minutes
2+	Mild	4 mm	10–15 seconds
1+	Trace	2 mm	Disappears rapidly

From Rhoads J: Advanced Health Assessment and Diagnostic Reasoning. Philadelphia: Lippincott Williams & Wilkins, 2006, p 253.

the components of the urine. Table 29-2 summarizes the components of the urinalysis.

Urine Volume
The difference between the glomerular filtration rate (GFR) and the amount of water reabsorbed determines the urine volume. A patient with a normal GFR of 180 L must reabsorb 179 L/day. This is the equivalent of roughly more than 99% of filtered volume. Patients with renal disease and impairment may actually excrete an appropriate amount of urine. For example, a patient with severe renal disease may have a GFR of 10 L but still excrete 1 L, or 90% reabsorption. Thus, urine volume is of little diagnostic importance in this setting. However, urine volume is important in the setting of acute anuria. In acute anuria, a patient may be making normal volume and experience an abrupt change in pattern. Causes of acute anuria include:

▶ Complete bilateral obstruction (i.e., abdominal compartment syndrome)
▶ Glomerulonephritis
▶ Bilateral vascular occlusion

However, trends in urine production can provide important clues to the body's recruitment of important compensatory responses, as in hypovolemia. The body initiates the renin–angiotensin–aldosterone system to maintain the crucial water balance (see Chapter 28).

Urine pH
Normal urinary pH is acidic, with a range between 5.0 and 6.5, depending primarily on dietary intake. The kidneys play a tremendous role in acid–base balance (see Chapter 28). Clinically, urinary pH is important in two settings. First, an alkaline urinary pH (above 7.5) suggests the presence of a urinary tract infection. Second, a low, or acidic, pH indicates the kidney may be compensating for a serum acidosis. Physiologically, in this state, the kidneys reabsorb more bicarbonate and excrete more hydrogen ions to buffer the serum acidosis. The urine becomes increasingly acidic (lower pH) when the body is attempting to conserve sodium, as in states of dehydration.

Urine Protein
Most proteins are large molecules and under normal conditions should not penetrate Bowman's capsule. Normal urinary protein levels, therefore, are zero to trace. Proteinuria usually indicates damage to the capillary structures, as in the case of glomerular diseases (glomerulonephritis) and intrarenal acute renal failure. For diagnostic purposes, a 24-hour sample of urine is used to assess for proteinuria. Single dipstick measurements are not as sensitive and may lead to false-positive values.

Urine Glucose and Ketones
Glucose, like most proteins, is not present in the urine under normal conditions. Unlike proteins, however, glucose is freely filtered but is reabsorbed in the proximal tubule. Glucose becomes detectable if the serum glucose is elevated (>200 mg/dL) as the filtered load exceeds the kidney's reabsorptive abilities. Findings of glucosuria should be confirmed with serum or capillary blood glucose measurement.

Ketone bodies are byproducts of fat metabolism and are formed in states of insulin deficiency. Three ketone bodies are formed: β-hydroxybutyric acid (the primary ketone formed), acetoacetic acid, and acetone. The latter two ketone bodies are detected in the urine. Acetone may be measured in the serum. A urine sample that is positive for ketones may indicate diabetic ketoacidosis.

Urinary Sediment
Sediment is particulate matter that, when examined, can reveal certain physiological conditions in the renal system. Sediment in general refers to casts, red cells, white cells, epithelial cells, and crystals. Casts are the breakdown products of cellular material formed in the collecting tubules. Urinary stasis, as in prerenal disease, may promote cast formation. Casts can be made up of different types of cells, and thus, the shape, composition, and size of the casts can help in the identification of the presence and etiology of a disease.

Red Blood Cells Red blood cells may be microscopic (microscopic hematuria) or grossly visible (macroscopic hematuria). Red blood cells enter the urine anywhere along the urinary tract. Any injury or damage to the structures making up the urinary tract can cause hematuria. Kidney stones, trauma, and prostatic disease are examples of extrarenal causes of hematuria (i.e., not related to the kidneys). Microscopic bleeding can be present in glomerular diseases, such as glomerulonephritis. When assessing the results of the urinalysis, take note of the presence of red blood cell casts and the red blood cell morphology. Glomerular bleeding is often associated with some type of fragmentation of the red

Table 29-2 • What Urinalysis Findings Mean

Test	Normal Values or Findings	Abnormal Findings	Possible Causes of Abnormal Findings
Color and odor	• Straw color	Clear to black	Dietary changes; use of certain drugs, metabolic inflammatory, or infectious disease
	• Slightly aromatic odor	Fruity odor	Diabetes mellitus, starvation, dehydration
	• Clear appearance	Turbid appearance	Renal infection
Specific gravity	• Between 1.005 and 1.030, with slight variations from one specimen to the next	Below-normal specific gravity	Diabetes insipidus, glomerulonephritis, pyelonephritis, acute renal failure, alkalosis
		Above-normal specific gravity	Dehydration, nephrosis
		Fixed specific gravity	Severe renal damage
pH	• Between 4.5 and 8.0	Alkaline pH (above 8.0)	Fanconi's syndrome (chronic renal disease) urinary tract infection, metabolic or respiratory alkalosis
		Acidic pH (below 4.5)	Renal tuberculosis, phenylketonuria, acidosis
Protein	• No protein	Proteinuria	Renal disease (such as glomerulosclerosis, acute or chronic glomerulonephritis, nephrolithiasis, polycystic kidney disease, and acute or chronic renal failure)
Ketones	• No ketones	Ketonuria	Diabetes mellitus, starvation, conditions causing acutely increased metabolic demands and decreased food intake (such as vomiting and diarrhea)
Glucose	• No glucose	Glycosuria	Diabetes mellitus
Red blood cells (RBCs)	• 0 to 3 RBCs/high-power field	Numerous RBCs	Urinary tract infection, obstruction, inflammation trauma, or tumor; glomerulonephritis; renal hypertension; lupus nephritis; renal tuberculosis; renal vein thrombosis; hydronephrosis; pyelonephritis; parasitis bladder infection; polyarteritis nodosa; hemorrhagic disorder
Epithelial cells	• Few epithelial cells	Excessive epithelial cells	Renal tubular degeneration
White blood cells (WBCs)	• 0 to 4 WBCs/high-power field	Numerous WBCs	Urinary tract inflammation, especially cystitis or pyelonephritis
		Numerous WBCs and WBC casts	Renal infection (such as acute pyelonephritis and glomerulonephritis, nephrotic syndrome, pyogenic infection, and lupus nephritis)
Casts	• No casts (except occasional hyaline casts)	Excessive casts	Renal disease
		Excessive hyaline casts	Renal parenchymal disease, inflammation, glomerular capillary membrane trauma
		Epithelial casts	Renal tubular damage, nephrosis, eclampsia, chronic lead intoxication
		Fatty, waxy casts	Nephrotic syndrome, chronic renal disease, diabetes mellitus
		RBC casts	Renal parenchymal disease (especially glomerulonephritis), renal infarction, subacute bacterial endocarditis, sickle cell anemia, blood dyscrasias, malignant hypertension, collagen disease
Crystals	• Some crystals	Numerous calcium oxalate crystals	Hypercalcemia
		Cystine crystals (cystinuria)	Inborn metabolic error
Yeast cells	• No yeast crystals	Yeast cells in sediment	External genitalia contamination, vaginitis, urethritis, prostatovesiculitis
Parasites	• No parasites	Parasites in sediment	External genitalia contamination
Creatinine clearance	• Males (age 20): 90 mg/min/173 m² of body surface • Females (age 20): 84 mL/min/1.73 m² of body surface • Older patients: normally decreased concentrations by 6 mL/min/decade	Above-normal creatinine clearance	Little diagnostic significance
		Below-normal creatinine clearance	Reduced renal blood flow (associated with shock or renal artery obstruction), acute tubular necrosis, acute or chronic glomerulonephritis, advanced bilateral renal lesions (as in polycystic kidney disease, renal tuberculosis, and cancer), nephrosclerosis, heart failure, severe dehydration

From Critical Care Nursing Made Incredibly Easy, 2nd ed. Philadelphia: Lippincott Williams & Wilkins, 2008, pp. 505–506.

blood cell, whereas extrarenal bleeding often leaves the cell intact. The presence of red blood cell casts is virtually diagnostic of glomerulonephritis.

Myoglobin in the urine makes the urine appear red; however, when the urine is inspected under the microscope, there is no evidence of red blood cells. Myoglobin is a component of skeletal muscle breakdown, or rhabdomyolysis. Crush injuries or protracted down times are the greatest predictors of this disease. When muscle begins to break down, it releases the myoglobin, which is similar in chemical structure to hemoglobin. Because of its large molecular size, myoglobin blocks the renal tubules, placing patients at very high risk for intrarenal failure.

White Blood Cells White blood cells in the urine (pyuria) usually indicate infection anywhere along the urinary tract. Leukocyte esterase is an enzyme that can be detected in the urine. This enzyme is present along the urinary tract as a component of the local immune response. High levels of this enzyme can indicate infection. The presence of nitrates may also aid in the diagnosis of a bacterial infection along the urinary tract.

Specific Gravity and Osmolality

The specific gravity of the urine tests the kidneys' ability to concentrate and dilute the urine. The specific gravity measures the buoyancy of a solution compared with water and depends on the number of particles in the solution and their size and weight. There are three methods used to obtain this measurement in clinical practice: a multiple-test dipstick that has a reagent area for specific gravity, the urinometer, and the refractometer (TS meter). The urinometer has been in clinical use for many years and requires enough urine to float the urinometer. Its results are questionable. The refractometer gives highly reproducible results and requires only one drop of urine for the measurement. In addition, this instrument can be used to measure the total solids in plasma (hence the name, TS meter), which is a good indicator of the plasma protein concentration and can be a useful indicator of a patient's fluid balance (especially if serial determinations are done).

The normal kidney has the capacity to dilute the urine to a specific gravity of 1.001 and to concentrate the urine to at least 1.022. For reference, the specific gravity of water is 1.000. Normally, a person's water balance determines whether the urine is concentrated or dilute; dilute urine is an indicator of water excess, and concentrated urine indicates water deficit. In many renal diseases, the ability of the kidneys to form concentrated urine is lost, and the specific gravity can become "fixed" at approximately 1.010. This finding is often seen in acute tubular necrosis, acute nephritis, and chronic renal disease. A falsely high specific gravity can be seen when high–molecular-weight substances, such as protein, glucose, mannitol, and radiographic contrast material, are present in the urine. Therefore, a greater degree of accuracy can be obtained by checking the urine osmolality in these cases.

Osmolality measures only the number of solute particles present in a solution. Recall that the main determinants of osmolality are the sodium, urea, and glucose. In states of volume depletion or excess, several neuroendocrine responses interact to maintain homeostasis, thereby affecting the urinary osmolality. Because of this dynamic interaction, particularly in critical illness, single measurements of the osmolality are of little diagnostic importance. The urinary osmolality is often followed for the evaluation of patients with hyponatremia.

Normal urine osmolality ranges from 300 to 900 mOsm/kg/24 hours. Because of this wide range, more information about renal function is obtained when simultaneous serum and urine samples are collected and interpreted. In renal disease, one of the first functions to be lost is the ability to concentrate urine. This can result in the urine osmolality becoming fixed within 150 mOsm of the simultaneously determined serum osmolality.

Urinary Sodium Concentration

The urinary sodium excretion is used as an indicator of renal function in differentiating the oliguria associated with acute renal failure from other prerenal causes. States of poor kidney perfusion are usually associated with a decrease in urinary sodium concentration (usually <10 mEq/L). This is a compensatory reaction generated by the activation of the renin–angiotensin–aldosterone system. Activation of this neuroendocrine response allows for increased reabsorption of sodium (reduced excretion) with a subsequent increase in water reabsorption. The root cause of kidney hypoperfusion can be anything that causes a reduction in effective circulating volume: Volume depletion and heart failure are two examples. Acute renal failure may develop if hypoperfusion persists. In acute renal failure, urine sodium concentration usually is greater than 30 to 40 mEq/L despite oliguria because of damage to the tubular transport mechanisms. However, when the urine pH is alkaline, urine sodium concentration does not reflect sodium balance accurately, and the chloride concentration becomes a better indicator of volume status.

Fractional Excretion of Sodium Test

The fractional excretion of sodium (FE_{Na}) test gives a more precise estimation of the amount of filtered sodium that remains in the urine and is more accurate in predicting tubular injury than the urinary sodium concentration.[2] One benefit of the FE_{Na} compared with the urinary sodium is that it removes the confounding effect of water. It can be calculated by using the following formula:

$$FE_{Na} = \frac{U_{Na} \times P_{Cr}}{P_{Na} \times U_{Cr}}$$

where U and P are the urinary and plasma concentrations of sodium and creatinine, respectively. (Although volume measurements are necessary to derive the absolute urinary excretion of both sodium and creatinine, these cancel out in deriving the formula.)

The Fe$_{Na}$ test requires the determination of both serum and urinary sodium and creatinine concentrations on simultaneously obtained samples. Values less than 1% indicate prerenal azotemia, or underperfusion. Values greater than 1% (and frequently greater than 3%) are indicative of acute renal failure.

Blood Studies

Creatinine and Creatinine Clearance

Creatinine is a byproduct of normal muscle metabolism and is excreted in the urine primarily as the result of glomerular filtration, with a small percentage secreted into the urine by the kidney tubules. Therefore, creatinine is currently the most useful indicator of GFR. The amount of creatinine excreted in the urine is directly related to muscle mass and normally remains constant unless significant muscle wasting (a catabolic state) occurs. Normal serum values for creatinine are 0.6 to 1.2 mg/dL.

The creatinine clearance can be defined as the amount of blood that is cleared of creatinine in 1 minute and is an excellent clinical indicator of renal function. As renal function diminishes, creatinine clearance decreases. To obtain an accurate creatinine clearance, the nurse collects all urine made in a 24-hour period and obtains a blood specimen at some point during the urine collection. Thus, it is essential for the nurse to communicate to other team members that a 24-hour collection is in progress. For consistency, the blood sample is usually collected at the midpoint of the urine collection. It is important to note the exact beginning and ending times of the urine collection.

The actual creatinine clearance is calculated by the following formula:

$$CrCl = \frac{U_{Cr} \times V}{P_{Cr}}$$

where U is the urine creatinine concentration; V, the urine volume; and P, the plasma creatinine concentration.

The product U multiplied by V tells how much creatinine appears in the urine during the period of collection. This can be converted readily to milligrams per minute, which is the standard reference point. Dividing this value by the plasma creatinine concentration (which must be converted from milligrams per 100 mL to milligrams per milliliter) tells the minimal number of milliliters of plasma that must have been filtered by the glomeruli to produce the measured amount of creatinine in the urine. The final result is usually expressed in milliliters per minute. The normal range varies between 80 and 120 mL/minute, depending on the person's size, age, and sex. The results can be adjusted to a standard body size of 1.73 m² (body surface area [BSA]), which can be derived from standard tables if the patient's height and weight are known; it averages between 120 and 125 mL/minute/1.73 m² BSA. After age 40 years, normal creatinine clearance values generally decrease 6.5 mL/minute per decade because of a decline in GFR.

There are also formulas that estimate creatinine clearance based on a single serum creatinine level. An estimate may be made when there is difficulty collecting a 24-hour urine sample or when spot-checking the creatinine clearance will assist prompt treatment (as in the case of drug nephrotoxicity). The estimate may be accurate only in patients with chronic renal failure with stable renal function who are not edematous or extremely overweight.

$$\text{Creatinine Clearance} = \frac{(140 - \text{age}) \times \text{weight (kg)}}{72 \times x \; P_{Cr} \, (\text{mg/dL})}$$

where P$_{Cr}$ is plasma creatinine; note that for women, the final result is multiplied by 0.85. Many labs are now routinely reporting the GFR using estimate formulas for creatine clearance.

When the kidneys are damaged by a disease process, the creatinine clearance decreases, and the serum creatinine concentration rises. The urine creatinine excretion decreases initially until the blood level rises to a point at which the amount of creatinine appearing in the urine is equal to the amount being produced by the body. Because men tend to have a higher proportion of muscle than women, the creatinine and creatinine clearance can be higher in men than women. A healthy person with a serum creatinine concentration of 1 mg/dL and a creatinine excretion of 1 mg/minute has a creatinine clearance of 100 mL/minute. When the person experiences a 50% loss of renal function, the serum creatinine rises to 2 mg/dL, and the person will continue to excrete 1 mg/minute of creatinine in the urine when balance is restored. When the person has rapidly changing renal function and oliguria (e.g., acute renal failure), the creatinine clearance is less reliable. Until renal function stabilizes, serum creatinine levels provide a better indication of the rate and direction of change. In patients with rhabdomyolysis, the serum creatinine is elevated out of proportion to the reduction of GFR as the result of chemical conversion of muscle creatine to creatinine. In this situation, the serum creatinine is less reliable as an indicator of renal function.

Blood Urea Nitrogen

The blood urea nitrogen (BUN) level has been used for many years as an indicator of kidney function, but unlike the serum creatinine, the BUN level can be influenced by many factors. At low urine flow rates, more sodium and water, and consequently more urea, are reabsorbed. Therefore, when the patient is volume depleted, the BUN tends to increase out of proportion to any change in renal function. A normal value for the BUN is considered to be 8 to 20 mg/dL.

Increased urea production can result from increased protein intake (tube feedings and some forms of hyperalimentation), increased tissue breakdown (as with crush injuries), febrile illnesses, steroid or tetracycline administration, and reabsorption of blood from the intestine in a patient with intestinal hemorrhage. The BUN also may be elevated in the dehydrated patient because the lack of fluid volume causes a concentrated value. The patient in shock and the patient with heart failure may have an elevated BUN secondary to decreased renal perfusion. The opposite is true for patients with decreased protein intake or liver disease (both of which reduce urea production) and for patients with large urine volumes secondary to excessive fluid intake.

However, the BUN can be of significant value when used as a comparison with the serum creatinine concentration. Normally, there is a urea/creatinine ratio of 10:1. Discrepancies in this ratio might suggest a potentially correctable situation, as Box 29-2 shows.

Osmolality

The osmolality of a solution is an expression of the total number (concentration) of particles in the solution and is independent of the size, molecular weight, and electrical charge of the molecules. All substances in solution contribute to the osmolality. For example, 1 mol (gram molecular weight) of sodium chloride dissociates incompletely into Na and Cl ions and produces 1.86 osm when dissolved in 1 kg of solvent (such as plasma). A mole of nonionic solute (e.g., glucose or urea) produces only 1 osm when dissolved in 1 kg of solvent. The total concentration of particles in a solution equals the osmolality and is normally reported in units of osmoles per kilogram of solvent. In the clinical setting (because of much smaller concentrations), the osmolality is reported in milliosmoles (thousandth of an osmole, abbreviated mOsm) per kilogram of solvent (plasma or serum).

The normal serum osmolality consists primarily of sodium and its accompanying anions, with urea and glucose contributing about 5 mOsm each. Therefore, when the serum sodium, urea, and glucose concentrations are known, the osmolality of plasma can be calculated by the following formula:

$$\text{Osmolality} = 2(\text{Na}) + \frac{\text{Glucose}}{18} + \frac{\text{BUN}}{2.8}$$

The normal adult average osmolality is 280 to 290 mOsm/kg and remains quite constant. Because water can move freely between the blood, interstitial fluid, and tissues, any change in the osmolality of one body compartment produces a shift in body fluids. Therefore, the osmolality of the plasma is the same as that of other body compartments except in rapidly changing conditions, when a slight lag may occur.

Box 29-2 • **Factors Affecting the Serum Urea: Creatinine Ratio**

Decreased Urea/Creatinine Ratio (<10:1)
- Liver disease
- Protein restriction
- Excessive fluid intake

Increased Urea/Creatinine Ratio (>10:1)
- Volume depletion
- Decreased "effective" blood volume
- Catabolic states
- Excessive protein intake

A decrease in the serum osmolality can occur only when the serum sodium is decreased. An increase in the serum osmolality can occur whenever the serum sodium, urea, or glucose is elevated or when abnormal compounds are present in the blood, such as drugs, poisons, or metabolic waste products, such as lactic acid. Symptoms usually do not occur until the osmolality is greater than 350 mOsm/kg. Coma can occur when the osmolality is 400 mOsm/kg or greater.

The calculated osmolarity normally is within 10 mOsm of the measured osmolality. Comparing the calculated and measured osmolality can be useful in determining potential substances present. An elevated osmolar gap provides evidence for the presence of a significant amount of abnormal solutes. Ethanol, methanol, and ethylene glycol are three examples of such solutes that, when present in appreciable amounts, cause an elevated osmolar gap. If ingestion of one of these substances is suspected, calculate the osmolar gap.

Nonspecific Studies

Hematocrit and Hemoglobin The normal hemoglobin for men is 13.5 to 17.5 g/dL and is 12 to 16 g/dL for women. The normal hematocrit should be 40% to 52% for adult men and 37% to 48% for adult women. False elevations of hematocrit can be seen with dehydration or after dialysis. Low hematocrits may be a dilutional value due to hypervolemia. The kidney is the primary site for the production of erythropoietin. It stimulates the bone marrow to release mature red blood cells. Many patients with CKD produce insufficient amounts of erythropoietin, which can result in chronic anemia. These patients may also have bleeding problems due to impaired platelet function and immunological abnormalities.

Uric Acid Uric acid is a nitrogenous end product of protein and purine metabolism. Humans produce only small quantities of uric acid under normal conditions, and the normal uric acid serum level is between 2 and 8.5 mg/dL. Uric acid is excreted primarily by the kidneys, with some in the stool. The value may be elevated because of excessive production from cell breakdown or inadequate excretion by the kidney.

DIAGNOSTIC STUDIES

Radiological Studies

Radiological studies of the kidneys that may be useful in evaluating renal abnormalities include roentgenography, ultrasonography, and radionuclide studies. Table 29-3 summarizes these studies and their purposes.

Renal Biopsy

Renal biopsy is the most invasive but most definitive diagnostic tool used in the comprehensive renal evaluation.[3] It is used to define the histological counter-

Table 29-3 • Radiological Study of Kidneys

Diagnostic Test	Definition	Purpose
Roentgenography		
Radiograph of kidney–ureter–bladder (KUB)	Also known as abdominal x-ray. Standard x-rays capture image.	Detects abnormal calcifications and renal size
Tomography	Standard x-rays capture series of cross-sectional scans made along single axis of bodily structure or tissue. Computer software is used to construct three-dimensional image of that structure.	Determines renal outlines and abnormalities
Intravenous pyelography (IVP)	X-ray of renal structures using contrast material. Images are captured on real-time basis. Contrast material is injected intravenously and then collected in renal system; this turns areas bright white, allowing assessment of anatomy and function of kidneys and lower urinary tract.	Detects anatomical abnormalities of kidneys and ureters
Retrograde pyelography	Similar to IVP, with use of x-ray and contrast material. Contrast material is injected through urinary catheter. This test is typically performed at the same time as cystoscopy.	Assesses renal size, evaluates ureteral obstruction, and localizes and diagnoses tumors as well as obstructions
Antegrade pyelography	Similar to IVP and retrograde pyelography, this x-ray test uses contrast material to visualize structures of urinary tract. Contrast dye, however, is injected into ureter. Thus, structures of upper urinary tract are well visualized.	Distinguishes cysts from hydronephrosis
Renal arteriography and venography	Vessel (artery or vein) is accessed and contrast dye is injected to visualize structures "downstream."	Evaluates possible renal arterial stenosis, renal mass lesions, renal vein thrombosis, and venous extension of renal cell carcinoma
Digital subtraction angiography	X-ray with a computer technique that compares x-ray image of kidney vessels before and after contrast dye is injected. Tissues and blood vessels on first image are digitally subtracted from second image, leaving clear picture of artery, which can then be studied independently from rest of the body.	Visualizes major arterial vessels
Ultrasonography	Imaging technique that is excellent means of visualizing tissues and organs to assess their size, structure, and possible pathology. Images are created by emission and receiving of sound waves.	Delineates renal outlines Measures longitudinal and transverse dimensions of the kidneys Evaluates mass lesions Examines perinephric area Detects and grades hydronephrosis
Radionuclide scintillation imaging (renal scan)	Nuclear medicine test that uses small amounts of radioactive materials (radioisotopes) to measure kidney function	
Static imaging	Gives information about the size, shape, and position of the kidneys; and whether there are scars on the kidney from a previous infection.	Evaluates location, size, and contour of functional renal tissue; may reveal areas of inhomogeneity or filling defects
Dynamic imaging	Gives information about the blood flow to the kidneys and how well each kidney is functioning for the production of urine	Monitors passage of radiopharmaceutical agent through vascular, renal parenchymal, and urinary tract compartments; also indicates whether there are any obstructions in urine output
Magnetic resonance imaging	Uses nonionizing radiofrequency signals (as opposed to computed tomography, which uses ionizing radiation) to acquire its images and is best suited for noncalcified tissue.	Determines anatomical abnormalities

Table 29-4 • Indications for Renal Biopsy

Clinical Condition	Biopsy Indicated	Expected Gain
Orthostatic proteinuria	No	–
Isolated hematuria and/or proteinuria	No*	–
Hematuria and/or proteinuria with ↓ GFR	Yes	D,P,T
Nephrotic syndrome	Yes	D,P,T
Systemic disease with renal abnormalities	Yes†	D,P,T
Classic ARF	No	–
ARF with		
1. azotemia >3 wk	Yes	D,P
2. moderate proteinuria	Yes	D,T
3. anuria	Yes	D,T
4. eosinophilia or eosinophiluria	Yes	D,T
Post-transplant ↓ in GFR	Yes	D,P,T

GFR, glomerular filtration rate; D, diagnosis; P, prognosis; T, therapy; ARF, acute renal failure

* Biopsy may be indicated for insurance, administrative reasons, and so forth.

† Biopsy may or may not be indicated, depending on clinical picture.

part of the clinical picture, provide etiological clues for diagnosis, assess prognosis, and guide therapy. Renal biopsy is also used as an assessment tool for insurability, employment, or disability. Table 29-4 lists the indications for renal biopsy. Contraindications to biopsy include serious bleeding disorders, excessive obesity, and severe hypertension.

Renal biopsies are usually performed percutaneously with a biopsy needle, but an open renal biopsy under general anesthesia still is performed. Preparation for a renal biopsy includes obtaining informed consent, prebiopsy clotting studies, preoperative blood typing, and sedation (usually diazepam, 5 to 10 mg). It is necessary to establish intravenous access to prevent or treat complications. After the biopsy, the patient's vital signs are checked every 15 minutes for the first 2 hours, hourly for 4 hours, and then every 4 hours for the first 24 hours. The patient's urine is examined for blood. The major complication is bleeding, which can occur either retroperitoneally or into the urinary tract. Other complications that can occur are biopsy of other abdominal viscera, such as bowel, pancreas, liver, spleen, or vessels, and tears in the diaphragm or pleura.

Renal Angiography

Assessment of the renal vasculature may be accomplished by ultrasonography. When precise measurements are required, evaluation of renal blood flow through angiography may be used. This procedure may be performed in conjunction with cardiac catheterization. Access is obtained by percutaneous technique: An introducer, or sheath, is inserted into the femoral artery, and a small catheter is passed to the bifurcation of the renal arteries. Contrast medium is injected to provide radiological visualization of blood flow. Preparation for a renal angiogram is similar to that for renal biopsy; it includes obtaining informed consent, preprocedure clotting studies, preoperative blood typing, and sedation (usually midazolam, 1 to 2 mg, or diazepam, 5 to 10 mg), as well as establishing intravenous access to prevent or treat complications. After the angiogram, the patient's vital signs are checked every 15 minutes for the first 2 hours, hourly for 4 hours, and then every 4 hours for the first 24 hours. Pressure is applied locally when the arterial access is removed. Because the artery has been accessed, life-threatening bleeding can ensue. Therefore, the access site is assessed for bleeding with the same frequency as the vital signs are assessed. Diligence in application of pressure to the site and conducting site assessment is imperative. Watch for development of bradycardia because pressure applied to the groin area may stimulate the vagus nerve.

• Assessment of Electrolytes and Acid–Base Balance

The role of the kidney is central in maintaining fluid volume and ionic composition of body fluids. When the kidneys properly regulate the excretion of water and ions, homeostasis is achieved. When they fail to adapt adequately, imbalances occur. Table 29-5 summarizes electrolyte values and signs and symptoms of imbalance. The critical care nurse needs to monitor closely all of the electrolytes because minor shifts can be lethal.

SODIUM BALANCE

Serum sodium concentration is normally 135 to 145 mEq/L. It is regulated by the kidneys and depends on the sodium concentration in the extracellular fluid. When the concentration of sodium rises, antidiuretic hormone (ADH) is secreted from the posterior pituitary gland and the kidneys retain water in response. When the concentration falls, aldosterone promotes sodium retention by the kidneys (see Chapter 42, Fig. 42-9). When the kidneys malfunction, this balance is not maintained. Low serum sodium usually indicates water intake in excess of sodium and is characterized by an increase in body weight. High serum sodium usually indicates water loss in excess of sodium and is reflected in weight loss. Sodium is essential for maintaining the osmolality of extracellular fluids, neuromuscular function, acid–base balance, and various other cellular chemical reactions.

Hyponatremia is important because it can produce a wide range of neurological symptoms, including death. The severity of symptoms depends on the degree of hyponatremia and the rate at which it has developed. Usually, symptoms do not occur until the

Table 29-5 • Disorders of Electrolyte Balance

Electrolyte Imbalance	Signs and Symptoms	Diagnostic Test Results
Hyponatremia	• Muscle twitching and weakness • Lethargy, confusion, seizures, and coma • Hypotension and tachycardia • Nausea, vomiting, and abdominal cramps • Oliguria or anuria	• Serum sodium <135 mEq/L • Decreased urine specific gravity • Decreased serum osmolality • Urine sodium >100 mEq/24 h • Increased red blood cell count
Hypernatremia	• Agitation, restlessness, fever, and decreased level of consciousness • Muscle irritability and convulsions • Hypertension, tachycardia, pitting edema, and excessive weight gain • Thirst, increased viscosity of saliva, rough tongue • Dyspnea, respiratory arrest, and death	• Serum sodium >145 mEq/L • Urine sodium <40 mEq/24 h • High serum osmolality
Hypokalemia	• Dizziness, hypotension, dysrhythmias, electrocardiogram (ECG) changes, and cardiac and respiratory arrest • Nausea, vomiting, anorexia, diarrhea, decreased peristalsis, abdominal distention, and paralytic ileus • Muscle weakness, fatigue, and leg cramps	• Serum potassium <3.5 mEq/L • Coexisting low serum calcium and magnesium levels not responsive to treatment for hypokalemia usually suggest hypomagnesemia • Metabolic alkalosis • ECG changes, including flattened T waves, elevated U waves, depressed ST segment
Hyperkalemia	• Tachycardia changing to bradycardia, ECG changes, and cardiac arrest • Nausea, diarrhea, and abdominal cramps • Muscle weakness and flaccid paralysis	• Serum potassium >5 mEq/L • Metabolic acidosis • ECG changes, including tented and elevated T waves, widened QRS complex, prolonged PR interval, flattened or absent P waves, depressed ST segment
Hypochloremia	• Muscle hyperexcitability and tetany • Shallow, depressed breathing • Usually associated with hyponatremia and its characteristic symptoms, such as muscle weakness and twitching	• Serum chloride <96 mEq/L • Serum pH >7.45 (supportive value) • Serum CO_2 >32 mEq/L (supportive value)
Hyperchloremia	• Deep, rapid breathing • Weakness • Lethargy, possibly leading to coma	• Serum chloride >108 mEq/L • Serum pH <7.35, serum CO_2 <22 mEq/L (supportive values)
Hypocalcemia	• Anxiety, irritability, twitching around the mouth, laryngospasm, seizures, positive Chvostek's and Trousseau's signs • Hypotension and dysrhythmias due to decreased calcium influx	• Serum calcium <8.5 mg/dL • Low platelet count • ECG changes: lengthened QT interval, prolonged ST segment, arrhythmias
Hypercalcemia	• Drowsiness, lethargy, headaches, irritability, confusion, depression, apathy, tingling and numbness of fingers, muscle cramps, and convulsions • Weakness and muscle flaccidity • Bone pain and pathological fractures • Heart block • Anorexia, nausea, vomiting, constipation, dehydration, and abdominal cramps • Flank pain	• Serum calcium >10.5 mg/dL • ECG changes: signs of heart block and shortened QT interval • Azotemia • Decreased parathyroid hormone level • Calcium stones in urine
Hypomagnesemia	• Nearly always coexists with hypokalemia and hypocalcemia • Hyperirritability, tetany, leg and foot cramps, positive Chvostek's and Trousseau's signs, confusion, delusions, and seizures • Dysrhythmias, vasodilation, and hypotension	• Serum magnesium <1.8 mEq/L • Coexisting low serum potassium and calcium levels

(continued)

Table 29-5 • Disorders of Electrolyte Balance (Continued)

Electrolyte Imbalance	Signs and Symptoms	Diagnostic Test Results
Hypermagnesemia	• Central nervous system depression, lethargy, and drowsiness • Diminished reflexes, muscle weakness to flaccid paralysis • Respiratory depression • Heart block, bradycardia, widened QRS, and prolonged QT interval • Hypotension	• Serum magnesium >2.5 mEq/L • Coexisting elevated potassium and calcium levels
Hypophosphatemia	• Muscle weakness, tremor, and paresthesia • Tissue hypoxia • Bone pain, decreased reflexes, and seizures • Weak pulse • Hyperventilation • Dysphagia and anorexia	• Serum phosphate <2.5 mg/dL • Urine phosphate >1.3 g/24 h
Hyperphosphatemia	• Usually asymptomatic unless leading to hypocalcemia, then evidenced by tetany and seizures • Hyperreflexia, flaccid paralysis, and muscular weakness	• Serum phosphate >4.5 mg/dL • Serum calcium <8.5 mg/dL • Urine phosphate <0.9 g/24 h

From Anatomical Chart Company: Atlas of Pathophysiology, 2nd ed. Ambler, PA, Lippincott Williams & Wilkins, 2006, pp 32–33.

serum sodium is below 120 mEq/L.[2] For patients with hyponatremia, the severity of symptoms encountered depends on how rapidly the sodium concentration was lowered, as well as the value. Hyponatremia requires further evaluation. Figure 29-5 illustrates the etiologies and evaluation for hyponatremia.

Symptoms of hypernatremia generally are the same as those of hyperosmolality and result from central nervous system dehydration. Mental confusion, stupor, seizures, coma, and death may occur, in addition to other signs of dehydration, such as fatigue, muscle weakness and cramps, and anorexia. The serum osmolality usually is above 350 mOsm/L before significant symptoms are noted. This corresponds to a serum sodium level of 165 to 170 mEq/L.

POTASSIUM BALANCE

Potassium is essential for regulating nerve impulse conduction and muscle contraction and is involved in numerous other body functions, including intracellular osmolality and acid–base balance. The normal serum potassium concentration is 3.5 to 5 mEq/L. Potassium balance is maintained by dietary intake and renal excretion. Ninety-eight percent of potassium is located in the skeletal muscle; therefore, the balance of this electrolyte also is strongly tied to the exchanges between the intracellular and extracellular compartments in the body.

Hypokalemia can result from inadequate potassium intake, excessive potassium loss through the kidneys, gastrointestinal loss, and extracellular-to-intracellular potassium shifts. Also, diuretic therapy can contribute to potassium excretion, further compounding the problem.

Hyperkalemia may be caused by a decrease in the renal excretion of potassium or transcellular shifts of potassium. This is seen most often in acidosis, cell injury or destruction, and hyperglycemia.

CALCIUM AND PHOSPHATE BALANCE

Calcium and phosphate are regulated reciprocally in the body by vitamin D, parathyroid hormone, and calcitonin. The calcium and phosphate salts are normally deposited in bone. When calcium levels are high, phosphate levels are low. Because in renal failure, the kidneys are unable to eliminate phosphate, patients with renal failure often have high phosphate and low calcium levels.

Calcium's primary function is maintenance of bone and tooth strength. It also plays an important role in myocardial and skeletal contractility. Calcium also maintains cellular permeability and assists in blood coagulation. The normal serum concentration of calcium is 8.5 to 10.5 mg/dL. The total serum calcium is composed of two major fractions: the diffusible or ultrafiltrable (or ionized) calcium and the nondiffusible or protein-bound (primarily to albumin) calcium. Many critically ill patients have low albumin, which will result in low serum calcium. This result does not necessarily mean that the patient's calcium is low. It is necessary to either assess the ionized calcium (if available) or to correct the serum calcium for the albumin level, using the following formula:

$$\text{Corrected calcium} = [0.8 \times (\text{normal albumin} - \text{patient's albumin})] + \text{serum}$$

Phosphate is essential for the formation of adenosine triphosphate (ATP). Phosphate also assists in the maintenance of cell membrane structure, oxygen delivery, and cellular immunity. The normal phosphate level is 3 to 4.5 mg/dL.

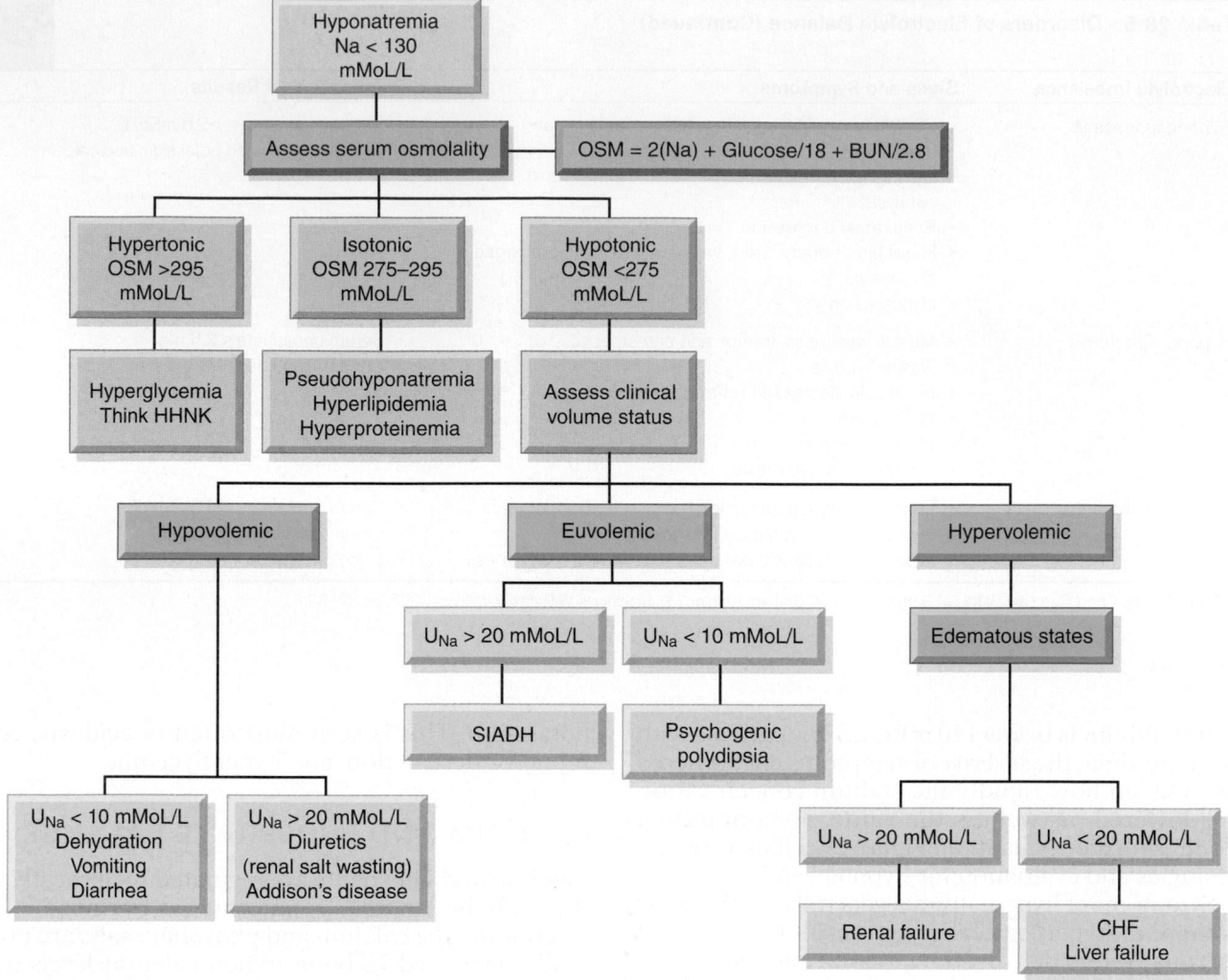

Figure 29-5 • Assessing hyponatremia. BUN, blood urea nitrogen; CHF, congestive heart failure; HHNK, hyperglycemic hyperosmolar nonketotic (coma); Na, sodium; OSM, osmolality; SIADH, syndrome of inappropriate antidiuretic hormone secretion; UNa, urine sodium.

MAGNESIUM BALANCE

The magnesium ion is the second major intracellular ion. The normal serum concentration is 1.4 to 2.1 mEq/L. Magnesium balance is necessary for the functional integrity of the neuromuscular system. The parathyroid glands regulate both magnesium and calcium. Sodium is necessary for magnesium reabsorption. Magnesium can accumulate in the serum, bone, and muscle in renal failure, causing numerous problems.

ACID–BASE BALANCE

A normal acidity or alkalinity (pH 7.35 to 7.45) of the body fluid is essential for life. The body maintains acid–base balance by the buffer system, the respiratory system, and the renal system. The buffer and respiratory systems are able to react quickly to changes in body pH. However, the kidneys take more time to adjust to changes in body pH.

Five major processes are associated with the regulation of acid–base balance by the renal system: hydrogen ion excretion; sodium ion reabsorption; bicarbonate ion generation and reabsorption; phosphate salt and titratable acid excretion; and ammonia synthesis and ammonium excretion. Acid–base imbalances may result when the kidneys are unable to perform those processes adequately. Table 29-6 summarizes acid–base balances.

The Anion Gap

To maintain chemical neutrality, the total concentration of cations and anions in the blood (and other body fluids) must be equivalent in terms of milliequivalents per liter. However, because there are a number of anions and cations present in blood that are not routinely measured, a "gap" exists between the total concentration of cations and anions and the concentration normally measured in the plasma.

Table 29-6 • Disorders of Acid–Base Balance

Disorder/Causes	Pathophysiology	Signs/Symptoms	Diagnosis
Respiratory Acidosis • Airway obstruction or parenchymal lung disease • Mechanical ventilation • Chronic metabolic alkalosis as respiratory compensatory mechanisms try to normalize pH • Chronic bronchitis • Extensive pneumonia • Large pneumothorax • Pulmonary edema • Asthma • Chronic obstructive pulmonary disorder (COPD) • Drugs • Cardiac arrest • Central nervous system (CNS) trauma • Neuromuscular diseases • Sleep apnea	When pulmonary ventilation decreases, partial pressure of carbon dioxide in arterial blood ($PaCO_2$) increases and CO_2 level rises. Retained CO_2 combines with water (H_2O) to form carbonic acid (H_2CO_3), which dissociates to release free hydrogen (H^+) and bicarbonate (HCO_3^-) ions. Increased $PaCO_2$ and free H^+ ions stimulate the medulla to increase respiratory drive and expel CO_2. As pH falls, 2,3-diphosphoglycerate (2,3-DPG) accumulates in red blood cells, where it alters hemoglobin (hgb) to release oxygen. The hgb picks up H^+ ions and CO_2 and removes them from the serum. As respiratory mechanisms fail, rising $PaCO_2$ stimulates kidneys to retain HCO_3^- and sodium (Na^+) ions and excrete H^+ ions. As the H^+ ion concentration overwhelms compensatory mechanisms, H^+ ions move into cells and potassium (K^+) ions move out. Without enough oxygen, anaerobic metabolism produces lactic acid.	• Restlessness • Confusion • Apprehension • Somnolence • Asterixis • Headaches • Dyspnea and tachypnea • Papilledema • Depressed reflexes • Hypoxemia • Tachycardia • Hypertension/hypotension • Atrial and ventricular dysrhythmias • Coma	• Arterial blood gas (ABG) analysis: $PaCO_2$ >45 mm Hg; pH <7.35 to 7.45; and normal HCO_3^- in the acute stage and elevated HCO_3^- in the chronic stage
Respiratory Alkalosis • Acute hypoxemia, pneumonia, interstitial lung disease, pulmonary vascular disease, or acute asthma • Anxiety • Hypermetabolic states such as fever and sepsis • Excessive mechanical ventilation • Salicylate toxicity • Metabolic acidosis • Hepatic failure • Pregnancy	As pulmonary ventilation increases, excessive CO_2 is exhaled. Resulting hypocapnia leads to reduction of H_2CO_3, excretion of H^+ and HCO_3^- ions, and rising serum pH. Against rising pH, the hydrogen–potassium buffer system pulls H^+ ions out of cells and into blood in exchange for K^+ ions. H^+ ions entering blood combine with HCO_3^- ions to form H_2CO_3, and pH falls. Hypocapnia causes an increase in heart rate, cerebral vasoconstriction, and decreased cerebral blood flow. After 6 hours, kidneys secrete more HCO_3^- and less H^+. Continued low $PaCO_2$ and vasoconstriction increases cerebral and peripheral hypoxia. Severe alkalosis inhibits calcium (Ca^{2+}) ionization; increasing nerve/muscle excitability.	• Deep, rapid breathing • Lightheadedness or dizziness • Agitation • Circumoral and peripheral paresthesias • Carpopedal spasms, twitching, and muscle weakness	ABG analysis showing $PaCO_2$ <35 mm Hg; elevated pH in proportion to decrease in $PaCO_2$ in the acute stage but decreasing toward normal in the chronic stage; normal HCO_3^- in the acute stage but less than normal in the chronic stage

(continued)

Table 29-6 • Disorders of Acid–Base Balance (Continued)

Disorder/Causes	Pathophysiology	Signs/Symptoms	Diagnosis
Metabolic Acidosis			
• Excessive acid accumulation • Deficient HCO_3^- stores • Decreased acid excretion by the kidneys • Diabetic ketoacidosis • Chronic alcoholism • Malnutrition or a low-carbohydrate, high-fat diet • Anaerobic carbohydrate metabolism • Underexcretion of metabolized acids or inability to conserve base • Diarrhea, intestinal malabsorption, or loss of sodium bicarbonate from the intestines • Salicylate intoxication, exogenous poisoning, or, less frequently, Addison's disease • Inhibited secretion of acid	As H^+ ions begin accumulating in the body, chemical buffers (plasma HCO_3^- and proteins) in cells and extracellular fluid (ECF) bind them. Excess H^+ ions decrease blood pH and stimulate chemoreceptors in the medulla to increase respiration. Consequent fall of partial pressure of $PaCO_2$ frees H^+ ions to bind with HCO_3^- ions. Respiratory compensation occurs but is not sufficient to correct acidosis. Healthy kidneys compensate, excreting excess H^+ ions, buffered by phosphate or ammonia. For each H^+ ion excreted, renal tubules reabsorb and return to blood one Na^+ ion and one HCO_3^- ion. Excess H^+ ions in ECF passively diffuse into cells. To maintain balance of charge across cell membrane, cells release K^+ ions. Excess H^+ ions change the normal balance of K^+, Na^+, and Ca^{2+} ions, impairing neural excitability.	• Headache and lethargy progressing to drowsiness, CNS depression, Kussmaul's respirations, hypotension, stupor, and coma and death • Associated gastrointestinal (GI) distress leading to anorexia, nausea, vomiting, diarrhea, and possibly dehydration • Warm, flushed skin • Fruity-smelling breath	• Arterial pH <7.35; $PaCO_2$ normal or <35 mm Hg as respiratory compensatory mechanisms take hold; HCO3- may be <22 mEq/L • Urine pH <4.5 in the absence of renal disease • Elevated plasma lactic acid in lactic acidosis • Anion gap >14 mEq/L in high–anion gap metabolic acidosis, lactic acidosis, ketoacidosis, aspirin overdose, alcohol poisoning, renal failure, or other disorder characterized by accumulation of organic acids, sulfates, or phosphates • Anion gap 12 mEq/L or less in normal anion gap metabolic acidosis from HCO_3^- loss, GI or renal loss, increased acid load, rapid intravenous (IV) saline administration, or other disorders characterized by HCO_3^- loss
Metabolic Alkalosis			
• Chronic vomiting • Nasogastric tube drainage or lavage without adequate electrolyte replacement • Fistulas • Use of steroids and certain diuretics (furosemide [Lasix], thiazides, and ethacrynic acid [Edecrin]) • Massive blood transfusions • Cushing's disease, primary hyperaldosteronism, and Bartter's syndrome • Excessive intake of bicarbonate of soda, other antacids, or absorbable alkali • Excessive amounts of IV fluids, high serum concentrations of bicarbonate or lactate • Respiratory insufficiency • Low serum chloride • Low serum potassium	Chemical buffers in ECF and intracellular fluid bind HCO_3^- in the body. Excess unbound HCO_3^- raises blood pH, depressing chemoreceptors in the medulla, inhibiting respiration and raising $PaCO_2$. CO_2 combines with H_2O to form H_2CO_3. Low oxygen limits respiratory compensation. When blood HCO_3^- rises to 28 mEq/L, the amount filtered by renal glomeruli exceeds reabsorptive capacity of the renal tubules. Excess HCO_3^- is excreted in urine, and H^+ ions are retained. To maintain electrochemical balance, Na^+ ions and water are excreted with HCO_3^- ions. When H^+ ion levels in ECF are low, H^+ ions diffuse passively out of cells and extracellular K^+ ions move into cells. As intracellular H^+ ion levels fall, calcium ionization decreases, and nerve cells become permeable to Na^+ ions. Na^+ ions moving into cells trigger neural impulses in peripheral nervous system and in CNS.	• Irritability, picking at bedclothes (carphology), twitching, and confusion • Nausea, vomiting, and diarrhea • Cardiovascular abnormalities due to hypokalemia • Respiratory disturbances (such as cyanosis and apnea) and slow, shallow respirations • Possible carpopedal spasm in the hand, due to diminished peripheral blood flow during repeated blood pressure checks	• Blood pH >7.45; HCO_3^- >26 mEq/L • Low potassium (<3.5 mEq/L), calcium (<8.9 mg/dL), and chloride (<98 mEq/L)

From Anatomical Chart Company: Atlas of Pathophysiology, 2nd ed. Ambler, PA, Lippincott Williams and Wilkins, 2006, pp 34–35.

The anion gap is composed primarily of an excess of unmeasured anions, including plasma proteins, inorganic phosphates and sulfates, and organic acids. The unmeasured cations that exist in smaller concentrations are primarily calcium and magnesium.

The anion gap usually is calculated by using the following formula:

$$Anion\ gap = [Na^+] + [K^+] - [Cl^-] - [HCO_3]$$

The normal mean is approximately 12 mEq/L (range, 8 to 16 mEq/L). However, departures from this "normal" anion gap may have important diagnostic significance in acid–base disorders, especially metabolic acidoses.

The most common abnormality of the anion gap is an increase that is associated with increased concentrations of lactate, ketone bodies, or inorganic phosphate and sulfate that are found in lactic acidosis, ketoacidosis, and uremia, respectively. Other forms of acidosis associated with ingestion of toxins, such as ethylene glycol, methanol, paraldehyde, and salicylates, also may produce significant increases in the anion gap.

Decreases in the anion gap are less common but equally important. They can occur because of increases in unmeasured cations or because of decreases in unmeasured anions. Table 29-7 lists the causes of altered anion gap.

• Assessment of Fluid Balance

The nurse's role in the assessment of problems of fluid balance includes accurate measurement of intake and output, weight, and vital signs. The most sensitive indices of changes in body water content are serial weights and intake and output patterns.[2]

Although vital signs can provide supporting data, they may not be abnormal until significant volume or water deficits occur. Assessment of fluid imbalance needs to be based on keen observation and recognition of pertinent symptoms.

WEIGHT

Weight is one of the single most important tests for critically ill patients. The admission weight is compared with that obtained in the history. Of note is whether the weight has changed significantly over the past 1 to 2 weeks. Weights should be carefully measured at the same time, with the same scale, and with the same linens daily. Variations in the procedure should be noted and made known to the physician. One liter of fluid equals 1 kg of body weight, equivalent to 2.2 pounds. A kilogram scale provides for greater accuracy because drug, fluid, and diet measurements can be calculated easily using the metric system. An increase in weight does not specify where the weight is gained. For example, a patient may be intravascularly volume depleted yet show an increase in weight because of third-spacing of fluid (i.e., movement of water to the interstitial space).

Rapid daily gains and losses of weight usually are associated with changes in fluid volume and not nutritional factors. Critically ill patients often experience unmeasured insensible losses, such as ventilation and wound losses. Fever can increase the amount of fluid lost through the skin and lungs by as much as 75 mL/1°F above baseline. Serial weights often are more reliable, and weight changes usually detect imbalances before any symptoms are apparent. In addition to the fluid balance perspective, weights are also used to calculate drug dosages and, for the patient receiving dialysis, determine the amount of fluid to be removed during therapy.

Table 29-7 • Causes of an Altered Anion Gap

Increased Anion Gap	Decreased Anion Gap
Increased unmeasured anions	Increased unmeasured cations
• Endogenous metabolic acidosis	• Normal cations
Lactic acidosis	Hypercalcemia
Ketoacidosis	Hyperkalemia
Uremic acidosis	Hypermagnesemia
• Exogenous anion ingestion	• Abnormal cations
Ethylene glycol	Increased globulins (e.g., myeloma)
Methanol	Lithium
Paraldehyde	
Salicylates	
Penicillin	
Carbenicillin	
• Increased plasma proteins	
Hyperalbuminemia	
Decreased unmeasured cations	Decreased unmeasured anions
• Hypokalemia	• Hypoalbuminemia
• Hypocalcemia	
• Hypomagnesemia	

INTAKE AND OUTPUT

An accurate intake and output record provides valuable data for evaluating and treating fluid and electrolyte imbalances. It is important that the nurse teach the patient or visitors to assist in this assessment. Intake and output are measured and recorded as they occur and totaled at the end of every shift. In the presence of excessive losses or deterioration of cardiac, hepatic, renal, or respiratory function, more detailed recording of every source of fluid intake and output is necessary, and calculations may be required every 1 to 4 hours.

In the critically ill patient, intake and output are monitored every 1 to 2 hours. The intake and output values are summed to provide an overall balance at the end of a 24-hour period. A net balance is calculated by subtracting the output from the intake:

$$\text{Fluid balance} = \text{total intake} - \text{total output}$$

Depending on the patient's condition, daily therapeutic goals, and response to interventions, the net balance may be neutral, positive, or negative. The 24-hour balance is compared with the daily weight to assess overall balance. If the net daily balance is positive, but the daily weight reflects a loss over the past 24 hours, insensible losses may be the cause of the discrepancy.

Intake should include all liquids, such as water, juices, or soup, and any foods that are high in water content (e.g., oranges, grapefruit, gelatin, and ice cream). It is useful to keep a list of equivalents for fruits, ice cubes and chips, and other sources of fluid. Output should include urinary and intestinal losses and estimates of respiratory and cutaneous losses when the patient's temperature or the ambient temperature is high. Also recorded are other sources of fluid loss that are present, such as ileostomy or other enteric drainage, wound drainage, or thoracic drainage.

In severe electrolyte and fluid imbalances, the time and type of fluid intake and the time and amount of each voiding must be recorded. In the event that renal function decreases, this information may aid immeasurably in the diagnosis and possible prevention of prerenal azotemia or acute renal failure. Box 29-3 gives risk factors for excessive fluid loss.

HYPOVOLEMIA AND HYPERVOLEMIA

The critical care nurse must be continually on the alert to detect early changes in the patient's volume status. Seldom is the diagnosis made on the basis of one parameter. The first clue may be the patient's general appearance; after observing this, the nurse seeks and notes more specific parameters.

Symptoms vary with the degree of imbalance; some are seen early in imbalance states, and others are not evident until severe imbalances are present. Table 29-8 lists the signs and symptoms of hypovolemia and hypervolemia.

In volume depletion, the patient may complain of orthostatic lightheadedness when assuming the sit-

Box 29-3 • RED FLAG: Risk Factors for Excessive Fluid Loss

- **Fever:** A patient with a body temperature of 40°C (104°F) and a respiratory rate of 40 breaths/min can lose as much as 2,500 mL of fluid in a 24-h period from the respiratory tract and from the skin.
- **Environment:** Hot, dry climates can increase evaporative sweat losses to 1,500 mL/h to maintain body evaporative heat loss. This can increase to between 2 and 2.5 L/h for short times in acclimatized people exercising in hot climates.
- **Hyperventilation:** Hyperventilation can increase respiratory water losses as a result of either disease or use of nonhumidified respirators or oxygen delivery systems.
- **Gastrointestinal tract:** Vomiting, nasogastric suction, diarrhea, and enterocutaneous drainage or fistulas can increase gastrointestinal losses.
- **Third-spacing:** Formation of pleural or peritoneal effusions and edema from liver, renal, or hepatic disease or from the diffuse capillary leak syndrome can result in a loss of effective intravascular volume. Drainage of peritoneal or pleural fluid, when formation of these third spaces still is occurring, can result in further effective intravascular losses because of continued fluid shifts from the vascular compartment to the third space.
- **Burns:** Fluid loss into burned tissues can result in a significant decrease in effective intravascular volume. Because both evaporative and transudative losses through the burned skin can result in very large losses of fluid daily, the burned patient requires special attention to maintain fluid and electrolyte balance. Formulas for determining burn area and fluid resuscitation are discussed in Chapter 53.
- **Renal losses:** Inappropriate solute and fluid loss from the kidneys can occur because of renal salt wasting. This is seen in the diuretic phase of acute tubular necrosis, in some rare patients with true renal salt wasting, and as a result of excessive diuretic administration. It also may occur as a result of solute diuresis from high-protein or high-saline enteral and parenteral alimentation and from administration of osmotic agents, such as mannitol and radiocontrast agents. Finally, fluid can be lost during the generation phase of metabolic alkalosis, in which compensatory urinary bicarbonate excretion obligates renal sodium excretion. This frequently results in volume depletion.

ting or standing position (this also can occur from inactivity and autonomic dysfunction). Development of tachycardia on assuming the upright position and a decrease in blood pressure (orthostatic hypotension), as opposed to the normal rise, are frequent early findings. Later, the pulse may become rapid, weak, and thready. There may be early dryness of the skin, with loss of elasticity, sunken eyes, loss of axillary sweating, and a dry, coated tongue. When severe volume depletion occurs, thirst, decreased urine volume, and weight loss may be noted; however, weight loss and orthostatic blood pressure and pulse changes may be the only findings.[2]

Laboratory studies, such as a high urine osmolality and low urinary sodium, may facilitate the diagnosis. Other guidelines, such as elevated hematocrit,

Table 29-8 • Signs and Symptoms of Hypovolemia and Hypervolemia

Parameters	Hypovolemia	Hypervolemia
Skin and subcutaneous tissues	Dry, less elastic	Warm, moist, pitting edema over bony prominences; wrinkled skin from pressure of clothing
Face	Sunken eyes (late symptom)	Periorbital edema
Tongue	Dry, coated (early symptom); fissured (late symptom)	Moist
Saliva	Thick, scanty	Excessive, frothy
Thirst	Present	May not be significant
Temperature	May be elevated	May not be significant
Pulse	Rapid, weak, thready	Rapid
Respirations	Rapid, shallow	Rapid dyspnea, moist rales, cough
Blood pressure	Low, orthostatic hypotension; small pulse pressure	Normal to high
Weight	Loss	Gain

decreased central venous pressure, and decreased pulmonary wedge pressure, may corroborate the diagnosis.

In fluid overload, the patient, if alert, may complain of puffiness or stiffness in the hands and feet. Later, periorbital edema or puffiness, followed by pitting edema of the dependent parts (feet and ankles if upright; sacral area and posterior thighs if supine) will occur, followed by dyspnea or ascites, depending on etiology (i.e., cardiac decompensation and systemic fluid overload versus hepatic disease). Urine volume and urine sodium may be normal, increased, or decreased, depending on the etiology. In most diseases with fluid retention, except for the syndrome of inappropriate ADH secretion, urine sodium is reduced. The hematocrit is decreased, reflecting hemodilution.

The pulse may be rapid, and auscultation of the heart may reveal the presence of a third heart sound (S_3), fourth heart sound (S_4), or murmur secondary to volume overload. Respirations may be increased because of pulmonary congestion, and auscultation of the chest may reveal rales. A chest film may reveal pulmonary vascular congestion, increased alveolar lung markings, cardiac dilation, frank pulmonary congestion, and pleural effusions.

All data should be evaluated in the light of other evidence. Trends usually are more significant than isolated values. For example, when a decrease in urine output is noted, a systematic assessment should be done to determine why this is happening and what nursing interventions are most appropriate. Depending on the stability of the patient, the health care team may use advanced physiological monitoring (e.g., pulmonary artery catheter) to guide assessment and management. Table 29-9 lists factors affecting water balance.

Table 29-9 • Factors Affecting Water Balance

	Water Excess	Water Deficiency
Intake		
Thirst	Decreased thirst threshold; Increased osmolality; Potassium depletion; Hypercalcemia; Fever; Dry mucous membranes; Poor oral hygiene; Unmisted O_2 administration; Hypotension; Psychiatric disorders	Increased thirst threshold; Decreased osmolality; Lack of access; Psychiatric disorders
Parenteral fluids	Excessive D_5W	Deficient replacement; Osmotic loads; Hyperalimentation; Hyperglycemia

(continued)

Table 29-9 • Factors Affecting Water Balance (Continued)

	Water Excess	Water Deficiency
		Mannitol
		Radiographic contrast agents
Output		
Sweating		High ambient temperature
		High altitude
		Fever
Renal excretion	Inappropriate ADH release	Excess excretion
	Appropriate ADH release	Central
	Congestive failure	Nephrogenic
	Decompensated cirrhosis	Potassium depletion
	Volume depletion	Hypercalcemia
	Adrenal insufficiency	Lithium administration
	Renal salt wasting	Demeclocycline (Declomycin)
	Hemorrhage	Methoxyflurane (Penthrane)
	Diuretics	
	Burns	
	Hypothyroidism	
	Renal disease	
	ARF	
	Chronic renal failure	
	Nephrotic syndrome	
	Acute glomerulonephritis	
	Nonsteroidal anti-inflammatory agents	

D₅W, Dextrose 5% in water; ADH, antidiuretic hormone; ARF, acute renal failure

HEMODYNAMIC MONITORING

Hemodynamic monitoring offers the clinician an improved assessment of the patient's overall status. For a detailed discussion, refer to Chapter 17. Although physical assessment may provide insight into the volume status, changes in physical assessment are reflected later than changes in hemodynamic assessment parameters, such as central venous pressure. Through improved monitoring, interventions are guided by information on a real-time basis. Table 29-10 provides an overview of the causes of altered parameters for the assessment of preload.

Based on data from the history, physical examination, and laboratory and diagnostic tests, nursing diagnoses are developed for the patient with renal problems. Box 29-4 lists possible nursing diagnoses.

• Clinical Applicability Challenges

Case Study

Mrs. R. is a 28-year-old woman who presented to the emergency department after being involved in a motor vehicle crash. There was a prolonged extrication time for Mrs. R. During her trauma evaluation, Mrs. R is noted to have bilateral lower extremity fractures and crush injuries. During physical examination, Mrs. R.'s vital signs are as follows: temperature, 35.6°C; heart

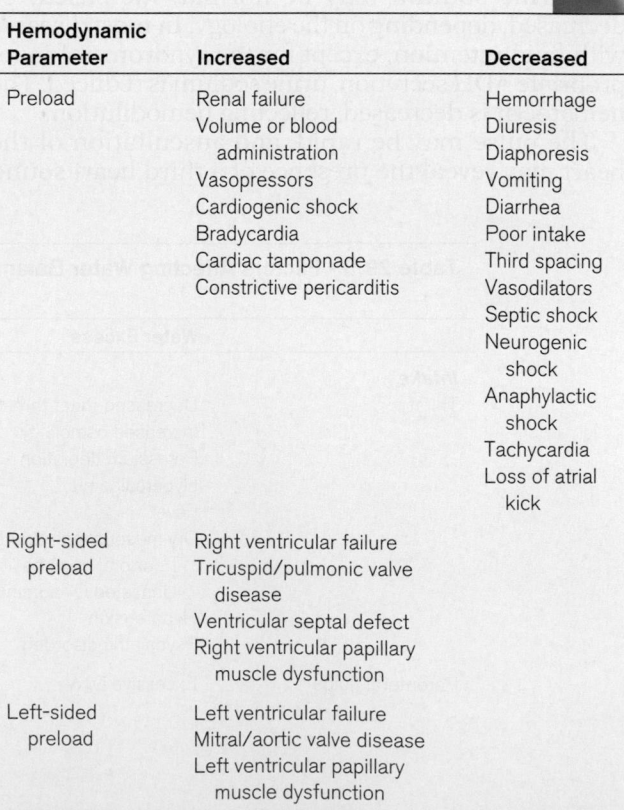

Table 29-10 • Etiologies of Altered Preload

Hemodynamic Parameter	Increased	Decreased
Preload	Renal failure	Hemorrhage
	Volume or blood administration	Diuresis
	Vasopressors	Diaphoresis
	Cardiogenic shock	Vomiting
	Bradycardia	Diarrhea
	Cardiac tamponade	Poor intake
	Constrictive pericarditis	Third spacing
		Vasodilators
		Septic shock
		Neurogenic shock
		Anaphylactic shock
		Tachycardia
		Loss of atrial kick
Right-sided preload	Right ventricular failure	
	Tricuspid/pulmonic valve disease	
	Ventricular septal defect	
	Right ventricular papillary muscle dysfunction	
Left-sided preload	Left ventricular failure	
	Mitral/aortic valve disease	
	Left ventricular papillary muscle dysfunction	

> **Box 29-4** **Examples of Nursing Diagnoses and Collaborative Problems for the Patient With Renal Problems**
>
> - Pain related to urinary retention
> - Acute Pain: Dysuria related to infection
> - Acute Pain: Dysuria related to urinary obstruction
> - Urinary Retention related to urinary tract obstruction
> - Impaired Urinary Elimination related to catheterization
> - Self-Concept Disturbance related to loss of bladder control
> - Alteration in Electrolyte Balance related to impaired kidney function
> - Excess Fluid Volume related to impaired kidney function
> - Impaired Urinary Elimination related to impaired kidney function

rate, 135 beats/minute; respiratory rate, 24 breaths/minute; and blood pressure, 102/68 mm Hg. Oxygen saturation is 95% on oxygen at 100% by non-rebreather mask. Additional injuries include a grade 2 splenic laceration, traumatic brain injury, and bilateral rib fractures. Her lower extremity fractures are repaired, and she is brought to the intensive care unit for further assessment and management.

Initial blood work obtained on arrival to the unit reveals the following: sodium, 135 mEq/L; chloride, 99 mEq/L; potassium, 3.4 mEq/L; carbon dioxide, 20 mEq/L; glucose, 156 mg/dL; blood urea nitrogen (BUN), 10 mg/dL; creatinine, 0.7 mg/dL; and hematocrit, 30%.

On post-trauma day 2, Mrs. R is endotracheally intubated and sedated. She has palpable distal pulses. Her vital signs are stable. Her urine is pink-tinged and over the past several hours has been averaging 20 to 25 mL/hour. Her blood work reveals a BUN of 22 mg/dL and a creatinine of 1.2 mg/dL. Other studies remain relatively unchanged. Mrs. R. is given a diagnosis of acute renal failure.

1. Explain why Mrs. R. is experiencing renal insufficiency. Describe the influence of Mrs. R.'s trauma on her renal function.
2. What interventions may be required to improve Mrs. R.'s renal function?
3. What other assessments or diagnostic tests may be indicated?

Review Questions

1. Mrs. S. is hospitalized for heart failure. In the morning, her patient care team examines her and then says that her kidney function is slightly abnormal and the plan is to continue to monitor her. After the patient care team leaves, Mrs. S. appears concerned and asks you, "Which test is for monitoring kidney function?" The nurse's best response would be:

a. "The potassium is checked every day. This way we know when the kidneys stop working."
b. "There are a lot of things we consider. You do not need to worry about the specifics."
c. "It sounds like you would like to know more detail. While there are a lot numbers to consider, we carefully look at the creatinine. This is a substance that is excreted by the kidneys and can give us a measure of how well they are doing their job."
d. "We check the uric acid every day because it has been shown to be the most specific in kidney failure."

2. Mr. F. is a patient in the intensive care unit and was admitted for sepsis. During the course of his 24 hours in the ICU, he has received multiple fluid boluses and has been started on low-dose vasopressors. Mr. F. has been having adequate urinary output (approximately 30 to 60 mL/hour); however, during the past hour, he had no urine out. Causes of acute anuria for Mr. F. include
a. administration of nephrotoxic antibiotics.
b. renal artery laceration.
c. volume depletion.
d. abdominal compartment syndrome.

3. Mr. V. is a patient in the ICU who was admitted following a heart attack. He has had a complicated course after percutaneous transluminal coronary angioplasty and stenting, requiring intra-aortic balloon counterpulsation, multiple vasoactive drips, and endotracheal intubation. On assessment, you notice the presence of periumbilical bruits. Based on this finding, you alert the medical team and anticipate which of the following diagnostic tests?
a. Computed tomography
b. Renal angiography
c. Plain radiograph
d. Costovertebral angle tenderness

4. Mrs. H. is a patient who presented to the emergency department with shortness of breath and fatigue. She is admitted to the intensive care unit with a diagnosis of cardiogenic shock and acute renal dysfunction. In addition to her routine home medications, she is started on a β-blocker, angiotensin-converting inhibitor, furosemide, oxygen, and lorazepam as needed for anxiety. Before initiating the new medications, the physician orders urinary studies to evaluate the cause of her kidney problem. Which of the following findings would you expect to see in Mrs. H.?
a. Low circulating levels of aldosterone
b. Increased urinary sodium
c. Decreased urinary potassium
d. Fractional excretion of sodium (FENa) less than 1%

5. You receive report from a nurse who mentions that your patient, Mr. J., has been receiving potassium replacements. On review of his medication administration record and laboratory studies, you notice that Mr. J. has been consistently hypokalemic and receiving multiple potassium replacements each day. You assess Mr. J. and determine that the

following condition is a likely a cause of persistent hypokalemia:

a. Nasogastric tube drainage
b. Administration of spironolactone
c. Acidosis
d. Constipation

6. You are examining Mrs. W., who was admitted to the intensive care unit (ICU) following surgery for trauma. She received multiple blood products during her resuscitation but has been stable in the ICU. You assess her blood pressure and notice that on inflation of the cuff, Mrs. W.'s wrist twitches. Given the presence of this sign, what additional findings would you expect?

a. Low potassium level
b. High calcium level
c. Muscle weakness, bone pain, hypertension
d. Cramps, tetany, positive Chvostek's sign

7. Which of the following is a cause of an increased anion gap?

a. Renal failure
b. Diarrhea
c. Hyperchloremic acidosis
d. Lactic acidosis

References

1. Kincaid-Smith P, Fairley K: The investigation of hematuria. Semin Nephrol 25(3):127–135, 2005
2. Elgart HN: Assessment of fluids and electrolytes. AACN Clin Issues 15(4): 607–621, 2004
3. Whittier WL, Korbet SM: Renal biopsy: Update. Curr Opin Nephrol Hypertens 13:661–665, 2004

Other Selected Readings

Hogan MA, Gingrich M, Ricci MJ, Oliver G: Prentice Hall Reviews & Rationales: Fluids, Electrolytes & Acid-Base Balance, 2nd ed. Upper Saddle River, NJ: Prentice Hall, 2006
McClelland RA: Chronic kidney disease: Risk factors, assessment and nursing care. Nurs Stand 20(10): 48–55, 2006
Molzahn AE (ed): Contemporary Nephrology Nursing: Principles and Practice, 2nd ed. Pitman, NJ: American Nephrology Nurses' Association, 2007
Rennke HG, Denker BM: Renal Pathophysiology: The Essentials, 2nd ed. Baltimore: Williams & Wilkins, 2006
Smilde TD, van Veldhuisen DJ, Navis G, et al: Drawbacks and prognostic value of formulas estimating renal function in patients with chronic heart failure and systolic dysfunction. Circulation 114:1572–1580, 2006

Patient Management: Renal System

Angela Muzzy • Kara Adams Snyder

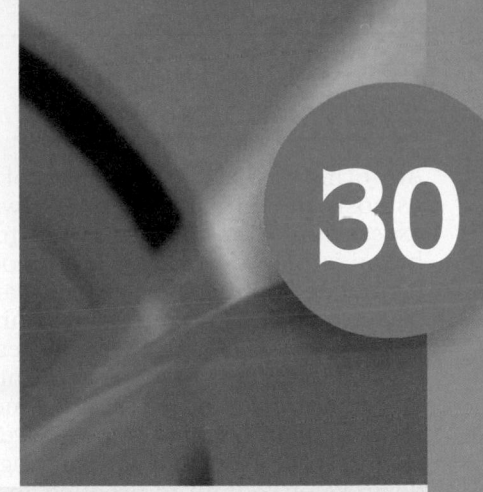

30

Objectives

Based on the content in this chapter, the reader should
be able to:

❶ Explain the physiological principles involved in renal
   replacement therapy: hemodialysis, continuous
   renal replacement therapies, and peritoneal dialysis.

❷ Analyze the differences in equipment and
   procedures used in renal replacement therapy.

❸ Explain the types of vascular access used in
   hemodialysis and continuous renal replacement
   therapies.

❹ Compare and contrast the indications, assessment
   and management, and complications for each renal
   replacement therapy.

❺ Discuss the psychosocial and teaching needs
   surrounding renal replacement therapy for patients
   and their families.

❻ Describe the nursing assessments and
   interventions for patients receiving fluid therapy.

❼ Analyze the specific fluid therapies chosen based
   on physiological alterations.

❽ Explain the nursing management of selected
   electrolyte disorders.

R enal function may be replaced by a process
   called dialysis, which is a life-maintaining
   therapy used in acute and chronic renal failure. Critical care nurses may encounter patients suffering from the effects of acute renal failure or
patients already on some form of chronic dialysis who
subsequently become critically ill. Critical care nurses

must be familiar with various dialysis therapies to
help care for patients with complex illnesses. This
chapter discusses the three most common forms of
renal replacement therapy: hemodialysis, continuous
renal replacement therapies [CRRTs], and peritoneal
dialysis. Common fluid and electrolyte imbalances
experienced by critically ill patients also are explored.

• Physiology

All forms of dialysis make use of the principles of osmosis and diffusion to remove waste products and excess fluid from the blood. A semipermeable membrane is placed between the blood and a specially formulated solution called dialysate. Dissolved substances, such as urea and creatinine, diffuse across the membrane from an area of greater concentration (blood) to an area of lesser concentration (dialysate). Water molecules move across the membrane by osmosis to the solution that contains fewer water molecules. Dialysate is formulated with varying concentrations of dextrose or sodium to produce an osmotic gradient, thereby pulling excess water from the circulatory system. This process of fluid moving across a semipermeable membrane in relation to forces created by osmotic and hydrostatic pressures is called ultrafiltration. These basic principles are the foundation of any dialysis therapy. The manner in which they are accomplished varies depending on the therapy.

• Extracorporeal Therapies

Hemodialysis and the CRRTs use an extracorporeal (outside the body) circuit. Therefore, they require access to the patient's circulation and anticoagulation of the circuit.

ACCESS TO CIRCULATION

The three most common methods used to access a patient's circulation are through a vascular catheter, an arteriovenous fistula, or a synthetic vascular graft. Patients who suddenly need hemodialysis or CRRT have a venous catheter, whereas patients already receiving chronic hemodialysis probably have either an arteriovenous fistula or a synthetic vascular graft. Box 30-1 lists nursing interventions for the patient with dialysis vascular access.

Venous Catheters

Dual-lumen catheters inserted into large central veins are used for acutely ill patients who need hemodial-

ysis, continuous venovenous hemofiltration (CVVH), or continuous venovenous hemofiltration with dialysis (CVVH/D). These catheters are also used for hemodialysis when there is no other means of access to the circulation. Veins commonly used are the femoral, internal jugular, and subclavian. The site chosen depends on the patient's anatomy and vein accessibility and the physician's experience and preference.

Dual-lumen venous catheters also are used temporarily for patients on acute dialysis who are critically ill or patients on chronic dialysis who are waiting for a more permanent access to mature. Tunneled dual-lumen central venous catheters are often used as a permanent means of access in patients in whom all other means of entry into the circulatory system have been exhausted. The tunneled catheter has an implantable Dacron cuff around which tissue grows and acts as a barrier against infection. If possible, the catheter should be placed in the right or left internal jugular vein because catheters placed in the subclavian vein can cause stenosis. The stenosis can cause increased venous pressure and edema that may thwart future efforts to create an arteriovenous fistula or place a graft.

Whenever venous catheters are used, care must be taken to avoid accidental slippage and dislodgment during hemodialysis. For example, femoral catheters are usually secured with sutures and also tape to the leg, whereas central venous catheters in the upper body are sutured to the skin. The length of time catheters are left in place depends on catheter function and institution policy. In general, central venous catheters may be used for up to 3 to 4 weeks. More permanent internal jugular vein catheters often function for many months before problems force their removal. Catheters left in place between dialysis treatments usually are filled with a concentrated heparin-saline solution after dialysis and plugged to prevent clotting. These catheters should never be used for any purpose other than hemodialysis without first checking with dialysis unit personnel. Cleansing and dressing of the insertion site are the same as with other central lines using strict aseptic technique.

If the catheters are removed at the end of dialysis, pressure is applied to the puncture sites until com-

---

 Box 30-1 • NURSING INTERVENTIONS for the Patient With Dialysis Vascular Access

Dual-Lumen Venous Catheter
- Verify central line catheter placement radiographically before use.
- Do not inject IV fluids or medication into the catheter. Both lumens of the catheter usually are filled with concentrated heparin.
- Do not unclamp the catheter unless preparing for dialysis therapy. This can cause blood to fill the lumen and clot.
- Maintain sterile technique in handling vascular access.
- Observe catheter exit site for signs of inflammation or catheter kinking.

Arteriovenous Fistula or Graft
- Do not take blood pressure or draw blood from the access limb.
- Listen for bruit, and palpate for thrill q8h.
- Make sure there is no tight clothing or restraints on the access limb.
- Check access patency more frequently when patients are hypotensive. Hypotension can predispose to clotting.
- In the event of postdialysis bleeding from the needle site, apply just enough pressure to stop the flow of blood and hold until bleeding stops. Do not occlude the vessel.

plete clotting occurs. The site is checked for several hours thereafter so that any recurrent bleeding can be detected. Removal of the more permanent tunneled catheter requires use of local anesthetic at the exit site and careful dissection around the Dacron cuff to free it from the attached subcutaneous tissue.

Catheter patency must be maintained. Thrombolytics may be used to dissolve clots in venous catheters. Thrombolytics are enzymes derived from streptococcal bacteria that are capable of activating the fibrinolytic system and dissolving intravascular thrombi. These agents can help preserve vascular access and reduce the need for surgery or catheter reinsertion. However, their use is associated with inherent risks and side effects, including bleeding and an allergic response.

In the early days of dialysis, vascular access was created at every treatment by cannulating an artery to remove blood from the body and a vein to return dialyzed blood to the patient. The lines carrying blood to the dialyzer were called arterial lines, and the lines returning blood to the body were called venous lines. The two lumens of the venous catheter used in dialysis are still designated as arterial and venous. The arterial lumen is longer than the venous lumen, so it can pull blood flowing by and allow it to be pumped out of the body and to the dialyzer. Blood is returned upstream from the arterial lumen to avoid pulling out the blood that has just been dialyzed and returned to the body. The lumens are distinguished by the presence of colored clamps: red on the arterial lumen and blue on the venous lumen.

Arteriovenous Fistulas

The arteriovenous fistula technique was developed in 1966 in an effort to provide long-term access for hemodialysis. To create the arteriovenous fistula, a surgeon anastomoses an artery and a vein, creating a fistula or artificial opening between them (Fig. 30-1A). Arterial blood flowing into the venous system results in a marked dilation of the vein, which can then be punctured easily with a 15- or 16-gauge dialysis fistula needle. Two venipunctures are made at the time of dialysis: one for blood outflow and one for blood return.

After the arteriovenous fistula incision has healed, the site is cleansed by normal bathing or showering. To avoid scar formation, excessive bleeding, or hematoma of the arteriovenous fistula, care is taken to avoid traumatic venipuncture, excessive manipulation of the needles, and repeated use of the same site for venipuncture. Adequate pressure must be put on the puncture sites after the needles are removed. In addition, blood pressure measurements and venipunctures should not be performed on the arm with the fistula.

Most arteriovenous fistulas are developed and ready to use 1 to 3 months after surgery. After initial healing has occurred, patients are taught to exercise the arm to assist in vessel maturation. They also are encouraged to become familiar with the quality of the "thrill" felt at the site of anastomosis so that they can report any change in its presence or strength. A loud, swishing sound termed a bruit indicates a func-

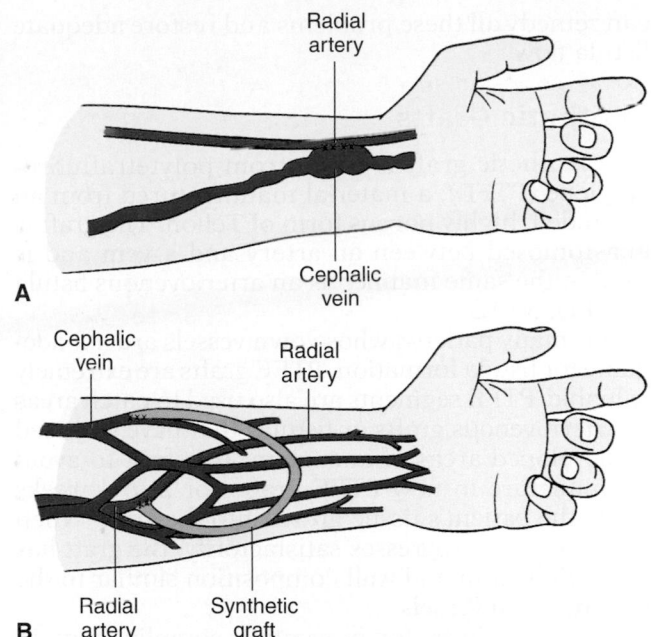

A: Arteriovenous fistula. **B:** Synthetic graft.

Figure 30-1 • Methods of vascular access for hemodialysis. **A:** Arteriovenous fistula. **B:** Synthetic graft.

tioning fistula. Box 30-2 presents a patient teaching guide for the care of arteriovenous fistulas.

Although arteriovenous fistulas usually have a long life, complications may occur. These include thrombosis, aneurysm or pseudoaneurysm, or arterial insufficiency causing a "steal syndrome." This syndrome occurs when shunting of blood from the artery to the vein produces ischemia of the hand, causing pain or coldness in the hand. Surgical intervention

---

Box 30-2 • TEACHING GUIDE:
Caring for an Arteriovenous Fistula

- Wash the fistula site with antibacterial soap each day and always before dialysis.
- Refrain from picking the scab that forms after completion of dialysis therapy.
- Check for redness, feeling of excess warmth, or the beginning of a pimple on any area of access.
- Ask the dialysis care team to rotate needles at the time of dialysis treatment.
- Check blood flow several times each day by feeling for a pulse or thrill. If this is not felt, or if there is a change, call your health care provider or dialysis center.
- Refrain from wearing tight clothes or jewelry on the access arm. Also avoid carrying anything heavy or doing anything that will put pressure on the access site.
- Avoid sleeping with your head on the arm where the access site is located.
- Remind caregivers and staff not to use a blood pressure cuff on, or draw blood from, the arm where the access site is located.
- Apply only gentle pressure to the access site after the needle is removed. Too much pressure stops flow of blood to the access site.

can remedy all these problems and restore adequate fistula flow.

Synthetic Grafts

The synthetic graft is made from polytetrafluoroethylene (PTFE), a material manufactured from an expanded, highly porous form of Teflon. The graft is anastomosed between an artery and a vein and is used in the same manner as an arteriovenous fistula (see Fig. 30-1B).

For many patients whose own vessels are not adequate for fistula formation, PTFE grafts are extremely valuable. PTFE segments are also used to patch areas of arteriovenous grafts or fistulas that have stenosed or developed areas of aneurysm. It is best to avoid venipuncture in new PTFE grafts for 2 to 4 weeks while the patient's tissue grows into the graft. When tissue growth progresses satisfactorily, the graft has an endothelium and wall composition similar to the patient's own vessels.

The procedures for preventing complications in grafts are the same as those used for arteriovenous fistulas. However, certain complications are seen more frequently with grafts than with fistulas, including thrombosis, infection, aneurysm formation, and stenosis at the site of anastomosis.

ANTICOAGULATION

Blood in the extracorporeal system, such as the dialyzer and blood lines, clots rapidly unless some method of anticoagulation is used. Heparin is most commonly used because it is simple to administer, increases clotting time rapidly, is monitored easily, and may be reversed with protamine. Citrate solutions may also be used for anticoagulation during dialysis. This agent chelates calcium, thereby inactivating the clotting cascade. Recent evidence suggests that the use of citrate in CRRTs is associated with fewer life-threatening bleeding complications than heparin.[1,2]

Specific anticoagulation procedures vary, but the primary goal of all methods is to prevent clotting in the dialyzer with the least amount of anticoagulation. Two methods of heparinization commonly used are intermittent and constant infusion.

Systemic Anticoagulation

Typically, the circuit is initially primed with a dose of heparin, followed by smaller intermittent doses of anticoagulant or heparin administered at a constant rate by an infusion pump. This results in systemic anticoagulation, in which the clotting times of the patient and the dialyzer essentially are the same.

Definitive guidelines are difficult to provide because methods and dialyzer requirements vary. The normal clotting time of 6 to 10 minutes may be increased to 30 to 60 minutes. The effect of heparin is generally monitored by the activated clotting time, prothrombin time (PT), or partial thromboplastin time (PTT).

The patient's need for heparinization and an appropriate beginning heparin dose should be assessed routinely before dialysis, especially in the critically ill patient who may be actively bleeding or at risk for bleeding. The patient's platelet count, serum calcium level, and results of coagulation studies are valuable in assessing current function of the clotting process. Often, little or no heparin can be used when the patient has serious alterations in one or more factors needed for effective clotting.

Regional Anticoagulation

Systemic heparinization does not usually present a risk unless the patient has overt bleeding (e.g., gastrointestinal bleeding, epistaxis, or hemoptysis), is 3 to 7 days postsurgery, or has uremic pericarditis. In these situations, other methods to prevent clotting of the extracorporeal system can be used. One method is regional heparinization, in which the patient's clotting time is kept normal while the clotting time of the dialyzer is increased. This is accomplished by infusing heparin at a constant rate into the dialyzer and simultaneously neutralizing its effects with protamine sulfate before the blood returns to the patient.

Like systemic heparinization, regional heparinization has no associated standard heparin/protamine ratio. Frequent monitoring of the clotting times with adjustment of the protamine sulfate rate is the best way to achieve effective regional heparinization. One patient safety concern is bleeding secondary to overheparinization. Causes of overheparinization include infusion pump malfunction, errors in setting delivery rates, and infrequent monitoring of clotting times. Because of these hazards, heparin delivery must be monitored carefully and frequently, with meticulous checking of pump rates.

Another way to prevent dialyzer clotting and reduce the risk for bleeding due to heparin is to infuse a small initial heparin dose and use frequent normal saline flushes of the extracorporeal system, or use saline flushes alone.

Some dialysis centers perform regional citrate anticoagulation in which citrate is infused into the system before the dialyzer binds calcium, obstructing the normal clotting pathway. The citrate-calcium complex is then cleared from the blood by the dialyzer, and the anticoagulant effect is reversed by infusing calcium chloride before the blood returns to the patient. The patient's sodium levels may rise because the citrate is administered in the form of sodium citrate.[3] Citrate has a higher pH, and therefore patients may also become metabolically alkalotic.

• Intermittent Hemodialysis

In hemodialysis, water and excess waste products are removed from the blood as it is pumped by the dialysis machine (Fig. 30-2) through an extracorporeal circuit (Fig. 30-3) into a device called a dialyzer, or artificial kidney. The blood is in one compartment,

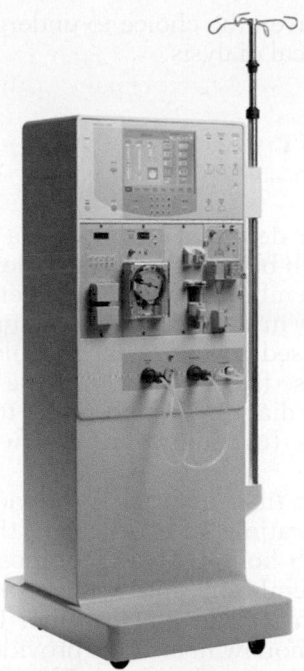

Figure 30-2 • Hemodialysis delivery unit, which includes an automatic blood pressure cuff, heparin infusion pump, and blood pump. This machine displays a continuous readout of ultrafiltration goal, rate, and total fluid removed and monitors dialysate temperature and conductivity. It can vary the sodium concentration of the dialysate. (Courtesy of Fresenius 2800K Fresenius VSA, Inc., Concord, CA.)

and the dialysate is in another compartment. There, the blood flows through a semipermeable membrane. The semipermeable membrane is a thin, porous sheet made of cellulose or a synthetic material. The pore size of the membrane permits diffusion of low-molecular-weight substances such as urea, creatinine, and uric acid. In addition, water molecules are small and move freely through the membrane, but most plasma proteins, bacteria, and blood cells are too large to pass through the pores of the membrane. The difference in the concentration of the substances in the two compartments is called the concentration gradient.

The blood, which contains waste products such as urea and creatinine, flows into the blood compartment of the dialyzer, where it comes into contact with the dialysate, which contains no urea or creatinine. A maximal gradient is established so that these substances move from the blood to the dialysate. These waste products fall to more normal levels as the blood passes through the dialyzer repeatedly at a rate ranging from 200 to 400 mL/minute over 2 to 4 hours.

Excess water is removed by a pressure differential created between the blood and fluid compartments. This pressure differential is aided by the action of the dialyzer pump and usually consists of positive pressure in the blood path and negative pressure in the dialysate compartment. This is the process of ultrafiltration.

Figure 30-3 • Hemodialysis system. (**A**) Blood from an artery is pumped into a dialyzer (**B**), where it flows through the cellophane tubes, which act as the semipermeable membrane (*inset*). The dialysate, which has the same chemical composition as the blood except for urea and waste products, flows in around the tubules. The waste products in the blood diffuse through the semipermeable membrane into the dialysate. (From Smeltzer SC, Bare BG, Hinkle JL, Cheever KH: Brunner & Suddarth's Textbook of Medical-Surgical Nursing, 11th ed. Philadelphia: Lippincott Williams & Wilkins, 2008., p 1538.)

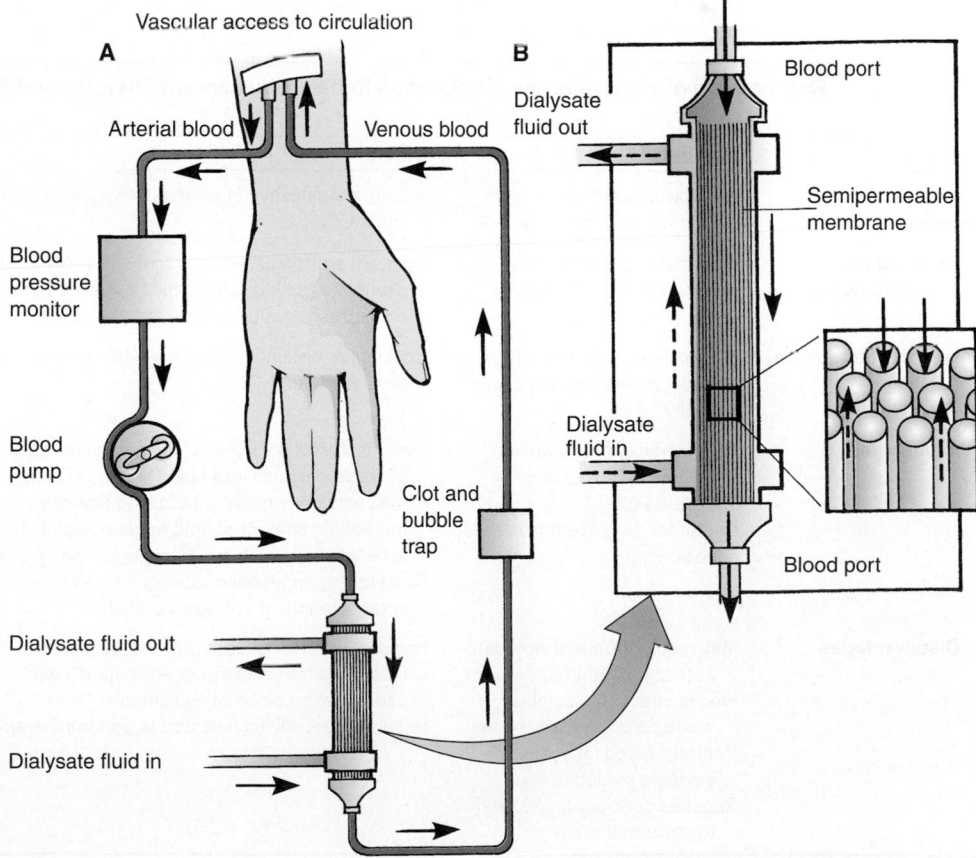

In summary, hemodialysis:

▶ Removes byproducts of protein metabolism, such as urea, creatinine, and uric acid
▶ Removes excess water
▶ Maintains or restores the body buffer system
▶ Maintains or restores the level of electrolytes in the body

INDICATIONS FOR HEMODIALYSIS

Hemodialysis is indicated in chronic renal failure and for complications of acute renal failure. These include uremia, fluid overload, acidosis, hyperkalemia, and drug overdose. Table 30-1 compares hemodialysis, CRRT, and peritoneal dialysis.

CONTRAINDICATIONS TO HEMODIALYSIS

Hemodialysis may be contraindicated in patients with coagulopathies because the extracorporeal circuit needs to be heparinized. Hemodialysis may also be difficult to perform in patients who are hypotensive, have extremely low cardiac output, or are sensitive to abrupt changes in volume status. For these critically ill patients, CRRT may be the optimal choice. In addition, intermittent hemodialysis may not keep up with the metabolic needs of a highly catabolic patient. In this case, CRRT would probably be chosen. Patients treated chronically for renal fail-

ure may be given the choice to undergo hemodialysis or peritoneal dialysis.

EQUIPMENT
Dialyzers

Dialyzers are designed to provide a parallel path through which blood and dialysate flow and to have a maximal membrane surface area between the two. Dialyzers vary in size, physical structure, and type of membrane used to construct the blood compartment. All these factors determine the potential efficiency of the dialyzer, which refers to its ability to remove water (ultrafiltration) and waste products (clearance).

The hollow-fiber dialyzer is the most commonly used configuration. In this design, the blood path flows through hollow fibers, composed of a semipermeable membrane, and the dialysate path, which is encased in a rigid plastic tube. Dialysate surrounds each hollow fiber. This provides a large surface area to cleanse the blood. Blood and dialysate flow in opposite directions from each other (countercurrent flow); as blood travels through the dialyzer, it is constantly exposed to a fresh flow of dialysate. This countercurrent flow maintains the concentration gradient between the two compartments and provides the most efficient dialysis.

Synthetic membranes are used most commonly because they are highly biocompatible. They remove waste products efficiently, and there is little reaction

Table 30-1 • Comparison of Hemodialysis, Continuous Renal Replacement Therapy, and Peritoneal Dialysis

	Hemodialysis	CRRT	Peritoneal Dialysis
Access	Arteriovenous fistula or graft; dual-lumen venous catheter	Arteriovenous fistula or graft; dual-lumen venous catheter	Temporary or permanent peritoneal catheter
Anticoagulation requirements	Systemic heparinization or frequent saline flushes	Systemic anticoagulation with heparin or trisodium citrate may be indicated depending on patient's coagulation studies before starting therapy	May only need heparin intra-peritoneally Not absorbed systemically
Length of treatment	3–4 h, three to five times per week, depending on patient acuity	Continuous throughout day; may last as many days as needed	Continuous (cycled) or intermittent exchanges; time between exchanges = 1–6 h
Advantages	Quick, efficient removal of metabolic wastes and excess fluid Useful for drug overdoses and poisonings	Best choice for patient who is hemodynamically unstable because less blood is outside body than with hemodialysis and blood flow rates are slower; amount of fluid removed can still be achieved but over a much longer period of time Good for hypercatabolic patients who receive large amounts of intravenous fluids	Continuous removal of wastes and fluid Better hemodynamic stability Fewer dietary restrictions
Disadvantages	May require frequent vascular access procedures Places strain on a compromised cardiovascular system Potential blood loss from bleeding or clotted lines Requires specially trained staff to perform therapy	Requires vascular access procedures; potential blood loss from clotting or equipment leaks; uses an extra piece of equipment Requires specially trained staff to perform therapy	Contraindicated after abdominal surgery or in presence of many scars Waste products may be removed too slowly in a catabolic patient Danger of peritonitis

between the blood and the membrane material. Because the synthetic membranes are highly permeable to water, they should be used only with a machine that controls the amount of ultrafiltration.

The size, efficiency, and metabolic needs of the patient are considered when choosing a dialyzer. A patient with a larger body surface area who has greater metabolic needs benefits from use of a larger and more efficient dialyzer, whereas a patient with a smaller body surface area and lower metabolic needs benefits from a smaller, less permeable dialyzer.

Dialysate

The dialysate, or "bath," is a solution composed of water and the major electrolytes of normal serum. It is made in a clean system with filtered tap water and chemicals. It is not a sterile system; bacteria are too large to pass through the membrane, and the potential for infection of the patient is minimal. However, because bacterial byproducts can cause pyrogenic reactions, especially in highly permeable membranes, water used to make dialysate must be bacteriologically safe. Dialysate concentrates usually are provided by commercial manufacturers. Generally, a standard bath is used for patients receiving chronic dialysis, but variations may be made to meet specific patient needs.

Dialysate Delivery System

A single delivery unit provides dialysate for one patient, whereas a multiple delivery system may provide dialysate for as many as 20 patient units. In either system, an automatic proportioning device and metering and monitoring devices ensure precise control of the water/concentrate ratio.

The single delivery unit is usually used in patients on acute dialysis. It is a mobile unit, and dialysate requirements are easily tailored to meet individual patient needs.

Accessory Equipment

Hardware used in most dialysis systems includes a blood pump, infusion pumps for heparin delivery, and monitoring devices for detection of unsafe temperatures, dialysate concentration, pressure changes, air, and blood leaks. All dialysis delivery systems consist of a single compact unit that includes the dialysate delivery equipment and blood monitoring components (see Fig. 30-2). Disposable items used in addition to the artificial kidney include dialysis tubing for transport of blood between the dialyzer and patient, pressure transducers for protection of monitoring devices from blood exposure, and a normal saline bag and tubing for priming the system before use.

Human Component

Expertise in the use of highly technical equipment is gained through theoretical and practical training in the clinical setting. However, the operation and monitoring of various kinds of dialysis equipment differ. Reference to the manufacturer's instruction manuals gives the nurse guidelines for the safe operation of equipment. The technical aspects of hemodialysis may seem overwhelming at first, but it is possible to learn them fairly rapidly. A more important aspect, the critical thinking and synthesis of patient assessment data that the nurse uses when caring for a patient during dialysis, takes longer to learn.

ASSESSMENT AND MANAGEMENT

The degree and complexity of problems arising during hemodialysis vary among patients and depend on many factors. Important variables are the patient's diagnosis, stage of illness, age, other medical problems, fluid and electrolyte balance, prior experience with hemodialysis, and emotional state. Because an increasing number of older adults are receiving dialysis, it also is important to consider the normal decreases in cardiac function and other system changes due to the aging process (Table 30-2).

Preprocedure

A predialysis assessment is the first step in managing the patient receiving hemodialysis. It consists of a review of the patient's history and clinical findings, response to previous dialysis treatment, laboratory results (such as electrolytes), consultation with other caregivers, and the nurse's direct assessment of the patient.

The nurse evaluates fluid balance before dialysis so that corrective measures may be initiated at the beginning of the procedure. Blood pressure, pulse, weight, intake and output, tissue turgor, and other symptoms assist the nurse in estimating fluid overload or depletion. Monitoring tools, such as pulmonary artery catheters and central venous pressures, also help determine cardiovascular fluid load.

The term *dry weight* or *ideal weight* is used to express the weight at which fluid volume is in a normal range for a patient who is free of the symptoms of fluid imbalance. It provides a guideline for fluid removal or replacement. The figure is not absolute. It requires frequent review and revision, especially in patients receiving dialysis in whom frequent weight changes occur.

After reviewing the data and while consulting with the physician, the dialysis nurse establishes objectives regarding fluid removal and restoration of electrolyte balance for the dialysis treatment. The objectives vary from one dialysis to the next in the patient whose condition may change rapidly. For example, fluid removal may take precedence over correction of an electrolyte imbalance, or vice versa.

Anxiety and apprehension, especially during the first dialysis, may contribute to change in blood pressure, restlessness, and gastrointestinal upset. The presence of a competent and caring nurse during dialysis may increase the patient's sense of security enough to avoid the need for an antianxiety drug that might precipitate changes in vital signs.

A basic explanation of the procedure and its place in the total plan of care for the patient may also allay

Table 30-2 • CONSIDERATIONS FOR THE OLDER PATIENT:
Normal Aging Changes That Affect Fluid Balance

Physiological Component	Normal Changes With Increasing Age	Nursing Implications
Total body water	About 6% reduction in total body water Decrease in ratio of intracellular fluid	Increased risk for fluid volume deficit
Renal function	Reduction in renal weight by 50 g between 40 and 80 y of age Loss of 30%–50% of glomeruli by 70 y of age Thickening of glomerular and tubular basement membranes from 20 to 90 y of age Decrease in GFR from 20 to 90 y of age Decrease in ability to concentrate urine (maximal ability to concentrate urine is urine specific gravity of 1.022–1.026)	Greater difficulty in eliminating heavy solute loads (drugs, glucose, protein, electrolytes) Slower conservation of fluids in response to fluid restriction
Regulatory functions	Decrease in secretion of aldosterone from adrenal cortex Decreased response of zona glomerulosa Decreased response of distal tubule to vasopressin Decreased ability to form and excrete ammonia Decreased glucose tolerance Decreased sensation of thirst	Diminished ability to conserve sodium and excrete potassium Reduced ability to correct acid–base imbalance Increased risk for hyperglycemia and osmotic diuresis Decreased ability to recognize fluid deficit
Skin changes	Decreased skin elasticity Atrophy of sweat glands Diminished capillary bed	Skin turgor is poor indicator of state of hydration Skin is less effective in cooling body temperature
Cardiovascular function	Decreased baroreceptor sensitivity Decreased cardiac output (1%/y from 20 to 80 y of age) Decreased stroke volume (0.7%/y from 20 to 80 y of age) Decrease in renal plasma flow from 600 mL/min in second decade to 300 mL/min by eighth decade Decreased elasticity of arteries Increased vascular rigidity, causing increased peripheral resistance	Diminished ability to manage hypotension associated with shock Increased frequency of peripheral edema Increased risk for orthostatic hypotension, dizziness, falls
Respiratory function	Decreased compliance of chest wall Decreased elasticity of lung tissue Decreased number of alveoli Decreased strength of expiratory muscles Decreased normal partial pressure of oxygen	Increased difficulty in regulating pH associated with major illness, surgery, burns, or trauma
Gastrointestinal function	Decreased volume of saliva Decreased volume of gastric juice Decreased calcium absorption	Mouth may be drier Increased risk for hyponatremia and hypokalemia during vomiting and gastric suction Increased need for dietary calcium and vitamin D

GFR, glomerular filtration rate.
Adapted from Metheny NM: Fluid and Electrolyte Balance: Nursing Considerations. Philadelphia: Lippincott Williams & Wilkins, 2000, p. 413, with permission.

some of the anxiety experienced by the patient and family. They must understand that dialysis is being used to support normal body function rather than to "cure" the kidney disease process.

Procedure

The nurse begins the procedure by checking the equipment (Box 30-3). After predialysis preparation and a safety check of equipment, the nurse is ready to begin hemodialysis. Access to the circulatory system is gained by one of several options: a dual-lumen catheter, an arteriovenous fistula, or graft. The dual-lumen catheter is opened under aseptic conditions according to institutional policy. Two large-gauge (15- or 16-gauge) needles are needed to cannulate a graft or fistula.

Figure 30-3 illustrates the hemodialysis circuit. After vascular access is established through strict aseptic technique, blood begins to flow, assisted by the blood pump. The part of the disposable circuit before the dialyzer is designated the arterial line, both to distinguish the blood in it as blood that has not yet reached the dialyzer and in reference to needle placement. The arterial needle is placed closest to the arteriovenous anastomosis in a graft or fistula to maximize blood flow. A clamped saline bag always is attached to the circuit just before the blood pump. In

Box 30-3 • NURSING INTERVENTIONS for Checking Hemodialysis and Continuous Venovenous Hemofiltration With Dialysis Equipment

- Prime lines and dialyzer or filter to expel all air before starting treatment.
- Test all alarms before connecting the patient to the circuit.
- Respond to all alarms immediately.

- Replace wet pressure transducers if they interfere with transmission of pressure reading.
- Inspect and tighten all connections before initiating treatment.

episodes of hypotension, blood flow from the patient can be clamped while the saline is opened and allowed to infuse rapidly to correct blood pressure. Blood transfusions and plasma expanders also can be attached to the circuit at this point and allowed to drip in, assisted by the blood pump. Heparin infusions may be located either before or after the blood pump, depending on the equipment in use.

The dialyzer is the next important component of the circuit. Blood flows into the blood compartment of the dialyzer, where exchange of fluid and waste products takes place. Blood leaving the dialyzer passes through an air detector that shuts down the blood pump if any air is detected. At this point in the pathway, any medications that can be given during dialysis are infused through a medication port. However, unless otherwise ordered, most medications are withheld until after dialysis.

Blood that has passed through the dialyzer returns to the patient through the venous (postdialyzer) line. After the prescribed treatment time, dialysis is terminated by clamping off blood from the patient, opening the saline line, and rinsing the circuit to return the patient's blood.

A dialysis nurse is in constant attendance during acute hemodialysis. Blood pressure and pulse are recorded at least every half hour when the patient's condition is stable. All machine pressures and flow rates are checked and recorded on a regular basis. The nurse assesses the patient's responses to fluid and solute removal and the condition and function of the patient's vascular access. A protective face shield and gloves are worn by the nurse performing hemodialysis because of the risk for exposure to blood. The dialysis nurse and critical care nurse work together to care for the patient because they must coordinate their specific patient care responsibilities.

Postprocedure

The results of a dialysis treatment can be determined by assessing the amount of fluid removed (as assessed by postdialysis weight) and the degree to which electrolyte and acid-base imbalances have been corrected. Blood drawn immediately after dialysis may show falsely low levels of electrolytes, urea nitrogen, and creatinine. The process of equilibration is thought to continue for some time after dialysis because these substances move from inside the cell to the plasma. To ensure accuracy of laboratory data after dialysis, a minimum of 2 to 3 hours should elapse before samples for laboratory tests are taken from the patient.

COMPLICATIONS

Dialysis Dysequilibrium

Uremia must be corrected slowly to prevent dysequilibrium syndrome, which is a set of signs and symptoms ranging from headache, nausea, restlessness, and mild mental impairment to vomiting, confusion, agitation, and seizures. This is thought to occur as the plasma concentration of solutes, such as urea nitrogen, is lowered. Blood urea and nitrogen play a role in calculating the serum osmolarity. Because of the blood-brain barrier, solutes are removed much more slowly from brain cells. Therefore, plasma becomes hypotonic in relation to the brain cells. This results in a shift of water from plasma to the brain cells and causes cerebral edema and symptoms of dysequilibrium syndrome. This syndrome can be avoided by dialyzing patients for short periods, such as 1 to 2 hours on 3 or 4 consecutive days.

Hypovolemia

Fluid overload is treated during dialysis by removing excess water. Because this removal depends on shifting fluid from other body compartments to the vascular space, clinicians must take care to avoid removing fluid so rapidly during dialysis that it leads to volume depletion. Excessive fluid removal may lead to hypotension, and little is gained if intravenous (IV) fluids are given to correct the problem. Therefore, it is better to reduce the volume overload over two or three dialyses, unless pulmonary congestion is life-threatening.

Hypotension

Normal saline in bolus amounts of 100 to 200 mL is used to correct hypotension. Dialysis machines now aid in preventing hypotension because the amount of ultrafiltration is controlled at the push of a button. It is also possible to vary the sodium concentration of dialysate. A higher sodium level in the dialysate means that less sodium is removed from the blood. A higher serum sodium assists the body as it shifts fluid from the interstitial to the intravascular compartment. Blood volume expanders, such as albumin, are sometimes used in patients with a low serum protein.

The use of antihypertensive drugs in patients who undergo dialysis may precipitate hypotension during dialysis. To avoid this, standard practice in many dialysis units is to omit antihypertensive drugs 4 to

6 hours before dialysis. Restriction of fluids and sodium before and during the dialysis phases is a more desirable method for control of hypertension. Sedatives and tranquilizers also may cause hypotension and should be avoided, if possible.

Hypertension

Fluid overload, dysequilibrium syndrome, renin response to ultrafiltration, and anxiety are the most frequent causes of hypertension during dialysis. Hypertension during dialysis is usually caused by sodium and water excess. This can be confirmed by comparing the patient's present weight to his or her ideal or dry weight. If fluid overload is the cause of hypertension, ultrafiltration usually brings about a reduction in the blood pressure.

Some patients who may be normotensive before dialysis become hypertensive during dialysis. The blood pressure rise may occur either gradually or abruptly. The cause is not well understood, but it may be the result of renin production in response to ultrafiltration and an increase in renal ischemia. Patients must be carefully monitored because the vasoconstriction caused by the renin response is limited. Once a decrease in blood volume surpasses the ability to maintain blood pressure through vasoconstriction, hypotension can occur precipitously.

Muscle Cramps

Muscle cramps may occur during dialysis as a result of excess fluid removal, which results in diminished intravascular volume and reduced muscle perfusion. During dialysis, cramps may be treated by lowering the rate of ultrafiltration and administering hypertonic solutions, normal saline boluses, mannitol, or glucose in an attempt to increase perfusion to the muscles.[4]

Dysrhythmias and Angina

Dysrhythmias and angina may occur in patients with underlying cardiac disease in response to fluid and electrolyte removal. Decreasing the rate of fluid removal may help. Medication may be needed to control cardiac rhythm.

• Continuous Renal Replacement Therapies

In CRRT, blood circulates outside the body through a highly porous filter similar to that used with hemodialysis. The process is similar to hemodialysis in that water, electrolytes, and small to medium-sized molecules are removed by ultrafiltration. CRRT is accompanied by a simultaneous reinfusion of a physiological solution, and it occurs continuously for an extended period. A pump, slightly different from that used in hemodialysis, is used and often incorporates a weighing system so that fluids can be intricately balanced hour to hour (Fig. 30-4).

CRRTs include continuous arteriovenous hemofiltration, continuous arteriovenous hemofiltration with dialysis, CVVH, and CVVH/D (Table 30-3). This discussion focuses primarily on CVVH and CVVH/D because these therapies are replacing the arteriovenous procedures. Access to the circulation for CVVH and CVVH/D is the same as that used for short-term hemodialysis. The extracorporeal circuit is similar to the hemodialysis circuit (Fig. 30-5). A pump is added to assist blood flow. The rate of blood flow is typically

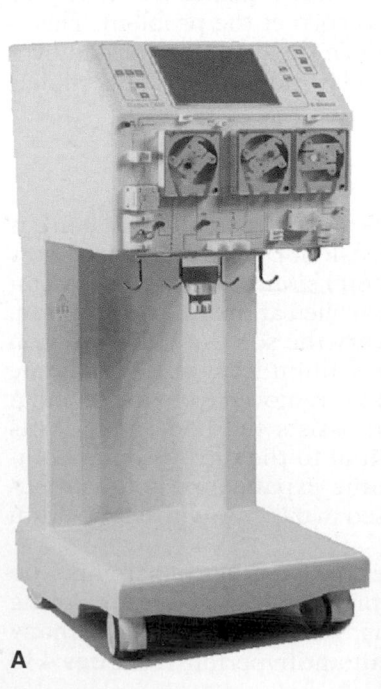

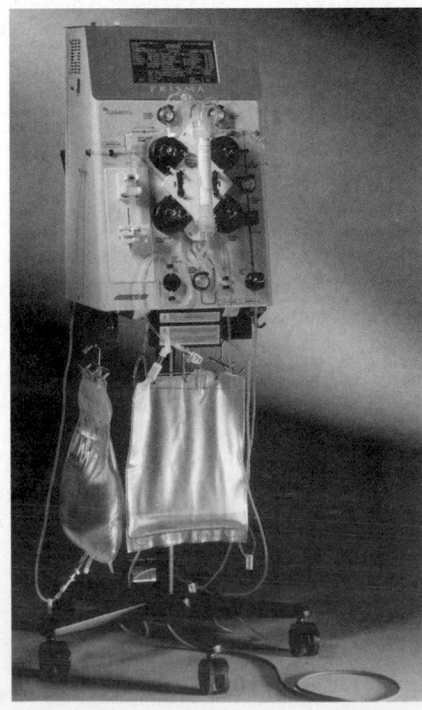

A   **B**

Figure 30-4 • Devices for administering continuous renal replacement therapy (CRRT) offer an integrated fluid warmer for the heating of infusion and dialysate fluids, a weighing system to reduce the possibility of error in assessing fluid balance, and a battery backup that allows treatments to continue when the patient is moved. **A:** Diapact pump, B-Braun McGraw Corporation. **B:** PRISMA, Gambro Corporation.

Table 30-3 • Continuous Renal Replacement Therapies

Type of Therapy	Mechanism of Action	Indications
Continuous venovenous hemodialysis	Blood is driven through low-permeability dialyzer, and countercurrent flow of dialysis solution is delivered on dialysate compartment. Ultrafiltrate produced during membrane transit corresponds to the patient's weight loss; solute clearance is mainly achieved by diffusion; replacement solution is not needed. Efficiency of clearance is limited to small molecules.	Fluid and solute clearance
Continuous venovenous hemofiltration	Blood is driven through highly permeable filter via extracorporeal circuit in venovenous mode. Ultrafiltrate produced during membrane transit is replaced partially or completely to achieve blood purification and volume control; ultrafiltration is in excess of patient weight loss; replacement solution is needed.	Fluid and solute clearance
Slow continuous hemofiltration	Blood is driven through highly permeable filter via extracorporeal circuit in venovenous mode. Ultrafiltrate produced during membrane transit is not replaced and corresponds exactly to patient weight loss.	Only for fluid control in overhydration status
Continuous venovenous hemofiltration with dialysis	Blood is driven through highly permeable dialyzer, and countercurrent flow of dialysis solution is delivered on the dialysate compartment. Ultrafiltrate produced during membrane transit is in excess of the patient's weight loss; solute clearance is obtained both by diffusion and convection; replacement solution is needed to obtain fluid balance (sometimes referred to as "push-pull" dialysis).	For combined convection and diffusion clearance

Adapted from Bellomo R, Ronco C: Continuous renal replacement therapy in the intensive care unit. Intensive Care Med 25:781–789, 1999, with permission.

much slower than in hemodialysis. The ultrafiltration rate is titrated to reach an hourly goal and is based on the patient's cardiac and pulmonary status.

When CVVH is used, a replacement fluid is ordered and is connected either before or after the filter, depending on patient characteristics and institutional practice. When dialysis is added to the CVVH process, it is called CVVH/D. Adding the dialysate increases the ability to remove wastes. Therefore, it is used when uremia must be aggressively managed, such as with the highly catabolic patient. CVVH and CVVH/D can be performed and managed by the critical care nurse. Typically, competency assessment and validation are performed before the nurse cares for patients with CRRT.

INDICATIONS FOR CONTINUOUS RENAL REPLACEMENT THERAPY

CRRT is indicated in the following circumstances: in patients with a high risk for hemodynamic instability who do not tolerate the rapid fluid shifts that occur with hemodialysis, in those who require large amounts of hourly IV fluids or parenteral nutrition, and in those who need more than the usual 3- to 4-hour hemodialysis treatment to correct the metabolic imbalances of acute renal failure. Table 30-4 presents criteria for initiating CRRT. CVVH is used when patients primarily need excess fluid removed, whereas CVVH/D is used when patients also need waste products removed because of uremia. For a comparison of CRRT with hemodialysis and peritoneal dialysis, see Table 30-1.

CONTRAINDICATIONS TO CONTINUOUS RENAL REPLACEMENT THERAPY

CRRT is contraindicated when patients become hemodynamically stable or no longer require continuous therapy, and intermittent hemodialysis should be used. It may be difficult to achieve access to circulation in some patients with coagulopathies, which may prolong initiation of therapy. Patient and family discussion is imperative before initiation of therapy; patients may not wish to receive CRRT, and it is essential that patient wishes be considered.

EQUIPMENT

A typical CVVH/D setup is shown in Figure 30-5. Blood exits the body through the arterial limb of the vascular access. The first infusion line shown is for anticoagulation. Located just before the blood pump is a line that measures pressure in the prefilter portion of the circuit, known as the arterial pressure. The blood pump, which propels blood into the filter, is next. An infusion port just after the blood pump is usually connected to normal saline for flushing the circuit or for attaching the replacement fluid. A bag of dialysate is shown flowing through the filter and surrounding the hollow fibers in which the blood travels. As the dialysate exits the filter, it passes through a sensor that detects microscopic amounts of blood, thereby warning of filter rupture. The dialysate and excess fluid removed from the patient are collected in a graduated collection device for easy measurement. Meanwhile, the blood exits

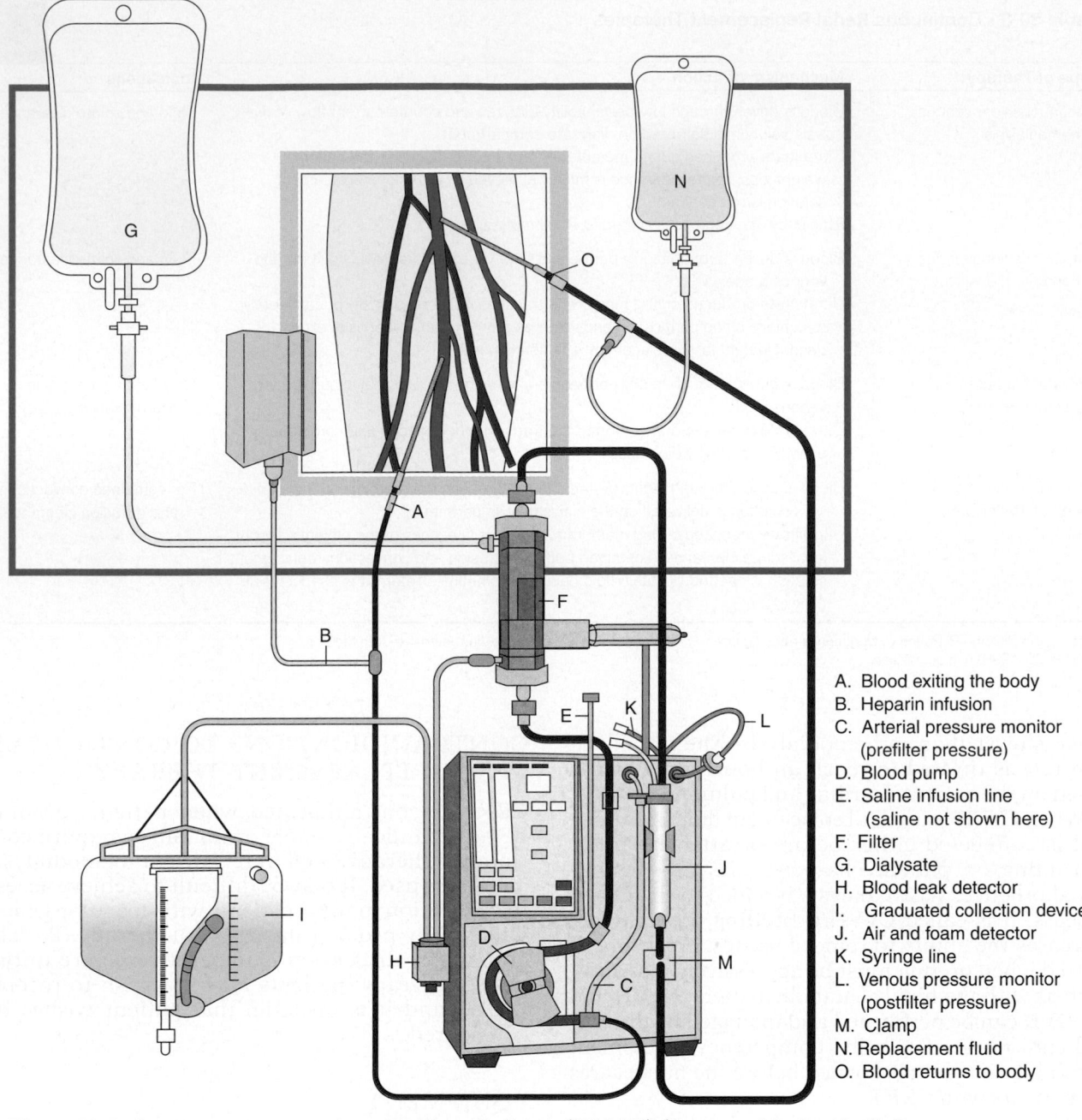

A. Blood exiting the body
B. Heparin infusion
C. Arterial pressure monitor
   (prefilter pressure)
D. Blood pump
E. Saline infusion line
   (saline not shown here)
F. Filter
G. Dialysate
H. Blood leak detector
I. Graduated collection device
J. Air and foam detector
K. Syringe line
L. Venous pressure monitor
   (postfilter pressure)
M. Clamp
N. Replacement fluid
O. Blood returns to body

Figure 30-5 • Continuous venovenous hemofiltration with dialysis (CVVH/D). (Courtesy of Baxter Health Care Corporation, Renal Division, McGaw Park, IL.)

the filter and passes into a drip chamber, where air and foam are trapped instead of entering the patient's circulation. The drip chamber also contains a line to which a syringe can be attached to raise and lower the blood level and another line that measures pressure in the postfilter section of the circuit, known as venous pressure. A clamp is located after the drip chamber and automatically engages if air tries to pass through it. The arterial and venous pressure transducers are protected by a disposable filter. As blood returns to the body, replacement fluid is infused. In some systems, the line for replacement fluid is placed before the blood pump so that it can be infused before the blood reaches the

filter. The total amount of blood in the circuit is about 150 mL.

ASSESSMENT AND MANAGEMENT

Preprocedure

Baseline hemodynamics, vital signs, and weight are obtained before initiation of therapy. The filters used in the continuous therapies are much more porous than those used in hemodialysis, and the circuit does not contain a mechanism to control the amount of fluid removed. Thus, the potential exists for uncontrolled losses of a large amount of fluid. Because of

Table 30-4 • Conditions That Warrant Continuous Renal Replacement Therapy (CRRT)*

Clinical Condition	Assessment Findings
Oliguria	Urine output <200 mL/12 h
Anuria	Urine output <50 mL/12 h
Severe acidemia due to metabolic acidosis	pH <7.1
Azotemia (urea)	>30 mmol/L
Hyperkalemia or rapidly rising serum potassium levels	Serum potassium >6.5 mEq/L
Suspected uremia organ involvement	Pericarditis, encephalopathy, neuropathy, myopathy
Severe alterations in serum sodium levels	Serum sodium >160 mmol/L or <115 mmol/L
Clinically significant organ edema	Pulmonary edema
Drug overdose with dialyzable toxin	Aspirin overdose
Coagulopathy requiring large amounts of blood products in patient at risk of pulmonary edema or acute respiratory distress syndrome	Disseminated intravascular coagulation

*One of these conditions is sufficient grounds for the initiation of CRRT. Two of these conditions make CRRT essentially mandatory. Combined derangements suggest the initiation of CRRT even before some of these conditions have been reached.
Adapted from Bellomo R, Ronco C: Continuous renal replacement therapy in the intensive care unit. Intensive Care Med 25:781–789, 1999, with permission.

this, an hourly fluid balance goal is set by the physician. Fluid is replaced each hour in varying amounts to achieve the goal (Box 30-4).

Procedure

Before therapy is initiated, the equipment is checked (see Box 30-3). The lines and filter are primed to expel air from the circuit. Arterial and venous lines are connected to the corresponding port of the access catheter, and the blood pump is turned on. Blood starts to flow through the tubing. Ultrafiltration begins to produce plasma water (ultrafiltrate) that starts to flow into the collection device. Most experts recommend controlling the amount of ultrafiltrate by raising or lowering the collection device until the desired hourly rate of ultrafiltration is achieved. Blood flow rates through the circuit average 100 mL/hour, and the standard dialysate flow rate is 1 L/hour. Substances are adequately cleared when ultrafiltration produces 500 to 600 mL/hour of ultrafiltrate.

Anticoagulation, if indicated, is administered as therapy begins. Low-dose heparin is the standard anticoagulant used in patients at risk for bleeding, and PTT values should be monitored frequently. It may also be used along with saline flushes to prevent circuit clotting, the most common mechanism for interruption of CRRT. Saline flushes without low-dose heparin may be used when the patient has a low platelet count. A typical protocol is to flush 100 mL through the circuit every half hour. Another method of anticoagulation is to infuse citrate before the filter. This anticoagulates only the extracorporeal part of the circuit. It chelates calcium, which is then replaced through infusion through the venous return line or peripherally to maintain normal ionized calcium levels.[4] Therefore, the patient needs to be closely monitored to prevent hypercalcemia or hypocalcemia.

Hourly maintenance of the CVVH/D system includes measuring blood and dialysate flows, calculating net ultrafiltration and replacement fluid, titrating anticoagulants, assessing the integrity of the vascular access, and monitoring hemodynamic parameters and blood circuit pressures. The nephrologist sets a goal for hourly fluid balance, and the critical care nurse is responsible to see that it is met. Box 30-5 lists interventions in monitoring fluid and electrolyte balance.

Box 30-4 • Example Showing Hourly Fluid Goal With Intake and Output in Fluid Replacement in CVVH/D

1. The patient needs to have 200 mL of fluid removed per hour.
2. The patient receives 500 mL/h of intravenous fluid (e.g., blood transfusions and parenteral nutrition).
3. The patient has 400 mL of nasogastric drainage and 100 mL of wound drainage in 1 hr.
4. Peritoneal dialysate is added at the rate of 1,000 mL/h to increase clearance.
5. The total amount of fluid in the collecting bag at the end of 1 hr is 2,500 mL. (Remember, 1,000 mL is peritoneal dialysate, so 1,500 mL has been filtered from the patient's plasma.)

To calculate the amount of replacement fluid, add the input fluid of 500 mL of IV fluid and 1,000 mL of peritoneal dialysate. Output is the 1,500 mL that has been filtered from the patient's plasma, 400 mL of nasogastric drainage, and the 100 mL of wound drainage. Total output is 2,000 mL, and the total input is 1,500 mL. The difference is 500 mL. The hourly fluid removal goal of 200 mL is subtracted, indicating 300 mL has been removed in excess of the goal and needs to be replaced this hour.

Box 30-5 • NURSING INTERVENTIONS for Monitoring Fluid and Electrolyte Balance During CVVH/D

- Draw electrolytes, blood urea nitrogen, and creatinine before initiating treatment and then at least twice daily.
- Assess vital signs, central pressure readings (if available), breath sounds, heart sounds, weight, intake, and output before initiating treatment and at least every half hour during treatment.
- Collaborate with nephrologist to determine hourly fluid balance.
- Record all intake and output when calculating replacement fluid for the next hour.

- Administer replacement fluid tailored to the patient's electrolytes, or obtain custom mixed dialysate from the pharmacy.
- If hypotension occurs, administer saline boluses (100–200 mL), reduce ultrafiltration by raising the collecting device, and, if necessary, obtain an order for 5% albumin.
- Observe patient for signs of electrolyte imbalances (i.e., electrocardiographic changes and muscle weakness, as with hypokalemia).

By comparing total intake and output, the hourly net fluid balance is calculated. The amount of replacement fluid is determined by the difference between desired and net fluid balance. Fluid balance and replacement should be carefully documented in the patient's medical record (i.e., intensive care unit flow sheet).

In CVVH, replacement fluid may be infused before or after the filter. Both techniques have advantages and disadvantages. When fluid is given before the filter, it decreases blood viscosity and increases blood flow through the filter. This enhances ultrafiltrate (plasma fluid) production and solute removal and decreases the frequency of clotting. The disadvantage is the increased need for fluid replacement. If replacement fluid is given after the filter, there is less total fluid loss and less need for replacement fluid. However, there is an increased incidence of filter clotting and decreased filter life. The method chosen depends on the system used and institutional preference.

Electrolytes, urea nitrogen, creatinine, and glucose levels are drawn before the procedure is started and then at least twice daily. Electrolyte imbalances can be corrected by altering the composition of the replacement fluid or by custom-mixing the dialysate. Anticoagulation is monitored by checking activated clotting times or PT and PTT. Although frequency is determined by each institution, it is not unusual to check clotting times every 1 or 2 hours to prevent clotting of the filter and blood lines.

No one policy delineates the optimal time to change the circuit. Many institutions put a 24- to 48-hour limit on circuit life, although there are reports of filters lasting an average of 4 days. System performance is monitored by checking the amount of urea nitrogen in the filtrate compared with the amount of urea nitrogen before the filter. A decreasing ratio indicates inadequate performance. A decreasing rate of ultrafiltration and increases in the venous pressure indicate clotting in the filter.

Treatment may be interrupted to transport the patient for a diagnostic test or to fix a mechanical problem with the circuit or vascular access. Treatment may be terminated if the patient shows signs of recovering renal function. When it is determined that continuous therapy can be terminated, the blood is returned to the patient. First, the ultrafiltrate outlet is clamped, and the dialysate is turned off.

Then, anticoagulation is turned off, and the blood is returned to the patient through a saline flush. Once the lines are clear, they are disconnected from the vascular access. Then the vascular access is heparinized per unit policy. Documentation includes fluid balance, condition of the access, and the patient's response to treatment. The tubing and filter are disposable. When working with the circuit and ultrafiltrate, the nurse uses Standard Precautions. Box 30-6 lists some nursing diagnoses and collaborative problems associated with hemodialysis and CRRT.

TECHNICAL COMPLICATIONS IN CONTINUOUS VENOVENOUS HEMOFILTRATION WITH DIALYSIS

Access Problems

Blood flows used in CVVH/D are much lower than for hemodialysis, making it more likely that a catheter will provide adequate flow. However, a poorly functioning access jeopardizes the entire CVVH/D procedure. Often, the position of the patient's extremity affects blood flow. If the access is in a limb, the limb should be gently immobilized. An obstruction, such as a clot or kink in the arterial lumen of the catheter, results in less blood being delivered to the circuit and manifests as lowered arterial and venous pressures. Clots or kinks in the venous lumen of the catheter raise venous pressures as blood tries to return against an obstruction. The treatment may be temporarily halted while the nurse manually flushes each lumen

Box 30-6 • Examples of Nursing Diagnoses for the Patient Undergoing Hemodialysis or Continuous Renal Replacement Therapy

- Excess Fluid Volume related to renal impairment
- Deficient Fluid Volume related to renal replacement fluid removal
- Ineffective Tissue Perfusion as manifested by decreased renal perfusion
- Risk for Infection related to invasive devices, malnutrition

to determine patency. If blood flow still cannot be established, the nephrologist is notified immediately to replace the catheter.

Clotting

An early sign of filter clotting is a reduced rate of ultrafiltration that cannot be corrected by increasing blood flow or by lowering the collection device. As clotting progresses, venous pressure rises, arterial pressure drops, and the blood lines appear dark. Clotting times are low. A saline bolus may help determine the location and extent of clotting. It may be possible to return some of the patient's blood before changing the circuit, but if clotting is extensive, this should not be attempted. Box 30-7 lists some nursing interventions for maintaining blood flow through a CVVH/D circuit.

Air in the Circuit

If the connections are loose, or a prefilter infusion line runs dry, air disrupts the system by collecting in the drip chamber and setting off the air detector alarm and triggering the clamp on the venous line to close. The nurse assesses the circuit's integrity to detect the source of air. Before resetting the line clamp, the nurse makes sure all bubbles have been tapped out of the drip chamber, all connections are tight, and there is no danger of air getting into the patient's bloodstream.

Blood Leaks

Blood appears in the ultrafiltrate if there is any rupture inside the filter. The blood leak alarm sounds, and the blood pump stops. Testing the ultrafiltrate with a dipstick can verify a microscopic leak. Blood can be safely returned to the patient as long as there is no gross blood in the ultrafiltrate. Then the circuit should be changed. A gross leak is readily identifiable. Blood should not be returned to the patient, and the patient's hematocrit should be checked to determine the need for transfusion.

PHYSIOLOGICAL COMPLICATIONS IN CONTINUOUS VENOVENOUS HEMOFILTRATION WITH DIALYSIS

Hypotension

If blood pressure and intravascular filling pressures fall below optimal, the nurse can increase the infusion rate of replacement fluid or give a normal saline bolus. At the same time, the ultrafiltrate collection device is raised to decrease ultrafiltration until pressures stabilize. An infusion of 5% albumin may also help stabilize blood pressure. If this situation persists, the physician is consulted to adjust the net ultrafiltration goal.

Hypothermia

Some patients experience chills and lowered body temperature while their blood is circulating outside the body. If this happens, it may be advisable to use a blood warmer to warm either the dialysate or the replacement fluid. Advancements in the technologies used to perform CRRT have improved the precision of fluid balance and reduced the hypothermia that can develop with any extracorporeal therapy.

PSYCHOLOGICAL ASPECTS OF RENAL REPLACEMENT THERAPIES

The psychological impact of short-term renal replacement therapy is different from that of lifelong therapy. Although the patient depends on a machine in both situations, in short-term therapy there is usually hope that the patient may recover renal function. Therefore, concerns usually focus on the discomfort associated with insertion of the temporary vascular access and the dialysis treatment. Once these situations are handled, the patient and family then must cope with the uncertainty of how long renal failure will last and how long dialysis will be necessary.

Patients who develop chronic renal failure must deal with the fact that renal replacement therapy will be necessary for the rest of their lives. At first, patients usually deny a great deal of what is happening to them. This may continue for some time and prevent some patients from accepting necessary aspects of their treatment regimen. Other patients who feel considerably better after starting dialysis may enter a "honeymoon phase" and appear quite euphoric for a while. Patients should progress through the normal grieving stages and develop healthy coping mechanisms to deal with their long-term treatment.

HEMODIALYSIS APPLIED TO OTHER THERAPIES

The technical equipment and knowledge needed to perform hemodialysis are often applied to other therapies that involve an extracorporeal blood process, such as hemoperfusion and therapeutic apheresis.

 Box 30-7 • NURSING INTERVENTIONS for Maintaining Blood Flow Through A Continuous Venovenous Hemofiltration With Dialysis Circuit

- Check clotting times at initiation and at the prescribed intervals throughout treatment.
- Flush system as often as needed with saline to assess appearance of filter and circuit.
- Monitor ultrafiltration rates, venous and arterial pressure, and color of blood in circuit.
- If system is clotting, return as much blood as possible to the patient before changing the system.

Hemoperfusion is used primarily for the treatment of drug overdose. Blood is pumped from the body and perfused through a column of charcoal or other absorbent materials that bind the drug. This leads to a rapid reduction in serum levels and avoids potential tissue damage caused by an abnormally high drug level. This therapy is particularly useful for drugs that are fat bound or whose molecular structure is too large to be removed by hemodialysis. With this in mind, critical care nurses may need to take the hemodialysis schedules of their patients into consideration when timing administration of medications. For a list of medications that are removed during dialysis, see Box 30-8.

Therapeutic plasma exchange, or apheresis, is another therapy that may be performed using standard hemodialysis equipment in conjunction with a plasma separator cell and replacement fluids. Apheresis is used to treat diseases caused or complicated by circulating immune complexes or their abnormal proteins. During the procedure, the patient's whole blood is separated into its major components, and the offending components are removed.

• Peritoneal Dialysis

Peritoneal dialysis and hemodialysis accomplish the same objective and operate on the same principle of diffusion. However, in peritoneal dialysis, the peritoneum is the semipermeable membrane, and osmosis is used to remove fluid, rather than the pressure differentials used in hemodialysis. To access the peritoneal cavity, a Tenckhoff (peritoneal) catheter is inserted (Fig. 30-6). Intermittent peritoneal dialysis is an effective alternative method of treating acute renal failure when hemodialysis is not available or when access to the bloodstream is not possible. It sometimes is used as an initial treatment for renal failure while the patient is being evaluated for a hemodialy-

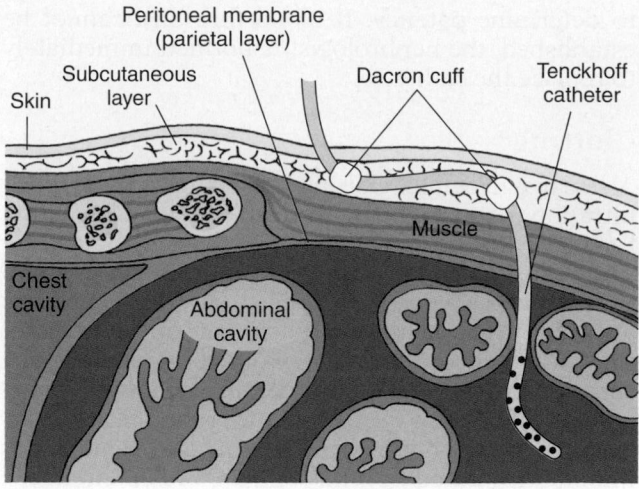

Figure 30-6 • A Tenckhoff (peritoneal) catheter is used to access the peritoneal cavity. A Dacron cuff wrapped around the catheter helps to reduce complications related to infection.

sis program. For a comparison of peritoneal dialysis with hemodialysis and CRRT, see Table 30-1.

Peritoneal dialysis has the following advantages over hemodialysis:

▶ The required technical equipment and supplies are less complicated and more readily available.

▶ There is less need for highly skilled personnel.

▶ The adverse effects associated with the more efficient hemodialysis are minimized. This may be important for patients with severe cardiac disease, who cannot tolerate rapid hemodynamic changes.

▶ Patients can learn to manage their own peritoneal dialysis at home.

Peritoneal dialysis also has a few disadvantages:

▶ It requires more time to remove metabolic wastes adequately and to restore electrolyte and fluid balance.

▶ Repeated treatments may lead to peritonitis.

▶ Long periods of immobility may result in complications such as pulmonary congestion and venous stasis.

Because fluid is introduced into the peritoneal cavity, peritoneal dialysis is contraindicated in patients who have existing peritonitis, in those who have undergone recent or extensive abdominal surgery, and in those who have abdominal adhesions. In the event of a cardiac arrest, the patient's abdomen is drained immediately to maximize the efficiency of chest compressions.

EQUIPMENT
Solutions

As in hemodialysis, peritoneal dialysis solutions contain "ideal" concentrations of electrolytes but lack urea, creatinine, and other substances that are to be removed. Unlike dialysate used in hemodialysis, solu-

---

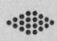 **Box 30-8 • Examples of Medications Commonly Hemodialyzed**

Acetaminophen, acyclovir, allopurinol, amoxicillin, ampicillin
Captopril, cefazolin, cefepime, cefoxitin, ceftazidime, cimetidine
Enalapril, esmolol
Fluconazole
Ganciclovir, gentamicin
Imipenem
Lisinopril, lithium
Mannitol, meropenem, metformin, methotrexate, methylprednisolone, metoprolol, metronidazole, morphine
Nitroprusside
Penicillin, phenobarbital, piperacillin, procainamide
Salsalate, sotalol, streptomycin, sulfamethoxazole
Theophylline, tobramycin
Valacyclovir

tions must be sterile. Dextrose concentrations of the solutions vary; a 1.5%, 2.5%, or 4.25% dextrose solution can be used. Use of 2.5% or 4.25% solutions usually is reserved for more fluid removal and occasionally for better solute clearance. If peritoneal dialysate does not contain potassium, a small amount of potassium chloride may have to be added to the dialysate to prevent hypokalemia. The patient's serum potassium must be monitored closely to regulate the amount of potassium to be added.

Automated Peritoneal Dialysis Systems

Automated peritoneal dialysis systems have built-in monitors and a system of automatic timing devices that cycle the infusion and removal of peritoneal fluid. For this reason, they are called cyclers, and they may be used in the intensive care setting. They are convenient because they eliminate the need to change solution bags constantly. Most cyclers also have a log that retains cycle-by-cycle information on ultrafiltration. Setting up the cycler requires attaching the appropriate strength of large-volume (5 L) solution bags to the cycler tubing, using aseptic technique. The cycler is programmed to deliver a set amount of dialysate per exchange for a certain length of time. When the time is up, the patient is automatically drained and then refilled. Cyclers are usually used when patients have a permanent peritoneal access device.

ASSESSMENT AND MANAGEMENT
Preprocedure

Before peritoneal dialysis begins, the nurse must perform the following interventions:

1. Prepare the patient for catheter insertion and the dialysis procedure by giving a thorough explanation of the procedure. Depending on hospital policy, a signed consent form may be necessary.
2. Ask the patient to empty his or her bladder just before the procedure to avoid accidental puncture with the trocar.
3. Give a preoperative medication, as ordered, to enhance relaxation during the procedure.
4. Warm the dialyzing fluid to body temperature or slightly warmer, using a device manufactured solely for this purpose. It is not recommended that peritoneal dialysate be warmed in microwave ovens because of uneven heating of the fluid and inconsistency from one microwave to another.
5. Take and record baseline vital signs, such as temperature, pulse, respirations, and weight. An in-bed scale is ideal for frequent monitoring of the patient's weight.
6. Take the patient's history, identifying abdominal surgery or trauma.
7. Examine the abdomen before the catheter is inserted.
8. Follow specific orders, obtained before the procedure, regarding fluid removal, replacement, and drug administration.

Procedure

The following items are needed for the procedure:

▶ Peritoneal dialysis administration set
▶ Peritoneal dialysis catheter set, which includes the catheter, a connecting tube for connecting the catheter to the administration set, and a metal stylet
▶ Trocar set of the physician's choice
▶ Ancillary drugs: local anesthetic solution (2% lidocaine), aqueous heparin (1,000 U/mL), potassium chloride, broad-spectrum antibiotics

The physician makes a small midline incision just below the umbilicus under sterile conditions. A trocar is inserted through the incision into the peritoneal cavity. The obturator is removed, and the catheter is inserted and secured.

The dialysis solution flows into the abdominal cavity by gravity as rapidly as possible (5 to 10 minutes; Fig. 30-7). If it flows in too slowly, the catheter may need to be repositioned. When the solution is infused, the tubing is clamped, and the solution remains in the abdominal cavity for 30 to 45 minutes. Next, the solution bottles or bags are placed below the abdominal cavity, and the fluid is drained out of the peritoneal cavity by gravity. If the system is patent and the catheter well placed, the fluid drains in a steady, forceful stream. Drainage should take no more than 20 minutes.

This cycle is repeated continuously for the prescribed time, which varies from 12 to 36 hours, depending on the purpose of the treatment, the patient's condition, and the proper functioning of the system. Dialysis effluent is considered a contaminated fluid, and gloves are worn while handling it.

Postprocedure

After the procedure, the nurse must perform the following interventions:

1. Maintain accurate records of intake and output and weights obtained from the same scale for assessment of volume depletion or overload.
2. Monitor blood pressure and pulse frequently. Orthostatic blood pressure changes and increased pulse rate are valuable clues that help the nurse evaluate the patient's volume status.
3. Detect signs and symptoms of peritonitis early. Low-grade fever, abdominal pain, and cloudy peritoneal fluid all are possible signs of infection.
4. Maintain sterility of the peritoneal system. Masks and sterile gloves must be worn while the abdominal dressing is being changed and when the catheter is being accessed or discontinued from the exchange. Solution bags or bottles are changed in as controlled a physical environment as possible to avoid contamination (e.g., avoiding areas of high traffic and high air flow).
5. Detect and correct technical difficulties early before they result in physiological problems. Slow outflow

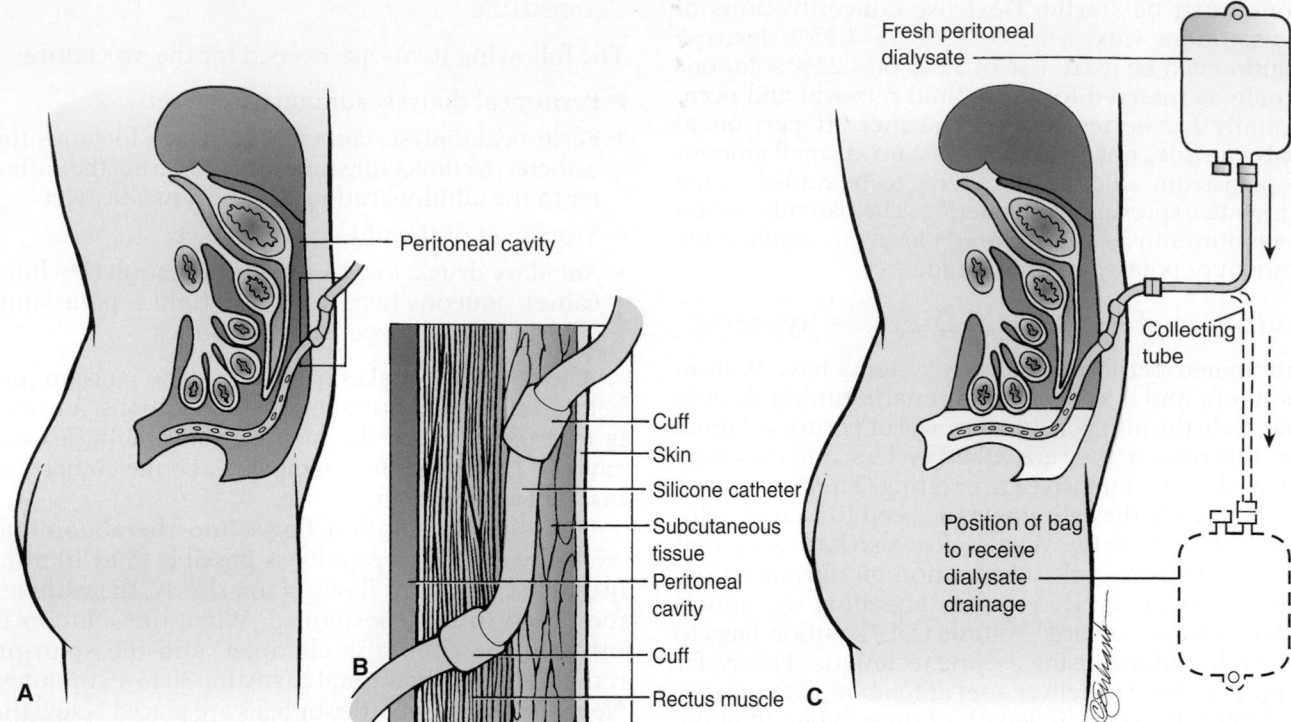

Figure 30-7 • Continuous ambulatory peritoneal dialysis. **A:** The peritoneal catheter is implanted through the abdominal wall. **B:** Dacron cuffs and a subcutaneous tunnel provide protection against bacterial infection. **C:** Dialysate flows by gravity into the peritoneal catheter and then into the peritoneal cavity. After a prescribed period of time, the fluid is drained by gravity and discarded. New solution is then infused into the peritoneal cavity until the next drainage period. Dialysis thus continues on a 24-hour-a-day basis during which the patient is free to move around and engage in his or her usual activities. (From Smeltzer SC, Bare BG, Hinkle JL, Cheever KH: Brunner & Suddarth's Textbook of Medical–Surgical Nursing, 11th ed. Philadelphia: Lippincott Williams & Wilkins, 2008, p 1546.)

of the peritoneal fluid may indicate early problems with the patency of the peritoneal catheter.

6. Prevent complications of bed rest and provide an environment that helps the patient in accepting bed rest for prolonged periods.

7. Prevent constipation. Difficult or infrequent defecation decreases the clearance of waste products and causes the patient more discomfort and distention.

TECHNICAL COMPLICATIONS

Incomplete Recovery of Fluid

The fluid that is removed should equal or exceed the amount inserted. Commercially prepared dialysate contains about 1,000 to 2,000 mL of fluid. If, after several exchanges, the volume drained is less (by 500 mL or more) than the amount inserted, an evaluation must be made. Signs of fluid retention include abdominal distention or complaints of fullness. The most accurate indication of the amount of unrecovered fluid is weight.

If the fluid drains slowly, the catheter tip may be buried in the omentum or clogged with fibrin. Turning the patient from side to side, elevating the head of the bed, and gently massaging the abdomen may facilitate drainage.

If fibrin or blood exists in the outflow drainage, heparin needs to be added to the dialysate. The specific dose, which is ordered by the physician, is 500 to 1,000 U/L.

Leakage Around the Catheter

Superficial leakage after surgery may be controlled with extra sutures and a decrease in the amount of dialysate instilled into the peritoneum. Increases in intra-abdominal pressure may also cause dialysate leaks. Therefore, continued vomiting, coughing, and jarring movements should be avoided during the initial postoperative period. The abdominal dressing must be checked frequently to detect leakage. Dialysate leaks can be distinguished from other clear fluids by checking with a dextrose test strip. Dialysate tests positive because of its dextrose content. A leaking catheter must be corrected because it acts as a pathway for bacteria to enter the peritoneum.

Blood-Tinged Peritoneal Fluid

Blood-tinged peritoneal fluid is expected in the initial outflow but should clear after a few exchanges. Gross bleeding at any time is an indication of a more serious problem and must be investigated immediately.

PHYSIOLOGICAL COMPLICATIONS

Peritonitis

Peritonitis is a serious, but manageable, complication of peritoneal dialysis. Signs of peritonitis include low-grade fever, abdominal pain when fluid is being inserted, and cloudy peritoneal drainage fluid. Early detection and treatment reduces the patient's discomfort and prevents more serious complications.

Treatment begins as soon as a sample of peritoneal fluid is obtained for culture and sensitivity. The patient is started on a broad-spectrum antibiotic, which is usually added to the dialysate solution, although it also can be given intravenously. Depending on the severity of the infection, the patient's condition should improve dramatically after 8 hours of antibiotic therapy.

Catheter Infection

During the daily dressing change, the nurse examines the exit site closely for signs of infection, such as tenderness, redness, and drainage around the catheter. In the absence of peritonitis, a catheter infection usually is treated with an oral, broad-spectrum antibiotic. Box 30-9 lists nursing interventions for preventing infections during peritoneal dialysis.

Hypotension

Hypotension may occur if excessive fluid is removed. Vital signs are monitored frequently, especially if a hypertonic solution is used. Lying and sitting blood pressure readings are especially useful for evaluating fluid status. Progressive drops in blood pressure and weight are signs of fluid deficit.

Hypertension and Fluid Overload

If all the dialysate solution is not removed in each cycle, hypertension and fluid overload may occur. If there is hypertension and a weight increase, the nurse assesses catheter patency and notes the exact amount of fluid in the dialysate bottle. Some manufacturers add 50 mL to a 1,000-mL bottle. Over a period of hours, this can make a considerable difference.

The nurse also observes the patient for signs of respiratory distress and pulmonary congestion. In the absence of other symptoms of fluid overload, hypertension may be the result of anxiety and apprehension. Nonpharmacological measures to reduce anxiety are preferable to administering sedatives and tranquilizers.

High Blood Urea Nitrogen and Creatinine

Blood urea nitrogen and creatinine levels are closely monitored because they help evaluate the effectiveness of the dialysis. When levels remain high, it indicates inadequate clearance of these waste products.

Hypokalemia

The serum potassium is monitored closely because hypokalemia is a common complication of peritoneal dialysis. When the serum potassium level is low, potassium chloride is added to the dialysate.

Hyperglycemia

Supplemental insulin can be added to the dialysate to control hyperglycemia. Blood glucose levels should be monitored closely in patients with diabetes mellitus and hepatic disease.

Pain

Patients may experience mild abdominal discomfort at any time during the procedure. It is probably related to the constant distention or chemical irritation of the peritoneum. If a mild analgesic does not provide relief, inserting 5 mL of 2% lidocaine directly into the catheter may help. The patient may be more comfortable if nourishment is given in small amounts, when the fluid is draining out rather than when the abdominal cavity is distended.

Severe pain may indicate more serious problems of infection or paralytic ileus. Infection is not likely in the first 24 hours. Aseptic technique and prophylactic antibiotics minimize the risk for infection. Periodic cultures of the outflowing fluid help in the early detection of pathogenic organisms.

Immobility

Immobility may lead to hypostatic pneumonia, especially in the debilitated or older patient. Deep breathing, turning, and coughing should be encouraged during the procedure. Leg exercises and the use of

---

Box 30-9 • NURSING INTERVENTIONS for Preventing Infection During Peritoneal Dialysis

- Maintain aseptic technique throughout dialysis procedure.
- Use sealed plastic dialysate bags.
- Change dialysis tubing regularly per protocol.
- Swab or soak tubing connections and injection ports with bactericidal solution before adding medications or breaking closed system.

- Assess patient continuously for signs and symptoms of peritonitis (pain, cloudy effluent, fever).
- Change exit site dressing daily using aseptic technique until healing occurs. Assess daily for increase in inflammation or drainage.
- If infection is suspected, obtain appropriate culture, and begin antibiotic according to protocol or physician's order.

elastic stockings may prevent the development of venous thrombi and emboli.

Discomfort

Peritoneal dialysis results in slower clearance of waste products than hemodialysis; therefore, it is rarely associated with the dysequilibrium seen with hemodialysis. However, boredom is a frequent problem because the treatment is longer. Nursing measures are directed toward making the patient as comfortable as possible. Diversions such as reading, watching television, and visitors should be encouraged. Educating the patient about peritoneal dialysis and involving the patient in the care may reduce some of the anxiety and discomfort.

PERITONEAL DIALYSIS AS A CHRONIC TREATMENT

Intermittent peritoneal dialysis (IPD) has been used for chronic therapy for some time, but it requires the patient to remain stationary for 10 to 14 hours, 3 times per week. Because of this inconvenience to the patient and increased staff time needed if this therapy is performed in-center, IPD seldom is used and is not available in many dialysis centers.

Peritoneal dialysis has gained popularity as a chronic form of dialysis therapy, especially since continuous ambulatory peritoneal dialysis (CAPD) has become available. CAPD is easily taught to patients and does not limit ambulation between dialysate fluid exchanges. It uses the dialysis fluid that is continuously present in the peritoneal cavity 24 hours a day, 7 days a week. Dialysis fluid is drained by the patient and replaced with fresh solution 3 to 5 times per day. The number of solution exchanges needed per day depends on the patient's individual needs. Although the patient is required to perform dialysis techniques every day, CAPD is attractive to many patients with end-stage renal disease (ESRD) because they can accomplish it easily and independently. CAPD may also be preferred in patients who benefit from a slow, continuous removal of sodium and water, such as in those with refractory congestive heart failure.

Continuous cyclic peritoneal dialysis (CCPD) is another variation of chronic peritoneal dialysis therapy. Patients who choose this form of therapy perform IPD at night during sleep using a cycling machine and in the morning instill dialysis fluid, which remains in the abdomen during the entire day. This is most convenient for patients who require the help of working family members to perform their exchanges.

As with acute peritoneal dialysis, peritonitis is the greatest potential problem associated with chronic forms of dialysis. Peritoneal catheters are permanent and inserted in the operating room. Such catheters have one or two Dacron cuffs that the surgeon sutures to the abdominal wall, subcutaneous tissue, or both to anchor the catheter and provide a permanent seal against invading bacteria. Patients are taught how to recognize any potential problem associated with the catheter or treatment and to seek help from the CAPD team when needed.

Patients who perform IPD, CAPD, or CCPD at home usually visit the dialysis unit every 4 to 8 weeks. At this time, a nursing assessment is performed, techniques are reviewed, and required blood studies are obtained. All health team members, including the physician, nurse, dietitian, and social worker, work together with the patient and family to ensure successful adaptation to the chosen mode of treatment. Box 30-10 presents a discharge planning guide for the patient undergoing chronic peritoneal dialysis.

• Pharmacological Management of Renal Dysfunction

When the kidneys fail, treatment such as dialysis may be used to achieve fluid and electrolyte balance. Pharmacological treatment may be initiated to enhance an

---

Box 30-10 • DISCHARGE PLANNING GUIDE: Peritoneal Dialysis

- Discuss basic information about normal kidney function.
- Discuss basic information about the disease process.
- Discuss the basic principles of peritoneal dialysis.
- Demonstrate catheter and exit site care.
- Demonstrate measurement of vital signs and weight measurement.
- Discuss monitoring and management of fluid balance.
- Discuss basic principles of aseptic technique.
- Demonstrate the CAPD exchange procedure using aseptic technique (CCPD patients should also demonstrate exchange procedure in case of failure or unavailability of cycling machine).
- Demonstrate cycler set-up procedure and maintenance if on CCPD.
- Discuss complications of peritoneal dialysis; prevention, recognition, and management of complications.
- Demonstrate procedure for adding medications to the dialysis solution.
- Demonstrate procedure for obtaining sterile dialysis fluid samples.
- Discuss routine laboratory work needed and implications of results.
- Discuss dietary restrictions and importance of maintaining normal weight.
- Discuss medications: name of medications, their actions, potential side effects, and when to contact the physician.
- Discuss ordering, storage, and inventory of dialysis supplies.
- Describe plan for follow-up continuing care.
- Demonstrate maintenance of home dialysis records, including daily weights.
- Describe actions in case of emergency.

CAPD, continuous ambulatory peritoneal dialysis; CPPD, continuous cyclic peritoneal dialysis.
Used with permission from Smeltzer SC, Bare BG: Brunner & Suddarth's Textbook of Medical–Surgical Nursing 10th ed. Philadelphia: Lippincott Williams & Wilkins, 2004, p 1296.

already functional kidney, attempt to recover renal function, or optimize fluid balance.

DIURETICS

Diuretics are drugs that promote fluid removal through increased urine production. There are three major classes of diuretics: loop, thiazide, and potassium sparing. Table 30-5 presents information about the various diuretics. In addition, acetazolamide and mannitol may be used to promote fluid removal. The ultimate goal of diuretic therapy is to improve cardiopulmonary status. It may be necessary to use combination therapy to achieve the desired therapeutic end point. Drugs from different classes are chosen to maximize urine production in combination therapy.

Diuretics may be administered orally or intravenously. The effect is more immediate with IV therapy. The patient is monitored for breath sounds, hemodynamic value changes (central venous and pulmonary pressures), weight, and peripheral edema to determine his or her response to therapy. Careful laboratory assessment of the blood urea nitrogen and creatinine level is required to monitor for development or worsening of acute renal failure. Ideally, the patient's pulmonary status and fluid balance improve while the glomerular filtration rate remains normal.

Diuretics have both desirable and undesirable effects (see Table 30-5). Overdiuresis is the most common side effect. The nurse must monitor for fluid volume depletion, especially when diuretic regimens are altered or initiated. Signs of volume depletion are discussed in Chapter 29. Other side effects include hyponatremia, hypokalemia, hyperkalemia, hypocalcemia, hypercalcemia, hypomagnesemia, and acid-base disturbances. A reduction in volume from vomiting, third-spacing of fluid, diuretic therapy, or other conditions may have the same consequences. A reduction in the effective circulatory volume can lead to acute renal failure, put increased work on the heart, and result in many metabolic derangements. The most effective management strategy is to replace only the volume required to achieve adequate perfusion. In

Table 30-5 • Diuretic Agents

Drug	Mechanism	Complication(s)	Management and Prevention
Loop diuretics Examples: furosemide (Lasix), ethacrynic acid (Edecrin), bumetanide (Bumex)	Powerful diuretics that act primarily in the thick segment of the medullary and cortical ascending limbs of loop of Henle Cause loss of sodium, chloride, and potassium Increase calcium excretion	Volume depletion Hypokalemia Hyponatremia Hypocalcemia Hypomagnesemia	Monitor daily weights, intake and output, signs and symptoms of volume depletion. Potassium supplements or extradietary potassium may be necessary when loop diuretics are used routinely. Monitor calcium levels and administer supplemental calcium as indicated. Usually no intervention is required because body stores of magnesium are quite high.
Thiazides Examples: chlorothiazide (Diuril), hydrochlorothiazide (HCTZ)	Act by inhibiting sodium reabsorption in distal tubule and, to a lesser extent, inner medullary collecting duct Cause loss of sodium, chloride, and potassium Decrease urinary calcium excretion	Hypercalcemia Hypokalemia Hypomagnesemia	Monitor calcium levels; loop diuretic may be indicated if calcium levels are persistently elevated. Potassium supplements or extradietary potassium may be necessary when these agents are used routinely. Usually no intervention is required because body stores of magnesium are quite high.
Potassium-sparing diuretics Examples: spironolactone (Aldactone), triamterene (Dyrenium), amiloride (Midamor)	Conserve potassium Spironolactone inhibits action of aldosterone, thereby reducing sodium reabsorption while increasing potassium reabsorption Triamterene acts on distal renal tubule to depress exchange of sodium Effects of amiloride are apparently due to inhibition of sodium entry into cell from luminal fluid	Hyperkalemia	Potassium supplements are contraindicated, as are salt substitutes containing potassium. Often combined with thiazides for effective diuresis; hypokalemic tendency of thiazides may offset hyperkalemic tendency of triamterene and spironolactone.
Carbonic anhydrase inhibitors Example: acetazolamide (Diamox)	Decrease proximal tubular sodium reabsorption Not very effective when administered alone Facilitate excretion of bicarbonate	Metabolic acidosis	Monitor pH and bicarbonate.
Osmotic diuretics Example: mannitol	Nonreabsorbable polysaccharide that pulls water into vascular space, thereby increasing glomerular flow	Hyperosmolarity	Monitor serum osmolarity. Withhold mannitol therapy if serum osmolarity is >300–305 mMol/L.

Adapted from Metheny NM: Fluid and Electrolyte Balance: Nursing Considerations. Philadelphia: Lippincott Williams & Wilkins, 2000, p 53, with permission.

cases in which a delicate balance exists between diuresis and overdiuresis, a pulmonary artery catheter may be inserted to guide therapy. Box 30-11 lists nursing diagnoses for patients taking diuretics.

Hypokalemia is another common side effect of diuretics, particularly the loop and thiazide diuretics. In general, hypokalemia is a benign condition that can be managed effectively with potassium supplementation. If left untreated, patients may experience harmful, sometimes life-threatening, cardiac dysrhythmias.

VASOACTIVE DRUGS

Sometimes the cause of decreased effective circulatory volume is reduced cardiac contractility. In such a case, an inotropic agent (e.g., dobutamine or milrinone) may be added to the plan of care to improve the forward flow of the heart, thereby improving the effective circulatory volume and stopping the cascade of counterproductive compensatory mechanisms. A failing heart, such as in congestive heart failure, can cause reduced blood flow to the kidney and potentiate acute renal failure. The same compensatory mechanisms used in volume depletion operate in an attempt to restore renal function. Namely, the renin–angiotensin–aldosterone system is activated to increase sodium and water retention and achieve renal and peripheral vasoconstriction. Other common inotropic agents are described in detail in Chapter 18.

Dopamine is a vasoactive drug at higher doses but can stimulate dopaminergic receptors in the kidneys when infused at lower doses (1–3 µg/kg/minute). Stimulation of dopamine receptors increases renal blood flow and promotes natriuresis. Although this practice is commonly used to prevent or treat acute renal failure in some settings, several studies have found that there is no improvement in clinical outcome and a lack of sufficient clinical evidence to support its routine use.[5,6]

• Disorders of Fluid Volume

Critically ill patients often have imbalances in fluid homeostasis related to their primary underlying disease. Fluid imbalance occurs when there is an excess or deficit of fluid and may be either absolute or relative. Medications, such as diuretics, put patients at increased risk for fluid imbalance. Infection increases metabolic demand and insensible loss, and fluid volume deficits may develop. Regardless of patient diagnosis, assessment of fluid balance (see Chapter 28) and careful management are mainstays of patient care in the critical care setting.

FLUID VOLUME DEFICIT

When fluid loss exceeds intake, a fluid volume deficit exists. A fluid volume deficit is a physiological situation in which fluids are lost in an isotonic fashion (both fluid and electrolytes are lost together). Dehydration is the loss of water alone, resulting in a hyperosmolar state. Although the critically ill patient typically can have both a fluid volume deficit and dehydration states simultaneously, this discussion is limited strictly to disorders of fluid volume deficit.

Several patient populations are particularly vulnerable to development of fluid volume deficits. Young children at prespeech developmental levels cannot communicate thirst; therefore, during times when fluid requirements increase, they do not increase their fluid intake of their own accord. Debilitated patients, such as patients after stroke, may not be able to communicate their needs or have swallowing disturbances and cannot manage their own intake of fluid. Elderly patients are at particular risk for a fluid volume deficit because of the multisystem changes associated with aging. For a review of the changes associated with aging and nursing implications for fluid volume assessment and management, see Table 30-2.

Causes

Gastrointestinal Loss
Physiologically, the body produces approximately 5 L of gastrointestinal fluid. In the gastrointestinal tract, fluids help act as a carrier of important enzymes and buffers to aid in digestion. In the distal small intestine and large intestine, fluid is reabsorbed, leaving only approximately 150 mL lost through the stool daily.

Excess loss from any site from which fluids are ordinarily lost may cause a fluid imbalance. Conditions such as vomiting and diarrhea may cause an increase beyond the typical 150 mL and result in a fluid volume deficit. In addition, surgically placed drainage tubes and nasogastric tubes used for suction may cause such a deficit.

Infection
Infection causes fluid deficits in several ways:

1. Infection can increase metabolic demand, increasing insensible water loss. When patients are not critically ill, they often mitigate this imbalance by increasing fluid intake. When they have widespread infections or a self-care deficit, which may occur in elderly people, fluid intake may not be sufficient to restore fluid balance.

2. Mediators are released as part of the immune response. These mediators cause a loosening of the capillary tight junctions, resulting in the third-spacing of fluids.

3. Carbon dioxide production increases due to increased metabolism. To maintain pH balance, tachypnea may develop. Although only a very small amount of fluid is lost daily through the respiratory tract, water loss may become clinically significant when the respiratory rate is greater than 35 breaths/minute.

Renal Loss
The kidneys filter approximately 180 L per day. However, urine output is only 1% to 2% of total blood volume filtered (see Chapter 28). Reabsorption of fluid is influenced by a complex regulatory system that includes the actions of aldosterone, angiotensin, and antidiuretic hormone (ADH). A defect in any one of the regulatory functions can cause a disruption in renal fluid balance.

Several endocrine disorders may disrupt the renal regulatory system. Adrenal insufficiency, the absence of glucocorticoids and aldosterone, can cause a reduction in the absorption of sodium, thereby promoting water loss. Diabetes insipidus is a profound reduction in ADH, which reduces the amount of fluid reabsorbed at the distal convoluted tubule. Water loss predominates in diabetes insipidus, and therefore volume imbalance is related to dehydration.

Serum osmolarity is predicted by sodium, glucose, and blood urea nitrogen. Normally, glucose does not influence the overall osmolarity. However, in profound hyperglycemia, the influence of glucose increases greatly. Serum osmolarity increases and is sensed by the osmoreceptors, thereby pulling fluids into the vascular space and initiating an osmotic diuresis. Two conditions that pathologically increase glucose are diabetic ketoacidosis (DKA) and hyperglycemic hyperosmolar nonketotic coma (HHNK). Both of these disorders are discussed in more detail in Chapter 44.

Diuretic therapy is intended to treat fluid volume excess. However, overadministration of diuretics may result in a fluid volume deficit. It is important to recognize the immediate onset that diuretics can have when administered intravenously, initiated for the first time, or adjusted in dosage (see Table 30-5 for more information).

Third-Spacing of Fluid
Third-spacing of fluid is the movement of fluid from the vascular space to the interstitial space. To create a movement of fluid between body compartments, there is an alteration in capillary permeability because of inflammation, ischemia, or injury. Causes of third-spacing of fluids are numerous and include infection; systemic inflammatory response syndrome, such as in pancreatitis; hypoalbuminemia, such as in liver failure; burns; intestinal obstruction; and surgery. The amount of fluid lost depends on the degree of the pathophysiological alteration. Regardless of cause, the fluid lost is not functioning to maintain vascular volume, and therefore a fluid volume deficit exists. When fluid leaks out of the vascular space, daily weights can increase, paradoxically, despite intravascular volume depletion.

Management: Fluid Volume Replacement
To correct a fluid volume deficit, it is necessary to treat the underlying cause and replace the lost fluid. The main purposes of fluid administration include replacement of lost fluid, maintenance of fluid balance, and replacement of lost electrolytes. Several types of fluids, which have different physiological effects, are available. Administration of fluids may occur using the gastrointestinal tract or an IV or intraosseous route. When chronic replacement is required, such as in patients with long-term tube feeding, the gastrointestinal approach is used. Enteral access is required when patients are unable to take fluids by mouth. When rapid restoration of fluid balance is required, the IV route is preferred. Occasionally, both routes are used.

Maintenance Fluids
Under normal conditions, the average healthy adult requires about 2.5 L/day. This volume replaces fluids lost through the feces, the respiratory tract, sweating, and the urine. Patients who are unable to consume their usual intake of fluid are often prescribed IV maintenance fluids of 2 to 3 L/day. When determining the rate of administration of maintenance fluid, factors such as medical history (renal failure), age (young or old), confounding water excesses (heart failure), and ongoing assessment parameters (edema formation) must be considered.

Replacement Fluids
Critically ill patients are often unable to consume the additional fluid required to replace the lost fluid. In this case, IV administration beyond baseline maintenance fluids is required for homeostasis. This is achieved by either administering a bolus of fluid or increasing the total daily fluid intake. When fluid loss occurs acutely, the loss must be replaced immediately to maintain tissue perfusion. The type of fluid given depends on the type of fluid lost. When whole blood is lost, such as in trauma or surgery, blood may be administered. When intravascular volume is depleted, such as in diarrhea, isotonic solutions may be administered. The rate of administration depends on the patient's medical history and amount of volume lost.

Crystalloids Crystalloid solutions are prepared with a specified balance of water and electrolytes. Box 30-12 provides a description of commonly used crystalloid solutions. These fluids are described separately, but they are most commonly used in combination. Fluids are classified as hypotonic (osmolarity < 250 mEq/L), isotonic (osmolarity approximately 310 mEq/L), or hypertonic (osmolarity > 376 mEq/L).

Box 30-12 • Common Crystalloid Solutions

5% Dextrose in water (D₅W): no electrolytes, 50 g dextrose
- Supplies about 170 cal/L and free water to aid in renal excretion of solutes
- Should not be used in excessive volumes in patients with increased antidiuretic hormone activity or to replace fluids in hypovolemic patients

0.9% NaCl (isotonic saline): Na^+ 154 mEq/L, Cl^- 154 mEq/L
- Isotonic fluid commonly used to expand the extracellular fluid in presence of hypovolemia
- Because of relatively high chloride content, it can be used to treat mild metabolic alkalosis

0.45% NaCl (½ strength saline): Na^+ 77 mEq/L, Cl^- 77 mEq/L
- A hypotonic solution that provides sodium, chloride, and free water (sodium and chloride provided in fluid allow kidneys to select and retain needed amounts)
- Free water desirable as aid to kidneys in elimination of solutes

0.33% NaCl (⅓ strength saline): Na^+ 56 mEq/L, Cl^- 56 mEq/L
- A hypotonic solution that provides sodium, chloride, and free water
- Often used to treat hypernatremia (because this solution contains a small amount of sodium, it dilutes the plasma sodium while not allowing the level to drop too rapidly)

3% Saline
- Grossly hypertonic solution used only to treat severe hyponatremia
- Use this solution only in settings where the patient can be closely monitored

Lactated Ringer's solution: Na^+ 130 mEq/L, K^+ 4 mEq/L, Ca^{2+} 3 mEq/L, Cl^- 109 mEq/L, lactate (metabolized to bicarbonate) 28 mEq/L
- Approximately isotonic solution that contains multiple electrolytes in about same concentrations as found in plasma (note that this solution is lacking magnesium and phosphate)
- Used in the treatment of hypovolemia, burns, and fluid lost as bile or diarrhea
- Useful in treating mild metabolic acidosis

Adapted from Metheny NM: Fluid and Electrolyte Balance: Nursing Considerations. Philadelphia: Lippincott Williams & Wilkins, 2000, p 181. with permission.

Dextrose solutions are given to provide free water and some calories to prevent protein catabolism. The 5% solution contains 50 g of dextrose for every liter of fluid and provides approximately 170 calories per liter. When pure dextrose solutions such as 5% dextrose in water (D₅W) are administered, the dextrose is metabolized, resulting in the administration of free water. When given intravenously, free water decreases the plasma osmolarity, thereby promoting the movement of water evenly into all body compartments. Free water does not stay in the vascular space; therefore, pure dextrose solutions should not be used when intravascular replacement of fluids is required.

Saline solutions are commonly used and are available in different strengths, such as 0.9% and 0.45%. Normal saline, or 0.9% saline, is an isotonic solution. Approximately one fourth of the fluid administered remains in the vascular space, and the remaining fluid moves into the extracellular space 1 hour after administration. During critical illness, the amount that exits into the extracellular space can increase owing to increased capillary permeability.

Half-strength saline, in comparison, is a hypotonic solution. Additional free water is administered with this solution, making it an ideal maintenance fluid. Occasionally, half-strength saline is administered to replace fluids lost when there is concurrent hypernatremia.

Saline solutions such as 3% saline are hypertonic and may be given for the treatment of symptomatic hyponatremia. The hypertonicity pulls fluid from the extravascular space to the vascular space. Hypertonic solutions should be administered only when patients may be closely monitored because fluid volume excess can develop rapidly. Some studies have shown that hypertonic saline solutions, such as 3% or 7.5% saline, may be beneficial during resuscitation.[7]

Colloids Colloids are high-molecular-weight substances and therefore do not cross the capillary membrane under normal conditions. Table 30-6 describes commonly prepared colloid solutions.

Albumin is the most abundant circulating protein in the body and accounts for 80% of the colloid oncotic pressure. For therapeutic uses, albumin is prepared from donor plasma. With albumin, there is no risk of blood-borne diseases, such as hepatitis or human immunodeficiency virus (HIV) infection. Albumin is available in two concentrations, 5% and 25%, and both preparations contain some sodium. The 5% solution is similar in osmolarity to plasma. In contrast, the 25% solution is hypertonic, thereby pulling extravascular water into the vascular space. Both preparations of albumin can cause the intravascular volume to expand beyond the volume of albumin infused because of the increased oncotic pressure generated. Care must be taken when administering albumin to patients at high risk for volume overload. Use of albumin should also be limited in patients with profound capillary leak syndrome (e.g., in sepsis, acute respiratory distress syndrome, and pancreatitis[7]). Although albumin is a protein, it is inefficient and expensive when used for malnutrition.

The starches dextran and hetastarch, which differ from each other only slightly, have an oncotic pressure similar to albumin. Both substances are used to expand plasma volume by exerting an oncotic pressure and thereby pulling water from the extravascular space to the vascular space. Hetastarch is metabolized by both the kidneys and liver. The diuresis that may occur with hetastarch is an osmotic diuresis and does not reflect an increase in effective renal circulatory volume. Both dextran and hetastarch may cause coagulopathies; however, dextran has a more profound effect on coagulation.

Table 30-6 • Common Colloid Solutions

Solution	Contents	Indications	Comments
Albumin	Available in two concentrations: 5%: oncotically similar to plasma 25%: hypertonic Both 5% and 25% solutions contain about 130–160 mEq/L of sodium	Used as volume expander in treatment of shock May be useful in treating burns and third-spacing shifts	Cost is approximately 25–30 times more than for crystalloid solutions. Increased interstitial oncotic pressure in disease states in which there is increased capillary leaking (e.g., burns, sepsis) may occur; this may result in increased vascular space loss of fluid. Use caution with rapid administration; watch for volume overload.
Hetastarch	Synthetic colloid made from starch (6%) and added to sodium chloride solution	May be used to expand plasma voume when volume is lost from hemorrhage, trauma, burns, and sepsis	Plasma volume expansion effects decrease over 24–36 h. Starch is eliminated by kidneys and liver; therefore, use caution in patients with liver and kidney impairment. Mild, transient coagulopathies may occur. Transient rise in serum amylase may occur.
Dextran	Glucose polysaccharide substance, available as low-molecular-weight dextran (dextran 40) or high-molecular-weight dextran (dextran 70) No electrolyte content	May be used to expand plasma volume when volume is lost from hemorrhage, trauma, burns, and sepsis	Has been associated with greater risk for allergic reaction than albumin or hetastarch. Interference with blood cross-matching may occur. May cause coagulopathy; has more profound effect on coagulation than hetastarch.

FLUID VOLUME EXCESS

Fluid volume excess occurs when there is retention of sodium, resulting in the reabsorption of water. Electrolytes typically remain unchanged when there is an increase in total body water and electrolytes increase in parallel. Many critically ill patients may have mixed disturbances with manifestations of the confounding compensatory mechanisms. Causes of fluid volume excess include overadministration of fluids, edematous disorder (e.g., congestive heart failure, kidney or liver failure), excessive sodium intake, and medications (e.g., steroids, desmopressin acetate).

When the kidneys are functioning normally and regulating fluid balance, the body typically rids itself of excess fluid, and fluid overload is not manifested clinically. When the kidneys sense a decrease in effective circulatory volume, the compensatory mechanisms prevent the excretion of excess water, such as in congestive heart failure.

Management of fluid volume excess is directed toward correction of the underlying disorder. If this is not feasible, efforts are geared to prevention of pulmonary compromise by attempting to rid the body of the excess sodium and water. In cases of volume overload, there is an increase in pulmonary hydrostatic pressure, which promotes movement of water into the alveoli, thereby impeding gas exchange. Sodium restriction reduces the amount of water reabsorption but does contribute to acute correction of volume overload. Diuretics are the mainstay of treatment for acute resolution of fluid volume excess (see Table 30-5).

• Management of Electrolyte Imbalances

Electrolyte disorders commonly occur in critically ill patients, typically in combination with other conditions. Management of the underlying problem ensures long-term restoration of balance. However, acute management of electrolyte disorders is often required to maintain cellular integrity.

SODIUM

Sodium is the major extracellular cation. It is a major predictor of serum osmolarity and controls movement of water. Disorders of sodium are typically associated with water disorders (Table 30-7).

Hyponatremia may be associated with volume excess, such as in edematous disorders (e.g., heart, kidney, or liver failure), or with volume deficit, such as when volume loss is exceeded by sodium loss (e.g., in gastrointestinal fluid, diuretic overuse, or adrenal insufficiency). Low sodium with euvolemia is manifested as the syndrome of inappropriate ADH secretion (SIADH; see Chapter 44). Pseudohyponatremia may occur in association with hyperlipidemia and hypoproteinemia; the total-body sodium remains unchanged, but the actual sodium measurement is altered.

Management of hyponatremia is aimed at correcting the underlying cause (see Table 30-7). When the hyponatremia is associated with hypervolemia, diuretics may be beneficial. When the disorder is

Table 30-7 • Management of Electrolyte Disorders

Electrolyte	Selected Medical Conditions Associated With Disturbance	Collaborative Interventions
Sodium		
Hyponatremia	Congestive heart failure Liver failure Kidney failure Hyperlipidemia Hypoproteinemia SIADH GI loss Adrenal insufficiency Thiazide diuretics Drugs: NSAIDs, tricyclic antidepressants, SSRIs, chlorpropamide, omeprazole Tumors associated with ectopic excessive ADH production: oat cell carcinoma, leukemia, lymphoma Pulmonary disorders: pneumonia, acute asthma AIDS	Review medication profile and patient history. Monitor for sites of fluid losses or gains. Monitor fluid balances and for signs and symptoms of electrolyte disturbance. Attempt to manage underlying cause. Correction of electrolyte may require sodium replacement (3% saline) or water restriction, depending on etiology of disorder.
Hypernatremia	Profound dehydration usually in patients not able to ask for water (e.g., debilitated elderly or children), in those with impaired thirst regulation (e.g., elderly), or in those with heatstroke Hypertonic tube feedings without water supplementation Increased insensible water loss (e.g., excessive sweating, second- and third-degree burns, hyperventilation) Excessive administration of sodium-containing fluids (3% saline, sodium bicarbonate) Diabetes insipidus	Assess in patients at particular risk for hypernatremia, including debilitated or elderly patients, acutely or critically ill children, and patients receiving tube feedings. Monitor laboratory values closely in patients with insensible fluid losses and in those receiving parenteral administration of sodium-containing fluids. For comprehensive review of management of diabetes insipidus, see Chapter 44. Administer therapeutic medications, including vasopressin, DDAVP. Administer hypotonic fluids (½ saline to free water, D_5W).
Potassium		
Hypokalemia	GI loss: diarrhea, laxatives, gastric suction Renal loss: potassium-losing diuretics, hyperaldosteronism, osmotic diuresis, steroids, some antibiotics Intracellular shifts: alkalosis, excessive secretion or administration of insulin, hyperalimentation Poor intake: anorexia nervosa, alcoholism, debilitation	Monitor laboratory values closely in patients at particular risk for hypokalemia. Pay particular attention to potassium level in patients receiving digoxin. Administer potassium either PO or IV (see Box 30-13). Monitor magnesium levels in patients who are refractory to potassium replacement.
Hyperkalemia	Pseudohyperkalemia: prolonged tight application of tourniquet; fist clenching and unclenching immediately before or during blood draws; hemolysis of blood sample Decreased potassium excretion: oliguric renal failure, potassium-sparing diuretics, hypoaldosteronism High potassium intake: improper use of oral potassium supplements; rapid IV potassium administration Extracellular shifts: acidosis, crush injuries, tumor cell lysis after chemotherapy	Ensure that minimal negative pressure is used to obtain all laboratory samples, particularly when drawn through small-gauge needles. Restrict potassium-sparing diuretics. Promote excretion: sodium polystyrene sulfonate PO or per rectum, dialysis, potassium-losing diuretics (e.g., furosemide) Emergency management measures: calcium IV, sodium bicarbonate, IV insulin with glucose, β_2-adrenergic agonists
Calcium		
Hypocalcemia	Surgical hypoparathyroidism Primary hypoparathyroidism Malabsorption (alcoholism) Acute pancreatitis Excessive administration of citrated blood Alkalotic states Drugs (loop diuretics, mithramycin, calcitonin) Hyperphosphatemia Sepsis Hypomagnesemia Medullary carcinoma of thyroid Hypoalbuminemia	Monitor for signs and symptoms associated with low calcium, especially for seizures, and stridor. Administer calcium IV for acute replacement (See Box 30-13). Ensure adequate dietary intake for patients at particular risk.

(continued)

Table 30-7 • Management of Electrolyte Disorders (Continued)

Electrolyte	Selected Medical Conditions Associated With Disturbance	Collaborative Interventions
Hypercalcemia	Hyperparathyroidism Malignant neoplastic disease Drugs (thiazide diuretics, lithium, theophylline) Prolonged immobilization Dehydration	Administer bisphosphonates, such as etidronate or mithramycin, especially when disorder is related to malignancy. Administer diuretics, such as loop diuretics, to promote renal excretion. Provide fluid replacement with 0.9% saline.
Magnesium Hypomagnesemia	Inadequate intake: starvation, total parenteral nutrition without adequate Mg^{2+} supplementation, chronic alcoholism Increased GI loss: diarrhea, laxatives, fistulas, nasogastric tube suction, vomiting Increased renal loss: drugs (loop and thiazide diuretics, mannitol, amphotericin B), diuresis (uncontrolled diabetes mellitus, hypoaldosteronism) Changes in magnesium distribution: pancreatitis, burns, insulin, blood products	Monitor for hypokalemia in patients with low magnesium because kidneys are not able to conserve potassium when magnesium level is low. Administer magnesium IV for acute replacement (see Box 30-13). Administer PO preparations for long-term replacement.
Hypermagnesemia	Renal failure Excessive intake of magnesium-containing compounds (e.g., antacids, mineral supplements, laxatives)	Avoid administration of magnesium-containing compounds to patients in renal failure. In extreme cases, dialysis may be indicated.
Phosphorus Hypophosphatemia	Refeeding syndrome Alcoholism Phosphate-binding antacids Respiratory alkalosis Administration of exogenous insulin IV Burns	Ensure nutritional intake. Monitor phosphorus for the first few days after initiation of enteral or parenteral nutrition. Administer by oral supplementation (Neutra-Phos capsules) or IV (see Box 30-13).
Hyperphosphatemia	Renal failure Chemotherapy Excessive administration of phosphate compounds	Prevention is mainstay of therapy; avoid administration of phosphorus to patients in renal failure. Administer calcium acetate. Administer IV fluids to promote renal excretion. In severe cases, administration of high levels of glucose with insulin may help shift phosphorus intracellularly.

ADH, antidiuretic hormone; AIDS, acquired immunodeficiency syndrome; DDAVP, desmopressin acetate; GI, gastrointestinal; NSAID, nonsteroidal anti-inflammatory drug; SIADH, syndrome of inappropriate antidiuretic hormone; SSRI, selective serotonin reuptake inhibitor.

associated with euvolemia, such as in SIADH, water restriction may be useful. In conditions in which there is both sodium loss and water loss, administration of hypertonic saline at slow rates may help improve clinically significant hyponatremia.

Hypernatremia may occur as an isolated condition when there is a loss of free water, which raises the sodium level. Increased insensible loss of fluid, such as occurs in sweating, hyperventilation, or fever, is the most common cause of this type of hypernatremia. The fluid volume deficit associated with the hypernatremia depends almost entirely on the degree of insensible loss. Endocrine disorders, such as hyperaldosteronism or Cushing's disease, can result in hypernatremia and are associated with total-body water excess. Administration of hypertonic fluids, such as sodium bicarbonate, 3% saline, or albumin, may also cause hypernatremia.

Management of hypernatremia is primarily aimed at restoring fluid balance (see Table 30-7). Correcting the underlying cause of the increased sodium is also important.

POTASSIUM

Potassium is the major intracellular ion. Potassium plays a key role in neuromuscular functioning, and high or low levels may result in alterations in the cardiac rhythm. Because of the narrow range of extracellular potassium balance, renal function is essential to regulation of potassium. In critically ill patients, disorders of potassium are common and have numerous causes (see Table 30-7).

Hypokalemia is most commonly caused by an absolute deficiency in potassium. Losses of potassium occur through the kidneys, gastrointestinal tract, sweat, and intracellular shifting. Although relative deficiencies may occur, such as in metabolic alkalosis, they are rare compared with the absolute deficits. Management of hypokalemia involves replacement of depleted potassium to restore potassium balance. It may be necessary to check the magnesium level in patients who do not respond to potassium replacement. Box 30-13 presents nursing considerations in potassium replacement.

Box 30-13 • NURSING INTERVENTIONS for Intravenous Electrolyte Replacement

Potassium

Dilution
- Do not administer undiluted potassium directly IV.
- Keep all vials of undiluted potassium away from patient care area.
- Dilution of potassium depends on the amount of fluid the patient can tolerate. Highly concentrated potassium solutions can cause irritation, pain, and sclerosing of vein.
- Typical concentrations of potassium are 10–40 mEq/100 mL. Premixed bags are available.

Peripheral IV Administration
- In collaboration with prescribing provider, consider the addition of small volume of lidocaine to minimize pain.
- Administer in central vein if available.
- For mild to moderate hypokalemia, rates of 10–20 mEq/h are recommended.
- Rates >40 mEq/h are not recommended.
- Use infusion pump to administer replacement.

Monitoring
- Monitor urinary output, blood urea nitrogen, and creatinine in patients receiving potassium replacement. Patients with impaired renal function or oliguric renal failure may experience transient hyperkalemia. Consider smaller replacement dosages and periodic reevaluation.
- When rate of administration exceeds 10 mEq/h, monitoring of cardiac rhythm is recommended.
- Assess magnesium level because correction of potassium may be refractory to potassium replacement with concurrent hypomagnesemia.

Calcium

Dilution
- Calcium can be delivered as calcium gluconate (4.5 mEq of elemental Ca^{2+}) or calcium chloride (13.5 mEq of elemental Ca^{2+}).

- Calcium can be irritating to veins. If peripheral administration is required, calcium gluconate is recommended because damage can occur to surrounding soft tissues.

Administration
- Administer by slow IV push through central vein or administer by mixing with compatible IV fluids.
- Administer slowly (over 1–2 h) for patients receiving digoxin.

Magnesium

Administration
- Administer with caution to patients with renal failure because magnesium is primarily excreted by the kidneys.
- During emergencies, such as torsades de pointes, magnesium may be injected directly.
- In mild to moderate hypomagnesemia, a rate of infusion of 1–2 g over 1 h is advisable.

Monitoring
- Monitor for hypotension or flushing during administration.
- Monitor deep tendon reflexes periodically during administration.

Phosphorus
- Phosphorus IV replacement is available as sodium or potassium phosphate. Note that phosphorus is dosed in millimoles, whereas sodium and potassium are dosed in milliequivalents.
- Administer sodium phosphate for patients with renal failure.
- Do not administer with calcium.
- Administer over several hours, typically 15–30 mmol phosphorus over 4–6 h.

Hyperkalemia is caused by reduced renal excretion, excessive administration of potassium replacements, transcellular shifts, and measurement error. Patients with renal failure are at particular risk. Dialysis is typically used to manage hyperkalemia in patients with ESRD. Noncompliance with dialysis can certainly cause hyperkalemia and is a frequent reason for hospital admission. Potassium replacement therapy, although performed frequently in critical care settings, must be performed carefully; particular attention should be paid to cardiac signs and laboratory reassessments. Acidosis of any cause can potentiate hyperkalemia; therefore, patients who are acidotic must be carefully monitored for potassium shifts.

The primary goal of management is resolution of the acidosis. However, clinically significant hyperkalemia must be resolved using the measures described in Table 30-7. Temporizing measures for hyperkalemia center on stabilization of cell membrane (calcium) and shifting potassium from the extracellular to the intracellular spaces (bicarbonate,

insulin). These measures resolve the potassium imbalance temporarily and give clinicians time to address the underlying problem. If it is anticipated that correction of this problem will take some time, the excretion of potassium is facilitated by administering sodium polystyrene, dialysis, and diuretics. Drawing laboratory samples can cause hemolysis of cells, which causes liberation of the abundant intracellular potassium. Evaluating trends and assessing the overall clinical picture prevent unnecessary treatment and therefore prevent hypokalemia.

CALCIUM

Almost all of the calcium in the body is contained in the bone, and the remaining 1% is either bound to albumin (50% plasma calcium) or in an ionized form. The primary function of calcium is promotion of the neuromuscular impulse. Several clotting factors also depend on calcium.

Hypocalcemia has numerous causes (see Table 30-7). Most hypocalcemia is a relative deficiency;

causes include intracellular shifting, decreased circulating protein, and binding with fatty acids (pancreatitis). The relative hypocalcemia that occurs with a massive transfusion of blood is common in the critical care setting. The blood is mixed with citrate to prevent coagulation; when the blood is infused, the citrate binds to calcium, causing a relative calcium deficiency. Citrate used for anticoagulation in CRRT also results in hypocalcemia. Other causes of hypocalcemia include increased renal excretion (loop diuretics) or decreased absorption (malabsorption syndromes).

Calcium is transported in its ionized form, provides some of the structural components in bone, and is also bound to albumin. A low albumin level can therefore be one cause of a low calcium level. The calcium level should be corrected for the low albumin before consideration of calcium replacement. Replacement of calcium is required to prevent complications of bleeding and decreased impulse transmission. For a review of nursing considerations in calcium replacement, see Box 30-13.

Hypercalcemia, which is less common in the critical care setting, is most often caused by malignancy. Treatment is supportive and involves administration of diuretics and IV fluids, sometimes simultaneously.

MAGNESIUM

About two thirds of the magnesium in the body is in the skeletal system, and the remaining one third is in the intracellular space. About 1% circulates in the extracellular space. Magnesium is a catalyst for hundreds of enzymatic reactions and plays a role in neurotransmission and cardiac contraction. Magnesium is primarily excreted by the kidneys.

Hypomagnesemia is caused by loss of magnesium through the gastrointestinal tract or (less commonly) the kidneys. Alcoholism is a significant cause. The etiological mechanism is not completely understood, but it is thought that decreased dietary intake due to malnutrition, decreased absorption, and increased gastrointestinal losses (due to periodic emesis) all play a role. Several drugs may also cause hypomagnesemia, including loop diuretics, aminoglycosides, amphotericin B, cis-platinum, cyclosporine, and citrate. For a review of the causes of hypomagnesemia, see Table 30-7.

Magnesium is available in a variety of preparations, including 50%, 20%, or 10% solutions. It is important to pay particular attention to how the replacement preparation is ordered; the replacement solution should be "dosed" in grams instead of milliliters. For a review of nursing considerations in magnesium replacement, see Box 30-13.

PHOSPHORUS

Phosphorus is the major intracellular anion. The source of adenosine triphosphate (ATP), phosphorus is implicated in many life-sustaining processes, such as muscle contraction, neuromuscular impulse conduction, and the regulation of several intracellular and extracellular electrolyte balances.

Hypophosphatemia may be caused by several metabolic disorders, including refeeding syndrome and alcoholism, intracellular shifting due to respiratory alkalosis, binding by medications, such as phosphate-binding magnesium-containing antacids, and excessive excretion of phosphate, such as in DKA (see Table 30-7). Refeeding syndrome occurs when the patient is fed, either enterally or parenterally, after some time of starvation. During starvation, protein catabolism occurs, depleting all of the intracellular phosphorus. When a large glucose load is administered, as occurs with refeeding, it is thought that the insulin response shifts the phosphorus intracellularly.

Management of hypophosphatemia may be problematic, particularly for patients on a mechanical ventilator. Contraction of all muscles, including the diaphragm, depends on ATP. Replacement of phosphorus is indicated in critically ill patients to achieve adequate pulmonary function. Once the critical illness abates, the hypophosphatemia typically resolves as well. However, replacement with either sodium or potassium phosphate is indicated in the meantime. For a review of nursing considerations in phosphorus replacement, see Box 30-13.

Hyperphosphatemia is commonly associated with renal failure due to reduced elimination of phosphorus. Because of the inverse relationship with calcium, the high phosphorus may also be associated with hypocalcemia. Administration of phosphate binders and calcium supplementation are indicated.

• Clinical Applicability Challenges

Case Study

Mr. D. is a 65-year-old man with a history of diabetes and hypertension. A year ago, he began experiencing some shortness of breath and was found to have heart failure. He has been treated with the following medications: furosemide, 20 mg orally (PO) once a day; KCl, 20 mEq PO once a day; metformin, 500 mg PO twice daily; enalapril, 10 mg PO once a day; and metoprolol, 25 mg PO twice daily. His shortness of breath has worsened over the past 2 days. He was seen in the clinic and was admitted for evaluation. Admission data are as follows: temperature, 97.3°F (36.3°C); pulse, 120 beats/minute; blood pressure, 87/50 mm Hg; respiratory rate, 18 breaths/minute; and oxygen saturation by pulse oximetry (SpO$_2$), 94% (on 50% fraction of inspired oxygen [FiO$_2$]). Laboratory test results are: Na$^+$, 130 mEq/L; K$^+$, 3.5 mEq/L; Cl$^-$, 100 mEq/L; CO$_2$, 18 mmol/L; blood urea nitrogen, 45 mg/dL; creatinine, 2.3 mg/dL; and glucose, 162 mg/dL. It is recommended that Mr. D. undergo a cardiac catheterization to rule out an ischemic component to his heart failure.

1. Explain the pathophysiological basis of Mr. D.'s symptoms.
2. What are Mr. D.'s risk factors for developing renal insufficiency?
3. What additional laboratory tests might you anticipate to be ordered to evaluate Mr. D.'s renal function?
4. What are some of the nursing care priorities for Mr. D.? What treatments could you anticipate for him?
5. Describe additional risk factors for a cardiac catheterization.
6. What are some interventions that may be initiated to reduce the risk factors?

Review Questions

1. The nurse is caring for a patient in the intensive care unit who is no longer tolerating traditional hemodialysis due to hypotension and has been ordered to receive continuous renal replacement therapy (CRRT). Which of the following statements best describes the difference between CRRT and hemodialysis?
   a. CRRT is a long-term therapy that can be continued as an outpatient, whereas hemodialysis is for inpatients only.
   b. Hemodialysis is reserved for hemodynamically stable patients, whereas CRRT is best for patients with potential hemodynamic instability.
   c. The patient's mean arterial pressure drives blood through the hemodialysis filter.
   d. CRRT requires placement of an arteriovenous fistula.

2. The nurse is caring for a patient who will be undergoing dialysis for the first time. The patient's family members are concerned and ask the nurse if this will "cure his kidney disease." As the nurse, you explain to the family in layman's terms that the major purpose of dialysis is to:
   a. remove proteins from the blood.
   b. correct imbalances of fluid and electrolytes.
   c. remove drugs from the blood.
   d. correct renal dysfunction.

3. A patient returns to the intensive care unit following the placement of a new peritoneal dialysis catheter. When performing peritoneal dialysis, the nurse understands that with this type of dialysis, the semipermeable membrane is the
   a. abdominal contents.
   b. filter in the tubing.
   c. peritoneal lining.
   d. renal lining.

4. The nurse is preparing to care for a patient receiving peritoneal dialysis. The nurse is aware that there is a risk for infection with this procedure. Which of the following signs and symptoms would cause the nurse to suspect peritonitis?
   a. Low-grade fever, abdominal pain, cloudy peritoneal drainage fluid
   b. Disequilibrium syndrome
   c. Urgency and frequency with voiding
   d. Confusion

5. During the peritoneal dialysis procedure, the nurse is aware that certain interventions may help facilitate drainage of peritoneal dialysis fluid. Which of the following actions by the nurse is most appropriate?
   a. Turning the patient from side to side, gently massaging the abdomen, elevating the head of bead
   b. Lying the patient flat in a prone position
   c. Increasing the flow of the dialysate
   d. Placing warm heating pads on the abdomen

6. The nurse is ordered to administer 40 mg IV furosemide, a loop diuretic, to the client at 9 a.m. Aware of the potential side effects of this medication, the nurse would want to assess for which of the following fluid and electrolyte imbalances that can occur as a result of loop diuretic therapy?
   a. Volume overload, hyperkalemia, hypomagnesemia, and metabolic alkalosis
   b. Volume depletion, hyperkalemia, hypercalcemia, and hypomagnesemia
   c. Volume overload, hypokalemia, hypocalcemia, and hypermagnesemia
   d. Volume depletion, hypokalemia, hypocalcemia, and hypomagnesemia

7. A man with end-stage renal failure arrives in the emergency department in acute respiratory distress, 3+ pitting edema in the lower extremities, and a potassium level of 5.5 mEq/L. He states that because of lack of transportation, he missed his last two appointments for dialysis this week. He is being admitted to the intensive care unit. As the nurse, you anticipate he will require dialysis soon. Which of the following types of dialysis is the preferred method when quick removal of water and toxins is needed?
   a. Continuous venovenous hemofiltration
   b. Hemodialysis
   c. Continuous venovenous hemofiltration with dialysis
   d. Peritoneal dialysis

8. A man with newly diagnosed renal failure is asking for salt with his meal. In addition to placing a consult with a dietitian, the nurse explains to the patient that a salt-restricted diet is necessary because increases in his sodium level may lead to
   a. hypotension.
   b. increases in fluid retention.
   c. alterations in acid-base balance.
   d. decreased circulating blood volume.

References

1. Brophy PD, Somers MJG, Baum MA, et al: Multi-centre evaluation of anticoagulation in patients receiving continuous renal replacement therapy (CRRT). Nephrol Dial Transplant 20:1416–1421, 2005

2. Cointault O, Kamar N, Bories P, et al: (2004). Regional citrate anticoagulation in continuous venovenous haemodiafiltration using commercial solutions. Nephrol Dial Transplant 19: 171–178, 2004

3. Kutsogiannis, Demetrios J, Gibney, R, et al: Regional citrate versus systemic heparin anticoagulation for continuous renal replacement in critically ill patients. Kidney Int 67(6): 2361–2367, 2005

4. Nissenson AR, Fine RN. Clinical Dialysis, 4th ed. New York: McGraw-Hill Medical, 2005

5. Friedrich JO, Adhikari N, Herridge MS, Beyenne J: Meta-analysis: Low-dose dopamine increases urine output but does not prevent renal dysfunction or death. Ann Intern Med 142(7):510–524, 2005

6. Debaveye YA, Van den Berghe GH: Is there still a place for dopamine in the modern intensive care unit? Anesth Analg 98(2):461–468, 2004

7. Cook D, Guyatt G: Colloid use for fluid resuscitation: Evidence and spin. Ann Intern Med 135:205–208, 2001

Other Selected Readings

Bellomo R, Baldwin I, Ronco C, et al (eds): Atlas of Hemofiltration. Philadelphia, WB Saunders, 2001

Daugirdis JT, Blake PG, Ing TS: Handbook of Dialysis, 4th ed. Philadelphia: Lippincott Williams & Wilkins, 2006

Denhaerynck K, Manhaeve D, Dobbels F, et al: Prevalence and consequences of nonadherence to hemodialysis regimens. Am J Crit Care 16(3):222–239, 2007

Dirkes S, Hodge K: Continuous renal replacement therapy in the adult intensive care unit: History and current trends. Crit Care Nurse 27(2):61–80, 2007

Gray RJ, Sands JJ (eds): Dialysis Access: A Multidisciplinary Approach. Philadelphia: Lippincott Williams & Wilkins, 2002

Pestans C: Fluids and Electrolytes in the Surgical Patient, 5th ed. Philadelphia: Lippincott Williams & Wilkins, 2000

Reilly L, Sullivan P, Ninni S, et al: Reducing Foley catheter device days in the intensive care unit: Using the evidence to change practice. AACN Clin Issues 17(3):272–283, 2006

Schrier RW: Manual of Nephrology: Diagnosis and Therapy, 6th ed. Philadelphia: Lippincott Williams & Wilkins, 2004

31

Renal Failure

Dorene Holcombe • Nancy Kern Feeley

Objectives

Based on the content in this chapter, the reader should be able to:

❶ Explain the causes of acute renal failure.

❷ Describe urine production during the nonoliguric, oliguric, and diuretic phases of acute tubular necrosis.

❸ Differentiate between the three types of acute renal failure based on history and physical examination, laboratory values, and diagnostic tests.

❹ Discuss the major causes and the clinical stages of chronic kidney disease.

❺ Explain factors that can contribute to the progression of chronic kidney disease.

❻ Discuss the clinical manifestations and management of renal failure.

• Acute Renal Failure

Acute renal failure occurs in 5% to 7% of hospitalized patients and in as many as 20% of the patients treated in intensive care units (ICUs).[1,2] In hospitalized patients with acute renal failure, the mortality rate exceeds 40% to 50%; in ICU patients who have multisystem organ failure and require dialysis, the mortality rate increases to 60% to 80%.[2–5] These discouraging mortality rates have not changed in the past three decades despite advances in technology and dialysis. However, the demographics of patients have changed, with patients in general being older and having an increased number of comorbid conditions.[2] On a more optimistic note, more than 70% of survivors of severe acute renal failure (those requiring renal replacement therapy) are independent of dialysis by discharge.[6–9]

Acute renal failure is a clinical syndrome in which there is a sudden loss of renal function (i.e., occur-

ring over hours to a few days) that results in derangements in fluid and electrolyte balance, acid–base homeostasis, calcium and phosphate metabolism, blood pressure regulation, and erythropoiesis. The hallmark of acute renal failure is a decreased glomerular filtration rate (GFR), reflected by an accumulation of blood urea nitrogen (BUN) and serum creatinine—a condition termed azotemia. Serum creatinine is the better marker because increases in serum creatinine are relatively unaffected by metabolic factors. Changes in serum creatinine levels that suggest acute renal failure include:

▶ An increase of 0.5 mg/dL or a doubling of creatinine from baseline in patients with a baseline creatinine level of less than 2.5 mg/dL

▶ An increase of more than 20% if the baseline serum creatinine is greater than 2.5 mg/dL[2]

▶ A 50% decrease in the measured creatinine clearance or calculated GFR[1]

Urine output patterns in acute renal failure can manifest as oliguria (<400 mL/day), nonoliguria (>400 mL/day), or anuria (<100 mL/day). Categorization of acute renal failure as oliguric or nonoliguric is diagnostically significant because the oliguric form is associated with higher morbidity and mortality rates. Anuria is rare and suggests obstructive uropathy, a vascular catastrophe resulting in a cessation of renal perfusion, severe acute tubular necrosis (ATN), or severe glomerulonephritis.[1] Any sudden and complete cessation of urinary flow in a patient with a Foley catheter should alert the nurse to inspect, flush, or change the urinary catheter.

CAUSES OF ACUTE RENAL FAILURE

Many pathophysiological pathways may lead to the syndrome of acute renal failure. To aid in the establishment of a diagnostic and management plan, acute renal failure is organized into three general categories according to precipitating factors and the symptoms manifested (Box 31-1).

Prerenal Acute Renal Failure

Prerenal acute renal failure accounts for 35% to 40% of inpatient cases and 70% of outpatient cases.[1] It is characterized by any physiological event that results in renal hypoperfusion. Most commonly, precipitating events include hypovolemia and cardiovascular failure; however, any other event that leads to an acute decrease in "effective renal perfusion" can fall into this category (see Box 31-1). For example, in sepsis, a systemic inflammatory response triggers a cascade of events that results in a vasodilated hypotensive state despite no net loss in body fluids.

Intrarenal Acute Renal Failure

The intrarenal category of acute renal failure is characterized by actual damage to the renal parenchyma and accounts for 55% to 60% of inpatient cases.[2] Intrarenal acute renal failure has many possible causes. One way to categorize these causes is by anatomical compartment: glomerular, vascular, interstitial, and tubular. The glomerular etiologies, which

---

Box 31-1 • Precipitating Causes of Acute Renal Failure

Prerenal
Decreased intravascular volume
  Dehydration
  Hemorrhage
  Hypovolemic shock
  Hypovolemia (gastrointestinal losses, diuretics, diabetes insipidus)
  Third-spacing (burns, peritonitis)
Cardiovascular failure
  Heart failure
  Myocardial infarction
  Cardiogenic shock
  Valvular heart disease
Renal artery stenosis or thrombosis
Drugs
  Angiotensin-converting enzyme (ACE) inhibitors
  Nonsteroidal anti-inflammatory drugs (NSAIDs)—inhibit prostaglandin-mediated afferent arteriolar vasodilation
  Calcineurin inhibitors (e.g., tacrolimus, cyclosporine)—cause preglomerular vasoconstriction
Decreased "effective renal perfusion"
  Sepsis
  Cirrhosis
  Neurogenic shock

Intrarenal
Acute glomerulonephritis
  Immune complex–mediated (postinfectious, lupus nephritis, cryoglobulinemia, immunoglobulin A [IgA] nephropathy)
  With vasculitis (Wegener's granulomatosis, antiglomerular basement membrane disease, polyarteritis nodosa)
Vascular disease
  Malignant hypertension
  Microangiopathic hemolytic–uremic syndrome (HUS)

Thrombotic thrombocytopenic purpura (TTP)
  Scleroderma
  Eclampsia
  Atheroembolic disease
  Acute cortical necrosis
Acute interstitial disease
  Allergic interstitial nephritis
  Acute pyelonephritis
Tubular obstruction
  Multiple myeloma
  Acute urate nephropathy
  Ethylene glycol or methanol toxicity
Acute tubular necrosis (ATN)
  Ischemia
  Nephrotoxins (contrast dye, drugs, heme pigments)
  Kidney transplant rejection

Postrenal
Ureteral obstruction
  Intrinsic (stones, transitional cell carcinoma of the ureter, blood clots, stricture)
  Extrinsic (ovarian cancer; lymphoma; metastatic cancer of the prostate, cervix, or colon; retroperitoneal fibrosis)
Bladder problems
  Tumors
  Blood clots
  Neurogenic bladder (spinal cord injury, diabetes mellitus, ischemia, drugs)
  Stones
Urethral obstruction
  Prostate cancer or benign prostatic hypertrophy
  Stones
  Stricture
  Blood clots
  Obstructed indwelling catheter

result in acute glomerulonephritis, include immune complex–mediated causes (e.g., as seen with post-streptococcal glomerulonephritis) and diseases that cause vasculitis, such as Wegener's granulomatosis and antiglomerular basement membrane disease. Interstitial causes include acute allergic interstitial nephritis, usually caused by pharmacological agents, and infectious causes such as pyelonephritis. Vascular etiologies include malignant hypertension as well as microangiopathic processes such as atheroembolic disease or hemolytic–uremic syndrome and thrombotic thrombocytopenic purpura. Finally, the tubules of the kidney can be primarily affected because of obstruction or ATN. Obstructive causes include multiple myeloma and acute urate nephropathy.

By far the most common cause of intrarenal hospital-acquired acute renal failure is ATN.[2] ATN results from either a prolonged prerenal condition (ischemic ATN) or the effects of toxins on the tubules (toxic ATN). Examples of potential toxins to the tubules include pharmacological agents, such as aminoglycosides, amphotericin B, and chemotherapeutic agents; heavy metals; organic solvents; heme pigments (e.g., myoglobin and hemoglobin); and radiocontrast dye (Box 31-2).

Postrenal Acute Renal Failure

Postrenal acute renal failure accounts for 5% of hospital cases.[2] Any obstruction in the flow of urine from the collecting ducts in the kidney to the external urethral orifice can result in postrenal acute renal failure. Postrenal obstruction can result from ureteral blockage (as with bilateral renal stones), urethral blockage (as from stricture and benign prostatic hypertrophy),

or an extrinsic source such as a retroperitoneal tumor or fibrosis. Another source of postrenal acute renal failure is a dysfunctional bladder (e.g., as might be caused by ganglionic blocking agents that interrupt autonomic supply to the urinary system). Elderly men and the young are populations particularly susceptible to postrenal acute renal failure. Children are at risk secondary to congenital anomalies and elderly men are at risk because of the high prevalence of benign or malignant prostatic hypertrophy.

PATHOPHYSIOLOGY OF ACUTE RENAL FAILURE

Prerenal Acute Renal Failure

The pathophysiology of prerenal acute renal failure is centered on the kidneys' response to inadequate perfusion. A decrease in renal perfusion results in the release of the enzyme renin from juxtaglomerular cells in the walls of the afferent arterioles. This activates the renin–angiotensin–aldosterone cascade, the end result being the production of angiotensin II and the release of aldosterone from the adrenal cortex. Angiotensin II causes profound systemic vasoconstriction, and aldosterone induces sodium and water retention. These effects help the body preserve circulatory volume so as to maintain adequate blood flow to essential organs such as the heart and brain. In the kidneys, angiotensin II also helps maintain the GFR by increasing efferent arteriolar resistance and by stimulating intrarenal vasodilator prostaglandins (which dilate the afferent arteriole), increasing hydrostatic pressure in the glomeruli.[10] In this way, the kidneys can preserve the GFR over a wide range of mean arterial pressures. However, when renal perfusion is severely compromised, the capacity for autoregulation is overwhelmed, and the GFR decreases.

It is of clinical importance that even with moderate hypovolemia or congestive heart failure, certain drugs, such as angiotensin-converting enzyme (ACE) inhibitors and nonsteroidal anti-inflammatory drugs (NSAIDs), can overwhelm the kidney's ability to autoregulate. These drugs disrupt some of the autoregulatory mechanisms such as prostaglandin-mediated afferent arterial vasodilation, in the case of NSAIDs, and increased efferent arteriolar resistance, in the case of ACE inhibitors. Predisposing factors for NSAID- and ACE inhibitor–induced prerenal failure are hypovolemia, baseline renal insufficiency, liver disease, heart failure, and diseases of the renal arteries.[1,10]

In prerenal acute renal failure, once autoregulatory capacity is overwhelmed and the GFR decreases, changes in urinary composition and volume occur in a predictable pattern. When the GFR decreases, the amount of tubular fluid is reduced, and the fluid travels through the tubule more slowly. This results in increased sodium and water reabsorption. Because of the reduced renal circulation, the solutes reabsorbed from the tubular fluid are removed more slowly than normal from the interstitium of the renal medulla. This results in increased medullary tonicity, further augmenting water reabsorption from the distal tubu-

---

Box 31-2 • Common Causes of Acute Tubular Necrosis

Ischemic
Hemorrhagic hypotension
Severe volume depletion
Surgical aortic cross-clamping
Cardiac surgery
Defective cardiac output
Septic shock
Pancreatitis
Immunosuppression (cyclosporine, tacrolimus)
Nonsteroidal anti-inflammatory drugs (NSAIDs)

Nephrotoxic
Drugs, including antimicrobials (aminoglycosides, amphotericin), cyclosporine, anesthetics, chemotherapeutic agents
Heavy metals (mercury, lead, cis-platinum, uranium, cadmium, bismuth, arsenic)
Radiological contrast agents
Heme/pigments (myoglobin, hemoglobin)
Organic solvents (carbon tetrachloride)
Fungicides and pesticides
Plant and animal substances (mushrooms, snake venom)

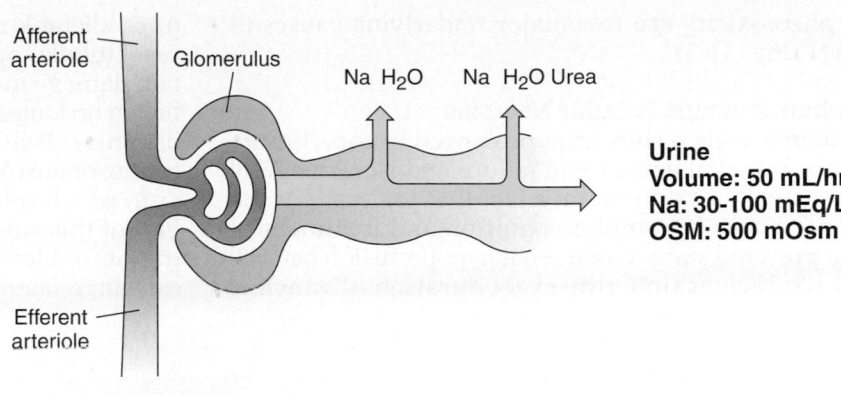

Afferent arteriole   Glomerulus

Na H₂O   Na H₂O Urea

**Urine
Volume: 50 mL/hr
Na: 30-100 mEq/L
OSM: 500 mOsm**

Efferent arteriole

A. Normal perfusion

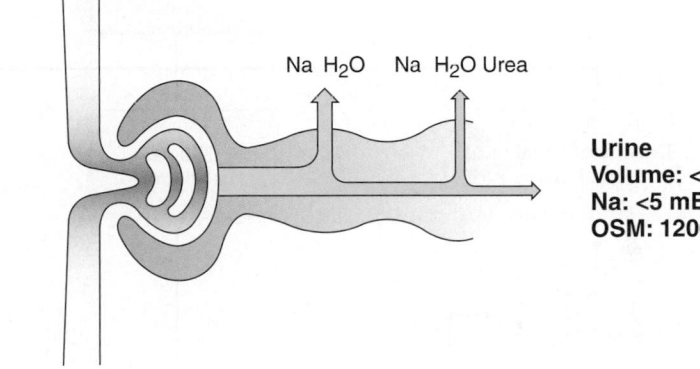

Na H₂O   Na H₂O Urea

**Urine
Volume: <17 mL/hr
Na: <5 mEq/L
OSM: 1200 mOsm**

Figure 31-1 • Normal perfusion (**A**) of the kidney compared with underperfusion (**B**), as seen in prerenal acute renal failure. Underperfusion of the kidney results in decreased renal blood flow and glomerular filtration, an increase in the fraction of filtrate reabsorbed in the proximal tubule, and low urine flow with low sodium (Na) content and increased concentration. H₂O, water; OSM, osmolarity.

B. Underperfusion

lar fluid. As a result of these events, the urinary volume is reduced to less than 400 mL/day (<17 mL/hour), the urine specific gravity is increased, and the urine sodium concentration is low (usually <5 mEq/L; Fig. 31-1). Because of these characteristic changes associated with renal underperfusion, measurement of urinary volume, urinary sodium, and specific gravity is a simple method of determining the effect of management on renal perfusion.

An increase in systemic blood pressure does not necessarily imply improvement in renal perfusion. This may be especially evident when drugs such as norepinephrine are used to correct the hypotension associated with states of volume depletion. These drugs may be associated with further reduction in renal blood flow as a consequence of constriction of the renal arteries. This is manifested by a further fall in urinary volume and rise in specific gravity.

In turn, if the hypoperfusion state is more appropriately and specifically treated by replacement of volume, improvement of cardiac output, correction of dysrhythmias, or a combination of these approaches, the improved renal perfusion is manifested as an increased urinary volume and urine sodium concentration and as a decreased specific gravity of the urine. This ability to reverse prerenal acute renal failure is the key to its diagnosis.

Intrarenal Acute Renal Failure

Just as there are many causes of intrarenal acute renal failure, there are also many pathophysiological

pathways that lead to it (Fig. 31-2). Because ATN is the most common hospital-acquired form of intrarenal acute renal failure, this discussion focuses on the pathophysiology of ATN. The pathophysiology of ATN is complex, but because of intense and ongoing research, there is an increased understanding of the factors contributing to this condition. Ischemia and

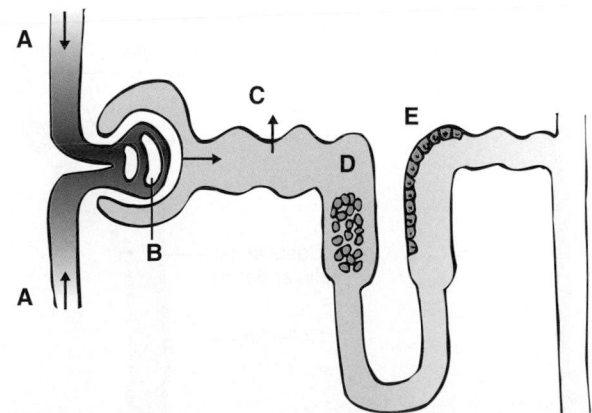

Figure 31-2 • Potential mechanisms of intrarenal acute renal failure include decreased filtration pressure because of constriction in the renal arterioles (**A**), decreased glomerular capillary permeability (**B**), increased permeability of the proximal tubules with back leak of filtrate (**C**), obstruction of urine flow by necrotic tubular cells (**D**), and increased sodium delivery to the macula densa (**E**), which causes an increase in renin–angiotensin production and vasoconstriction at the glomerular level.

nephrotoxicity are two major underlying causes of ATN (Fig. 31-3).

Ischemic Acute Tubular Necrosis

Ischemic ATN results from prolonged hypoperfusion. Thus, prerenal acute renal failure and ischemic ATN are actually a continuum, a fact that underscores the importance of prompt recognition and treatment of the prerenal state. When renal hypoperfusion persists for a sufficient time (the exact duration of which is unpredictable and varies with clinical circumstances), renal tubular epithelial cells become hypoxic and sustain damage to the point that restoration of renal perfusion no longer effects an improvement in glomerular filtration. Ischemia results in decreased adenosine triphosphate (ATP) production in renal cell mitochondria, which robs the cells of a needed energy supply. Part of this energy is used to keep the proper concentration of electrolytes in the cell through electrolyte exchange channels. Some of the cellular electrolyte

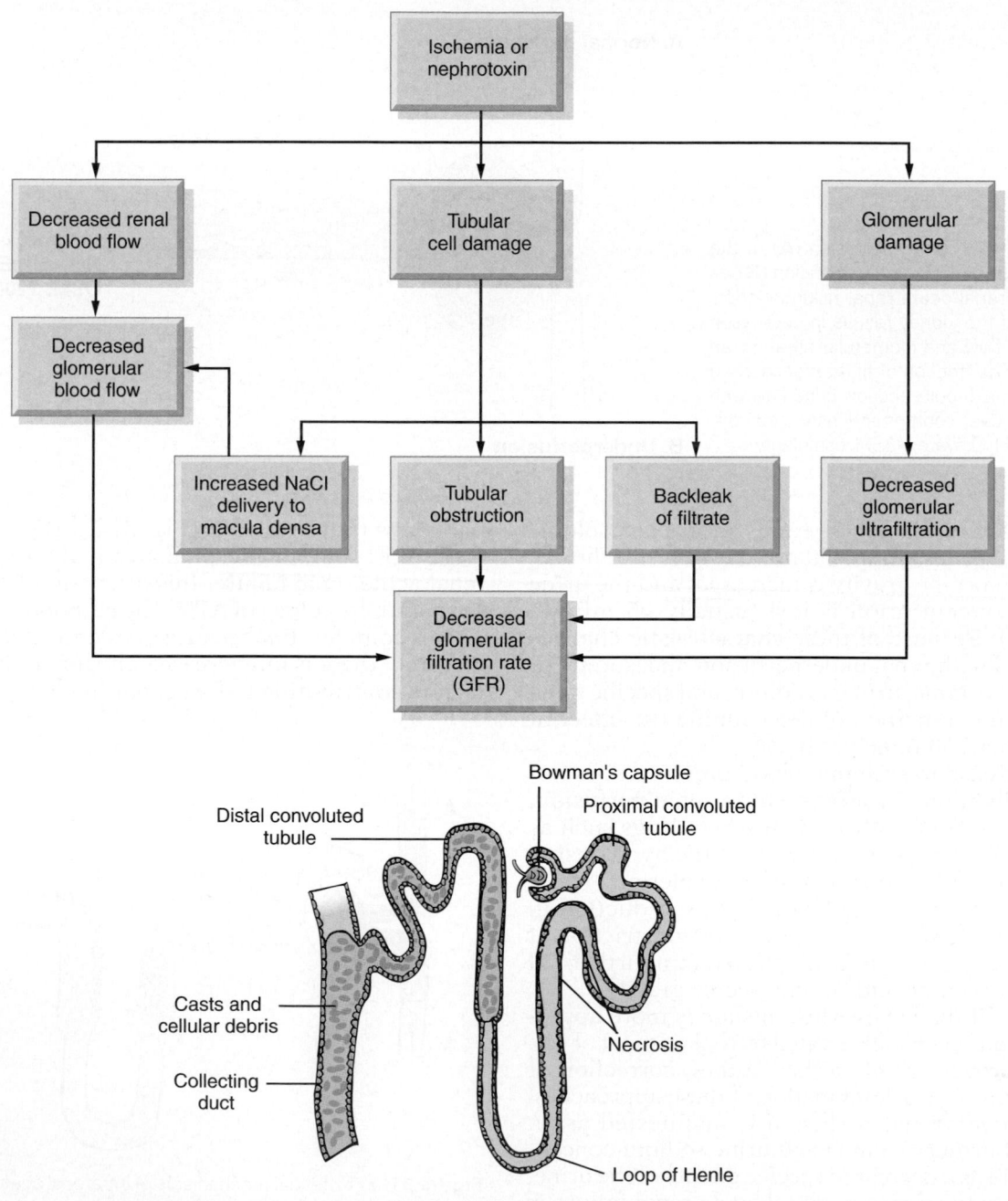

Figure 31-3 • Ischemic acute tubular necrosis (ATN) results from prolonged hypoperfusion. A sequence of pathophysiological processes results in the sloughing off of necrotic cells that block the tubular lumen. Toxic ATN occurs when a nephrotoxin becomes concentrated in the renal tubular cells and causes necrosis. The necrotic cells slough off and obstruct the tubular lumen, similar to ischemic ATN. In toxic ATN, the basement membrane of the renal cells usually remains intact, and the necrotic areas are more localized.

disturbances from ischemia are decreased intracellular potassium, magnesium, and phosphate, and increased intracellular sodium, chloride, and calcium. Increased intracellular calcium specifically has been shown to predispose the cells to injury and dysfunction.[10,11]

Cellular insults also occur during reperfusion from the formation of oxygen free radicals. Eventually, these cellular insults cause the tubular cells to swell and become necrotic. The necrotic cells then slough off and may obstruct the tubular lumen. These sloughed cells also allow back leak of tubular fluid because of altered function of their basement membrane, contributing to the decreased GFR seen in this disorder.

A final contributor to the pathophysiology of ischemic ATN is profound renal vasoconstriction, which reduces renal blood flow by as much as 50%.[10] These hemodynamic disturbances further compromise renal oxygen delivery and add to the ischemic damage. Vasoconstrictors involved include norepinephrine from sympathetic nervous system activation, angiotensin II, thromboxane A_2, adenosine, leukotrienes C4 and D4, prostaglandin H_2, and endothelin, a powerful vasoconstrictor released by damaged vascular endothelial cells of the kidney.[10]

Toxic Acute Tubular Necrosis

The pathophysiology of toxic ATN begins with a concentration of a nephrotoxin in the renal tubular cells, which causes necrosis. These necrotic cells then slough off into the tubular lumen, possibly causing obstruction and impairing glomerular filtration in a manner similar to that of ischemic ATN. However, significant differences between toxic ATN and ischemic ATN include the fact that in toxic ATN, the basement membrane of the renal cells usually remains intact, and the injured necrotic areas are more localized. In addition, nonoliguria occurs more often with toxic ATN, and the healing process is often more rapid.

Although the potential nephrotoxins in toxic ATN are many (see Box 31-2), aminoglycoside antibiotics and radiocontrast dye deserve special mention because of the frequency with which they are seen as causes in hospitalized patients. Nephrotoxicity occurs in 10% to 20% of patients treated with aminoglycosides for 10 days or more.[11] The onset of acute renal failure secondary to aminoglycosides is usually delayed, often beginning 7 to 10 days after the onset of therapy. The toxicity of these agents is dose dependent, and because these agents are primarily eliminated by the kidneys, dosage must be adjusted in patients with preexisting renal impairment. To ensure that the correct therapeutic range is being achieved, peak and trough blood levels are drawn frequently. Offending agents (listed in decreasing order of the severity with which they produce dose-dependent proximal tubule damage) are neomycin, gentamicin, amikacin, tobramycin, and streptomycin. Several studies have suggested that a single daily dose of an aminoglycoside may result in less nephrotoxicity than giving the same total amount of medication in three daily doses.[12,13] Besides dosage, increased risk

factors for aminoglycoside toxicity are volume depletion, advanced age, concurrent use of other nephrotoxic agents, and hepatic dysfunction.[11,13]

Contrast-induced nephropathy (CIN), the sudden decline of renal function following intravascular injection of contrast media, is the third leading cause of hospital-acquired acute renal failure.[14,15] It usually begins within 48 hours of intravenous (IV) radiocontrast administration, peaks in 3 to 5 days, and returns to baseline in another 3 to 5 days. Typically, CIN is nonoliguric, transient, and reversible; however, in high-risk patients, it can cause severe renal failure that necessitates permanent dialysis or kidney transplantation.[14] Patients at greatest risk for CIN are those with diabetes, especially those with diabetes and underlying renal impairment. In these patients, the incidence of CIN may be as high as 50%.[14] Other patients at risk are elderly patients; those with intravascular volume depletion, congestive heart failure, or multiple myeloma; and those who receive a large contrast load.[15,16]

An important way to reduce the risk for CIN is by aggressive hydration with IV saline or sodium bicarbonate before and after contrast dye administration. Because CIN is believed to involve the production of oxygen free radicals, it is postulated that alkalinization of the urine with sodium bicarbonate may confer greater protection than IV saline alone. This is supported in one prospective, randomized, non-blinded study of 119 patients by Merten and colleagues in which CIN occurred in 1.7% in the patients hydrated with bicarbonate compared with 13.6% of the patients hydrated with isotonic saline.[17] Although promising, further more rigorous studies need to be conducted.

Other interventions to reduce the incidence of CIN include using the minimal necessary dose of contrast media, using low or iso-osmolar nonionic contrast media instead of ionic hyperosmolar agents, stopping the intake of nephrotoxic drugs 24 hours before contrast media injection, and avoiding short intervals between contrast procedures.[15,16] N-Acetylcysteine (NAC), an antioxidant and a potent vasodilator, is part of the protocol in many hospitals to prevent CIN based on clinical trials demonstrating its renoprotective effects in patients receiving IV contrast. However, NAC has been the subject of many recent meta-analyses, and, overall, there has been insufficient evidence to support the universal use of NAC to prevent CIN.[16,18–20] Studies have shown that other pharmacological interventions such as calcium channel blockers, dopamine, mannitol, and atrial natriuretic peptide do not consistently reduce the incidence of CIN and may even be harmful.

Of course, avoiding any use of iodinated contrast media in high-risk patients is the best prevention, and alternative studies such as ultrasonography, computerized tomography (CT) scanning without contrast, and contrast-enhanced magnetic resonance imaging (MRI) should be considered. The MRI contrast agents in use are mostly chelates of gadolinium and have been found to have little or no nephrotoxicity. Because of this, gadolinium-based chelates are also being used for digital subtraction angiography or other interventions, particularly in high-risk patients or in those with an iodinated contrast allergy.[21,22] One important caveat regarding the use of gadolinium in patients with advanced kidney disease (GFR < 30 mL/min) is the rare but serious risk for developing nephrogenic systemic fibrosis (NSF). NSF, a fibrosing disorder seen only in patients with kidney disease, is characterized by thickening and hardening of the skin overlying the extremities and trunk. Occasionally fibrosis of deeper structures (such as muscles, the lungs, and the heart) occurs as well. Because the condition can be devastating to a patient (resulting in significant loss of mobility and even death), gadolinium agents should be avoided in patients with a GFR less than 30 mL/min.[23]

Postrenal Acute Renal Failure

Obstruction can occur at any point in the urinary tract. When urine cannot get around the obstruction, resulting congestion causes retrograde pressure through the collecting system and nephrons. This slows the rate of tubular fluid flow and lowers the GFR. As a result, the reabsorption of sodium, water, and urea is increased, leading to a lowered urine sodium concentration and increased urine osmolality and BUN. Serum creatinine levels also increase. With prolonged pressure from urinary obstruction, the entire collecting system dilates, compressing and damaging nephrons. This results in dysfunction of the concentrating and diluting mechanism, and the urine osmolality and urine sodium concentration become similar to that of plasma. This circumstance can be avoided by prompt removal of the obstruction.

Because a single well-functioning kidney is adequate to maintain homeostasis, the development of acute renal failure from obstruction requires blockage of both kidneys (i.e., urethral or bladder neck obstruction or bilateral ureteral obstruction) or unilateral ureteral obstruction in patients with a single kidney. After relief of the obstruction, there is often a profound diuresis that may be as great as 5 to 8 L/day.[11] If electrolytes and water are not replenished as needed, this diuresis can lead to hemodynamic compromise, dysrhythmias, and ATN.

CLINICAL COURSE OF ACUTE TUBULAR NECROSIS

The course of ATN can be divided into four clinical phases: onset phase, oliguric or nonoliguric phase, diuretic phase, and recovery phase.

Onset Phase

The onset (initiating) phase begins with an initial insult and lasts until cell injury occurs. During this phase, injury is evolving, and the health care team members need to attempt to prevent disease progression. The onset phase lasts from hours to days, depending on the cause, and is heralded by an increase in serum creatinine. The major goal during this phase is to determine the cause of the ATN and initiate treatment to prevent irreversible tubular damage.

Oliguric or Nonoliguric Phase

The second phase of ATN is characterized as either oliguric or nonoliguric. Patients who present with oliguric ATN are less likely to recover renal function and have a higher associated mortality rate.[11] This presentation of ATN is most commonly the result of ischemic insult. Oliguric ATN is marked by fluid overload, azotemia, electrolyte abnormalities (i.e., hyperkalemia, hyperphosphatemia, and hypocalcemia), metabolic acidosis, and symptoms of uremia. The main goal during this period is to support renal function and keep the patient alive until renal injury heals. Complications during this period are from hyperkalemia, hypoxemia, gastrointestinal bleeding, and infection. Oliguric ATN lasts approximately 7 to 14 days, although it may persist for weeks depending on the extent of renal injury.[11]

The nonoliguric presentation of ATN is most commonly associated with toxic injury (e.g., from aminoglycoside antibiotics). It is characterized by a renal concentrating defect rather than the impaired urinary flow seen in oliguric ATN. Urine volume in nonoliguric ATN ranges from normal to as much as 2 liters/hour.[11] Because of the higher volume of urine output, fluid complications are minimized. However, because potassium excretion parallels that seen in oliguria, hyperkalemia remains a major risk. The duration of nonoliguric ATN is typically short, lasting an average of 5 to 8 days.

Diuretic Phase

The diuretic phase lasts 1 to 2 weeks and is characterized by a gradual increase in urine output as renal function starts to return. The degree of diuresis, which can exceed 10 L/day, is primarily determined by the state of hydration at the time the patient enters this stage. Thus, patients who are receiving hemodialysis or who are nonoliguric tend to diurese less. The diuresis is thought to result from the osmotic pull of retained substances (i.e., urea and sodium), which act as osmotic agents. Although the urine output may be normal or elevated, renal concentrating ability is still impaired. This puts patients at risk for fluid volume deficits and electrolyte abnormalities such as hyponatremia and hypokalemia. Primary goals during this stage are maintenance of hydration, prevention of electrolyte depletion, and continued support of renal function.

Recovery Phase

The recovery phase of ATN lasts from several months to a year. It is the time it takes for renal function to return to normal or near-normal levels. If significant renal cell damage has occurred, especially to the basement membrane (which cannot regenerate), residual renal impairment may result. Major goals of the health care team in this phase revolve around patient education. To foster and maintain the return of renal function, it is critical that patients and family members understand what precipitated the acute renal failure episode as well as what follow-up care and preventive measures are necessary to prevent a recurrence.

DIAGNOSIS OF ACUTE RENAL FAILURE

Diagnosis of acute renal failure begins with a determination of whether the acute renal failure is prerenal, intrarenal, or postrenal. The assessment tools used to make this determination include the history and physical examination, laboratory tests, and diagnostic studies. Special considerations for assessing renal function in older patients are given in Box 31-3.[24]

Box 31-3 • CONSIDERATIONS FOR THE OLDER PATIENT: Physiological Changes Affecting the Renal System

As the body ages, physiological systemic and kidney-specific changes occur that are important to take into consideration when addressing the kidney.

- Vascular changes: At 30 years of age, arteriosclerosis starts to develop, including in the renal arteries; this can result in significant damage.
- Musculoskeletal changes: In elderly people, there is a decreased muscle mass and body weight. These changes must be kept in mind when assessing renal function because of the possibility of a consequent decreased baseline serum creatinine value. A minimum rise in serum creatinine in elderly patients, which may be within normal limits for a young adult, may actually signify major renal impairment.
- Kidney-specific changes: With aging, there is a decrease in the total number of functioning glomeruli, a decrease in renal blood flow, and a decrease in glomerular filtration rate (GFR) of about 7 to 10 mL/min per decade after 40 years of age.[24]

In view of these systemic and kidney-specific changes, an accurate assessment of GFR using a 24-hour urine study or an isotopic study is essential. The Cockroft-Gault formula or the Modification of Diet in Renal Disease (MDRD) formulas below, which take into account gender and age, can also be used. It is important to realize that these formulas are not extensively validated in patients older than 70 years. After true GFR is realized, therapy (e.g., drug dosages) can be guided more safely.

Cockcroft-Gault Formula for Creatinine Clearance (mL/min)

Men = (140 − age) × weight in kg/72 × serum creatinine
Women = 0.85 × creatinine clearance for men

MDRD Formula for GFR (adults; mL/min)

$175 \times$ Serum creatinine concentration$^{-1.154}$
$\times$ Age$^{-0.203}$
$\times 0.742$ (if female)
$\times 1.210$ (if black)

Websites are available to aid in the calculation of the GFR through these formulas. These include http://www.kidney.org and http://www.nephron.com.

History and Physical Examination

Essential to any assessment is the history and physical examination. By taking a detailed history, clues to the categorization and exact cause of the acute renal failure can be obtained. Important indications in the history that suggest prerenal acute renal failure include any event or condition that may have contributed to decreased renal perfusion (e.g., acute myocardial infarction, cardiovascular surgery, cardiac arrest, high fever, any shock state, and the use of certain drugs, such as NSAIDs). Also, a history of atherosclerotic disease may be a clue to renal artery stenosis, another precipitant of prerenal acute renal failure. Clues to an intrarenal cause provided by the history include any prolonged prerenal event or condition as well as exposure to nephrotoxins, especially aminoglycoside antibiotics and radiocontrast dye. It is also important to collect information regarding systemic diseases such as lupus or vasculitis, recent streptococcal infections, and causes for heme pigment toxicity such as rhabdomyolysis (i.e., a history of trauma or a patient found unconscious for an unknown amount of time). In addition, a history of cardiac catheterization, anticoagulation, and thrombolytic therapy increases the possibility of atheroembolic intrarenal diseases. Findings that may point to postrenal acute renal failure include any history of abdominal tumors or calculi, and especially a history of benign prostatic hypertrophy in elderly men. A family history of urolithiasis or benign prostatic hypertrophy may be contributory.

The physical examination, particularly fluid status, is critical to the diagnosis of acute renal failure. In prerenal acute renal failure, a state of decreased renal perfusion related to dehydration or hypovolemia is heralded by poor skin turgor, dry mucous membranes, weight loss, and reduced jugular venous distention. In contrast, when decreased perfusion is related to vasodilation, third-spacing, cardiovascular disease (e.g., heart failure), liver disease, or a combination of these factors, findings of increased extracellular fluid may be manifested. These findings include edema, ascites, and weight gain. For critical care patients, hemodynamic monitoring values help determine intravascular fluid status as well as cardiac functioning. Surveillance values include central venous pressure, pulmonary artery wedge pressure (PAWP), and cardiac output (or cardiac index). By correlating physical examination findings with the history, hemodynamic values, and laboratory tests, potential prerenal etiologies can be narrowed down further.

Although no specific physical examination finding prompts consideration of intrarenal acute renal failure, many examination findings are helpful clues to potential causes of intrarenal acute renal failure. For example, signs of a streptococcal throat infection, lupus (e.g., a butterfly mask rash), or embolic phenomena (e.g., discolored toes and livido reticularis, a semipermanent bluish mottling of the skin in the extremities) may all suggest an intrarenal cause. Again, correlation with the history and laboratory studies helps narrow the list of potential causes.

Table 31-1 • Acute Renal Failure: Comparison of Laboratory Findings in Prerenal Failure, Postrenal Failure, and Acute Tubular Necrosis

Value	Prerenal	Postrenal	Acute Tubular Necrosis
Urine volume	Oliguria	May alternate between anuria and polyuria	Anuria, oliguria, or nonoliguria
Urine osmolality	Increased (>500 mOsm/kg H_2O)	Varies, increased or equal to serum	250–300 mOsm/kg H_2O
Urine specific gravity	Increased (>1.020)	Varies	Approximately 1.010
Urine sodium	<20 mEq/L	Varies	>40 mEq/L
Urine sediment	Normal, few casts	Normal, may be crystals	Granular casts, tubular epithelial cells
FE_{Na}	<1%	>1%	>1% (often >3%)
BUN:Cr	>20:1	10:1 to 15:1	10:1 to 15:1

FE_{Na}, fractional excretion of sodium; BUN:Cr, blood urea nitrogen/creatinine ratio.

Findings on physical examination that may suggest a postrenal cause include a distended bladder, an abdominal mass, an enlarged or nodular prostate gland, and, most obviously, a kinked or obstructed Foley catheter.

Laboratory Studies

Laboratory assessment, critical to the diagnosis and categorization of acute renal failure, includes both serum and urinary values. For a basic comparison of laboratory values in prerenal acute renal failure, postrenal acute renal failure, and ATN, see Table 31-1. In addition to helping differentiate between prerenal, intrarenal, and postrenal acute renal failure, blood and urine tests are also helpful for diagnosing the underlying etiology of the acute renal failure (Box 31-4).

Urinary Values

Obtaining a urine specimen for diagnostic chemistries and indices is invaluable in establishing the diagnosis and determining the type of acute renal failure. The urine specimen should be obtained before a diagnostic challenge of diuretics is administered because these agents may alter the urine's chemical composition. The urine sodium concentration, osmolality, and specific gravity are especially helpful in distinguishing between prerenal acute renal failure and ATN because these values reflect the concentrating ability of the kidney. In prerenal failure, the hypoperfused kidney actively reabsorbs sodium and water in an attempt to increase circulatory volume. Consequently, the urine sodium level and the fractional excretion of sodium (FE_{Na}) are low (<20 mEq/L and <1%, respectively), whereas the urine osmolality and concentration of nonreabsorbable solutes are high. In contrast, in ATN where there is parenchymal damage to the kidney, the tubular cells can no longer effectively reabsorb sodium or concentrate the urine. As a result, the urine sodium concentration is often greater than 40 mEq/L, the FE_{Na} is greater than 1%, and the urine osmolality is close to that of plasma (isosthenuria). Unfortunately, there is a limit to the usefulness of these indices because of overlap in these values for prerenal acute renal failure and

Box 31-4 • Diagnostic Clues in Acute Renal Failure

Urine
- Urate crystals: tumor lysis, especially lymphoma (urate nephropathy)
- Oxalate crystals: ethylene glycol nephrotoxicity, methoxyflurane nephrotoxicity
- Eosinophils: allergic interstitial nephritis, especially methicillin
- Positive benzidine without red blood cells: hemoglobinuria or myoglobinuria
- Pigmented casts: hemoglobinuria or myoglobinuria
- Massive proteinuria: acute interstitial nephritis, thiazide diuretics, hemorrhagic fevers (i.e., Korean, Scandinavian)
- Abnormal urine protein electrophoresis: multiple myeloma
- Anuria: renal cortical necrosis, bilateral obstruction, renal vascular catastrophe

Plasma
- Marked hyperkalemia: rhabdomyolysis, tissue necrosis, hemolysis
- Marked hypocalcemia: rhabdomyolysis
- Hypercalcemia: hypercalcemic nephropathy
- Hyperuricemia: tumor lysis, rhabdomyolysis, toxin ingestion
- Marked acidosis: ethylene glycol, methyl alcohol
- Elevated creatine kinase or myoglobin levels: rhabdomyolysis
- Low complement levels: systemic lupus erythematosus (SLE), postinfectious glomerulonephritis, subacute bacterial endocarditis
- Abnormal serum protein electrophoresis: multiple myeloma
- Positive antibody/glomerular basement membrane ratio: Goodpasture's syndrome
- Positive antineutrophilic cytoplasmic antibody: small vessel vasculitis (Wegener's granulomatosis or polyarteritis nodosa)
- Positive antinuclear antibody (ANA) or antibody to double-stranded DNA: SLE
- Positive antibodies to streptolysin O: poststreptococcal glomerulonephritis
- Elevated lactate dehydrogenase (LDH) level, elevated serum bilirubin level, or decreased haptoglobin level: hemolytic–uremic syndrome (HUS) or thrombotic thrombocytopenic purpura (TTP)

ATN (i.e., urine sodium concentration values in the 20- to 40-mEq/L range). Values at the extremes thus are most useful.

One test that may be helpful in distinguishing prerenal acute renal failure from ATN in patients who have already been given diuretics is the fractional excretion of urea nitrogen (FE_{UN}). Urea, like sodium, is reabsorbed in a prerenal hypoperfused kidney, but unlike sodium, its reabsorption is primarily dependent on passive forces and is not inhibited by loop and thiazide diuretic administration.[25] In prerenal acute renal failure, the FE_{UN} is less than 35%, whereas in ATN and normally, it is greater than 50%.

The sediment in a urinalysis is also very helpful in diagnosing and distinguishing the types of acute renal failure. In prerenal acute renal failure, the urinary sediment is normal with only a few hyaline casts, whereas in ATN, coarse, muddy-brown granular casts and tubular epithelial cells are typically found. In postrenal acute renal failure, the sediment is often normal but can be helpful in diagnosing stones.

Blood Urea Nitrogen and Creatinine Levels

Serum tests for BUN and creatinine are essential not only for diagnosing acute renal failure but also for helping to distinguish between prerenal acute renal failure and ATN or postrenal acute renal failure. In prerenal acute renal failure, the BUN-to-creatinine ratio is increased from the normal ratio of 10:1 to more than 20:1. This finding is caused by a state of dehydration and by the fact that as the tubules become more permeable to sodium and water in prerenal acute renal failure, urea is also passively reabsorbed. In ATN and postrenal acute renal failure, when the concentrating ability of the kidneys is impaired, both the BUN and creatinine increase proportionally, maintaining the normal 10:1 ratio.

Diagnostic Studies

One important diagnostic test in the evaluation of acute renal failure is renal ultrasonography. This test is especially useful in ruling out an obstruction and has the advantage of being noninvasive. With a high-grade obstruction, dilation of the urinary collecting system is detectable on ultrasonography within 1 to 2 days of the onset of the obstruction. Ultrasonography may also reveal proximal renal calculi as a cause of postrenal obstruction. In addition, it can be used to estimate renal size, which is helpful in distinguishing between acute renal failure and advanced chronic kidney disease. In advanced chronic kidney disease, the kidneys are often small (<9 cm) and echogenic.

Other studies may be useful in diagnosing acute renal failure. These include CT and MRI to evaluate for masses, vascular disorders, and filling defects in the collecting system, as well as renal angiography to evaluate for renal artery stenosis. It is important to keep in mind that the iodinated contrast dyes used in some studies are allergenic and nephrotoxic, and thus benefits of the study must be weighed against potential risks. Fortunately, new technology and the use of carbon dioxide and gadolinium as contrast agents now allow most studies to be performed with little risk of nephrotoxicity.[21,22,26] Finally, renal biopsy may be helpful in patients thought to have intrarenal acute renal failure that is not ATN, especially if significant proteinuria or unexplained hematuria is revealed on urinalysis. In addition to having diagnostic value, the results of a biopsy may help determine prognosis and therapy.

• Chronic Kidney Disease

Chronic kidney disease is a slow, progressive, irreversible deterioration in renal function that results in the kidney's inability to eliminate waste products and maintain fluid and electrolyte balance. Ultimately, it leads to end-stage renal disease (ESRD) and the need for renal replacement therapy or renal transplantation to sustain life.

Currently there are more than 450,000 dialysis and renal transplant recipients in the United States, and in 2004 alone, more than 100,000 patients were newly diagnosed with ESRD. The prevalence rate of ESRD per million population in 2004 was more than 5 times higher than in 1980. Among patients receiving dialysis, incidence rates are 52% higher in men than in women and are higher with increasing age. The incidence rates in patients on dialysis are 268% higher in the African American population than in the white population. Hispanics and Native Americans also have higher incidence rates than whites, but the difference in rates is not as dramatic.[27] These differences in incidence rates are important to remember when considering patient risk factors and populations to which increased health education regarding prevention should be targeted.

Although the exact reason for the growth in ESRD is unclear, it is postulated that changes in the demographics of the population, differences in disease burden among racial groups, underrecognition and undertreatment of earlier stages of chronic kidney disease, and underrecognition of the risk factors for chronic kidney disease may partially explain this growth.[28] Increasing evidence shows that early detection and treatment of chronic kidney disease may prevent or at least delay progression to ESRD.[29] Consequently, it is important that opportunities to prevent and treat chronic kidney disease are not lost secondary to underdiagnosis, undertreatment, or both.

DEFINITION AND CLASSIFICATION OF CHRONIC KIDNEY DISEASE

In an effort to address the growing public health problem of chronic kidney disease, the Kidney Disease Outcome Quality Initiative (K/DOQI) of the National Kidney Foundation published clinical practice guidelines for chronic kidney disease in 2002. The goals of the working group that developed these guidelines were as follows: to define chronic kidney disease and classify its stages, to evaluate laboratory measurements for clinical assessment of kidney disease, to associate the level of kidney function with the com-

Box 31-5 • Definition of Chronic Kidney Disease

1. Kidney damage for ≥3 months as defined by structural or functional abnormalities of the kidney, with or without decreased glomerular filtration rate (GFR), manifested by *either:*
   a. Pathological abnormalities; *or*
   b. Markers of kidney damage, including abnormalities in the composition of the blood and urine, or abnormalities in imaging tests.
2. GFR < 60 mL/min/1.73 m^2, with or without kidney damage

From National Kidney Foundation: K/DOQI clinical practice guidelines for chronic kidney disease: Evaluation, classification, and stratification. Am J Kidney Dis 39(2 Suppl 1): S1–S266, 2002.

plications of chronic kidney disease, and to stratify risk for the loss of kidney function and the development of cardiovascular disease.[28]

The K/DOQI defines chronic kidney disease as either kidney damage with or without decreased GFR for 3 or more months *or* a GFR of less than 60 mL/min/1.73 m^2 for greater than 3 months (Box 31-5). Markers of damage include abnormalities in the blood or urine tests or imaging studies. Examples are proteinuria, abnormalities in the urine sediment, increased serum creatinine, and multiple renal cysts detected on ultrasound in a patient with a family history of polycystic kidney disease. A GFR (considered to be the best overall measure of kidney function) of less than 60 mL/min/1.73 m^2 was chosen for two reasons: (1) it represents a loss of half or more of the adult level of normal kidney function; and (2) below this level, the prevalence of complications due to chronic kidney disease increases.

Because predictable complications and management issues are based on the level of kidney dysfunction, regardless of the specific underlying etiology of

chronic kidney disease, the K/DOQI working group also developed a classification system for chronic kidney disease based on the measured GFR (Table 31-2). This classification system provides a common language for practitioners and patients to improve communication, enhance education, and promote research. Most importantly, it also provides a framework for evaluation and development of a treatment plan for patients with various stages of chronic kidney disease, as outlined below.[11]

▶ Stage 1 is characterized by the lack of a clear filtration deficit and is defined as normal or increased kidney function (GFR greater than or equal to 90 mL/min/1.73 m^2) in association with evidence of kidney damage. This damage most often is represented by persistent albuminuria defined as two spot urine albumin-to-creatinine ratios (mg/g) of greater than 17 mg/g in men and greater than 25 mg/g in women.

▶ Stage 2 is a mild reduction in kidney function (GFR, 60 to 89 mL/min/1.73 m^2) that occurs in association with kidney damage.

▶ Stages 3 and 4 are defined as moderately decreased kidney function (GFR, 30 to 59 mL/min/1.73 m^2) and severely decreased kidney function (GFR, 15 to 29 mL/min/1.73 m^2), respectively. These degrees of reduced GFR are classified as chronic kidney disease regardless of the presence of any additional evidence of kidney damage.

▶ Stage 5 chronic kidney disease is defined as a GFR of less than 15 mL/min/1.73 m^2 or the need for dialysis therapy. The term ESRD, widely used in regulatory and administrative circles, continues to be used by K/DOQI to represent those patients receiving or eligible for renal replacement therapy by dialysis or transplantation.

It is important to note (see Table 31-2) that stage 5, which basically correlates to patients who are classified as having ESRD, represents only the tip of

Table 31-2 • Stages and Prevalence of Chronic Kidney Disease in the U.S. Adult Population

Stage*	Description	GFR (mL/min/1.73 m^2)	Prevalence* No. of Patients (×100)	Percentage of Patients
1	Kidney damage with normal or increased GFR	≥90	5,900	3.3
2	Kidney damage with mild or decreased GFR	60–89	5,300	3
3	Moderately decreased GFR	30–59	7,600	4.3
4	Severely decreased GFR	15–29	400	0.2
5	Kidney failure	<15 or dialysis	300	0.1

GFR, glomerular filtration rate.
*Data for stages 1 through 4 from National Health and Nutrition Examination Survey (HANES) III (1988–1994). Population: 177 million adults aged ≥ 20 years. Data for stage 5 from United States Data System (1998) include approximately 230,000 patients treated by dialysis, assuming 70,000 additional patients not on dialysis. GFR estimated from serum creatinine using Modification in Diet and Renal Disease (MDRD) Study equation based on age, gender, race, and calibration for serum creatinine. For stages 1 and 2, kidney damage estimated by spot albumin-to-creatinine ratio of >17 mg/g in men or >25 mg/g in women on two measurements.
From National Kidney Foundation: K/DOQI clinical practice guidelines for chronic kidney disease: Evaluation, classification, and stratification. Am J Kidney Dis 39(2 Suppl 1):S1–S266, 2002.

the iceberg of the total number of people who have chronic kidney disease. According to the Third National Health and Nutrition Examination Survey (NHANES III), conducted between 1988 and 1994, which examined the health and nutritional status of 15,624 participants age 20 years or older, the prevalence of adults in the United States with stage 1 to 4 chronic kidney disease was 19.2 million (11%), and 8.3 million (4.7%) had stage 3 to 5 chronic kidney disease, with a GFR of less than 60 mL/min/m²; this is when most of the complications of chronic kidney disease begin or have already occurred.[30] The most recent NHANES data collected in 1999 to 2000 reveal stable high prevalence rates for stage 1 to 4 chronic kidney disease and a twofold increase in the prevalence rate for stage 5.[31] Compounding these grave statistics is the fact that chronic kidney disease is associated with a twofold to threefold higher risk for death and a higher risk for cardiovascular disease.[31]

CAUSES OF CHRONIC KIDNEY DISEASE

The causes of chronic kidney disease are numerous (Box 31-6). By far, the two most common causes are diabetes mellitus and hypertension, which account for more than 36% and 24% of cases of ESRD, respectively.[27] Other causes include glomerulonephritis (both primary and secondary to systemic diseases), interstitial nephritis, congenital malformations, genetic disorders, neoplasms, hepatorenal syndrome, obstructive uropathy, and microangiopathic etiologies such as scleroderma and atheroembolic disease.

PATHOPHYSIOLOGY OF CHRONIC KIDNEY DISEASE

Although many diseases can cause chronic kidney disease, there appear to be common pathophysiologic pathways for disease progression. The outstanding

Box 31-6 • Causes of Chronic Kidney Disease

- Diabetes mellitus
- Hypertension
- Glomerulonephritis
  - Primary (immunoglobulin A nephropathy, postinfectious glomerulonephritis)
  - Secondary (HIV nephropathy, lupus, cryoglobulinemia, Wegener's granulomatosis, Goodpasture's syndrome, polyarteritis nodosa, amyloidosis)
- Interstitial nephritis (allergic interstitial nephritis, pyelonephritis)
- Microangiopathic vascular disease (atheroembolic disease, scleroderma)
- Congenital disease
- Genetic disease (polycystic kidney disease, medullary cystic kidney disease)
- Obstructive uropathy
- Neoplasms or tumors
- Transplant rejection
- Hepatorenal syndrome

common morphologic features seen in chronic kidney disease include fibrosis, loss of native renal cells, and infiltration by monocytes and macrophages. The mediators of the process are many and include abnormal glomerular hemodynamics, hypoxia, proteinuria, and vasoactive substances, such as angiotensin II.[31]

In discussing glomerular hemodynamics, it is important to understand intact nephron theory. Because each of the more than 1 million nephrons in each kidney is an independent functioning unit, as renal disease progresses, nephrons can lose function at different times. When an individual nephron becomes diseased, nephrons in close proximity increase their individual filtration rates by increasing the rate of blood flow and hydrostatic pressure in their glomerular capillaries. This hyperfiltration response in the nondiseased nephrons enables the kidneys to maintain excretory and homeostatic functions, even when up to 70% of the nephrons are damaged. However, eventually, the intact nephrons reach a point of maximal filtration, and any additional loss of glomerular mass is accompanied by an incremental loss in GFR and subsequent accumulation of filterable toxins.

Although hyperfiltration is an adaptive measure to nephron loss, over time it actually can accelerate the loss of nephrons because the hyperfiltration causes endothelial injury, stimulation of profibrotic cytokines, infiltration by monocytes and macrophages, and detachment of glomerular epithelial cells. In addition, hypertrophy of the nondiseased nephrons due to hyperfiltration leads to increased wall stress and even more injury.[11] This is why many interventions to slow down the progression of renal failure involve measures that reduce glomerular hydrostatic pressure. One such example is the use of ACE inhibitors and angiotensin receptor blockers (ARBs), which prevent angiotensin II–mediated efferent arteriolar vasoconstriction and subsequent nephron hyperfiltration.

Other possible mediators of chronic kidney disease progression are hypoxia and angiotensin II. In chronic kidney disease, the loss of peritubular capillaries by various causes results in reduced capillary perfusion of the tubules. The resultant hypoxia favors the release of proinflammatory and profibrotic cytokines, leading to fibrosis and cell injury. Angiotensin II stimulates growth factors and cytokines that contribute to fibrosis aside from its hemodynamic effects on the glomerulus.[11,31]

Proteinuria, the result of glomerular hypertension and abnormal glomerular permeability, also contributes to chronic kidney disease progression. Abnormally filtered protein is reabsorbed by proximal tubular cells through endocytosis and accumulates in the cells, causing the production of cytokines. These proinflammatory factors ultimately cause fibrosis and scarring of the tubulointerstitium.[31] Proteinuria is a very strong predictor of chronic kidney disease progression, consistent with its role in the pathophysiology of chronic kidney disease.

Diabetic Nephropathy

Because of the extremely high prevalence of diabetes and hypertension as causes of chronic kidney disease, an understanding of the renal pathophysiology specific to these entities and knowledge of interventions designed to slow down or even prevent progression to stage 5 chronic kidney disease is imperative. Kidney failure is a major complication of diabetes, with an incidence of approximately 30% in patients with type 1 diabetes mellitus and 10% to 40% in patients with type 2 diabetes mellitus.[33]

In diabetes, the microvasculature in the organ systems of the body, including the kidneys, is damaged. In the kidneys, primarily the afferent and efferent arterioles and the glomerular capillaries are affected. Glomerular changes include thickening of the basement membrane, mesangial expansion from overproduction and underdegradation of extracellular matrix proteins, and diffuse glomerulosclerosis. Late in diabetic nephropathy, tubular atrophy and interstitial fibrosis also occur. The exact physiological mechanism for these structural alterations is unclear, but hyperglycemia is a major contributor. In the classic Diabetes Control and Complications Trial (DCCT)—a prospective, randomized, multicenter trial performed to assess the effectiveness of tight blood glucose control on the complications of type 1 diabetes—researchers found that strict blood glucose control delayed and possibly even prevented the progression of diabetic nephropathy.[34] More recently, the follow-up study to the DCCT, called the Epidemiology of Diabetes Interventions and Complications (EDIC) study, revealed that the benefits of tight control persist for a number of years.[35] In addition, the classic United Kingdom Prospective Diabetes Study (UKPDS) reached conclusions in people with type 2 diabetes that were similar to those of the DCCT.[36]

At the onset of diabetic nephropathy, patients may have an increased GFR (as high as 140 mL/minute) because of hyperfiltration, slightly enlarged kidneys, and microalbuminuria (30 to 300 mg/day of albumin in the urine). Over the course of approximately 10 to 15 years, hypertension and protein leakage increase. Eventually protein leakage is massive, with consequent hypoalbuminemia and edema as well as mild azotemia. At this point kidney damage is extensive, often requiring dialysis therapy within a few years.

Hypertensive Nephrosclerosis

The effect of systemic hypertension on the kidneys results in a condition known as nephrosclerosis. Hypertensive nephrosclerosis involves the development of sclerotic lesions in the renal arterioles and glomerular capillaries that cause them to become thickened, narrowed, and eventually necrotic. Hypertensive nephrosclerosis can be benign or malignant. In benign nephrosclerosis, associated with chronic mild or moderate hypertension, renal impairment occurs over many years. Malignant nephrosclerosis, associated with malignant hypertension, can lead to permanent renal failure rapidly if blood pressure is not immediately reduced. Often symptoms such as blurred vision and a severe headache accompany this crisis situation.

Because hypertensive nephrosclerosis is directly caused by hypertension, its incidence is greater in populations with a higher incidence of primary hypertension (e.g., elderly people, African Americans). Among African Americans, the risk for hypertension-induced renal failure is nearly 8 times that of Caucasians.[37] The signs of hypertensive nephrosclerosis vary depending on the severity of the renal damage and the acuteness of the hypertension. Some signs that may be present include proteinuria, azotemia, and hematuria with red blood cell casts. Unfortunately, like those with hypertension, patients often remain asymptomatic until extensive damage has occurred. To prevent or delay the progression of hypertensive nephropathy, blood pressure control is essential, and often multiple different antihypertensive medications are required. This is an area in which patient education can have a great impact in decreasing the incidence of ESRD. Educating patients about the complications of uncontrolled hypertension is particularly important and may foster the patient's active involvement in controlling his or her blood pressure.

PREVENTING THE PROGRESSION OF CHRONIC KIDNEY DISEASE

An important characteristic of chronic kidney disease is continuous progression. Slowing the rate of progression after chronic kidney disease is diagnosed is a focus of extensive and ongoing research. Regardless of the primary cause of chronic kidney disease, specific identifiable secondary insults to the kidney can rapidly accelerate the loss of nephrons. Such secondary insults include an alteration in renal perfusion, as observed in congestive heart failure or intravascular volume depletion; the administration of nephrotoxic agents; urinary obstruction; and urinary infections. Consequently, monitoring for and avoiding these insults or aggressively treating them if they occur is paramount.

It is also important to educate patients and their families about the dangers of these insults. Patients and families should be instructed, for instance, about the signs and symptoms and the need for prompt treatment of urinary infections as well as common nephrotoxic drugs to avoid. Common over-the-counter and prescription analgesics, such as NSAIDs, can cause rapid deterioration in renal function and should be avoided in patients with chronic kidney disease.

Strict control of blood glucose levels is critical to preventing and retarding the progression of renal failure in people with diabetes. The targets for key parameters of glucose control set by the American Diabetes Association for people with diabetes are a glycosylated hemoglobin of less than 7.0%, a preprandial plasma glucose of 90 to 130 mg/dL, and a peak postprandial plasma glucose of less than 180 mg/dL.[38] Blood pressure control is also essential for preventing the progression of renal failure from almost any primary etiology, not just hypertension or diabetes. According to the K/DOQI Clinical Practice Guidelines on Blood Pressure Management and Use of Antihypertensive Agents in Chronic Kidney Disease (2004), the target of therapy is a blood pressure of less than 130/80 mm Hg.[39] Control of hypertension entails lifestyle changes (e.g., exercise, salt restriction, smoking cessation, and avoidance of excessive alcohol) as well as pharmacological therapy if necessary. Regarding pharmacological therapy, ACE inhibitors and ARBs have been shown to offer a selective advantage in slowing the progression of diabetic and other proteinuric syndromes. Both drugs have been proved to lower blood pressure, reduce proteinuria, and slow the progression of kidney disease,[11,32] presumably because of their ability to decrease intraglomerular pressure by blocking the effect of angiotensin II on the afferent and efferent arterioles.

A protein-restricted diet as a means to slow the progression of renal failure is controversial, but the evidence appears to support the view that moderate protein restriction of 0.6 to 0.8g/kg/day in patients may help.[40] However, caution with protein restriction, especially in critically ill patients who are in a catabolic state, is important to prevent malnutrition. Malnutrition itself is a major determinant of morbidity and mortality in patients with renal failure.[11] Ways to avoid malnutrition include providing protein with high biological value, ensuring that adequate caloric requirements are met, and closely monitoring nutritional assessment parameters (i.e., body weight, serum albumin and prealbumin levels, and total protein levels). Because of the complexity of nutritional requirements in critically ill patients, collaboration with a dietitian is essential.

Finally, controlling serum lipids may slow the progression of renal failure. Hyperlipidemia is commonly seen in patients with chronic kidney disease, particularly those with diabetes and nephrotic syndrome, and is hypothesized to contribute to renal failure. Several animal studies support this. In addition, numerous secondary analyses of data from lipid trials suggest that high lipid levels are associated with a faster rate of progression and that statins slow this rate. The mechanisms by which dyslipidemias may contribute to renal failure are unclear, but the formation of oxygen free radicals, the expression of growth factors and cytokines, the proliferation of mesangial cells, and the inhibition of nitric oxide have been postulated.[41] Because the use of lipid-lowering agents is safe in diverse renal diseases, their use may be prudent, especially because lowering lipids decreases the risk for cardiovascular events (the primary cause of mortality in patients with ESRD).

• Management of Renal Failure

Although some distinct differences exist between the ways acute renal failure and chronic kidney disease are managed, many of the clinical manifestations and complications encountered are the same. Thus, the general management of renal failure is addressed here, noting any differences between acute renal failure and chronic kidney disease as necessary. In either type of renal failure, management begins with treating the primary insult. Common nursing diagnoses and collaborative problems for patients with acute renal failure are given in Box 31-7. An overview of the management of patients with acute renal failure is provided in the accompanying Collaborative Care Guide (Box 31-8).

MANAGING FLUID BALANCE ALTERATIONS

Clinical management of fluid balance is of primary importance in patients with renal failure and is the area in which differences in the management of acute renal failure and chronic kidney disease are perhaps most dramatic.

Acute Renal Failure

In prerenal acute renal failure and the early stages of ischemic ATN, the cause of the renal failure is inadequate renal perfusion, often due to intravascular volume deficits. After using laboratory, physical assessment, and hemodynamic clues to make a rapid diagnosis of intravascular volume depletion, therapy involves prompt administration of replacement fluids, such as blood and crystalloids. The replacement solutions used should reflect the type of losses (e.g., for a patient with a hemorrhagic condition, blood would be the replacement fluid of choice). Often in acute renal failure, even if signs and symptoms of intravascular volume deficits are not present, large boluses of IV fluid challenges are given. Reversal of acute renal failure after such a bolus is therapeutic as well as diagnostic of prerenal acute renal failure.

Box 31-7 — **Nursing Diagnoses and Collaborative Problems for the Patient With Acute Renal Failure**

- Fluid Volume, Excess, related to decreased kidney function
- Cardiac Output, Decreased, related to fluid volume excess, disturbances in renin–angiotensin system
- Nutrition, Imbalanced, Less Than Body Requirements, related to anorexia, nausea and vomiting, dietary restrictions, and altered oral mucous membranes
- Skin Integrity, Risk for Impaired, related to poor nutritional status, immobility, and edema
- Anxiety related to unexpected serious illness and uncertain prognosis, unfamiliar environment, and current symptoms
- Activity Intolerance related to shortness of breath, fatigue, anemia, uremia, and dialysis procedure
- Sleep Pattern, Disturbed, related to fragmented sleep in hospital environment
- Infection, Risk for, related to decreased functioning of immune system
- Knowledge, Deficient, related to pathophysiology and etiology of acute episode, dietary restrictions, medications, complications, prognosis, and follow-up care

Box 31-8 • COLLABORATIVE CARE GUIDE for the Patient With Acute Renal Failure

OUTCOMES	INTERVENTIONS
Coordination of Care All appropriate team members and disciplines will be involved in the plan of care.	• Develop the plan of care with the patient, family, primary physician, nephrologist, pulmonologist, cardiologist, registered nurse, advanced practice nurse, social worker, respiratory therapist, physical therapist, occupational therapist, dietitian, chaplain, and dialysis staff.

Oxygenation/Ventilation
Patient will have adequate gas exchange as evidenced by:
• Arterial blood gases (ABGs) within normal limits
• Functional oxygen saturation (SpO_2) greater than 92%
• Clear breath sounds
• Normal respiratory rate and depth
• Normal chest x-ray
	• Monitor ABGs and continuous pulse oximetry.
	• Monitor acid–base status.
	• Monitor for signs and symptoms of pulmonary distress from fluid overload.
	• Provide routine pulmonary toilet, including the following:
	  • Airway suctioning
	  • Chest percussion
	  • Incentive spirometer
	  • Frequent turning
	• Mobilize out of bed to chair.
	• Support patient with oxygen therapy, mechanical ventilation, or both as indicated. Involve respiratory therapist.

Circulation/Perfusion Patient's blood pressure, heart rate, and hemodynamic parameters will be within normal limits. Patient will have adequate tissue perfusion as evidenced by: • Adequate hemoglobin levels • Euvolemic status • Optimal urine output depending on phase of acute renal failure • Appropriate level of consciousness	• Monitor vital signs every 1 to 2 hours. • Monitor pulmonary artery wedge pressure (PAWP) and right atrial pressure every hour and cardiac output, systemic vascular resistance, and peripheral vascular resistance every 6 to 12 h if pulmonary artery catheter is in place. • Assess vital signs continuously or every 15 min during dialysis. • Monitor hemoglobin and hematocrit levels daily. • Assess evidence of tissue perfusion (pain, pulses, color, temperature, and signs of decreased organ perfusion such as an altered level of consciousness, ileus, and decreasing urine output). • Administer intravascular crystalloids or blood products as indicated.
Fluids/Electrolytes Patient will be euvolemic. Patient will achieve normal electrolyte balance. Patient will achieve optimal renal function.	• Monitor fluid status, including input and output (fluid restriction), daily weight, urine output trends, vital signs, central venous pressure (CVP), and PAWP. • Monitor for signs and symptoms of hypervolemia (hypertension, pulmonary edema, peripheral edema, jugular venous distention, and increased CVP). • Monitor serum electrolytes daily. • Monitor renal parameters, including urine output, blood urea nitrogen (BUN), serum creatinine, acid–base status, urine electrolytes, urine osmolality, and urine specific gravity. • Administer fluids and diuretics to maintain intravascular volume and renal function, per order. • Replace electrolytes as ordered. • Treat patient with, and monitor response to, dialysis therapies if indicated. • Monitor and maintain dialysis access for chosen intermittent or continuous dialysis method: *Continuous Veno–Veno Dialysis* • Monitor and regulate ultrafiltration rate hourly based on patient's response and fluid status. • Provide fluid replacements as ordered.

Box 31-8 • COLLABORATIVE CARE GUIDE for the Patient With Acute Renal Failure (Continued)

OUTCOMES	INTERVENTIONS
	• Assess and troubleshoot hemofilter and blood tubing hourly. • Protect vascular access from dislodgment. • Change filter and tubing per protocol. • Monitor vascular access for infection.
	Peritoneal Dialysis • Slowly infuse warmed dialysate. • Drain after appropriate dwell time. • Assess drainage for volume and appearance. • Send cultures daily. • Assess access site for infection.
	Intermittent Hemodialysis • Assess shunt for thrill and buzzing sound (bruit) every 12 h. • Avoid constrictions (i.e., blood pressures), phlebotomy, and intravenous fluid administration in arm with shunt. • Assess for infection. • Monitor perfusion of related extremity.
Mobility Patient will remain free of complications related to bed rest and immobility.	• Initiate deep venous thrombosis prophylaxis. • Reposition frequently. • Mobilize to chair when possible. • Consult physical therapist. • Conduct range-of-motion and strengthening exercises.
Protection/Safety Patient will be protected from possible harm.	• Assess need for wrist restraints if patient is intubated, has a decreased level of consciousness, is unable to follow commands, or is acutely agitated, or for affected extremity during hemodialysis. Explain need for restraints to patient and family members. If restrained, assess response to restraints and check every 1 to 2 h for skin integrity and impairment in tissue perfusion. Follow hospital protocol for use of restraints. • Use siderails on bed and safety belts on chairs as appropriate. • Follow seizure precautions.
Skin Integrity Patient will have intact skin.	• Assess skin integrity and all bony prominences every 4 h. • Turn every 2 h. • Consider a pressure relief/reduction mattress. Use Braden Scale to assess risk for skin breakdown. • Use superfatted or lanolin-based soap for bathing and apply emollients for pruritus. • Treat pressure ulcers according to hospital protocol. Involve enterostomal nurse in care.
Nutrition Patient will be adequately nourished as evidenced by: • Stable weight not less than 10% below, or greater than 20% above, ideal body weight • An albumin level of 3.5 to 4.0 g/dL • A total protein level of 6 to 8 g/dL • A total lymphocyte count of 1,000 to 3,000 × 10^6/L	• Consult dietitian to direct and coordinate nutritional support. • Observe sodium, potassium, protein, and fluid restriction as indicated. • Provide small, frequent feedings. • Provide parenteral or enteral feeding as ordered. • Monitor albumin, prealbumin, total protein, hematocrit, hemoglobin, and white blood cell counts, and monitor daily weights to assess effectiveness of nutritional therapy.
Comfort/Pain Control Patient will be as comfortable and as pain free as possible as evidenced by: • No complaints of discomfort • No objective indicators of discomfort	• Monitor for signs and symptoms of respiratory distress related to fluid overload and support oxygenation as needed. Keep head of bed elevated and teach breathing techniques to minimize oxygen distress, such as pursed-lip breathing.

(continued)

Box 31-8 • COLLABORATIVE CARE GUIDE for the Patient With Acute Renal Failure (Continued)

OUTCOMES	INTERVENTIONS
	• Plan fluid restrictions over 24 h, allowing for periodic sips of water and ice chips to minimize thirst. • Provide frequent mouth and skin care. • Assess quantity and quality of discomfort. • Provide a quiet environment and frequent reassurance. • Observe for complications that may cause discomfort, such as infection of vascular access device, peritonitis or inadequate draining during peritoneal dialysis, and gastrointestinal disturbances (nausea, vomiting, diarrhea, constipation). • Administer analgesics, antiemetics, antidiarrheals, laxatives (non–magnesium and non–phosphate containing), stool softeners, antihistamines, sedatives, or anxiolytics as needed and monitor response.
Psychosocial Patient will demonstrate a decrease in anxiety as evidenced by: • Vital signs within normal limits • Level of consciousness within normal limits • Subjective reports of decreased anxiety levels • Objective assessment of decreased anxiety level	• Assess vital signs. • Explore patient and family concerns. • If the patient is intubated, develop interventions for effective communication. • Arrange for flexible visitation to meet needs of the patient and family. • Provide for adequate rest and sleep. • Provide frequent information and updates on condition and treatment, and explain equipment. Answer all questions. • Consult social services and clergy as appropriate. • Administer sedatives and antidepressants as appropriate and monitor response.
Teaching/Discharge Planning Patient and family members will understand procedures and tests needed for treatment during the acute phase and maintenance of a patient with chronic disease. Patient and family members understand the severity of the illness, ask appropriate questions, and anticipate potential complications. In preparation for discharge to home, the patient and family members will demonstrate an understanding of renal replacement therapy, fluid and dietary restrictions, and the medication regimen.	• Prepare the patient and his or her family members for procedures, such as insertion of dialysis access, dialysis therapy, or laboratory studies. • Explain the causes and effects of renal failure and the potential for complications, such as hypertension and fluid overload. • Encourage family members to ask questions related to the pathophysiology of renal failure, dialysis, and dietary or fluid restrictions. • Make appropriate referrals and consults early during hospitalization. • Initiate family education regarding home care of the patient on dialysis, what to expect, maintenance of renal function, and when to seek medical attention.

Fluid administration in acute renal failure is also indicated in the diuretic phase of ATN, when extensive diuresis may occur, and for the prevention or alleviation of tubular obstruction seen in obstructive causes of acute renal failure, including ATN and many postrenal etiologies. However, in any oliguric state, caution must be taken to prevent fluid overload. In a sustained oliguric state, such as the oliguric stage of ATN, fluid is restricted to the previous day's urine output amount plus 500 to 800 mL to account for insensible losses.

Diuretics are often used in acute renal failure to increase urinary flow and thereby help alleviate conditions of fluid overload or to prevent tubular obstruc-tion. Furosemide, a loop diuretic, and mannitol, an osmotic diuretic, are often used with hydration to prevent tubular obstruction in certain obstructive causes of acute renal failure, such as acute urate nephropathy, and in heme pigment nephropathy, such as rhabdomyolysis. In states of fluid overload, such as pulmonary edema and heart failure, diuretics are also useful. Often in these situations, furosemide is administered every 6 hours, with the initial dose ranging between 20 and 100 mg depending on whether the patient has taken furosemide regularly. If within an hour the response is inadequate, the dose may then be doubled. This process may be repeated until adequate urine output is achieved. Sometimes even a continuous furosemide drip is required. In addition, a thiazide diuretic, such as chlorothiazide, may be administered with furosemide because of the synergistic action of these diuretics in promoting urinary excretion.

With the use of diuretics, caution must be taken to avoid complications of dehydration, electrolyte imbalances, and side effects. Tinnitus and hearing impairment (reversible and irreversible) have been reported after IV furosemide administration. Ototoxicity is associated with rapid injection, excessively high doses, or concomitant therapy with other ototoxic drugs. The manufacturer recommends controlled IV infusion (not to exceed 4 mg/minute) for high-dose parenteral furosemide therapy.

The use of diuretics to convert oliguria to nonoliguria, unlike the aforementioned uses of diuretics, has not been substantiated in medical research and may even be harmful. Additionally, research has not shown that the use of loop diuretics in acute renal failure reduces mortality, shortens the duration of renal failure, or helps avoid or reduce the requirements for renal replacement therapy.[42,43] Hence, based on the literature, it is reasonable to use diuretics for a short length of time for volume control but not for therapy for established oliguric acute renal failure.

Dopamine is another agent that has been traditionally used in acute renal failure because of its ability to theoretically cause renal vasodilation at "renal doses" (1 to 3 μg/kg/minute), thereby increasing renal perfusion. However, the efficacy of this agent to affect the course of acute renal failure has not been substantiated despite many clinical trials, and some studies have even shown deleterious effects.[1,2,44] Nevertheless, some clinicians may institute a trial of dopamine, particularly in combination with fluid resuscitation, in patients with prerenal acute renal failure.

If fluid complications arise and cannot be controlled by fluid restrictions and pharmacological agents, dialysis (discussed in detail in Chapter 30) or isolated ultrafiltration may be necessary. This is often the case in oliguric patients who are receiving large amounts of IV fluids hourly in the form of medications and nutritional supplements. People in whom acute renal failure develops secondary to hypoperfusion or tubular injury may have a delayed recovery time, necessitating maintenance dialysis until the tissue repairs itself and normal function returns. For these patients, discharge planning should take into consideration the need for outpatient dialysis therapy (which may last for several weeks to months), the need to modify the person's diet and consumption of fluids, and the psychosocial implications of these measures for the patient and his or her family members.

Chronic Kidney Disease

In chronic kidney disease, fluid and salt restriction is a mainstay of therapy to prevent fluid overload. Sodium is restricted to less than 2,400 mg/day, and fluid intake is limited to 500 mL plus the patient's previous day's 24-hour urine output. Diuretics are also used to manage volume overload. Patients usually are able to respond to diuretics until they reach stage 5 chronic kidney disease, at which point extensive renal damage prevents an adequate response. By the time chronic kidney disease progresses to stage 5, oliguria is typically manifested, and signs and symptoms of fluid overload such as edema, hypertension, pulmonary edema, heart failure, and jugular vein distention occur unless dialysis therapy is instituted. In these patients, an ongoing assessment of fluid status, including obtaining accurate intake and output measurements with daily weights and monitoring for fluid complications, is imperative.

MANAGING ACID–BASE ALTERATIONS

Acute renal failure and chronic kidney disease typically result in metabolic acidosis because of the nephrons' inability to secrete and excrete hydrogen ions and reabsorb bicarbonate ions as renal failure progresses. In critically ill patients, this acid–base disturbance may be intensified because of concurrent conditions such as lactic acidosis or diabetic ketoacidosis and because such patients are in a high catabolic state, which increases the release of intracellular acids into the circulation. Clinical manifestations of metabolic acidosis include headaches, nausea and vomiting, deep and rapid respirations (Kussmaul respirations), altered mental status, hyperkalemia, and tachycardia. In severe metabolic acidosis, bradycardia and hypotension may manifest because of myocardial depression and vasodilation. There is also a dramatic depression of the patient's level of consciousness, often resulting in a stuporous or comatose state.

In chronic kidney disease, metabolic acidosis begins to manifest as the patient reaches stage 3 and the GFR falls below 60 mL/min/1.73 m^2. Although the metabolic acidosis associated with chronic kidney disease is usually mild (CO_2, 16 to 22 mEq/L), it is associated with many adverse consequences, including fatigue, protein catabolism, and bone demineralization. The bones become demineralized because bone phosphate and carbonate are used as buffers against excess hydrogen ion.

Laboratory assessments of acid–base status using arterial blood gases (ABGs) and venous carbon dioxide content guide therapy. Patients with a plasma bicarbonate level less than 22 mEq/L warrant treatment. Therapy involves the administration of alkaline medications (e.g., Bicitra, sodium bicarbonate tablets), dialysis, or both. When using citrate-containing medications, such as Bicitra, it is important that these medications not be given with aluminum-containing phosphate binders. Using these agents together would put the patient at risk for aluminum toxicity because citrate significantly increases aluminum absorption from the gastrointestinal tract.

The use of IV sodium bicarbonate is reserved for severe acidosis (evidenced by a blood pH < 7.2 or a plasma bicarbonate level < 12 to 14 mEq/L) because of potential complications of extracellular volume excess, metabolic alkalosis, and hypokalemia. Intractable acidosis is an indication for dialysis, which removes excess hydrogen ions and adds a buffer to the body. In hemodialysis, the buffer is bicarbonate, and in peritoneal dialysis, it is lactate, which is metabolized to bicarbonate. An important caveat to keep in mind when correcting metabolic acidosis is that rapid correction may result in a suppressed respiratory drive and hypoventilation. Rapid correction can also lead to acute hypocalcemia and tetany because the amount of ionized calcium decreases in an alkalotic state owing to increased binding of calcium with albumin and inorganic substances such as phosphate. Throughout any kind of acid–base therapy, it is necessary to monitor serum bicarbonate, pH, and calcium and potassium levels closely.

MANAGING CARDIOVASCULAR ALTERATIONS

Alterations in the cardiovascular system can cause or accelerate acute renal failure and chronic kidney disease. In addition, cardiovascular complications can arise as a result of renal failure itself. Common cardiovascular complications in acute renal failure and chronic kidney disease include hypertension and hyperkalemia. Pericarditis, another cardiovascular complication of renal disease, is primarily seen with chronic kidney disease.

Hypertension

Hypertension as a complication of renal failure results from excess retention of water and sodium, overactivation of the sympathetic nervous system, and stimulation of the renin–angiotensin–aldosterone system. Because controlling blood pressure is essential to prevent end-organ damage and reduce the risk for life-threatening cardiovascular events, adequate treatment is essential. Management may include fluid and sodium restrictions, diuretic administration, antihypertensive therapy, and dialysis to remove excess fluid. Extensive patient teaching regarding nonpharmacological and pharmacological treatment and the potential complications of uncontrolled hypertension is an integral part of management.

Hyperkalemia

Hyperkalemia is a life-threatening condition seen in patients with acute renal failure and chronic kidney disease. As the GFR decreases, the ability of the kidneys to excrete excess potassium diminishes. In critically ill patients, this renal impairment is frequently compounded by states of increased catabolism, acidosis, cellular injury, administration of potassium-based medications, and blood transfusions, all of which can raise serum potassium levels. If not recognized and treated, hyperkalemia leads to fatal dysrhythmias.

Assessment of hyperkalemia involves close monitoring of serum potassium levels as well as monitoring the effects of potassium on the electrical conduction system of the heart. Characteristic electrocardiogram (ECG) changes occur as potassium levels rise (Fig. 31-4). The first ECG changes that occur, usually when serum potassium is in the range of 6 to 7 mEq/L, are the appearance of tall, tented T waves and a prolonged PR interval. Next, there is a loss of the P wave and a slight widening of the QRS complex. At this point, the serum potassium is usually in the range of 8 to 9 mEq/L. From here, the QRS complex continues to widen until a sine wave (wavy line) pattern develops. This ominous sign is closely followed by ventricular fibrillation or standstill.

In evaluating hyperkalemia, it should be noted that patients with long-standing elevations in serum potassium are more refractory to its effects on the heart than patients in whom hyperkalemia develops suddenly. Thus, potassium and ECG changes must be evaluated together to determine the acuteness of the situation. Other effects of hyperkalemia that are monitored include paresthesias, hyporeflexia, and muscle weakness (which typically begins in the lower extremities and ascends to the trunk and upper extremities).

Mild hyperkalemia (a serum potassium level < 6 mEq/L without ECG changes) may be treated with dietary potassium restriction, diuretics, and potassium-binding resins (e.g., sodium polystyrene sulfate). Sodium polystyrene is given orally or as an enema. The oral dose of 15 to 30 g in 60 to 120 mL of a 20% sorbitol solution (to prevent constipation) may be repeated every 4 to 6 hours as needed. The rectal dose of 50 g in 50 mL of 70% sorbitol and 150 mL tap water should be retained in the colon for at least 30 to 60 minutes. This drug must be used with caution in critically ill patients with decreased colonic motility, such as postsurgical patients and patients taking large amounts of opiates, because of its association

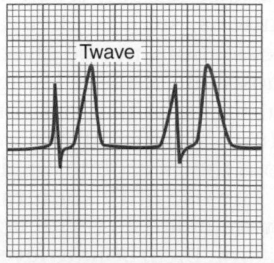

A. Peaked T waves, prolonged PR interval, depressed ST segment

B. Lost P wave

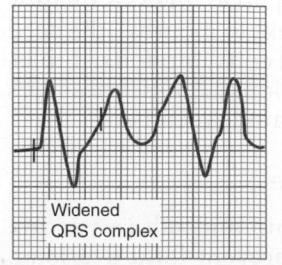

C. Widened QRS complex

Figure 31-4 • Typical electrocardiogram (ECG) findings indicative of various degrees of hyperkalemia. **A:** When the serum potassium (K^+) level is about 6–7 mEq/L, the T waves become peaked, the PR interval is prolonged, and the ST segment is depressed. **B:** At about 8–9 mEq/L, the P wave is lost. **C:** At about 10–11 mEq/L, the QRS complex widens.

with colonic necrosis in this population. To reduce this risk, a cleansing enema may be given after rectal administration.[11] Sodium polystyrene should never be used in a patient with a gastrointestinal obstruction, and bowel sounds should always be assessed before its administration.

Treatment of life-threatening hyperkalemia entails taking steps to antagonize the effects of potassium on the heart, promote intracellular shifting of potassium, and remove potassium from the body. Antagonizing the effects of potassium on the heart is achieved with IV calcium gluconate or chloride and is the first priority for patients with substantial ECG changes. Intracellular shifting of potassium is done next to bridge the gap until potassium removal from the body can be executed. Means to shift potassium into the cell include IV insulin and dextrose administration and IV bicarbonate administration. β_2-Adrenergic therapy can also effect transcellular potassium shifting but is less commonly used because of the requirement for 10 to 20 times the dose used for reactive airway disease. Removal of potassium from the body entails, as previously mentioned, diuretic administration and the use of potassium exchange resins. If these measures do not control hyperkalemia, dialysis must be initiated. Obviously, in a patient with stage 5 chronic kidney disease, who is likely already receiving dialysis therapy, dialysis is initiated immediately along with other emergent therapy in life-threatening hyperkalemia.

Pericarditis

Pericarditis due to uremia (uremic pericarditis) is a complication that can be seen primarily in stage 5 chronic kidney disease. This type of pericarditis is characterized by an inflammation of the pericardial membrane, which causes the pericardial capillaries to become permeable to fluid, red blood cells, fibrinogen, and albumin. In most cases, the inflammation is aseptic, although it may also result from bacterial or viral infections. The consequent serous or serosanguineous fluid in the pericardial cavity (pericardial effusion) can increase the intrapericardial pressure and compromise ventricular contractility, stroke volume, and cardiac output. Pericardial tamponade, which results when the accumulation of pericardial fluid is so large that adequate cardiac output cannot be maintained, is a life-threatening emergency. The exact etiology of uremic pericarditis is unknown, but it is associated with prolonged inadequate dialysis therapy, uremic toxins, infectious agents, treatment with the antihypertensive agent minoxidil, and heparin administration.

Chest pain, fever, and a pericardial friction rub are the classic triad of findings associated with pericarditis. The chest pain is characteristically sharp and steady and is relieved by sitting forward and intensified by breathing deeply. The pericardial friction rub (a harsh, leathery sound heard over the precordium) may precede the pain, may persist after the pain has subsided, and may disappear when the volume of effusion increases.[11] In addition to these findings, there are typical ECG changes in pericarditis. The most notable are new-onset atrial dysrhythmias and widespread ST elevations with an upward concavity (versus the upward convexity typical in an acute myocardial infarction). In a large pericardial effusion, signs and symptoms are more dramatic and include dyspnea, tachycardia, mental confusion, weakness, increased jugular venous distention, peripheral edema, and a paradoxical pulse greater than 10 mm Hg during inspiration. Tamponade results in distended neck veins, tachypnea, a narrowed pulse pressure, an increased PAWP, muffled heart sounds, diminished peripheral pulses, and a decreased level of consciousness.

Therapy for uremic pericarditis includes aggressive dialysis therapy, usually daily, until symptoms disappear. Also, because anticoagulation during dialysis may precipitate or enhance bleeding into the pericardial space, low-dose, regional, or no heparin may be prescribed. Systemic steroids and NSAIDs, such as indomethacin, may also be used but have variable results. Cardiac tamponade is an emergency that requires urgent pericardiocentesis to relieve the pressure on the heart. For the patient in whom recurrent pericarditis develops or the pericardium becomes constrictive, surgical creation of a pericardial window or pericardiectomy may be necessary.

Cardiovascular Disease in Chronic Kidney Disease

In patients with ESRD, cardiovascular disease is the leading cause of morbidity and mortality. It accounts for almost 40% to 45% of deaths in the ESRD population,[11] which equates to a mortality rate 10 to 30 times higher than in the general population. Increasingly, earlier stages of chronic kidney disease are also associated with high rates of cardiovascular morbidity and mortality. In fact, patients with chronic kidney disease are much more likely to suffer from cardiac disease resulting in cardiovascular death than to eventually require renal replacement therapy.[45] The predominant cardiac disorders in chronic kidney disease are left ventricular hypertrophy (found in 75% of patients on dialysis), coronary artery disease, cardiomyopathy, congestive heart failure, and valvular dysfunction.

Because these disorders develop over a period of at least a few years, they usually present early in chronic kidney disease and continue to progress as renal function declines. This association between chronic kidney disease and cardiovascular disease may occur for the following reasons: (1) cardiovascular disease causes renal dysfunction (i.e., heart failure), (2) chronic kidney disease causes an increased risk for cardiovascular disease, or (3) other factors (i.e., hypertension, diabetes mellitus, anemia, or hyperlipidemia) cause or accelerate both renal dysfunction and cardiovascular disease. In any case, monitoring for cardiovascular disease, reducing modifiable risk factors, and treating specific cardiovascular conditions when present are essential to decrease mortality in patients with chronic kidney disease.

Diagnostic tests useful in assessing for cardiovascular disease in these high-risk patients include routine ECGs, echocardiography, and cardiac stress testing. Pharmacological rather than exercise stress testing is the stress test of choice because patients with chronic kidney disease are often unable to attain the level of exercise needed to make exercise stress tests useful. More invasive tests for symptomatic patients include a thallium scan and coronary angiography.

Modifiable risk factors that can contribute to cardiovascular disease and that should be addressed as part of the management of patients with chronic kidney disease include hypertension, hyperlipidemia, hypervolemia, anemia, smoking, hyperglycemia, calcium and phosphate imbalances, vitamin D deficiency, hyperhomocysteinemia, and metabolic acidosis. Regarding blood pressure control, the Joint National Committee for the Prevention, Detection, Evaluation and Treatment of High Blood Pressure (JNC-7) and the K/DOQI Clinical Practice Guidelines recommend strict blood pressure control with a goal of less than 130/80 mm Hg in all patients with chronic kidney disease.[39,46] Similarly, the K/DOQI Clinical Practice Guidelines recommend that all patients with chronic kidney disease be included in the highest risk group, justifying strict lipid control with a target low-density lipoprotein cholesterol level of less than 100 mg/dL.[47] As with the general population, disease-specific treatment (e.g., antiplatelet therapy and β-blocker administration for coronary artery disease) must be instituted as appropriate.

MANAGING PULMONARY ALTERATIONS

A frequent complication in patients with oliguric acute renal failure or stage 5 chronic kidney disease is the development of pulmonary edema. This complication results from fluid overload, heart failure, or both. Clinical manifestations include dyspnea; the presence of crackles on auscultation; the production of pink, frothy sputum; tachypnea; tachycardia; decreased arterial oxygen saturation (SaO_2); and evidence of fluid overload on chest radiograph. Management involves fluid and sodium restriction, treating underlying cardiac disease, and possibly the use of diuretics if the patient's kidneys can respond to them. Frequently, pulmonary edema becomes life-threatening, necessitating intubation, emergent dialysis, or both to improve arterial oxygenation and restore fluid balance.

Other pulmonary complications in renal failure include pleural effusions, pleuritic inflammation and pain, uremic pneumonitis, and pulmonary infections. Pleuritic inflammation and uremic pneumonitis are seen more frequently with stage 5 chronic kidney disease and are due to the effect of uremic toxins on the lungs and inadequate dialysis. Pulmonary infections, on the other hand, are common in both acute renal failure and chronic kidney disease, especially in critically ill patients. Factors associated with renal failure that contribute to pulmonary infections include decreased pulmonary macrophage activity, a generalized immunocompromised state, tenacious sputum, and a depressed cough reflex. Collaborative management includes culturing sputum, administering broad-spectrum antibiotics until organism-specific sensitivities are available, and teaching and encouraging pulmonary toilet measures (i.e., coughing and deep breathing).

MANAGING GASTROINTESTINAL ALTERATIONS

A potentially life-threatening gastrointestinal complication in both acute renal failure and chronic kidney disease is gastrointestinal bleeding. Proposed etiologies for gastrointestinal bleeding as it relates to renal failure include platelet and blood-clotting abnormalities; anticoagulation use associated with dialysis, access patency, or both; ingestion of irritating drugs (e.g., NSAIDs, aspirin); and increased ammonia production in the gastrointestinal tract from urea breakdown. Ammonia is known to be irritating to mucosal surfaces. Physiological stress, especially in critically ill patients, is another proposed contributor. Assessment parameters include examining all vomitus and stool for gross and occult blood; monitoring iron, hemoglobin, hematocrit, and red blood cell indices; and paying close attention to signs of intravascular volume depletion. If gastrointestinal bleeding is suspected, radiographic and endoscopic examinations are often required to diagnose and treat specific lesions. Management depends on the specific lesion but often includes volume restoration with crystalloids and blood products as well as the administration of histamine-2 receptor (H_2) blockers, proton pump inhibitors (PPIs), or both.

Other gastrointestinal complications associated with renal failure primarily occur in chronic kidney disease and include anorexia, nausea, vomiting, diarrhea, constipation, gastroesophageal reflux disease (GERD), and oral cavity alterations such as stomatitis, a metallic taste in the mouth, and uremic fetor (the smell of urine and ammonia on the breath). Oral alterations and symptoms of anorexia, nausea, and vomiting are partially attributable to high levels of uremic toxins, which affect the intestinal mucosa and stimulate vomiting centers in the brain. The reason GERD is common is unclear but may be due to alterations in the hormones that affect lower esophageal sphincter tone and a higher occurrence of hiatal hernias in patients with chronic kidney disease.[11] Collaborative management involves initiating (or providing) adequate dialysis, providing prophylactic antacids and H_2 blockers or PPIs, and administering antiemetics. Good oral hygiene is also essential.

The complication of constipation is seen frequently in patients with renal failure owing to decreased bulk and fluid in the diet and the administration of oral iron supplements and calcium-based phosphate binders. Diarrhea may also occur as a result of intestinal irritation from uremia. Collaborative management includes increasing dietary bulk; administering bulk-forming laxatives, stool softeners, or both; administering antidiarrheal agents; or a combination of these therapies. For patients with stage 5 chronic kidney disease, magnesium-containing medications, including cathartics such as magnesium citrate, should be avoided because of the risk for hypermagnesemia in these patients. In addition, Fleet enemas, which contain large amounts of phosphate that could be absorbed systemically, should not be used.

MANAGING NEUROMUSCULAR ALTERATIONS

Neuromuscular alterations include sleep disturbances, cognitive process disturbances, lethargy, muscle irritability, and peripheral neuropathies, including restless leg syndrome and burning feet syndrome. Restless leg syndrome is characterized by a discomfort in the legs, especially at night, which is sometimes relieved by continuous movement of the extremities. Burning feet syndrome consists of paresthesias and numbness in the soles of the feet and lower parts of the legs. These neuromuscular complications are associated primarily with stage 4 and 5 chronic kidney disease and are thought to be the result of electrolyte imbalances, metabolic acidosis, and the effect of uremic toxins on motor and sensory nerves. Cognitive process disturbances, such as difficulty concentrating and impaired short-term memory, are linked to elevations of BUN in the cerebral vasculature, which can result in cerebral edema. Extensive cerebral edema can result in seizures, projectile vomiting, and even coma or death.

Frequent assessments for cognitive disturbances, seizure activity, and other neuromuscular alterations are important. In addition to thorough neuromuscular examinations, nerve conduction studies and diagnostic tests, including electroencephalograms and head CT scans, may be used. Collaborative management involves implementing emergency treatment, as in the case of sustained seizure activity; maintaining electrolyte balance; correcting metabolic acidosis; using regular dialysis; and providing extensive patient teaching. Specific points that need to be included during patient teaching are the importance of preventing injury to the extremities by heat or trauma when paresthesias are present and that alterations in neuromuscular function often improve with regular dialysis or transplantation. However, if components of the patient's neuropathies are due to other comorbid conditions, such as diabetes, the problem may respond only minimally to dialysis or renal transplantation.

Cognitive alterations encountered are important to remember during any patient teaching. Because of difficulties in concentrating and impairments in short-term memory, teaching should be provided in short, frequent sessions with reinforcement of material and should include the family as much as possible. These points are especially true for critically ill patients who are, by definition, in a crisis situation.

MANAGING HEMATOLOGICAL ALTERATIONS

Hematological system alterations are major complications in acute renal failure and chronic kidney disease. These alterations include an increased bleeding tendency, an impaired immune system, and anemia.

Increased Bleeding Tendency

The increased bleeding tendency in renal failure is attributable to impaired platelet aggregation and adhesion and an altered platelet response to clotting factor VII (von Willebrand's factor). These alterations are thought to be due to uremia, but their exact pathophysiological mechanisms are unknown. Assessment involves the monitoring of platelet counts and bleeding times, coagulation studies, and assessing for bleeding, especially gastrointestinal bleeding. Collaborative management includes administering blood products as needed, protecting the patient from injury, and avoiding medications that alter platelet function, such as NSAIDs and aspirin. Often heparin (for dialysis) and aspirin (for myocardial infarction prevention) are indicated in patients with renal failure. In such cases, the effects of these medications on platelets must be closely monitored. One potential and serious complication of heparin is heparin-induced thrombocytopenia; the development of this complication mandates discontinuation of the drug.

Impairments in the Immune System

Patients with renal failure are in an immunocompromised state, which sets the stage for infections (a major cause of mortality in acute renal failure and chronic kidney disease). The impairments in the immune system are thought to be due to malnutrition and the effects of uremia on white blood cells. These effects include, among others, depressed T-cell– and antibody-mediated immunity, impaired phagocytosis, and decreased chemotaxis and adherence of white blood cells.[11]

Assessing the patient for infection and monitoring laboratory indicators of infection must be done continuously. Regarding temperature as a gauge of infection, the baseline body temperature in uremic patients is decreased, and thus any increase in temperature above baseline is significant. Collaborative management includes frequent handwashing, removing invasive catheters as soon as possible (or avoiding their use altogether), and obtaining cultures of blood and other body fluids that may be infected to identify specific organisms and determine appropriate antimicrobial therapy.

Anemia

Anemia associated with renal failure is attributable to three main mechanisms: erythropoietin deficiency, decreased red blood cell survival time, and blood loss due to an increased bleeding tendency. Of these three mechanisms, erythropoietin deficiency has the most dramatic effect.

More than 90% of the hormone erythropoietin is produced in the kidneys. It is a glycoprotein that stimulates red blood cell production in response to hypoxia and is essential to maintaining normal red blood cell counts. As kidney disease progresses and nephrons are damaged, this hormone is inadequately synthesized and a hypoproliferative anemia, resulting in normocytic normochromic red blood cells, results. Before the production of erythropoietin by human recombinant techniques, this hormone deficiency caused most patients with chronic kidney disease to be in a severely anemic state, requiring frequent blood transfusions.

Decreased red blood cell survival time in renal failure occurs in the form of a mild hemolysis. The exact mechanism for this hemolysis is unclear, but it may be related to dialysis therapy or the effect of uremia on red blood cells. The average survival of red blood cells in uremia is only 70 days, which contrasts with the normal 120-day life span of a red blood cell in the general population.

In addition to the three aforementioned mechanisms of anemia, other factors can contribute to anemia in patients with renal failure, particularly those who are critically ill. Examples are malnutrition, frequent laboratory blood sampling, dialyzer malfunction and sequestration of blood in the dialyzer, and infectious states. Treating anemia in patients with renal failure is extremely important for many different reasons, including increasing the oxygen-carrying capacity of the blood, increasing intravascular volume, and preventing the negative consequences of anemia on the cardiovascular system. Concerning the cardiovascular system, anemia exacerbates myocardial, cerebral, and peripheral ischemia and increases the risk for development (or acceleration) of left ventricular hypertrophy. Correcting anemia has also been shown to have a positive impact on quality-of-life issues in patients with renal failure, including increases in appetite, energy, and work capacity. In addition, chronic kidney disease anemia is associated with increased hospitalization rates and increased mortality in patients with chronic kidney disease.[11]

A thorough evaluation of anemia involves both diagnostic studies and a history and physical examination. Diagnostic metabolic parameters that should be obtained and monitored include hemoglobin, hematocrit, red blood cell indices, and reticulocyte counts. In addition, the stool or vomitus should be tested for occult blood. Iron studies also need to be obtained because iron deficiency itself can cause anemia and because adequate iron stores are needed for erythropoietin to be effective. Specific iron indices that should be obtained include total serum iron, total iron-binding capacity, and serum ferritin levels. Finally, nutritional parameters and levels of folic acid, pyridoxine, and vitamin B_{12}, all of which affect red blood cell production, need to be monitored.

A thorough history and physical examination involves questioning patients about potential sites of bleeding (e.g., by asking about stool color), assessing for signs and symptoms of anemia (i.e., angina, tachycardia, skin and mucous membrane pallor, appetite suppression, weight loss, decreased energy levels, fatigue), assessing for sources of blood loss, assessing for inflammation or infection, and assessing for other diseases that can cause anemia (e.g., lupus, sickle cell anemia).

Collaborative management of anemia includes minimizing blood loss, administering oral or IV iron supplements, providing vitamin supplementation, aggressively treating infections, ensuring adequate nutrition, and administering human erythropoietin (rHuEPO) or darbepoetin (an analogue of rHuEPO), blood products, or both. Goals for iron therapy and rHuEPO or darbepoetin administration in the chronic kidney disease population are a transferrin saturation greater than 20%, serum ferritin levels greater than 100 ng/mL (greater than 200 ng/mL for dialysis patients), and a hemoglobin level of 11 to 12 g/dL. These goals and guidelines to achieve them are detailed in the K/DOQI guidelines on anemia.[48]

Certain points regarding rHuEPO or darbepoetin therapy and the management of anemia deserve special mention. One is that the full effect of these medications takes weeks to achieve, and hence in patients with profound anemia, blood administration is indicated. In addition, rHuEPO or darbepoetin administration may result in an elevation of blood pressure. In some cases, modification of antihypertensive therapy may be needed. When there is an inadequate response to rHuEPO or darbepoetin despite increased dosages, reasons for erythropoietin resistance need to be explored. These include occult infections, inflammatory states, human immunodeficiency virus infection, hyperparathyroidism, aluminum toxicity, malnutrition, iron deficiency, and bone marrow malignancy.

Important clinical features regarding iron preparations should also be considered by the nurse. One is that oral iron is poorly absorbed if taken with phosphate binders, antacids, H_2 blockers, or PPIs, all of which are commonly prescribed to patients with renal failure. On the other hand, IV iron has much better bioavailability but carries the risk for an allergic, sometimes life-threatening, reaction.

Extensive patient teaching about anemia is crucial. At minimum, teaching should include information about medication therapy; timing of iron supplements; potential causes, signs, and symptoms of worsening anemia; and energy conservation techniques. Instruction about measures to decrease bleeding, such as use of a soft toothbrush and avoidance of NSAIDs, is also helpful.

MANAGING ALTERATIONS IN DRUG ELIMINATION

Because many pharmacological agents, their metabolites, or both are excreted by the kidneys, extreme caution must be used when administering medication to patients with renal failure. Depending on the patient's GFR, adjustments may need to be made in drug dosage, the interval between drug dosages, or both. Important to consider, especially in acute renal failure, is that the GRF is often unstable, and thus the GFR must be monitored frequently to determine dosages accurately. As in patients without renal failure, monitoring serum levels of certain medications to be sure they are within the therapeutic range is essential. For patients receiving dialysis, the health care team must be cognizant of which drugs are dialyzed out during therapy to ensure appropriate timing of drug administration. For a listing of frequently encountered antimicrobial agents in critical care that are affected by renal failure, hemodialysis, or both, see Table 31-3.

MANAGING SKELETAL ALTERATIONS

In renal failure, disturbances in calcium and phosphate balance occur and set the stage for secondary hyperparathyroidism and high-turnover renal osteodystrophy (renal bone disease). As the GFR declines, glomerular filtration of phosphate also decreases, and serum phosphate levels begin to rise. This results in decreased serum ionized calcium levels because of binding of the calcium with the phosphate. Calcium levels also decrease because of the failing kidneys' inability to convert vitamin D to its active form (1,25-dihydroxycholecalciferol, or vitamin D_3), which is needed for adequate intestinal absorption of calcium. In response to decreased ionized calcium levels, elevations in serum phosphorus, and reduced vitamin D_3 synthesis, the parathyroid glands secrete parathyroid hormone (PTH). Over time, the continuous PTH stimulation leads to hyperplasia and proliferation of the parathyroid cells, resulting in secondary hyperparathyroidism. PTH causes the reabsorption of calcium and phosphate salts from bones, thus increasing the serum calcium level at the expense of bone density and mass. PTH also causes calcium reabsorption and phosphate excretion in the kidneys; however, as renal failure progresses, this effect of PTH is not realized. Eventually, as calcium and phosphate continue to be reabsorbed from bones, both levels rise in the serum concomitantly. This results in an elevation in the normal calcium–phosphate product (serum calcium multiplied by serum phosphate) of less than 40 mg/dL. When the product exceeds 55 mg/dL, calcium phosphate crystals can form and precipitate in various parts of the body (a condition known as metastatic calcifications), including the brain, eyes, gums, valves of the heart, myocardium, lungs, joints, blood vessels, and skin. Other insults to bones that can occur in renal disease include bone demineralization in response to metabolic acidosis and low-turnover renal osteodystrophy due to aluminum deposits in the bone or overuse of vitamin D_3 therapy. The events related to high-turnover renal osteodystrophy in renal failure are summarized in Figure 31-5.

Complications resulting from renal bone disease include bone pain, fractures, pseudogout from deposits of calcium oxalate in synovial fluid, periarthritis from calcifications of the joints, proximal muscle weakness, spontaneous tendon rupture, and pruritus. Metastatic calcifications can result in calcified blood vessels and valves, skin lesions, red-eye syndrome from crystal deposition in the conjunctiva, and, most seriously, ischemic ulcers. Laboratory data, including levels of calcium, phosphate, aluminum, alkaline phosphatase, and intact PTH, help make the diagnosis. Radiographic findings also may be helpful, particularly in high-turnover bone disease; images may reveal subperiosteal bone thinning, most easily seen in the hands and clavicles. A bone biopsy, considered the gold standard for obtaining a definitive diagnosis of renal bone disease, is not routinely performed secondary to patient discomfort and controversy surrounding the indications for this invasive test.

Management involves phosphate regulation, maintenance of normal calcium levels, treatment of vitamin D deficiency, suppression of PTH, prevention of aluminum toxicity, and controlling metabolic acidosis. Measures to control phosphate levels include dietary restrictions and phosphate-binding medications. Commonly used phosphate binders are calcium acetate (Phos-lo), calcium carbonate (Tums), sevelamer hydrochloride (Renagel), and lanthanum carbonate (Fosrenol). Sevelamer and lanthanum carbonate are calcium-free phosphate binders and are preferred over calcium-based binders in patients with high calcium levels because they lessen the risk for hypercalcemia and further elevations in the calcium–phosphate product. Aluminum hydroxide binders, once a mainstay of therapy, are now infrequently used because of the effects of aluminum toxicity on the bones as well as the nervous system. Aluminum toxicity causes erythropoietin resistance as well.

According to the K/DOQI Clinical Practice Guidelines, calcium levels should be maintained in the normal range, preferably toward the lower end of normal (8.4 to 9.5 mg/dL).[49] This is accomplished with diet and calcium supplements. If calcium levels exceed 10.2 mg/dL, therapies that may be contributing to hypercalcemia (e.g., administering calcium or vitamin D supplements) should be adjusted to reduce the risk for extraskeletal calcifications.

Vitamin D supplements are administered to suppress PTH secretion. Besides causing a decrease in PTH indirectly through the elevation of serum calcium, active vitamin D also directly inhibits PTH secretion by binding to vitamin D receptors on the parathyroid gland. Active vitamin D may be given orally (calcitriol) or intravenously (Calcijex). In either case, caution must be exercised with the administration of these agents to avoid hypercalcemia and hyperphosphatemia, as well as to avoid oversuppression of the parathyroid gland. Two synthetic analogues of active vitamin D that can also be used are paricalcitol (Zemplar) and doxercalciferol (Hectorol). These drugs have the advantage of causing less dramatic increases in serum calcium and phosphate levels while still causing PTH suppression.

The most recent therapeutic agents developed to help suppress PTH and the development of secondary hyperparathyroidism are calcimimetics, which work by increasing the sensitivity of the calcium-sensing receptor in the parathyroid gland to extracellular calcium. In the United States, the Food and Drug Administration approved the calcimimetic cinacalcet hydrochloride (Sensipar) for patients with ESRD. Thus far, it has been shown to be both safe and efficacious, with the most common side effects being nausea and vomiting and hypocalcemia.[50] Rarely, for patients who are refractory to available treatments for secondary hyperparathyroidism, including vitamin D

Table 31-3 • Impact of Renal Failure and Hemodialysis on Commonly Used Antimicrobials in Critical Care

Drug	Drug Renally Excreted (%)	Adjustment for Renal Failure (Glomerular Filtration Rate [mL/min/1.73 m²])		Effect of Hemodialysis
		10–50	<10	
*Aminoglycosides**				
Amikacin†	95	100% of normal dose q24–48h	100% of normal dose q48–72h	Dialyzed
Gentamicin†	95	100% of normal dose q24–48h	100% of normal dose q48–72h	Dialyzed
Tobramycin†	95	100% of normal dose q24–48h	100% of normal dose q48–72h	Dialyzed
Cephalosporins				
Cefazolin†	75–95	100% of normal dose q12h	100% of normal dose q24–48h	Dialyzed
Cefepime†	85	100% of normal dose q16–24h	100% of normal dose q24–48h	Dialyzed
Cefotaxime (active metabolite in end-stage renal disease)	60	100% of normal dose q8–12h	100% of normal dose q24h	Dialyzed
Cefotetan	75	50% of normal dose	25% of normal dose	Dialyzed
Ceftazidime	60–85	100% of normal dose q24–48h	100% of normal dose q48h	Dialyzed
Ceftriaxone	30–65	Normal dose	Normal dose	Dialyzed
Penicillins				
Amoxicillin	50–70	100% of normal dose q8–12h	100% of normal dose q24h	Dialyzed
Ampicillin	30–90	100% of normal dose q6–12h	100% of normal dose q12–24h	Dialyzed
Mezlocillin	65	100% of normal dose q6–8h	100% of normal dose q8h	Not dialyzed
Nafcillin	35	Normal dose	Normal dose	Not dialyzed
Penicillin G	60–85	75% of normal dose	20%–50% of normal dose	Dialyzed
Piperacillin	75–90	100% of normal dose q6–8h	100% of normal dose q8h	Dialyzed
Ticarcillin†	85	1–2 g q8h	1–2 g q12h	Dialyzed
Quinolones				
Ciprofloxacin	50–70	50%–75% of normal dose	50% of normal dose	Slightly dialyzed
Levofloxacin	67–87	250 mg q24–48h (500 mg initial dose)	250 mg q48h (500 mg initial dose)	No data
Tetracyclines				
Doxycycline	35–45	Normal dose	Normal dose	Not dialyzed
Tetracycline†	48–60	100% of normal dose q12–24h	100% of normal dose q24h	Not dialyzed
Miscellaneous Antibacterials				
Azithromycin	6–12	Normal dose	Normal dose	Not dialyzed
Aztreonam	75	50%–75% of normal dose	25% of normal dose	Moderately dialyzed
Clarithromycin	15–25	75% of normal dose	50%–75% of normal dose	No data; give after dialysis
Erythromycin	15	Normal dose	50%–75% of normal dose	Not dialyzed
Imipenem	20–70	50% of normal dose	25% of normal dose	Dialyzed
Metronidazole	20	Normal dose	50% of normal dose	Dialyzed
Sulfamethoxazole	70	100% of normal dose q18h	100% of normal dose q24h	Dialyzed
Trimethoprim	40–70	100% of normal dose q18h	100% of normal dose q24h	Dialyzed
Vancomycin†	90–100	1.0 g q24–96h	1.0 g q4–7d	Not dialyzed
Linezolid‡	30	Normal dose	Normal dose	Not dialyzed
Antifungals				
Amphotericin B	5–10	Normal dose	100% of normal dose q24–36h	Not dialyzed
Fluconazole	70	Normal dose	Normal dose	Dialyzed
Ketoconazole	13	Normal dose	Normal dose	Not dialyzed
Antiviral				
Acyclovir	40–75	100% of normal dose q12–24h	50% of normal dose q24h	Dialyzed
Ganciclovir	90–100	100% of normal dose q24–48h	100% of normal dose q48–96h	Dialyzed
Antitubercular				
Amantadine†	90	100% of normal dose q48–72h	100% of normal dose q7d	Not dialyzed
Ethambutol	75–90	100% of normal dose q24–36h	100% of normal dose q48h	Dialyzed
Isoniazid	5–30	Normal dose	Normal dose	Dialyzed
Rifampin	15–30	50%–100% of normal dose	50%–100% of normal dose	Not dialyzed

*Aminoglycosides are nephrotoxic and ototoxic and have a narrow therapeutic window. Serum levels must be monitored frequently for efficacy and toxicity.

†These drugs have adjustment in dose and/or frequency when a patient's GFR is > 50 mL/min as well.

‡Metabolites may accumulate in renal failure; significance unknown.

Modified from Aronoff G, Berns J, Brier M, et al: Drug Prescribing in Renal Failure, 4th ed. Philadelphia: American College of Physicians, 1999. Updates from The Renal Drug Book online edition providing dose guidelines for adult drug prescriptions in renal failure. Available at: http://www.kdp-baptist.louisville.edu/renalbook/. Accessed 2006.

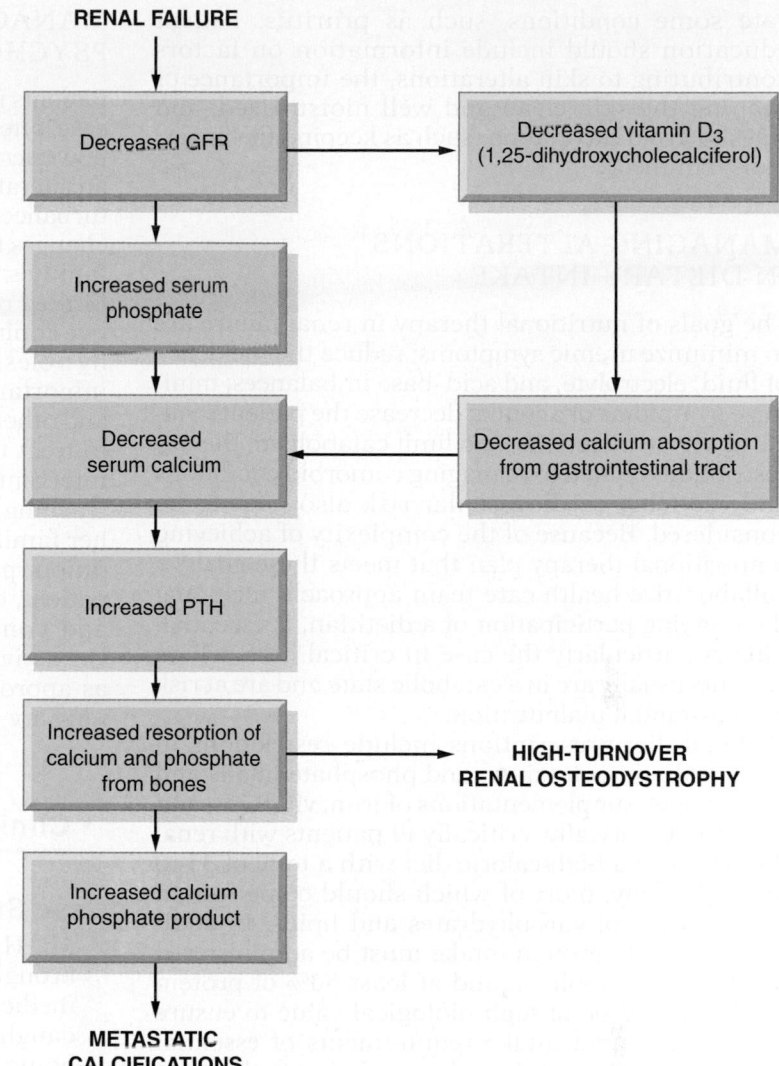

RENAL FAILURE

Decreased GFR → Decreased vitamin D₃ (1,25-dihydroxycholecalciferol)

Decreased GFR → Increased serum phosphate

Increased serum phosphate → Decreased serum calcium

Decreased vitamin D₃ (1,25-dihydroxycholecalciferol) → Decreased calcium absorption from gastrointestinal tract → Decreased serum calcium

Decreased serum calcium → Increased PTH

Increased PTH → Increased resorption of calcium and phosphate from bones → **HIGH-TURNOVER RENAL OSTEODYSTROPHY**

Increased resorption of calcium and phosphate from bones → Increased calcium phosphate product → **METASTATIC CALCIFICATIONS**

Figure 31-5 • Effects of renal failure on the skeletal system.

therapy and calcimimetics, a parathyroidectomy may be necessary.

Patient teaching concerning bone disease and its management is complex and needs to be continually reinforced. Particular areas that should be included are the purpose and timing of medications (e.g., phosphate binders must be given with meals to be effective), dietary modifications, and the complications of untreated bone disease.

MANAGING INTEGUMENTARY ALTERATIONS

Alterations in the integumentary system in renal failure include xerosis (dryness), pruritus, pallor, ecchymosis and purpura, and a pale bronze skin discoloration. Contributing factors to these alterations are anemia, decreased activity of sweat and sebaceous glands, retained skin pigments, platelet dysfunction and capillary fragility, deposition of calcium phosphate crystals into the skin, hyperparathyroidism, hyperphosphatemia, and possibly increased mast cell activity and histamine secretion.

In patients with an arteriovenous fistula or graft, pseudo-Kaposi's sarcoma may develop in the area of the fistula, graft, or hands due to overflow of blood or insufficient blood drainage from the area. Patients with stage 5 chronic kidney disease may also experience bullous lesions and bullous dermatosis, especially male patients who have been on dialysis for long periods.[11] Uremic frost, a white, powdery substance composed of urates on the skin, is due to crystallization of urea. It is usually seen only in severely uremic patients for whom needed dialytic therapy is being withheld. These skin alterations, particularly pruritus and xerosis, may lead to localized infection from excoriation. In addition, substantial patient discomfort and psychological disturbances from skin disfigurement may occur.

Collaborative management for skin alterations includes phosphate regulation, active vitamin D administration, correction of anemia, antihistamine medications, and meticulous skin care and turning to prevent skin breakdown. Dialysis therapy helps as well by removing metabolic waste products. However, because of potential allergies to the dialysis system components, dialysis therapy can also aggravate some conditions, such as pruritus. Patient education should include information on factors contributing to skin alterations, the importance of keeping the skin clean and well moisturized, and ways to avoid excoriation (such as keeping the fingernails trimmed).

MANAGING ALTERATIONS IN DIETARY INTAKE

The goals of nutritional therapy in renal failure are to minimize uremic symptoms; reduce the incidence of fluid, electrolyte, and acid–base imbalances; minimize symptoms of anemia; decrease the patient's vulnerability to infections; and limit catabolism. Dietary restrictions related to managing comorbid conditions and reducing cardiovascular risk also need to be considered. Because of the complexity of achieving a nutritional therapy plan that meets these goals, a collaborative health care team approach, including the ongoing participation of a dietitian, is essential. This is particularly the case in critical care, where patients usually are in a catabolic state and are at risk for substantial malnutrition.

Renal diet prescriptions include restrictions in fluid, sodium, potassium, and phosphate intake and may include supplementations of iron, vitamins, and calcium. Calorically, critically ill patients with renal disease need a high-calorie diet with a total of 35 to 45 kcal/kg/day, most of which should come from a combination of carbohydrates and lipids. In addition, adequate protein intake must be administered to prevent catabolism, and at least 50% of protein intake should be of high biological value to ensure that the minimal intake requirements of essential amino acids are met. Protein restriction to decrease symptoms of uremia and slow the progression of renal failure is controversial (refer to the section on preventing the progression of chronic kidney disease) but may be beneficial. However, protein restriction should never compromise meeting anabolic goals, which would expose the patient to the risk for malnutrition. For patients with chronic kidney disease, the K/DOQI guidelines recommend a moderate protein restriction of 0.6 to 0.8 g/kg/day in patients not yet receiving dialysis and from 1.2 to 1.3 g/kg/day in patients on dialysis.[51] In critically ill patients, parenteral nutrition may need to be instituted because of impaired bowel function or severe malnutrition. In oliguric patients, the high hourly volume requirements needed for parenteral nutrition often must be offset by dialysis or isolated ultrafiltration.

To determine the effectiveness of nutritional therapy, continual laboratory monitoring of serum protein, cholesterol, albumin and prealbumin, electrolytes, hemoglobin, hematocrit, and urea and creatinine levels is essential. Patient weight, volume status, and energy levels are additional monitoring parameters. Nutritional education, including information on dietary restrictions, the use and timing of phosphate binders, vitamin and mineral supplements, and measures of nutritional status should be provided.

MANAGING ALTERATIONS IN PSYCHOSOCIAL FUNCTIONING

Patients in acute renal failure and chronic kidney disease often experience feelings of fear, anxiety, and powerlessness. In addition, patients frequently have an alteration in self-concept as well as body image disturbances because of both physical and functional changes that occur in renal failure. Patients and their families may have difficulty coping owing to stress, limited resources or support, inadequate or ineffective coping mechanisms, interruptions in usual family roles, or a combination of these factors. It is important that the health care team attend to these and other psychosocial complications of renal failure to treat the patient and family holistically. Specific interventions include thorough patient and family teaching, active involvement of the patient and his or her family members in the management of the condition, provision of adequate rest and sleep to the patient, exploring the patient's and family's feelings and concerns, providing support, and obtaining the active involvement of social services and clergy as appropriate. Considerations for discharge planning are given in Box 31-9.

• Clinical Applicability Challenges

Case Study

Mr. H., a 72-year-old African American, is brought to the emergency department by paramedics. According to the paramedics, Mr. H.'s daughter found her father unconscious in his home. Two days ago, when she last saw him, he "seemed slightly more confused than normal but otherwise okay." His past medical history is notable for hypertension, type 2 diabetes mellitus, chronic kidney disease (stage 3), "mild" dementia, and benign prostatic hypertrophy. Every day he takes the following medications: aspirin, 81 mg; lisinopril, 5 mg; Norvasc, 10 mg; atorvastatin, 20 mg; glipizide XL, 5 mg; and tamsulosin, 0.4 mg. His baseline serum creatinine and estimated glomerular filtration rate, determined in a routine clinic visit less than 2 weeks ago, are 2.0 mg/dL and 56 mL/min/1.73 m², respectively.

On presentation, Mr. H. is responsive to painful stimuli. Vital signs are: blood pressure, 80/40 mm Hg; heart rate, 130 beats/minute and regular; respirations, 28 breaths/minutes; and rectal temperature, 101.3°F (38.5°C). Physical examination shows temporal wasting; dry mucous membranes; clear bilateral breath sounds; tachycardia without any rubs, gallops, or murmurs; a soft abdomen, but grimacing on deep palpation, normal active bowel sounds in all quadrants, and no organomegaly or masses; no edema in the extremities or diminished distal pulses; and no tenting or rashes on the skin.

Box 31-9 • DISCHARGE PLANNING GUIDE: Acute Renal Failure

- Explain the pathophysiology of acute renal failure in understandable terms. Use appropriate teaching aids (e.g., pictures, kidney models).
- Explain the etiology of acute renal failure and ways to decrease risk for further or future kidney damage, including control of hypertension, strict control of blood glucose levels (in patients with diabetes), the maintenance of normal serum lipid levels, and the avoidance of nephrotoxins.
- Explain the level of renal function the patient can expect to have after the acute phase is over.
- Explain and provide written guidelines on diet and fluid restrictions. Teach the patient how to reduce thirst (e.g., by sucking on sour, hard candy) and stress that any substance that is liquid at room temperature counts as fluid intake.
- Demonstrate how to check blood pressure, pulse, respirations, and weight. Teach the patient about the importance of weighing himself or herself at the same time, on the same scale, and with similar amounts of clothing to monitor weight accurately.
- Provide instruction on how to monitor for and avoid infections. Instruct the patient to report any occurrence of an infection to a health care professional.
- Describe the purpose, action, and adverse effects of medications. Point out when medications need to be taken (e.g., phosphate binders are taken with meals) and what medications should not be taken together.
- Explain the importance of rest during the recovery phase; assist the patient in planning for exercise as tolerated.
- Teach the patient ways to minimize the risk for bleeding.
- Explain the purpose of dialysis and the importance of regular treatments.
- Explain the need for ongoing follow-up with health care professionals.

Initial laboratory studies are notable for the following: sodium, 158 mEq/L; potassium, 5.8 mEq/L; chloride, 98 mEq/L; carbon dioxide, 14 mEq/L; blood urea nitrogen (BUN), 127 mg/dL; creatinine, 8.5 mg/dL; white blood cell count, 20,000/mm³ with 85% neutrophils; hemoglobin, 14g/dL; hematocrit, 47%; urinalysis—specific gravity, 1.030, +1 protein, +1 blood; and urine microbiology—too numerous to count white blood cells, 3 to 5 red blood cells and dark muddy casts, and renal tubular epithelial cells. Arterial blood gases on room air show: pH, 7.2, $PaCO_2$, 25 mm Hg; and PaO_2, 75 mm Hg. A chest radiograph shows no infiltrates. An electrocardiogram shows sinus tachycardia, left ventricular hypertrophy, and no ischemic changes. Additional diagnostic testing reveals a normal total creatine phosphokinase and serum troponin, urine sodium of 45 mEq/L, FE_{Na} of greater than 2%, and FE_{UN} of 66%.

Mr. H. is admitted to the intensive care unit (ICU). His blood pressure remains tenuous despite 2.5 L of normal saline, and he is placed on a dopamine infusion to keep his mean arterial pressure greater than 65 mm Hg. His first hospital day is notable for persistent fever ($T_{max} = 102.2°F$ [$39°C$]) and hemodynamic instability. Blood and urine cultures return positive for *Escherichia coli* sensitive to piperacillin/tazobactam. Repeat laboratory studies on ICU day 1 reveal the following: sodium, 148 mEq/L; potassium, 6 mEq/L; chloride, 105 mEq/L; carbon dioxide, 12 mEq/L; BUN, 134 mg/dL; and creatinine 8.7 mg/dL. Urine output for the first 24 hours is only 50 mL.

Renal ultrasound reveals no hydronephrosis. Kidneys are 9 cm bilaterally and echogenic. Repeat arterial blood gases on 50% oxygen are now pH, 7.2; $PaCO_2$, 33 mm Hg; and PaO_2, 83 mm Hg. Mr. H. is intubated. A chest radiograph obtained after intubation shows prominent pulmonary arteries with diffuse alveolar infiltrates consistent with pulmonary edema. The nephrologist who is consulted recommends continuous renal replacement therapy.

1. What is the cause of Mr. H.'s acute renal failure?
2. Is Mr. H.'s acute renal failure prerenal or intrarenal?
3. What acid–base disorder does Mr. H. have? Explain your answer.
4. Why does the nephrologist recommend dialysis for Mr. H?

Review Questions

1. A male patient has been diagnosed with acute renal failure post–myocardial infarction. Laboratory and urine values before diuretic administration are: blood urea nitrogen–to-creatinine ratio of 20:1, benign urinary sediment, and FE_{Na} less than 1%. These results are reflective of what type of acute renal failure?
   a. Prerenal
   b. Intrarenal
   c. Postrenal
   d. Cannot determine type

2. A female patient is in the oliguric phase of acute tubular necrosis due to ischemia secondary to sepsis. Which of the following potential complications is she most at risk for developing?
   a. Hyponatremia, hypokalemia, infection, and vascular volume overload
   b. Hypercalcemia, gastrointestinal bleeding, vascular volume depletion, and infection
   c. Hyperkalemia, gastrointestinal bleeding, infection, and vascular volume overload
   d. Hyperkalemia, hyponatremia, vascular volume depletion, and infection

3. A woman with stage 5 chronic kidney disease is admitted to the intensive care unit for an arterio-

venous graft infection. Before admission, her hemoglobin has been stable at 11.0 mg/dL on 10,000 units of intravenous erythropoietin with every hemodialysis treatment. The nurse notices her hemoglobin is now 9.7 mg/dL despite increases in erythropoietin dosage. What are the most common causes that may account for her resistant anemia?

a. Low iron stores, infection, and elevated folic acid levels
b. Low iron stores, infection, and gastrointestinal losses
c. Metabolic acidosis, bone marrow suppression, and gastrointestinal losses
d. Frequent phlebotomy, vitamin D_3 deficiency, and gastrointestinal losses

4. A woman presents to the emergency department with a potassium level of 8.5 mEq/L and a widened QRS interval on electrocardiography after missing two previous dialysis treatments. What emergency treatment for hyperkalemia may be given to antagonize the effects of potassium on her heart?

a. 1 ampule of intravenous calcium gluconate
b. 10 units of intravenous regular insulin and 1 ampule of D_{50}
c. 1 ampule of intravenous sodium bicarbonate
d. 30 g of oral sodium polystyrene

5. A woman is diagnosed with acute renal failure secondary to aminoglycoside toxicity. She complains of nausea, vomiting, and lethargy and is noted to have deep, rapid respirations. What acid–base disturbance would you expect to see based on her diagnosis and these clinical findings?

a. Respiratory alkalosis secondary to hyperventilation
b. Respiratory acidosis secondary to hyperventilation
c. Metabolic alkalosis secondary to acute renal failure
d. Metabolic acidosis secondary to acute renal failure

6. A male patient with chronic kidney disease has secondary hyperparathyroidism. He is managed with phosphate binders and vitamin D_3 therapy. He has trouble with medication compliance, and his wife asks what he risks if he stops taking the medications?

a. Progressive loss of appetite
b. Hypercalcemia
c. Bone demineralization
d. Metabolic acidosis

7. During her hospitalization, a woman is found to have proteinuria and subsequently is diagnosed with stage 2 chronic kidney disease due to diabetes. She confides in the nurse that she is afraid of the possibility that she may need dialysis in the future and asks how she can slow disease progression. Which of the following would be an appropriate response as to how she may slow progression of chronic kidney disease?

a. Maintain a low-potassium diet, compliance with an angiotensin-converting enzyme inhibitor drug, and daily exercise
b. Maintain a high-protein diet, compliance with an angiotensin-converting enzyme inhibitor drug, and weight loss
c. Maintain a low-phosphorus diet, compliance with an angiotensin-converting enzyme inhibitor drug, and strict glycemic control
d. Strict glycemic control, compliance with an angiotensin-converting enzyme inhibitor drug, and strict blood pressure control

References

1. Needham E: Management of acute renal failure. Am Fam Physician 72(9):1739–1746, 2005
2. Singri N, Ahya S, Levin M: Acute renal failure. JAMA 289(6): 747–751, 2003
3. Schrier R, Wang W, Poole B, Mitra A: Acute renal failure: Definitions, diagnosis, pathogenesis, and therapy. J Clin Invest 114(1):5–14, 2004
4. Ympa Y, Sakr Y, Reinhart K, et al: Has mortality from acute renal failure decreased? A systematic review of the literature. Am J Med 118(8):827–832, 2005
5. Joannidis M, Metnitz P: Epidemiology and natural history of acute renal failure in the ICU. Crit Care Clin 21(2):239–249, 2005
6. Bagshaw S, Laupland K, Doig C, et al: Prognosis for long-term survival and renal recovery in critically ill patients with severe acute renal failure: A population-based study. Crit Care 9(6):R700–R709, 2005
7. Wald R, Deshponde R, Bell C, et al: Survival to discharge among patients treated with continuous renal replacement therapy. Hemodial Int 10(1):82–87, 2006
8. Uchino S, Kellum J, Bellomo R, et al: Acute renal failure in critically ill patients: A multinational, multicenter study. JAMA 294(7):813–818, 2005
9. Manns B, Doig C, Lee H, et al: Cost of acute renal failure requiring dialysis in the intensive care unit: Clinical and resource implication of renal recovery. Crit Care Med 31(2):449–455, 2003
10. Lameire N: The pathophysiology of acute renal failure. Crit Care Clin 21(2):197–210, 2005
11. Molzahn A, Butera E (eds): Contemporary Nephrology Nursing: Principles and Practice, 2nd ed. Pitman, NJ: AJ Jannetti, 2006
12. Olsen K, Rudis M, Rebuck J, et al: Effect of once-daily dosing vs multiple daily dosing of tobramycin on enzyme markers of nephrotoxicity. Crit Care Med 32(8):1678–1682, 2004
13. Rougier F, Claude D, Maurin M, et al: Aminoglycoside nephrotoxicity. Curr Drug Targets Infect Disord 4(2):153–162, 2004
14. Finn W: The clinical and renal consequences of contrast-induced nephropathy. Nephrol Dial Transplant 21(Suppl 1): i2–i10, 2006
15. Toprak O, Cirit M: Risk factors and therapy strategies for contrast-induced nephropathy. Ren Fail 28(5):365–381, 2006
16. Lameire N: Contrast-induced nephropathy: Prevention and risk reduction. Nephrol Dial Transplant 21(Suppl 1):i11–i23, 2006
17. Merten G, Burgess W, Gray L, et al: Prevention of contrast-induced nephropathy with sodium bicarbonate: A randomized controlled trial. JAMA 291(19):2328–2334, 2004
18. Fishbane S, Durham J, Marzo K, et al: N-acetylcysteine in the prevention of radiocontrast-induced nephropathy. J Am Soc Nephrol 15(2):251–260, 2004
19. Kshirsagar A, Poole C, Mottl A, et al: N-acetylcysteine for the prevention of radiocontrast induced nephropathy: A meta-analysis of prospective controlled trials. J Am Soc Nephrol 15(3):761–769, 2004

20. Nallamothu B, Shajaniak K, Saint S, et al: Is acetylcysteine effective in preventing contrast-related nephropathy? A meta-analysis. Am J Med 117(12):938–947, 2004

21. Rieger J, Sitter T, Toepfer M, et al: Gadolinium as an alternative contrast agent for diagnostic and interventional angiographic procedures in patients with impaired renal function. Nephrol Dial Transplant 17(5):824–828, 2002

22. Erley C, Bader B, Berger E, et al: Gadolinium-based contrast media compared with iodinated media for digital subtraction angiography in azotaemic patients. Nephrol Dial Transplant 19(10):2526–2531, 2004

23. Galan A, Cowper S, Bucala R, et al: Nephrogenic systemic fibrosis (nephrogenic fibrosing dermopathy). Curr Opin Rheumatol 18(6):614–617, 2006

24. Lamb E, O'Riordan S, Delaney M: Kidney function in older people: Pathology, assessment and management. Clin Chim Acta 334(1–2):25–40, 2003

25. Carvounis C, Nisar S, Guro-Razuman S: Significance of the fractional excretion of urea in the differential diagnosis of acute renal failure. Kidney Int 62(6):2223–2229, 2002

26. Liss P, Eklof H, Hellberg O, et al: Renal effects of CO_2 and iodinated contrast media in patients undergoing renovascular intervention: A prospective, randomized study. J Vasc Intervent Radiol 16(1):57–65, 2005

27. U.S. Renal Data System: USRDS 2006 Annual Data Report: Atlas of End-Stage Renal Disease in the United States, National Institutes of Health, National Institute of Diabetes and Digestive and Kidney Diseases, Bethesda, MD, 2006.

28. National Kidney Foundation: K/DOQI clinical practice guidelines for chronic kidney disease: Evaluation, classification, and stratification. Am J Kidney Dis 39(2 Suppl 1):S1–S266, 2002

29. Remuzzi G, Ruggenenti P, Perico N: Chronic renal diseases: Renoprotective benefits of renin-angiotensin system inhibition. Ann Intern Med 136(8):604–615, 2002

30. Coresh J, Astor B, Greene T, et al: Prevalence of chronic kidney disease and decreased kidney function in the adult US population: Third National Health and Nutrition Examination Survey. Am J Kidney Dis 41(1):1–12, 2003

31. Coresh J, Byrd-Holt D, Astor B, et al: Chronic kidney disease awareness, prevalence, and trends among U.S. adults, 1999–2000. J Am Soc Nephrol 16(1):180–188, 2005

32. Yu H: Progression of chronic renal failure. Arch Intern Med 163(12):1417–1429, 2003

33. National Kidney Foundation: Diabetes and Kidney Disease, 2006. Retrieved August 4, 2006, from http://www.kidney.org/atoz/atozltem.cfm?id=37

34. Diabetes Control and Complications Trial Research Group: The effect of intensive treatment of diabetes on the development and progression of long-term complications in insulin-dependent diabetes mellitus. N Engl J Med 329(14):977–986, 1993

35. Sustained effect of intensive treatment of type I diabetes mellitus on development and progression of diabetic nephropathy: The Epidemiology of Diabetes Interventions and Complications (EDIC) study. JAMA 290(16):2159–2167, 2003

36. UK Prospective Diabetes Study (UKPDS) Group: Intensive blood-glucose control with sulphonylureas of insulin compared with conventional treatment and risk of complications in patients with type 2 diabetes (UKPDS 33). Lancet 352(9131):837–853, 1998

37. Toto R: Hypertensive nephrosclerosis in African Americans. Kidney Int 64(6):2331–2341, 2003

38. American Diabetes Association: Standards of medical care. Diabetes Care 28(Suppl 1):S4–S36, 2005

39. National Kidney Foundation: K/DOQI clinical practice guidelines on blood pressure management and use of antihypertensive agents in chronic kidney disease. Am J Kidney Dis 43(Suppl 1):S1–S268, 2004

40. Mitch W, Remuzzi G: Diets for patients with chronic kidney disease, still worth prescribing? J Am Soc Nephrol 15(1):234–237, 2004

41. Zandi-Nejad K, Brenner B: Strategies to retard the progression of chronic kidney disease. Med Clin North Am 89(3):489–509, 2005

42. Davis A, Gooch I: Best evidence topic report: The use of loop diuretics in acute renal failure in critically ill patients to reduce mortality, maintain renal function, or avoid the requirements for renal support. Emerg Med J 23(7):569–570, 2006

43. Cantarovich F, Rangoonwala B, Lorenz H, et al: High-dose furosemide for established ARF: A prospective, randomized, double-blind, placebo-controlled, multicenter trial. Am J Kidney Dis 44(3):402–409, 2004

44. Friedrich J, Adnikari N, Herridge M, et al: Meta-analysis: Low-dose dopamine increased urine output but does not prevent renal dysfunction or death. Ann Intern Med 142(7):510–524, 2005

45. Sarnak M, Levey A, Schoolwerth A, et al: Kidney disease as a risk factor for development of cardiovascular disease: A statement from the American Heart Association Councils on Kidney in Cardiovascular Disease, High Blood Pressure Research, Clinical Cardiology, and Epidemiology and Prevention. Circulation 118(17):2154–2169, 2003

46. Chobanian A, Bakris G, Black H, et al: National Heart, Lung and Blood Institute Joint National Committee on Prevention, Detection, Evaluation and Treatment of High Blood Pressure; National High Blood Pressure Education Program Coordinating Committee. The Seventh Report of the Joint National Committee on Prevention, Detection, Evaluation, and Treatment of High Blood Pressure: The JNC 7 report. JAMA 289(19):2560–2572, 2003

47. National Kidney Foundation: K/DOQI clinical practice guidelines on managing dyslipidemias in chronic kidney disease. Am J Kidney Dis 41(Suppl 3):S1–S77, 2003

48. National Kidney Foundation: K/DOQI clinical practice guidelines and clinical practice recommendations for anemia in chronic kidney disease in adults. Am J Kidney Dis 47(5 Suppl 3):S16–S85, 2006

49. National Kidney Foundation: K/DOQI clinical practice guidelines for bone metabolism and disease in chronic kidney disease. Am J Kidney Dis 42(Suppl 3):S1–S210, 2003

50. Brommage D, Gallgano C: The role of cinacalcet in treating secondary hyperparathyroidism. Nephrol Nurs J 32(2):229–231, 2005

51. National Kidney Foundation: K/DOQI clinical practice guidelines for nutrition in chronic renal failure. Am J Kidney Dis 35(6 Suppl 2):S1–S140, 2000

Other Selected Readings

Bro S: How abnormal calcium, phosphate, and parathyroid hormone relate to cardiovascular disease. Nephrol Nurs J 30(3):275–283, 2003

Broscious S, Castagnola J: Chronic kidney disease: Acute manifestations and role of critical care nurses. Crit Care Nurse 26(4):17–29, 2006

Burrows-Hudson S: Chronic kidney disease: An overview. Am J Nurs 105(2):40–49, 2005

Chikotas N, Gunderman A, Oman T: Uremic syndrome and end-stage renal disease: Physical manifestations and beyond. J Acad Nurse Practitioner 18(5):195–202, 2006

Gill N, Nally J, Fatica R: Renal failure secondary to acute tubular necrosis: Epidemiology, diagnosis, and management. Chest 128(4):2847–2863, 2005

McCarley P, Salai P: Cardiovascular disease in chronic kidney disease: Recognizing and reducing the risk of a common chronic kidney disease comorbidity. Am J Nurs 105(4):40–52, 2005

Michael M, Garcia D: Secondary hyperparathyroidism in chronic kidney disease: Clinical consequences and challenges. Nephrol Nurs J 31(2):185–196, 2004

Molzahn A, Butera E (eds): Contemporary Nephrology Nursing: Principles and Practice, 2nd ed. Pitman, NJ: AJ Jannetti, 2006

Redmond A, McClelland H: Chronic kidney disease: risk factors, assessment and nursing care. Nurs Stand 20(10):48–55, 2006

INTERNET RESOURCES

Topic	Web Page Address
American Academy of Physical Medicine and Rehabilitation	www.aapmr.org
American Association of Neuroscience Nurses	www.aann.org
American Association of Spinal Cord Injury Nurses	www.aascin.org
American Spinal Injury Association	www.asia-spinalinjury.org
Brain Injury Association of America	www.biausa.org
Brain Injury Resource Center	www.headinjury.com
Brain Trauma Foundation	www.braintrauma.org
British Trauma Society	www.trauma.org
The Center for Neuro Skills: Traumatic Brain Injury Resource Guide	www.neuroskills.com
Center for Paralysis Research	www.vet.purdue.edu/cpr
Guillain-Barre Syndrome and Chronic Inflammatory Demyelinating Polyneuropathy	www.gbs-cidp.org
The International Brain Injury Association	www.internationalbrain.org
International Spinal Development & Research Foundation	www.spine-research.org
Miami Project to Cure Paralysis	www.miamiproject.med.miami.edu
Myasthenia Gravis Foundation of America	www.myasthenia.org
National Institute of Neurological Disorders and Stroke	www.ninds.nih.gov
National Spinal Cord Injury Association	www.spinalcord.org
National Stroke Association	www.stroke.org
NeuroLand	www.NeuroLand.com
Paralyzed Veterans of America	www.pva.org
The Perspectives Network	www.tbi.org
Society of Trauma Nurses	www.traumanurses.org
Spinal Cord Injury Network	www.spinalcordinjury.net
The Spinal Cord Injury Resource Center	www.spinalinjury.net
Spinal Cord Society	http://members.aol.com/scsweb/

Anatomy and Physiology of the Nervous System

32

Mary Ciechanowski • Donna Mower-Wade
Sandra W. McLeskey

Objectives

Based on the content in this chapter, the reader should be able to:

❶ Describe the cellular units of the nervous system.

❷ Briefly explain the physiology of a nerve impulse.

❸ Discuss two functions of cerebrospinal fluid.

❹ Describe the circle of Willis.

❺ Explain the functions of the thalamus.

❻ Define the reticular activating system.

❼ Briefly define the sensory system and the motor system.

❽ Explain the baroreceptor reflex, and list three spinal cord reflexes.

❾ Explain the anatomy and physiology of pain.

❿ Explain the concept of homeostasis.

⓫ Describe the acute stress response.

⓬ Discuss why the stress response could be helpful or harmful, depending on the situation.

We now know that the brain is a central organ that coordinates activity of most, if not all, body systems through its influence on the endocrine and immune systems as well as its more generally appreciated influence on skeletal muscle and autonomic function. Its influence is modulated by sensory perceptions that convey a picture of the external and internal environments, and also by internal circuits having to do with emotional state and levels of arousal. Therefore, the brain can be thought of as the integrative organ that drives our responses to environmental influence. Moreover, separation of the brain and spinal cord from the periphery is more anatomical than conceptual, and modern nurses must always keep in mind that the brain has a profound influence on almost everything that happens in the periphery, and vice versa.

Traditionally, the nervous system is discussed with reference to both anatomical and functional divisions. Anatomical components are the central nervous system (CNS), comprising the brain and spinal cord, and the peripheral nervous system

(PNS), comprising the cranial and spinal nerves. The nervous system is functionally separated into the sensory, integrative, and motor (somatic and autonomic) divisions. Content in this chapter is ordered according to both divisions. However, first cell anatomy and physiology are discussed.

• Cells of the Nervous System

The cellular units are the neuron—the basic functional unit—and its attendant cells, the neuroglia.

NEUROGLIA

Neuroglia constitute the supportive tissue associated with the neurons. In the CNS, there are four types of neuroglia: microglia, astrocytes, ependymal cells, and oligodendroglia. The microglia are phagocytic cells of the nervous system similar to macrophages in the periphery. The astrocytes are supportive cells of the nervous system and make up the blood–brain barrier. The ependymal cells line the ventricles and aid in the production and circulation of the CSF. The oligodendroglia are mostly found in the white matter and produce the myelin that covers nerve fibers in the CNS. In the PNS, the counterpart of the myelin-producing oligodendroglial cell is the Schwann cell.

Under most circumstances, neurons lose their ability to undergo mitosis early in the life of the individual. However, neuroglia retain mitotic abilities throughout a person's life span. Because of this, malignant or benign proliferative lesions originating in the CNS involve neuroglia rather than neurons. However, as the neuroglial tumor enlarges, it adversely affects adjacent neurons—early by exerting pressure and later by promoting an inflammatory reaction along with the pressure.

NEURONS

The basic functional unit of the nervous system is the neuron (or nerve cell), and all information and activity, whether sensory, motor, or both, is accomplished by neurons. The neuron consists of a nerve cell body or soma that contains nuclear and cytoplasmic material, and processes, either axons or dendrites, that arise from the soma (Fig. 32-1). Axons normally carry nerve impulses away from the cell body, whereas dendrites conduct impulses toward the cell body. Axons and dendrites may be merely microscopic knobs or areas on the cell body surface, or they may be cylindrical processes that can extend to more than 1 m (3.25 ft) in length. A specialized structure at the end of the axon is called the axon terminal. This is a bulbous ending (sometimes called a bouton) that forms a synapse with another neuron. The axon terminal contains vesicles of neurotransmitter that is released into the synapse, diffuses across to the postsynaptic neuron, and binds to specific receptors on the membrane of the postsynaptic cell. Binding of a particular neurotransmitter to its specific receptor on the postsynaptic neu-

ron either depolarizes or hyperpolarizes the postsynaptic neuron in the area of the synapse. Axons and dendrites are referred to collectively as nerve fibers. A bundle of nerve fibers together with their coverings is called a tract in the CNS and a nerve in the periphery.

Some nerve fibers are covered with a white lipid–protein sheath termed the myelin sheath. This covering is what differentiates white matter from gray matter in the CNS. The myelin sheath is formed in the CNS by the oligodendrocytes. Other fibers remain unmyelinated. All nerve fibers in the PNS are covered by a neurilemma. This is a sheath formed by the Schwann cells, which wrap themselves around the fiber. Some Schwann cells around particular fibers secrete myelin; others do not (see Fig. 32-1). The neurilemma of a myelinated fiber comes in contact with the axon at periodic intervals. These periodic constrictions of the neurilemmal sheath are termed the nodes of Ranvier. The nodes of Ranvier produce faster nerve impulse conduction by allowing the impulse to jump from one node to the next (saltatory conduction).

Neurons are very diverse, with many specialized anatomical features that are important to their function. Some neurons are extremely large or may give rise to extremely long nerve fibers. Transmission velocities in long, myelinated fibers may be as high as 100 m/second, whereas unmyelinated neurons with very short, unmyelinated processes demonstrate velocities of 1 m/second. Some neurons connect to many different neurons, perhaps thousands of other neurons, in a "network," whereas others have relatively few connections to other cells of the nervous system.

It has been estimated that there are 12 billion neurons in the human CNS. Three fourths of these neurons are located in the cerebral cortex, where conscious thought and feeling reside, along with integrative processing and smoothing of planned motor movements. This processing includes not only the determination of appropriate and effective responses but also the storage of memory and the development of associative motor and thought patterns.

• Characteristics of Neurons

RESTING MEMBRANE POTENTIAL

As is true of all cells, the neuronal cell membrane contains sodium–potassium pumps that keep the inside of the neuron more negatively charged than the outside interstitial fluid. The cytoplasm of all cells contains anions (negatively charged ions) that are too large to leave the cell. Many ions, including sodium, potassium, and chloride, are small enough to diffuse through tiny pores in the cell membrane. If it were not for the sodium–potassium pump, the concentrations of these ions would be equal on the inside of the cell compared with the outside. However, the sodium–potassium pump in the cell membrane pumps sodium ions out of the cell almost as fast as they enter. For every two sodium ions that are pumped out, one potassium ion is pumped into the cell. Because

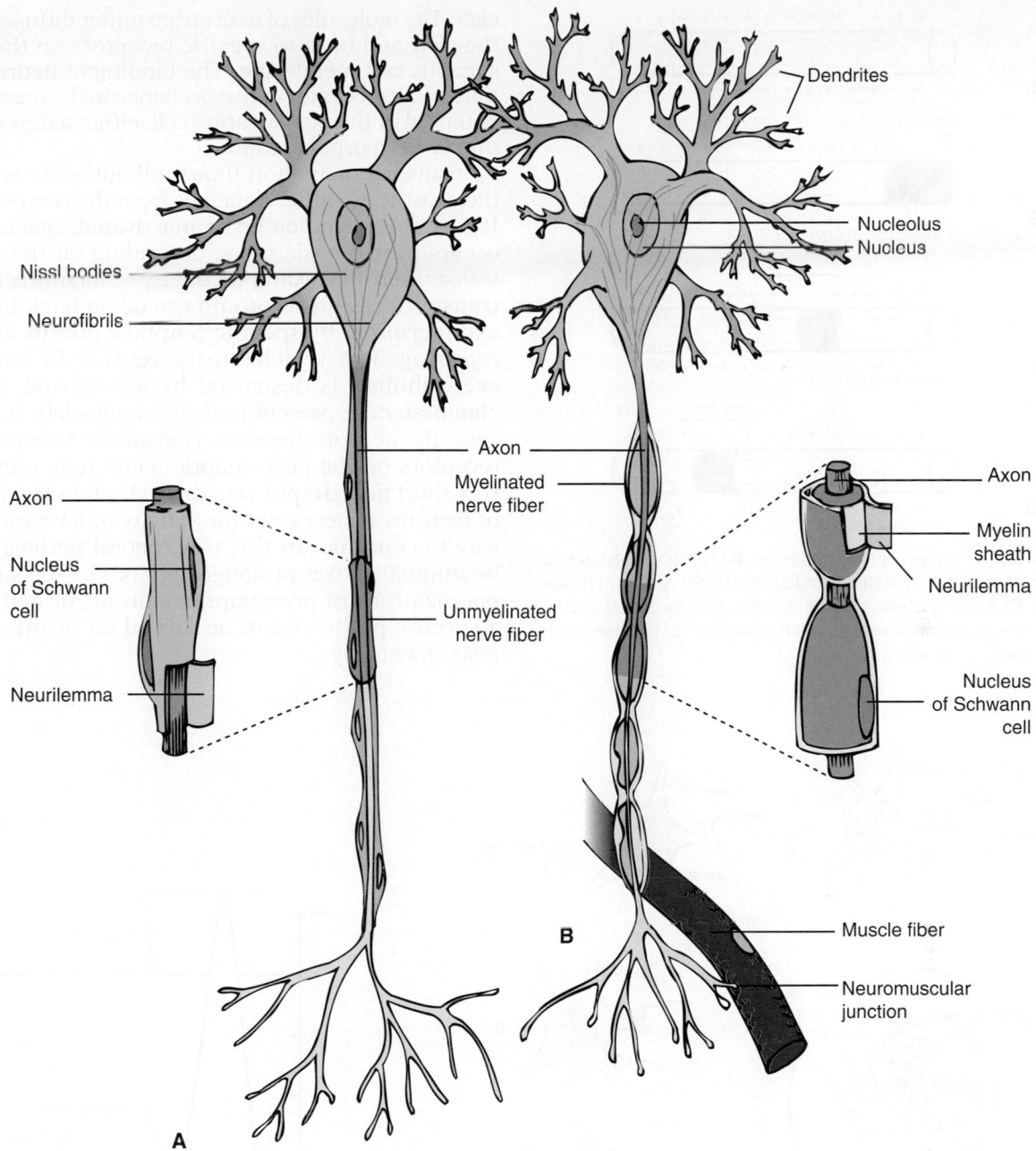

Figure 32-1 • Typical efferent neurons. **A:** Unmyelinated fiber. **B:** Myelinated fiber.

of this, there is a net positive charge leaving the cell, and the large anions cannot be counterbalanced. Thus, under resting conditions when no impulse is being conducted, the inside of the neuron is negative with respect to the outside. This internal relative negativity is the resting membrane potential of the neuron and typically measures about −85 mV.

In addition, as a result of activity of the sodium–potassium pump, sodium ion concentration inside the cell is much lower than outside, and potassium ion concentration is much higher inside the cell than outside. These concentration gradients are important for depolarization produced by synaptic transmission and also for conduction of the action potential down the axon (Fig. 32-2).

SYNAPTIC TRANSMISSION

CONCEPTS in action **ANIMATION**

Submicroscopic spaces between the axon (or axons) of one neuron and the dendrite (or dendrites) or soma of another are called synapses. Axons or dendrites may branch, enabling the axon of one neuron to synapse with dendrites or somas of several neurons. A synapse consists of a presynaptic axon terminal, a postsynaptic neuron, and the small (150 to 1000 Å) space between elements called a synaptic cleft (Fig. 32-3A). When an action potential is conducted down the presynaptic axon and depolarizes the axon terminal, vesicles of neurotransmitter fuse with the plasma membrane, releasing neurotransmitter into the synaptic

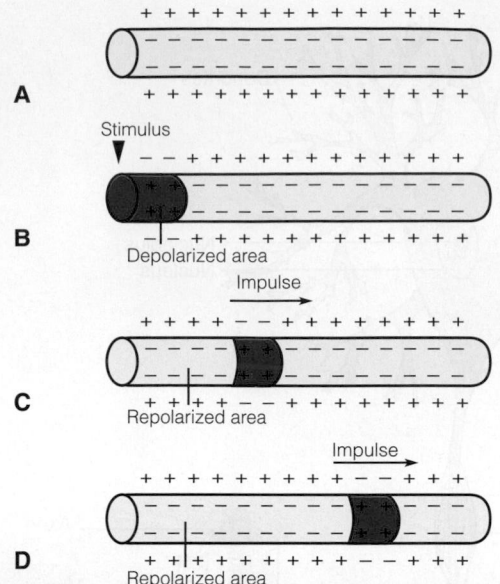

Figure 32-2 • Propagation of impulses. **A:** Resting membrane. **B:** Action potential, first stage: stimulation of fiber results in depolarization. **C:** Action potential, second stage: repolarization occurs as the resting potential is restored. **D:** Propagation of impulses continues in direction of arrow.

cleft. The molecules of neurotransmitter diffuse across the cleft and bind to specific receptors on the postsynaptic cell membrane. The binding of neurotransmitter to its receptor causes a change in the membrane potential of the postsynaptic cell, either a depolarization or a hyperpolarization.

In an extremely short time (millionths of a second), the neurotransmitter detaches from the receptor site. It may then reattach or be inactivated. Inactivation occurs in two basic ways, depending on the neurotransmitter. For example, the catecholamine neurotransmitters and serotonin are taken back into the axon terminal by specific reuptake pumps and are repackaged in vesicles to be reused. In contrast, acetylcholine is destroyed by an enzyme, acetylcholinesterase, present in the synaptic cleft. In either case, the neurotransmitter is available to bind to its receptors on the postsynaptic membrane only for a very short time. Rapid, repetitive, discrete stimulation of neurons is necessary for activity of a neural pathway to continue. In this way, neural pathways can be stimulated over prolonged periods by repeated depolarizations of presynaptic neurons, or activity of a specific pathway can be turned on or off almost instantaneously.

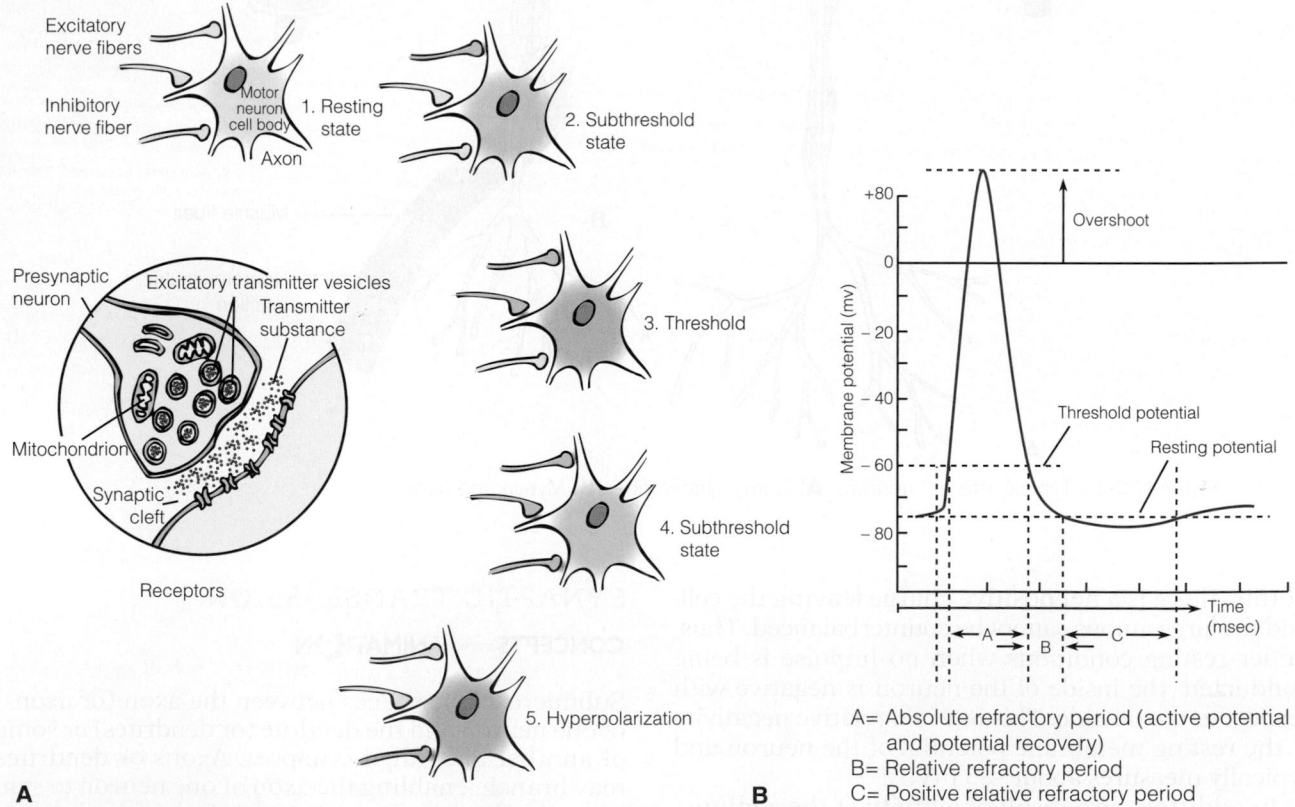

Figure 32-3 • Conduction at synapses. **A:** A neuron may be excited or inhibited by transmitter substances liberated by presynaptic nerve fiber endings. Two excitatory fibers and one inhibitory fiber are shown. (1) During the resting state, no impulses are received. (2) During the subthreshold state, impulses from only one excitatory fiber cannot cause the postsynaptic neuron to mount an action potential. (3) The threshold is reached by the addition of impulses from a second excitatory fiber. This enables the postsynaptic neuron to mount an action potential. (4) The subthreshold state is restored by impulses from an inhibitory fiber. (5) When the inhibitory fiber alone is carrying impulses, the postsynaptic neuron is in a state of hyperpolarization and is unable to fire. **B:** The time course of a neural action potential.

From the preceding discussion, it can be seen that synaptic transmission is a one-way street—from the axon across the synaptic cleft to the dendrite or soma of the next neuron. It cannot proceed in the opposite direction. It also can be seen that decreased destruction or decreased reuptake of a transmitter can increase the effect of this transmitter on the postsynaptic membrane. Similarly, increased destruction or increased reuptake of a transmitter reduces its postsynaptic effects. Several classes of pharmacological agents take advantage of these facts. For instance, acetylcholinesterase inhibitors such as neostigmine are used to increase the amount of acetylcholine remaining in the synapse of the neuromuscular junction to counteract the effects of paralytic drugs given during anesthesia. Serotonin or norepinephrine reuptake pump inhibitors increase the amount of serotonin or norepinephrine in the synapse and have therapeutic effects in depressed patients.

Each neuron synthesizes and stores only one major neurotransmitter in its axon terminal. Major neurotransmitters include serotonin, acetylcholine, γ-aminobutyric acid (GABA), glycine, glutamate, and the catecholamines, dopamine, norepinephrine, and epinephrine. Examples of neuropeptide neurotransmitters are the endogenous opioids (endorphins and enkephalins) and substance P, all of which appear to be involved in pain sensation. The endorphins and enkephalins, often described as the body's own morphine, contribute to a decrease in pain sensation. Substance P excites sensory neurons that respond to painful stimuli, so it is thought to be involved in transmission of pain information from the periphery to the CNS.

Each major neurotransmitter has multiple receptors. For instance, epinephrine can bind to α_1, α_2, β_1, and β_2 receptors, and acetylcholine can bind to neuronal nicotinic, skeletal muscle nicotinic, or muscarinic receptors, which are further subdivided into m_1, m_2, and m_3. The postsynaptic membrane of each synapse contains only one receptor type for the particular neurotransmitter synthesized by the presynaptic neuron. The receptor subtype dictates the effects of a neurotransmitter in a particular synapse on the postsynaptic cell (hyperpolarization or depolarization). Therefore, the same neurotransmitter might be either hyperpolarizing or depolarizing to a given postsynaptic neuron, depending on the receptor subtype present on the postsynaptic cell. However, all GABA receptor types are hyperpolarizing, and GABA is the most important inhibitory neurotransmitter in the nervous system. Likewise, glutamate and glycine are always depolarizing (excitatory) neurotransmitters.

NEURONAL THRESHOLDS AND THE ACTION POTENTIAL

A depolarizing impulse that reaches a neuron's dendrites or soma through action of a neurotransmitter binding to its receptors causes the membrane to depolarize locally through action of the receptor. The local depolarization causes voltage-sensitive sodium channels locally in the membrane to open, and sodium ions are transmitted down their concentration gradient from outside the neuron to inside, causing further local depolarization. If enough sodium channels open locally, the resulting depolarization is large enough to open sodium channels in adjacent areas, depolarizing a larger area of the membrane. Conversely, release of an inhibitory neurotransmitter such as GABA at a synapse may cause hyperpolarization of the postsynaptic neuron through receptor action.

As mentioned, for a given nerve cell, there typically are many other neurons that synapse with its soma or dendrites. Some of these synapsing neurons release an excitatory neurotransmitter that interacts with the nerve cell's receptors to depolarize the postsynaptic neuron. Other synapsing neurons release inhibitory neurotransmitters that interact with their receptors to hyperpolarize the postsynaptic neuron. The nerve cell body algebraically sums the positive depolarizing (excitatory) and negative hyperpolarizing (inhibitory) influences. If the depolarizing influences outweigh the hyperpolarizing influences, the membrane potential of the nerve cell body may reach a value called threshold. At that point, an action potential is generated at the point where the axon leaves the soma. The action potential is propagated down the length of the axon by the process of sodium channel openings in the area of the advancing action potential, followed by complete depolarization of that area. After this process, sodium channels close, and the membrane in that area can repolarize through activity of the sodium–potassium pump and through opening of voltage-sensitive potassium channels. As potassium accumulates within the cell, either by entry through the voltage-sensitive potassium channels or the sodium–potassium pump, the membrane potential is reestablished.

The action potential is normally propagated down the entire length of the axon to the axon terminal. At that point, depolarization of the axon terminal causes neurotransmitter to be released, which diffuses across the synapse and binds to specific receptors, causing a depolarizing or hyperpolarizing change in the postsynaptic neuron.

Neuronal activity can be influenced by hormones. For example, thyroxine lowers thresholds of certain neurons, and one sign of hyperthyroidism is the presence of exaggerated spinal reflexes, such as the knee jerk and ankle jerk.

Figure 32-3B depicts the time course of a neuronal action potential as monitored by electrodes inserted into an axon. Compared with cardiac action potentials, neuronal action potentials are quite short, with durations of approximately 5 to 15 milliseconds. Like the cardiac action potential, there are absolute and relative refractory periods during which the neuron cannot easily be re-excited. However, these refractory periods are very short because repeated impulse conduction is necessary to maintain tonic activity of particular neural pathways. For instance, the motor pathways that supply muscles of posture must be tonically active to maintain a steady contraction in these muscles that keep us erect. Other pathways that have tonic activity include the autonomic motor pathways

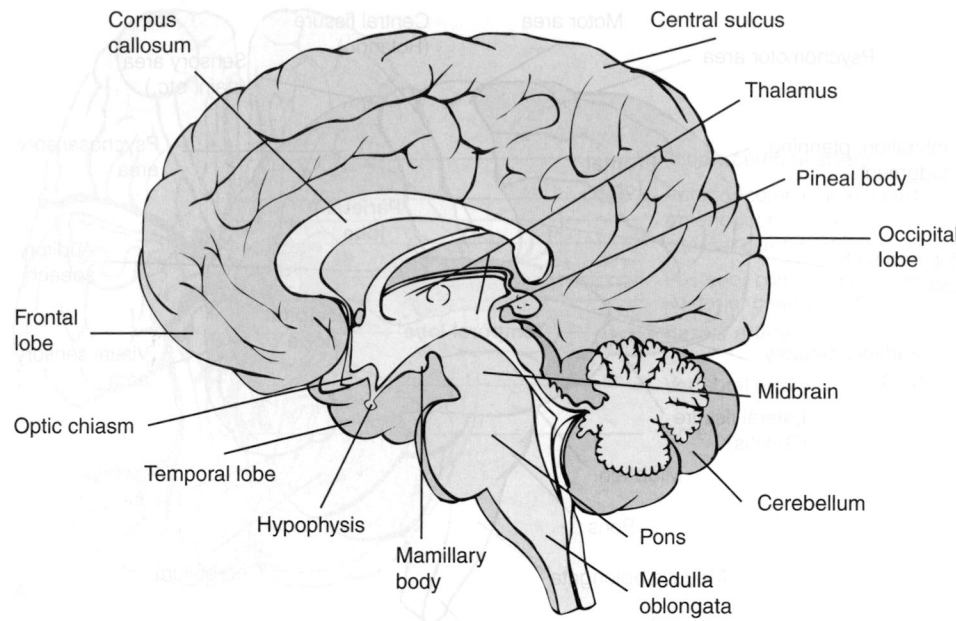

Corpus callosum
Central sulcus
Thalamus
Pineal body
Occipital lobe
Frontal lobe
Optic chiasm
Midbrain
Temporal lobe
Cerebellum
Hypophysis
Pons
Mamillary body
Medulla oblongata

Figure 32-10 • Lateral view of the human brain, showing the parts of the brainstem, the cerebellum, and other major landmarks. (From Cohen H: Neuroscience for Rehabilitation, 2nd ed. Philadelphia: Lippincott Williams & Wilkins, 1999.)

Midbrain

The midbrain lies between the diencephalon and the pons. It contains the aqueduct of Sylvius, many ascending and descending nerve fiber tracts (white matter), and centers for auditory and visually stimulated nerve impulses. The Edinger-Westphal nucleus in the midbrain contains the autonomic reflex centers for pupillary accommodations to light. It receives sensory fibers from the retina through cranial nerve II and sends motor impulses by way of sympathetic and parasympathetic fibers (cranial nerve III) to the smooth muscles of the iris. Impaired pupillary accommodation means that at least one of these inputs or outputs is damaged or that the midbrain is suffering insult (often from tentorial herniation or stroke). Cranial nerve IV also originates in the midbrain.

Pons

The pons lies between the midbrain and the medulla and has cell bodies of fibers contained in cranial nerves V, VI, VII, and VIII. It contains respiratory centers and fiber tracts connecting higher and lower centers, including the cerebellum.

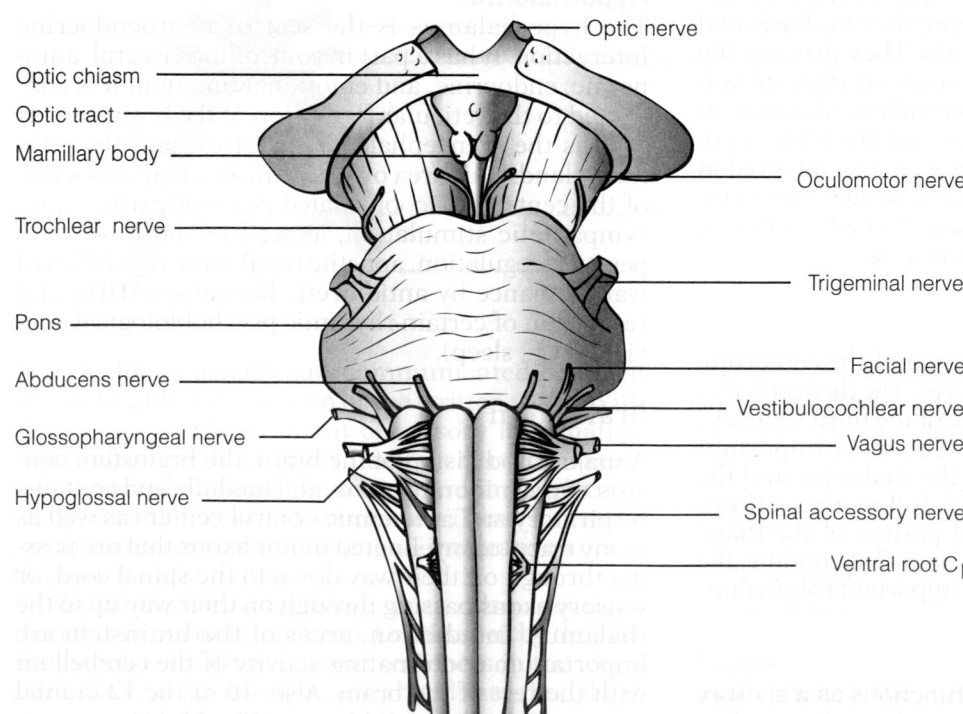

Optic nerve
Optic chiasm
Optic tract
Mamillary body
Oculomotor nerve
Trochlear nerve
Trigeminal nerve
Pons
Abducens nerve
Facial nerve
Vestibulocochlear nerve
Glossopharyngeal nerve
Vagus nerve
Hypoglossal nerve
Spinal accessory nerve
Ventral root C$_I$

Figure 32-11 • Anterior surface of the brainstem, showing the emergence and entrance of most of the cranial nerves. (From Parent A: Carpenter's Human Neuroanatomy, 9th ed. Baltimore: Williams & Wilkins, 1996.)

Medulla Oblongata

The medulla lies between the pons and the spinal cord. It contains centers that regulate vital functions such as breathing, cardiac rate, and vasomotor tone, as well as centers for swallowing, vomiting, gagging, coughing, and sneezing reflex behaviors. It also contains the fourth ventricle. Cranial nerves IX, X, XI, and XII originate in the medulla. Impairment of any of the vital functions or reflexes involving these cranial nerves suggests medullary damage.

Functionally Integrated Brainstem Systems

Four networks of neurons in the brainstem should be mentioned. They are the integrated systems responsible for posture and equilibrium, consciousness, emotional reactions, and sleep.

Bulboreticular Formation The bulboreticular formation is a network of neurons in the brainstem that helps maintain balance and erect posture. This area receives sensory information from a variety of sources, including the peripheral sensory receptors that are relayed from the spinal cord, the cerebellum, the inner ear vestibular apparatus, the motor cortex, and the basal ganglia. Therefore, the bulboreticular formation is an integrative network for sensory information and motor information that has to do with body posture and balance. Output from the bulboreticular formation travels down descending fibers to internuncial neurons in the spinal cord, which synapse with motor neurons. This output alters the tonus of muscles maintaining balance and erect posture and positions of major body parts (trunk, appendages) necessary for the performance of discrete actions (e.g., writing at a table, walking).

Reticular Activating System The RAS is an ascending nerve fiber system originating in the midbrain and thalamus. The RAS is stimulated by sensory impulses from various sources. These include input from the optic and acoustic cranial nerves, somesthetic impulses from the dorsal column and spinothalamic pathways, and fibers from the cortex. Therefore, the RAS is an integrative system that receives sensory information concerning light, sound, and touch that may indicate a need for alertness. Excitatory output of the RAS extends to a variety of higher centers, including the cortex. In this way, the RAS can stimulate these centers to maintain alertness. The stimulation of the cortex by the RAS seems to be the major physiological basis for consciousness, alertness, and attention to various environmental stimuli. Decreased activity of the RAS produces decreased alertness or levels of consciousness, including stupor and coma. Inactivation of the RAS can result from anything that interrupts the entry of a critical amount of sensory input or from any damage that prevents the RAS fibers from sending impulses to the cortex.

Limbic System The hypothalamus, the cingulate gyrus of the cortex, the amygdala and hippocampus in the temporal lobes, and the septum and interconnecting nerve fiber tracts among these areas compose a functional unit of the brain called the limbic system. This system provides a neural substrate for emotions (e.g., terror, intense pleasure, eroticism). This region of the brain is involved in emotional experience and in the control of emotion-related behavior. Also, it is here that neural pathways provide a connection between higher brain functioning and endocrine or autonomic activities.

Sleep Centers The release of stored serotonin from axon terminals in the diencephalon, medulla, thalamus, and a small forebrain area, collectively called DMTF, results in inactivation of the RAS and activation of the DMTF. DMTF activity results in the four stages of sleep. During sleep stages III and IV, parasympathetic activity (with decreased heart rate, respiratory rate, and so forth) predominates, and sleepwalking, sleep talking, and nocturnal enuresis occur.

Rhythmic discharges (about 4 to 8 times per night, from 10 to 20 minutes per episode) from the pontine nuclei during sleep result in rapid eye movement sleep, during which approximately 80% of all dreaming occurs and sympathetic nervous system activity predominates. Based on circadian rhythmicity and decreasing cerebral serotonin levels, the RAS is reactivated in the morning, after 6 to 8 hours of sleep. See Chapter 2, Box 2-2, for a review of the stages and characteristics of sleep.

Cerebellum

The cerebellum (see Fig. 32-10) is located just superior and posterior to the medulla. It receives "samples" of all ascending somesthetic sensory input and all descending motor impulses. Use of these connections enables the cerebellum to match intended motor stimuli (before they reach the muscles) with actual sensory data. This ensures an optimal match for voluntary motor "intention" with actual motor action, with time to alter the motor message in case of error. It sends its own messages to the basal ganglia and cortex and to parts of the brainstem.

The cerebellum functions to produce smooth, steady, harmonious, and coordinated skeletal muscle actions; maintain equilibrium; and control posture without any jerky or uncompensated movements or swaying. The cerebellum is also involved in motor learning and is responsible for reflexive activities that occur when motor learning is complete, such as correcting one's balance when riding a bike. Cerebellar disease can produce typical symptoms, the most prominent of which are disturbances of gait, equilibrium ataxia (overstability or understability of the walk), inability to perform rapid repetitive movements, and characteristic intention tremors.

SPINAL CORD

The spinal cord lies within the neural canal of the vertebral column for protection from traumatic injury. The bony structures of the spine, along with those of the skull, are one mechanism for protection of the delicate structures of the CNS (see Fig. 32-5; Fig. 32-12). The vertebral column of the spine is composed of 33 vertebrae: 7 cervical, 12 thoracic, 5 lumbar, 5 sacral (fused into one), and four coccygeal (fused into one). Each vertebra is composed of two essential parts, an anterior body and a posterior arch, which form a protective ring (vertebral foramen) around the spinal cord. The arch has two pedicles and two laminae to support seven processes (four articular, two transverse, and one spinous), on which muscles and ligaments can attach (Fig. 32-13).

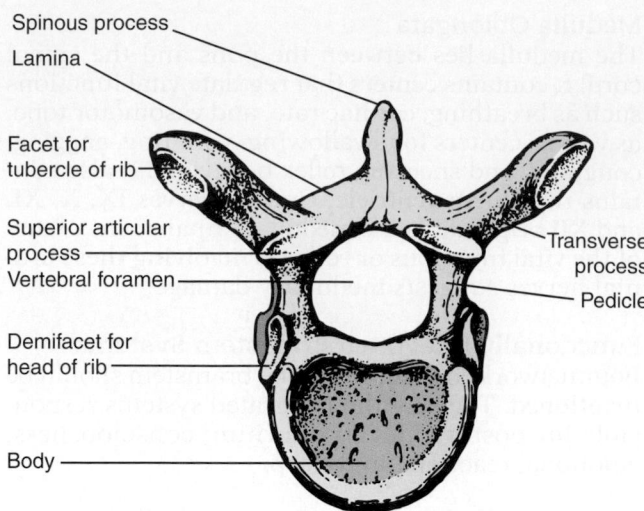

Figure 32-13 • The sixth thoracic vertebra with anatomical markings. The vertebral foramen is the site of the spinal cord, and the spinous and transverse processes serve as places for attachments for muscles. The articular processes form synovial joints between the vertebrae. The vertebral body is opposed to superior and inferior intervertebral disks. (From Hickey JV: The Clinical Practice of Neurological and Neurosurgical Nursing, 5th ed. Philadelphia: Lippincott Williams & Wilkins, 2003.)

The first cervical vertebra, the atlas, supports the weight of the head by articulating with the occiput of the skull. The second cervical vertebra, the axis, has a perpendicular projection called the odontoid process that the atlas sits on; this allows for lateral rotation of the head (Fig. 32-14).

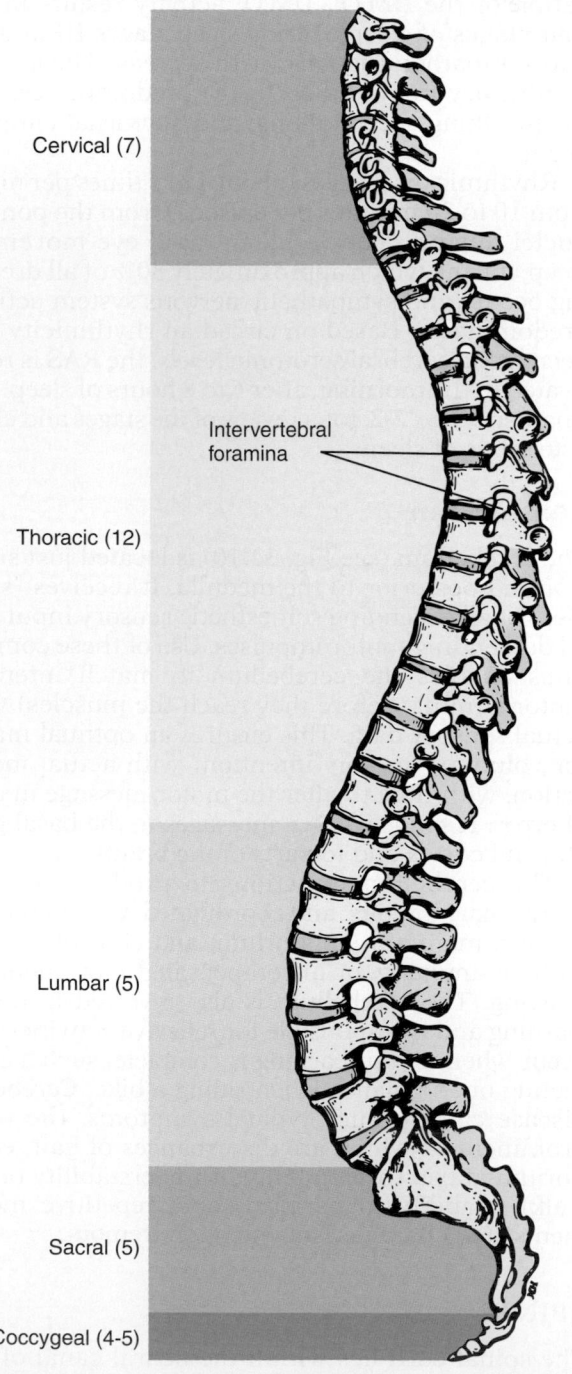

Figure 32-12 • Lateral view of the adult vertebral column. (From Hickey JV: The Clinical Practice of Neurological and Neurosurgical Nursing, 5th ed. Philadelphia: Lippincott Williams & Wilkins, 2003.)

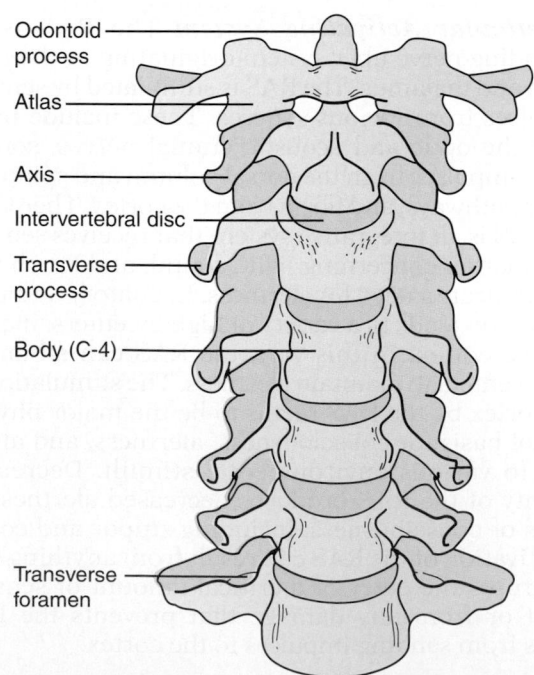

Figure 32-14 • The cervical spine. Note odontoid process of C2 and the atlas, C1, positioned on top of C2. (From Hickey JV: The Clinical Practice of Neurological and Neurosurgical Nursing, 5th ed. Philadelphia: Lippincott Williams & Wilkins, 2003.)

In addition to the bony structures of the spinal column, ligaments and the intervertebral disks also protect the spinal cord by providing support and stability to the vertebral column. The anterior longitudinal ligament and the posterior longitudinal ligament hold the disks and vertebral bodies in position. The intervertebral disks are fibrocartilaginous, disk-shaped structures located between the vertebral bodies from the second cervical vertebra to the sacrum. These disks, which act as shock absorbers between the vertebrae, have a central core known as the nucleus pulposus surrounded by a fibrous capsule known as the anulus fibrosus (Fig. 32-15).

The spinal cord extends down and fills the neural canal to the level of about the second lumbar vertebra in an adult. Over the entire length of the vertebral column, a pair of spinal nerves exits between adjacent vertebrae at its respective level (e.g., C5, T11, L1, S1). However, because the cord is shorter than the spinal column, the level of the cord that gives rise to a particular pair of spinal nerves is above the vertebra of that level. For instance, the two spinal nerves that leave the spinal column between the L4 and L5 vertebrae have to travel down the neural canal from the cord level L4, which is actually up at about vertebral level T12. Below the point at which the cord terminates, the neural canal is filled with descending spinal nerves collectively known as the cauda equina (horse's tail), which exit the neural canal at the vertebra that corresponds to the cord level from which they arose (Fig. 32-16). Because neurons occupy less space in the canal at lower lumbar levels, it is here that spinal taps may be performed safely. This anatomical fact also explains why injuries to lumbar and lower thoracic vertebrae can produce impairment at disproportionately lower body levels.

Within the cord lie ascending sensory fibers and descending motor fibers, many of which are myelinated and appear as white matter. Interneurons, and the nerve cell bodies and dendrites of the second-order somatic (voluntary) and first-order autonomic motor neurons, are not myelinated and appear as gray matter. The central area of the cord contains nerve cell bodies and internuncial neurons (i.e., nerve cells contained entirely within the cord) and also appears as gray matter. The gray matter has left and right dorsal and ventral projections, giving it an H-shaped appearance (Fig. 32-17). Nerve cell bodies of motor neurons supplying skeletal muscles lie in the ventral horns. Nerve cell bodies of the sympathetic preganglionic neurons lie in left and right lateral projections or horns of gray matter referred to as

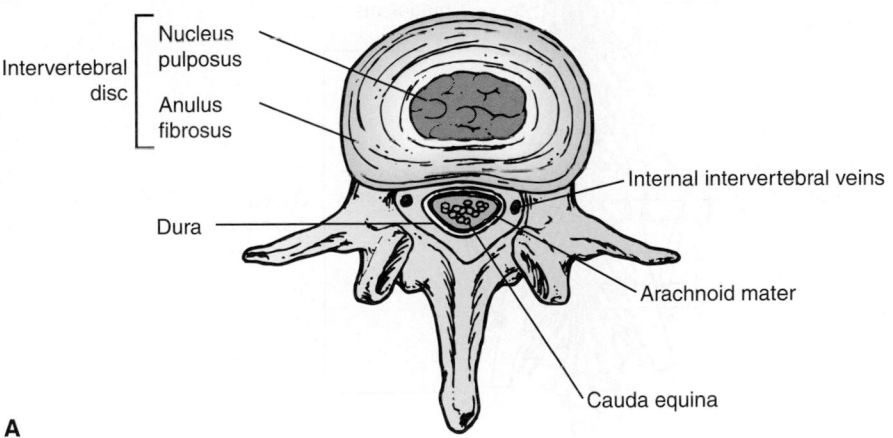

Figure 32-15 • A: Third lumbar vertebra seen from above, showing the intervertebral disk. **B:** Sagittal section through three lumbar vertebrae, showing the ligaments and the intervertebral disks. (From Hickey JV: The Clinical Practice of Neurological and Neurosurgical Nursing, 5th ed. Philadelphia: Lippincott Williams & Wilkins, 2003.)

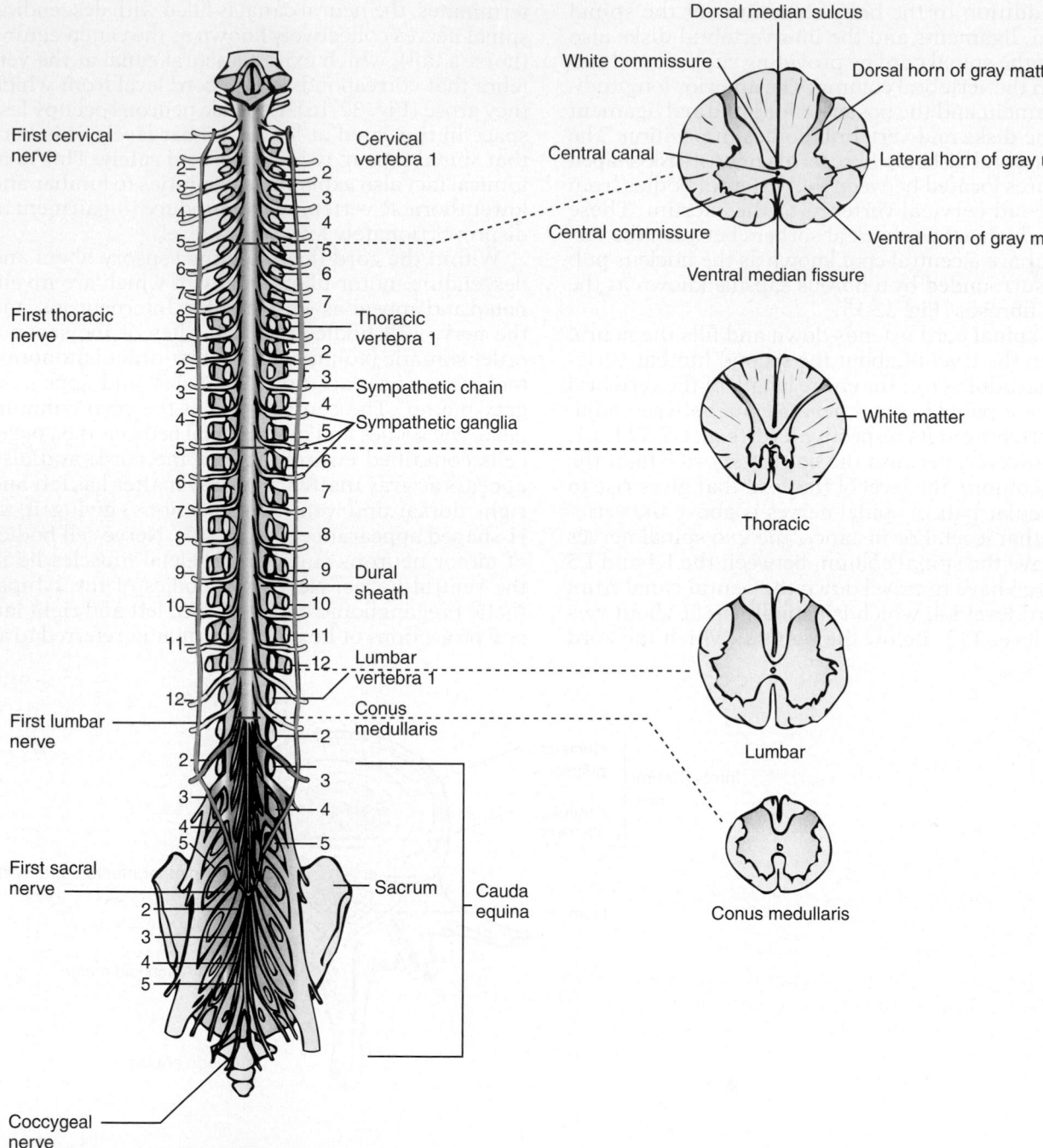

First cervical nerve

Cervical vertebra 1

First thoracic nerve

Thoracic vertebra 1

Sympathetic chain

Sympathetic ganglia

Dural sheath

Lumbar vertebra 1

Conus medullaris

First lumbar nerve

First sacral nerve

Sacrum

Cauda equina

Coccygeal nerve

Dorsal median sulcus

White commissure

Dorsal horn of gray matter

Central canal

Lateral horn of gray matter

Central commissure

Ventral horn of gray matter

Ventral median fissure

White matter

Thoracic

Lumbar

Conus medullaris

Figure 32-16 • The spinal cord within the vertebral canal. The spinal canal and meninges have been opened. The spinal nerves and vertebrae are numbered on the left. Cross (transverse) sections with regional variations in gray matter and increasing proportions of white matter as the cord ascends appear on the right. (From Hickey JV: The Clinical Practice of Neurological and Neurosurgical Nursing, 5th ed. Philadelphia: Lippincott Williams & Wilkins, 2003.)

the intermediolateral cell column in the thoracic and upper lumbar cord.

It is important to realize that the spinal cord is really an extension of the brain and contains many integrative and processive functions. For instance, the substantia gelatinosa contains nerve terminals of descending neurons, and also interneurons, which function to moderate ascending pain impulses (see later).

• Peripheral Nervous System

The PNS consists of 12 pairs of cranial nerves and 31 pairs of spinal nerves and includes all neural structures lying outside the pia mater of the spinal cord and brainstem. The parts of the PNS inside the neural canal and attached to the ventral and dorsal surfaces of the cord are called the spinal nerve roots. Those

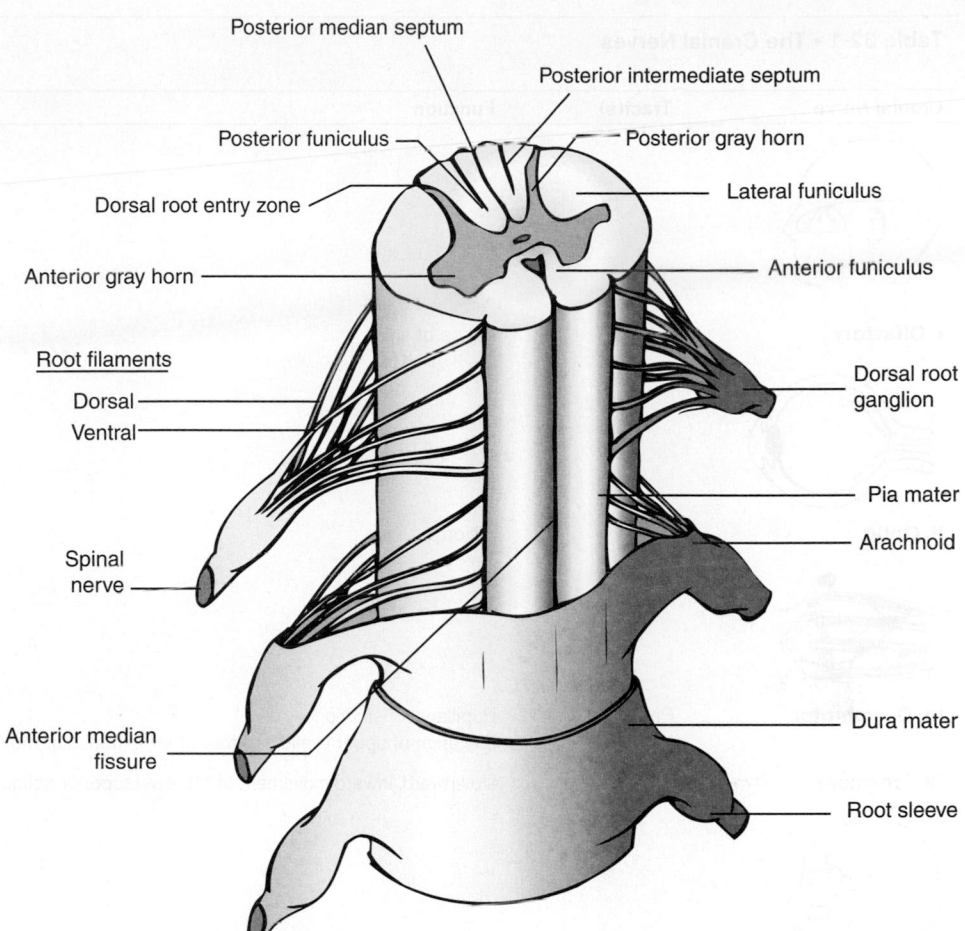

Posterior median septum

Posterior intermediate septum

Posterior funiculus

Posterior gray horn

Dorsal root entry zone

Lateral funiculus

Anterior gray horn

Anterior funiculus

Root filaments

Dorsal

Ventral

Dorsal root ganglion

Pia mater

Arachnoid

Spinal nerve

Anterior median fissure

Dura mater

Root sleeve

Figure 32-17 • Spinal cord, nerve roots, and meninges. (From Parent A: Carpenter's Human Neuroanatomy, 9th ed. Baltimore: Williams & Wilkins, 1996.)

attached to the ventrolateral surface of the brainstem are the cranial nerve roots.

Functionally, the PNS is separated into sensory and motor divisions. The sensory division includes sensory neurons that innervate the skin, muscles, joints, and viscera and provide sensory information about the environment outside and inside the body to the CNS. The motor division includes motor neurons that innervate skeletal muscles and the autonomic nervous system (ANS) that innervates smooth and cardiac muscle and glands. The ANS is responsible for regulating the ongoing functions of many organ systems, such as blood pressure, heart rate, and gastrointestinal activity.

CRANIAL NERVES

The 12 pairs of cranial nerves supply motor and sensory fibers mostly to the structures of the head, neck, and upper back, although cranial nerve X, the vagus nerve, supplies the viscera to about the level of the waist (Table 32-1). Most cranial nerves originate in the brainstem (see Fig. 32-11), except cranial nerves I and II, which originate in the diencephalon. Cranial nerves are classified as either sensory, motor, or mixed (carrying both sensory and motor signals). They bring input from the special senses (vision, hearing, smell)

and somatic sensory input from the face and head into the brain. They also send motor commands out to the muscles and glands of the head and neck to control facial expression, eye movements, movements of the structures in the mouth and throat, movements of the head and neck, and autonomic functions of the eyes, salivary glands, and viscera in the chest and upper abdomen. Most cranial nerves contain fibers of more than one functional type; thus, most cranial nerves are associated with more than one nucleus in the brainstem (see Table 32-1).

SPINAL NERVES

Spinal nerves are attached to the spinal cord in pairs; there are 8 cervical, 12 thoracic, 5 lumbar, 5 sacral, and 1 coccygeal pair of spinal nerves (see Fig. 32-16). In the cervical spine, the spinal nerves exit above the vertebrae. At C7, an extra spinal nerve exists below C7, giving rise to the C8 spinal nerve. All of the rest of the spinal nerves (i.e., the thoracic, lumbar, sacral, and coccygeal spinal nerves) exit below the vertebrae. Spinal nerves contain both sensory and motor fibers. Each spinal nerve attaches to the cord by a dorsal and a ventral root. The dorsal root houses the nerve cell bodies of sensory neurons. Motor axons, whose nerve cell bodies lie in the gray matter of the ventral horn of

Table 32-1 • The Cranial Nerves

Cranial Nerve	Tract(s)	Function	Location of Origin
I. Olfactory	Sensory	Sense of smell	Diencephalon
II. Optic	Sensory	Vision	Diencephalon
III. Oculomotor	Parasympathetic Motor	Pupillary constriction Elevation of upper eyelid and four of six extraocular movements	Midbrain
IV. Trochlear	Motor	Downward, inward movement of the eye (superior oblique)	Midbrain
V. Trigeminal	Motor Sensory	Muscles of mastication and opening jaw Tactile sensation to the cornea, nasal and oral mucosa, and facial skin	Pons
VI. Abducens	Motor	Lateral deviation of eye (lateral rectus)	Pons
VII. Facial	Parasympathetic Motor Sensory	Secretory for salivation and tears Movement of the forehead, eyelids, cheeks, lips, ears, nose, and neck to produce facial expression and close eyes Tactile sensation to parts of the external ear, auditory canal, and external tympanic membrane Taste sensation to the anterior two thirds of the tongue	Pons
VIII. Vestibulocochlear (also known as acoustic or cochlear)	Sensory	*Vestibular branch:* Equilibrium *Cochlear branch:* Hearing	Pons

(continued)

Table 32-1 • The Cranial Nerves (Continued)

Cranial Nerve	Tract(s)	Function	Location of Origin
IX. Glossopharyngeal	Parasympathetic	Salivation	Medulla
	Motor	Voluntary muscles for swallowing and phonation	
	Sensory	Sensation to pharynx, soft palate, and posterior one third of tongue	
		Stimulation elicits gag reflex	
X. Vagus	Parasympathetic	Autonomic activity of viscera of thorax and abdomen	Medulla
	Motor	Voluntary swallowing and phonation	
		Involuntary activity of visceral muscles of the heart, lungs, and digestive tract	
	Sensory	Sensation to the auditory canal and viscera of the thorax and abdomen	
XI. Spinal accessory	Motor	Sternocleidomastoid and trapezius muscle movements	Medulla
XII. Hypoglossal	Motor	Tongue movements	Medulla

Artwork from Evans MJ: Neurologic Neurosurgical Nursing, 2nd ed. Springhouse, PA: Springhouse, 1995, pp 7–8.

the cord, traverse the ventral root. Thus, damage to the dorsal root may impair sensory function without impairing motor function, and vice versa. However, a spinal nerve injury distal to the roots could damage both sensory and motor functioning. A dermatome is the area of skin innervated by sensory fibers from a particular spinal nerve emanating from a particular segment of the spinal cord (see Chapter 37, Fig. 37-3).

SENSORY DIVISION

The sensory division of the nervous system is composed of sensory receptors, sensory neurons whose axons form sensory pathways, and perceptive areas of the brain.

Sensations and Sensory Receptors

Sensations often are divided into the special senses (e.g., vision, hearing, and smell) and those termed somesthetic sensations (e.g., pain, touch, and stretch). In this section, only somesthetic sensations are discussed. Such sensations provide information about, for example, body position and conditions of the external and internal environment. These are called proprioceptive, exteroceptive, and visceral sensations, respectively.

Proprioceptive sensations describe the physical position state of the body, such as muscle tension, joint flexion or extension, tendon tension, and deep pressure in dependent parts, such as the feet while one is standing or the buttocks while one is sitting. Exteroceptive sensations monitor conditions on the body surface, such as temperature and pain. Visceral sensations are similar to exteroceptive sensations, except that they originate from within the body and monitor pain, pressure, and fullness from internal organs.

The sensory receptors for somesthetic sensations are basically dendrites, which can have the form of free nerve endings or specialized receptors. Free nerve endings are nothing more than small, filamentous branches of dendrites. They detect crude sensations of touch, pain, heat, and cold. The precision is crude because different neurons have overlapping distributions of their dendrites. These nerve endings are the most widely distributed and most numerous of sensory receptors and perform the general discriminatory functions. The more specialized sensory receptors discriminate between very slight differences in degrees of touch, pain, heat, and cold. Indeed, the special exteroceptive end organs for detecting light touch, warmth, and cold differ structurally from one another and are specific in their function. The physiological basis for this specific function has not been determined but is presumed to be based on some specific physical effect on the receptor itself.

Sensation from the internal organs may come from specialized sensory receptors, such as baroreceptors and chemoreceptors that reside in arterial walls, or stretch receptors in sphincters. In contrast, visceral pain is the result of stimulation of unmyelinated, raw sensory nerve endings, usually by stretch, as might happen during swelling or distention, or by pressure on the organ as might happen from compression by a tumor. For both specialized and unspecialized visceral receptors, the sensory fibers run within the autonomic nerves (sympathetic or parasympathetic) back to CNS centers that are closely associated with autonomic motor responses. For this reason, these sensory fibers are sometimes referred to as autonomic afferent fibers. This is a somewhat misleading name because the autonomic nervous system is purely a motor system (see later), and the name refers only to the anatomical location of sensory fibers within the nerves that also carry autonomic motor fibers.

Stimulation of a sensory receptor initiates an electrical charge (generator potential) that depolarizes the sensory dendrite, causing a series of nerve impulses to travel along the sensory dendrite to the cell body. As mentioned, the sensory neuron cell body is contained in the dorsal root ganglion just outside the spinal cord. The sensory neuron sends axons into the spinal cord (or brain in the case of cranial nerves), where it synapses with projection neurons in either brain or spinal cord that carry impulses to the appropriate centers in the brain, including the thalamus, where the sensation finally may be perceived consciously. The projection neuron may synapse in the thalamus with another neuron, which relays the sensory impulse to the sensory cortex.

When the sensation first stimulates the sensory receptor in the periphery, there is a burst of impulses; if the stimulus persists, the frequency of impulses transmitted begins to decrease. All sensory receptors show this phenomenon of adaptation to varying degrees and at different rates. Adaptations to light touch and pressure occur in a few seconds, whereas pain and proprioceptive sensations adapt very little, if at all, and at a very slow rate. This adaptation results in our being unaware of the touch of our clothing to our skin or the pressure on our buttocks while we are seated. Determination of the intensity of the sensation is made on a relative rather than an absolute basis.

Although there are structurally different receptors for detecting each type of sensation, the area of the brain to which the information is transmitted determines the modality, or type of sensation, a person feels. The thalamus and sensory cortex operate together to attribute various sensory qualities and intensities to nerve impulse information they receive.

Sensory Pathways

As mentioned, sensory neurons that enter the cord synapse with projection neurons that carry the sensory information up the spinal cord. There are a number of pathways by which sensory information is transmitted up the cord by axons of the projection neurons. Depending on the type of somesthetic receptor involved, fibers of sensory neurons may, on entering the cord, do one of three things.

First, they may send axons up the cord to the medulla on the same side of the body as the sensory receptor. This tract of myelinated axons (white matter) is called the dorsal column. In the medulla, the sensory neurons synapse with projection neurons that cross over to the opposite side of the brain and travel to the thalamus. This tract is called the medial lemniscus (Fig. 32-18). It is used for the conduction of impulses originating from stimulation of joint, muscle, and tendon proprioceptors; vibration-sensitive receptors; and receptors in the skin involved in precise localization of touch.

Second, the sensory neurons may synapse immediately on entering the cord with projection neurons that immediately cross over to the opposite side of the cord. Fibers from these projection neurons then travel up the white matter of the cord to the thalamus. This is called the spinothalamic pathway (see Fig. 32-18). It conducts impulses concerned with pain, temperature, poorly localized touch, and sex organ sensations. Both the dorsal column–medial lemniscus pathway and the spinothalamic pathway involve crossing of the sensory information from each side of the body to the opposite side of the CNS. Therefore, sensations on each side of the body are perceived by the thalamus and sensory cortex on the opposite side. In the thalamus, neurons of both the dorsal column pathway and the spinothalamic pathway synapse with other neurons that transmit impulses to the appropriate area of the sensory cortex. Because of their final destination in the cortex, impulses from either pathway give rise to consciously perceived sensations. The sensory homunculus (Fig. 32-19) is a pictorial representation of the number of neurons in the sensory cortex that are devoted to receiving sensations from various areas of the body. It should be noted that very sensitive areas, such as the lips, have a large representation in the sensory cortex, whereas less sensitive areas, such as the trunk, have a smaller representation.

Third, certain sensory neurons may synapse with a projection neuron belonging to the spinocerebellar pathway. Spinocerebellar neurons do not cross over. They carry impulses only as far as the cerebellum (and possibly lower brainstem). This pathway carries impulses originating from stimulation of joint, muscle, and tendon proprioceptors. Because this pathway ends at the cerebellum, it transmits sensory information that is not perceived consciously. Instead, these data are used in reflex postural adjustments.

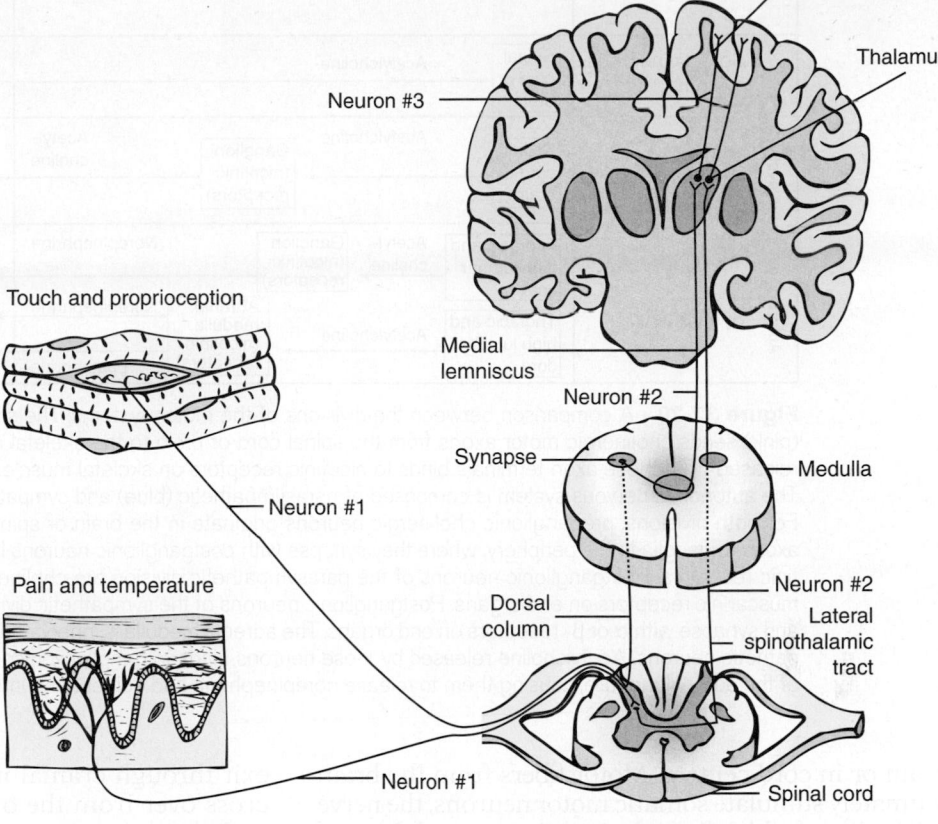

Figure 32-18 • Pathways of ascending tracts. Sensory neurons enter the cord at the dorsal horn. Axons of sensory neurons for touch and proprioception ascend in the dorsal columns to the medulla, where they synapse with second-order projection neurons that cross (decussate) to the opposite side before ascending to the thalamus in the tract called the medial lemniscus. First-order neurons for pain and temperature enter the dorsal gray matter of the cord, where they synapse with second-order projection neurons that cross to the opposite side and ascend in the lateral spinothalamic tract to the thalamus. Third-order neurons connect both pathways from thalamus to the sensory cortex.

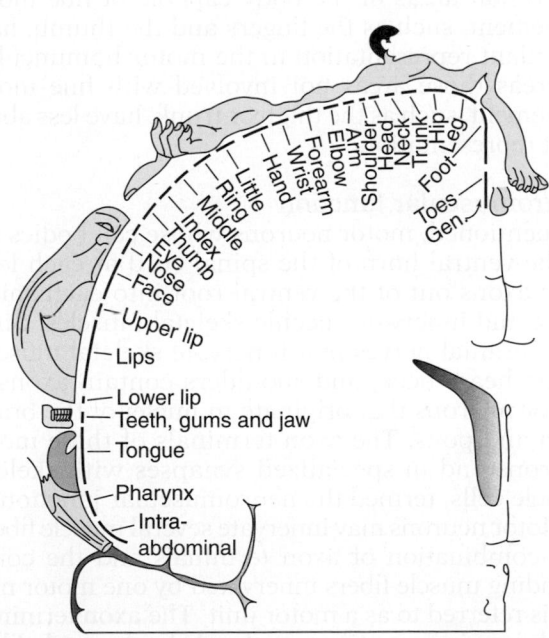

Figure 32-19 • The sensory homunculus, a representation of the relative extent of the somatosensory cortex devoted to various body regions, as determined by stimulation studies on the human somatosensory cortex during surgery. (From Penfield E, Rasmussen T: The Cerebral Cortex of Man. New York: Macmillan, 1955. Copyright © by MacMillan Publishing Co., Inc., renewed 1978 by Theodore Rasmussen.)

MOTOR DIVISION AND THE NEUROMUSCULAR JUNCTION

The motor division comprises the areas of the brain, descending fiber tracts, and motor neurons involved in producing or altering movement or adjusting tonus of skeletal, cardiac, and smooth muscles and in regulating the secretions of the various exocrine and certain endocrine gland cells. Muscle and glandular tissues are referred to as the effector organs of this system.

The motor division can be divided on the basis of motor neurons and effector organs into somatic and autonomic subdivisions (Fig. 32-20). The former involves skeletal muscles and the motor neurons innervating them. The latter is composed of smooth muscle, cardiac muscle, and gland cells plus the sympathetic and parasympathetic fibers innervating them.

Somatic Motor Division

Figure 32-21 depicts the major descending fiber tracts from motor areas of the cortex. The most prominent of these tracts is the corticospinal tract, often called the pyramidal tract because it originates from pyramid-shaped nerve cell bodies in the cortex. The corticospinal tract is heavily myelinated and appears as white matter in the brain and spinal cord. The fibers cross to the opposite side in an area of the medulla referred to as the decussation (crossing over) of the pyramids. Several other motor tracts originate in the cortex or in the cerebellum. These tracts may cross over in the

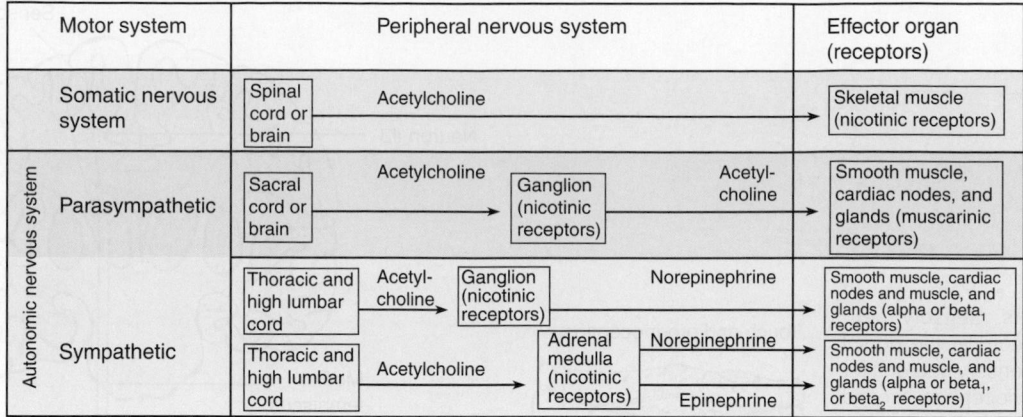

Motor system	Peripheral nervous system				Effector organ (receptors)
Somatic nervous system	Spinal cord or brain	Acetylcholine			Skeletal muscle (nicotinic receptors)
Autonomic nervous system — Parasympathetic	Sacral cord or brain	Acetylcholine →	Ganglion (nicotinic receptors)	Acetylcholine	Smooth muscle, cardiac nodes, and glands (muscarinic receptors)
Sympathetic	Thoracic and high lumbar cord	Acetylcholine	Ganglion (nicotinic receptors)	Norepinephrine	Smooth muscle, cardiac nodes and muscle, and glands (alpha or beta₁ receptors)
	Thoracic and high lumbar cord	Acetylcholine	Adrenal medulla (nicotinic receptors)	Norepinephrine / Epinephrine	Smooth muscle, cardiac nodes and muscle, and glands (alpha or beta₁, or beta₂ receptors)

Figure 32-20 • A comparison between the divisions of the motor systems. The somatic nervous system (pink) sends cholinergic motor axons from the spinal cord or brain to the skeletal muscles. Acetylcholine released from these axon terminals binds to nicotinic receptors on skeletal muscles to cause contraction. The autonomic nervous system is composed of parasympathetic (blue) and sympathetic (green) divisions. For both divisions, preganglionic cholinergic neurons originate in the brain or spinal cord and send their axons to ganglia in the periphery, where they synapse with postganglionic neurons having ganglionic nicotinic receptors. Postganglionic neurons of the parasympathetic division are cholinergic and synapse with muscarinic receptors on end organs. Postganglionic neurons of the sympathetic division are noradrenergic and synapse with α or β_1 receptors on end organs. The adrenal medulla is innervated by preganglionic sympathetic neurons. Acetylcholine released by these neurons binds to ganglionic nicotinic receptors on cells of the adrenal medulla, causing them to release norepinephrine and epinephrine into the bloodstream.

brain or in cord centers. Motor fibers from the brain ultimately stimulate somatic motor neurons, the nerve cell bodies of which lie in the anterior (ventral) horn of the gray matter in the cord. The axons of these motor neurons travel within spinal nerves and terminate at the neuromuscular junction, the synapse between the somatic motor neuron axon and the muscle cell. When a motor neuron depolarizes, acetylcholine is released into the synapse at the neuromuscular junction. It binds to nicotinic receptors on the skeletal muscle membrane, causing depolarization of the muscle cell, which stimulates contraction.

Figure 32-21 also shows several extrapyramidal (not part of the pyramidal [corticospinal] tracts) tracts arising from the brainstem centers (e.g., bulboreticular formation, midbrain). Some of these cross over; others do not. Fibers in these tracts descend the cord and ultimately stimulate either somatic motor neurons, which stimulate skeletal muscle contraction, or other motor neurons (gamma efferent) that alter the tensions of stretch receptor organelles (muscle spindles) in the skeletal muscles. Alteration of spindle tension provokes a spinal reflex arc that efficiently alters skeletal muscle tonus. These extrapyramidal pathways conduct impulses that produce the automatic coordinated alterations in skeletal muscle tonus and movement that are necessary for gross motor movements (e.g., walking) and for appropriate posture for conduction of finer movements (e.g., sitting at a desk with arm flexed in preparation for writing).

Not shown in Figure 32-21 are descending fiber tracts that stimulate motor neurons responsible for the movement of skeletal muscles of the head (e.g., tongue, face, jaw). The general pattern and myoneural transmitter are the same, except the somatic motor neuron nerve cell bodies lie in particular areas of the brain and

exit through cranial nerves. These fibers must also cross over from the opposite side before synapsing with the motor neurons.

The motor homunculus (Fig. 32-22) is a pictorial representation of the number of neurons in the motor cortex devoted to each area of the body. It should be noted that areas of the body capable of fine motor movement, such as the fingers and the thumb, have abundant representation in the motor homunculus, whereas those areas not involved with fine motor movement, such as the thigh or trunk, have less abundant representation.

Neuromuscular Junction

As mentioned, motor neurons whose cell bodies are in the ventral horn of the spinal cord at each level send axons out of the ventral root into each spinal nerve and innervate specific skeletal muscles. Similarly, cranial nerves that innervate skeletal muscles of the head, neck, and shoulders contain axons of motor neurons that originate in nuclei of the brainstem and pons. The axon terminals of these motor neurons end in specialized synapses with skeletal muscle cells, termed the neuromuscular junction.

Motor neurons may innervate several muscle fibers. The combination of axon terminals and the corresponding muscle fibers innervated by one motor neuron is referred to as a motor unit. The axon terminals reach into invaginations on the skeletal muscle fiber, called motor end plates, and form the highly structured synapses that compose the neuromuscular junctions (Fig. 32-23). The cell membrane of the skeletal muscle contains abundant nicotinic skeletal muscle receptors concentrated in the area of the motor end plate. These receptors bind acetylcholine, which is released from the motor neuron in response to an arriv-

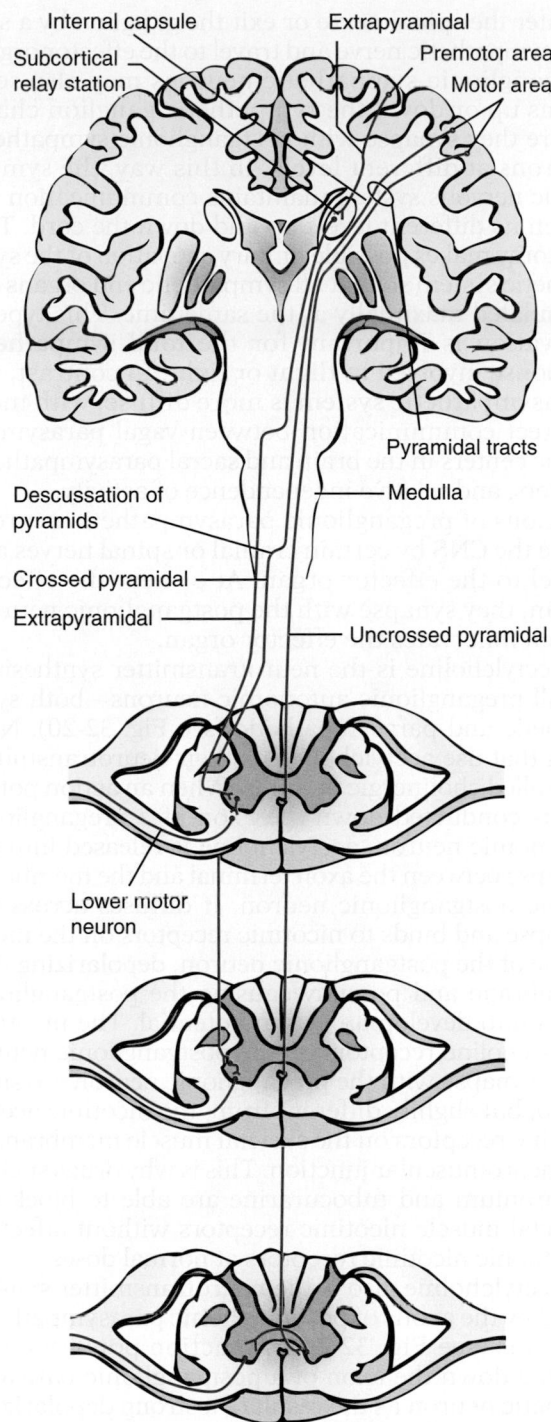

Figure 32-21 • Diagram of motor pathways between the cerebral cortex, one of the subcortical relay centers, and lower motor neurons in the spinal cord. Decussation (crossing) of fibers dictates that each side of the brain controls skeletal muscles on the opposite side of the body.

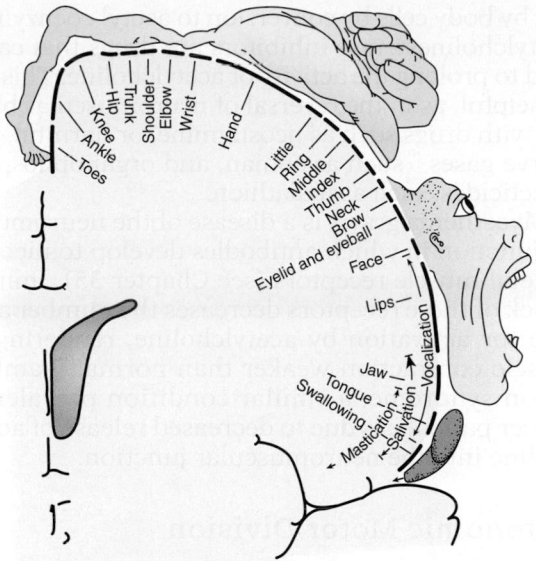

Figure 32-22 • The motor homunculus, a representation of the relative extent of the primary motor cortex devoted to various body regions. (From Penfield E, Rasmusen T: The Cerebral Cortex in Man: A Clinical Study of Localization of Function. New York: MacMillan, 1968.)

Also located within the neuromuscular junction, similar to other cholinergic synapses, are many molecules of acetylcholinesterase, an enzyme that degrades acetylcholine into acetate and choline with great rapidity. This enzyme is responsible for terminating the activity of acetylcholine in the synapse. Following the degradation of acetylcholine, choline is quickly taken back up into the motor nerve terminal and used to resynthesize acetylcholine. Acetate can be used for

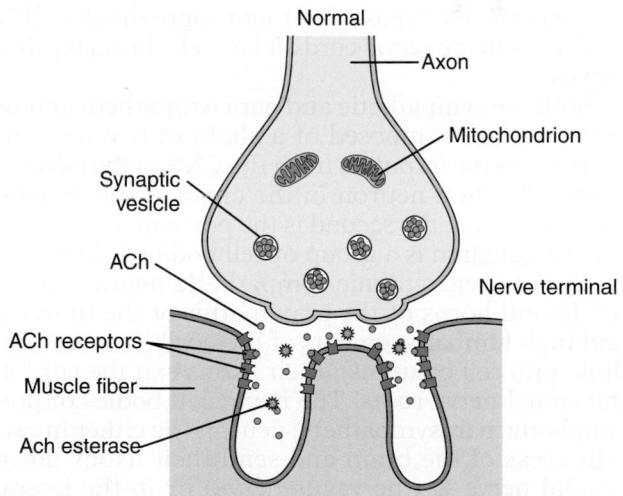

Figure 32-23 • The neuromuscular junction. Acetylcholine (Ach), released from the motor neuron, crosses the synaptic cleft to bind to and activate Ach receptors that are concentrated in folds of the muscle end plate. These activated receptors depolarize the muscle, causing a contraction. Once released, Ach is rapidly broken down by the enzyme acetylcholinesterase (Ach esterase), which terminates the activity of Ach in the synapse. (From Porth CM: Essentials of Pathophysiology, 2nd ed. Philadelphia: Lippincott Williams & Wilkins, 2006.)

ing action potential. These nicotinic receptors are slightly different from those located at ganglionic synapses of the autonomic nervous system, making it possible to design drugs that bind only to skeletal muscle nicotinic receptors, not ganglionic ones. These drugs, such as tubocurarine, are used for neuromuscular blockade during anesthesia or in the intensive care unit.

fuel by body cells by conversion to acetyl coenzyme A. Acetylcholinesterase inhibitors are drugs that can be used to prolong the activity of acetylcholine. This may be helpful, as in the reversal of neuromuscular blockade with drugs such as neostigmine, or harmful, as in "nerve gases," such as soman, and organophosphate insecticides, such as malathion.

Myasthenia gravis is a disease of the neuromuscular junction in which antibodies develop to nicotinic skeletal muscle receptors (see Chapter 35). Immune attack of these receptors decreases the number available for activation by acetylcholine, rendering the muscle contraction weaker than normal. Lambert-Eaton syndrome, a similar condition prevalent in cancer patients, is due to decreased release of acetylcholine into the neuromuscular junction.

Autonomic Motor Division

The autonomic division contains both sympathetic and parasympathetic motor fibers. They are responsible for contraction and relaxation of smooth muscle, rate and strength of contraction of cardiac tissue, secretion by exocrine glands, and secretion by the adrenal medulla. They also influence the secretion by the islets of Langerhans in the pancreas.

The sympathetic and parasympathetic sections differ on the basis of the anatomical distribution of nerve fibers, the secretion of two different neurotransmitters by the postganglionic fibers of the two divisions, and the antagonistic effects of the two divisions on some of the organs they innervate (Table 32-2). Figure 32-24 shows the anatomy of the sympathetic and parasympathetic nervous systems. The CNS center immediately responsible for sympathetic outflow resides in the thoracic cord. In contrast, 80% of parasympathetic activity originates in the brain and travels through cranial nerve X (the vagus nerve), and approximately 20% originates in the sacral cord and travels through pelvic nerves.

Both the sympathetic and parasympathetic motor pathways are composed of a chain of two neurons carrying nerve impulses from the CNS to the effector organ. The first neuron in the chain is the preganglionic neuron; the second is the postganglionic neuron. (A ganglion is a group of cell bodies.) Nerve cell bodies of preganglionic sympathetic neurons lie in the lateral horns of the gray matter of the thoracic and high lumbar segments of the cord (the intermediolateral cell columns); their axons exit the cord in the spinal nerve roots. The nerve cell bodies of preganglionic parasympathetic neurons lie either in certain areas of the brain and send their axons down cranial nerve X (the vagus nerve) or in the lateral horns of gray matter in the sacral cord and send their axons down the pelvic nerves.

As mentioned, axons of preganglionic sympathetic neurons exit the cord and enter the ventral roots of spinal nerves. They then leave the spinal nerve to enter a nearby sympathetic ganglion by a connecting pathway termed a ramus. In a sympathetic ganglion, the preganglionic neuron synapses with a postganglionic one. The postganglionic sympathetic neuron then may reenter the spinal nerve or exit the ganglion by a special sympathetic nerve and travel to the effector organ. Preganglionic sympathetic neurons may also send axons up or down the sympathetic ganglion chain, where they synapse with postganglionic sympathetic neurons at different levels. In this way, the sympathetic nervous system maintains communication between its different levels up and down the cord. This anatomy makes possible unitary activation of the sympathetic system so that all sympathetic end organs are stimulated maximally at the same time. This type of activation is important for the total sympathetic response involved in flight or fight. In contrast, the parasympathetic system is more diffuse, with more indirect communication between vagal parasympathetic centers in the brain and sacral parasympathetic centers, and relative independence of activity.

Axons of preganglionic parasympathetic neurons leave the CNS by certain cranial or spinal nerves and travel to the effector organ. At or near the effector organ, they synapse with the postganglionic neuron, which innervates the effector organ.

Acetylcholine is the neurotransmitter synthesized by all preganglionic autonomic neurons—both sympathetic and parasympathetic (see Fig. 32-20). Neurons that use acetylcholine as their neurotransmitter are called cholinergic neurons. When an action potential is conducted down the axon of a preganglionic autonomic neuron, acetylcholine is released into the synapse between the axon terminal and the membrane of the postganglionic neuron. It diffuses across the synapse and binds to nicotinic receptors on the membrane of the postganglionic neuron, depolarizing that membrane and possibly causing the postganglionic neuron to develop an action potential. The nicotinic acetylcholine receptors on the postganglionic neuron at its synapse with the preganglionic neuron are similar to, but slightly different from, the nicotinic acetylcholine receptors on the skeletal muscle membrane at the neuromuscular junction. This is why drugs such as vecuronium and tubocurarine are able to block the skeletal muscle nicotinic receptors without affecting ganglionic nicotinic receptors at normal doses.

Acetylcholine also is the neurotransmitter synthesized by the axons of postganglionic parasympathetic neurons (see Fig. 32-20). An action potential conducted down the axon of a postganglionic parasympathetic neuron as the result of a strong depolarizing influence received from the preganglionic neuron causes acetylcholine to be released from the axon terminal into the synapse. The acetylcholine diffuses across the synapse and binds to muscarinic acetylcholine receptors on the parasympathetic end organ. These receptors cause changes in the end organ cell that result in smooth muscle contraction, glandular secretion, hyperpolarization of the sinoatrial node of the heart (causing a decrease in heart rate), or slowing in the speed of conduction in the atrioventricular node of the heart. Table 32-2 shows the effects of acetylcholine on the muscarinic receptors in the various effector organs of the parasympathetic nervous system. As noted previously, the activity of the acetylcholine is terminated by acetylcholinesterase, an

Table 32-2 • Responses of Effector Organs to Autonomic Nerve Impulses and Circulating Catecholamines

Effector Organs	Muscarinic Response	Adrenergic & Noradrenergic Responses	
		Receptor Type	Response*
Eye			
Radial muscle of iris	—	α	Contraction (mydriasis)
Sphincter muscle of iris	Contraction (miosis)		
Ciliary muscle	Contraction for near vision	β	Relaxation for far vision
Heart			
Sinoatrial node	Decrease in heart rate; vagal arrest	β_1	Increase in heart rate
Atria	Decrease in contractility	β_1	Increase in contractility and conduction velocity
AV node and conduction system	Decrease in conduction velocity; atrioventricular block	β_1	Increase in conduction velocity
Ventricles	—	β_1	Increase in contractility and conduction velocity
Arterioles			
Coronary, skeletal muscle, pulmonary, abdominal viscera, renal	—	α β_2	Constriction Dilation
Skin and mucosa, cerebral, salivary glands	—	α	Constriction
Systemic Veins	—	α β_2	Constriction Dilation
Lung			
Bronchial muscle	Contraction	β_2	Relaxation
Bronchial glands	Stimulation	?	Inhibition (?)
Stomach			
Motility and tone	Increase	α, β_2	Decrease (usually)
Sphincters	Relaxation (usually)	α	Contraction (usually)
Secretion	Stimulation		Inhibition (?)
Intestine			
Motility and tone	Increase	α, β_2	Decrease
Sphincters	Relaxation (usually)	α	Contraction (usually)
Secretion	Stimulation		Inhibition (?)
Gallbladder and Ducts	Contraction		Relaxation
Urinary Bladder			
Detrusor	Contraction	β	Relaxation (usually)
Trigone and sphincter	Relaxation	α	Contraction
Ureter			
Motility and tone	Increase (?)	α	Increase (usually)
Uterus	Variable†	α, β_2	Variable†
Male Sex Organs	Erection	α	Ejaculation
Skin			
Pilomotor muscles	—	α	Contraction
Sweat glands	Generalized secretion	α	Slight, localized secretion‡
Spleen Capsule	—	α β_2	Contraction Relaxation
Adrenal Medulla	—		—
Liver	—	α, β_2	Glycogenolysis
Pancreas			
Acini	Secretion	α	Decreased secretion
Islets	Insulin and glucagon secretion	α β_2	Inhibition of insulin and glucagon secretion Insulin and glucagon secretion
Salivary Glands	Profuse, watery secretion	α β_2	Thick, viscous secretion Amylase secretion
Lacrimal Glands	Secretion		—
Nasopharyngeal Glands	Secretion		—
Adipose Tissue		β_1	Lipolysis
Juxtaglomerular Cells	—	$\beta(\beta_1?)$	Renin secretion
Pineal Gland	—	β	Melatonin synthesis and secretion

*α and β_1—norepinephrine and epinephrine; β_2—epinephrine only.
†Depends on stage of menstrual cycle, amount of circulating estrogen and progesterone, pregnancy, and other factors.
‡On palms of hands and in some other locations ("adrenergic sweating").
From Ganong WF: Review of Medical Physiology: Los Altos, CA: Lange Medical Publications, 2003

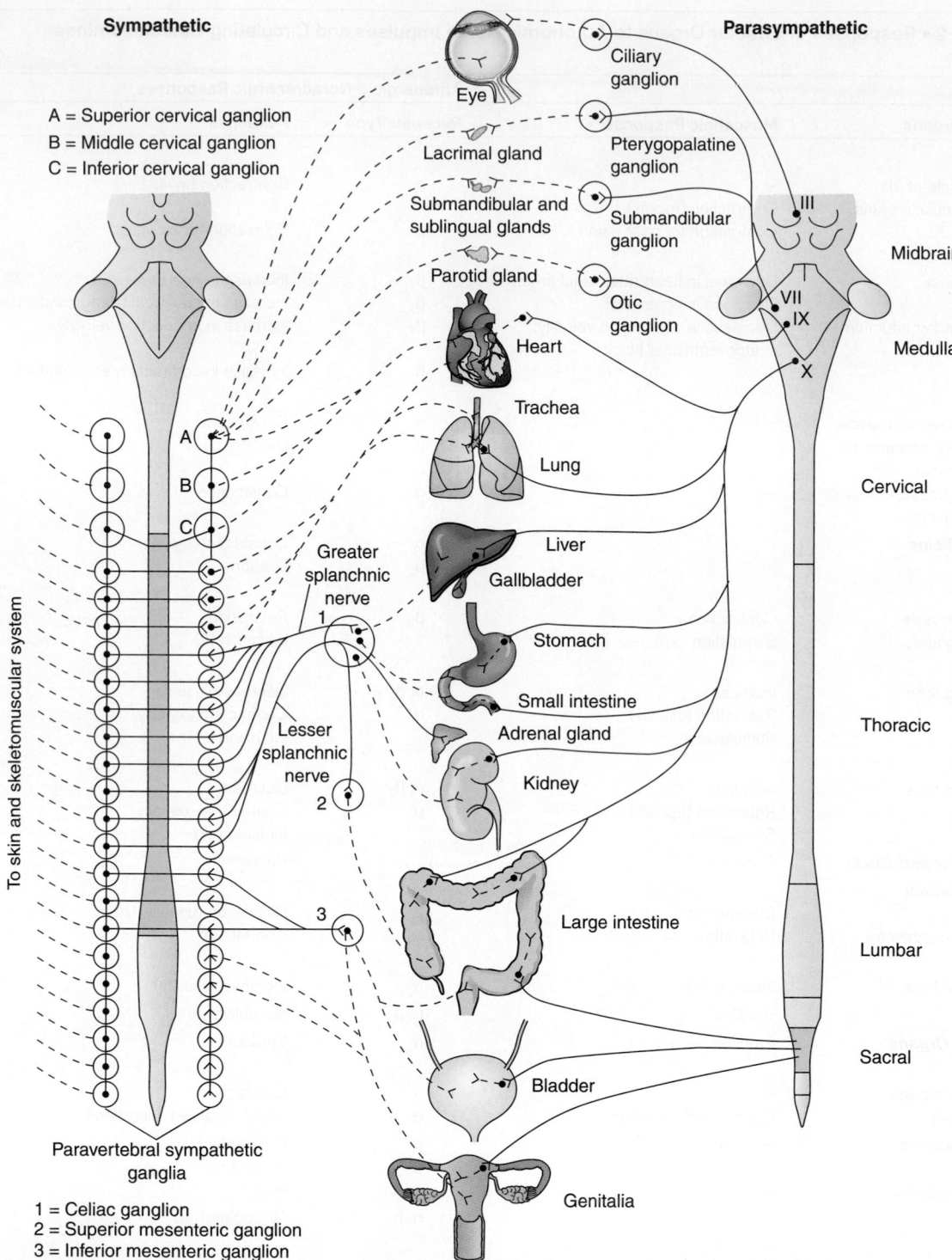

Sympathetic

A = Superior cervical ganglion
B = Middle cervical ganglion
C = Inferior cervical ganglion

To skin and skeletomuscular system

A
B
C

Greater
splanchnic
nerve
1

Lesser
splanchnic
nerve
2

3

Paravertebral sympathetic
ganglia

1 = Celiac ganglion
2 = Superior mesenteric ganglion
3 = Inferior mesenteric ganglion

Parasympathetic

Eye
Ciliary ganglion
Lacrimal gland
Pterygopalatine ganglion
Submandibular and sublingual glands
Submandibular ganglion
Parotid gland
Otic ganglion
Heart
Trachea
Lung
Liver
Gallbladder
Stomach
Small intestine
Adrenal gland
Kidney
Large intestine
Bladder
Genitalia

III
VII
IX
X

Midbrain
Medulla
Cervical
Thoracic
Lumbar
Sacral

Figure 32-24 • The autonomic nervous system and the organs it affects. The left side illustrates the actions of the sympathetic nervous system. The right side illustrates the parasympathetic nervous system. (From Porth CM: Pathophysiology: Concepts of Altered Health States, 6th ed. Philadelphia: Lippincott Williams & Wilkins, 2002.)

enzyme in the synapse. Because muscarinic receptors are structurally different from nicotinic receptors, although both can bind acetylcholine, drugs have been developed that affect only muscarinic receptors and not nicotinic receptors. An example of such a drug is atropine, which blocks muscarinic receptors and prevents the binding of acetylcholine. This and similar drugs are called muscarinic antagonists (also known

as anticholinergics), and their effects are opposite to those of acetylcholine at muscarinic receptors.

Most postganglionic sympathetic neurons synthesize norepinephrine, also called noradrenaline. For this reason, they and other neurons that use norepinephrine as their neurotransmitter are called noradrenergic neurons. When an action potential is conducted down a postganglionic sympathetic neuron because of a strong depolarizing influence received from the preganglionic neuron, norepinephrine is released from the axon terminal into the synapse. It diffuses across the synapse and binds to receptors on the cell membrane of the effector organ. These receptors may be α or β receptors. α Receptors may be α_1 or α_2 receptors, and β receptors may be β_1 or β_2 receptors. The heart has mostly β_1 receptors, and the smooth muscle of the arteries and veins has mostly α_1 and α_2 receptors. The sympathetic nervous system innervates organs with α_1, α_2, and β_1 receptors, and norepinephrine activates these receptors to cause changes in the effector organs that have them. For instance, activation of β_1 receptors in the sinoatrial node by norepinephrine released from sympathetic axon terminals results in depolarization of the sinoatrial node and an increase in heart rate. Activation of α_1 or α_2 receptors in the arteries results in increased contraction by arteriolar smooth muscle and an increase in blood pressure. Table 32-2 shows effects of activation of α and β receptors on various effector organs.

The adrenal medulla is innervated by the sympathetic nervous system through preganglionic (cholinergic) sympathetic neurons. When an action potential is conducted down their axons, these neurons release acetylcholine from their axon terminals into their synapses. The acetylcholine diffuses across the synapse and binds to nicotinic receptors on the cell membranes of the adrenal medullary cells, triggering the release of some norepinephrine but mostly epinephrine from the adrenal cells into the bloodstream. Circulating norepinephrine and epinephrine can both bind to α and β receptors on sympathetic effector organs, similar to synaptic norepinephrine that is released from sympathetic nerve terminals. However, there is one important difference between norepinephrine and epinephrine. As mentioned, β_2 receptors are not innervated by the sympathetic nervous system, and norepinephrine does not bind or activate β_2 receptors to any degree. However, epinephrine is a powerful stimulator of β_2 receptors, which it reaches through the bloodstream after being secreted by the adrenal medulla. Thus, dilation of bronchiolar smooth muscle and dilation of blood vessels in skeletal muscles are important effects of β_2 receptors that are mediated by circulating epinephrine rather than by norepinephrine released from sympathetic nerve terminals or the adrenal medulla.

Although the sympathetic nerves originate in the thoracic and high lumbar cord, and parasympathetic nerves originate with nuclei that send axons down various cranial nerves or sacral spinal nerves, inputs into the patterns of autonomic function are regulated or triggered by centers in the hypothalamus, medulla, and bulboreticular formations. These centers in the CNS send impulses along descending fibers to the appropriate preganglionic autonomic neuron. In the cord, such fibers travel by special descending tracts in the white matter until they reach the appropriate level of the cord. Thus, any interruption of these descending fibers (e.g., transection of cervical tracts) impedes or prevents stimulation of preganglionic autonomic neurons in the thoracic, lumbar, and sacral regions of the cord.

Inputs into the centers in the brainstem and hypothalamus that regulate sympathetic or parasympathetic outflow come from diffuse areas throughout the brain, including visual or auditory centers and areas of the brain associated with conscious thought or planning. Therefore, when we see an alarming sight, such as a car bearing down on us, or hear a frightening noise, sympathetic centers are stimulated and sympathetic outflow increases. Conversely, if we smell food, parasympathetic outflow might increase to prepare the digestive glands for secretion.

In many organ systems, the sympathetic and parasympathetic systems are antagonistic. For instance, the sympathetic system increases the rate of firing of the sinoatrial node and increases the speed of conduction in the atrioventricular node of the heart, whereas the parasympathetic system does the opposite. The parasympathetic system activates the gastrointestinal tract, whereas the sympathetic system inhibits it. Although this is a recurring theme, it is not an absolute rule. Thus, sympathetic stimulation constricts blood vessels (through α receptors), but blood vessels are not innervated by the parasympathetic system, so an opposite effect is not produced by the parasympathetic system. The sympathetic system stimulates cardiac ventricular contractility (through β_1 receptors), but the ventricles are not innervated by the parasympathetic system, so contractility is not affected by it. The two systems actually work together in the male genitalia, where the parasympathetic system mediates erection while the sympathetic system mediates ejaculation.

Both the sympathetic and parasympathetic systems are tonically active most of the time. One or the other may be more active at a given time, but it is rare that either of them is completely silent. Therefore, a person's heart rate at any given time is a summation of the positive effects of the sympathetic system and the negative effects of the parasympathetic system. At rest, parasympathetic influence is strongest, and the heart rate is slow. With exertion or strong emotion, sympathetic activation increases, and the heart rate speeds up.

• Reflexes

Basically, a reflex is a motor response to a sensory input. Reflexes have three components. There is a sensory component, which may consist of only one sensory input or multiple inputs. There is an integrative CNS component that processes the sensory component and "decides" whether it is strong enough to warrant a motor response. Finally, the motor component executes the response. The motor component can consist of one motor nerve and one muscle, or several motor nerves and several muscles. The three components together constitute a "reflex arc" (Fig. 32-25). Reflexes are mediated by lower areas of the brain or by the spinal cord, so that they happen without conscious thought. We become aware of the sensory

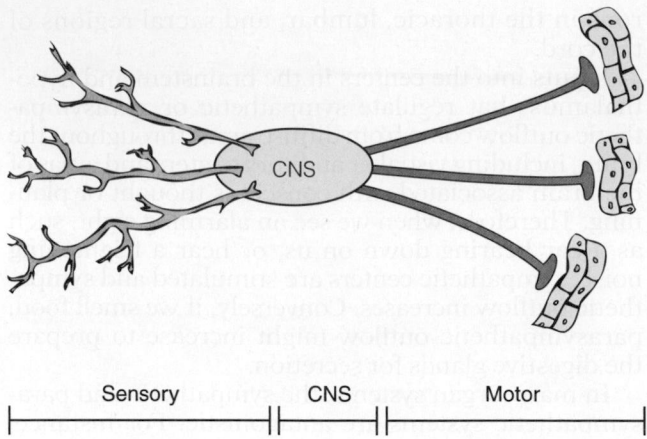

Figure 32-25 • Schematic representation of a reflex arc. CNS, central nervous system.

input and the motor response when they are communicated to our cortex, but by then, the reflex is over. However, if we know that a reflexive action is likely, such as when we see someone about to strike our knee with a reflex hammer, we can often suppress a reflex by willing ourselves not to perform the motor action. This capability illustrates that the cortex has input into the integrative CNS component of the reflex. If higher centers are damaged, the reflex still occurs. For example, people with spinal cord transections still have reflexes in areas supplied by spinal nerves below the transection. Of course, they are unaware that these reflexes are taking place because they cannot receive sensory input to their cortex from below the level of the transection.

BRAIN REFLEXES

Brain reflexes include those involving the cardio-regulatory and vasomotor centers of the medulla, plus the pupillary adjustment center, which involves the midbrain. Additional reflexes mediated by brain centers include the gag reflex, blink reflex, vomiting, and swallowing.

Because of its importance to critical care, the baroreceptor reflex will be used as an illustration of a brain reflex. The sensory components of the baroreceptor reflex are stretch receptors in various arteries, the most important of which are in the carotid sinuses and the aortic arch. These stretch receptors are actually specialized dendrites of sensory nerves that sense the stretch in the arterial wall produced by the pulse. If the blood pressure is high, the stretch receptors are highly stimulated, whereas if the blood pressure is low, the stretch receptors are not stimulated very much. The stretch receptors send nerve impulses down their dendrites to sensory ganglia near the brain in their respective nerves (cranial nerve IX—the glossopharyngeal nerve—in the case of the carotid sinuses, and cranial nerve X—the vagus nerve—in the case of the aortic arch) that are proportional to the degree of stretch. This information is communicated by sensory axons to autonomic centers in the medulla that process the information and compare it with a

"set point" that represents the degree of stimulation they should receive if blood pressure were normal. If the medullary centers receive too little stimulation from the baroreceptors, they send impulses to sympathetic centers to increase sympathetic outflow. This stimulates sympathetic nerves supplying the heart to increase their release of norepinephrine, which binds to β_1 receptors in the sinoatrial node to increase heart rate and β_1 receptors in the ventricles to increase contractility. Sympathetic nerves supplying the veins release norepinephrine, which binds to α receptors, causing constriction of the veins, which increases venous return to the heart. Sympathetic nerves supplying the arteries release norepinephrine, which binds to α receptors, causing constriction of the arteries, which raises the blood pressure. The combination of increased venous return to the heart, increased heart rate, and increased contractility raises the cardiac output, which also increases the blood pressure. Finally, sympathetic nerves supplying the juxtaglomerular apparatus in the kidney release norepinephrine, which binds to β_1 receptors there, stimulating renin release. Through a series of events, renin stimulates the formation of angiotensin II, which is a potent arterial constrictor, increasing blood pressure directly; it also acts on the kidney (through aldosterone) to cause sodium and water retention. Increased retention of sodium and water further increases venous return to the heart, causing additional increased cardiac output and blood pressure. Therefore, activation of the sympathetic nervous system in response to decreased stimulation of the baroreceptors produces many consequences at the effector organs, all of which separately and together cause a rise in blood pressure. If the stretch on the baroreceptors is too high (according to the normal set point), the sympathetic nervous system is inhibited, sympathetic outflow decreases, and consequences at the effector organs are diminished.

SPINAL CORD REFLEXES

In one type of cord reflex, the sensory component of the reflex is the sensory neurons that send their axons to the cord through one of the spinal nerves, the CNS integrative component is the spinal cord, and the motor component is the motor neurons that supply skeletal muscles. Deep tendon reflexes belong in this classification, as does the withdrawal reflex (Fig. 32-26A). These reflexes are present at each level of the spinal cord, bilaterally.

The sensory component of the withdrawal reflex is pain that originates in nociceptors, specialized dendrites of sensory neurons. Impulses are conducted through dendrites of the sensory neurons to the dorsal root ganglia next to the spinal cord and from there along sensory axons into the cord. These impulses stimulate cord interneurons, which, if the sensory input is strong enough, stimulate motor neurons whose axons innervate skeletal muscles, causing contraction. When contracted, the skeletal muscles produce withdrawal of the body part from the painful stimulus. The withdrawal reflex depends on the appropriate anatomical connections between sensory

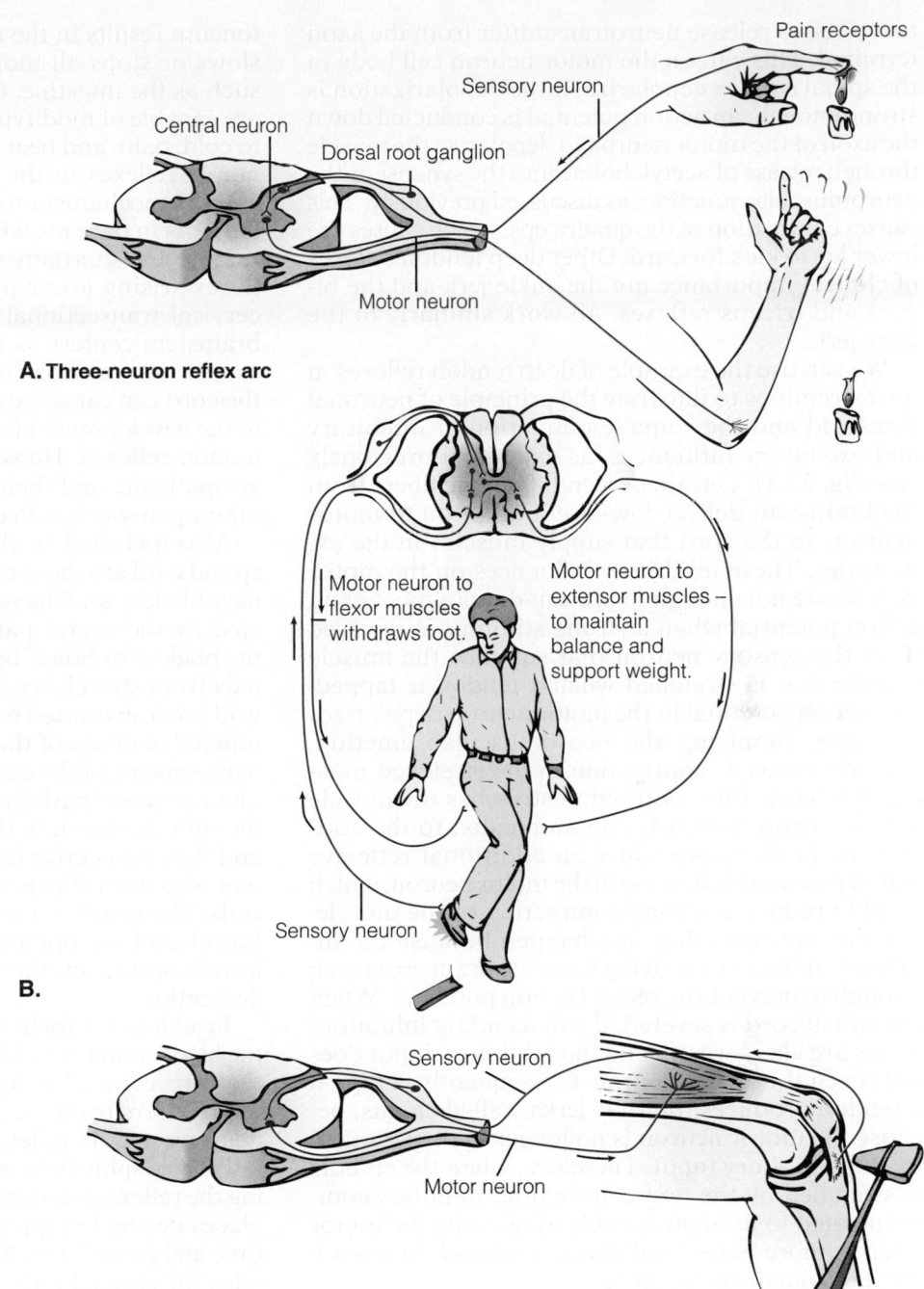

A. Three-neuron reflex arc

Central neuron
Dorsal root ganglion
Motor neuron

Pain receptors
Sensory neuron

B.

Motor neuron to flexor muscles withdraws foot.

Motor neuron to extensor muscles — to maintain balance and support weight.

Sensory neuron

Figure 32-26 • Reflex arcs showing pathways of impulses in response to a stimulus. **A:** The withdrawal reflex involves a three-neuron reflex arc: sensory, central, and motor neurons. **B:** The flexor and crossed extensor reflexes. **C:** Example of a stretch reflex, involving only a two-neuron reflex arc: sensory and motor neurons.

Sensory neuron
Motor neuron

C. Two-neuron reflex arc

neurons, interneurons, and motor neurons in the cord. If these become nonfunctional (e.g., spinal shock or physical trauma), this and other spinal reflexes do not occur.

The withdrawal reflex of one foot is associated with another reflex, the crossed extensor reflex (see Fig. 32-26B). This reflex involves stimulation of various extensor muscles in the opposite leg so that a person's weight is fully supported by the other leg while one lower extremity is withdrawn from a painful stimulus. Such a reflex is complex and involves many levels of the cord. Any imbalance, however slight, during the operation of this reflex in a normal person triggers the occurrence of additional reflexes involving the bulboreticular formation, cerebellum, and various muscles of arms and trunk to maintain balance and posture.

Another cord reflex is the stretch reflex or deep tendon reflex, most commonly illustrated by the clinical test of the knee jerk response (see Fig. 32-26C). In the deep tendon reflex, the sensory component is a specialized sense organ, the muscle spindle, which sends its signals along a spinal nerve to the dorsal horn of the spinal cord. The CNS component is a single synapse of the sensory axon terminal with the motor nerve cell body. The motor component is the motor axon supplying the skeletal muscle. In the knee jerk test, a reflex hammer blow stretches the quadriceps tendon, which stretches the muscle spindle, which sends impulses through the dendrite and axon of its nerve cell to release neurotransmitter from the axon terminal. This causes the motor neuron cell body in the spinal cord to depolarize. If the depolarization is strong enough, an action potential is conducted down the axon of the motor neuron to depolarize the muscle through release of acetylcholine into the synapse at the neuromuscular junction, as discussed previously. This causes contraction of the quadriceps, which causes the lower leg to kick forward. Other deep tendon reflexes of clinical importance are the ankle jerk and the biceps and triceps reflexes. All work similarly to the knee jerk.

We can use the example of deep tendon reflexes in the extremities to illustrate the principle of neuronal threshold and the soma's summation of inhibitory and excitatory influences, as explained previously (see Fig. 32-3). Certain descending nerve fibers from the brainstem deliver low-level inhibition to motor neurons in the cord that supply muscles in the extremities. These inhibitory influences on the motor neuron are not enough to prevent development of an action potential when a strong stimulus is received from the sensory neuron that supplies the muscle spindle that is stretched when a tendon is tapped. The action potential in the motor neuron depolarizes the axon supplying the neuromuscular junction, causing a muscle contraction in the stretched muscle. However, this contraction stretches the muscle spindle again, which is communicated to the cord and might therefore cause an additional reflexive action potential to develop in the motor neuron, which would produce a second contraction of the muscle. Yet this normally does not happen because the inhibitory influences arriving from the brain are strong enough to prevent the second action potential. When the spinal cord is severed, the descending inhibitory axons are also severed, and the inhibitory input does not reach the motor neuron. Consequently, a tap on a tendon produces multiple jerks, called clonus, because the motor neuron is no longer hyperpolarized by the inhibitory input. Therefore, when the spindle is stretched by the first contraction, impulses communicated to its axon are able to re-excite the motor neuron more easily and cause a second, or even a third or fourth contraction.

An important feature of all cord reflexes involving skeletal muscles is reciprocal inhibition, which occurs in the antagonist muscle of the one stimulated. For example, when a flexor reflex stimulates the biceps, it also inhibits its antagonist, the triceps, and provides for more efficient performance of motor activities in the upper arm.

Spinal cord activities also include autonomic reflex circuits, which aid in the control of visceral functions of the body. Sensory input arises from visceral sensory receptors and is transmitted to the spinal cord, where reflex patterns appropriate to the sensory input are determined. The signals are then transmitted to autonomic motor neurons in the gray matter of the spinal cord, which send impulses to the sympathetic nerves innervating visceral motor end organs.

A most important autonomic reflex is the peritoneal reflex. Tissue damage in any portion of the peritoneum results in the activation of this reflex, which slows or stops all motor activity in nearby viscera, such as the intestine. Other autonomic cord reflexes are capable of modifying local blood flow in response to cold, pain, and heat. This vascular control by autonomic reflexes in the spinal cord can operate as a backup mechanism for the usual brainstem control patterns in patients with transectional injuries at the brainstem. Alternatively, because the autonomic reflexes arising lower in the cord of a patient with a cervical transectional injury are not modulated by brainstem centers as they are in patients without a transection, sensory input to autonomic centers in the cord can cause extreme motor responses, similar to the development of clonus with unmodulated deep tendon reflexes. However, these motor reflexes are sympathetic, and their out-of-control state in spinal injury patients is called autonomic hyperreflexia.

Also included in the autonomic reflexes of the spinal cord are those causing the emptying of the urinary bladder and the rectum. These reflexes are mediated by the sacral parasympathetic system. When the bladder or bowel becomes distended, sensory signals from stretch receptors in the bladder or bowel wall are transmitted by sensory neurons to the internuncial neurons of the upper sacral and lower lumbar segments of the cord. These neurons in turn stimulate parasympathetic motor neurons innervating the smooth muscle in the wall of the bladder or bowel, and their respective internal smooth muscle sphincters also are reflexively inhibited by the internuncials. The result is a reflex contraction of bladder or bowel and an opening of the respective smooth muscle sphincter, thereby permitting micturition or defecation.

In addition to their smooth muscle sphincters, both the bladder and bowel have skeletal muscle sphincters that are controlled by motor neurons. Descending motor fibers from the cortex synapse with the motor neurons, and, in toilet-trained people, keep the skeletal muscle sphincters in a state of contraction, inhibiting the reflex emptying of bladder or bowel at times or places deemed inappropriate. When an appropriate time and place is reached, the person can consciously relax the skeletal muscle sphincter and either void or defecate reflexively. Toilet training of infants must await the functional maturation of these descending motor fibers. Cord transection or other damage above the level of the cord housing the neurons for the bladder or bowel evacuation reflexes interrupts some or all of these descending fibers. This produces a condition in which the patient cannot consciously control (prevent) the emptying of the bladder or bowel, or both. As long as the sacral cord and associated spinal nerves are functioning, voiding or defecation proceeds reflexively in such a patient. Damage to or interrupted function of the level of the cord housing the anatomical neuronal connections for these reflexes (as in, for example, spina bifida, spinal shock, or severe injuries to the lower sacral or lumbar cord) or damage to the spinal nerves supplying the bladder or rectum prevents reflex evacuation of bladder or bowel, or both. Such a patient may exhibit retention with overflow and does not possess any effective mechanism for emptying the bladder or bowel.

• Pain

The sensation of pain warrants special consideration because it plays such an important protective role. Whenever there is tissue damage, pain receptors, called nociceptors, are stimulated and send impulses back to the spinal cord. These impulses are transmitted up to the brain, where they are perceived, as previously explained. Stimulation of the nociceptors is caused by the release of substances from damaged tissue and from activation of the inflammatory response. Damaged cells release potassium and hydrogen ion, both of which can stimulate nociceptors. However, the inflammatory response that is evoked in response to tissue damage is responsible for much of the stimulation of nociceptors. For instance, histamine can stimulate nociceptors and prostaglandins, and leukotrienes can sensitize nociceptors to other stimuli. All of these substances are released by inflammatory cells (macrophages, neutrophils, and other white blood cells) that are attracted to the area of tissue injury. In addition, activated platelets participating in clot formation in response to tearing of blood vessels release serotonin, which also stimulates nociceptors. Finally, the nociceptor itself may release substance P when it is stimulated, which sensitizes it to other activating substances. Thus, pain may be due to actual tissue injury or to the inflammatory response evoked by the injury.

PAIN PATHWAYS AND THEIR MODULATION

The sensation of pain is transmitted to the spinal cord and up to the brain in the same manner as previously described for sensations in general. To review, the nociceptor is actually a specialized dendrite of a sensory neuron, whose cell body is in the dorsal root ganglion of the spinal nerve. When the nociceptor is stimulated enough to mount an action potential, the impulse travels to the dorsal root ganglion, and then down the sensory nerve's axon into the dorsal horn, where it synapses with one or more projection neurons. The projection neurons carry the pain message to the thalamus, where pain is first perceived. The projection neurons synapse in the thalamus with neurons that carry the message to the sensory cortex, where the pain is perceived as a localized sensation.

However, there is an important difference in how pain messages are transmitted to the thalamus and cortex compared with other sensations. This difference is in the way the pain impulse can be modulated by spinal influences before it ascends the cord. In brief, gating mechanisms exist in an area in the gray matter called the substantia gelatinosa at all levels of the dorsal cord. These mechanisms, which are described in the following text, are capable of regulating the number of pain impulses that can enter the ascending tracts and travel to the brain.

To regulate ascending pain impulses, an area of the brainstem called the periaqueductal gray sends axons to the nucleus raphe magnus in the medulla. These axons synapse with neurons that send axons from the nucleus raphe magnus back down to all levels of the cord in the substantia gelatinosa. These neurons regulate the ability of pain-stimulated sensory neurons to stimulate projection neurons of the spinothalamic tract. Thus, the descending fibers of the substantia gelatinosa control the entry of pain impulses into the spinal pain conduction system at the level of the cord where the particular sensory neuron enters (Fig. 32-27). Sensory stimuli cannot be conducted and, at least to the thalamus, cannot be perceived.

How do the descending fibers modulate stimulation of the projection neurons by the sensory neurons? When researchers answered this question, we also obtained the answer to another perplexing question: How do the opioid drugs relieve pain? The neurons that descend from the nucleus raphe magnus in the medulla, as well as the modulating internuncial neurons, use previously undiscovered small protein neurotransmitters collectively referred to as the endogenous opioid peptides:

▶ Leucine-enkephalin

▶ Methionine-enkephalin

▶ β-Endorphin

▶ Dynorphin

▶ α-Neoendorphin

When the endogenous opioid peptides are released into a synapse and bind to their receptors on the postsynaptic cell, they produce hyperpolarization of the postsynaptic cell. As explained previously, that makes the postsynaptic cell less likely to be able to conduct an action potential along its axon. Therefore, the descending fibers that synapse with the projection neurons can produce hyperpolarization in the projection neurons, lessening or perhaps even eliminating the pain messages that would otherwise be conducted upward by the projection neurons. Therefore, the endogenous opioid neurotransmitters, by binding to their receptors on the projection neurons, lessen the perception of pain in the thalamus and cortex. Under extreme circumstances, these descending pathways may be so inhibitory to projection neurons that they eliminate all ascending pain messages, producing complete analgesia to pain. This phenomenon is sometimes seen in victims of automobile crashes or in wounded soldiers, who continue to function, oblivious to their wounds.

What stimulates areas of the periaqueductal gray and nucleus raphe magnus to send these descending inhibitory messages to the substantia gelatinosa, resulting in the release of opioid neurotransmitters and diminution of ascending pain signals? Unfortunately, very little is known about this, but it is possible that acupuncture and electrical stimulation devices for pain control are stimulating these pathways, causing inhibition of the projection neurons by the descending neurons' release of opioid neurotransmitters.

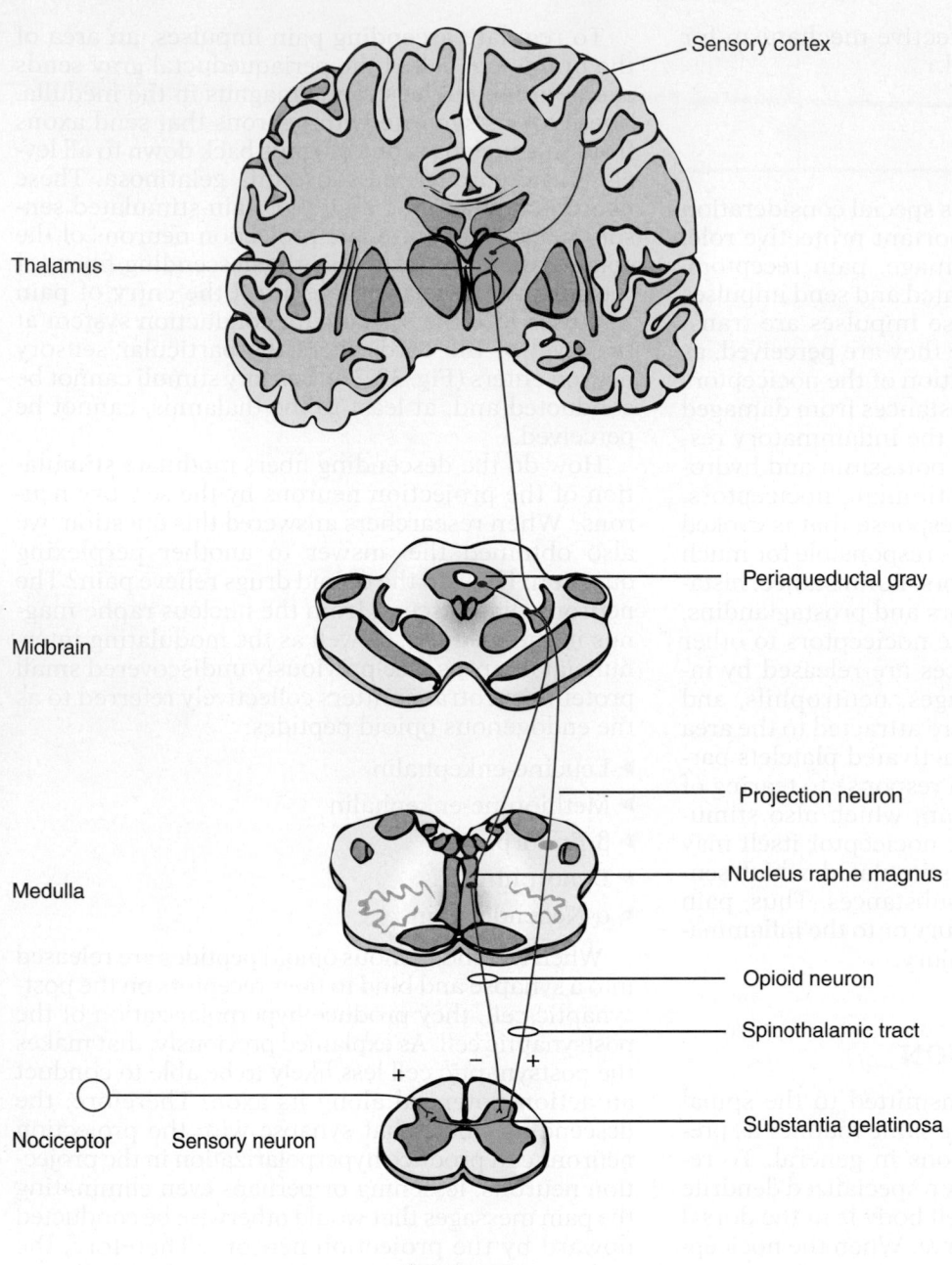

Sensory cortex

Thalamus

Midbrain

Periaqueductal gray

Medulla

Projection neuron

Nucleus raphe magnus

Opioid neuron

Spinothalamic tract

Substantia gelatinosa

Nociceptor   Sensory neuron

Spinal cord

Figure 32-27 • Modulation of ascending pain impulses by descending opioid neurons with origins in the nucleus raphe magnus and input from the periaqueductal gray. The sensory neuron's influence on the projection neuron is stimulatory (depolarizing), designated by the plus sign, but the influence of the opioid neuron is inhibitory (hyperpolarizing), designated by the minus sign. Therefore, if the strength of impulses descending in the opioid neuron is high, the projection neuron will experience fewer action potentials and send fewer pain impulses up to the thalamus.

The opioid drugs work in the same way as the endogenous opioid neurotransmitters. They bind to opioid receptors on the projection or internuncial neuron, producing hyperpolarization and a decrease in the amount of pain stimulus reaching the thalamus and the cortex. There are neurons that use the endogenous opioids as neurotransmitters in the brain as well, and opioid drugs also bind to the receptors that these neurons supply. These effects may increase the analgesic effects of the drug, or they may be responsible for other effects, such as the somnolence or dizziness that opioid drugs produce. In addition, there are opioid receptors in the intestinal tract that are stimulated by endogenous opioids and by opioid drugs. These receptors inhibit peristalsis in the intestinal tract, and this effect is responsible for the constipation and nausea often seen with opioid drugs.

Pain is a complex sensation. There is great variation in pain thresholds among different people and within the same person at different times. These variations can partly be explained by the modulation of pain pathways by endogenous opioid neurotransmitters. In addition, the amount of tissue injury and presence of chemical mediators can increase the pain experience qualitatively, quantitatively, temporally, and spatially. However, pain perception is also influenced by expectations and by cultural influences. It is helpful to remember that pain is a perception and that we have to take a person's word in describing that perception to us. It is impossible to judge a patient's pain by his or her appearance or actions, or physical or laboratory signs. The complexity of the pain pathways can make the clinical management of pain difficult, but every patient's description of his or her pain should be taken seriously. Opioid addiction is practically unknown in patients without a history of drug abuse who receive opioids for pain relief. Pain medication should be administered to most patients based on their own self-report of their pain.

REFERRED PAIN

Referred pain is pain perceived as arising from a site that is different from its true point of origin. The "true point of origin" for this type of pain usually is some visceral organ or deep somatic structure, and the "point of reference" is some area of the body surface. Well-known examples include the referring of pain from severe cardiac ischemia to the left arm or the referring of diaphragmatic pain to the neck and shoulder.

The most generally accepted theory for referred pain is that the two sensory neurons, one from the region of the true point of origin and one from the point of reference, enter the same segment of the spinal cord and synapse with the same projection neuron. There is no way for the cortex to know whether a given projection neuron was originally stimulated by pain from the true point of origin or from the referred area. In localizing the source of the pain stimulus, the cortex relies on prior experience regarding the person's geographical knowledge of his or her own body. Because surface areas are more familiar to a person than the locations of the visceral or deep somatic structures, the referred locale is used preferentially over the more unfamiliar but true point of origin (Fig. 32-28).

• The Neurohormonal Stress Response

HOMEOSTASIS

In the middle of the 19th century, the French physiologist Claude Bernard (1813–1878) coined the term milieu intérieur to mean the internal environment to which body cells are exposed. He stated that to maintain proper cell functioning, the milieu intérieur must be constant and proper.[1,2]

> The living body, though it has need of the surrounding environment, is nevertheless relatively independent of it. This independence which the organism has of its external environment, derives from the fact that in the living being, the tissues are in fact withdrawn from direct external influences and are protected by a veritable internal environment which is constituted, in particular, by the fluids circulating in the body.
>
> *Opening lecture in general physiology given to the College de France, as quoted in Scultz SG: The internal environment. In Johnson LR (ed): Essential Medical Physiology, 2nd ed. New York, Raven Press, 1998.*

Although Bernard thought the blood constituted the milieu intérieur, we now realize that each tissue and cell type probably has its own environment that

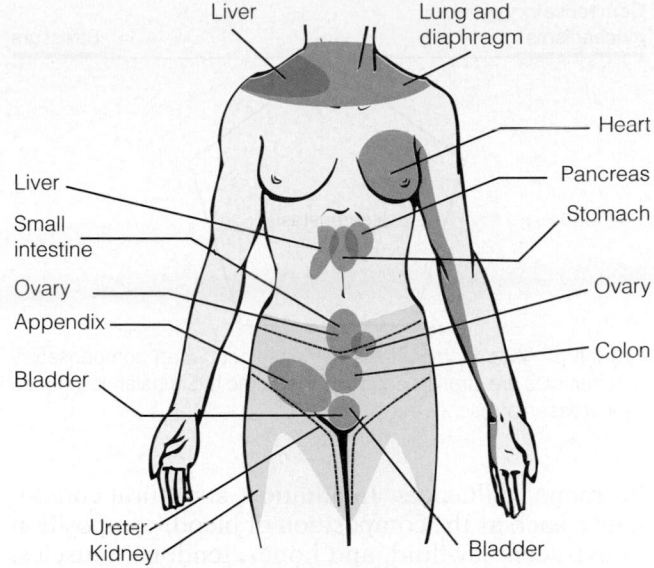

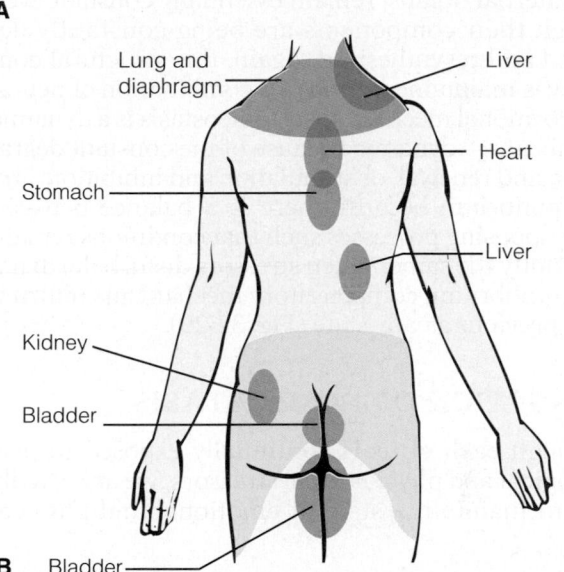

Figure 32-28 • Areas of referred pain. **A:** Anterior view. **B:** Posterior view.

may be different from that of other tissues or cell types. However, the idea of a constant and appropriate internal environment remains valid to this day. Bernard was the first to advance the concept that bodily processes are constantly responding to the external environment with mechanisms that maintain constancy of the milieu intérieur: "The constancy of the internal environment requires such a perfection in the organism that external variations are instantly compensated for and balanced."[1] The concept of a constant internal environment was expanded by Walter Canon in the early 20th century to include all bodily process and structures, and was termed homeostasis.

Homeostasis is defined as the situation in which attributes of the body such as blood pressure, level of alertness, and muscle tone remain constant or change appropriately for different situations. The constant nature of these attributes is due to the right balance between stimulatory and inhibitory neuronal and

Compensatory
mechanisms   Stressors

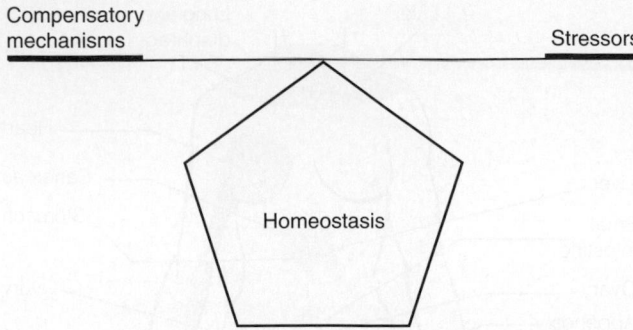

Figure 32-29 • Homeostasis is maintained when compensatory mechanisms are strong enough to overcome the imbalance induced by increased stress.

hormonal influences. In addition, structural components, such as the composition of blood, composition of extracellular fluid, and bones, tendons, muscles, and internal organs, remain essentially constant even though their components are being constantly degraded and resynthesized. Again, this structural constancy is maintained through a combination of neural and hormonal mechanisms. Homeostasis is a dynamic equilibrium—dynamic because of the constant degradation and renewal, or stimulation and inhibition, and an equilibrium because there is a balance between these opposing processes such that conditions remain constantly the same. When stressors disturb the dynamic equilibrium, compensatory mechanisms return it to its previous steady state (Fig. 32-29).

DISRUPTION OF HOMEOSTASIS

Although each of us is continually exposed to psychological and physiological stressors, we are usually able to maintain a state of emotional and physical health through compensatory mechanisms that maintain homeostasis. In fact, it has been shown that some level of stress is beneficial to health. However, in the event of stress that overwhelms compensatory mechanisms, we can become ill (Fig. 32-30). Overwhelming stressors may become so because of their large magnitude over time, or because of their sudden onset. People who present as patients in critical care settings have usually experienced recent, severe physiological stressors, but these are superimposed on their level of chronic physiological and psychological stress. In addition, the patient is exposed to continuous stressors that are byproducts of the critical care setting, such as monitoring devices, invasive procedures, and the continual presence of devices for intravenous access, endotracheal intubation, and others.[3]

Although others, especially Walter Cannon (who also coined the term homeostasis), presented some of these theories earlier, Dr. Hans Selye was the most prolific researcher and author on the topic of stress.[4,5] Stress is "any external or internal factor that affects the normal state of dynamic equilibrium in an individual." These factors, or stressors, can be either physical or psychological. Regardless of whether the person consciously perceives a threat, the body responds with certain intrinsic reactions. When the effects are realized by the conscious mind, the person perceives a stressful experience. The stress response is how a person reacts to the stressors that he or she encounters (i.e., the person's physiological adaptation or psychological coping mechanisms). One person may have compensatory mechanisms with a large capacity to handle stressors, whereas another person may not. Therefore, exposure to a given stressor does not elicit the same response in all people. This difference may be based on internal conditioning factors, such as age, sex, and genetics, and on external factors, such as culture, pre-

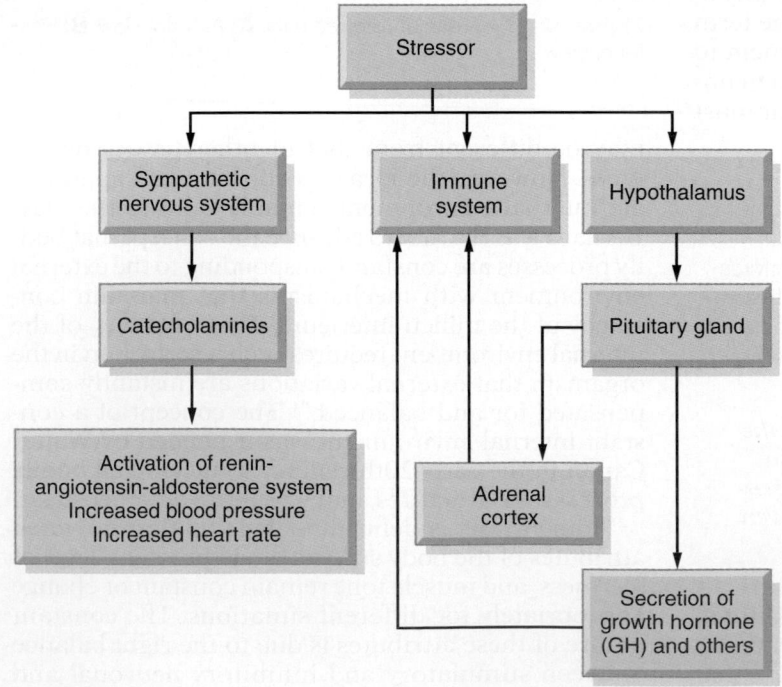

Figure 32-30 • The stress response induces increased activity in the sympathetic nervous system, including the adrenal medulla, which activates the renin–angiotensin–aldosterone system and increases the blood pressure and heart rate, among other things. The stress response also activates the pituitary gland, which secretes increased growth hormone; the adrenal cortex, which secretes increased cortisol; and the immune system.

vious life events, exposure to this or similar stressors, diet and nutrition, and medications.

Stressors may be either psychological or physiological in origin. Psychological stressors are additive in nature (e.g., life events such as a job change, divorce, marriage) and have a physiological impact. Physiological stressors, such as injury or infection, disrupt homeostasis, eliciting the stress response in an attempt to restore it. If homeostasis is not restored quickly, illness results.

General Adaptation Syndrome

Selye and his collaborators noted commonalities in responses to different stressors in different individuals. They termed these commonalities the general adaptation syndrome. Although this term has fallen from favor, and the changes they noted are probably not as general as they thought, the concept of a generalized response to stress remains. They also defined the three basic stages of the stress syndrome as the alarm reaction, stage of resistance, and stage of exhaustion.

▶ *Alarm reaction.* During this initial stage, the threat is perceived, either consciously or subconsciously, and body processes are modified to counteract it. The sympathetic nervous system is stimulated by the stressor, and there is a subsequent response through the release of norepinephrine and epinephrine. Additionally, adrenocorticotropic hormone (ACTH) and ADH are released by the anterior and posterior pituitary. Stimulation of the sympathetic nervous system raises heart rate and blood pressure and stimulates the renin–angiotensin–aldosterone system, which results in sodium and water retention, increasing the blood pressure further. ACTH stimulates the release of cortisol by the adrenal cortex, which produces numerous adaptations to stress, outlined below. ADH raises blood pressure mainly by causing the kidney to retain water. These effects are additive to those elicited by the sympathetic nervous system and the renin–angiotensin–aldosterone system.

▶ *Stage of resistance.* During the second stage, the stress is being compensated for by increased activity of the stress responses evoked during the alarm phase. Cortisol secretion, the sympathetic nervous system, and other mechanisms triggered in the alarm reaction may continue to be activated at a lower, more constant level. This phase may continue for a long time, even years, if the increased levels of stress response mechanisms are maintained. However, the increased levels of stress response mechanisms come at a price—the use of additional resources of energy and nutrients. It is during this stage that symptoms of disease may become chronic if the compensatory responses are not adequate to control them.

▶ *Stage of exhaustion.* The ability to mount a stress response has limits. Therefore, the stress response can be activated only for a finite time or to a finite degree. If the stressor is not removed or adaptation does not occur, the person is no longer able to resist the stressor. At this point, homeostasis is no longer achievable. A shock state may occur (see Chapter 54), and, without appropriate intervention, organ failure and death may rapidly ensue.

The Stress Response

Acute Stress

Consider a prehistoric man walking on the African veldt. Suddenly, a lion springs from behind some vegetation. The man's eyes capture an image of the lion, which is communicated to the visual areas in his occipital cortex. From there, the image is sent to and processed by his prefrontal and frontal cortex and perceived as a threat. This information of threat is communicated to many centers in his brain, including those supplying the ANS. Immediately, sympathetic outflow is greatly increased by activation of brainstem sympathetic centers and through unitary activation of the sympathetic nervous system (remember the autonomic ganglia that communicate with each other at all levels of the spinal cord), increasing the rate of firing of his sympathetic nerves, releasing norepinephrine into sympathetic synapses. At the same time, parasympathetic outflow is greatly inhibited, decreasing activity of the gastrointestinal system and the need of those organs for blood. The man's heart rate and cardiac contractility (β_1 receptors) are greatly increased, both of which increase his cardiac output, and his resistance arterioles constrict (α receptors). Increased cardiac output and increased arteriolar resistance raise his blood pressure. At the same time, veins also constrict (α receptors), increasing venous return to his heart and increasing cardiac output still more. The adrenal medulla is stimulated by sympathetic outflow (neuronal nicotinic receptors) to secrete some norepinephrine, but mostly epinephrine, into the bloodstream. The epinephrine stimulates α and β_1 receptors all over the man's body, causing the same effects as norepinephrine does at those receptors. It also stimulates β_2 receptors on his bronchiolar smooth muscle, causing relaxation and dilation of the bronchioles, enabling him to inspire and expire greater volumes of air. In addition, it stimulates β_2 receptors on arterioles in his skeletal muscle beds, causing profound dilation, increasing the capacity of these beds for blood flow. Because arterioles to digestive and other internal organs are constricted by virtue of α-receptor activation, the greatly increased cardiac output is directed to skeletal muscle beds, supplying the muscle cells with increased amounts of oxygen and glucose to sustain increased contraction. Blood flow to the brain is also greatly increased by the increased cardiac output because arterioles supplying the brain have few α receptors, so they remain fully dilated. Stimulation of β_1 receptors in the juxtaglomerular apparatus of the kidney by norepinephrine (from sympathetic nervous system nerve terminals and the adrenal medulla) and epinephrine (from the adrenal medulla) causes the release of renin, which activates the renin–angiotensin–aldosterone system. Renin acts on circulating angiotensinogen to angiotensin I, which is further converted to angiotensin II by angiotensin-converting enzymes. Angiotensin II causes additional arteriolar constriction, increasing blood pressure still further. It also causes the release of aldosterone, which causes the kidney to retain sodium and water. Sodium and water retention increases the preload to the heart, increasing cardiac output still further.

In addition, communication of the threatening sight to the hypothalamus activates many neurohormonal mechanisms controlled by the pituitary. We consider only three of these. First, the hypothalamus increases its synthesis and release of ADH from the posterior pituitary. ADH causes the kidney to retain water, further increasing the preload and thereby the cardiac output. Second, the hypothalamus increases its secretion and release of corticotropin-releasing hormone, which causes the anterior pituitary to secrete additional ACTH, which in turn causes the adrenal cortex to release increased quantities of cortisol. Cortisol has far-reaching effects on many organs that increase their ability to respond to stress. Third, through increased synthesis and release of growth hormone–releasing hormone by the hypothalamus, growth hormone (GH) synthesis and release by the anterior pituitary is increased. Like cortisol, GH has many far-reaching effects on many organs, but its overall effect is to increase the activity of tissue repair mechanisms and utilization of nutrients.

Finally, the man's immune system is activated by the stress response. This activation is achieved by multiple influences, only a few of which are mentioned here. First, GH increases the ability of many cells of the immune system, such as neutrophils and T and B lymphocytes, to carry out their functions, including phagocytosis, antigen presentation, and antibody production. In addition, the physiologically high levels of cortisol affect the immune system's ability to respond to foreign antigens. (Levels produced by pharmacological doses of corticosteroids are much higher than those produced by stress and are immunosuppressive.) The effects of physiologically elevated levels of cortisol in response to stress on immune function are complex and may involve effects on the ability of immune cells to exit the circulation and go to sites of tissue injury, or their ability to respond to antigen presentation. Finally, catecholamines also affect the immune system's ability to respond to tissue injury or foreign antigens. The net response of the immune system to acute influences of the stress response is generally considered to be an increased ability to mount an inflammatory response and respond to a foreign antigen. Figure 32-30 summarizes the effects on various body systems.

Returning to our prehistoric man threatened by a lion, the changes produced in his body by the threatening sight of a lion all have the effect of increasing the ability of his muscles to help him run faster or fight harder to escape the lion, and increasing his ability to respond to tissue injury that might result from his encounter with the lion. These changes constitute the alarm reaction characterized by Selye. The lion threat represents an acute stressor that would end very quickly, either because the man escaped or was killed. If the man was successful in escaping the lion, the stress response would extinguish itself very

rapidly, and his physiological state would gradually return to normal.

The question that arises for modern humans is, "How are the changes of the alarm reaction beneficial for stresses encountered in modern times?" If one is running to get away from a dangerous situation or to catch a bus, is injured in an automobile crash, or contracts an acute illness, the acute stress response is very likely still beneficial. However, if one undergoes an acute emotional stress, such as an intense argument or the death of a loved one, the alarm reaction is invoked, the same as it would be for a more physiologically oriented stress. In such circumstances, we do not need increased ability to fight or run away, decreased activity of our gastrointestinal system, or increased ability for tissue repair. Therefore, in these circumstances, the acute stress response is at best superfluous, and at worst consumes resources and unnecessarily creates wear and tear on body systems.

Chronic Stress

Selye's "stage of resistance" describes our ability to handle chronic stress. Chronic stressors that affected prehistoric humans included starvation or extreme heat or cold. Responses to these stressors included some of the same mechanisms as outlined earlier for acute stress, but at diminished levels that are more sustainable over a long period. However, responses to these stressors also included additional mechanisms that conserve body stores of nutrients and energy. These responses include cortisol, but also insulin, glucagon, and GH. The chronic stress response in prehistoric times probably did not include response to diseases. Because disease processes could not be treated, affected people quickly died during the acute stress response. The mechanisms that evolved prehistorically to handle chronic stress may or may not be appropriate to handle modern stressors such as chronic disease or the chronic emotional stress associated with constant deadlines or commuting in heavy traffic. Moreover, with modern medical care, we now have the ability to maintain people with extremely high levels of chronic stress due to disease, their emotional state, and the stress induced by our interventions. In intensive care units we measure many aspects of homeostasis, such as electrolyte levels, blood cell counts, cardiac functioning, and hormonal levels, and adjust our care to preserve homeostasis (a proper milieu intérieur).

In many such situations, the chronic stress responses as they have been handed down to us from prehistoric times may actually be counterproductive and decrease our ability to maintain homeostasis. In addition, increased activity of stress responses may increase the likelihood of degenerative diseases of the circulatory system, such as atherosclerosis, leading to vascular events in the heart, periphery, or brain; disorders of glucose metabolism that lead to type 2 diabetes; or, perhaps, disorders of the immune system that lead to inflammatory diseases. These types of diseases are all the result of a complex interplay between a person's genetic makeup, his or her life experiences (including exposure to antigens and infectious diseases), and level of both physiological and psychological stress.

• Age-Related Changes

Because of age-related changes in the nervous system, older people are at higher risk for injury and have less chance for survival after a severe injury. Impairment of sensation, proprioception, gait, vision, and hearing and delayed response time are a few factors that predispose older people to injury. Considerations for the older patient are given in Box 32-1.

 Box 32-1 • CONSIDERATIONS FOR THE OLDER PATIENT: Anatomical and Physiological Changes in the Nervous System That Occur With Aging

- Cerebral atrophy results in a decrease in total brain weight and volume, especially in the frontal and temporal lobes, enlargement of the ventricles, and a loss of gray matter.
- Cerebral atrophy causes the dura mater and bridging veins to become tightly adherent to the skull; thus, they are easily torn with significant movement of the cranial contents, leading to subdural hematoma formation.
- Cerebral atrophy creates more space for intracranial blood to be concealed, so the older patient may manifest only subtle symptoms, which may lead to a delay in diagnosis.
- Axonal loss or decreases in myelination result in a loss of white matter.
- There is atrophy of the hippocampus, which correlates with a decline in learning and memory and cognitive impairments.
- A decreased number of neuronal cells and degeneration of dendrites and dendritic spines in cortical pyramidal cells leads to declining synaptic transmission and slowed impulse conduction.
- There is decreased production, release, and metabolism of neurotransmitters.
- Altered circulation in the inner ear and fewer functional cochlear cells lead to reduced hearing.
- A decreased number of olfactory cells in nasal mucosa leads to a reduced sense of smell.
- There is an increase in wakefulness and arousal from sleep and a decrease in slow-wave sleep, leading to changes in sleep patterns.
- The odontoid process in the cervical spine is most commonly fractured because of osteoporosis and degenerative joint disease.
- Central cord syndrome occurs more frequently because of spinal stenosis.
- The patient is more prone to severe brain injury and may have less reserve to survive a severe injury.
- The incidence of dementia somewhat increases. Those who develop dementia have a decline in cognitive and emotional abilities, which can affect memory, language, visuospatial skills, complex cognition, emotion, and personality.

• Clinical Applicability Challenges

Short-Answer Questions

1. A male patient is newly admitted to the intensive care unit with a stroke that has left him partially paralyzed and mute. He looks around wildly and continually moves his unaffected limbs. His heart rate, blood pressure, and respiratory rate are elevated. Describe the stressors and mechanisms of the stress response in this patient.

2. A 45-year-old female patient with a subarachnoid hemorrhage is admitted to the intensive care unit for close observation. Describe the flow of the cerebrospinal fluid circulation and how a subarachnoid hemorrhage could cause hydrocephalus, one of the complications that can develop from such a hemorrhage.

3. A 52-year-old male patient is brought to the emergency department after sustaining a stab wound to the neck. He has active arterial bleeding at the lateral side of his neck, and he is brought to the operating room where he undergoes ligation of the right internal carotid artery. Postoperatively, he is neurologically intact. Explain what symptoms a patient can display after ligation of the right internal carotid artery. Also, explain why only some people are symptomatic.

Review Questions

1. A patient has sustained a traumatic head injury. The nurse knows that it is important to examine the patient's extraocular movements. Which cranial nerves are assessed?
   a. Third, fourth, and fifth
   b. Third, fourth, and sixth
   c. Fourth, fifth, and sixth
   d. Second, third, and fourth

2. The nurse is performing a history and physical examination and notes that the patient has intention tremors, no fine motor coordination, and ataxia. What part of the brain is affected?
   a. Basal ganglia
   b. Frontal lobe
   c. Cerebellum
   d. Reticular activating system

3. The nurse is completing a head-to-toe assessment on a spinal cord injury patient. The nurse finds that the patient has no movement in the lower extremities. What tract is involved?
   a. Spinothalamic tract
   b. Corticospinal tract
   c. Posterior columns
   d. Spinocerebellar tract

4. A patient is admitted to a neurointensive care unit with an elevated heart rate. The nurse knows that this could be the result of increased activity at which

of the following receptors of the autonomic nervous system?

a. α Receptors
b. β_1 Receptors
c. β_2 Receptors
d. Muscarinic receptors

5. A patient with a spinal cord injury at T3 is unable to feel pain from a deep decubitus ulcer on the foot. This results because of interruption of the pain signal at which of the following locations in the sensory pathway?

a. The first-order neuron
b. The second-order neuron
c. The third-order neuron
d. The sensory homunculus

6. A patient is brought into the trauma unit from a fiery automobile crash in which he sustained fractures of his arm and fibula. He reports that he was able to run away from the burning wreck despite his broken leg and did not feel pain until after the ambulance arrived. This phenomenon is most likely due to activation of which neuronal pathway?

a. The parasympathetic nervous system
b. The reticular activating system
c. The descending pathways in the substantia gelatinosa
d. The spinal reflexes

References

1. Conti F: Claude Bernard: Primer of the second biomedical revolution. Nat Mol Cell Biol 2:703–708, 2001
2. Conti F: Claude Bernard's Des Fonctions du Cerveau: An ante litteram manifesto of the neurosciences? Nat Neurosci 3:979–985, 2002
3. Hickey JV: The Clinical Practice of Neurological and Neurosurgical Nursing, 5th ed. Philadelphia: Lippincott Williams & Wilkins, 2003
4. Selye H: The general adaptation syndrome and the diseases of adaptation. J Clin Endocrinol 6:117, 1946
5. Selye H: Stress Without Distress. Philadelphia: JB Lippincott, 1974

Other Selected Readings

Baer MF, Connors BW, Paradiso MA: Neuroscience: Exploring the Brain, 3rd edition. Philadelphia: Lippincott Williams & Wilkins, 2007

Burton H: Visual cortex activity in early and late blind people. J Neurosci 23(10):4005–4011, 2003

Burton H: Visual cortex activation in late onset, Braille naïve blind individuals: An fMRI study during semantic and phonological tasks with heard words. Neurosci Lett 392(1–2):38–42, 2006

Eigsti J, Henke K: Anatomy and physiology of neurological compensatory mechanisms. Dimens Crit Care Nurs 25(5):197–204, 2006

Gattey D: The pupil examination in the trauma patient. J Emerg Nurs 30:512–513, 2004

Haines DE: Neuroanatomy: An Atlas of Structures, Sections, and Systems, 6th ed. Philadelphia: Lippincott Williams & Wilkins, 2004

Haymore J: A neuron in a haystack. AACN Clin Issues 15(4): 568–581, 2004

Horner A, VanDemark M, Jensen GA: The challenge of assessing a patient with dementia and head injury. AACN Clin Issues 13(1):73–83, 2002

Kiernan JA: Barr's The Human Nervous System: An Anatomical Viewpoint, 8th ed. Philadelphia: Lippincott Williams & Wilkins, 2005

Lower J: Facing neuro assessment fearlessly. Nursing 32(2):58–65, 2002

Pudelek B: Geriatric trauma: Special needs for a special population. AACN Clin Issues 13(1):61–72, 2002

Siegel A, Sapru HN: Essential Neuroscience. Philadelphia: Lippincott Williams & Wilkins, 2006

Snell RS: Clinical Neuroanatomy, 6th ed. Philadelphia: Lippincott Williams & Wilkins, 2006

White A: Neurologic assessment: Vital in prioritizing emergency department interventions. Am J Nurse Practitioner 10(9):57–67, 2006

Patient Assessment: Nervous System

Genell Hilton

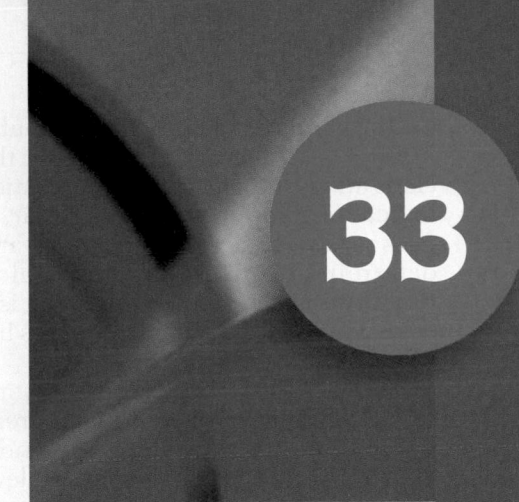

33

History
Physical Examination
  Mental Status
  Motor Function
  Pupillary Changes
  Vital Signs
  Cranial Nerve Function
  Reflexes
  Sensation
  Signs of Trauma or Infection
  Signs of Increased Intracranial Pressure
  Evaluation of Dysfunction in the Patient's
    Living Patterns
Neurodiagnostic Studies
  Neuroradiological Techniques
  Computed Tomography
  Magnetic Resonance Imaging
  Positron Emission Tomography and Single-Photon
    Emission Computed Tomography
  Angiography and Digital Subtraction Angiography
  Cerebral Blood Flow Studies
  Myelography

Ultrasonography and Noninvasive
  Cerebrovascular Studies
Electrophysiological Studies
Lumbar Puncture for Cerebrospinal Fluid Examination

Objectives

Based on the content in this chapter, the reader should
be able to:

❶ Perform a comprehensive neurological assessment.

❷ Identify abnormal assessment findings consistent
   with neurological compromise.

❸ Analyze assessment findings and identify potential
   nursing diagnoses.

❹ Evaluate the effect of neurological dysfunction on
   the patient.

❺ Identify preprocedure and postprocedure nursing
   interventions appropriate to selected
   neurodiagnostic tests.

Assessment and care of a patient with a neurological problem constitute one of the biggest
challenges for critical care nurses. Basic nursing education and critical care courses may not
address the assessment of the nervous system to
the depth or complexity of other body systems. In
addition, a comprehensive neurological assessment
involves the use of techniques not commonly performed in the assessment of other body systems.
Therefore, it is not uncommon for even the experienced nurse to feel uncertain when gathering data
about the nervous system.

There are four major objectives in the nursing
assessment of a patient with a real or potential neurological problem. The first objective is to gather data
about the functioning of the nervous system in an
unbiased and orderly manner, avoiding inconsistencies in data collection or inadequate data collection.
It is essential that examination results be recorded
clearly so that changes in findings can be easily identified. A standard neurological check sheet should

be used by all the nursing staff, with clearly defined
grading scales or terms listed as appropriate.

The second objective of neurological assessment
is to follow the data over time, discovering correlations and trends. For such correlations to be of value,
it is necessary to interrelate the results of history,
physical assessment, and diagnostic tests. Use of a
patterned format helps establish medical and nursing diagnoses and guides the nurse in choosing and
evaluating therapy.

The third objective of neurological assessment
is to analyze the data to develop a list of potential
or actual diagnoses. Minor changes in neurological
status may be the first indication that the patient's
physical condition is worsening. It is the responsibility of the nurse providing care to the patient
to recognize these changes, correlate these findings to the pathophysiological process, and intervene appropriately.

The fourth objective of the neurological nursing
assessment is to determine the effect of dysfunction

on the patient's daily living and ability to care for himself or herself. Up to this point, the goals of physicians and nurses in the care of a patient with a neurological problem have been similar. Each discipline uses many of the same questions and techniques to determine normal and abnormal nervous system functioning. The focus of nursing is to help patients cope with real or potential changes in daily living and self-care.

These objectives of neuroassessment are the same for all patients. However, in children, aspects of this process may be difficult, and findings may differ depending on the child's stage of development. Likewise, in older patients, it is necessary to take the normal changes of aging into account when assessing for neurological problems. Older adults are at increased risk for certain medical conditions that predispose them to neurological problems. These same medical conditions or their prescribed treatment may also alter neurological assessment findings. Special considerations for older adults are given in Box 33-1.

• History

Neurological assessment begins with the nurse's first encounter with the patient. Conversation with the patient and family is a vital source of data needed to evaluate overall functioning. The nurse ascertains the reason for the patient's visit and obtains data regarding symptoms. In addition, the nurse evaluates the patient's past medical history, family history, and

Box 33-1 • CONSIDERATIONS FOR THE OLDER PATIENT: Neuroassessment

When assessing an older adult, it is necessary to ascertain the person's previous level of functioning to adequately assess the person's status. The following should be taken into consideration when the nurse assesses an older adult's neurological function:

- Motor function may be affected by decreased strength, alterations in gait, changes in posture, and increased tremors.
- Vision may be decreased, pupils may be less reactive, color discrimination may be decreased, gaze may be impaired, and night vision may be diminished.
- Hearing may be diminished and changes in Rinne test findings may be noted. The nurse should bear in mind that an undetected hearing impairment can lead to the erroneous assumption that a person has more neurological deficits than he or she actually has.
- Changes in sensory function may include decreased reflexes, decreased vibratory and position sense, and decreased two-point discrimination.
- Older adults are at increased risk for depression, nutritional abnormalities, stroke, transient ischemic attacks (TIAs), and dementia.
- Older adults may have impaired sleep patterns.

personal and social history. A comprehensive review of systems is also performed as part of the initial assessment (Box 33-2).

• Physical Examination

MENTAL STATUS

The mental status examination includes tests to evaluate level of consciousness and arousal, orientation to the environment, and thought content. The quality of a patient's level of consciousness is the most basic and critical parameter requiring assessment. Level of consciousness evaluates the functioning of the cerebral hemispheres as well as that of the reticular activating system, which is responsible for arousal. The degree of a patient's awareness of, response to, and interaction with the environment is the most sensitive indicator of nervous system dysfunction. Responsiveness may be categorized according to the patient's arousal to external stimuli, and gradations of response include terms such as lethargic, stuporous, and semicomatose (Box 33-3).

Orientation to the environment involves assessing not only the patient's ability to respond but also the content of his or her response. This is assessed by asking the patient questions such as, "What is your name? Where are you right now? What is the month/year/date/time?" An increase in the number of wrong answers indicates increasing confusion and possible deterioration in neurological status. Likewise, an increase in the number of correct answers may indicate neurological improvement.

In instances in which brain injury is suspected, the Glasgow Coma Scale (GCS) has proved a reliable tool for assessing arousal and level of consciousness (Box 33-4). The GCS allows the examiner to record objectively the patient's response to the environment in three major areas: eye opening, verbalization, and movement. In each category, the best response is scored. The GCS uses two responses, best eye-opening response and best verbal response, to assess arousal and level of consciousness. Best eye-opening response is scored from 1 to 4, with 1 as no response and 4 as spontaneous eye opening. Best verbal response addresses orientation and ranges from 1 to 5, with 1 again indicating no response and 5 indicating a fully oriented patient. The intubated patient is usually noted to have a verbal score of 1T, which should be added into the total score. In this way, recognition is given to the patient's inability to speak secondary to the presence of the endotracheal tube. Best motor responses ranges from 1 to 6, with 1 indicating no motor response and 6 representing a patient with movement of all extremities to command.

The maximal total score for a fully awake and alert person is 15. A minimal score of 3 is consistent with complete lack of responsiveness. An overall score of 8 or below is associated with coma. If maintained over time, a low GCS score may be a predictor of poor functional recovery. This scoring system was designed

Box 33-2 • Neurological Health History

Chief Complaint
- One-sentence description, in patient's own words, of why the patient is seeking care

History of Present Illness
- Complete analysis of the following signs and symptoms (using the NOPQRST format; see Box 17-1 in Chapter 17)
- Dizziness, syncope, or seizures
- Headaches
- Vision or auditory changes, including sensitivity to light and tinnitus
- Difficulty swallowing or hoarseness
- Slurred speech or word finding difficulty
- Confusion, memory loss, or difficulty concentrating
- Gait disturbances
- Motor symptoms, including weakness, paresthesia, paralysis, decreased range of motion, and tremors

Past Health History
- Relevant childhood illnesses and immunizations: febrile seizures, birth injuries, physical abuse or trauma, meningitis
- Past acute and chronic medical problems, including treatments and hospitalizations: tumors, traumatic head injuries, hypertension, thrombophlebitis or deep venous thrombosis, coagulopathies, sinusitis, meningitis, encephalitis, diabetes, cancer, psychiatric disorders
- Risk factors: diabetes, smoking, hypercholesterolemia, hypertension, drug use, alcohol use, cardiovascular disease
- Past surgeries: peripheral vascular surgeries; carotid endarterectomy; aneurysm clipping; evacuation of hematoma; head, eyes, ears, nose, or throat (HEENT) procedures
- Past diagnostic tests and interventions: electroencephalography, brain scan, carotid Doppler, head and neck computed tomography, magnetic resonance imaging, thrombolytic therapy, cardiac catheterization
- Medications: anticonvulsants, anticoagulants, psychotropic agents, oral contraceptives, β-blockers, calcium channel blockers, antihyperlipidemics, hormone replacement therapy
- Allergies and reactions: contrast dye, medications
- Transfusions including type and date

Family History
- Health status or cause of death of parents and siblings: coronary artery disease, peripheral vascular disease, cancer, hypertension, diabetes, stroke, hyperlipidemia, coagulopathies, seizures, psychiatric disturbances

Personal and Social History
- Tobacco, alcohol, and substance use
- Family composition
- Occupation and work environment: exposure to chemicals and toxins
- Living environment: physical, verbal, and emotional abuse
- Diet
- Sleep patterns
- Exercise
- Cultural beliefs
- Spiritual and religious beliefs
- Coping patterns and social support systems
- Leisure activities
- Sexual activity
- Recent travel

Review of Systems
- HEENT: visual changes, tinnitus, headache
- Cardiovascular: hypertension, syncope, palpitations, intermittent claudication
- Respiratory: shortness of breath, infections, cough, dyspnea
- Gastrointestinal: weight loss, change in bowel habits, nausea/vomiting/diarrhea
- Genitourinary: change in bladder habits, painful urination, sexual dysfunction
- Musculoskeletal: sensitivity to temperature changes, varicosities, loss of hair on extremities, change in sensation

Box 33-3 • Clinical Terminology for Grading Responsiveness

Alert (full consciousness): normal
Awake: may sleep more than usual or be somewhat confused on first awakening, but fully oriented when aroused
Lethargic: drowsy but follows simple commands when stimulated
Obtunded: arousable with stimulation; responds verbally with a word or two; follows simple commands; otherwise drowsy
Stuporous: very hard to arouse; inconsistently may follow simple commands or speak single words or short phrases; limited spontaneous movement
Semicomatose: movements are purposeful when stimulated; does not follow commands or speak coherently
Comatose: may respond with reflexive posturing when stimulated or may have no response to any stimulus

as a guide for rapid evaluation of the acutely ill or severely injured patient whose status may change quickly. It is not useful as a guide for evaluation of patients in long-standing comas or during prolonged recovery from severe brain injury.

More complex information about nervous system functioning can be obtained by gathering data about the patient's ability to integrate attention, memory, and thought processes (Table 33-1). Such a mental status examination also may uncover clues about the presence of additional problems affecting the patient's lifestyle. The Mini-Mental State Examination (MMSE) is a widely used cognitive assessment tool that is easy and rapid to administer and has good interrater reliability. It is frequently used to monitor disease progression in patients with dementia or other progressive disease states. The MMSE is composed of questions related to orientation, recall/memory, attention, calculation, language, and spatial insight. Points are assigned for correct answers, with a maximum

Box 33-4 • The Glasgow Coma Scale

Best Eye-Opening Response	Score
Spontaneously	4
To speech	3
To pain	2
No response	1

Best Verbal Response	Score
Oriented	5
Confused conversation	4
Inappropriate words	3
Garbled sounds	2
No response	1

Best Motor Response	Score
Obeys commands	6
Localizes stimuli	5
Withdrawal from stimulus	4
Abnormal flexion (decorticate)	3
Abnormal extension (decerebrate)	2
No response	1

A total score of 3 to 8 suggests severe impairment, 9 to 12 suggests moderate impairment, and 13 to 15 suggests mild impairment.

of 30 points. Scores of less than 20 may indicate neurological disease. Examples of specific deficits are presented in Table 33-2.

When gathering such a wealth of data, assessment of the patient's ability to communicate becomes paramount. Use of language requires comprehension of verbal and nonverbal symbols and the ability to use those symbols to communicate with others. Evaluation of the patient's understanding normally is accomplished through the spoken word. However, speech dysfunctions can make such evaluations exceedingly difficult (Table 33-3).

MOTOR FUNCTION

Evaluation of motor function consists of two components—motor response to stimuli and motor strength and coordination. Assessment of motor response involves evaluating the type of stimuli necessary to elicit a motor response. This gives the health care team information regarding the level of awareness necessary to obtain a motor response as well as the patient's ability to follow commands. Evaluation of motor strength and coordination gives an indication of potential problems with motor neuron pathways or the cerebellum.

Motor Response to Stimuli

The nurse first attempts to elicit a motor response by asking the patient to move an extremity. If no response is forthcoming, the patient is unable to carry out verbal commands, and noxious stimuli should be used to elicit a motor response. When noxious stimuli are needed to evoke a response, the nurse pays careful attention to where the painful stimulus is applied. A misplaced examiner's hand may cause serious skin or tissue injury. Areas to avoid include the skin of the nipples and genital area. Instead, one should apply pain to the big toenail, the knuckles or nails of the fingers, or the supraorbital ridge. All provide sufficient stimuli to elicit a patient's response to pain. When stimulating the supraorbital ridge, one should take care not to compress the eye itself.

Localization to painful stimuli is characterized by an organized attempt to remove the stimulus, which entails movement of the extremity across midline. This contrasts to withdrawal, in which the patient simply pulls away from the noxious stimulus, rather than attempting to remove it (Fig. 33-1). Appropriate responses, such as localization or withdrawal, mean that the sensory and corticospinal pathways are func-

Table 33-1 • Mental Status Examination

Functions	Test	Implications
Orientation	*Time:* state year, month, date, season, day of week *Place:* indicate state, county, city of residency State hospital name, floor or room number	May be altered by a multitude of neurologic conditions
Attention	Digit span; serial 7's; recitation of months of the year in reverse order	May be impaired in delirium, frontal lobe damage, and dementia
Memory	*Short-term:* recall of three items after 5 minutes *Long-term:* recall of such items as mother's maiden name, events of previous day	May be impaired in conditions such as dementia, cerebrovascular accident, and delirium
Language	*Naming:* point to three objects and have patient name them *Comprehension:* give simple and complex commands *Repetition:* repeat phrases such as "no if's, ands, or buts" *Reading:* have patient read and explain a short passage *Writing:* have patient write a brief sentence	Requires integration of visual, semantic, and phonological aspects of knowledge Dysfunction may be associated with lesions of Broca's area; may be dependent on educational level
Spatial/perceptual	Copy drawings such as cross or square; draw a clock face Point out right and left side of self Demonstrate such actions as putting on a coat or blowing out a match	May be associated with parietal lobe lesions

Table 33-2 • Selected Deficits in Higher Intellectual Function

Type	Characteristics
Anomia	Inability to name objects or recognize written or spoken names of objects
Phonemic paraphasia	Substitutes parts of words (e.g., pan opener instead of can opener)
Semantic paraphasia	Substitutes whole words (e.g., apple for orange)
Dyslexia	Inability to recognize and comprehend written words
Alexia	Reading letter by letter instead of whole words
Neglect dyslexia	Omissions or substitutions of letters confined to initial part of the word
Surface dyslexia	Difficulty reading words with irregular spelling
Dysgraphia	Difficulty with writing
Central dysgraphia	Affects both written and oral spelling
Neglect dysgraphia	Misspelling the initial part of the word
Agnosia	Failure to recognize objects despite intact sensory input; may be visual, auditory, or sensory
Prosopagnosia	Inability to recognize familiar faces
Achromatopsia	Inability to discriminate colors
Acalculia	Inability to read, write, and comprehend numbers

tioning (see Fig. 33-1A, B). There may be monoplegia or hemiplegia, indicating that the corticospinal pathways are interrupted on one side.

Inappropriate responses include decorticate rigidity and decerebrate rigidity. Flexion of the arms, wrists, and fingers; adduction of the upper extremities; and extension, internal rotation, and plantar flexion of the lower extremities characterize decorticate rigidity (see Fig. 33-1C). Such rigidity results from lesions of the internal capsule, basal ganglia, thalamus, or cerebral hemisphere, interrupting corticospinal pathways.

Decerebrate rigidity consists of extension, adduction, and hyperpronation of the upper extremities and extension of the lower extremities, with plantar flexion of the feet (see Fig. 33-1D). Many times, the person also has clenched teeth. Injury to the midbrain and pons results in decerebration. At times, the inappropriate responses of decortication and decerebration may switch back and forth. If there is no response to noxious stimuli or only very weak flexor responses (i.e., flaccidity), the patient likely has extensive brainstem dysfunction (see Fig. 33-1E). Additional abnormal motor responses in a comatose patient include tonic contraction, which is consistent muscular contraction, and clonus, which is alternating muscle spasticity and relaxation.

Motor Strength and Coordination

The second component of the motor assessment addresses strength and coordination. Muscle weakness is a cardinal sign of dysfunction in many neurological disorders. The nurse tests extremity strength by offering resistance to various muscle groups, using his or her own muscles or gravity. As a quick test to detect weakness of the upper extremities, have the patient hold the arms straight out with palms upward and eyes closed and observe for any downward drift or pronation of the forearms. This is referred to as pronator drift. A similar test for the lower extremities

Table 33-3 • Patterns of Speech Defecits

Type	Deficit Locations	Speech Patterns
Fluent dysphasia	Left parietal–temporal lobes (Wernicke's area)	• Fluent speech that lacks coherent content • Impaired understanding of spoken word despite normal hearing • May have normal-sounding speech rhythm but no intelligible words • May use invented, meaningless words (neologism), word substitution (paraphasia), or repetition of words (perseveration, echolalia)
Nonfluent dysphasia	Left frontal area (Broca's area)	• Slow speech with poor articulation • Inability to initiate sounds • Comprehension usually intact • Usually associated with impaired writing skills
Global dysphasia	Diffuse involvement of frontal, parietal, and occipital areas	• Nonfluent speech • Inability to understand spoken or written words
Dysarthria	Corticobulbar tracts; cerebellum	• Loss of articulation, phonation • Loss of control of muscles of lips, tongue, palate • Slurred, jerky, or irregular speech but with appropriate content

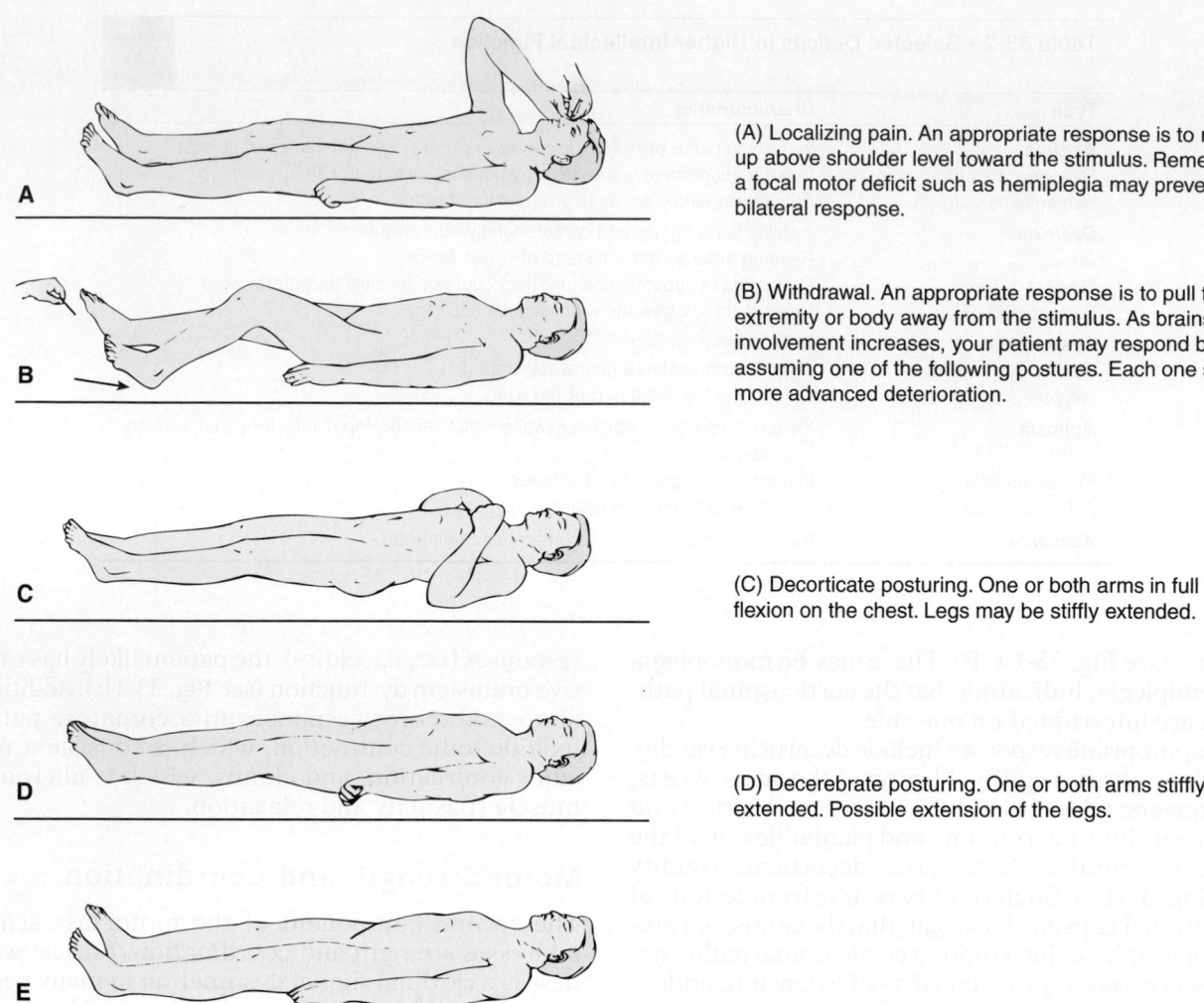

(A) Localizing pain. An appropriate response is to reach up above shoulder level toward the stimulus. Remember, a focal motor deficit such as hemiplegia may prevent a bilateral response.

(B) Withdrawal. An appropriate response is to pull the extremity or body away from the stimulus. As brainstem involvement increases, your patient may respond by assuming one of the following postures. Each one shows more advanced deterioration.

(C) Decorticate posturing. One or both arms in full flexion on the chest. Legs may be stiffly extended.

(D) Decerebrate posturing. One or both arms stiffly extended. Possible extension of the legs.

(E) Flaccid. No motor response in any extremity.

Figure 33-1 • Motor responses to pain. When a painful stimulus is applied to an unconscious patient's supraorbital notch, the patient responds in one of these ways.

involves having the patient lie in bed and raise the legs, one at a time, straight off the bed against the examiner's resistance. Weakness noted in any of these tests can indicate damage to the motor neuron pathways of the pyramidal system, which transmits commands for voluntary movement. Motor function for each extremity is reported as a fraction, with 5 as the denominator, as shown in Box 33-5.

Box 33-5 • A Motor Function Scale

Score	Interpretation
0/5	No muscle contraction
1/5	Flicker or trace of contraction
2/5	Moves but cannot overcome gravity
3/5	Moves against gravity but cannot overcome resistance of examiner's muscles
4/5	Moves with some weakness against resistance of examiner's muscles
5/5	Normal power and strength

Muscle groups are assessed individually, initially without resistance and then against resistance, to obtain a thorough evaluation. Upper extremity muscle strength is evaluated by asking the patient to shrug the shoulders (trapezius and levator scapulae muscles), raise the arms (deltoid muscle), flex the elbow (biceps muscle), extend the arm (triceps muscle), and extend the wrist (extensor carpi radialis longus muscle). Lower extremity muscle strength is evaluated by asking the patient to raise the leg (iliopsoas muscle), extend the knee (quadriceps muscle), dorsiflex and plantar flex the foot (anterior tibialis and gastrocnemius muscles, respectively), and flex the knee (hamstring muscle).

Assessment of movement and strength in a patient who cannot follow commands or is unresponsive can be difficult because participating in muscle strength testing against gravity requires the patient's understanding and cooperation. Unless the patient is able to mount a motor response secondary to painful stimuli, the nurse may not have the opportunity to test for muscle strength in any sort of reliable manner. Therefore, for comatose patients, it is important to note what, if any, stimuli initiate a response and to describe or grade the type of response obtained.

The nurse may also assess each extremity for size, muscle tone, and smoothness of passive movement. Abnormal responses may indicate problems in the basal ganglia (also called the extrapyramidal system). These pathways normally suppress involuntary movements through controlled inhibition. Assessment findings may include the "clasp-knife" phenomenon, in which initially strong resistance to passive movement suddenly decreases. Alternatively, "lead-pipe" rigidity may be present, which is steady, continuous resistance to passive movement and is characteristic of diffuse hemispheric damage. "Cogwheel" rigidity, which is a series of small, regular, jerky movements felt on passive movement, is characteristic of Parkinson's disease. The nurse also should be alert to involuntary movements, from mild fasciculation (muscle twitching) to violent, flailing movement of an extremity. Descriptive terms for involuntary movements are given in Box 33-6.

Hemiparesis (weakness) and hemiplegia (paralysis) are unilateral symptoms resulting from a lesion contralateral to the corticospinal tract. Paraplegia results from a spinal cord lesion below the first thoracic spinal nerve or from peripheral nerve dysfunctions. Quadriplegia (also known as tetraplegia) is associated with cervical spinal cord lesions, brainstem dysfunction, and large bilateral lesions in the cerebrum.

The cerebellum is responsible for smooth synchronization, balance, and ordering of movements. It does not initiate any movements, so a patient with cerebellar dysfunction is not paralyzed. Instead, ataxia, dysmetria, and lack of synchronization of movement are common manifestations. Some of the more common tests for cerebellar synchronization of movement with balance include the following:

▶ **Romberg test.** This test is performed by having the patient stand with his or her feet together, first with the eyes open, then with the eyes closed. The nurse looks for sway or direction of falling and is prepared to catch the patient if necessary.

▶ **Finger-to-nose test.** This test is performed by having the patient touch one finger to the examiner's finger, then touch his or her own nose. Overshooting or past-pointing the mark is called dysmetria. Both sides are tested individually.

▶ **Rapidly alternating movement (RAM) test.** The patient's ability to perform RAMs is checked on each side by having the patient oppose each finger and thumb in rapid succession or by performing rapid pronation and supination of the hand on the leg. Inability to perform RAMs is termed adiadochokinesia; performing RAMs poorly or clumsily is termed dysdiadochokinesia.

▶ **Heel-to-shin test.** This test is performed by having the patient extend the heel of one foot down the anterior aspect of the shin, moving from the knee to the ankle.

PUPILLARY CHANGES

Assessment of pupillary response is an important component of the neurological examination. Pupils are examined for size (specified in millimeters) and shape (Fig. 33-2). The patient focuses on a distant point in the room. To isolate the eye being examined, the examiner places the edge of one hand along the patient's nose. A bright light is directed into one eye, and the briskness of pupillary constriction (direct response) is noted. The other pupil also should constrict (consensual response). The procedure is then repeated with the other eye. Anisocoria (unequal pupils) is normal in a small percentage of the population but can also indicate neural dysfunction. If it is a normal variant, the difference in pupil size should be less than 1 mm.

Box 33-6 • Types of Voluntary Movements	
Tremor	Purposeless movement
Resting	Lesion in basal ganglia
Intention	Lesion in cerebellum
Asterixis	Metabolic derangement
Physiological	Due to fatigue or stress
Fasciculation	Twitching of resting muscles due to peripheral nerve or spinal cord lesion or to metabolic influences such as cold or anesthetic agents
Clonus	Repetitive movement; elicited with stretch reflex and implies lesion of the corticospinal tracts
Myoclonus	Nonrhythmic movement; single jerk-like movements; symmetrical; unknown etiology
Hemiballismus	Flailing movement of extremity; violent movement; not present during sleep; lesion in subthalamic nuclei of basal ganglia
Chorea	Irregular movements; involves limbs and facial muscles; asymmetrical movements at rest; involuntary movements may increase when purposeful movement is attempted
Athetosis	Slow, writhing movements

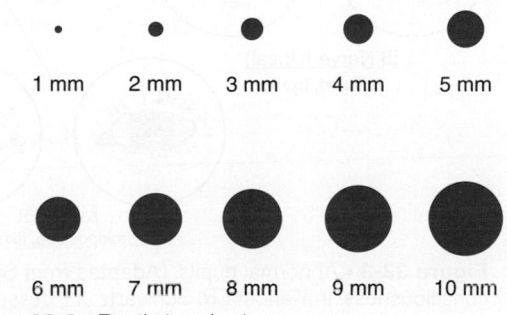

Figure 33-2 • Pupil size chart.

Pupil reactivity is also assessed with respect to accommodation. To test accommodation, an object is held 8 to 12 inches in front of the patient's face. The patient focuses on the object as the examiner moves it toward the patient's nose. The pupils should constrict as the object gets closer, and the eyes turn inward to maintain a clear image. The normal response to testing is documented as PERRLA, or **p**upils **e**qual, **r**ound, **r**eactive to **l**ight and **a**ccommodation.

Some important pupillary abnormalities are shown in Figure 33-3. Causes of small, reactive pupils include metabolic abnormalities and bilateral dysfunction in the diencephalon. Large, fixed pupils (5 to 6 mm) that may show slight rhythmic constriction and dilation when stimulated may indicate midbrain damage. Midposition, fixed pupils (4 to 5 mm) also may indicate midbrain dysfunction, with sympathetic and parasympathetic pathways interrupted. Pinpoint, non-reactive pupils are seen after damage to the pons area of the brainstem (thus the phrase "pontine pupils are pinpoint"), with selected eye medications, and with opiate administration. A unilaterally dilated, non-reactive ("blown") pupil is seen with third cranial (oculomotor) nerve damage when the uncal portion of the temporal lobe herniates through the tentorium.

> ### Box 33-7 • Quick Guide to Causes of Pupil Size Change
>
> **Pinpoint pupils**
> - Drugs: opiates
> - Drops: medications for glaucoma
> - "Nearly dead": damage in the pons area of the brainstem
>
> **Dilated pupils**
> - Fear: panic attack, extreme anxiety
> - "Fits": seizures
> - "Fast living": cocaine, crack, phencyclidine (PCP)

When structures are compressed around the opening in the tentorium or fold of dura that separates the cerebrum from the cerebellum and brainstem, loss of functioning of the parasympathetic nerves to the pupil on that side results in ipsilaterally (same side) dilated pupils. A quick guide to changes in pupil size is given in Box 33-7.

The assessment of pupillary response for comatose patients is the same as for conscious patients. Pupil

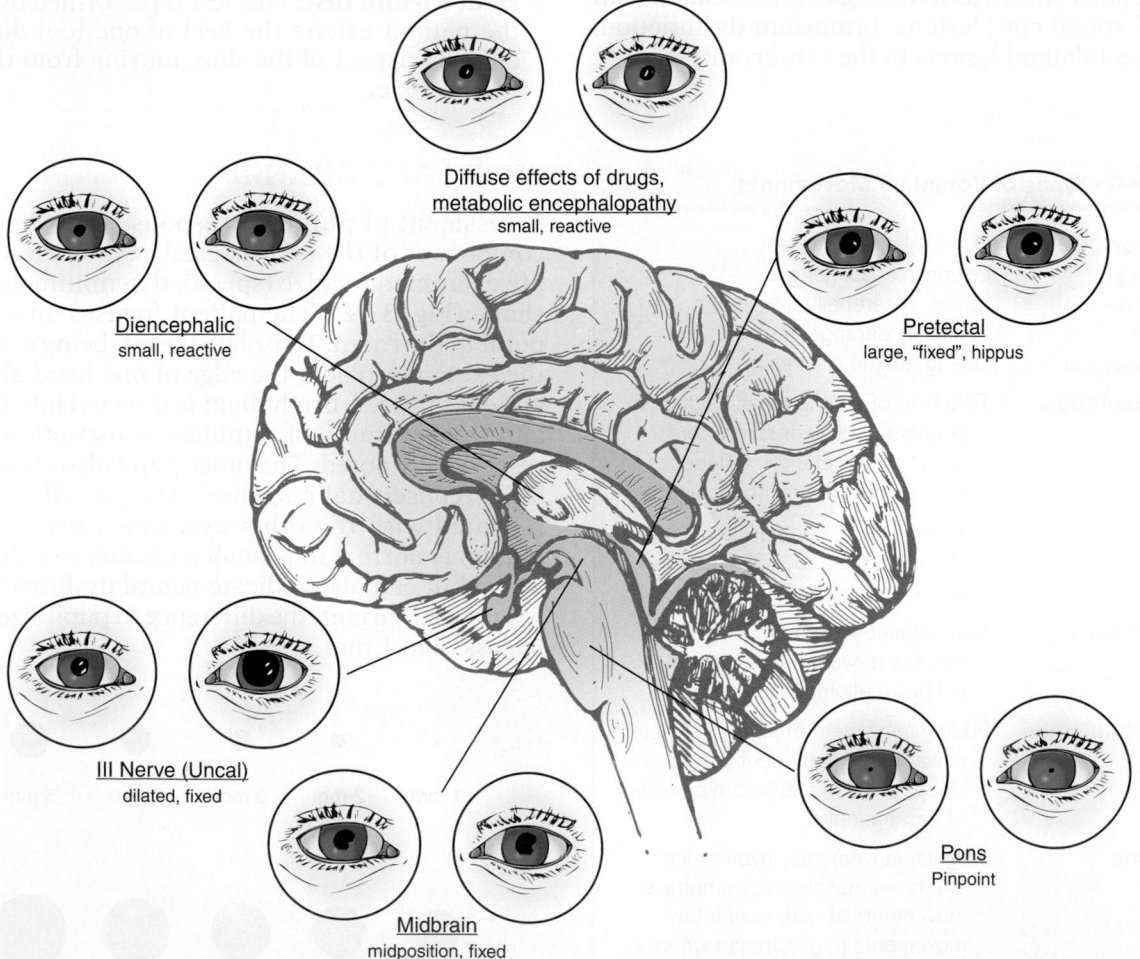

Diffuse effects of drugs, metabolic encephalopathy
small, reactive

Diencephalic
small, reactive

Pretectal
large, "fixed", hippus

III Nerve (Uncal)
dilated, fixed

Midbrain
midposition, fixed

Pons
Pinpoint

Figure 33-3 • Abnormal pupils. (Adapted from Saper C: Brain stem modulation of sensation, movement, and consciousness. In Kandel ER, Schwartz JH, Jessel TM (eds): Principles of Neural Science, 4th ed. New York: McGraw-Hill, 2000, pp 871–909. By permission of McGraw-Hill.)

reactivity to light, by direct and consensual response, is easily obtained. It may be impossible to ascertain reactivity to accommodation because the patient may be unable to cooperate.

VITAL SIGNS

Vital sign assessment is crucial to the neurological examination. Changes in temperature, heart rate, and blood pressure are considered late findings in neurological deterioration. Changes in respiratory rate, on the other hand, can indicate progression of neurological impairment and are frequently seen early in neurological deterioration.

Respirations

Variations in respiratory pattern are commonly associated with neurological injury. Shallow, rapid respirations can indicate a problem with maintenance of a patent airway or the need for suctioning. Snoring respirations or stridor can also indicate a partially obstructed airway. The inability to maintain an effective airway may be associated with a high cervical spinal cord lesion or progressive diaphragmatic paralysis (seen with neurodegenerative diseases), or it may be seen with a decreasing level of consciousness.

Changes in respiratory pattern can also be a direct indication of increasing intracranial pressure (ICP) (see Chapter 36, Fig. 36-6). Cheyne-Stokes respirations (crescendo–decrescendo respirations alternating with periods of apnea) are frequently noted in neurological disease.

Hypoventilation after cerebral trauma can lead to respiratory acidosis. As the blood carbon dioxide increases and blood oxygen decreases, cerebral hypoxia and edema can result in secondary brain injury, thereby extending the degree of damage. Hyperventilation after cerebral trauma produces respiratory alkalosis with decreased blood carbon dioxide levels. This causes vasoconstriction of cerebral vessels, contributing to decreased cerebral blood flow.

Temperature

Normal regulation of temperature occurs in the hypothalamus. Diffuse cerebral damage can result in alterations in temperature. Central nervous system (CNS) fevers may be very high and differentiate themselves from other causes of fever by their resistance to antipyretic therapy. Hypothermia occurs with metabolic causes, pituitary damage, and spinal cord injuries.

Pulse

Variations in heart rate and rhythm may also be associated with neurological injury. An increase in ICP may lead to episodes of tachycardia and can predispose the patient to alterations in electrocardiogram (ECG) pattern, such as ventricular or atrial dysrhythmias. As the ICP increases, bradycardia results, and the combination of the two is indicative of impending herniation.

Blood Pressure

Blood pressure is controlled at the level of the medulla. Therefore, specific damage to this area or encroaching edema secondary to injury in other areas results in alterations in blood pressure. Hypotension is not normally associated with neurological injury except in instances of impending cerebral herniation. On the other hand, hypotension must be avoided in the post-injury stage because it can lead to decreased cerebral perfusion, hypoxia, and extension of the initial injury.

Hypertension is much more commonly seen. In the intact brain, the mechanism of cerebral autoregulation (on which cerebral perfusion depends) maintains constant blood flow to the brain, despite wide variations in systemic pressure. However, after injury, autoregulatory mechanisms fail, and cerebral blood flow varies dramatically with variations in systemic pressure. As blood pressure increases, cerebral blood flow increases, resulting in an increase in ICP. Likewise, as blood pressure decreases, cerebral blood flow decreases, resulting in ischemia.

CRANIAL NERVE FUNCTION

The performance of a cranial nerve assessment varies depending on whether the patient is conscious or unconscious. Assessment of the cranial nerves in the unconscious patient is important because it provides data regarding brainstem function. Many components must be eliminated, but a significant number of the cranial nerves can still be assessed. For specific physiological information about the cranial nerves, see Chapter 32.

Cranial Nerve I (Olfactory Nerve)

The first cranial nerve contains sensory fibers for the sense of smell. This test usually is deferred unless the patient complains of an inability to smell. The nurse tests the nerve, with the patient's eyes closed, by placing aromatic substances near the nose for identification. Items that have a distinct smell (e.g., soap, coffee, or cinnamon) should be used. Ammonia should not be used because the patient will respond to irritation of the nasal mucosa rather than to the odor. Each nostril is checked separately by closing off one nostril at a time. Loss of smell may be caused by a fracture of the cribriform plate or a fracture in the ethmoid area. The patient may also have anosmia (loss of sense of smell) from a shearing injury to the olfactory bulb after a basilar skull fracture or from cerebrospinal fluid (CSF) leak.

Cranial Nerve II (Optic Nerve)

Assessment of the optic nerve involves evaluation of visual acuity and visual fields. Gross visual acuity is checked by having the patient read ordinary newsprint, noting the patient's preinjury need for glasses. Visual fields are tested by having the patient look straight ahead with one eye covered. The examiner moves a finger from the periphery of each quadrant

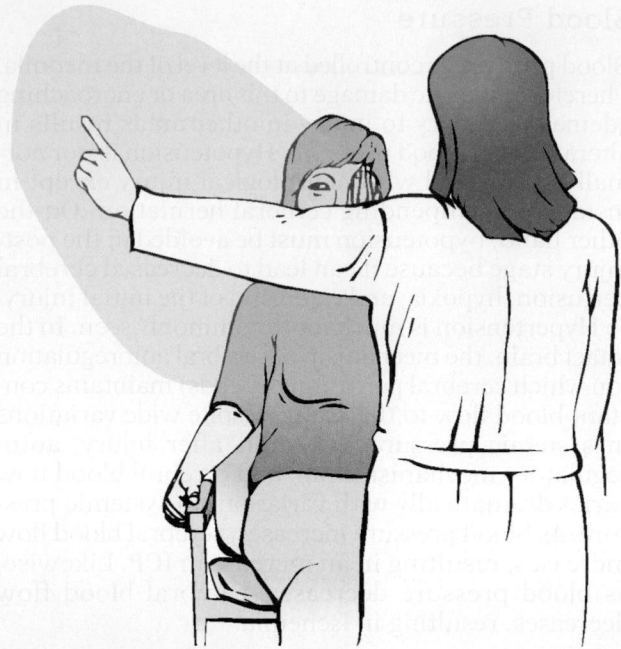

Figure 33-4 • Confrontational method of testing visual fields.

Cranial Nerves III (Oculomotor Nerve), IV (Trochlear Nerve), and VI (Abducens Nerve)

Cranial nerves III, IV, and VI are checked together because they innervate extraocular muscles involved in eye movement. The parasympathetic fibers of the oculomotor nerve are responsible for lens accommodation and pupil size through control of the ciliary muscles. This is the nerve tested when a nurse elicits a pupillary response. The motor fibers of the oculomotor nerve innervate the muscles that elevate the eyelid and those that move the eyes up, down, and medially. These include the superior rectus, inferior oblique, inferior rectus, and medial rectus muscles. The trochlear nerve innervates the superior oblique muscle to move the eyes down and in. The lateral rectus muscle moves the eyes laterally and is innervated by the abducens nerve. Diplopia, nystagmus, conjugate deviation, and ptosis may indicate dysfunction of these cranial nerves. In the conscious patient, these nerves are tested by having the patient follow the examiner's finger as he or she moves it in all directions of gaze (Fig. 33-5).

Ocular position and movement are among the most useful guides to the site of brain dysfunction in the comatose person. When observing the eyes at rest, it is not uncommon to note a slight divergence of gaze. If both eyes are conjugately deviated to one side, there is possible dysfunction either in the frontal lobe on that side or in the contralateral pontine area of the brainstem. Downward deviation suggests a dysfunction in the midbrain.

Although the unconscious patient cannot participate in the examination by voluntarily moving the eyes through fields of gaze, the examiner still can test the range of ocular movement by assessing the oculocephalic ("doll's eyes" test) and oculovestibular (caloric ice-water test) reflexes. The oculocephalic reflex can be assessed by quickly rotating the patient's head to one side and observing the position of the eyes (Fig. 33-6). This maneuver must never be performed in

of vision toward the patient's center of vision. The patient should indicate when the examiner's finger is seen. This is done for both eyes, and the results are compared with the examiner's visual fields, which are assumed to be normal (Fig. 33-4). Damage to the retina produces a blind spot. An optic nerve lesion produces partial or complete blindness on the same side. Damage to the optic chiasm results in bitemporal hemianopsia, blindness in both lateral visual fields (Table 33-4). Pressure on the optic tract can cause homonymous hemianopsia, half-blindness on the opposite side of the lesion in both eyes. A lesion in the parietal or temporal lobe may produce contralateral blindness in the upper or lower quadrant of vision, respectively, in both eyes (quadrant deficit). Damage in the occipital lobe can cause homonymous hemianopsia with central vision sparing.

Table 33-4 • Visual Field Defects Associated With Defects of the Visual System			
Visual Field Defect			
	Left	Right	Description
Anopsia	○	●	Blindness in one eye; due to complete lesion of the right optic nerve.
Bitemporal hemianopsia (central vision)	◑	◐	Blindness in both lateral visual fields; due to lesions around the optic chiasm such as pituitary tumors or aneurysms of the anterior communicating artery. Affected fibers originate in the nasal half of each retina.
Homonymous hemianopsia	◑	◑	Half-blindness involving both eyes with loss of visual field on the same side of each eye; due to lesion of temporal or occipital lobe with damage to the optic tract or optic radiations (blindness occurs on the side opposite the lesion; here, the lesion occurred in the right side of the brain, resulting in loss of vision in the left visual field of both eyes)
Quadrant deficit	◔	◔	Blindness in the upper or lower quadrant of vision in both eyes, resulting from a lesion in the parietal or temporal lobe

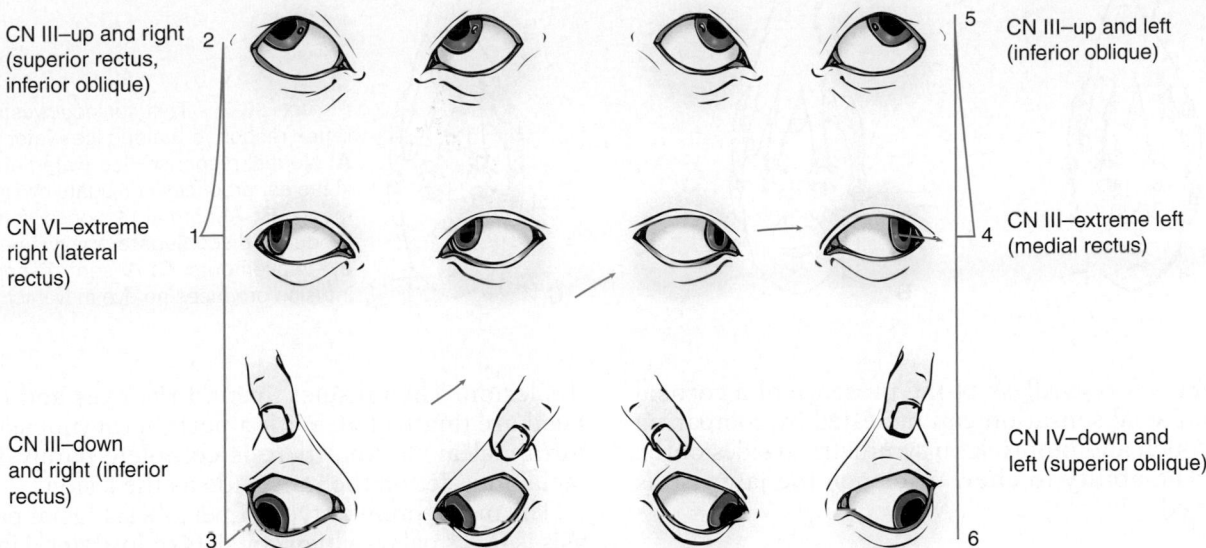

CN III—up and right (superior rectus, inferior oblique)

CN VI—extreme right (lateral rectus)

CN III—down and right (inferior rectus)

CN III—up and left (inferior oblique)

CN III—extreme left (medial rectus)

CN IV—down and left (superior oblique)

Figure 33-5 • Muscles used in conjugate eye movements in the six cardinal directions of gaze. Lead the patient's gaze in the sequence numbered 1 through 6. CN III, oculomotor nerve; CN IV, trochlear nerve; CN VI, abducens nerve.

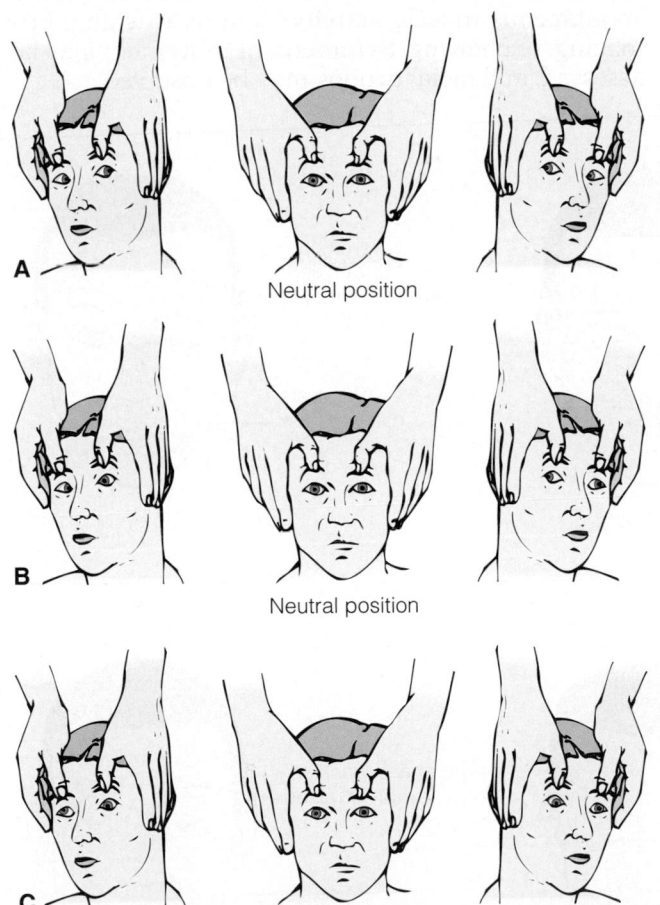

Neutral position

Neutral position

Neutral position

Figure 33-6 • Test for oculocephalic reflex response (doll's eyes phenomenon). **A:** Normal response—when the head is rotated, the eyes turn together to the side opposite to the head movement. **B:** Abnormal response—when the head is rotated, the eyes do not turn in a conjugate manner. **C:** Absent response—as head position is changed, eyes do not move in the sockets.

a person with possible cervical spine injury. A normal response consists of initial conjugate deviation of the eyes in the opposite direction, then, within a few seconds, smooth and simultaneous movement of both eyes back to midline position. This response indicates an intact brainstem. An abnormal reflex response occurs when one eye does not follow the normal response pattern. Absence of any ocular movement when the head is rotated briskly to either side or up and down indicates an absent reflex and portends severe brainstem dysfunction.

The examiner tests the oculovestibular reflex by elevating the patient's head 30 degrees and irrigating each ear separately with 30 to 50 mL of ice water (Fig. 33-7). This test should never be performed in a patient who does not have an intact eardrum or who has blood or fluid collected behind the eardrum. Also, the external ear canal should be unobstructed by cerumen or debris. In an unconscious patient with an intact brainstem, the eyes exhibit horizontal nystagmus with slow, conjugate movement toward the irrigated ear followed by rapid movement away from the stimulus. When the reflex is absent, both eyes remain fixed in midline position, indicating midbrain and pons dysfunction.

Cranial Nerve V (Trigeminal Nerve)

Cranial nerve V has three divisions: ophthalmic, maxillary, and mandibular. The sensory portion of this nerve controls sensation to the cornea and face. The motor portion controls the muscles of mastication. This nerve is partially tested by checking the corneal reflex; if it is intact, the patient blinks when the cornea is stroked with a wisp of cotton or when a drop of normal saline is placed in the eye. Care must be taken not to stroke the eyelash because this can cause the

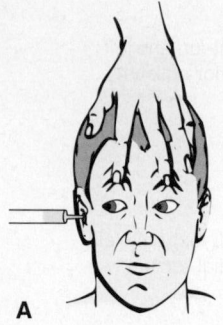
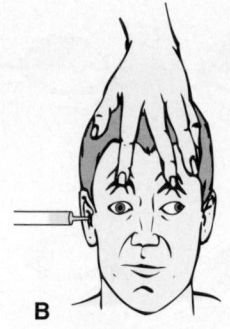
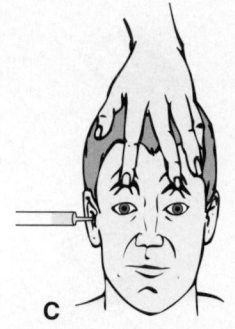

Figure 33-7 • Test for oculovestibular reflex response (caloric ice-water test). **A:** Normal response—ice-water infusion in the ear produces conjugate eye movements. **B:** Abnormal response—infusion produces disconjugate or asymmetrical eye movements. **C:** Absent response—infusion produces no eye movements.

eye to blink regardless of the presence of a corneal reflex. Facial sensation can be tested by comparing light touch and pinprick on symmetrical sides of the face. The ability to chew or clench the jaw also is observed.

Cranial Nerve VII (Facial Nerve)

The sensory portion of cranial nerve VII is concerned with taste on the anterior two thirds of the tongue. The motor portion controls muscles of facial expression (Fig. 33-8). Testing is performed by asking the patient to raise the eyebrows, smile, or grimace. With a central (supranuclear) lesion, there is muscle paralysis of the lower half of the face on the side opposite

the lesion. The muscles around the eyes and forehead are unaffected. With a peripheral (nuclear or infranuclear) lesion, there is complete paralysis of facial muscles on the same side as the lesion.

The most common type of peripheral facial paralysis is Bell's palsy, which consists of ipsilateral facial paralysis. There is drooping of the upper lid with the lower lid slightly everted. Facial lines on the same side are obliterated, with the mouth drawn toward the normal side.

In the comatose patient, motor function of the facial muscles and jaw can be ascertained by observing spontaneous muscle activity such as yawning, grimacing, or chewing. Symmetry of movement may be assessed, and facial droops may be observed.

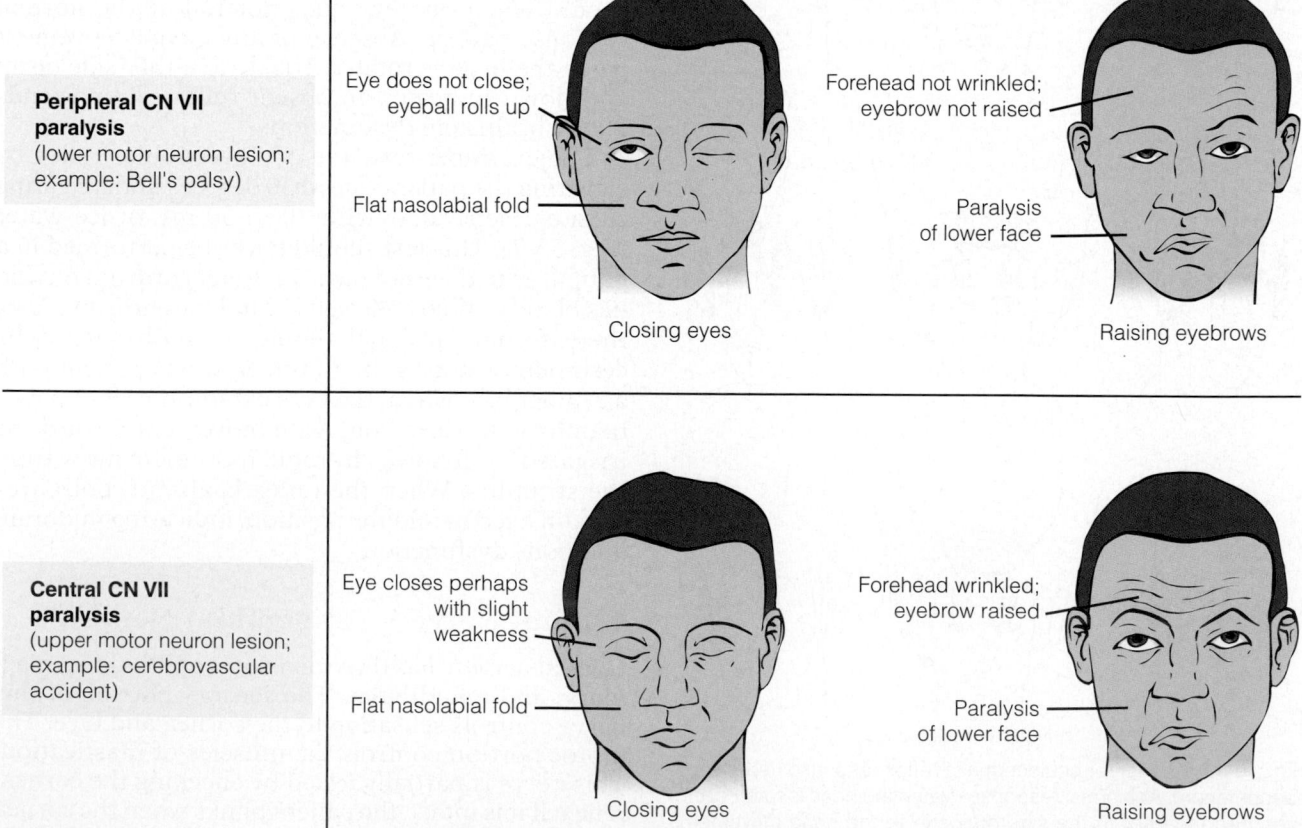

Figure 33-8 • Facial movements with upper and lower motor neuron facial paralysis. CN VII, facial nerve.

Cranial Nerve VIII (Acoustic Nerve)

Cranial nerve VIII is divided into the cochlear and vestibular branches, which control hearing and equilibrium, respectively. The cochlear nerve is tested by air and bone conduction. A vibrating tuning fork is placed on the mastoid process; after the patient can no longer hear the fork, he or she should be able to hear it for a few seconds longer when it is placed in front of the ear (Rinne test). The patient may complain of tinnitus or decreased hearing if this nerve is damaged. The vestibular nerve may not be evaluated routinely. However, the nurse should be alert to complaints of dizziness or vertigo from the patient.

Cranial Nerves IX (Glossopharyngeal Nerve) and X (Vagus Nerve)

Cranial nerves IX and X usually are tested together. The glossopharyngeal nerve supplies sensory fibers to the posterior third of the tongue and the uvula and soft palate. The vagus nerve innervates the larynx, pharynx, and soft palate and conveys autonomic responses to the heart, stomach, lungs, and small intestine. These nerves can be tested by eliciting a gag reflex, observing the uvula for symmetrical movement when the patient says "ah," or observing midline elevation of the uvula when both sides are stroked. Inability to cough forcefully, difficulty with swallowing, and hoarseness may be signs of dysfunction. Autonomic vagal functions usually are not tested because they are checked during the general physical examination.

Cranial Nerve XI (Spinal Accessory Nerve)

Cranial nerve XI controls the trapezius and sternocleidomastoid muscles. The examiner tests this nerve by having the patient shrug the shoulders or turn the head from side to side against resistance.

Cranial Nerve XII (Hypoglossal Nerve)

Cranial nerve XII controls tongue movement. This nerve can be checked by having the patient protrude his or her tongue. The examiner checks for deviation from midline, tremor, and atrophy. If deviation is noted secondary to nerve damage, it will be to the side of the cerebral lesion.

Testing cranial nerve function completely is time consuming and exacting. A partial, quicker screening assessment may be performed, focusing on nerves in which dysfunction may indicate serious problems or interfere with activities of daily living (Table 33-5). The cranial nerves of primary importance in a screening examination are the optic, oculomotor, trigeminal, facial, glossopharyngeal, and vagus nerves.

REFLEXES

A reflex occurs when a sensory stimulus evokes a motor response. Cerebral control and consciousness are not required for a reflex to occur. Superficial and deep reflexes are tested on symmetrical sides of the body and compared by noting the strength of contraction elicited on each side.

Cutaneous, or superficial, reflexes occur when certain areas of skin are lightly stroked or tapped, causing contraction of the muscle groups beneath. Such reflexes are graded simply as normal, abnormal (pathological), or absent. An example is the plantar reflex. A sensory stimulus is applied by briskly stroking the outer edge of the sole and across the ball of the foot with a dull object, such as a tongue blade or key. The normal motor response is downward or plantar flexion of the toes. An abnormal response (Babinski's sign) is upward or dorsiflexion of the big toe, with or without fanning of the other toes. A positive Babinski's sign can indicate a lesion in the pyramidal tract.

Muscle stretch reflexes, also called deep tendon reflexes, are elicited by a brisk tap with a reflex hammer on the appropriate tendon insertion site. The target for this sensory stimulus is a stretched tendon of a muscle group. Deep tendon reflexes are tested on the biceps, brachioradial, triceps, patellar, and Achilles tendons. The desired motor response is contraction of the stimulated muscle group. Deep tendon reflexes are commonly graded on a scale of 0 to 4:

4+: A very brisk response; evidence of disease, electrolyte imbalance, or both; associated with clonic contractions

---

Table 33-5 • A Quick Screening Test for Cranial Nerve Function

	Nerve	Reflex	Procedure
II III	Optic Oculomotor	Pupil constriction (protection of the retina)	Shine a light into each eye and note if the pupil on that side constricts (direct response). Next, shine a light into each eye and note if the opposite pupil constricts (consensual response).
V VII	Trigeminal Facial	Corneal reflex (protection of the cornea)	Approaching the eye from the side and avoiding the eyelashes, touch the cornea with a wisp of cotton. Alternatively, a drop of sterile water or normal saline may be used. A blink response should be present.
IX X	Glossopharyngeal Vagus	Airway protection	Touch the back of the throat with a tongue depressor. A gag or cough response should be present.

3+: A brisk response; possibly indicative of disease

2+: A normal response

1+: A response in the low-normal range

0: No response; possibly evidence of disease or electrolyte imbalance

Hyperreflexia is associated with upper motor neuron disease, whereas areflexia (absence of reflexes) is associated with lower motor neuron dysfunction, such as spinal cord lesions. Reflexes can be tested on the comatose patient. It is anticipated that, depending on the severity and location of the neuronal damage, either hyperreflexia or areflexia will be present.

SENSATION

The last component of the neurological examination involves a sensory assessment. Normal sensory findings depend on an intact spinal cord, sensory pathways, and peripheral nervous system. The primary forms of sensation are tested first. These include perception of touch (cotton wisp), pain (pinprick), temperature (hot, cold), proprioception (limb position), and vibration. With the patient's eyes closed, multiple and symmetrical areas of the body are tested, including the trunk and extremities.

The nurse assesses the perception of touch by asking the patient to close the eyes and identify when and where he or she feels a cotton wisp or cotton swab on the skin. Pain is assessed with the use of a pin or the sharp edge of a cotton swab, moving in a head-to-toe direction on both sides of the body. Temperature, if tested, uses glass tubes of hot and cold water and proceeds in the manner described previously. Two-point discrimination may also be tested and refers to the patient's ability to distinguish between two closely located points. Discrimination of sharp versus dull is also a commonly used test.

Proprioception is tested by asking the patient, again with the eyes closed, to identify the direction of movement (e.g., moving a finger upward and then asking the patient if the finger is up or down). The same test is performed on the other hand, as well as both lower extremities. The nurse assesses vibration using a tuning fork placed over a bony prominence. The patient is asked to identify when vibration is felt.

The patient's ability to perceive the sensation is noted, with distal areas compared with proximal areas and right and left sides compared at corresponding points. The nurse also determines whether sensory change involves one entire side of the body. Abnormal results may indicate damage somewhere along the pathways of the receptors in the skin, muscles, joints and tendons, spinothalamic tracts, or sensory area of the cortex (Table 33-6).

Cortical forms of sensation also should be tested. When primary sensation is intact, but interpretation of the sensory input is altered, then damage to the parietal lobe may be anticipated. Problems with discriminative sensation include those involving stereognosis, graphesthesia, and point localization. The ability to recognize and identify objects by touch is called stereognosis and is a function of the parietal lobe. The inability to recognize objects by touch, sight, or sound is termed agnosia. This may be tested by placing an object in a patient's hand and asking him or her, with the eyes closed, to identify the object solely based on touch. Identification of an object by the sense of sight is a function of the parieto-occipital junction. The temporal lobe is responsible for identification of objects by sound. Each of these senses should be tested separately. For example, a patient may not be able to

Table 33-6 • Testing Superficial and Deep Sensations

Sensation	Stimuli	Dysfunction
Spinothalamic Tracts Carry Impulses for		
Pain	Alternate sharp and dull ends of a pin, asking patient to discriminate between the two (superficial pain). Squeeze nail beds; apply pressure on the orbital rim; rub sternum (deep pain).	• Ipsilateral sensory loss implies a peripheral nerve lesion. • Contralateral sensory loss is seen with lesions of the spinothalamic tract or in the thalamus.
Light touch	Use a wisp of cotton on skin and ask patient to identify when it touches.	• Bilateral sensory loss may indicate a spinal cord lesion. • Paresthesia is an abnormal sensation, such as itching or tingling.
Temperature	Use test tubes filled with hot and cold water or use small metal plates of varying temperatures. (Test only if pain and light touch sensations are abnormal.)	• Causalgia is a burning sensation that can be caused by peripheral nerve irritation.
Posterior Columns Carry Impulses for		
Vibration	Apply a vibrating tuning fork on bony prominences, and note patient's ability to sense and locate vibrations bilaterally.	• Ipsilateral sensory loss may be due to spinal cord injury or to peripheral neuropathy.
Proprioception	Move the patient's finger or toe up and down and ask patient to identify final resting position.	• Contralateral loss may occur from lesions of the thalamus or of the parietal lobes.

identify a whistle by its sound but may recognize it immediately if he or she holds it or looks at it.

Graphesthesia is the ability to recognize numbers or letters traced lightly on the skin. Bilateral sides are compared. Point localization refers to the ability to locate the precise spot on the body touched by the examiner. One version of dysfunction in this area is called extinction phenomenon, the inability to recognize bilateral sensations when the examiner simultaneously touches two symmetrical areas on opposite sides of the body.

In a comatose patient, it is impossible to perform a complete test for sensation because patient cooperativeness is required. However, use of painful stimuli to elicit a response gives a gross indication that some degree of sensory function remains intact. More detailed data would be unavailable, though.

SIGNS OF TRAUMA OR INFECTION

Signs of trauma or infection may be evident on examination:

▶ **Battle's sign** (bruising over the mastoid areas) suggests a basal skull fracture.

▶ **Raccoon's eye** (periorbital edema and bruising) suggests a frontobasilar fracture.

▶ **Rhinorrhea** (drainage of CSF from the nose) suggests fracture of the cribriform plate with herniation of a fragment of the dura and arachnoid through the fracture.

▶ **Otorrhea** (drainage of CSF from the ear) usually is associated with fracture of the petrous portion of the temporal bone.

▶ **Signs of meningeal irritation** include nuchal rigidity (i.e., pain and resistance to neck flexion), fever, headache, and photophobia. A positive Kernig's sign (i.e., pain in the neck when the thigh is flexed on the abdomen and the leg is extended at the knee) also may be present. Brudzinski's sign (involuntary flexion of the hips when the neck is flexed toward the chest) is another indication of meningeal inflammation. Kernig's sign and Brudzinski's sign are shown in Figure 33-9.

SIGNS OF INCREASED INTRACRANIAL PRESSURE

The prevention of increased ICP, or intracranial hypertension, is of key importance to the nurse's role when caring for a patient with a neurological injury. It is first essential for the nurse to establish a baseline neurological assessment on the patient, on which further deterioration can be based. In general terms, increased ICP is manifested by deterioration in all aspects of neurological functioning.

Level of consciousness decreases as ICP rises. Initially, the patient may present with evidence of restlessness, confusion, and combativeness. This then decompensates into lower levels of consciousness,

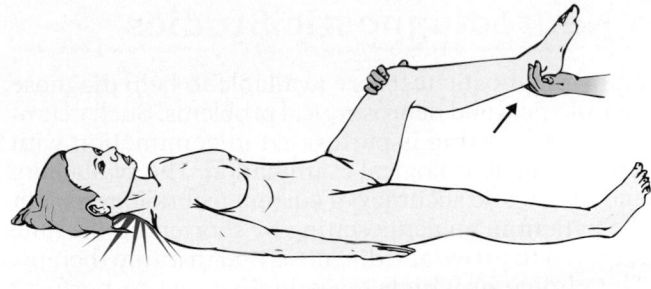

A. Kernig's sign

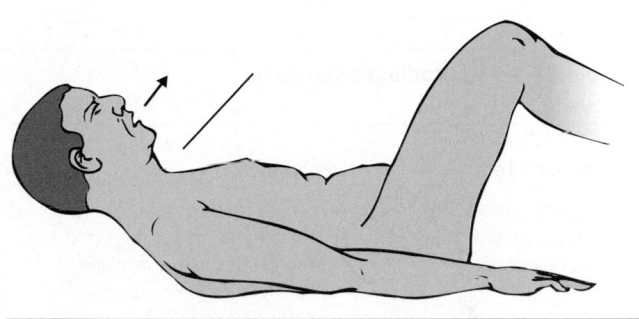

B. Brudzinksi's sign

Figure 33-9 • Two signs of meningeal irritation.

ranging from lethargy to obtundation to coma. Pupillary reactions begin to diminish, with sluggishly reactive pupils and eventually fixed, dilated pupils. Frequently, because of the potential for injury to be ipsilateral, one pupil dilates before the other one does, resulting in unequal pupils.

Motor function also declines, and the patient begins to show abnormal motor activity. For example, the patient who initially may have localized to painful stimuli now shows either abnormal flexion or extension. Changes in vital signs are considered a late finding. Variations in respiratory patterns occur, eventually resulting in complete apnea. Cushing's triad is considered a sign of impending herniation (see Chapter 36). This triad consists of an increased systolic pressure (resulting in an increased pulse pressure), bradycardia, and decreased irregular respirations.

EVALUATION OF DYSFUNCTION IN THE PATIENT'S LIVING PATTERNS

Neurological nursing assessment would be incomplete if the process consisted solely of gathering data and identifying abnormal functions. Nursing expertise should expand the scope to include an evaluation of the impact of dysfunction on the patient's living patterns and ability to care for self. For example, diplopia (double vision) is an abnormal finding and may be an indicator of problems with the ocular muscles or with the nervous system; however, it also may be a clue suggesting difficulty in carrying out daily activities.

• Neurodiagnostic Studies

Many diagnostic tests are available to help diagnose neurological and neurosurgical problems. Such neurodiagnostic testing is performed in conjunction with a thorough neurological examination. The availability and diagnostic accuracy of current technology benefit the patient in an acute setting by shortening the time required to arrive at a diagnosis and institute therapy. The choice of which investigative test to perform should be based on the examiner's ability to integrate the findings with neurological assessment and locate the cause of the abnormality.

The nurse's role in neurodiagnostic testing involves patient and family preparation and monitoring the critically ill patient for potential complications during and after the procedure. Although there has been a definite increase in the number of tests that can be performed at the bedside, many still require that the patient be transported to the imaging department or even out of the institution, further expanding the role of the critical care nurse. Table 33-7 summarizes

Table 33-7 • Neurodiagnostic Tests

Diagnostic Test	Description	Information Obtained	Nursing Considerations and Interventions
Computed tomography, or CT scan (invasive and noninvasive)	A scanner takes a series of radiographic images all around the same axial plane. A computer then creates a composite picture of various tissue densities visualized. The images may be enhanced with the use of IV contrast dye.	CT scans give detailed outlines of bone, tissue, and fluid structures of the body. They can indicate shift of structures due to tumors, hematomas, or hydrocephalus. A CT scan is limited in that it gives information only about structure of tissues, not about functional status.	Instruct the patient to lie flat on a table with the machine surrounding, but not touching, the area to be scanned. Patient also must remain as immobile as possible; sedation may be required. The scan may not be of the best quality if the patient moves during the test or if the x-ray beams were deflected by any metal object (i.e., traction tongs, ICP monitoring devices).
Magnetic resonance imaging (MRI)	A selected area of the patient's body is placed inside a powerful magnetic field. The hydrogen atoms inside the patient are temporarily "excited" and caused to oscillate by a sequence of radiofrequency pulsations. The sensitive scanner measures these minute oscillations, and a computer-enhanced image is created.	An MRI scan creates a graphic image of bone, fluid, and soft tissue structures. It gives a more defined image of anatomical details and may help one diagnose small tumors or early infarction syndromes.	Risk factors for this technique are not well identified. This test is contraindicated in patients with previous surgeries where hemostatic or aneurysm clips were implanted. The powerful magnetic field can cause such clips to move out of position, placing the patient at risk for bleeding or hemorrhage. Other contraindications include cardiac pacemakers, prosthetic valves, bullet fragments, and orthopedic pins. Inform patient that the procedure is very noisy. Use caution if patient is claustrophobic. The patient (and caregivers) must remove all metal objects with magnetic characteristics (e.g., scissors, stethoscope).
Positron emission tomography (PET); single-photon emission computed tomography (SPECT)	The patient either inhales or receives by injection radioactively tagged substances, such as oxygen or glucose. A gamma scanner measures the radioactive uptake of these substances, and a computer produces a composite image, indicating where the radioactive material is located, corresponding to areas of cellular metabolism.	These diagnostic tests are the only ones to measure physiological and biochemical processes in the nervous system. Specific areas can be identified as to functioning and nonfunctioning. Cerebral metabolism and cerebral blood flow can be measured regionally. PET and SPECT scans help diagnose abnormalities (tumors, vascular disease) and behavioral disturbances, such as dementia and schizophrenia, that may have a physiological basis.	The patient receives only minimal radiation exposure because the half-life of the radionuclides used is from a few minutes to 2 h. Testing may take a few hours. The patient must remain very still and immobile. Procedure is very expensive.

(continued)

Table 33-7 • Neurodiagnostic Tests (Continued)

Diagnostic Test	Description	Information Obtained	Nursing Considerations and Interventions
Cerebral angiography (invasive)	This is a radiographic contrast study in which radiopaque dye is injected by a catheter into the patient's cerebral arterial circulation. The contrast medium is directed into each common carotid artery and each vertebral artery, and serial radiographs are then taken.	The contrast dye illuminates the structure of the cerebral circulation. The vessel pathways are examined for patency, narrowing, and occlusion, as well as structural abnormalities (aneurysms), vessel displacement (tumors, edema), and alterations in blood flow (tumors, arteriovenous malformations).	In preparation for this test, inform the patient as to the location of the catheter insertion (femoral artery is a common site) and that a local anesthetic will be used. Also warn that a warm, flushed feeling will occur when the dye is injected. After this procedure, assess the puncture site for swelling, redness, and bleeding. Also check the skin color, temperature, and peripheral pulses of the extremity distal to the site for signs of arterial insufficiency due to vasospasm or clotting. A large amount of contrast medium may be needed during this test, with resulting increased osmotic diuresis and risk for dehydration and renal tubular occlusion. Other complications include temporary or permanent neurological deficit, anaphylaxis, bleeding or hematoma at insertion site, and impaired circulation to the extremity used for injection.
Digital subtraction angiography (invasive)	In this test, a plain radiograph is taken of the patient's cranium. Then, radiopaque dye is injected into a large vein, and serial radiographs are taken. A computer converts the images into digital form and "subtracts" the plain radiograph from the ones with the dye. The result is an enhanced radiographic image of contrast medium in the arterial vessels.	Extracranial circulation (arterial, capillary, and venous) can be examined. Vessel size, patency, narrowing, and degree of stenosis or displacement can be determined.	There is less risk to the patient for bleeding or vascular insufficiency because the injection of dye is intravenous rather than intra-arterial. The patient must remain absolutely motionless during the examination (even swallowing will interfere with the results).
Radioisotope brain scan (noninvasive)	In this test, radioactive isotope is usually injected intravenously. The scanning device produces films of areas of concentration of the isotope within the patient's head.	Because damaged brain tissue absorbs more isotope, the presence of an intracranial lesion can be diagnosed, as well as cerebral infarction or contusion. Lack of uptake of the isotope may indicate cerebral brain death.	Minimal patient preparation is required. The isotope may not be readily available within the institution. Movement will make the test difficult to interpret. This test is less commonly used than CT scan or MRI.
Myelography (invasive)	A myelogram is a radiographic study in which a contrast substance (either air or dye) is injected into the lumbar subarachnoid space. Fluoroscopy, conventional radiographs, or CT scans are used to visualize selected areas.	The spinal subarachnoid space is examined for partial or complete obstructions due to bone displacements, spinal cord compression, or herniated intervertebral disks.	Instruct the patient as for a lumbar puncture. In addition, advise that a special table will tilt up or down during the procedure. Postprocedure care is determined by the type of contrast material used. Oil-based contrast dye: • flat in bed for 24 h • force fluids • observe for headache, fever, back spasms, nausea, and vomiting Water-based contrast dye: • head of bed elevated for 8 h • keep patient quiet for first few hours • do not administer phenothiazines • observe for headache, fever, back spasms, nausea, vomiting, and seizures

(continued)

Table 33-7 • Neurodiagnostic Tests (Continued)

Diagnostic Test	Description	Information Obtained	Nursing Considerations and Interventions
Electroencephalogram, or EEG (noninvasive)	An EEG is a recording of electrical impulses generated by the brain cortex that are sensed by electrodes on the surface of the scalp.	Analysis of the resulting tracings helps detect and localize abnormal electrical activity occurring in the cerebral cortex. It aids in seizure focus detection, localization of a source of irritation such as a tumor or abscess, and diagnosis of metabolic disturbances and sleep disorders.	Reassure the patient that he or she will not feel an electrical shock or pain during this test. The nurse also may need to clarify for the patient that the machine cannot "read minds" or indicate the presence of mental illness. The patient's scalp and hair should be free of oil, dirt, creams, and sprays because they can cause electrical interference and thus an inaccurate recording. Inform the EEG technician of electrical devices around the patient that may cause interference during the procedure (e.g., cardiac monitor, ventilator).
Cortical evoked potentials (noninvasive) Somatosensory evoked potentials (SSEPs) Brainstem auditory evoked response (BAER) Visual evoked potentials (VEPs)	In this test, a specialized device senses central or cortical cerebral electrical activity by skin electrodes in response to peripheral stimulation of specific sensory receptors. The sensory receptors stimulated can be those for vision, hearing, or tactile sensation. The signals are graphically displayed by a computer, and characteristic peaks, and the intervals between them, are measured.	Cortical evoked potentials provide a detailed assessment of neuron transmission along particular pathways. It has value in determining the integrity of visual, auditory and tactile pathways in patients with multiple sclerosis and spinal cord injury. This test also may be used in the assessment of a sensory pathway before, during, and after surgery.	This test may be used in conscious as well as unconscious patients and can be performed at the bedside. The patient must be as motionless as possible during some phases of this test to minimize musculoskeletal interference. Depending on the sensory pathway being tested, the patient may be instructed to watch a series of geometric designs or listen to a series of clicking noises.
Transcranial Doppler sonography (TCD)	This is a test in which high-frequency ultrasonic waves are directed from a probe toward specific cerebral vessels. The ultrasonic energy is aimed through cranial "windows," areas in the skull where the bony table is thin (temporal zygoma) or where there are small gaps in the bone (orbit or foramen magnum). The reflected sound waves are analyzed for shifts in frequency, indicating flow velocity.	The speed or velocity at which blood travels through cerebral vessels is an indicator of the size of the vascular channel and the resistance to blood flow. An approximation of cerebral blood flow may be determined. Cerebral autoregulation can be monitored by observing the response of intracranial vessels to changes in arterial carbon dioxide and to the partial occlusion of the proximal vessels, as may occur in vasospasm.	The test is noninvasive and may be performed at the bedside by the physician or ultrasound technician in 30–60 min. There are no known adverse effects, and the procedure may be repeated as often as necessary. The testing is accomplished with the patient initially supine, and later on his or her side, with the head flexed forward.
Lumbar puncture (invasive)	A hollow needle is positioned in the subarachnoid space at L3–4 or L4–5 level, and CSF is sampled. The pressure of the CSF also is measured. Normal pressure varies with age from 45 mm H_2O in full-term newborns to 120 mm H_2O in adults.	The CSF is examined for blood and for alterations in appearance, cell count, protein, and glucose. The opening pressure is roughly equivalent to the ICP for most patients, if done recumbent and no block is present.	This test is contraindicated in patients with suspected increased ICP because a sudden reduction in pressure from below may cause brain structures to herniate, leading to death. In preparation for this test, position the patient on side with knees and head flexed. Explain to the patient that some pressure may be felt as the needle is inserted and not to move suddenly or cough. After this procedure, keep the patient flat for 8 to 10 h to prevent headache. Encourage liberal fluid intake.

some of the diagnostic tests and outlines nursing implications.

NEURORADIOLOGICAL TECHNIQUES

Conventional radiographs of the skull and spine are used to identify fractures, dislocations, and other bony anomalies, especially in the setting of acute trauma. In addition, radiographs may be diagnostic when displacement of the calcified pineal gland is visible, which is an immediate clue to the presence of a space-occupying lesion. Air inside the skull also suggests an open skull fracture, such as a frontal or basilar skull fracture, that may not be readily apparent externally. However, the use of plain films has decreased in recent years as computed tomography (CT) and magnetic resonance imaging (MRI) have proved to be better diagnostic tools.

Spinal films are still used as an initial screening in suspected vertebral or spinal cord trauma. They allow for visualization of the spine to evaluate complaints of pain or noted motor and sensory impairment. In the suspected spinal cord injured–patient, visualization of the cervical spine through C7 is indicated to rule out a cervical spine injury. However, frequently it is difficult to visualize through C7; therefore, it is sometimes necessary for another individual to pull down on the patient's arms to drop the shoulders low enough for the film to be taken. In addition, visualization of C1-2 is indicated, which may be obtained by an odontoid or Waters' view. This film is taken through the open mouth of the patient and necessitates patient cooperation. In instances in which complete clearance is impossible, CT must be used to rule out cervical spinal injury.

The procedure for plain films of the skull and spine requires careful patient positioning and is relatively painless. The nurse's role involves monitoring the patient and attendant equipment during the procedure and being alert for complications related to patient position and the length of the procedure. In the spinal cord injured–patient, care should be taken to ensure stabilization of the neck by a hard cervical collar and logrolling during testing.

COMPUTED TOMOGRAPHY

CT scanning has been in use in the United States since 1973. CT scanning uses intersecting x-ray beams through the brain and skull to measure the density of tissues through which the x-ray beams pass. The denser the material (i.e., skull), the whiter it appears on the film (Fig. 33-10). The less dense the material (i.e., air), the darker it appears on the film. With mathematical reconstruction, multiple views or slices of the brain can be seen, which allows for a very precise, detailed picture of the brain and its contents.

The CT scan permits more refined measurement of the density of tissues, blood, and bone in the body compared with that afforded by conventional radiographs. For example, cerebral edema appears less dense and therefore is of a lighter color than normal tissue. The value of this technique is illustrated best in the trauma setting, where the ability to image rapidly and accurately the intracranial contents and position of vertebrae and spinal cord has dramatically changed the treatment of neurological patients. CT scans are recommended in the initial workup of seizures, headache, and loss of consciousness, and for the diagnosis of suspected hemorrhage, tumors, and other lesions. CT scanning can reliably detect conditions such as skull fractures, tissue swelling, hematomas, tumors, and abscesses. However, it has been noted that some vascular lesions are not as reliably documented using CT scan as they are with MRI. Therefore, MRI is indicated if these lesions are suspected.

Use of a contrast medium can enhance a CT scan. Using radiographic contrast material allows better visualization of vascular areas and enhances lesions previously seen on noncontrast films. Serial CTs may allow the health care team to follow neurological

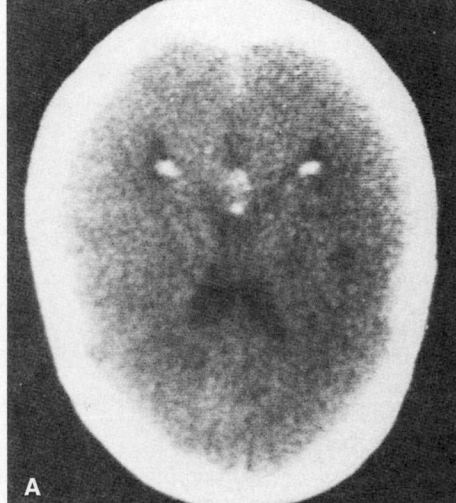
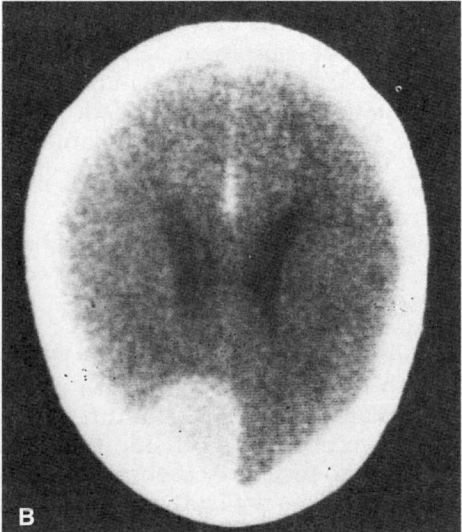

Figure 33-10 • Computed tomography scan of the brain. **A:** Normal scan. **B:** Scan showing a large mass in the left frontal lobe. (Reprinted with permission from Hickey J: The Clinical Practice of Neurological and Neuroscience Nursing, 5th ed. Philadelphia: Lippincott Williams & Wilkins, 2003, p 97.)

progression and therefore to intervene in a rapid manner. Care should be taken in the patient with renal failure or renal insufficiency because contrast clearance by the kidneys may be impaired.

Sometimes two technologies are used in combination, such as myelography with CT scanning, to provide a more refined image of anatomical structures of the spinal cord and vertebral column. With current technology, a routine scan now takes less than 5 minutes to survey the patient, analyze the data, and display a finished image.

Nursing management is focused on patient education to obviate any potential complications, such as poor patient tolerance. The patient should be aware that he or she must lie very still during the procedure and that he or she may experience feelings of claustrophobia. In addition, the nurse ascertains whether the patient has any preexisting allergies, particularly if contrast is to be used. The nurse may need to remain with the patient during the procedure to continue to monitor neurological status and vital signs.

MAGNETIC RESONANCE IMAGING

MRI, known in the past as nuclear magnetic resonance imaging, has become widely available in medium and large medical centers. This modality uses non-ionizing forms of radiation to produce computerized cross-sectional images in much the same fashion as a CT scan. However, it provides more finely detailed images that look remarkably like anatomical slices of the body. MRI is superior to a CT scan in the early diagnosis of cerebral infarction and the detection of demyelinating disorders, such as multiple sclerosis. It is also helpful in diagnosing small lesions, such as tumors and hemorrhages, that might not appear on a CT scan. However, traditional CT scanning is superior for scanning for bony abnormalities, which are visualized poorly on MRI.

Although superior in many ways to CT scanning, MRI has its limitations. Its powerful magnetic fields interfere with the functioning of devices such as cardiac pacemakers. Patients with surgical clips and prosthetic implants made of ferrous metal cannot be scanned. It is also difficult to study patients on life-support equipment because most ventilators and monitors are constructed in part of ferrous metal. If emergency therapy is needed, the patient must be removed from the scanning chamber and the imaging suite before resuscitation can begin.

POSITRON EMISSION TOMOGRAPHY AND SINGLE-PHOTON EMISSION COMPUTED TOMOGRAPHY

Positron emission tomography (PET) is a process in which molecules labeled with radioactive isotopes are located in the brain and recorded by radiation-sensitive detectors outside the head. PET has the capacity to measure cerebral blood flow and cerebral metabolism as the isotope-labeled glucose or oxygen is used in the body. It is superior to previous technologies that could image structure only, not function. It currently assists in the diagnosis of Alzheimer's disease, which shows a characteristic pattern of glucose consumption, as well as in Parkinson's disease, Huntington's disease, and Tourette's syndrome. However, the complexity of the testing, the comparatively high cost per scan, and the need to have a cyclotron nearby to produce the short-lived radioactive isotopes make this modality impractical and unwieldy in the clinical setting.

Single-photon emission computed tomography (SPECT) combines the imaging ability of conventional nuclear medicine scanners with the technology of transaxial CT scanning to overcome some limitations. Using more stable radioisotopes, SPECT scanning has been able to detect diminished perfusion in an area of stroke before there is conventional CT evidence of infarction, as well as alterations in regional blood flow in patients with Alzheimer's disease.

ANGIOGRAPHY AND DIGITAL SUBTRACTION ANGIOGRAPHY

Cerebral angiography remains the study of choice for evaluating cerebrovascular problems (Fig. 33-11). It is the only test that can reveal large and small aneurysms and arteriovenous malformations and their relationship to adjacent structures and vessels. It involves the passage of a radiographic catheter through a large artery (usually femoral) to each of the arterial vessels bringing blood to the brain and spinal cord. Radiopaque contrast dye is then injected into each vessel. A rapid sequence of films is taken after the dye has passed through small arterial branches and capillaries and into the venous circulation. In this way, the vessel lumen and size and the presence of any occlusions can be visualized. Cerebral angiography has been used before surgery to help decide the appropriateness of medical versus surgical management. It has also been combined with balloon angioplasty

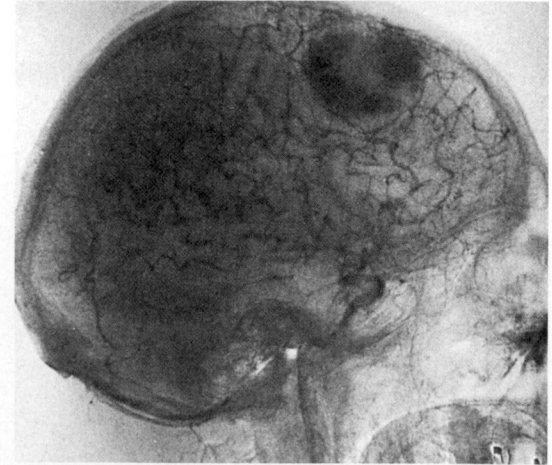

Figure 33-11 • Cerebral angiogram showing an abnormal, large, space-occupying lesion at 1 o'clock. (Reprinted with permission from Hickey J: The Clinical Practice of Neurological and Neuroscience Nursing, 5th ed. Philadelphia: Lippincott Williams & Wilkins, 2003, p 108.)

in instances of vascular occlusion or coiling in the treatment of aneurysms.

Digital subtraction angiography makes use of radiographic contrast to illuminate the cerebral circulation, but in considerably smaller quantities than required for conventional angiography. The dye may be injected into the arterial or the venous systems. Films are taken before and after the dye injection and converted into digital information in the accompanying computer. The images are "subtracted" from each other, removing all images in common. The resultant image displays only the enhanced circulatory system, free of other anatomical distortion.

The major complications associated with angiography include stroke, vasospasm, or renal failure secondary to the contrast load. Contraindications to angiography include identified allergies to contrast, anticoagulant therapy, and kidney and liver disease.

CEREBRAL BLOOD FLOW STUDIES

In the diagnostic setting, cerebral blood flow is evaluated most commonly by a radioisotope brain scan. A radioactive isotope is injected intravenously. In unusual circumstances, the isotope can also be administered orally or intra-arterially. The brain is then scanned to determine which areas show an accumulation of the radioactive substance. If there is blood flow to the brain, damaged areas absorb more of the isotope than areas without damage. A newer technique, perfusion CT, involves scanning before, during, and after infusion of the contrast agent to obtain "real time" data with respect to blood flow. Cerebral blood flow studies are indicated in the detection of either increased or decreased blood flow during operative procedures or to assess for vasospasm. They may also be used after carotid endarterectomy. The test may be used to determine brain death, which is evidenced if there is no flow to the cerebral hemispheres. In certain disorders, such as carbon monoxide poisoning, there may be increased blood flow to the brain, yet anoxic brain death may still occur. The measurement of cerebral flow assists with decision making regarding treatment and in the identification of complications.

MYELOGRAPHY

Myelography is a contrast study of the spinal cord and surrounding structures. It involves the introduction of water-soluble material into the CSF through a lumbar or cisternal puncture, performed under fluoroscopy, after about 10 mL of CSF has been removed. Myelography is indicated in the evaluation of herniated intervertebral disks, spinal cord tumors, and congenital problems and in the assessment of spinal cord trauma. It allows for better visualization of nerve roots and surrounding structures because it uses a contrast agent that is lighter than CSF. However, the agent disperses rapidly into the subarachnoid space, which means that the patient's position cannot be adjusted. The contrast agent does not require removal; therefore, the patient should be kept well hydrated to facilitate dye excretion. A heavier, oil-based preparation is sometimes used, which must be removed at the end of the procedure.

The contrast agents are potentially toxic to cerebral tissue and may cause grand mal seizures. Thus, the patient must remain with the head up at least 30 to 45 degrees, and phenothiazine medications, which increase the toxic symptoms, must be avoided.

ULTRASONOGRAPHY AND NONINVASIVE CEREBROVASCULAR STUDIES

Transcranial Doppler ultrasonographic studies are a noninvasive means of monitoring intracranial hemodynamics at the bedside. The examination is performed through cranial "windows," areas in the skull where the bone is relatively thin, such as the temporal area, or where there are small spaces between bones, such as the orbit. The ultrasonic probe transmits sound waves at certain frequencies to a specified depth. The resultant reflected signal from blood traveling through cerebral vessels is interpreted for speed or velocity. As resistance or vascular size changes, it is reflected as a change in blood flow velocities. The data may be used to monitor therapy, aid in determining prognosis, and provide early recognition of cerebral vasospasm in patients after subarachnoid hemorrhage or severe head injury. Serial Doppler studies in patients with an aneurysm provide data regarding postoperative vasospasm and alleviate the need for repeat angiograms.

Carotid and vertebral artery duplex scans provide anatomical imaging of blood vessels combined with hemodynamic information. Doppler studies at the cranial window provide information about direction of flow, pulsatile rhythmicity, and resistance to flow of the cerebral vasculature. Carotid duplex scans are routinely used as a screening tool in patients at risk for atherosclerotic disease. The nurse should be aware of whether the patient has any history of dysrhythmias or cardiac disease because these may alter the hemodynamic profile and findings of the test.

ELECTROPHYSIOLOGICAL STUDIES

Electroencephalography

Using electroencephalography (EEG), a record is made of the brain's electrical activity. Small plate electrodes are placed in specific locations on the patient's scalp, and 16 to 21 channels transcribe the electrical potentials generated by the brain. Waveforms are classified in terms of voltage and amplitude. EEG is most valuable in the diagnosis and treatment of patients with seizures. In addition, it may help localize structural abnormalities, such as tumors and abscesses, and aid in the differentiation of structural and metabolic abnormalities. It also may provide confirmatory criteria in the diagnosis of brain death. In recent years, a modified form of EEG has been used at the bedside in critical care to monitor the effects of pharmacological agents that reduce cerebral blood flow and hence reduce electrical activity. This is termed continuous EEG monitoring and is rapidly becoming a standard of care in many facilities. It is intended to detect subclinical or nonconvulsive seizure activity in patients who are taking medications that suppress electrical activity.

A computerized technique that dramatically compresses standard EEG data and converts them into a more easily interpreted and colorized form is compressed spectral array. This technique is also seen at the bedside in neurological intensive care units to monitor patients with severe head injuries.

Evoked Potentials

An evoked potential is an electrical manifestation of the brain's response to an external stimulus: auditory, visual, somatic, or a combination of these. The measurement of such a response provides an assessment of the function of neuropathways from the periphery through the spinal cord and brainstem and finally to cortical structures (Fig. 33-12). This technique has been most helpful in the diagnosis of multiple sclerosis and Guillain-Barré syndrome and in determining the prognosis for reversibility of coma in the brainstem-injured patient. It also may be used during surgery to monitor potential injury during manipulations of spinal nerves and structures.

The three most frequently used techniques in head trauma evaluation are somatosensory evoked potentials (SSEPs), which use electrical shock as a stimulus; brainstem auditory evoked response, which uses click or sound stimulus; and visual evoked potentials, which use light stimulus. SSEPs assess neurological function in specific neural pathways postinjury and detect further CNS insults from secondary processes, such as hypoxia and hypertension.

LUMBAR PUNCTURE FOR CEREBROSPINAL FLUID EXAMINATION

A lumbar puncture for CSF analysis may be performed to help diagnose autoimmune disorders or infections. Occasionally, it is performed to verify subarachnoid hemorrhage, although a CT scan is the procedure of choice and is safer for such a patient. CSF is obtained by the insertion of an 18- to 22-gauge needle between the vertebrae at the L3–4 or L4–5 levels. The fluid is sent for content analysis and for culture, sensitivity, and other serological tests (Table 33-8). Pressure readings may also be obtained for diagnostic use.

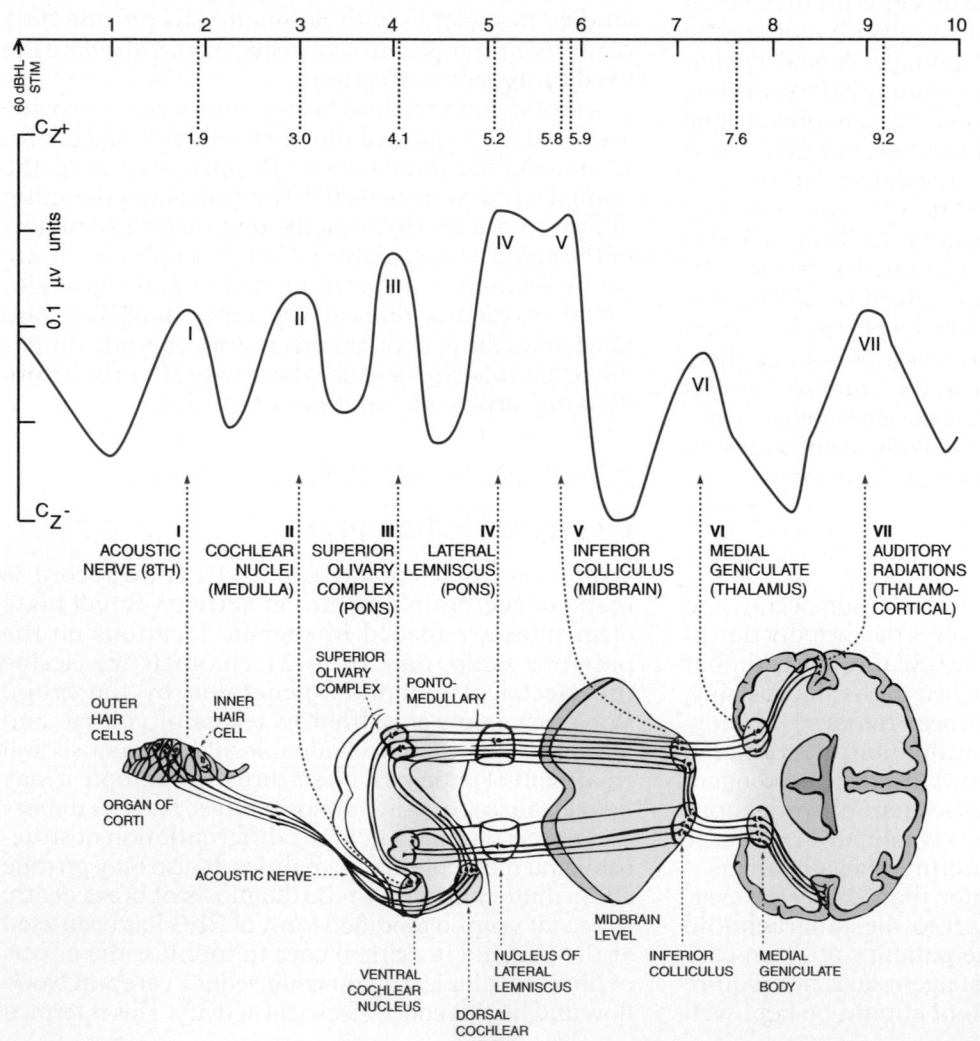

Figure 33-12 • The waveform of a normal brainstem auditory evoked response. (Courtesy of Grass-Telefactor, an Astro-Med, Inc. Product Group, West Warwick, RI.)

Table 33-8 • Normal and Abnormal Values for Cerebrospinal Fluid

Characteristic	Normal	Abnormal
Color	Clear, colorless	Cloudy often due to presence of WBC or bacteria Xanthochromic due to presence of RBC
WBC	0–5/mm^3, all mononuclear	Elevated count accompanies many conditions (tumor, meningitis, subarachnoid hemorrhage, infarct, abscess)
RBC	None	Presence may be due to traumatic tap or subarachnoid hemorrhage
Chloride	120–130 mEq/L	Low concentration associated with meningeal infection and tuberculous meningitis Elevated level not neurologically significant
Glucose	50–75 mg/100 mL	Decreased level associated with presence of bacteria in CSF Elevated level not neurologically significant
Pressure	70–180 mm H$_2$O	Low pressure associated with inaccurate placement of needle, dehydration, or block along subarachnoid space or at foramen magnum Elevated pressure associated with benign intracranial hypertension; cerebral edema; CNS tumor, abscess, or cyst; hydrocephalus; muscle tension or abdominal compression; subdural hematoma
Protein	14–45 mg/100 mL	Decreased level not neurologically significant Increased level associated with demyelinating or degenerative disease, Guillain-Barré syndrome, hemorrhage, infection, spinal block, tumor

From Cammermeyer M, Appeldorn C [eds]: Core Curriculum for Neuroscience Nursing, 4th ed. Chicago: American Association of Neuroscience Nurses, 1996.

If a lumbar puncture is performed in a patient with elevated ICP, herniation can be a life-threatening complication. Complications that can result from a CSF leak include a postprocedure headache, nuchal rigidity, fever, and difficulty voiding. Treatment involves the injection of blood into the dura, called a blood patch, to stop the leak.

• Clinical Applicability Challenges

Case Study

Ms. J., a 66-year-old woman, is admitted to the critical care unit after she presented to the emergency department with a complaint of sudden-onset dizziness, unsteady gait, and weakness in her left arm and leg. She also complains of a severe temporal headache. She has a positive past medical history of hypertension, diabetes, hypercholesterolemia, and smoking. Your initial neurological examination reveals a pleasant, anxious woman who answers questions appropriately and follows all commands. However, she exhibits questionable mild weakness of the left arm when performing hand grasps.

An hour later, the nurse observes that Ms. J. is somewhat somnolent and difficult to arouse. Her pupils are equal and reactive to light and accommodation. However, she is able to open her eyes only to repeated verbal stimuli. She does not follow commands and only moves her extremities to painful stimuli by pulling away from the stimuli. She is oriented only to self.

1. After the initial neurological examination, what additional neurological assessment might the nurse perform in order to better characterize the extremity weakness?

2. What is Ms. J.'s Glasgow Coma Scale score and what might this suggest?

3. What diagnostic tests might be ordered?

4. What nursing interventions are appropriate?

Review Questions

1. A normal response to the oculocephalic reflex is
   a. initial conjugate deviation of the eyes in the opposite direction, with simultaneous movement of both eyes back to midline.
   b. midline positioning of both eyes when the head is rotated briskly.
   c. initial disconjugate deviation of the eyes in the direction of movement, with simultaneous movement of both eyes to the opposite direction.
   d. horizontal nystagmus with conjugate movement of the eyes toward the direction of movement.

2. Fluent speech that lacks coherent content associated with impaired understanding of the spoken word in spite of normal hearing is called
   a. nonfluent dysphasia.
   b. global dysphasia.
   c. dysarthria.
   d. fluent dysphasia.

3. Extension, adduction, and hyperpronation of the upper extremities and extension of the lower extremities with plantar flexion of the feet is termed
   a. clonus.
   b. decerebrate rigidity.
   c. athetosis.
   d. decorticate rigidity.

4. On examination, you note that the patient has a negative corneal reflex. What cranial nerve does this reflex test and what other tests might the nurse perform to fully explore the response of this cranial nerve?
   a. Facial nerve; have patient clench the jaw
   b. Facial nerve; have patient raise eyebrows or smile
   c. Trigeminal nerve; have patient clench the jaw
   d. Trigeminal nerve; have patient raise eyebrows or smile

5. A patient with a suspected spinal cord lesion will most likely be scheduled for which of the following diagnostic tests?
   a. Evoked potential
   b. Myelogram
   c. Subtraction angiography
   d. Positron emission tomography

Selected Readings

American Association for Neuroscience Nursing: AANN Core Curriculum for Neuroscience Nursing, 4th ed. St. Louis: Elsevier, 2004

Arbour R: Intracranial hypertension: Monitoring and nursing assessment. Crit Care Nurse 24:19–32, 2004

Barker E: Neuroscience Nursing: A Spectrum of Care, 2nd ed. St. Louis: Mosby–Year Book, 2002

Bickley BS, Szilagyi PG: Bates' Guide to Physical Examination and History Taking, 9th ed. Philadelphia: Lippincott Williams & Wilkins, 2006

Gray JT, Gavin CM: Assessment and management of neurological problems. Emerg Med J 22(6):440–445, 2005

Harris MD, Sethi RK: The initial assessment and management of the multiple trauma patient with an associated spine injury. Spine 31(11 Suppl):S9–15, 2006

Haymore J: A neuron in a haystack: Advanced neurological assessment. AACN Clin Issues 15(4):568–581, 2004

Henneman LA, Karras GE: Determining brain death in adults: A guideline for use in critical care. Crit Care Nurse 24:50–56, 2004

Hickey JV: The Clinical Practice of Neurological and Neurosurgical Nursing, 5th ed. Philadelphia: Lippincott Williams & Wilkins, 2002

Hoeffner EG: Cerebral perfusion imaging. J Neuroophthalmol 25(4):313–320, 2005

Kipps CM, Hodges JR: Cognitive assessment for clinicians. J Neurol Neurosurg Psychiatry 76(1 Suppl):i22–30, 2005

Kirkness CJ, Arbour R: Cerebral blood flow monitoring in clinical practice. AACN Clin Issues 16(4):476–487, 2005

McQuillan KA, Von Rueden KT, Hartsock R, et al (eds): Trauma Nursing From Resuscitation to Rehabilitation, 3rd ed. St. Louis: WB Saunders, 2002

Newberg AB, Alavi A: The role of PET imaging in the management of patients with central nervous system disorders. Radiol Clin North Am 43(10):49–65, 2005

Olson DM, Graffagnino C: Consciousness, coma and caring for the brain injured patient. AACN Clin Issues 16(4):441–455, 2005

Rowe VL, Tucker SW: Advances in vascular imaging. Surg Clin North Am 84(5):1189–1202, 2004

Stevens RD, Bhardwaj A: Approach to the comatose patient. Crit Care Med 34(1):31–41, 2006

Teasdale G, Jennett W: Assessment of coma and impaired consciousness: A practical scale. Lancet 2(7872):81–84, 1974

Patient Management: Nervous System

34

Mona N. Bahouth • Karen L. Yarbrough

Physiological Principles
  Intracranial Dynamics
  Volume–Pressure Curve
  Cerebral Perfusion Pressure
Increased Intracranial Pressure
  Cushing's Triad
  Cerebral Edema
  Herniation
Intracranial Pressure Monitoring
  Indications for Intracranial Pressure Monitoring
  Intracranial Pressure Monitoring Devices
  Intracranial Pressure Measurements
Management of Increased Intracranial Pressure
  Clinical Management
  Nursing Considerations

Objectives

Based on the content in this chapter, the reader should be able to:

❶ Define intracranial pressure and intracranial hypertension.

❷ Discuss several physiological principles affecting intracranial pressure, including the Monro-Kellie doctrine, compliance, autoregulation, and cerebral perfusion.

❸ Discuss indications for intracranial pressure monitoring.

❹ Describe currently available methods of monitoring intracranial pressure.

❺ Explain three possible complications associated with intracranial pressure monitoring and discuss troubleshooting strategies.

❻ Identify various strategies to manage increased intracranial pressure.

❼ Describe the pharmacological agents used for patients experiencing a neurological emergency.

Intracranial pressure (ICP) is defined as the pressure in the cranial vault relative to atmospheric pressure. Understanding general principles regarding the concepts of ICP provides the critical care nurse with a framework that he or she can then apply to multiple neurological conditions. In addition, a working knowledge of the pharmacological agents used in neurological emergencies, such as steroids, antihypertensive agents, diuretics, analgesics, sedatives, barbiturates, and anticonvulsants, better prepares the nurse to handle these situations.

• Physiological Principles

INTRACRANIAL DYNAMICS

Concepts of ICP management and intervention strategies are based on the principle that the skull is a rigid box, a nonexpansile, noncontractile space. Its contents are divided into three intracranial sections: blood maintained in the blood vessels, cerebrospinal fluid (CSF), and brain parenchyma. The brain's ability to self-regulate is based on the Monro-Kellie doctrine of fixed intracranial volume. This doctrine states that the volume of the intracranium is equal to the volume of the cerebral blood (3% to 10%); plus the volume of the CSF (8% to 12%); plus the volume of brain tissue, which consists of more than 80% water. As long as the total intracranial volume remains the same, ICP remains constant. To maintain equilibrium, there cannot be any increase in volume of one of these components without a compensatory decrease in the other two. Any alterations in the volume of any of these three components within the cranial vault, without a response from the other two components, may lead to a change in ICP. A normal ICP measurement ranges between 0 and 15 mm Hg. An ICP measurement greater than 15 mm Hg is considered intracranial hypertension, or increased ICP. Basic physiological responses to illness in any of the three components in the intracranial vault can cause increased ICP (Table 34-1).

Cerebral Blood Flow

Autoregulation is defined as the ability of an organ to maintain consistent blood flow despite marked changes in arterial circulatory and perfusion pressures. The normal brain has the ability to autoregulate cerebral blood flow (CBF). Normally, autoregulation ensures a constant blood flow through the cerebral vessels over a range of perfusion pressures by changing the diameter of vessels in response to changes in arterial pressures. This mechanism is the brain's protective device against the constantly fluctuating changes of blood pressure. When autoregulation is impaired, the CBF fluctuates in direct correlation with the systemic blood pressure. In patients with impaired autoregulation, any activity that causes an increase in blood pressure, such as coughing, suctioning, or restlessness, can cause an increase in CBF that could also increase ICP.

The first of three components that may undergo changes as the body attempts to maintain a consistent intracranial volume is the CBF. Normal CBF is provided by a cerebral perfusion pressure (CPP) in the range of 60 to 100 mm Hg. The brain receives approximately 750 mL/minute of arterial blood (15% to 20% of total cardiac output when at rest). For autoregulation to be functional, carbon dioxide levels must be in an acceptable range and hemodynamic pressure targets must be within the following ranges: CPP greater than 60 mm Hg, mean arterial pressure (MAP) less than 160 mm Hg, systolic pressure between 60 and 140 mm Hg, and ICP less than 30 mm Hg.[1] Factors that alter the ability of the cerebral vessels to constrict or dilate, such as hypoxia, hypercapnia, and brain trauma, also interfere with autoregulation. Carbon dioxide is a potent vasodilator of cerebral vessels, causing increased CBF and increased volume, leading to increased ICP.

Cerebrospinal Fluid Circulation

CSF also contributes to fluctuations in intracranial hemodynamics. CSF is a clear fluid produced predominantly in the choroid plexus in the lateral, third, and fourth ventricles. It fills the ventricles and subarachnoid space and protects the brain and spinal cord from injury. Circulation of CSF occurs in a closed system; it is predominantly reabsorbed by the arachnoid villi located in the subarachnoid space and dispersed into the venous system through the superior sagittal sinus (see Chapter 32, Fig. 32-6). Along the entire CSF cycle, potential disturbances in production, circulation, and absorption can contribute to changes in ICP. For instance, overproduction of CSF in the choroid plexus overwhelms the circulatory system. Obstruction of CSF circulation through the ventricles leads to dilation of the ventricular system (obstructive hydrocephalus). Marked slowing of absorption in the arachnoid villi caused by blood or infectious debris interferes with the reabsorption of CSF, thereby leading to systemic overload (communicating hydrocephalus).

Parenchyma

The third and most difficult intracranial component to manipulate without surgical intervention is the brain parenchyma. However, the brain tissue does respond to increased ICP and changes within the other two intracranial components. The brain can accommodate or compensate for minimal changes in volume by partial collapse of the cisterns, ventricles, and vascular systems, in turn decreasing production and increasing reabsorption of CSF. Compensatory mechanisms to maintain normal ICP include:

▶ Shunting of CSF into the spinal subarachnoid space
▶ Increased CSF absorption
▶ Decreased CSF production
▶ Shunting of venous blood out of the skull

Table 34-1 • Potential Causes of Increased Intracranial Pressure

Contributing Physiology	Intracranial Component Involved	Potential Cause	Potential Treatment
Overproduction of CSF	CSF space	Choroid plexus papilloma	Surgical removal, diuretics
Inadequate CSF reabsorption (communicating hydrocephalus)	CSF space	Subarachnoid hemorrhage, infection	Drainage of CSF from lumbar intrathecal site, shunt placement
Blockage of CSF circulation (obstructive hydrocephalus)	CSF space	Posterior fossa tumor, brain injury, birth defects (spina bifida)	Ventricular drainage, surgical removal of obstruction
Edema (vasogenic, cytotoxic)	Brain tissue	Tumor, infection, infarction, hypoxia, arteriovenous malformation	Drainage of CSF, removal of lesion, adequate oxygenation
Expansile mass	Brain tissue	Tumor, abscess, intracerebral hemorrhage	Surgical removal, steroids
Vasospasm	Intracranial circulation	Subarachnoid hemorrhage	Hypervolemia, hypertensive therapy, calcium channel antagonists
Vasodilation	Intracranial circulation	Elevated $PaCO_2$, systemic vasodilators (α-adrenergic agents)	Hyperventilation, removal of offending agent

During the compensatory period, ICP remains fairly constant. However, when these compensatory mechanisms have been exhausted, pressure increases rapidly until shifting of brain tissue toward open spaces in the skull occurs, and the blood supply to the medulla is cut off. The ability of the intracranial content to compensate depends on the location of the lesion, the rate of expansion, and cranial compliance.

VOLUME–PRESSURE CURVE

The intracranial volume–pressure curve, also called a pressure–volume index, demonstrates the relationship between changes in intracranial volume and changes in ICP. An awareness of the patient's position on this curve is useful in monitoring and selecting appropriate interventions. The rate at which ICP increases in response to a change in intracranial volume depends on the compliance of the brain. *Compliance* is a change in volume resulting from a change in pressure. *Elastance* is a change in pressure resulting from a change in volume and is often used interchangeably with the term compliance. When compliance in the intracranial compartment is low, a small volume change causes a large increase in ICP. In Figure 34-1, the curve illustrates compliance, as the compensatory mechanisms maintain ICP in the normal range during increases in intracranial volume. Little change occurs in ICP during the initial increase in volume because the volume added to the cranium is compensated for by volume displacement. As the compensatory mechanisms become exhausted, the volume added becomes greater than the volume displaced, and there is a larger increase in ICP with any incremental volume increase. Free communication of CSF between the lateral ventricles and infratentorium is lost as a result.

A major reason for controlling and decreasing ICP is the maintenance of cerebral oxygenation by adequate CBF, which is estimated clinically by the measurement of CPP. Many factors contribute to increased ICP along the volume–pressure curve. Drastic increases in ICP may result from hypercarbia, hypoxia, rapid eye movement sleep, pyrexia, or the administration of certain anesthetics. Additionally, ICP is affected by environmental stimulation and increased metabolic rates.[2]

CEREBRAL PERFUSION PRESSURE

Cerebral perfusion pressure is the blood pressure gradient across the brain. CPP is calculated by subtracting the mean ICP from the mean systemic arterial pressure (MAP): CPP = MAP – ICP. When the CPP is greater than 100 mm Hg, there is a potential for hyperperfusion and increased ICP. When the CPP is less than 60 mm Hg, blood supply to the brain is inadequate, and neuronal hypoxia and cell death may occur. If MAPs and ICPs are equal, CPP is zero, indicating no CBF. CBF may also cease totally at pressures somewhat greater than zero. Patients with hypotension, such as postcardiac resuscitation or trauma patients, with normal ICPs (0 to 15 mm Hg), may have impaired CPP.

The autoregulation system for maintenance of constant blood flow does not function at pressures less than 40 mm Hg. Because an acutely injured brain requires a higher CPP than a normal brain, a minimum CPP of 70 mm Hg is required for maintenance of adequate cerebral perfusion and potentially improved outcomes in patients with brain injuries.[2] When CPP decreases, the cardiovascular response is an increase in systemic pressure.

When brain damage is severe, as with widespread brain edema or when blood flow has been arrested in the brain, CBF may be reduced at relatively normal levels of CPP. The cause is impedance to the flow of blood across the cerebrovascular bed. If autoregulation is impaired, CBF may not increase despite increases in CPP. Increased ICP leads to ischemia, anoxic injury, decreased compliance, and possible herniation.

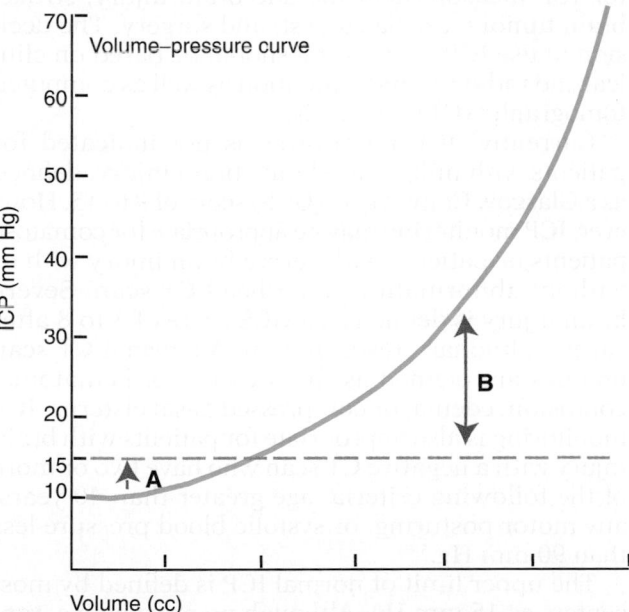

Figure 34-1 • Volume–pressure curve. Volume–pressure response (VPR), also referred to as the pressure–volume index (PVI), provides a method of estimating the compensatory capacity of the intracranial cavity. Note that the intracranial pressure (ICP) remains within the normal limit of 0–15 mm Hg as long as compliance is normal and fluid can be displaced by the additional volume (**A**). Once the compensatory system is exhausted, a small additional volume causes a greater increase in pressure (**B**). Acute changes can cause serious and sometimes fatal neurological deterioration.

• Increased Intracranial Pressure

CUSHING'S TRIAD

Cushing's triad is the classic syndrome of increased ICP and includes increased pulse pressure, decreased pulse, and change in respiratory pattern with pupillary changes. This syndrome usually occurs only in association with posterior fossa lesions and seldom with the more commonly observed supratentorial mass lesions, such as subdural hematomas. When these classic signs do accompany a supratentorial lesion, they are associated with a sudden pressure increase and usually herald a state of decompensation. Brain damage usually is irreversible if prolonged, and death is imminent without emergent intervention.

CEREBRAL EDEMA

Cerebral edema leading to increased ICP is a process common to multiple neurological illnesses. Its presence leads to secondary complications related to the expansion of brain tissue within the closed space of the cranium. Independently, cerebral edema can cause marked increases in ICP and must be treated aggressively. In general, once edema begins, its progression is rapid and difficult to control.

Treatment of cerebral edema may include the use of corticosteroids as well as osmotic diuretics directed at the reduction of ICP. These agents work by increasing plasma osmolarity, which draws fluid out of the brain tissue and into the bloodstream. The goal of therapy is to maintain plasma osmolarity up to 320 mOsm/L. See Chapter 36 for further information about cerebral edema.

Vasogenic Edema

The most common type of cerebral edema is vasogenic edema, which is characterized by a disruption in the blood–brain barrier and the inability of the cell walls to control movement of water in and out of the cells. Capillary permeability is affected, and fluid and protein are allowed to leak from the plasma into the extracellular space, resulting in increased extracellular fluid volume predominantly in the white matter. Common processes leading to vasogenic edema include brain tumors, cerebral abscess, and both ischemic and hemorrhagic stroke.

Cytotoxic Edema

Cytotoxic edema is characterized by swelling of the individual neurons and endothelial cells, which increases fluid in the intracellular space and reduces available extracellular space, affecting the gray matter. Eventually the cell membrane cannot maintain an effective barrier, and both water and sodium enter the cell, causing swelling and loss of function. Cytotoxic edema occurs after injuries such as anoxia or hypoxic injury.

HERNIATION

Herniation is defined as the displacement of tissue through structures within the skull. Transtentorial or uncal shifting of brain tissue through rigid openings in the skull or dura leads to displacement of midline brain structures and compression of structures in the central nervous system (CNS), causing traditional clin-

ical herniation syndromes. See Chapter 36 for more information about herniation syndromes.

• Intracranial Pressure Monitoring

Monitoring ICP provides information that facilitates interventions to prevent secondary cerebral ischemia and brainstem distortion. For ICP monitoring to be safe and effective, the indications for monitoring, methods of monitoring, and ethical considerations for patient care and nursing practice must be taken into account for each patient. Factors that affect patient selection include the potential benefit from invasive ICP monitoring and therapy, the patient's diagnosis and prognosis, and the availability of the appropriate level of critical care. ICP monitoring helps improve patient outcome by providing information about the likelihood of cerebral herniation and facilitating calculation of CPP. It is also helpful in guiding the use of potentially harmful treatments, such as hyperventilation, mannitol, and barbiturates.

INDICATIONS FOR INTRACRANIAL PRESSURE MONITORING

ICP monitoring is primarily used for guiding therapy. General guidelines exist to provide direction in therapy for patients at risk for and with increased ICP. Diagnostic conditions that may be indications for ICP measurement include brain injury, stroke, brain tumors, cardiac arrest, and surgery. The decision to use ICP monitoring should be based on clinical and radiographic evaluation as well as computed tomography (CT) diagnosis.

Currently, ICP monitoring is not indicated for patients with mild to moderate brain injury, defined as a Glasgow Coma Scale (GCS) score of 9 to 15. However, ICP monitoring may be appropriate for comatose patients or patients with severe brain injury with or without abnormalities on a head CT scan. Severe brain injury is defined as a GCS score of 3 to 8 after cardiopulmonary resuscitation. Abnormal CT scan findings are defined as the presence of hematoma, contusion, edema, or compressed basal cisterns. ICP monitoring is also appropriate for patients with brain injury with a negative CT scan who have two or more of the following criteria: age greater than 40 years, any motor posturing, or systolic blood pressure less than 90 mm Hg.[3,4]

The upper limit of normal ICP is defined by most centers as 15 mm Hg. Although no prospective, randomized trial has been completed, a summary of the literature suggests that ICP monitors are beneficial in:

▶ Providing earlier detection of intracranial mass lesions

▶ Limiting indiscriminate use of therapies with potentially harmful consequences

▶ Reducing ICP through CSF drainage, thereby improving CPP

▶ Assisting in determining prognosis

▶ Possibly improving outcomes[4]

Nontraumatic neurological disorders that may benefit from ICP monitoring are subarachnoid hemorrhage, intracerebral hemorrhage, ischemic infarction, infection, hydrocephalus, and, rarely, brain tumors with associated edema or with significant lesion volume.

Coagulopathy, systemic infection, CNS infection, and infection at the site of device insertion are relative contraindications to the placement of ICP monitors.

INTRACRANIAL PRESSURE MONITORING DEVICES

Various devices, such as intraventricular catheters, fiberoptic devices, and epidural monitors, are used to monitor ICP. A chosen ICP device should have pressure range capability of 0 to 100 mm Hg, accuracy within the ICP range of 0 to 20 mm Hg ± 2 mm Hg, and a maximal error of 10% in the range of 20 to 100 mm Hg of ICP.[4] The type of monitor used depends on several clinical factors, the type of neurological process, and the patient's symptoms on presentation (Fig. 34-2). A variety of advantages and disadvantages exist with each of the devices; therefore, an awareness of potential complications is essential in the bedside management of the patient undergoing such monitoring (Table 34-2). Guidelines provided by the Brain Trauma Foundation consortium rank available devices by consensus preference (http://www.braintrauma.org/guidelines).

Intraventricular catheters (IVCs) provide accurate, low-cost, and reliable ICP monitoring, and they are widely used. The catheter is a tubular instrument that is placed inside fluid-filled cavities in the ventri-

cles. CSF is synthesized in these cavities and flows out to circulate over the surface of the brain. IVCs allow for simultaneous monitoring and treatment of ICP by intermittently draining CSF (Fig. 34-3). IVCs can be inserted under sterile conditions at the bedside in the intensive care unit (ICU) or in the operating room during surgical cases. Unlike parenchymal monitors, the IVC can be recalibrated *in situ*.

Fiberoptic monitors use fiberoptic technologies to measure ICP. The tip of the fiberoptic probe has a transducer, which is inserted into brain parenchyma, the ventricles it surrounds, or the subdural space. Fiberoptic monitors are easily inserted, and their use is increasing. Fiberoptic ventricular catheters provide benefits similar to those of IVCs, but at a higher cost. Of similar precision are parenchymal ICP monitors with fiberoptic or strain gauge catheter tip transduction; however, these devices are subject to potential measurement drift.

Subarachnoid, subdural, and epidural monitors are less accurate and less frequently used than the other types of monitors.[5] The subarachnoid bolt or screw is inserted through a twist drill hole to the level of the subarachnoid space and secured to a saline-filled pressure tubing transducer system. Epidural monitors are placed into the epidural space between the inner surface of the skull and the dura mater to monitor ICP.

Complications of Intracranial Pressure Monitoring Devices

Each type of monitoring system has potential complications. To ensure accurate measurements and reduce morbidity, the nurse must be alert to problems associated with ICP monitoring systems that could cause incorrect ICP measurements and complications. When the monitor indicates a change in ICP, the nurse must first determine whether the reading is accurate. If the reading is accurate, an attempt is then made to determine the reason for the pressure change. Table 34-3 provides a guide to troubleshooting ICP lines.

As with any invasive procedure, complications may occur. In critically ill patients with neurological problems, the risk/benefit ratio for any therapy must be considered before the implementation of that therapy. For instance, IVCs carry the potential risks for catheter misplacement, obstruction, infection, and hemorrhage. Use of antibiotic-impregnated IVCs is on the rise as a promising technology for reduction in device-related infection rates. There are few published data about this practice as of yet; however, studies are ongoing.

Because drainage holes responsible for the collection of excessive CSF are very small, it is easy for the catheter to become obstructed; the nurse must monitor for this complication. Malfunction or obstruction occurs at a rate of 6% to 10% in patients with an IVC and is significantly higher in patients with parenchymal or ventricular fiberoptic catheter tip devices, at a rate of 9% to 40%.[6] Higher rates of obstruction have been correlated with malignant elevations of ICP

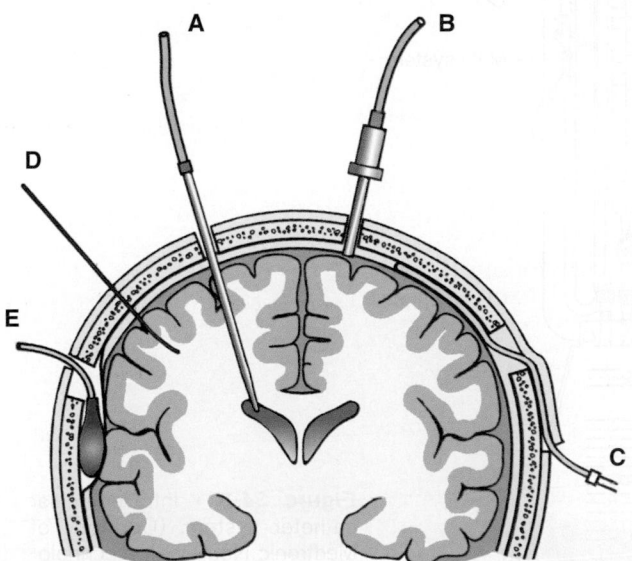

Figure 34-2 • Intracranial pressure (ICP) monitoring systems: intraventricular (**A**); subarachnoid (**B**); subdural (**C**); parenchymal (**D**); and epidural (**E**).

Table 34-2 • Advantages and Disadvantages of Intracranial Pressure Monitoring Devices

Monitoring Site	Advantages	Disadvantages
Intraventricular (ventriculostomy)	• Very accurate • True central direct measure of ICP • Can withdraw CSF to decrease ICP or measure compliance • Ease of CSF sampling	• Need transducer repositioned with every change in head position • High risk for serious infection • Difficult insertion in patients with small or displaced ventricles • Risk for intracerebral bleeding or edema along the cannula track
Intraventricular (fiberoptic catheter)	• Versatile; may be placed in ventricle or subarachnoid space • No adjustment of transducer with head movement	• Separate monitoring system required • Fragile catheter • Unable to recalibrate once device is placed
Intraparenchymal	• Ease of insertion • True brain pressures	• Infections rare, but serious
Lumbar/subarachnoid	• Simple-to-do single readings • No penetration of the brain parenchyma • Decreased risk for infection • Can sample CSF • Direct pressure management	• Contraindicated with evidence of increased ICP • Requires intact skull • Transducer repositioned with head movement
Subdural	• Ease of insertion	• Risk for serious infection
Epidural	• Low risk for infections • No transducer adjustment with head movement	• Imperfect correlation with intradural pressure (sensing through dura) • Operating room for placement • Unable to recalibrate once device is placed • Unable to drain CSF

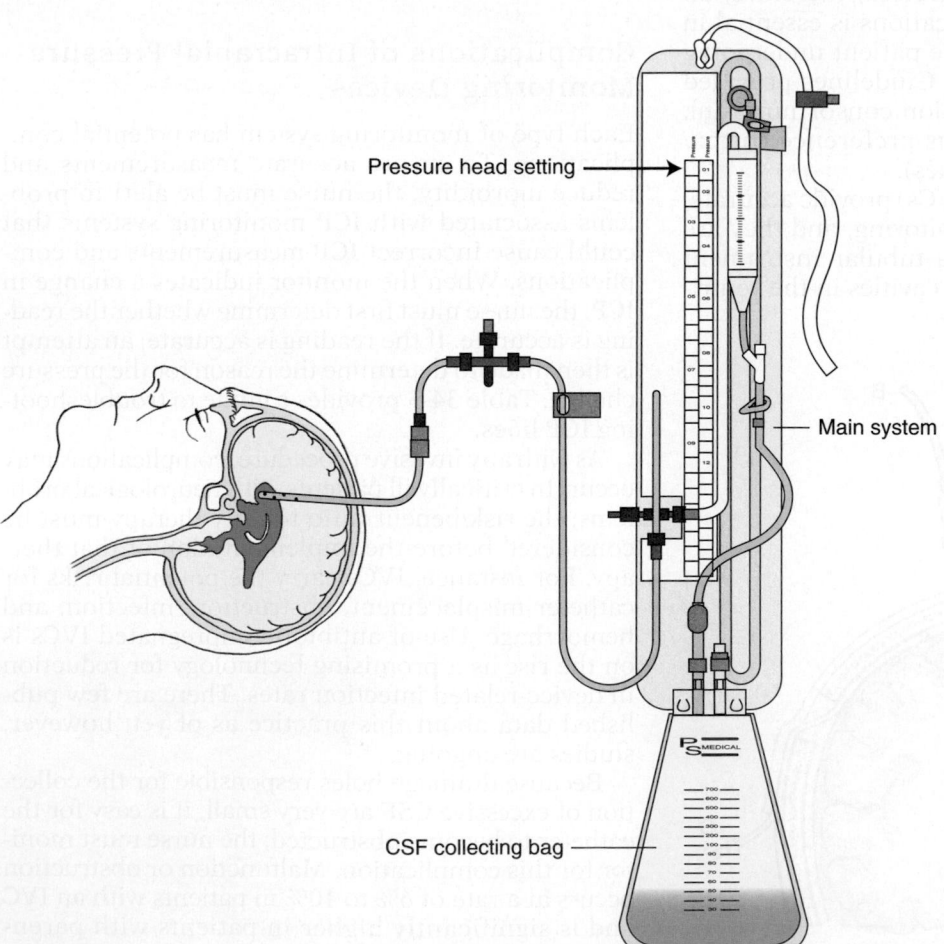

Pressure head setting

Main system

CSF collecting bag

Figure 34-3 • Intraventricular catheter system. (Courtesy of Medtronic Neurologic Technologies, Goleta, California.)

Table 34-3 • Troubleshooting Intracranial Pressure Lines

Problem	Cause	Nursing Considerations and Interventions
No ICP waveform	Air between the transducer diaphragm and pressure source	Eliminate air bubbles with sterile saline.
	Occlusion of intracranial measurement device with blood or debris	Flush intracranial catheter or screw as directed by physician: 0.25 mL sterile saline is often used.
	Transducer connected incorrectly	Check connection, and be sure the appropriate connector for amplifier is in use.
	Fiberoptic catheter bent, broken	Replace fiberoptic catheter.
	Incorrect gain setting for pressure or patient having plateau waves	Adjust gain setting for higher pressure range.
	Trace turned off	Turn power on to trace.
False high-pressure reading	Transducer too low	Place the venting port of the transducer at the level of the foramen of Monro. For every 2.54 cm (1 in) the transducer is below the pressure source, there is an error of approximately 2 mm Hg.
	Transducer incorrectly balanced	With transducer correctly positioned, rebalance. Transducer should be balanced every 2 to 4 h and before the initiation of treatment based on a pressure change.
	Monitoring system incorrectly calibrated	Repeat calibration procedures.
	Air in system: air may attenuate or amplify pressure signal	Remove air from monitoring line.
High-pressure reading	Airway not patent: an increase in intrathoracic pressure may increase $PaCO_2$	Suction patient. Position. Initiate chest physiotherapy.
	Ventilator setting incorrect	Check ventilator settings.
	Positive end-expiratory pressure (PEEP)	Draw arterial blood gases because hypoxia and hypercarbia cause increases in ICP.
	Posture	Head should be elevated 15–30 degrees unless contraindicated by other problems, such as fractures.
	Head and neck	The head should be positioned to facilitate venous drainage.
	Legs	Limit knee flexion. Avoid acute hip flexion.
	Excessive muscle activity during decerebrate posturing in patients with upper brainstem injury may increase ICP.	Muscle relaxants or paralyzing agents sometimes are indicated.
	Hyperthermia	Initiate measures to control muscle movement, infection, and pyrexia.
	Excessive muscle activity	
	Increased susceptibility to infection	
	Fluid and electrolyte imbalance secondary to fluid restrictions and diuretics	Draw blood for serum electrolytes, serum osmolality. Note pulmonary artery pressure. Evaluate input and output with specific gravity.
	Blood pressure: vasopressor responses occur in some patients with elevating ICP.	Use measures to maintain adequate continuous positive pressure.
	Low blood pressure associated with hypovolemia, shock, and barbiturate coma may increase cerebral ischemia.	
False low-pressure reading	Air bubbles between transducer and CSF	Eliminate air bubbles with sterile saline.
	Transducer level too high	Place the venting port of the transducer at the level of the foramen of Monro. For every 2.54 cm (1 in) the transducer is above the level of the pressure source, there will be an error of approximately 2 mm Hg.
Low-pressure reading	Zero or calibration incorrect	Rezero and calibrate monitoring system.
	Collapse of ventricles around catheter	If ventriculostomy is being used, there may be inadequate positive pressure. Check to make sure a positive pressure of 15 to 20 mm Hg exists. Drain CSF slowly.
	Otorrhea or rhinorrhea	These conditions cause a false low-pressure reading secondary to decompression. Document the correlation between drainage and pressure changes.
	Leakage of fluid from connections	Eliminate all fluid leakage.
	Dislodgment of catheter from ventricle into brain	Contact physician regarding appropriate diagnostic studies and intervention. Use soft catheter designed for intraventricular measurement.
	Occlusion of the end of a subarachnoid screw by the necrotic brain	In most cases, remove screw.

greater than 50 mm Hg. A reduction in catheter infections has been reported with recent changes in insertion techniques, antibiotic prophylaxis, and improved CSF sampling methods.[6] Hemorrhage associated with IVC placement is poorly described in the literature, prompting the reporting of a 1.1% to 2.8% risk for hematoma formation. The hemorrhage rate is highly dependent on the choice of device.

INTRACRANIAL PRESSURE MEASUREMENTS

Normal measurements of ICP range between 0 and 10 mm Hg, with an upper limit of 15 mm Hg. During coughing or straining, a normal ICP may increase to 100 mm Hg. In acute situations, patients often become symptomatic at pressures ranging from 20 to 25 mm Hg.

A patient's tolerance of a change in ICP varies with the acuteness of its onset. A patient with a slower buildup of ICP (for example, as the result of an expanding brain tumor) is typically more tolerant of elevations in ICP than a patient whose ICP increases rapidly (for example, as the result of an acute subdural hematoma). Uncontrolled ICP between 20 and 25 mm Hg is considered extremely dangerous for the patient with brain injury. Sustained ICP greater than 60 mm Hg usually is fatal. ICP may rise to the level of the MAP. The greater the variations in the mean ICP, the more nearly exhausted are the compensatory mechanisms for intracranial volume increases.

CPP is the main indicator of the circulatory system's ability to infuse the brain. However, CPP has limitations; it measures only a single parameter that influences oxygen delivery and the neurons' ability to sustain injury. Neuronal demand for oxygen is governed by the cell's metabolic needs, which increase during neuronal activity or injury. Therefore, to understand the metabolic status of the neuron, both CBF and oxygen content in the blood must be measured. The equation $CBF \times OEF \times SaO_2$ is commonly used to calculate the cerebral metabolic rate for oxygen ($CMRO_2$). The oxygen extraction fraction (OEF), which is measured using both the arterial and venous oxygen content, describes how much oxygen is extracted. SaO_2 represents the oxygen saturation in the arterial blood. Necessary information can be obtained using multimodality monitoring, including blood flow studies such as jugular venous bulb oximetry, as well as positron emission tomography and single-photon emission computed tomography.

Jugular Venous Bulb Oximetry

Jugular venous bulb oximetry is an invasive technique that involves placing a sampling catheter in the internal jugular vein, with the tip of the jugular venous bulb at the base of the brain. Blood samples from this location measure the mixed venous oxygen saturation (SjO_2) of blood leaving the brain. This is normally 50% to 75%. The SjO_2 decreases when there is an imbalance between oxygen consumption and delivery. If the SjO_2 decreases to less than 50% (without a decrease in SaO_2), this implies either a decrease in CBF or an increase in oxygen utilization (higher $CMRO_2$). If CPP is maintained, a decrease in CBF is due to an increase in cerebrovascular resistance (CVR). Vascular spasm and an increase in CVR are very common after brain injury and are significantly worsened by hyperventilation. Jugular venous bulb oximetry should be used whenever there is prolonged hyperventilation. An increase in SjO_2 greater than 85% implies either a hyperemia with an increase in CBF, shunting of blood away from neurons, or a decrease in $CMRO_2$ (impending cell death or brain death). It should be emphasized that SjO_2 is a measure of global cerebral oxygenation and is not sensitive to small areas of focal ischemia. However, SjO_2 may be of assistance in guiding some therapies for the patient with brain injury, including barbiturate-induced cerebral metabolic suppression and the rare use of induced hyperventilation.

Transcranial Doppler Ultrasound

Transcranial Doppler is a noninvasive method of assessing the state of the intracranial circulation. The velocity of flow can be measured in the middle, anterior, and posterior cerebral arteries, the ophthalmic artery, and internal carotid artery. Flow cannot be measured from velocity because the cross-sectional area of the arteries cannot be measured directly. However, the Doppler shift measured is inversely proportional to the diameter of the vessel, so that if all other factors remain constant, vascular spasm leads to an increase in flow velocity. Doppler waveform analysis can provide further information about the state of blood flow, but the value and utility of these and other multimodality techniques are as yet unknown.

Intracranial Pressure Waveforms

Waveforms of ICP provide an index of ICP dynamics, such as changes in intracerebral compliance. The appearance of ICP waveforms varies according to the measurement technique being used, the patient's pathological status and activities, interventions, or environmental changes. Hemodynamic and respiratory oscillations can be observed in ICP traces. Computerized systems are being developed to analyze waveforms and integrate ICP, CPP, and other relevant parameters.

Sometimes the waveforms closely resemble arterial pressure waveforms; at other times they resemble central venous pressure waveforms. To varying degrees, oscillations corresponding to intracranial arterial pulsations with retrograde venous pulsations are seen with each heartbeat (Fig. 34-4). In patients with ICP less than 20 mm Hg, a slower waveform, synchronous with respiration and caused by changes in intrathoracic pressure, can be seen (see Fig. 34-4, middle). Alterations in arterial driving force, disturbance of venous outflow, and cerebral vasodilation correlate with changes in waveform appearances. At times, a small "a" wave is superimposed on diastole, reflecting right arterial pressure.

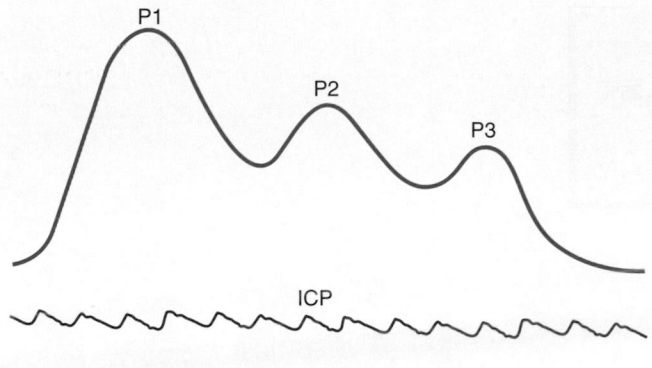

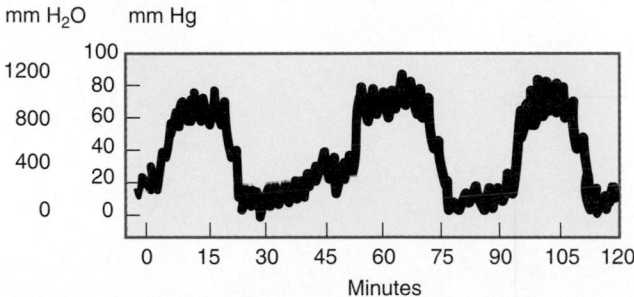

Figure 34-4 • Intracranial pressure (ICP) waveforms. **Top:** A normal ICP pulse waveform may demonstrate three or more descending peaks. P1, the pressure wave, originates from choroid plexus pulsations. P2, the tidal wave, is more variable in shape and amplitude and ends on the dicrotic notch. P3, the dicrotic wave, follows the dicrotic notch and tapers down to the diastolic position unless retrograde venous pulsations cause a few more peaks. The P2 portion of the waveform most directly reflects the state of intracerebral compliance. As mean ICP rises, P2 progressively elevates, causing the pulse wave to appear more rounded. When a state of decreased compliance exists, the P2 component is equal to or higher than P1. **Middle:** An ICP waveform demonstrating hemodynamic and respiratory oscillations. Note the vascular pressure-type notches in the waveforms and the baseline variations that reflect respirations. **Bottom:** "A," or plateau, waves, associated with decreased intracranial compliance, may be secondary to an increase in blood volume with a simultaneous decrease in blood flow.

Some patients exhibit waveform variation, most commonly A, B, and C waves. A waves, also known as plateau waves, are spontaneous, rapid increases of pressure ranging from 50 to 200 mm Hg, occurring at variable intervals (see Fig. 34-4, bottom). They tend to occur in patients with moderate elevations of ICP, last 5 to 20 minutes, and fall spontaneously. Plateau waves usually are accompanied by a temporary increase in neurological deficit.

Although the mechanism of A waves has not been established firmly, it is thought that they indicate decreased intracranial compliance; therefore, these waveforms should be identified and treated quickly. They may result from an increase in blood volume with a simultaneous decrease in blood flow. The sudden reversal of high pressure may be caused by increased CSF absorption. Falls in CPP with intact autoregulation and low intracranial compliance have been correlated with the initiation of plateau waves. Plateau waves may also be set off by a vasodilating

stimulus or by nonspecific stimuli, such as hypoventilation or hyperventilation, pain, and aroused mental activities.

B waves are small, sharp, rhythmic waves with ICPs up to 50 mm Hg, occurring at a frequency of 0.5 to 2 per minute. They correspond to changes in respiration, providing clues to periodic respiration related to poor cerebral compliance or pulmonary dysfunction. B waves often are seen with Cheyne-Stokes respirations (see Chapter 36). They may precede A waves and increase as compliance decreases. At times, they occur in patients with normal ICP and no papilledema. They may be secondary to oscillations of cerebral blood volume.

C waves are small, rhythmic waves with ICPs up to 20 mm Hg, occurring at a rate of approximately six per minute. They are related to blood pressure. Like A waves, they indicate severe intracranial compression, with limited remaining volume residual in the intracranial space.

• Management of Increased Intracranial Pressure

In the stage between the onset of increased ICP and herniation, many treatments are available to reduce ICP and maintain adequate cerebral perfusion. No single management routine is appropriate for all patients. In addition to clinical pathways and nursing care protocols, algorithms for the incremental application and weaning of ICP management have been developed. Figure 34-5 provides an algorithm for first-tier (conventional) and second-tier (refractory) treatments of increased ICP. First-tier therapy includes ventricular CSF drainage (as discussed previously), mannitol administration, respiratory support, and sedation and analgesia. Second-tier therapy includes hypothermia, barbiturate coma, optimized hyperventilation, hypertensive CPP therapy, and decompressive craniectomy.

Although no one therapeutic regimen has been accepted universally, the goals of treatment for the patient with increased ICP are as follows: reduce ICP, optimize CPP, and avoid brain herniation. Most management techniques are oriented toward control of cerebral blood volume and CSF circulation, the two major mechanisms responsible for the regulation of ICP. Measures to reduce ICP are usually initiated when the patient's ICP increases to approximately 15 mm Hg.

CLINICAL MANAGEMENT
Mannitol Administration

Mannitol, a hypertonic crystalloid solution that decreases cerebral edema, is also used as first-tier therapy for reducing ICP after brain injury. It is typically administered as a bolus intravenous (IV) infusion over 10 to 30 minutes in doses ranging from 0.25 to 2 g/kg body weight. Studies have demonstrated

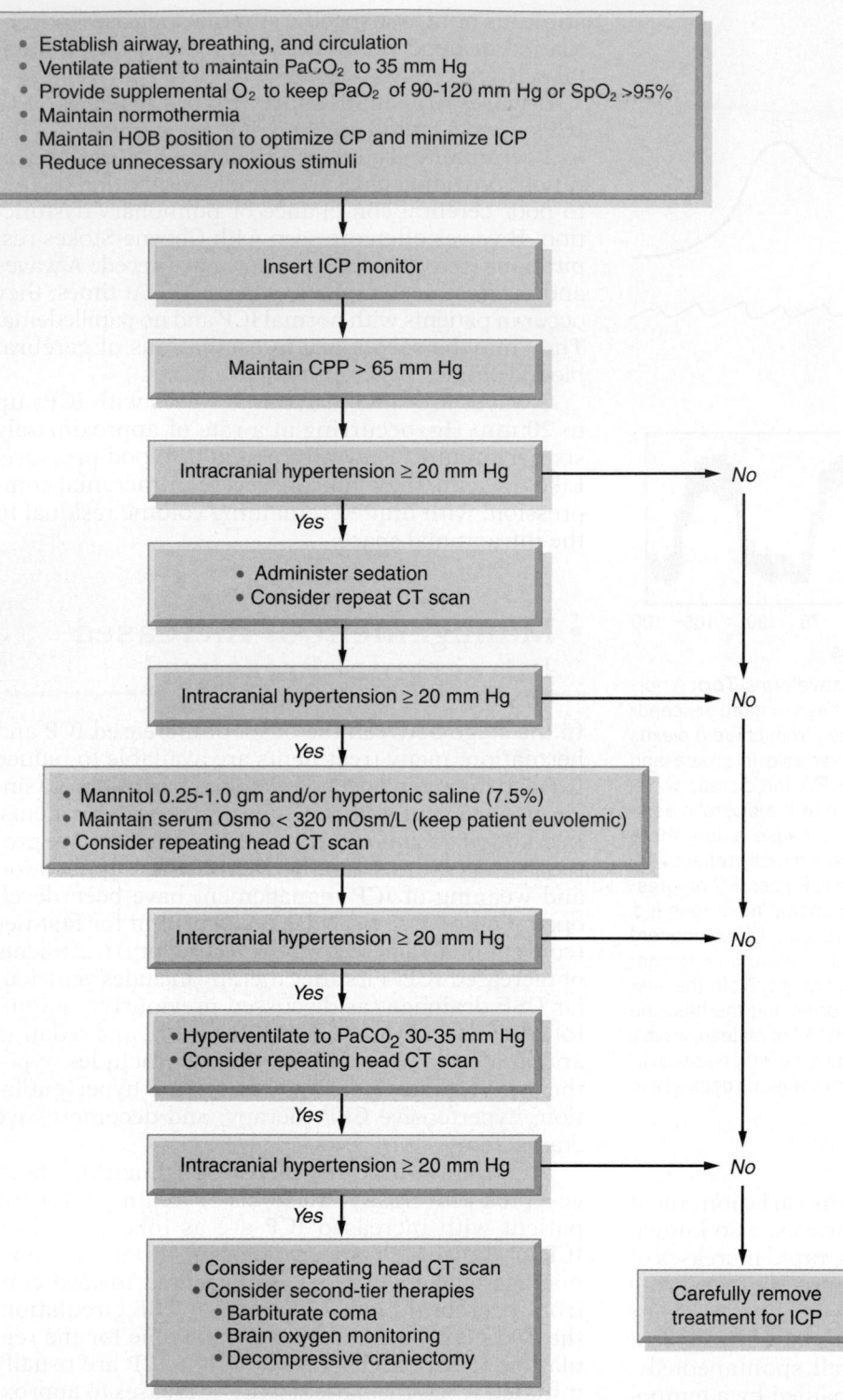

- Establish airway, breathing, and circulation
- Ventilate patient to maintain $PaCO_2$ to 35 mm Hg
- Provide supplemental O_2 to keep PaO_2 of 90-120 mm Hg or SpO_2 >95%
- Maintain normothermia
- Maintain HOB position to optimize CP and minimize ICP
- Reduce unnecessary noxious stimuli

Insert ICP monitor

Maintain CPP > 65 mm Hg

Intracranial hypertension ≥ 20 mm Hg — No

Yes

- Administer sedation
- Consider repeat CT scan

Intracranial hypertension ≥ 20 mm Hg — No

Yes

- Mannitol 0.25-1.0 gm and/or hypertonic saline (7.5%)
- Maintain serum Osmo < 320 mOsm/L (keep patient euvolemic)
- Consider repeating head CT scan

Intercranial hypertension ≥ 20 mm Hg — No

Yes

- Hyperventilate to $PaCO_2$ 30-35 mm Hg
- Consider repeating head CT scan

Yes

Intracranial hypertension ≥ 20 mm Hg — No

Yes

- Consider repeating head CT scan
- Consider second-tier therapies
  - Barbiturate coma
  - Brain oxygen monitoring
  - Decompressive craniectomy

Carefully remove treatment for ICP

Figure 34-5 • Management of increased intracranial pressure (ICP). CP, cerebral perfusion; CPP, cerebral perfusion pressure; HOB, head of bed. (Courtesy of the Brain Trauma Foundation, New York, 2000.)

the effect of mannitol on ICP, CPP, CBF, and brain metabolism and have also shown a beneficial effect on long-term neurological outcome. More recently, research has shown that hypertonic saline is also effective.[7-9] The immediate plasma-expanding effect of mannitol, which reduces blood viscosity, increases CBF and cerebral oxygen metabolism, permitting cerebral arterioles to decrease in diameter. This lowers cerebral blood volume and ICP, while maintain-ing constant CBF. Ideally, to reduce potential side effects and optimize the risk/benefit ratio, mannitol administration should be based directly on ICP mea-surements. However, mannitol may be safely admin-istered when it is not possible to measure ICP.

Mannitol is excreted in the urine. If it is adminis-tered in large doses and serum osmolarity is greater than 320 mOsm, there is a significant risk for acute tubular necrosis and renal failure. Therefore, it is customary to measure serum osmolarity every 6 to 8 hours to a target of less than 320 mOsm.

A Foley catheter must be inserted when mannitol is administered. When mannitol is used during the early resuscitation phase in hypovolemic patients with brain injuries, crystalloid solutions are infused simultaneously to correct hypovolemia. Adjunct crystalloid fluid administration facilitates rapid renal excretion of mannitol, preventing renal failure. In the early phases of acute brain injury, mannitol is recommended as monotherapy. When mannitol is combined with furosemide, there is a risk for excessive diuresis, causing depletion of intravascular volume and electrolytes.

Furosemide is a loop diuretic that is frequently used for the critically ill patient experiencing congestive heart failure. It is also used in patients who are experiencing fluid retention because of poorly functioning kidneys. A critically ill patient who is hypovolemic or has poor blood flow to the kidneys experiences renal dysfunction and low urinary output. Furosemide increases reabsorption of sodium in the loop of Henle, and the result is increased urinary output. This drug is indicated in adults, infants, and children for the treatment of edema associated with congestive heart failure, cirrhosis of the liver, and renal disease.

Furosemide is particularly useful when an agent with greater diuretic potential is desired. Excessive diuresis may cause dehydration and blood volume reduction with circulatory collapse and possible vascular thrombosis and embolism, particularly in older patients. As with any effective diuretic, electrolyte depletion may occur during furosemide therapy, especially in patients receiving higher doses and a restricted salt intake. Symptoms of electrolyte imbalance include dryness of mouth, thirst, weakness, lethargy, drowsiness, restlessness, muscle pains or cramps, muscular fatigue, hypotension, oliguria, tachycardia, dysrhythmias, or gastrointestinal disturbances such as nausea and vomiting.

Respiratory Support

Mean airway pressure is the leading factor affecting ICP in the patient who is ventilated. Positive airway pressure is transmitted to the intracranial cavity through the mediastinum. Therefore, any condition decreasing pulmonary compliance or use of positive end-expiratory pressure increases the mean airway pressure and decreases the MAP and CPP.

Normocapnia is essential for the maintenance of stable ICP. Hyperventilation remains controversial in the management of increased ICP. Hyperventilation decreases the arterial carbon dioxide tension ($PaCO_2$) and results in cerebral vasoconstriction. As a result, the CBF is reduced because of the strong vasoconstrictive effect of hypocarbia on the cerebral arteries. The $PaCO_2$ should be lowered gradually to avoid a rebound effect of vasodilation from overcorrection. When hyperventilation is discontinued, ventilation rates should be gradually returned to

normal. Severe, prolonged hyperventilation has been conclusively shown to worsen the outcome of patients with a severe brain injury. Severe hyperventilation is defined as a $PaCO_2$ of less than 25 mm Hg by jugular venous oxygen saturation monitor. Extreme hyperventilation is believed to cause secondary ischemia by constricting cerebral vasculature.[4]

In the absence of a malignant increase in ICP, hyperventilation therapy ($PaCO_2$ < 25 mm Hg) should be avoided after a traumatic brain injury. Also, the use of prophylactic hyperventilation therapy ($PaCO_2$ < 35 mm Hg) during the first 24 hours after a traumatic brain injury should be avoided because it can compromise cerebral perfusion during a time of critically reduced CBF.[4,10] Hyperventilation may become necessary for brief periods when there is acute neurological deterioration, or if increased ICP is refractory to sedation, paralysis, CSF drainage, and osmotic diuretics. Therefore, the literature suggests avoiding hyperventilation during the first 5 days after a traumatic injury and most directly during the first 24 hours after trauma.[4]

Suctioning should be approached thoughtfully to avoid hypoxemia as well as increased intrathoracic pressures. Limiting the duration of passes of the suction catheter to no more than 5 to 10 seconds and limiting the number of passes to one or two avoids overstimulation of the cough reflex and decreases the incidence of increased intrathoracic pressure and ICP.

Analgesics, Sedatives, and Paralytics

Before starting patients on analgesics or sedatives, every effort should be made to implement nonpharmacological management techniques for pain, agitation, anxiety, and confusion. However, patients with impaired neurological function may require analgesia, sedation, or neuromuscular blockade to decrease anxiety and diminish awareness of noxious stimuli (Table 34-4). The treatment of pain lowers energy expenditures, facilitating healing. Further, analgesics and sedatives may potentiate each other, allowing patients to be calm and comfortable at lower doses.[11]

In patients with a severe brain injury (GCS score < 8), pain medications and sedatives are used to:

▶ Reduce agitation, discomfort, and pain
▶ Facilitate mechanical ventilation by suppressing coughing
▶ Limit responses to stimuli, such as suctioning, which may increase ICP

A patient with a neurological emergency must be treated for pain and provided sedation. The patient with a brain injury does require frequent neurological assessments that may be affected by pain medications; however, the patient has a right to adequate pain relief. A neurologist should be consulted early in the patient's hospital course to assist in the proper dosing of medications so that frequent neurological assessments can be performed.

Table 34-4 • Major Classes of Pharmacological Agents Used to Treat Neurological Emergencies

Class	Medication	Mechanism of Action/Dosage	Comments
Direct vasodilators	Sodium nitroprusside Nitroglycerin Hydralazine	Directly dilate the peripheral vasculature and lower vascular resistance Sodium nitroprusside: start at 0.3 µg/kg/min, maximal continuous IV infusion 10 µg/kg/min Nitroglycerin: start at 5 µg/min, then titrate as needed upward q 5 min (max 100 µg/min) Hydralazine: 10–20 mg IV, may be repeated as needed	• Dilate the cerebral vasculature • Increase cerebral blood volume and ICP, decrease MAP and CPP • Sodium nitroprusside: at high doses may cause cyanide toxicity, check thiocyanate levels, protect infusion from light • Nitroglycerin: venous dilation, caution with high doses; may cause hypotension • Hydralazine: used in hypertensive emergency, may cause hypotension and headache
β-Adrenergic antagonists	Metoprolol Esmolol	β-Adrenergic receptor antagonist Metoprolol: 5 mg IV q 3–5 min in 3 doses, followed by PO administration 25–50 mg PO twice daily and may increase to 50–100 mg PO twice daily Esmolol: for hypertensive emergency, bolus dose 500 µg/kg over 1 min, then 50–200 µg/kg/min	• Do not affect cerebral blood flow (CBF) • Use with caution with Cushing's response, can potentiate bradycardia
Mixed α- and β-adrenergic antagonists	Labetalol	Selective α- and nonselective β-adrenergic receptor antagonist Labetalol: for hypertensive emergency, start 20 mg IV over 3–5 min, followed by 40–80 mg IV every 10 min PRN up to 300 mg, or IV infusion 0.5–2 mg/min	• Reduce SVR • Improve CPP and do not increase ICP • May slow heart rate
Calcium channel antagonists	Verapamil Diltiazem	Prevent transport of calcium ions in vascular smooth muscle, resulting in vasodilation, decreased myocardial contractility, decreased heart rate Verapamil: for supraventricular tachycardia, 5–10 mg IV over 2 min, followed by 40–80 mg three to four times a day Diltiazem: 20 mg over 2 min, continuous infusion 5–15 mg/h	• Use with caution, may cause cerebral vasodilation with increased ICP • Contraindicated in patients with tumors and cerebral edema
Angiotensin-converting enzyme (ACE) inhibitors	Lisinopril	Shift the upper and lower limits of blood brain autoregulation by inhibiting angiotensin II–mediated vascular tone in large cerebral arteries, while small vessels vasoconstrict Lisinopril: start 10 mg/d, titrate to 80 mg/d PRN	• Preserve CBF after single dose • Increase CBF with chronic treatment • Have the potential to increase ICP in patients with intracranial hypertension by increasing CBF
Osmotic diuretic	Mannitol	Indicated for intracranial hypertension Mannitol: 0.25–2 g/kg IV over 30–60 min	• If infused too quickly, may contribute to renal insufficiency
Loop diuretic	Furosemide	Indicated for pulmonary edema and adjunct therapy for hypertension Furosemide: 20–80 mg IV, increase dose 20–40 mg IV q6–8h until desired effect	• May cause potassium loss; check electrolytes q8–12h with initial therapy
Nondepolarizing muscle blockading agents	Pancuronium	Skeletal muscle paralysis Bolus 0.04–0.1 mg/kg Continuous infusion	• May cause tachycardia and dysrhythmias • Patient must be mechanically ventilated
	Atracurium	Skeletal muscle paralysis Bolus 0.4–0.5 mg/kg IV Continuous infusion 4–12 µg/kg/min IV	• Rare occurrence of prolonged weakness after discontinuation of drug infusion • Patient must be mechanically ventilated • Use in patients with hepatic and renal impairment • Neuromuscular blockade should be preceded by adequate sedation and analgesia, which should be maintained during course of blockade
	Cisatracurium	Skeletal muscle paralysis Bolus 0.1–0.2 mg/kg Continuous infusion 2.5–3 µg/kg/min IV	• Rare incidence of prolonged weakness after continuous IV infusion • Patient must be mechanically ventilated • Use in patients with hepatic and renal impairment

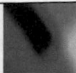

Table 34-4 • Major Classes of Pharmacological Agents Used to Treat Neurological Emergencies (Continued)

Class	Medication	Mechanism of Action/Dosage	Comments
Sedatives	Diazepam Lorazepam Midazolam	Benzodiazepines are sedatives and hypnotics that induce anterograde amnesia Diazepam and lorazepam are also used to stop seizure activity Diazepam: 10–20 mg IV no faster than 2 mg/min, then repeat q4h Lorazepam: 0.05–0.2 mg/kg/dose, up to 8 mg, may repeat every 15 min, continuous infusion 1 mg/h and titrate to goal, not to exceed 8 mg/h Midazolam: 0.1–0.3 mg/kg bolus, no faster than 4 mg/min, continuous infusion 0.05 mg/kg/h up to 1.0 mg/kg/h	• May cause somnolence, hypotension, delirium, hallucinations, respiratory depression • Titrate to goal using sedation scale • Lorazepam/midazolam: use with caution in patients with hepatic/renal failure, contraindicated in patients with acute narrow-angle glaucoma or in shock, and in older patients
Anticonvulsants	Phenytoin Carbamazepine	Indicated for tonic-clonic seizures and partial seizures Phenytoin: loading dose 15–20 mg/kg for status epilepticus, no faster than 50 mg/kg; maintenance dose 200–500 mg daily or in divided doses three times a day Carbamazepine: 200 mg twice daily, maintenance 200–400 three times a day	• May cause ataxia, lethargy, movement disorders, rash, coarse facies, lymphadenopathy • May decrease theophylline, oral contraceptive, and warfarin levels • Phenytoin levels may increase with methsuximide and alcohol • Phenytoin levels may decrease when used with valproic acid and Tegretol • Contraindicated with alcohol ingestion, sinus bradycardia, heart block
Analgesics	Morphine Fentanyl Hydromorphone	Opiate analgesics blunt the pain response by interfering with central and peripheral pain pathways Morphine: bolus 1–4 mg, continuous infusion 0.07–0.5 mg/kg/h Fentanyl: bolus 50–100 µg over 1–2 min, continuous infusion 0.7–10 µg/kg/h Hydromorphone: continuous infusion 7–15 µg/kg/h	• May cause respiratory depression; must have naloxone readily available • Have resuscitation equipment nearby at all times • Use the lowest dose that provides adequate pain relief • Use a 1–10 pain scale to assess effectiveness of pain relief • For severe pain, around-the-clock administration or a continuous infusion of pain medication provides more efficient pain relief than PRN dosing • Use lower doses in older patients • Use nonpharmacological approaches to pain management • Side effects: decrease gastric motility; nausea/vomiting, tremulousness
Anesthetic	Propofol	Propofol is an intravenous general anesthetic agent that can be used to treat agitation in the ICU Propofol: bolus not necessary, continuous infusion 5–50 µg/kg/min	• Patient must be mechanically ventilated • Must have dedicated IV line • Must use aseptic technique • May cause hypotension • Must provide analgesics and sedation • Use for the shortest period possible
Barbiturates	Phenobarbital Pentobarbital	Used to produce CNS depression and reduce the spread of an epileptic focus Phenobarbital: loading dose 6–8 mg/kg IV; maintenance dose 1–3 mg/kg/24 h IV Pentobarbital: loading dose 3–10 mg/kg over 30 min; maintenance dose 0.5–3.0 mg/kg/h	• May cause respiratory depression and cardiac depression • Patient must be mechanically ventilated • Continuous EEG monitoring for barbiturate-induced coma

Analgesics

Opioid narcotics primarily affect the CNS. Fentanyl and morphine are two of the most frequently used opiate narcotics (see Table 34-4). They:

► Limit pain caused by injuries and nursing interventions

► Facilitate mechanical ventilation
► Potentiate the effect of sedatives[11]

Potentially life-threatening adverse effects of narcotics include respiratory depression, depression of the cough reflex, mood changes, nausea, and vomiting. As a result, a patient may experience hypoxia;

therefore, intubation equipment must be readily available at all times when a patient is receiving narcotics. Naloxone reverses CNS depression, which can occur with the administration of fentanyl and morphine and therefore must also be readily available whenever narcotics are administered. Vital signs, including pulse oximetry, must be monitored diligently when a patient receives IV pain medication. With proper dosing and diligent nursing observation, narcotics can be used effectively in the critically ill patient.

The basic principles of narcotic administration are adequate pain relief and safe administration. It is necessary to begin with the lowest possible dose, which is titrated until pain relief is obtained. When a patient with a brain injury also has severe pain caused by multiple traumatic injuries, a continuous infusion of fentanyl or morphine is indicated. A typical pain management regimen may include a continuous morphine infusion starting at 1 to 2 mg/hour, or fentanyl, 50 to 100 μg/hour, and titrated every 15 to 30 minutes until the patient appears comfortable. For a patient with moderate pain, a 24-hour regimen of opiate narcotic administration has been proved to provide increased pain relief versus a PRN schedule of opiate dosing.

For the patient who is able to communicate, a verbal pain scale is used to assess pain. Standardized rating scales, such as a 1 to 10 pain scale, should be used to quantify and evaluate pain status and response to therapy. In addition to location, quality, and duration of pain, the nurse must document the effectiveness of analgesics every hour for 4 hours with initial administration, then every 4 hours, and 15 minutes after each dose change.[11] All hospitals have a pain management protocol that identifies analgesics that should be used, dosing titration guidelines, and documentation requirements. In addition, most protocols address sedation recommendations.

For the patient who is unable to communicate, physiological parameters are used to determine the effectiveness of pain management. The nurse assesses heart rate, respiratory rate, use of accessory muscles for breathing, and blood pressure. Adequate pain management leads to less patient movement, such as thrashing, which increases metabolic activity. The following clues can be used to determine whether adequate pain relief has been obtained for the patient who cannot communicate:

▶ Ease of breathing
▶ Mechanically ventilated patient whose breathing is synchronous with the ventilator
▶ Possible decrease in heart rate
▶ Less agitation as indicated by restful sleep state
▶ Cooperation with nursing interventions without excessive physical activity

Narcotics can be safely administered to the older patient. However, the older critically ill patient may be especially susceptible to respiratory depression and therefore may require lower dosages. Also, narcotics decrease gastric motility and may cause constipation. For the patient confined to bed, prophylactic administration of a stool softener is normal practice. For all patients receiving narcotics, documentation of the number of bowel movements is essential. Patients may also be susceptible to nausea and vomiting with the administration of narcotics. Protection of the airway is especially important in the patient with a neurological diagnosis. Mechanically ventilated patients require the insertion of a nasogastric or orogastric tube to decompress the stomach and prevent vomiting.

Sedatives

The most commonly used sedatives in the ICU are benzodiazepines, which potentiate the effects of analgesic agents. Midazolam, diazepam, and lorazepam are used frequently for sedation before ICU procedures and as needed to treat anxiety (see Table 34-4). Lorazepam is frequently used for alcohol withdrawal and anticonvulsant therapy. Midazolam, in combination with fentanyl, is most often used for sedation before procedures to produce amnesia of immediate events. Benzodiazepines cause little change in CBF, ICP, and cerebral metabolic rate. Side effects of sedatives include respiratory depression, hypotension, and somnolence. It is mandatory that resuscitation equipment be available at all times when IV benzodiazepines are used. Benzodiazepines should be administered at the lowest possible dose that produces effective sedation, without causing somnolence. As with analgesic agents, frequent vital signs must be obtained with the administration of sedatives. Recommended minimal documentation of vital signs should be every hour for 4 hours, then every 4 hours, and 15 minutes after every dosage change.[11]

Various scales may be used to document the patient's response to sedation. The target sedation level for a patient with a critical neurological illness is one that allows easy arousal of the patient with light touch or voice.[11] For the patient who cannot communicate (as discussed earlier with analgesic use), the assessment of physiological parameters can be used to determine the patient's response to sedation in order to achieve maximal comfort. Pharmacological management of sedation is only one strategy to treat anxiety. Nursing measures to provide comfort must be offered in addition to medications.

Anesthetics

Propofol is a fat-soluble anesthetic that is administered as a continuous infusion to decrease agitation in the critically ill patient. Studies have shown that propofol may decrease CBF, ICP, CPP, and cerebral metabolic function.[12] Propofol is easily titrated based on patient response. It also has a short half-life and can be discontinued for frequent neurological assessments. Propofol can cause a decreased level of consciousness in 2 minutes. Common side effects include hypotension; therefore, frequent blood pressure monitoring must be performed, especially if the patient has increased ICP. Also, diligent airway protection must be provided for the patient receiving propofol. The patient must be intubated and mechanically ventilated when propofol is administered to prevent respiratory depression. For these reasons, the patient who is provided a continuous infusion of propofol must be cared for in the ICU, with constant surveillance by the critical care nurse. Only an anesthesia provider may administer an IV bolus dose of propofol.

Other cautions with propofol are related to the handling of the drug. Propofol is manufactured by using a fat emulsion, making it a powerful medium for bacterial growth. Propofol must be handled meticulously to prevent the risk for bacterial or fungal infection associated with its use. Propofol IV lines should be changed every 12 hours. In addition, the ICU team calculates the number of fat calories provided by propofol and includes these in the total number of calories required by the patient. It may be necessary to monitor the triglyceride level for patients receiving propofol longer term.

Neuromuscular Blockade

Neuromuscular blockading (NMB) agents (see Table 34-4) are used to induce muscle paralysis and remain a "last resort" therapy. An NMB agent blocks the transmission of acetylcholine at the motor end plate, producing skeletal muscle paralysis. Reversal of NMB agents is provided by acetylcholinesterase inhibitors such as neostigmine, edrophonium, and pyridostigmine. The use of an NMB agent requires mechanical ventilation with full support. Resuscitation equipment must be present at all times when a patient is treated with an NMB agent. For a conscious patient, the inability to move and communicate is frightening; therefore, concurrent administration of analgesia and sedation is mandatory.[13] Analgesia and sedation provide the added benefit of producing amnesia.

Complications common with most NMB agents are tachycardia, hypotension, and dysrhythmias. Cardiac medications such as antidysrhythmics, diuretics, and calcium channel and β-blockers can potentiate the action of NMB drugs. Certain antibiotics such as aminoglycosides and clindamycin can potentiate the action of paralytic agents. Alterations in body temperature or acid–base balance and electrolyte disturbances also alter the action of NMB agents.[13]

A troubling complication of paralytic therapy is prolonged polymyopathy. A condition known as acute quadriplegic myopathy syndrome (AQMS), or postparalytic quadriparesis, is one of the most devastating complications caused by prolonged use of an NMB agent.[13] This condition is manifested by prolonged weakness of the upper and lower extremities. The extraocular motor muscles are usually spared in this condition, so patients with AQMS can move their eyes. A patient may also experience painful muscle fasciculations. For this reason, the smallest dosage of an NMB agent should be used to obtain adequate respiratory support.

Peripheral nerve stimulation monitoring is mandatory with NMB therapy[13]; its use every 4 hours, with a dosage change as necessary, may help prevent complications associated with NMB therapy. A peripheral nerve stimulator is a small hand-held device used in the ICU to monitor the depth of NMB in the patient receiving prolonged paralytic therapy. This device delivers a small jolt of energy to the ulnar surface of the wrist, causing the thumb to twitch. The train-of-four method is used to measure the efficacy and depth of NMB. The peripheral nerve stimulator delivers four 2-Hz stimuli of 0.2 millisecond delivered at intervals of 0.5 second to the ulnar nerve at the wrist. Normally, the thumb twitches 4 times when the peripheral nerve stimulator is activated. The nurse observes thumb movements after peripheral nerve stimulation. If the thumb twitches 2 or 3 times, NMB dosing is usually sufficient. If 4 thumb twitches occur, paralysis is ineffective. If no twitches occur, paralysis is excessive, and the dose of the NMB agent must be reduced.

Excellent nursing care also can help prevent some of the complications caused by NMB agents. A rigid turning schedule must be maintained to prevent the development of pressure ulcers. Aspiration precautions must be maintained at all times. Also, deep venous thrombosis prophylaxis must be implemented before induction of paralysis.

Barbiturate Coma

For the patient with severe and refractory elevated ICP, an induced barbiturate coma may be attempted to decrease systemic metabolic activity in an attempt to preserve brain function. It must be understood that induction of a barbiturate coma is a rare therapy and is used only as a last resort to save brain function. Criteria for the induction of a barbiturate coma includes a GCS score of less than 7; ICP greater than 25 mm Hg at rest for 10 minutes; and failed maximal interventions, including drainage of CSF, mannitol, analgesia, and sedation. Barbiturate coma is typically used for less than 72 hours.

Barbiturates suppress seizure activity and reduce cerebral metabolic activity and cerebral oxygen demand (see Table 34-4). Barbiturates affect CBF, metabolic demand, electroencephalographic (EEG) activity, and systemic hemodynamics. CBF may decrease by 50%. The barbiturate appears to have a direct restrictive effect on cerebral vasculature by diverting small amounts of blood from well-perfused areas to ischemic areas, thereby improving cerebral pressure.

Before the administration of barbiturates, the following must be provided for the patient: a secure airway with mechanical ventilation; ICP, blood pressure, cardiac, and pulmonary artery monitoring; and continuous EEG monitoring. An EEG is obtained before administration of a barbiturate so that spontaneous electrocortical activity is documented. The EEG pattern of burst suppression is the most common method to establish barbiturate dosing. The barbiturate is dosed until EEG burst suppression is achieved. The initial dose may be supplemented by an IV bolus to achieve burst suppression. Barbiturate serum levels alone are poor guides to measure therapeutic efficacy and systemic toxicity.

Barbiturates should be discontinued with any of the following clinical findings:

▸ ICP less than 15 mm Hg for 24 to 72 hours
▸ Systolic blood pressure less than 90 mm Hg despite the use of vasopressors

▶ Progressive neurological impairment, as evidenced by deterioration of brainstem auditory evoked responses

▶ Cardiac arrest

At the time of discontinuation, the barbiturate is tapered gradually over 24 to 72 hours. Arousal is gradual and prolonged, even after blood levels have been zero for several days. The patient must be weaned slowly and carefully from mechanical ventilation, monitoring for residual muscle weakness that occurs with barbiturate therapy. Patients may experience facial weakness for several days after the barbiturate has been discontinued. Occasionally the patient may experience dysarthria, related to weakness of the muscles of speech. During the first 24 hours of barbiturate withdrawal, slow, abnormal muscle movements may be observed.

Blood Pressure Management

The regulation of blood pressure is an important aspect of managing the patient with increased ICP. Pharmacological management of increased ICP includes the aggressive administration of vasopressors or antihypertensives to manipulate systolic and mean arterial blood pressures to maintain effective CPP.

Blood pressure is directly related to cerebral blood volume, perfusion pressure, ischemia, and compliance. For patients with brain injuries, the preservation of CPP and maintenance of systemic oxygenation are two important goals. Also, patients with the most severe brain injuries are at risk for secondary injury caused by hypotension and hypoxia. Patients with brain injury may have increased metabolic oxygen consumption, mild hypertension, and increased cardiac indices. Invasive blood pressure monitoring is routinely used to provide continuous and accurate blood pressure measurement during the acute management phase of patients with brain injuries. MAP is the parameter used for evaluating CPP and the efficacy of antihypertensive or vasopressor therapies.

Patients with brain injuries must be monitored continuously for any adverse effect from drug therapies. In addition to the MAP, the cardiac output may be monitored in the acute management of patients with head injuries. See Chapter 17 for further description of hemodynamic monitoring. Drug therapies to manage blood pressure may cause a precipitous increase or decrease in cardiac output. When the cardiac output is low, patients with head injuries are in jeopardy of further ischemic injury. When the cardiac output is too high, excess myocardial work may lead to myocardial injury. The cardiac output is individualized to patients' weight, creating the cardiac index. The cardiac index is usually maintained at 3 L/minute/m^2 because patients with head injuries frequently have increased metabolic needs. The pulmonary artery capillary wedge pressure is usually maintained at 12 to 15 mm Hg in patients with head injuries. In addition, noninvasive continuous pulse oximetry and arterial blood gas measurement are used to determine arterial oxygen content.

Different classes of antihypertensive medications can be used to treat systemic hypertension in the critically ill patient.[14] An agent that will not cause acute hypotension must be carefully chosen. A patient with neurologic illness may also experience myocardial ischemia/infarction and be at risk for developing dysrhythmias. The danger exists that if a dysrhythmia is not managed aggressively, hypotension may develop. Antidysrhythmics can be safely used in a patient with a head injury. As with any medication, the patient must be assessed for the development of adverse effects associated with cardiovascular medications, including bradycardia, hypotension, myocardial ischemia, tachycardia, and decreased cardiac output.

For patients with acute ischemic stroke, acute hypertension is defined as a systolic blood pressure greater than 185 mm Hg and a diastolic blood pressure greater then 110 mm Hg. The blood pressure must be gently decreased to avoid problems with cerebral autoregulation dysfunction. In the emergency department or ICU, IV hydralazine and IV labetalol are frequently used to treat acute hypertension. Both agents must be administered slowly to avoid hypotension. If the patient remains hypertensive after hydralazine or labetalol administration, nicardipine or nitroprusside may be used (see Table 34-4). Both nicardipine and nitroprusside are potent vasodilators and can lower the blood pressure quickly. They are administered as continuous infusions, are easily titrated, and have relatively short half-lives. These medications must be used in the ICU or emergency department, where continuous blood pressure monitoring can be provided. Hypotension may occur if the infusion is increased too quickly.

For patients with hemorrhagic brain injury, a more rigorous blood pressure range is maintained. An MAP greater than 110 mm Hg is avoided in these patients.[15] Angiotensin-converting enzyme (ACE) inhibitors and β-blockers are often used to treat hypertension in the head-injured patient with systemic hypertension. β-Blockers are most often used because of their safe side-effect profile, although they may cause bradycardia. Calcium channel blockers are usually avoided in head-injured patients because of their potential to exacerbate cerebral edema. See Table 34-4 for additional information.

Seizure Prophylaxis

Seizure activity markedly elevates the cerebral metabolic rate and CBF. It can lead to hypoxia and hypercapnia. In a patient with increased ICP, seizure prophylaxis should be considered to prevent additional neurological injury. Anticonvulsant therapy may be used to prevent early post-traumatic seizure, especially in patients at risk for seizure. Phenytoin and carbamazepine are considered in the treatment panel for prevention of early (<7 days) post-traumatic seizure.

The treatment of choice for acute-onset seizures (such as tonic-clonic seizures) in the critically ill patient remains diazepam. The patient should be placed on his or her side and an oxygen mask applied. When seizure activity has subsided, the nurse should obtain a serum glucose to determine whether hypoglycemia is a contributing cause. An EEG may also be ordered to determine whether the patient is continuing to experience subclinical seizures and to determine seizure focus.

Hypothermia

Hypothermia continues to be explored as a means for reducing the brain's metabolic demands during peak times of cerebral edema and brain injury. This technique remains controversial but is widely studied. One difficulty is cooling the patient adequately to achieve optimal neuroprotection. The degree of coolness has also not yet been established, although it continues to be investigated in multicenter clinical trials. However, control of fever is essential and is being more aggressively addressed using different types of cooling devices (both surface cooling and intravascular cooling devices).[16]

Decompressive Craniectomy

Another strategy used for the management of refractory intracranial hypertension is decompressive craniotomy. This surgery is based on the theory that ICP can be reduced through surgical release of the rigid skull. Although surgical decompression remains an option for patients with uncontrollable ICPs, studies of patients suffering massive cerebral edema and refractory intracranial hypertension after ischemic stroke have shown varying results when comparing postdecompression outcomes and outcomes after best medical management.[17–25] However, the procedure remains widely used for patients with malignant cerebral edema after traumatic brain injury. Further studies are in progress to evaluate the risks and benefits of craniectomy for patients with traumatic brain injury. Evaluation of long-term morbidity and mortality as well as the best timing for this procedure continues.[17–25]

NURSING CONSIDERATIONS

Nursing care activity can compound primary and secondary intracranial insults, contributing to rapid deterioration in the unstable patient who has lost intracranial compliance, autoregulation, and vasomotor tone.[22] Patient positioning, agitation, pain, hemodynamic and respiratory status, and seizures can all contribute to a patient's elevated ICP. The following sections describe a few patient management strategies for the reduction of ICP (Table 34-5).

Positioning

Primary positioning strategies for the patient with impending or increased ICP include placement of the head and neck in a neutral position. Extreme neck flexion, extension, or rotation restricts venous drainage from the head through the internal jugular venous system and the vertebral venous plexus, increasing the total intracranial content. Decerebrate or decorticate posturing may also increase ICP. In addition, head of bed elevation has been shown to promote venous drainage and decrease ICP. The head is elevated 15 to 30 degrees, unless contraindicated by spine or limb fractures.

Tracheostomy ties and cervical collars are frequently checked for proper fit. Flexion of the hips greater than 90 degrees is avoided because it contributes to both intra-abdominal and thoracic pressures, also impairing venous outflow.

Environmental Considerations

Environmental stimuli contributing to pain, stress, or anxiety can increase cerebral metabolic rates and blood flow, confounding the management of increased ICP. Pain control and sedation are essential to reduce environmental overload, with consideration for the need for serial neurological assessments in the critically ill patient. Anxiety and discomfort in the ICU cannot be underestimated and should be considered in the patient who is neurologically impaired. Periods of uninterrupted sleep and rest should be provided between activities. Only essential interventions are performed during times of poor intracranial compliance, and activities are spaced to avoid a cumulative effect. Also, avoiding unnecessary painful procedures, such as frequent blood draws, is helpful.

• Clinical Applicability Challenges

Case Study

Mr. H., a 56-year-old retired man, collapsed while watching television. Before collapsing, he experienced the acute onset of right arm and leg weakness, right facial weakness, and difficulty speaking. Mr. H. was transported to the closest hospital and evaluated for suspected acute stroke. In the emergency room, the stroke work-up suggests a large ischemic infarct involving the middle cerebral artery (MCA). Mr. H. is ineligible for thrombolytic therapy because the time of symptom onset was unknown. His wife gives the following history:

- Allergies: none
- Medical history: nonmodifiable stroke risk factors—family history of stroke; modifiable stroke risk factors—obesity, cigarette smoking, hypertension, hypercholesterolemia
- Surgical history: none
- Social history: retired military computer analyst, married with supportive wife, three biological children, ages 28, 26, and 25, and all healthy; social ingestion of alcohol; smoking history 1 pack per day for 35 years
- Medications: lisinopril, 20 mg/day; atorvastatin (Lipitor), 10 mg/day

Table 34-5 • Nursing Considerations for Patients at Risk for Increased Intracranial Pressure

Problem	Nursing Action	Rationale
Adequate ventilation	• Assess respiratory patterns and rate • Suctioning: Preoxygenate with 100% O_2, one or two catheter passes, no more than 10 sec per catheter insertion • Monitor continuous pulse oximetry and blood gases	• Indicates neurological changes, pain status, and patency of airway • Prevents increased CO_2 (vasodilator that increases ICP); decreases coughing stimulation and increased intrathoracic pressure • Alerts nurse to airway problems; good indicator of hemodynamics of respiration
Neurological assessment	• Evaluate patient baseline neurological status at beginning of shift (preferably with previous shift RN)—mental status; pupil shape, size, and response; motor function • Assess vital signs—note trends (review ordered parameters for notification of physician) • Review nursing actions and emergency algorithm for neurologic deterioration (available medications—mannitol, hyperventilation, etc)	• Subtle changes from baseline indicate deterioration and the need for early intervention • Mean arterial pressure directly correlates with ICP in patient with loss of autoregulation • Ensures optimal benefit to patient and decreases secondary injury from prolonged ICP
Positioning	• Place head of bed flat or at 30 degrees elevation per orders • Maintain head in neutral position • Avoid hip flexion • Assess agitation in restrained patients • Turn patient q2h, instructing patient to exhale with turn • Carry out passive range-of-motion exercises • Avoid clustering of patient activities (e.g., turning, bathing, suctioning) • Use therapeutic interventions for emotional upset—speak with soft voice, use caution with unpleasant conversations, decrease noxious stimuli (noise), use therapeutic touch	• Promotes cerebral perfusion or facilitates venous drainage; orders based on physiological process • Promotes jugular outflow • Decreases intrathoracic pressure • Increases ICP • Prevents skin breakdown and avoids Valsalva maneuver during repositioning • Prevents contractures while avoiding Valsalva-inducing isometric contractions • Produces prolonged ICP spikes • Causes elevations in ICP; comatose patients still respond to unpleasant environmental stimuli
Transport of patient with invasive ICP monitor	• Confirm time of test or possibility of completing as portable study • Prepare respiratory therapy and other assistants during transport • Gather transport supplies (sedation if ordered, transport monitor, antihypertensives) • Assist with transfer of patient to diagnostic table with RN at head of bed monitoring device • Monitor and record hemodynamics and ICP dynamics during study	• Avoids excessive delays in uncontrolled and potentially overstimulating environment • Adequate oxygenation remains a priority; multiple lines necessitate additional manpower • Prepare for intervention with any adverse patient response during travel specific to contributors of increased ICP • Ensures patient protection and provides for monitor equipment recalibration for accuracy of monitoring • Monitors patient response to procedure
Temperature control	• Frequent temperature checks (oral or rectal preferred if no contraindications) • Confirm orders for early treatment of fever and aggressively treat • Provide gradual cooling with cooling blanket, closely monitored	• Cerebral metabolic rate increases with elevated body temperature • Increased cerebral blood flow increases ICP • Shivering increases ICP
Glycemic control	• Monitor serum glucose and fingersticks as ordered (q4–6h)—adhere closely to sliding scale protocols in nondiabetic patients • Maintain euvolemia with normal saline	• Alterations in glucose can produce neurological changes (i.e., changes in metabolic rate) • Hypotonic glucose intravenous solutions should be avoided
Bowel and bladder regimens	• Administer daily stool softeners as ordered • Avoid enemas • Assess patency of Foley catheters • Document strict intake and output	• Reduces risk for straining and increased intra-abdominal pressure, which increases ICP • Prevents Valsalva maneuver • Important to monitor amount of diuresis, especially in patients treated with osmotic diuretics • Important to maintain euvolemia
Seizure precautions	• Seizure precautions per hospital protocol (padding, etc.) • Monitor serum anticonvulsant drug levels	• Prevents injury in high-risk patients • Maintains therapeutic levels

Mr. H. is admitted to the neuroscience ICU for acute stroke management. Because of his large left MCA stroke, he is at risk for cerebral edema, seizure, and worsening of his stroke. During the first 24 hours, he shows no change in neurological status, and his vital signs remain stable. On day 2, his neurological examination shows a decrease in level of consciousness, a decrease in heart rate to 55 beats/minute, and an increase in blood pressure to 200/110 mm Hg. He requires immediate intubation for airway protection. The nurse suspects that Mr. H. is experiencing increased intracranial pressure (ICP) due to either cerebral edema or hemorrhagic conversion of the ischemic stroke territory. Laboratory samples are sent for testing, and a "stat" computed tomography (CT) scan is obtained. The neurology specialist and neurosurgeon are notified of the rapid change in Mr. H.'s status.

The CT scan reveals massive cerebral edema with midline shift (no hemorrhage noted). On arrival back at the neuroscience intensive care unit, Mr. H. is given his first dose of mannitol, and based on osmolarity levels, the dose is repeated every 6 hours. The neurosurgeon places an intraventricular drainage device under sterile conditions at the bedside. Mr. H.'s initial ICP is 32 mm Hg. The nurse monitors his ICP and mean arterial pressure on an hourly basis. Nursing interventions to assist in decreasing ICP include maintaining a quiet environment, limiting nursing activities, and avoiding flexion and extension of the neck. The patient's blood pressure decreases, and he does not require antihypertensive medications.

On day 3, Mr. H. experiences a generalized tonic-clonic seizure, which is treated with diazepam and a phenytoin load, with daily phenytoin administration. He is taken to CT, and the scan is negative for hemorrhage. On day 4, his ICP has been less than 15 mm Hg for more than 24 hours, and the intraventricular catheter is removed. On day 5, he is extubated. He is alert enough to understand what is being said to him. At this time, Mr. H. is formally evaluated by physical, speech, and occupational therapists. He fails a swallowing evaluation; therefore, he requires a percutaneous gastrostomy tube.

During his hospital stay, Mr. H. receives prophylaxis for stress ulcers and deep venous thrombosis, as well as aspirin for stroke prevention. His lipid panel reveals that his atorvastatin needs to be increased. He remains on lisinopril for hypertension. Diagnostic studies to determine the stroke etiology include a transthoracic echocardiogram, which reveals a normal ejection fraction, no right-to-left shunting, and no valvular abnormalities or vegetation. A carotid duplex does not reveal significant carotid stenosis.

Until discharge, Mr. H.'s vital signs and clinical status remain stable. His residual neurologi-

cal deficits include significant hemiparesis on the right side and dysarthria. Mr. H. is transferred to a stroke rehabilitation facility for aggressive stroke rehabilitation.

1. Describe other noninvasive approaches that the nurse might incorporate into Mr. H.'s care in order to reduce ICP.
2. Describe the potential complications that Mr. H. might experience while the intraventricular catheter for ICP monitoring is in place.
3. Does the neurological worsening that Mr. H. experiences on day 2 occur at a "typical" time point for patients with neurological injury? Explain your answer.

Review Questions

1. Your patient has an intraventricular catheter in place for intracranial pressure (ICP) monitoring after a subarachnoid hemorrhage. What other conditions may require monitoring of ICP?
   a. Escalating headache and fever
   b. Hemiplegia for 1 hour
   c. Normal brain computed tomography (CT) scan; Glasgow Coma Scale (GCS) score of 13; and orientation to person, place, and time
   d. Abnormal brain CT scan, GCS < 8, and inability to obey commands

2. Your patient is demonstrating restlessness, is complaining of a severe headache, and has an intracranial pressure (ICP) of 22 to 24 mm Hg after a closed head injury. Which intervention is effective to reduce increased ICP?
   a. Giving mannitol
   b. Using hypoventilation
   c. Placing the head of bed flat
   d. Giving a 500-mL bolus of normal saline

3. A patient in the neuroscience ICU has refractory elevated intracranial pressure (ICP). Nondepolarizing neuromuscular blockading (NMB) agents are used as last-effort therapy for managing mechanical ventilation and increased ICP. Which of the following statements regarding NMB agents made by a student nurse is incorrect?
   a. The patient must be mechanically ventilated.
   b. The patient requires adjunctive analgesia therapy.
   c. Sedation should be avoided for patients receiving NMB agents.
   d. Depth of neuromuscular blockade is measured using a peripheral nerve stimulator.

4. A patient with traumatic brain injury requires opiate administration for pain management. When educating a new nurse about administration of opiates to a patient with neurological injury, it is important to include which of the following statements?
   a. Opiate analgesics cannot be administered to a patient with a brain injury because frequent neurological examinations will not be possible.

b. A visual or verbal pain score should be used to assess pain frequently.

c. For the patient with a brain injury, PRN dosing (aliquot) of opiates is the only effective method of pain relief.

d. The maximal dose possible of an opiate analgesic should be administered as first-line therapy to provide adequate pain relief.

References

1. March K: Intracranial pressure monitoring and assessing intracranial compliance in brain injury. Crit Care Nurs Clin North Am 12(4):429–436, 2000

2. Ter Minassian A, Dube L, Guilleux AM, et al: Changes in intracranial pressure and cerebral autoregulation in patients with severe traumatic brain injury. Crit Care Med 30(7):1616–1622, 2002

3. Ghajar J: Intracranial pressure monitoring techniques. New Horiz 3(3):395–399, 1995

4. Brain Trauma Foundation, American Association of Neurological Surgeons, Joint Section on Neurotrauma and Critical Care: Guidelines for the management of severe traumatic brain injury. J Neurotrauma 17(6/7):449–554, 2000

5. Brain Trauma Foundation: Guidelines for the Management of Severe Traumatic Brain Injury, 3rd ed. New York: McGraw-Hill, 2007

6. Kapadia F, Rodriguez C, Jha AN: A simple technique to limit ICP catheter infection. Br J Neurosurg 11:335–336, 1997

7. Adelson PD, Bratton S, Carney N, et al: Guidelines for the acute medical management of severe traumatic brain injury in infants, children, and adolescents: Use of hyperosmolar therapy in the management of severe pediatric traumatic brain injury. Pediatr Crit Care Med 4:S40–S44, 2003

8. Roberts I, Schierhout G, Wakai A: Mannitol for acute traumatic brain injury. Cochrane Database 2:CD001049, 2003

9. Vialet R, Albanese J, Thomachot L, et al: Isovolume hypertonic solutes in the treatment of refractory posttraumatic intracranial hypertension. Crit Care Med 31(6):1683–1687, 2003

10. Cruz J: Low clinical ischemic threshold for cerebral blood flow in severe acute brain trauma. J Neurosurg 80:143–147, 1994

11. Jacobi J, Fraser G, Coursin D: Clinical practice guidelines for the sustained use of sedatives and analgesics in the critically ill adult. Crit Care Med 30(1):119–141, 2002

12. Wagner BK, O'Hara DA: Pharmacokinetics and pharmacodynamics of sedatives and analgesics in the treatment of agitated critically ill patients. Clin Pharmacokinet 33(6):426–453, 1977

13. Murray MJ, Cowen J, DeBlock H, et al: Clinical Practice Guidelines for Sustained Neuromuscular Blockade in the Adult Critically Ill Patient. Crit Care Med 30(1):142–156, 2002

14. Joint National Committee on Prevention, Detection, and Evaluation and Treatment of High Blood Pressure: The Sixth Report of the Joint National Committee on Prevention, Detection, and Evaluation and Treatment of High Blood Pressure. Arch Intern Med 157(21):2413–2446, 1997

15. Broderick JP, Adams HP, Barsan W, et al: Guidelines for the management of spontaneous intracerebral hemorrhage. Stroke 30:905–915, 1999

16. Harris OA, Colford JM, Good MC, et al: The role of hypothermia in the management of severe brain injury: A meta-analysis. Arch Neurol 59(7):1077–1083, 2002

17. Albanese J, Leone M, Alliez J, et al: Decompressive craniectomy for severe traumatic brain injury: Evaluation of the effects at one year. Crit Care Med 31(10):2535–2538, 2003

18. Figaji A, Fieggen A, Peter J: Early decompressive craniotomy in children with severe traumatic brain injury. Childs Nerv Syst 19(9):666–673, 2003

19. Jaeger M, Sochle M, Meixensberger J: Effects of decompressive craniectomy in brain tissue oxygen in patients with intracranial hypertension. J Neurol Neurosurg Psychiatry 74(4):513–515, 2003

20. Vahedi K, Hofmeijer J, Juettler E, et al: Early decompressive surgery in malignant infarction of the middle cerebral artery: a pooled analysis of three randomised controlled trials. Lancet Neurol 6(3):215–222, 2007

21. Vahedi K, Vicaut E, Mateo J, et al: Sequential-design, multicenter, randomized controlled trial of early decompressive craniectomy in malignant middle cerebral artery infarction (DECIMAL trial). Stroke 38:2506–2517, 2007

22. Cho DY, Chen TC, Lee HC: Ultra-early decompressive craniectomy for malignant middle cerebral artery infarction. Surg Neurol 60(3):227–232, 2003

23. Juttler E, Schwab S, Schmidek P, et al: Decompressive surgery for the treatment of malignant infarction of the middle cerebral artery (DESTINY): A randomized, controlled trial. Stroke 38(9):2518–2525, 2007

24. Morik K, Nakao Y, Yamamoto T, Maeda M: Early external decompressive craniectomy with duraplasty improves functional recovery in patients with massive hemispheric embolic infarction: Timing and indication of decompressive surgery for malignant cerebral infarction. Surg Neurol 62(5):420–429, 2004

25. Schwab S, Steiner T, Aschoff A, et al: Early hemicraniectomy in patients with complete middle cerebral artery infarction. Stroke 29(9):1888–1893, 1998

Other Selected Readings

Arbour R: Aggressive management of intracranial dynamics. Crit Care Nurse 18(3):30–40, 1998

Caplan L: Caplan's Stroke: A Clinical Approach. Boston, Butterworth Heinemann, 2000

Cruz J, Minoja G, Okuchi K: Major clinical and physiological benefits of early high doses of mannitol for intraparenchymal temporal lobe hemorrhages with abnormal papillary widening: A randomized trial. Neurosurgery 51(3):628–637, 2002

Deray M, Resnick T, Alvarez L: Complete Pocket Reference for the Treatment of Epilepsy. Miami, C.P.R. Educational Services, 2001

Dunn LT: Raised intracranial pressure. J Neurol Neurosurg Psychiatry 73:23–27, 2002

Haltiner AM, Newell DW, Temkin NR: Side effects and mortality associated with use of phenytoin for early post-traumatic seizure prophylaxis. J Neurosurg 91:588–592, 1999

Kidd KC, Criddle L: Using jugular venous catheters in patients with traumatic brain injury. Crit Care Nurse 21(6):17–22, 2001

Kolb S, Litt B: Management of epilepsy and co-morbid disorders in the emergency room and intensive care unit. In Ettinger A, Devinsky O (eds): Managing Epilepsy and Co-Existing Disorders. Woburn, MA: Butterworth-Heinemann, 2002, pp 515–533

Krauss JJ, Metzler MD, Coplin WM: Critical care issues in stroke and subarachnoid hemorrhage. Neurol Res 24:S47–S57, 2002

Mokri B: The Monro-Kellie hypothesis: Applications in CSF volume depletion. Neurology 56:1746–1748, 2001

Phillips J: Neuroscience critical care: The role of the advanced practice nurse in patient safety. AACN Clin Issues 16(4):581–592, 2005

Sahjpaul R, Girotti M: Intracranial pressure monitoring in severe traumatic brain injury. Can J Neurol Sci 27:143–147, 2000

Segal S, Gallagher AC, Shefler AG, et al: Survey of the use of intracranial pressure monitoring in children in the United Kingdom. Intensive Care Med 27:236–239, 2001

VanderSchaaf IC, Ruigrok YM, Rinkel GJ, et al: Study design and outcome measures in studies on aneurysmal subarachnoid hemorrhage. Stroke 33(8):2043–2046, 2002

Wong F: Prevention of secondary brain injury. Crit Care Nurse 20:18–27, 2000

Common Neurosurgical and Neurological Disorders

Barbara Fitzsimmons • Eileen Bohan

35

Neurological Surgery
  Brain Tumors
  Aneurysms
  Arteriovenous Malformations
  Surgical Approaches
Neurological Disorders
  Stroke
  Seizures
  Guillain-Barré Syndrome
  Myasthenia Gravis

Objectives

Based on the content in this chapter, the reader should be able to:

❶ Discuss the surgical management of the patient with a brain tumor.

❷ Name the medical and surgical options for the patient with a cerebral aneurysm or arteriovenous malformation.

❸ Describe the classification of stroke.

❹ Discuss the nursing management of a patient who has experienced an acute ischemic stroke.

❺ Differentiate between partial and generalized seizures.

❻ Review the current antiepileptic drugs used to manage epilepsy.

❼ Describe the pathophysiological basis of Guillain-Barré syndrome.

❽ Explain the pharmacological management of myasthenia gravis.

During the course of their illness, many patients with neurological diseases require critical care management. Routine neurosurgical procedures usually involve a short intensive care unit (ICU) admission. In addition, complications of the tumor or treatments may necessitate readmission. ICU admission follows the use of thrombolytic therapy for stroke and may be required to treat the patient with stroke and increased intracranial pressure (ICP). Patients with myasthenia gravis or Guillain-Barré syndrome may require an ICU stay for respiratory sequelae of their disease. The critical care nurse is better prepared to manage the acute and chronic needs of this patient population if the nurse understands the course of the disease, as well as the medical and surgical tools available for these disorders. This chapter provides an overview of the etiology, clinical manifestations, diagnostic tests, and current management of the neurosurgical and neurological disorders most often encountered in the ICU environment.

• Neurological Surgery

Surgery is indicated for several neurological disorders. Neurological surgery is a common and integral part of the management of patients with brain tumors, arteriovenous malformations, and aneurysms. Craniotomy is the most common procedure performed for these problems. The following section reviews the etiology and pathophysiology of these conditions and describes surgical approaches used for the management of these patients.

BRAIN TUMORS

A brain tumor is broadly described as any neoplasm arising within the cranium. Tumors may originate in the brain (primary) or seed in the brain from other organs (metastatic). Pathological examination of a tumor is used to classify the tumor by cell type. Tumors are further graded based on the degree of malignancy. Classification and grade are used to predict patient outcome. Table 35-1 outlines the

Table 35-1 • Classification and Grading of Brain Tumors (Most Common Intracranial Tumors)*

Classification/Grade	Description	Symptoms	Treatment/Prognosis
Neuroepithelial (approximately 50% of primary tumors)			
Gliomas			
Astrocytic			
WHO grade I—pilocytic astrocytoma	Pediatric; 85% cerebellar; slow growing; well circumscribed; cystic; benign	Increased intracranial pressure (ICP); focal neurologic signs	Curable with surgery (craniotomy for tumor removal)
WHO grade II—astrocytoma	Infiltrative; slow growing	Seizures; acute or subtle onset of symptoms	Radiation therapy (RT) for residual tumor; may withhold RT after gross total resection; young age is good prognostic factor
WHO grade III—anaplastic astrocytoma	Hypercellular; anaplasia	May have acute onset of symptoms	RT with or without chemotherapy; high recurrence rate; age and overall health affect prognosis
WHO grade IV—glioblastoma multiforme	Poorly differentiated, with high mitotic rate; highly malignant; most common glioma in adults	Rapid onset of symptoms; increased ICP or focal signs	Infiltrative nature: complete removal of all cells not possible; RT with chemotherapy; experimental protocols; recurrence in virtually all cases; median survival: 12–18 mo
Oligodendroglioma	Well differentiated; calcified; infiltrative; slow growing; some tumors are malignant (anaplastic)	Seizures; headaches; subtle onset of symptoms	RT with residual tumor; may withhold after gross total resection; RT with or without chemotherapy for anaplastic oligodendroglioma
Mixed glioma (oligoastrocytoma)	May behave more or less aggressively, depending on features	Dependent on location and degree of malignancy	Variable outcome
Ependymoma	Pediatric and young adult patients; originates from lining of the ventricles; frequently in posterior fossa; usually benign	May present with hydrocephalus; symptoms related to location	RT for residual or recurrent disease; craniospinal RT for evidence of spinal disease only; good prognosis
Embryonal (primitive neuroectodermal tumor) medulloblastoma, most common	Primarily pediatric; malignant; occurs mainly in posterior fossa; cerebrospinal fluid (CSF) metastasis in 33% of patients	Symptoms by location; hydrocephalus common	Craniospinal RT; poor prognosis, particularly with CSF dissemination
Peripheral Nerve Tumors (approximately 8% of primary brain tumors)			
Vestibular schwannoma (acoustic neuroma)	Cerebellopontine angle; benign; encapsulated; seen in association with neurofibromatosis, type 2	Decreased hearing; tinnitus; balance problems; may have other cranial nerve deficits	Curable with surgery; excellent prognosis; cranial nerve deficits may be permanent or temporary; affect quality of life
Meningeal Tumors (approximately 30% of primary brain tumors)			
Meningioma	Composed of arachnoid cells; attached to dura; usually benign; well circumscribed; may be vascular; common locations: falx convexity; olfactory groove; sphenoid ridge; parasellar region; optic nerve	Headaches may occur from dural stretching; seizures and focal neurologic signs	Degree of resection (and recurrence) associated with location; excellent prognosis with gross total resection; atypical and malignant meningiomas have more aggressive features and less favorable outcomes
Lymphomas and Hematopoietic Tumors (approximately 3% of primary brain tumors)			
Malignant central nervous system lymphoma	Arise in central nervous system without systemic lymphoma; commonly suprasellar; diffuse brain infiltration; may be periventricular and may involve leptomeninges; solitary or multiple	Neurologic or neuropsychiatric symptoms	Diagnosis commonly via stereotactic biopsy or CSF cytology; steroids may decrease or temporarily obliterate lesion on computed tomography or magnetic resonance imaging (MRI); RT with or without chemotherapy; high-dose methotrexate used as single agent; some studies defer RT;

(continued)

Table 35-1 • Classification and Grading of Brain Tumors (Most Common Intracranial Tumors)* (Continued)

Classification/Grade	Description	Symptoms	Treatment/Prognosis
			increasing incidence in immuno-competent persons; decreasing in AIDS patients; possible improved survival with newer treatments
Germ Cell Tumors (approximately 1% of primary brain tumors)			
	Developmental tumors—from gonads and extragonadal sites; germinoma (solid, enhancing on MRI) and teratoma (cystic, with fat and calcification) most common	Symptoms are location dependent; germinomas are often suprasellar—diabetes insipidus	RT for germinomas; curable; teratoma has less favorable prognosis; gross total resection means improved survival; chemotherapy in some cases
Sellar Tumors (approximately 7% of primary brain tumors)			
Pituitary adenoma	6.3% of sellar tumors; benign; originate from adenohypophysis; classification by hormonal content; microadenoma ≤ 1 cm; macroadenoma ≥ 1 cm	Hypersecretion • Prolactin: amenorrhea, galactorrhea • Growth hormone: acromegaly • Adrenocorticotropic hormone: Cushing's syndrome • Thyroid-stimulating hormone: hyperthyroidism (rare) Hyposecretion caused by compression of the pituitary gland Visual field deficits (bitemporal hemianopia); headache; pituitary apoplexy: acute hemorrhage or infarct of gland—emergency treatment indicated	*Surgical:* transsphenoidal for approximately 95% of surgical cases; *medical:* appropriate in some cases of prolactin-secreting and growth hormone–secreting tumors; RT for recurrence or for hypersecretory tumors, when medical management has failed
Craniopharyngioma	Benign, calcified, cystic tumors	Endocrine abnormalities; visual impairment; cognitive and/or personality changes; may have increased ICP	Gross total resection affects prognosis; RT for residual tumor
Metastatic Tumors (approximately 150,000 new cases yearly; occur in 20%–40% of cancer patients)			
	Originate from primary systemic tumors; discrete, round, ring-enhancing; 50% are solitary; lung and breast are most common primary sites	Symptoms are location dependent	Prognosis dependent on number of tumors, tumor location, systemic disease, and patient age; improved prognosis with gross total resection and RT

*For all tumors, biopsy or craniotomy for tumor removal is necessary to establish a definitive diagnosis.

most common brain tumors designated by the World Health Organization system.[1-3] Other predictors of outcome include patient age and general health, early detection, and tumor location.

Although many brain tumors are low grade or "benign," their location may impede surgical removal and cause brain edema as well as shifting of the surrounding structures. This causes increased ICP. Untreated ICP can lead to brain herniation and can be fatal. Early diagnosis and symptom management, in addition to histological diagnosis, are important prognostic factors.

Etiology

The cause of most brain tumors is still unknown. As research improves in the area of genetics, there has been increased interest in identifying chromosomal abnormalities in many types of cancer, including brain tumors. Cytogenetic studies of glioblastoma multiforme, the most common primary brain tumor, have shown multiple chromosomal changes, with both gain and loss of certain chromosomes. It is hypothesized that this information will, at the very least, aid in the development of individualized therapies for patients with primary brain tumors. Some hereditary diseases, such as neurofibromatosis and polyposis, are associated with the development of certain types of brain tumors.[4]

Data from a familial brain tumor registry of primary brain tumors have been collected in the United States and Canada. These data showed a number of cases of first-degree relatives with gliomas. More than 50% of these cases involved high-grade gliomas. One noticeable difference from common familial tumors, such as colon and breast cancer, was that the gliomas were reported for two generations only, unlike multi-generational reporting in the other cancers. Of note, the incidence of husband-and-wife gliomas suggests that environmental factors may play a role in the development of these tumors.[5]

Other environmental factors currently being studied are electric and magnetic fields, foods (particularly those that are broken down in the stomach or bladder to form *N*-nitroso compounds), occupational exposure, and chemical exposure.[4]

Ionizing radiation has been shown to increase the occurrence of some brain tumors (nerve sheath tumors, meningiomas, and gliomas) when given in high doses. Low-dose radiation exposure is a topic of discussion and controversy.[6]

To further evaluate these and other possible causes of brain tumors, large, multi-institutional collaborative studies are needed.

Epidemiology

Recent statistics indicate that there are approximately 44,000 new cases of primary brain tumors diagnosed in the United States each year. The Central Brain Tumor Registry of the United States identifies 18,500 of these as high-grade or malignant.[1] More than 150,000 new cases of metastatic brain tumors are diagnosed in the United States yearly.[7]

Epidemiological studies have confirmed certain patterns of brain tumor incidence. There has been a significant increase in the incidence of brain tumors in developed countries over the past several decades. Some of this increase can be attributed to improved diagnostic techniques, access to medical care, and an increasing elderly population. However, it is suspected that some of these increases are also attributable to environmental and lifestyle factors, as previously outlined.

Other patterns of incidence have been documented by age, ethnicity, and sex. For example, the average age of onset for glioblastomas and meningiomas is approximately 60 years. Gliomas are diagnosed more often in the white population and in men. African Americans and women have higher rates of meningiomas.[6]

Pathophysiology

The brain has its own distinct protective mechanism in the form of the blood–brain barrier. Studies undertaken in the mid-19th century showed that dyes injected intravenously were not observed in brain tissue as they were in other body organs. However, when injected directly into the cerebrospinal fluid (CSF), they were absorbed into the brain but not disseminated through the brain's vascular system to the rest of the body. These studies confirmed the restricted permeability between the blood and the brain and between the blood and the CSF, but not between the brain and CSF. Tumors are able to cause disruption of this blood–brain barrier, as evidenced by computed tomography (CT) and magnetic resonance imaging (MRI) scans, which show contrast uptake at the site of many tumors. Studies by Long and others

confirmed that a tumor's capillary system becomes increasingly abnormal, and permeable, with increasing malignancy, therefore causing blood–brain barrier disruption.[8,9]

Vasogenic edema, caused by increased capillary permeability and commonly seen in association with brain tumors and other brain lesions, is the direct result of blood–brain barrier disruption. As outlined in the Monro-Kellie doctrine, the contents of the cranial vault—brain, CSF, and blood—have a fixed volume. Any addition to this volume must be balanced by reduction in one of the other components. When this compensatory mechanism is no longer able to function, edema develops and ICP increases. In Figure 35-1, an MRI scan shows brain edema and mass effect (shifting of brain structures) caused by a glioblastoma multiforme. Some slow-growing tumors (e.g., meningiomas) can become quite large as a result of this compensatory mechanism and the brain's plasticity. This plasticity allows the brain to accommodate to slow tumor growth over a long period of time.

Clinical Manifestations

The patient with a brain neoplasm may present with one or more signs of tumor growth. The signs may be general or focal. The most common general signs of brain tumors are headaches, seizures, or mental status changes. These are related to increasing ICP.

The triad of symptoms associated with increased ICP includes headache, nausea with or without vomiting, and papilledema (swelling of the optic discs). Symptoms are typically treated with corticosteroids, which are discussed later in this chapter. Clinical evidence of herniation (shifting of brain tissue by masses, increased ICP, or both) often requires critical care management using fluid restriction, hyperventilation, osmotic agents, and diuretics. Some situations necessitate the use of CSF drainage through an intraventricular catheter (see Chapter 34).[10,11]

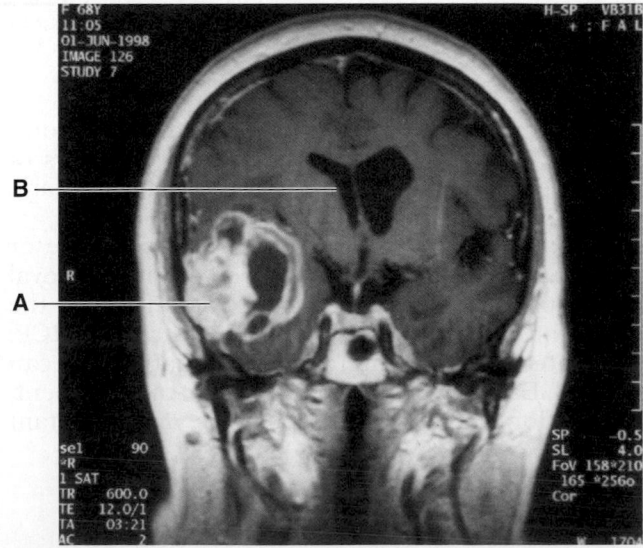

Figure 35-1 • Coronal magnetic resonance imaging view of ring-enhancing glioblastoma multiforme (**A**) with evidence of mass effect (**B**). (Courtesy of Henry Brem, MD, Johns Hopkins University, Baltimore, MD.)

The frequency of seizures depends on tumor location as well as tumor histology. More than 60% of patients experience seizures over the course of their disease. Seizure activity is more common in patients with low-grade tumors. Tumors in the cerebral hemispheres are much more likely to cause seizure activity than posterior fossa tumors. Seizures may be focal or generalized, as discussed later in this chapter.[12]

Mental status changes occur as the result of mass effect on the brain caused by increased ICP or hydrocephalus. Patients may become drowsy and mentally slower as ICP increases. Cognitive changes occur in the form of problems concentrating, memory difficulties, personality changes, confusion, or disorientation. Although mental status changes are associated with frontal lobe tumors, they are also the result of increased ICP.[13]

Focal neurological deficits may be the temporary result of tumor compression, or may be permanent, as a result of tumor destruction. These deficits are directly related to tumor location, as outlined in Chapter 34. Figure 35-2 outlines site-specific signs and symptoms of brain tumors.

Diagnosis

History taking is a key element in the process of diagnosing a brain neoplasm. The duration, frequency, and severity of symptoms are ascertained. It is important to assess whether there is a particular time of day or series of activities that initiate symptoms. Are they intermittent or continuous? Do they resolve with pharmacological management? Morning headaches and headaches that increase with Valsalva maneuver or are associated with nausea and vomiting are seen

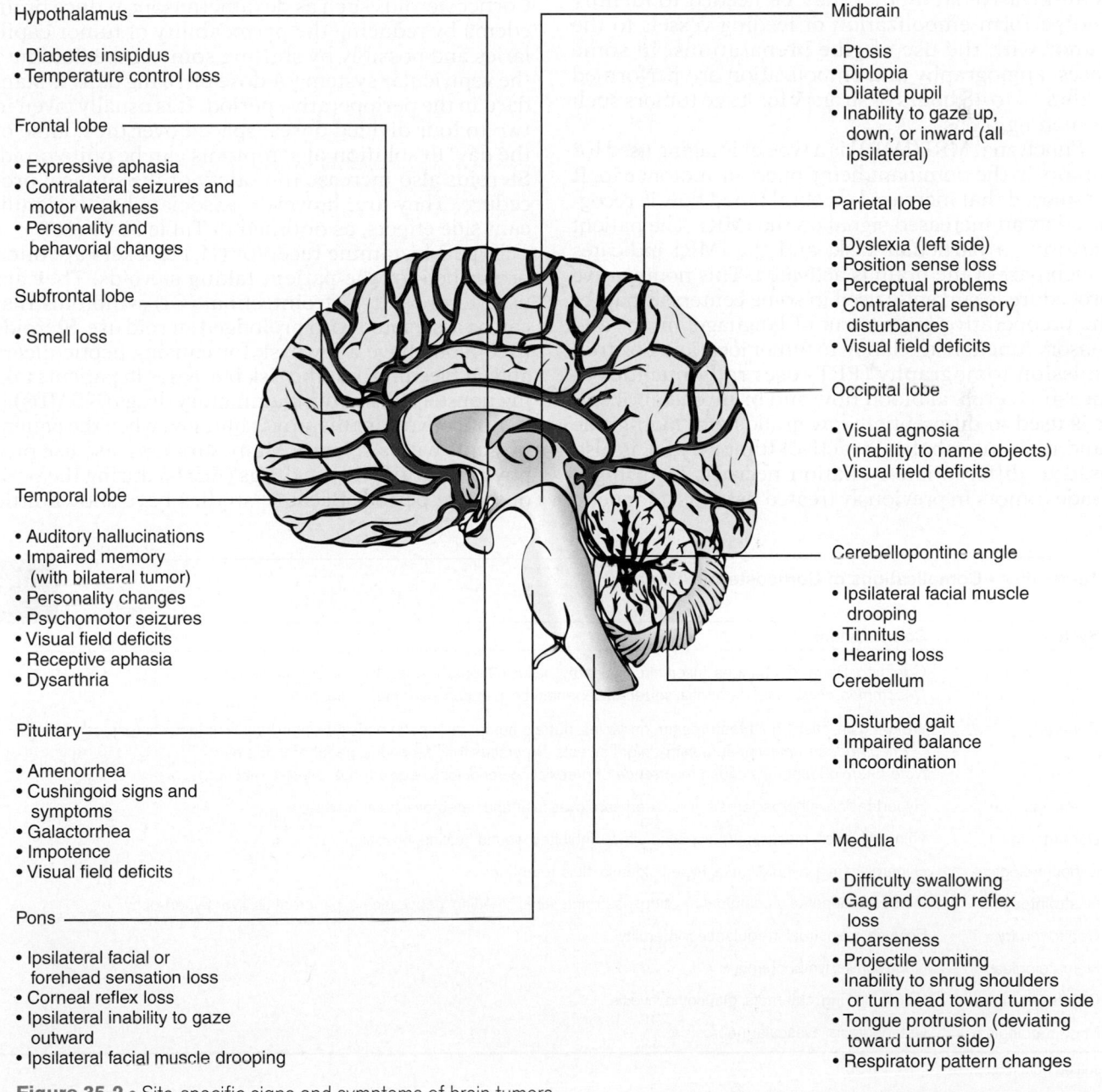

Hypothalamus

• Diabetes insipidus
• Temperature control loss

Frontal lobe

• Expressive aphasia
• Contralateral seizures and motor weakness
• Personality and behaviorial changes

Subfrontal lobe

• Smell loss

Temporal lobe

• Auditory hallucinations
• Impaired memory (with bilateral tumor)
• Personality changes
• Psychomotor seizures
• Visual field deficits
• Receptive aphasia
• Dysarthria

Pituitary

• Amenorrhea
• Cushingoid signs and symptoms
• Galactorrhea
• Impotence
• Visual field deficits

Pons

• Ipsilateral facial or forehead sensation loss
• Corneal reflex loss
• Ipsilateral inability to gaze outward
• Ipsilateral facial muscle drooping

Midbrain

• Ptosis
• Diplopia
• Dilated pupil
• Inability to gaze up, down, or inward (all ipsilateral)

Parietal lobe

• Dyslexia (left side)
• Position sense loss
• Perceptual problems
• Contralateral sensory disturbances
• Visual field deficits

Occipital lobe

• Visual agnosia (inability to name objects)
• Visual field deficits

Cerebellopontine angle

• Ipsilateral facial muscle drooping
• Tinnitus
• Hearing loss

Cerebellum

• Disturbed gait
• Impaired balance
• Incoordination

Medulla

• Difficulty swallowing
• Gag and cough reflex loss
• Hoarseness
• Projectile vomiting
• Inability to shrug shoulders or turn head toward tumor side
• Tongue protrusion (deviating toward tumor side)
• Respiratory pattern changes

Figure 35-2 • Site-specific signs and symptoms of brain tumors.

in patients with tumor-induced increased ICP. The physical examination aids in further localizing the lesion. Patients may minimize or are often unaware of subtle neurological deficits. Family involvement in this discussion is useful.

Imaging studies such as CT scans and MRI are typically ordered to localize the lesion and assess the amount of edema and mass effect on surrounding structures. CT scans are often obtained to establish a differential diagnosis when a patient is seen in the emergency department. Because MRI shows tumors in three dimensions (axial, coronal, and sagittal), it is the preferred diagnostic tool. An electroencephalogram (EEG) is used to confirm the presence of seizure discharges, which may be useful in determining whether anticonvulsants are needed. Magnetic resonance angiography (MRA) images the vascular anatomy and vessels that feed certain tumors. It can be a noninvasive alternative to the angiogram, which is an invasive study that may be needed to identify and perform embolization of feeding vessels to the tumor with the use of glue preparations. In some cases, angiography and embolization are performed within 24 to 48 hours of surgery for large tumors such as meningiomas.

Functional MRI (fMRI) is a type of imaging used for tumors in the dominant hemisphere or motor strip. It is believed that increased cerebral blood flow is recognized as an increased signal on the fMRI. The patient performs a particular task, and the fMRI indicates which part of the brain is activated. This noninvasive procedure is currently used in some centers as part of the preoperative assessment of language, motor and sensory function in relation to tumor location. Positron emission tomography (PET) uses radionuclides to measure cerebral blood flow and brain metabolism. It is used to differentiate low-grade from high-grade (and more metabolically active) tumors. PET is also used to differentiate radiation necrosis from high-grade tumors in previously treated patients. Magnetic resonance spectroscopy (MRS) is a noninvasive radiographic technique that measures metabolite levels in brain tumors. Biological compounds such as choline can be quantitated in brain tumors. Because MRS is obtained at the same time as MRI, the anatomic and metabolic characteristics of the tumor are obtained with little additional inconvenience to the patient.[14-18]

Clinical Management

Once the differential diagnosis of brain tumor is obtained through history, physical examination, and imaging studies, decisions are made regarding appropriate treatment modalities. A medical and surgical plan of care is discussed with the patient and family members.

Pharmacological Management

Tumors and tumor treatments are known to cause increased ICP, which is treated with corticosteroids. Corticosteroids such as dexamethasone reduce brain edema by reducing the permeability of tumor capillaries and possibly by shifting some of the fluid into the ventricular system.[8] A dose of 16 mg daily is standard in the perioperative period. It is usually given in two to four divided doses, spaced over the course of the day. Resolution of symptoms can be quite rapid. Steroids also increase the safety of the surgical procedure. They are, however, associated with significant side effects, as outlined in Table 35-2.[12,19,20]

Type 2 histamine receptor (H$_2$) blockers are often prescribed for the patient taking steroids. They are used to prevent gastrointestinal (GI) symptoms that can be associated with prolonged steroid use. Steroids used alone have a low risk for causing peptic ulcers and GI bleeding, but the risk increases in patients taking nonsteroidal anti-inflammatory drugs (NSAIDs).[12]

Anticonvulsant therapy is initiated when the patient presents with a seizure. Many surgeons also use prophylactic antiepileptic drugs (AEDs) during the perioperative period. Because studies have shown little

Table 35-2 • Complications of Corticosteroid Therapy

System	Complications
Neurological	*Common:* Behavior changes, insomnia, myopathy, hallucinations, hiccups, tremor, cerebral atrophy *Uncommon:* Psychosis, dementia, seizures, dependence, paraparesis (epidural lipomatosis)
General	Weight gain, cushingoid features (moon facies, buffalo hump, centripetal obesity), opportunistic infections (e.g., candidiasis, *Pneumocystis carinii* pneumonitis), night sweats, hypersensitivity reactions, peripheral edema *Note:* Steroid taper may cause recurrence of preexisting conditions (e.g., arthritis, allergic reaction)
Cardiovascular	Hypertension, atherosclerosis, increased cardiovascular and cerebrovascular disease
Dermatological	Thin skin, ecchymoses, purpura, acne, striae, inhibited wound healing, hirsutism
Endocrinological	Hyperglycemia, hypokalemia, hyperlipidemia, fluid retention
Gastrointestinal	Increased appetite, abdominal bloating, gastrointestinal bleeding, peptic ulcers, pancreatitis, liver hypertrophy
Genitourinary	Polyuria, menstrual irregularities, infertility
Hematological	Neutrophilia, lymphopenia
Ophthalmological	Visual blurring, cataracts, glaucoma, uveitis
Rheumatological	Osteoporosis, avascular necrosis

Modified from references 12, 19, and 20.

difference in the occurrence of postoperative seizures in patients receiving AEDs compared with control groups without such drugs, some physicians are limiting the use of postoperative and prophylactic AED therapy.[21,22] However, 70% of members of the American Association of Neurological Surgeons who responded to a survey stated that they continue to prescribe prophylactic AEDs for their patients with brain tumors.[23] Seizures are extensively discussed later in this chapter.

Surgical Management

Clinical and radiographic evaluations are useful in obtaining a differential diagnosis. However, pathologic examination of tumor tissue produces the definitive diagnosis. There are two distinct surgical approaches to diagnosing and treating brain tumors. Stereotactic biopsy is used to obtain small samples of tumor tissue under CT or MRI guidance. Craniotomy is performed when tumor removal is feasible and provides both a pathological diagnosis and surgical resection of the lesion. These approaches are discussed in the "Surgical Approaches" section of this chapter.

During the past several decades, improvements in anesthesia, microsurgical equipment, intraoperative monitoring techniques, and pharmacological management have significantly improved intraoperative mortality rates. Postoperative morbidity has also significantly decreased. The perioperative management of the patient with a brain tumor involves a multidisciplinary team approach, as outlined in Table 35-3.[24]

Despite substantial improvements in the management of the patient with a brain tumor, surgical complications may be severe and require critical care monitoring and management. The most common complications include brain edema, infection, hyponatremia or other electrolyte imbalances, hemorrhage, venous thromboembolism (including deep venous thrombosis [DVT] and pulmonary embolism [PE]), and seizures (Table 35-4).

Radiation Therapy

Many brain tumors are treated with adjuvant therapies, either because they are not able to be surgically resected or because of their aggressive nature. For most brain tumors, radiation therapy (RT) is the first-line treatment after biopsy or craniotomy. The energy produced by radiation damages tumor DNA at the time of cell division. Three-dimensional conformal radiation is generally used to treat those tumor cells that are not surgically resectable. This form of RT treats the shape and the volume of tumor while normal brain tissue is protected.[25] A standard dose of up to 6,000 centigray (cGy; also referred to as radiation absorbed dose, or rad) is administered to primary brain tumors 5 days a week over a period of 6 weeks. Multiple metastatic tumors receive a dose of approximately 3,000 cGy divided over 10 treatments. Some metastases may be treated with higher radiation doses with or without a boost of focused radiation.[26,27]

There are other approaches to applying RT. Intensity-modulated radiation therapy (IMRT) modifies the radiation beam so that a more focused dose can be given, without exposing surrounding brain tissue. Stereotactic radiosurgery (e.g., gamma knife and linear accelerator) is applied under MRI guidance. A three-dimensional image is obtained, and radiation is given in one large dose to residual tumor, sparing normal brain tissue. Brachytherapy uses radioactive isotopes in seeds or liquid-filled balloons inserted into residual tumor. Radiosensitizers are agents given in addition to RT. It is postulated that some substances increase oxygen delivery to hypoxic tumors. The oxygen enhances the effects of radiation. Hyperthermia is also being applied with the same goal of increasing oxygen to tumors to maximize the effects of radiation.[27–32]

Chemotherapy

Malignant brain tumors require multiple treatment modalities. Chemotherapy is given in conjunction with radiation or at the time of tumor recurrence. Drugs may be administered orally or intravenously but can cause systemic toxicities and have difficulty crossing the blood–brain barrier in sufficient amounts to provide benefit. An approach using RT in conjunction with temozolomide chemotherapy has shown survival benefit in the most malignant primary brain tumor, glioblastoma multiforme.[33]

Chemotherapy can also be placed in the tumor resection cavity at the time of craniotomy. A biodegradable polymer wafer that delivers a continuous infusion of carmustine (BCNU) chemotherapy over a period of 2 to 3 weeks is being used for primary malignant and metastatic brain tumors. The wafer is surgically implanted at the time of initial diagnosis or when the tumor recurs.[34,35]

Research Initiatives

Radiation and chemotherapy are targeted at damaging cell DNA, thereby killing the cell or preventing it from dividing. Other approaches have been used in an effort to address different aspects of tumor growth:

▶ Glioma cells are deficient in a protein that suppresses tumor growth (–p53). Gene therapy is being explored using adenoviruses, for example, which are engineered to replicate in and inactivate these cells. They are designed not to replicate in normal (+p53) cells.

▶ Antiangiogenic factors are used to prevent tumors from forming their own blood supply, crucial to tumor growth.

▶ Immunotherapy is designed to stimulate the immune system to eliminate tumors. Targeted toxins are injected into and infiltrate tumor cells. Cytokines, such as interferon and interleukin, are proteins produced by the body to stimulate an immune response. They are being combined with inactivated tumor cells as the basis for tumor vaccines.

▶ Cancer cells have enzymes that resist chemotherapy. Certain drugs called resistance modifiers are being used to inhibit these enzymes and to increase the effectiveness of chemotherapy.[36,37]

Nursing Management

Assessment Some tumors are cured with surgery, whereas others have a protracted course involving

Table 35-3 • Multidisciplinary Management Guide for the Patient With a Brain Tumor

Stage	Management Team	Interventions	Nursing Considerations
Preoperative			
• History and physical	• Neurosurgeon, nurse practitioner, RN	• Baseline history and physical examination; neurological evaluation: mental status, cranial nerves, motor and sensory function, coordination, reflexes	• Preoperative teaching to begin • Involve family as much as possible
• Medications	• Physician, pharmacist, nurse practitioner, RN	• Steroids; histamine type 2 receptor (H_2) blockers, as needed; anticonvulsants for supratentorial lesions • Prescribe new medications; medication review; discuss interactions or contraindications	• Anticoagulants, nonsteroidal anti-inflammatory drugs (NSAIDs) to be discontinued (with consent of prescribing physician)
• Diagnostic testing	• Neuroradiologist	• Baseline magnetic resonance imaging (MRI) or computed tomography (CT) scan • Electrocardiogram, chest x-ray • Other diagnostic studies as indicated	• Most preoperative testing performed within 1 week of surgery
• Preoperative teaching	• By speciality: RN, neurosurgeon, neuroanesthesiologist	• Informed consent • Obtain all test results before admission day	• A written teaching pamphlet is recommended for patient and family use
• Hospital admission	• Admitting office, OR staff	• Obtain/confirm demographics	• Most patients are admitted the day of surgery
Intraoperative			
• Stereotactic biopsy	• OR team, surgeon, anesthesiologist, radiologist, pathologist	• Stereotactic frame placed; samples taken through catheter inserted under MRI/CT guidance • Histological evaluation	• May be performed in radiology suite or OR • Teaching regarding stereotactic frame • May also be done as a frameless procedure
• Craniotomy	• OR team, surgeon, anesthesiologist, pathologist	• Tumor tissue obtained for biopsy; tumor resected • Histological evaluation	• Teaching regarding general anesthesia
Postoperative			
• Critical care unit	• Critical care staff, neurosurgeon	• Hemodynamic monitoring; frequent neurological evaluations	• If possible, it is useful for patient and family to see the unit before surgery
• Nursing unit	• Floor nurses, surgeon, consulting physicians, rehabilitation medicine, pharmacist, clergy, nutritionist	• Postoperative care to include vital signs, neurological exam, wound care, cough, and deep breathing; increase activity as tolerated; advance diet as tolerated • Rehabilitation medicine consult • Evaluate for deficits and complications and provide consultations, as indicated	• More family participation in care when possible • Patients are usually out of bed within 24 hours of surgery • Recently, short hospital stays cause increased family involvement and responsibility; begin teaching while patient is on the nursing unit
Discharge Planning	• Social worker, nursing staff, consulting physicians, radiation oncologist, medical oncologist (when indicated)	• Inpatient/outpatient rehabilitation as needed (occupational therapy, physical therapy, speech, cognitive) • Outpatient therapies as needed (e.g., radiation, chemotherapy) • Hospice care (inpatient or home hospice) may be indicated, particularly in cases of recurrent malignant gliomas, refractory to conventional treatments	• Ideally, planning begins as soon as the patient arrives on the nursing unit • Family takes on greater role because patient is often discharged from the hospital 2–3 days postoperatively, particularly in cases of highly malignant tumors where home hospice is indicated

Adapted from Bohan E, Macenka DG: Surgical management of patients with brain tumors. Semin Oncol Nurs 20(4):240–252, 2004.

adjuvant therapies and treatment for recurrent disease. As part of the multidisciplinary team, the nurse plays a central role in patient care and family support throughout the course of the patient's illness. The nurse participates in the diagnosis, treatment, and follow-up care of the patient with a brain tumor.

Plan Careful history taking and symptom evaluation contribute to the accurate diagnosis of a brain tumor. Once medications are prescribed, patient education includes discussion of dose, side effects, and contraindications. The results of tests leading to a differential diagnosis are reviewed with the patient

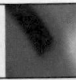

Table 35-4 • Critical Care Management of the Patient With Brain Tumor Complications

Diagnosis	Management
Increased intracranial pressure (ICP)	• Corticosteroids and antacids or histamine type 2 receptor (H_2) blockers • IV fluids: Avoid hypotonic solutions • Elevate head of bed and maintain adequate body alignment • Avoid hypotension and control hypertension; arterial line useful; if ICP monitor is available, titrate BP to maintain a continuous positive pressure of 70–80 mm Hg • Keep well oxygenated; may need to intubate • Judicious use of osmotic therapy: mannitol to expand plasma volume and draw fluid out of the brain; may be used in conjunction with furosemide • Sedation to reduce activity and decrease hypertension • Intraventricular catheter may be necessary to monitor ICP and drain CSF • Cautious use of hyperventilation for short periods only to reduce arterial carbon dioxide pressure (PCO_2) (6–24 h) • May require surgical intervention for hematoma
Wound infection, intracranial abscess, or bone flap infection	• Blood work, including complete blood count (CBC) and blood cultures • CT scan, MRI, and in some cases magnetic resonance spectroscopy to identify abscess • Surgical removal of abscess or bone flap, when feasible • Appropriate wound cultures, when possible • Antibiotic therapy • Infectious disease consultation for appropriate drug, dose, and duration
Hyponatremia or hypernatremia	• Possible diabetes insipidus, salt-wasting syndrome, or syndrome of inappropriate antidiuretic hormone secretion • For hyponatremia: fluid restriction, hypertonic saline • For hypernatremia: fluids, vasopressin
Intracranial hemorrhage	• Immediate CT scan to evaluate for early signs of a bleed • Monitor blood pressure • Check laboratory values: prothrombin time, partial thromboplastin time, platelets • Management of increased ICP, as described above • May need to intubate and ventilate • Surgery may be necessary to remove blood clot
Thromboembolism: deep venous thrombosis and pulmonary embolus (PE)	• Diagnosed through transcranial Doppler study or ventilation-perfusion scan • Heparinization *only after* CT scan has ruled out intracranial blood • Alternatively, vena cava filter (Greenfield filter) may be used • Large PEs require ICU care for further medical treatment
Seizures	• Potential for status epilepticus • Protect patient from injury • Titrate antiepileptics to therapeutic levels

Courtesy of Michael Torbey.

and family. When a decision has been made to proceed with surgery, extensive teaching is required in the perioperative period. Table 35-3 outlines the nurse's role in the plan of care for this patient population. Patient teaching is better retained if it is both verbal and written. Teaching sheets are useful and can be referred to at different times during the treatment period.

Although surgery and follow-up therapies are disruptive to patient and family activities, it is important to encourage a return to normalcy as soon as possible. Continuing with activities of daily living that encourage a positive and motivated attitude contributes to recovery.

Hospice

Multiple surgical procedures and adjuvant therapies are often successful in containing malignant brain tumors for a period of time. Inevitably, these tumors recur and become resistant to all treatment modalities. In addition, patient quality of life may be so compromised that further therapy is not feasible. Palliative care services are now available in many hospitals. Home and inpatient hospice are available in most communities and provide dedicated and supportive end-of-life care.[38,39]

ANEURYSMS

An aneurysm is a weakening in the arterial wall that causes either a ballooning effect or overall distention of the affected vessel. Aneurysms may be congenital or degenerative arterial lesions. Concern arises if the outpouching of the vessel wall ruptures or becomes large enough to exert pressure on surrounding brain structures.[40]

Approximately 20% to 40% of patients die from the initial bleed of their aneurysm before reaching medical care. Rebleeding is the leading cause of death in patients with a history of ruptured aneurysm. Of those who survive the initial bleeding, 35% to 40%

bleed again if left untreated, with a mortality rate of about 42%. Some recent data suggest that the mortality rate from initial hemorrhage is as high as 60%. Rebleeding most often occurs around the seventh day after the original bleed. Predictors of good recovery by 1 month after the bleed include a high score on the admission Glasgow Coma Scale (GCS) and an absence of blood on the first CT scan.[41]

Etiology

The etiology of aneurysms is unclear but is probably a combination of congenital and degenerative factors. Carmichael described the combination hypothesis of aneurysm formation. Of the three layers of an artery— tunica intima (innermost), tunica media (middle), and tunica adventitia (outer layer)—he found that congenital focal defects of the tunica media are common. However, degenerative changes are also necessary for the formation of aneurysms. Histological investigation of the normal vessel wall into the aneurysmal sac shows that the tunica media usually ends at the neck of the aneurysm and the internal elastic lamina becomes fragmented as it enters the sac. Consistent with this hypothesis, aneurysms are rare in childhood but are common into late adulthood.[41]

Although the exact cause of intracranial aneurysms is not understood, there is evidence to support that acquired and genetic factors contribute to the development of aneurysms. Genetic factors include heredity and genetically transmitted diseases. Acquired factors include traumatic brain injury, sepsis, cigarette smoking, and hypertension.[41]

Epidemiology

Intracranial aneurysms are common lesions, with autopsy reports indicating a prevalence of 1% to 5% of the adult population. Most of these aneurysms are small and do not rupture during the patient's lifetime, and some people have more than one aneurysm. In the United States, approximately 27,000 new cases of subarachnoid hemorrhage (SAH) each year are attributed to aneurysmal rupture. The incidence of SAH is 1 case per 10,000 persons.[42] The annual risk for rupture is about 1.34% per year.[43]

Aneurysm may also be associated with other pathological processes, such as polycystic kidney disease. Screening with MRI is warranted for patients with two immediate relatives with a history of intracranial aneurysm and for all patients with autosomal dominant polycystic kidney disease. The incidence of aneurysms increases with age, with peak incidence occurring between 55 and 60 years. They occur more often in women than in men and, as noted earlier, can be linked to cigarette smoking.[42] Seasonal variability is another epidemiological feature. Clinicians observed that there may be a seasonal variability, with increases occurring in spring and fall.

The Cooperative Study of Intracranial Aneurysms and Subarachnoid Hemorrhage reported that in 32% of cases, the hemorrhage occurred during physical activity. The study also reported that a similar proportion occurred during sleep. In summary, the incidence of SAH can be roughly divided into thirds: sleeping, active, and at rest.

Pathophysiology

Arterial vessels are composed of three layers: endothelial lining, smooth muscle, and connective tissue. A defect in the smooth muscle layer, or tunica media, allows the endothelial lining to bulge through, creating an aneurysm. Most aneurysms arise from larger arteries around the anterior section of the circle of Willis. The most frequent sites of occurrence in the anterior circulation are the anterior communicating artery, the posterior communicating artery, the middle cerebral artery bifurcation, and the internal carotid artery bifurcation. In the posterior circulation, the most common locations are the basilar artery apex and the posterior inferior cerebellar artery.[40]

As the intimal layers of the vessel weaken, high-velocity blood begins to flow to create a whirlpool effect, thus stretching the wall of the vessel. This creates an abnormal pocket or sac of blood. As the wall of the vessel expands, it begins to weaken and may eventually rupture. Compression by the sac on surrounding brain structures may result in focal neurologic deficits. Rupture of the aneurysm may result in subarachnoid, intracerebral, or intraventricular hemorrhage.[40]

Aneurysms may be classified according to shape. *Saccular* aneurysms are also known as "berry" because of a well-defined stem and berry-like outpouching of the medial layer of the arterial wall. Berry aneurysms are usually located on major cerebral arteries at the apex of branch points, which is where maximal hemodynamic stress occurs in the vessel (Fig. 35-3). *Fusiform* aneurysms are another type of aneurysm that occur more commonly in the vertebrobasilar system. Fusiform aneurysms are dilated circumferentially and usually occur secondary to atherosclerosis.[40] A third type of aneurysm is known as *mycotic*, which is due to infection.[44]

Aneurysms may also be categorized according to size. A small aneurysm is smaller than 10 mm, a large one is 10 to 20 mm, and a giant one is larger than 25 mm.[44] Giant aneurysms are a cause for great concern because they may compress surrounding brain tissue or compromise the existing circulation to that area.[40] Controversy exists about size and relationship to rupture.[44] Seven millimeters is the average size of a ruptured aneurysm, but smaller lesions routinely hemorrhage.

Hemorrhage from an aneurysm usually occurs in the subarachnoid space because aneurysm-forming vessels usually lie in the space between the arachnoid layer of the meninges and the brain. The force of the rupturing vessel can be so great that it can push blood through the pia mater and into the brain substance, causing an intracerebral hemorrhage. It can also push through the arachnoid into the subdural space, causing a subdural hemorrhage.

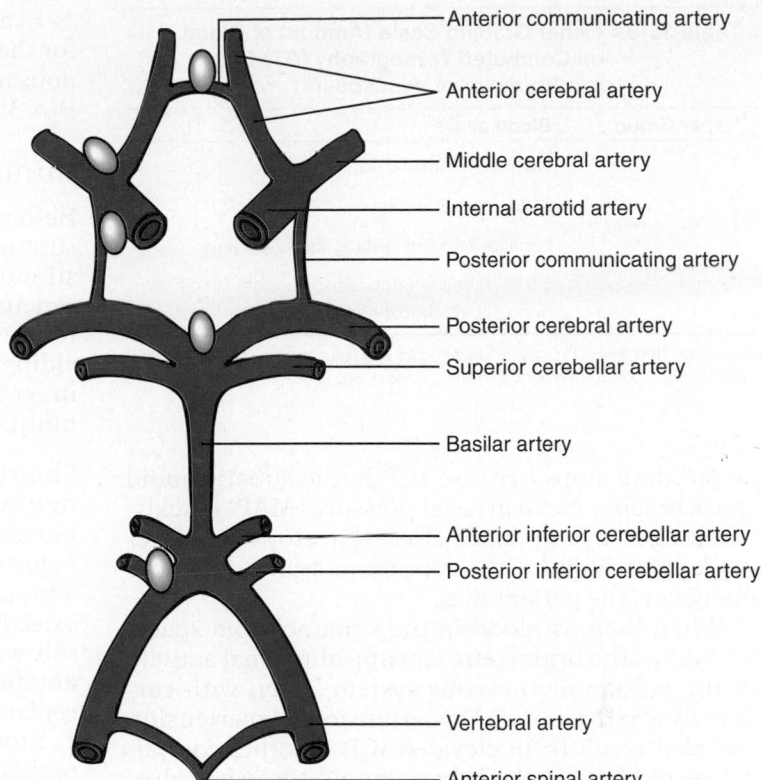

Anterior communicating artery

Anterior cerebral artery

Middle cerebral artery

Internal carotid artery

Posterior communicating artery

Posterior cerebral artery

Superior cerebellar artery

Basilar artery

Anterior inferior cerebellar artery

Posterior inferior cerebellar artery

Vertebral artery

Anterior spinal artery

Figure 35-3 • Circle of Willis with common aneurysm sites.

Clinical Manifestations

Many aneurysms are silent and never cause a problem but may be discovered on postmortem examination. An aneurysm that does cause problems typically does so between the ages of 35 and 60 years. Use of a grading scale can enhance the ability to determine clinical outcome.[40] Aneurysmal SAHs are graded according to their severity on the Hunt and Hess scale. In this grading system, grade 0 is the unruptured aneurysm, and grade V is a hemorrhage with severe neurological sequelae (Table 35-5).[45,46] However, the Hunt and Hess scale is not the only grading system that has been developed for SAH. The World Federation of Neurological Surgeons grading scale is also used for SAH. The Fisher scale is another grading scale that is used to estimate the density of subarachnoid blood on CT scan at the time of a patient's admission to the hospital (Table 35-6). A score of 3 or 4 on the Fisher scale has been found to increase the likelihood of poor clinical outcomes. A score of 1 to 2 has not been shown to increase mortality rates.[47]

Approximately half of patients have some warning signs before an aneurysm ruptures. These signs may include headache, lethargy, neck pain, a "noise in the head," and optic, oculomotor, or trigeminal cranial nerve dysfunction.

After an aneurysm has bled or ruptured, the patient usually complains of a horrific headache. The classic description is "the worst headache of my life," which is often abbreviated as WHOL in the medical record.[44] Other symptoms that may accompany SAH or aneurysms that present with mass effect are nausea, vomiting, focal neurologic deficits, or coma.

Aneurysms presenting with mass effect typically show symptoms associated with increased ICP.[40] With an SAH, there are also signs of meningeal irritation, such as a stiff and painful neck, photophobia, blurred vision, irritability, fever, positive Kernig's sign, and positive Brudzinski's sign. Exactly which deficits are present depends on the location of the aneurysm, the subsequent hemorrhage, and the severity of the bleeding.

Table 35-5 • Hunt and Hess Grading Scale for Aneurysms	
Grade 0	Unruptured aneurysm
Grade I	Asymptomatic Minimal headache Slight nuchal rigidity (neck stiffness)
Grade II	Moderate to severe headache Nuchal rigidity Cranial nerve deficits
Grade III	Lethargy Mental confusion Mild focal neurological deficit
Grade IV	Stupor Moderate to severe motor deficit Possible posturing
Grade V	Deep coma Posturing Declining appearance

Adapted from Mower-Wade D, Cavanaugh MC, Bush C: Protecting a patient with ruptured cerebral aneurysm. Nursing 2001 31(2):52–58, 2001.

Table 35-6 • Fisher Grading Scale (Amount of Blood on Computed Tomography (CT) Scan Is a Predictor of Vasospasm)	
Fisher Group	**Blood on CT**
1	No subarachnoid blood detected
2	Diffuse or vertical layers <1 mm thick
3	Localized and/or vertical layers ≥1 mm
4	Intracerebral or intraventricular clot with diffuse or no subarachnoid hemorrhage

Hickey JV: The Clinical Practice of Neurological and Neurosurgical Nursing, 5th ed. Philadelphia: Lippincott Williams & Wilkins, 2003.

Bleeding stops because ICP in the subarachnoid space reaches mean arterial pressure (MAP) quickly, resulting in a tamponade effect that stops the bleeding long enough for the rupture to seal. If this does not occur, the patient dies.

When there is blood in the subarachnoid space, it irritates the brainstem, causing abnormal activity in the autonomic nervous system, often with cardiac dysrhythmias and hypertension. Hypertension can also result from elevated ICP. Another complication of blood in the subarachnoid space is hydrocephalus. Blood in the subarachnoid space impedes reabsorption of CSF by the arachnoid villi. Hydrocephalus results in enlargement of the lateral and third ventricles.

Diagnosis

The diagnosis of a cerebral aneurysm usually is made on the basis of history, physical examination, CT scan, lumbar puncture, and cerebral angiogram. When the nurse takes the patient's history, he or she identifies risk factors such as genetic predisposition, hypertension, and cigarette smoking. Patients with an SAH may present with a headache, neck discomfort, or both without any neurological signs. The headache may range in severity from mild to severe. A CT scan reveals hemorrhage in most cases when it is obtained within 24 hours of the hemorrhage. It has the most sensitivity when obtained within 24 hours of onset. There is a steady decline over ensuing days, with approximately 50% of CTs being positive 5 days after an SAH occurs.[44]

If the results of a CT scan are negative and there are signs and symptoms indicating that a patient has experienced an SAH, a lumbar puncture is typically performed to confirm the diagnosis. After a positive lumbar puncture, a cerebral angiogram is obtained to determine the source of the SAH. Different types of angiography may be used for this purpose, including CT angiography, MRA, or digital subtraction angiography (DSA). Although all of these studies can determine vascular anatomy, DSA is the gold standard if surgery is planned.[40] Transcranial Doppler (TCD) ultrasonography can also be used to diagnose and treat vasospasm, a common complication of an SAH.

Examples of diagnoses and collaborative problems for the patient with a cerebral aneurysm or arteriovenous malformations (discussed later) are presented in Box 35-1.

Clinical Management

Before repair, the management of a patient with a ruptured or leaking aneurysm focuses on minimal stimulation of the patient. Some institutions initiate "aneurysm precautions" as precautionary measures to prevent rebleeding. These measures include providing a quiet environment, establishing a bowel regimen to prevent straining (Valsalva maneuver), and limiting visitors.[40]

Pharmacological Management
Antihypertensive medications may be used to manage blood pressure before procedures or surgery.[40] Plasma volume should not be allowed to fall. Frequently, abnormalities of electrolytes, notably hyponatremia, exist. Hyponatremia, usually associated with cerebral salt wasting rather than syndrome of inappropriate antidiuretic hormone, must be managed with sodium replacement and euvolemia.[44]

Stool softeners are used in the management of patients with an aneurysm to prevent straining. Mild analgesics can be used to relieve headaches. An antipyretic, usually acetaminophen, and hypothermia blankets can be used to manage fever; acetaminophen can be used without masking neurological signs. Judicious use of narcotics is appropriate in these patients. Blood in the subarachnoid space causes an elevated temperature.

Surgical Management
Clipping Surgical clipping may be considered if the aneurysm is in an accessible area. The goal of surgery is complete obliteration of the aneurysm. Aneurysms of the vertebrobasilar system often present the problem of surgical inaccessibility. The accepted surgical treatment is the placement of a clip across the neck of the aneurysm. These clips, which are made of titanium, come in a variety of shapes and sizes. For

---

> **Box 35-1**
> **Examples of Nursing Diagnoses and Collaborative Problems for the Patient With Cerebral Aneurysm or Arteriovenous Malformations**
>
> - Altered Cerebral Tissue Perfusion related to interruption in cerebral blood flow or intracranial hypertension
> - Pain related to meningeal irritation
> - Risk for Sensory/Perceptual Alterations (visual, auditory, kinesthetic, and tactile) related to altered level of consciousness, disorientation, impaired communication skills, restricted or unfamiliar environment, photophobia
> - Risk for Fluid Volume Excess related to hypervolemia used to treat vasospasm
> - Risk for Fluid Volume Deficit related to fluid restriction and use of osmotics to control intracranial hypertension

larger or wider aneurysms, more than one clip can be used to ensure complete occlusion of the neck of the aneurysm.[40] Once clipped, the aneurysm may be punctured to allow it to collapse and relieve mass effect if present.[44]

Some aneurysms may be wrapped in a gauzelike material or coated with an acrylic substance that gives the aneurysm support. Although wrapping or coating should not be the goal of surgery, there may be conditions, as with a fusiform aneurysm, in which there is no other option.

In the past several years, there has been controversy over when surgical intervention should occur. The current philosophy is that surgery should occur sooner rather than later. Thus, surgery is generally performed 24 to 48 hours after the bleed occurs (Fig. 35-4).

After aneurysm clipping, the patient is managed in a critical care environment. Maintenance of an adequate airway is vital. If the patient is intubated and suctioning is needed, it is important that the suction catheter be passed and removed quickly to prevent desaturation.

Signs of vasospasm, such as hemiparesis, visual disturbance, seizures, or a decreasing level of consciousness, should be noted and reported so that medical interventions can be rapidly implemented. Control of ICP is a collaborative effort. Nurses should keep the head of the patient's bed elevated without neck flexion or severe rotation. Nursing care activities should be spaced to avoid causing a sharp rise in ICP.

Coiling One of the most valuable recent developments in the management of aneurysms has been the technique of endovascular thrombosis of aneurysms with Guglielmi detachable coils (GDCs). These are thrombogenic platinum alloy microcoils. They are soft to allow the coil to conform to the shape of the aneurysm. Coils are available in various shapes, dimensions, lengths, and diameters to provide maximal occlusion.[48]

The procedure used to introduce the coil into the aneurysm is similar to that used for a cerebral angiogram, using the femoral artery and fluoroscopic equipment. In this procedure, a microcatheter is passed through the aorta, around the aortic arch, and then into the vessel specific to the aneurysm. Once the catheter is in position, the coil system is advanced through the catheter into the aneurysm sac. The coil is then in position, and if placement is satisfactory, a low-voltage current is applied. The current causes the coil to detach. If the coil is successfully placed, it occludes the aneurysm and separates it from the cerebral circulation. The number of coils placed is individualized to the patient. Through this coiling procedure, the risk for hemorrhage or rehemorrhage is decreased.[48]

Complications of this treatment are embolic stroke, coil migration, failure to obliterate the aneurysm, and aneurysm rupture. Stroke may occur because the parent artery feeding the aneurysm becomes occluded or because of the introduction of air or particles into the catheter system. Coil migration occurs because of

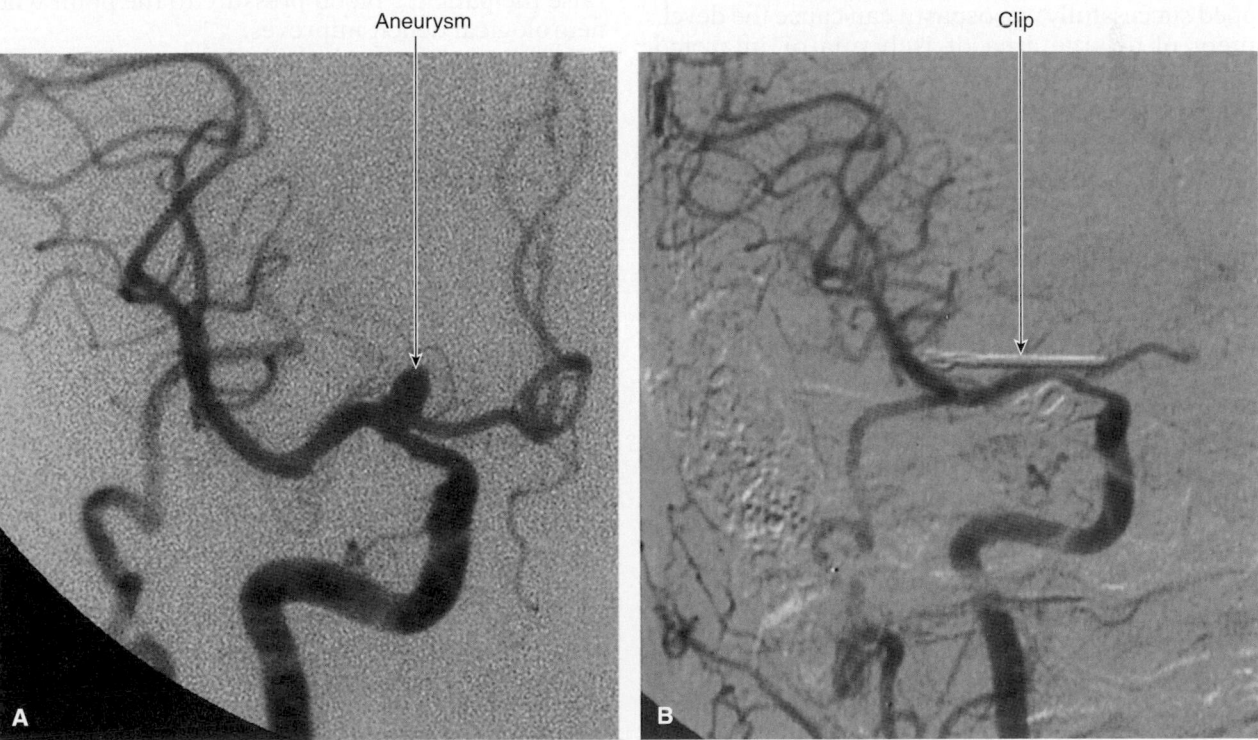

Figure 35-4 • Preoperative (**A**) and postoperative (**B**) angiography: clipping of right internal carotid artery termination aneurysm. (Courtesy of Rafael Tamargo, MD, and Richard Clatterbuck, MD, Johns Hopkins University, Baltimore, MD.)

reintroduction of blood into the sac. The coils become repositioned outside the fundus of the sac and can then flow to other anatomic areas of the brain, creating disturbances. Failure to obliterate the aneurysm is also a possibility. If the coils fail to obliterate the aneurysm, the sac may grow larger, cause more symptoms, and may even rupture. Further intervention with another endovascular procedure or surgery is then warranted.[40]

Although clipping is the preferred treatment or gold standard for most aneurysms, GDC coiling is an option for patients who are considered to be surgically high risk because of medical instability, or those who would otherwise be treated conservatively. With the rapidly evolving technology, endovascular embolization of cerebral aneurysms is a safe alternative to surgical clipping in the treatment of ruptured and unruptured cerebral aneurysms. Long-term outcomes require further study.[49] Some experts currently consider coiling to be the preferred treatment, although this is still a matter of controversy.

Medical Management of Complications

As previously noted, vasospasm can occur after, as well as before, surgery in the patient with an aneurysm. Angiographic vasospasm is seen early. Vasospasm may be recognized clinically through frequent neurological assessment. The patient's signs and symptoms can fluctuate but may include changes in level of consciousness, headache, language impairment, hemiparesis, and seizures.[46]

Vasospasm usually occurs 3 to 12 days after an SAH. The peak incidence is between postbleed days 7 and 10. Although the aneurysm may have been clipped successfully, vasospasm can cause the development of a large area of ischemia or infarcted brain, with severe deficits. Vasospasm is of clinical significance because it decreases cerebral blood flow, depriving brain tissue of oxygen and promoting accumulation of metabolic waste products, such as lactic acid. "The reduced size of the vessel lumen restricts blood flow to the brain tissue, causing temporarily irreversible vasoconstriction."[46]

TCD imaging is a valuable noninvasive technique used to diagnose vasospasm. This technique, which can be performed at the bedside, measures the velocity of blood flow through segments of the arterial vessels. Monitoring trends in flow velocity allows prompt identification of patients at risk for the development of vasospasm. The results of the neurological examination can be correlated with TCD findings for prompt diagnosis and treatment of vasospasm. This technique is highly reliable in predicting vasospasm of the middle cerebral and internal carotid arteries.[46]

The exact etiology of vasospasm is not clear. Apparently, there is a positive correlation between the size of the hemorrhage seen on CT scan and the subsequent development of spasm. Vasospasm is likely caused by inflammatory processes. There has been some success in using nimodipine, a calcium antagonist, after an SAH to improve patient outcomes. It is recommended that nimodipine be used from onset through day 21.[50] Nimodipine reduces the contraction of smooth and cardiac muscles without affecting skeletal muscles. The dose is 60 mg every 4 hours. The theory is that nimodipine improves outcomes by limiting collateral cerebral damage that is mediated by calcium.

"Triple H" therapy is the standard for the prevention and treatment of vasospasm. It consists of hypervolemic expansion, hemodilution, and induced hypertension in postoperative patients.[50] Nimodipine is used with this therapy. These measures reduce smooth muscle spasm and maximize perfusion when spasm does occur.

Hypervolemia is accomplished by volume expansion, using both intravenous (IV) colloid and crystalloid solutions. They are given to increase intravascular volume and decrease blood viscosity. Through hypervolemia, the cerebral vessels dilate and the MAP increases, thereby improving cerebral perfusion pressure (CPP). During this therapy, the patient should be monitored for pulmonary edema and heart failure. A pulmonary artery catheter helps monitor the patient's hemodynamic status.

Hemodilution through the administration of IV fluids decreases blood viscosity, increases regional cerebral blood flow, and may decrease infarction size and increase oxygen transport. The goal of hemodilution is to reduce the hematocrit by 15%. The patient's hematocrit level should be maintained between 30% and 33%, which helps improve cerebral blood flow (CBF) without causing hypoxia.

Vasopressors are used to induce hypertension. The objective is to maintain systolic blood pressure at greater than 20 mm Hg over normal. Vasopressors raise the patient's blood pressure to the point where neurological deficit improves.

When conventional medical therapy is not effective, acute arterial vasospasm secondary to an SAH can be managed by balloon angioplasty in centers where this technology is available. Recent advances in microballoon technology now allow access to the cerebral vasculature with soft, flexible angioplasty balloons, which mechanically dilate and improve CBF through the major arterial segments affected by vasospasm. Balloon angioplasty allows direct widening of the stenotic segment.[46]

Another complication after aneurysmal rupture is hydrocephalus. Hydrocephalus indicates an imbalance between the production and absorption of CSF. It may occur in patients who have experienced an SAH. When there is blood in the subarachnoid space, the red blood cells can occlude the very small channels leading from one ventricle to another. If this occurs, an obstructive hydrocephalus develops. In this case, there is an obstruction of the normal flow of CSF, often between the third and fourth ventricles, or at the exits from the fourth ventricle. There is also the potential for a reabsorption problem, whereby red blood cells occlude the arachnoid villi, impeding reabsorption and resulting in a communicating hydrocephalus. The patient may require a shunt. With a ventriculoperitoneal shunt, the proximal tip of the catheter is placed in a lateral ventricle, and the distal tip is placed in the peritoneum. The shunt drains into the peritoneal cavity to treat the hydrocephalus.

Seizures may occur from blood in the subarachnoid space acting as an irritant. Typically, patients are placed on an anticonvulsant to minimize seizure risk.

Rebleeding is another complication in patients with an SAH if the aneurysm is not repaired. At least 10% of all patients with an SAH have another bleed within hours of the initial hemorrhage. Without intervention, the risk for rebleeding in the remaining patients is at least 30% during the subsequent 3 weeks. The immediate mortality rate of rebleeding is about 60%.

Nursing Management

Assessment One of the nurse's primary responsibilities is to obtain a baseline neurological assessment and perform subsequent assessments to monitor for changes. After surgery, the nurse must be alert to the development of new deficits or a worsening of preoperative deficits. The severity and duration of any postoperative disability depend largely on the location and extent of the vascular lesion and resultant ischemia. The patient must also be carefully monitored for the development of cerebral edema.

Plan Before surgery, the nurse implements aneurysm precautions by providing a quiet environment with limited stimulation. The nurse does a bowel assessment and implements individualized interventions.

A patent airway is required. Management of the patient's fluid and electrolytes includes careful monitoring for hyponatremia, which can cause an increase in cerebral edema. Accurate intake and output measurements are imperative.

The nurse also monitors vital signs to avoid any significant change, especially in blood pressure. Hypotension must be treated immediately to prevent a drop in cerebral perfusion. Cardiac dysrhythmias may be present, especially if there was bleeding into the subarachnoid space. Dysrhythmias require prompt management because they may precipitate a drop in cardiac output and a consequent drop in cerebral perfusion.

A patent IV site is maintained for hydration. Continuous fluids are a part of the management of vasospasm. The IV site is monitored frequently, and fluids are not interrupted for any reason. In the event of an infiltrate, the nurse restarts the line immediately.

Measures also need to be taken to manage increased ICP if it develops. Measures such as hyperventilation and osmotic diuretics are valuable tools in managing cerebral edema.

Emotional support is also a crucial part of the overall nursing care of the patient with a ruptured aneurysm. Because of an aneurysm's abrupt onset, the hospital admission cannot be planned. Often the rupture suddenly interrupts the patient's daily life and perhaps leaves the patient with neurological impairment. The patient's support system needs to be organized to tend to daily activities and responsibilities in his or her absence. Families require assistance when confronting the financial, physical, and emotional burden of caring for a patient after an SAH.[50] A social worker can be instrumental in helping to organize the support of friends and family.

Patient Education and Discharge Planning

Smoking and hypertension are both preventable risk factors associated with intracranial aneurysm and SAH. Patients can be instructed that cessation of smoking and control of hypertension can reduce the incidence of aneurysm formation and rupture.

Patients who have undergone clipping of cerebral aneurysms should be carefully screened before MRI. Titanium clips used after 1996 are "MRI friendly." It is necessary to ascertain the composition of the clip before MRI.

If a patient has experienced a seizure and is being maintained on anticonvulsant therapy, instructions should be given about medication monitoring and the need for compliance. In addition, the patient should be instructed about seizure safety.

Patients who have experienced SAH face a lengthy recovery. Rehabilitation for specific deficits should begin early. Also, family participation in the rehabilitation plan is encouraged. Members of the health care team, such as physical, occupational, and speech therapists, can help restore independence.[50] Services can be coordinated either for inpatient or outpatient settings, depending on the extent of impairment and insurance coverage.

ARTERIOVENOUS MALFORMATIONS

Arteriovenous malformations (AVMs) are lesions consisting of dilated arteries and veins without a capillary system. Arterial blood flows directly into the venous system. AVMs are usually described as a "tangle" of blood vessels with a well-defined nidus that does not involve brain parenchyma. Presumably, AVMs are congenital, and they typically enlarge with age. Although they are found throughout the central nervous system (CNS), approximately 90% of AVMs are located in the cerebrum. Of these, the most common locations are the frontal and temporal lobes, most often supplied by the middle cerebral artery.[51,52]

Epidemiology

AVMs are relatively uncommon brain lesions. Population-based studies have estimated an occurrence rate of 1.1 per 100,000 persons. However, autopsy studies report a 1% to 4% occurrence rate. There is no statistically significant predisposition by sex. AVMs are diagnosed most often in young adults, and average age at diagnosis is 33 years, with 64% of AVMs being detected in people younger than 40 years. In cases in which the patient has both an AVM and an aneurysm (7%), the symptomatic lesion is treated initially. In some instances, both can be surgically treated at the same time. Of the two, aneurysms are more likely to be the cause of hemorrhage.[52,53]

Pathophysiology

AVMs develop as an atypical preservation of embryonic connections between arteries and veins, most likely between the fourth and eighth weeks of embryo development. This is the period in which cells begin to differentiate and capillary components to the brain develop. AVMs are most likely to arise at this time because of the failure of the primitive vasculature to develop an adequate capillary system. Because blood is shunted directly from the arterial to the venous circulation without benefit of a capillary bed, there is less resistance, and AVMs receive significant blood flow. Arteries and veins enlarge to carry this increased flow, and their walls are characteristically quite thin. Arteries providing blood to the malformation and draining veins also become enlarged with increased flow volume in the lesion.[54,55]

Clinical Manifestations

Hemorrhage, the most common presenting sign of AVMs, occurs in 50% to 70% of affected patients. These hemorrhages may be intracerebral, subdural, or subarachnoid. Opinions differ regarding whether the size of the lesion affects the likelihood of a bleed. Small size may be associated with an increased risk for hemorrhage, which may be caused by higher flow and pressure from the feeding vessels.[52] Conversely, according to the results of a prospective study, large and deep lesions are more likely to cause hemorrhage.[56] The location of the AVM also affects the risk for a bleed. Periventricular, intraventricular, and posterior fossa lesions have a higher risk for bleeding.[53]

There is an approximate 30% to 50% morbidity rate and 10% mortality rate after a bleed. The risk for a rebleed is higher in the first year after the initial hemorrhage and declines over subsequent years. Cerebral AVMs cause about 4% to 5% of SAHs. An SAH caused by an AVM is less lethal than one caused by an aneurysm rupture but is associated with significant neurological morbidity.[52]

Seizures are another common presenting sign (>25%) of an AVM. The risk for a seizure increases with the size of the lesion. Patients are treated with AEDs after presentation with a seizure, but AEDs are not routinely used prophylactically for AVMs. Seizures are more likely to occur in patients who have large and more superficial AVMs.[55]

Other presenting signs include headache (1% to 11%), increased ICP, neurological deficits (5% to 7%) referable to the location of the lesion, bruit, and visual symptoms. Cognitive decline is seen particularly in older patients with large AVMs. This may be related to cerebral steal, which can cause ischemic changes by diverting arterial blood away from normal brain tissue to the AVM.[53]

AVMs are graded based on features, location, and venous drainage. The Spetzler-Martin grading system assigns 1 point for lesions less than 3 cm, 2 points for 3- to 6-cm lesions, and 3 points for lesions greater than 6 cm. If the AVM is located in an eloquent area of the brain, it is given 1 point. No points are given for noneloquent areas. Deep venous drainage associated with the malformation is allotted 1 point, with no points for superficial venous drainage. A low score is associated with better outcomes and a higher score with increased morbidity from surgery.[57]

Diagnosis

CT and MRI are used to evaluate the presence of an AVM. The lesion is differentiated from tumors and other brain lesions by the presence of a hemosiderin ring around the lesion. Three-dimensional imaging is useful in establishing the malformation in relation to the surrounding anatomy. MRA is a noninvasive method of evaluating feeding and draining vessels in relation to the nidus of the AVM. Although MRA does provide useful information, it is not consistently able to replace the more invasive angiography that is also used to evaluate feeding arteries and draining veins. Rarely, the AVM is not angiographically evident. This may be true of lesions that have bled, have small feeding and draining vessels, or have low flow. TCD, single-photon emission computed tomography (SPECT), and PET are also used to image blood flow changes. To identify the AVM in relation to eloquent areas of the brain (sensory, motor, speech, visual, brainstem), fMRI is useful.[51]

Clinical Management

AVMs can be managed in a number of ways. Management decisions are based on the patient's age and medical condition, flow associated with the malformation, history of hemorrhage, other symptoms, and the location of the lesion. Table 35-7 outlines procedures, indications, outcomes, and possible complications.

Interventional, Surgical, and Radiosurgical Management

Endovascular embolization of feeding arteries is used for small, low-grade malformations. The cure rate is low (10% to 15%), and one or more procedures may be needed to occlude the abnormal vessels. Embolization is used as an adjunct to surgery and radiosurgery. In this procedure, particles, liquids, balloons, or coils are inserted into the AVM nidus before surgery or radiosurgery.[58]

Stereotactic radiosurgery provides good outcomes for relatively small lesions. This can be accomplished by gamma knife, linear accelerator, or heavy ion radiation. When radiosurgery is used for lesions less than 3 cm in diameter, the cure rate is estimated at 65% to 85%. However, complete obliteration of the malformation takes 2 to 3 years, and there is a risk for hemorrhage during this time.[52]

Surgery is the preferred treatment for most AVMs. Surgery can reduce the risk for both hemorrhage and seizure. Brain mapping, fMRI, and intraoperative evoked potentials may be used in surgical planning for lesions in eloquent areas of the brain. Outcomes are positive, particularly in the case of Spetzler-Martin grade I and II lesions. Not only are neurological complications low, but also surgery provides

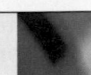

Table 35-7 • Management of the Patient With an Arteriovenous Malformation

Procedure	Indication	Outcome	Complications and Comments
Surgery	Surgically accessible arteriovenous malformation (AVM)	Removal of lesion Decreased risk for bleed Improved seizure control Preoperative propranolol believed to minimize postoperative bleed and edema Labetalol used to keep mean arterial pressure (MAP) 70–80 mm Hg perioperatively	Inability to remove lesion Risks for surgery: cerebral edema; hemorrhage; neurological deficits Inpatient hospital stay Excellent results in Spetzler-Martin grade I–III lesions
Radiation: stereotactic radiosurgery (SRS) (external beam radiation effective in only a small percentage of cases; gamma knife, proton beam, or linear accelerator used)	≤ 3 cm AVM Surgery not indicated	Reduction in size of lesion Noninvasive Outpatient, no recovery period	Lesion not removed May take years for complete obliteration May require multiple treatments Continued risk for bleed for 2–3 y Used for small AVMs or as part of multimodality treatment
Embolization	Injection of substance to occlude the feeder vessels	Facilitates other therapies (surgery; radiation) by reducing AVM Useful for larger AVMs Short hospital stay	Does not typically cure AVM May need more than one procedure Need to wait days or weeks before surgery or SRS Risk for stroke or hemorrhage

Data from references 53, 56, 59, and 86.

an immediate cure. Intraoperative angiography is recommended.[52,53]

Treatment approaches vary between surgery and radiosurgery for Spetzler-Martin grade III lesions. For large AVMs or lesions in eloquent areas of the brain, multimodality therapy with embolization, radiosurgery, or microsurgery is preferred.[59] The most appropriate treatment approach for Spetzler-Martin grade IV and V lesions is a matter of controversy. Some practitioners recommend the multimodality approach, and others opt for no treatment.

Nursing Management

Assessment The nursing management of the patient with an AVM is similar to that described for a patient with a cerebral aneurysm. Baseline and follow-up neurological assessments are necessary to monitor for subtle changes or evidence of hemorrhage.

Plan Careful evaluation of focal neurological signs or evidence of cerebral edema minimizes significant postoperative morbidity.

Patient Education and Discharge Planning

Patients who have experienced a hemorrhage or seizures secondary to an AVM are managed in much the same way as patients with aneurysms. Safeguards and family teaching include a discussion of signs of increased ICP; seizure control and safety; anticonvulsant therapy; postoperative complications; and side effects of radiation, when appropriate.

SURGICAL APPROACHES

Neurological surgery may be performed in a number of situations:

1. To obtain tissue for pathological diagnosis
2. To remove an abnormal mass or space-occupying lesion (e.g., tumor, cyst, hemorrhage) and, consequently, to reduce mass effect
3. To repair an abnormality (e.g., aneurysm)
4. To place a device (e.g., shunt, reservoir)

A number of factors are considered when making the appropriate surgical decision. Diagnostic studies are first performed to establish a differential diagnosis. Patient age, neurological status, and concurrent medical conditions are factors in the decision to proceed with surgery and the decision regarding the appropriate approach. The most commonly used surgical procedures are briefly described in the following sections.

Stereotactic Biopsy

A stereotactic biopsy is used to obtain tissue for definitive pathological diagnosis. It is often used when a tumor is suspected but the lesion is too small or deep for surgical removal. It is used for tumors in eloquent areas of the brain, lesions crossing the corpus callosum, and multiple lesions that are not resectable. A stereotactic biopsy is also used to confirm the diagnosis of previously treated tumors—for example, when a malignant glioma has been treated with multiple therapies, tissue is obtained and analyzed to differentiate active tumor from treatment effect (i.e., necrosis). In addition, some patients may have multiple medical problems and be too ill to proceed with a craniotomy. Others may opt to have the less invasive biopsy.

The goal of stereotactic surgery is to locate a target using a trajectory. Stereotactic biopsies with a frame require placement of a rigid head frame to establish the appropriate coordinates. Next, a contrast-enhanced CT scan or MRI is obtained in the radiology suite by using the localizing frame. An axial image of the tumor is displayed, with a number of coordinates to indicate entry points. After the imaging is completed, the patient is usually transferred from the radiology suite to the operating room for completion of the procedure. The biopsy can be performed under general or local anesthesia. After the skin is shaved and prepared, a small hole (twist drill or burr hole) is made, a needle is passed to the lesion, and one or more biopsies are obtained and immediately evaluated by a pathologist. Once sufficient tissue or cyst fluid is obtained for diagnostic purposes, the procedure is complete. Because of the possibility of sampling error, it is not unusual for the neurosurgeon to take multiple specimens from various areas of the tumor, when feasible.[60,61]

A stereotactic biopsy may also be performed without a frame. Frameless stereotaxy is a navigational system used to generate a three-dimensional tumor image. A CT or MRI scan is taken before the procedure, and markers (fiducials) are placed on the scalp. The markers are evident on the scan and are used to determine the actual target. A computer image is then generated from the imaging data.[60]

Craniotomy

A craniotomy is performed to remove a space-occupying abnormality such as a tumor, cyst, or vascular malformation. This procedure may also be needed on an emergency basis to evacuate a hematoma or reverse a herniation syndrome. When appropriate, a craniotomy is used to clip an aneurysm.

In this procedure, a skin incision is made, the bone flap is elevated, the dura is opened, and the lesion is subjected to biopsy or resection. The neurosurgical patient has quite distinct intraoperative pharmacological needs. The neuroanesthesiologist administers agents that provide the needed anesthetic effect while minimizing risks for increasing ICP or lowering seizure threshold. Rapid reversibility is also particularly important in patients receiving a craniotomy because their postoperative neurological status needs to be assessed quickly.

In addition to the equipment used during surgery to maximize safety and efficiency, specific tools for intraoperative monitoring may enhance the outcome for these patients. During the past 10 to 15 years, significant advances have taken place. Ultrasonography has been a standard of neurosurgical monitoring for some years because it can distinguish abnormal lesions from normal brain tissue and edema. Residual abnormal tissue may be identified before closing. Frameless stereotaxy, as described previously, is also used during craniotomy. It is thought that this procedure enhances surgical safety and effectiveness by reducing craniotomy size, minimizing brain manipulation, and maximizing tumor resection. Cortical mapping is used for masses in eloquent areas of the brain. Somatosensory evoked potentials are recorded during surgery under general anesthesia to assess the relationship between the motor strip and the lesion to be resected. Direct cortical stimulation provides for localization of the sensory-motor cortex and is also used to minimize neurological deficits and maximize tumor removal. In some cases, greater seizure control is accomplished with these procedures. Direct cortical stimulation requires local anesthesia and the patient to be conscious during much of the procedure.[62-66]

Craniotomies have been enhanced by the use of microscopes, operating loupes, self-retaining retractors, high-speed drills, ultrasonic aspirators (using sound waves), and laser (using light beams). Bipolar coagulation is used to minimize bleeding.[63]

Postoperative management of the patient who has undergone a craniotomy or stereotactic biopsy for a brain tumor focuses on assessment of and intervention for a number of potential complications. In the immediate postoperative period, patients may be slow to respond because of the effects of general anesthesia. Temporary changes in mental status or new focal neurological signs should resolve rather quickly in this situation. If there is a significant change from the baseline examination, radiographic documentation of hemorrhage or cerebral edema is performed. A CT scan or MRI is obtained to rule out postoperative complications. Edema is expected and can often be treated with corticosteroids. If significantly increased ICP occurs, the patient is medically managed in an intensive care environment under close observation. Occasionally, surgical intervention is required for acute postoperative hemorrhage.

Other postoperative monitoring includes evaluation of vital signs and neurological vital signs; early ambulation to avoid pulmonary and cardiovascular complications; physical and occupational therapy evaluations; speech and cognitive assessment when indicated; DVT and PE prophylaxis; and wound evaluation and care.

Transsphenoidal and Transnasal Surgeries

Transsphenoidal and transnasal surgeries are being used in many centers to remove pituitary tumors and cysts. The transnasal and transsphenoidal approaches replace transcranial surgery, when appropriate. An estimated 75% to 95% of cases are treated in this way. The patient is positioned on the operating table under general anesthesia. The sphenoid sinus is opened, the sella is opened, and the tumor is removed using the surgical microscope. If there is evidence of a CSF leak at the time of surgery, the sellar cavity is packed with fat tissue, typically taken from the patient's abdomen. The mucosal incision is closed with reabsorbable sutures. Nasal septal splints are applied.

This procedure is usually well tolerated. Postoperative care is aimed at increasing mobility, monitoring respiration, evaluating fluid and electrolyte balance, and observing for evidence of CSF leak. The major risks of intracranial surgery—cerebral edema and intracerebral hemorrhage—are avoided.[67] Nasal splints are removed 2 to 4 days after surgery.

Neuroendoscopy as a Surgical Tool

Endoscopic microsurgical techniques are being used with increasing frequency. This surgical tool provides improved visualization of normal anatomy and of abnormal lesions. It is most often used for smaller, avascular lesions of soft consistency. Colloid and choroid plexus cysts, ependymomas, some skull base tumors, and certain gliomas are amenable to this approach. The technique involves the use of an angled, flexible scope, thus enhancing the approach to tumor removal and aneurysm clipping. Additionally, it allows for improved inspection during transsphenoidal surgery, providing closer evaluation of the pituitary tumor versus the normal gland.

In selected endoscopic cases, frameless stereotaxy is used to increase accuracy and minimize brain trauma. It should be noted that surgeon experience and expertise are crucial to minimizing morbidity and maximizing the effectiveness of this approach.[68,69]

• Neurological Disorders

STROKE   CONCEPTS in action ANIMATION

Cerebrovascular disease includes any pathological process that involves the blood vessels of the brain. It is the most frequent neurological disorder that affects adults. Most cerebrovascular disease is caused by thrombosis, embolism, or hemorrhage. The mechanism of each of these etiologies is different, but the ultimate result is damage to a focal area of the brain.

A stroke may be defined as a neurological deficit that has a sudden onset, results in permanent damage to the brain, and is caused by cerebrovascular disease. A stroke occurs when there is a disruption of blood flow to a region of the brain. Blood flow is disrupted because of an obstruction of a vessel, a thrombus or embolus, or the rupture of a vessel. The clinical features seen depend on the location of the event and region of the brain perfused by the vessel.[70]

A stroke is now referred to as a "brain attack" to encourage health care professionals and the public to think about stroke with the same urgency as a "heart attack." A "brain attack" must be viewed as a medical emergency. To reverse cerebral ischemia, patients must be evaluated promptly. Ischemic brain injury occurs when arterial occlusion lasts longer than 2 to 3 hours. Delay in seeking medical care may eliminate the potential for tissue-saving therapy with thrombolytic agents. Stroke is the third leading cause of death in the United States, and even if it is not fatal, it often results in serious long-term disability.

During the past several years, advances have been made in the treatment of stroke. Early recognition and prompt entry into the emergency medical system are essential to reduce death and disability from stroke. Media campaigns have been launched to increase public awareness about the signs and symptoms of stroke so that care may be sought promptly.

A recent innovation in the way stroke care is delivered has involved the establishment of the Joint Commission's certified stroke centers. The Joint Commission implemented a Disease-Specific Care Certification program in 2002, and stroke was one of the disease-specific categories in which program certification could be achieved. In this voluntary program, organizations have disease management programs reviewed by the Joint Commission. Criteria for the program include compliance with consensus-based national standards, effective use of established clinical practice guidelines to manage and optimize care, and an organized approach to monitor performance improvement activities.[70] Achievement of Primary Stroke Center certification denotes clinical excellence in the management of stroke provided by a multidisciplinary team from several departments. This designation is attractive to many institutions that aspire to be recognized for their care of stroke patients.

Etiology

Approximately three fourths of strokes in the United States are due to vascular obstruction (thrombi or emboli), resulting in ischemia and infarction. About one fourth of strokes in the United States are hemorrhagic, resulting from hypertensive vascular disease (which causes an intracerebral hemorrhage), a ruptured aneurysm, or an arteriovenous malformation. Figure 35-5 outlines stroke classification.

Epidemiology

Approximately 700,000 people have a new or recurrent stroke each year, with a mortality rate of 22%. Even though the average age of stroke is 70 years, 40% of all strokes occur in people younger than 60 years. "Women have overtaken men in stroke incidence, with about 40,000 more women than men experiencing strokes annually. Because the life expectancy for women is longer than men, more women actually die of stroke, accounting for 61% of stroke deaths."[70] It is estimated that there are 3 million stroke survivors and that stroke is a leading cause of disability and a leading diagnosis for long-term care.[47] Risk factors for stroke include smoking, hypertension, obesity, cardiac disease, hypercholesterolemia, diabetes, cancer, use of birth control pills, and patent foramen ovale with atrial septal aneurysm.[71] Prevention efforts focus on lifestyle changes that can modify risk factors. In addition, the appropriate use of warfarin in patients at risk for cardiac sources of emboli (e.g., atrial fibrillation) and use of aspirin in patients at risk for thrombotic stroke constitute primary prevention.

Pathophysiology

When blood flow to any part of the brain is impeded as a result of a thrombus or embolus, oxygen deprivation

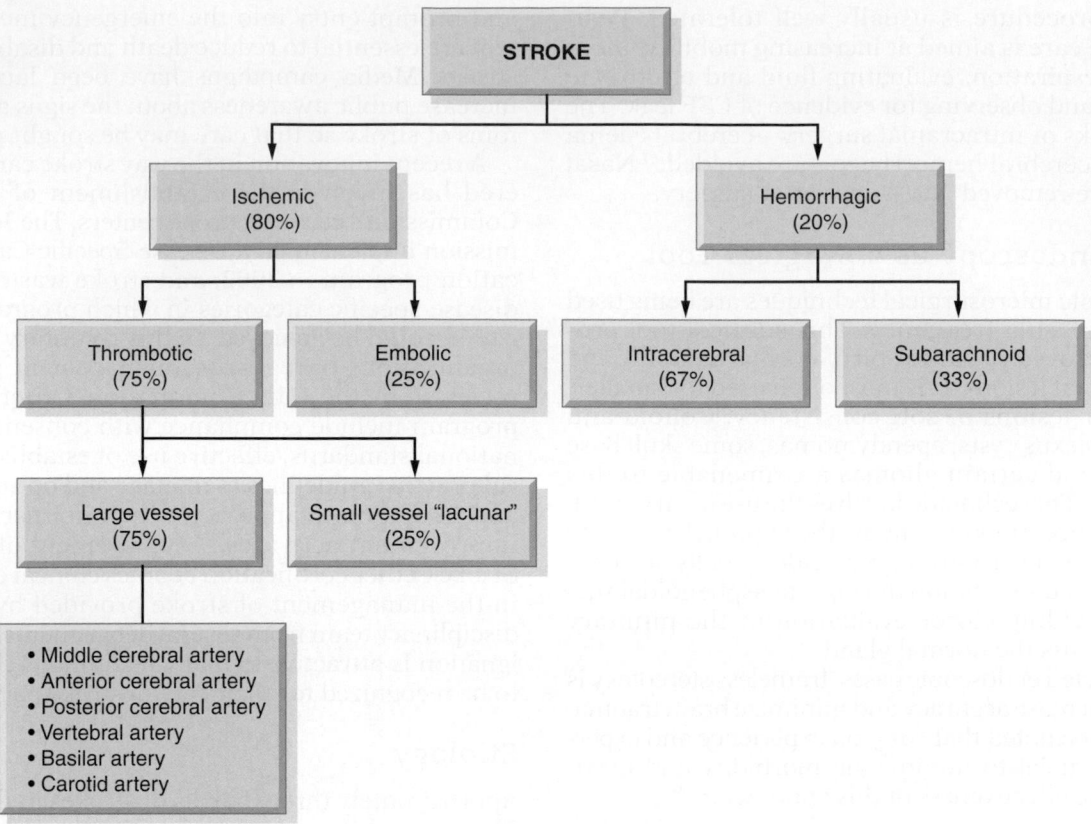

Note: Generated/simplified data

Figure 35-5 • Classification of stroke. (Courtesy of Eric Aldrich, MD, PhD, Johns Hopkins University, Baltimore, MD.)

of the cerebral tissue begins. Deprivation for 1 minute can lead to reversible symptoms, such as loss of consciousness. Oxygen deprivation for longer periods can produce microscopic necrosis of the neurons. The necrotic area is then said to be infarcted.

The initial oxygen deprivation may be caused by general ischemia (from cardiac arrest or hypotension) or hypoxia (from an anemic process or high altitude). If the neurons are ischemic only and have not yet necrosed, they may be saved. This situation is analogous to the focal injury caused by a myocardial infarction. An occluded coronary artery can produce an area of infarcted (dead) tissue. Surrounding the infarcted zone is an area of ischemic tissue, which has been marginally deprived of oxygen. This ischemic tissue, as in the brain, may be either salvaged with appropriate treatment or killed by secondary events.

Cerebral ischemia is a complex process that depends on the severity and duration of the decline in cerebral blood flow. The ischemic cascade begins within seconds to minutes after perfusion failure, creating a zone of irreversible infarction and a surrounding area of potentially salvageable "ischemic penumbra." The goal of acute stroke management is to salvage the ischemic penumbra, or the territory at risk. Without prompt intervention, the entire ischemic penumbra can eventually become an infarcted region.[47]

A stroke caused by an embolus may be a result of blood clots, fragments of atheromatous plaques, lipids,

or air. Emboli to the brain most often have a cardiac source, secondary to myocardial infarction or atrial fibrillation. If hemorrhage is the etiology of a stroke, hypertension often is a precipitating factor. Vascular abnormalities, such as AVMs and cerebral aneurysms, are more prone to rupture and cause hemorrhage in the presence of hypertension.

The most frequent neurovascular syndrome seen in thrombotic and embolic strokes is due to involvement of the middle cerebral artery. This artery supplies mainly the lateral aspects of the cerebral hemisphere. Infarction to that area of the brain can cause contralateral motor and sensory deficits. If the infarcted hemisphere is dominant, dysphasia may be present. It is difficult to predict the amount of brain ischemia and infarction resulting from a thrombotic or embolic stroke. There is a possibility that the stroke will extend after the initial insult. There can be massive cerebral edema and an increase in ICP to the point of herniation and death after a huge thrombotic stroke. The area of the brain involved and the extent of the insult influence the prognosis. Because thrombotic strokes often are caused by atherosclerosis, there is risk for a future stroke in a patient who already has had one. With embolic strokes, patients also may have subsequent episodes of stroke if the underlying cause is not treated. If the extent of brain tissue destroyed from a hemorrhagic stroke is not excessive and is in a nonvital area, the patient may recover with minimal deficits. If the hemorrhage is large or in a vital area of the brain, the patient may not recover; however, if the intracerebral hemorrhage is less massive, survival is possible. For the purposes of this discussion, the focus is on the diagnosis and management of ischemic stroke.

Clinical Manifestations

A stroke is usually characterized by the sudden onset of focal neurological impairment. The patient may experience signs such as weakness, numbness, visual changes, dysarthria, dysphagia, or aphasia. The manifestations of a stroke depend on the anatomical location of the lesion; an infarct in a certain portion of the brain results in loss of function of the body part that it controlled or skill for which it was responsible.[70] Table 35-8 presents the correlation of blood supply to symptomatology in a brain attack.[72]

If symptoms resolve in less than 24 hours, the event is classified as a transient ischemic attack (TIA), which is defined as a "neurological deficit lasting less

Table 35-8 • Anterior and Posterior Blood Supply

Artery	Brain Structure	Signs/Symptoms of Occlusion
Anterior Blood Supply		
Anterior choroidal	Globus pallidus, lateral geniculate body, posterior limb of internal capsule, medial temporal lobe	Contralateral hemiplegia Hemihypesthesia Homonymous hemianopia
Ophthalmic	Orbit and optic nerve	Transient mononuclear blindness or complete unilateral blindness
Anterior cerebral	Anterior three fourths of medial surface of cerebral hemispheres, caudate nucleus, globus pallidus, and the internal capsule	Contralateral sensory and motor deficits greater in leg than arm Incontinence Deviation of the eyes and head toward the lesion Contralateral grasp reflex Abulic symptoms Arm apraxia Expressive aphasia (in dominant hemisphere occlusion) Motor or sensory aphasia (distal occlusion)

Middle cerebral	Cortical surfaces of the parietal, temporal, and frontal lobes
	Basal ganglia and internal capsule
		Complete:
		  Spatial neglect and homonymous hemianopia
		  Global aphasia (left lesion)
		Superior trunk:
		  Contralateral hemiplegia and hemianesthesia in face and arm
		  Ipsilateral deviation of eyes and head
		  Broca's aphasia (usually left sided)
		Inferior trunk:
		  Contralateral hemianopia or upper quadrantanopia
		  Wernicke's aphasia (left lesion)
		  Left visual neglect (right lesion)

Posterior Blood Supply		
Vertebral	Anterolateral parts of the medulla	Contralateral impairment of pain and temperature sensation
Posterior cerebral	Occipital lobe, medial and inferior surface of temporal lobe, the midbrain, third and lateral ventricles	Contralateral hemiplegia, sensory loss, and ipsilateral visual field deficits

Posterior inferior cerebellar	Medulla and cerebellum	Medial branch:
		  Vertigo, nystagmus, ataxia, persistent dizziness
		Lateral branch:
		  Unilateral clumsiness with gait and limb ataxia
		  Inability to stand
		  Sudden falling
		  Vertigo, dysarthria, oculomotor signs

Anterior inferior cerebellar	Cerebellum and pons	Horner's syndrome and contralateral loss of pain and temperature sense of the arm, trunk, and leg
Superior cerebellar	Upper part of cerebellum, midbrain	Slurred speech and contralateral loss of pain and thermal sensation
Basilar	Pons and midbrain	Limb paralysis, bulbar or pseudobulbar paralysis of cranial nerve motor nuclei, nystagmus, coma, or locked-in syndrome

From Testani-Dufour L, Morrison CAM: Brain attack: Correlative anatomy. J Neurosci Nurs 29(1):213–224, 1997.

than 24 hours that is attributed to focal cerebral or retinal ischemia." Most TIAs last for only minutes to less than an hour, which further clouds recognition and prompt treatment. Approximately 30% of people who experience a TIA will have a stroke within 5 years. An aggressive workup following TIA is encouraged.[73]

Diagnosis

Rapid diagnosis of a stroke is essential so that appropriate patients can receive thrombolytic therapy, the goal of which is to save damaged brain tissue and minimize permanent deficits. The patient should be taken to an emergency department where a neurologist can perform an initial screening and obtain appropriate neuroimaging studies. The time of symptom onset to administration of thrombolytic therapy (or "time to needle") should be within a 3-hour window. Emergency departments need to have services streamlined so that testing may be performed and treatment initiated promptly.

The patient's history helps determine what has happened to the person. It is important to obtain a description of the neurological event; how long it lasted; and whether the symptoms are resolving, completely gone, or the same as at the time of onset. The differential diagnosis of stroke includes ruling out intracerebral hemorrhage, SAH, subdural or epidural hematoma, neoplasm, seizure, or migraine headache. Identifying the type of symptoms can help determine the diagnosis and locate a possible vascular distribution. Determination of risk factors for stroke, such as hypertension, chronic atrial fibrillation, elevated serum cholesterol, smoking, oral contraceptive use, or a familial history of stroke, also aids in diagnosis.

In the emergency department, some of the tests that are frequently used to evaluate the patient with acute ischemic stroke are a CT scan of the brain without contrast, blood studies, neurological examination, and a screening performed using the National Institutes of Health Stroke Scale (NIHSS). This tool allows a score to be given for the severity of the stroke. Table 35-9 summarizes the NIHSS.[47]

There is no definitive laboratory study currently available that determines whether a patient has experienced a stroke. Rather, the results are viewed in conjunction with the history, neurological examination, and neuroimaging studies. Laboratory tests, including complete blood cell count, electrolytes, glucose, and coagulation parameters, are obtained.

An urgent CT scan should be performed to rule out intracerebral hemorrhage. Ideally, the CT scan is obtained within 60 minutes of arrival in the emergency department so that treatment decisions can be made. A CT scan can be useful in differentiating between cerebrovascular and nonvascular lesions. For example, a subdural hemorrhage, brain abscess, tumor, SAH, or intracerebral hemorrhage is visible on the CT scan. However, an area of infarction may not show on the CT scan for 48 hours.

Newer neuroimaging techniques also provide valuable information. MRI, including T1- and T2-weighted, fluid-attenuated inversion recovery (FLAIR), and diffusion-weighted techniques, has become widely available and is better at detecting infarction than a CT scan. The earliest changes normally appear within the first 24 hours.

Other studies that may be performed, based on availability of the technology, are MRI diffusion-weighted imaging (DWI) and perfusion-weighted imaging (PWI). These techniques help identify the infarct core and penumbra, which is important because the presence of viable tissue directs interventions such as reperfusion. The ischemic penumbra surrounds the infarcted tissue. It is the marginally perfused area of the brain that has been damaged by the insult but is potentially salvageable. DWI detects acute infarction as early as a few hours after the onset of symptoms. It can reveal changes associated with infarcted tissue hours before a CT scan or conventional MRI can detect any abnormality. It also differentiates acute from chronic ischemic changes. PWI shows the regional abnormalities of cerebral blood flow. The difference between the diffusion defect and the perfusion defect represents the ischemic penumbra, or the "territory at risk." DWI-PWI identifies patients who are ideal candidates for thrombolytic therapy.[47]

Cerebral angiography has been the gold standard for evaluating cerebral vasculature. There is an estimated 1.5% to 2% associated risk for morbidity or mortality with this procedure. However, it can demonstrate an arterial occlusion or embolus. Because of the time that it takes to perform cerebral angiography, the window of opportunity to treat a patient with IV thrombolytics may be missed. However, angiography is necessary for intra-arterial thrombolysis in which tissue plasminogen activator (t-PA) or another thrombolytic is administered at the site of the clot by catheter into the artery. The vasculature can be evaluated noninvasively by the use of TCD, ultrasonography, MRA, or CT angiography.

An electrocardiogram (ECG) should be obtained to assess for evidence of dysrhythmia or cardiac ischemia. The ECG helps determine whether a dysrhythmia is present, which may have caused the stroke. Atrial fibrillation is a dysrhythmia in which clots form in the heart and may travel to the brain (hence a cardioembolic etiology). Other changes that might be found on an ECG are an inverted T wave, ST elevation or depression, and QT prolongation. Transesophageal echocardiography and Holter monitoring may also be performed.

In summary, prompt performance of a CT scan and subsequent interpretation are crucial to acute stroke management. Head CT and TCD provide vital information and allow the physician to make the decision to use thrombolytic therapy. An alternate approach is urgent MRI with PWI and DWI.[47]

Clinical Management

The management of an ischemic stroke has four primary goals: restoration of cerebral blood flow (reperfusion), prevention of recurrent thrombosis, neuroprotection, and supportive care. The timing

Table 35-9 • National Institutes of Health Stroke Scale

1.a.	Level of consciousness (LOC)	Alert	0
		Drowsy	1
		Stuporous	2
		Comatose	3
1.b.	LOC questions	Answers both correctly	0
		Answers one correctly	1
		Answers neither correctly	2
1.c.	LOC commands	Performs both correctly	0
		Performs one correctly	1
		Performs neither correctly	2
2.	Best gaze	Normal	0
		Partial gaze palsy	1
		Forced deviation	2
3.	Visual	No visual loss	0
		Partial hemianopia	1
		Complete hemianopia	2
		Bilateral hemianopia	3
4.	Facial palsy	Normal	0
		Minor paralysis	1
		Partial paralysis	2
		Complete paralysis	3
5.	Motor arm	No drift	0
		Drift	1
		Some effort against gravity	2
		No effort against gravity	3
		No movement	4
		Amputation, joint fusion explain:	9
6.	Motor leg	No drift	0
		Drift	1
		Some effort against gravity	2
		No effort against gravity	3
		No movement	4
		Amputation, joint fusion explain:	9
7.	Limb ataxia	Absent	0
		Present in one limb	1
		Present in two limbs	2
8.	Sensory	Normal	0
		Mild to moderate loss	1
		Severe to total loss	2
9.	Best language	No aphasia	0
		Mild to moderate	1
		Severe	2
		Mute	3

of each element of clinical management should be implemented in a decisive manner.

Optimally, patients are initially evaluated at a center that has a stroke program, perhaps even a Joint Commission Primary Stroke Center. Decisions in the emergency department determine the patient's treatment plan. Emergency departments may have standardized orders, clinical pathways, or protocols that have been developed by a multidisciplinary team to guide care.[70]

The focus of initial treatment is to save as much of the ischemic area as possible. Three ingredients necessary to this area are oxygen, glucose, and adequate blood flow. The oxygen level can be monitored through arterial blood gases or pulse oximetry, and oxygen can be given to the patient if indicated. Hypoglycemia can be evaluated with serial checks of blood glucose. Reperfusion may be accomplished by the use of IV t-PA.

CPP is a reflection of the systemic blood pressure and ICP. Regional perfusion is influenced by autoregulation in the brain, and MAP is influenced by cardiac output and heart rate (CPP = MAP − ICP). The parameters most easily controlled externally are the blood pressure and cardiac rate and rhythm. Dysrhythmias can reduce cardiac output and blood pressure but usually can be corrected. There is a loss of autoregulation in the ischemic penumbra, so that reducing blood pressure can further reduce blood flow in the penumbra and can lead to infarction.

If the patient is a candidate for IV thrombolytic therapy, treatment with t-PA begins in the emergency department, and he or she is then moved to the ICU for further monitoring. If the patient is not a candidate for thrombolytic therapy, the complexity of the patient's problems determines his or her placement in the ICU, medical unit, or stroke specialty unit.

Currently, two emergency treatments are available for stroke management: IV t-PA and the mechanical embolus removal for cerebral ischemia (MERCI) retriever.[70] IV t-PA is an approved U.S. Food and Drug Administration (FDA) treatment. The MERCI retriever was approved by the FDA in 2004 for other uses and is currently being used in trials to determine its efficacy, but is not approved as a treatment for stroke management.

Thrombolytic Agents

Thrombolytic agents are exogenous drugs that dissolve clots. IV t-PA dissolves the clot and permits reperfusion of the brain tissue. IV thrombolytic therapy should be initiated within 3 hours or less of the onset of neurological symptoms. The clock begins for the patient from the time he or she was last seen well. For example, a patient retires to bed at 11:00 p.m. and awakens at 5:00 a.m. to go to the bathroom. As he attempts to rise from the bed, he feels weak and has difficulty standing up. As he calls out for his wife's help, his speech is garbled. The last time he was awake and functioning normally was 11:00 p.m. Even if his symptoms started only a few minutes ago, the time he was last seen well was 6 hours ago. Therefore, he is already outside of the treatment window for IV t-PA.

Candidate selection for IV t-PA must be done carefully. The neurological examination, NIHSS score, and results of neuroimaging studies assist the physician with the decision to offer thrombolytic therapy. Box 35-2 outlines eligibility criteria for this treatment. The standards for the administration of IV t-PA to treat stroke are a result of the National Institute of Neurologic Disorders and Stroke t-PA Stroke Study. A dose of IV t-PA, 0.9 mg/kg (maximal dose, 90 mg), is administered as 10% of the total dose as a bolus over 1 to 2 minutes, with the remainder infused over 60 minutes. The t-PA activates plasminogen, a naturally occurring enzyme present in the intravascular endothelium that protects against excessive clotting. Activating plasminogen initiates the process of dissolving the clot through fibrinolysis. No other antithrombotic therapy should be given for the next 24 hours. A major risk of this therapy is intracerebral hemorrhage. However, it is encouraging that this agent may prove effective in reversing a neurological deficit and improving quality of life after a stroke.

The direct administration of a thrombolytic into an artery is an alternative to IV t-PA. Such administration is effective in acute ischemic stroke and can

> **Box 35-2 • Eligibility Criteria for Thrombolytic Therapy**
>
> **Inclusion Criteria**
> 1. Symptom onset of less than 3 h
> 2. Clinical diagnosis of ischemic stroke with measurable deficit on the National Institutes of Health Stroke Scale (NIHSS)
> 3. Older than 38 y
> 4. Computed tomography (CT) criteria: absence of high-density lesion consistent with intracerebral hemorrhage; absence of significant mass effect or midline shift; absence of parenchymal hypodensity; or effacement of cerebral sulci in more than 33% of the middle cerebral artery territory
>
> **Exclusion Criteria**
> 1. Stroke or serious head trauma within past 3 mo
> 2. Systolic blood pressure (BP) more than 185 mm Hg or diastolic BP more than 110 mm Hg, or BP readings that require aggressive treatment
> 3. Conditions that could precipitate or suggest parenchymal bleeding (subarachnoid and intracerebral hemorrhage; recent-onset myocardial infarction; seizures at onset; major surgery within past 14 days; gastrointestinal or urinary tract hemorrhage within previous 21 days; and arterial puncture of a noncompressible site or lumbar puncture within previous 7 days)
> 4. Glucose less than 50 mg/dL or more than 400 mg/dL; international normalized ratio (INR) more than 1.7; platelet count less than 100,000/mm³
> 5. Rapidly improving or deteriorating neurological signs or minor symptoms
> 6. Recent myocardial infarction
> 7. Recent treatment with IV or subcutaneous heparin within past 48 hours and elevated partial thromboplastin time
> 8. Women of childbearing age who have a positive pregnancy test result
>
> *From Hock NH: Brain attack: The stroke continuum. Nurs Clin North Am 34(3):718, 1999.*

be given up to 6 hours after the onset of symptoms. A limiting factor is that the patient must be admitted to a specialty center in which localized intra-arterial infusion of thrombolytic agents is possible. Through this approach, an occluded cerebral artery can be reopened. For intra-arterial therapy, a femoral arterial sheath is usually inserted, through which a microcatheter can be threaded, under fluoroscopy. The catheter tip is positioned into the clot and advanced as the clot dissolves. The femoral sheath usually remains in place for 24 hours in case of recurrent vessel occlusion. The advantage of this approach is that the medication can be delivered directly to its target.[47]

MERCI Retriever

The MERCI system (a mechanical clot retriever) can be used for up to 8 hours after stroke onset to remove blood clots from vessels. If a patient arrives at the hospital too late to receive IV t-PA, the MERCI device presents another treatment option if the patient meets strict criteria. Inclusion criteria include diagnosis of acute ischemic stroke; NIHSS greater than 8; and occlusion of internal carotid artery, basilar artery, or vertebral artery on cerebral angiography. Some exclusion criteria include blood glucose less than 50 mg/dL, excessive vessel tortuosity, hemorrhagic tendency, elevated international normalized ratio (INR), decreased platelets, sustained hypertension, CT revealing large areas of hypodensity, and arterial stenosis on angiography proximal to the embolus.[74]

The MERCI retriever works like a corkscrew to retrieve the clot. During cerebral angiography, an interventional radiologist passes the microcatheter into the femoral artery. It is advanced into the carotid until it reaches the clot. A wire is then pushed through the catheter, causing it to return to a corkscrew shape. It then snares the embolus.

Potential hazards from use of the MERCI retriever include bleeding and vascular dissection or perforation. The patient needs to be closely monitored for the first 24 hours to detect adverse effects. The nurse, who plays a key role in postprocedure monitoring, performs neurological assessments and carefully monitors the patient for signs of intracranial hemorrhage, new stroke, or myocardial infarction.[74]

Anticoagulation

Aside from thrombolytic therapy and mechanical clot retrieval, secondary treatment options for stroke include anticoagulation with antithrombotic and antiplatelet agents. If a patient experiences atrial fibrillation, anticoagulation with warfarin (Coumadin) may be warranted. The patient will need instruction about bleeding precautions. Education also includes the purpose of the medication, information about moderate consumption of leafy green vegetables containing vitamin K, and the importance of having blood drawn regularly to monitor prothrombin time and the INR. In addition, for safety, patients should be instructed to obtain Medic Alert cards and bracelets so that they can be identified as taking an anticoagulant in the event of a medical emergency.

Antiplatelet drugs include dipyridamole-ER, ticlopidine, clopidogrel, and aspirin. These agents deter platelets from adhering to the wall of an injured blood vessel or other platelets and are given to prevent a future thrombotic or embolic event. The modified-release formula of dipyridamole increases the effect of specific factors that act as antiaggregates to reduce platelet aggregation. Ticlopidine inhibits platelet function by suppressing adenosine diphosphate–induced platelet aggregation and aggregation due to other factors. The recommended dose of ticlopidine is 250 mg twice a day. Neutropenia and thrombocytopenia are known serious adverse effects, so it is now rarely used. Clopidogrel also inhibits the activity of adenosine diphosphate but is not associated with an increased risk for neutropenia. Aspirin limits platelet adhesion and aggregation. The suggested dose of aspirin is 81 to 325 mg per day. The administration of these agents plays a role in stroke prevention by decreasing the risk for future strokes.[73]

Control of Hypertension and Increased Intracranial Pressure

The control of hypertension, increased ICP, and CPP takes the efforts of both the nurse and the physician. The nurse must assess for these problems, recognize them and their significance, and ensure that medical interventions are initiated.

Patients with moderate hypertension usually are not treated acutely. If their blood pressure decreases after the brain becomes accustomed to the hypertension needed for adequate perfusion, the brain's perfusion pressure falls along with the blood pressure. If the diastolic blood pressure is above approximately 105 mm Hg, it needs to be lowered gradually. This can be accomplished effectively with labetalol.

If ICP is elevated in a patient who has had a stroke, it usually occurs after the first day. Although this is a natural response of the brain to some cerebrovascular lesions, it is destructive to the brain. The usual methods of controlling increased ICP can be instituted: hyperventilation; fluid restriction; head elevation; avoidance of neck flexion or severe head rotation that would impede venous outflow from the head; and the use of osmotic diuretics (mannitol) to decrease cerebral edema (see Chapter 34 for more information).

Surgical Management

In patients with carotid stenosis, carotid endarterectomy may be performed to prevent a stroke. Carotid endarterectomy is a surgical procedure in which atherosclerotic plaque that has accumulated inside the carotid artery is surgically removed. Once the plaque is removed, blood flow is restored. The North American Symptomatic Carotid Endarterectomy Trial and the European Carotid Surgery Trial were designed to examine the benefit of surgery for patients with symptomatic carotid stenosis. These studies determined that carotid endarterectomy is justifiable in patients with high-grade stenosis (>70%) if the operation is performed by a skilled surgeon. The benefit of surgery increases for male patients with a prior history of stroke. Patients with less than 50% stenosis do not benefit from surgery.[47]

Nonsurgical Management

Although the gold standard for managing carotid artery stenosis has been carotid endarterectomy, another management option has become available. Carotid stenting is a newer, minimally invasive procedure that is attractive to patients in whom traditional surgery is contraindicated, such as in people with severe cardiac or pulmonary disease. Carotid artery stenting opens vessels that have been narrowed by plaque accumulation. An interventional radiologist passes a catheter through the femoral artery to the narrowed artery. Once the catheter crosses the area of stenosis, a small filter may be deployed to catch any pieces of plaque that may be dislodged during the procedure. Angioplasty, in which plaque is pressed against the artery wall, may be performed, and a stent is placed in the artery.

Following carotid stenting, there is a risk for stroke and hyperperfusion syndrome. Postprocedure, the nurse monitors the patient's neurological status and assesses the groin site for bleeding and hematoma formation.[75,76]

Nursing Management

Assessment A thorough neurological assessment is essential to identify deficits the patient is experiencing. As previously discussed, the NIHSS is a valuable tool that can be used in the emergency department to rate severity of the stroke and determine whether the patient is a candidate for t-PA (see Table 35-9).[77] The brevity and reliability of the tool make it ideal for use in the emergency department. The NIHSS is also helpful for making subsequent assessments and should be performed in conjunction with the neurological examination.[47]

As a member of a large multidisciplinary team, the nurse must be prepared to assume a critical role to assist with the administration of thrombolytic therapy, optimize acute patient care, and move the patient to rehabilitation quickly to maximize the patient's outcome. The nurse is in the unique position to identify problems and collaborate with the physician to initiate appropriate referrals to rehabilitation medicine specialists, social workers, speech-language pathologists, or dietitians. Because of the nature of the patient's problems, the multidisciplinary approach provides comprehensive care by addressing all needs.

In addition, the nurse must carefully monitor the patient for infection, changes in temperature, and changes in glucose level, all of which have potentially deleterious effects in people who have had a stroke. "Hyperglycemia in acute stroke patients increases cerebral infarct size and worsens neurologic outcomes with and without preexisting diabetes mellitus."[78] In a critical care unit, the upper limit of glycemic control should be 110 mg/dL. Strict glycemic control in the intensive care setting may be achieved with a continuous insulin infusion or sliding-scale regimen.[78]

Plan The nurse plays a significant role in preventing complications associated with immobility, hemiparesis, or any neurological deficit produced by a stroke. Preventive measures are particularly important in the areas of urinary tract infections, aspiration, pressure ulcers, contractures, and thrombophlebitis. Patients in critical care units are at risk for DVT and its resultant complications. Mechanical prophylactic measures for DVT prevention include range-of-motion exercises, antiembolism stockings, and pneumatic compression devices. Additionally, pharmacological measures such as unfractionated heparin, low-molecular-weight heparin, or warfarin may be ordered to prevent blood coagulability.[79] Effective interventions for the treatment of acute stroke help lower the mortality rate and reduce the morbidity of patients who have had a stroke. The Collaborative Care Guide (Box 35-3) delineates the specific outcomes and interventions for the patient who has had a stroke.[77]

Emotional and Behavioral Modification Patients who have experienced a stroke may display emotional problems, and their behavior may be different from

baseline. Emotions may be labile; for example, the patient may cry one moment and laugh the next, without explanation or control. Tolerance to stress may also be reduced. A minor stressor in the prestroke state may be perceived as a major problem after the stroke. Families may not understand the behavior. Patients may show frustration or agitation with the nursing staff or their family members.

It is the nurse's role to help the family understand these behavioral changes. The nurse can help modify the patient's behavior by controlling stimuli in the environment, providing rest periods throughout the day to prevent fatigue, giving positive feedback, and providing repetition when the patient is trying to relearn a skill.

Communication Patients can demonstrate much frustration with their deficits. Probably no deficit produces more frustration for the patient and those trying to communicate with him or her than the one involving the production and understanding of language. Dysphasia can involve motor abilities, sensory function, or both. If the area of brain injury is in or near the left Broca's area, the memory of motor patterns of speech is affected. This results in an expressive or nonfluent dysphasia, in which the patient understands language but is unable to use it appropriately.

Receptive or fluent dysphasia usually is a result of injury to the left Wernicke's area, which is the control center for recognition of spoken language. The patient therefore is unable to understand the meaning of the spoken word (and usually the written word). The presence of both expressive and receptive dysphasia is referred to as global dysphasia. Box 35-4 summarizes differences between expressive and receptive problems.

It is important for the nursing staff to inform families that having dysphasia does not mean that a person is intellectually impaired. Communication at some level should be attempted, whether it is by writing, using picture boards, or gestures.

Patient Education and Discharge Planning

Education provides information to patients about modifying risk factors and teaches people to recognize the signs and symptoms of a stroke. Information can be presented regarding medication and other lifestyle modifications to manage blood pressure. Patients can be referred to smoking cessation programs. Education can also be provided about glucose control, weight management, and exercise programs. Compliance with medication regimens should also be stressed.

Hospitals need to organize community outreach programs regarding stroke prevention, the recognition of signs and symptoms of a stroke, its emergent nature, and the need to contact 911 at the onset of symptoms. There must be public awareness about the signs and symptoms, such as sudden onset of numbness or weakness of the face, arm, or leg; confusion; trouble speaking or understanding; vision problems;

Box 35-3 • COLLABORATIVE CARE GUIDE for the Patient Who Has Experienced a Stroke

OUTCOMES	INTERVENTIONS
Oxygenation/ventilation Adequate airway is maintained. Oxygen saturation (SpO_2) is maintained within normal limits. Atelectasis is prevented.	• Monitor breath sounds every shift. • Check oxygen saturation every shift. • Instruct to cough and deep-breathe and use incentive spirometry every 2 h while awake. • Assist with removal of airway secretions as needed.
Circulation/perfusion Patient is free of dysrhythmias.	• Monitor vital signs closely. • Manage blood pressure carefully; avoid sharp drops in blood pressure that could result in hypotension and cause an ischemic event secondary to hypotension. • During cardiac monitoring, identify dysrhythmias. • Treat dysrhythmias to maintain adequate perfusion pressure and reduce chance of neurological impairment.
Neurological Adequate perfusion pressure is maintained. Effective communication is established.	• Obtain vital signs and perform a neurological assessment to establish a baseline and to monitor for the development of additional deficits. • Use the NIHSS for detection of early changes suggesting cerebral edema or extension of stroke. • Position head of bed at 30 degrees to promote venous drainage. • Assess ability to speak and to follow simple commands. • Arrange for consultation with speech-language pathologist to differentiate language disturbances. • Use communication aids such as picture cards, pantomime, erase board, or computer to enhance communication. • Provide a calm, unrushed environment. Listen attentively to the patient. Speak in a normal tone.
Fluids/electrolytes Electrolytes are within normal limits.	• Monitor laboratory results, especially glucose. • Monitor intake and output.
Mobility/safety Safety is maintained. Complications of immobility are avoided.	• Initiate deep venous thrombosis precautions to include TED hose, sequential compressive devices, and subcutaneous heparin, as ordered. • Perform fall risk assessment. • Consult with physical therapy. • Provide active or passive range-of-motion exercises to all extremities every shift. • Establish splinting routine for affected limbs. • Instruct in use of mobility aids and fall prevention strategies. • For visual field cuts, teach scanning techniques.
Skin integrity Skin is intact.	• Perform skin assessment using the Braden scale. • Provide pressure relief mattress as indicated by Braden scale. • Turn and reposition every 2 h. • Consult with wound nurse specialist for skin issues and concerns.

(continued)

Box 35-5 • Classification of Seizure Types

1. **Generalized:** involves both hemispheres; loss of consciousness; no local onset in the cerebrum
   a. *Tonic-clonic* (grand-mal)—loss of consciousness; stiffening; forced expiration (cry); rhythmic jerking
   b. *Clonic*—symmetrical, bilateral semirhythmic jerking
   c. *Tonic*—sudden increased tone and forced expiration
   d. *Myoclonic*—sudden, brief body jerks
   e. *Atonic* ("drop attacks")—sudden loss of tone; falls
   f. *Absence* (petit mal)—brief staring, usually without motor involvement
2. **Partial:** involves one hemisphere
   a. *Simple partial seizure*—no change in level of consciousness, jacksonian
      i. Motor—frontal lobe
      ii. Somatosensory—parietal lobe
      iii. Visual—occipital lobe
      iv. May involve: autonomic (e.g., respiratory changes, tachycardia, flushing); psychic (e.g., déjà vu); cognitive (without change in level of consciousness)
   b. *Complex partial seizures*—altered level of consciousness; with or without automatisms: lip-smacking, swallowing, aimless walking, verbalizations
      i. Simple partial followed by change in level of consciousness
      ii. Starts with change in consciousness
      iii. Typically of temporal lobe origin
   c. *Partial with secondary generalization*
      i. Simple partial → generalization
      ii. Complex partial → generalization
      iii. Simple partial → complex partial → generalization
      iv. Continuous electroencephalogram monitoring may be necessary to differentiate from generalized seizures
3. **Unclassified**

with a description of the event by the patient or witnesses. This description should include:

1. What the patient was doing at the time of the seizure
2. Duration of the episode
3. Unusual symptoms or behaviors before the seizure
4. Specific features, including movements, sensations, sounds, tastes, smells, and incontinence
5. Level of consciousness during and after the event
6. Duration and description of symptoms after the seizure
7. Reporting of any similar previous episodes and age of onset

Inquiry should be made about:

1. Sleep patterns
2. Alcohol or drug abuse
3. History of illnesses or injuries
4. Family seizure history

5. Other possible variables: menstrual cycle, stress, fevers, metabolic disorders
6. If other seizures have occurred, similarities in symptoms, duration, frequency, and time of day

After the first seizure occurrence, a CT scan or MRI is taken to assess for a structural lesion. An EEG is obtained to screen for interictal seizure discharges (electrical abnormalities present in between seizures) and to measure cerebral excitability. These techniques can help determine whether the seizures have focal origins or are more generalized. During the EEG, scalp electrodes are placed to measure neuronal membrane activity in the underlying cerebral cortex. Rhythms may be obtained when the patient is both awake and asleep. The EEG localizes the region from which the patient's seizure arises at one time point.

If additional information regarding seizure patterns and characteristics is needed, an inpatient hospital stay may be recommended in an epilepsy monitoring unit, as discussed in the following section. Also, continuous EEG monitoring is now being used in the ICU, where it has helped identify subtle seizures in critically ill patients. Because it is not uncommon for these patients (e.g., brain injured or comatose patients) to suffer nonconvulsive seizures, this tool is becoming more widespread in the ICU.[88]

Other diagnostic studies that may be obtained include PET to identify abnormal hypometabolic cortical areas that correlate with the epileptogenic area; SPECT to identify cerebral blood flow and perfusion differences during and after a seizure; bilateral carotid amobarbital (Amytal) testing to assess speech dominance and memory; fMRI to localize seizure focus and identify its relationship to a structural lesion; and neurocognitive testing to obtain a baseline evaluation.[89,90]

Epilepsy Monitoring Unit

Patients who require more detailed seizure characterization or localization are admitted for video EEG monitoring to an appropriate unit, where scalp electrodes are placed. Video EEG monitoring is continuous and involves audiovisual observations. Monitoring occurs while the patient is awake and asleep. Medications may be tapered or withdrawn during these observations. Because video EEG monitoring captures ictal, postictal, and interictal data, seizures are documented and localized and the patient's clinical symptoms are observed. Video EEG can often localize seizures for possible epilepsy surgery. It is also very helpful for identifying pseudoseizures and other disorders that are mistaken for epileptic disorders. Neuropsychological and psychiatric evaluations may be part of the assessment, particularly if surgery is being anticipated.[89]

In situations in which localization is not obtained or is questionable, a more invasive approach using surgical electrodes to localize seizure activity may be necessary. Three different types of electrodes can be implanted for intracranial recording.

Depth electrodes are typically placed bilaterally, targeting the hippocampus and other common seizure sites in the amygdalae and frontal lobes. Multiple electrodes are placed under local or general anesthesia through twist drill or burr holes for simultaneous recording. The electrode cables exit the skull, and patients have continuous video monitoring over several days in the epilepsy monitoring unit. Hemorrhage, headache, and infection are possible complications. This procedure is most often used to show which regions are involved at seizure onset.

Subdural and epidural electrodes are typically placed unilaterally, under general anesthesia. Strips are placed through burr holes. Grids require a craniotomy and allow for a larger region to be monitored (Fig. 35-6). They are secured to the dura, and the electrode leads exit through an incision for continuous monitoring. Infection, hemorrhage, and mass effect from cerebral edema are possible risks. The bone flap can be replaced at the end of the procedure or after the strips or grids are removed. Intracranial monitoring may be initiated before seizure surgery.[89,91]

Clinical Management

Pharmacological Management

In most cases, the patient with epilepsy can be medically treated. Some AEDs are known to be more appropriate for specific classes of seizures. Certain drugs are found most useful in the pediatric patient population. Some AEDs are preferred as monotherapy, and others are more appropriate as adjunctive therapy with other drugs. Table 35-10 describes current AEDs with general indications, doses, side effects, and nursing considerations.[12,80,92]

Status epilepticus is an emergency situation and requires rapid pharmacological management. Parenteral drugs are given to provide fast absorption. Drugs are given intravenously, intramuscularly, or rectally. Many fast-acting drugs are lipid soluble and have a tendency to redistribute from the plasma to the fat and muscle, thereby leading to an initial drop in blood and brain concentrations. This may lead to recurrence of seizures. The administration of repeat boluses or a continuous infusion must be done judiciously because the drugs saturate fat, and muscle and plasma levels will increase. This may result in prolonged decreased mental status, obtundation, and even death. Emergency management of status epilepticus is summarized in Box 35-6.[86,89,93]

Surgical Management

There are situations in which AEDs are unable to control epilepsy. Attempts at monotherapy and adjunctive therapy have been exhausted and multiple drug regimens have failed; seizure activity has compromised a patient's quality of life. In these cases, seizures are intractable, and surgery is considered to obtain seizure control. It may also be considered in situations in which the side effects of therapy are so debilitating that the patient is unable to function at an acceptable capacity.

In many cases, the patient is monitored before surgery in an epilepsy monitoring unit using a video EEG. Grid or strip placement to localize seizure focus and identify functional areas is often used. After surgery, the nurse performs regular, intermittent neurological examinations and has the patient attempt to perform certain tasks. Language deficits and motor weakness are observed. The goals of this procedure are to localize epileptiform discharges in relation to speech, memory, and sensory or motor function. It is also useful in identifying the relationship between seizure discharges and a focal lesion, such as a tumor, when present. This enhances the safety and accuracy of tumor surgery.

The decision to proceed with surgery depends on a thorough discussion among the multidisciplinary team members. The neurologist, neurosurgeon, patient, and family review the medical treatment used to date and establish that therapy has been maximized. They evaluate the likelihood of seizure control with surgery. Preoperative neuropsychological testing is obtained, and other appropriate testing is established and discussed. Some or all of the diagnostic studies previously outlined may be indicated.

The goal of seizure surgery is to remove or disrupt the seizure focus. Patients are often maintained on AEDs for 2 years postoperatively because seizure recurrence is most likely during this period. Table 35-11 summarizes the most commonly performed surgical procedures, along with expected outcomes, possible complications, and nursing considerations.[86,89,94–96]

Nursing Management

Assessment Careful history taking is a central component of the accurate diagnosis and management of epilepsy. Family history, age at onset, frequency, and a description of symptoms and their duration all aid in the development of a plan of care tailored to the patient's particular situation. AEDs are prescribed based on all these data. Changes in severity or frequency of symptoms require modification of the treatment regimen. Drug therapy may last indefinitely;

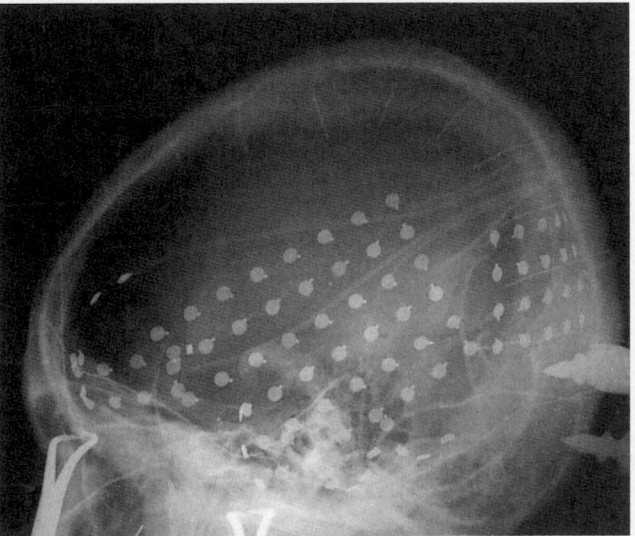

Figure 35-6 • Radiograph of a grid for seizure monitoring. (Courtesy of Frederick Lenz, MD, and Ira Garonzik, MD, Johns Hopkins University, Baltimore, MD.)

⋯⋯⋯ Table 35-10 • Clinical Application: Drug Therapy—Current Antiepileptic Drugs

Drug Name (Brand)	Indications	Daily Adult Dose	Side Effects	Nursing Considerations
Carbamazepine (Tegretol, Tegretol XR, Carbitrol)	Mono/adjunctive therapy Partial and generalized seizures	400–2000 mg; serum levels of 4–12 µg/mL	Drowsiness, fatigue, dizziness, blurred vision, rash, hyponatremia, bone marrow dyscrasia	Interactions with other antiepileptic drugs (AEDs); rare aplastic anemia, hepatic failure; obtain blood levels
Clobazam	Adjunctive therapy Partial and generalized seizures	10–30 mg	Drowsiness, fatigue, dizziness, blurred vision	Benzodiazepine; used as second-line therapy for resistance to other AEDs
Clonazepam (Klonopin)	Adjunctive therapy Partial and generalized seizures	0.5–4 mg	Sedation, cognitive, ataxia, behavior changes, leukopenia	Helpful in children with severe epilepsy
Ethosuximide (Zarontin)	Mono/adjunctive Absence seizures	250–1,500 mg; serum levels of 40–100 mcg/ml	Nausea, somnolence	Levels affected by other AEDs
Felbamate (Felbatol)	Mono/adjunctive Partial or secondarily generalized seizures	1,200–3,600 mg	Nausea, anorexia, headache, insomnia	Effective in severe, resistant epilepsy; affects other AEDs; aplastic anemia (Food and Drug Administration alert); liver failure
Gabapentin (Neurontin)	Adjunctive Partial and secondary generalized seizures	900–4,800 mg	Sedation, dizziness, weight gain	No significant drug interactions; minimal side effects
Lamotrigine (Lamictal)	Mono/adjunctive Partial in adults and partial and generalized seizures in children	200–700 mg	Rash Nausea, dizziness, ataxia	Affected by other AEDs
Levetiracetam (Keppra)	Adjunctive therapy for partial seizures	1,000–3,000 mg	Somnolence, asthenia, irritability, dizziness, infection	Can be administered IV
Oxcarbazepine (Trileptal)	Mono/adjunctive therapy Partial and secondarily generalized seizures	1,200–2,400 mg	Cognitive, headaches, somnolence, dizziness, rash, hyponatremia	Increase dose over several weeks
Phenobarbital	Mono/adjunctive therapy Partial or generalized (myoclonus/absence)	90–180 mg	Sedation, depression, ataxia, rash, impotence, hyperactivity	Potential central nervous system toxicity, especially in children; taper slowly
Phenytoin (Dilantin)	Mono/adjunctive therapy Partial and generalized (not absence/myoclonus)	300–600 mg; serum levels of 10–20 mg/L	Ataxia, dizziness, sedation, rash, gum hyperplasia	Interactions with multiple other drugs; dose guided by blood levels; less expensive
Fosphenytoin	Replacing IV phenytoin	Loading dose 15–20 mg IV or IM; administered 100–150 mg/min		
Pregabalin (Lyrica)	Adjunctive therapy for partial and secondary generalized seizures	150–600 mg	Drowsiness, dizziness, poor concentration, weight gain and edema, blurred vision, ataxia	This drug can cause dependency
Primidone (Mysoline)	Adjunctive therapy Partial and secondarily generalized seizures	500–1,500 mg	Dizziness, nausea, those seen with phenobarbital	Converted to phenobarbital in the body
Tiagabine (Gabitril)	Adjunctive therapy Partial seizures	32–56 mg	Fatigue, somnolence, dizziness, incoordination	Promising for refractory partial seizures
Topiramate (Topomax)	Adjunctive therapy Partial and generalized seizures	400 mg 750–4,000 mg; serum levels of 50–100 mg/L	Cognitive, somnolence, dizziness, tremor, anorexia, paresthesias, kidney stones	Highly effective; titrate up very slowly; daily dose divided

(continued)

Table 35-10 • Clinical Application: Drug Therapy—Current Antiepileptic Drugs (Continued)

Drug Name (Brand)	Indications	Daily Adult Dose	Side Effects	Nursing Considerations
Valproate (Depakote)	Mono/adjunctive therapy Generalized seizures; childhood epilepsy; febrile convulsions	1,000–3,000 mg	Nausea, weight gain, endocrine, thrombocytopenia, hair loss	Interactions with other AEDs; can be administered IV
Vigabatrin (Sabril)	Adjunctive therapy Partial and secondarily generalized seizures	200–600 mg	Somnolence, dizziness, headache, mood changes, visual fields, weight gain	Effective; use limited by neuropsychiatric and visual symptoms
Zonisamide (Zonegran)	Adjunctive therapy Partial seizures; myoclonic epilepsy		Cognitive, psychiatric, somnolence, fatigue, kidney stones, rash	Does not affect other AEDs

therefore, treatment should address both efficacy and tolerability. Side effects can compromise quality of life, necessitating the use of different, and possibly less effective, medications or multiple AEDs.

Plan Inpatient nursing care includes monitoring the patient during the seizure (the patient is never left alone) and providing support and protection without attempting to restrain the individual. Turning the patient to his or her side during a generalized seizure, if possible, helps maintain a patent airway.

Patient Education and Discharge Planning

Patient education should provide instructions for independent functioning. The following patient education points are critical parts of discharge planning:

Box 35-6 • Emergency Treatment of Status Epilepticus

- **Goals:** maintain airway, breathing, circulation; stop seizures; stabilize patient; identify and treat cause
- **Treatment:** airway; O_2; intubation, if necessary; electroencephalogram (EEG) monitoring; monitor electrocardiogram and blood pressure; catheter for incontinence; computed tomography scan; lumbar puncture if CNS infection is suspected; CPR if needed
- **Blood work:** electrolytes; magnesium; calcium; anticonvulsant levels; blood gases; complete blood count; renal and liver function studies; coagulation studies; toxicology studies may be needed
- **Medications:**
  - Benzodiazepines (lorazepam, 1–2 mg/min over 8 min or diazepam to total of 20 mg). These are short-acting drugs, and simultaneous loading with phenytoin at 50 mg/min or fosphenytoin at equivalent of 150 mg phenytoin/min is necessary; may total 20 mg/kg
  - For persistent seizures, add 5–10 mg/kg phenytoin or phenobarbital at 50–100 mg/min to total of 20 mg/kg
  - If ineffective, barbiturate anesthesia: pentobarbital and intubation. Benzodiazepines (e.g., midazolam) may be attempted prior to barbiturate anesthesia. Continuous EEG monitoring in ICU environment.

---

1. Make the home environment safe, particularly in the case of tonic-clonic epilepsy.
2. Assess for injury after each seizure.
3. Keep a log to record a description of the seizure and postictal period, duration, time of day, severity, and any new characteristics.
4. Know the specifics of a ketogenic (high-fat, low-carbohydrate) diet, when appropriate, for children with intractable seizures.
5. Be aware of state laws on driving restrictions related to epilepsy.
6. Wear a Medic Alert bracelet.
7. Monitor serum antiepileptic drug levels when appropriate.
8. Be aware of circumstances when emergency treatment is required.
9. Consult seizure experts for intractable epilepsy.

GUILLAIN-BARRÉ SYNDROME

Guillain-Barré syndrome, also known as acute inflammatory demyelinating polyneuropathy, is a rapidly evolving illness that commonly presents as symmetrical weakness, sensory loss, and areflexia.[97] This condition is an inflammatory peripheral neuropathy in which lymphocytes and macrophages strip myelin from axons. The diffuse inflammatory reaction may be seen in the peripheral nervous system, cranial nerves, and spinal nerve roots. It is referred to as a syndrome, as opposed to a disease, because of the combination of signs and symptoms seen in the patient.

Etiology

Guillain-Barré syndrome is an immune-mediated neuropathy that is associated with a broad range of symptoms, severity, and length of progression. This disorder follows an antecedent infection in some patients.[98] Approximately half of the people who develop Guillain-Barré syndrome have a mild febrile illness 2 to 3 weeks before the onset of symptoms. The febrile infection is usually respiratory or gastrointestinal. *Campylobacter jejuni* and cytomegalovirus are causes of the most frequent antecedent infections,

Table 35-11 • Clinical Applications: Seizure Surgery: Indications and Outcomes

Procedure	Indications	Expected Outcomes	Possible Complications	Nursing Considerations
Temporal lobectomy: removal of 6 cm of temporal lobe in the nondominant hemisphere and 4–5 cm in the dominant hemisphere	Intractable anterior temporal lobe seizures > 5 years' duration Significant quality-of-life compromise	60%–70% seizure free 20% greatly improved seizure control	Visual (superior quadrantanopsia) field defects Dysphasia (usually temporary) Mild memory problems Depression Transient psychiatric disturbance Infection and/or bleeding	At 1 year postoperatively, it is expected that seizure status will not change Medication management continues for 2–3 years postoperatively
Hemispherectomy: surgical removal (or disconnection) of a hemisphere in children and adolescents	Severe seizures Often multiple seizure types and daily seizures	90%–95% improvement in seizure activity 70%–85% resolution of seizures	Contralateral neurological deficits Late hydrocephalus Chronic bleeding into surgical cavity → neurological disability and death	Careful patient selection required May see improved behavior and social development
Corpus callosectomy: transection of the corpus callosum (or anterior two thirds)	Cases of severe secondarily generalized epilepsy; drop attacks	Reduces number of generalized seizures Seizure-free periods usually temporary and occur in only 5%–10% of patients	Hemiparesis Transient syndrome of mutism, urinary incontinence, and bilateral leg weakness	Used when other options have failed Many patients have learning disabilities Wada test recommended for left-handed patients
Vagal nerve stimulator: implanted programmable signal generator in the chest with stimulating electrodes to the left vagus nerve	Refractory to medication Often partial seizures	Reduction in seizure frequency: high stimulation 25%; low stimulation 15%	Changes in voice Dyspnea Tingling in neck during stimulation Rare cases of bradycardia or asystole	Does not generally resolve seizures Used when resective surgery is not an option
Deep brain stimulator: Electrodes placed in deep brain structures (thalamus, hippocampus, internal capsule) and programmed to activate when seizure activity is recorded	Uncontrolled epilepsy	Reduction in seizures	Bleeding Infection Neurological deficits	Has been used for tremor in Parkinson's disease Relatively new use in refractory seizures with unknown long-term outcomes

which usually occur 1 to 4 weeks before the onset of symptoms of Guillain-Barré syndrome.[99] Occasionally, vaccinations have been known to induce Guillain-Barré syndrome.[100] Although previously administered vaccinations, including swine flu and rabies, have been linked to the development of Guillain-Barré syndrome, no current vaccination has been conclusively demonstrated to induce the disease.

The attack on the immune system is extensive and occurs proximally at the nerve roots and distally at the motor axon terminal. Both cellular and humoral immune mechanisms appear to be implicated. Lymphocytes and macrophages are the effector cells that result in damage to myelin and adjacent axons. Motor, sensory, and autonomic nerves are involved. Weakness and sensory disturbances result from blockage of nerve fiber action potentials (secondary to demyelination or axon damage).[99]

In affected patients, the immune system most likely is first primed as it responds to a virus or bacteria.

Then, the immune system inappropriately attacks host tissue that shares an epitope (surface portion of an antigen capable of triggering an immune response). This process is referred to as molecular mimicry.[99]

Epidemiology

Guillain-Barré syndrome occurs with equal frequency in both sexes and all races. It can develop at any age. The annual incidence is approximately 2 cases per 100,000 population.[97]

Pathophysiology

In Guillain-Barré syndrome, the myelin sheath surrounding the axon is lost. The myelin sheath is quite susceptible to injury by many agents and conditions, including physical trauma, hypoxemia, toxic chemicals, vascular insufficiency, and immunological reactions. Demyelination is a common response of neural tissue to any of these adverse conditions.

Myelinated axons conduct nerve impulses more rapidly than nonmyelinated axons. Along the course of a myelinated fiber are interruptions in the sheath (nodes of Ranvier), where there is direct contact between the cell membrane of the axon and the extracellular fluid. The membrane is highly permeable at these nodes, resulting in especially good conduction. The movement of ions into and out of the axon can occur rapidly only at the nodes of Ranvier; therefore, a nerve impulse along a myelinated fiber may jump from node to node (known as saltatory conduction) quite rapidly. Loss of the myelin sheath makes saltatory conduction impossible, and nerve impulse transmission is aborted.

A current theory regarding the disease process of Guillain-Barré syndrome speculates that a primary lymphocytic T-cell mechanism is the cause of the inflammation. Cells migrate through the vessel walls to the peripheral nerve. The result is edema and perivascular inflammation. Macrophages then break down the myelin.

Another theory of causation is that the process of demyelination is initiated by an antibody attack on the myelin early in the course of the disease. Demyelination causes axon atrophy, which results in slowed or blocked nerve conduction.

Clinical Manifestations

Guillain-Barré syndrome may develop rapidly over the course of hours or days, or it may take up to 3 to 4 weeks to develop. Most patients demonstrate the greatest weakness in the first weeks of the disorder and are weakest by the third week of the illness.

In the beginning, a flaccid, ascending paralysis develops quickly. The patient is most commonly affected in a symmetrical pattern. The patient may first notice weakness in the lower extremities that may quickly extend to include weakness and abnormal sensations in the arms. Deep tendon reflexes are usually lost, even in the earliest stages. The trunk and cranial nerves may become involved. Respiratory muscles can become affected, resulting in respiratory compromise.[97]

Autonomic disturbances such as urinary retention and orthostatic hypotension may also occur. Some patients experience tenderness and pain on deep pressure or movement of some muscles.

Sensory symptoms of paresthesias, including numbness and tingling, may occur. Pain is a complaint in a large number of patients. It is aching in nature and often compared with the feeling of muscles that have been overexerted. If there is cranial nerve involvement, cranial nerve VII, the facial nerve, is most often affected. Guillain-Barré syndrome does not affect level of consciousness, pupillary function, or cognitive functioning.

Symptoms may progress for several weeks. The level of paralysis may stop at any point. Progression usually occurs in three stages: acute, plateau, and recovery. The acute stage starts at the onset of symptoms and rapidly progresses until no additional deterioration occurs. The plateau stage, during which patients are symptomatic, lasts for a few days up to a few weeks. The recovery phase can take up to 2 years. It is thought that the recovery phase coincides with remyelination and axonal regeneration.[101] Although demyelination occurs rapidly, the rate of remyelination is approximately 1 to 2 mm per day. Motor function returns in a descending fashion.

Diagnosis

The diagnosis of Guillain-Barré syndrome depends greatly on the patient's history and clinical progression of symptoms. As noted, onset is usually sudden, and the history often reveals an upper respiratory or GI disorder occurring 1 to 4 weeks before onset of the neurological manifestations. The history of the onset of symptoms can be revealing because symptoms of Guillain-Barré syndrome usually begin with weakness or paresthesias of the lower extremities and ascend in a symmetrical pattern.[97]

A lumbar puncture may be performed and reveals increased protein. However, negative results from this test should be interpreted cautiously because only 50% of patients in the first week of illness have increased protein. By 3 weeks, this percentage increases to greater than 90%.[102] Also, nerve conduction studies record impulse transmission along the nerve fiber. In the patient with Guillain-Barré syndrome, the velocity of conduction is reduced.[99]

Pulmonary function tests are performed when Guillain-Barré syndrome is suspected to establish a baseline for comparison as the disease progresses. Declining pulmonary function capacity may indicate the need for mechanical ventilation and management in an ICU.

Clinical Management

Because of the risks associated with respiratory failure, bulbar symptoms, and autonomic dysfunction, all patients with Guillain-Barré syndrome, except those with mild disease, should be admitted to a hospital that has specialized ICUs. Progression to mechanical ventilation is expected in patients with rapid disease progression, bulbar involvement, bilateral facial weakness, or dysautonomia. ICU admission is recommended for patients with vital capacity below 20 mL/kg, vital capacity checks that are required more than every 4 hours, aspiration, autonomic instability, or rapid progression or weakness.[97] Patients who are older, have rapid progression or prior GI infection, or are ventilator dependent tend to have a poor prognosis and need to be monitored closely.

Certain strategies can lessen the severity of the illness and hasten recovery. A useful clinical sign of respiratory compromise is the strength of the neck flexor muscles. When the head cannot be lifted against gravity, the phrenic nerves are also affected, causing diaphragm paralysis and reduction of the forced vital capacity (FVC)—the amount of air a patient can forcefully exhale after maximal inhalation. Under these circumstances, the airway cannot be successfully managed without intubation.

Preventive measures need to be established so that DVT and subsequent PE do not develop. DVT prophylaxis includes subcutaneous heparin, 5,000 units twice daily, along with antiembolism stockings and sequential compression devices. Also, autonomic nervous system fluctuations need to be evaluated by checking blood pressure and monitoring for cardiac dysrhythmias.

Plasmapheresis was the first therapy proved to benefit patients with Guillain-Barré syndrome. It is the only therapy that has been proved superior to supportive treatment alone.[98] This procedure mechanically removes humoral factors. Currently, it is recommended that patients with Guillain-Barré syndrome receive plasmapheresis. A dual-lumen central vascular access device and a specially trained team are needed to perform the plasmapheresis treatments. The physician may order plasmapheresis when the patient's condition is worsening in an attempt to lessen the severity of the disease. Of note, two prominent risks associated with plasmapheresis are catheter-related infections and hemorrhage during line placement.

Intravenous immunoglobulin (IVIG) is also useful in managing Guillain-Barré syndrome. A blood product that has been derived from large pools of plasma donors, IVIG has the potential to bind many common pathogens and modulate a wide range of effectors in autoimmune disease such as Guillain-Barré syndrome.[103] The major component is immunoglobulin G, with a trace amount of immunoglobulin A. Immunoglobulins can be infused easily, even in the home setting, without expensive equipment. The optimal dosages and frequency of administration are individualized. Immunoglobulin, which binds to receptors on T cells or receptors on nerves, induces only a temporary improvement because of the turnover of T cells or the loss of antibodies from the receptors. Daily treatments with IVIG may be helpful in acute Guillain-Barré syndrome when the patient is rapidly deteriorating.

The dose of IVIG is set at 2 g/kg, and usually the total dose is divided into five daily infusions of 400 mg/kg each. Neurologists who use IVIG for Guillain-Barré syndrome are familiar with the side effects, which include low-grade fever, chills, myalgia, diaphoresis, fluid overload, hypertension, nausea, vomiting, rash, headaches, aseptic meningitis, and neutropenia. The most serious adverse effect is acute tubular necrosis, which occurs with any concomitant disease that compromises renal glomerular filtration.[100]

Currently there are no efficacy data that favor IVIG rather than plasmapheresis in the management of Guillain-Barré syndrome. IVIG and plasma exchange have a similar ability to speed a patient's recovery. The individual patient's circumstances, such as availability of resources to perform plasmapheresis and underlying medical conditions, dictate the specific treatment for each patient. IVIG is an attractive treatment because it can be easily administered in the critical care setting.[98]

Nursing Management

Assessment For the patient with Guillain-Barré syndrome, careful assessment and the resultant plan help minimize the complications of immobility and move the patient toward rehabilitation without deficits. Although patients are critically ill, their chances of returning to a productive life are good if they survive the acute stages and avoid the complications of immobility. Most deaths are due to preventable respiratory complications or autonomic dysfunction.[99]

Once Guillain-Barré syndrome is suspected, the patient is hospitalized so that frequent assessments can be performed to monitor the patient for deterioration. Because of the progressive nature of the disease, assessment should focus on the neurological examination (i.e., cranial nerve involvement, motor weakness, and sensory changes). Cranial nerve deficits identify if the patient is at risk for aspiration. The patient's level of numbness, tingling, and pain should be assessed.

Cardiovascular assessment is done to monitor blood pressure and heart rate. The autonomic nervous system is frequently involved in Guillain-Barré syndrome. Dysautonomia manifests itself as sinus tachycardia but may result in other cardiac dysrhythmias or labile blood pressures that require close monitoring because they may be life threatening.[99] The patient's respiratory status should be monitored, and FVC should be assessed at least once every shift. GI and urinary function should come under surveillance as well. The patient is at risk for constipation and urinary tract infections due to urinary retention. Other complications of immobility are the potential for pressure ulcers and DVT.

Plan When caring for a patient with Guillain-Barré syndrome, the major goals are to prevent infections and complications of immobility, provide functional maintenance of the body systems, treat life-threatening crises promptly, and provide psychological support for the patient and family. In terms of the patient's neurological status, weakness results in impaired mobility. Range-of-motion exercises should be performed at least once per shift to minimize the patient's risk for contractures. Families are encouraged to help with this beside therapy.[101]

Also, steps are taken to maintain proper body alignment. Measures such as splint placement are implemented to prevent wrist hyperflexion and footdrop. Physical therapy is initiated early in the course of hospitalization and continued throughout the recovery period.

Cranial nerve involvement places the patient at risk for aspiration, and adequate nutrition must be maintained. If the patient is unable to take oral feedings, enteral tube feedings are initiated. A nutritional consult should occur with a registered dietitian to provide adequate calories for remyelination. Enteral nutritional support that supplies at least 1,500 to 2,000 kcal/day should be instituted.[97]

Additionally, because of intubation or impaired verbal communication, alternate methods to facilitate communication are important. Alternate ways to communicate are established using communication boards as well as nonverbal means such as gestures and eye blinking. Being unable to communicate can be frustrating for the patient and cause undue anxiety.[97]

Respiratory failure is the most severe complication of Guillain-Barré syndrome. Weakened respiratory muscles put the patient at great risk for hypoventilation and repeated pulmonary infections. Fifty percent of patients with Guillain-Barré syndrome have some respiratory compromise, resulting in reduced tidal volume and vital capacity or perhaps complete respiratory arrest. A tracheostomy may be indicated if the patient requires long-term mechanical ventilation.

If there is autonomic nervous system involvement, drastic changes in blood pressure (hypotension or hypertension), heart rate, or both can occur. Labile hypertension and dysrhythmias occur frequently, prompting admission and management in the ICU.[99] Cardiac monitoring allows quick identification and treatment of dysrhythmias. Valsalva maneuver, coughing, and suctioning may trigger an autonomic nervous system disturbance. The patient is monitored closely.

Comfort measures are used. For instance, frequent position changes may be helpful. When remyelination occurs, it is often uncomfortable, and the patient may complain of numbness and pain. This can be an encouraging sign to the patient because the disease process is reversing.

Although the patient is incapacitated physically, he or she is fully aware of the surroundings. The patient may experience a sense of helplessness and hopelessness. Frequent explanations of the interventions and of progress are useful. The patient should be allowed to participate in care as much as functionally possible. It is essential that the nurse in the critical care setting provide empathy, compassion, sensitivity, and active listening to the patient with Guillain-Barré syndrome so that his or her emotional concerns can be addressed. In addition, the nurse can provide positive reinforcement for achievement of physical gains.[101]

Patient Education and Discharge Planning

Education of the patient and family about all issues of care is important. Knowledge is power and is helpful in a situation in which the patient is powerless. The nurse can provide information about the disease process, course, and recovery. Patients need to know that the disease may progress to the point at which mechanical ventilation is required. In addition, they should understand that they may be discharged to a rehabilitation facility where recovery can continue. Many months of rehabilitation may be required for them to regain strength and previous level of functioning. Patients may continue to show improvement for up to 2 years. The nurse can tell patients and their families about the Guillain-Barré Syndrome International Foundation, which provides information and resources. Before discharge to home, the patient can be referred to a support group so that he or she can interact with other people who have had Guillain-Barré syndrome.

MYASTHENIA GRAVIS

Myasthenia gravis is an autoimmune disorder of the neuromuscular junction transmission that presents with fatigue and muscle weakness in the ocular, bulbar, diaphragm, or limb muscles. Myasthenia is derived from the Greek words for "muscle" and "weakness," whereas gravis means "grave" in Latin. Because of the high mortality related to diaphragmatic muscle weakness, the disorder was called "grave muscle weakness." However, myasthenia gravis is not a grave disease today because of advancements with immunomodulatory treatments and the ability to manage respiratory failure.

Etiology

Myasthenia gravis is an autoimmune disorder that is characterized by weakness and fatigability of skeletal muscles. The disease involves a reduction in the number of acetylcholine receptors (AChRs) at the neuromuscular junction caused by antibodies against the AChR.[104] The factors that trigger the autoimmune process are not known, but the thymus gland plays an important role. The thymus gland lies behind the sternum and may extend down to the diaphragm and up to the neck. This gland plays a role in the responsiveness of T cells to foreign antigens. The thymus gland is large in children and small in adults. By adulthood, the gland has shrunken and has nearly been replaced by fat. Abnormalities in the thymus gland frequently occur in patients with myasthenia gravis. Eighty percent of patients with myasthenia gravis have thymal hyperplasia, and approximately 12% have tumor of the thymus gland.[104]

Epidemiology

Myasthenia gravis is seen more often in women than in men at a ratio of 3:2. It is primarily a disease of young women and older men. Symptoms most commonly appear in the third decade of life, although any age group may be affected. It is estimated that the prevalence of the disease is 1 case per 10,000 population. During the past 40 years, prevalence has increased because of improved recognition of the disorder, medical management, and survival.[105] Myasthenia gravis is not hereditary in the mendelian sense; however, there may be a history of autoimmune disorders in the family, including thyroid disorders or lupus. It should be remembered that approximately 10% of women with myasthenia gravis may transmit a transient type of neonatal myasthenia to the infant that resolves within days after birth.[106]

Pathophysiology

Myasthenia gravis is a result of circulating antibodies directed toward the AChRs in the skeletal muscle. The AChR is a protein composed of five subunits situated in a specialized surface of the muscle membrane termed the end plate. When acetylcholine is released from the nerve after depolarization, it binds to the AChR and causes the ion channel to open. This passage of ions moving through the channel leads to depolarization of the end plate, action potential generation, and subsequent muscle fiber contraction. With this process, the depolarization of the end plate is 3 to 4 times greater than what is required for action potential generation. Therefore, fluctuations in end plate depolarization do not affect action potential generation or the overall strength of muscle contraction.

The AChR antibodies in myasthenia gravis lead to the loss of AChRs by increased internalization of the receptor and complement-based lysis of the muscle membrane. Compromise of ion flow through AChR occurs, leading to a decrease in end plate depolarization, which may be insufficient to generate an action potential. This results in a failure of the muscle to contract. Often, at rest, the compromise of neuromuscular transmission is mild, and action potentials are still generated. However, with exercise or with repetitive nerve stimulation, the end plate potential is further reduced, the action potential is not generated, and muscle weakness occurs. In summary, antibodies attack the AChRs of the neuromuscular junction, thereby blocking the transmission of nerve impulses to muscle.

Clinical Manifestations

Myasthenia gravis can be characterized as ocular myasthenia or generalized myasthenia, depending on whether the symptoms are limited to the eye muscles or are spread elsewhere.

In ocular myasthenia, patients may present with problems such as droopy eyelids or double vision. More than 90% of patients have ocular symptoms. In only 16% of the patients, the symptoms remain confined to the eye muscles. In the rest, the symptoms spread to other muscles (bulbar, limb, diaphragm) within a year of the onset of eye symptoms.

In generalized myasthenia gravis, patients may demonstrate ocular manifestations as well as bulbar symptoms, presenting as difficulty with chewing, swallowing, talking, and handling secretions, and neck weakness. The voice may have a nasal quality. Prolonged talking brings on slurred speech. Weakness of jaw closure (masseter muscle) may lead to the jaw hanging open. Muscle weakness in the limbs is also apparent and can vary among patients. Patients often demonstrate more proximal than distal weakness. They often report increased weakness with sustained activity and improvement with rest. Patients may also demonstrate respiratory compromise due to weakness of the respiratory muscles. The most serious potential complication of myasthenia gravis is respiratory failure (myasthenic crisis) secondary to intercostal and diaphragmatic muscle weakness.[105] Respiratory failure may result in death.

Diagnosis

Similar to other neurological disorders, the patient's history along with other diagnostic tests aids in an accurate diagnosis. Patients may present with complaints of double vision or drooping eyelids. Also, myasthenia gravis causes weakness of the shoulder girdle muscles. Therefore, the patient may complain of the inability to perform a variety of self-care activities, such as drying the hair with a blow dryer.

The neurological examination is also valuable in making the diagnosis. The cranial nerve examination may reveal ptosis and diplopia as well as other cranial nerve involvement. Motor weakness may be exhibited.

In addition, laboratory studies are obtained. Blood is drawn for AChR antibodies, which are present in up to 80% of patients.

Repetitive nerve conduction study during electromyography (EMG) is helpful in the diagnosis of myasthenia gravis. In EMG, a needle electrode is inserted into a skeletal muscle and a recording of the electrical activity at rest, during voluntary activity, and with electrical stimulation is displayed on an oscilloscope. The patient should be informed that the needle causes some discomfort. In myasthenia gravis, the loss of functional AChRs results in a decrease in action potential size with repeated stimulation.[105] Repetitive muscle stimulation produces a rapid decline in muscle action potential because of the deficient numbers of AChRs. Single-fiber EMG is a very sensitive test to assess the functioning of neuromuscular junction transmission.

The Tensilon, or edrophonium, test is a classic diagnostic tool for confirming a diagnosis of myasthenia gravis. A positive test result lends strong support for the diagnosis of myasthenia gravis. In this test, 10 mg of IV Tensilon, a short-acting anticholinesterase agent, is given over an approximately 1-minute period. When injected, it transiently inhibits the breakdown of acetylcholine at the neuromuscular junction. A response is anticipated within 2 to 3 minutes. The test is most useful if there is improvement of ptosis or strength of the extraocular muscles. Limb strength or improved bulbar function may be difficult to interpret. When Tensilon is administered, atropine should be readily available in the event that the patient develops bradycardia.[106] Because there have been reports of ventricular tachycardia and death as well, Tensilon should be administered in a monitored setting.

A CT scan or MRI of the chest may also be performed to rule out thymoma or thymal hyperplasia. As noted earlier, patients with myasthenia gravis may have thymic tumors and should be screened. Thyroid function tests and vitamin B_{12} levels should also be checked, along with antinuclear antibodies, parietal cell antibodies, and antimicrosomal antibodies.

Clinical Management

The clinical management of myasthenia gravis includes the following strategies: use of medications to enhance neuromuscular transmission; long-term immunosuppression with corticosteroids, mycophenolate mofetil (CellCept), azathioprine (Imuran), or cyclosporine; cyclophosphamide (Cytoxan); short-term immunomodulation with plasmapheresis or IVIG; or thymectomy.

Pharmacological Management

Pharmacological management includes the use of anticholinesterases, steroids, or other immunosuppressive agents. Pyridostigmine (Mestinon) is available in three formulations: liquid, a 60-mg tablet, or as a 180-mg time-span formula. If the patient is unable to swallow the tablet or has a nasogastric tube or percutaneous endoscopic gastrostomy, the 60-mg tablet may be crushed, or the liquid form of pyridostigmine may be used.[107] This agent inhibits the enzymatic elimination of acetylcholine, thus prolonging its action at the postsynaptic membrane and enhancing neuromuscular transmission.[104] As a result of this action, more acetylcholine is available at the neuromuscular junction, and the patient has improved muscle strength. Medication onset is 30 minutes after administration, peaks in 1 hour, and lasts for 3 to 4 hours.

Pyridostigmine should always be administered promptly as prescribed. It should be given every 3 to 4 hours when the patient is awake. If there is difficulty with chewing and swallowing, timing the medication 30 minutes before meals is helpful. The 180-mg time-span tablet is administered at bedtime and should never be crushed.[108] Because the medication is given at night, the patient will have the benefit of sleep. Muscarinic side effects include diarrhea, abdominal cramping, increased salivation, blurred vision, bradycardia, and increased perspiration. Nicotinic side effects include muscle twitching, weakness, and fatigue.[106]

If the patient cannot take oral pyridostigmine because of NPO status or intubation, a comparable approach is to use IV neostigmine. IV neostigmine bromide 1 mg is equivalent to pyridostigmine 60 mg. Neostigmine can be infused as a continuous infusion, and care should be taken to ensure the patency of the IV access. Cardiac monitoring is essential.

Steroids and other immunosuppressive medications may be used in conjunction with pyridostigmine in the management of myasthenia gravis. A summary of the mechanism of action, onset of immunosuppression, usual dosage, and nursing considerations can be found in Table 35-12.[104,107]

There are some medications the patient should not receive. For example, D-penicillamine is contraindicated in patients with myasthenia gravis. Other agents, including some antibiotics, can cause an increase in myasthenic weakness (Table 35-13).[106] Both patients and health care professionals need to be cognizant of these medications. Although physicians and nurses working in the neuroscience arena are often familiar with these agents, patients may face potential difficulties in settings such as the emergency department or surgery, where health care professionals do not encounter patients with myasthenia gravis on a regular basis and may not be familiar with these medications.

Table 35-12 • Immunosuppressive Agents for the Treatment of Myasthenia Gravis

Drug Mechanism of Action	Onset of Immunosuppression	Dose	Adverse Effects	Considerations and Patient Teaching
Corticosteroid (Prednisone): reduces amount of antibodies produced, blocks immune mechanism and restores chemical reaction at neuromuscular junction	3 wk	60 mg daily	Steroid-induced diabetes Osteoporosis Weight gain Fluid retention Hirsutism Moon facies Insomnia Mood changes Gastric ulcers Susceptibility to infection	Starting with high dose may increase motor weakness temporarily
Azathioprine (Imuran): reduces the level of circulating acetylcholine receptor (AChR) antibodies	3–6 mo Maximal improvement in 36 mo	2–3 mg/kg/day	Bone marrow depression Increased risk for carcinoma Hepatotoxicity	Should be taken with food Pregnancy precautions Nurse to follow safe handling of hazardous drugs
Mycophenolate mofetil (CellCept): inhibition of purine synthesis by the de novo pathway	3–6 mo	1 g bid	Neutropenia; anemia; thrombocytopenia; leukopenia GI hemorrhage/perforation	Cautious use in digestive system disorders
Cyclosporine: suppresses T-cell function that decreases circulating AChR antibodies	4 wk	2–3 mg/kg/day; after morning and evening meals	Hypertension Nephrotoxicity	Traditionally used to provide immunosuppression after organ transplantation More costly than azathioprine
Cyclophosphamide (Cytoxan): chemotherapeutic agent; potent immunosuppressant	4 wk	2–3 mg/kg/day	Hair loss Hemorrhagic cystitis Bone marrow suppression Jaundice Kidney failure	Chemotherapy administration protocol to be followed Nurses to follow safe handling principles Education about reproductive risks

Table 35-13 • Medications to Avoid in Myasthenia Gravis

Category	Drug
Antibiotics	Aminoglycosides "Mycins" Tetracycline Polymyxin B and E Colistin
Antiepileptic drugs	Phenytoin Mephenytoin Trimethadione
Cardiovascular medications	Quinidine Procainamide β-blockers
Psychotropics	Lithium carbonate Phenothiazines
Muscle relaxants	Curare Succinylcholine
Others	Magnesium preparations Quinine D-Penicillamine Chloroquine

Adapted from Kernich C, Kaminski H: Myasthenia gravis: Pathophysiology, diagnosis and collaborative care. J Neurosci Nurs 27(4):207–215, 1995.

Plasmapheresis

Plasmapheresis may be indicated for patients in crisis or who are otherwise refractory to treatment. Plasmapheresis is initiated to remove circulating anti-AChR antibodies from the plasma, which results in clinical improvement. This procedure is performed through a dual-lumen central vascular access device, which is similar to a dialysis catheter. A specialized team of nurses, trained in plasmapheresis, performs the treatment, usually 3 times a week, while the patient is an inpatient. Treatments may continue on an outpatient basis. The patient's circulating blood volume is removed through one of the lumens, filtered, and then returned through the second lumen. The patient's plasma is removed and albumin is returned, along with the solid components of the patient's blood. The procedure takes several hours, and the patient is monitored for hypotension. Electrolytes and clotting factors are evaluated after each treatment.[106]

The catheters must be managed appropriately because they are a potential source of infection. They can pose a special challenge because the patient with myasthenia gravis may be receiving steroids or other immunosuppressive therapy. The nurse must also be aware that plasmapheresis removes medications, including pyridostigmine, which the patient has taken. The nurse must obtain an order from the physician to hold the medication.

Intravenous Immunoglobulin

Another treatment in place of plasma exchange is IVIG. It is used either for acute disease management or as a long-term treatment for patients with myasthenia gravis who do not respond to other types of treatments. It is often used before thymectomy to stabilize the patient. The patient's dose is individualized. Patients may exhibit clinical improvement in 2 to 4 days, and it may last for weeks or months. The mechanism of action of IVIG is unknown. The patient needs to be monitored for fever and chills, leukopenia, headache, fluid overload, and renal failure. Approximately 70% of patients receiving IVIG have been shown to improve rapidly in 4 to 5 days.[106]

Thymectomy

Thymectomy is a standard treatment for patients younger than 52 years with generalized myasthenia gravis. This surgical procedure promotes sustained remission and improvement, although no controlled studies have been performed. However, the fall in antibody titers after surgery supports the use of thymectomy. Patients must be aware that this procedure is performed for its long-term benefit so that they do not expect a dramatic improvement immediately after surgery. Clinical improvement may not be realized for 6 to 12 months after thymectomy. In some cases, benefit may not be seen for several years.[105] Patients may demonstrate enough improvement so that their medications may be reduced, thereby reducing adverse side effects.

Post-thymectomy care involves a short stay in the ICU. Epidural analgesia is used to manage pain after the procedure. The patient is usually extubated immediately after the surgery. Intermittent positive-pressure breathing may be used to minimize postoperative respiratory complications. After the critical care stay, patients are transferred to an inpatient setting, where they are monitored for complications.

Management of Myasthenic Versus Cholinergic Crisis

Factors such as stress, respiratory infection, too rapid a steroid taper, or medication affecting the neuromuscular junction may predispose the patient to a crisis. A myasthenic crisis needs to be differentiated from a cholinergic crisis because the management of each is different.

A myasthenic crisis is characterized by respiratory failure along with sudden exacerbation of weakness in other muscle groups. It is usually caused by lack of medication or lack of responsiveness at the neuromuscular junction to cholinergic treatment, as well as a worsening of the disease process. The patient is unresponsive to an increase in anticholinesterase medications and can experience severe weakness, dysphagia, and respiratory compromise. Frequent FVC checks should be performed, and when it falls below 15 mL/kg, the patient should be intubated. Any patient with myasthenia gravis with uncertain respiratory status should be admitted to an ICU to permit close monitoring of FVC, negative inspiratory force, and anxiety, as well as to facilitate a physical examination.[109]

The hallmarks of cholinergic crisis are muscarinic or nicotinic side effects, namely, increased perspiration, abdominal cramping, and diarrhea. Cholinergic crisis results from too much medication that causes neuromuscular blockage (which prevents muscle depolarization because of excess acetylcholine). The patient may also experience respiratory failure.

Indeed, respiratory failure may be seen in both types of crises.

Patients should be managed intensively. Admission to the ICU includes DVT prophylaxis and ulcer prevention.[109] Providers need to be aware that patients in myasthenic crisis are not intubated due to lung or systemic problems. It is due to difficulties with muscle strength.[108]

In the past, the Tensilon test was used to determine whether the patient was in a myasthenic or cholinergic crisis. If there was an improvement in muscle strength when Tensilon was administered, it indicated a myasthenic crisis. If there was no improvement or further deterioration of muscle strength, the patient was most likely experiencing a cholinergic crisis.[107] This test is no longer required because the withdrawal of cholinesterase drugs is necessary for improvement in both crises. Respiratory and nutritional support is provided in both situations.

Nursing Management

Assessment The nurse must focus the neurological assessment on cranial nerve involvement, motor strength, and the extent of respiratory involvement. The patient should be monitored for ptosis and double vision. The patient's motor strength should be evaluated by the use of arm abduction times up to 5 minutes. One valuable tool in monitoring respiratory function is the use of a hand-held spirometer to measure FVC. The nurse must be vigilant in monitoring the patient's respiratory status because the patient's diaphragm and intercostal muscles may become weak. If the patient's FVC falls below 1 liter, it usually indicates respiratory failure, and intubation and mechanical ventilation are necessary. An easy bedside test involves counting out numbers in one breath. Most patients should be able to count out up to 50 in one breath. In summary, useful clinical assessment involves arm abduction times, FVC, range of eye movements, and time to the development of ptosis on upward gaze. Muscle strength testing is also valuable.[108]

Plan The patient with myasthenia gravis may need assistance with activities of daily living. Adaptive equipment can help him or her perform self-care activities. Short rest periods are planned throughout the day, so the patient does not fatigue easily.

Nutrition also needs to be addressed. Meals should be planned when pyridostigmine is at its peak. Aspiration precautions should be established. Thin liquids should be given only if the patient can tolerate them well. If the patient chokes when swallowing water, oral intake should cease. If the patient has a wet, gurgling, or stridorous voice, intubation may be necessary for airway protection, and nutrition may need to be offered through the enteral route. Caloric intake must be sustained to prevent a negative energy balance that interferes with weaning from the ventilator.[109]

Skin care also needs to be incorporated into the care routine, and measures should be taken to avoid pressure ulcers. Pressure relief devices can be used in bed or on chairs.

An effective method of communication should also be developed. It may be difficult to understand the patient because of the nasal quality of the voice. A communication board may be helpful as an alternate communication device.

Patient Education and Discharge Planning

Support and education about myasthenia gravis are crucial for the successful management of the disease. The patient needs to learn about the purpose of medications, medication schedules, and side effects. Patients should be instructed to adhere to their medication schedules and to contact the physician for modification if needed. Doses of medication should be kept at home and work so that they are readily available. During travel, the patient should always carry his or her medication (e.g., in a purse or camera case) so that it does not become lost with luggage.

It is also helpful for the patient to obtain a Medic Alert bracelet and card so that rapid identification can occur in the event of a medical emergency. If the patient is unable to communicate, successful management may hinge on health care professionals recognizing that the person has myasthenia gravis.

The patient and family are taught to recognize signs and symptoms of a crisis. In addition, the importance of avoiding potential triggers for a crisis, such as respiratory infection or undue stress, is emphasized. During the winter months, when colds and flu occur, the patient should be instructed to stay away from places where large groups of people gather, such as movies or concerts.

The patient should also be educated about community support groups. The Myasthenia Gravis Foundation can provide valuable resources. Box 35-7 lists patient teaching guidelines for myasthenia gravis. Long-term outcomes in myasthenia gravis have improved markedly because of the availability of immune-modulating therapies, and patients need to be educated on how to live with their disease. A discharge planning guide for the patient with neurological dysfunction is provided in Box 35-8.

• Clinical Applicability Challenges

Case Study

Mrs. S. is a 35-year-old school librarian who lost consciousness while moderating the fifth grade reading group. Her students report seeing her "eyes roll back in her head and then she started to shake all over." She is taken by ambulance to the emergency department of the local hospital, where a computed tomography scan reveals a nonenhancing left frontal lobe tumor consistent with a low-grade glioma. Steroids are initiated for brain edema, and anticonvulsants are ordered to control seizures. Magnetic resonance imaging (MRI) further delineates the lesion.

Box 35-7 • TEACHING GUIDE: Living With Myasthenia Gravis

Safety
- Obtain a Medic Alert bracelet and wear it at all times. Always carry personal identification in your wallet or purse.
- Avoid respiratory infections. Stay away from concert halls and movie theaters in the winter.
- Avoid stress and stressful situations.
- Consider grinding or pureeing foods to make them easier to eat. Choose calorie-rich, nutritious snacks. Request a consultation with a dietitian if you have difficulty maintaining your weight.

Activity
- Plan frequent rest periods during the day.
- Conserve energy as much as possible.
- Avoid shopping at peak times or substitute "on-line" shopping so items can be delivered directly to your door.

Medications
- Mestinon should be taken as directed by your physician. Adjustments should be made only under the direction of your physician. Remember not to crush Mestinon Timespan.
- Mestinon should be stored at home and at work. Do not store medication in your car where it could be exposed to extreme heat and cold. When traveling, keep medication with you; do not store it in your luggage.
- Avoid medications (certain antibiotics such as aminoglycosides, anticonvulsants, and muscle relaxants) that could exacerbate myasthenia gravis.
- Do not take any over-the-counter preparations or complementary medications without first contacting your physician.
- If you are taking Imuran or cyclophosphamide, you need to follow precautions about hazardous drugs. Be certain to discuss family planning issues with your physician.

When to Call the Physician
- Call your physician if you are experiencing increased weakness, swallowing problems, or respiratory difficulties.
- Contact your physician immediately if you are hospitalized for any reason.

The Myasthenia Gravis Foundation of America is a valuable resource. Contact them for additional information and to find local support groups.

Box 35-8 • DISCHARGE PLANNING GUIDE: Neurological Dysfunction

- Arrange for a safety assessment of the home environment to identify potential hazards to ambulation.
- Review the patient's medication profile to reinforce compliance and to ensure therapeutic monitoring.
- If the patient cannot care for himself or herself or if the family cannot provide care, consider the services of a home health agency.
- Provide resources to take home, such as written materials about neurological dysfunction, information about medications, and the name of the person to contact with questions. The home care nurse will be able to reinforce patient teaching and answer questions.
- Arrange for resources such as speech therapy, occupational therapy, and physical therapy.

Several days later, Mrs. S. is taken to the operating room, where she undergoes a gross total resection of the tumor. Final pathology reveals a grade II astrocytoma. No further therapy is recommended, and she is followed with MRI scans every 3 months for the first year and semiannually thereafter.

After 6 years, follow-up MRI reveals a "ring-enhancing lesion with peritumoral edema." Mrs. S. has no neurologic symptoms. She undergoes a repeat craniotomy and receives the appropriate mechanical and pharmacological venous thromboembolism prophylaxis during her hospitalization. She is discharged on a steroid taper and anticonvulsant therapy. The final pathology reveals that the lesion has progressed to grade IV (glioblastoma multiforme). After appropriate consultations, she starts a 6-week course of radiation therapy with concomitant low-dose temozolomide. After this treatment, she is to receive monthly temozolomide for an additional 6 months.

During the third week of treatment, Mrs. S. develops moderate to severe headaches. She also has leg and chest discomfort, which she does not report, suspecting that they are related to her medications. Brain MRI reveals treatment-related edema; steroids (dexamethasone) are increased from 2 mg twice a day to 4 mg four times a day. The headaches resolve within 24-hours.

However, the following afternoon, Mrs. S. is found by her husband, unconscious and with irregular respirations. He calls 911, and she is taken to the nearest emergency department, where she is pronounced dead. Autopsy reveals a massive pulmonary embolus.

Short-Answer Questions

1. Seizures are experienced by approximately 50% of patients during the course of treatment for a brain tumor. Which patients are most likely to experience seizures?
2. Would giving radiation therapy after the initial surgery for a low-grade tumor have decreased the likelihood of tumor recurrence and progression to a higher grade?
3. What is the risk for venous thromboembolism in patients with brain tumors?

Review Questions

1. The nurse educator in the neuroscience critical care unit is teaching an introductory brain tumor course

to newly hired nurses. Which statement accurately describes the classification of brain tumors?
  a. Metastatic brain tumors arise in the brain and disseminate to distant sites.
  b. The most common sites of origin for primary brain tumors are lung and breast.
  c. Metastatic brain tumors seed to the brain from distant sites.
  d. Primary brain tumors occur more frequently than metastatic brain tumors.

2. The neurosurgeon and neurosurgical nurse are describing the necessity of surgery to the patient and her family members. Which statement best describes the treatment plan for a suspected glioblastoma multiforme (GBM)?
  a. "Surgery is needed for diagnosis and tumor removal. No additional treatment is necessary."
  b. "Once surgery is performed, if the diagnosis of GBM is confirmed, you will require further therapy in the form of radiation and chemotherapy."
  c. "Because your MRI scan shows a tumor consistent with GBM, you do not need surgery. You do need radiation and chemotherapy."
  d. "Although we think this is a malignant tumor, we expect you to live a normal life after aggressive treatment."

3. When teaching family members to care for a patient with a seizure disorder, the nurse should reinforce which of the following instructions?
  a. "Put your finger in the patient's mouth during the seizure to keep him from choking."
  b. "Once the seizure is over, give the patient extra medicine to prevent another seizure. Then call the doctor."
  c. "Turn the patient to his side if possible and move sharp objects out of the way."
  d. "Take the patient to the emergency department immediately."

4. A patient is seen in the emergency department for prolonged seizure activity. Which of the following describes status epilepticus?
  a. A period of continued and/or repetitive seizures lasting at least 30 minutes
  b. An episode of abnormal and excessive discharges of cerebral neurons with change in level of consciousness
  c. Recurrent seizures involving loss of consciousness
  d. A nonepileptic event that may involve either asymmetrical motor activity or physical collapse

5. Mr. C. is a 68-year-old man who is outdoors working in his garden at 12:00 noon on a sunny July day. Suddenly, he begins to experience right-sided weakness, numbness, and blurred vision. When he calls out to his wife who is sitting on a nearby porch, his speech is slurred and difficult to understand. He states that he is feeling weak and his vision is fuzzy. Based on these symptoms, Mrs. C. should:
  a. Offer her husband some lemonade because he is dehydrated.
  b. Call emergency medical personnel and tell them that she thinks her husband is having a stroke.

  c. Drive her husband to their local physician's office.
  d. Instruct her husband to lie in the shade and rest.

6. Mr. B. is a 65-year-old retired car salesman with a history of uncontrolled hypertension, type 2 diabetes, and hypercholesterolemia. While mowing his lawn on a hot August afternoon, he develops right-sided numbness and tingling at 1:00 p.m., but he continues to work outdoors. When his wife returns from shopping at 5:00 p.m., she is concerned about her husband's garbled speech and his dragging right leg. She immediately calls 911. Mr. B. is transported by emergency medical personnel to the emergency department. What factors determine whether Mr. B. is a candidate for thrombolytic therapy?
  a. Age and sex
  b. Witnessed time last seen well
  c. Length of diagnosis of diabetes
  d. History of prostate cancer

7. A female patient is transferred from the emergency department to the neurological intensive care unit with a diagnosis of subarachnoid hemorrhage. A cerebral angiogram reveals the presence of an intracranial aneurysm. On examination, she is difficult to arouse but follows commands. She is disoriented to time and place. Motor strength in her right arm is 3/5, and she has right facial weakness. Based on these findings, the patient has what grade of aneurysm?
  a. Grade I
  b. Grade II
  c. Grade III
  d. Grade IV

8. Ms. K. is a 30-year-old woman with a 2-year history of myasthenia gravis. She has been home ill with the flu for 2 days. She presents to the emergency department complaining of increasing weakness, vomiting, difficulty swallowing, and ptosis. On initial assessment, her forced vital capacity is 0.9 L. When obtaining the history, the nurse would expect the patient to give which of the following responses?
  a. Her fatigue is constant.
  b. Her weakness improves with rest.
  c. Her strength improves with constant activity.
  d. Her swallowing improves when she drinks only liquids.

References

1. Central Brain Tumor Registry of the United States: Primary Brain Tumors in the United States, 1998–2002. Statistical Report, 2005–2006
2. Burger PC, Scheithauer BW, Vogel FS: The brain: Tumours. In Surgical Pathology of the Nervous System and Its Coverings, 4th ed. New York: Churchill Livingstone, 2002, pp 160–378
3. World Health Organization: Classification of tumours. In Kleihues P, Cabenne WK (eds): Pathology and Genetics of Tumours of the Nervous System. Lyon, France: IARC Press, 2000
4. Bondy ML, El-Zein R, Wrensch M: Epidemiology of brain cancer. In Schiff D, O'Neill P (eds): Principles of Neuro-oncology. New York: McGraw-Hill, 2005, pp 3–16

5. Grossman S: Familial gliomas. In Berger MS, Wilson CB (eds): The Gliomas. Philadelphia: WB Saunders, 1999, pp 12–14

6. Wrensch N, Fisher JL, et al: The molecular epidemiology of gliomas in adults. Neurosurg Focus 19(5):E5, 2005

7. American College of Surgical Oncology CNS Working Group: The management of brain metastases. In Schiff D, O'Neill P (eds): Principles of Neuro-oncology. New York: McGraw-Hill, 2005, pp 553–580

8. Papadopoulos MC, Saadoun S, Binder DK, et al: Molecular mechanisms of brain tumor edema. Neuroscience 129(4):1011–1020, 2004

9. Long D: Capillary ultrastructure and the blood-brain barrier in human malignant brain tumors. J Neurosurg 32:127–144, 1970

10. Kaal EC, Vecht CJ: The management of brain edema in brain tumors. Curr Opin Oncol 16(6):593–600, 2004

11. Layon AJ, Gabrielli A: Elevated intracranial pressure. In Layon AJ, Gabrielli A, Friedman WA (eds): Textbook of Neurointensive Care. Philadelphia: WB Saunders, 2004, pp 709–732

12. Wen PY, Schiff D, Kesari S, et al: Medical management of patients with brain tumors. J Neurooncol PMID:16807780, 2006

13. Farace E, Shaffrey ME: Neuropsychological issues. In Shiff D, O'Neill BP (eds): Principles in Neuro-oncology. New York: McGraw-Hill, 2006, pp 201–216

14. Aronen HJ, Perkio J: Dynamic susceptibility contrast MRI of gliomas. Neuroimaging Clin North Am 12(4):501–523, 2002

15. Bullitt E, Zeng D, Gerig G, et al: Vessel tortuosity and brain tumor malignancy: A blinded study. Acad Radiol 12(10):1232–1240, 2005

16. Gujar SK, Maheshwari S, Bjorkman-Burtscher I, et al: Magnetic resonance spectroscopy. J Neuroophthalmol 25(3):217–226, 2005

17. Spence AM, Mankoff DA, Muzi M: Positron emission tomography of brain tumors. Neuroimaging Clin North Am 13:715–739, 2003

18. Wilkinson ID, Romanowski CA, Jellinek DA, et al: Motor functional MRI for preoperative and intraoperative neurosurgical guidance. Br J Radiol 76:98–103, 2003

19. Sills AK: Current treatment approaches to surgery for brain metastases. Neurosurg Online 57(5):S4-24–S4-32, 2005

20. Nahaczewski AE, Fowler SB, Hariharan S: Dexamethasone therapy in patients with brain tumors—a focus on tapering. J Neurosci Nurs 36(6):340–343, 2004

21. Forsyth PA, Weaver S, Fulton D, et al: Prophylactic anticonvulsants in patients with brain tumor. Can J Neurol Sci 30(2):102–112, 2003

22. De Santis A, Villani R, Sinisi M, et al: Add-on phenytoin fails to prevent early seizures after surgery for supratentorial brain tumors: A randomized controlled study. Epilepsia 43(2):175–182, 2002

23. Siomin V, Angelov L, Li L, et al: Results of a survey of neurosurgical practice patterns regarding the prophylactic use of anti-epilepsy drugs in patients with brain tumors. J Neurooncol 74:211–215, 2005

24. Bohan E, Macenka DG: Surgical management of patients with brain tumors. Semin Oncol Nurs 20(4):240–252, 2004

25. Khatua S, Jalali R: Recent advances in the treatment of childhood brain tumors. Pediatr Hematol Oncol 22(5):361–371, 2005

26. Martin JJ, Kondiolka D: Indications for resection and radiosurgery for brain metastases. Curr Opin Oncol 17(6):584–587, 2005

27. Fiveash JB, Spencer SA: Role of radiation therapy and radiosurgery in glioblastoma multiforme. Cancer J 9(3):222–229, 2003

28. Pang LJ: Radiation oncology update. Hawaii Med J 62(5):109–110, 2003

29. Yu C, Shepard D: Treatment planning for stereotactic radiosurgery with photon beams. Technol Cancer Res Treat 2(2):93–104, 2003

30. Vitaz TW, Warnke PC, Tabar V, Gutin PH, et al: Brachytherapy for brain tumors. J Neurooncol 73:71–86, 2005

31. Chan TA, Weingart JD, Parisi M, et al: Treatment of recurrent glioblastoma multiforme with GliaSite brachytherapy. Int J Radiat Oncol Biol Phys 62(4):1133–1139, 2005

32. Kleinberg L, Grossman SA, Carson K, et al: Survival of patients with newly diagnosed glioblastoma multiforme treated with RSR13 and radiotherapy: Results of a phase II New Approaches to Brain Tumor Consortium safety and efficacy study. J Clin Oncol 20(14):3149–3155, 2002

33. Stupp R, Mason WP, van den Bent MJ, et al: Radiotherapy plus concomitant and adjuvant temozolomide for glioblastoma. N Engl J Med 352:987–996, 2005

34. Brem H, Piantadosi S, Burger PC, et al: Placebo-controlled trial of safety and efficacy of intraoperative controlled delivery by biodegradable polymers of chemotherapy for recurrent gliomas. Lancet 345:1008–1012, 1995

35. Gallia GL, Brem S, Brem H: Local treatment of malignant brain tumors using implantable chemotherapeutic polymers. J Natl Compr Cancer Netw 3(5):721–728, 2005

36. Chiocca EA, Broaddus WC, Gillies GT, et al: Neurosurgical delivery of chemotherapeutics, targeted toxins, genetic and viral therapies in neuro-oncology. J Neurooncol 69:101–117, 2004

37. Steiner HH, Bonsanto MM, Beckhove P, et al: Antitumor vaccination of patients with glioblastoma multiforme: A pilot study to assess feasibility, safety, and clinical benefit. J Clin Oncol 22(21):4272–4281, 2004

38. Fairbrother CA, Paice JA: Life's final journey: The oncology nurse's role. Clin J Oncol Nurs 9(5):575–579, 2005

39. Braunack-Mayer THN, Beilby J: The impact of the hospice environment on patient spiritual expression. Oncol Nurs Forum 32(5):1049–1055, 2005

40. Brettler S: Endovascular coiling for cerebral aneurysms. AACN Clinical Issues 16(4):515–525, 2005

41. Tamargo RJ, Walter KA, Oshiro EM: Aneurysmal subarachnoid hemorrhage: Prognostic features and outcomes. New Horizon 5:364–375, 1997

42. Brisman JL, Song JK, Newell DW: Cerebral aneurysms. N Engl J Med 333(9):928–939, 2006

43. Juvela S, Porras M, Poussa K: Natural history of unruptured intracranial aneurysms: Probability and risk factors for aneurysm rupture. Neurosurg Focus 8(5):preview 1, 2000

44. David CA: Cerebral aneurysms and subarachnoid hemorrhage. In Netter's Neurology. Philadelphia: Saunders Elsevier, 2005, pp 248–261

45. Mower-Wade D, Cavanaugh MC, Bush C: Protecting a patient with ruptured cerebral aneurysm. Nursing 31(2):52–58, 2001

46. Oyama K, Criddle, L: Vasospasm after aneurysmal subarachnoid hemorrhage. Crit Care Nurse 24(5):58–67, 2004

47. Hickey J (ed): The Clinical Practice of Neurological and Neurosurgical Nursing, 5th ed. Philadelphia: Lippincott Williams & Wilkins, 2003

48. Pope WL: Cerebral vessel repair with coils & glue . . . Gentler on the mind. Nursing 32(7):46–49, 2002

49. Tara MM, Nakahara I, Higashi T, et al: Endovascular embolization vs surgical clipping in treatment of cerebral aneurysms: morbidity and morality with short-term outcome. Surg Neurol 66:277–284, 2006

50. Twedell D: Aneurysmal subarachnoid hemorrhage. J Contin Educ Nurs 35(4):150–151, 2004

51. Yamada S, Brauer FS, Colohan AR, et al: Concept of arteriovenous malformation compartments and surgical management. Neurol Res 26:288–300, 2004

52. Greenberg MS: Vascular malformations. In Handbook of Neurosurgery. New York: Thieme, 2006, pp 835–848

53. Graham GD: Arteriovenous malformations in the brain. Curr Treat Options Neurol 4:435–444m, 2002

54. Garretson HD: Vascular malformations and fistulas. In Wilkins RH, Rengachary SS (eds): Neurosurgery. New York: McGraw-Hill, 1991, pp 1448–1458

55. Parsa AT, Solomon RA: Vascular malformations affecting the nervous system. In Rengachary SS, Ellenbogen RG (eds): Principles of Neurosurgery, 2nd ed. Philadelphia: Elsevier Mosby, 2005, pp 241–258

56. Stefani MA, Porter PJ, ter Brugge KG, et al: Large and deep brain arteriovenous malformations are associated with risk of future hemorrhage. Stroke 33:1220–1224, 2002

57. Spetzler RF, Martin NA: A proposed grading system for arteriovenous malformations. J Neurosurg 65:476–483, 1986

58. Gailloud P: Endovascular treatment of cerebral arteriovenous malformations. Tech Vasc Interv Radiol 8(3):118–128, 2005

59. Fleetwood IG: Arteriovenous malformations. Lancet 359:863–873, 2002

60. Zonenshayn M, Rezai A: Stereotactic surgery. In Rengachary SS, Ellenbogen RG (eds): Principles of Neurosurgery, 2nd ed. Philadelphia: Elsevier Mosby, 2005, pp 785–817

61. Woodworth G, McGirt MJ, Samdani A, et al: Accuracy of frameless and frame-based image-guided stereotactic brain biopsy in the diagnosis of glioma: comparison of biopsy and open resection specimen. Neurol Res 27(4):358–362, 2006

62. Whittle IR: Surgery for gliomas. Curr Opin Neurol 15:663–699, 2002

63. Weingart J, Brem H: Basic principles of cranial surgery for brain tumors. In Winn HR (ed): Youmans Neurosurgical Surgery, 5th ed. Philadelphia: WB Saunders, 2003, pp 899–907

64. Nakao N, Nakai K, Itakura T, et al: Updating of neuronavigation on images intraoperatively acquired with a mobile computerized tomographic scanner: Technical note. Minim Invasive Neurosurg 46:117–20, 2003

65. Amundson EW, McGirt MJ, Olivi A: A contralateral, transfrontal, extraventricular approach to stereotactic brainstem biopsy procedures. J Neurosurg 102(3):565–570, 2005

66. Meyer FB, Bates LM, Goerss SJ, et al: Awake craniotomy for aggressive resection of primary gliomas located in eloquent brain. Mayo Clin Proc 76:677–687, 2001

67. Oyesiku NM: Nonfunctioning pituitary adenomas. In Rengachary SS, Ellenbogen RG (eds): Principles of Neurosurgery, 2nd ed. Philadelphia: Elsevier Mosby, 2005, pp 593–602

68. Teo C, Mobb R: Neuroendoscopy. In Rengachary SS, Ellenbogen RG (eds): Principles of Neurosurgery, 2nd ed. Philadelphia: Elsevier Mosby, 2005

69. Schwartz TH, Stieg PE, Anand VK: Endoscopic transsphenoidal pituitary surgery with intraoperative magnetic resonance imaging. Neurosurgery 58(1 Suppl):ONS44–51, 2006

70. Morrison K: The road to JCAHO disease specific care certification. Dimens Crit Care Nurs 24(5):221–227, 2005

71. Claves CJ, Jones HR: Ischemic stroke. In Netter's Neurology. Philadelphia: Saunders Elsevier, 2005, pp 195–217

72. Testani-Dufour L, Morrison CAM: Brain attack: Correlataive anatomy. J Neurosci Nurs 29(1):213–224, 1997

73. Hinkle J: An update on transient ischemic attacks. J Neurosci Nurs 37(5):243–248, 2005

74. Barker E: A new weapon to combat stroke. RN 69(3):26–30, 2006

75. Macari-Hinson M, Moore, C, Morley, M: Carotid artery stenting: New hope for blocked vessels. Crit Care Insider, 14–20, 2006

76. Pope W: Angioplasty and stenting the carotid? RN 65(6):54–60, 2002

77. Hock NH: Brain attack: The stroke continuum. Nurs Clin North Am 34(3):689–723, 1999

78. Paolino AS, Garner KM: Effects of hyperglycemia on neurologic outcome in stroke patients. J Neurosci Nurs 37(3):130–135, 2005

79. Kehl-Pruett W: Deep vein thrombosis in hospitalized patients a review of evidence-based guidelines for prevention. Dimens Crit Care Nurs 25(2):53–59, 2006

80. Oster JM, Gutrecht JA, Gross PT: Epilepsy and syncope. In Jones HR (ed): Netter's Neurology. Philadelphia: Saunders Elsevier, 2005, pp 264–280

81. O'Brien MD, Gilmour-White SK: Management of epilepsy in women. Postgrad Med J 81(955):278–285, 2005

82. Bhatia MS, Sapra D: Pseudoseizures in children: A profile of 50 cases. Clin Pediatr (Phila) 44:617–621, 2005

83. Benbadis SR: Practical management issues for idiopathic generalized epilepsies. Epilepsia 46(Suppl 9):125–132, 2005

84. Tatum WO, Liporace J, Benbadis SR, Kaplan PW: Updates on the treatment of epilepsy in women. Arch Intern Med 164(2):137–145, 2004

85. Benbadis SR, Tatum WO 4th: Advances in the treatment of epilepsy. Am Fam Physician 64:91–98, 2001

86. Greenberg MS: Seizures. In Handbook of Neurosurgery. New York: Thieme, 2006, pp 256–288

87. Spencer SS, Spencer DD: Surgery for Epilepsy. Boston: Blackwell Scientific, 1991, pp 54–65

88. Wittman JJ Jr, Hirsch LJ: Continuous electroencephalogram monitoring in the critically ill. Neurocrit Care 2(3):330–341, 2005

89. Arle JE: Surgical treatments for epilepsy. In Netter's Neurology. Philadelphia: Saunders Elsevier, 2005, pp 281–286

90. Akanuma N, Koutroumanidis M, Adachi N, et al: Presurgical assessment of memory-related brain structures: The Wada test and functional neuroimaging. Seizure 12:346–358, 2003

91. Hamer HM, Luders HO, Knake S, et al: Electrophysiology of focal clonic seizures in humans: A study using subdural and depth electrodes. Brain 126(Pt 3):547–555, 2003

92. Krauss G, Betts T, Abou-Khalil B, et al: Levetiracetam treatment of idiopathic generalised epilepsy. Seizure 12(8):617–620, 2003

93. Kaplan P: The EEG of status epilepticus. J Clin Neurophysiol 23(3):221–229, 2006

94. Engel J Jr, Wiebe S, French S, et al: Practice parameter: Temporal lobe and localized neocortical resections for epilepsy. Report of the Quality Standards Subcommittee of the American Academy of Neurology, in association with the American Epilepsy Society and the American Association of Neurological Surgeons. Neurology 60:538–547, 2003

95. Siegel AM: Presurgical evaluation and treatment of medically refractory epilepsy. Neurosurg Rev 27:1–18, 2004

96. Handforth A, DeSalles AAF, Krahl SE: Deep brain stimulation of the subthalamic nucleus as adjunct treatment for refractory epilepsy. Epilepsia 47:1239–1242, 2006

97. Green DM: Weakness in the ICU: Guillain-Barre syndrome, myasthenia gravis, and critical illness polyneuropathy/myopathy. Neurologist 11(6):338–347, 2005

98. Van Doorn PA: Treatment of Guillain-Barre syndrome and CIDP. J Peripheral Nervous Syst 10:113–127, 2005

99. Burns TM, Russell JA, Jones HR: Acquired demyelinating polyradiculoneuropathies: Guillain-Barre syndrome and chronic inflammatory demyelinating polyradiculoneuropathy. In Netter's Neurology. Philadelphia: Saunders Elsevier, 2005, pp 818–826

100. Sheikh KA: Peripheral nerve disease: Guillain-Barre syndrome. In Johnson RT, Griffin JW, McArthur JC (eds): Current Therapy in Neurologic Disease. St. Louis: Mosby, 2002, pp 366–370

101. Haldeman D, Zulkosky K: Treatment and nursing care for a patient with Guillain-Barre syndrome. Dimens Crit Care Nurs 24(6):267–272, 2005

102. Ropper AH: The Guillain-Barre syndrome. N Engl J Med 326:1130–1136, 1992

103. Koski CL, Patterson JV: Intravenous immunoglobulin use for neurologic diseases. J Infusion Nurs 29(35):S21–S28, 2006

104. Chaudhry V, Drachman DB: Disorders of neuromuscular junction transmission. In Asbury A, McKhann G, McDonald W, Goadsby, P, McArthur J (eds): Diseases of the Nervous System: Clinical Neuroscience and Therapeutic Principles. Cambridge, UK: Cambridge University Press, 2002, pp 1143–1162

105. Burns T, Ryan M, Jones H: Myasthenia gravis. In Netter's Neurology. Philadelphia: Saunders Elsevier, 2005, pp 864–870

106. Kernich C, Kaminski H: Myasthenia gravis: Pathophysiology, diagnosis and collaborative care. J Neurosci Nurs 27(4): 207–215, 1995

107. Lisak R: Neuromuscular and muscle disease: Myasthenia gravis. In Johnson RT, Griffin JW, McArthur JC (eds): Current Therapy in Neurologic Disease. St. Louis: Mosby, 2002, pp 407–409

108. Kirmani JF, Yahia AM, Qureshi AI; Myasthenic crisis. Curr Treat Options Neurol 6(3):3–15, 2004

109. Green D: Weakness in the ICU: Guillain-Barre syndrome, myasthenia gravis, and critical illness polyneuropathy/myopathy. Neurologist 11(6):338–347, 2005

Other Selected Readings

Atkinson SB, Carr RL, Maybee P, Haynes D: The challenges of managing and treating Guillain-Barre syndrome during the acute phase. Dimens Crit Care Nurs 25(6):256–263, 2006

Bader MK, Palmer S: What's the "hyper" in hyperacute stroke? Strategies to improve outcomes in ischemic stroke patients presenting within 6 hours. AACN Adv Crit Care 17(2):194–214, 2006

Blissitt PA, Mitchell PH, Newell DW, et al: Cerebrovascular dynamics with head-of-bed elevation in patients with mild or moderate vasospasm after aneurysmal subarachnoid hemorrhage. Am J Crit Care 15(2):206–216, 2006

Brettler S: Endovascular coiling for cerebral aneurysm. AACN Clin Issues 16(4):515–525, 2005

Bullock MR, Chesnut R, Ghajar D, et al: Surgical management of traumatic brain injury group: Surgical management of subdural hematomas. Neurosurgery 58(3 Suppl):S2-16–S2-24, 2006

Dunleavy K, et al: Improving care for patients with subarachnoid hemorrhage. Nursing 35(11):26–27, 2005

Frizzell JP: Acute stroke: Pathophysiology, diagnosis, and treatment. AACN Clin Issues 16(4):421–440, 2005

Mahanes D, Lewis R: Weaning of the neurologically impaired patient. Crit Care Nurs Clin North Am 16(3):387–393, 2004

Nieves J, Capone-Swearer D: Stroke: The clot that changes lives. Men in Nursing 1(5):18–27, 2006

Owens D, Flom J: Integrating palliative and neurological critical care. AACN Clin Issues 16(4):542–550, 2005

Sharma M, Clark H, Armour T, et al: Acute stroke: Evaluation and treatment. Summary, evidence report/technology assessment: Number 127. Rockville, MD: Agency for Healthcare Research and Quality. AHRQ Publication Number 05-E023-1, July 2005. Available at: http://www.ahrq.gov/clinic/epcsums/acstrokesum.htm

ACKNOWLEDGMENTS

We would like to thank the following people for their advice and support: Drs. Henry Brem, Vinay Chaudhry, Richard Clatterbuck, Argye Hillis, Gregory Krauss, and Brett Morrison.

Traumatic Brain Injury

36

Elizabeth Zink

Objectives

Based on the content in this chapter, the reader should be able to:

❶ Explain the significance of the mechanism of injury when assessing the patient with traumatic brain injury.

❷ Describe various types of head injuries and typical patient presentation.

❸ Differentiate between primary and secondary brain injury.

❹ Explain the importance and process of serial neurological assessment in the patient with traumatic brain injury.

❺ Discuss the rationale for medical and nursing management in the care of the patient with a traumatic brain injury.

❻ Describe the roles of multidisciplinary health care team members in caring for the patient with traumatic brain injury.

Traumatic brain injury (TBI) affects as many as 1.4 million Americans each year and has devastating effects on patients and their families. More than one million (1.1 million) people, or 79.6% of those with TBIs, are evaluated and discharged from emergency departments each year, 235,000 (16.8%) are admitted to hospitals, and 50,000 (3.6%) die. It is suspected that a large number of people who sustain TBIs do not seek health care. Falls are the leading cause of TBIs, constituting 28% of all cases, followed by motor vehicle crashes, which account for 20% of all TBIs.[1] The incidence of TBI is 1.5 times greater in men than in women, and TBIs occur most frequently in children younger than 4 years of age and in adolescents between 15 and 19 years of age.[1] TBIs in adults older than 65 years of age most often result from falls (52%) (Box 36-1). Critical care nurses play a role in reducing the incidence of head injury through patient and family teaching as well as participation in primary prevention efforts (e.g., helmet safety, violence prevention, fall prevention, and drug and alcohol awareness).

TBI can have a profound and lasting effect on the patient and family. Neurologic deficits may affect the patient's ability to resume his or her chosen career, or to return to work at all. Emotional and behavioral changes may affect interpersonal relationships and family roles. A thorough understanding of the pathophysiology of TBI enables the critical care nurse to individualize nursing care and positively affect patient and family outcomes. Critical care nurses play a key role in planning and implementing the multidisciplinary care of these complex patients and their families.

Box 36-1 • CONSIDERATIONS FOR THE OLDER PATIENT: Preventing Falls in the Older Adult

- Screen patients 75 years of age and older for history of falling or at age 70 if they are deemed to be at a higher risk for falling
- Consider the following factors, which may need to be evaluated and/or modified in patients found to be at a greater risk for future falls:
  - Impaired vision
  - Medications
  - Blood pressure (postural hypotension)
  - Balance and gait
  - Hazards in living environment

Tinchi ME: Preventing falls in elderly persons. N Engl J Med 384(1):42–49, 2003.

• Mechanisms of Traumatic Brain Injury

Typical mechanisms of injury include acceleration, acceleration–deceleration, coup–contre coup, rotational injury, and penetrating injury (Fig. 36-1):

▶ Acceleration injuries occur when a moving object strikes the stationary head (e.g., a bat striking the head or a missile fired into the head).

▶ Acceleration–deceleration injuries occur when the head in motion strikes a stationary object. For example, a motor vehicle crash in which the head strikes the windshield produces an acceleration–deceleration injury. Acceleration–deceleration injuries can also occur with falls or physical assaults.

▶ Coup–contre coup injuries occur when the brain "bounces" back and forth within the skull, striking both sides of the brain. Coup refers to the brain tissue where impact initially occurred, and contre coup refers to the brain tissue on the opposite side. For example, when assessing a patient struck in the back of the head, the clinician evaluates for injury to posterior structures (i.e., the occipital lobes and cerebellum) as well as anterior brain structures (i.e., the frontal lobes).

▶ Rotational forces cause the brain to twist within the meninges and the skull, resulting in stretching and tearing of blood vessels and shearing of neurons. Physical assaults and motor vehicle crashes are examples of situations in which rotation and torsion may be a mechanism of injury.

▶ Penetration injuries may be caused by a bullet, shrapnel, or another sharp object traveling at a velocity substantial enough to disrupt the integrity of the skull. Depending on the speed and trajectory of the object, underlying brain structures may or may not be injured.

Cervical spine injury must be automatically assumed and systematically excluded with all types of TBIs before immobilization devices are removed. TBI is categorized by severity based on radiographic injury and the Glasgow Coma Scale (GCS) (Table 36-1).

• Primary and Secondary Brain Injury

The term *primary brain injury* describes injury occurring at the time of trauma. Injury occurring after the traumatic event is referred to as *secondary brain injury*. The initial injury causes immediate disruption of the skull, brain structures (i.e., meninges, blood vessels, brain tissues, neurons), and functions (blood flow, oxygenation, cellular metabolism). Secondary injury describes the physiological response to brain injury, including cerebral edema, cerebral ischemia, and biochemical changes. Current research and existing therapies are aimed at preventing and mitigating secondary brain injury to maximize chances for positive functional outcomes.

PRIMARY BRAIN INJURY

Scalp Laceration

A scalp laceration frequently causes significant bleeding due to the vascularity of the scalp and may be associated with other underlying injuries to the skull and brain. The scalp should be carefully palpated assessing for deformation. Skull fractures may be present even if deformities are not palpable; therefore, care must be exercised in applying pressure to scalp wounds. Scalp lacerations can be sutured at the bedside or may require surgical repair, depending on the size and extent of injury. Avulsion of areas of the scalp may require surgical reimplantation to address injured vascular structures.

Skull Fracture

The skull protects the brain by distributing forces outward, lessening direct impact to the brain. Skull fractures are categorized by location; the fractured bones may be located in the anterior, middle, or posterior fossae, or the base of the skull. Skull fractures may be compound (i.e., occurring with an open wound), displaced (closed wound in which the edges of the fracture no longer meet), or linear. Depressed skull fractures are fractures in which bone fragments are driven into the underlying meninges or brain tissue; this often presents as a depression or dip on palpation. Patients with depressed skull fractures may require surgical management to débride bone fragments, repair the skull or dura, evacuate a hematoma, or repair other adjacent structures such as sinuses or blood vessels.[2] Blood vessels travel along bony grooves on the inside surface of the skull; as a result, they are vulnerable to injury during a direct blow to the skull. Injury to the dura places the patient at risk for meningitis; therefore, careful monitoring for signs and symptoms of infection is important.

Basilar skull fractures occur at the base, or floor, of the skull, typically in the areas of the anterior and middle fossae. Basilar skull fractures are linear or displaced. Assessment of extraocular movements is important in detecting impingement of cranial nerves. Nasogastric and nasotracheal intubation are avoided

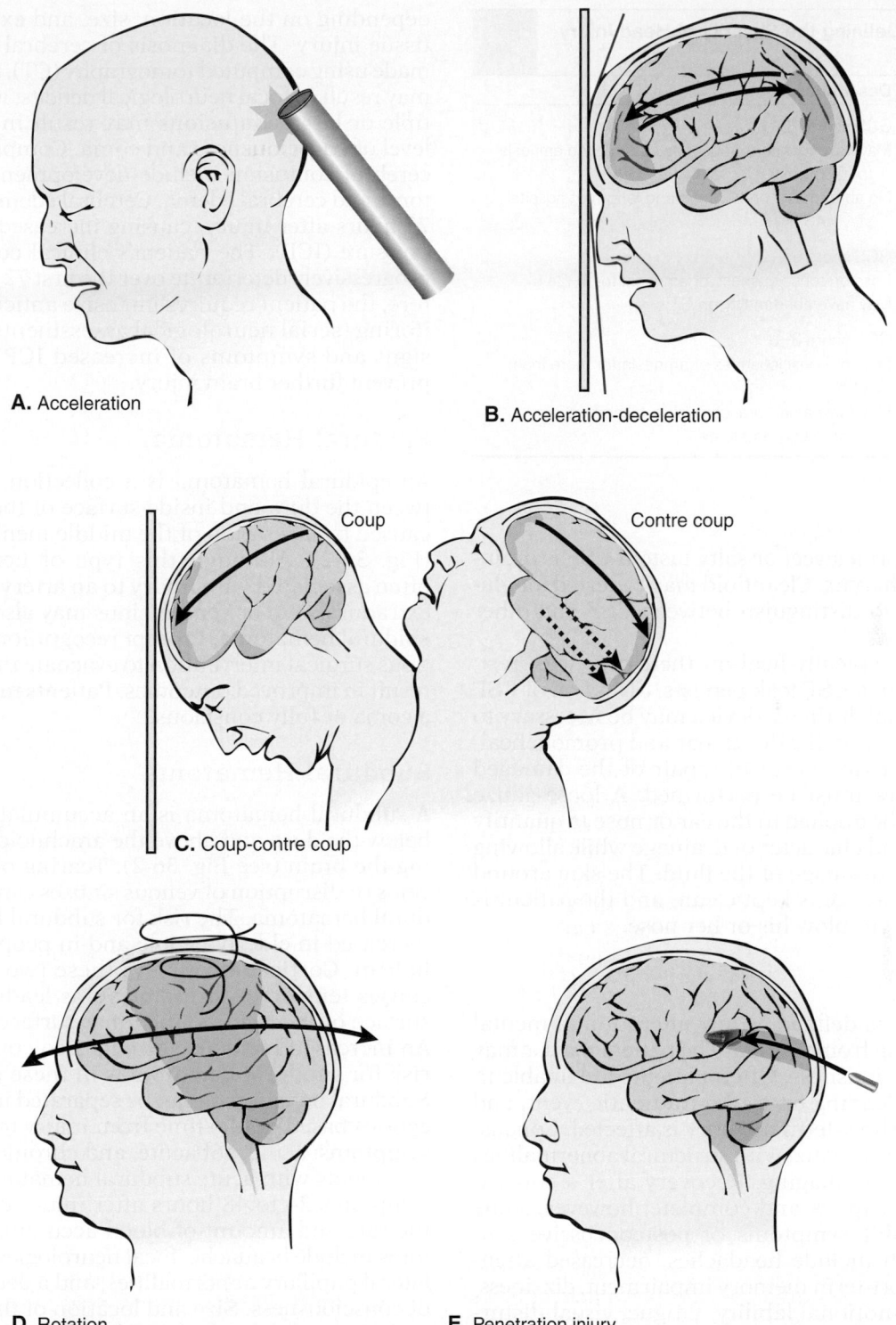

A. Acceleration

B. Acceleration-deceleration

Coup

Contre coup

C. Coup-contre coup

D. Rotation

E. Penetration injury

Figure 36-1 • Typical mechanisms of head injury. **A:** Acceleration. **B:** Acceleration–deceleration. **C:** Coup-contre coup. **D:** Rotation. **E:** Penetration.

to reduce the risk for passing the tube through the fractured areas into the brain.

Drainage of cerebrospinal fluid (CSF) from the ear or nose indicates injury to the dura. Drainage from the ear, otorrhea, typically signifies a fracture in the middle fossa. Ecchymosis (bruising) behind the ear (Battle's sign) is a delayed sign of a basilar skull fracture in the middle fossa. Rhinorrhea, CSF drainage

from the nose, occurs with a fracture in the anterior fossa. "Raccoon eyes," a ring-like pattern of bruising around the eyes, is a late sign of this type of fracture.

Drainage from the ear or nose may be mixed with blood, making identification of CSF difficult. A layering of fluids, with blood on the inside and CSF in a yellowish ring on the outside (the "halo sign"), should appear when the area is wiped with gauze. Patients

Table 36-1 • Defining the Severity of Head Injury

Severity	Description
Mild	GCS score 13–15
	May have lost consciousness or exhibited amnesia for 5–60 min
	No abnormality on CT scan and length of hospital stay <48 h
Moderate	GCS score 9–12
	Loss of consciousness or amnesia for 1–24 h
	May have abnormality on CT scan
Severe	GCS score 3–8
	Loss of consciousness or amnesia for more than 24 h
	May have a cerebral contusion, laceration, or intracranial hematoma

GCS, Glasgow Coma Scale.

may also report a sweet or salty taste if CSF is draining into the pharynx. Clear fluid may be tested for glucose content to distinguish between CSF and other body fluids.

CSF leaks typically heal on their own with rest; however, when a CSF leak persists, diversion of CSF into an external drainage device may be necessary to reduce pressure on the dural tear and promote healing. In some cases, surgical repair of the damaged region of dura must be performed. A loose gauze dressing can be applied to the ear or nose to quantify the amount and character of drainage while allowing unobstructed drainage of the fluid. The skin around the site of drainage is kept clean, and the patient is instructed not to blow his or her nose.

Concussion

A concussion is defined as any alteration in mental status resulting from trauma. The patient may or may not lose consciousness. Often patients are unable to recall events leading up to the traumatic event, and occasionally short-term memory is affected. Concussions are not associated with structural abnormalities on radiographic imaging. Recovery after a concussion is usually quick and complete; however, some patients exhibit symptoms of postconcussive syndrome, which include headaches, decreased attention span, short-term memory impairment, dizziness, irritability, emotional lability, fatigue, visual disturbances, noise and light sensitivity, and difficulties with executive functions.[3] These symptoms can last for months to 1 year and can be alarming to the patient and the family. Discharge teaching must include a review of these signs and symptoms as well as criteria for obtaining medical follow-up.

Contusion

Contusions in the brain are the result of laceration of the microvasculature. They are focal and superficial, occasionally spreading to deeper layers of the brain. Cerebral contusions can range from mild to severe depending on the location, size, and extent of brain tissue injury. The diagnosis of cerebral contusion is made using computed tomography (CT). Small lesions may result in focal neurological deficits, whereas multiple or large contusions may result in a depressed level of consciousness and coma. Complications of a cerebral contusion include development of a hematoma and cerebral edema. Cerebral edema peaks 24 to 72 hours after injury, causing increased intracranial pressure (ICP). The patient's clinical condition may progressively deteriorate over the first 72 hours; therefore, the patient requires intensive anticipatory monitoring (serial neurological assessments) to identify signs and symptoms of increased ICP quickly and prevent further brain injury.

Epidural Hematoma

An epidural hematoma is a collection of blood between the dura and inside surface of the skull, often caused by laceration of the middle meningeal artery (Fig. 36-2). Although this type of hemorrhage is often associated with injury to an artery, injury to an extradural vein or venous sinus may also produce an epidural hematoma. Prompt recognition and expeditious surgical intervention to evacuate the hematoma result in improved outcomes. Patients may present in a coma or fully conscious.

Subdural Hematoma

A subdural hematoma is an accumulation of blood below the dura and above the arachnoid layer covering the brain (see Fig. 36-2). Tearing of the surface veins or disruption of venous sinuses can cause a subdural hematoma. The risk for subdural hematoma is increased in elderly people and in people with alcoholism. Cortical atrophy in these two populations causes tension on bridging veins leading from the surface of the brain to the inner surface of the dura. An increased incidence of falls also compounds the risk for subdural hematomas in these populations. Subdural hematomas can be separated into three categories based on the time from injury to the onset of symptoms: acute, subacute, and chronic.

Patients with acute subdural hematomas manifest symptoms 24 to 48 hours after injury depending on the rate and amount of blood accumulation. Symptoms include headache, focal neurological deficit, unilateral pupillary abnormalities, and a decreasing level of consciousness. Size and location of the hematoma and the degree of neurological dysfunction are considered in making the decision to surgically evacuate the hematoma.

Patients with subacute subdural hematomas have a delayed onset of symptoms, 2 days to 2 weeks after injury. The delay in symptom onset may be explained by a slower accumulation of blood caused by disruption of smaller blood vessels. In some cases, cerebral atrophy may allow for a greater amount of fluid to collect before symptoms of increased ICP manifest. Surgical clot evacuation may be performed on an elective basis with respect to the degree of neurologic dysfunction.

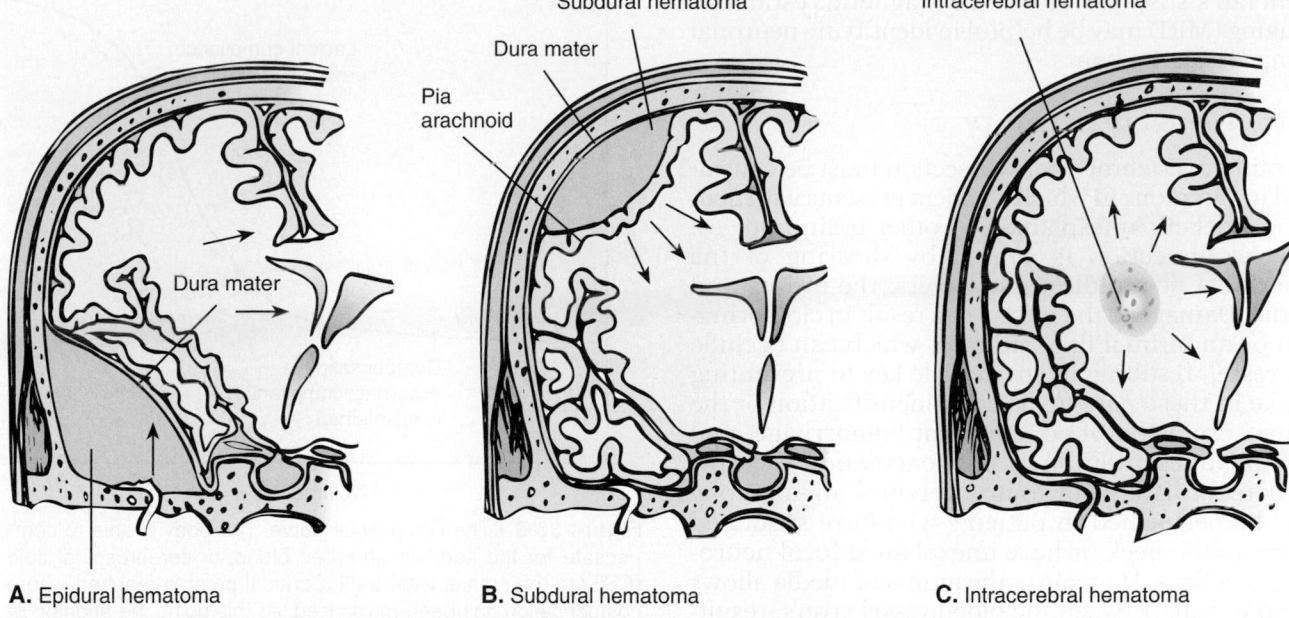

Subdural hematoma

Dura mater

Pia arachnoid

Intracerebral hematoma

Dura mater

A. Epidural hematoma   **B.** Subdural hematoma   **C.** Intracerebral hematoma

Figure 36-2 • Cerebral hematomas. **A:** An epidural hematoma. **B:** A subdural hematoma. **C:** An intracerebral hematoma. (Used with permission from Hickey JV: The Clinical Practice of Neurological and Neurosurgical Nursing, 5th ed. Philadelphia: Lippincott Williams & Wilkins, 2002, p 381.)

Patients with chronic subdural hematomas may initially experience a small bleed that does not cause symptoms. Over time, slow capillary leaking of proteinaceous fluid causes expansion of the mass and produces symptoms of increased ICP. Chronic subdural hematomas are often seen in elderly patients with a history of falling. The slow accumulation of fluid accounts for delayed presentation of signs and symptoms of increased ICP.[4] Common symptoms include headache, lethargy, confusion, and seizures. Surgical intervention may include drilling burr holes into the skull or craniotomy to remove the hematoma. Drains may be placed intraoperatively to prevent reaccumulation of fluid. A Jackson-Pratt–like drain connected to a skull bolt may also be used to treat this type of fluid collection. This drainage procedure may be preferred to a surgical procedure because it may be performed at bedside under local anesthesia. It is necessary to keep the head of the patient's bed flat to decrease tension placed on bridging veins. When the head is elevated, the brain settles downward. Therefore, the head of the patient's bed must be raised slowly to prevent rebleeding.

Intracerebral Hematoma

An intracerebral hematoma is a collection of blood within brain tissue caused by disruption of blood vessels (see Fig. 36-2). Traumatic causes of intracerebral hematoma include depressed skull fractures and penetrating injuries. Surgical management of intraparenchymal hematomas is indicated in patients with a deteriorating neurologic examination referable to the injured region of brain tissue or patients with increased ICP that is uncontrolled with maximal medical therapies (e.g., osmotic therapy, hyperventi-

lation, and sedation). Medical therapy aims to manage cerebral edema and promote adequate cerebral perfusion.

Traumatic Subarachnoid Hemorrhage

Traumatic subarachnoid hemorrhage occurs with tearing or shearing of microvessels in the arachnoid layer where CSF flows around the brain. A traumatic subarachnoid hemorrhage often accompanies other severe brain injuries and appears to be associated with poor neurologic outcome and increased mortality.[5,6] Additional complications such as hydrocephalus and cerebral vasospasm add to the complexity of the injury.

Diffuse Axonal Injury

Diffuse axonal injury (DAI) is characterized by a direct tearing or shearing of axons, which worsens during the first 12 to 24 hours as local edema and diffuse edema develop. DAI prolongs or disables signal conduction from the white matter to gray matter in the brain and is thought to occur with rotational and acceleration–deceleration forces. DAI can be classified as mild, moderate, or severe based on length of coma and degree of neurological dysfunction. Mild DAI is associated with a coma lasting no longer than 24 hours. Moderate DAI is characterized by a coma lasting longer than 24 hours with transient flexor or extensor posturing. Severe DAI is characterized by prolonged coma, fever, diaphoresis, and severe extensor posturing. DAI is not easily identified through radiographic imaging in the first 24 hours; however, small punctate hemorrhages may be visualized deep in the white matter, a finding that increases the clinician's suspicion for DAI. Magnetic resonance imaging (MRI) may be helpful in identifying neuronal damage after 24 hours.

Cerebrovascular Injury

Carotid or vertebral artery dissection must be considered in situations in which a patient presents with neurologic deficits unexplained by other brain injuries. Arterial dissection is caused by shearing of the innermost or middle vessel layers, the intima and media. Damage to the intima can result in clot formation or an intimal flap, either of which can occlude the vessel, resulting in stroke. The key to preventing stroke in these patients is early identification of the injury, exclusion of concomitant hemorrhage, and may include initiation of anticoagulation therapy. To detect this type of injury, cerebral angiography may be performed in patients who have sustained injury to the neck or have unexplained focal neurological deficits. Damage to the intima or media allows blood to leak between the blood vessel layers, resulting in a ballooning of the outermost vessel layers and creating an aneurysm. This type of aneurysm is referred to as a traumatic intracerebral aneurysm and may also be called a pseudoaneurysm.

SECONDARY BRAIN INJURY

Secondary brain injury events occur after the initiating traumatic event and cause additional brain injury. Examples of conditions causing or exacerbating secondary brain injury are uncontrolled increased ICP, cerebral ischemia, hypotension, hypoxemia, and local or systemic infection. Secondary brain injury occurs as a function of the inflammatory response, reduced cerebral blood flow, and dysfunctional cerebral autoregulation causing damage to neurons. These secondary processes can result in cerebral infarction, coma, and increased cerebral edema.[7] Prevention of hypotension, hypercarbia, hypoxemia, and seizures is extremely important in attempting to prevent further injury.[7,8]

Understanding intracranial dynamics and the nature of cerebral blood flow is essential to preventing and treating secondary brain injury (see Chapter 34 for a complete discussion of intracranial dynamics and the Monro-Kellie hypothesis).

Compensation for increased volume in the cranium occurs when CSF is channeled through the foramen magnum into the spinal canal, CSF production is decreased, and venous blood is channeled out of the cranium into the jugular veins.[9] The compliance curve (Fig. 36-3) illustrates the body's ability to compensate for additions of water, CSF, or blood into the cranial vault and the point at which intracranial compliance is maximized. Decreased intracranial compliance results in a small addition of volume causing disproportionate increases in ICP. Examples of conditions causing decreased intracranial compliance are cerebral edema (an increase in brain water), expansion of a hematoma (an increase in blood), and hydrocephalus (an increase in CSF). An understand-

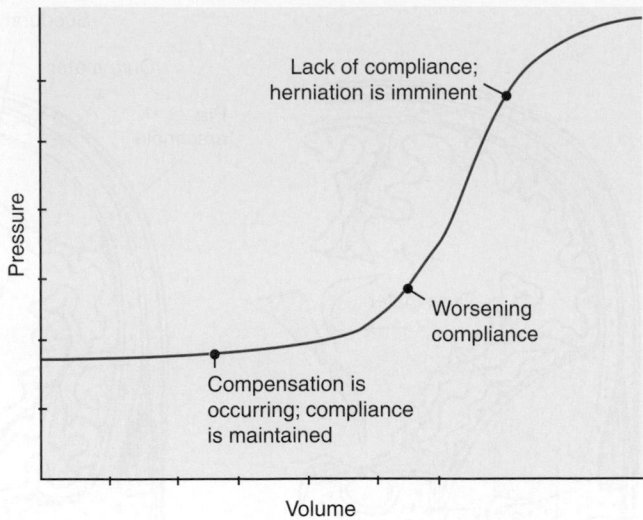

Figure 36-3 • The compliance curve. The body is able to compensate for the addition of water, blood, or cerebrospinal fluid (CSF) to the cranial vault until a critical point is reached where compensation has been maximized. At this point, the addition of a small amount of volume will cause a disproportionate increase in intracranial pressure (ICP).

ing of pressure–volume relationships allows the nurse to anticipate deterioration of the patient's clinical condition, tailor nursing interventions, and anticipate potential medical or surgical treatments.

Cerebral autoregulation is a protective mechanism that enables the brain to receive a constant blood flow over a range of systemic blood pressures (see Chapter 34 for a complete discussion). Several studies have suggested that cerebral blood flow may decrease up to 50% during the first 24 to 48 hours after TBI.[10]

Biochemical mechanisms also play a significant role in causing secondary brain injury. The inflammatory response has been implicated as a potential cause or exacerbating factor in many disease processes, and its role in secondary brain injury is the subject of scientific investigation.

Cerebral Edema

Cerebral edema commonly occurs in patients with TBIs 24 to 48 hours after the primary insult and typically peaks at 72 hours.[11] Patients require increased observation during this period owing to the increased risk for neurological deterioration. It is helpful to inform families about the course of cerebral edema so that they can be aware of the potential for deterioration over the first 72 hours, even if the patient appears to be progressing well. If cerebral edema is not aggressively treated, herniation syndrome may ensue. The treatment of cerebral edema is discussed in Chapter 34.

The two most common types of edema occurring after TBI are cytotoxic and vasogenic edema. Cytotoxic edema occurs as the result of failure of the intracellular sodium–potassium pump, allowing an influx of sodium and water into the cell and an efflux of potassium. Vasogenic edema occurs as a result of a disruption to the blood–brain barrier.[11]

Ischemia

Cerebral ischemia, a major cause of morbidity and mortality, may be a result of direct vascular injury or cerebral edema that causes compression or occlusion of blood vessels within the brain. Ischemia in the brain may occur at the time of injury or during the period subsequent to the injury. Cerebral ischemia occurs whenever blood flow is inadequate to meet metabolic demands of the brain. If the cause of cerebral ischemia is not controlled, cerebral infarction (stroke) may result (see Chapter 35 for further information on cerebral ischemia and stroke).

Herniation Syndrome

Herniation syndrome occurs when pressure builds within the cranium, exceeding the brain's ability to compensate for the increase in pressure and causing brain tissue to be displaced. Cushing's triad refers to the three late signs of herniation: increased pulse pressure, decreased heart rate, and an irregular respiratory pattern. It is of critical importance to identify early signs of increased ICP (such as change in level of consciousness) in order to prevent herniation syndrome. The examination findings of a patient with increased ICP is in sharp contrast with those of a patient with herniation syndrome (Table 36-2).

Cerebral herniation syndrome is classified according to the compartment in which it is occurring. The most common syndromes in the setting of critical care and trauma are uncal and central herniation (Table 36-3).

Herniation of the medial temporal lobe (uncus) through the tentorium and into the brainstem is called uncal herniation. Herniation of the uncus through the tentorium results in pressure on the midbrain where the third cranial nerve exits, producing ipsilateral pupillary dilation. Contralateral hemiparesis occurs during uncal herniation. Central or tonsillar herniation describes the downward displacement of the cerebellar tonsils through the foramen magnum, causing compression of the brainstem. Clinical signs

of central herniation syndrome include loss of consciousness, bilateral pupillary dilation, respiratory pattern changes or respiratory arrest, and flaccid paralysis. Central herniation may be caused by bilateral expanding lesions or a centrally located mass lesion causing downward displacement of the cerebral hemispheres and midline structures (i.e., the basal ganglia, diencephalon, and the midbrain) through the tentorium (Fig. 36-4).

Critical care nurses have the opportunity to make a significant contribution to patient outcome by performing thorough serial neurological examinations, taking into account subtle changes. Once thought to be immediately fatal, herniation syndrome may be reversible in certain circumstances if it is identified early and aggressive therapies are administered.

Coma

Coma is an alteration in consciousness caused by damage to both hemispheres of the brain or the brainstem. Coma results from disruption of the reticular activating system (RAS), which is a physiological region encompassing nuclei from the medulla to the cerebral cortex. The RAS is responsible for wakefulness, heightened arousal, and alertness. Consciousness can be placed on a continuum from full consciousness to coma, and states of coma can be subdivided into light coma, coma, and deep coma (see Chapter 33, Box 33-3).

Persistent Vegetative State

Several terms describe a persistent vegetative state, such as irreversible coma or coma vigil. A persistent vegetative state is characterized by a period of sleeplike coma followed by a return to the awake state with an inability to respond to the environment. In a persistent vegetative state, higher cortical functions of the cerebral hemispheres have been damaged permanently, but the lower functions of the brainstem remain intact. The patient's eyes open spontaneously and may appear as if they are opening in response to verbal stimuli. Sleep–wake cycles exist, and the patient maintains normal cardiovascular and respiratory control. Also seen are involuntary lip smacking,

Table 36-2 • Increased Intracranial Pressure Versus Herniation Syndrome

	Increased Intracranial Pressure	Herniation Syndrome
Level of arousal	Increased stimulus required	Unarousable
Motor function	Subtle motor weakness or pronator drift	Dense motor weakness, posturing or absent response
Pupillary response	Sluggish pupillary response	Unilateral dilated and fixed pupil ("blown pupil")
Vital signs	May be stable or labile	Cushing's triad (increased systolic blood pressure, decreased heart rate, irregular respiration)

Used with permission from an unpublished lecture, Lower J, 1997.

result of activation of a spinal cord reflex. A painful stimulus should be applied for 15 to 30 seconds before the patient is considered not to have a motor response. Patients with brain injury may exhibit delayed responses to stimuli.

Assessment of the Eyes

Assessment of the eyes includes evaluation of the pupils and extraocular movements, which assists in localizing cranial nerve dysfunction.

Testing of cranial nerve II (the optic nerve) involves detection of gross visual field defects and visual acuity. Visual fields can be adequately assessed by the patient's ability to detect movement of the evaluator's finger in each field of vision (see Chapter 33 for technique). Visual acuity can be grossly assessed by asking the patient to read printed words on a page or by using a Snellen eye chart. If there is concern about optic nerve impairment, a full evaluation by an ophthalmologist is recommended.

Evaluation of cranial nerve III (the oculomotor nerve) involves inspection of the pupil, including size, shape, equality, and reaction to light. Increased ICP can cause irregularities in shape, pupillary inequality (anisocoria), and sluggish or absent reaction to light. Cranial nerves III, IV, and VI (the oculomotor, trochlear, and abducens nerves) enable movement of the eyes. Cranial nerves III and IV exit at the level of the midbrain, and cranial nerve VI exits at the level of the pons. Assessment of these nerves is accomplished by asking the patient to follow the evaluator's finger while it is moved in an "H" pattern. Double vision (diplopia) is a sign of eye muscle weakness and cranial nerve impairment.

In the comatose patient, the following tests are performed to evaluate cranial nerves III, VI, and VIII (the oculomotor and abducens nerves, and the vestibular portion of the acoustic nerve). The oculocephalic reflex (i.e., the "doll's eyes" phenomenon; see Chapter 33, Fig. 33-6) is tested by moving the head from side to side in a horizontal plane (after confirming the absence of cervical spinal fracture). If the oculocephalic response is present, the eyes move together in the opposite direction of the head as it is turned from side to side. Absence of eye movement on head turning reflects brainstem dysfunction. The oculovestibular reflex (see Chapter 33, Fig. 33-7) is tested by instilling cold water into each ear and observing the eyes for movement. A normal oculovestibular response is characterized by movement of the eyes toward the stimulus with nystagmus. The absence of movement signals loss of function of the vestibular portion of the eighth cranial nerve as well as the brainstem.

Assessment of Brainstem Responses

The brainstem can be further assessed in the unconscious patient by testing corneal, cough, and gag reflexes. The corneal reflex reflects function of cranial nerves V and VII (the trigeminal and facial nerves), which exit the brain at the level of the pons. This reflex is tested by passing a wisp of cotton over the lower conjunctiva of each eye. Movement of the lower lid indicates the presence of the reflex. Sensation of the irritating stimulus represents gross function of one branch of the trigeminal nerve, and movement of the lower lid represents motor function of the facial nerve. Care must be taken in testing the corneal reflex to avoid causing corneal abrasions.

Cranial nerves IX and X (the glossopharyngeal and vagus nerves) exit at the level of the medulla and are responsible for the cough and gag reflexes and protection of the airway from aspiration. The cough and gag reflexes should be evaluated in the awake and unconscious patient.

Assessment of Motor Function

Motor function is evaluated by using the staged approach described earlier. Further detailed assessment of motor function is tested in the awake and cooperative patient by having the patient move his or her extremities against gravity and with passive resistance, grading the movement on a scale of 1 to 5 (see Chapter 33).

The unresponsive patient may exhibit localization, withdrawal, flexor posturing, or extensor posturing in response to noxious stimuli. Localization of a painful stimulus is observed as a purposeful response in which the patient is able to locate the source of pain and move toward it with one or both extremities crossing the midline of the body. A patient may try to remove the evaluator's hand when he or she performs a trapezius squeeze, or the patient may attempt to grab medical equipment (e.g., catheters or endotracheal tubes). A withdrawal response is characterized by movement away from a painful stimulus. Flexor (decorticate) posturing is indicative of diffuse cortical injury and is characterized by the bending or flexing of the upper extremities and extension of the lower extremities and feet. Extensor (decerebrate) posturing indicates injury to the brainstem and is observed as extension and internal rotation of the upper extremities and extension of the lower extremities and feet (see Chapter 33, Fig. 33-1). It is possible that a patient may exhibit one type of movement in one extremity and another type of movement in another extremity. Presence of the Babinski reflex may also be observed in the patient with severe TBI.

Assessment of Respiratory Function

Assessment of respiratory patterns is important in detecting worsening neurologic injury and the need for airway management and mechanical ventilation. Numerous locations in both cerebral hemispheres regulate voluntary control over the muscles used in breathing. The cerebellum synchronizes and coordinates the muscles involved in respiration. The cerebrum controls the rate and rhythm of respiration. Nuclei in the pons and midbrain regulate the automaticity of respiration.

Abnormal respiratory patterns may be correlated with injured regions of the brain (Fig. 36-6). Cheyne-Stokes breathing is periodic breathing in which the depth of each breath increases to a peak and then decreases to apnea. The hyperpneic phase usually

Type	Respiratory Pattern	Neuroanatomical Lesion

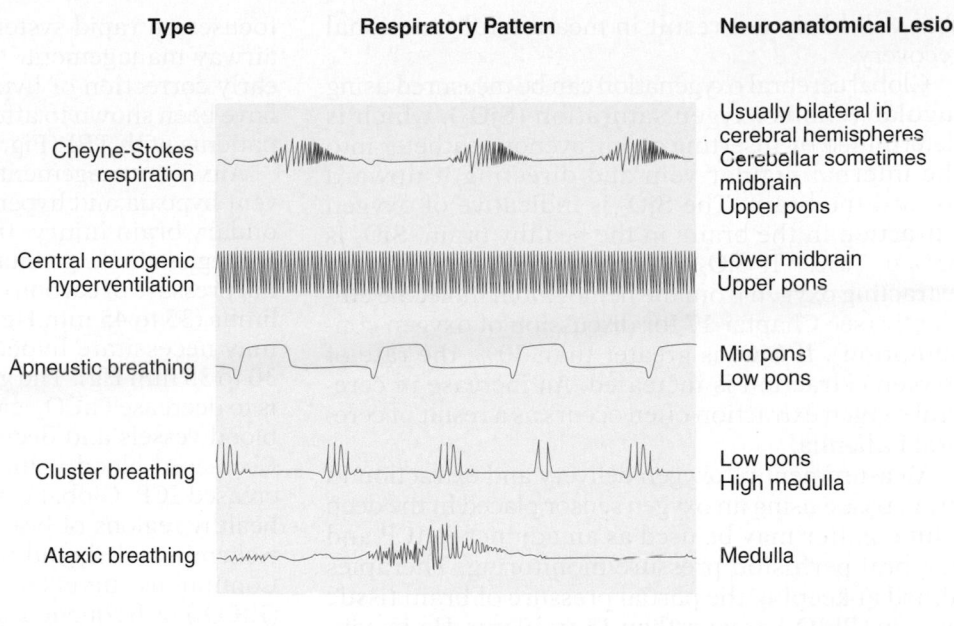

Cheyne-Stokes respiration — Usually bilateral in cerebral hemispheres Cerebellar sometimes midbrain Upper pons

Central neurogenic hyperventilation — Lower midbrain Upper pons

Apneustic breathing — Mid pons Low pons

Cluster breathing — Low pons High medulla

Ataxic breathing — Medulla

⊢ One minute ⊣

Figure 36-6 • Injury to the brainstem can result in various abnormal respiratory patterns.

lasts longer than the apneic phase. This breathing pattern may be seen in patients with bilateral lesions located deep in the cerebral hemispheres. Compression of the midbrain can cause central neurogenic hyperventilation. Hyperventilation is sustained, regular, rapid, and deep. It usually is caused by a lesion above the midbrain. Apneustic breathing is characterized by respiration with a long pause at full inspiration or full expiration. The etiology of this pattern is loss of all cerebral and cerebellar control of breathing, with respiratory function at the brainstem level only. Cluster breathing may be seen in a patient when the lesion is high in the medulla or low in the pons. This pattern of respiration is seen as gasping breaths with irregular pauses.

The critical centers of inspiration and expiration are located in the medulla oblongata. Rapidly expanding intracranial lesions, such as cerebellar hemorrhage, can compress the medulla, resulting in ataxic breathing. This irregular breathing consists of both deep and shallow breaths with irregular pauses. This pattern of respiration signals the need for definitive airway control (i.e., endotracheal intubation).

Assessment of Other Body Systems

In addition to thorough assessment of the central nervous system, comprehensive assessment of all other body systems is crucial in the early identification of complications in patients with TBI. Organ dysfunction, particularly respiratory failure, is common in patients with severe TBI.[13]

DIAGNOSTIC TESTING

CT is performed as an initial diagnostic test to identify structural injuries in the brain and intracranial bleeding. A CT scan can be obtained quickly. One disadvantage of the CT scan is that it is unable to image the cerebelli and brainstem adequately. An initial CT scan is performed without contrast. CT scans performed with intravenous contrast are used to investigate suspected masses (i.e., tumors or abscesses). MRI is useful to assess structures in the posterior fossa and spinal cord. Magnetic resonance angiography may be used to evaluate cerebral vascular injuries such as carotid or vertebral dissection.

Cerebral angiography is the gold standard diagnostic test to investigate injuries to cerebral blood vessels. A cerebral angiogram may also be obtained to confirm the absence of cerebral blood flow in brain death.

Transcranial Doppler (TCD) ultrasonography indirectly evaluates cerebral blood flow and autoregulatory mechanisms by measuring the velocity at which blood travels through blood vessels. TCD may also be used as a confirmatory test when diagnosing brain death to document cessation of blood flow to the brain.

Other diagnostic tests are used to assess electrical impulse transmission in the brain. These tests are often obtained to provide information for physicians to make prognoses for patient recovery. Neurophysiological tests include the electroencephalogram (EEG), brainstem auditory evoked responses (BAERs), and somatosensory evoked potentials (SSEPs). The EEG measures electrical activity in all regions of the cortex and is useful in identifying seizures and correlating the abnormal neurological examination with abnormal cortical function. The EEG is necessary in ruling out subclinical or nonconvulsive seizures in the comatose patient. It may also be used as a confirmatory test in brain death to demonstrate cessation of electrical conduction to the cerebral cortex. The most common finding in the patient with TBI is a slowing of electrical activity in the area of injury. BAER and SSEP are useful prognostic tests in a patient with TBI. Abnormal results of either of these tests may help confirm a diagnosis of severe brainstem or cortical dysfunction that will likely not result in meaningful functional recovery.

Global cerebral oxygenation can be measured using jugular venous oxygen saturation (SjO_2), which is determined by inserting an intravenous catheter into the internal jugular vein and directing it upward toward the brain. The SjO_2 is indicative of oxygen extraction in the brain; in the healthy brain, SjO_2 is 55% to 70%.[14] If SjO_2 is less than 55%, cells are not extracting oxygen from the hemoglobin molecule efficiently (see Chapter 17 for discussion of oxygen consumption). If SjO_2 is greater than 70%, the rate of oxygen extraction is increased. An increase in cerebral oxygen extraction often occurs as a result of cerebral ischemia.

Measurement of oxygen delivery and extraction in brain tissue using an oxygen sensor placed in the deep white matter may be used as an adjunct to ICP and cerebral perfusion pressure monitoring. Therapies aimed at keeping the partial pressure of brain tissue oxygen ($PbtO_2$) greater than 15 to 20 mm Hg in conjunction with ICP and cerebral perfusion pressure management may optimize the patient's chances for maximal functional recovery.[15,16]

In addition, microdialysis is used to measure cellular metabolites such as glutamate as markers of cellular dysfunction and injury. A small microdialysis catheter is inserted into the brain tissue through a hole made in the skull. Small amounts of CSF-like fluid are infused at very slow rates by a specialized infusion pump, and extracellular fluid is pumped out into a collection chamber. Currently, this monitoring modality primarily is used in the context of research.

• Management

Guidelines for the management of severe TBI have been developed by the Brain Trauma Foundation and the American Association of Neurological Surgeons to disseminate evidence-based recommendations.[17] The goal of these guidelines is to create a consistent standard for the care and treatment of patients with severe TBI. Several studies have suggested the benefit of evidenced-based standardization of care in improving functional outcomes after TBI.[17] Specific guidelines for the management of severe TBI in infants, children, and adolescents are available, outlining the unique needs of the pediatric population.[18] The focus of the discussion in this chapter is the management of severe TBI in adults.

INITIAL MANAGEMENT

Initial assessment and treatment of the patient with TBI begins immediately after the insult, often with prehospital care providers. Specific guidelines for prehospital management of TBI were developed and published by the Brain Trauma Foundation in 2002. Prehospital treatment of the patient with a head injury focuses on rapid systems assessment and definitive airway management.[19] These guidelines emphasize early correction of hypoxia and hypercarbia, which have been shown to affect morbidity and mortality in patients with TBI (Fig. 36-7).[7]

Airway management is a crucial initial step to prevent hypoxia and hypercarbia, which exacerbate secondary brain injury. Initial mechanical ventilation strategies aim to maintain normal ventilation or a partial pressure of carbon dioxide ($PaCO_2$) within normal limits (35 to 45 mm Hg). Signs of cerebral herniation may necessitate hyperventilation therapy ($PaCO_2$, 30 to 35 mm Hg). The goal of hyperventilation in TBI is to decrease $PaCO_2$, causing constriction of cerebral blood vessels and decreased cerebral blood volume. Decreased blood volume in the brain results in decreased ICP. Global cerebral vasoconstriction places healthy regions of brain tissue at risk for developing ischemia and should not be used prophylactically.[16] Continuous surveillance of end tidal carbon dioxide ($EtCO_2$) or frequent assessment of $PaCO_2$ is essential to prevent cerebral ischemia. Monitoring cerebral oxygenation (i.e., SjO_2 or $PbtO_2$) is an option for identifying cerebral ischemia. Research suggests that the brain experiences decreased blood flow in the first 24 hours after injury; therefore, hyperventilation should be avoided during this period.[16]

Diagnostic testing is performed subsequent to the initial resuscitation to evaluate the need for immediate surgical intervention. Typical tests include radiographs of the cervical spine and a CT scan of the brain, which is useful in diagnosing intracranial bleeding that may require surgical intervention. Additional imaging and blood tests may be obtained to rule out systemic injuries and assist in treating complications. The mechanism of injury helps clinicians determine appropriate diagnostic testing.

Continuing management seeks to control ICP, promote cerebral perfusion, and correct the primary pathological process. Examples of nursing diagnoses and collaborative problems for the patient with TBI are given in Box 36-2. General management of the patient with TBI requires a holistic, multisystem, multidisciplinary approach, taking into consideration the unique physiological and psychosocial characteristics of the patient (Box 36-3).

MONITORING AND CONTROLLING INTRACRANIAL PRESSURE

ICP monitoring, which is discussed in depth in Chapter 34, allows the health care team to make rapid treatment decisions based on pressure displays and ICP waveform analysis. ICP monitors are typically inserted by neurosurgeons at the bedside or in the operating room. ICP monitoring is recommended for patients with severe head injury (GCS score < 8) and CT scan abnormalities on admission. ICP monitoring may also be considered when the CT scan is normal but the patient meets two or more of the following criteria: older than 40 years, posturing, or a systolic blood pressure less than 90 mm Hg.[16]

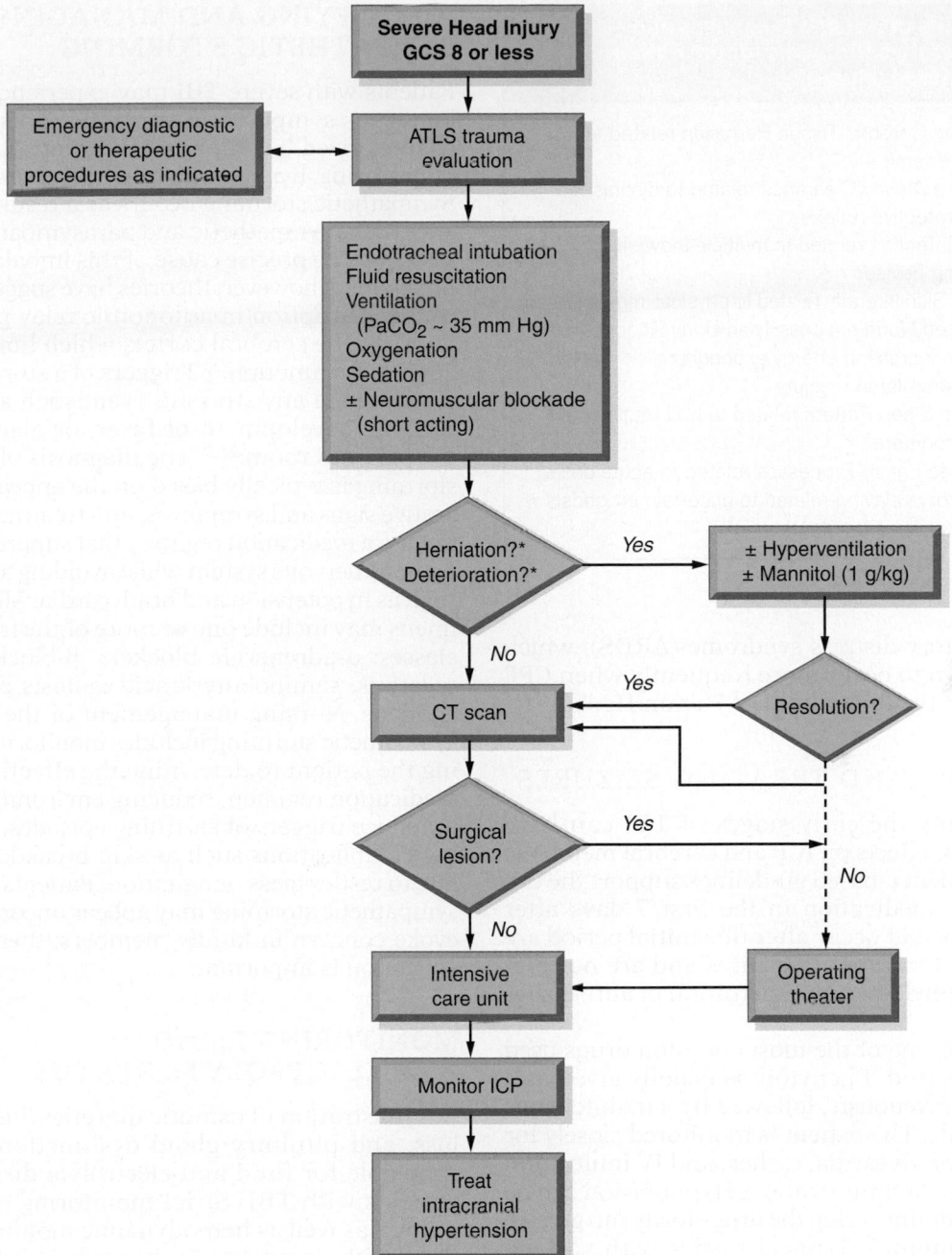

**Severe Head Injury
GCS 8 or less**

Emergency diagnostic
or therapeutic
procedures as indicated

ATLS trauma
evaluation

Endotracheal intubation
Fluid resuscitation
Ventilation
   (PaCO$_2$ ~ 35 mm Hg)
Oxygenation
Sedation
± Neuromuscular blockade
   (short acting)

Herniation?*
Deterioration?*

Yes → ± Hyperventilation
± Mannitol (1 g/kg)

No

CT scan ← Yes ← Resolution?

Yes

Surgical
lesion? Yes →

No   No

Intensive
care unit ← Operating
theater

Monitor ICP

Treat
intracranial
hypertension

Figure 36-7 • Flowchart for resuscitation of the patient with a severe head injury before intracranial pressure (ICP) monitoring. *Presence or signs of herniation (pupillary dilation or motor posturing) or progressive neurological deterioration are not attributable to external factors. GCS, Glasgow Coma Scale; ATLS, advanced trauma life support; CT, computed tomography; ICP, intracranial pressure. (Used with permission from Chestnut RM: Medical management of severe head injury: Present and future. New Horiz 3[3]:583, 1995.)

Nursing interventions to manage increased ICP include maintaining body alignment as well as avoiding sharp turning of the head to one side and sharp hip flexion. Turning the head to one side causes compression of the jugular vein, preventing drainage of venous blood from the head and increasing ICP. Sharp hip flexion increases intra-abdominal pressure, decreasing venous outflow and causing an increase in ICP.

MAINTAINING CEREBRAL PERFUSION

Management of cerebral perfusion involves control of ICP and maintenance of mean arterial pressure. Cerebral perfusion pressure (CPP) is calculated by subtracting ICP from mean arterial pressure (MAP): CPP = MAP – ICP. Maintenance of CPP within the range of 50 to 70 mm Hg prevents cerebral ischemia at the lower end and mitigates the risk for acute respiratory distress syndrome (ARDS), which has been shown to occur more frequently when CPP is pushed over the upper limit of 70 mm Hg.[16]

PREVENTING AND TREATING SEIZURES

Seizures during the early stages of TBI can have severe negative effects on ICP and cerebral metabolic demands. Evidence-based guidelines support the use of antiseizure medication in the first 7 days after TBI.[16] Seizures that occur after this initial period are called late post-traumatic seizures and are not prevented by prophylactic administration of antiseizure medications.[8,16]

Phenytoin is one of the most common drugs used in the acute period. Phenytoin is usually given as a bolus dose intravenously, followed by a maintenance dosing schedule. The patient is monitored closely for hypotension, bradycardia, rashes, and IV infiltration during and after administration. Hypotension can be mitigated by administering the drug slowly (no greater than 50 mg/minute). Truncal rashes with varying severity, including Stevens-Johnson syndrome, can occur with administration of phenytoin. The drug should be discontinued at the appearance of rash.

MAINTAINING A NORMAL BODY TEMPERATURE

Hyperthermia (body temperature > 37.5°C) in a patient with severe TBI increases cerebrometabolic demands and may compound secondary brain injury. Frequent monitoring of body temperature is necessary to maintain normothermia (35°C to 37.5°C). Infection must be ruled out as the cause of fever, and cooling methods are used as needed to maintain a normal body temperature. Inducing hypothermia in patients with TBI may be beneficial in improving functional outcome, although further research is required before this practice is recognized as a standard.[16]

IDENTIFYING AND MANAGING SYMPATHETIC STORMING

Patients with severe TBI may experience a condition known as sympathetic storming. This condition is characterized by diaphoresis; agitation, restlessness, or posturing; hyperventilation; tachycardia; and fever. Sympathetic storming occurs as a result of an imbalance of the sympathetic and parasympathetic nervous systems. The precise cause of this imbalance is poorly understood; however, theories have suggested that TBI causes disruption in autonomic relay pathways and injury to the cerebral cortex, which limits control of autonomic function.[20] Triggers of a storming episode may include any stressful event such as suctioning, turning, development of fever, or alarm sounds in the patient's room.[20,21] The diagnosis of sympathetic storming is typically based on the appearance of suggestive signs and symptoms, and treatment focuses on finding a medication regimen that suppresses the sympathetic nervous system while avoiding adverse effects such as hypotension and bradycardia. Medication regimens may include one or more of the following drug classes: α-adrenergic blockers, β-blockers, opiates, sedatives, γ-aminobutyric acid agonists, and dopamine agonists. Nursing management of the patient with sympathetic storming includes monitoring and assessing the patient to determine the effectiveness of the medication regimen, reducing environmental stimuli to reduce triggers of storming episodes, and preventing complications such as skin breakdown or injury due to restlessness or agitation. Patients experiencing sympathetic storming may appear uncomfortable and evoke concern in family members; therefore, family education is important.

MONITORING FLUID AND ELECTROLYTE STATUS

Administration of osmotic diuretics, insensible fluid loss, and pituitary gland dysfunction may be responsible for fluid and electrolyte disturbances in patients with TBI. Strict monitoring of intake and output, as well as hemodynamic monitoring, guides the health care team in prescribing adequate fluid replacement. Routine monitoring of serum osmolality is helpful in preventing excessive systemic dehydration when administering osmotic diuretics or hypertonic saline. Surveillance of serum electrolytes allows for early identification and treatment of electrolyte abnormalities.

Disorders of sodium imbalance are common in the patient with TBI (Table 36-4). Hyponatremia most commonly occurs as a result of the syndrome of inappropriate antidiuretic hormone secretion (SIADH), in which antidiuretic hormone (ADH) is released in excessive amounts, resulting in hemodilution. Hemodilution leads to a lower concentration of sodium in the blood. SIADH often is a transient phenomenon that can be treated with fluid restriction.

Cerebral salt-wasting syndrome may also cause hyponatremia. The precise physiologic mechanism of cerebral salt-wasting syndrome is poorly understood

Box 36-3 • COLLABORATIVE CARE GUIDE for the Patient With a Head Injury

OUTCOMES	INTERVENTIONS
Oxygenation/Ventilation Patient will maintain a patent airway. Lungs will be clear to auscultation. Arterial pH, PaO_2, and SaO_2 will be maintained within normal limits. $ETCO_2$ or PCO_2 will be maintained within prescribed range. There will be no evidence of atelectasis or pneumonia on chest x-ray.	• Auscultate breath sounds every 2–4 h and PRN. • Hyperoxygenate before and after each suction pass. • Avoid suction passes greater than 10 s. • Monitor intracranial pressure (ICP) and cerebral perfusion pressure (CPP) during suctioning and chest physiotherapy. • Provide meticulous oral hygiene. • Monitor for signs of aspiration. • Encourage nonintubated patients to use incentive spirometer, cough, and deep breathe every 4 h and PRN. • Turn side-to-side every 2 h. • Move patient out of bed to chair 1 to 2 times per day when ICP has been controlled.
Circulation/Perfusion Patient will exhibit normal sinus rhythm without ectopy or ischemic changes. Patient will not experience thromboembolic complications.	• Monitor for myocardial ischemia and dysrhythmias due to sympathetic activation and catecholamine surges. • Prevent deep venous thrombosis with the use of pneumatic compression devices, antiembolic stockings, and subcutaneous heparin. • Implement early mobilization. Facilitate moving to a chair 1 to 2 times per day. • Monitor blood pressure continuously by arterial line or frequently by noninvasive cuff. • Monitor oxygen delivery (hemoglobin, SaO_2, cardiac output). • Administer red blood cells, inotropes, intravenous fluids as indicated.
Cerebral Perfusion/Intracranial Pressure CPP will be greater than 60 mm Hg. ICP will be less than 20 mm Hg. Patient will not experience seizure activity.	• Monitor ICP and CPP every hour. • Make neurological checks every 1–2 h. • Elevate the head of bed to 30 degrees unless contraindicated. • Maintain proper body alignment, keeping the head in a neutral position, and avoiding sharp hip flexion. • Maintain normothermia. • Maintain a quiet environment, cluster care, and provide rest periods. • Provide sedation as necessary and as prescribed. • Administer prophylactic antiepileptic agents as prescribed to prevent seizure activity.
Fluids/Electrolytes Serum electrolytes will be within normal limits. Serum osmolality will remain within prescribed range.	• Strict documentation of input/output, consider insensible losses due to intubation, fever, and the like. • Monitor serum electrolytes, glucose, and osmolality as ordered. • Consider need for electrolyte replacement therapy and administer per physician order or protocol.
Mobility/Safety There will be minimal and transient changes in ICP/CPP during treatments or patient care activities. ICP/CPP will return to baseline within 5 min. Patient will not experience complications related to prolonged immobilization (e.g., DVT, pneumonia, ankylosis). Patient will not harm self by dislodging medical equipment or falling.	• Provide range of motion and functional splinting for paralyzed limbs or patients in a coma. • Position patient off of pressure points at least every 2 h. • Consider use of specialty mattresses based on skin and risk factor assessments. • Keep bed rails in the upright position. • Provide restraints if necessary to prevent dislodgment of medical devices as hospital policies permit.

Table 36-4 • Disorders of Sodium Imbalance: Comparison of Diabetes Insipidus, the Syndrome of Inappropriate Antidiuretic Hormone Secretion, and Cerebral Salt-Wasting Syndrome

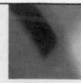

	Diabetes Insipidus	Syndrome of Inappropriate Antidiuretic Hormone Secretion	Cerebral Salt-Wasting Syndrome
Urinary output	Increased	Decreased	Increased
Specific gravity	Decreased	Increased	Decreased
Volume status	Decreased	Mildly increased	Decreased
Serum sodium	Increased	Decreased	Decreased
Treatment	Administration of exogenous vasopressin, fluid replacement	Fluid restriction, judicious sodium replacement	Fluid and sodium replacement

but involves a primary loss of sodium and free water through the kidneys. Treatment of this disorder requires fluid and sodium replacement in amounts that equal losses.[22]

Diabetes insipidus (DI) is a cause of hypernatremia and hypovolemia that occurs commonly in patients with injury or ischemia in the pituitary gland. Herniation syndrome often causes direct compression of the pituitary gland or compression to the supplying blood vessels. Damage to the pituitary gland prevents or decreases the secretion of ADH. Diabetes insipidus is diagnosed by an increasing serum sodium level, a low urine specific gravity, and an increased urine output. Treatment of DI includes aggressive fluid replacement that matches hourly fluid losses and the administration of exogenous ADH (vasopressin). Vasopressin may be given intravenously, subcutaneously, or intranasally, depending on the severity of the disorder.

MANAGING CARDIOVASCULAR COMPLICATIONS

Myocardial stunning and a transient decrease in cardiac function may occur in severe TBI. Inversion of T waves and ST-segment elevation or depression may be noted. Serum cardiac enzymes, electrocardiography, and echocardiography may be used to evaluate myocardial function. Hemodynamic monitoring devices, such as arterial and central lines and pulmonary artery catheters, may be used to guide medical therapies in the critical phases of TBI.

Disorders of coagulation are a significant concern in patients with TBI owing to the release of large amounts of thromboplastin in response to brain injury. Disseminated intravascular coagulation may result. If hypothermia is employed, it is important to recognize that coagulopathies may be exacerbated as the body temperature decreases.

Prophylaxis of deep venous thrombosis (DVT) is an essential component in the care of patients with head injuries, who are often immobile for extended periods. Sequential compression devices provide intermittent pulsatile pressure to the lower extremities, increasing venous return and promoting systemic

fibrinolysis. Antiembolic stockings, anticoagulant administration, and early mobilization are recommended to prevent DVT and pulmonary emboli.[16]

MANAGING PULMONARY COMPLICATIONS

Pulmonary complications in the patient with TBI include pneumonia, ARDS, neurogenic pulmonary edema, and pulmonary embolus. Pulmonary toilet, vigilant oral hygiene, and monitoring of endotracheal tube cuff pressure are necessary to prevent nosocomial pneumonia and mitigate pulmonary complications in patients with head injuries who require prolonged mechanical ventilation (see Chapter 25 for a discussion of the causes and prevention of ventilator-associated pneumonia).

Early mobility is critical in facilitating pulmonary toilet, preventing atelectasis, and preventing pulmonary emboli due to DVT. Early consideration of extubation to reduce the number of days on mechanical ventilation as well as early planning for tracheostomy in patients unable to protect their airway may prevent additional pulmonary complications.[17]

ARDS is a hypoxic lung disease resulting from the activation of the inflammatory cascade, causing leakage of protein-rich fluid from the pulmonary capillaries into the interstitium of the lungs as well as destruction of alveolar cells. There are many causes of ARDS in patients with head injuries, including concomitant pulmonary contusion, aspiration pneumonia, sepsis, and massive blood transfusion. Medical management of ARDS may involve the use of pressure modes of mechanical ventilation to decrease the volume needed to deliver each breath (high volumes have been implicated in furthering alveolar injury); see Chapter 27 for a complete discussion of the management of ARDS.

Neurogenic pulmonary edema may result from injury to the brainstem, increased ICP, or an increase in sympathetic tone that causes a catecholamine surge at the time of trauma. Neurogenic pulmonary edema often presents as "flash pulmonary edema" because it has a sudden onset. This type of pulmonary edema is thought to be caused by massive vasoconstriction secondary to activation of the sympathetic nervous system, which causes a marked increase in left ventricular afterload resulting in left ventricular failure. Pulmonary edema due to left ventricular failure is exacerbated by an increase in pulmonary capillary permeability, causing further edema.[23] Treatment includes judicious use of low-dose diuretics. The condition is typically self-limiting in patients without cardiac disease.

Multidisciplinary care of the patient with TBI with respect to pulmonary complications requires the involvement of the nursing and the physician teams; the respiratory therapist; the occupational therapist, the physical therapist (for early mobilization); and the speech–language pathologist (to address issues with aspiration).

MANAGING NUTRITION AND MAINTAINING GLYCEMIC CONTROL

Head injury is thought to cause hypermetabolic and hypercatabolic states as well as a decrease in immunocompetency.[24] Morbidity and mortality may significantly increase if nutritional requirements are not met. Indirect calorimetry is useful in determining resting energy expenditure (REE).[24] Indirect calorimetry is performed using a machine (metabolic cart) that interfaces with the ventilator to measure oxygen consumption and carbon dioxide production.

Nutrition in the form of enteral or parenteral nutrition is administered in amounts that meet metabolic needs within 7 days of the injury.[16] Enteral feeding may prevent the translocation of bacteria from the gut to the bloodstream as well as prevent gastrointestinal ulceration and bleeding.[24] Current recommendations suggest replacement of 140% of REE in patients who are not paralyzed and 100% of REE in patients who are paralyzed.[16] Recognition of the importance of nutrition and multidisciplinary collaboration with a nutrition support team are essential to optimize patient outcome. Research suggests a detrimental effect of hyperglycemia on morbidity and mortality of patients with TBI; however, specific treatment thresholds have not been established. Hyperglycemia should be avoided in patients with TBI.[16,25,26]

MANAGING MUSCULOSKELETAL AND INTEGUMENTARY COMPLICATIONS

Comprehensive assessment of the musculoskeletal and integumentary systems is necessary to prevent skin breakdown and other complications such as contractures. Collaboration with other disciplines, such as occupational and physical therapy, is also essential in developing a plan of care to prevent or mitigate the effects of immobility on the skin and musculoskeletal systems. Splinting of the hands and feet in an unresponsive patient is necessary to preserve musculoskeletal function and ensure the best conditions for future rehabilitation. Functional splint-

ing and range-of-motion exercises also help reduce dependent edema in immobile extremities. Frequent turning of patients, even in the critical phase of the illness, is integral in maintaining skin integrity and facilitating pulmonary drainage.

CARING FOR THE FAMILY

Caring for families in crisis, as well as coordinating available services (such as social work and pastoral care), is an important function of the critical care nurse. Bond and colleagues[27] surveyed the needs of family members of patients with severe TBI and found the following four needs:

▶ The need for specific truthful information
▶ The need for information to be consistent
▶ The need to be actively involved in the care
▶ The need to make sense of the entire experience

Critical care nurses have an opportunity to meet all of these specific needs and to change unit culture to meet these needs. Encouraging family members to touch the patient or allowing family members to assist in providing sensory stimulation (Box 36-4) may be helpful and comforting to some family members. Finding opportunities to involve family members in the patient's plan of care may also be therapeutic for the patient and the family. The Ranchos Los Amigos Scale can be used by the critical care nurse to describe the stages of coma as they relate to rehabilitative methods and interventions (Table 36-5). Attention is given to including both spiritual and cultural needs in the plan of care.

A patient with TBI may be discharged to home, a rehabilitation program, or a nursing facility depending on the severity of his or her neurologic deficits. Families must be informed and educated about the expected course of events and potential scenarios for continued care after the acute hospitalization, especially when the patient has severe TBI. Family resources, as well as other support systems and services available to the patient, should be assessed early in all patients with TBI to facilitate a smooth transition into the next stage of care. Social workers and case managers play an integral role in obtaining information and communicating with the patient, the family, and the multidisciplinary team.

• Brain Death

A patient's condition may be so severe that brain death is the final outcome. The critical care nurse continues to provide nursing care to the patient as treatment is continued or life support measures are withdrawn.

In the past, the declaration of brain death was controversial with regard to the standardization of tests needed to make the decision and ethical considerations. The Uniform Determination of Death Act was developed in 1981 by the President's Commission for

---

Box 36-4 • NURSING INTERVENTIONS for Sensory Stimulation

Sound
- Explain to the patient what you are going to do.
- Play the patient's favorite television or radio program for 10–15 min. Alternatively, play a tape recording of a familiar voice of a friend or family member.
- During the program, do not converse with others in the room or perform other activities of patient care. The goal is to minimize distractions so the patient may learn to attend to the stimulus selectively.
- Another approach is to clap your hands or ring a bell. Do this for 5–10 seconds at a time, moving the sound to different locations around the bed.

Sight
- Place a brightly colored object in the patient's view. Present only one object at a time.
- Alternatively, use an object that is familiar, such as a family photo or favorite poster.

Touch
- Stroke the patient's arm or leg with fabrics of various textures. Alternatively, the back of a spoon can simulate smooth texture and a towel rough texture.
- Rubbing lotion over the patient's skin will also stimulate this sense. For some, firm pressure may be better tolerated than very light touch.

Smell
- Hold a container of a pleasing fragrance under the patient's nose. Use a familiar scent, such as perfume, aftershave, cinnamon, or coffee.
- Present this stimulation for very short periods (1–3 min maximum).
- If a cuffed tracheostomy or endotracheal tube is in place, the patient will not be able to appreciate this stimulation fully.

---

the Study of Ethical Problems in Medicine and Biomedical Behavior Research and adopted by all 50 states. This act states: "An individual, who has sustained either (1) irreversible cessation of circulatory and respiratory functions, or (2) irreversible cessation of all functions of the entire brain, including the brainstem, is dead. A determination of death must be made in accordance with accepted medical standards."[28]

The brain death examination seeks to confirm the following three cardinal findings: coma or unresponsiveness, absence of brainstem reflexes, and apnea.[29,30] Tests specific for brain death include, but are not limited to, motor testing; evaluation of pupillary responses; evaluation of the oculocephalic reflex ("doll's eyes" phenomenon); evaluation of the oculovestibular reflex (caloric ice-water test); evaluation of the corneal, cough, and gag reflexes; and apnea testing. Electrolyte abnormalities, hypothermia or hyperthermia, severe hypotension, or the presence of medications in amounts that could cause coma must be resolved before brain death testing can be performed. Apnea testing is performed by removing the patient from the ventilator, inspecting the chest for spontaneous respiratory effort while providing supplemental oxygen, and monitoring the increase in $PaCO_2$. Baseline acid–base balance is established with an arterial blood gas (ABG) following removal from the ventilator, and then serial ABGs are obtained. A $PaCO_2$ greater than 60 mm Hg or an increase in the $PaCO_2$ of 20 mm Hg or more above the patient's baseline $PaCO_2$ is regarded as a positive test, supporting the diagnosis of brain death.[29,30] The patient is simultaneously observed for spontaneous respiration and hemodynamic instability, which may cause the test to be aborted. An increased $PaCO_2$ is the single strongest stimulus for the initiation of

breathing; therefore, the absence of respiratory effort in the presence of severe hypercarbia constitutes strong evidence of brain death. Confirmatory tests for brain death, such as cerebral angiography (to test for the absence of cerebral blood flow), TCD ultrasonography, EEG, BAER, and SSEP, can be used if any doubt exists after a full clinical examination has been completed.

The American Academy of Neurology recommends repeating the clinical evaluation for brain death after 6 hours.[30] Time of death is recorded at the time that brain death is declared. Different institutions specify requirements based on state laws and statutes for physicians declaring brain death. Brain death determination in pediatric patients differs from that in adults owing to the increased viability of the immature brain.[31] Specific guidelines for the determination of brain death in children were developed by a federal task force in 1987. These guidelines delineate physical examination features unique to pediatric patients as well as specific time frames for observation when brain death is suspected, depending on the age of the child.[31]

The concept of brain death is often confusing for families because death is so commonly associated with cardiopulmonary death. Therefore, the language used in discussions is very important. Some family members may interpret the term "brain dead" to mean that the rest of the body can continue to live, so care must be taken to assess the understanding and coping mechanisms of family members.[32]

The discussion of brain death should be separated in time from conversations regarding the opportunities for organ donation. It is essential to work closely with an organ procurement organization in order to provide the most complete and accurate information regarding organ donation.

Table 36-5 • Ranchos Los Amigos Scale

Level	Guidelines for Interacting With Patient
1. **No response** to any stimuli occurs.	• Assume that the patient can understand all that is said. Converse with, not about, the patient.
2. **Generalized response.** Stimulus response is incoherent, limited, and nonpurposeful with random movements or incomprehensible sounds.	• Do not overwhelm the patient with talking. Leave some moments of silence between verbal stimuli.
3. **Localized response.** Stimulus response is specific but inconsistent; patient may withdraw or push away, may make sounds, may follow some simple commands, or may respond to certain family members.	• Manage the environment to provide only one source of stimulation at a time. If talking is taking place, the radio or television should be turned off. • Provide short, random periods of sensory input that are meaningful to the patient. A favorite television program or tape recording or 30 minutes of music from the patient's favorite radio station will provide more meaningful stimulation than constant radio accompaniment, which becomes as meaningless as the continual bleep of the cardiac monitor.
4. **Confused–agitated.** Stimulus response is primarily to internal confusion with increased state of activity; behavior may be bizarre or aggressive; patient may attempt to remove tubes or restraints or crawl out of bed; verbalization is incoherent or inappropriate; patient shows minimal awareness of environment and absent short-term memory.	• Be calm and soothing when handling the patient. Approach with gentle touch to decrease the occurrence of defensive emotional and motor reflexes. • Watch for early signs that the patient is becoming agitated (e.g., increased movement, vocal loudness, resistance to activity). • When the patient becomes upset, do not try to reason with him or her or "talk him or her out of it." Talking will be an additional external stimulus that the patient cannot handle. • If the patient remains upset, either remove him or her from the situation or remove the situation from him or her.
5. **Confused, inappropriate–nonagitated.** Patient is alert and responds consistently to simple commands; however, patient has a short attention span and is easily distracted; memory is impaired and patient exhibits confusion of past and present events; patient can perform previously learned tasks with maximal structure but is unable to learn new information; may wander off with vague intention of "going home."	• Present the patient with only one task at a time. Allow time to complete it before giving further instructions. • Make sure that you have the patient's attention by placing yourself in view and touching the patient before talking. • If the patient becomes confused or resistant, stop talking. Wait until he or she appears relaxed before continuing with instruction or activity.
6. **Confused–appropriate.** Patient shows goal-directed behavior but still needs external direction; can understand simple directions and reasoning; follows simple directions consistently and requires less supervision for previously learned tasks; has improved past memory depth and detail and basic awareness of self and surroundings.	• Use gestures, demonstrations, and only the most necessary words when giving instructions. • Maintain the same sequence in routine activities and tasks. Describe these routines to the patient and relate them to time of day.
7. **Automatic–appropriate.** Patient is able to complete daily routines in structured environment; has increased awareness of self and surroundings but lacks insight, judgment, and problem-solving ability.	• Supervision is still necessary for continued learning and safety. • Reinforce the patient's memory of routines and schedules with clocks, calendars, and a written log of activities.
8. **Purposeful–appropriate.** Patient is alert, oriented, and able to recall and integrate past and recent events; responds appropriately to environment; still has decreased ability in abstract reasoning, stress tolerance, and judgment in emergencies or unusual situations.	• The patient should be able to function without supervision. • Consideration should be given to job retraining or a return to school.

• Clinical Applicability Challenges

Case Study

Ms. S., a 20-year-old woman, arrives at the emergency department (ED) after a motor vehicle crash. Emergency medical personnel have immobilized her using a long spine immobilization board and a rigid cervical collar. On arrival at the ED, she is unresponsive. Her vital signs are blood pressure, 96/64 mm Hg; heart rate, 110 beats/minute; and respiratory rate (snoring respirations), 24 breaths/minute. On neurologic examination, the following findings are evident: flexor (decorticate) posturing in both upper extremities with extension of both legs to painful stimuli and no eye opening; large right pupil (bigger than the left pupil) that is sluggishly reactive to light (cranial nerve III); moderate-sized left pupil that is briskly reactive to light; intact corneal reflex in each eye (cranial nerves V and VII); and intact cough and gag reflexes (cranial nerves IX and X). The Glasgow Coma Scale (GCS) score is 5.

Because of Ms. S.'s depressed level of consciousness and GCS score, she is intubated using rapid-sequence intubation technique and placed on a ventilator. A secondary survey is performed to detect other obvious traumatic injuries and does not reveal additional deformities. An emergency CT scan is obtained and reveals a large right parietotemporal subdural hematoma with shifting of the midline brain structures and a right frontal contusion. Radiographs of the patient's cervical spine are obtained to rule out vertebral fracture and do not reveal fracture or dislocation of the vertebrae.

Based on the patient's clinical neurologic examination and CT findings, neurosurgeons take her emergently to the operating room to evacuate the subdural hematoma. The hematoma is evacuated, and an intraventricular catheter is placed.

Ms. S. is admitted to the intensive care unit (ICU) postoperatively. The GCS score is 7T (eye opening = 2, best motor response = 4, best verbal response = 1T). The right pupil remains larger than the left and is briskly reactive to light.

Over the next 2 days, Ms S. experiences periods of increased intracranial pressure (ICP) to 25 to 30 mm Hg. After aggressive treatment to reduce the ICP, her clinical neurologic examination improves. The patient is localizing to noxious stimuli and opening her eyes to voice. During the next 7 days, she remains stable, and at the end the week, she begins to follow simple commands, is oriented to person only, demonstrates short-term memory loss, and left arm and leg hemiparesis. She is also opening her eyes spontaneously and tracking her caregivers from side to side. On ICU day 9, she is extubated to a face mask. She is confused and moves her left arm and leg in a horizontal plane, not against gravity.

Physical and occupational therapy are consulted to begin the rehabilitation process. On day 13, Ms. S. is transferred to an acute rehabilitation facility specializing in the care of patients with traumatic brain injury.

1. Based on your knowledge of the functions of the parietal, temporal, and frontal lobes, list at least four potential problems or deficits Ms. S. might experience as a result of her brain injury.

2. Using the radiological findings and your knowledge of the pathophysiology of head injury, explain why Ms. S. initially has a dilated right pupil that is sluggishly reactive to light. (Hint: State which cranial nerve is affected.)

3. Name at least three postoperative complications that Ms. S. may experience.

4. State the rationale for the placement of an intraventricular catheter versus an intraparenchymal or subarachnoid monitor in this patient.

5. Using the description of the patient's neurologic status at the end of the case study, place the patient into the appropriate level on the Ranchos Los Amigos Scale (see Table 36-5). Name two interventions that could be used when interacting with patients in this category.

Review Questions

1. The critical care nurse responds to a high intracranial pressure (ICP) of 25 mm Hg. Which of the following actions is the most appropriate next step?
   a. Quickly assess the patient's neurologic examination, compare it to the last examination, and ensure that the patient's head is in a midline position.
   b. Notify the physician, recalibrate the ICP monitor, and prepare to administer an osmotic diuretic.
   c. Recalibrate the ICP monitor, ensure that the patient's head is in a midline position, and notify the physician.
   d. Monitor the ICP to see if it will decrease over the next 5 minutes, ensure that the patient's head is in a midline position, and raise the head of bed to 90 degrees.

2. An epidural hematoma is typically caused by injury to a cerebral artery, which causes blood to accumulate between which of the following?
   a. The skull and pia mater
   b. The dura and arachnoid layer
   c. The skull and dura mater
   d. The pia mater and brain tissue

3. Secondary brain injury occurs after the onset of the initial injury. To mitigate secondary brain injury, the multidisciplinary critical care team should perform which of following sets of interventions?
   a. Monitor blood pressure closely, preventing decreases of systolic blood pressure below 90 mm Hg; and maintain normothermia.
   b. Monitor oxygenation closely, preventing decreases of PaO_2 below 50 mm Hg; and maintain a patent airway.
   c. Monitor cerebral perfusion pressure closely, keeping it greater than 80 mm Hg; and maintain normothermia.
   d. Monitor oxygenation closely, preventing acute respiratory distress syndrome; and administer antiepileptic drugs, preventing seizures.

4. A patient with a subdural hematoma should lie flat for 12 to 24 hours after surgical evacuation of the hematoma and then have the head of bed raised gradually for which one of the following reasons?
   a. To promote cerebral blood flow, reducing the risk for cerebral ischemia
   b. To reduce tension on bridging veins, reducing the risk for rebleeding
   c. To decrease tension on the dura, reducing risk for blood clot reaccumulation
   d. To decrease intracranial pressure, reducing the risk for herniation syndrome

References

1. Langlois JA, Rutland-Brown W, Thomas KE: Traumatic Brain Injury in the United States: Emergency Department Visits, Hospitalizations, and Deaths. Atlanta, GA: Centers for Disease Control and Prevention, National Center for Injury Prevention and Control, 2006

2. Bullock MR, Chestnut R, Ghajar, J, et al: Surgical management of depressed cranial fractures. Neurosurgery 58(3): S2-56–S2-60, 2006

3. Gouvier, WD, Cubic B, Jones G, et al: Post concussion symptoms and daily stress in normal and head-injured college populations. Arch Clin Neuropyschol 7:193–211, 1992

4. Lee KS: Natural history of chronic subdural haematoma. Brain Injury 18(4):351–358, 2004

5. Mattioli C, Beretta L, Gerevini S, et al: Traumatic subarachnoid hemorrhage on the computerized tomography scan obtained at admission: A multicenter assessment of the accuracy of diagnosis and the potential impact on patient outcome. J Neurosurg 98(1):37–42, 2003

6. Servadei F, Murray GD, Teasdale GM, et al: Traumatic subarachnoid hemorrhage: Demographic and clinical study of 750 patients from the European Brain Injury Consortium survey of head injuries. Neurosurgery 50(2):261–267, 2002

7. Jeremitsky E, Omert L, Dunham CM, et al: Harbingers of poor outcome the day after severe brain injury: Hypothermia, hypoxia, and hypoperfusion. J Trauma 54(2):312–319, 2003

8. Chang BS, Lowenstein DH: Practice parameter: Antiepileptic drug prophylaxis in severe traumatic brain injury. Report of the Quality Standards Subcommittee of the American Academy of Neurology. Neurology 60(1):10–16, 2003

9. March K, Wellwood J: Intracranial pressure concepts and cerebral blood flow. In Bader M, Littlejohns L (eds): AANN Core Curriculum for Neuroscience Nursing, 4th ed. St. Louis: Elsevier, 2004, pp 87–93

10. Ng SC, Poon WS, Chan MT: Cerebral hemisphere asymmetry in cerebrovascular regulation in ventilated traumatic brain injury. Acta Neurochir Supplement 96:21–23, 2006

11. Unterberg AW, Stover J, Kress, B, Kiening KL: Edema and brain trauma. Neuroscience 129(4):1021–1029, 2004

12. Quality Standards Subcommittee of the American Academy of Neurology: Practice parameters: Assessment and management of patients in the persistent vegetative state [summary statement]. Report of the Quality Standards Subcommittee of the American Academy of Neurology. Neurology 45:1015–1018, 1995

13. Zygun DA, Kortbeek JB, Fick GH, et al: Non-neurologic organ dysfunction in severe traumatic brain injury. Crit Care Med 33(3):654–660, 2005

14. Kidd KC, Criddle L: Using jugular venous catheters in patients with traumatic brain injury. Crit Care Nurse 21(6):17–22, 2001

15. Littlejohns LR, Bader MK, March K: Brain tissue oxygen monitoring in severe brain injury I. Crit Care Nurse 23(4):17–27, 2003

16. Brain Trauma Foundation: Guidelines for the management of severe traumatic brain injury, 3rd ed. J Neurotrauma 24(Suppl 1):s1–s106, 2007

17. Fakhrysm, Trask AL, Waller MA, Watts DD, for the IRTC Neurotrauma Taskforce: Management of brain-injured patients by an evidence-based medicine protocol improves outcomes and decreases hospital charges. J Trauma 56(3):492–299, 2004

18. Society of Critical Care Medicine: Guidelines for the acute medical management of severe traumatic brain injury in infants, children, and adolescents. Crit Care Med 31(6 Suppl):407–491, 2003

19. Gabriel EJ, Ghajar J, Jagoda A, et al: Guidelines for prehospital management of traumatic brain injury. J Neurotrauma 19:117–174, 2002

20. Lemke DM: Sympathetic storming after severe traumatic brain injury. Crit Care Nurse 27(1):30–37, 2007

21. Lemke DM: Riding out the storm: Sympathetic storming after traumatic brain injury. J Neurosci Nurs 36(1):4–9, 2004

22. Agha A, Thornton, E, O'Kelly P, et al: Posterior pituitary dysfunction after traumatic brain injury. J Clin Endocrinol Metab 89(12):5987–5992, 2004

23. Bahloul M, Chaari AN, Kallel H, et al: Neurogenic pulmonary edema due to traumatic brain injury: Evidence of cardiac dysfunction. Am J Crit Care 15(5):462–470, 2006

24. Krakau K, Omne-Ponten M, Karlsson T, Borg J: Metabolism and nutrition in patients with moderate and severe traumatic brain injury: A systematic review. Brain Injury 20(4):345–367, 2006

25. Diaz-Parejo P, Stahl N, Xu W, et al: Cerebral energy metabolism during transient hyperglycemia in patients with severe brain trauma. Intensive Care Med 29(4):544–550, 2003

26. Song EC, Chu K, Jeong SW, et al: Hyperglycemia exacerbates brain edema and perihematomal cell death after intracerebral hemorrhage. Stroke 34(9):2215–2220, 2003

27. Bond AE, Draeger CRL, Mandleco B, et al: Needs of family members of patients with severe traumatic brain injury: Implications for evidenced-based practice. Crit Care Nurse 23(4): 63–71, 2003

28. Uniform Determination of Death Act. Presented and approved at the 89th Annual Conference of Commissioners on Uniform State Laws, July 26–August 1, 1980, Kauai, Hawaii. Chicago, IL: National Conference of Commissioners on Uniform State Laws, 1980

29. Wijdicks EFM: Determining brain death in adults. Neurology 45:1003–1011, 1995

30. Quality Standards Subcommittee of the American Academy of Neurology: Practice parameters for determining brain death in adults (summary statement). Report of the Quality Standards Subcommittee of the American Academy of Neurology. Neurology 45:1012–1014, 1995

31. Task Force for the Determination of Brain Death in Children: Guidelines for the determination of brain death in children. Arch Neurol 44(6):587–588, 1987

32. Arnold RM: Discussing brain death with families; declaring brain death: The neurologic criteria. J Palliative Med 8(3): 639–640, 2005

Other Selected Readings

Bader MK, Littlejohns LR, Mack K: Brain tissue oxygen monitoring in severe brain injury, II: Implications for critical care teams and case study. Crit Care Nurse 23(4):29–44, 2003

Blissitt PA: Care of the critically ill patient with penetrating head injury. Crit Care Nurs Clin North Am 18(3):321–332, 2006

Bullock MR, Chestnut R, Ghajar J, et al: Guidelines for the surgical management of traumatic brain injury. Neurosurgery 58(Suppl): s2–s61, 2006

Jacobs DG, Plaisier BR, Barie PS, et al: Practice management guidelines for geriatric trauma: The EAST Practice Management Guidelines Work Group. J Trauma 54:391–416, 2003

Kirkness CJ, Burr RL, Cain KC, et al: Effect of continuous display of cerebral perfusion pressure on outcomes in patients with traumatic brain injury. Am J Crit Care 15(6):600–610, 2006

Littlejohns L, Bader MK: Prevention of secondary brain injury: Targeting technology. AACN Clin Issues 16(4):501–514, 2005

McIlvoy LH: The effect of hypothermia and hyperthermia on acute brain injury. AACN Clin Issues 16(4):488–500, 2005

Mitchell I, Nikolic G: Peaked waves after head injury. Heart Lung 35(2):117–118, 2006

O'Connor KJ, Wood KE, Lord K: Intensive management of organ donors to maximize transplantation. Crit Care Nurse 26:94–100, 2006

Olson DM, Graffagnimo C: Consciousness, coma, and caring for the brain-injured patient. AACN Clin Issues 16(4):441–455, 2005

Presciutti M: Nursing priorities in caring for patients with intracerebral hemorrhage. J Neurosci Nurs 38(4):296–300, 2006

Sadovich I, Rehman Z, Yunen J, Coritsidis G: Propofol infusion syndrome: A case of increasing morbidity with traumatic brain injury. Am J Crit Care 16(1):72–81, 2007

37

Spinal Cord Injury

Kathy A. Hausman

Objectives

Based on the content in this chapter, the reader should be able to:

❶ Describe the mechanism of spinal cord injury.

❷ Discuss the various classification systems for spinal cord injuries.

❸ Differentiate between the following syndromes: central cord syndrome, Brown-Séquard syndrome, anterior cord syndrome, and posterior cord syndrome.

❹ Differentiate between spinal shock, neurogenic shock and orthostatic hypotension.

❺ Perform an assessment of a patient with a spinal cord injury.

❻ Develop a collaborative plan of care for a patient with an acute spinal cord injury.

❼ Describe immediate nursing actions when the patient develops autonomic dysreflexia.

❽ Explain other typical complications that occur after a spinal cord injury.

Each year in the United States, there are approximately 11,000 new spinal cord injuries. Fortunately, progress in neurological research and advances in technology have led to a dramatic increase in the number of people who survive a traumatic spinal cord injury. The number of people alive today who have a spinal cord injury is estimated at between 225,000 and 296,000.[1]

Spinal cord injury is most common in young adults between the ages of 16 and 30 years.

Among this age group, spinal cord injury is more common in men than women, although the number of men affected is decreasing slightly. The most common causes of spinal cord injuries include motor vehicle crashes (MVCs), falls, acts of violence, and sports. Falls are the most common cause of spinal cord injuries in older adults. Since 2000, the percentage of people with such injuries who are older than 60 years of age has increased to 11.5%.[1]

The overwhelming majority of people with spinal cord injuries discharged from health care facilities return to their homes or to noninstitutional settings. Slightly more than 34% of patients discharged have incomplete tetraplegia, followed by complete paraplegia, complete tetraplegia, and then incomplete paraplegia.[1] Unfortunately, fewer than 1% of these patients have complete return of neurological function.[1] Many of those discharged home require partial or total care. The economic consequences of this type of injury, especially if repeated hospitalizations are necessary, can be staggering. Cost of care in the first year after injury for a person with a complete spinal cord injury is estimated at $121,600 and $42,100 for a person with an incomplete injury.[2] Pneumonia, pulmonary embolism, and septicemia are the leading causes of death that appear to have the greatest impact on decreased life expectancy for a person with a spinal cord injury.[1]

• Classification of Injury

Spinal cord injuries can be classified by mechanism, type of vertebral injury, level of injury, or cause. Spinal cord injuries occur as a result of penetrating injury or mechanical forces. Penetrating injuries, which are most often caused by gunshot or stab wounds, damage the spinal cord and cause loss of neurological functioning.

MECHANISM OF INJURY

Mechanical forces that can result in spinal cord injury include hyperflexion, hyperextension, axial loading (compression), and rotational forces (Fig. 37-1):

1. Hyperflexion, depicted in Figure 37-1A, is caused by a sudden deceleration of the head and neck. Hyperflexion injuries are often seen in patients

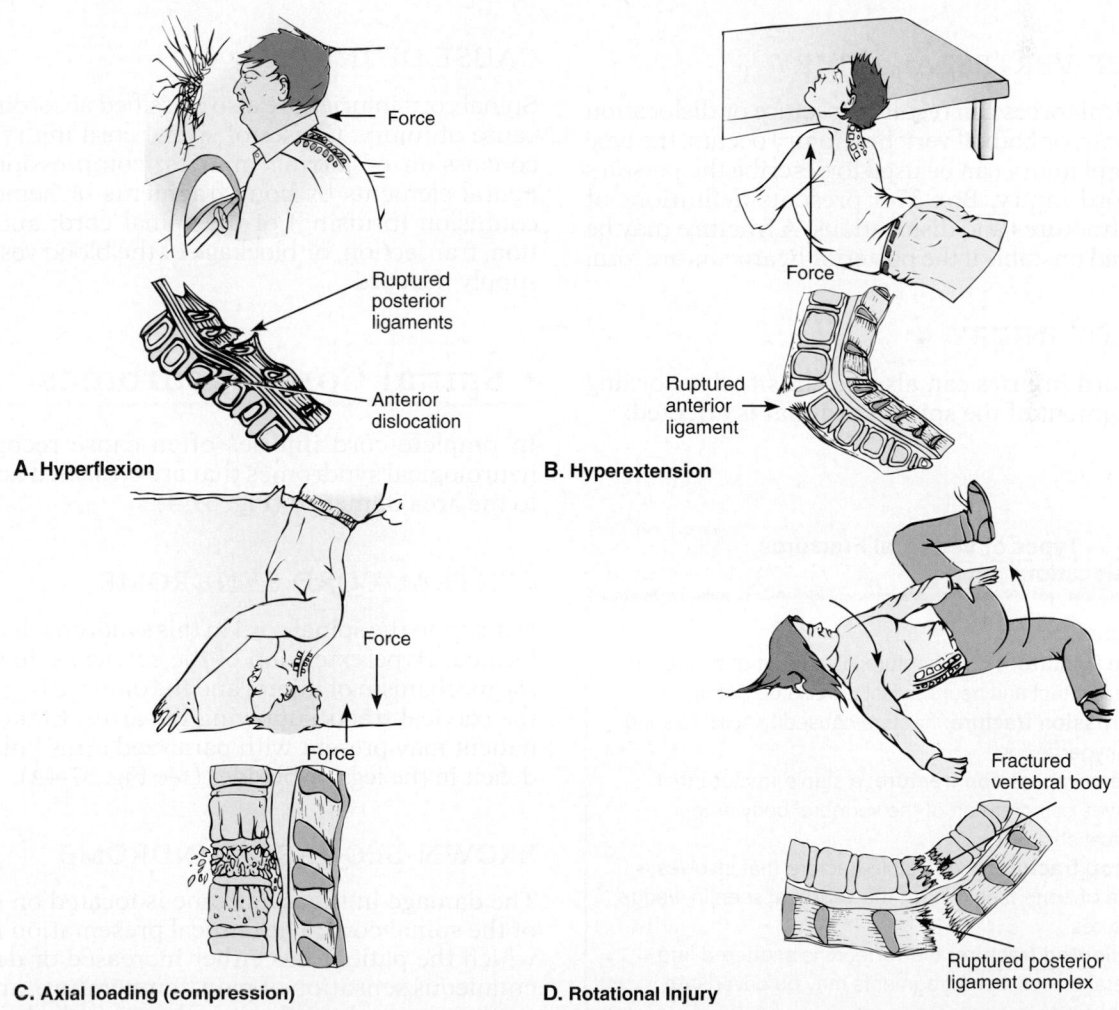

A. Hyperflexion

B. Hyperextension

C. Axial loading (compression)

D. Rotational Injury

Figure 37-1 • Spinal cord injuries can be classified according to the mechanism of injury. **A:** With hyperflexion to the cervical spine, there may be tearing of the posterior ligamentous complex, resulting in anterior dislocation. **B:** Hyperextension injury can result in rupture of the anterior ligament. **C:** Axial loading (compression) of the spine results in fracture and subsequent spinal cord damage. **D:** When rotational force occurs, there is concurrent fracture and tearing of the posterior ligamentous complex. (From Hickey JV: Clinical Practice of Neurological and Neurosurgical Nursing, 5th ed. Philadelphia: Lippincott Williams & Wilkins, 2003, pp 409–412.)

who have sustained trauma from a head-on MVC or diving accident. The cervical region is most often involved, especially at the C5–C6 level.

2. Hyperextension (see Fig. 37-1B) is the most common type of injury. Hyperextension injuries can be caused by a fall, a rear-end MVC, or getting hit in the head (e.g., during a boxing match). Hyperextension of the head and neck may cause contusion and ischemia of the spinal cord without vertebral column damage. Whiplash injuries are the result of hyperextension.

3. Axial loading, also known as compression (see Fig. 37-1C), typically occurs when a person lands on the feet or buttocks after falling or jumping from a height. It may also occur when there is a direct blow to the head. The vertebral column is compressed, causing a fracture that results in damage to the spinal cord.

4. Rotational injuries result from forces that cause extreme twisting or lateral flexion of the head and neck (see Fig. 37-1D). Fracture or dislocation of vertebrae may also occur.

TYPE OF VERTEBRAL INJURY

Mechanical forces can result in fracture or dislocation of vertebrae, or both. If vertebral injury occurs, the type of vertebral injury can be used to describe the person's spinal cord injury. Box 37-1 presents definitions of types of fractures and dislocations. A fracture may be considered unstable if the posterior ligaments are torn.

LEVEL OF INJURY

Spinal cord injuries can also be classified according to the segment of the spinal cord that is affected:

---

1. Upper cervical (C1–C2) injuries (atlas fractures, atlantoaxial subluxation, odontoid fractures, and hangman's fractures)
2. Lower cervical (C3–C8) injuries
3. Thoracic (T1–T12) injuries
4. Lumbar (L1–L5) injuries
5. Sacral (S1–S5) injuries

The degree of functional recovery depends on the location and extent of the injury. The level of spinal cord injury is determined by the effect of the injury on sensory and motor function (Table 37-1). Retention of all or some of the motor or sensory function below the level of injury implies that the lesion is incomplete. Total loss of voluntary muscle control and sensation below the level of injury suggests that the lesion is complete. Complete lesions involving spinal cord regions C1 to T1 result in tetraplegia (Fig. 37-2). Complete lesions involving spinal cord regions T2 to L1 result in paraplegia (see Fig. 37-2). A person with a complete cord injury follows the dermatome pathways for the level of sensory loss shown in Figure 37-3.

CAUSE OF INJURY

Spinal cord injuries are also classified according to the cause of injury. Causes of spinal cord injury include concussion or jarring injuries; compression of the neural elements by bony fragments or hemorrhage; contusion (bruising) of the spinal cord; and laceration, transection, or blockage of the blood vessels that supply the cord.

• Spinal Cord Syndromes

Incomplete cord injuries often cause recognizable neurological syndromes that are classified according to the area damaged (Fig. 37-4).

CENTRAL CORD SYNDROME

Damage to the spinal cord in this syndrome is centrally located. Hyperextension of the cervical spine often is the mechanism of injury, and the damage is greatest to the cervical tracts supplying the arms. Clinically, the patient may present with paralyzed arms but with no deficit in the legs or bladder (see Fig. 37-4A).

BROWN-SÉQUARD SYNDROME

The damage in this syndrome is located on one side of the spinal cord. The clinical presentation is one in which the patient has either increased or decreased cutaneous sensation of pain, temperature, and touch on the same side of the spinal cord at the level of the lesion. Below the level of the lesion on the same side, there is complete motor paralysis. On the patient's opposite side, below the level of the lesion, there is loss of pain, temperature, and touch because the spinothalamic tracts cross soon after entering the

---

> **Box 37-1 • Types of Vertebral Fractures and Dislocations**
>
> **Fractures**
> **Simple fracture:** single fracture; alignment of the vertebrae is intact and neurological deficits do not occur
> **Compression fracture:** fracture caused by axial loading and hyperflexion
> **Wedge compression fracture:** a stable fracture that involves compression of the vertebral body in the cervical area
> **Teardrop fracture:** an unstable fracture that involves a piece of bone breaking off the vertebra; seen in wedge fractures
> **Comminuted fracture:** the vertebra is shattered into several pieces; bone fragments may be driven into spinal cord
>
> **Dislocations**
> **Dislocation:** one vertebra overrides another
> **Subluxation:** partial or incomplete dislocation
> **Fracture–dislocation:** fracture and dislocation

Table 37-1 • Functional Loss From Spinal Cord Injury (Based on Complete Lesions)

Level of Spinal Injury	Motor Function	Deep Tendon Reflexes	Sensory Function	Respiratory Function	Voluntary Bowel and Bladder Function	Rehabilitative Potential
C1–C4	Quadriplegia: loss of all motor function from the neck down	All lost	Loss of all sensory function in the neck and below (C4 supplies the clavicles)	Loss of involuntary (phrenic) and voluntary (intercostals) respiratory function; ventilatory support and a tracheostomy needed	No bowel or bladder control	May be discharged home on a ventilator with home care
C5	Quadriplegia: loss of all function below the upper shoulders **Intact:** sternomastoids, cervical paraspinal muscles, and the trapezius; can control head	C5, C6 biceps	Loss of sensation below the clavicle and most portions of arms, hands, chest, abdomen, and lower extremities **Intact:** head, shoulders, deltoid, clavicle, portion of forearms (C5 supplies the lateral aspect of the arm)	Phrenic nerve intact, but not intercostal muscles	No bowel or bladder control	Use of extremity-powered devices to achieve some upper limb control Head control facilitates wheelchair (W/C) balance Adaptive tools, held in mouth, for typing and writing Some adaptive tools and use of special computer technology
C6	Quadriplegia: loss of all function below the shoulders and upper arms; lacks elbow, forearm, and hand control **Intact:** deltoid, biceps, and external rotator muscles of shoulders	C5, C6 brachioradialis	Loss of everything listed for a C5 lesion, but greater arm and thumb sensation **Intact:** head, shoulders, arms, palms of hands, and thumbs (C6 supplies the forearm and thumb)	Phrenic nerve intact, but not intercostal muscles	No bowel or bladder control	Needs assistive devices to use arms (may be able to help feed, groom, and dress self) Needs a motorized W/C Dependent for all transfers
C7	Quadriplegia: loss of motor control to portions of the arms and hands **Intact:** voluntary strength in shoulder depressors, shoulder abductors, internal rotators, and radial wrist extensors	C7, C8 triceps	Loss of sensation below the clavicle and portions of arms and hands **Intact:** head, shoulders, most of arms and hands (C7 supplies the middle finger)	Phrenic nerve intact, but not intercostal muscles	No bowel or bladder function	Can perform some activities of daily living (ADLs) Can use wrist extensor with a special splint to induce finger flexion Can push a W/C with special handgrasps May be able to drive a specially equipped car
C8	Quadriplegia: loss of motor control to portions of the arms and hands **Intact:** some voluntary control of elbow extensors, wrist, finger extension, and finger flexors		Loss of sensation below the chest and in portions of hands **Intact:** sensation to face, shoulders, arms, hands, and part of chest (C8 supplies the little finger)	Phrenic nerve intact, but not intercostal muscles	No bowel or bladder function	Able to push up in the W/C Improved sitting tolerance Can grasp and release hands voluntarily Independent in most ADLs from W/C Independent in use of W/C

(continued)

Table 37-1 • Functional Loss From Spinal Cord Injury (Based on Complete Lesions) (Continued)

Level of Spinal Injury	Motor Function	Deep Tendon Reflexes	Sensory Function	Respiratory Function	Voluntary Bowel and Bladder Function	Rehabilitative Potential
						Can use hands for catheterization and rectal stimulation for bowel movements
T1–T6	Paraplegia: loss of everything below the midchest region, including the trunk muscles **Intact:** control of function to the shoulders, upper chest, arms, and hands		Loss of sensation below the midchest area **Intact:** everything to the midchest region, including the arms and hands (T1 and T2 supply the inner aspect of the arm; T4 supplies the nipple area)	Phrenic nerve functions independently Some impairment of intercostal muscles	No bowel or bladder function	Full control of upper extremities and completely independent in W/C Full-time employment possible Independent in managing urinary drainage and inserting suppositories Able to live in a dwelling without major architectural changes
T6–T12	Paraplegia: loss of motor control below the waist **Intact:** shoulders, arms, hands, and long trunk muscles		Loss of everything below the waist **Intact:** shoulders, chest, arms, and hands (T10 supplies the umbilicus; T12 supplies the groin area)	No interference with respiratory function	No bowel or bladder control	In addition to the previously described capabilities, there is complete abdominal and upper back control. Good sitting balance (allows for greater ease of W/C operation and athletics)
L1–L3	Paraplegia: loss of most control of legs and pelvis **Intact:** shoulders, arms, hands, torso, hip rotation and flexion, and some leg flexion	L2–L4 (knee jerk)	Loss of sensation to the lower abdomen and legs **Intact:** all of the above plus some sensation to the inner and anterior thigh (L3 supplies the knee)	No interference with respiratory function	No bowel or bladder control	Independent for most activities from W/C
L3–L4	Paraplegia: loss of control of portions of lower legs, ankles, and feet **Intact:** all of the above, plus increased knee extension		Loss of sensation to portions of the lower legs, feet, and ankles **Intact:** all of the above, plus sensation to the upper legs	No interference with respiratory function	No bowel or bladder control	Voluntary control of hip extensors; weak abductors Walking with braces possible

(continued)

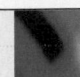

Table 37-1 • Functional Loss From Spinal Cord Injury (Based on Complete Lesions) (Continued)

Level of Spinal Injury	Motor Function	Deep Tendon Reflexes	Sensory Function	Respiratory Function	Voluntary Bowel and Bladder Function	Rehabilitative Potential
L4 to S5	Paraplegia: incomplete Segmental motor control L4 to S1: abduction and internal rotation of hip, ankle dorsiflexion, and foot inversion L5 to S1: foot eversion L4 to S2: knee flexion S1–S2: plantar flexion (ankle jerk) S2–S5: bowel/bladder control	S1–S2 (ankle jerk)	Lumbar sensory nerves innervate the upper legs and portions of the lower legs L5: medial aspect of foot S1: lateral aspect of foot S2: posterior aspect of calf/thigh Sacral sensory nerves innervate the lower legs, feet, and perineum	No interference with respiratory function	Bowel and bladder control possibly impaired S2–S4 segments control urinary continence S3–S5 segments control bowel continence (perianal muscles)	Can walk with braces or may use W/C Can be relatively independent

From Hickey JV: The Clinical Practice of Neurological and Neurosurgical Nursing, 5th ed. Philadelphia: Lippincott Williams & Wilkins, 2003, pp 424–425.

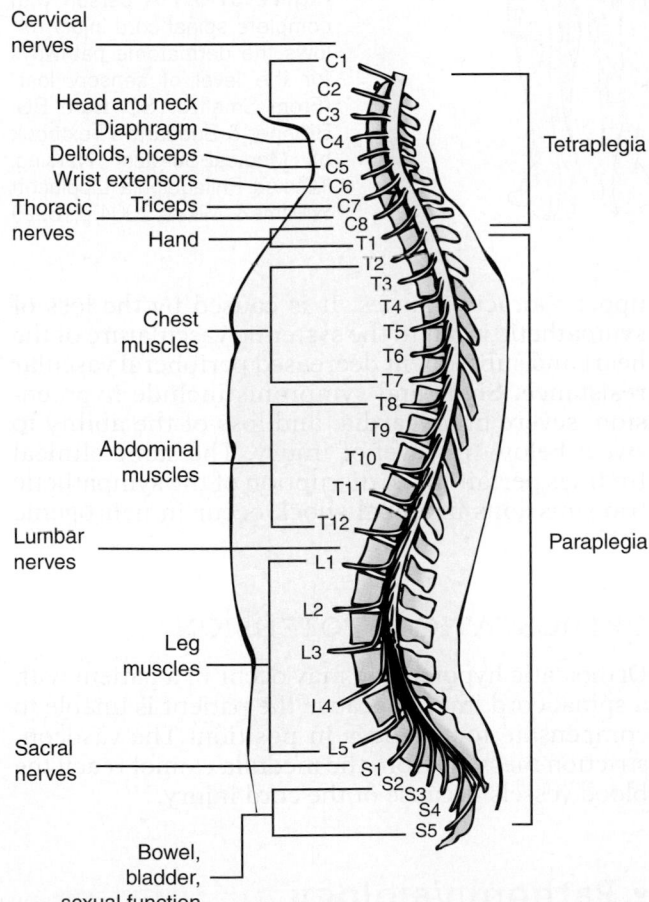

Figure 37-2 • The level of spinal cord injury relates to functional loss. The higher the spinal cord injury, the more motor, sensory, and autonomic functional losses are incurred. (From Hickey JV: Clinical Practice of Neurological and Neurosurgical Nursing, 5th ed. Philadelphia: Lippincott Williams & Wilkins, 2003, p 408.)

cord. The posterior columns are interrupted ipsilaterally (on the same side), but this does not cause a major deficit because some fibers cross instead of running ipsilaterally. Clinically, the patient's limb with the best motor strength has the poorest sensation. Conversely, the limb with the best sensation has the poorest motor strength (see Fig. 37-4B).

ANTERIOR CORD SYNDROME

The area of damage in this syndrome is, as the name suggests, the anterior aspect of the spinal cord. Clinically, the patient usually has complete motor paralysis below the level of injury (corticospinal tracts) and loss of pain, temperature, and touch sensation (spinothalamic tracts), with preservation of light touch, proprioception, and position sense (see Fig. 37-4C).

POSTERIOR CORD SYNDROME

Posterior cord syndrome is usually the result of a hyperextension injury at the cervical level and is not commonly seen. Position sense, light touch, and vibratory sense are lost below the level of the injury.

• Autonomic Nervous System Syndromes

SPINAL SHOCK

Spinal shock is a condition that occurs immediately or within several hours of a spinal cord injury and is caused by the sudden cessation of impulses from the higher brain centers (Fig. 37-5). Charac-

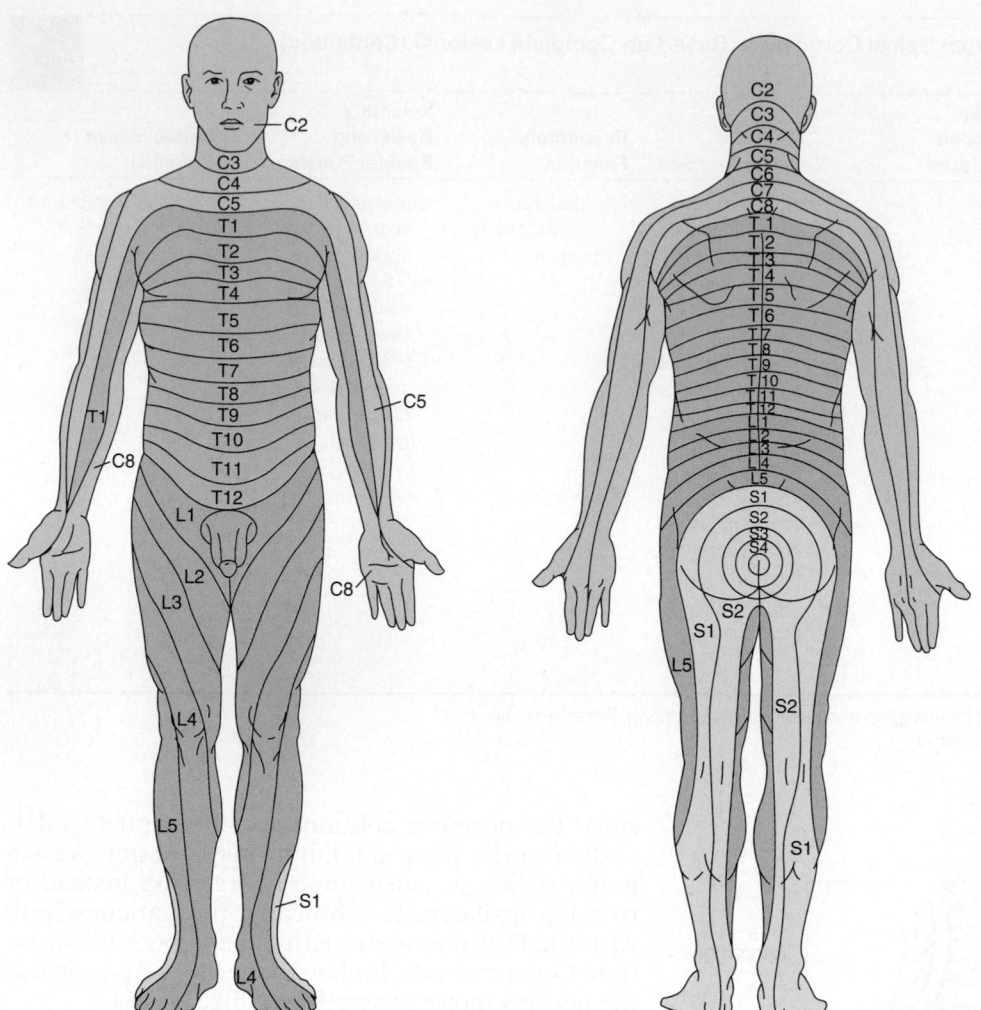

Figure 37-3 • A person with complete spinal cord injury follows the dermatome pathways for the level of sensory loss. (From Smeltzer SC, Bare BG: Brunner & Suddarth's Textbook of Medical-Surgical Nursing, 10th ed. Philadelphia: Lippincott Williams & Wilkins, 2004, p 1829.)

teristics include the loss of motor, sensory, reflex, and autonomic function below the level of the injury, with resultant flaccid paralysis (Box 37-2). Loss of bowel and bladder function also occurs. In addition, the body's ability to control temperature (poikilothermia) is lost, and the patient's temperature tends to equilibrate with that of the external environment. There is no treatment for spinal shock.

If the spinal cord injury produces an incomplete transection, the suppression of function below the level of injury is temporary, lasting a few days to weeks or months. The duration of spinal shock is variable, depending on the severity of the insult and the presence of other complications. The return of perianal reflex activity signals the end of the period of spinal shock. Reflexes associated with the area surrounding the injured cord return last. The skeletal muscles become spastic, and there is increased muscle tone and exaggerated flexor muscle movement.

NEUROGENIC SHOCK

Neurogenic shock, a form of distributive shock, is a condition seen in patients with severe cervical and upper thoracic injuries. It is caused by the loss of sympathetic input to the systemic vasculature of the heart and subsequent decreased peripheral vascular resistance. Signs and symptoms include hypotension, severe bradycardia, and loss of the ability to sweat below the level of injury. The same clinical findings pertaining to disruption of the sympathetic transmissions in spinal shock occur in neurogenic shock.

ORTHOSTATIC HYPOTENSION

Orthostatic hypotension may occur in a patient with a spinal cord injury because the patient is unable to compensate for changes in position. The vasoconstriction message from the medulla cannot reach the blood vessels because of the cord injury.

• Pathophysiology

The spinal cord extends from the base of the brain to approximately the level of the first or second lumbar vertebra. Blood is supplied to the cord by the anterior and posterior spinal arteries. Extending off of

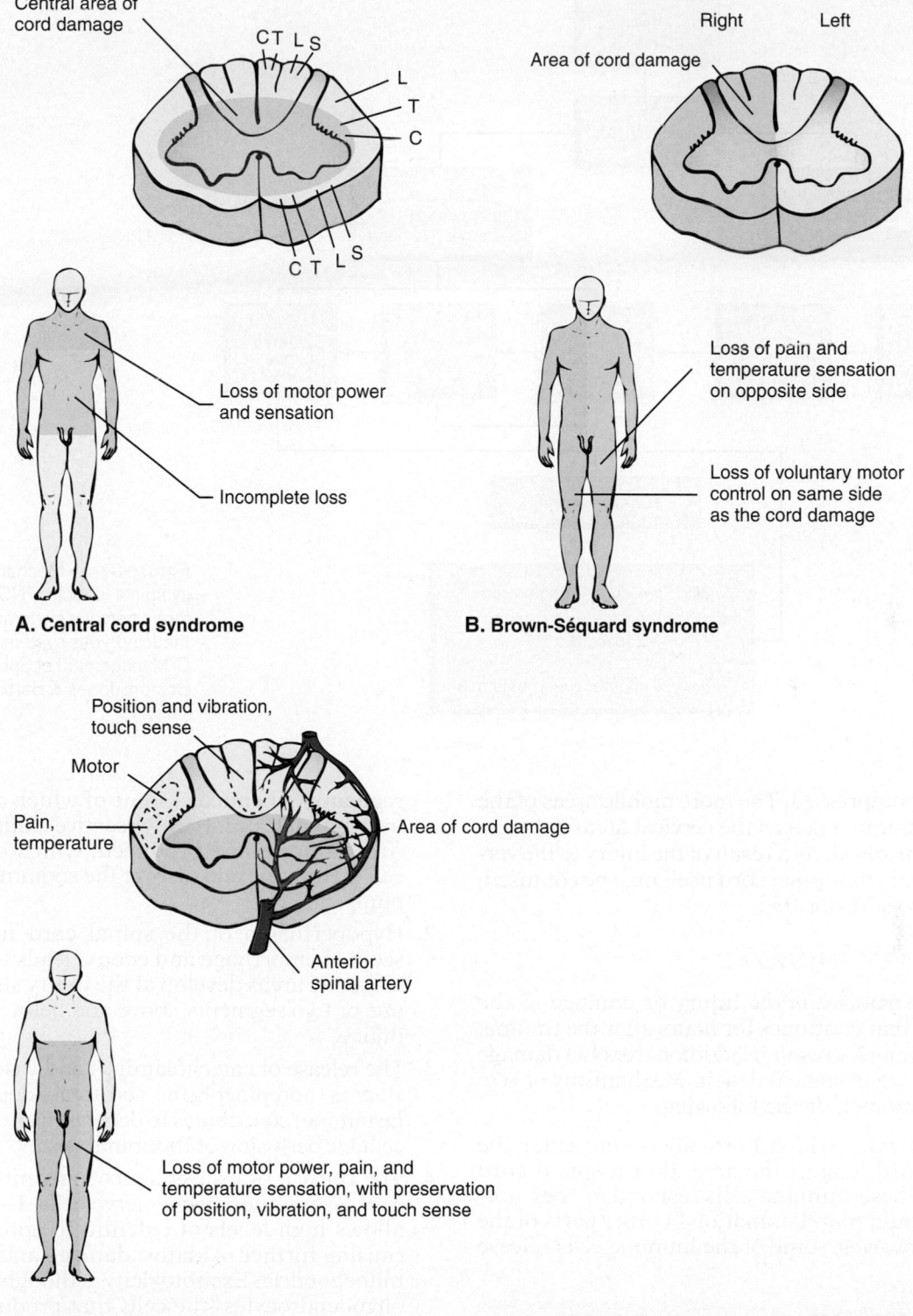

Figure 37-4 • Selected syndromes related to spinal cord injury. C, cervical; L, lumbar; S, sacral; T, thoracic. (From Hickey JV: Clinical Practice of Neurological and Neurosurgical Nursing, 5th ed. Philadelphia: Lippincott Williams & Wilkins, 2003, pp 420–421.)

the spinal cord are the spinal nerve roots. The spinal cord is enclosed in the vertebral canal, which consists of 33 vertebrae: 7 cervical, 12 thoracic, 5 lumbar, 5 sacral (fused), and 4 coccygeal (fused). The vertebrae are held in place by ligaments, muscles, and other supporting structures.

PRIMARY INJURY

Injury to the spinal cord that occurs at impact is referred to as the primary injury. Damage to the spinal cord is most often associated with damage to the vertebral column. The vertebrae may be fractured, dis-

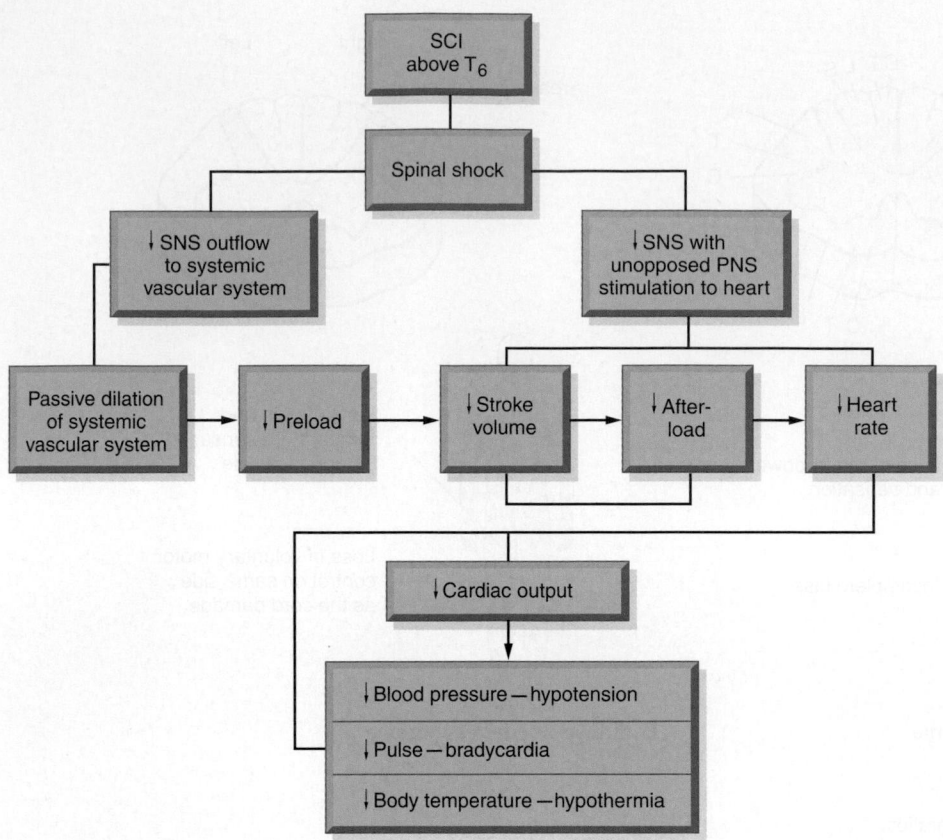

Figure 37-5 • Mechanisms involved in spinal shock. PNS, parasympathetic nervous system; SNS, sympathetic nervous system. (From Zejdlik C: Management of Spinal Cord Injury. Boston: Jones & Bartlett Publishers, 1992.)

located, or compressed. The more mobile areas of the vertebral column (such as the cervical area) are most frequently involved. As a result of the injury to the vertebral column, the spinal cord itself may be contused, compressed, or dislocated.

SECONDARY INJURY

Equally destructive is the injury or damage to the spinal cord that continues for hours after the trauma. Secondary injuries result in additional axonal damage and further neurological deficit. Mechanisms of secondary injury include the following:

1. Immune cells, which normally do not enter the spinal cord, engulf the area after a spinal cord injury. These immune cells respond as they normally would to inflammation in other parts of the body. However, some of the immune cells release

regulatory chemicals, some of which are harmful to the spinal cord. Highly reactive oxidizing agents (free radicals) are produced, which damage the cell membrane and disrupt the sodium–potassium pump.

2. Hypoperfusion of the spinal cord from microscopic hemorrhage and edema leads to ischemia. Ischemic areas develop at the injury site as well as one or two segments above and below the level of injury.

3. The release of catecholamines and vasoactive substances (norepinephrine, serotonin, dopamine, and histamine) contributes to decreased circulation and cellular perfusion of the spinal cord.

4. The release of excess neurotransmitters results in overexcitation of the nerve cells. Excitotoxicity allows high levels of calcium to enter the cells, causing further oxidative damage and damage to mitochondria. Excitotoxicity is thought to damage oligodendrocytes (the cells that produce myelin), leading to demyelinated axons that are unable to conduct impulses.

• Initial Assessment and Management

PREHOSPITAL MANAGEMENT

A spinal cord injury should be suspected at the scene of an accident any time the patient has decreased

---

Box 37-2 • Clinical Manifestations of Spinal Shock

- Flaccid paralysis below the level of injury
- Absence of cutaneous and proprioceptive sensation
- Hypotension and bradycardia
- Absence of reflex activity below the level of injury; may cause urinary retention, bowel paralysis, and ileus
- Loss of temperature control; vasodilation and inability to shiver make it difficult for the patient to conserve heat in a cool environment, and the inability to perspire prevents normal cooling in a hot environment

or absent movement or sensation. An unconscious patient or one with a head injury is treated as though a spinal cord injury has occurred until proved otherwise. Because elapsed time from injury significantly affects prognosis, the patient with a spinal cord injury is transported as safely and rapidly as possible to a specialized trauma center or a hospital with adequate diagnostic and treatment facilities to handle such trauma. A primary survey performed at the scene of an accident includes a rapid assessment of airway, breathing, and circulation (ABCs). Airway patency is assessed, and the cervical spine is immobilized and stabilized. It is important to remember that a cervical collar increases the level of stability but does not provide complete immobilization, especially in the case of complete ligamentous disruption, in which the collar has a minimal immobilization effect on spinal stability.[3]

IN-HOSPITAL MANAGEMENT

After the patient has been admitted to the emergency department, assessment of the patient's airway is a priority. Facial, mandibular, or laryngeal injuries, as well as the presence of broken teeth or a swollen tongue, may be a cause of airway obstruction. Based on assessment findings, the medical staff promptly initiates appropriate ventilation support. Ventilation support may include elective intubation and mechanical ventilation followed by a chest radiograph. Breathing is assessed after an airway is established. Absence of breath sounds or hyperresonance on chest percussion may indicate an open or tension pneumothorax, flail chest, or hemothorax. These injuries are promptly treated to prevent exacerbation of the patient's respiratory status.

In addition, the patient's circulatory status is assessed. Hypotension generally occurs secondary to volume loss from hemorrhage. Fluid resuscitation is accomplished by the use of intravenous fluids, crystalloids, or blood. Early administration of blood enhances oxygenation and may minimize the secondary ischemic injury to the spinal cord, as discussed later.[4] The clinical staff completes a thorough neurological and orthopedic assessment and assesses the patient for additional injuries. They then move the patient off the backboard as soon as possible to minimize the development of pressure ulcers. Finally, the emergency department team stabilizes the patient before transfer to the intensive care unit (ICU) or a specialized trauma center occurs.

The administration of high-dose methylprednisolone in the emergency department remains controversial. The drug reduces swelling and helps minimize secondary injury by reversing the intracellular accumulation of calcium, reducing the risk for cord degeneration and ischemia. However, steroid use has been associated with severe pneumonia and sepsis. The physician determines whether to prescribe methylprednisolone based on assessment of the patient, past medical history, and diagnostic testing.[5]

Physical Examination

Respiratory Assessment

The nurse assesses and records the patient's respiratory rate and arterial oxygen saturation (by pulse oximetry). Clinical manifestations other than those associated with concomitant injuries may include hypoventilation or respiratory failure, particularly with high cervical injuries. Hypoventilation from inadequate innervation of respiratory muscles is a common problem after spinal cord injury. It is important to assess whether the intercostal muscles are functioning, or whether the patient has only diaphragmatic breathing. Spinal cord edema can act like an ascending lesion and may compromise function of the diaphragm. Assessment of tidal volume and vital capacity and auscultation of breath sounds are frequent.

The patient with a spinal cord injury may have additional respiratory compromise because of preexisting pulmonary disease or coexistent chest, laryngeal, tracheal, or esophageal injuries. Major cranial nerves and surrounding arteries and veins may also be injured. Pulmonary collapse or consolidation from retained secretions or aspiration of vomitus may directly affect alveolar ventilation. Pulmonary edema may also result from incorrect management of intravenous fluids. Paralytic ileus and gastric dilation may increase the pressure on the diaphragm and cause further respiratory compromise. Consequently, insertion of a nasogastric tube may be necessary.

Cardiovascular Assessment

The trauma team immediately places the patient on a cardiac monitor, takes vital signs, and completes a cardiovascular assessment. Hypotension and bradycardia may be due to neurogenic shock or hemorrhagic shock. Causes of hemorrhagic shock (manifested by hypotension, tachycardia, and cold, clammy skin) include intrathoracic, intra-abdominal, or retroperitoneal injury, or pelvic or long bone fractures. Examination of the patient determines whether other injuries are present. The rate of intravenous infusion is adjusted based on the patient's presenting signs and symptoms and past medical history. Insertion of an indwelling Foley catheter allows for strict monitoring of the patient's intake and output. Chest injury often accompanies thoracic spinal cord trauma. It is important to examine the chest, head, and abdomen for evidence of concomitant injuries.

Neurological Assessment

Frequent assessment of neurological status determines the extent of the spinal cord injury and monitors for changes in level of consciousness that may occur secondary to traumatic brain injury. The trauma team uses the Glasgow Coma Scale (GCS) or other standardized tools to determine patient's level of consciousness. Most spinal cord injury centers use a specialized flow sheet, such as the Standard Neurological Classification of Spinal Cord Injury flow sheet, to assess and document the patient's level of functioning (Fig. 37-6). Cranial nerve testing is necessary, particularly if the cause of the injury was

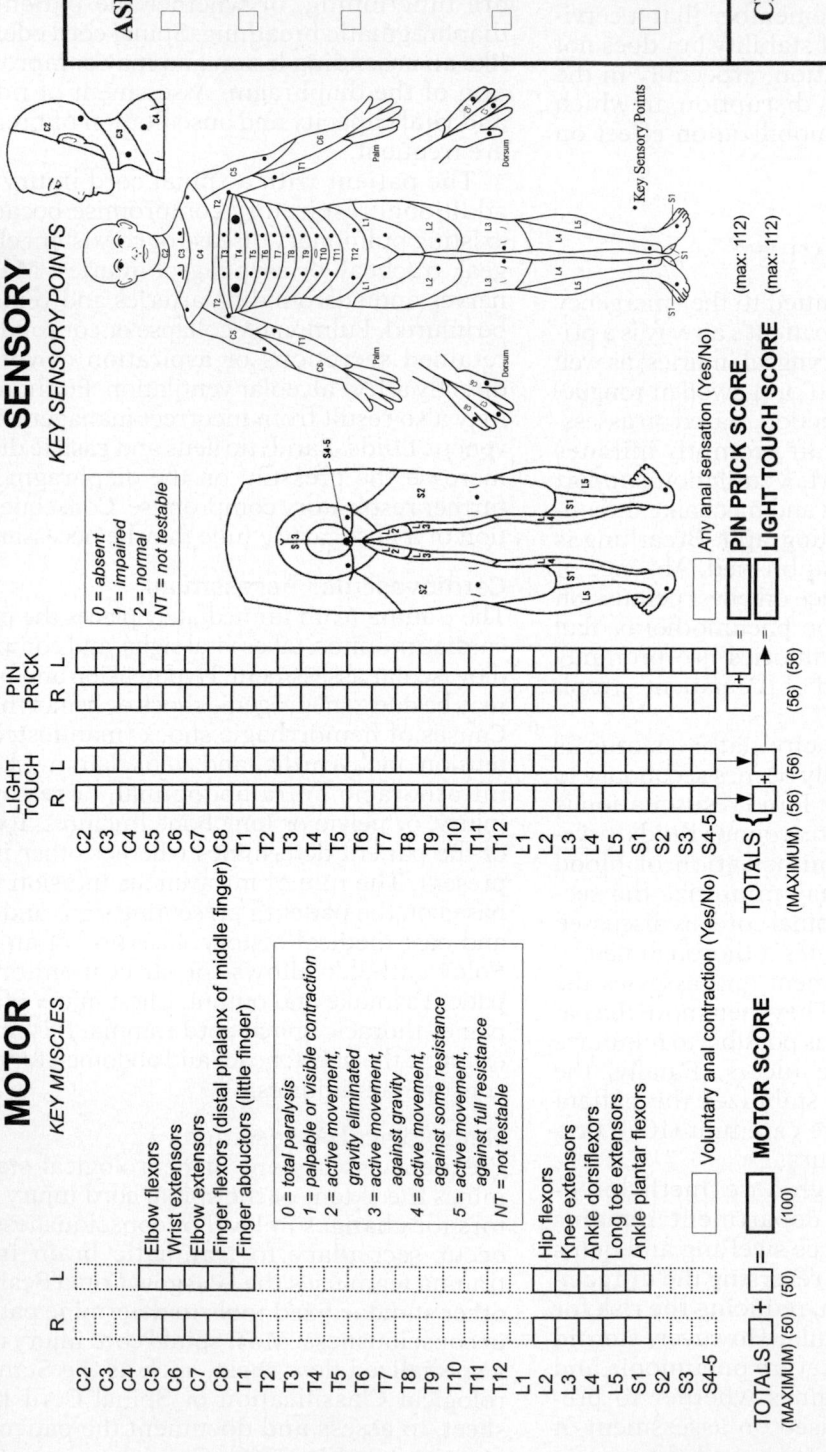

Figure 37-6 • This Standard Neurological Classification of Spinal Cord Injury flow sheet defines key motor and sensory impairments and clinical syndromes and also includes a functional assessment scale. Motor movement of the major muscle groups is scored on a scale of 0 to 5, with 0 indicating total paralysis and 5 indicating active movement against full resistance or normal movement. Sensation testing is done starting at the area of absent or decreased sensation and proceeding to the area of normal sensation, following the sensory distribution of the skin dermatomes. Each spinal cord segment is tested for sensation and is scored as 0 for absent, 1 for impaired, or 2 for normal. (Courtesy of the American Spinal Injury Association.)

penetrating trauma or involved a head injury. For a further discussion of the care of patients with a head injury, see Chapter 36.

During the early assessment of the patient, a digital rectal examination is important to determine whether the injury is incomplete or complete. The lesion is incomplete if the patient can feel the palpating finger or can contract the perianal muscles around the finger voluntarily. Sensation may be present in the absence of voluntary motor activity. Sensation seldom is absent when voluntary perianal muscle contraction is present. In either case, the prognosis for further motor and sensory return is good. Preservation of sacral function might be the only finding that indicates an incomplete lesion, and significant neurological recovery may occur in the patient with an incomplete cord injury. Rectal tone by itself, without the presence of voluntary perianal muscle contraction or rectal sensation, is not evidence of an incomplete cord injury.

Bowel and Bladder Assessment

Incontinence of urine and possibly feces may have occurred at the scene of the accident. To prevent the bladder from becoming distended secondary to an atonic bladder, insertion of an indwelling urinary catheter is necessary. There may be an imbalance between parasympathetic and sympathetic innervation to the bowel and therefore a loss of voluntary control.

Diagnostic Studies

When the patient is stabilized, it is possible to perform definitive diagnostic tests safely. The diagnostic workup consists of radiographs of the spine, chest, and other structures as clinically indicated. A computed tomography (CT) scan provides additional information concerning bony structures and fractures. Soft tissue injury is more easily diagnosed with magnetic resonance imaging (MRI). Typical laboratory tests ordered include a complete blood count (CBC), electrolytes, glucose, blood urea nitrogen (BUN), creatinine, blood type and crossmatch, arterial blood gases (ABGs), and coagulation studies.

Although rare, the incidence of missed spinal fractures varies between 0.001% and 4.6%.[6] Consequences of a missed injury include chronic pain, deformity, and a delayed injury to the spinal cord or adjacent nerve root. The factors most associated with a missed injury are high-energy trauma, older age, closed head injury, and insufficient imaging.[6] Ideally, flexion extension views or an MRI is necessary in patients with altered mental status and in those who complain of pain, even when plain radiographs and CT are negative.

When the patient is in the critical care or acute care environment, a physician often orders somatosensory evoked potential (see Chapter 33). This test measures the ability of the spinal cord to carry messages along the neural pathways to the higher centers in the brain, and it is used as a tool to help determine treatment and patient outcome. In this test, a peripheral nerve in the arm or leg below the level of injury is stimulated, and the neurological response (evoked potential) is recorded. If the injury is complete, there is no response. In incomplete injuries, a varying response occurs.

• Ongoing Assessment and Management

Box 37-3 presents examples of nursing diagnoses and collaborative problems for the patient with a spinal cord injury. Based on the assessment data, the interdisciplinary team develops an individual treat-

---

Box 37-3 | **Examples of Nursing Diagnoses and Collaborative Problems for the Patient With Spinal Cord Injury**

Respiratory
- Impaired Gas Exchange
- Ineffective Airway Clearance
- Ineffective Breathing Pattern

Cardiovascular
- Cardiac Output, Decreased

Neurological
- Acute Pain
- Autonomic Dysreflexia, Risk for
- Body Temperature, Risk for Imbalanced
- Impaired Comfort
- Impaired Mobility, Wheelchair
- Tissue Perfusion, Ineffective

Gastrointestinal/Genitourinary
- Bladder Incontinence
- Bowel Incontinence
- Constipation

Psychosocial
- Anxiety
- Body Image Disturbance, Risk for
- Fear
- Impaired Adjustment, Risk for
- Ineffective Coping: Individual and Family

Activities of Daily Living
- Activity Intolerance, Risk for
- Nutrition, Imbalanced: Less Than Body Requirements
- Impaired Skin Integrity, Risk for Complications
- Infection, Risk for
- Injury, Risk for
- Self Care Deficit, Bathing/Hygiene
- Self Care Deficit, Dressing/Grooming
- Self Care Deficit, Feeding
- Self Care Deficit, Toileting
- Sexual Dysfunction, Ineffective Sexuality Pattern

Collaborative Problems
- Potential for atelectasis, pneumonia
- Potential for deep vein thrombosis
- Potential for hypoxemia
- Potential for sepsis

ment plan (Box 37-4). Management of the patient is based on the type and severity of injury. Collaboration of all health care disciplines is necessary to enable the patient to achieve his or her fullest potential after injury. The goals of ongoing management are to realign or stabilize the spine to prevent further neurological deterioration, to prevent complications, and to initiate prompt interventions to treat any complications that do occur.

REALIGNMENT AND STABILIZATION OF THE SPINE

The trauma team carefully evaluates the patient to determine the most effective treatment based on the type and cause of injury. The surgeon must balance the risks of surgery against the possible benefits associated with eventual patient outcome. For example, adolescents with low-velocity gunshot injuries are usually managed medically because of the increased risk for complications.[7] These complications include spinal fluid fistulas, infections, and wound dehiscence. If the bullet fragments remain in place, serum lead levels monitoring occurs, and surgery is necessary if the lead level increases. Surgical decompression is indicated in patients with cauda equine injuries.

Medical Management

Regardless of the treatment approach, medical management of the patient is an important cornerstone of initial treatment.[8]

Closed reduction of a cervical fracture often involves skeletal traction. Cervical traction is used when the fracture is unstable or if subluxation has occurred. Gardner-Wells, Vinke, or Crutchfield tongs are common forms of cervical traction; however, because of the complications that accompany prolonged immobility, long-term traction with tongs is seldom used, especially since the advent of the halo vest (Fig. 37-7). Boxes 37-5 and 37-6 present collaborative care guides for the patient in cervical traction and for the patient in a halo vest, respectively.

A halo device, Miami J, or Aspen collar is used for cervical immobilization. Immobilization devices for cervical and thoracic injuries may involve the use of a metal and plastic (Minerva) brace. Thoracolumbar-sacral orthosis may be accomplished using a fiberglass and plastic canvas corset or Jewett brace. Each of these devices is fitted to the patient to provide support and stabilization of the spine. Surgical stabilization may also be necessary. Bed rest is the recommended treatment for sacral and coccygeal injuries.

Surgical Management

The goal of surgical management is to stabilize and support the spine. Emergency surgery may be necessary to remove bone fragments, a hematoma, or a penetrating object such as a bullet. If the patient's motor status continues to decline, a surgeon may perform a laminectomy to allow for swelling of the spinal cord secondary to edema. Rod placement, laminec-

tomy and fusion, and anterior fusion are types of surgical stabilization. Bone for fusion usually comes from the iliac crest, tibia, or ribs. A tissue bank may also be a source of bone grafts; strict standards for sterilization are necessary to ensure viability of the allograft tissue.

After surgery, the patient receives routine postoperative care. The nurse monitors the patient's neurological status at least every hour for the first 24 hours and then every 4 hours. He or she notifies the surgeon immediately if deterioration in neurological status occurs.

A major complication of surgery is postoperative infection. This is especially true in older patients and in those with preexisting comorbidities who have open wounds, injuries to the thoracolumbar spine, or complete injuries.[9] The causative organisms are typically gram-positive organisms, although other concurrent organisms may include *Enterococcus faecalis*, *Enterobacter cloacae*, *Pseudomonas* species, *Klebsiella* species, and *Escherichia coli*.

PREVENTION OF RESPIRATORY PROBLEMS

Patients with a spinal cord injury, especially injuries above T6, are at risk for respiratory problems such as ineffective airway clearance, ineffective breathing patterns, and impaired gas exchange. The degree of respiratory compromise is determined primarily by the level of the injury, although not entirely. For example, a 28-year-old patient with C5 tetraplegia with no lung disease may have better ventilation than a 65-year-old patient with C8 tetraplegia with a long history of smoking and chronic obstructive pulmonary disease.

Normally, ventilation is accomplished through a complex interaction between muscles of the chest, the abdominal wall, and the diaphragm. A spinal cord injury results in paralysis of the inspiratory and expiratory muscles. Dysfunction of the intercostal and accessory muscles decreases ventilation and predisposes the patient to atelectasis. Dysfunction of the abdominal muscles and expiratory intercostal muscles diminishes the patient's ability to generate a cough to clear secretions. The intercostal muscles also normally provide support to the lateral chest wall. When the intercostals are impaired, this part of the chest wall collapses during inspiration as the abdomen expands. This breathing pattern is easily discernible and results in ineffective ventilation.

Respiratory complications are the leading cause of death in the acute and chronic phases of spinal cord injury, especially among tetraplegic patients. The nurse and respiratory therapist auscultate breath sounds and measure respiratory parameters (e.g., tidal volume and vital capacity) frequently. Respiratory failure is anticipated if the patient's vital capacity is less than 15 to 20 mL/kg and the respiratory rate is greater than 30 breaths/minute. Other interventions include measuring the patient's pulse oximetry; if the value is less than 85 mm Hg or if the arterial carbon dioxide tension ($PaCO_2$) is above 45 mm Hg, intubation may

Box 37-4 • COLLABORATIVE CARE GUIDE for the Patient With Spinal Cord Injury

OUTCOMES	INTERVENTIONS

Oxygenation/Ventilation
Arterial blood gas values will be within normal limits.
No evidence of atelectasis is demonstrated.
	• Assess need for mechanical ventilation.
	• Provide routine pulmonary toilet, including:
	  Airway suctioning
	  Chest percussion, couth and deep breathing
	  Incentive spirometer, nebulizer treatment
	• Turn frequently.
	• Mobilize out of bed to chair.
	• Apply abdominal binder when out of bed.
	• Consult pulmonologist as needed.
	• Obtain pulmonary function tests.

Circulation/Perfusion There will be no evidence of neurogenic (spinal) shock (T10 injuries and higher). Blood pressure will be adequate to maintain vital organ function. There will be no development of deep venous thrombosis (DVT) or pulmonary embolism. There will be no evidence of orthostatic hypotension.	• Monitor for bradycardia, vasodilation, and hypotension. • Assess for arrhythmias. • Prepare to administer intravascular volume, vasopressors, and positive chronotropic agents. • Begin DVT prophylaxis on admission (e.g., external compression device, low-dose heparin). • Measure calf and thigh circumference daily and at same location; report increase. • Apply Ace wraps to lower extremities before mobilizing out of bed. • Monitor for orthostatic hypotension when raising head of bed and getting out of bed. • Consult cardiology as needed.
Neurological There will be no evidence of deterioration in neurological status.	• Perform neurological check and spinal cord function checks every 2–4 h. • Monitor for deterioration in neurological status and report to the physician or nurse practitioner. • Monitor for and prevent complications. • Provide patient and family education concerning injury, effects of injury, and rehabilitation.
Fluids/Electrolytes Serum electrolytes will be within normal limits. Fluid balance will be maintained as evidenced by stable weight, absence of edema, normal skin turgor.	• Monitor laboratory studies as indicated by patient condition. • Assess for dehydration. • Administer mineral/electrolyte replacement as ordered. • Monitor gastrointestinal and insensible fluid loss. • Make accurate daily fluid intake and output measurements. • Weigh weekly. • Monitor results of laboratory studies, particularly albumin and electrolyte levels.
Mobility/Safety Joint range of motion will be maintained and contractures prevented. Skin integrity will be maintained under or around stabilization devices (e.g., cervical collar, Yale brace, halo vest).	• Position in correct alignment. • Consult with wound care specialist to determine correct type of bed. • Begin range-of-motion exercises early after admission. • Use high-top tennis shoes, moon boots, extremity splints routinely. • Consult with physical and occupational therapists. • Maintain splint, brace, and adaptive device schedule; check for pressure ulcers every 4 h or more often if indicated. • Monitor skin or pin sites of stabilization devices. • Use meticulous skin care/pin care under or around stabilization devices.

(continued)

Box 37-4 • COLLABORATIVE CARE GUIDE for the Patient With Spinal Cord Injury (Continued)

OUTCOMES	INTERVENTIONS
Skin Integrity Skin will remain intact.	• Consult with wound care specialist to determine correct type of bed. • Reposition at least every 2 h while in bed. • Position to prevent pressure on bony prominences. • Use upright, straight-backed chair when out of bed (not a reclining chair). Use felt pad on chair seat. • Reposition/shift weight every hour when sitting upright. • Use Braden scale to monitor risk for skin breakdown.
Nutrition Protein, carbohydrate, fat, and calorie intake will meet minimal daily requirements.	• Consult dietitian. • Encourage fluids, high-fiber diet. • Monitor fluid intake and output, calorie count. • Administer parenteral and enteral nutrition as appropriate. • Assist with feeding/feed as needed.
Comfort/Pain Pain will be less than "4" on visual analog scale.	• Assess and differentiate pain from anxiety or stress response. • Administer appropriate analgesic or sedative to relieve pain and monitor patient response. • Use nonpharmacological pain relief techniques (e.g, distraction, music, relaxation therapies).

Psychosocial
Patient will adapt to loss of motor and sensory function.
 	
Therapeutic strategies will be used to cope with anxiety and chronic pain syndrome.
 	
Integration will be made into prior social role.
	• Provide emotional support by:
	  Encouraging ventilation of sadness, fears, and the like.
	  Arranging for social services, clergy, neuropsychologist, or support groups to see patient.
	• Provide information and counseling regarding:
	  Personal resources
	  Nonpharmacological pain management techniques
	  Stress management strategies
	  Appropriate use of prescribed pharmacological agents
	• Provide patient/family counseling regarding:
	  Stages of grief
	  Sexual function and management techniques
	  Social services and community resources

Teaching/Discharge Planning
Patient will adapt to loss of bowel/bladder control.
Patient will participate in bowel and bladder program.
 	
Complications of immobility will be prevented.
 	
Patient will be placed in appropriate postacute setting.
	• Teach patient/family:
	  Bowel program and training
	  Dietary habits to maintain bowel function
	  Bladder training/intermittent catheterization
	  Prevention of, and signs/symptoms of autonomic dysreflexia
	• Teach patient/family:
	  Positioning to prevent skin breakdown
	  Physical therapy exercises
	  Pulmonary toilet
	• Consult rehabilitation/discharge planner/social services early after admission to initiate placement arrangements.

be required. Other interventions include oxygen per nasal canula and ensuring that the patient is well hydrated.

Kinetic therapy involves placing the patient on a special bed that rotates a minimum of 40 degrees on a continuous basis. This stabilizes the spine and the continuous slow rotation prevents pulmonary complications.

The nurse encourages the patient to take deep breaths and to use an incentive spirometer every 2 hours, or more frequently if tolerated. For example, every time there is a television or radio commercial,

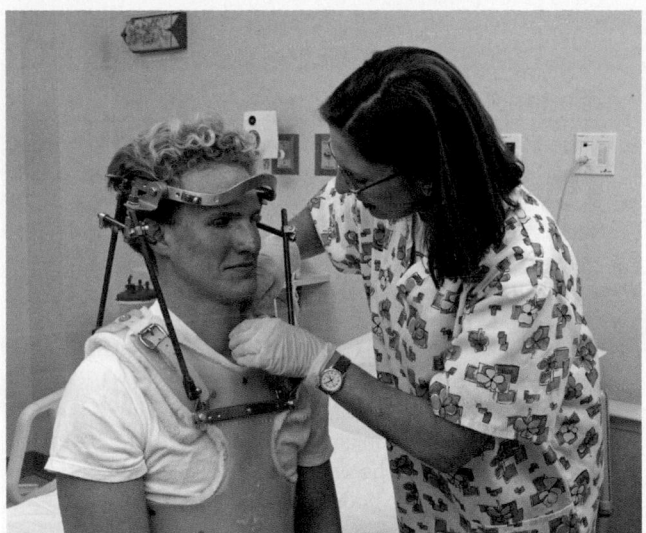

Figure 37-7 • A lightweight fleece-lined vest with a halo may be used to stabilize the cervical vertebrae. Note that the vest comes in various sizes and does not need to be removed for magnetic resonance imaging studies. (Courtesy of Bremer Medical, Inc., Dawin Road, Jacksonville, FL 32207).

the patient can take four to five deep breaths or use the incentive spirometer independently or with the assistance of the nurse or a family member. Assisting the patient with the quad coughing technique may help clear airways more effectively despite weakness or loss of the respiratory muscles that produce the automatic cough reflex. The quad coughing technique involves compressing the sides of the patient's chest (if patient is on his or her side or abdomen) or the diaphragm (if the patient is supine) during exhalation. This technique often is most helpful after postural drainage or vibration of the chest.

Suctioning may be necessary if the patient's airway cannot be cleared effectively with other techniques. Nurses should remember that suctioning (or nasogastric tube insertion) might trigger an abnormal vasovagal response, resulting in bradycardia.

When turning a patient to the prone position on a Stryker frame, the nurse needs to remain at the bedside for the first few turns to evaluate the patient's respiratory tolerance of the turn. Patients with high-level tetraplegia can experience respiratory arrest in the prone position because movement of the diaphragm

---

Box 37-5 • COLLABORATIVE CARE GUIDE for the Patient in Cervical Traction

OUTCOMES	INTERVENTIONS
Equipment Management The orthopedic frame will remain intact. Tongs will not slip. Traction weights will hang freely. There will not be any extension of cord injury secondary to slippage of the traction apparatus.	• Check the orthopedic frame and traction daily to ensure that nuts and bolts are secure. • Check tongs daily to be sure that they are secure. • Be sure that traction weights are hanging freely and not resting on the floor or frame. (Releasing the traction is dangerous because cord injury could be extended.)
Oxygenation/Ventilation Airway patency will be maintained. The patient will not aspirate. The patient will not develop a respiratory infection.	• Have suction available to maintain a patent airway. • Provide respiratory care. • Provide for deep breathing, assistive coughing, and incentive spirometer exercises every 1 to 2 h.
Circulation/Perfusion Air boots and thigh-high elastic hose (TEDs) will be worn at all times. Vital signs will be maintained within normal limits. The patient will be observed for deep venous thrombosis (DVT) and pulmonary emboli.	• Maintain TEDs and sequential compression boots. • If the patient is receiving heparin, observe for signs and symptoms of bleeding. • Monitor for DVT and pulmonary emboli. (May be receiving minidoses of subcutaneous heparin every 12 h, if not contraindicated.)
Mobility/Safety The patient will be free from pain. Contractures will not develop. Strategies will be used to manage spasticity if it occurs.	• Provide comfort measures. • Provide range-of-motion exercises four times per day. • Position the patient in proper body alignment. • Reposition the patient frequently. • Stretch the patient's heel cord with exercises.
Skin Integrity The pin site will remain free of infection. Skin integrity will be maintained. The vertebral column will be maintained in a neutral position and in proper alignment.	• Inspect tong sites, and clean and dress daily as ordered (may be referred to as "pin care"). • Turn the patient every 2 h from side to back to other side using a triple log-roll technique as described below if a patient is on a regular hospital bed:

(continued)

Box 37-5 • COLLABORATIVE CARE GUIDE for the Patient in Cervical Traction (Continued)

OUTCOMES	INTERVENTIONS
	Nurse #1 stands behind the head of the bed and places hands firmly on the patient's head and neck, maintaining them in a neutral position; the head and neck are turned as a unit.
	Nurse #2 stands at the patient's side and moves the patient's shoulders.
	Nurse #3 stands at the patient's side and moves the patient's hips and legs.
	Plan ahead, identifying desired position and pillow placement *before* moving the patient. When all three nurses are ready, turn the patient as a log on the count of three. Leave the patient positioned in the middle of the bed (if not, he or she will be uncomfortable); use pillows to support the patient's body in alignment.
	Nurse #1 should hold the head and neck until the patient is supported adequately (if traction slips, manual traction can be supplied by Nurse #1).
Nutrition	
A diet high in protein and carbohydrates, which includes a fluid intake of up to 3,000 mL, will be provided.	• Encourage an adequate diet.
Aspiration will be prevented.	• Ask the dietitian to see the patient.
	• Provide for adequate fluid intake up to 3,000 mL daily.
	• Encourage the patient to take small portions of food into the mouth and chew well to prevent aspiration.
	• Keep suction equipment handy.
Elimination	
Pattern of bowel evacuation every 1 to 2 days will be established.	• Institute a bowel retraining program.
Intake will be 3,000 mL unless contraindicated.	• Auscultate the abdomen for bowel sounds.
Postvoid residuals will be less than 100 mL.	• Record the frequency and consistency of stool.
Strict aseptic technique will be used for catheter protocols.	• Monitor intake and output.
	• Force fluids.
	• If an intermittent catheterization protocol is initiated, use aseptic technique.
	• If the patient is voiding on his or her own, monitor postvoid residuals.
Psychosocial	
The patient's mental health will be supported.	• Provide for social interaction and diversion based on the patient's functional level.
Social interaction and diversion will be provided based on the patient's ability to participate.	• Reinforce a positive self-image.
A positive body image will be supported.	• Allow the patient to participate in decision making as much as possible.
Necessary information will be provided.	• Provide for patient teaching.
Sexual function and spinal cord injury are discussed with the patient when he or she is ready.	• Provide information about sexual function.

is compromised. Bradycardia in the prone position also is common.

RESTORATION OF HEMODYNAMIC STABILITY

The management of arterial oxygenation and blood pressure support is critical in optimizing the potential for neurological recovery. Continuous hemodynamic monitoring is essential to measure cardiac output and systemic perfusion. Insertion of a pulmonary artery catheter and central venous line may be necessary if this was not done in the emergency department. It is important to maintain mean arterial pressure between 85 and 90 mm Hg for the first week after injury. The systolic blood pressure should be above 90 mm Hg.[10] The patient is at risk for cardiovascular compromise because of disruption in the autonomic nervous system. Bradycardia, hypotension, and dysrhythmias may occur. Hypotension and tachycardia may indicate hemorrhage from intra-abdominal bleeding or bleeding around fracture sites. Sequential compression devices, antiembolism stockings, or an abdominal binder may be used to promote venous return.

Left ventricular dysfunction may occur secondary to release of β-endorphins. Cardiac enzymes should

Box 37-6 • COLLABORATIVE CARE GUIDE for the Patient in a Halo Vest

OUTCOMES	INTERVENTIONS
Equipment Management The patient will be comfortable and without signs of skin irritation. Proper body alignment will be maintained.	• Check the pins on the halo ring to be sure they are secure and tight. • Check the edges of the fiberglass vest for comfort and fit by inserting the small finger or index finger between the vest and the patient's skin. If the vest is too tight, skin breakdown, edema, and possible nerve injury can occur. • The vest should be supported while the patient is in bed. • Place a rubber cork over the tips of the halo device to diminish magnification of sound if the pin is bumped.
Oxygenation/Ventilation The patient will not develop a respiratory infection.	• Provide for deep-breathing exercises at least 4 times daily.
Circulation/Perfusion Risk for thrombus or embolus formation will be decreased.	• Apply thigh-high elastic hose to the legs to improve blood return to the heart. • Observe the legs for development of thrombophlebitis or deep venous thrombosis.
Mobility/Safety The patient will maintain muscle tone. The patient will ambulate in a safe manner to the best of his or her ability.	• If the patient's neurological function is intact, he or she will be able to ambulate in the halo vest. • Start to assess the patient's tolerance of the upright position by having him or her sit on the edge of the bed ("dangle"). Check vital signs. (Orthostatic hypotension may be a problem to overcome in the early stages.) • Teach the patient to compensate for lost head and neck movement by making increased use of eye movement to scan the area. • Accompany patients when ambulating because they are more accident prone owing to a displaced center of gravity, a tendency for loss of balance, and decreased peripheral vision. • Consider the patient's use of a walker for ambulation as a means of support and greater safety.
Skin Integrity The patient will maintain skin integrity. The patient will maintain proper body alignment without injuries. Early signs of skin irritation or breakdown will be detected.	• Inspect and cleanse the pin site once or twice daily, as prescribed, to prevent infection. • Turn the patient in bed every 2 h by means of the triple log-roll technique to prevent the development of hypostatic pneumonia, atelectasis, and skin breakdown. • Provide sponge pads to prevent pressure on prominent body areas, such as the forehead and shoulder, while the patient is in bed. • Inspect under the vest, and keep all areas of skin dry.
Elimination Pattern of bowel elimination every 1 to 2 days will be established. Intake will be 3,000 mL unless contraindicated; postvoid residuals will be less than 100 mL.	• Institute a bowel retraining program. • Monitor intake and output.
Comfort/Pain Control The patient will be comfortable, with pain controlled.	• Administer mild analgesics to control headache and discomfort, which are common, around the pin site. • Provide a soft diet, because many patients have jaw pain if they attempt to chew.

(continued)

Box 37-6 • COLLABORATIVE CARE GUIDE for the Patient in a Halo Vest (Continued)

OUTCOMES	INTERVENTIONS
Psychosocial The patient's emotional well-being will be supported.	• Help the patient adjust to the distorted body image that the halo device can create. • Encourage self-care as much as possible.
Teaching/Discharge Planning The patient will be provided the necessary information to ensure competent home care. The patient will use equipment in a safe manner.	• If the patient is to go home with the halo vest, begin a patient and family teaching plan using a booklet or other printed material. Review any written material prepared by the manufacturer for accuracy before giving it to the patient or family.

be obtained if there are electrocardiographic (ECG) changes. Dysrhythmias and heart block may occur. It is necessary to address adequate tissue perfusion to the spinal cord and other vital organs, such as the kidneys. Careful intravenous fluid replacement provides hydration without fluid overload. Vasopressors may not be necessary to maintain blood pressure during spinal shock, but when the blood pressure is not high enough to sustain vital organ perfusion, usually low-dose dopamine is useful. Bradycardia also may not need treatment, but if necessary, atropine may be used to speed up the heart rate. A transcutaneous or transvenous pacemaker may be essential if the patient remains bradycardic despite atropine.

NEUROLOGICAL MANAGEMENT

While in the ICU, the patient requires neurological assessment every hour until stable, then every 4 hours. The patient's motor and sensory states warrant particular attention. If there is any deterioration in the patient's condition, the frequency of assessment increases, and the nurse notifies the physician or nurse practitioner.

Depending on the patient's motor function, an adapted nurse call system may be necessary. Useful devices include low-pressure, voice-controlled, and sip-and-puff straw-like call systems. Other communication systems can be developed in conjunction with the speech language pathologist for the patient on a mechanical ventilator.

PAIN MANAGEMENT

It is not unusual for the patient to complain of pain, frequently severe pain. The source of the pain may be neuropathic, musculoskeletal, central, or visceral. Abnormal sensation may occur at the level of the lesion in injuries causing diverse nerve root damage, such as occurs with gunshot or knife wounds. Pain resulting from either the spinal cord injury, surgery, or both is treated aggressively following institutional protocol and within the pain management standards of the institution.

MEDICATION ADMINISTRATION

Medications used in the treatment of the patient with spinal cord injury are listed in Table 37-2. Nurses administering medications to patients with spinal cord injuries must take into account several special considerations. Subcutaneous and intramuscular injections are not absorbed well because of the lack of muscle tone. Sterile abscesses may result, causing autonomic dysreflexia or an increase in spasms. Injection sites are the deltoid area, the anterior thigh, and the abdominal area. Rotation of injection sites is necessary, and the volume injected should not exceed 1 mL at any one site.

Nurses often start peripheral intravenous lines, but the intravenous site of choice is the subclavian vein. In this area of high blood flow, there is less chance of thrombosis secondary to vasomotor paralysis, especially during spinal shock. For this reason, the veins of the lower extremities should never be used for intravenous administration.

THERMOREGULATION

Ineffective thermoregulation is a common problem seen in patients with spinal cord injuries above the thoracolumbar area. Interruption of the sympathetic nervous system prevents the thalamic thermoregulatory mechanisms. As a result, the patient fails to sweat to get rid of body heat, and there is an absence of vasoconstriction, resulting in an inability to shiver to increase body heat. The degree of thermal control and dysfunction is directly proportional to the extent of body area with loss of thermal regulation. Hence, a tetraplegic patient has more difficulty with thermoregulation than a paraplegic patient.

Hypothermia is usually managed by using warmed blankets. The room temperature is adjusted to maintain patient comfort. Electric heating blankets or hot water bottles may present a danger for body parts with no sensation. An attempt is made to stabilize the patient's temperature above 96.5°F (35.8°C). Ideally, the patient is placed in a private room so that the room temperature does not adversely affect the other patient in the room. Over the long term, thermal con-

Table 37-2 • Drugs Used in the Treatment of the Patient With a Spinal Cord Injury

Drug	Description	Administration*
Drugs to Minimize Injury		
Methylprednisolone	Synthetic adrenal corticosteroid used as an anti-inflammatory agent	Loading dose: 30 mg/kg IV over 15 min Pause for 45 min; infuse normal saline or other IV fluid Maintenance dose: 5.4 mg/kg/h IV for 23 h if loading dose given within 3 h of injury 5.4 mg/kg/h IV for 47 h if loading dose given within 3–8 h of injury Loading dose must be given within 8 h of injury. Maintenance dose must begin within 1 h of loading dose.
Tirilazad	Used as an anti-inflammatory agent; inhibits lipid peroxidation without glucocorticoid activity; associated with a lower incidence of sepsis and pneumonia (compared with methylprednisolone)	Dosage: 25 mg/kg bolus infusion every 6 h for 48 h Limit use to those patients who received an initial bolus of methylprednisolone 3–8 h after injury
Drugs for Cardiovascular Stabilization		
Atropine	Anticholinergic used to treat symptomatic bradycardia	Dosage: 0.4–1.0 mg IV slowly; maximum dose 2 mg
Dobutamine (Dobutrex)	β-Adrenergic agent that enhances myocardial contractility, stroke volume, and cardiac output; improves perfusion to the spinal cord	Dosage: 2.5–10 µg/kg/min up to maximum dosage of 40 µg/kg/min; usually given for a total of 72 h if needed
Dopamine (Intropin)	α- and β-Adrenergic agent used to treat hypotension related to neurogenic shock	Dosage: 3–5 µg/kg/min; increase gradually at 10- to 30-min intervals up to 20–50 µg/kg/min until optimum blood pressure achieved Start the older adult on lower doses; use with caution if the patient is on a monoamine oxidase inhibitor
Drugs for Paralytic Ileus and Stress Ulcers		
Proton pump inhibitors (lansoprazole, omeprazole, pantoprazole)	Suppress gastric acid secretion; used to prevent or treat gastric ulcers	Dosage: dependent on medication prescribed
Histamine blockers (cimetidine, famotidine, nizantine, ranitidine hydrochloride)	Inhibit histamine action at H_2 receptor sites; used to treat and prevent ulcers and gastric reflux	Dosage: dependent on medication prescribed
Drugs for Autonomic Hyperreflexia		
Nitroglycerin	Organic nitrate used if systolic blood pressure above 140 mm Hg	Dosage: 1 inch of nitroglycerin paste placed above the level of injury
Nifedipine (Procardia)	Calcium channel blocker used to decrease systemic vascular resistance and blood pressure	Dosage: 10–20 mg PO every 20–30 min if necessary
Hydralazine, trimethaphan, diazoxide	Antihypertensive agents	Dosage: dependent on medication prescribed Trimethaphan: dilute per hospital protocol (usually 500 mg in 500 mL D5W); usual dose 0.5–1 mg/min Hydralazine: 25 mg PO 4 times per day or 10–20 mg IV every 4–6 h Diazoxide: 1–3 mg/kg, up to 150 mg, IV; repeat at 5- to 15-min intervals if needed
Drugs for Skeletal Muscle Spasm		
Dantrolene (Dantrium)	Skeletal muscle relaxant used to treat spasticity	Dosage: Initial dose 25 mg/day; increase to 25 mg 2 to 4 times per day; may increase up to 100 mg 2 to 4 times per day over 4–7 days
Baclofen (Lioresal)	Skeletal muscle relaxant used to treat spasticity	Dosage: Initially 5 mg 2 to 3 times per day; may increase slowly to range of 40–80 mg per day; total dose not to exceed 80 mg/day
Tizanidine hydrochloride (Zanaflex)	Central acting skeletal muscle relaxant used to treat acute and intermittent increased muscle tone associated with spasticity	Dosage: Initially 4 mg; gradually increase to 8 mg every 6–8 h for a maximum dose of 36 mg/24 h
Investigational Drugs		
Fampridine-SR ("4-AP," "4-aminopyridine")	In previous phase II studies, evidence of benefit has been seen in several areas—reduced muscle spasticity, improved sexual function, increased bladder control and bowel function	

*Follow hospital protocol. Refer to an up-to-date drug guide for updated information. Doses listed here are guidelines only.

trol can be facilitated by use of clothing appropriate for the weather conditions.

NUTRITION

The possibility of inadequate nutrition is of significant concern during the acute phase of injury and must not go unnoticed while the focus is on hemodynamic stability. Negative nitrogen balance contributes to skin breakdown, poor wound healing, and lack of energy for rehabilitative efforts. Along with other required blood work, a serum albumin test is necessary. A value less than 3.5 g/dL and/or total lymphocyte count less than 1,500/mm² to 2,000/mm² is indicative of clinical malnutrition. A dietary consult should be obtained as early as possible. Caloric requirements are calculated to ensure adequate, but not excessive, nutritional support. If the patient must remain NPO for more than a few days, total parenteral nutrition should be initiated.

Patients with spinal cord injuries often have increased energy needs secondary to metabolic stress response. This can lead to a severe catabolic state and malnutrition. It is not unusual to see a significant weight loss within the first few days of injury. Total parental nutrition or enteral feedings are instituted until the patient is able to start on an oral diet. The patient's intake and output are strictly monitored.

Ensuring adequate nutrition is a collaborative problem involving the patient, family, dietitian, occupational therapist, and nurse. The dietitian meets with the patient and family to identify the foods the patient enjoys and develops a menu that incorporates patient preference into the required dietary plan. Family members learn what foods they can bring from home to include in the patient's prescribed diet. The occupational therapist assesses the patient's need for assistive devices to use during mealtimes and teaches the patient and family how to use the adapted silverware. The nurse reinforces the information provided by the dietitian and occupational therapist. The nurse may teach family and friends how to assist the patient with meals and about the importance of allowing the patient as much independence as possible at mealtime. It is necessary to encourage fluid and a high-roughage diet, unless contraindicated. Before meals, the nurse assists the patient with mouth care and ensures that the patient has not been incontinent.

MOBILIZATION AND SKIN CARE

Rehabilitation begins in the critical care unit and is a collaborative effort involving the patient, physician, physical therapist (PT), occupational therapist (OT), nurse, and the patient's family. Initially, the nurse assists the patient with range-of-motion exercises. When the patient is stable, family members may be taught to assist the patient with these exercises. Based on their assessment findings, the PT and OT develop an individualized treatment plan to begin mobilization of the patient.

Positioning is not simply based on the usual every-2-hour turn schedule. Development of proper positioning protocols occurs in conjunction with the physical and occupational therapist to maximize range of motion and prevent joint contractures. When turning the patient, the nurse places a pillow under the patient's head but not under the forearms. When the patient is on his or her side, most of the upper body weight should be over the scapula that rests on the bed.[10] Flexing of the hips and knees allows the patient to remain on the side with minimal support. The nurse places pillows and foam cushions between the knees and against the back.

Pressure is a common cause of structural damage to a muscle and its peripheral nerve supply. Preventing skin breakdown is a priority for the nurse in the critical care unit. There is a definite time–pressure relationship in the development of pressure ulcers. Microscopic tissue changes secondary to local ischemia occur in less than 30 minutes. Pressure interferes with arteriolar and capillary blood flow. When the pressure is prolonged, there is definite damage to superficial circulation and tissue. The damage may be associated with congestion and induration of the area or blistering and loss of the superficial epidermal layers of the skin. As the pressure continues, the deeper skin layers are lost, leading to necrosis and ulceration. Serous drainage from such ulceration can constitute a continuous protein loss of as much as 50 g/day. Prolongation of the pressure results in deep penetrating necrosis of the skin, subcutaneous tissue, fascia, and muscle. The destruction may progress to gangrene of the underlying bony structure. Pressure necrosis can begin from within the tissue over a bony prominence, where the body weight is greatest per square inch.

A turn schedule for the patient is important, even if the patient has not had stabilizing surgery. It may take three staff members to accomplish this safely, particularly in the patient with a cervical injury. One person stabilizes the neck, and the other two flex the hips, knees, and ankles and hold the feet flat on the bed surface while turning the patient's trunk. To maintain alignment, the nurse uses foam wedges, pillows, or air-filled rolls. Turning occurs a minimum of every 2 hours. Use of an air or egg-crate mattress does not preclude the need to turn. The nurse checks the condition of the skin before and after the position change, paying particular attention to the patient's earlobes, back of head, elbows, inner aspects of the knees, heels, and sacral area. The posterior thigh and ischial tuberosities are prone to skin breakdown from prolonged lying on the back with the head of bed elevated or when sitting in a chair. The nurse documents any change in skin integrity, notifies the wound care specialist, and implements a plan of care. Numerous kinetic beds and air beds are available for patient comfort, preventing skin breakdown and treating complications of immobility.

Together with the PT and the OT, the nurse develops a plan to prevent foot drop. Initially, the heels are placed in "bunny boots." Frequently, high-top tennis shoes are worn. It is important to ensure that the boots or shoes are the correct size, to check for signs of skin breakdown, and to ensure that the patient's feet are dry. It is necessary to develop an "on and off" schedule with the PT. When the boots or shoes are off, the nurse pays careful attention to foot positioning and assesses for pressure ulcers.

The OT determines the need for splints or braces for the patient's wrists and hands. The nurse must assess the patient's skin frequently to identify pressure areas early. If necessary, the splints are modified to prevent skin breakdown.

URINARY MANAGEMENT

Acute tubular necrosis may occur within 48 hours of injury as a result of hypotension. An indwelling urinary catheter is necessary to allow for hourly measurement of urinary output during this phase, with the goal of keeping it at least 30 mL/hour. The nurse closely monitors fluid and electrolyte balance. Removal of the indwelling catheter as soon as spinal shock has resolved reduces the risk for infection.

The long-range objective of bladder management, regardless of the level of the injury, is to achieve a means whereby the bladder consistently empties, the urine is sterile, and the patient remains continent. The ultimate goal is to have the patient catheter free, with consistent low residual urine checks, no urinary tract infection, and no evidence of damage to the upper urinary tract structures.

One method of bladder management involves intermittent catheterization, and it may begin in the early recovery phase after spinal shock is resolved. The purpose of this program is to exercise the detrusor muscle, again with the goal of keeping the patient catheter free. The advantage of this method is that no irritant remains in the bladder; consequently, the risk for urinary tract infection, periurethral abscess, and epididymitis is reduced.

BOWEL MANAGEMENT

Before the initiation of a bowel program, it is necessary to perform a systematic, comprehensive evaluation of the type of cord injury, bowel function, impairment, and possible problems. This includes an abdominal assessment, a rectal examination, and evaluation of anal sphincter tone. In addition, the anocutaneous reflex (contraction of the anal sphincter secondary to cutaneous stimulation) and bulbocavernosus reflex (also referred to as the penile reflex; compression or tapping on the dorsum of the glans penis, which leads to contraction of the bulbocavernosus muscle at the tip of the penis) warrant assessment to determine whether the patient has upper motor neuron or lower motor neuron dysfunction. Equally important, a bowel program must consider the ability of the patient and caregivers to carry out the planned interventions at discharge.

Simple steps can prevent constipation and begin progress toward bowel continence. It is necessary to maintain appropriate intake, either through intravenous or oral fluids and diet. The nurse records bowel movements in an area that is easily accessible for review and administers stool softeners daily. Development of a consistent schedule for the bowel program is warranted. The timing of the program is usually after meals to coincide with peristalsis that occurs after meals to move food through the gastrointestinal tract. Rectal stimulation may be necessary to trigger defecation.

PSYCHOLOGICAL SUPPORT

As soon as the patient is medically stable, the nurse begins to focus on the psychosocial issues that are of concern to the patient and family. Questions often asked of the nurse include: Am I going to die? Will I walk or use my arms again? What is going to happen to me? There are no easy answers to these questions. It can be difficult for patients and family members to accept this uncertainty. Most of us are accustomed to receiving treatment for illnesses or conditions that have a predictable course of treatment and outcome. For example, antibiotics are prescribed for 10 days and the infection clears up, or surgery is performed and we are discharged home and able to return to our normal activities within an expected timeframe.

Answer questions to the best of your knowledge. Never predict the future, tell stories about patients who made a complete recovery, or ignore a question or a concern. Listen to the patient and the family. Let the patient and family talk about their fears and anxieties. Detailed patient education in a critical care unit is not generally appropriate. However, providing information the patient and family need to know while they are being cared for in the critical care unit is important. Focus on the patient care issues that present each day and on the patient's abilities. Do not minimize the patient's disabilities. Refer questions to other members of the health care team as appropriate. If indicated, ask for an order for a psychiatric consult.

Incorporate the use of technology to help the patient stay connected with family and friends. For example, place a "hands free" telephone in the room. Use a laptop computer and web cam if wireless Internet is available. Explore other enhancements that may be on the patient's personal laptop that will enable continued support with others and provide a means for helping the long days in the critical care unit pass.

Psychological transition from the loss of previous physical abilities to their current state is unique to each person. Feelings of grief, loss, anger, and frustration are common. Certain emotions are characteristic after a cord injury, whatever names are given to the stages of grief (Box 37-7). The rate at which a person works through this process varies, and none of the stages is static. A person can move back and forth between stages. The emotions felt and displayed by someone with a spinal cord injury are no different from the emotions felt by everyone at one time or another, and recognition of that fact may help promote empathy with the patient.

Box 37-7 • Stages of Grief in a Patient With a Spinal Cord Injury

STAGE	DESCRIPTION	IMPLICATIONS FOR THE NURSE
1. **Shock and disbelief**	During this phase, the patient does not request an explanation of what has happened. The patient is overwhelmed by the injury. There may be more concern with whether he or she will live than with whether he or she will walk again. This period may result in extreme dependence on the staff members.	The nurse may feel that the patient does not understand the ramifications of the injury. The nurse may identify with the feelings of being overwhelmed because he or she is often over-whelmed with the acute medical management of this catastrophic illness.
2. **Denial**	The process of denial is an escape mechanism. Usually, the whole disability is not denied, but particular aspects of it are. For instance, the patient may say he or she cannot walk now but will be able to in 6 mo. Bargaining, instead of being a separate stage, can be considered a form of denial. Bargains with God may be in the form of offering Him the legs if He will just return function of the arms.	The nurse often finds it difficult to deal with patients in this stage. A helpful approach is to focus on the present problems. This is not the stage to discuss long-term changes, such as ordering a wheelchair or making modifications to the home. More appropriate matters to deal with would be skin care and range-of-motion exercises.
3. **Reaction**	During this stage, instead of denying the impact of the injury, the patient expresses this impact. There may be severe depression and loss of motivation and involvement. Previous hobbies or interests lose their meaning. There is great helplessness during this period, and there may be suicidal statements.	The nurse can help at this stage by listening to the patient as feelings are verbalized. The nurse should avoid setting up failure situations, which could happen if he or she pushes the patient too fast. It is important to note that both the sudden absence of muscular activity and sensations in the patient with a spinal cord injury and the mental state of helplessness appear to alter central nervous system metabolism. Depression coincides with a fall in a brain metabolite excreted in the urine as tryptamine. Thus, it is important for the nurse to understand that depression in some patients with spinal cord injury might have a metabolic basis and that a trial of pharmacological therapy might be beneficial.
4. **Mobilization**	Problem-solving behavior is seen during this stage. The patient is looking toward the future and wants to learn about self-care. In fact, the patient may become very possessive of the therapist or nurse and resent the time spent with other patients. This is a time of sharing and planning between patient and staff.	
5. **Coping**	Some authorities think that patients do not accept the disability *per se* but instead learn to cope with it. Disability still is an inconvenience, but it is no longer the center of the patient's life. Life is again meaningful to the patient, and the patient is again involved with others.	

All staff members should have an understanding of the types of feelings and reactions the patient with a spinal cord injury may exhibit. They can share this process of recovery with family members in helping them to support the injured person and participate in recovery. It is necessary to provide psychological support for family members, who no doubt have many concerns, such as finances, role changes, and long-term prognosis. It is important to be supportive of them and help them and the patient with coping strategies.

ADDRESSING CONCERNS ABOUT SEXUALITY

After a spinal cord injury, patients have concerns about their ability to function sexually, although they may not verbalize this issue immediately. Critical care nurses probably will not deal with this problem specifically, but it is important to have some knowledge of the functional potential of the patient to begin to manage the patient's fears and concerns in this area. By avoiding discussion of this important issue, professionals validate the patient's fear that there can be no sex after a spinal cord injury, which is certainly not true.

Male Sexuality

Many men with a spinal cord injury believe that their total sexuality is tied to erection and ejaculation. There are three general types of erection in men: psychogenic, reflexogenic, and spontaneous. A psychogenic erection can result from sexual thoughts. The area of the cord responsible for this type of erection is between T11 and L2. Therefore, if the lesion is above this level, the message from the brain cannot get through the damaged area.

Reflexogenic erections are a direct result of stimulation to the penis. Some patients may get this type of erection when changing their catheter or pulling the pubic hairs. The length of time the erection can be maintained is variable; therefore, its usefulness for sexual activity is variable. Reflexogenic erections are better with higher cervical and thoracic lesions. Damage to lumbar and sacral regions may destroy the reflex arc.

The third type of erection is spontaneous. This may occur when the bladder is full, and it comes from some internal stimulation. How long the spontaneous erection lasts will determine its usefulness for sexual activity. The ability to achieve a reflexogenic or spontaneous erection comes from nerves in the S2, S3, and S4 segments of the cord.

Female Sexuality

In 50% of women with a spinal cord injury, the menstrual pattern is interrupted for approximately 6 months after injury but then is reestablished. Women are able to become pregnant and seem to have no increase in rate of miscarriage. There are potential complications for the pregnant woman, such as urinary tract infection, pressure sores, and anemia, but with careful medical attention, complications usually can be avoided or minimized.

Labor may be painless, or the woman may experience other signs that indicate labor is occurring (e.g., abdominal or leg spasms, back pain, difficulty breathing). Autonomic dysreflexia is a complication of labor in women with injuries above T4 to T6 and should be anticipated so that it can be controlled. Women may breast-feed if they wish.

• Complications

AUTONOMIC DYSREFLEXIA

Autonomic dysreflexia, or hyperreflexia, is a syndrome that sometimes occurs after the acute phase in patients with a spinal cord lesion at T7 or above. Autonomic dysreflexia constitutes a medical emergency. The syndrome presents quickly and can precipitate a seizure or stroke. Death can occur if the cause is not relieved.

Triggering conditions include bladder or intestinal distention, spasticity, pressure ulcers, or stimulation of the skin below the level of the injury. In men, ejaculation can initiate the reflex, and in pregnant women, strong uterine contractions can elicit it. Box 37-8 lists potential precipitating factors.

These stimuli produce a sympathetic discharge that causes a reflex vasoconstriction of the blood vessels in the skin and splanchnic bed below the level of the injury. The vasoconstriction produces extreme hypertension and a throbbing headache. Vasoconstriction of the splanchnic bed distends the baroreceptors in the carotid sinus and aortic arch. These baroreceptors in turn stimulate the vagus nerve, producing a bradycardia, in an attempt to lower the blood pressure. The body also attempts to reduce the hypertension by superficial vasodilation of vessels above the spinal cord injury. As a result, there is flushing, blurred vision, and nasal congestion. Because the spinal cord injury interrupts transmission of the vasodilation message below the level of the injury, the vasoconstriction continues below the level of the injury until the stimulus is identified and interrupted. The vasoconstriction results in pallor below the injury, whereas flushing occurs above the injury. Box 37-9 summarizes the signs and symptoms of autonomic dysreflexia.

When autonomic dysreflexia is recognized, there are several things the nurse can do quickly to relieve the patient's condition. The nurse can elevate the head of the bed and make frequent checks of blood pressure. In addition, he or she quickly checks the bladder drainage system for kinks in the tubing. The urine collection bag should not be overly full. Some protocols for checking the patency of the urinary drainage system include irrigating the catheter with 10 to 30 mL of irrigating solution. Absolutely no more than that amount is used because the addition of the fluid may aggravate the massive sympathetic outflow already present. If the symptoms persist, the catheter is changed so that the bladder can empty. Foley catheter

---

Box 37-8 • Precipitating Factors in Autonomic Dysreflexia

- Bladder distention or urinary tract infection
- Bladder or kidney stones
- Distended bowel
- Pressure areas or decubitus ulcers
- Thrombophlebitis
- Acute abdominal problems (e.g., ulcers, gastritis)
- Pulmonary emboli
- Menstruation
- Second stage of labor
- Constrictive clothing
- Heterotopic bone
- Pain
- Sexual activity; ejaculation by a man
- Manipulation or instrumentation of bladder or bowel
- Spasticity
- Exposure to hot or cold stimuli

Box 37-9 • RED FLAG: Signs and Symptoms of Autonomic Dysreflexia

- Paroxysmal hypertension
- Pounding headache
- Blurred vision
- Bradycardia
- Profuse sweating above the level of the injury
- Flushing or splotching of the face and neck
- Piloerection
- Nasal congestion
- Nausea
- Pupil dilation

placement may be necessary for patients on a bladder management program and those who have not voided in the past 4 to 6 hours.

If the urinary system does not appear to be the cause of the stimulus, it is necessary to check the patient for bowel impaction. Removal of the impaction should not occur until the symptoms subside. Rectal application of dibucaine or lidocaine ointment anesthetizes the area until symptoms disappear. If the patient's blood pressure does not return to normal, sublingual nifedipine (Procardia) may be very effective. A sympathetic ganglionic blocking agent such as atropine sulfate, guanethidine sulfate (Ismelin), reserpine, or methyldopa (Aldomet) may be useful. Hydralazine (Apresoline) and diazoxide (Hyperstat) also may help. Box 37-10 presents nursing intervention guidelines for managing autonomic dysreflexia.

PULMONARY COMPLICATIONS

Pulmonary complications are the most common cause of death in people with spinal cord injury, both in the acute and chronic phases. These pulmonary complications are especially prevalent in people injured above T10. If there is concomitant chest trauma or preexisting pulmonary disease, a history of smoking, or older age, there is higher risk for these complications.

Atelectasis and Pneumonia

Atelectasis is possible in any immobilized patient. Early mobilization, ensuring the airways are clear of secretions, and bronchial hygiene may be useful in minimizing or preventing atelectasis. Pneumonia may also result from hypoventilation and an inability to keep the airways clear. Adequate hydration helps keep secretions liquefied for ease of removal, and bronchoscopy may be necessary to remove mucus plugs. Supplemental oxygen administration is used to treat hypoxia. Ventilator-dependent patients need exquisite pulmonary care (see Chapter 25).

Deep Venous Thrombosis and Pulmonary Embolus

The Virchow triad for venous thrombosis—venous stasis, vein injury, and hypercoagulability—is found in the patient with a spinal cord injury. As a result, the patient is at increased risk for deep venous thrombosis (DVT) and pulmonary embolus. In addition to swelling and pain, obstruction to venous return can lead to compartment syndrome and limb ischemia. Although it is infrequent, hypovolemic shock can occur if enough blood and interstitial fluid pool in the

Box 37-10 • NURSING INTERVENTIONS for Managing Autonomic Dysreflexia

1. Elevate the head of bed.
2. Apply blood pressure cuff, and check blood pressure every 1 to 2 min.
   - If BP is above 180/90, proceed to step 5.
   - If BP is below 180/90, proceed as follows.
3. Quickly insert bladder catheter or check bladder drainage system in place to detect possible obstruction.
   - Check to make sure plug or clamp is not in catheter or on tubing.
   - Check for kinks in catheter or drainage tubing.
   - Check inlet to leg bag to make sure it is not corroded.
   - Check to make sure leg bag is not overfull.
   - If none of these are evident, proceed to step 4.
4. Determine whether catheter is plugged by irrigating the bladder slowly with no more than 30 mL of irrigation solution. Use of more solution may increase the massive sympathetic outflow already present. If symptoms have not subsided, proceed to step 5.
5. Change the catheter and empty the bladder.
6. When you are sure the bladder is empty and if BP is:
   - Above 180/90, call physician immediately.

- Below 180/90, proceed as follows: Give sublingual nifedipine (Procardia) if protocol calls for it. Give atropine according to physician's order. If BP rises or fails to subside, call physician immediately. Guanethidine monosulfate (Ismelin), hydralazine (Apresoline), or inhaled amyl nitrate may then be ordered by the physician. Dibenzylene may be used for chronic dysreflexia.
7. Ideally, this procedure requires three people: one to check the BP, one to check the drainage system, and one to notify the physician.

If bladder overdistention does not seem to be the cause of the dysreflexia,

- Check for bowel impaction. Do not attempt to remove it, if present. Apply Nupercainal ointment or Xylocaine jelly to the rectum and anal area. As the area is anesthetized, the BP should fall. After the BP is again stable, using a generous amount of anesthetizing ointment or jelly, manually remove impaction.
- Change the patient's position. Pressure areas may be the source of dysreflexia.

extremity.[11] (If the thrombus breaks off, pulmonary emboli can obstruct venous return and lead to cardiovascular collapse and death.) Patients particularly at risk for a fat embolus are those with long bone fractures. Signs of chest or neck petechiae and low-grade fever may be early indications.

Leg veins should not be used as sites from which to draw blood, lest the trauma to the vessel wall enhance platelet aggregation and clot formation. It is important to encourage smokers to quit because nicotine causes vasoconstriction, thereby slowing blood flow through the periphery.

There is some controversy about the effectiveness of serial leg measurements in monitoring for DVT. A standard measurement protocol is necessary, and all staff should follow it. For example, use a special measuring tape rather than a sewing tape, mark the area where the tape is placed, and use running averages.

Treatment of DVT and pulmonary embolus includes heparin infusion, insertion of an intravenous vena cava filter, or dissolving the clot with thrombolytic agents. Measures to prevent DVT may include the administration of low–molecular-weight heparin and the use of antiembolic stockings. Other modalities include sequential compression devices, passive range-of-motion exercises, and early mobilization. In addition, a kinetic bed can be useful; this device works by keeping the patient in continuous motion.

PARALYTIC ILEUS AND STRESS ULCERS

Early medical management for paralytic ileus and stress ulcers includes NPO status, particularly for cervical spinal cord–injured patients. Nasogastric tube placement with intermittent suction is useful for treatment of the paralytic ileus that frequently accompanies spinal cord injury. Nasogastric tube placement also decreases the risk for aspiration and decreases abdominal distention. As soon as bowel sounds are present, safe stimulation of peristalsis may occur using stool softeners, mild laxatives, or suppositories. It is important to avoid enemas, other than the oil-retention type, because the risk for intestinal perforation is high.

Patients with cervical injuries are more likely to experience gastrointestinal bleeding as a result of stress ulcers. Medical treatment includes histamine-2 (H_2) receptor blockers, proton pump inhibitors, antacids, or a combination of the three.

HETEROTROPIC OSSIFICATION

Calcification around a joint, especially the hip joint, may occur within 12 weeks of injury. Clinical manifestations include limited range of motion, swelling of the affected joint, and an elevated alkaline phosphatase level. Pain may or may not be present. The goal of treatment is to prevent further damage and progression. Additional treatment includes irradiation, nonsteroidal anti-inflammatory drugs, and disodium etidronate.

SPASTICITY

Spasticity develops after recovery from the period of spinal shock and affects the flexor muscles of the arms and the extensor muscles of the legs. An interdisciplinary approach is the hallmark of treatment. A physical therapy consult is warranted to develop an exercise, stretching, and positioning program for the patient. A variety of medications such as baclofen, dantrolene sodium, diazepam, and clonidine may be useful.

• Research in the Treatment of Spinal Cord Injuries

Recent progress in clinical investigations may contribute to the treatment of spinal cord injury.

▶ Stem cell research holds promise for a number of neurological disorders, including spinal cord regeneration. Small studies have advanced to phase I clinical trials.

▶ Medications are under investigation to identify agents that may be useful in the treatment of the primary and secondary effects of the cord injury itself. Other studies are focusing on the development of medications to treat complications such as spasticity or neuropathic pain. Other research is focusing on designing DNA vaccines for the treatment of axonal degeneration and demyelination. The goal is to improve motor function.

▶ Medical devices and assistive devices continue to be developed and older tools improved to enable the person with a spinal cord injury to function at the maximal level possible. With the increased numbers of military personnel suffering spinal cord injuries, this area will continue to expand.

• Patient Teaching and Discharge Planning

Usually, the patient is discharged to a rehabilitation setting to learn the skills needed for activities of daily living and, when possible, independent living. The nurse helps the family find a rehabilitation program specific for patients with spinal cord injury. When searching for an appropriate rehabilitation program, the family should obtain answers to the following questions:

1. How many patients with spinal cord injury are treated in the program each year?
2. What is the average age of the patients in the program?
3. Does the treatment plan identify both long-term and short-term goals?
4. Will the patient be assigned an experienced case manager to coordinate the transition between the rehabilitation center and home?

5. How much time is spent teaching the patient and family about sexuality, bowel and bladder care, and other activities of daily living?

The family should also ask if the staff has specialized training in spinal cord injury. Rehabilitation therapies should be available for a minimum of 3 hours per day. There should be activities or programs for the patients on weekends and in the evenings. Most important, the facility should have 24-hour staffing with registered nurses and respiratory therapists. Box 37-11 contains a discharge planning guide for a person with a spinal cord injury. Box 37-12 provides a patient teaching guide for patients living with a spinal cord injury.

• Clinical Applicability Challenges

Case Study: Spinal Cord Injury

A coworker finds Mr. S., a 60-year-old man, lying injured on the floor in the service station where he works as a mechanic. It appears that he slipped on the grease on the floor while working on the transmission of a small truck. Paramedics arrive at the scene of the accident within 10 minutes. Mr. S. is able to move his extremities, and he complains of neck pain of 6 on a pain scale of 10. He is awake, alert, and oriented to his current location; the date and day of the week; and details of the accident. His pupils are equal and reactive to light. He shows no other signs of injury except for a cut on his forehead. Vital signs are blood pressure, 170/102 mm Hg; heart rate, 86 beats/minute; and respiratory

Box 37-11 • DISCHARGE PLANNING GUIDE: Spinal Cord Injury

- Arrange for representatives from physical and occupational therapy to evaluate the patient's home for the following:
  Wheelchair accessibility
  Clearance for maneuvering a wheelchair within the home
  Necessary adaptations to the bedroom, bathroom, and kitchen
  Smoke and fire alarms
- Obtain needed equipment for home care, depending on patient's level of injury. Be sure the equipment is delivered before the patient leaves the rehabilitation facility. Also be sure that the patient and his or her family members know how to operate the equipment.
- Make arrangements for home health care, physical therapy, occupational therapy, and job training or vocational rehabilitation, as necessary.
- Notify the electric company if there will be life-saving equipment in the home, such as a respirator.
- Carry out patient and family education (see Box 37-12).
- Locate community support groups.

rate, 28 breaths/minute (unlabored and regular). The paramedics apply a cervical collar, place the patient on a backboard, and transport him to the medical center by helicopter. He arrives in the emergency department within 45 minutes of the accident.

On initial examination, the patient's vital signs are blood pressure, 180/90 mm Hg; heart rate, 88 beats/minute; respiratory rate, 24 breaths/minute and respirations somewhat shallow; and temperature, 98.6°F (37°C). Mr. S. is sweating and mildly confused. His arm veins are quite distended. According to the paramedics, his motor and sensory function has decreased since his initial evaluation at the scene of the accident. Although he could originally tighten his biceps, now he cannot overcome gravity to raise his arms. Deep tendon reflexes are markedly decreased.

The emergency trauma team starts intravenous lactated Ringer's solution, inserts a Foley catheter into Mr. S.'s bladder, and inserts a nasogastric tube, which is connected to low intermittent suction. The trauma physician orders full spine, skull, and chest radiographs. The radiographs reveal that the patient has a dislocated fracture of C5 and C6. The chest film shows a lack of full lung field expansion. Blood work results are normal with the exception of arterial blood gases, which show respiratory acidosis (pH 7.30).

Mr. S. is admitted to the critical care unit, where he is placed in a halo fixation device to realign the cervical vertebrae and stabilize the fracture. Neurogenic shock treatment includes careful intravenous fluid replacement to avoid overhydration, the use of dopamine or a similar drug when hypotension compromises adequate perfusion of vital organs, and atropine to correct bradycardia if he becomes symptomatic.

Nursing interventions include monitoring neurological signs and vital signs every hour for the first 24 hours, then every 2 hours until the patient is stabilized. The nurses who are caring for Mr. S. pay particular attention to the patient's respiratory status. He is at risk for respiratory failure due to spinal cord edema. They turn him every 2 hours and measure and record the output of his Foley catheter and nasogastric tube every 4 hours. They make every effort to prevent complications of immobility, both in the critical care and acute care units. After consulting physical and occupational therapy, Mr. S.'s health care team initiates a treatment plan. Once past the acute phase of his injury, the patient is transferred to a rehabilitation facility for further recovery and adaptation to his injury.

1. What additional information is needed about Mr. S. to provide him with appropriate care while hospitalized?

2. Based on the information from the case study, list the five priorities of care for Mr. S. Include the reason/rationale these priorities were selected.

Box 37-12 • TEACHING GUIDE:
Living With a Spinal Cord Injury

Nutritional Management
- Eat a well-balanced diet that includes protein (lean meat, dairy foods, legumes), fresh fruits, vegetables, and liquids.
- Maintain ideal body weight.

Skin Management
- You and your helper should check your skin twice a day. Look for redness, bruises or scrapes, blisters, and rashes. Pay particular attention to bony areas. Check your groin for rashes and reddened areas.
- Keep your skin clean and dry, especially in areas where skin touches skin (e.g., between the toes, underneath the breasts). Do not use antimicrobial or harsh soaps. Apply moisturizing lotion. Avoid lotions or creams that dry the skin.
- Check your feet whenever you wear new shoes. Check for ingrown toenails. Keep your nails trimmed and filed smooth, and have calluses treated by a podiatrist.
- Use the wheelchair and cushion prescribed by your physical therapist.
- Change positions frequently to relieve pressure on bony areas.
- Be sure you are not sitting or lying on anything. Avoid putting objects in your pockets.
- Check to be sure braces, leg bags, and other adaptive equipment is not too tight.
- When in bed, use padding over bony areas. Use a firm mattress. If possible, sleep on your stomach.
- Notify your health care provider of any skin breakdown.

Urinary Tract Management
- Follow the bladder program developed by the rehabilitation team.
- Drink plenty of fluids unless contraindicated.
- If you have a Foley catheter, keep it free of kinks and change it as directed by your health care provider.
- Watch for signs and symptoms of urinary tract infection (e.g., cloudy urine with a foul odor, sediment in the urine).

Bowel Management
- Follow the bowel program developed by your rehabilitation team. Avoid the regular use of laxatives. Schedule sufficient time to complete the required activities. Notify your health care provider if you have not had a bowel movement in 3 or 4 days.
- Drink plenty of fluids, unless contraindicated.
- Monitor your diet to see what foods cause constipation and diarrhea.
- Prevent constipation through diet and fluid intake and medications as needed.
- Avoid foods that cause gas, such as beans, corn, and apples.
- Be aware of the potential for the development of autonomic dysreflexia during your bowel program.

Respiratory Management
- Cough and deep-breathe routinely.
- Drink plenty of fluids, unless contraindicated.
- Use postural drainage or chest physiotherapy.
- Because you are at risk for pneumonia, be careful around anyone with a cold and get an annual influenza vaccination.

Complications
Autonomic Dysreflexia
- This complication occurs in patients with injury at T5 or above.
- The most common cause is overfilling of the bladder. Other causes include constipation or gas, skin irritations, pressure sores, wounds, and ingrown toenails.
- Autonomic dysreflexia can be a life-threatening emergency. You or a helper must take immediate action to correct this problem.
- Signs and symptoms include a severe headache, nasal congestion, goose pimples, and restlessness.
- Be sure your head is up. If you are sitting in a chair, stay there; if you are in bed, get your head elevated.
- If you have an indwelling catheter:
  Check for kinks along the tubing.
  Empty the Foley bag; if there is no drainage, the Foley may be obstructed—change the Foley.
  Check the catheter and drainage bag for deposits.
  Check urine for color.
- If you are on intermittent catheterization, catheterize yourself.
- If the problem is related to the bowel, perform a digital stimulation and empty the bowel.
- If it is not related to a bladder or bowel problem, check for a pressure sore, ingrown toenail, or possible bone fracture.
- If none of the above actions relieve the signs and symptoms, get emergency medical treatment.

Deep Venous Thrombosis
- Prevention is important.
- Signs and symptoms include leg swelling, chest pain, and cough.
- Call your health care provider immediately if signs or symptoms develop.

Hypothermia and Hyperthermia
- To prevent hyperthermia:
  Drink lots of fluids.
  Dress according to the temperature you will be in.
  Watch for signs and symptoms of hyperthermia.
  Use sun block.
- To prevent hypothermia:
  Dress appropriately for the weather.
  Watch for signs and symptoms of hypothermia and frostbite.

Heterotopic Ossification
- Check for development of abnormal bone in soft tissue, usually around the hip or knee.
- Signs and symptoms include a change in range of motion, decreased ability to perform activities of daily living, swelling, warmth, redness over the hip or knee, spasticity, and fever.
- Notify your health care provider immediately if any of these signs or symptoms develop.

Medication-Related Complications
- Select a pharmacy that will keep your medication profile on record, including any allergies you may have.

(continued)

Box 37-12 • TEACHING GUIDE:
Living With a Spinal Cord Injury (Continued)

- Be sure the pharmacy has a system to check for and identify drug and food interactions.
- Have all of your prescriptions filled at the same pharmacy.
- Follow the directions on the label.
- Take all the medication that is ordered.
- Keep a current list of all medications.
- Know the important side effects of the medication; if any occur, notify your health care provider.

Pain
- Prevention of other problems such as pressure ulcers, stress ulcers, and infections is important.
- Maintain your activity program, range-of-motion exercises, and a healthy diet.
- Notify your health care provider of the type of pain you are experiencing.
- Medications and stress reduction techniques may be used.

Orthostatic Hypotension
- Know that this is a drop in blood pressure when you first sit up.
- Wear elastic hose or an abdominal support.
- Sit up slowly.
- If you experience orthostatic hypotension while you are sitting up, ask someone to tilt your wheelchair back until your head is parallel to the floor.
- Be sure to drink plenty of fluids.

Spasticity
- Prevention is crucial. Watch for and immediately treat skin problems such as an ingrown toenail. Prevent pressure ulcers. Maintain your bowel and bladder program.
- Notify your health care provider if spasticity develops.

---

3. What nursing interventions should be implemented based on the priorities of care listed above?

Review Questions

1. While driving down the street, you arrive at the scene of an automobile accident. The driver's head hit the steering wheel; you suspect a cervical cord injury. Which of the following is an assessment priority?
   a. Stabilizing the patient's neck
   b. Cardiac assessment
   c. Neurological assessment
   d. Respiratory assessment

2. The patient is on a cardiac monitor with continuous blood pressure (BP) recording. The alarm on the monitor sounds because the patient's BP is now 86/70 mm Hg. The nurse's first response is to
   a. check the monitor to ensure there is no interference.
   b. ask the nursing assistant/technician to check the patient's BP with a manual cuff.
   c. assess the patient including vital signs.
   d. lower the head of the bed if it is elevated.

3. A patient asks the nurse if he will ever walk again. The correct response is:
   a. "You should ask the physician."
   b. "What do you think?"
   c. "Because of the location of your injury, it is unlikely."
   d. "It is too early to tell; we just have to wait and see."

4. The patient has been kept flat in bed since surgery to stabilize his spine and for the placement of a halo vest. Today there is an order for the patient to sit up in a chair. What is the most important priority of care?

   a. Monitor the patient's vital signs.
   b. Raise the head of the bed slowly to prevent orthostatic hypotension.
   c. Educate the patient—tell him what will be done and how.
   d. Dangle on the side of the bed before transfer to chair.

5. A significant weight loss may occur during the first few days after a spinal cord injury. An important nursing intervention is to
   a. increase the amount of calories consumed by the patient.
   b. perform a 24-hour calorie count.
   c. Maintain strict intake and output.
   d. Obtain a dietary consult and a serum albumin.

6. Mr. Smith, a 75-year-old man with a history of diabetes mellitus and hypertension, has just returned to the critical care unit after thoracic spine surgery. He is at risk for which of the following complications of this surgery?
   a. Hypertensive crisis
   b. Hypoglycemia
   c. Infection
   d. Urinary incontinence

7. The patient is complaining of headache and nasal congestion. He tells the nurse that he must be getting a cold. The nurse's best response is to
   a. administer nifedipine, which is ordered PRN.
   b. notify the health care provider immediately.
   c. take the client's vital signs.
   d. raise the head of the bed.

References

1. The National Spinal Cord Injury Statistical Center: SCI: Facts and figures at a glance. Available at: http://www.spinalcord.uab.edu

2. Dryden DM, Saunders LD, Jacobs P, et al: Direct health care costs after traumatic spinal cord injury. J Trauma 59(2): 441–447, 2005

3. Rechtine GR: Nonoperative management and treatment of spinal injuries. Spine 31(11 Suppl):SP22–27, 2006

4. Harris MB, Sethi RK: The initial assessment and management of the multiple trauma patient with an associated spine injury. Spine 31(11 Suppl):S9–15, 2006

5. Hurlbert RJ: Strategies of medical intervention in the management of acute spinal cord injury. Spine 31(11 Suppl):16–21, 2006

6. Levi D, Hurlbert J, Anderson P, et al: Neurological deterioration secondary to unrecognized spinal instability following trauma: A multicenter study. Spine 31(4):451–458, 2006

7. Aryan HE, Amar AP, Ozgur BM, Levy ML: Gunshot wounds to the spine in adolescents. Neurosurgery 57(4):748–752, 2005

8. Fisher C, Harris M, Hurlbert J, et al: Summary statement: Early management of spinal cord and column injury. Spine 31(11 Suppl):S36, 2006

9. Lim MR, Lee JY, Vaccaro AR: Surgical infections in the traumatized spine. Clin Orthop 444(3):114–119, 2006

10. Fries J: Critical rehabilitation of the patient with a spinal cord injury. Crit Care Nurs Q 28(2):179–187, 2005

11. Yang JC: Prevention and treatment of deep vein thrombosis and pulmonary embolism in critically ill patients. Crit Care Nurs Q 28(1):72–79, 2005

Other Selected Readings

Bartley MK: Keep venous thromboembolism at bay. Nursing 2006 36(10):36–41, 2006

Donovan WH: Donald Munro Lecture: Spinal cord injury past, present and future. J Spinal Cord Med 30(2):85–100, 2007

Evans RW: Neurology and Trauma, 2nd ed. New York: Oxford University Press, 2006

Fehlings MG, Rerrin AR: The timing of surgical intervention in the treatment of spinal cord injury: A systematic review of recent clinical evidence. Spine 31(11 Suppl):S28–35, 2006

Frederickson MD: Acute spinal cord injury management. J Trauma 62(6 Suppl):S9, 2007

Furlan JC, Krassioukov AV, Fehlings MG: Hematologic abnormalities within the first week after acute isolated traumatic cervical spinal cord injury: A case-control cohort study. Spine 31(23): 2674–2683, 2006

Harvey CV: Spinal surgery patient care. Orthop Nurs 24(6): 426–440, 2005

Hughes R, Fintan S, McCourt F: Identifying and defining the problems, interventions, and outcomes of spinal cord injured patients in the Irish Spinal Cord Injury Service using standardized nursing language: A Delphi study. Int J Nurs Terminol Classif 17(1):38–39, 2006

Leypold BG, Flanders AE, Schwartz ED, et al: The impact of methylprednisolone on lesion severity following spinal cord injury. Spine 32(3):373–378, 2007

McLain RF, et al: Summary statement: Thoracolumbar spine trauma. Spine 31(11 Suppl):103, 2006

Myers J, Lee M, Kiratli J: Cardiovascular disease in spinal cord injury: An overview of prevalence, risk, evaluation, and management. Am J Phys Med Rehabil 86(2):142–152, 2006

Nelson A, Baptiste A: Evidence-based practices for safe patient handling and movement. Orthop Nurs 25(6):366–379, 2006

Powers J, Daniels D, McGuire C, Hilbish C: The incidence of skin breakdown associated with use of cervical collars. J Trauma Nurs 13(4):198–200, 2006

Sherwood PR, Crago EA, Spiro RM, Okonkwo D: Cervical spine injuries: Preserving function, improving outcomes. Am Nurse Today 2(9):26–29, 2007

Sipski ML, Scott RJ: Spinal cord injury rehabilitation: State of the science. Am J Phys Med Rehabil 85(4):310–342, 2006

Tator CH: Review of treatment trials in human spinal cord injury: Issues, difficulties, and recommendations. Neurosurgery (On Line) 59(5):957–987, 2006

Gastrointestinal System

PART 9

INTERNET RESOURCES

Topic	Web Page Address
American College of Gastroenterology	www.acg.gi.org
American Diabetes Association	www.diabetes.org
American Gastroenterological Association	www.gastro.org
American Liver Foundation	www.liverfoundation.org
American Society for Clinical Nutrition	www.ascn.org
American Society for Parenteral and Enteral Nutrition	www.clinnutr.org
American Society of Gastrointestinal Endoscopy	www.asge.org
Canadian Association of Gastroenterology	www.cag-acg.org
Canadian Enteral-Parenteral Nutrition Association	www.cpena.ca
Canadian Society of Gastroenterology Nurses and Associates	www.csgna.com
Center for Science in the Public Interest	www.cspinet.org
The Centers for Disease Control and Prevention	www.cdc.gov
Children's Liver Disease Foundation	www.childliverdisease.org
The Digestive Disorders Foundation	www.digestivedisorders.org.uk
Electronic Enteral and Parenteral Nutrition	http://epen.kumc.edu/
Gastro Online	www.gastronews.com
Hepatitis Foundation International	www.hepfi.org
The Hepatitis Information Network	www.hepnet.com
Medline Plus Website	www.nlm.nih.gov/medlineplus
National Institute of Diabetes, Digestive and Kidney Diseases	www.niddk.nih.gov
The National Pancreas Foundation	www.pancreasfoundation.org
The Nutrition Source	www.hsph.harvard.edu/nutritionsource/
Pancreatitis Information	www.pancreatitis.org.uk
Society of Gastroenterology Nurses and Associates	www.sgna.org
Texas Virtual Clinic	www.utsurg.th.tmc.edu/digestive
Virtual Hospital	www.vh.org

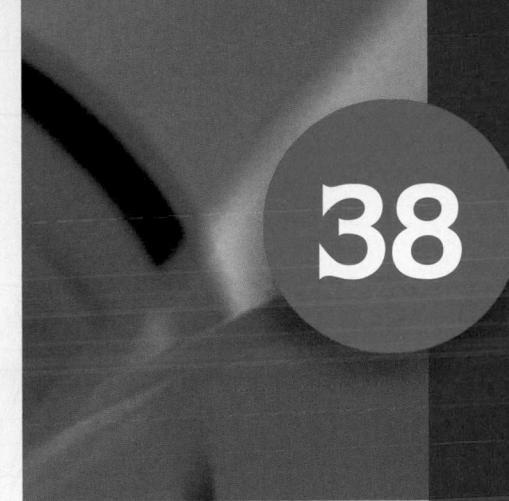

Anatomy and Physiology of the Gastrointestinal System

38

Allison G. Steele • Valerie K. Sabol

Objectives

Based on the content in this chapter, the reader should be able to:

❶ Examine the processes of ingestion, digestion, absorption, and elimination.

❷ Describe the functions of the major structures of the gastrointestinal system.

❸ Explain digestion and absorption of carbohydrates, proteins, fats, vitamins, and minerals.

❹ Discuss the processes involved in emesis and defecation.

❺ Describe bile production, secretion, and excretion.

The gastrointestinal system consists of the gastrointestinal tract and the accessory glandular organs that empty their contents into the gastrointestinal tract. The major structures of the gastrointestinal tract are the mouth, pharynx, esophagus, stomach, small intestine (duodenum, jejunum, ileum), and large intestine (colon, rectum, anus). The accessory glandular organs include the salivary glands, liver, gallbladder, and pancreas.

The primary physiological functions of the gastrointestinal system are to take in nutrients for cell maintenance and growth and to eliminate waste. Cell maintenance and growth are accomplished through the processes of ingestion (taking in food), motility (mixing and propelling food through the gastrointestinal tract), digestion (breaking down food), and absorption (movement of food particles into the bloodstream). Elimination is the process by which waste is eliminated from the body.

Gastrointestinal function is regulated and coordinated by the autonomic nervous system and a variety of peptides, which are further classified as endocrines (hormones), paracrines, and neurocrines. Endocrines are released in the general circulation and

reach all tissues. Endocrine cells release paracrines, which target specific tissues. Neurocrines, or neurotransmitters, diffuse across a synaptic gap and can stimulate or inhibit the release of endocrines and paracrines.

• Structure of the Gastrointestinal System

MACROSCOPIC ANATOMY OF THE GASTROINTESTINAL SYSTEM

The gastrointestinal system is composed of the gastrointestinal tract (also called the alimentary canal), a hollow tube about 8 m (25 ft) long that begins at the mouth and ends at the anus (Fig. 38-1). The accessory glands (e.g., salivary glands) and organs (e.g., liver and pancreas) release secretory products into the gastrointestinal tract.

The oral cavity opens into the pharynx, a structure that allows the passage of nutrients and air. The anterior pharynx, divided into the oropharynx

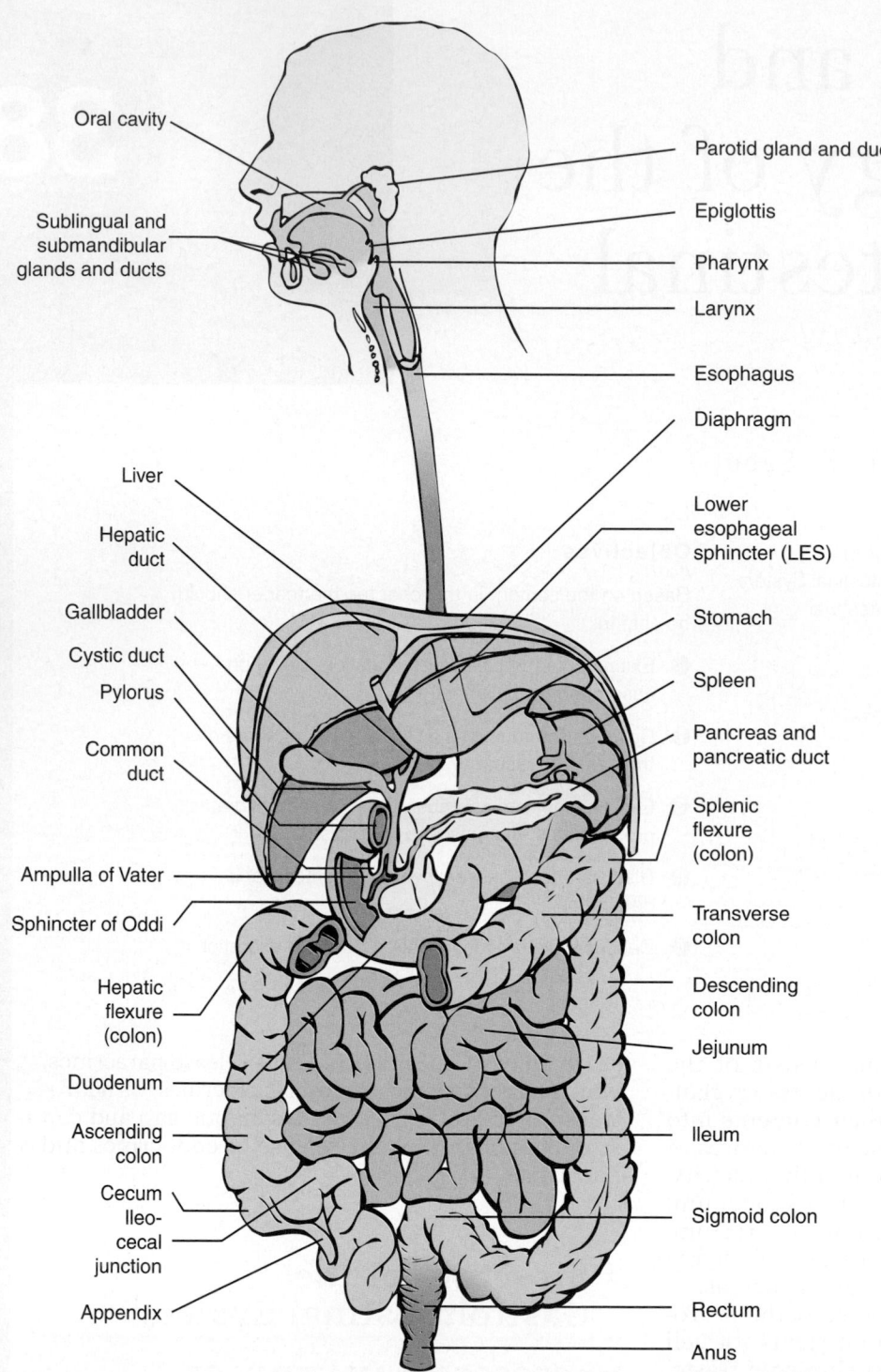

- Oral cavity
- Sublingual and submandibular glands and ducts
- Parotid gland and duct
- Epiglottis
- Pharynx
- Larynx
- Esophagus
- Diaphragm
- Liver
- Hepatic duct
- Gallbladder
- Cystic duct
- Pylorus
- Common duct
- Lower esophageal sphincter (LES)
- Stomach
- Spleen
- Pancreas and pancreatic duct
- Splenic flexure (colon)
- Ampulla of Vater
- Sphincter of Oddi
- Hepatic flexure (colon)
- Transverse colon
- Descending colon
- Jejunum
- Duodenum
- Ascending colon
- Ileum
- Cecum Ileo-cecal junction
- Sigmoid colon
- Appendix
- Rectum
- Anus

Figure 38-1 • The gastrointestinal tract.

and nasopharynx, connects the oral and nasal cavities. The posteroinferior end of the pharynx (at about the level of the sixth cervical vertebra) connects to the esophagus and larynx. The epiglottis, a thin cartilaginous flap covered by soft tissue, reflexively covers the larynx during swallowing and prevents the passage of food and water into the trachea.

The esophagus, a 25-cm (10-in) collapsible tube, connects the pharynx to the stomach at the cardiac orifice (Fig. 38-2). The esophagus is posterior to the trachea, in the posterior mediastinum, and crosses through the diaphragm. Its main function is to deliver food to the stomach. Two muscular rings, the upper and lower esophageal sphincters, border the esophagus. The upper esophageal sphincter (UES) prevents aspiration and swallowing of excessive air. The lower esophageal sphincter (LES), a muscular ring at the gastroesophageal junction, prevents reflux of gastric contents into the esophagus.

The stomach is a flask-shaped organ that lies in the upper abdomen below the diaphragm (Fig. 38-3). The main function of the stomach is storage; it acts as a reservoir for chewed food. The stomach also mixes ingested food with gastric secretions to form a semi-

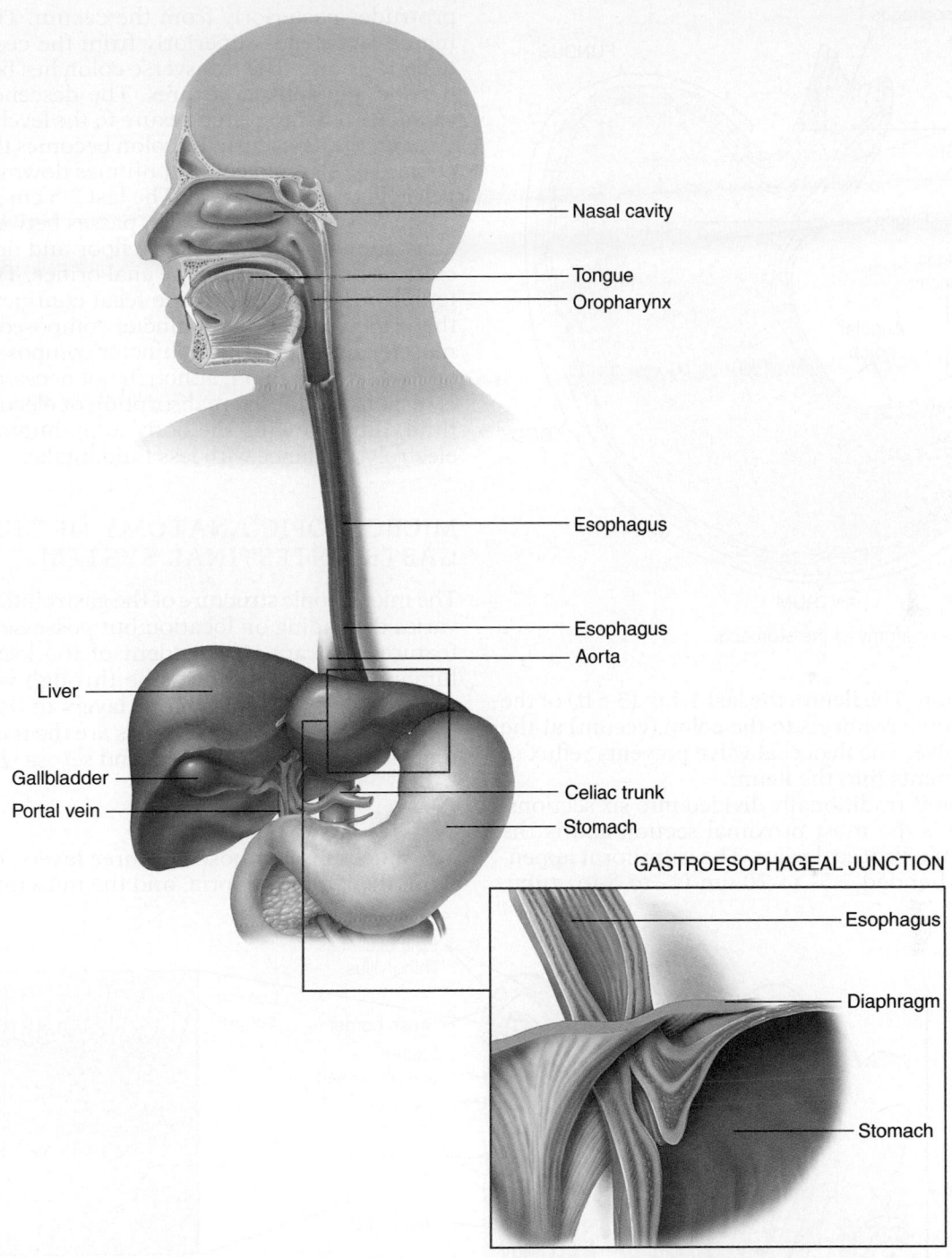

Nasal cavity

Tongue
Oropharynx

Esophagus

Esophagus
Aorta

Liver

Gallbladder
Portal vein

Celiac trunk
Stomach

GASTROESOPHAGEAL JUNCTION

Esophagus

Diaphragm

Stomach

Figure 38-2 • Gastroesophageal junction. (From Anatomical Chart Company: Atlas of Human Anatomy. Springhouse, PA: Springhouse, 2001, p 203.)

solid liquid called chyme and regulates the release of chyme into the duodenum at a controlled rate. The esophagus joins the stomach at the cardia of the stomach. The cells of the cardia secrete mucus that helps protect the esophagus from the acidic secretions of the stomach. The dome-shaped fundus, located to the left of the cardia, acts as a reservoir. The body and the fundus have coarse folds called rugae that allow for expansion of the stomach. Gastric pits, which contain the acid-secreting cells of the stomach, are located mainly in the body of the stomach. The antrum, the most distal area of the stom-

ach, is the site of G cells, which secrete gastrin. The antrum narrows into the pyloric channel, or pylorus, ending in the gastroduodenal junction at the pyloric sphincter. The pyloric sphincter, a muscular structure between the stomach and the duodenum, minimizes intestinal reflux.

Most digestion and absorption take place in the small intestine. The duodenum, the first 25 to 30 cm (10 to 12 in) of the small intestine, begins at the pylorus. The common bile duct opens into the duodenum at the duodenal papilla through the ampulla of Vater. The next 2.6 m (8.5 ft) of the small intestine

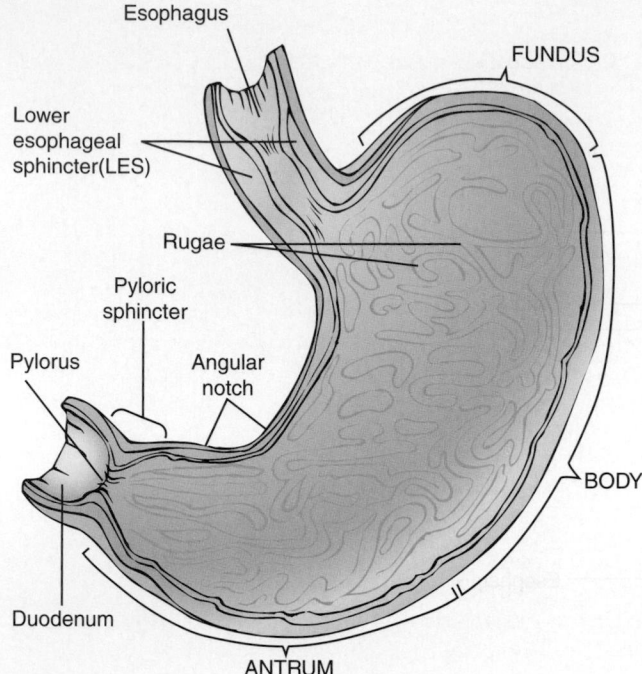

Figure 38-3 • Anatomy of the stomach.

is the jejunum. The ileum, the last 1.1 m (3.6 ft) of the small intestine, connects to the colon (cecum) at the ileocecal valve. The ileocecal valve prevents reflux of colonic contents into the ileum.

The colon is traditionally divided into six sections. The cecum is the most proximal section and is the location of the ileocecal valve. The vermiform appendix, a blind-ended 2.5- to 20-cm (1- to 8-in) tube,

protrudes posteriorly from the cecum. The ascending colon extends superiorly from the cecum to the hepatic flexure. The transverse colon lies between the hepatic and splenic flexures. The descending colon extends from the splenic flexure to the level of the iliac crest. At the iliac crest, the colon becomes the sigmoid colon. The sigmoid colon continues downward to the pelvic floor as the rectum. The last 2.5 cm (1 in) or so of the rectum, the anal canal, passes between the levator ani muscles of the pelvic floor and opens to the exterior body surface as the anal orifice. Two sphincters, which work to provide fecal continence, guard this orifice: an internal sphincter composed of smooth muscle and an external sphincter composed of skeletal muscle. The colon, although not necessary for life, is responsible for the reabsorption of electrolytes and fluid, thus allowing the body to maintain fluid and electrolyte balance with less fluid intake.

MICROSCOPIC ANATOMY OF THE GASTROINTESTINAL SYSTEM

The microscopic structure of the gastrointestinal tract varies depending on location but possesses common features that are independent of the location. The lumen, a central hollow tube through which food passes, is surrounded by four layers of tissue. From the lumen outward, these layers are the mucosa, submucosa, muscularis propria, and serosa (Fig. 38-4).

Mucosa

The mucosa is composed of three layers: the epithelium, the lamina propria, and the muscularis muco-

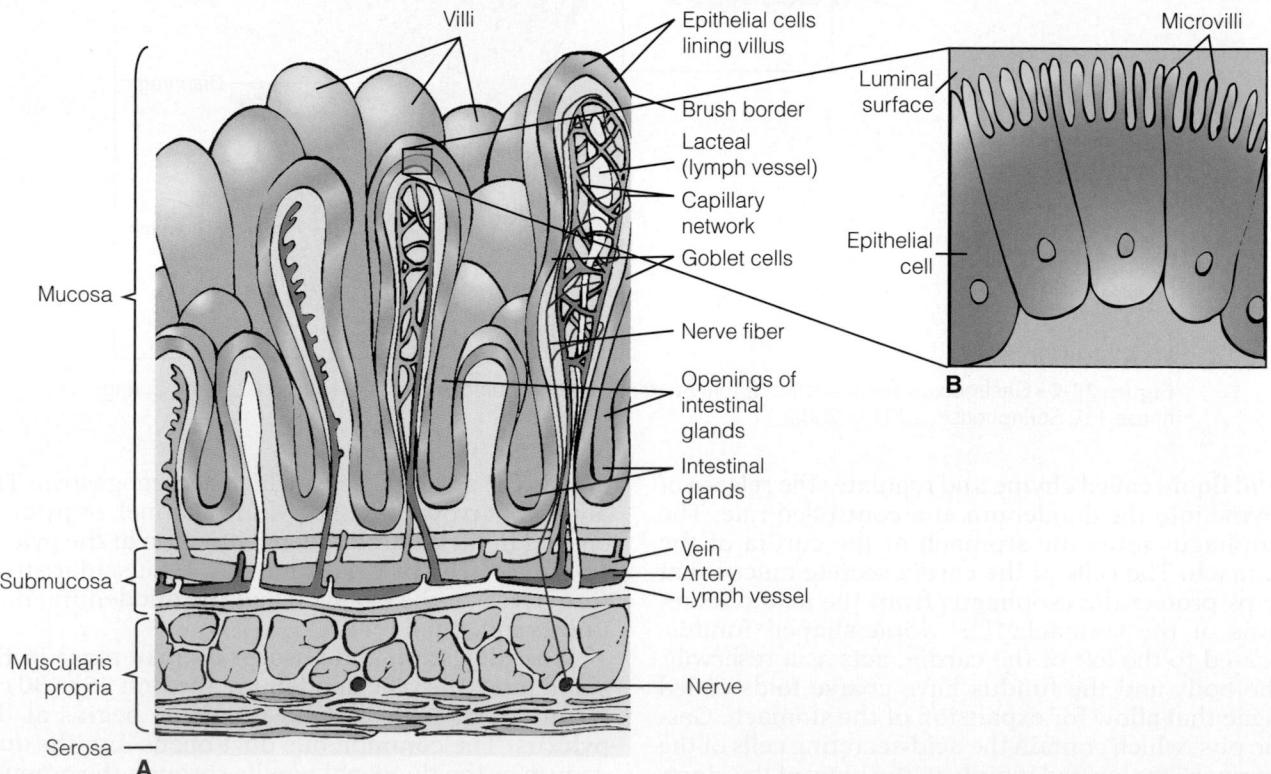

Figure 38-4 • A: Layers of tissue in the gastrointestinal tract. **B:** Microvilli on the luminal surface of intestinal epithelial cells.

sae. A single layer of epithelial cells lines the mucosa. The tight junctions between the epithelial cells act as a barrier to bacteria and other large molecules. In the small intestine, this layer is more convoluted and possesses finger-like projections called villi (see Fig. 38-4). Such structural modifications dramatically increase the surface area of the small intestine, thereby facilitating absorption. The lamina propria, a layer of connective tissue, contains capillaries and lymph vessels. The muscularis mucosae, the innermost layer, is composed of two layers of smooth muscle. The mucosa contains cells that produce gastrointestinal secretions and cells that are sensitive to chemical and mechanical stimuli.

Submucosa

The submucosa contains blood vessels, nerve networks, and connective tissue. The submucosa of the small intestine contains aggregates of lymphatic tissue (Peyer's patches), which are especially numerous in the ileum. Specialized mucosal cells that lie superiorly to the patches of lymphatic tissue in the small intestine absorb viral and bacterial antigens. These specialized cells sensitize the lymphatic cells to antigens and manufacture and secrete antibodies of immunoglobulin class A (IgA). The antibodies protect the body from the antigen the next time (or times) it enters the small intestine.

Muscularis Propria

The muscularis propria consists of two layers of smooth muscle, an inner circular muscle layer and an outer longitudinal layer. The two smooth muscle layers function in the two major types of gastrointestinal motility: propulsive motion and mixing movements. The stomach has an additional layer of smooth muscle to facilitate its food-mixing movements.

Serosa

The serosa, or adventitia, is the outermost layer of the gastrointestinal tract. The serosa is continuous with the mesentery and forms part of the visceral peritoneum.

INNERVATION

The gastrointestinal tract is innervated by the autonomic nervous system (ANS). The ANS can be divided into the extrinsic nervous system and the intrinsic (enteric) nervous system.

Extrinsic Nervous System

The extrinsic nervous system is further divided into parasympathetic and sympathetic branches (Fig. 38-5). Supplied primarily by the vagus and pelvic nerves,

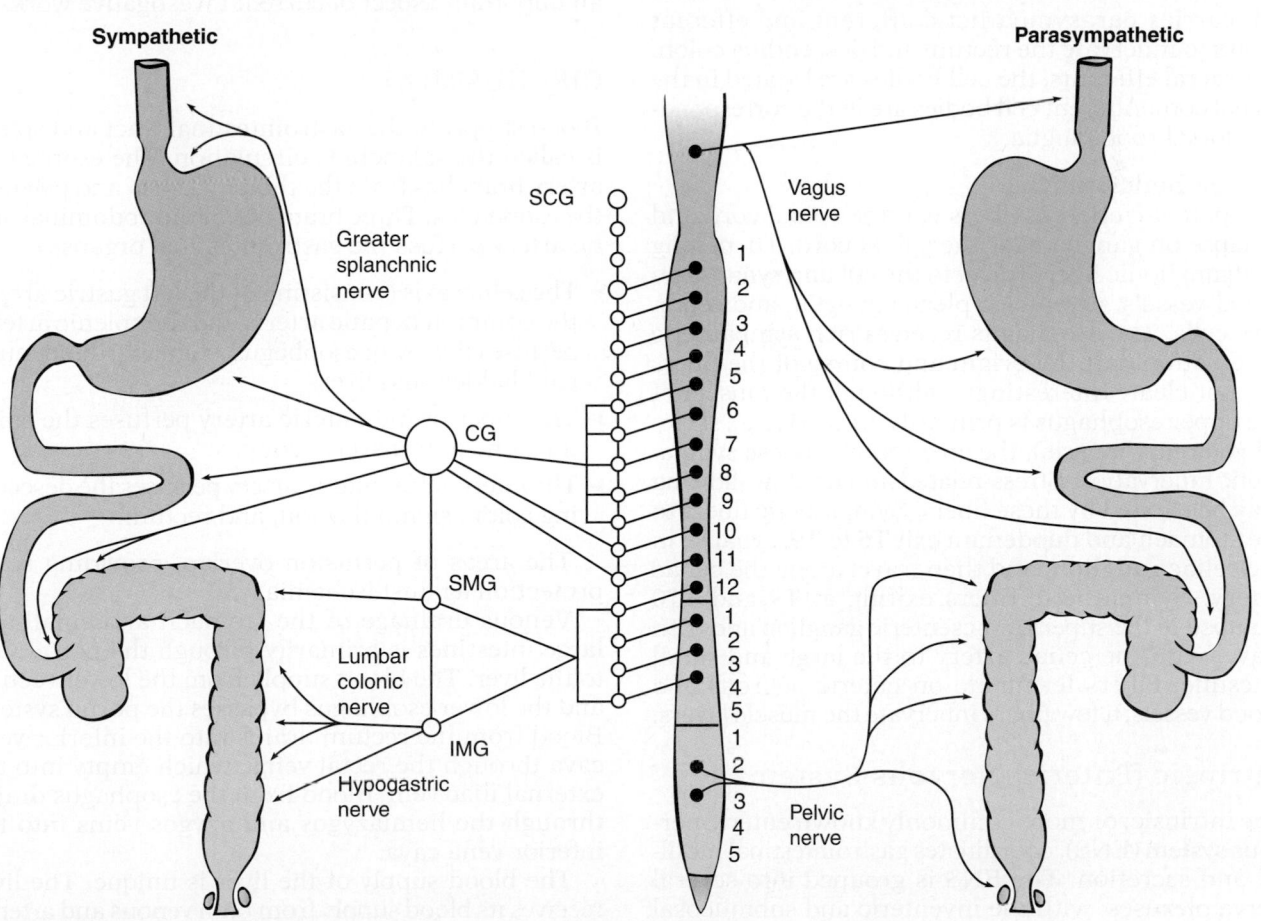

Figure 38-5 • Extrinsic efferent innervation of the gastrointestinal tract. CG, celiac ganglion; IMG, inferior mesenteric ganglion; SCG, superior cervical ganglion; SMG, superior mesenteric ganglion. (Redrawn from Johnson LR [ed]: Physiology of the Gastrointestinal Tract. New York: Raven Press, 1987, p 508.)

parasympathetic stimulation increases gastrointestinal activity through sensory and motor fibers to promote motility, relax sphincters, and promote secretion. Activation of the sympathetic nerves usually inhibits the motor and secretory activities of the gastrointestinal system.

Parasympathetic Branch

Parasympathetic efferent (motor) fibers of the gastrointestinal tract are preganglionic fibers carried primarily by the vagus and pelvic nerves. Vagal parasympathetic efferent preganglionic fibers richly innervate the gastrointestinal tract, including the esophagus, stomach, and small intestine. It is generally accepted that vagal efferents innervate the colon, but their distribution and function are controversial. Cell bodies for the vagal efferents are located primarily in the dorsal motor nucleus of the vagus. Vagal efferents synapse onto neurons in the myenteric plexus, or Auerbach plexus, which lies between the circular and longitudinal layers of smooth muscle cells in the muscularis propria. Postganglionic fibers then synapse with secretory and smooth muscle cells.

Vagal afferent (sensory) fibers originate in the esophagus, stomach, small intestine, and possibly the large intestine. The cell bodies are located in the nodose ganglion (in the neck) and join the vagus high in the neck. Afferent fibers relay information about pain and distention to the brain and spinal cord.

The pelvic nerve, issuing from spinal routes S2 to S4, carries parasympathetic afferent and efferent fibers to innervate the rectum and descending colon. For sacral efferents, the cell bodies are located in the spinal cord. Afferent cell bodies are in the corresponding dorsal root ganglia.

Sympathetic Branch

Sympathetic efferent fibers exit the spinal cord and synapse on ganglia near the spinal cord. Then, long postganglionic fibers travel to the gut and synapse on blood vessels, myenteric plexus ganglia, and secretory cells. The esophagus receives rich sympathetic innervation, but the origin and course of the fibers are not clear. Interestingly, although the muscle of the upper esophagus is primarily striated (e.g., skeletal voluntary muscle), the area receives dense sympathetic innervation. Stress-related impaired swallowing may be elicited by these fibers. Sympathetic fibers to the stomach and duodenum exit T6 to T9, synapse in the celiac ganglion, and then travel along the celiac artery. Sympathetic fibers exiting at T9 and T10 synapse in the superior mesenteric ganglion and then travel with the celiac artery to the large and small intestine. Fibers terminate on enteric neurons and blood vessels; a few fibers innervate the muscle layers.

Intrinsic (Enteric) Nervous System

The intrinsic, or more commonly known enteric nervous system (ENS), coordinates gastrointestinal motility and secretion. The ENS is grouped into several nerve plexuses, with the myenteric and submucosal plexuses being the most prominent. The nerves in these plexuses receive input from receptors in the gastrointestinal tract and from the ENS. When integrated into the intrinsic system, this input helps coordinate function. Peripheral fibers innervate the voluntary muscles responsible for chewing, swallowing, and defecating.

The ENS is a complex network embedded in the wall of the gastrointestinal tract from the pharynx to the anus. It includes enteric neurons and the processes of afferent and efferent extrinsic neurons. There are two main ganglionic plexuses containing the cell bodies of enteric neurons: the myenteric plexus (between the longitudinal and circular muscle layers) and the submucosal plexus, or Meissner plexus (between the circular muscle and the mucosa). From these two ganglionic plexuses emerge smaller bundles of fibers forming nonganglionic plexuses in longitudinal and circular muscle, around blood vessels, in the muscularis mucosae, at the base of mucosal glands, and within the villi.

Enteric neuronal neurotransmitters include acetylcholine, norepinephrine, serotonin, and dopamine. Neuropeptides form the largest group of potential enteric neurotransmitters. These include substance P, vasoactive intestinal polypeptide, gastric inhibitory peptide (GIP), and opioid peptides. There is evidence that these neuropeptides participate in the control of all gastrointestinal functions (secretion, motility, and absorption). How actions of these substances integrate with those of more classic neurotransmitters is an important aspect of current investigative work.

CIRCULATION

Blood supply to the gastrointestinal tract and spleen is called the splanchnic circulation. The esophageal artery branches from the thoracic aorta and perfuses the esophagus. Three branches of the abdominal aortic artery perfuse the gastrointestinal organs:

▶ The celiac axis (consisting of the left gastric artery, the common hepatic artery, and the splenic artery) perfuses the lower esophagus, stomach, duodenum, gallbladder, and liver.

▶ The superior mesenteric artery perfuses the small intestine to transverse colon.

▶ The inferior mesenteric artery perfuses the descending colon, sigmoid colon, and rectum.

The areas of perfusion overlap, providing some protection against ischemia.

Venous drainage of the stomach and small and large intestines is primarily through the portal vein to the liver. The blood supply from the lower rectum and the lower esophagus bypasses the portal system. Blood from the rectum drains into the inferior vena cava through the rectal veins, which empty into the external iliac vein. Blood from the esophagus drains through the hemiazygos and azygos veins into the inferior vena cava.

The blood supply of the liver is unique. The liver receives its blood supply from both venous and arterial sources. The venous blood is supplied by the portal vein, which drains most of the blood from the gastrointestinal tract (Fig. 38-6). The portal vein forms behind the spleen at the confluence of the superior mesenteric and splenic veins and leads to the liver. The arterial supply is by the common hepatic artery, which branches from the celiac trunk near the aorta and then perfuses the liver. Both sets of vessels form capillaries and then drain into the hepatic vein, which in turn feeds into the inferior vena cava.

The gastrointestinal system receives about one fourth of the resting cardiac output, more than any other organ system. When circulation is impaired (as in shock), perfusion to the splanchnic bed is shunted to the systemic circulation. Because splanchnic organs normally extract only about 20% of the oxygen from the perfusing blood, splanchnic perfusion can be reduced without compromising the organs. However, a severe reduction in splanchnic perfusion can damage the mucosal lining of the gut.

• Function of the Gastrointestinal System

The main function of the gastrointestinal tract is to break down nutrients into a form of usable energy. Food is ingested in the form of macromolecules that cannot be absorbed. These macromolecules are converted into usable forms of energy by mixing with di-gestive enzymes and secretions as they move through the gastrointestinal tract. These processes will be discussed in relationship to the various parts of the gastrointestinal tract and the secretions and motility that make digestion possible.

OROPHARYNX

Secretions

The salivary glands of the oropharynx produce saliva. There are three pairs of salivary glands: the submaxillary glands, the sublingual glands, and the parotid glands. These glands are drained by ducts into the mouth. Saliva is composed of mucus (a lubricant that facilitates swallowing), lingual lipase (a fat-digesting enzyme secreted by tongue glands), salivary amylase (an enzyme that breaks down starch), and class A (IgA) antibodies (which provide a first line of defense against bacteria, viruses, and bacteriostatic and carcinogenic chemicals; Table 38-1). A moist oral cavity also facilitates speech. The pH of saliva is 7 and contains bicarbonate, which allows saliva to neutralize acid substances that enter the oral cavity, including regurgitated gastric acid. Lingual lipase digests about 30% of the dietary fat in the stomach. The salivary glands secrete about one half of the digestive amylase used in digestion; the rest is secreted by the pancreas.

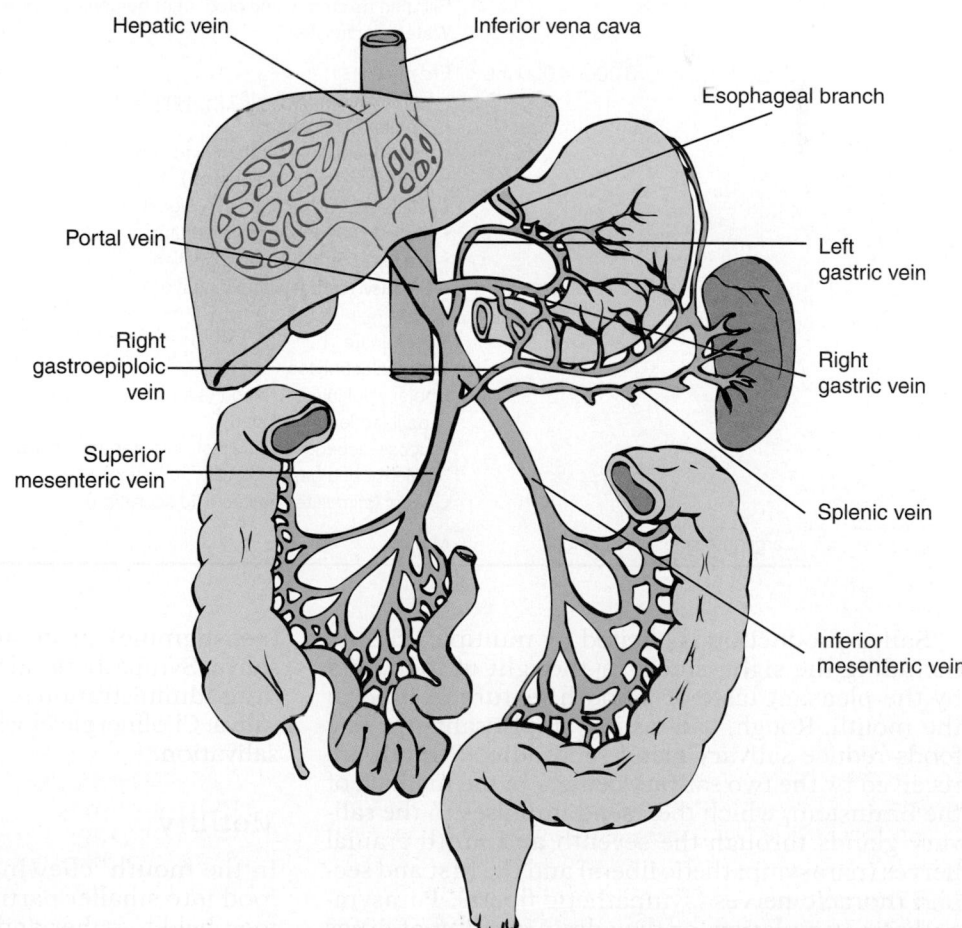

Figure 38-6 • Portal circulation. Blood from the gastrointestinal tract, spleen, and pancreas travels to the liver by way of the portal vein before moving into the inferior vena cava for return to the heart.

980

Table 38-1 • Major Gastrointestinal Secretions

Location	Daily Volume	Composition (and Action)
Mouth	1,000–2,000 mL	Amylase (carbohydrate digestion) Lipase (fat digestion) Immunoglobulins Mucus Water, electrolytes
Esophagus	300–800 mL	Mucus
Stomach	2,000 mL	Intrinsic factor (vitamin B_{12} absorption) Hydrochloric acid (activates pepsinogen) Pepsinogen (protein digestion) Mucus Water, electrolytes Gastrin (stimulates hydrochloric acid release; trophic effects on mucosa, especially in stomach)
Pancreas	1,200–1,800 mL	Enzymes • Amylase (carbohydrate digestion) • Trypsinogen (protein digestion) • Chymotrypsin (protein digestion) • Elastase (protein digestion) • Carboxypeptidase (protein digestion) • Lipase (fat digestion) • Colipase (fat digestion) • Esterase (cholesterol digestion) • Phospholipase (phospholipid digestion) • Nucleases (RNA and DNA digestion) Bicarbonate (protects luminal wall by neutralizing acid) Water, electrolytes
Liver	500–1,000 mL	Bile salts (emulsify fats) Bilirubin (excretory end product of hemoglobin breakdown) Water, electrolytes
Small intestine	3,000–4,000 mL	Enzymes • Enterokinase (activates trypsinogen) • Lipase (fat digestion) • Enteropeptidase (protein digestion) • Peptidase (protein digestion) • Nucleases (RNA and DNA digestion) • Maltase (carbohydrate digestion) • Lactase (carbohydrate digestion) • Sucrase (carbohydrate digestion) Mucus Bicarbonate Water, electrolytes Cholecystokinin into blood (stimulates pancreatic secretion and gallbladder contraction) Glucose-dependent insulinotropic peptide into blood (stimulates insulin release and gastric motility, secretion) Gastrin (stimulates gastric acid secretion)
Large intestine	Variable	Mucus

Saliva production is elicited by multiple stimuli, including the sight, smell, or thought of food, and by the pleasant taste or smooth texture of food in the mouth. Rough, bad-tasting, unpleasant-smelling foods reduce salivary gland secretions. Stimuli are received by the two salivary centers in the medulla of the brainstem, which then send impulses to the salivary glands through the seventh and ninth cranial nerves (parasympathetic fibers) and the first and second thoracic nerves (sympathetic fibers). Parasympathetic stimulation, or the administration of drugs that mimic stimulation (cholinergics) or enhance it (neostigmine), promotes copious secretion of watery saliva. Sympathetic stimulation or sympathomimetic drug administration produces a scanty output of thick saliva. Cholinergic blockers (e.g., atropine) also inhibit salivation.

Motility

In the mouth, chewing mechanically breaks down food into smaller particles. This produces a bolus of food held together and lubricated by saliva that can then be propelled into the stomach by the process of

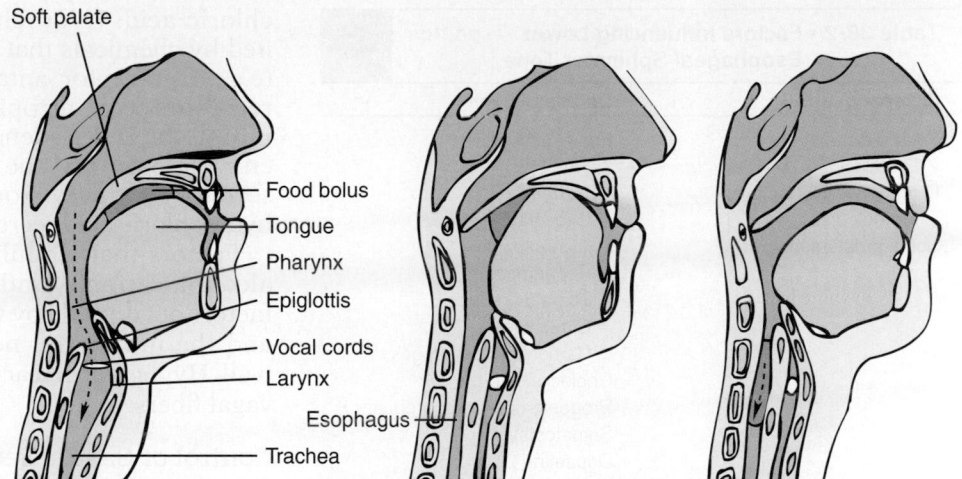

Figure 38-7 • Swallowing. Passage of bolus of food from the mouth through the pharynx. (From Rhoades RA, Pflanzer RG (eds): Human Physiology, 3rd ed. Philadelphia: WB Saunders, 1996. Reprinted with permission of Brooks/Cole, a division of Thomson Learning: http://www.thomson rights.com. Fax 800-730-2215.)

Labels: Soft palate, Food bolus, Tongue, Pharynx, Epiglottis, Vocal cords, Larynx, Esophagus, Trachea

swallowing. Swallowing is a complex process that has several phases (Fig. 38-7). During the oral phase, the tongue propels the food or fluid bolus to the posterior pharynx. This is a voluntary process. During the involuntary pharyngeal phase, the presence of food or fluid in the pharynx stimulates pharyngeal sensory receptors that initiate impulses through cranial nerve V (the trigeminal nerve) to the swallowing center in the medulla. Sensory impulses reflexively trigger the outflow of impulses down motor fibers in cranial nerve IX (the glossopharyngeal nerve) and cranial nerve X (the vagus nerve) to pharyngeal and laryngeal structures. This causes the following coordinated events, which propel the solid or fluid substance into the esophagus:

1. The soft palate elevates and retracts, sealing off the nasopharynx to prevent regurgitation.
2. The vocal cords close, and the epiglottis closes over the larynx to prevent aspiration.
3. The UES relaxes.
4. The larynx pulls up and increases the opening of the esophagus and UES.
5. The pharyngeal muscles contract, propelling food or fluid into the opened esophagus.

During this phase, respiration is reflexively inhibited. Damage to sensory or motor fibers (in cranial nerves V, IX, or X) or to the swallowing center in the brainstem weakens or eliminates the ability to swallow or causes poorly coordinated swallowing, wherein food or fluid enters the nasopharynx or larynx, or both.

ESOPHAGUS

Secretions

Esophageal mucosal cells secrete mucus (see Table 38-1). The mucus protects the esophageal lining from damage by gastric secretions or food and acts as a lubricant to facilitate the passage of food.

Motility

The esophageal phase of swallowing begins once food or fluid enters the esophagus (Fig. 38-8). Swallowing-induced contractions of the esophagus are called primary peristalsis. The wave of peristalsis causes the LES to relax, thereby allowing food to enter the stomach. If primary peristalsis is unable to clear the esophagus, food or fluid distends the esophagus. This distention stimulates stretch receptors that reflexively promote relaxation of the esophageal muscles ahead of the area of distention as well as contraction of the esophageal muscles in and behind it. This propels the food or fluid ahead into the newly relaxed area, which then becomes distended. This is called secondary peristalsis. The peristalsis reflex repeatedly recurs until the food or fluid arrives at the LES.

The tone of the LES can be altered by a variety of agents (Table 38-2). Some people suffer from a hypertrophic LES, which impedes esophageal emptying (and can lead to overdistention of the lower

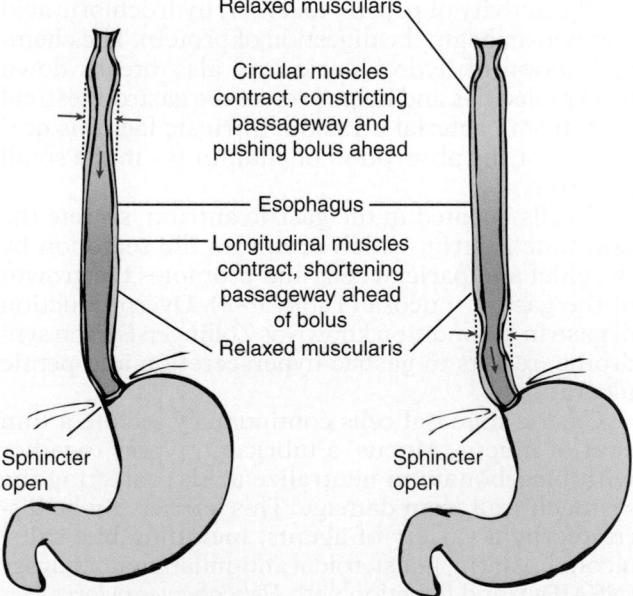

Figure 38-8 • Movement of a bolus of food through the esophagus by a peristaltic contraction. (From Rhoades RA, Pflanzer RG (eds): Human Physiology, 3rd ed. Philadelphia: WB Saunders, 1996. Reprinted with permission of Brooks/Cole, a division of Thomson Learning: http://www.thomsonrights.com. Fax 800-730-2215.)

Labels: Relaxed muscularis; Circular muscles contract, constricting passageway and pushing bolus ahead; Esophagus; Longitudinal muscles contract, shortening passageway ahead of bolus; Relaxed muscularis; Sphincter open; Sphincter open

Table 38-2 • Factors Influencing Lower Esophageal Sphincter Tone	
Increased Tone	**Decreased Tone**
Food substances:	Food substances:
Protein	Fats
Drugs:	Coffee
Metoclopramide	Chocolate
Some prostaglandins (F₂)	Alcohol
	Peppermint
	Tomato products
	Citrus juices
	Carbonated beverages
	Cholecystokinin
	Progesterone (as in pregnancy)
	Somatostatin
	Dopamine
	Some prostaglandins (E₂, A₂)
	Cigarette smoking

esophagus), whereas others have an incompetent LES, which results in repeated episodes of gastric reflux (which can lead to lower esophageal strictures).

STOMACH

Secretions

The major secretions of the stomach are hydrochloric acid, intrinsic factor, pepsinogen, gastrin, and mucus (see Table 38-1).

The oxyntic glands contain parietal cells that secrete hydrochloric acid and intrinsic factor. Hydrochloric acid converts pepsinogen, which is secreted by the chief cells of the stomach, to pepsin, a proteolytic enzyme. The hydrochloric acid provides an ideal pH for the activity of pepsin; together, hydrochloric acid and pepsin begin the digestion of protein. The chemical action of hydrochloric acid also breaks down food molecules and helps protect the gastrointestinal tract from bacterial invasion. Intrinsic factor is necessary for the absorption of vitamin B_{12} in the small intestine.

G cells, located in the gastric antrum, secrete the hormone gastrin, which promotes the secretion by the chief and parietal cells and promotes the growth of the gastric mucosa (Table 38-3). Overproduction of gastrin, a condition known as Zollinger-Ellison syndrome, results in gastric hypersecretion and peptic ulceration.

Gastric mucosal cells continuously secrete a thin coat of mucus. Mucus, a lubricant, works together with bicarbonate to neutralize acid, protecting the stomach wall from damage. This barrier can be disrupted by a variety of agents, including bile salts, alcohol, aspirin, nonsteroidal anti-inflammatory drugs (NSAIDs), and infection with *Helicobacter pylori*.

Factors Affecting Gastric Secretions

The gastric parietal cells contain receptors for acetylcholine, histamine, and gastrin. Stimulation of these receptors prompts the parietal cells to secrete hydrochloric acid. Hydrochloric acid secretion is inhibited by chemicals that block the histamine receptors (e.g., H_2-receptor antagonists) or the acetylcholine receptors (e.g., atropine). Proton pump inhibitors inhibit the H^+/K^+-adenosine triphosphatase (ATPase) enzyme pathway, the final common step in the acid secretory pathway. Some prostaglandins also inhibit hydrochloric acid secretion.

Factors that stimulate gastric secretions include alcohol, caffeine, and hypoglycemia. The first two factors act directly by way of gastric chemoreceptors and the intramural nerve plexuses in the stomach wall. Hypoglycemia acts by way of the brainstem and vagal fibers.

Control of Gastric Secretions

Gastric secretions are regulated in three phases: the cephalic phase, the gastric phase, and the intestinal phase (Table 38-4). These phases are controlled by neural and hormonal mechanisms.

In the cephalic phase, the sight, smell, taste, or thought of food stimulates brainstem centers, reflexively prompting parasympathetic (vagal) stimulation of salivation, pancreatic secretion, bile release, and gastric secretions of pepsinogen and hydrochloric acid by the chief and parietal cells, respectively. Sympathetic stimulation can alter the cephalic phase response. This is the mechanism by which emotions can influence gastrointestinal secretions. Fear, anger, and depression decrease secretions.

During the gastric phase, distention of the stomach by food stimulates stretch receptors in the stomach wall. Chemicals, mainly proteins, stimulate chemoreceptors in the mucosa. The stretch receptors and chemoreceptors in turn activate neurons in the submucosal plexus, which then stimulate neurons in the myenteric plexus, which in turn stimulate secretion by the parietal and chief cells. Proteins in the chyme also directly promote gastrin secretion by G cells; the gastrin provides an additional stimulus for parietal and chief cell secretion. A combination of events eventually brings the gastric phase to a halt: the stretch receptors and chemoreceptors in the wall of the stomach become refractory to stimulation, the acidity of the chyme inhibits further gastrin secretion, and GIP decreases hydrochloric acid secretion and gastric motility.

The intestinal phase begins after chyme reaches the duodenum. The acidity of the chyme stimulates duodenal mucosal cells to release secretin into the bloodstream; proteins and fat trigger the release of cholecystokinin (CCK) into the blood from similar cells, and glucose and fat stimulate the secretion of GIP. Secretin and CCK cause pancreatic secretion and release of gallbladder contents into the duodenum. GIP stimulates the release of insulin from the islets of Langerhans and decreases gastric motility and secretions (see Table 38-3). Stretch receptors in the duodenum trigger peristalsis so that chyme is degraded, mixed with enzymes and diluents, and moved past the highly absorbent small intestinal lumen. If the chyme is less acidic, gastrin is released.

Table 38-3 • Hormones Controlling Secretion and Motility

Hormone	Source	Stimulation of Release	Major Function
Gastrin	Stomach, small intestine	Gastric distention, presence of partially digested protein near pylorus	Stimulates • Gastric acid secretion • Gastric intrinsic factor secretion • Gastric motility • Intestinal motility • Mucosal growth • Pancreatic growth • Pancreatic insulin release • Lower esophageal tone
Secretin	Small intestine	Acid entering small intestine	Stimulates • Pancreatic bicarbonate secretion • Pancreatic enzyme secretion • Pancreatic growth • Gastric pepsin secretion • Bile bicarbonate secretion • Gallbladder contraction Inhibits • Gastric emptying • Gastric motility • Intestinal motility
Cholecystokinin	Small intestine	Fatty acids and amino acids in small intestine	Stimulates • Gastric acid secretion • Gastric motility • Intestinal motility • Colonic motility • Gallbladder contraction and sphincter of Oddi relaxation (thus increasing bile flow into small intestine) • Pancreatic bicarbonate secretion • Pancreatic enzyme release • Pancreatic growth Inhibits • Lower esophageal tone • Gastric emptying
Gastric inhibitory peptide	Small intestine	Fatty acids and lipids in small intestine	Inhibits • Gastric acid secretion • Gastric emptying • Gastric motility Stimulates • Insulin release • Intestinal motility
Motilin	Small intestine	Acid and fat in small intestine	Stimulates • Gastric motility • Intestinal motility

Under neural control, motilin is another hormone that is cyclically released during fasting. Motilin stimulates stomach and small intestine motility.

Motility

The passage of food from the esophagus into the stomach reflexively initiates receptive relaxation. After the stomach has filled with food, peristaltic contractions mix the food and propel gastric contents toward the pylorus, where small amounts enter the duodenum. The pyloric sphincter plays a minor role in gastric emptying; its main function is to prevent duodenal reflux. The bile acids in the chyme that reenters the stomach through duodenal reflux damage the chemical barrier that coats the surfaces of gastric mucosal cells. Mild peristaltic contractions that persist after the stomach has completely emptied are called hunger contractions; however, they play no role in appetite regulation. Gastric emptying can be retarded by vagotomy; by the presence of fats, proteins, or hydrochloric acid in the duodenal chyme; by duodenal distention; and by intestinal hormones.

Emesis, or vomiting, is the regurgitation of food from the stomach through the mouth. During vomiting, the abdominal muscles and diaphragm contract,

Table 38-4 • Phases of Gastric Secretion

Phase	Stimulus to Secretion	Effect
Cephalic (neuronal)	Sight, smell, taste of food initiates central nervous system impulse mediated by vagus nerve	Gastric effects: 　Hydrochloric acid (from parietal cells) 　Pepsinogen (from chief cells) 　Mucus secretion Other effects: 　Salivation 　Pancreatic secretion 　Bile release
Gastric (neuronal and hormonal)	Food in antrum initiates central nervous system impulse mediated by vagus nerve	Gastrin release Hydrochloric acid release Pepsinogen release
Intestinal (hormonal)	Chyme in small intestine	pH of chyme <2: release of secretin, gastric inhibitory polypeptide, cholecystokinin (decreases gastric acid secretion) pH of chyme >3: release of gastrin (increases gastric acid secretion)

and the LES relaxes, allowing reflux of gastric content into the esophagus and propulsion of gastric contents out of the mouth. The reflex elevation of the palate prevents expulsion through the nasopharynx. Respiratory inhibition and closure of the glottis prevent pulmonary aspiration. In addition, irritation of the small intestine (by materials in the chyme, by inflammation, or by a disease process) can cause reverse peristalsis. These movements move chyme toward the pyloric valve. If strong enough to force open the pylorus, intestinal contents may be vomited. When yellow bile from the duodenum is exposed to acid in the stomach, the interaction turns the vomitus green. Occasionally, vomiting of intestinal contents can be so rapid that the vomitus contains yellow bile. When blood is exposed to acid in the stomach, the exposure results in a brownish-black "coffee-ground" emesis. If the rapidity of vomiting does not allow sufficient time for this interaction between acid and blood to occur, blood in the vomitus has its normal red color (hematemesis).

PANCREAS

The pancreas is composed of both exocrine and endocrine tissue. The islets of Langerhans, endocrine tissue scattered throughout the pancreas, secrete insulin, glucagon, and pancreatic polypeptide hormones, which aid in the digestive process. The exocrine pancreas is composed of acinar cells, which are arranged in lobules. The acinar cells empty secretions into an internal pancreatic ductal system (Fig. 38-9). These internal ducts drain into progressively larger ducts that terminate in the duct of Wirsung, the main pancreatic duct. This pancreatic duct then joins the common bile duct to form a shared short duct called the ampulla of Vater. This ampulla, carrying bile and pancreatic secretions, opens into the duodenum. A smooth muscle ring, the sphincter of Oddi, encircles the ampulla. Because of the anatomical arrangements between the common bile duct and the duct of Wirsung, a gallstone that obstructs the ampulla of Vater can ob-

struct the normal flow of bile and pancreatic secretions. (Such obstruction, although rare, can lead to a stasis of pancreatic secretion, resulting in acute pancreatitis.) Some people have a second external pancreatic duct (duct of Santorini) that opens into the duodenum near the pylorus.

The exocrine acinar cells secrete both a watery alkaline bicarbonate solution and enzymes (see Table 38-1). The large amount of water secreted by the pancreas is instrumental in diluting chyme before absorption. In addition, the bicarbonate neutralizes the highly acidic chyme from the stomach. The pancreatic enzymes digest proteins (trypsin, chymotrypsin, elastase, and carboxypeptidase), fats (lipase, colipase, and esterase), phospholipase and nucleic acids (nucleases), and starch (amylase). Although pancreatic enzymes require a pH close to neutrality for optimal activity, they are capable of nearly completing the digestion of food in the absence of all other digestive secretions.

Pancreatic enzymes are secreted from the pancreas in their inactive forms. Trypsin inhibitor prevents the premature activation of trypsinogen into its active form, trypsin. Once the pancreatic secretions arrive in the duodenum, trypsinogen is activated by an intestinal mucosal enzyme, enterokinase, into its active form, trypsin. Trypsin then activates the other pancreatic enzymes.

Regulation of pancreatic secretion occurs by neural and hormonal means. Vagal stimulation results in the secretion of pancreatic enzymes. Hormonal regulation occurs as a result of duodenal mucosal responses to chyme and is discussed later.

GALLBLADDER

In the duodenum, chyme mixed with pancreatic secretions is watery. The fat in chyme is not water soluble and requires a solvent enzyme mixture from the liver to render it absorbable by intestinal cells. Hepatocytes, among many other metabolic functions, make bile. Bile is a mixture of bile salts, cholesterol, biliru-

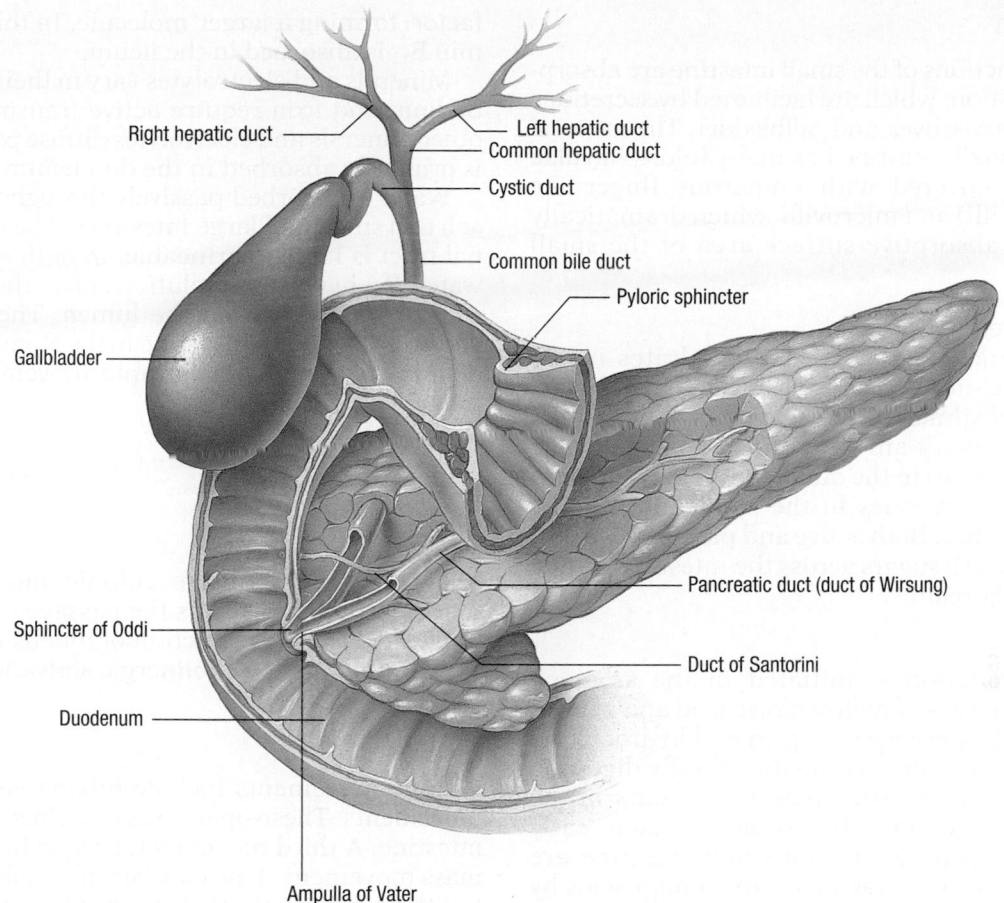

Figure 38-9 • Biliary system. (From Anatomical Chart Company: Atlas of Human Anatomy. Springhouse, PA: Springhouse, 2001, p 217.)

bin, and acids suspended in water. This solution emulsifies the fat in chyme, breaking the fat into small globules that can be absorbed across the intestinal lumen. The action of bile ionizes fat-soluble vitamins into absorbable forms. Bile also suspends cholesterol, triglycerides, and multiple-density lipoproteins in the bloodstream, thus preventing precipitation and deposition of these molecules in the vasculature until they can be catabolized.

Bile is stored and concentrated in the gallbladder. Gallbladder secretion is greatest during the intestinal phase of digestion. This activity is stimulated by CCK, which is secreted by the intestinal mucosa when fatty acids or amino acids are present. CCK causes gallbladder contraction and relaxation of the sphincter of Oddi, allowing the release of bile into the duodenum to mix with chyme.

SMALL INTESTINE

Secretions

In the duodenum, chyme mixes with pancreatic digestive enzymes, alkaline substances, water, mucus, and bile. When the mucosa of the small intestine is exposed to acid in the chyme, secretin is released. Secretin stimulates bicarbonate release by cells that line the bile ducts. The intestinal enzymes secretin, CCK, and enterokinase are added to this mixture, along with mucus, bicarbonate, and water. The small intestine secretes 3 to 4 liters a day of alkaline secretions. These intestinal secretions help maintain the liquidity of chyme and can dilute noxious agents.

Motility

The small intestine has two types of characteristic movements, propulsive and mixing. The intramural plexuses initiate and coordinate these movements, but the movements can be enhanced or retarded by extrinsic autonomic stimulation, as discussed previously. Propulsive movements propel food forward, allowing for digestion and absorption. This peristalsis is stimulated by distention. During mixing movement, localized concentric contractions of the intestinal wall called segmentation promote mixing of food particles. These segments have the appearance of linked sausages. Repetition of this process continually kneads the chyme, which increases the exposure of the molecules to the absorptive surfaces of the intestinal mucosa.

Emptying of the small intestine into the colon occurs in the same way as gastric emptying. Peristaltic waves build pressure in the ileum behind the ileocecal valve and push the chyme through the valve into the colon. The ileocecal valve then prevents backflow. Ileal emptying can be retarded by intramural reflexes, which are initiated by a full (distended) colon.

Absorption

The major functions of the small intestine are absorption and digestion, which are facilitated by secretions from the pancreas, liver, and gallbladder. The mucosal layer of the small intestine has many folds (valvulae conniventes) covered with numerous finger-like projections (villi) and microvilli, which dramatically increase the absorptive surface area of the small intestine.

Carbohydrates

The three major sources of carbohydrates in the human diet are sucrose, lactose, and starch. The breakdown of carbohydrates begins in the mouth when food mixes with salivary amylase during chewing. The digestion continues in the duodenum. Conversion to simple sugars continues in the small intestine by intestinal enzymes. Both active and passive transport are used to absorb sugars across the intestinal lumen into the bloodstream.

Proteins

Protein degradation is initiated in the stomach through the actions of hydrochloric acid and pepsin. However, in the absence of pepsin and hydrochloric acid, the small intestine is capable of fully digesting all available protein. Most digestion occurs in the duodenum and jejunum by proteolytic pancreatic enzymes. Polypeptides in the small intestine are degraded into peptide fragments and amino acids by trypsin, chymotrypsin, and carboxypeptidase. Amino acids are absorbed into the blood by active and passive diffusion.

Fats

Triglycerides, lipids, and phospholipids are first degraded in the small intestine. Bile salts, in a process called emulsification, facilitate the creation of small droplets of fats from larger globules. Pancreatic enzymes then degrade the fats into fatty acid chains and monoglycerides. These smaller molecules form into even smaller globules, called micelles. Fatty acids and monosaccharides are transported across the intestinal mucosa from a micelle passively, leaving bile behind.

In the submucosa, free fatty acids are passed into the blood directly, if small enough. If too large for direct passive diffusion, the free fatty acid is reorganized into a triglyceride, coupled with lipoproteins and cholesterol, and passed into the lymph fluid as chylomicron.

The bile left behind in the intestine after absorption of fats from a micelle is reabsorbed in the ileum. If bile salts enter the colon, they decrease the reabsorption of sodium and water, thereby increasing the liquidity of the undigested food residues in the colon. Most fat is absorbed by the time chyme reaches the middle of the jejunum.

Vitamins, Minerals, and Water

Most vitamins, whether fat or water soluble, diffuse across the intestinal mucosa and submucosa into the blood. Fat-soluble vitamin B_{12} couples with intrinsic factor, forming a larger molecule. In this form, vitamin B_{12} is absorbed in the ileum.

Minerals and electrolytes vary in their absorption. Sodium and iron require active transport, whereas other minerals and electrolytes diffuse passively. Iron is primarily absorbed in the duodenum.

Water is absorbed passively throughout the stomach and small and large intestines. The gastrointestinal tract is highly permeable, in both directions, to water. If a hypertonic solution enters the duodenum, osmosis occurs within the lumen. The converse is also true: a hypotonic chyme in the stomach and duodenum causes extremely rapid movement of water into the bloodstream.

LARGE INTESTINE

Secretion

The goblet cells of the colonic mucosa secrete mucus, which lubricates the passage of chyme (see Table 38-1). The production of mucus is stimulated by irritation and by cholinergic activation.

Motility

Colonic movements include mixing and peristaltic movements. These operate as described for the small intestine. A third movement, unique to the colon, is mass movement. This consists of simultaneous contractions of colonic smooth muscle over large portions of the descending and sigmoid portions of the colon. Mass movement rapidly moves the undigested food residue (feces) from these areas into the rectum.

Humans cannot digest the cellulose, hemicellulose, or lignin in plant tissues. These plant materials form a large portion of the undigested food residue. They are usually termed vegetable fiber or dietary bulk. These fibers attract and hold water, creating a larger, softer stool. Low quantities of bulk result in a relatively inactive colon, leading to bowel movements that are relatively infrequent and feces that are relatively small, dry, and difficult to pass. Epidemiological reports suggest that high-fiber diets are associated with a decreased incidence of diverticulitis and colon cancer.

Filling of the rectum triggers the defecation reflex by stimulating stretch receptors in the rectal wall. Stimulation of the stretch receptors causes sensory (afferent) nerve fibers to transmit impulses to the lower spinal cord. Because of anatomical arrangements of neurons in this part of the cord, these afferent impulses reflexively cause nerve impulses to travel out of the cord along parasympathetic motor fibers that innervate the smooth muscles of the descending and sigmoid colon, the rectum, and the internal anal sphincter. The afferent impulses also reflexively cause nerve impulses to be sent out of the cord along somatic motor neurons that innervate the skeletal muscle of the external anal sphincter. The total effect of these events is to produce coordinated expulsive contractions of the colon and rectum, relaxation (opening) of the sphincters, and expulsion of feces from the anus.

The urge to defecate begins after the pressure within the rectum reaches 18 mm Hg. After intrarectal pressure reaches 55 mm Hg, reflex bowel evacuation occurs. This defecation reflex is inhibited in a continent person by descending neuronal impulses from higher brain centers that inhibit the actions of the somatic motor neurons that innervate the external sphincter. Such inhibition keeps the external anal sphincter closed, thereby averting inappropriate defecation. After a few minutes, the defecation reflex subsides, but it usually becomes active again a few hours later. Defecation is a spinal cord reflex that does not require intact pathways between the sacral cord and the brain. In the early post-traumatic phase of spinal shock, the reflex does not work. After cord shock is ended, reflex defecation occurs once again, but voluntary inhibition is not possible (neurogenic bowel).

Absorption

In the large intestine, most of the water and potassium are absorbed from the chyme. This produces a semisolid residue of undigested food (feces) that can be eliminated from the body. Diarrhea can reduce the transit time for chyme, thereby limiting such potassium and water reabsorption. This can result in hypokalemia and dehydration. Diarrhea can be caused by materials that hold water in the chyme (e.g., magnesium sulfate), resulting in semiliquid stool.

At birth the colon is sterile, but large colonic bacterial populations become established soon afterward. Some of these organisms produce vitamin K and a number of B vitamins. Other bacteria produce ammonia, which is absorbed. Normally, ammonia is removed from the blood once it reaches the liver. However, in people with seriously impaired liver function or with collateral circulatory routes that bypass the liver (usually the result of portal hypertension), ammonia can remain in the circulation and lead to hepatic encephalopathy.

LIVER

The liver lies in the right upper quadrant of the abdomen. It has two lobes (right and left) and lies just below the diaphragm, with its greatest portion located on the right side of the body. Its superior (rounded) surface fits into the curve of the diaphragm and is in contact with the anterior wall of the abdominal cavity. The inferior surface is molded over the stomach, the duodenum, the pancreas, the hepatic flexure of the colon, the right kidney, and the right adrenal gland.

The liver is covered with a thin layer of peritoneum over a thin fibrous coat called Glisson's capsule. This fibrous capsule encases and partitions the liver, sending inward fibrous sheets that divide the liver into functional units called lobules. Each lobule consists of sheets of hepatocytes organized around a core cluster of vessels called the portal triad (Fig. 38-10). The portal triad includes the two sets of afferent vessels (portal vein and hepatic artery) and a small bile duct. The afferent vessels lead to the liver sinusoids, which drain into the efferent hepatic vein, lying at the periphery of each lobule.

The lobule measures approximately 1.5 mm in diameter and 8 mm in length. Each lobe of the liver

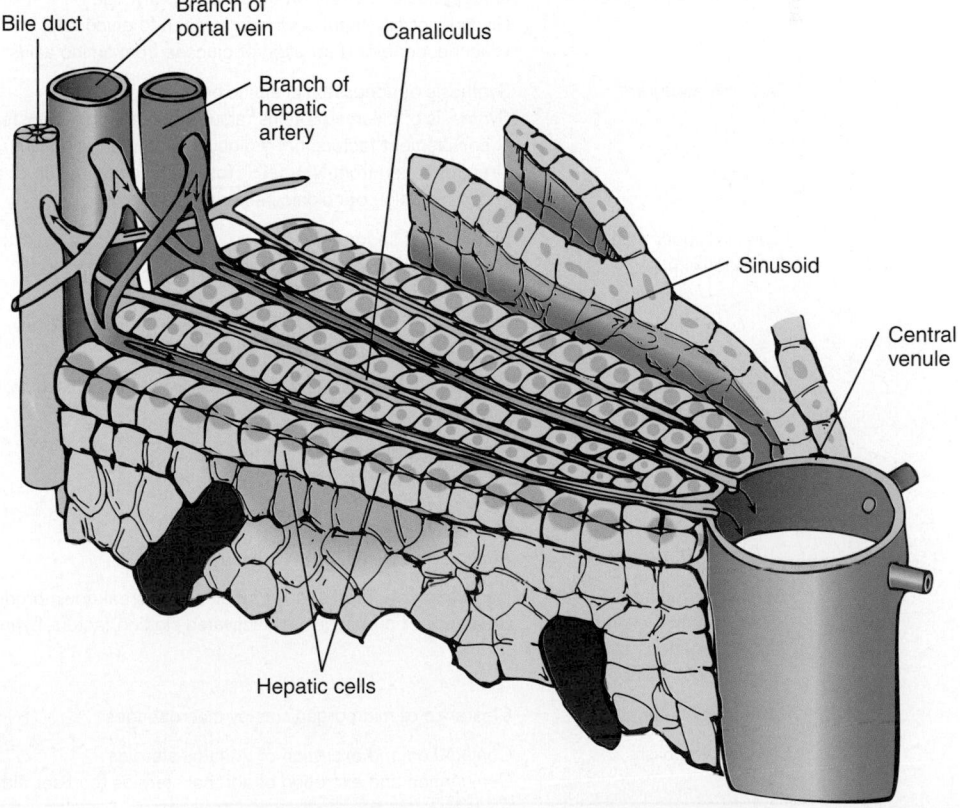

Figure 38-10 • A section of the liver lobule showing the location of the hepatic veins, hepatic cells, liver sinusoids, and branches of the portal vein and hepatic artery.

contains between 50,000 and 100,000 lobules. Rows of hepatocytes radiate from a central venule like spokes of a wheel. Branches of the hepatic artery and the hepatic portal vein lie at the periphery of the wheel. Blood from these branches is poured into open channels (hepatic sinuses) that run between alternate rows of hepatocytes. Kupffer's cells, specialized white cells of the reticuloendothelial system, phagocytize bacteria, debris, and other foreign matter in the sinus blood. The sinuses drain into the central venule, which in turn carries blood to the hepatic vein.

Blind-ended bile canaliculi arise between the other rows of hepatocytes. They carry newly secreted bile to larger ducts located at the periphery. These smaller ducts eventually drain into the common bile duct. Bile that is leaving the liver is concentrated and stored in the gallbladder. Fluid and electrolyte reabsorption in the gallbladder can increase the concentration of bile salts, cholesterol, and bilirubin 12-fold.

The gallbladder has a maximum capacity of 50 mL and can hold a 24-hour output of bile (600 mL) from the liver. The intestinal hormone CCK (secreted by the duodenal mucosa) and vagus nerve activity stimulate gallbladder contraction as a part of food digestion, particularly lipids. CCK and local reflexes initiated by duodenal peristalsis open the sphincter of Oddi. These events permit an outflow of bile down the common bile duct into the duodenum.

The common bile duct and the main duct from the pancreas usually unite just before the duct enters the lumen of the duodenum. There is often a dilation of the tube after this junction (the ampulla of Vater). The opening of the common bile duct in the duodenum is about 8 to 10 cm from the pylorus.

The liver cells perform many vital functions, as described in the sections that follow and summarized in Table 38-5.

Carbohydrate Metabolism

The liver participates in carbohydrate metabolism. The liver and skeletal muscle are the two primary sites of glycogen storage. Serum glucose levels are maintained by hepatic glycostatic function, involving two mechanisms. When plasma glucose levels are high, hepatocytes remove glucose from the plasma. Some of this glucose is then stored in the liver as glycogen. If plasma glucose levels decline, hepatocytes convert the glycogen back into glucose through a process called glycogenolysis, and the glucose is released into the bloodstream. Although many body tissues have the requisite cellular enzymes for glycogenolysis, hepatocytes are one of the few cell types that can release this intracellular glucose into the bloodstream. Hepatocytes do not simply respond directly to plasma glucose. These glycostatic functions are mediated by several

Table 38-5 • Hepatic Function

General Category	Specific Description
Carbohydrate metabolism	Glycogenesis (conversion of glucose to glycogen) Glycogenolysis (breakdown of glycogen to glucose) Gluconeogenesis (formation of glucose from amino acids or fatty acids)
Protein metabolism	Synthesis of nonessential amino acids Synthesis of plasma proteins (albumin, prealbumin, transferrin, clotting factors, complement factors; not γ-globulin or immunoglobulins) Urea formation from NH_3 (NH_3 formed by deamination of amino acids in liver and by action of colonic bacteria on proteins)
Lipid and lipoprotein metabolism	Synthesis of lipoproteins Breakdown of triglycerides into fatty acids and glycerol Formation of ketone bodies Synthesis of fatty acids from amino acids and glucose Synthesis and breakdown of cholesterol
Bile acid synthesis and excretion	Bile formation (containing bile salts, bile pigments [bilirubin, biliverdin]), cholesterol Bile excretion
Storage	Glucose (as glycogen) Vitamins (A, D, E, K, B_1, B_2, B_{12}, folic acid) Fatty acids Minerals (Fe, Cu) Amino acids (as albumin, β-globulins)
Biotransformation, detoxification, excretion of endogenous and exogenous compounds	Inactivation of drugs and excretion of the breakdown products Clearance of procoagulants, activated clotting factors, byproducts of coagulation
Removal of pathogens	Clearance of microorganisms by macrophages
Steroid catabolism	Conjugation and excretion of gonadal steroids Conjugation and excretion of adrenal steroids (cortisol, aldosterone)

hormones; some (e.g., insulin) promote hepatic glucose uptake, and others (e.g., glucagon, growth hormone, and epinephrine) stimulate glycogenolysis and the release of glucose from liver cells.

The liver does not contain enough glycogen reserves to be able to buffer plasma glucose during prolonged fasting or severe exercise. During these times, low plasma glucose levels stimulate the secretion of one or more hormones (glucagon, glucocorticoids, or thyroxine) that trigger the biochemical conversion of intracellular fatty and amino acids into glucose (gluconeogenesis), which the liver cell can then release into the bloodstream or store as glycogen. Only hepatocytes possess the enzyme that is critical for gluconeogenesis. Glycogen storage is important for other functions of liver cells. A glycogen-rich hepatocyte conjugates bilirubin at a faster rate and is more resistant to toxins and infectious agents.

Protein Metabolism

The liver plays an essential role in the metabolism of proteins. The amino acids that result from the breakdown of proteins are deaminated to form ammonia by the liver and then converted to urea. The liver also synthesizes plasma proteins, including albumins, globulins, fibrinogens, plasma lipoproteins, and other proteins involved in clotting. The albumins maintain normal plasma oncotic pressure. A fall in this pressure leads to edema (both systemic and pulmonary) and contributes to ascites. The globulins bind thyroid and adrenal hormones. Bound, the hormones are inactive. Decreased hepatic protein levels can lead to a clinical excess of these hormones.

Lipid and Lipoprotein Metabolism

The liver contributes to adipose stores through the metabolism of triglycerides, fatty acids, and cholesterol. During fasting, triglycerides from adipose tissue are catabolized by the liver into fatty acids and glycerols. The free fatty acids in prolonged fasting are further catabolized into acetyl coenzyme A and then into ketone bodies. Ketone bodies provide an energy source for some (non-neuronal) tissues.

Bile Acid Synthesis and Excretion

Hepatocytes make bile, which contains water, bile salts, cholesterol, bilirubin, gluconate, and inorganic acids. Bile salts aid digestion by emulsifying dietary fats and fostering their absorption and the absorption of fat-soluble vitamins through the intestinal mucosa. They also prevent the cholesterol in the bile from precipitating out of solution and forming calculi. More than 90% of the daily output of bile is reabsorbed for recycling by an active transport process of the ileal mucosa.

Another hepatic function is elimination of bilirubin from the body. Old or defective erythrocytes are phagocytosed by large reticuloendothelial cells that line the large veins and the sinuses of the liver and spleen. These phagocytes degrade the hemoglobin of these cells into biliverdin, iron, and globulin molecules. The last two components are recycled by the body and used for future erythropoiesis. The biliverdin is almost immediately converted to free bilirubin. Because free bilirubin is an insoluble compound, it is transported bound to plasma albumin molecules. The hepatocytes convert this insoluble bilirubin into a soluble (and thus excretable) form by conjugating it with glucuronic acid to form bilirubin gluconate. This soluble form of bilirubin is then added to the bile and is eliminated from the body by the feces. Bilirubin gluconate gives the bile its normal golden yellow color. Organisms in the intestine convert most of the bilirubin gluconate into a darker brown compound, urobilinogen, which gives the feces its natural brown color. Because it is soluble in water, urobilinogen can also be absorbed from the colon back into the bloodstream and can be excreted by the kidneys. Excess plasma levels of either conjugated (direct) or unconjugated (indirect) bilirubin produce jaundice. Excess unconjugated bilirubin can cross the immature or damaged blood–brain barrier and bind with the basal ganglia, resulting in kernicterus.

Storage

Fat-soluble vitamins and many minerals are stored in the liver. These vitamins and minerals are released under the influence of hormones and serum concentrations of inorganic elements.

Biotransformation

Hepatocytes possess a mixed-function oxidase (MFO) system of enzymes that degrade certain drugs, including alcohol, benzodiazepines, tranquilizers, phenobarbital, phenytoin, and sodium warfarin, among others. This system operates in addition to other intracellular systems that also degrade some of these drugs. Its clinical significance lies in the nature of the drugs that this system catabolizes and in the fact that MFO system activity can be either inhibited or augmented (induced) by these same drugs, depending on when they are taken.

Administration of two MFO system–catabolized drugs within a few hours of one another or together causes each agent to act competitively, slowing down the degradation of the other. For example, simultaneous ingestion of diazepam (Valium) and alcohol can result in slower degradation of each drug. The outcome is higher blood levels of both chemicals for a longer time after administration.

The repeated administration of one MFO system–catabolized drug for several days causes the MFO system to enlarge physically and to possess more enzymes. This is called induction. Once induced, the MFO system degrades drugs more rapidly (including the drug that initiated the induction). If administration of a second MFO system–catabolized drug is begun after MFO system induction, a larger dose of this drug is required to produce a given effect. For example, induction of the MFO system by diazepam increases the dosage of warfarin needed to produce a given therapeutic effect. Other drugs are degraded by various hepatic systems.

Steroid Catabolism

The liver cells degrade steroid hormones, thereby preventing excess serum levels of estrogen, testosterone, progesterone, aldosterone, and glucocorticosteroids.

• Clinical Applicability Challenges

Short-Answer Questions

1. Mr. T. is an overweight 53-year-old male truck driver. He complains of daily heartburn that is accompanied by a sour taste in his mouth. His symptoms are worse after heavy meals, particularly after a cup of coffee and a cigarette. What is the most likely etiology of this patient's symptoms? What lifestyle modifications would you recommend, if any?

2. Mrs. M. is a 75-year-old woman with a history of bleeding gastric ulcers. Approximately 20 years ago, she had a partial gastrectomy. She now receives the diagnosis of vitamin B_{12} deficiency anemia (vitamin B_{12} deficiency). What is the likely etiology of this vitamin deficiency?

3. Mr. S. is an 82-year-old man who takes non-steroidal anti-inflammatory drugs as needed for his osteoarthritic pain. This self-treatment would put him at risk for what potential gastrointestinal problem?

Review Questions

1. Which anatomical structure increases the surface area available for food absorption?
   a. Villi
   b. Ampulla of Vater
   c. Rugae
   d. Muscularis propria

2. Gallbladder contraction is stimulated by which hormone?
   a. Gastric inhibitory peptide
   b. Gastrin
   c. Secretin
   d. Cholecystokinin

3. Which enzyme, once activated in the duodenum, activates other pancreatic enzymes?
   a. Motilin
   b. Acetylcholine
   c. Trypsin
   d. Cholecystokinin

4. One of the functions of the liver includes
   a. storage of chyme.
   b. detoxification of drugs.
   c. water regulation and reabsorption.
   d. formation of platelets.

5. The pancreas secretes
   a. lactase.
   b. amylase.
   c. gastrin.
   d. immunoglobulins.

Selected Readings

Andreoli TE, Carpenter CCJ, Griggs RC, Loscalzo J: Cecil Essentials of Medicine, 6th ed. Philadelphia: WB Saunders, 2004

Braunwald E, Fauci AS, Kasper DL, et al (eds): Harrison's Principles of Internal Medicine, 16th ed. New York: McGraw-Hill, 2005

Feldman M, Friedman LS, Sleisenger MH (eds): Sleisenger and Fortran's Gastrointestinal and Liver Disease: Pathophysiology, Diagnosis, and Management, 7th ed., Vols. 1 and 2. Philadelphia: WB Saunders, 2002

Johnson LR (ed): Encyclopedia of Gastroenterology. San Diego: Elsevier, 2004

Rhoades RA, Tanner GA (eds): Medical Physiology, 2nd ed. Philadelphia: Lippincott Williams & Wilkins, 2003

Yamada T, Alpers DH, Laine L, et al (eds): Textbook of Gastroenterology, 4th ed. Philadelphia: Lippincott Williams & Wilkins, 2003

Patient Assessment: Gastrointestinal System

JoAnn Coleman

Objectives

Based on the content in this chapter, the reader should be able to:

❶ Explain the nursing role in assessing the critical care patient with gastrointestinal compromise.

❷ Discuss important health history components that provide information about gastrointestinal system status.

❸ Describe a systematic approach for conducting a complete gastrointestinal physical examination.

❹ Discuss the importance of referred pain patterns in an abdominal assessment.

❺ Differentiate between normal and abnormal findings detected on physical assessment of the gastrointestinal system.

❻ Identify the data used to make judgments about nutrition and metabolism in a critical care patient.

❼ Discuss appropriate studies and procedures used to diagnose gastrointestinal disorders.

The gastrointestinal system is a long tube with glands and accessory organs (salivary glands, liver, gallbladder, and pancreas). The gastrointestinal tract begins at the mouth; extends through the pharynx, esophagus, stomach, small intestine, colon, and rectum; and ends at the anus. It is an unsterile system filled with bacteria and other flora. These organisms can cause superinfection from antibiotic therapy, and they can infect other systems when an organ of the gastrointestinal tract ruptures. A malfunction along the gastrointestinal tract can produce a variety of metabolic effects, which eventually may be life-threatening.

Assessment of the gastrointestinal system in a critically ill patient provides essential information. Early identification and treatment of gastrointestinal disorders is necessary and serves as a foundation for developing a holistic plan of care for the patient. Ongoing assessment of the gastrointestinal system in the critical care patient may help identify new complications. The ability to complete a comprehensive assessment of the gastrointestinal system depends on the status of the patient. In an intensive care environment, the dynamic nature of the patient may dictate a more focused assessment of the patient. The nurse must be perceptive in obtaining information and timely in soliciting critical information. For example, a ventilated patient cannot converse in an intensive care area, and neither can a comprehensive assessment of the gastrointestinal system be obtained nor would it be necessary at that time.

When a patient is critically ill, assessment of the gastrointestinal system helps determine whether assessment findings relate to the current clinical problem or herald a new complication. The nurse correlates and integrates presenting gastrointestinal signs and symptoms, whether they are isolated entities or related to another underlying problem: Is the bright red blood in the stool a result of gastrointestinal bleeding or from external bleeding hemorrhoids? Is the abdominal pain due to recent bowel surgery or to a distended stomach? The nurse must be aware of the patient's changing metabolic state and nutritional status because this information may directly affect other health outcomes such as length of stay, morbidity, and even mortality.[1]

• History

Unless emergency conditions require immediate action to preserve life, an assessment of the gastrointestinal system begins with the history. A thorough and accurate history greatly enhances the assessment process. The patient's history provides information that can lay the foundation and set the direction for the rest of the assessment.

The history is the major subjective data source about a patient's health status and provides insight into actual or potential health problems. It guides the physical assessment. The history organizes pertinent physiological, psychological, cultural, and psychosocial information as it relates to the patient's current health status and accounts for factors such as lifestyle, family relationships, and cultural influences.[2] Box 39-1 lists elements for a comprehensive gastrointestinal health history.

The initial presentation of the patient in the intensive care area determines how quickly the history will be obtained as well as the focus of the interview. If the patient is in acute distress, the history must focus on obtaining answers to pertinent questions about the patient's chief complaint and precipitating events. Information may be more readily obtained from family members or friends. The nurse can obtain a more thorough history from a patient in no obvious distress by focusing on the patient's current symptoms, medical history, and family history. Information that is fixed and needs to be obtained only once includes data about personal health, preexisting gastrointestinal conditions, previous gastrointestinal or abdominal surgeries or injuries, and hospitalizations. The critical care nurse must also consider the present nutritional status of the patient, the projected length of illness, and its impact on future nutritional needs or adjustments.[3]

The gastrointestinal assessment may change over the course of the illness. The data gathered during the initial history may have focused on the pressing issues facing the patient at that time, but these issues can change in a short or protracted amount of time. The critical care nurse must be vigilant, and he or she must maintain data and incorporate additional information to provide individualized and holistic nursing care as the status of the patient continually evolves.

Because pain is often the chief complaint of patients presenting with abdominal disorders, it must be dealt with in detail.[4] A thorough assessment of pain must include details about the onset, progression, migration, character, localization, radiation, and duration of the pain, as well as information about factors that exacerbate or alleviate the pain. To help understand the potential origin, location, and radiation of the pain, the nurse mentally divides the abdomen into regions using either the quadrant method or the nine regions method (Fig. 39-1). Figure 39-2 summarizes common causes of pain by location.

With many gastrointestinal problems, the pain is referred, which makes diagnosis especially difficult. Referred pain is pain felt at a site different from that of the involved organ. Pain results because nerves that supply an organ also supply the body surface.[4] Figure 39-3 identifies common sites of referred abdominal pain.

• Physical Examination

The physical examination helps establish baseline information about the physical dimensions of the patient's present situation. The physical assessment begins by observing the patient's overall appearance. Motor activity, body position, gait, hair (pattern, loss), skin color (jaundice, cyanosis, pallor) and quality (edema), facial expression, level of consciousness, and signs of depression, anxiety, confusion, or irritability are noted. It is important to note that changes in fluid and electrolyte balance, severe infection, drug toxicity, and hepatic disease may cause a change in behavior such as confusion, lethargy, or agitation. Next, a focused examination of the gastrointestinal system is necessary. A focused examination of the gastrointestinal system includes evaluation of the oral cavity and throat, abdomen, and rectum. Assessment of the abdomen includes assessment of the liver, gallbladder, and pancreas.[5]

ORAL CAVITY AND THROAT

Adequate nutrition is related to good dental health and the general condition of the mouth. Any disorders of the upper gastrointestinal tract (lips, mouth, teeth, pharynx, and esophagus) can prevent adequate nutritional intake. Changes in the oral cavity may influence the type and amount of food ingested and the extent to which food is properly mixed with salivary enzymes. Esophageal problems can also adversely affect food and fluid intake, jeopardizing a patient's health.

Examination of the oral cavity includes inspection and palpation using a good light source, a tongue depressor, an examining glove, and a mask (Fig. 39-4). The nurse should explain the procedure to the patient. The patient assumes a comfortable position that facilitates examination. Sitting upright is the best position for this part of the examination.

Inspection of the lips and jaws for abnormal color, texture, lesions, symmetry, and swellings is essential. Palpation of the temporomandibular joints for mobility, tenderness, and crepitus is also warranted. The nurse retracts the lips to allow adequate visualization. It is necessary to inspect dentures for fit and to remove them for the oral examination. The nurse should use a good light source to inspect all structures inside the mouth and the buccal mucosa (see Fig. 39-4). The nurse identifies missing, broken, loose, and decayed

Box 39-1 • Gastrointestinal Health History

Chief Complaint
- Patient's description of the problem

History of the Present Illness
- Complete analysis of the following signs and symptoms (using the NOPQRST format; see Box 17-1)
- Abdominal pain
- Anorexia
- Indigestion (heartburn)
- Dysphagia
- Eructation
- Nausea
- Vomiting
- Hematemesis
- Fever and chills
- Jaundice
- Pruritus
- Diarrhea
- Constipation
- Flatulence
- Bleeding
- Hemorrhoids
- Melena
- Change in appetite
- Recent weight gain or weight loss
- Mouth lesions
- Anal discomfort
- Fecal incontinence
- Change in abdominal girth

Past Health History
- Relevant childhood illnesses and immunizations: hepatitis, influenza, pneumococcal, meningococcal
- Past acute and chronic medical problems: treatments and hospitalizations—diabetes, cancer, inflammatory bowel disease (Crohn's disease, ulcerative colitis, irritable bowel syndrome, diverticulitis), peptic ulcer, gallstones, polyps, pancreatitis, hepatitis or cirrhosis of the liver, previous gastrointestinal bleeding, cancers or tumors of the gastrointestinal tract, spinal cord injury; for women, episiotomy or fourth-degree laceration during delivery
- Risk factors: age, heredity, gender, race, tobacco use, physical inactivity, obesity, diabetes mellitus, tattoos, exposure to infectious diseases—hepatitis, influenza
- Past surgeries: previous gastrointestinal surgeries (mouth, pharyngeal, esophageal, stomach, small intestine, colon, gallbladder, liver, gallbladder, pancreas), abdominal surgeries or trauma
- Past diagnostic tests and interventions: upper endoscopy, colonoscopy, upper GI, barium enema, rectal manometry

- Medications (prescription drugs, over-the-counter drugs, vitamins, herbs and supplements): aspirin, steroids, anticoagulants, nonsteroidal anti-inflammatory drugs, laxatives, stool softeners
- Allergies and reactions to medications, foods, contrast dye, latex or other materials
- Transfusions, including type and date

Family History
- Health status or cause of death of parents and siblings: inflammatory bowel disease, Hirschsprung's disease, aganglionic megacolon, malabsorption syndrome, cystic fibrosis, celiac disease, gallbladder disease, Peutz-Jeghers syndrome, familial adenomatous polyposis, familial Mediterranean fever, any cancers of the gastrointestinal tract

Personal and Social History
- Tobacco, alcohol, and substance use
- Family composition
- Occupation and work environment
- Living environment, water source
- Diet: food intolerances, taste sensations, coffee intake, special diet
- Oral hygiene: dental status, pattern of dental care, dentures, braces, bridges, crowns, caries
- Bowel habits
- Sleep patterns
- Exercise
- Cultural beliefs
- Spiritual/religious beliefs
- Coping patterns and social support systems
- Leisure activities
- Sexual activity
- Recent stressful events: physical or psychological
- Recent travel, overseas military duty

Review of Other Systems
- HEENT: visual changes, headaches, tinnitus, vertigo, epistaxis, sore throat, mouth lesions, swollen glands, lymphadenopathy
- Respiratory: shortness of breath, dyspnea, cough, sputum, lung disease, recurrent infections
- Cardiovascular: chest pain, palpitations, orthopnea, edema, hypertension, congestive heart failure, arrhythmia, angina, valvular disease
- Genitourinary: incontinence, erectile dysfunction, dysuria, frequency, nocturia
- Musculoskeletal: pain, weakness, varicose veins, change in sensation
- Neurological: transient ischemic attacks, stroke, change in level of consciousness, syncope, seizures, cerebrovascular disease

teeth while noting redness, pallor, white patches, plaques, ulcers, petechiae, bleeding, and masses. A pool of saliva under the tongue helps assess hydration. Palpation of the parotid and submaxillary ducts is necessary. The nurse palpates suspect areas with a gloved finger to determine tenderness or induration. The patient sticks out his or her tongue while the nurse checks for symmetry of movement, swelling, lesions, and any abnormal coating. While depressing the tongue with a tongue blade, the nurse observes the movement of the soft palate and uvula as the patient says "ah." These structures should rise symmetrically. This is a good time to inspect the hard and soft palates, uvula, tonsils, pillars, and posterior pharynx (Fig. 39-5). Note decreased or absent gag reflex, which suggests possible neurological dysfunction and

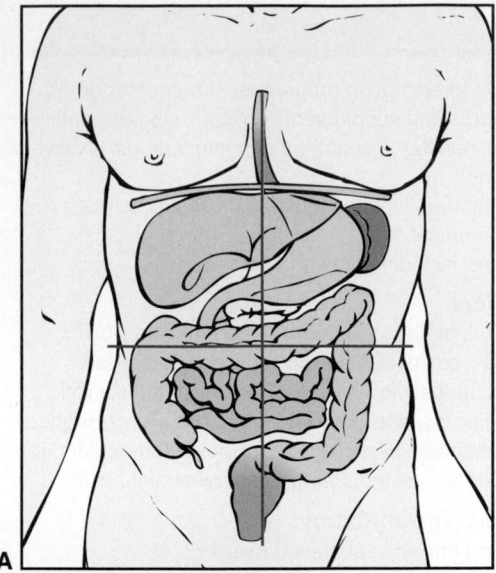

Right upper quadrant (RUQ)

Liver and gallbladder
Pylorus
Duodenum
Head of pancreas
Hepatic flexure of colon
Portions of ascending and
transverse colon

Left upper quadrant (LUQ)

Left liver lobe
Stomach
Body and tail of pancreas
Splenic flexure of colon
Portions of transverse and
descending colon

Right lower quadrant (RLQ)

Cecum and appendix
Portion of ascending colon

Left lower quadrant (LLQ)

Sigmoid colon
Portion of descending colon

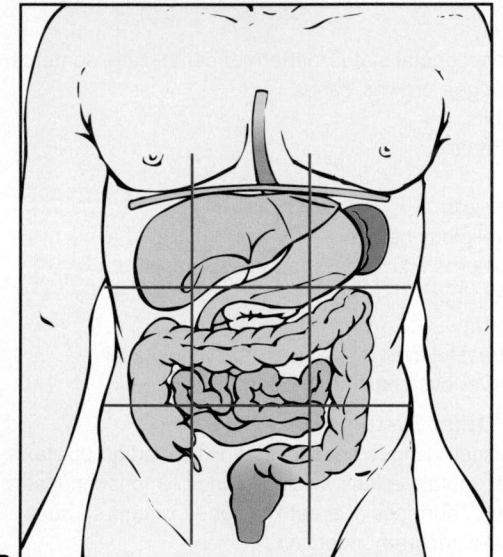

Right hypochondriac

Right liver lobe
Gallbladder

Epigastric

Pyloric end
  of stomach
Duodenum
Pancreas
Portion of liver

Left hypochondriac

Stomach
Tail of pancreas
Splenic flexure of colon

Right lumbar

Ascending colon
Portions of duodenum
  and jejunum

Umbilical

Omentum
Mesentery
Lower part
  of duodenum
Jejunum and ileum

Left lumbar

Descending colon
Portions of jejunum
  and ileum

Right inguinal

Cecum
Appendix
Lower end of ileum

**Suprapubic or
hypogastric**

Ileum

Left inguinal

Sigmoid colon

Figure 39-1 • To aid accurate abdominal assessment and documentation of findings, the nurse can mentally divide the patient's abdomen into regions. **A:** The quadrant method. **B:** The nine regions method.

increases the patient's risk for aspiration. Deviation of the uvula to one side when the patient says "ah" may indicate pathology of cranial nerve IX (the glossopharyngeal nerve) or cranial nerve X (the vagus nerve).[6] Unusual breath odors may indicate serious gastrointestinal disease, such as esophageal cancer. Fecal breath odor may be caused by a bowel obstruction or hepatic failure; a fruity breath odor may be the result of diabetic or starvation ketoacidosis. Table 39-1 reviews oral assessment, normal and abnormal findings, and possible causes of abnormal findings.

Examination of the oral cavity in an intubated patient is very important, even though the tube may hinder vision during the assessment. The condition of the mouth of a critically ill patient can change rapidly, and the nurse must conduct a periodic assessment to initiate treatment and intervene to prevent complications. It is necessary to assess the presence of any secretions, oral odor, or changes in odors coming from the oral cavity promptly. Studies have indicated that microbial colonization of the oropharynx and dental plaque are associated with pneumonia in patients who are receiving mechanical ventilation. Evidence now shows that implementing a standardized oral care protocol and providing the appropriate tools at the bedside increase the frequency and comprehensiveness of the oral care provided.[7]

The patient with a nasogastric, orogastric, or long tube for intestinal decompression warrants close observation because these tubes prevent the lower esophageal sphincter from closing completely. Gastric reflux or even reflux into the oropharynx may

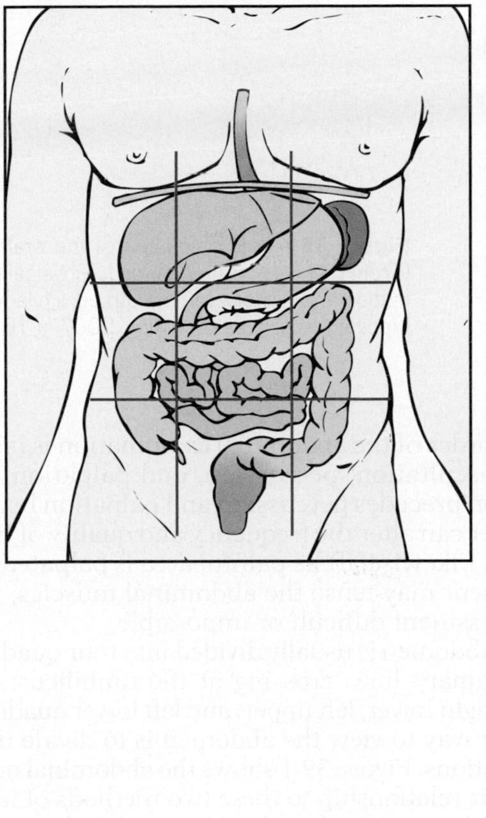

Right hypochondriac	Epigastric	Left hypochondriac
Cholecystitis/ cholangitis	Duodenal or gastric ulcer	Pleurisy, lower lobe pneumonia, or pneumothorax
Hepatitis	Duodenitis or gastritis	Myocardial infarction or angina
Metastatic disease to the liver	Pancreatitis	Pericarditis
Pleurisy, lower lobe pneumonia, or pneumothorax	Myocardial infarction or angina	Pyelonephritis
Congestive hepatomegaly	Pericarditis	Renal colic
Pyelonephritis	Gastroenteritis	Splenic injury
Renal colic	Mesenteric embolus or thrombus	
Duodenal ulcer	Small bowel obstruction	

Right lumbar	Umbilical	Left lumbar
Pancreatitis	Appendicitis	Pancreatitis
Pyelonephritis	Small bowel obstruction	Pyelonephritis
Renal colic	Rectus sheath hematoma	Renal colic
Colon obstruction/ gangrene	Gastroenteritis	Sigmoid diverticulitis
	Umbilical hernia	Colon obstruction/ gangrene
	Abdominal aortic aneurysm	
	Aortic dissection	
	Mesenteric embolus or thrombus	

Right inguinal	Suprapubic or hypogastric	Left inguinal
Meckel's diverticulum	Rectus sheath hematoma	Sigmoid diverticulitis
Appendicitis	Salpingitis	Groin hernia
Cecal perforation	Ectopic pregnancy	Colon obstruction/ gangrene
Groin hernia	Tubo-ovarian torsion	Ectopic pregnancy
Colon obstruction/ gangrene	Mittelschmerz	Spigelian hernia
Ectopic pregnancy	Regional enteritis	Regional enteritis
Spigelian hernia	Endometriosis	
Regional enteritis	Abdominal aortic aneurysm	

Figure 39-2 • Common causes of pain by location.

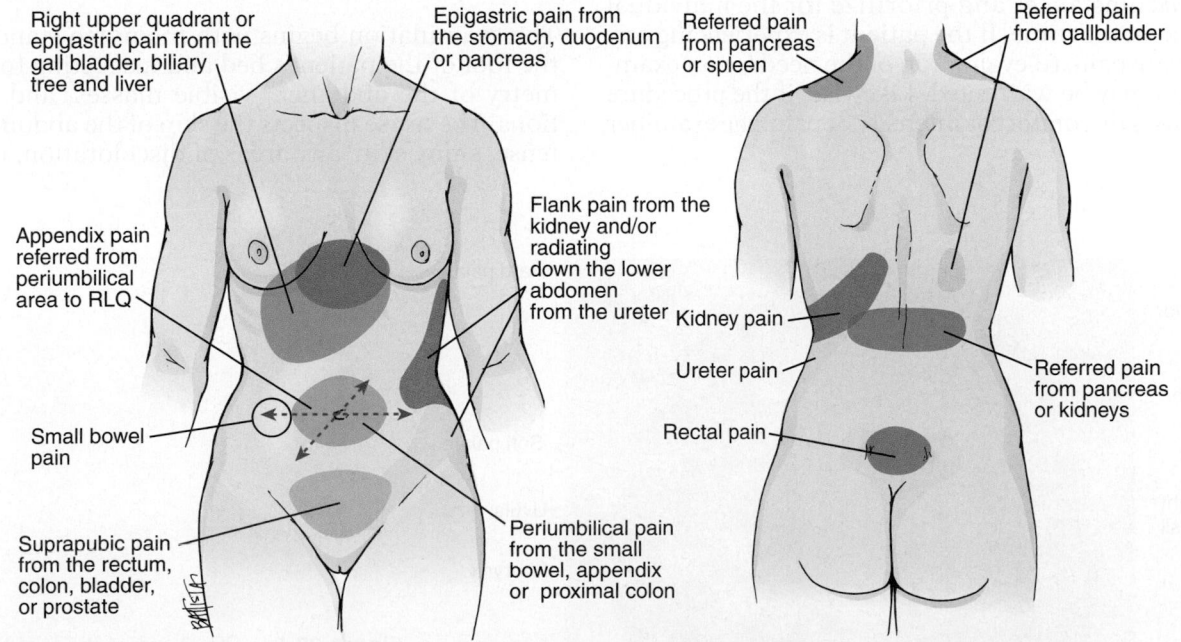

Right upper quadrant or epigastric pain from the gall bladder, biliary tree and liver

Epigastric pain from the stomach, duodenum or pancreas

Referred pain from pancreas or spleen

Referred pain from gallbladder

Appendix pain referred from periumbilical area to RLQ

Flank pain from the kidney and/or radiating down the lower abdomen from the ureter

Kidney pain

Ureter pain

Referred pain from pancreas or kidneys

Small bowel pain

Rectal pain

Suprapubic pain from the rectum, colon, bladder, or prostate

Periumbilical pain from the small bowel, appendix or proximal colon

Figure 39-3 • Mechanisms and sources of abdominal pain. Abdominal pain may be described as visceral, parietal, or referred. (From Weber J, Kelley J: Health Assessment in Nursing, 3rd ed. Philadelphia: Lippincott Williams & Wilkins, 2007, p 431.)

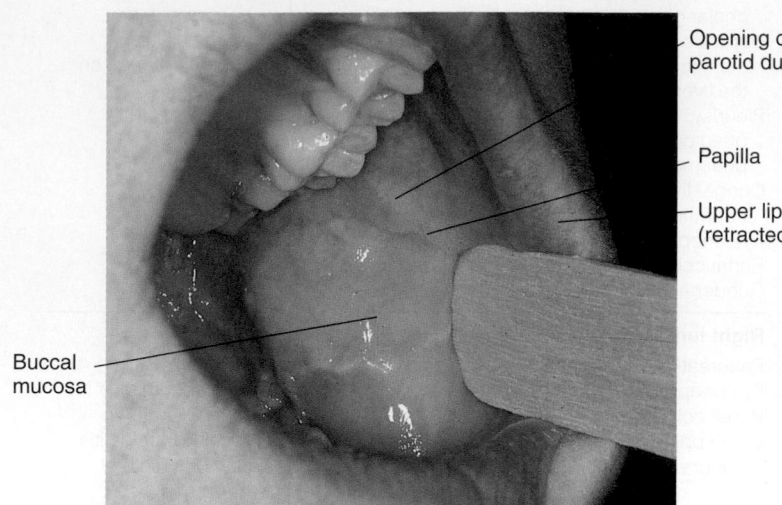

Opening of the parotid duct

Papilla

Upper lip (retracted)

Buccal mucosa

Figure 39-4 • Examination of the oral cavity. (From Bickley L: Bates' Guide to Physical Examination and History Taking, 9th ed. Philadelphia: Lippincott Williams & Wilkins, 2007, p 167.)

occur, which can cause erosive damage to the esophagus as well as a noxious odor in the mouth. Delayed gastric emptying may also exacerbate the reflux.

ABDOMEN

The patient's comfort should be preserved as the nurse performs the abdominal examination (Table 39-2). The patient should empty his or her bladder before the examination. A supine position with arms down and knees slightly bent is preferred because this position relieves tension on the abdominal wall. Draping exposes the abdomen and protects the patient's modesty.[5] This is the ideal situation for performing an abdominal examination, but it may not always be possible in a critically ill patient. The nurse must assess the circumstances and prioritize for the individual patient at that time. If the patient is experiencing any or severe pain, re-evaluation of the need for an examination may be warranted. Likewise, if the procedure increases discomfort or intensity of pain, the examiner stops.

The order of the abdominal examination is inspection, auscultation, percussion, and palpation. Auscultation precedes percussion and palpation because the latter can alter the frequency and quality of bowel sounds. Likewise, if the painful area is palpated first, the patient may tense the abdominal muscles, making assessment difficult or impossible.

The abdomen is usually divided into four quadrants by imaginary lines crossing at the umbilicus: right upper, right lower, left upper, and left lower quadrants. Another way to view the abdomen is to divide it into nine sections. Figure 39-1 shows the abdominal organs and their relationship to these two methods of identifying abdominal landmarks. Figure 39-3 shows common causes of pain by location.

Inspection

The examination begins with the nurse standing at the foot of the patient's bed and inspecting for symmetry of the abdomen, visible masses, and pulsations. The nurse inspects the skin of the abdomen for tense, shiny skin, any areas of discoloration, rashes,

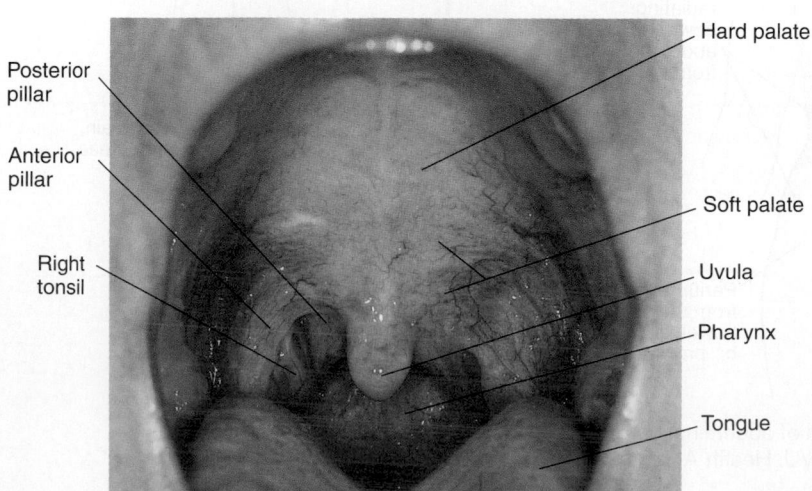

Posterior pillar

Anterior pillar

Right tonsil

Hard palate

Soft palate

Uvula

Pharynx

Tongue

Figure 39-5 • Structures of the mouth. (From Bickley L: Bates' Guide to Physical Examination and History Taking, 9th ed. Philadelphia: Lippincott Williams & Wilkins, 2007, p 167.)

Table 39-1 • Oral Assessment

Structure	Normal	Abnormal Findings	Possible Cause
Lips	Smooth, pink, and moist	Dry or cracked	Febrile illness
		Asymmetrical, cracked, fissured, or bleeding	Cheilitis
		Cyanotic	Cold or hypoxia
		Cracks at corner of lips	Possible vitamin B deficiency or poor hygiene
Tongue	Pink, moist with papillae present	Coated or loss of papilla and a shiny appearance (with or without redness); blistered or cracked; altered taste	Infection
		Deviation to one side	Cranial nerve XII (hypoglossal nerve) problem
		Nodules or ulcers on base of tongue	Cancerous lesion
Saliva	Watery	Thick, ropy, or absent	
Mucous membranes	Pink and moist	Reddened without ulcerations	Infection
		Ulcerations with or without bleeding	Poor nutrition
		Inflammation	Ill-fitting dentures
		Leukoplakia on buccal membrane	Precancerous lesion
		Cyanosis	Hypoxia
		Pale mucosa	Anemia
		Small areas of white scar tissue	Chronic irritation from friction of irregular tooth surfaces or biting when chewing
		Inflamed or painful Stensen's duct opening	Parotid gland infection
Gingiva	Pink, stippled, and firm	Edematous with or without redness; spontaneous bleeding or bleeding with pressure; soreness	Gingivitis
Teeth or dentures	Clean without debris	Plaque or debris in between teeth; plaque or debris along gum line or denture-bearing area	
		Toothache, tooth abscess	
		Misfit of dental appliances	
		Absent or broken teeth, cavities	
		Malocclusion, worn or flattened tooth edges	Bruxism
Voice	Normal	Deeper or raspy; difficulty talking or painful to talk	Vocal cord paralysis
Throat/swallowing	Normal	Some pain on swallowing or unable to swallow; sore throat	Cancerous lesion
Glands	Nonpalpable	Inflammation and lumps	Stones or cysts

striae (lines resulting from rapid or prolonged skin stretching), ecchymoses, petechiae, lesions, scars, and prominent or dilated veins. Then the nurse moves to the patient's side and assumes a position to obtain an eye-level view across the abdomen. Size, shape, asymmetry, and movements from respirations, peristalsis, vascular pulsations, and exaggerated movement are noteworthy. It is necessary to inspect the umbilicus for position, contour, and color (Fig. 39-6). Pulsation of the aorta is normally apparent in the epigastric area. In a thin person, the femoral pulses may be visible. When ascites or abdominal bleeding is suspected, the nurse should measure the abdominal girth.[6] Measure abdominal girth at the same time of day, ideally in the morning just after voiding, or at a designated time for bedridden patients and those with indwelling catheters. The patient will normally be supine in the intensive care unit. Place the tape measure behind the patient and measure at the umbilicus. Record the distance in designated units (inches or centimeters). Take all future measurements from the same location. The abdomen may be marked with a pen to help identify the correct site.

Auscultation

Auscultation provides information on bowel motility and the vessels and organs that lie beneath the abdominal wall. The nurse applies light pressure on the diaphragm of the stethoscope when auscultating the four quadrants of the abdomen. The nurse starts below and to the right of the umbilicus and proceeds in a methodical direction through all four quadrants. To prevent contraction of the abdominal muscles that

Table 39-2 • Abnormal Abdominal Findings

Finding	Characteristic	Possible Cause
Abdominal contour	Concave (scaphoid)	Malnutrition
	Distention	Tumor; excessive fluid (ascites, perforation); gas accumulation; severe malnutrition
Skin abnormalities	Bulging around old scar	Incisional hernia
	Striae	Obesity; pregnancy; abdominal tumor; Cushing's syndrome (purple striae)
	Pink or blue	Recently developed striae
	White or silver	Older striae
	Tense, glistening	Ascites
	Dilated, tortuous veins	Inferior vena cava obstruction
Umbilicus	Everted	Increased intra-abdominal pressure
	Bluish ecchymosis surrounding umbilicus (Cullen's sign)	Intra-abdominal bleeding; pancreatitis; ectopic pregnancy
Peristaltic wave	Strong	Intestinal obstruction
Abdominal aortic pulsations	Obvious and pronounced	Increased intra-abdominal pressure (from tumor or ascites)
Murphy's sign	Sharp pain that stops respiration when palpating under liver border	Cholecystitis
Grey Turner's sign	Flank ecchymosis	Intra-abdominal bleeding; hemorrhagic pancreatitis
Blumberg's sign	Rebound tenderness	Peritoneal irritation; inflamed or perforated appendix
Iliopsoas muscle	Right lower quadrant pain when right leg elevated against tension	Inflamed or perforated appendix from inflamed psoas muscle
Obturator muscle	Abdominal pain when right leg rotated at hip (internal or external rotation)	Inflamed or perforated appendix

can obscure sounds, the nurse lifts the stethoscope completely off the abdominal wall when changing its location. Normally, air and fluid moving through the bowel by peristalsis create a soft, bubbling sound with no regular pattern, often with soft clicks and gurgles interspersed, approximately every 5 to 15 seconds. Colonic sounds are low pitched with a rumbling feature. A hungry patient may exhibit a "growling stomach" resulting from hyperperistalsis, called borborygmi. High-pitched, rapid, loud, and gurgling

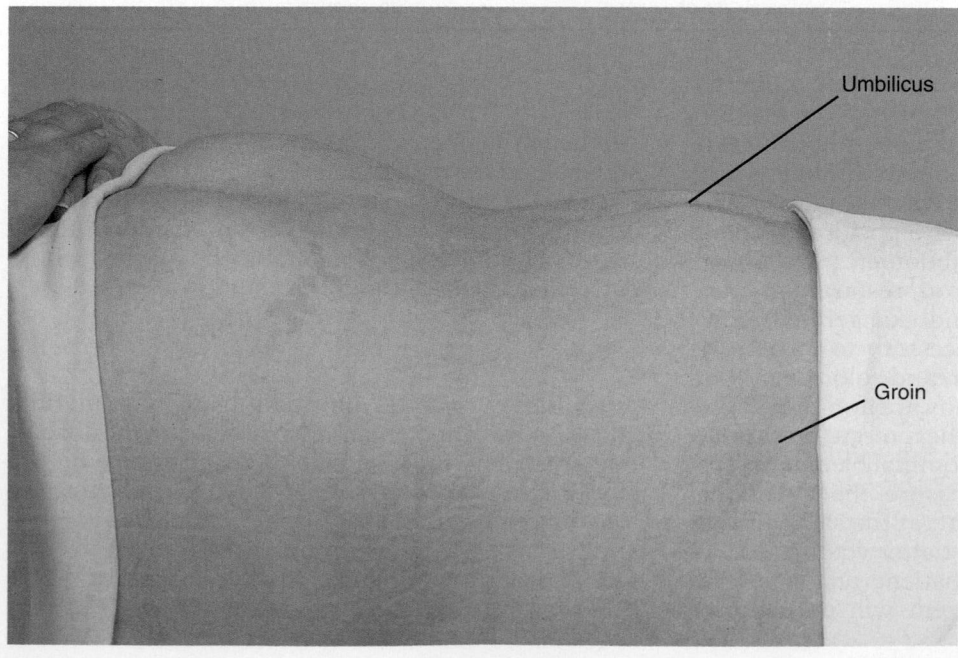

Figure 39-6 • Inspection of the abdomen. (From Bickley L: Bates' Guide to Physical Examination and History Taking, 9th ed. Philadelphia: Lippincott Williams & Wilkins, 2007, p 375.)

bowel sounds are hyperactive and may occur in a hungry patient. High-pitched tinkling and rushes of high-pitched sounds with abdominal cramping usually indicate obstruction. Bowel sounds that occur once every minute or less frequently are hypoactive and usually occur after bowel surgery or when feces fill the colon.[8] Absent bowel sounds may be associated with peritonitis or paralytic ileus.

Edema of the abdominal wall can be detected when an imprint of the diaphragm remains after light auscultation. The nurse uses the bell of the stethoscope to listen for vascular sounds over the abdominal aorta and the renal and femoral arteries. Figure 39-7 illustrates auscultation sites of the abdomen for vascular sounds. If the nurse hears a bruit (a continuous purring, blowing, or humming sound), percussion and palpation do not follow. If a bruit is a new finding, it is necessary to notify the physician. Table 39-3 describes abnormal abdominal sounds.

Percussion

The nurse percusses the abdomen lightly in all four quadrants of the abdomen, listening for the location and distribution of tympany and dullness (Fig. 39-8A). The percussion may proceed clockwise or up and down over the abdomen (see Fig. 39-8B and C). Abdominal percussion helps identify air, gas, and fluid in the abdomen and helps determine the size and location of abdominal organs. The percussion sound depends on the density of the underlying structure. The sound is dull over solid organs (e.g., liver), a stool-filled colon, abdominal masses, or pleural effusions. The sound is tympanic over air, such as in the gastric bubble or air-filled intestine. To determine the size of the liver, the nurse percusses along the right mid-clavicular line (Fig. 39-9A). One method is to begin at the iliac crest and work upward. The point at which the sound becomes dull is marked. It

is necessary to perform percussion down from the clavicle. The dull sound of the rib should not be mistaken for the superior edge of the liver. After marking the superior edge, the nurse measures the distance between the marks in centimeters. The normal liver measures 6 to 12 cm in height at the mid-clavicular line (see Fig. 39-9B).[6]

It may be necessary to postpone performing abdominal percussion on a critically ill patient, especially if there is abdominal guarding. The nurse percusses areas where the patient is not experiencing pain before examining painful areas. Abdominal percussion or palpation is contraindicated in a patient with suspected appendicitis, abdominal aortic aneurysm, or polycystic kidneys or in a patient who has received an abdominal organ transplantation to prevent rupture of the organs or aorta.

Palpation

Abdominal palpation is necessary to establish the character of the abdominal wall, including the size, condition, and consistency of abdominal organs; the presence of abdominal masses; and the presence, location, and degree of abdominal pain. Abdominal palpation includes light palpation, deep palpation, and ballottement.

Light palpation, which is performed first, identifies muscular resistance and areas of tenderness (Fig. 39-10). Fingertips are used to depress the abdominal wall 1 cm (0.5 in). The nurse notes skin temperature, muscle resistance, tender areas, and masses. The femoral artery is subject to bilateral palpation. To ensure patient cooperation and relaxed muscles, the nurse always palpates a symptomatic area last.

When disease is present, palpation may result in somatic or organ pain. Somatic pain is localized and reflects inflammation of the skin, fascia, or abdominal surfaces. Guarding of the abdominal muscles

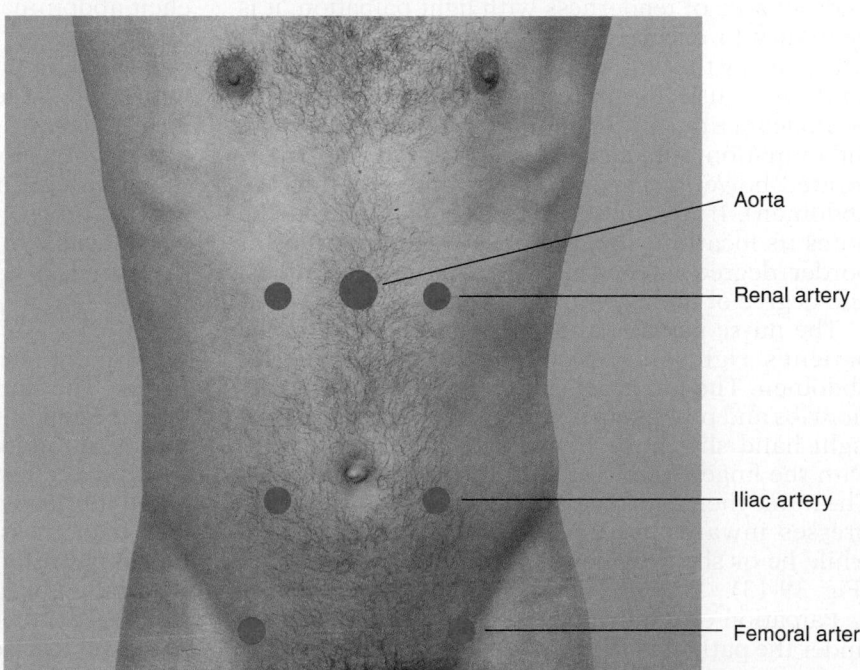

Figure 39-7 • Auscultation sites for vascular sounds. (From Bickley L: Bates' Guide to Physical Examination and History Taking, 9th ed. Philadelphia: Lippincott Williams & Wilkins, 2007, p 376.)

Table 39-3 • Abnormal Abdominal Sounds

Sound and Description	Location	Sound	Possible Cause
Bowel sounds	All four quadrants	Hypoactive sounds unrelated to hunger	Diarrhea or early intestinal obstruction
		Hypoactive, then absent, sounds	Paralytic ileus or peritonitis
		High-pitched "tinkling" sounds	Intestinal air and fluid under tension in a dilated bowel; early intestinal obstruction
		High-pitched "rushing" sounds coinciding with an abdominal cramp	Intestinal obstruction
		Hyperactive sounds, long and prolonged (borborygmi)	Hunger, gastroenteritis
		Absence of sounds over 5 min in all four quadrants	Temporary loss of intestinal motility; occurs with ileus
Systolic bruits (vascular "blowing" sounds resembling cardiac murmurs)	Abdominal aorta	Partial arterial obstruction or turbulent blood flow	Dissecting abdominal aneurysm
	Renal artery		Renal artery stenosis
	Iliac artery		Hepatomegaly
Venous hum (continuous, medium-pitched tone created by blood flow in a large, engorged vascular organ such as the liver)	Epigastric area and umbilicus	Increased collateral circulation between portal and systemic venous systems	Hepatic cirrhosis
Friction rub (harsh, grating sound resembling two pieces of sandpaper rubbing together)	Hepatic	Inflammation of the peritoneal surface of an organ	Liver mass

accompanies somatic pain. Organ pain is visceral in nature and is usually dull, diffuse, and generalized.

Deep palpation is used to locate abdominal organs (enlarged spleen, edge of the liver, pole of the right kidney; the left kidney is usually not palpable) and large masses (Fig. 39-11). The fingertips are used to depress the abdominal wall firmly to a depth of 7.5 cm (3 in). Palpation in the epigastric area for the pulse of the aorta is warranted (Fig. 39-12). If the nurse finds an area of tenderness with light palpation, it is necessary to check rebound tenderness by quickly withdrawing the fingertips after depression. Rebound tenderness usually indicates inflammation of the peritoneum from an abdominal process such as organ inflammation, infection, abscess formation, or perforated bowel (release of bowel contents into the abdomen). If the nurse palpates a mass, he or she notes its location, size, shape, consistency, type of border, degree of tenderness, presence of pulsations, and degree of mobility (fixed or mobile).[9]

The nurse palpates the spleen by standing at the patient's right side, reaching over the patient's abdomen. The left hand should be under the posterior ribs and pulling up gently on the patient, and the right hand should be below the left costal margin with the fingers pointing toward the patient's head. The nurse then asks the patient to inhale as the nurse presses inward and upward with the right hand while he or she provides support with the left hand (Fig. 39-13).

Palpation of the liver is easiest when one hand is under the patient at the level of the 11th rib while the other hand is on the abdomen at the level of the percussed liver edge dullness (Fig. 39-14). With the abdominal fingers pointing upward to lift the organ, the upper hand pushes down and upward to palpate the lower border of the liver. The liver edge should be firm and smooth. Finding an enlarged, nodular, or irregularly shaped liver warrants reporting.

Ballottement is the light, rapid tapping of the fingertips against the abdominal wall. This is used to elicit abdominal muscle resistance or guarding that may be missed with deep palpation or to detect the movement or bounce of a movable mass. In a patient with ascites, deep ballottement may be warranted. It is necessary to push the fingertips deeply inward in a rapid movement and then quickly release them, maintaining fingertip contact with the abdominal wall. Any movement of an organ lying beneath is felt, or a movable mass moves toward the fingertips.[5]

ANUS AND RECTUM

Assessment of the anus involves inspection and palpation. The skin around the anus is normally darker than the surrounding area. The nurse should inspect for inflammation, lesions, skin tags or warts, obvious fissures, and hemorrhoids. Palpation of the area with a well-lubricated gloved finger for outpouchings, nodules, tenderness, irregularities, and fecal impaction is necessary. Alteration in elimination due to immobility, limited or no gastrointestinal intake, opioids, or decreased intestinal peristalsis may result from a patient's disease or its treatment. Constipation may

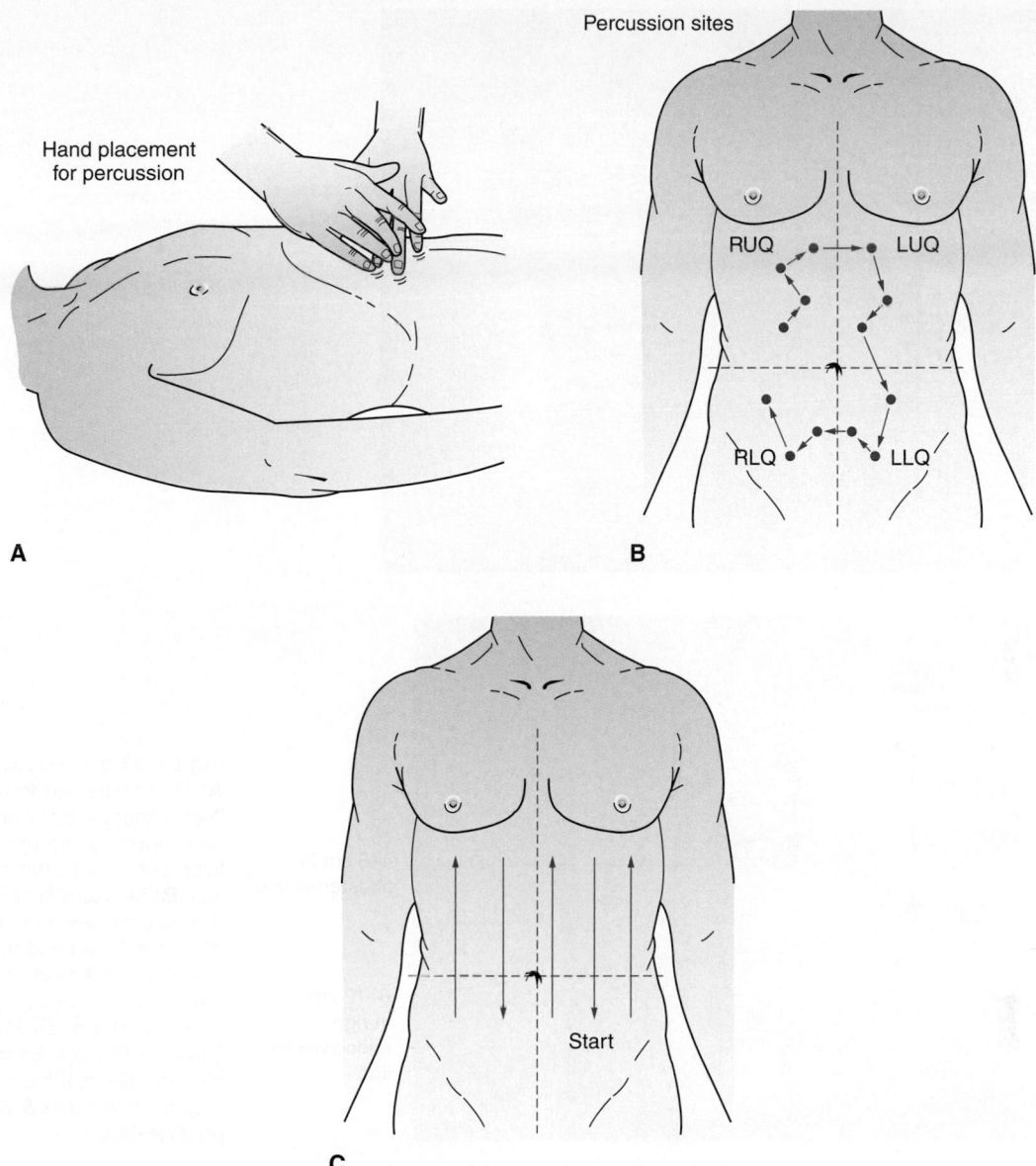

Hand placement for percussion

Percussion sites

RUQ   LUQ

RLQ   LLQ

A

B

Start

C

Figure 39-8 • Percussing the abdomen. Percuss the abdomen systematically, starting with the right upper quadrant and moving clockwise to the percussion sites in each quadrant. If the patient complains of pain in a particular quadrant, adjust the percussion sequence to percuss that quadrant last. Remember when tapping to move your right finger away quickly so you do not inhibit vibrations. Abdominal percussion sequences may proceed clockwise or up and down over the abdomen. (From Weber J, Kelley J: Health Assessment in Nursing, 3rd ed. Philadelphia: Lippincott Williams & Wilkins, 2007, p 445).

compound matters and, if left untreated, can lead to fecal impaction.[9] Astute nursing assessment is critical in preventing and treating constipation or fecal impaction in any patient.

To assess anal sphincter tone, it is necessary to slip a well-lubricated tip of the index finger of a gloved hand into the anal canal. The nurse asks the patient who can cooperate to bear down to tighten the external sphincter around the inserted finger. He or she assesses the tone; it should tighten, exert even pressure all around, feel smooth, and cause no discomfort to the patient. A lax sphincter may indicate a neurological deficit. A very tight sphincter may result from scarring, spasticity caused by a fissure or other lesion, inflammation, or anxiety about the examination. Inserting the finger farther allows palpation of the walls of the rectum. It is necessary to assess the walls for any nodules, masses, irregularities, polyps, or tenderness. The wall should feel smooth, even, and uninterrupted.[5]

• Nutritional Assessment

A critically ill patient's nutritional status may fall anywhere on a continuum ranging from optimal nutrition to malnutrition. The critical care patient may have an inadequate dietary intake because of illness or the disorder that caused the hospitalization, particularly if

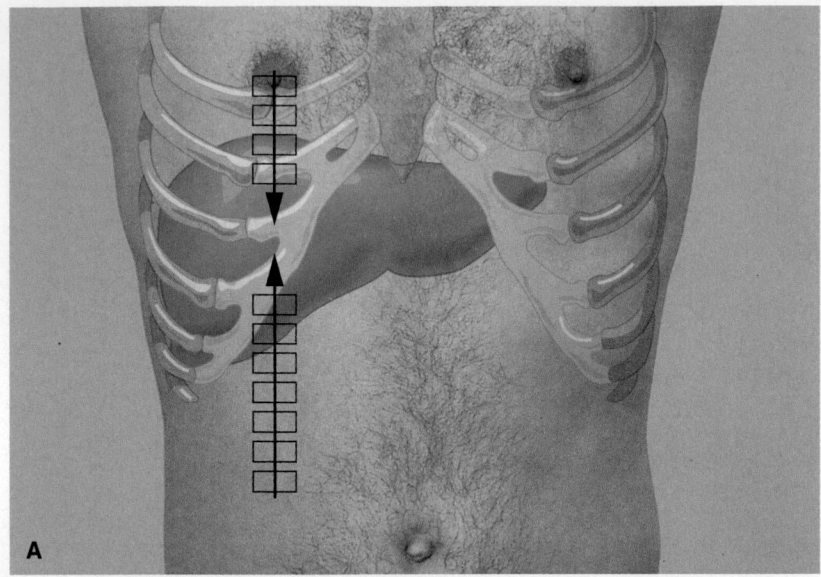

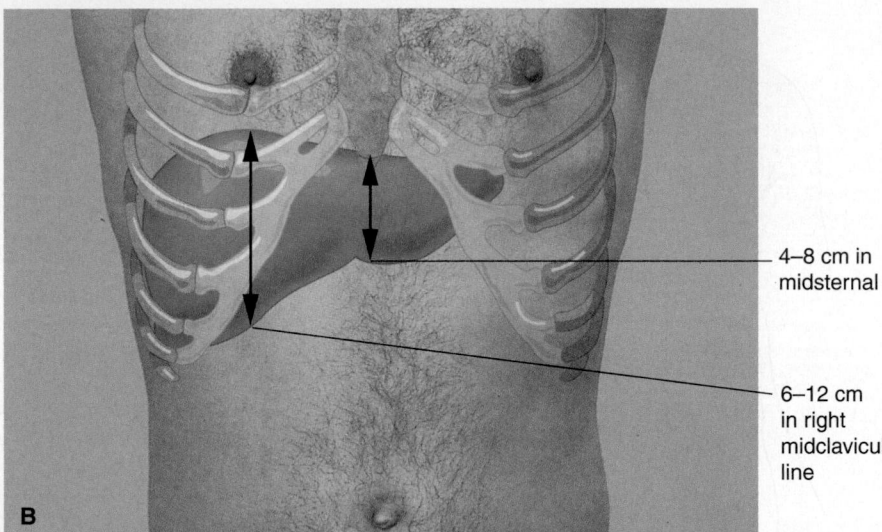

4–8 cm in
midsternal line

6–12 cm
in right
midclavicular
line

Figure 39-9 • Percussing the liver.
A: Determine the lower border of
liver dullness in the midclavicular line.
Next, identify the upper border of
liver dullness in the midclavicular
line. B: Measure in centimeters the
distance between the lower border
of liver dullness and the upper border of liver dullness. The distance is
known as the vertical span of liver
dullness. (From Bickley L: Bates'
Guide to Physical Examination and
History Taking, 9th ed. Philadelphia:
Lippincott Williams & Wilkins, 2007,
pp 379–380.)

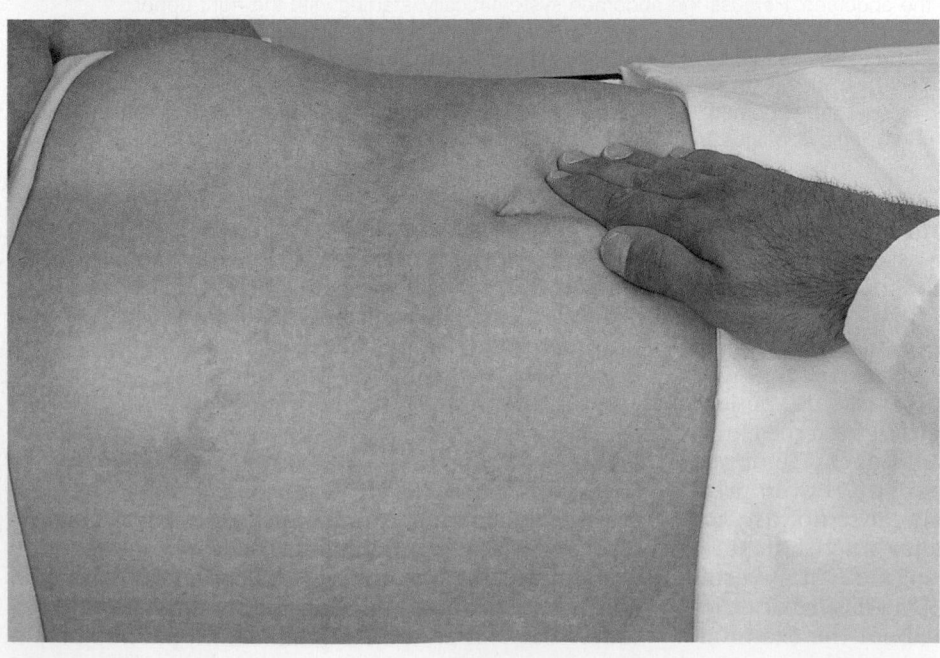

Figure 39-10 • Performing light
palpation. (From Bickley L: Bates'
Guide to Physical Examination and
History Taking, 9th ed. Philadelphia:
Lippincott Williams & Wilkins, 2007,
p 378.)

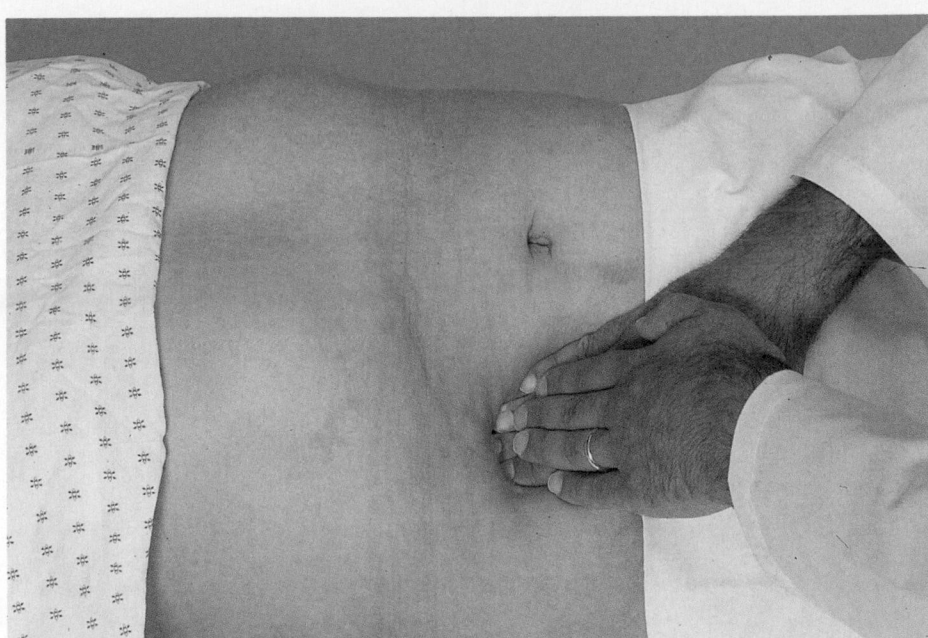

Figure 39-11 • Two-handed deep palpation. (From Bickley L: Bates' Guide to Physical Examination and History Taking, 9th ed. Philadelphia: Lippincott Williams & Wilkins, 2007, p 378.)

the disorder is gastrointestinal. In addition, critically ill patients are at risk for gastrointestinal problems due to treatments that cause damage to the gastrointestinal system and reduce the body's ability to absorb nutrients. Optimal nutrient intake provides adequate energy and can protect from complications of disease.[10]

The nurse plays an important role in evaluating the nutritional status of the patients under his or her care. Certain signs and symptoms that suggest possible nutritional deficiency are easy to note because they are specific. Conversely, fluid changes, such as edema or effusions, can mask protein and fat loss. The fact that nutritional disturbances can be subtle and are frequently nonspecific makes the need for assessment important.[10]

An initial nutritional screening may begin with cursory data, as dictated by the patient's condition. A registered dietitian or nutritionist or a nutritional support team may perform a more comprehensive assessment. The parameters of the nutritional assessment include anthropometric measurement, laboratory studies, physical examination, and dietary evaluation. Anthropometric measurements include height, weight, body mass index, triceps skinfold thickness, and midarm and arm muscle circumference. Table 39-4 lists laboratory studies performed to evaluate nutritional status. Table 39-5 presents information about the physical examination and its interpretation in nutritional disorders.

The dietary evaluation may consist of a 24-hour recall to elicit all the foods and beverages consumed in the preceding 24 hours. However, this method may overestimate or underestimate a patient's usual caloric intake because the patient's recollection may not reflect long-term dietary habits. The nurse assesses the quantity and quality of food ingested by asking the patient to recall his or her normal daily intake pattern. This approach provides more information about intake patterns and tends to reflect long-term

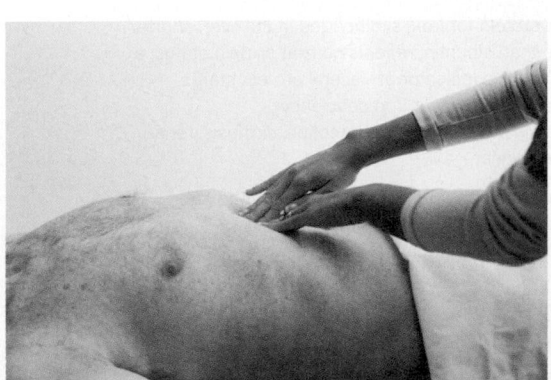

Figure 39-12 • Palpating the aorta. (From Weber J, Kelley J: Health Assessment in Nursing, 3rd ed. Philadelphia: Lippincott Williams & Wilkins, 2007, p 451).

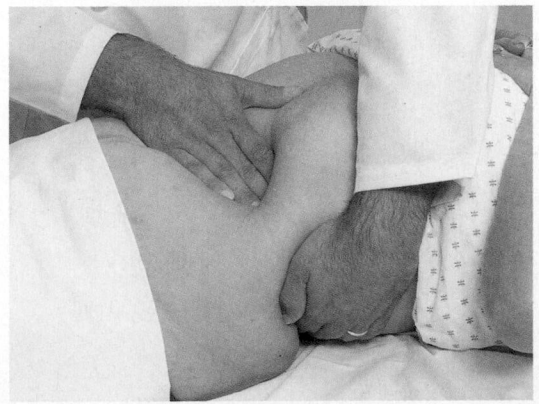

Figure 39-13 • Palpating the spleen. (From Weber J, Kelley J: Health Assessment in Nursing, 3rd ed. Philadelphia: Lippincott Williams & Wilkins, 2007, p 452.)

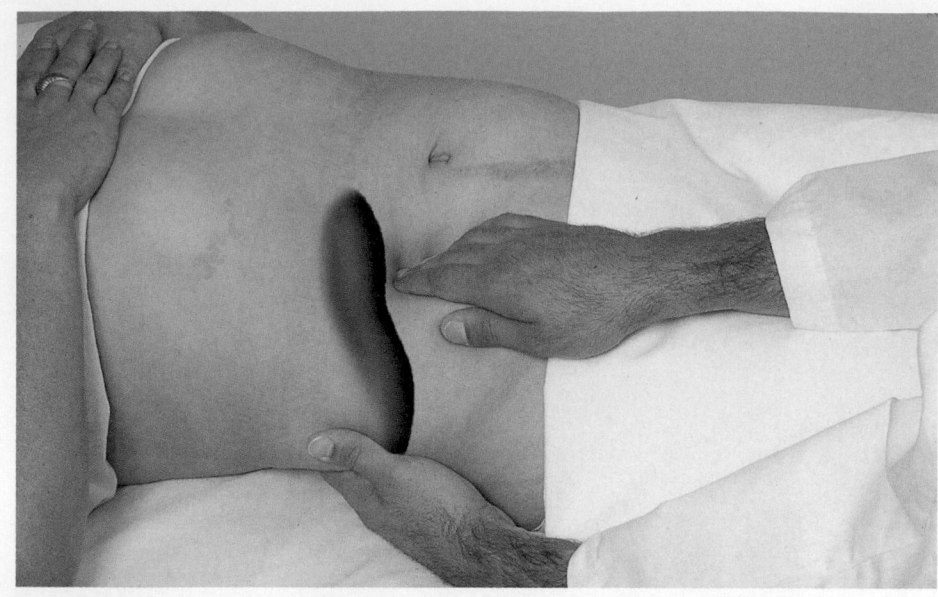

Figure 39-14 • Bimanual technique for liver palpation. (From Bickley L: Bates' Guide to Physical Examination and History Taking, 9th ed. Philadelphia: Lippincott Williams & Wilkins, 2007, p 380.)

Table 39-4 • Laboratory Studies to Evaluate Nutritional Status

Study	Normal Findings	Clinical and Nursing Significance
Hemoglobin	Males: 13–18 g/dL Females: 12–16 g/dL	Main component of RBCs used to transport oxygen; identifies iron carrying capacity of the blood Helps identify anemia, protein deficiency, excessive blood loss, hydration status Elevated with dehydration; decreased in overhydration
Hematocrit	Males: 40%–52% Females: 36%–48%	Identifies volume of RBCs Decreased value with overhydration, blood loss, poor dietary intake of iron, protein, certain vitamins
Albumin	3.5–5.5 g/dL	Assesses protein levels in the body; requires functioning liver cells Decreased with protein deficiency, blood loss secondary to burns, malnutrition, liver/renal disease, heart failure, major surgery, infections, cancer Elevated with dehydration
Total protein	6–8 g/dL	Decreased with overhydration, malnutrition, liver disease
Prealbumin	15–30 mg/dL	Transport protein for thyroxine (T_4) Short half-life makes it more sensitive than albumin to changes in protein stores Decreased in malnutrition in critically ill or those with chronic disease
Transferrin	200–400 mg/dL	Transport protein for iron; synthesized in the liver; shorter half-life than albumin; reflects current protein status; a more sensitive indicator of visceral protein stores Elevated in pregnancy or iron deficiency Decreased in acute or chronic infection, cirrhosis, renal disease, cancer
Retinol-binding protein	3–6 mg/L	Rapidly responds to nutritional depletion due to short half-life Decreased in overhydration and liver disease
Total lymphocyte count	>2,000 mm³	Indicator of immunocompetence Mild: 1,200–2,000 Moderate: 800–1,199 Severe: <800 May indicate malnutrition when no other cause apparent; may point to infection, leukemia, or tissue necrosis

Table 39-5 • Physical Assessment Interpretation in Nutritional Disorders

Body System or Region	Sign or Symptom	Implications
General	Weakness and fatigue	Anemia or electrolyte imbalance, decreased calorie intake, increased calorie use, or inadequate nutrient intake or absorption
	Weight loss	
Skin, hair, and nails	Dry, flaky skin	Vitamin A, vitamin B complex, or linoleic acid deficiency
	Dry skin with poor turgor	Dehydration
	Rough, scaly skin with bumps	
	Petechiae or ecchymoses	Vitamin A deficiency
	Sore that will not heal	Vitamin C or K deficiency
	Thinning, dry hair	Protein, vitamin C, or zinc deficiency
	Spoon-shaped, brittle, or rigid nails	Protein deficiency / Iron deficiency
Eyes	Night blindness; corneal swelling, softening, or dryness; Bitot's spots (gray triangular patches on the conjunctiva)	Vitamin A deficiency
	Red conjunctiva	Riboflavin deficiency
Throat and mouth	Cracks at the corner of mouth	Riboflavin or niacin deficiency
	Magenta tongue	Riboflavin deficiency
	Beefy, red tongue	Vitamin B_{12} deficiency
	Soft, spongy, bleeding gums	Vitamin C deficiency
	Swollen neck (goiter)	Iodine deficiency
Cardiovascular	Edema	Protein deficiency
	Tachycardia, hypotension	Fluid volume deficit
Gastrointestinal	Ascites	Protein deficiency
Musculoskeletal	Bone pain and bow leg	Vitamin D or calcium deficiency
	Muscle wasting	Protein, carbohydrate, and fat deficiency
Neurological	Altered mental status	Dehydration and thiamine or vitamin B_{12} deficiency
	Paresthesia	Vitamin B_{12}, pyridoxine, or thiamine deficiency

From Nutrition Made Incredibly Easy. Philadelphia: Lippincott Williams & Wilkins, Springhouse, 2006.

dietary habits with greater accuracy. It is also necessary to consider a patient's past or current patterns of food intake, or both, such as vegetarian or kosher diet practices, as well as cultural background and social situation.[11] Special consideration of the geriatric patient is warranted; age-related changes in the gastrointestinal system may affect dietary intake and maintenance of adequate nutrition (Box 39-2).

Serial weight measurement is perhaps the single most important indicator of nutritional status and is the evaluation that the nurse performs most often. In addition, a number of quick and efficient screening instruments have been developed. The Subjective Global Assessment (SGA) is an example of a screening instrument (Fig. 39-15).

An important factor that influences nutritional status is nitrogen balance, a sensitive indicator of the body's gain or loss of protein. An adult is in nitrogen balance when the nitrogen intake equals the nitrogen output (in urine, feces, and perspiration). Nitrogen balance is a sign of health. A positive nitrogen balance exists when nitrogen intake exceeds nitrogen output and indicates tissue growth, such as

occurs during recovery from surgery, and rebuilding of wasted tissue. A negative nitrogen balance indicates that the tissue is breaking down faster than it is being replaced. In the absence of an adequate intake of protein, the body converts protein to glucose for energy. This can occur with fever, starvation, surgery, burns, and debilitating diseases. Malnutrition occurs when a patient is in negative nitrogen balance. Malnutrition, in turn, interferes with wound healing, increases susceptibility to infection, and contributes to an increased incidence of complications, a protracted hospitalization, and an extended bed confinement.[12]

The nutritional assessment directs the nutritional prescription and assists in the development of the interventions. Enteral or parenteral nutrition may be initiated if oral intake is prohibited or threatened for longer than a week. If the gastrointestinal tract of the patient is functioning, enteral feeding is the intervention of choice. For people without a functioning gastrointestinal tract, total parenteral nutrition may be the nutritional treatment of choice. See Chapter 40 for a discussion of enteral and parenteral nutrition. The level of interventions is dictated by the patient's baseline nutritional state, disease status,

Box 39-2 • CONSIDERATIONS FOR THE OLDER PATIENT: Age-Related Changes of the Gastrointestinal System

Oral Cavity and Pharynx
- Injury/loss or decay of teeth
- Atrophy of taste buds
- Decreased saliva production
- Reduced ptyalin and amylase in saliva

Esophagus
- Decreased motility and emptying
- Weakened gag reflex
- Decreased resting pressure of lower esophageal sphincter

Stomach
- Degeneration and atrophy of gastric mucosal surfaces with decreased production of HCl
- Decreased secretion of gastric acids and most digestive enzymes
- Decreased motility and emptying

Small Intestine
- Atrophy of muscle and mucosal surfaces
- Thinning of villi and epithelial cells

Large Intestine
- Decrease in mucus secretion
- Decrease in elasticity of rectal wall
- Decreased tone of internal anal sphincter
- Slower and duller nerve impulses in rectal area

From Smeltzer SC, Bare BG, Hinkle JL, Cheever KH (eds): Brunner & Suddarth's Textbook of Medical-Surgical Nursing, 11th ed. Philadelphia: Lippincott Williams & Wilkins, 2008, p 1126.

risk for malnutrition from treatment, and anticipated response to therapy.[13]

• Laboratory Studies

Because the oral cavity is the only part of the gastrointestinal tract that is visible, it is essential to combine the information gleaned from the history and physical examination with the results of laboratory and diagnostic studies to assess the rest of the gastrointestinal tract. Many laboratory studies help in the diagnosis of gastrointestinal and abdominal disorders in the critically ill patient. Parameters evaluated include serum electrolytes; levels of end products of metabolism, enzymes, and proteins; and hematological parameters.

LABORATORY STUDIES RELATING TO LIVER FUNCTION

The liver is responsible for many functions, the most significant being bile formation and secretion, protein and fat metabolism, detoxification of many substances, and the production of clotting factors and enzymes. Table 39-6 summarizes common laboratory studies relating to liver function.

A single laboratory test or single value from any laboratory test does not give an accurate assessment of an organ's function. A series of values from a laboratory study and combinations of studies provide a

(Select appropriate category with a checkmark, or enter numerical value where indicated by "#.")

A. History
1. Weight change
   Overall loss in past 6 months: amount = #_____kg; % loss = #_____
   Change in past 2 weeks _____increase,
   　　　　　　　　　_____no change,
   　　　　　　　　　_____decrease.
2. Dietary intake change (relative to normal)
   _____No change
   _____Change _____duration = #_____weeks.
   　　　　　　_____type: _____suboptimal solid diet, _____full liquid diet,
   　　　　　　　　　_____hypocaloric liquids, _____starvation.
3. Gastrointestinal symptoms (that persisted for > 2 weeks)
   _____none, _____nausea, _____vomiting, _____diarrhea, _____anorexia.
4. Functional capacity
   _____No dysfunction (e.g., full capacity)
   _____Dysfunction _____duration = #_____weeks.
   　　　　　　_____type: _____working suboptimally,
   　　　　　　　　　_____ambulatory,
   　　　　　　　　　_____bedridden.
5. Disease and its relation to nutritional requirements
   Primary diagnosis (specify)_____
   _____
   Metabolic demand (stress): _____no stress, _____low stress,
   　　　　　　　_____moderate stress, _____high stress.

B. Physical (for each trait specify: 0 = normal, 1+ = mild, 2+ = moderate, 3+ = severe)
　#_____loss of subcutaneous fat (triceps, chest)
　#_____muscle wasting (quadriceps, deltoids)
　#_____ankle edema
　#_____sacral edema
　#_____ascites

C. SGA rating (select one)
　_____A = Well-nourished
　_____B = Moderately (or suspected of being) malnourished
　_____C = Severely malnourished

Figure 39-15 • The Subjective Global Assessment (SGA), used to assess nutritional status. The final SGA rating is based on clinical judgment of the items and not a specific number. (Reprinted from the American Society for Parenteral and Enteral Nutrition [ASPEN]: J Parenter Enter Nutr 11[1]:8–13, 1987. ASPEN does not endorse the use of this material in any form other than its entirety.)

Table 39-6 • Laboratory Studies Used to Evaluate Liver Function

Study	Normal Findings	Clinical and Nursing Significance
Bile Formation and Secretion		
Serum bilirubin		
Direct (conjugated)—soluble in water	0–5.1 µmol/L	Abnormal in biliary and liver disease; causes clinical jaundice
Indirect (unconjugated)—insoluble in water	0–14 µmol/L	Abnormal in hemolysis and in functional disorders of uptake or conjugation
Urine bilirubin	0	Urine is mahogany in color; shaking the specimen results in a light yellow foam; confirmed with Ictotest tablet or dipstick; false-positive results possible if patient is taking phenazopyridine (Pyridium)
Urobilinogen		Increased in cirrhosis; biliary obstruction with biliary tract infection; hemorrhage; and hepatoxicity; decreased in biliary obstruction without biliary tract infection; hepatocellular damage; and renal insufficiency
Urine urobilinogen	Up to 0.09–4.23 µmol/24 h	Urine specimen is collected over a 2-h period after lunch; must be placed in a dark brown container and sent to the laboratory immediately to prevent decomposition
Fecal urobilinogen	Up to 0.068–0.34 mmol/24 h	
Protein Studies		
Albumin	35–55 g/L	Decreased in cirrhosis, chronic hepatitis
Globulin	15–30 g/L	Increased in cirrhosis, chronic obstructive jaundice, viral hepatitis
Albumin/globulin ratio	1.5:1 to 2.5:1	Ratio reverses with chronic hepatitis or other chronic liver disease
Total serum protein	60–80 g/L	Individual protein measurements are of greater significance than total protein measurements
Transferrin	220–400 µg/dL	Decreased in cirrhosis, hepatitis, and malignancy; increased in severe iron deficiency anemia
Prothrombin time (PT)	11.0–14.0 sec or 100% of control	Prolonged PT in liver disease will not return to normal with vitamin K administration, whereas prolonged PT resulting from malabsorption of fat and fat-soluble vitamins will return to normal with vitamin K administration
Partial thromboplastin time (PTT)	25.0–36.0 sec	Increased with severe liver disease or therapy with heparin or other anticoagulants
α-Fetoprotein (AFP)	6–20 ng/mL	Elevated in primary hepatocellular carcinoma
Fat Metabolism		
Cholesterol	< 200 mg/dL (adults)	Decreased in parenchymal liver disease; increased in biliary obstruction
High-density lipoprotein (HDL)		
Men	35–70 mg/dL	
Women	35–85 mg/dL	
Low-density lipoprotein (LDL)	<130 mg/dL	
Very-low-density lipoprotein (VLDL)	25%–50%	
Liver Detoxification		
Serum alkaline phosphatase (AP)	20–90 U/L at 30°C	Level is elevated to more than 3 times normal in obstructive jaundice, intrahepatic cholestasis, liver metastasis, or granulomas; also elevated in osteoblastic diseases, Paget's disease, and hyperparathyroidism
Ammonia	15–49 µg/dL	An elevation indicates hepatocyte damage (liver converts ammonia to urea)
Enzyme Production		
Aspartate aminotransferase (AST)	8–20 U/L	Any elevation indicates hepatocyte damage
Alanine aminotransferase (ALT)	10–32 U/L	Any elevation indicates hepatocyte damage
Lactate dehydrogenase (LDH)	200–500 U/L	Any elevation indicates hepatocyte damage
γ-Glutamyl transferase (GGT)	0–30 U/L at 30°C	An elevation in GGT along with an elevated alkaline phosphatase usually indicates biliary disease; helpful in the diagnosis of chronic liver disease

more precise picture. For example, if a patient's liver enzymes and bilirubin are elevated but the alkaline phosphatase level is normal, this usually indicates injury to the hepatocytes, such as in hepatitis and cirrhosis. If the liver enzymes are within normal range and the bilirubin and alkaline phosphatase levels are elevated, this usually indicates an extrahepatic biliary obstruction, such as in a distal common bile duct obstruction from pancreatic cancer or a clip occluding the common bile duct from a laparoscopic cholecystectomy misadventure.

LABORATORY STUDIES RELATING TO PANCREATIC FUNCTION

Table 39-7 lists serum laboratory tests that relate to pancreatic function. Amylase and lipase are digestive enzymes secreted by the pancreas. Serum amylase is found in the pancreas, parotid glands, intestine, liver, and fallopian tubes. Lipase is found primarily in the pancreas. In acute pancreatitis, serum amylase and lipase can be elevated 4 to 6 times the normal level, whereas in chronic pancreatitis, serum amylase and lipase levels may be normal or very low because the pancreas may no longer be producing the enzymes.

The pancreas produces insulin and glucagon, hormones that aid in the regulation of serum glucose levels. A disruption in normal pancreatic function or the presence of a tumor may alter the production of these hormones. Frequent blood glucose monitoring is warranted. Any elevation in the serum and urine glucose levels has a cascading effect on multiple body systems, which in turn affects the patient's overall condition.[14]

OTHER LABORATORY STUDIES

Table 39-8 provides information about other selected laboratory studies that are used in the evaluation of gastrointestinal disorders.

• Diagnostic Studies

The nurse caring for the critically ill patient coordinates the preparation for, and possibly the timing of, many diagnostic tests. The nurse prepares the patient, the family members, or both for the test by providing a thorough explanation of how the test is performed and what information the test is expected to yield. In addition, the nurse explains the need for informed consent to perform the test and answers any questions the patient or family members may have about the test. Table 39-9 summarizes the diagnostic studies for evaluating the gastrointestinal tract, which can be divided into two categories, noninvasive and invasive.

RADIOLOGICAL AND IMAGING STUDIES

Body tissue has different densities that produce different shades of black and white on an x-ray. Bone tissue is high in density and appears white; air appears black; and soft tissue results in shades of gray. The stomach and intestines usually contain some air and appear darker. Solid organs, such as the pancreas, spleen, kidneys, or liver, appear grayer.[15]

ENDOSCOPIC STUDIES

The use of an endoscope is an important adjunct to radiographic studies because it allows direct observation of portions of the intestinal tract. A flexible fiberoptic endoscope, designed with a movable tip, can be manipulated through the intestinal tract by the operator. It also includes an instrument channel that allows for biopsy of lesions, such as tumors, ulcers, or areas of inflammation. Fluids can be aspirated from the lumen of the intestinal tract, and air can be insufflated to distend the intestinal tract for better observation. Cytology brushes and electrocautery snares can be passed through the scope. Special studies of the

(text continues on page 1012)

Table 39-7 • Laboratory Studies Used to Evaluate Pancreatic Function

Study	Normal Findings	Clinical and Nursing Significance
Serum amylase	25–125 U/L	In acute pancreatitis, the serum levels peak between 4–8 h after onset of condition, then fall to normal within 48–72 h; low levels usually indicate pancreatic insufficiency.
Urine amylase	2 h: 2–34 units 24 h: 24–408 units	Urine values 6–10 h behind serum values; low levels indicate pancreatic insufficiency.
Serum lipase	10–40 U/L (adults)	Elevated only in pancreatitis, markedly in acute pancreatitis and pancreatic duct obstruction; remains elevated after amylase returns to baseline.
Serum glucose	65–110 mg/dL (fasting)	Patient must fast for 12 h before drawing of specimen.
Serum triglycerides	50–250 mg/dL	Patient must fast for 12 h before drawing of specimen; levels increased in alcoholic cirrhosis, diabetes mellitus (untreated), high-carbohydrate diet, hyperlipoproteinemia, and hypertension; levels decreased in malnutrition, vigorous exercise.

Serum calcium
  Total
  Ionized
	
	8.2–10.2 mg/dL
	4.65–5.28 mg/dL
		
		High total calcium levels seen in cancer of the liver, pancreas, and other organs.
		Useful in tracking the course of disorders such as cancer and acute pancreatitis.

Fecal fat	2–5 g/24 h	Content of greater than 6 g/24 h is suggestive of a decrease in the body's ability to absorb foods; indicative of pancreatic exocrine insufficiency as in chronic pancreatitis.

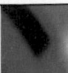

Table 39-8 • Other Selected Laboratory Studies Used in the Diagnosis of Gastrointestinal Disorders

Study	Normal Findings	Clinical and Nursing Significance
Stool specimen		
Occult blood	None	Positive test suggests possible malignancy.
Fat	2–5 g/24 h	Screening test for steatorrhea when malabsorption syndrome or pancreatic insufficiency is suspected.
Ova and parasites	None	Positive test suggests infection.
Pus	None	Increased amount of pus may indicate ulcerative colitis, abscess, or anal or rectal fissure.
Pathogens	None	Common pathogens are *Salmonella typhi* (typhoid fever), *Shigella* (dysentery), *Vibrio cholerae* (cholera), *Yersinia* (enterocolitis), *Escherichia coli* and *Aeromonas* (gastroenteritis), *Staphylococcus aureus, Clostridium botulinum,* and *Clostridium perfringens* (food poisoning).
Urea breath test	Negative	Detects the presence of *Helicobacter pylori*
Hydrogen breath test	Negative	Determines the amount of hydrogen expelled in the breath after it is produced in the colon and absorbed into the blood; aids in the diagnosis of bacterial overgrowth in the intestine and short bowel syndrome.

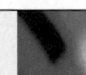

Table 39-9 • Diagnostic Studies Used to Evaluate the Gastrointestinal Tract

Study	Description	Indications	Invasiveness	Preparation	Contrast
Abdominal film "flat plate of the abdomen"	Radiology test used to visualize a single flat plane; shows organ size, position, intactness, and normal gas patterns in the stomach, small intestine, and colon	Aids in diagnosis of intestinal obstruction, organ rupture, masses, foreign bodies, abnormal fluid or air ("stones, bones, gas, masses")	Noninvasive	None	No
Upper gastrointestinal (GI) series (barium swallow)	Radiology test used to visualize the esophagus, stomach, and duodenum; barium enhances image; double-contrast study administers barium first followed by a radiolucent substance, such as air, to help coat bowel mucosa for better visualization of any type of lesion	Aids in diagnosis of hiatal hernia, ulcers, tumors, foreign bodies, bowel obstruction	Noninvasive	NPO	Yes
Upper GI series with small bowel follow-through	Radiology test used to visualize the jejunum, ileum, and cecum	Aids in the diagnosis of tumors, Crohn's disease, Meckel's diverticulum	Noninvasive	NPO	Yes
Enteroclysis	Radiology test used to visualize entire small intestine; continuous infusion (through a duodenal tube) of air in a barium sulfate suspension along with methylcellulose fills the intestinal loops; transit of contrast filmed at intervals for progress through jejunum and ileum	Aids in diagnosis of partial bowel obstruction or diverticula	Invasive	NPO	Yes
Barium enema	Radiology test used to visualize the colon; barium enhances image; air may be introduced after the barium to provide a double-contrast study	Aids in diagnosis of polyps, tumors, fistulas, obstruction, diverticula, and stenosis	Noninvasive	Bowel cleansing	Yes
Gastric lavage	Aspiration of stomach contents and washing out of the stomach by a large gastric tube	Aids in diagnosis of upper GI bleeding, also used to arrest hemorrhage and prepare for further tests	Invasive	None	No

(continued)

Table 39-9 • Diagnostic Studies Used to Evaluate the Gastrointestinal Tract (Continued)

Study	Description	Indications	Invasiveness	Preparation	Contrast
Paracentesis	Aspiration of peritoneal fluid	Laboratory studies (such as amylase and lipase to assess for pancreatitis); cytologic studies (to detect tumors); comfort measure (to alleviate accumulation of ascitic fluid)	Invasive	None	No
Peritoneal lavage	Irrigation of peritoneal cavity to examine irrigating fluid for blood	Blunt or penetrating trauma to the abdomen	Invasive	None	No
Biopsy					
Percutaneous	A needle is placed through the skin to obtain tissue specimen for pathology evaluation	Aids in diagnosis of malignancy	Invasive	NPO	No
Fine-needle aspiration (FNA)	A thin needle is used to obtain cells or minute tissue fragments from a suspect area for examination by light microscopy; usually guided by radiologists with fluoroscopy, ultrasound, computed tomography, or magnetic resonance imaging	Aids in diagnosis of malignancy	Invasive	NPO	No
Ultrasonography (sonogram)	Use of high-frequency sound waves over an abdominal organ to obtain an image of the structure	Aids in diagnosis of masses, dilated bile ducts, gallstones, and ascites	Noninvasive	NPO	No
Hepatobiliary scan	Intravenously injected radioisotope is primarily taken up by the liver and then secreted into the bile, allowing visualization of the biliary system, gallbladder, and duodenum (size, function, vascularity, and blood flow)	Aids in the diagnoses of common bile duct obstruction, acute and chronic cholecystitis, bile leaks, biliary dyskinesia, and biliary atresia; also used to evaluate liver transplant function	Noninvasive	NPO	Yes
Tagged red blood cell scan (technetium-labeled red blood cell scintigraphy)	Red blood cells are labeled with technetium and injected intravenously; images are obtained with a gamma camera that can identify areas of increased radioactivity as a site of slow or intermittent GI hemorrhage	Aids in the diagnosis of GI bleeding	Noninvasive	None	Yes
Computed tomography (CT) scan	A radiological procedure that uses narrow x-ray beams to produce cross-sectional images of organs and tissues; can be performed with or without contrast medium; multidetector-row CT (MDCT) now provides more exact information	Excellent for visualizing the abdomen, retroperitoneal structures, tumors, cysts, collection of fluid, air in a cavity, bleeding or pulmonary embolism	Noninvasive	NPO	Yes/No

(continued)

Table 39-9 • Diagnostic Studies Used to Evaluate the Gastrointestinal Tract (Continued)

Study	Description	Indications	Invasiveness	Preparation	Contrast
Magnetic resonance imaging (MRI)	Diagnostic study that does not use radiation; obtains images by passing the patient through a tubular device that generates a powerful electromagnetic field; radiofrequency waves are transmitted into the patient in a controlled manner so that the patient's hydrogen ions (protons) emit radiofrequency signals that are processed by a computer to produce an image	Useful in evaluating abdominal soft tissue and blood vessels, abscesses, fistulas, tumors, and sources of bleeding	Noninvasive	No metal devices attached to or implanted in the patient; patient must be able to lie quietly for a period of time	No
Magnetic resonance cholangiopancreatography (MRCP)	Similar to MRI; because no contrast agent is required, MRCP is ideal for patients with allergies to iodine-based contrast medium	Aids in the diagnosis of disorders affecting the pancreatic ducts and biliary tree	Noninvasive	No metal devices attached to or implanted in the patient	No
Percutaneous transhepatic cholangiography (PTC)	Radiological procedure done under fluoroscopy to examine the intrahepatic and extrahepatic biliary ducts after injection of contrast medium into the biliary tree through percutaneous needle injection	Helps to distinguish obstructive jaundice caused by liver disease from jaundice caused by biliary obstruction (e.g., from a tumor, common bile duct injury, stones within the bile ducts, or sclerosing cholangitis)	Invasive	NPO	Yes
Percutaneous transhepatic biliary drainage (PTBD)	A biliary catheter is placed during a PTC; the biliary catheter may be placed to the obstruction or it may bypass the obstruction to allow the free flow of bile; catheter relieves jaundice and pruritus; improves nutritional status; allows easy access into the biliary tree for further procedures; can be used as an anatomical landmark and stent at the time of surgery	Biliary obstruction resulting in jaundice, cholangitis, sepsis, or pain	Invasive	NPO	Yes
Positron emission tomography (PET)	A computerized radiographic technique that uses radioactive substances to examine the metabolic activity of body structures	Useful for precisely locating a tumor	Noninvasive	None	Yes
Angiography	A radiographic study of selected arteries and veins to see defects in the walls of the vessels; also used to evaluate blood flow through the vessels	Usually done when initial, noninvasive procedures are insufficient in revealing the cause of a suspected vascular defect	Invasive	NPO	Yes

common bile duct and the pancreatic duct, or endoscopic retrograde cholangiopancreatography, use a side-viewing upper intestinal endoscope.[16] Table 39-10 describes endoscopic procedures used to evaluate the gastrointestinal tract.

OTHER DIAGNOSTIC STUDIES

In addition to radiological and imaging studies and endoscopic procedures, other studies are specifically designed to aid in the diagnosis of gastrointestinal disorders.[13] Table 39-11 provides information about

selected diagnostic studies used to diagnose specific gastrointestinal disorders.

• Clinical Applicability Challenges

Case Study

Mrs. A is a 79-year-old woman with a history of coronary artery disease, hypertension, gastroesophageal reflux disease, irritable bowel syndrome, and a left modified radical mastectomy

Table 39-10 • Endoscopic Studies Used to Evaluate the Gastrointestinal Tract

Study	Description	Indications	Invasiveness	Preparation	Contrast
Esophagogastro-duodenoscopy (EGD)	Endoscope passed through the mouth and advanced to visualize the esophagus, stomach, and duodenum; any abnormalities can be photographed and biopsied; bleeding areas may be cauterized and varices may be injected with sclerosing agents	Helps to diagnose acute or chronic upper GI bleeding, esophageal or gastric varices, polyps, tumors, ulcers, esophagitis, gastritis, esophageal stenosis, and gastroesophageal reflux	Invasive	NPO	No
Colonoscopy	Flexible fiberoptic endoscope passed through the rectum and advanced to visualize the large intestine; any abnormalities can be photographed and biopsied; polyps can be removed and bleeding areas may be cauterized	Helps to diagnose bleeding, diverticulosis, polyps, stricture, tumor, or inflammatory bowel disease (Crohn's disease or ulcerative colitis)	Invasive	Bowel cleansing	No
Proctoscopy (anoscopy)	Rigid scope passed through the rectum to visualize the mucosal surface of the anus and rectum	Helps to diagnose polyps, bleeding, tumors, and other defects	Invasive	None	No
Sigmoidoscopy	Flexible fiberoptic endoscope passed through the rectum and advanced to visualize the rectum, sigmoid colon, and proximal colon; any lesions can be biopsied	Helps to diagnose tumors, polyps, diverticula, or bleeding	Invasive	Enema	No
Endoscopic retrograde cholangiopancreatography (ERCP)	Flexible fiberoptic endoscope inserted into the esophagus, passed through the stomach, and into the duodenum to visualize the common bile duct, hepatic bile ducts, and pancreatic ducts; the common bile duct and pancreatic duct are cannulated and contrast medium is injected into the ducts, permitting visualization and radiographic evaluation	Can detect extrahepatic biliary obstruction (e.g., from stones, tumors of the bile duct, strictures or injuries to the bile duct); intrahepatic biliary obstruction caused by stones or tumor; and pancreatic disease, such as chronic pancreatitis, pseudocysts, or tumors	Invasive	NPO	Yes
Endoscopic ultrasonography	Endoscopy and ultrasonography are used to visualize the GI tract; an ultrasonic transducer built into the distal end of the endoscope allows for high-quality resolution of the walls of the GI tract	Useful in evaluating and staging tumors of the GI tract	Invasive	NPO	No

Table 39-11 • Other Selected Diagnostic Studies Used in the Diagnosis of Gastrointestinal Disorders

Study	Description	Normal Findings
Gastric emptying studies	Liquid and solid components of a meal are tagged with a radionuclide marker. After ingesting the meal, the rate of passage of the radioactive substance out of the stomach is measured by a scintiscanner. Useful in diagnosing gastric motility disorders	Normal transit
Gastric analysis	Analysis of gastric juice yields information about the secretory activity of the gastric mucosa and the presence or degree of gastric retention, which is useful to help diagnose patients with pyloric or duodenal obstruction.	Normal contents
Gastric acid stimulation (usually performed in conjunction with gastric analysis)	Histamine or pentagastrin is given subcutaneously to stimulate gastric secretions. Gastric specimens are collected at intervals for analysis. Helps to determine the presence or absence of malignant cells.	11–20 mEq/h after stimulation
Manometry	Measurement of pressures using a water-filled catheter connected to a transducer passed into the esophagus, stomach, colon, or rectum to evaluate contractility; useful in detecting motility disorders of the esophagus and lower esophageal sphincter; gastroduodenal, small intestine, and colonic manometry are used to evaluate delayed gastric emptying and gastric and intestinal motility disorders such as irritable bowel syndrome or atonic colon; anorectal manometry measures the resting tone of the internal anal sphincter and the contractility of the external anal sphincter, which is helpful in evaluation of chronic constipation or fecal incontinence	Values differ at various levels of the intestine
Gastric tonometry	Monitoring modality used to determine the perfusion status of the gastric mucosa using measurements of local PCO_2. The CO_2 diffuses from the mucosa of the stomach into the lumen of the stomach and then into the silicone balloon of the tonometer. The PCO_2 within the balloon serves as a proxy measure for gastric mucosal CO_2 ($PgCO_2$). In a normally perfused gastric mucosa, $PgCO_2$ is nearly equivalent to the $PaCO_2$. With hypoperfusion, the $PgCO_2$ increases and the gap between the $PgCO_2$ and the $PaCO_2$ increases. The gap is a very sensitive indicator of gastric hypoperfusion.	The $PgCO_2$ and the $PaCO_2$ are nearly equal.

and adjuvant therapy for breast cancer 5 years earlier who develops jaundice, pruritus, and abdominal pain. The pain begins in the mid-epigastric area of the abdomen and radiates around both sides to the back. The woman's family noted yellowing of her sclera 2 weeks ago when she complained of severe itching all over her body. She has taken over-the-counter medications for the pruritus with minimal effect and has self-inflicted multiple scratches over her torso and extremities. In addition, she has also noted a decrease in her appetite, a 10-pound weight loss, very dark urine, and clay-colored stools.

An evaluation by her primary care physician included laboratory values significant for the following: total bilirubin, 8.6 µmol/L; alanine aminotransferase, 129 U/L; aspartate aminotransferase, 120 U/L; alkaline phosphatase, 700 U/L; total protein, 4.8 g/L; and albumin, 2.3 g/L. Complete blood count and coagulation studies were within normal limits. Multidetector-row computed tomography revealed a 3.5-cm mass in the head of the pancreas, intrahepatic and extrahepatic bile duct dilation with an enlarged gallbladder, no vessel involvement, and no evidence of metastatic lesions.

The patient's physician referred her to an interventional gastroenterologist for endoscopic retrograde cholangiopancreatography and decompression of her biliary tree by placement of an endoscopic stent. This procedure was not successful. Interventional radiologists then saw her, and she had a percutaneous transhepatic cholangiogram with placement of an internal-external percutaneous transhepatic biliary drain. This procedure immediately allowed the free flow of dark bile to exit into a dependent external bile bag for biliary decompression. The patient experienced rigor and chills, along with a temperature of 103.5°F (39.7°C) after the procedure. She was transferred from the interventional radiology department directly to the intensive care unit.

1. Discuss the risk factors for malnutrition for the patient in the case study.
2. What would be included in an educational plan for the patient and her family?
3. What directed abdominal assessment would the nurse perform when the patient in the case study is admitted to the intensive care unit?

Review Questions

1. Laboratory studies are performed for a patient who is admitted to the hospital. What laboratory

value provides the best initial information about the patient's nutritional status?
   a. Albumin
   b. Protein
   c. Prealbumin
   d. Transferrin

2. The nurse performs an oral assessment of a patient in the intensive care unit who is mechanically ventilated and has a nasogastric tube in place. What abnormal findings require prompt intervention?
   a. Copious secretions and foul oral odor
   b. Missing and broken teeth
   c. Saliva under the tongue
   d. Pink and moist mucous membranes

3. A patient is admitted to the intensive care unit with nausea, vomiting, distended abdomen, and no bowel movements in the past 3 days. The order of the abdominal assessment is
   a. inspection, percussion, palpation, auscultation.
   b. inspection, auscultation, percussion, palpation.
   c. inspection, auscultation, palpation, percussion.
   d. inspection, percussion, auscultation, palpation.

4. The patient with obstructive jaundice from an extrahepatic bile duct obstruction would most likely have the following laboratory values:
   a. Elevated alanine aminotransferase and aspartate aminotransferase
   b. Elevated bilirubin and alkaline phosphatase
   c. Elevated alanine aminotransferase and alanine phosphatase
   d. Elevated bilirubin and aspartate aminotransferase

5. The patient arrives in the intensive care unit after surgery for wound dehiscence and evisceration. An important assessment of the patient's abdomen would include
   a. assessing abdominal symmetry.
   b. percussion of the abdomen.
   c. auscultation of bowel sounds.
   d. deep palpation of the abdominal wall.

References

1. Ignatavicius DD, Workman ML: Medical-Surgical Nursing: Critical Thinking for Collaborative Care, 5th ed. Philadelphia: WB Saunders, 2005
2. Tierney LM, Henderson MC: The Patient History: Evidence-Based Approach. New York: Lange Medical Books/McGraw Hill, 2005
3. Higgins PA, Daly BJ, Lipson AR, Guo S: Assessing nutritional status in chronically critically ill adult patients. Am J Crit Care 15(2):166–176, 2006
4. Silen W: Cope's Early Diagnosis of the Acute Abdomen, 20th ed. Oxford: Oxford University Press, 2000
5. D'Amico D, Barbarito C: Health & Physical Assessment in Nursing. Englewood Cliffs, New Jersey, Prentice Hall, 2006
6. Leblond RF, DeGowin RL, Brown DD: DeGowin's Diagnostic Examination. New York, McGraw Hill, 2004
7. Cutler CJ, Davis N: Improving oral care in patients receiving mechanical ventilation. Am J Crit Care 14(5): 389–384, 2005
8. Estes MEZ: Health Assessment and Physical Examination, 3rd ed. Canada: Thomson Delmar Learning, 2006
9. Goolsby MJ, Grubbs L: Advanced Assessment: Interpreting Findings and Formulating Differential Diagnoses. Philadelphia: FA Davis, 2006
10. Rodriguez L: Nutritional status: Assessing and understanding its value in the critical care setting. Crit Care Nurs Clin North Am 16(4):509–514, 2004
11. Hark L, Morrison G: Medical Nutrition and Disease: A Case-Based Approach, 3rd ed. Malden, MA: Blackwell Science, 2003
12. Harrington L: Nutrition in critically ill adults: Key processes and outcomes. Crit Care Nurs Clin North Am 16(4):459–465, 2004
13. Griffiths RD, Bongers T: Nutrition support for patients in the intensive care unit. Postgrad Med J 81:629–636, 2005
14. Finney SJ, Zekveld C, Elia A, Evans TW: Glucose control and mortality in critically ill patients. JAMA 290:2041–2047, 2003
15. Federle MP, Jeffrey RB, Desser TS, et al: Diagnostic Imaging: Abdomen, 1st ed. Canada: Amirsys, Inc., Elsevier Saunders, 2005
16. Cotton PB, Leung J: Advanced Digestive Endoscopy: ERCP. Malden, MA: Blackwell Publishing, 2005

Other Selected Readings

Andreoli TE, Carpenter CCJ, Griggs RC, Loscalzo J: Cecil's Essentials of Medicine, 6th ed. Philadelphia: WB Saunders, 2003
Bickley LS: Bates' Guide to Physical Examination and History Taking, 9th ed. Philadelphia: Lippincott Williams & Wilkins, 2007
Chernecky CC, Berger BJ: Laboratory Tests and Diagnostic Procedures, 4th ed. Philadelphia: Saunders, 2004
Craven RF, Hirnle CJ: Fundamentals of Nursing: Human Health and Function, 5th ed. Philadelphia: Lippincott Williams & Wilkins, 2007
Determann RM, Wolthius EK, Spronk PE, et al: Reliability of height and weight estimation in patients acutely admitted to intensive care units. Crit Care Nurse 27(5):48–55, 2007
Gibson RS: Principles of Nutritional Assessment, 2nd ed. New York: Oxford University Press, 2005
Halpert RD: Gastrointestinal Imaging: The Requisites, 3rd ed. Philadelphia: Mosby Elsevier, 2006
Heard SO. Gastric tonometry: The hemodynamic monitor of choice.
Higgins PA, Daily BJ, Lipson AR, Guo, SE: Assessing nutritional status in chronically critically ill adult patients. Am J Crit Care 15(2):166–177, 2006
Kasper DL, Fauci AS, Longo DL, et al: Harrison's Principles of Internal Medicine, 16th ed. New York: McGraw Hill, 2005
Lee M: Basic Skills in Interpreting Laboratory Data, 3rd ed. Bethesda, MD: American Society of Health-System Pharmacists, 2004
Munro CL, Grap MJ: Oral health and care in the intensive care unit: State of the science. Am J Crit Care 13:25–33, 2004
Pagana KD, Pagana TJ: Mosby's Diagnostic and Laboratory Test Reference, 7th ed. St. Louis: Elsevier Mosby, 2005
Pineda LA, Saliba RG, El Sohl AA: Effect of oral decontamination with chlorhexidine on the incidence of nosocomial pneumonia: A meta-analysis. Crit Care 10:R25, 2006
Runge MS, Greganti MA: Netter's Internal Medicine. Teterboro, NJ: Icon Learning Systems LLC, 2003
Sabol VK: Nutrition assessment of the critically ill adult. AACN Clin Issues 15(4):595–606, 2004
Shils ME, Shike M, Ross AC, et al: Modern Nutrition in Health and Disease, 10th ed. Philadelphia: Lippincott Williams & Wilkins, 2006
Stonesifer E: Common laboratory and diagnostic testing in patients with gastrointestinal disease. AACN Clin Issues 15(4):582–594, 2004
Weber J, Kelley J: Health Assessment in Nursing, 3rd ed. Philadelphia: Lippincott Williams & Wilkins, 2007

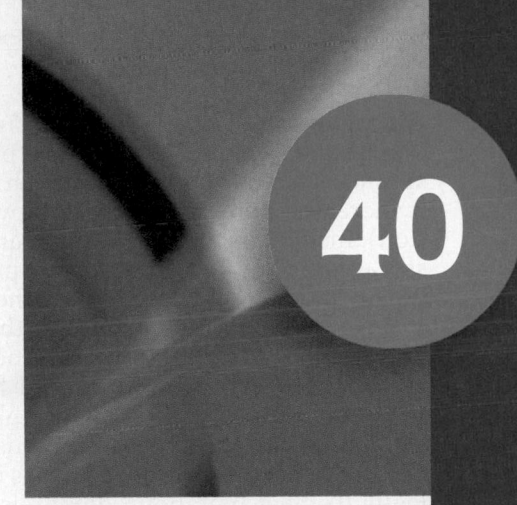

Patient Management: Gastrointestinal System

Valerie K. Sabol • Allison G. Steele

40

Malnutrition
Nutritional Support
    Enteral Nutrition
    Parenteral (Intravenous) Nutrition
    Role of the Nurse in Nutritional Support
Pharmacological Management of Gastrointestinal Disorders

Objectives

Based on the content in this chapter, the reader should be able to:

1 Explain how the physiological stressors of illness and injury alter the body's needs for energy.

2 Describe the different forms of malnutrition.

3 Discuss enteral and parenteral nutrition with regard to indications, assessment, management, and complications.

4 Discuss common medications used for patients with gastrointestinal disorders.

Health and nutrition have a symbiotic relationship. Physiological stressors, such as illness and injury, alter the body's metabolic and energy demands. Although early identification and nutritional intervention can lessen morbidity and mortality risks in critically ill patients, the underlying disease process must be identified and corrected before the body can reverse abnormal nutrient metabolism. This chapter presents an overview of physiological stress and its effect on metabolism, types of malnutrition, and the indications, assessment, and management of enteral and parenteral nutrition support therapies and the complications associated with these therapies. The chapter also provides an overview of commonly used medications for patients with gastrointestinal disorders.

• Malnutrition

According to the laws of thermodynamics, energy can be neither created nor destroyed. Through the processes of metabolism, people obtain energy from the foods (or organic fuels) they consume. Metabolism has two parts: anabolism and catabolism. Anabolism is a building-up and repair process that requires energy. Catabolism consists of breaking down food and body tissues for the purpose of liberating energy.

Glucose is the obligatory fuel of the body, and it is the primary fuel of the brain and nervous system in particular. The nervous system cannot store or synthesize glucose as a fuel source, so it relies on glucose extraction from the bloodstream. The liver regulates glucose entry into the circulatory system because it has the ability to both store and synthesize glucose. Excess glucose is converted and stored as either glycogen or fatty acids (triglycerides). Although glucose can be converted to fatty acids for storage, there is no pathway for converting fatty acids back to glucose. Instead, fatty acids are used directly as a fuel source or are converted to ketones by the liver. After prolonged starvation, the body adapts to preserve vital proteins by using ketones, rather than glucose, as energy. Ketoacidosis occurs when ketone production exceeds utilization.

The pancreatic hormones glucagon and insulin have opposing functions in metabolic processes.

Glucagon stimulates glycogenolysis (glycogen breakdown) and gluconeogenesis (the process of glucose synthesis from other sources such as proteins), and it increases lipolysis (fat breakdown and mobilization). Insulin, in contrast, helps transport glucose for storage into the cells and tissues, prevents fat breakdown, and increases protein synthesis.

Glycogenolysis is controlled by the hormone glucagon and the catecholamines epinephrine and norepinephrine, which are released from the adrenal medulla in times of stress. Once glucose and glycogen stores have been exhausted (usually within 8 to 12 hours), hepatic gluconeogenesis increases dramatically to meet metabolic demands. Hormones that stimulate gluconeogenesis include glucagon and the glucocorticoid hormone cortisol. If catabolic processes continue without the support of energy, amino acids, and essential nutrients, depletion of existing body stores compromises overall bodily health and function. In this event, without intervention, malnutrition may develop.

Approximately 30% to 55% of hospitalized patients have evidence of malnutrition.[1–3] Forty percent of patients experience considerable weight loss (>10 kg) during and after a stay in the intensive care unit (ICU).[4] This unintentional weight loss may deplete vital nutrient reserves, which may predispose the patient to malnutrition. Malnutrition is associated with increased morbidity and mortality, delayed wound healing, increased length of hospitalization, increased complications, immunosuppression, and organ impairment.[5] Malnutrition from starvation alone can usually be corrected by replacing body stores of essential nutrients. However, malnutrition resulting from critical illness and disease processes that alter metabolism is not as easily rectified.

The degree of starvation and physiological stress determines the extent and type of malnutrition. The three major types of protein-energy malnutrition are marasmus, kwashiorkor, and protein–calorie malnutrition. Marasmus is a severe, cachectic process, whereby virtually all of the available fat stores have been exhausted from prolonged calorie deficiency. Severe muscle wasting is evident in marasmus; however, serum albumin levels may be within normal limits or only slightly reduced. Treatment requires nutrition and fluid volume replacement at slow rates to prevent the complications associated with sudden fluid shifts, electrolyte abnormalities, and cardiorespiratory failure.

In contrast to the adaptive response of relative protein sparing in marasmus, kwashiorkor and protein–calorie malnutrition are typically caused by an acute, life-threatening illness, such as surgery, trauma, or sepsis. Kwashiorkor is usually seen in children in developing countries who have had prolonged periods of protein malnutrition. Protein–calorie malnutrition is more commonly seen in developed countries and is due to depletion of fat, muscle wasting, and micronutrient deficiencies from acute and chronic illness. Typically, during periods of critical illness when the patient is relegated to NPO status (*nil per os*, nothing by mouth) for surgery, diagnostic testing, or a number of other medical complications, hypermetabolism and catabolism increase protein and energy demands. Although the critically ill patient may appear nourished, this is often due to the masking effects of generalized edema—the result of extracellular fluid shifts caused by low-protein oncotic pressures in the intravascular space. Other than edema, clinical signs of protein malnutrition include skin breakdown, poor wound healing, surgical dehiscence, or a combination of the three. Additionally, hair can easily be plucked, and hair remnants are often noted on the patient's pillowcase and sheets. Laboratory data reveal low serum albumin levels, and treatment requires aggressive repletion of protein stores. The fact that protein malnutrition is much easier to prevent than to treat reinforces the need for intense nursing vigilance over the patient's nutritional status.

Marasmus and kwashiorkor can coexist. Typically, this is seen when a patient with marasmus is exposed to an acute stressor such as surgery, trauma, or sepsis. Although each situation must be evaluated individually, aggressive protein and calorie replacement is often indicated. Regardless of the type (or types) of malnutrition, vigilant monitoring is crucial to the success of nutrition therapy.

A nutritional assessment should be completed on all critically ill or injured patients early in their hospitalization to determine the need for nutritional support. Nutritional support delivered within 24 to 48 hours of admission, once patients are hemodynamically stable, is advocated.[2,6–10] Goals of care in nutritional support include the following: prevention and treatment of macronutrient and micronutrient deficiencies, maintenance of fluid and electrolyte balance, prevention of infection and other complications associated with nutritional support, and improvement of patient morbidity and mortality. Meeting these goals involves a multidisciplinary approach that includes the nurse, physician, dietitian, and pharmacist. Sample nursing diagnoses and collaborative problems are given in Box 40-1. After a dietitian determines nutri-

---

Box 40-1 — Examples of Nursing Diagnoses and Collaborative Problems for the Patient With Gastrointestinal Problems

- Imbalanced Nutrition: Less Than Body Requirements
- Imbalanced Nutrition: More Than Body Requirements
- Risk for Aspiration related to reduced level of consciousness, depressed cough and gag reflexes, incompetent lower esophageal sphincter, delayed gastric emptying, displaced feeding tube
- Diarrhea related to altered dietary intake, malabsorption, concomitant drug therapy, type of formula, bacterial contamination, stress/anxiety
- Risk for Infection related to invasive procedure and delivery of high concentrations of glucose parenterally
- Disturbed body image
- Bowel incontinence
- Risk for Imbalanced Fluid Volume
- Impaired Swallowing

tional needs, a method of delivering nutritional supplementation must be selected. In patients unable to meet their nutritional needs with oral intake, nutritional supplementation may be delivered by either enteral or parenteral routes. Figure 40-1 outlines the decision-making process. Considerations for elderly patients are given in Box 40-2.

• Nutritional Support

ENTERAL NUTRITION

Enteral nutrition refers to any form of nutrition delivered to the gastrointestinal tract. For those patients with an intact gastrointestinal tract, the enteral route is the preferred method of nutritional support. A clinical rule of thumb is, "If the gut works, use it."

The gastrointestinal mucosa depends on nutrient delivery and adequate blood flow to prevent atrophy, thereby maintaining the absorptive, barrier, and immunological functions of the intestine.[11] Enterocytes are tightly packed epithelial cells that line the intestinal lumen and function as a barrier to bacterial invasion. Gut-associated lymphoid tissue (GALT) lines the gastrointestinal tract and is associated with maintenance of the immunological function of the mucosa.[12] GALT produces immunoglobulin A (IgA), which is secreted across the gastrointestinal mucosa, preventing bacterial adherence to the enterocytes. Without food, the gastrointestinal mucosa atrophies. In the event of atrophy, the tissue available to absorb nutrients decreases, and GALT is impaired.[7] Preservation of the intestinal mucosal integrity is also essential to preserve its function as a barrier. With atrophy, there is a loss of the tight junctions between enterocytes, resulting

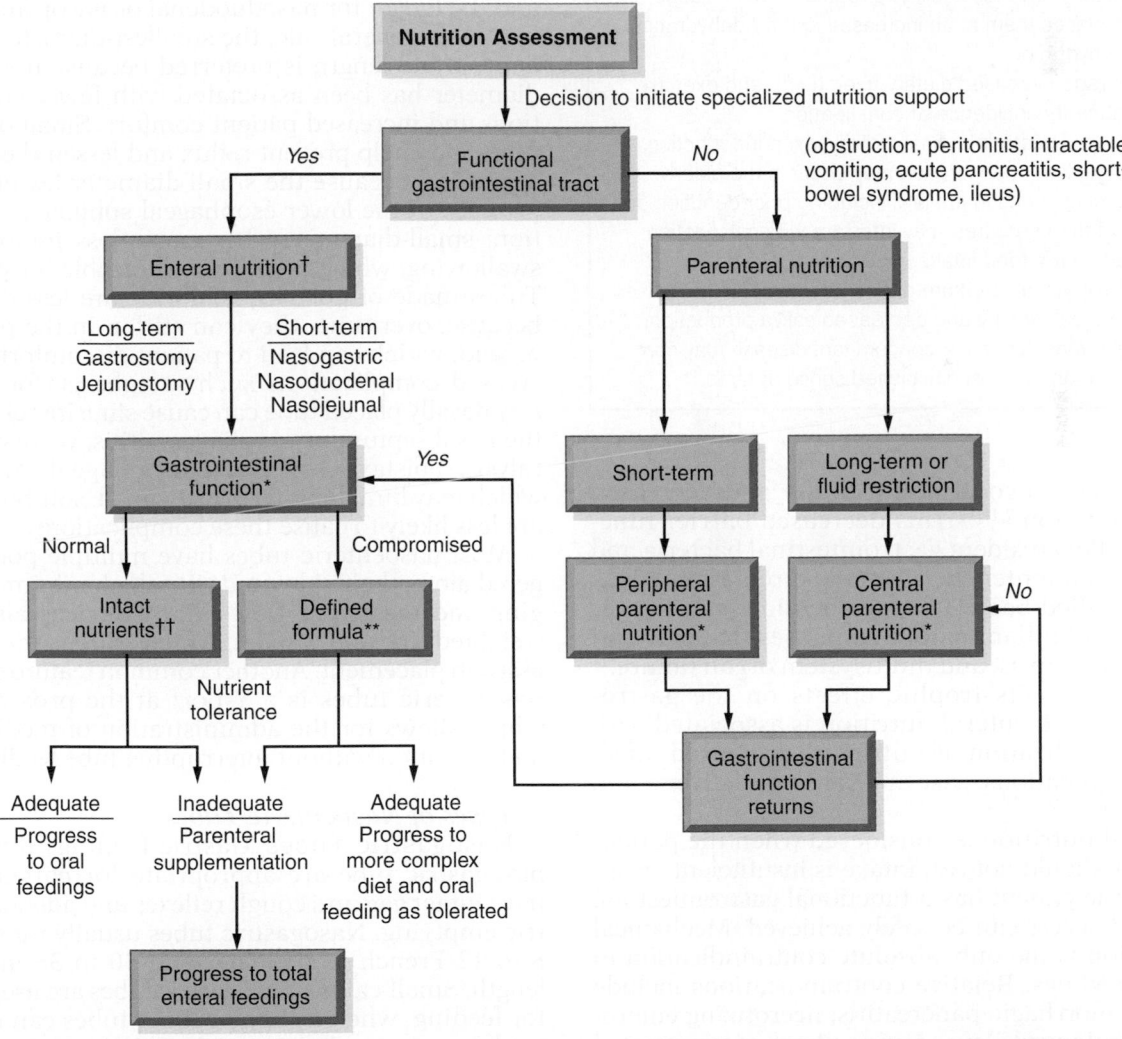

Figure 40-1 • Route of administration of specialized nutrition support. *Formulation of enteral and parenteral solutions should be made considering organ function (e.g., cardiac, renal, respiratory, hepatic). †Feeding may be more appropriate distal to the pylorus if the patient is at increased aspiration risk. **Elemental low-/high-fat content, lactose-free, fiber-rich, and modular formulas should be provided according to the patient's gastrointestinal tolerance. ‡Polymeric, complete formulas, or pureed diets are appropriate. (Adapted from ASPEN Clinical Pathways and Algorithms for Delivery of Parenteral and Enteral Nutrition Support in Adults. Jacobs D [ed]: Section II: Nutrition care process. J Parent Enter Nutr 26[1 Suppl]:85A, 2002.)

Box 40-2 • CONSIDERATIONS FOR THE OLDER PATIENT: Nutritional Requirements

- The risk for malnutrition increases as functional abilities decrease.
- The caloric needs of the elderly are generally less, secondary to decreased metabolism.
- Although protein requirements remain the same, it is important to monitor renal function.
- There is decreased ability to tolerate glucose loads.
- Atrophic gastritis occurs frequently in the elderly, which can result in decreased gastric acid secretion. The resultant achlorhydria or hypochlorhydria can lead to bacterial overgrowth and altered absorption of iron, vitamin B_{12}, folate, calcium, vitamin K, and zinc.
- Lactose intolerance increases with age; this intolerance to dairy products can contribute to osteopenia.
- Vitamin D deficiency in the elderly can be due to decreased dietary intake, decreased synthesis, or decreased exposure to sunlight.
- The elderly have less ability to regulate fluid balance, which places them at an increased risk for dehydration or overhydration.
- Encourage increased dietary fiber, fluids, and exercise to reduce the incidence of constipation.
- Decreased gastrointestinal motility, exocrine function, and digestion or absorption may occur in the elderly.
- Physical changes in the jaw, including poor dentition or poorly fitting dentures, may interfere with mastication and adequate food intake.
- Swallowing may be more difficult because of decreased esophageal motility and decreased saliva production.
- Multiple medications or concomitant disease may contribute to anorexia or diminished sense of taste.

in increased mucosal permeability and decreased barrier function.[7,11,13] This decreased barrier function can allow resident gastrointestinal bacteria and endotoxins to enter the systemic circulation.[9] This process, called bacterial translocation, can trigger immune and inflammatory responses that can lead to infection, sepsis, and multisystem organ failure.[11] In addition to its trophic effects on the gastrointestinal tract, enteral nutrition is associated with enhanced utilization of nutrients, decreased infectious complications, ease and safety of delivery, and lower cost.

Enteral nutrition is considered when the patient cannot or should not eat, intake is insufficient or unreliable, the patient has a functional gastrointestinal tract, and access can be safely achieved. Mechanical obstruction is the only absolute contraindication to enteral feedings. Relative contraindications include severe hemorrhagic pancreatitis, necrotizing enterocolitis, prolonged ileus, severe diarrhea, protracted vomiting, enteric fistulas, intestinal dysmotility, and intestinal ischemia.[14] Each patient situation should be evaluated individually.

Enteral nutrition can be delivered through feeding tubes placed into the stomach or the small intestine. The expected duration of nutritional support, patient's overall condition, risk for aspiration, function of the gastrointestinal tract, and placement technique should all be considered when deciding on which type of feeding tube to place. For most patient populations, nasoenteric tubes are widely used.

Methods of Enteral Nutrition Delivery

Nasoenteral Feeding Tubes

A nasoenteric tube is indicated for short-term use, usually less than 4 to 6 weeks. Nasoenteral tubes are inserted through the nose and advanced through the esophagus into the stomach (nasogastric tube), duodenum (nasoduodenal tube), or jejunum (nasojejunal tube). The tube is identified by the distal location of its tip. Most nasoenteric tubes are soft, flexible, small-bore polyurethane or silicone tubes that are 8 to 14 French in diameter and 20 to 60 inches in length, have markers to aid measurement, and are radiopaque to allow for radiographic confirmation of placement.[1] The shorter lengths are used for nasogastric feedings, and the longer for nasoduodenal or nasojejunal feedings. As a general rule, the smallest-diameter tube of appropriate length is preferred because the smaller diameter has been associated with fewer complications and increased patient comfort. Small-diameter tubes may help prevent reflux and lessen the risk for aspiration because the small diameter lessens compromise of the lower esophageal sphincter. In addition, small-diameter tubes cause less inhibition of swallowing, which is more comfortable for patients. Tubes made of polyvinyl chloride are less desirable because, over time, they can stiffen in the presence of acid, which can lead to patient discomfort and increased complications such as tube perforation.[1,15] Any nasally placed tube can cause sinusitis, erosion of the nasal septum or esophagus, otitis, vocal cord paralysis, epistaxis, or distal esophageal strictures, which may limit long-term use. Small, soft-bore tubes are less likely to cause these complications.

Most nasoenteric tubes have multiple ports staggered along their sides and tip, which minimize clogging and maximize flow. Many devices also have weighted tips and a stylet, which stiffens the tube to assist in placement. Another common feature of many nasoenteric tubes is a Y-port at the proximal tip, which allows for the administration of medications and irrigation without interrupting tube feeding.

Types of Nasoenteric Tubes

Nasogastric Tubes Gastric feedings through a nasogastric tube are appropriate for patients who have intact gag and cough reflexes and adequate gastric emptying. Nasogastric tubes usually range from 8 to 12 French in diameter and 30 to 36 inches in length. Small-caliber nasogastric tubes are used solely for feeding, whereas large-caliber tubes can be used to decompress the stomach, monitor gastric pH, and deliver medications and feedings. Large-caliber nasogastric tubes are usually made of stiffer material and are often less comfortable for patients, possibly triggering self-extubation. These tubes are usually used to decompress and drain the stomach temporarily and are therefore typically for short-term use.

Advantages to gastric feeding include the ease of placement, the ease of checking residuals, and patient tolerability during enteral infusions. However, patients with nasogastric tubes are at the greatest risk for aspiration, especially when they are unconscious, mechanically ventilated, or otherwise unable to protect their airway. In a conscious patient, the mere physical appearance of the tube and associated discomfort may limit the clinical use of nasogastric tubes.

Nasoduodenal Tubes and Nasojejunal Tubes

Nasoduodenal tubes and nasojejunal tubes are thought to be better suited for long-term use than nasogastric tubes. Nasoduodenal tubes and nasojejunal tubes are advanced through the stomach, past the pylorus, and into the small intestine, usually in the third portion of the duodenum beyond the ligament of Treitz. In theory, the pyloric sphincter provides a barrier that lessens the risk for aspiration or regurgitation.

Transpyloric feeding can be given without regard to gastric emptying, providing an additional advantage over intragastric feeding. Candidates for transpyloric feedings include critically ill patients with a prior history of gastric aspiration, patients at risk for aspiration (such as ventilated patients), those with gastroparesis, and patients with neurological conditions who are unable to protect their airway.

A common misconception is that enteral feedings should not be started if bowel sounds are absent. Bowel sounds are an indication of gastrointestinal motility, not of absorption. After injury and postoperatively, bowel sounds may not be detected for 3 to 5 days owing to gastric atony. The small bowel is less prone to ileus than the stomach or the colon and retains its absorptive and digestive capabilities, making it possible to accept enteral feedings immediately after surgery or trauma.[9]

Nasoduodenal tubes and nasojejunal tubes range from 8 to 16 French in diameter and 152 to 240 cm in length.[16,17] The length and diameter make it more difficult to check feeding residual because the lumen is smaller and tends to collapse on itself when aspirated. In addition, clogging of medications is more common than with nasogastric tubes. The primary disadvantage associated with nasoduodenal and nasojejunal tubes relates to the difficulty in initially placing the tubing tip past the pyloric sphincter.

Placement of Nasoenteric Tubes

In most ICUs, trained nurses or physicians routinely place nasoenteric tubes. Before placing a feeding tube, institutional policy and protocol should be reviewed because nasoenteric tube placement has many potential complications. Patients with a decreased level of consciousness, poor cough or gag reflex, or an inability or unwillingness to cooperate are at increased risk for pulmonary intubation. When a patient cannot cooperate or cough when the tube enters the bronchial tree, extra precautions must be taken to ensure proper placement. Feeding tubes placed in the bronchial tree can cause pulmonary hemorrhage or pneumothorax. A cuffed endotracheal tube does not preclude accidental pulmonary intubation. Nasoenteric tubes can also be accidentally placed in the esophagus or, in patients with basilar skull fractures, in the intracranial space.

Nasogastric tube placement is usually easier than nasoduodenal or nasojejunal tube placement. When placing a nasoenteric feeding tube in the stomach, the nurse determines the length of tube insertion by measuring the distance from the tip of the nose, to the earlobe, to the tip of the xiphoid process. Before insertion, the nurse considers using a topical anesthetic or water-soluble lubricant to assist in placement. After placing the patient's bed in a high Fowler's position, the nurse slightly flexes the patient's head (if not clinically contraindicated) and passes the lubricated tip through the nares into the nasopharynx. While advancing the tube, the nurse asks the patient to swallow repeatedly. Having the patient sip water through a straw may also assist in tube placement (if not clinically contraindicated). Rotating the tube as it is advanced may also ease advancement.

When attempting to pass the nasoenteric tube tip past the pylorus, the nurse follows the same procedure described previously, and then turns the patient to the right lateral decubitus position with the head of the bed at a 30- to 45-degree angle to take advantage of gravity and peristalsis.[9] Nasoduodenal and nasojejunal tubes depend on gastric motility to carry the tip through the pylorus, but they have a tendency to coil in the stomach. Some nasoduodenal tubes and nasojejunal tubes have weights to aid in passage through the pylorus; however, the utility of the weighted tip is dubious. A promotility agent such as metoclopramide or erythromycin may be ordered before insertion because such a medication increases upper gastrointestinal motility while relaxing the pylorus. Air insufflation, the process of inserting large amounts of air into the stomach, may also be helpful by distending the stomach and facilitating tube passage though the pylorus. If attempts to pass a nasoduodenal or nasojejunal tube are not successful within 24 hours, endoscopic or radiological assistance should be sought to advance the tip of the tube.

Before initiating tube feeding, proper tube placement must be confirmed by an abdominal radiograph. Feeding tubes placed surgically, by endoscopy, or under fluoroscopy do not require radiographic confirmation of placement. The external length of the tube is documented after placement is confirmed. The nurse marks the tube with tape or indelible ink at the point it enters the nares, rechecks tube placement before initiating intermittent feedings or medication administration and at least once each shift, and monitors tube placement during continuous tube feeding according to the institution's policy.

Auscultation, aspiration and inspection of aspirate, and pH testing have been used to monitor tube placement after initial placement is confirmed by an abdominal radiograph. No one method is infallible, so using a combination of these methods is advised. Injecting air into the tube and auscultating the gastric bubble, although commonly used, is not an accurate method to verify initial tube placement. An air bubble sound can be transmitted to the epigastrium when the tube is in the esophagus. Although auscultation of insufflated air is not a reliable method to confirm initial feeding tube placement, it may still provide useful information. If no resistance is met, the tube is unlikely to be kinked, and if the patient immediately burps back air, the tip of the tube is probably in the esophagus.

Aspiration and inspection of the aspirate may help differentiate between gastric and intestinal placement, but not between intestinal and pulmonary placement. Fluid aspirated from the stomach is usually green, tan, brown, or bloody.[15,18] Small intestinal aspirate is usually golden yellow, clear, or bile colored and is often thicker than gastric aspirate.[18] Pulmonary fluid is usually tan, white, clear, or pale yellow and can closely mimic gastric or intestinal aspirates.[15,19] However, it is necessary to keep in mind that the diameter of small intestinal tubes may not allow withdrawal to check aspirate.

Measuring the pH of fluid aspirated from the feeding tube is another method of monitoring tube placement. The pH of esophageal secretions is usually 6.0 to 7.0, gastric aspirates 1.0 to 4.0, and intestinal contents 6.0 to 7.0.[9,19,20] However, the pH of gastric aspirate can be elevated with the infusion of enteral formulas, the use of acid-modifying medications, and the presence of bile reflux. The pH of both small intestinal aspirate and pulmonary fluid is usually greater than 6.0; therefore, if the pH of the aspirate is greater than 4.0, tube position cannot be determined based on pH alone.[9,15] For optimal results with pH testing, nothing that may alter the pH should be instilled in the tube for 60 minutes.[19]

Capnometry and capnography detect carbon dioxide; these noninvasive monitoring techniques are used to monitor and evaluate respiratory function and ventilation. Observation of the presence or absence of a waveform is used to evaluate for accidental pulmonary placement of feeding tubes.[19]

Suctioning and patient movement or coughing may potentially dislodge a feeding tube. If at any time tube location is in question, the nurse holds the tube feeding and requests an order for an abdominal radiograph to confirm placement.

Securing Nasoenteric Tubes

Before securing any feeding tube, the nurse cleans the skin with alcohol to remove oils and dirt and considers applying a skin protectant to maintain skin integrity. Nasoenteric tubes should be secured in a way that avoids irritation or pressure of the nares, thus preventing necrosis. The nurse allows the tube to hang straight from the nares and secures it to the bridge of the nose or the cheek with tape (or one of the many commercially available devices). For agitated or uncooperative patients, the nurse considers soft wrist restraints or mitts to avoid accidental self-extubation (refer to your institution's policy and procedure regarding the use of restraints). It is necessary to inspect the skin and nostrils every 4 to 8 hours for signs and symptoms of irritation, erythema, or skin

breakdown. Patient comfort can be maximized by providing frequent mouth care and moistening of the nares.

Enterostomal Feeding Tubes

If therapy is expected to last a month or more, a more permanent enterostomal device can be inserted through the abdomen into the stomach (gastrostomy) or jejunum (jejunostomy) (Fig. 40-2). Enterostomal feeding tubes are also indicated when the nasal route is contraindicated and in patients with impaired swallowing or obstruction of the oropharynx, the larynx, or esophagus. Enterostomal tubes are 18 to 28 French in diameter, made of silicone and polyurethane, and very durable.[17]

Types of Enterostomal Feeding Tubes

Gastrostomy Tubes Gastrostomy tubes have an internal retention bolster to prevent accidental dislodgment. Gastrostomy tubes may be used temporarily or for permanent feeding. If a gastrostomy tube is intended for permanent feedings, it may need to be replaced as the tube material deteriorates over time. Gastrostomy tubes may also be used for chronic gastric decompression. A low-profile gastrostomy device (LPGD), often referred to as a button, may be used to replace gastrostomy tubes in a mature gastrostomy tract, usually 3 to 6 months after initial placement or as an initial placement. LPGDs are anchored in the stomach and protrude through the abdomen, flush with the skin. These devices require a special extension adapter to connect with the tube-feeding bag, to check for residuals, and to use for decompression. This adapter may then be removed after use. Some LPGDs are equipped with a one-way antireflux valve to prevent leakage of gastric contents onto the skin. These devices are usually well accepted because they are durable, unlikely to irritate the skin, and difficult to dislodge. With agitated or confused adults who have a tendency to pull on their tubes, these advantages may be of benefit.

Jejunostomy Tubes When gastric feedings are not possible or desired, jejunostomy tubes (J-tubes) are preferred for long-term feeding because they deliver enteral formula past the duodenum into the jejunum, decreasing pancreatic stimulation. J-tubes are indicated in patients who will benefit from jejunal feeding, particularly those with gastric disease, abnormal gastric emptying, upper gastrointestinal obstruction or fistula, pancreatitis, or decreased gag reflex with significant risk for aspiration. J-tubes are contraindicated in patients with primary diseases of the small bowel (such as Crohn's disease) or radiation enteritis because of the increased risk for enterocutaneous fistula formation. A limitation of J-tubes is the potential for obstruction due to the small diameter of the lumen.

Placement of Enterostomal Tubes

Percutaneous endoscopic, open surgical, laparoscopic, and fluoroscopic techniques may be used to place a gastrostomy tube. J-tubes may be placed by percutaneous endoscopy or surgical methods. The

EVIDENCE-BASED PRACTICE HIGHLIGHT: VERIFICATION OF FEEDING TUBE PLACEMENT

Expected Practice:

- Obtain radiographic confirmation of correct tube placement on all critically ill patients who are to receive feedings or medications via blindly inserted gastric or small bowel tubes prior to initial use.
- Mark and document the tube's exit site from the nose or mouth immediately after radiographic confirmation of correct tube placement; observe the mark to assess for a change in length of the external portion of the tube.
- Use bedside techniques to assess tube location at regular intervals to determine if the tube has remained in its intended position. No one single technique has been shown to be reliable for continually assessing tube placement:
  - Review routine chest and abdominal x-rays to determine if they refer to tube location
  - Helpful bedside techniques include measuring the pH and observing the appearance of fluid withdrawn from the tube.
  - Do not rely on the auscultatory method to determine tube location.

Supporting Evidence:

- Radiographic confirmation is the only reliable method to date of confirming enteral tube placement. The pH and appearance of an aspirate from the newly inserted tube, while not 100% reliable, are highly suggestive of gastric or small bowel placement and can be used as an initial indicator of placement. However, radiographic confirmation should always be done.
  - An aspirate from a gastric tube often has a pH of 5 or less and is usually grassy-green or clear and colorless, with off-white to tan mucus shreds.[1-10]
  - An aspirate from a small bowel tube often has a pH of 6 or greater and is usually bile-stained (ranging in color from light to golden yellow or brownish-green). In addition, the aspirate is usually thicker and more translucent than fluid withdrawn from a gastric tube.[1-10]
  - An aspirate from a tube inadvertently positioned in the tracheobronchial tree or the pleural space typically has a pH of 6 or greater. An aspirate from a tube in the tracheobronchial tree usually has the appearance of fluid obtained during tracheal suctioning. An aspirate from a tube in the pleural space is usually straw-colored and watery, perhaps tinged with bright-red blood (caused by perforation of the pleura by the tube).[1-10]

- There are numerous anecdotal reports of blindly inserted tubes entering the respiratory tract undetected. In most of these cases, the auscultatory method falsely ensured that the tube was correctly positioned in the stomach.[11-16] There is also a report of the auscultatory method failing to detect inadvertent placement of a nasogastric tube in the brain.[17] The auscultatory method was found to have a sensitivity of only 34% in differentiating between gastric and small bowel tube placement in 85 acutely ill adults.[18] In another study auscultation for insufflated air was found to have a sensitivity of only 45% in determining whether 134 tube insertions resulted in placement above or below the diaphragm.[19]
- It is not uncommon for a feeding tube to dislocate from its intended site, either after being tugged at by a confused patient or during the delivery of care.[20,21] An increase in the external portion of tubing extending from the nose or mouth can signal that the tube's distal tip has dislocated upward in the gastrointestinal tract (such as from the small bowel into the stomach or esophagus, or from the stomach into the esophagus).[22]
- Measuring the pH of fluid aspirated from tubes of fasting patients is helpful in differentiating between gastric and respiratory placement, and gastric and small bowel placement.[1-7]
- Observing the appearance of fluid aspirated from tubes of fasting patients is helpful in differentiating between gastric and respiratory placement, and gastric and small bowel placement.[7-10]
- Observing the pH and appearance of aspirates from feeding tubes when continuous feedings are in progress is less helpful than when the patient is fasting; nonetheless, these methods are occasionally of benefit in distinguishing between gastric and small bowel tube location.[23]
- A sudden increase in residual volume from a feeding tube in the small bowel may signal upward displacement of the tube into the stomach. Aspirates from small bowel feeding tubes are usually less than 10 mL; an increase to 50 mL or higher may signal upward displacement of the tube into the stomach.[22]
- Injecting 30 mL of air into the tube via a 60-mL syringe immediately before pulling back on the plunger facilitates the withdrawal of fluid from small-diameter tubes.[24]
- Flushing the tube with 30 mL of water (or normal saline, if indicated for patients with hyponatremia) after residual volume measurements prevents the tube from clogging.[25,26]

References

1. Metheny NA, Williams P, Wiersema L, et al: Effectiveness of pH measurements in predicting feeding tube placement. Nurs Res; 38(5):280–285, 1989

2. Metheny NA, Reed L, et al: Effectiveness of pH measurements in predicting feeding tube placement: An update. Nurs Res; 42(6):324–331, 1993

3. Metheny NA, Stewart BJ, Smith L, et al: pH and concentrations of pepsin and trypsin in feeding tube aspirates as predictors of tube placement. JPEN; 21(5):279–285, 1997

4. Metheny NA, Clouse RE, Clark JM, et al: Techniques and procedures: pH testing of feeding-tube aspirates to determine placement. Nutr Clin Pract; 9(5):185–190, 1994

5. Metheny NA, Stewart BJ, Smith L, et al: pH and concentration of bilirubin in feeding tube aspirates as predictors of tube placement. Nurs Res; 48(4):189–197, 1999

6. Griffith DP, McNally AT, Battey CH, et al: Intravenous erythromycin facilitates bedside placement of postpyloric feeding tubes in critically ill adults: A double-blind, randomized, placebo-controlled study. Crit Care Med; 31(1):39–44, 2003

(continued)

EVIDENCE-BASED PRACTICE HIGHLIGHTS: VERIFICATION OF FEEDING TUBE PLACEMENT (Continued)

7. Gharpure V, Meert KL, Sarnaik AP, Metheny NA: Indicators of postpyloric feeding tube placement in children. Crit Care Med; 28(8):2962–2966, 2000

8. Metheny N, Reed L, Berglund B, Wehrle MA: Visual characteristics of aspirates from feeding tubes as a method for predicting tube location. Nurs Res; 43(5):282–287, 1994

9. Harrison AM, Clay B, Grant MJ, et al: Nonradiographic assessment of enteral feeding tube position. Crit Care Med; 25(12):2055–2059, 1997

10. Welch SK, Hanlon MD, Waits M, Foulks CJ: Comparison of four bedside indicators used to predict duodenal feeding tube placement with radiography. JPEN; 18(6):525–530, 1994

11. Metheny NA, Dettenmeier P, Hampton K, et al: Detection of inadvertent respiratory placement of small-bore feeding tubes: A report of 10 cases. Heart Lung; 19(6):631–638, 1990

12. Lipman TO, Kessler T, Arabian A: Nasopulmonary intubation with feeding tubes: Case reports and review of the literature. JPEN; 9(5):618–620, 1985

13. Hendry PJ, Akyurekli Y, McIntyre R, et al: Bronchopleural complications of nasogastric feeding tubes. Crit Care Med; 14(10):892–894, 1986

14. Metheny NA, Meert K: Invited Review: Monitoring feeding tube placement. Nutr Clin Pract. 19(5):487–496, 2004

15. el Gamel A, Watson DC: Transbronchial intubation of the right pleural space: A rare complication of nasogastric intubation with a polyvinylchloride tube–a case study. Heart Lung; 22(3):224–225, 1993

16. Nakao MA, Killam D, Wilson R: Pneumothorax secondary to inadvertent nasotracheal placement of a nasoenteric tube past a cuffed endotracheal tube. Crit Care Med; 11(3):210–211, 1983

17. Metheny NA: Inadvertent intracranial nasogastric tube placement. Am J Nurs; 102(8):25–27, 2002

18. Metheny NA, McSweeney M, Wehrle MA, Wiersema L: Effectiveness of the auscultatory method in predicting feeding tube location. Nurs Res; 39(5):262–267, 1990

19. Kearns PJ, Donna C: A controlled comparison of traditional feeding tube verification methods to a bedside, electromagnetic technique. JPEN; 25(4):210–215, 2001

20. Metheny NA, Spies M, Eisenberg P: Frequency of nasoenteral tube displacement and associated risk factors. Res Nurs Health; 9(3):241–247, 1986

21. Ellett MLC, Maahs J, Forsee S: Prevalence of feeding tube placement errors and associated risk factors in children. MCN; 23(5):234–239, 1998

22. Metheny NA, Schnelker R, McGinnis J, et al: Indicators of tube site during feedings. J Neurosc Nurs; (in press)

23. Metheny NA, Stewart BJ: Testing feeding tube placement during continuous tube feedings. Appl Nurs Res; 15(4):254–258, 2002

24. Metheny NA, Reed L, Worseck M, Clark J: How to aspirate fluid from small-bore feeding tubes. Am J Nurs;93(5):86–88, 1993

25. Metheny NA, Eisenberg P, McSweeney M: Effect of feeding tube properties and three irrigants on clogging rates. Nurs Res; 37(3):165–169, 1988

26. Schallom L, Stewart J, Nuetzel G, et al: Testing a protocol for measuring gastrointestinal residual volumes in tube-fed patients (abstract). Am J Crit Care; 13(3):265–266, 2004

*Excerpted from American Association of Critical-Care Nurses Practice Alert.

patient's underlying disease and physician expertise need to be considered when selecting the appropriate placement technique.

Percutaneous Endoscopic Gastrostomy Percutaneous endoscopic gastrostomy (PEG) has rapidly become the preferred method for placement of gastrostomy devices. A PEG may be performed at the bedside or in the endoscopy suite, using minimal sedation. Placement is through an abdominal incision using direct endoscopic visualization. Gastric decompression allows feeding to be administered soon after placement.[14] Other advantages of PEG include increased comfort, decreased cost, and decreased recovery time. A candidate for a PEG must have an intact oropharynx and an esophagus free from obstruction. The only absolute contraindication to PEG is the inability to bring the gastric wall into apposition with the abdomen. Prior abdominal surgeries, ascites, hepatomegaly, and obesity may impede gastric transillumination and preclude placement of a PEG.

Complications of PEG are infrequent but include wound infection related to bacterial contamination by oral flora during insertion, necrotizing fasciitis, peritonitis, and aspiration. Pneumoperitoneum, a common finding after PEG placement, is not clinically significant unless accompanied by signs and symptoms of peritonitis. Prophylactic antibiotics are usually given 30 to 60 minutes before the procedure. Correct placement is then verified by endoscopy.

In patients with severe gastroesophageal reflux disease, gastroparesis, or increased risk for aspiration related to tube feeding, a PEG can be modified with a jejunal extension tube known as a PEG/J tube.

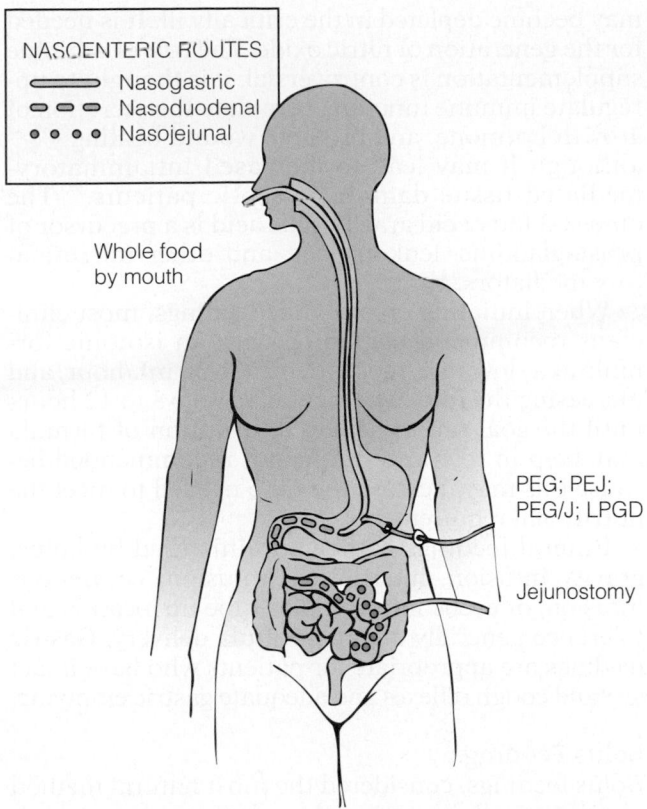

NASOENTERIC ROUTES
━━━ Nasogastric
━ ━ ━ Nasoduodenal
• • • • Nasojejunal

Whole food
by mouth

PEG; PEJ;
PEG/J; LPGD

Jejunostomy

Figure 40-2 • Possible routes for feeding. LPGD, low-profile gastrostomy device; PEG, percutaneous endoscopic gastrostomy; PEG/J, PEG modified with a jejunal extension tube; and PEJ, percutaneous endoscopic jejunostomy.

The gastric lumen of a PEG/J tube is usually used for gastric decompression, and the jejunal lumen is used for the simultaneous delivery of enteral feeding. PEG/J tubes may decrease the risk for gastric aspiration; however, they do not necessarily provide the same protection against aspiration as jejunal tubes because the pylorus is compromised by the large catheter. The jejunal portion of a PEG/J tube may migrate back into the stomach and increase the risk for occlusion, gastric reflux, or aspiration. Both PEG and PEG/J tubes are held in place by internal and external retention devices. The internal device rests in the stomach, which prevents migration and leakage of gastric contents. The external retention device anchors the tube to the abdomen. These tubes have a high rate of mechanical dysfunction, which limits their long-term use.[14]

Surgical Gastrostomy Surgical gastrostomy tubes are inserted through an incision in the abdominal wall under general anesthesia. The stomach is usually sutured to the abdominal wall to create a permanent connection between the gastric and abdominal walls. Surgical placement of a gastrostomy is usually chosen if the surgeon wants to view the gastric anatomy clearly or as a secondary procedure during abdominal surgery. Disadvantages of surgical placement include the need for general anesthesia, increased recovery time, decreased comfort, and increased cost.

Laparoscopic Gastrostomy A laparoscopically placed gastrostomy tube also requires general anesthesia or intravenous (IV) conscious sedation. Laparoscopic placement is usually reserved for patients with head, neck, or esophageal cancer. It is less invasive, less painful, and usually involves fewer complications than a surgical gastrostomy.

Fluoroscopic Gastrostomy Direct percutaneous catheter insertion of a gastrostomy tube under fluoroscopy is indicated with high-grade pharyngeal or esophageal obstruction. Disadvantages to the use of fluoroscopy to place enterostomal devices include the inability to detect mucosal disease, the potential for prolonged exposure to radiation, the necessity of transport to the fluoroscopy suite, and increased cost.

Securing Enterostomal Tubes and Caring for the Enterostomy Site

Enterostomal tubes are secured to the abdominal wall to prevent dislodgment or migration of the tube, to avoid tension on the tubing, and to prevent the external retention device from digging into the skin. The length of the external tubing is documented to monitor for migration of the tubing.

To avoid maceration, the insertion site is kept clean and dry by leaving it open to air (unless draining), and lifting or adjusting the tube is avoided for several days after the initial insertion. To avoid pulling the internal retention device taut against the gastric or intestinal mucosa, the amount of dressing between the device and the skin is limited. Any accumulated drainage may be cleaned with water.[1] Serosanguineous drainage may be expected for 7 to 10 days after insertion.[1] If no drainage is present, cleansing with soap and water is adequate. The skin around the insertion site and the retention device is assessed at least daily for skin breakdown, erythema, or drainage. The tissue usually heals within a month.

In-and-out play on the tubing is checked; it should be able to move ¼ inch to prevent erosion of gastric or abdominal tissue. If the anchor is too tight, the nurse should notify the physician immediately because this may indicate "buried bumper syndrome," a situation in which the retention device is imbedded in the tissue, thereby leading to mucosal or skin erosion. If a gastrostomy tube becomes accidentally dislodged, the nurse should notify the physician immediately so that the tube can be reinserted quickly before the tract closes.

Types and Delivery of Enteral Formulas

When selecting a tube feeding formula, nutrient requirements, the patient's clinical status, location of enteral access, gastrointestinal function, cost, and duration must all be considered. Numerous tube feeding solutions are available for enteral nutrition, with many designed to assist in the management of specific disease processes; however, no single formula is ideal for all patients. All contain proteins, carbohydrates, fats, vitamins, minerals, trace elements, and water. The difference lies in how these nutrients are structured and delivered. The dietary formula selected is based on the patient's ability to digest and absorb major nutrients, the total nutrient requirements, and fluid and electrolyte restrictions.

Polymeric solutions are isotonic and can provide enough protein, carbohydrate, fat, vitamins, trace elements, and minerals to prevent nutritional deficiencies. They are considered nutritionally complete if given in enough volume to meet caloric needs. Standard formulas deliver 1 kcal/mL, but some concentrated formulas may provide 2 kcal/mL.[2,3] The carbohydrates in polymeric solutions are oligosaccharides and polysaccharides that require pancreatic enzymes for digestion. All polymeric solutions contain intact proteins (most often meat, whey, milk, or soy proteins) that require normal pancreatic enzymes for digestion. Several disease-specific formulas are available.

Peptide (elemental) formulas provide proteins as dipeptides, tripeptides, or oligopeptides and free amino acids from hydrolysis of whey, milk, or soy proteins. Because peptides do not require pancreatic enzymes for digestion, elemental solutions are used when digestion is impaired, such as in pancreatic insufficiency, radiation enteritis, Crohn's disease, or short bowel syndrome secondary to surgical resection. Elemental solutions have no proven advantage in patients with normal gut function, are usually more expensive than polymeric formulas, and have an unpleasant taste.

Modular formulas contain individual nutrient components such as protein, carbohydrates, and fat that can be mixed or added to other formulas to individualize feedings to a patient's specific nutritional needs. The involvement of a dietitian is essential in the selection of these formulas.

Attention has recently been focused on the role of enteral formulas that contain additional nutrients purported to enhance immune function. These formulas, referred to collectively as immunonutrition or immune-enhancing diets, have been reported to decrease infection rates, duration of mechanical ventilation, and length of hospitalization, but they have not been shown to affect mortality.[21] Several nutrients that have attracted attention are glutamine, arginine, and omega-3 polyunsaturated fatty acids. Studies have suggested that formulas supplemented with one or a combination of these nutrients may have immune-enhancing properties. The benefit of these formulas is a subject of controversy because several studies have not clearly identified positive effects on infectious complications.[6]

Among these additives is glutamine, a nonessential amino acid that is synthesized and released from skeletal muscle.[22] A precursor of nucleotide synthesis, it is an important fuel source for rapidly dividing cells such as enterocytes, lymphocytes, and macrophages.[7,21-23] Glutamine availability is limited in catabolic illness, and low levels of this amino acid have been associated with mortality.[21,22] In addition, glutamine may improve immune function and reduce intestinal permeability.[22] Another additive is arginine, which is also a nonessential amino acid that

may become depleted in the critically ill. It is needed for the generation of nitric oxide. The role of arginine supplementation is controversial: it is thought to up-regulate immune function, stimulate the secretion of growth hormone, and promote wound healing,[3,22-26] although it may lead to increased inflammatory-mediated tissue damage in septic patients.[25] The omega-3 fatty acid arachidonic acid is a precursor of prostaglandins, leukotrienes, and other inflammatory mediators.

When initiating enteral tube feedings, most clinicians recommend beginning with an isotonic formula at a slow rate, most often 20 to 30 mL/hour, and increasing the rate incrementally every 8 to 12 hours until the goal rate is achieved.[2] Dilution of formula may help in tolerance but is not recommended because this may increase the time needed to meet the nutritional requirements.[2]

Enteral feedings can be administered by bolus, gravity infusion, intermittent infusion, continuous infusion, or cyclic infusion. The tube tip location and tolerance generally dictate formula delivery. Gastric feedings are appropriate for patients who have intact gag and cough reflexes and adequate gastric emptying.

Bolus Feedings

Bolus feedings, considered the most natural method physiologically, are given by a large syringe in volumes as high as 400 mL over 5 to 10 minutes, 5 to 6 times a day. The stomach is the preferred site for bolus feedings. The stomach and pyloric sphincter regulate the outflow of feeding from the stomach. Bolus feedings allow for increased patient mobility because the patient is free from a mechanical device between feedings. Unfortunately, as a result of high residuals, bolus feedings are usually not well tolerated and are often accompanied by nausea, bloating, cramping, diarrhea, or aspiration.

Intermittent Feedings

Intermittent feedings of 300 to 400 mL are administered by slow gravity drip 4 to 6 times a day over a period of 30 to 60 minutes.[23] The stomach is the preferred site for intermittent infusion because of its capacity. Intermittent feedings are associated with a decreased risk for osmotic diarrhea. Advantages of intermittent feedings include freedom from dependence on a mechanical device and a power source, which can decrease cost and increase patient mobility.

Continuous Feedings

If the tip of the nasoenteric tube is in the duodenum or jejunum, tube feedings must be delivered by infusion. Continuous infusions are administered over 24 hours with the aid of a feeding pump to ensure a constant flow rate. Continuous pump feedings are the preferred method for intestinal feeding because delivery that is too rapid may lead to "dumping syndrome," characterized by osmotic diarrhea, abdominal distention, cramps, hyperperistalsis, lightheadedness, diaphoresis, and palpitations. When the tube is placed in the third portion of the duodenum, past the ligament of Treitz, continuous pump feedings are associated with decreased risk for aspiration. If the feeding is advanced slowly, the small bowel can usually tolerate feedings at a rate of 150 mL/hour. The continuous method is best suited to the critically ill patient because it allows more time for nutrients to be absorbed in the intestine. Continuous infusion is also often used in the ICU because there is decreased incidence of gastric distention and potential for aspiration. Continuous infusion tube feeding may also act prophylactically to prevent stress ulcers and metabolic complications. As with intermittent feedings, disadvantages include the dependence on a mechanical device and a power source.

Cyclic Feedings

Cyclic feedings are continuous feedings that deliver the total daily nutritional requirements in a shorter time frame, typically over 8 to 12 hours, to allow the patient freedom from 24-hour continuous feedings.[11] Cyclic feedings of high density and high volume are typically given at night to allow hunger to develop during the day, but may be given during the day if a patient has difficulty with regurgitation while supine. This schedule may assist the patient in progressing from enteral to oral consumption.

The ultimate goal is for patients to resume adequate oral intake. Enteral feeding may be discontinued when patients can drink enough liquid to maintain hydration and can eat two thirds of their nutritional requirements.

Complications of Enteral Nutrition

Although enteral nutrition is in general associated with fewer complications than parenteral nutrition, complications may still occur. These complications generally fall into gastrointestinal, mechanical, metabolic, and infectious categories. Many of these complications can be prevented or treated by closely observing residuals and watching for signs and symptoms of gastric intolerance.

Gastrointestinal Complications

The patient's tolerance to enteral feeding depends on the rate of flow and the osmolality of the formula. Signs and symptoms of gastrointestinal intolerance to enteral feeding include diarrhea, nausea, vomiting, abdominal discomfort, distention, and high residual returns. Food normally passes through the stomach at a rate of 2 to 10 mL/minute; however, gastric emptying is delayed or absent in many critically ill patients. Unlike the stomach, the small intestine cannot act as a reservoir. If large residuals are withdrawn through a nasoduodenal tube or nasojejunal tube, the tube may have moved back into the stomach, and placement should be confirmed with an abdominal radiograph.

High Residuals

Monitoring gastric residual volumes (GRVs) is based on the assumption that GRVs are useful in predicting the risk for aspiration and pneumonia.[27,28]

However, high GRVs can be problematic because consensus about what constitutes high GRVs ranges from 100 to 400 mL. High GRVs do not indicate aspiration, and low GRVs do not preclude aspiration.[27–30] GRV is an imprecise measure of gastric emptying and may not take into account the volume of gastric and salivary secretions.[27,30] In addition, it is difficult to determine whether gastric contents have been completely removed. Many clinicians stop tube feeding inappropriately, based on a single GRV of less than 400 to 500 mL.[27,30–33] Although a high GRV should raise suspicion of intolerance, one high value does not mean feeding failure, and automatic cessation of feeding can delay the patient's ability to meet his or her nutritional goals. The nurse must be sure to evaluate the clinical status of his or her patient before stopping tube feeding solely on the basis of one high GRV; the key is to monitor trends in GRV.[27,30] Residuals should be checked every 4 to 6 hours during continuous feedings and before initiating intermittent feedings.[20]

Tube feeding should be held if a patient demonstrates overt signs of regurgitation, vomiting, or aspiration. A common intervention involves holding the feeding for 1 to 2 hours and rechecking GRV every 1 to 2 hours until the GRV is less than 200 to 250 mL from a nasogastric tube or less than 100 mL from a gastrostomy tube, at which point feedings can be resumed.[10,20] Promotility agents may also be useful if high GRVs persist. This allows time for normal gastric emptying and reduces the risk for aspiration. It is necessary to remember that high infusion rates result in higher GRVs and to be aware of the institution's policy and protocol regarding high GRV.

Nausea, Vomiting, and Bloating

Nausea, vomiting, and bloating are commonly associated with enteral feedings. Medications, rapid infusion rate, or improper tube placement may cause both nausea and vomiting. Nausea, vomiting, and bloating are most likely to occur when gastric emptying is delayed. The nurse carefully assesses medications that may contribute to these symptoms, and the medications should be eliminated, if possible. A change of formula, reduction in rate, or addition of a prokinetic medication may also help.

Diarrhea

Diarrhea is the most common complication of enteral feedings; however, it is important to consider other etiologies before assuming that enteral feedings are the cause of diarrhea. Diarrhea in a patient receiving enteral feeding may result from the use of antibiotics or other diarrhea-inducing medications; altered bacterial flora; formula composition; intolerance to lactose, fat, or osmolality; a rate of infusion that is too high; hypoalbuminemia; or enteral formula contamination.

The liquid form of many medications may contain hypertonic sorbitol, which can have laxative effects. Antibiotics, antacids, magnesium, and prokinetic medications can also contribute to diarrhea. Antibiotics can contribute to diarrhea by causing overgrowth of *Clostridium difficile*. To assess for *C. difficile* infection, a stool sample is assessed for *C. difficile* toxin. Treatment options include antibiotic therapy with oral metronidazole, vancomycin, or cholestyramine (a bile acid sequestrant that binds the toxin). A patient who has received antibiotics should not receive antidiarrheals until *C. difficile* infection has been ruled out because diarrhea helps eliminate the toxin from the intestinal mucosa.

Bacterial overgrowth may cause diarrhea. Reduced gastric and small bowel motility may lead to small intestinal overgrowth, which can alter intestinal microflora. Acid suppression may also permit bacterial overgrowth because bacteria can colonize the gastrointestinal tract when the gastric pH is greater than 6.0.

The infusion of enteral feedings too rapidly may cause diarrhea. Intolerance of lactose, fat, or osmolality may also lead to diarrhea. Reducing the infusion rate, changing to a peptide-based formula that is easier to digest, and giving an absorbing product, such as Metamucil, may help. The use of a fiber-containing formula may be helpful in bulking stools and correction of the diarrhea.

The composition of enteral formulas makes them an ideal medium for bacterial growth, which may result in diarrhea.[8,30,34] Many organisms have been associated with enteral feedings, including coagulase-negative staphylococci, *C. difficile*, and gram-negative bacilli such as *Serratia*, *Klebsiella*, *Enterobacter*, *Proteus*, and *Pseudomonas* species.[8,35] Bacterial contamination from the surface of the can, or even water added when the preparations are mixed or poured, may lead to diarrhea. Contamination of enteral feeds may also occur as a result of retrograde movement of bacteria from the patient's own gastrointestinal tract.[8,30] In addition, the aspiration of gastric residuals and the removal of guide wires may contribute to contamination.

Contamination of the administration set may also cause diarrhea. Breaks in the system should be minimized, and the use of a closed, prefilled, ready-to-hang solution should be considered to minimize contamination from pathogens. To prevent bacterial contamination, the nurse hangs no more than 4 hours of feeding solution in the container at one time and uses any open solution within 24 hours.[8] The nurse checks the expiration date of the formula and discards the formula if it has expired. Changing of administration sets is a daily practice, and rinsing occurs between bolus feedings. All practitioners use good handwashing technique when handling equipment and wear gloves when handling feeding systems.

In patients receiving enteral feedings, a hyperosmotic formula may also contribute to diarrhea. If diarrhea decreases when the feedings are held, the formula may be the cause. After consultation with the dietitian, the nurse may consider changing the formula. Also, the nurse collects a stool sample to evaluate for an osmotic gap; this may help identify osmotic diarrhea.

Hypoalbuminemia may predispose patients to diarrhea by decreasing the osmotic pressure gradient. This decrease may lead to bowel edema and mal-absorption. Any formula that is not absorbed may contribute to the diarrhea. Prealbumin is monitored because it is a more reliable indicator of current nutritional status than serum albumin.

Constipation

Constipation associated with enteral feedings may be related to poor hydration, lack of fiber, bed rest, impaction, obstruction, and narcotics. Adequate hydration is ensured, and adding a stool softener should be considered, along with minimizing narcotics, encouraging ambulation, and considering the addition of fiber to relieve constipation.

Mechanical Complications

Mechanical complications occur when the tube becomes dislodged, occluded, or malpositioned.

Tube Dislodgment

Tube dislodgment by either patients or staff accounts for most tube removals. Soft restraints or hand mitts should be considered for agitated patients to prevent accidental self-extubation (refer to your institution's policy regarding the use of restraints).

Tube Clogging

Precipitation of medications, clogging of pill fragments, or coagulation of formula may cause obstruction of any feeding tube, delaying the administration of nutrients and medications. To avoid clogging, the nurse flushes enteral feeding tubes every 4 to 6 hours during continuous feeds, before and after medication administration, after checking residuals, and when turning off feedings. For flushing nasoenteric tubes, the nurse always uses a large, 30- to 60-mL syringe to avoid rupturing the tube with excessive pressure and irrigates with 20 to 30 mL of tepid water.

The nurse frequently checks the enteral solution container for precipitation. Crushed tablets may leave a residual that blocks the tube. To prevent clogging, the nurse administers liquid medications when available. Flushing the tube before and after each medication administration also helps avoid incompatibilities between medications and feedings and reduces the incidence of clogging.

An obstruction may exist if the formula does not flow by gravity, flushing an aspirate from the tube is not possible, or the occlusion alarm of the feeding pump sounds repeatedly. If an occlusion is suspected, the nurse uses a large piston syringe to flush the tube with warm water, using a gentle push–pull motion. Although many solutions have been proposed to assist in clearing an obstructed feeding tube, they offer no demonstrable benefit over tap water.[15,36] A stylet should never be used to unclog a tube because of the risk for rupturing the feeding tube and perforating the esophagus, stomach, or small intestine. Recent studies have shown that pancreatic enzymes have been effective in unclogging a tube when water is unsuccessful, as long as the enzymes are activated before instillation.[36]

Metabolic Complications

Multiple metabolic complications can accompany enteral nutrition. Fluid and electrolyte imbalance may occur because of fluid excess, fluid depletion by gastrointestinal or renal losses, wound drainage, diuresis, fever, or inadequate free water intake. If dehydration is due to inadequate fluid intake, the nurse may need to give the patient extra fluid by bolus or by automatic flush using specialized feeding pumps. The average patient with good renal function needs 30 to 35 mL/kg of free water per day, if not otherwise medically contraindicated. Conversely, if cardiac or hepatic function is impaired, overhydration from enteral feedings may occur. The determination of the patient's baseline fluid requirements and accurate measurement of intake and output can help maintain fluid balance. The nurse should keep in mind that many of the patients seen in the ICU are often unable to convey feelings of thirst, secondary to diminished levels of consciousness or intubation.

Hyperglycemia may occur if patients are being overfed, during hypermetabolic states, and as a result of steroid medications. Blood glucose is monitored during enteral therapy; a decrease in formula rate or concentration may help if hyperglycemia occurs. Bolus feeding may exacerbate hyperglycemia in patients with diabetes. If feedings are abruptly stopped, hypoglycemia is assessed, especially in patients receiving insulin.

Infectious Complications

Aspiration of enteral feeding resulting in hypoxia or pneumonia is one of the most dreaded complications of enteral feeding. The incidence of aspiration of enteral formulas is as high as 50% to 75% in patients with endotracheal tubes (ETTs).[29,37] Loss of consciousness, mechanical ventilation, and many medications used in critically ill patients increase the risk for aspiration. To reduce this risk, the head of the bed should be maintained at a 30- to 45-degree angle.[10,37,38] If head of the bed elevation is medically contraindicated, a reverse Trendelenburg position is used unless medically contraindicated.[10,39] Intermittent or continuous feedings are used rather than rapid boluses because they allow the restoration of gastric pH, which can minimize gastric colonization. GRV is checked frequently, and signs of feeding intolerance are assessed. Feedings are discontinued at least 30 minutes before any procedure for which the patient must lay flat.[29] If a patient is intubated, ETT cuff pressure is maintained at 20 to 30 cm H_2O, and secretions above the cuff are cleared before deflating the tube.[29,37]

Pulmonary aspiration, although often subclinical, may be indicated by a low-grade fever, coughing, shortness of breath, rhonchi during or after enteral feeding infusions, and presence of a "sweet" formula odor emanating from the tracheal or oral secretions during suctioning. The addition of Food, Drug, and Cosmetic (FD&C) blue dye No. 1 to enteral feeding formula to help visually identify aspirated feeding formula was a common practice for years. However, in 2003, the U.S. Food and Drug Administration (FDA) issued an FDA Public Health Advisory after several reports of toxicity, including bacterial colonization, diarrhea, systemic absorption, and death.[40] As a result, the American Association of Critical-Care Nurses Practice Alert advises that FD&C No. 1 dye should not be used in enteral feedings.[41] It is necessary that each nurse check his or her institution's policy and protocol regarding blue dye administration.

Checking tracheal suction fluid with a glucose strip and glucometer has been used to test for formula aspiration. Tracheobronchial secretions usually contain less than 5 mg/dL of glucose, so a reading greater than 20 to 25 mg/dL suggests aspiration, although controversy concerning this procedure exists.[37,39]

PARENTERAL (INTRAVENOUS) NUTRITION

Parenteral nutrition is indicated when oral or enteral nutrition is not possible or when absorption or function of the gastrointestinal tract is not sufficient (or is unreliable) to meet the nutritional needs of the patient. Before the inception of parenteral nutrition in the early 1960s, bowel rest was thought to be the cornerstone of treatment for many gastrointestinal disorders. Today, except in cases of severe hemorrhagic pancreatitis, necrotizing enterocolitis, prolonged ileus, and distal bowel obstruction, some enteral nutrition is recommended to maintain gut integrity and function.[14] If the patient has a functioning gastrointestinal tract, if the treatment is anticipated to last for less than 5 days, or if prognosis does not warrant aggressive nutrition support, an alternative form of nutritional therapy is suggested.

There are two types of parenteral (IV) nutrition: central and peripheral. Central parenteral nutrition, also known as total parenteral nutrition (TPN), is infused through a large central vein (Fig. 40-3). TPN has sometimes been referred to as "hyperalimentation" or "hyperal." These are not preferred terms because they imply that parenteral nutrition gives more nutrients than the patient may actually require. If TPN is expected to be needed for more than a few weeks, a more permanent device such a subcutaneously tunneled Hickman catheter or Port-a-Cath can be placed. Another central venous access device that can be used for long-term nutritional support is the peripherally inserted central catheter (PICC). A PICC is inserted peripherally into the basilic vein and advanced so that the tip of the catheter rests in the superior vena cava. Peripheral parenteral nutrition (PPN), unlike TPN, is infused into smaller, peripheral veins (e.g., basilic vein) and is often used for short-term nutrition support (e.g., 7 to 10 days) or as a supplement during transitional phases to enteral or oral nutrition (see Fig. 40-3). Because of the risks for phlebitis, concentrations of PPN formulas must not exceed 900 mOsm/L.[42]

TPN differs from standard IV fluids in that all daily required nutrients are delivered to the patient in the form of macronutrients (carbohydrates, proteins, and fats) and micronutrients (electrolytes, vitamins, and trace minerals). Typically, the solution is infused at a constant rate over a 24-hour period to

EVIDENCE-BASED PRACTICE HIGHLIGHT: DYE IN ENTERAL FEEDING*

Expected Practice:
- Dye should not be added to enteral feeding as a method for identifying aspiration of gastric contents.

Supporting Evidence:
- Research and case reports of aspiration have shown that dye in enteral feedings is not visually detectable in situations similar to aspiration pneumonia.[1–4] A recent consensus statement on methods for identifying aspiration in critically ill patients recommended that dye be eliminated from enteral feeding because it lacks sensitivity for identifying aspiration of gastric contents.[5]

- The addition of dye to enteral feeding has been associated with several adverse events, including gastric bacterial colonization and diarrhea, systemic dye absorption, and death.[6–9] The FDA recently issued a Public Health Advisory based on reports of toxicity and death associated with dye in enteral feeding, though a direct causal relationship has not yet been definitively confirmed.[9] The majority of reported cases of toxicity and/or death occurred in patients with sepsis.
- Use of glucose testing of tracheal aspirates,[1,10] once proposed as a method for identification of gastric aspiration, is no longer recommended as a viable strategy.[5]

References:

1. Potts R, Zaroukian M, Guerrero P, Baker C: Comparison of blue dye visualization and glucose oxidase test strip methods for detecting pulmonary aspiration of enteral feedings in intubated adults. Chest;103:117–121, 1993

2. Thompson-Henry S, Braddock B: The modified Evan's blue dye procedure fails to detect aspiration in the tracheostomized patients: Five case reports. Dysphagia;10:172–174, 1995

3. Metheny N, Dahms T, Stewart B, et al: Efficacy of dye-stained enteral formula in detecting pulmonary aspiration in intubated adults. Chest;122:276–281, 2002

4. McClave S, Lukan J, Stefater J, et al: Poor validity of residual volumes as a marker for risk of aspiration in critically ill patients. Crit Care Med;33(2):324–330, 2005

5. McClave S, DeMeo M, DeLegge M, et al: North American Summit on Aspiration in Critically Ill Patients: Consensus statement. JPEN;26:S80–85, 2002

6. File T, Tan J, Thomson R, et al: An outbreak of Pseudomonas aeruginosa ventilator-associated respiratory infection and the significance of gastric colonization preceding nosocomial pneumonia. Infect Control Hosp Epidemiol;16:417–418, 1995

7. Maloney J, Halbower A, Fouty R, et al: Systemic absorption of food dye in patients with sepsis (letter). N Engl J Med;343:1047–1048, 2000

8. Bell R, Fishman S: Eosinophilia from food dye added to enteral feedings (letter). N Engl J Med;322:1822, 1990

9. Acheson D: FDA Public Health Advisory: Reports of blue discoloration and death in patients receiving enteral feedings tinted with the dye, FD&C Blue No. 1. FDA Web site. Accessed September 29, 2003, from http://www.cfsan.fda.gov/~dms/col-ltr2.html

10. Metheny N, St John R, Clouse R: Measurement of glucose in tracheobronchial secretions to detect aspiration of enteral feedings. Heart Lung;27:285–292, 1998

Excepted from American Association of Critical-Care Nurses Practice Alert.

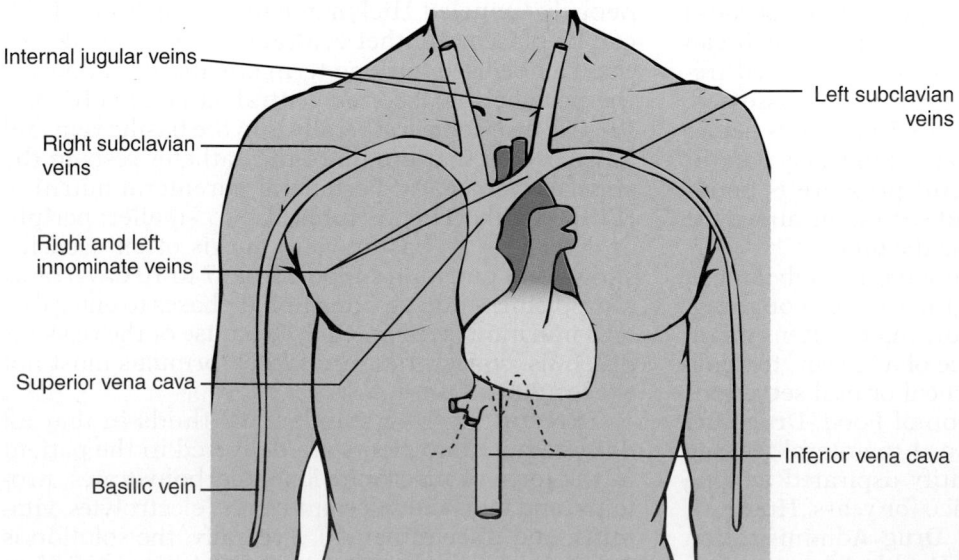

Internal jugular veins

Left subclavian veins

Right subclavian veins

Right and left innominate veins

Superior vena cava

Basilic vein

Inferior vena cava

Figure 40-3 • Venous anatomy for parenteral nutrition routes.

achieve maximal assimilation of the nutrients and to prevent hyperglycemia (or hypoglycemia). The aim of treatment is a continuous infusion that meets the caloric and nutritional requirements of the patient.

Critically ill patients often have issues with reliable IV access. TPN must be infused separately from other IV fluids, medications, and blood products, because of the high risk for formula contamination and precipitation. Fortunately, the introduction of multiple-lumen catheters has greatly facilitated the care of patients who require multiple IV therapies by providing separate infusion ports and corresponding distal exit sites staggered along the catheter tubing. This separation prevents direct mixing of solutions before high blood volume dilution of the central veins. One port must be dedicated to exclusive use of TPN, whereas the remaining ports can be used for the administration of IV fluids and blood sampling. When the central line is a single lumen, this lumen should be used exclusively for the infusion of TPN.

Composition of Parenteral Nutrition Formulas

TPN formulas typically contain three primary macronutrients: carbohydrates, lipids (fats), and amino acids (protein). This combination is called a mixed fuel source. When all three fuel sources are combined together in one TPN bag, it is often referred to as a "3 in 1" admixture. The desired proportions of these nutrients are prepared by a pharmacist under a laminar flow hood to maintain strict sterility. Because of differences in pharmacy equipment used to mix TPN, some agencies infuse lipids separately, usually in a glass bottle. Medications are not to be added to a TPN bag after it has been prepared by the pharmacist because of the risk for contamination or precipitation of its contents. The current trend in TPN formulation is based on the specific needs of each patient; standard formulas are no longer widely prescribed.

Carbohydrates

The primary source of energy in the body is carbohydrates (e.g., dextrose). This macronutrient usually provides 40% to 60% of daily caloric requirements and is essential to central nervous system function. The most common and preferred source of carbohydrates is dextrose (D-glucose) because it is readily metabolized, stimulates the secretion of insulin, and is usually well tolerated in large quantities. Dextrose provides 3.4 kcal/g in IV form and contributes to most of the osmolality (or concentration) of the TPN solution. Initial TPN concentrations of dextrose may range from 50% to 70%, but final concentrations are diluted to approximately 25% to 30% after the addition of amino acids, lipid emulsions, and water.[42]

Despite dilution, this concentration remains very high and requires delivery through a central venous catheter so that the higher blood volumes in the larger central veins are able to further dilute and disperse the solution. The superior vena cava is an excellent site for such delivery. Passage of a central venous catheter, by way of the subclavian vein into the superior vena cava, is the route of choice because it allows the patient the greatest freedom of movement without disturbing the insertion site. Jugular veins can also be used but may make it more difficult to keep dressings sterile, and these are not as comfortable for the patient because of limitations in neck movement. Regardless of the site, strict adherence to insertion and infection protocols must be followed, and radiologic verification of catheter tip placement is necessary before initial infusion (refer to your institution's central line care and infection control policies and procedures).

The amount of dextrose prescribed in TPN is based on metabolic needs, which, once met, allows utilization of amino acids for protein synthesis rather than solely as an energy source. Adults require a minimum of 100 g/day of dextrose to perform vital metabolic activities; however, the maximal dose of dextrose varies based on an individual's needs, medical condition, and glucose tolerance. Recommendations suggest that dextrose must not exceed 7 g/kg/day[14] or 5 to 7 mg/kg/min.[43] One of the most common metabolic side effects of excessive dextrose concentrations is hyperglycemia, which often requires the use of insulin. In addition, excessive dextrose administration may put certain patients, such as those with pulmonary compromise, at risk for carbon dioxide retention and subsequent respiratory acidosis. Because one of the end products of dextrose metabolism is carbon dioxide, elevated levels may increase minute ventilation and hence the work of breathing. Overfeeding carbohydrates may make ventilator weaning difficult, if not impossible.

Lipids

Parenteral IV lipids, or fat emulsions, primarily contain long-chain linoleic and α-linolenic acids (essential fatty acids) from safflower and soybean vegetable oils. Lipid solutions also contain egg yolk phospholipids as emulsifiers, so it is important to check food allergy history before administration. Lipids provide a concentrated source of calories, 9 kcal/g, and are important in the maintenance of connective tissue integrity and prevention of fatty acid deficiency. Patients should receive 1% to 2% of their daily energy requirements as linoleic acid and 0.5% of their daily energy requirements from α-linolenic acid.[14] The usual dose is 0.5 to 1.0 g/kg/day (not to exceed 2.5 g/kg/day) to supply up to 30% of the patient's caloric intake; however, only 500 mL of a 20% lipid emulsion given once per week prevents essential fatty acid deficiency in adults.[14,43] Symptoms of essential fatty acid deficiency include rough, dry, scaly skin; nasolabial seborrhea; dull or dry hair, soft or brittle nails, poor wound healing, and diarrhea.[44,45]

Lipid emulsions are isotonic and concentrations are available in 10%, 20%, and 30% solutions, providing 1.1, 2.0, and 2.9 kcal/mL, respectively.[42] The benefit of higher concentrations is that they provide a greater concentration of calories in less total fluid volume, an important consideration for many patients. In situations in which hyperglycemia has become problematic, dextrose solution concentrations and volumes may be reduced, and unless contraindicated, lipids concentrations and volumes can be increased. Lipids typically provide 15% to 30% of daily caloric intake; if delivery of lipids is higher than 30% of total caloric intake, vigilant monitoring for metabolic side effects is especially important. Baseline and weekly triglyceride trends monitor lipid tolerance. Elevated triglyceride levels exceeding 400 mg/dL suggest impaired lipid clearance and an increased risk for pancreatitis, so it is recommended that lipid emulsions be held until levels return to normal.[46]

Lipid concentrations may need to be adjusted for patients who may also be receiving additional lipids from sources other than TPN (e.g., continuous infusion of propofol, a sedative delivered as a lipid emulsion). Lipid emulsions provide an excellent medium for bacterial growth, so increased manipulation and prolonged hang times are avoided. Adverse lipid reactions include, but are not limited to, fever, chills, chest or back tightness, dyspnea, tachycardia, headache, nausea, and vomiting. If such reactions occur, the nurse stops the infusion immediately and reports the reaction to the physician and pharmacist. Long-term lipid reactions include concerns over immune system suppression.[42]

Before infusion, the nurse inspects lipid-containing TPN solutions for separation of the lipid solution, also know as cracking and coalescence. This loss of emulsion can be identified by yellow-brown marbling of the entire solution or as layering of oil at the surface of the TPN bag. Such solutions are not safe for infusion and should be returned to the pharmacy for replacement.

Amino Acids

All tissues require protein to maintain structure and facilitate wound healing. If protein intake is inadequate, the body becomes catabolic, seeking protein from skeletal muscle and vital organs. In TPN, protein is provided as a mixture of essential and nonessential crystalline amino acids, which are available in concentrations ranging from 5% to 15%. These concentrations supply approximately 15% to 20% of daily caloric needs. One gram of amino acids is equivalent to 1 g of protein, which provides 4 kcal/g.[47] Adult amino acid requirements can range widely from 0.8 to 2.0 g/kg/day, and those patients with burns, wounds, draining fistulas, renal failure, or hepatic failure may need frequent adjustments in the amount of amino acids they receive.[48] For patients with renal disease, solutions with a higher concentration of essential amino acids are available. For patients with hepatic failure or hypercatabolic conditions, formulas with branched-chain amino acids, which spare the breakdown of other muscle proteins to use as energy, possibly reducing the incidence of hepatic encephalopathy, may be used.

Micronutrients

Vitamins, trace minerals, and electrolytes are considered micronutrients. Unfortunately, the U.S. Recommended Dietary Allowance requirements do not apply to parenteral nutrition for several reasons. First, the liver and gastrointestinal tract absorptive processes are bypassed, resulting in elimination of these micronutrients through the urine without their being utilized. Second, many diseases alter the gut's ability to absorb fat-soluble vitamins and vitamin B_{12}. Finally, many nutrients adhere to the plastic tubing and IV solution bags or are destroyed by light and oxygen exposure (especially vitamin A) before reaching the bloodstream.

With these factors in mind, standard aqueous multivitamin preparations have been created, and according to recent recommendations by the FDA, provide higher levels of thiamine, pyridoxine, ascorbic acid, and folic acid.[49] Unfortunately, hypermetabolic conditions of critical illness can exacerbate deficiencies that require additional monitoring and potential supplementation; individual vitamin products are available for supplements as needed. Until recently, vitamin K was the only vitamin not included in the multivitamin preparation; it is provided by adding up to 10 mg/week of the vitamin to the TPN solution (unless contraindicated by anticoagulation treatment). Because some parenteral formulas may now contain vitamin K, weekly supplementation is no longer necessary, but it is important to continue to monitor coagulation studies, especially if the patient is receiving anticoagulation treatment. Unlike patients who require additional nutrients, patients with liver or kidney disease may need to receive lower doses of certain vitamins.

Trace mineral elements are required to maintain biochemical homeostasis and come in a variety of commercial mixtures but typically include chromium, copper, manganese, selenium, and zinc. Parenteral iron is not added to TPN solutions because of stability issues and the potential for adverse effects, and it may need to be supplemented in long-term therapy.

Most electrolyte standard mixtures contain sodium, potassium, calcium, magnesium, phosphorus, chloride, and acetate. Sodium bicarbonate is not added to TPN; precipitation with the other electrolytes may occur. Instead, acetate is used because it can be converted by the liver to bicarbonate. Depending on the patient's underlying disease process and physical assessment findings, specific electrolyte concentrations can be adjusted daily in the TPN solution. If an electrolyte deficiency is detected after the TPN solution has already been prepared or while infusing, additional IV supplements can be given as a separate IV piggyback. Electrolyte supplements should never be added to the TPN bag after the pharmacist has formulated it because this would break the sterility of the solution and may cause the solution to precipitate.

Medications

During the process of preparing the TPN solution, the pharmacist can add medications, many of which are often necessitated by the TPN therapy itself. For instance, although insulin drips are now the current trend in management of hyperglycemia, insulin can be added to the TPN solution. Additionally, heparin can be added to reduce fibrin buildup along the catheter tip. The clinician ordering the medications consults with the pharmacist to ensure compatibility.

Complications of Parenteral Nutrition

Complications can be divided into three main categories: metabolic, infectious, and mechanical.

Metabolic Complications

Hepatic dysfunction may occur in patients receiving parenteral nutrition; abnormal liver enzymes can occur in as many as 40% to 70% of patients.[50] This is often related to the infusion amount and flow rate. Specific complications include hepatic steatosis (fatty liver), intrahepatic and extrahepatic cholestasis (suppression of bile flow), and cholelithiasis (formation of gallstones). Although the exact mechanisms of these hepatic disorders are still not completely understood, it has been observed that cholestasis is less likely to occur if some form of enteral feeding is maintained.[51] Gastrointestinal atrophy, and all of its associated complications, may occur from disuse. If not contraindicated, oral or enteral feedings should be initiated as soon as possible.

It is important to understand that many metabolic complications stem from the patient's underlying disease processes or from imprudent formula administration. Some metabolic disturbances can be prevented by checking each bag of parenteral nutrition solution for transcription accuracy, monitoring the IV pump for infusion accuracy, and monitoring the patient's response to therapy. Virtually any metabolic disturbance can occur during parenteral nutrition infusion: the most common metabolic complications include hyperglycemia, hypoglycemia, hypophosphatemia, hypokalemia, hypomagnesemia, and hypocalcemia. These metabolic disturbances, coupled with rapid fluid shifts and imbalances, may lead to a disorder called refeeding syndrome, which is discussed later.

Hyperglycemia

Hyperglycemia, or a blood sugar elevated over 220 mg/dL, can occur if the pancreas does not respond to the increased glucose load. Although hyperglycemia can be caused by either enteral or parenteral feedings, it is more commonly seen in patients receiving parenteral nutrition. Even slightly elevated blood glucose levels can impair the function of lymphocytes, leading to immunosuppression and increased risk for infection. Elevated glucose concentrations have been shown to reduce neutrophil chemotaxis and phagocytosis and may be an independent risk factor for short-term infections.[52] If the renal threshold for glucose reabsorption is exceeded, osmotic diuresis results in subsequent dehydration and electrolyte imbalances. Glycemic control can be achieved by increasing the amount of insulin in the TPN solution, by maintaining a continuous insulin drip during TPN administration, or by administering sliding-scale insulin subcutaneously at regular intervals. Once TPN is discontinued, insulin requirements become notably less or nonexistent. If new TPN solution is temporarily unavailable, administration of 10% dextrose in water ($D_{10}W$) is recommended to prevent rebound hypoglycemia. In addition, if a solution is "behind schedule," it is not recommended that the infusion rate be increased to make up time because this may cause sudden metabolic fluctuations and fluid overload.

Refeeding Syndrome

Refeeding syndrome is one of the most critical complications that occurs with the initiation of TPN. This condition is characterized by rapid shifts in electrolytes (phosphorus, potassium, magnesium, and calcium), glucose, and volume status within hours to days of nutrition implementation. Parenterally delivered glucose loads stimulate insulin release, which in turn stimulates intracellular uptake of phosphorus, glucose, and other electrolytes for anabolic processes. Despite relatively normal serum phosphorus levels

on standard laboratory reports, intracellular stores are markedly depleted in malnourished catabolic patients; severe hypophosphatemia (<1 mg/dL) can lead to neuromuscular, respiratory, and cardiac dysfunction. Low serum levels of potassium, magnesium, and calcium can precipitate cardiac dysrhythmias. The increased intravascular fluid volumes associated with parenteral nutrition can strain the viscerally depleted heart and possibly induce heart failure and myocardial damage. Risk factors for refeeding syndrome include marasmus, chronic alcoholism, anorexia nervosa, rapid refeeding, and excessive dextrose infusion.

Prevention of refeeding syndrome includes repletion of phosphorus, potassium, magnesium, and calcium before TPN initiation, limiting initial dextrose dosing, and titrating total volume and rate to evaluate for fluid overload and potential cardiac decompensation. Daily monitoring of phosphorous, potassium, and magnesium is recommended.[53] Weight-based phosphorus repletion algorithms (e.g., 0.32 to 1.0 mmol/kg) have been shown to be highly efficacious in correcting hypophosphatemia during nutrition support therapy.[54] It is of paramount importance that the critical care nurse take accurate intake and output measurements and daily weights because adequate parenteral nutrition often means giving 1.5 to 3 L of fluid per day in addition to other therapies. Progressive weight gain could be an early indicator of poor fluid tolerance.

Infectious Complications

Both the solution and the indwelling catheter are prime sites for infection because of the high glucose content. Any break in the system is a nidus for infection that can progress to a systemic infection if left unchecked. After initial preparation by a pharmacist, the access hubs on the bag of TPN are often covered with tape as a reminder that no additional solutions or medications are to be added.

At the bedside, the nurse changes the TPN solution bag and tubing according to institution policy, usually every 24 hours. He or she redresses the catheter insertion site per institution policy as well, usually every 24 to 72 hours, using either a sterile transparent or gauze dressing. Although transparent dressings allow for easier observation of the catheter entrance site, these dressings have a tendency to trap moisture and hence have a higher incidence of infection and sepsis than traditional, sterile dry gauze dressings; however, this is still under investigation (check your institution's policies and procedures regarding central and peripheral line dressing changes).[51] At the time of the dressing change, a clinician examines the site for signs of leakage, erythema, edema, and inflammation. The nurse cleanses the site with an antibacterial solution to remove pathogenic organisms. Researchers have shown that chlorhexidine solution is a more effective local antiseptic than povidone-iodine solutions,[55] and use of impregnated chlorhexidine/silver sulfadiazine or minocycline/rifampin catheters could reduce the incidence of central venous catheter–related infections.[56] The presence of a tracheostomy or other open draining wounds near the IV insertion site requires special precautions to prevent site contamination.

Potential for infection can be minimized by meticulous catheter care. In critically ill patients, catheter-related infections range from local inflammation to systemic bloodstream infection and sepsis. Systemic catheter-related infections are associated with a 35% mortality rate, and hospital stays are reportedly longer and more expensive as a result of complications and associated treatment.[51] If fever, rigors, or chills coincide with parenteral infusion, catheter-related sepsis should be suspected; slowing or stopping the infusion may cause defervescence. Treatment of an infection may involve local topical antibiotics, systemic antibiotics, and, in many cases, catheter removal. If catheter sepsis is suspected, the catheter tip is usually cultured to identify the offending organism to ensure appropriate antibiotic coverage.

Mechanical Complications

Mechanical complications include those associated with central venous catheter insertion, such as trauma to the vessel, pneumothorax, catheter occlusion, thrombosis, and venous air embolism. After insertion of a central catheter, a chest radiograph is the standard of care to confirm correct placement. If there is a clinical suspicion of catheter tip migration or other potential complications, further diagnostic testing is indicated.

Trauma to vessels and pneumothorax are complications that may warrant surgical intervention, insertion of a chest tube or tubes, or both. Catheter occlusion can simply be a result of the catheter tip lodging against the vessel wall or being physiologically "pinched" between the clavicle and first rib. Occlusion can also occur from fibrin buildup, blood or lipid deposition, drug precipitates, and catheter breakage.[57] Another type of occlusion, "withdrawal occlusion," is an occlusion that allows infusion of a solution but prevents blood withdrawal. Although more research is needed to determine optimal methods for catheter maintenance and patency during parenteral nutrition infusions, routine flushing of catheters with diluted heparin (10 to 100 units/mL in those without heparin sensitivities) is recommended.[45]

Thrombosis formation in the lumen of the vessel often results from mechanical irritation (such as from traumatic catheter insertion), a small lumen, an extended duration of catheter use, the catheter material, or malpositioning. Nurses need to be aware that patients may have a thrombosis and may be asymptomatic, yet complain of vague head and eye swelling on the affected side.[45] Vigilant assessments during parenteral nutrition administration are recommended. Treatment includes catheter removal, systemic anticoagulation, and thrombolytic therapy.

A venous air embolism is another serious complication, with a mortality rate of up to 32%.[58] Use of a filter, no smaller than 1.2 microns, can reduce the incidence of particulates and air being transfused, thus reducing the risk for pulmonary embolism. However, there is no evidence to suggest that these filters reduce the risk for infection.[59] Any disruption of the closed catheter system (usually during line connection changes, when hanging a new bag of TPN, or in an accidental tubing disconnection) can increase the risk for an air embolism. If such an incident occurs, the patient will most likely experience acute, centrally located chest pain, dyspnea, and hypotension. Immediate nursing interventions include clamping the tubing of the catheter or occluding the catheter hub, attempting to aspirate air directly from the venous line, administering 100% oxygen, and placing the patient in steep Trendelenburg position with the left lateral side down. This position allows air to rise to the level of the right ventricle, away from the pulmonary vasculature.[45] Prevention of an air embolism can be facilitated by having the patient perform the Valsalva maneuver or simply hum audibly during line changes. In ventilator-dependent patients, positive intrathoracic pressure can be created by initiating mechanical lung inflations or "breaths." Finally, use of sterile occlusive dressings (e.g., petroleum gauze) over the catheter entrance site is an effective measure in preventing air from entering the track after the catheter has been discontinued.[45]

Tapering Parenteral Nutrition

Tapering TPN is often initiated for those patients who are able to resume safely (and tolerate) approximately 50% to 75% of their nutritional needs by enteral or oral nutrition. In such instances, a calorie count is essential to ascertain that the patient's nutritional needs are being met. Before the parenteral nutrition is discontinued, the infusion rate is decreased by half for 30 to 60 minutes. This allows for a plasma glucose response and prevention of rebound hypoglycemia.[45] Checking blood sugars for 30 to 60 minutes after discontinuation helps the nurse identify and manage immediate glucose abnormalities.

In situations in which poor prognosis does not warrant aggressive nutritional support, emotional and ethical dilemmas may surface for many nurses because feeding and hydration have long been basic tenets of nursing care. Although many institutions may have protocols in place regarding parenteral nutrition, treatment decisions and plans of care should be discussed on an individual basis. Frequent, ongoing discussions between the patient, family, and the health care team are imperative to providing the best possible care to each patient.

ROLE OF THE NURSE IN NUTRITIONAL SUPPORT

Nurses are responsible for obtaining initial "dry weight" and weekly weight measurements, vital signs, intake and output measurements, and laboratory data, and for providing enteral tube and IV catheter care throughout the duration of nutrition support therapies. Many complications, whether from enteral or parenteral nutrition, can be prevented by vigilant observation and care. If the patient is awake and alert, the patient's subjective assessment of tolerance can be very informative. The nurse obtains more objective signs of feeding tolerance through abdominal examinations, which assess bowel sounds and changes in abdominal girth. Also, the nurse monitors and records volume and frequency of both urine and stool.

In addition, the nurse must monitor for clinical signs of dehydration (thirst, dry mucous membranes, tachycardia, and poor skin turgor), and fluid excess (peripheral edema and adventitious lung sounds). Early detection and subsequent interventions may prevent the occurrence of excessive fluid shifts and cardiac compromise. This is of special concern if the patient is severely malnourished, which may precipitate refeeding syndrome and other untoward complications. Meticulous feeding tube and IV catheter care is critical to preventing local and systemic forms of infection.

Care also includes providing information and emotional support to the patient and family. Examples include explaining the procedure, what to expect, risks, and expected outcomes (Box 40-3). Guidelines for discharge planning are given in Box 40-4.

Box 40-3 • TEACHING GUIDE: Living With Nutritional Support

General Care: Enteral Nutrition
- Administer enteral formulas as prescribed.
- Know potential complications and appropriate treatments.
- Avoid activities that may result in high impact or stress at the insertion site and report any activity that may have damaged the enteral access site.
- Return to previous activities (e.g., work, leisure, sexual activity) after obtaining physician consent.

General Care: Parenteral Nutrition
- Administer parenteral formulas as prescribed.
- Monitor blood sugars closely to help determine tolerance of parenteral solutions.
- Know the potential complications and appropriate treatments.
- Avoid activities that may result in high impact or stress at the insertion site and report any activity that may have damaged the parenteral access site.
- Return to previous activities (e.g., work, leisure, sexual activity) after obtaining physician consent.

Signs of Infections
- Understand the rationale for aseptic technique.
- Notify the nurse of symptoms of fever, localized warmth, redness, pain, or drainage at the feeding tube or intravenous insertion site.

Medications
- Follow instructions regarding medications.
- Know the names of medications and the dose, frequency of administration, side effects, and use of each medication.
- Know the proper technique of administering medications through the feeding tube and proper flushing technique.
- Never add medications to TPN solutions—they should be added by the supplier because of risk for contamination or precipitation of the formula.

Safety Measures
- Inform other health care providers of either enteral or parenteral access devices and notify them of any medications that the patient may be taking.

Follow-up Care
- Report any problems to the home care nurse.
- Adhere to schedule for follow-up visits with patient's physician or clinic.

Box 40-4 • DISCHARGE PLANNING GUIDE: Nutritional Therapy

- Assess patient/caregiver ability to deliver home nutritional therapy, including physical and cognitive abilities.
- Identify health care team members who will be responsible for the management of home therapy.
- Assess patient's home environment for safety.
- Evaluate support system available in home.
- Identify an in-home caretaker who is willing and able to learn and carry out the home care regimen. If the patient does not have a caretaker at home and there are concerns about patient's ability to become independent, reevaluate discharge plan.
- Ensure that patient/caregiver learning includes determining procedures and risks, picking up patient and equipment problems early, troubleshooting, and following up with the health care provider.
- Refer to and communicate with home care services.
- Provide written instructions for patient.
- If possible, do not change the amount or rate of nutrition support on the day of discharge to home.

• Pharmacological Management of Gastrointestinal Disorders

Table 40-1 summarizes many of the common gastrointestinal medications administered to critically ill patients who are concurrently receiving nutrition support therapy.

• Clinical Applicability Challenges

Case Study

Mr. P. is a 62-year-old executive who is status post cerebrovascular accident with severe dysphagia (impaired swallowing). He has a past medical history of gastroesophageal reflux disease, coronary artery disease, hypertension, hypercholesterolemia, and type 2 diabetes mellitus. He is currently prescribed pantoprazole (Protonix), 40 mg daily; aspirin, 81 mg daily; clopidogrel (Plavix), 75 mg daily; metoprolol (Lopressor), 50 mg twice daily; simvastatin (Zocor), 20 mg daily; and 15 units Lantus insulin subcutaneously at bedtime. Because of Mr. P.'s severe dysphagia, swallowing studies and calorie counts are ordered to determine whether he will be able to resume safe and adequate oral nutrition. In the meantime, to ensure that Mr. P.'s nutritional needs are met, he is receiving enteral nutrition 400 mL every 4 hours through a small-bore nasogastric tube.

Physical examination reveals a nontender, nondistended, obese abdomen with positive bowel sounds. However, before the instillation of a scheduled feeding, the gastric residual volume (GRV) is found to be 300 mL. Subsequently, the

Table 40-1 • Common Gastrointestinal Medications

Agent	Mechanism of Action	Indication	Common Adverse Effects	Comments
Antacids				
Aluminum carbonate	Neutralization of gastric acid; binding phosphates in the gastrointestinal tract	Symptomatic relief of gastric irritation, prevention of urinary phosphate stone development, binding of phosphate in chronic renal failure	Fecal impaction, cramps, constipation, hypophosphatemia (when given in excessive doses)	Monitor phosphorus levels.
Aluminum hydroxide (Amphojel, AlternaGEL)	Neutralization of gastric acid; binding phosphates in the gastrointestinal tract	Symptomatic relief of gastric irritation, hyperphosphatemia in chronic renal failure	Constipation, hypophosphatemia (when given in excessive doses)	Less phosphate binding than aluminum carbonate. Monitor phosphorus levels.
Calcium carbonate (Tums, Caltrate)	Neutralization of gastric acid	Symptomatic relief of gastric irritation, calcium supplementation	Headaches	Usually well tolerated. Monitor calcium and phosphorus levels.
Magnesium hydroxide (Milk of Magnesia)	Neutralization of gastric acid	Symptomatic relief of gastric irritation, hypomagnesemia, constipation	Hypermagnesemia, abdominal cramping and diarrhea (with high doses)	Monitor magnesium levels.
Dihydroxyaluminum, sodium carbonate (Rolaids)	Neutralization of gastric acid; reduction of pepsin	Symptomatic relief of gastric irritation	Constipation	Use with caution in sodium-restricted patients.
Histamine Type 2 (H₂) Receptor Antagonists				
Cimetidine (Tagamet)	Inhibition of histamine at H_2 receptor sites on gastric parietal cells, which inhibits gastric acid secretion	GERD, PUD, acid hypersecretory states	Confusion, headaches, diarrhea	May cause rare blood dyscrasias. Monitor CBC.
Ranitidine (Zantac)	Inhibition of histamine at H_2 receptor sites on gastric parietal cells, which inhibits gastric acid secretion	GERD, PUD, acid hypersecretory states	Headaches, dizziness, constipation	May cause hepatotoxicity and rare blood dyscrasias.
Famotidine (Pepcid)	Inhibition of histamine at H_2 receptor sites on gastric parietal cells, which inhibits gastric acid secretion	GERD, PUD, acid hypersecretory states	Headaches, dizziness	May cause seizures, bronchospasm, constipation, or thrombocytopenia. Monitor CBC.
Nizatidine (Axid)	Inhibition of histamine at H_2 receptor sites on gastric parietal cells, which inhibits gastric acid secretion	GERD, PUD, acid hypersecretory states	Dizziness, headaches, diarrhea	
Proton Pump Inhibitors				
Omeprazole (Prilosec), lansoprazole (Prevacid), rapeprazole (Aciphex), pantoprazole (Protonix), esomeprazole (Nexium)	Suppression of gastric acid secretion by inhibition of H^+, K^+-ATPase pump (proton pump) of parietal cells, blocking final step in acid production	Reflux esophagitis, treatment of gastric and duodenal ulcers, pathological hypersecretory states (Zollinger-Ellison syndrome)	Headaches, diarrhea, abdominal pain	Less common side effects include nausea, vomiting, and dizziness.
Pancreatic Enzymes				
Pancreatin (Creon, Donnazyme, Ultrase)	Assistance in the digestion of carbohydrates, fats, and proteins	Replacement in pancreatic enzyme deficiencies, cystic fibrosis	Nausea, diarrhea, cramping, anorexia, hypersensitivity reactions, perianal irritation	

(continued)

Table 40-1 • Common Gastrointestinal Medications (Continued)

Agent	Mechanism of Action	Indication	Common Adverse Effects	Comments
Pancrealipase (Pancrease, Viokase)	Assistance in the digestion of carbohydrates, fats, and proteins	Replacement in pancreatic enzyme deficiencies, steatorrhea of malabsorption, cystic fibrosis, postgastrectomy, or postpancreatectomy	Nausea, diarrhea, cramping, anorexia, hypersensitivity reactions, perianal irritation	
Antidiarrheals				
Attapulgite (Kaopectate)	Absorption of toxins produced by bacterial and gastrointestinal irritants; decrease in gastric motility and stool water content	Diarrhea	Increased potassium loss, interference with absorption of medications	
Bismuth subsalicylate (Pepto Bismol)	Slowing of motility; antimicrobial activity against gastrointestinal microbes; antisecretory sensitivity	Diarrhea, prophylaxis of traveler's diarrhea	Tongue discoloration, dark stools	Assess electrolytes if diarrhea persists. Use cautiously in patients using other salicylates.
Cholestyramine (Questran)	Absorption of bile salts, which can cause diarrhea; absorption of *Clostridium difficile* toxin	Diarrhea caused by bile salts or *C. difficile*	Constipation	Because it may alter absorption of other medications, administer other medications at least 1 h before cholestyramine.
Loperamide (Imodium)	Slowing intestinal motility, including peristalsis	Acute and chronic diarrhea	Abdominal distention, constipation, drowsiness, dizziness, nausea, vomiting	
Tincture of opium (Paregoric, DTO)	Decrease in gastrointestinal motility and peristalsis, decrease in digestive secretions	Acute diarrhea, relief of abdominal cramping	Drowsiness, lightheadedness, bradycardia	Side effects are related to opioid content. Other possible reactions include allergic reactions, vomiting, dizziness, sweating, constipation, and habituation.
Laxatives				
Bowel Evacuants				
Polyethylene glycol with electrolytes (Colyte, NuLytely, GoLYTELY)	Nonabsorbable solution that acts like an osmotic agent	Bowel cleansing before colonoscopy or bowel surgery	Transient bloating, nausea, cramping	
Bulk-Forming Agents				
Calcium polycarbophil (Fibercon), methylcellulose (Citracel), psyllium (Metamucil)	Nondigestable plant cell wall draws water into the feces and softens stool; absorption of excess water in the stool	Diarrhea, constipation	Flatulence, impaction (if feces is obstructed)	Generally well tolerated.
Lactulose (Cephulac, Enulose)	Hyperosmolality draws water into the intestinal lumen, increasing stool water content and softening stool; prevention of absorption of ammonia in the colon	Constipation, prevention and treatment of hepatic encephalopathy	Flatulence, cramping, impaction (if feces is obstructed)	For use in prevention and treatment of hepatic encephalopathy, titrate dose to two to three loose stools a day. Monitor serum ammonia levels.
Polyethylene glycol (MiraLax)	Nonabsorbable solution that acts like an osmotic agent	Constipation	Nausea, abdominal bloating, cramping, diarrhea	

(continued)

Table 40-1 • Common Gastrointestinal Medications (Continued)

Agent	Mechanism of Action	Indication	Common Adverse Effects	Comments
Saline Laxatives				
Magnesium citrate (Citrate of Magnesium)	Magnesium and sodium salts are poorly absorbed, drawing water into the intestinal lumen	Constipation, cleansing of the colon before examination	Cramps, flatulence, nausea, vomiting	Do not use in renal disease. Observe for hypermagnesemia (watching for thirst, drowsiness, dizziness).
Sodium biphosphate (Fleet Phospha-soda, Fleet Enema)	Increase in water absorption in the small intestine through osmosis	Constipation, acute bowel evacuation before a bowel or colon examination	Nausea, cramps	May precipitate or exacerbate cardiac, renal, or seizure disorder.
Stimulants				
Bisacodyl (Dulcolax)	Increase in peristalsis by direct effect on nerve endings in colonic mucosa	Constipation, evacuation of bowel before examination		Can cause habituation with gradual lessening effect in long-term use. PO onset is 6 to 10 h; PR onset is 15 to 60 min.
Cascara	Increase in propulsive movements through chemical irritation of the colon	Constipation	Discoloration of urine (red or yellow-brown)	May cause habituation. Onset is 6 to 10 h.
Senna (Senokot, SenokotXTRA)	Stimulation of propulsion	Constipation	Discoloration of urine	Natural product from cassia
Phenolphthalein (Ex-Lax)	Stimulation of peristalsis (similar to bisacodyl)	Constipation		May cause an allergic reaction; discontinue use if rash develops.
Stool Softeners				
Docusate sodium (Surfak, Colace)	Increase in the penetration of the feces by water and fat; softening of the stool	Constipation	Cramping, diarrhea	Prolonged or excessive use may cause habituation or electrolyte abnormalities.
Stimulant/Stool Softeners				
Glycerin	Drawing water into the colon (by high osmotic pressure)	Constipation	Headaches, nausea, vomiting	
Antiemetics				
Trimethobenzamide (Tigan)	Inhibition of the chemoreceptor trigger zone, which then inhibits the vomiting center	Symptomatic relief of nausea and vomiting	Hypersensitivity, drowsiness, hypotension, diarrhea, depression, vertigo	
Prochlorperazine (Compazine)	Blocking of dopamine receptors in the chemoreceptor trigger zone in the brainstem	Nausea, vomiting	Extrapyramidal side effects such as drowsiness, blurred vision, tachycardia, and respiratory depression	
Promethazine (Phenergan)	Competition with histamine in blood vessels and gastrointestinal and respiratory systems to decrease allergic responses	Nausea, vomiting, motion sickness, sedation	Dizziness, drowsiness, constipation, urinary retention	Other reactions may include thrombocytopenia, agranulocytosis, and hemolytic anemia.

(continued)

Table 40-1 • Common Gastrointestinal Medications (Continued)

Agent	Mechanism of Action	Indication	Common Adverse Effects	Comments
Dolasetron (Anzemet)	Blocking serotonin (5-HT$_3$) receptors in the chemoreceptor trigger zone and gastro-intestinal tract	Nausea and vomiting associated with chemotherapy, prevention and treatment of postoperative nausea and vomiting	ECG changes, hypertension, abdominal pain, diarrhea, urinary retention	
Granisetron (Kytril)	Blocking serotonin (5-HT$_3$) receptors in the chemoreceptor trigger zone and gastro-intestinal tract	Nausea and vomiting associated with chemotherapy and radiation	Headache, constipation, asthenia	Use with caution in patients with liver disease.
Ondansetron (Zofran)	Blocking serotonin (5-HT$_3$) receptors in the chemoreceptor trigger zone and gastro-intestinal tract	Nausea and vomiting associated with chemotherapy, prevention of postoperative nausea and vomiting	Diarrhea, bronchospasm, fatigue, constipation	
Other				
Sucralfate (Carafate)	Formation of a protective covering at ulcer site	Short-term treatment of peptic ulcers	Constipation	Because it may alter absorption of other medications, patient should take other medications at least 2 h before sucralfate.
Metoclopramide (Reglan)	Stimulation of upper gastrointestinal motility; decrease in inhibitory tone	Diabetic gastroparesis, delayed gastric emptying, short-term treatment of GERD, prevention of postoperative nausea and vomiting, facilitation of small bowel feeding tube placement	Diarrhea, constipation, drowsiness, restlessness	May occasionally have extrapyramidal side effects.
Misoprostol (Cytotec)	Prostaglandin analog increases bicarbonate and mucus release and decreases acid secretions	Prevention of aspirin- and NSAID-induced ulcers	Diarrhea, nausea, vomiting, flatulence	Use with caution in pregnant women and in women of child-bearing age; it increases uterine contractions, which may cause abortion.
Octreotide (Sandostatin)	Synthetic analog of somostatin, inhibition of the secretion of gastrin, vasoactive intestinal peptide (VIP), insulin, glucagon, motilin, secretin, and pancreatic polypeptides	Secretory diarrhea, acute variceal hemorrhage	Edema, flushing, dizziness, headache, abdominal pain, constipation, diarrhea, hyperglycemia, hypoglycemia	Monitor blood sugar and adjust insulin requirements.

CBC, complete blood count; ECG, electrocardiogram; GERD, gastroesophageal reflux disease; NSAIDs, nonsteroidal anti-inflammatory drugs; PUD, peptic ulcer disease.

nurse decides to hold the enteral feedings for the remainder of the day. The following morning, Mr. P. resumes his scheduled enteral bolus feeds of 400 mL every 4 hours, and he is found to have minimal gastric residuals. However, Mr. P. now complains of abdominal cramps, bloating, and diarrhea after each bolus feeding; abdominal examination reveals positive bowel sounds with mild abdominal distention.

Because of these multiple issues, the nurse recommends to the physician that a central line be placed and that the patient should be started on total parenteral nutrition (TPN) to meet his long-term nutritional requirements.

1. Initially the nurse held the enteral tube feedings for one high GRV. Was this an appropriate action to take? Why or why not?

2. What was the most likely etiology of the patient's diarrhea? What interventions are needed, if any?

3. Is TPN appropriate for this patient? Why or why not?

Review Questions

1. A 68-year-old woman is 3 weeks status post cerebrovascular accident; the stroke has impaired her ability to swallow safely without aspirating. The patient has no other past medical history. She currently has bowel sounds and is passing flatus. What is the most appropriate method to provide nutrition to this patient?
   a. Nasogastric tube placement for enteral nutrition
   b. Surgical gastrostomy tube placement for enteral nutrition
   c. Jejunostomy tube placement for enteral nutrition
   d. Central line placement for total parenteral nutrition

2. A 59-year-old cancer patient with cachexia and a distal bowel obstruction is to be started on total parenteral nutrition (TPN) after successful subclavian central line placement. His most recent laboratory results indicate a glucose level of 61 mg/dL, a potassium level of 3.0 mEq/L, and a phosphorus level of 1.9 mEq/L. As the nurse who is managing this patient, what would be the appropriate intervention?
   a. Insist that the patient be started on oral supplements
   b. Insist that the patient be started on enteral nutrition
   c. Because of his cachexia, make sure the total TPN calories are more than required
   d. Replace potassium and phosphorus before initiation of TPN

3. Which of the following is *not* a benefit of enteral nutrition?
   a. Better glucose control
   b. Fewer fluid and electrolyte disturbances
   c. Decreased protein synthesis
   d. Preserved gastrointestinal mucosa

4. A 57-year-old man with a history of diabetes mellitus is admitted with pneumonia requiring mechanical ventilation. A nasogastric feeding tube is placed to initiate enteral nutrition support, but 3 days after reaching his goal infusion rate of 50 mL/hour, the patient develops high gastric residuals. A radiograph confirms the tip of the tube is in the stomach. What is the most appropriate nursing intervention?
   a. Discontinue tube feedings and reinsert another feeding tube
   b. Discontinue tube feedings and request the initiation of total parenteral nutrition
   c. Hold tube feedings for the remainder of the day to allow the stomach a chance to digest current volume
   d. Hold tube feedings for 2 hours, request a prokinetic agent, and restart at lower infusion rate

5. A 32-year-old man is admitted after a gunshot wound to his chest and requires mechanical ventilation. A nasogastric tube is placed to initiate enteral nutrition, and the patient is at goal infusion rate of 65 mL/hour without residuals. The patient develops diarrhea. What is the most appropriate nursing intervention?
   a. Discontinue tube feedings and request maintenance intravenous fluids
   b. Discontinue tube feedings and request the initiation of total parenteral nutrition
   c. Review the medication list to determine whether the patient is taking anything that may induce diarrhea (e.g., prokinetic agents, sorbitol-containing elixirs)
   d. Dilute the tube feedings with tap water to reduce their osmolarity

References

1. Holmes S: Enteral feeding and percutaneous endoscopic gastrostomy. Nurs Stand 18(20):41–43, 2004
2. Marshall AP, West SH: Enteral feeding in the critically ill: Are nursing practices contributing to hypocaloric feeding? Intensive Crit Care Nurs 22(2):95–105, 2006
3. Sloane DS: Nutritional support of the critically ill and injured patient. Crit Care Clin 20(1):135–157, 2004
4. Krale R, Ulvik A, Flaaten H: Follow-up after intensive care: A single center study. Intensive Care Med 29:2149–2156, 2003
5. Kudsk KA, Tolley EA, DeWitt RC, et al: Preoperative albumin and surgical site identify surgical risk for major postoperative complications. J Parenter Enter Nutr 27(1):1–9, 2003
6. Dhaliwal R, Heyland DK: Nutrition and infection in the intensive care unit: What does the evidence show? Curr Opin Crit Care 11(5):461–467, 2005
7. Jacobs DG, Jacobs DO, Kudsk KA, et al: Practice management guidelines for nutritional support of the trauma patient. J Trauma Injury Infect Crit Care 57(3):660–679, 2004
8. Padula CA, Kenny A, Planchon C, Lamoureux C: Enteral feedings: What the evidence says. Avoid contamination of feedings and its sequelae with this research-based protocol. Am J Nurs 104(7):62–69, 2004
9. Ellet MLC: Important facts about intestinal feeding tube placement. Gastroenterol Nurs 29(2):112–124, 2006
10. Kattelmann KK, Hise M, Russell M, et al: Preliminary evidence for a medical nutrition therapy protocol: Enteral feedings for critically ill patients. J Am Diet Assoc 106(8):1226–1241, 2006
11. Lin L, Cohen NH: Early nutritional support for the ICU patient: Does it matter? Contemp Crit Care 2(9):1–10, 2005
12. Posthauer ME: When is enteral nutrition support an effective strategy? Adv Skin Wound Care 19(5):257–261, 2006
13. Okamato K, Fukatsu K, Ueno C, et al: T-lymphocyte numbers in human gut associated lymphoid tissue are reduced without enteral nutrition. J Parenter Enter Nutr 29(1):56–58, 2005
14. ASPEN Board of Directors and the Clinical Guidelines Taskforce: Guidelines for the use of parenteral and enteral nutrition in adult and pediatric patients. J Parenter Enter Nutr 26 (1 Suppl):1138, 2002.
15. Best C: Caring for the patient with a nasogastric tube. Nurs Stand 20(3):59–65, 2005
16. Fang J: Appendix-enteral feeding devices. J Parenter Enter Nutr 30(1):S96–97, 2006
17. Bosco JJ, Barkun AN, Isenberg GA, et al: Endoscopic enteral nutrition access devices. Gastrointest Endosc 56(6):796–802, 2002
18. American Association of Critical Care Nurses: 2005 Practice alert: Verification of feeding tube placement. Retrieved November 13, 2006, from http://www.aacn.org/AACN/practiceAlertnsf/Files/VOFTP/$file/Verificationoffeedingtubeplacement.pdf

19. Williams TA, Leslie GD: A review of the nursing care of enteral feeding tubes in critically ill adults: Part II. Intensive Crit Care Nurs 21(1):5–15, 2005

20. Pullen R: Clinical do's and don'ts: Measuring gastric residual volume. Nursing 2006 34(4):18, 2004

21. Zaloga GP: Improving outcomes with specialized nutrition support. J Parenter Enter Nutr 29(Suppl 1):49–52, 2005

22. Baudouin SV, Evans TW: Nutritional support in critical care. Clin Chest Med 24(4):633–644, 2003

23. Klein S, Rubin DC: Enteral and parenteral nutrition. In Feldman M, Friedman LS, Sleisenger MH (eds): Sleisenger & Fordtran's Gastrointestinal and Liver Disease: Pathophysiology/Diagnosis/Treatment, 7th ed. Philadelphia: Saunders, 2002, pp 287–309

24. Ochoa JB, Caba D: Advances in surgical nutrition. Surg Clin North Am 86:1483–1493, 2006

25. Marik PE: Arginine: Too much of a good thing may be bad! Crit Care Med 34(11):2844–2847, 2006

26. Fuhrman MP: Clinical Nutrition Practice: Wound healing and nutrition. Top Clin Nutr 18(2):100–110, 2003

27. McClave SA, Lukan JK, Stefater JA, et al: Poor validity of residual volumes as a marker for risk of aspiration in critically ill patients. Crit Care Med 33(2):324–330, 2005

28. Zalaga GP: The myth of the gastric residual volume. Crit Care Med 33(2):449–450, 2005

29. Serna ED, McCarthy MS: Heads up to prevent aspiration during enteral feeding. Nursing 2006 36(1):76–77, 2006

30. Williams TA, Leslie GD: A review of the nursing care of enteral feeding tubes in critically ill adults: Part 1. Intensive Crit Care Nurs 20:330–343, 2004

31. Metheny NA, Schallom ME, Edwards SJ: Effect of gastrointestinal motility and feeding tube site on aspiration risk in critically ill patients: A review. Heart Lung 33(3):131–145, 2004

32. McClave SA, Snider HL: Clinical use of gastric residual volumes as a monitor for patients on enteral tube feeding. J Parenter Enter Nutr 26(6 Suppl):43–48, 2002

33. Woien H, Bjork IT: Nutrition of the critically ill patient and effects of implementing a nutritional support algorithm in the ICU. J Clin Nurs 15:168–177, 2006

34. Segal R, Pogoreliuk I, Dan M, et al: Gastric microbiota in elderly patients fed via nasogastric tubes for prolonged periods. J Hosp Infect 63(1):79–83, 2006

35. Mathus-Vliegen EMH, Bredius MWJ, Binnekade JM: Analysis of sites of bacterial contamination in an enteral feeding system. J Parent Enter Nutr 30(6):519–525, 2006

36. Reising DL, Neal RS: Enteral tube flushing: What you think is the best practice may not be. Am J Nurs 105(3):58–63, 2005

37. Sanko JS: Aspiration assessment and prevention in critically ill enterally fed patients: Evidence-based recommendations for practice. Gastroenterol Nurs 27(6):279–285, 2004

38. Parrish CR, McCray SF: Nutrition support for the mechanically ventilated patient. Crit Care Nurse 23(1):77–80, 2003

39. Metheny NA, Dahms TE, Stewart BJ, et al: Verification of inefficacy of the glucose method for detecting aspiration associated with tube feedings. MedSurg Nurs 14(2):112–119, 2005

40. U.S. Food and Drug Administration Center for Food Safety and Applied Nutrition: FDA Public Health Advisory: 2003. Reports of blue discoloration and death in patients receiving enteral feeding tinted with the dye, FD&C blue No. 1. Retrieved November 13, 2006, from http://www.cfsan.fda.gov/%7Edms/col-ltr2.html

41. American Association of Critical Care Nurses: 2005 Practice alert: Dye in enteral feeding. Retrieved November 13, 2006, from http://www.aacn.org/AACN/practceAlertnsf/Files/DEF/$files/dyeinenteralfeeding.pdf

42. Miller SJ: Parenteral nutrition. U.S. Pharmacist 31(7):10–20, 2006

43. Martarese LE: Metabolic complications of parenteral nutrition therapy. In Gottschlich MM, Fuhrman MP, Hammond KA, et al (eds): The Science and Practice of Nutrition Support: A Core-Based Curriculum. Dubuque, Iowa, Kendall Hunt, 2001, p 273

44. Halsted CH: Malnutrition and nutritional assessment. In Kasper DL, Fauci AS, Longo DL, et al (eds): Harrison's Principles of Internal Medicine, 16th ed. New York: McGraw-Hill, 2005, pp. 411–415

45. Worthington P, Gilbert KA, Wagner BA: Parenteral nutrition for the acutely ill. AACN Clin Issues 11(4):559–579, 2000

46. Koretz RL, Lipman TO, Klein S: AGA technical review on parenteral nutrition. Gastroenterology 121(4):970–1001, 2001

47. McGinnis C: Parenteral nutrition focus: Nutritional assessment and formula composition. J Infusion Nurs 25(1):54–64, 2002

48. Huckleberry Y: Nutritional support and the surgical patient. Am J Health-System Pharm 61(7):671–684, 2004

49. U.S. Food and Drug Administration: Parenteral vitamin products: Drugs for human uses. Drug efficiency implementation: Amendment. Fed Reg 65(77):21200–21201, 2000

50. Kwan V, George J: Liver disease due to parenteral and enteral nutrition. Clin Liver Dis 8:893–913, 2004

51. Howard L: Enteral and parenteral nutrition therapy. In Kasper DL, Fauci AS, Longo DL, et al (eds): Harrison's Principles of Internal Medicine, 16th ed. New York: McGraw-Hill, 2005, pp 415–422

52. Braunschweig CL, Levy P, Sheean PM, Wang X: Enteral compared with parenteral nutrition: A meta-analysis. Am J Clin Nutr 75:534–542, 2001

53. Lafrance JP, Leblanc M: Metabolic, electrolyte, and nutritional concerns in critical illness. Crit Care Clin 21:305–327, 2005

54. Brown KA, Dickerson RN, Morgan LM, et al: A new graduated dosing regimen for phosphorus replacement in patients receiving nutrition support. J Parenter Enter Nutr 30(3):209–214, 2004

55. Chaiyakunapruk N, Veenstra DL, Lipsky BA, Saint S: Chlorhexidine compared with povidone-iodine solution for vascular catheter-site care: A meta-analysis. Ann Intern Med 136:792–801, 2002

56. Centers for Disease Control and Prevention: Guidelines for the prevention of intravascular catheter-related infections. MMWR Morb Mortal Wkly Rep 51:1–29, 2002

57. Wingerter L: Vascular access device thrombosis. Clin J Oncol Nurs 7(3):345–348, 2001

58. Spinello I, Balk RA: An infrequent but life-threatening complication of a simple procedure. J Intensive Care Med 17:92–94, 2002

59. Mermel LA: Prevention of intravascular catheter-related infections. Ann Intern Med 132:391–402, 2000

Other Selected Readings

Ackerman MH, Mick DJ: Technologic approaches to determining proper placement of enteral feeding tubes. AACN Clin Issues 17(3):246–249, 2006

Ali S, Robert PR: Nutrients with immune-modulating effects: What role should they play in the intensive care unit? Curr Opin Anaesthesiol 19(2):132–139, 2006

Bistrina BR, McCowen KC: Nutritional and metabolic support in the adult intensive care unit: key controversies. Crit Care Med 34(5):1525–1531, 2006

Bowman A, Greiner JE, Doerschug KC, et al: Implementation of an evidence-based feeding protocol and aspiration risk reduction algorithm. Crit Care Nurs Q 28(4):324–333, 2005

Burns SM, Carpenter R, Blevins C, et al: Detection of inadvertent airway intubation using gastric tube insertion: Capnography versus a colorimetric carbon dioxide detector. Am J Crit Care 15(2):188–193, 2006

Conner TM, Carver D: The role of gastric pH testing with small-bore feeding tubes: In the intensive care unit. Dimens Crit Care Nurs 43(5):210–214, 2005

Dwyer KM, Watts DD, Thurber JS, et al: Percutaneous endoscopic gastrostomy: The preferred method of elective feeding tube placement in trauma patients. J Trauma 52(1):26–32, 2002

Eisenberg P: An overview of diarrhea in the patient receiving enteral nutrition. Gastroenterol Nurs 25(3):95–104, 2002

Hildebrandt LA, Fracchia J, Driscoll J, Giroux P: Comparison of post-pyloric vs. gastric enteral formula administration. Top Clin Nutr 17(3):44–51, 2002

Martindale RG, Cresci G: Preventing infectious complications with nutrition intervention. J Parenter Enter Nutr 29(1):S53–S56, 2003

Metheny NA: Preventing respiratory complications of tube feedings: Evidence-based practice. Am J Crit Care 15(4):360–369, 2006

Novak F, Heyland DK, Avenell A, et al: Glutamine supplementation in serious illness: A systematic review of the evidence. Crit Care Med 30(9):2022–2029, 2002

Radich K, Hildebrandt LA: Use of colored dyes in enteral formulas. Top Clin Nutr 21(3):226–233, 2006

Sabol VK, Carlson KK. Diarrhea: Applying research to bedside practice. AACN Clin Issues 18(1):32–44, 2007

Steele A, Carlson KK: Nausea and vomiting: Applying research to bedside practice. AACN Clin Issues 18(1):61–75, 2007

Trujillo MH, Fragachan CF, Tortoledo F, Ceballos F: "Lariat loop" knotting of a nasogastric tube: An ounce of prevention. Am J Crit Care 15(4):413–414, 2006

Wiesen P, Van Gossum A, Preiserr J: Diarrhoea in the critically ill. Curr Opin Crit Care 12(2):149–154, 2006

Common Gastrointestinal Disorders

41

Allison G. Steele • Valerie Sabol

Objectives

Based on the content in this chapter, the reader should be able to:

❶ Examine the pathophysiological concepts that help define acute gastrointestinal bleeding, obstruction and ileus, acute pancreatitis, hepatitis, and complications of liver disease.

❷ Compare and contrast the pertinent history, physical examination, and diagnostic study findings for acute gastrointestinal bleeding, obstruction and ileus, acute pancreatitis, hepatitis, and cirrhosis.

❸ Discuss laboratory studies that are useful in the diagnosis and management of acute gastrointestinal bleeding, obstruction and ileus, acute pancreatitis, hepatitis, and complications of liver disease.

❹ Analyze the similarities and differences in caring for patients with acute gastrointestinal bleeding, obstruction and ileus, hepatitis, and complications of liver disease.

❺ Explore the nursing role in assessing, managing, and evaluating a plan of care for patients with acute gastrointestinal bleeding, obstruction and ileus, acute pancreatitis, hepatitis, and complications of liver disease.

• Acute Gastrointestinal Bleeding

Acute gastrointestinal bleeding (GIB) is a common, and potentially lethal, medical emergency seen in people admitted to the intensive care unit (ICU). There are 300,000 hospital admissions each year in the United States as a result of acute GIB.[1-3] The 10% mortality rate associated with acute GIB has remained constant over the past half century despite advances in diagnosis and treatment.[1,3] This constant mortality rate may result from the prevalence of comorbid disease in older adults and the widespread use of nonsteroidal anti-inflammatory drugs (NSAIDs). The cause of death is rarely from exsanguination but rather from the exacerbation of other medical illnesses. Prompt recognition and treatment of patients experiencing acute GIB requires a team approach.

Acute GIB is differentiated into upper and lower GIB. The ligament of Treitz at the junction of the duodenum and jejunum is the anatomic division between the upper and lower gastrointestinal (GI) tracts. Upper GIB occurs from a source in the esophagus, stomach, or duodenum. Lower GIB occurs from a source in the jejunum, ileum, colon, or rectum. GIB from a lower GI source is less common than upper GIB.

UPPER GASTROINTESTINAL BLEEDING

Etiology

The possible causes of acute upper GIB are listed in Box 41-1. A complete discussion of this list is beyond the scope of this chapter. The most commonly seen causes of acute GIB in the ICU are discussed below.

Peptic Ulcer Disease

Peptic ulcer disease, which includes both gastric and duodenal ulcers, accounts for approximately 50% to 75% of acute upper GIB.[1,4] The epithelial cells of the gastroduodenal mucosa are protected from the potentially damaging effects of gastric secretions, medications, alcohol, and bacteria by several protective mechanisms. These cells secrete mucins, phospholipids, and bicarbonate, which create a pH gradient between the acidic gastric lumen and the cell surface. Prostaglandins enhance this mucosal protection by increasing mucosal secretion, increasing bicarbonate production, maintaining mucosal blood flow, and

---

Box 41-1 • **Common Causes of Acute Gastrointestinal Bleeding**

Upper Gastrointestinal Bleeding

Esophageal Source
- Varices
- Esophagitis
- Ulcers
- Tumors
- Mallory-Weiss tears

Gastric Source
- Peptic ulcers
- Gastritis
- Tumors
- Angiodysplasia
- Dieulafoy's lesions

Duodenal Source
- Peptic ulcers
- Angiodysplasia
- Crohn's disease
- Meckel's diverticulum

Lower Gastrointestinal Bleeding
- Malignant tumors
- Polyps
- Ulcerative colitis
- Crohn's disease
- Ischemic colitis
- Infectious colitis
- Angiodysplasia
- Diverticulosis
- Hemorrhoids
- Massive upper gastrointestinal hemorrhage

---

enhancing the resistance of gastroduodenal cells to injury. In addition, the tight junctions of the epithelial cells resist diffusion. When these protective factors are overwhelmed by aggressive factors, the integrity of the gastric or duodenal mucosal is interrupted, which can result in peptic ulcer disease. Bleeding from peptic ulcer disease occurs when the ulcer erodes into the wall of a blood vessel.

The primary risk factor for peptic ulcer disease is infection with the bacterium *Helicobacter pylori*. *H. pylori* infection has been associated with 90% of duodenal ulcers and 75% of gastric ulcers. *H. pylori* is a gram-negative, spiral, flagellated rod that colonizes the mucus layer overlying the gastric epithelium. The flagellum of *H. pylori* facilitates the bacterium's ability to move and adhere to the mucus layer. *H. pylori* produces urease, which converts urea to ammonia and carbon dioxide. The ammonia buffers the acid surrounding the bacterium, creating a more hospitable environment that allows the bacterium to thrive in the acidic stomach. *H. pylori* infection predisposes the mucosa to damage by disrupting the mucus layer, liberating enzymes and toxins, and adhering to the epithelium. Inflammation is furthered by a host immune response. This chronic inflammation usually results in an asymptomatic chronic gastritis. However, in some instances, ulceration develops.

In the absence of *H. pylori* infection, the ingestion of aspirin or NSAIDs accounts for most cases of peptic ulcer disease. The ingestion of aspirin and NSAIDs may directly injure the mucosal layer. Ingestion enhances mucosal permeability and allows back-diffusion of acid. Systemic effects of chronic aspirin or NSAID use include inhibition of prostaglandin synthesis by the gastroduodenal mucosa, which decreases mucus and bicarbonate production, as well as mucosal blood flow. This alteration in mucosal cytoprotection may lead to the development of an ulcer. Upper GIB related to NSAIDs is more common in older patients. Cigarette smoking may also predispose to peptic ulcer disease, and it is linked to prolonged healing rates and high ulcer reoccurrence.

Stress-Related Erosive Syndrome

Stress-related erosive syndrome, also called erosive gastritis, stress ulceration, and hemorrhagic gastritis, is a common cause of acute GIB in critically ill patients. Stress ulcers are different from the ulcers of peptic ulcer disease; they tend to be more numerous, more shallow, and more diffuse. These ulcers may develop in the stomach, duodenum, and esophagus within hours of injury. They are usually shallow and cause oozing from superficial capillaries but may erode into the submucosa and cause massive hemorrhage.

The risk for development of a stress ulcer depends on the severity and type of illness (Box 41-2). The common feature of these risk factors is the relationship to physiological stress. Decreased perfusion of the stomach mucosa is probably the main mechanism of ulcer development. This contributes to impaired mucus secretion, low mucosal pH, poor mucosal cell regeneration, and decreased tolerance to acidic gastric secretions. Acute GIB from stress-related erosive syndrome is associated with a high mortality rate.

Esophageal Varices

Portal hypertension usually develops as a result of cirrhosis, from increased resistance in the portal venous system caused by disruption of the normal liver lobular structure. This resistance impedes blood flow into, through, and out of the liver. In response to portal hypertension, collateral veins develop to bypass the increased portal resistance in an attempt to return blood to systemic circulation. As pressure rises in these veins, they become tortuous and distended, forming varicose veins or varices.

Varices may develop in the esophagus, stomach, duodenum, colon, rectum, or anus. The most clinically significant site of varices is the gastroesophageal junction because of the propensity of varices in this area to rupture, resulting in massive GI hemorrhage. Esophageal varices account for 10% to 15% of all cases of acute upper GIB.[1] In patients with cirrhosis, 60% of upper GIB is the result of varices.[5] The mortality rate associated with variceal bleeding is 30% to 50% with each episode.[6,7]

Mallory-Weiss Tears

Mallory-Weiss tears account for approximately 10% to 15% of acute upper GIB.[1] Mallory-Weiss tears are lacerations that occur in the distal esophagus, at the gastroesophageal junction, and in the cardia of the stomach. Bleeding from Mallory-Weiss tears occurs when the tear involves the underlying venous or arterial bed. Mallory-Weiss tears are strongly associated with heavy alcohol use or recent binge drinking and a prior history of forceful vomiting or retching, or violent coughing. Patients with portal hypertension have an increased risk for bleeding from Mallory-Weiss tears.

Dieulafoy's Lesions

Dieulafoy's lesions are vascular malformations of unusually large submucosal arteries, which lie in close contact with the mucosal surface. They can be found anywhere in the GI tract but are most likely to be found in the proximal stomach. Because of the large size of the artery, bleeding from a Dieulafoy's lesion may be massive and recurrent. When bleeding ceases, a Dieulafoy's lesion can be difficult to identify because there is no associated ulcer, and it is likely to be the origin of many upper GIBs of unknown cause.[8]

Clinical Presentation

Regardless of the cause, patients with acute upper GIB have a clinical presentation consistent with the amount of blood loss. A patient's response to blood loss depends on the amount and rate of blood loss, age, degree of compensation, comorbidities, and rapidity of treatment. Patients with minimal loss may present with anemia and no further symptoms, whereas patients with rapid and severe loss may present with signs and symptoms of shock. If blood loss is moderate, the sympathetic nervous system responds with a release of the catecholamines epinephrine and norepinephrine, which initially cause an increase in heart rate and peripheral vascular vasoconstriction in an attempt to maintain an adequate blood pressure. Orthostatic changes (a decrease in blood pressure greater than 10 mm Hg with a corresponding heart rate increase of 20 beats/minute in the sitting or standing position) imply volume depletion of 15% or more.[1,2,9]

With severe blood loss, signs and symptoms of shock appear. The release of catecholamines triggers the blood vessels in the skin, lungs, intestines, liver, and kidneys to constrict, thereby increasing the volume of blood flow to the brain and heart. Because of the decreased flow of blood in the skin, the patient's skin is cool to the touch. With decreased blood flow to the lungs, hyperventilation occurs to maintain adequate gas exchange.

The classic hallmarks of GIB are hematemesis, hematochezia, and melena. Patients with upper GIB usually present with hematemesis, the vomiting of fresh, unaltered blood or "coffee-ground" material; melena, the passage of foul-smelling, black, tarry, sticky stool; or both. A patient who presents with hematemesis is usually bleeding from a source above the ligament of Treitz. Reverse peristalsis is seldom sufficient to cause hematemesis if the bleeding point is below this area. The classic coffee-ground emesis associated with upper GIB results from the partial decomposition of the blood from contact with gastric secretions. Gastric acid converts bright red hemoglobin to brown hematin, accounting for the coffee-ground appearance of the drainage. Maroon or bright red blood results from profuse bleeding and little contact with gastric juices.

Melena is black from the breakdown of the blood in transit and suggests a long transit time through the GI tract. Melena is indicative of upper GIB in 90% of cases. It may take several days after bleeding cessation for melenic stools to clear. After upper GIB, stool may remain Hemoccult positive for 1 to 2 weeks. Melena should not be confused with greenish stool that results from iron ingestion or black stool caused by the ingestion of bismuth subsalicy-late (Pepto-Bismol).

Hematochezia, the passage of maroon or bright red blood that may be mixed with stool, usually indicates bleeding from a lower GI source. Uncommonly, hematochezia can occur in the setting of massive, rapid hemorrhage from the upper GI tract, where the large amount of blood acts as a cathartic, resulting in rapid transit through the GI tract.

Occult GIB refers to small amounts of blood loss, which is not apparent to the patient. Obscure GIB refers to obvious bleeding with no easily identifiable source on routine examination.

Assessment

History

A prompt, careful, focused history may suggest the underlying cause of GIB. A history of epigastric pain or dyspepsia or a past medical history of peptic ulcer disease is suggestive of peptic ulcer disease. A past medical history of GIB should be elicited because most upper GI bleeds rebleed from the same site. Heavy alcohol use increases the likelihood of cirrhosis and bleeding from esophageal varices. Patients with a history of tobacco use have a greater risk for duodenal ulcers. Underlying medical conditions may suggest an underlying cause; patients with renal failure frequently bleed from arteriovenous malformations. Vomiting, coughing, or retching before bleeding suggests a Mallory-Weiss tear. Prior use of NSAIDs or aspirin increases the risk for gastroduodenal ulcers and the likelihood of bleeding from these ulcers.

Physical Examination

The physical examination is directed initially to the assessment of hemodynamic stability with ongoing assessment of vital signs. Tachycardia and orthostatic hypotension indicate dehydration secondary to blood loss or vomiting. Orthostatic hypotension and tachycardia are suggestive of a greater than 15% blood volume loss and are predictive of a poor outcome.[2,10,11] If 39% of blood volume is lost, hypovolemia occurs, with decreased perfusion of the brain and heart.[11] Therefore, assessing for signs and symptoms of poor tissue perfusion such as angina, cyanosis, and altered mental status is important. A baseline electrocardiogram is critical in patients with known cardiac disease because blood loss may precipitate cardiac ischemia. A loss of circulating blood volume may result in decreased cerebral perfusion. The nurse should be alert to signs of agitation or confusion, which may signal cerebral hypoperfusion. The abdomen is assessed for bowel sounds; abdominal tenderness; the presence of guarding, rigidity, or abdominal masses; and the stigmata of liver disease. Splenomegaly, ascites, and caput medusae suggest liver disease. A tender, board-like abdomen is suggestive of peritonitis, possibly as a result of perforation. A rectal examination is essential to assess for hematochezia and melena.

Laboratory Studies

Laboratory studies can help determine the extent of bleeding and can often provide a clue to the etiology.

Common laboratory abnormalities for the patient with acute GIB are listed in Box 41-3. The initial hematocrit and hemoglobin may not accurately reflect initial blood loss because plasma volume is lost in the same proportion as red blood cells (RBCs). Within 24 to 48 hours of the initial bleed, redistribution of plasma from the extravascular to the intravascular space results in a decreased hematocrit. Fluids administered during resuscitation contribute to the hemodilution. Leukocytosis and hyperglycemia may reflect the body's response to stress. Hypokalemia and hypernatremia may result from loss through emesis. An elevated blood urea nitrogen (BUN) level reflects a large protein load from the breakdown of blood. A high BUN/creatinine ratio suggests an upper GI source of bleeding.[9] Coagulopathy with a prolonged prothrombin time (PT) can indicate liver disease or concurrent long-term anticoagulant therapy. Thrombocytopenia may be present in patients with cirrhosis and portal hypertension with splenomegaly. If large amounts of blood are lost, metabolic acidosis occurs as a result of anaerobic metabolism. Severe blood loss can result in hypoxemia because of decreased circulating hemoglobin with impairment of oxygen transport to cells.

Management

Resuscitation

The initial management of any patient with acute upper GIB is directed at fluid resuscitation to reverse the effects of blood loss. Supplemental oxygen is provided to any patient with acute GIB to promote oxygen saturation and transport as well as to prevent ischemia and dysrhythmias. Intubation may be required for actively bleeding patients at high risk for aspiration, those with a diminished mental status, and those in respiratory distress. Patients with acute upper GIB should be given nothing by mouth (NPO) because urgent endoscopy or surgery may be required. A Foley catheter is inserted to monitor urine output as an indication of the adequacy of fluid resuscitation. All patients with hemodynamic instability, a drop in hematocrit, transfusion requirements greater than 2 units of packed red blood cells (PRBCs), or active bleeding may warrant an ICU admission.

Volume Resuscitation Patients with acute GIB require immediate intravenous (IV) access with at least two large-bore (14- to 16-gauge) IV catheters or

---

Box 41-3 • Typical Laboratory Abnormalities in a Patient With Acute Gastrointestinal Bleeding

- Decreased hemoglobin and hematocrit
- Mild leukocytosis and hyperglycemia
- Elevated blood urea nitrogen level
- Hypernatremia
- Hypokalemia
- Prolonged prothrombin time/partial thromboplastin time
- Thrombocytopenia
- Hypoxemia

central access. A type and cross-match should be sent early in the course of the bleed because blood losses of greater than 1,500 mL require blood replacement in addition to fluids. While awaiting cross-matched blood, Ringer's lactate or normal saline is infused to restore circulating volume and to prevent the progression to hypovolemic shock. PRBCs are often transfused to reestablish the oxygen-carrying capacity of the blood. Other blood products, such as platelets and clotting factors, are ordered according to results of laboratory tests and the patient's underlying condition. Calcium replacement may be necessary if large numbers of banked RBCs are transfused because the citrate in banked blood products can bind calcium and lead to hypocalcemia. A pulmonary artery catheter or central venous catheter may be useful to help avoid over-resuscitation in patients with underlying renal or cardiac disease. In patients with a coagulopathy, vitamin K can be given in the form of phytonadione (AquaMEPHYTON), 10 mg intramuscularly or very slowly intravenously, in an attempt to restore the PT to normal. Fresh frozen plasma is ordered to correct the abnormality if rapid correction of the abnormality is warranted.

Vasoactive drugs may be used until fluid balance is restored to maintain blood pressure and perfusion to vital body organs. Dopamine, epinephrine, or norepinephrine may be ordered to stabilize the patient until definitive treatment can be undertaken.

Nasogastric Intubation A large-bore nasogastric tube is placed in all patients with GIB to aspirate and lavage gastric contents. A nasogastric tube documents the presence and activity of bleeding. The color of gastric aspirate is prognostically significant. Coffeeground or black nasogastric drainage with melenic stools indicates a slow bleed and has a corresponding 9% mortality rate, whereas bright red nasogastric drainage and bright red blood in the stools signify a rapidly bleeding upper GI source, with a corresponding mortality rate of 30%.[12]

A nasogastric tube is also useful for decompression and lavage. Lavage helps clear blood from the stomach, which allows better visualization to identify the source of bleeding during endoscopy. Iced lavage should be avoided because it is uncomfortable, fails to control bleeding, can significantly decrease core body temperature, and can trigger cardiac dysrhythmias. Lavage should be performed with tap water or saline. A total of 250 to 500 mL is instilled through the nasogastric tube and then removed with a syringe or by intermittent wall suction until gastric secretions are clear. Nasogastric tubes are usually removed after lavage of stomach contents unless the patient is actively bleeding or is experiencing severe nausea and vomiting because a nasogastric tube may injure the gastric mucosa and contribute to bleeding.

Acid-Suppressive Therapy Patients with acute upper GIB are often treated with acid-suppressive therapy to decrease the risk for recurrent bleeding, particularly from peptic ulcers. The use of high-dose proton pump inhibitors (omeprazole, lansoprazole, esomeprazole, pantoprazole, rabeprazole) to maintain a gastric pH greater than 4.0 has been shown to be beneficial in this setting. Acid-suppressive therapy with histamine (H_2)-antagonistic drugs (cimetidine, ranitidine, famotidine, nizatidine) may be used as prophylactic therapy in patients at high risk for stress-related erosive syndrome.

Antacids are also ordered. Antacids act as a direct alkaline buffer and are administered to control gastric pH. Sucralfate, a basic aluminum salt of sucrose octasulfate, acts locally as a cytoprotective drug and can be ordered for stress-related erosive syndrome prophylaxis.

Pharmacotherapy for Decreasing Portal Hypertension Even before a bleeding source is identified, decreasing portal pressure with vasopressin or octreotide should be considered for patients in whom variceal hemorrhage is suspected. Vasopressin (Pitressin) decreases portal hypertension by constriction of the splanchnic arteries, which reduces portal blood flow. Vasopressin should be administered through a central line. Complications of vasopressin therapy can limit its use. Vasopressin reduces coronary blood flow and increases blood pressure, which increases oxygen demand, and causes coronary artery constriction, which can potentially result in multiple cardiac dysrhythmias. Because vasopressin also reduces blood flow to the mesenteric circulation, bowel ischemia can develop. To minimize these potential side effects, vasopressin should be given concurrently with IV, sublingual, or topical nitroglycerin, which reduces its systemic effects.

Somatostatin is a natural polypeptide that lowers portal venous pressure by vasoconstriction of splanchnic circulation. Somatostatin causes selective vasoconstriction of the splanchnic circulation and is associated with fewer systemic side effects than vasopressin. IV infusion is necessary because of its short half-life.

Octreotide (Sandostatin), a synthetic analog of somatostatin with similar hemodynamic properties but a longer half-life, is available in the United States. Octreotide causes a decrease in splanchnic blood flow and a decrease in intravariceal pressure. Octreotide is usually given as a 50-μg IV bolus followed by 50 μg/hour for 3 to 5 days. The effects of octreotide are similar to vasopressin with concurrent nitroglycerin infusion without the impact on hemodynamics or cardiac output.

Definitive Diagnosis

After patients with acute upper GIB are resuscitated, endoscopy is considered. Endoscopy can be performed urgently at the bedside and is the procedure of choice for the diagnosis and treatment of acute upper GIB. Endoscopy within 12 to 24 hours of the initial bleed has the best results. Early endoscopy is essential in acute GIB because the treatment is directed by the cause. Endoscopy allows the identification of the site of the bleed because direct mucosal inspection is possible. The endoscopic appearance provides prognostic value for the risk for rebleeding based on the presence of stigmata of recent bleeding and the patient's hemodynamic status. Vital signs must be monitored closely during endoscopy. The left lateral decubitus position decreases the risk for aspiration from active bleeding.

When diagnostic endoscopy is unsuccessful because of massive hemorrhage, angiography can be used to define the site of bleeding or abnormal vasculature. Angiography can detect bleeding rates as low as 1.0 mL/minute.[13]

Barium studies, such as an upper GI series, are of no value in acute upper GIB. These studies lack therapeutic capability and preclude endoscopy and angiography because of retained barium. Barium studies are also often inconclusive if there are clots in the stomach or if there is superficial bleeding.

Therapeutic Intervention

Endoscopy In addition to its use in diagnosis, endoscopy is the procedure of choice for the treatment of a GIB. In 90% of cases, endoscopic therapy results in hemostasis, although 20% to 25% of sites may rebleed within 72 hours.[1,2,14] Multiple therapeutic options are available, including injection sclerotherapy, thermal coagulation, the placement of hemostatic clips, and endoscopic variceal ligation (EVL). The optimal technique depends on multiple variables, including the type and appearance of the lesion and the experience of the endoscopist.

The primary methods of endoscopic control of upper GI hemorrhage from peptic ulcers include injection therapy and thermal methods. Injection therapy consists of the injection of an agent such as epinephrine around and into the bleeding vessel. Thermal methods include heater probe and bipolar electrocoagulation (where a probe is applied with pressure to heat and seal the bleeding vessel). Hemostatic clips, called endoclips, have also been used successfully to ligate bleeding blood vessels within a lesion.

EVL is the treatment of choice for variceal bleeding. In EVL, a rubber band is placed endoscopically around the base of each varix. This causes coagulative necrosis and sloughing of thrombosed varices. EVL can control acute variceal bleeding in 90% of cases, with a reduction in the rate of rebleeding to 30%.[14] An alternative to EVL is sclerotherapy. Injection sclerotherapy involves injecting the varices with a sclerosing agent to stop the bleeding. These agents cause local tamponade and vasoconstriction, causing necrosis and eventual sclerosis of the bleeding vessel. Acute hemostasis rates are similar to those with EVL, but sclerotherapy is associated with a higher complication rate.

Angiography Most cases of GIB resolve spontaneously or can be controlled during endoscopy. However, those patients with persistent bleeding may require angiography to control the source of bleeding. During angiography, arterial GIB can be controlled by the infusion of intra-arterial vasopressin or by the embolization of the artery by an interventional radiologist. If therapeutic endoscopy fails, this is a useful therapeutic option, particularly in those who are critically ill and poor surgical candidates.

Intra-arterial vasopressin causes a generalized vasoconstriction that produces a rapid reduction in local blood flow. Patients should be monitored closely for dysrhythmias and fluid retention with resultant hyponatremia. Repeat angiography is performed after the initial infusion, and the dose can then be titrated as needed. Once bleeding is controlled, this infusion may be continued in the ICU for 24 to 36 hours and then tapered over 24 hours. Patients should have cardiac monitoring during vasopressin therapy to watch for cardiac dysrhythmias. Nitroglycerin patches or drips may be used to counteract any ischemic changes.

Embolization of a bleeding vessel consists of occluding the vessel with material that can be either temporary or permanent. Biodegradable long-acting gelatin sponges are commonly used. These sponges cause hemostasis on contact when injected into the vessel. Steel coils, balloons, and silk thread can be used to block an artery mechanically, resulting in permanent occlusion.

Balloon Tamponade Variceal bleeding unresponsive to endoscopic therapy can be temporarily controlled with balloon tamponade in 60% to 90% of cases.[14] Most esophagogastric tubes have two balloons, one for the stomach and one for the esophagus, and a distal port for gastric drainage. The Sengstaken-Blakemore tube is the most widely used (Fig. 41-1).

With the use of balloon tamponade, pressure is exerted on the cardia of the stomach and against the bleeding varices. The tube is inserted to at least 50 cm to ensure gastric intubation. The gastric balloon is then slowly inflated with 250 to 300 mL of air, and gentle traction is applied, until the gastric balloon fits snugly against the cardia of the stomach. Position is then confirmed by radiography. Traction is then placed on the tube where it enters the patient by means of a piece of sponge rubber, as shown in Figure 41-1, or by traction fixed to a head helmet device or the foot of the bed. If chest pain occurs, the gastric balloon must be deflated immediately because it may have shifted into the esophagus.

If bleeding continues, the esophageal balloon is inflated to a pressure of 25 to 39 mm Hg and maintained at this pressure for 24 to 48 hours. Although pressure for longer than 24 hours may be needed to control bleeding, it can cause edema, esophagitis, ulcerations, or perforation of the esophagus. After bleeding is controlled, the balloon is maintained and inflated for no longer than 12 to 24 hours to decrease the risk for gastric ischemia and necrosis. Unfortunately, rebleeding often occurs after balloon deflation unless additional therapeutic measures are taken.

A nasogastric tube should be placed in patients with a Sengstaken-Blakemore tube to aspirate oral and nasopharyngeal secretions that collect above the esophageal balloon, preventing aspiration of these secretions into the lungs. The Minnesota esophagogastric tamponade tube (see Fig. 41-1) has a suction port above the esophageal balloon in addition to the usual ports (two balloon, one gastric suction) of the Sengstaken-Blakemore tube. Nursing interventions

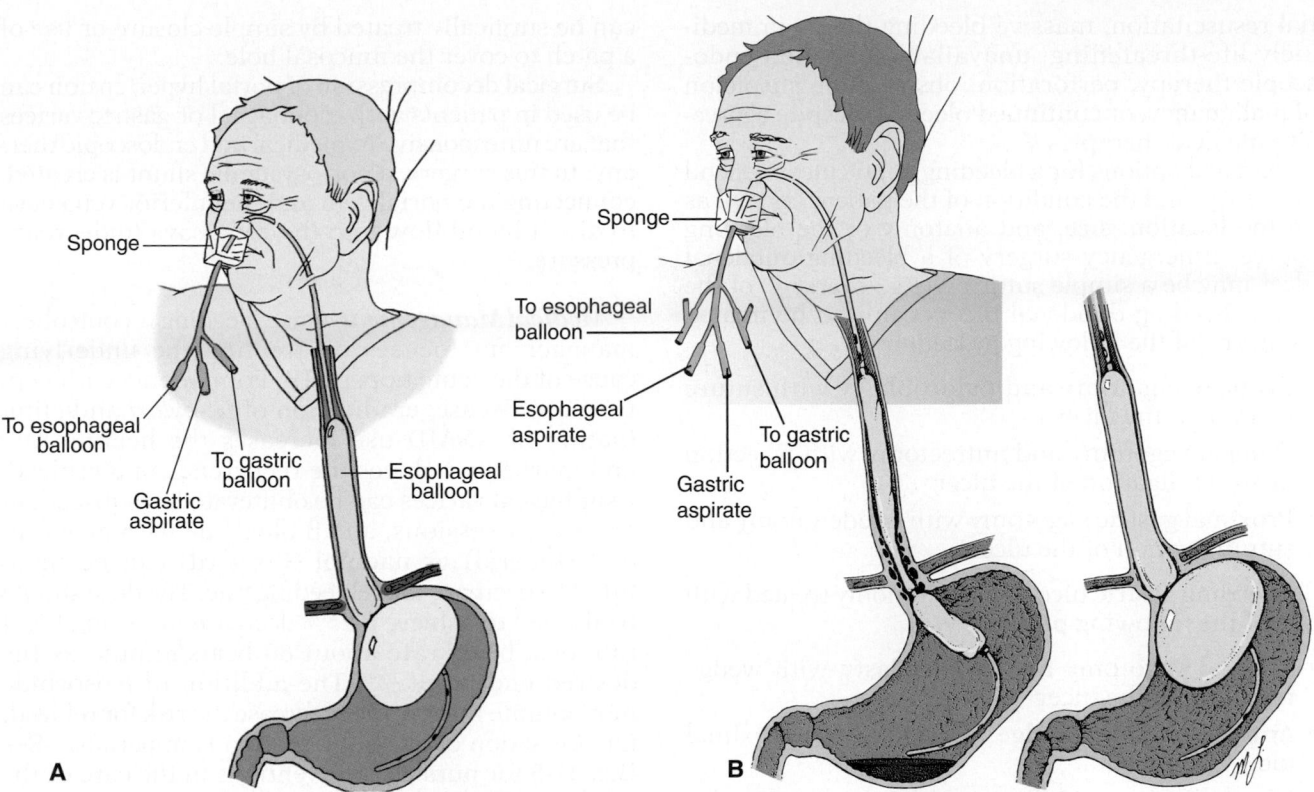

Figure 41-1 • Comparison of two types of esophageal tamponade tubes. **A:** The Sengstaken-Blakemore tube is the best known. An additional tube must be placed in the proximal esophagus. **B:** The Minnesota esophagogastric tamponade tube includes an esophageal aspirate lumen.

for the patient with an esophageal tamponade tube are given in Box 41-4.

Transjugular Intrahepatic Portosystemic Shunt
A transjugular intrahepatic portosystemic shunt (TIPS) is a radiologic procedure that creates an intrahepatic shunt in an attempt to decrease portal pres-

sure. The placement of a TIPS may be considered if other methods of managing esophageal varices fail.

Surgery In the era of endoscopic therapy and proton pump inhibitors, surgery is rarely used for the control of GIB. The indications for surgical intervention are severe hemorrhage unresponsive to ini-

---

Box 41-4 • NURSING INTERVENTIONS for the Patient With an Esophagogastric Balloon Tamponade Tube

- Explain the purpose of the tube and the procedure to the patient.
- Lubricate and chill the tube as directed by the manufacturer.
- Identify and label the lumens of the tube.
- Check the patency of each lumen before insertion of the tube.
- Lavage the patient's stomach before insertion of the tube.
- Monitor the patient while the physician inserts the tube.
- Elevate the head of the bed to 30 degrees to prevent reflux.
- When a Sengstaken-Blakemore tube is in place, perform oropharyngeal suction frequently to prevent aspiration, *or* place a second nasogastric tube if ordered above the esophageal balloon to control secretions and prevent aspiration.
- Suction the esophageal port when a Minnesota tube is used.
- Maintain balloon pressure and traction.
- Maintain balloon position.
- Clean and lubricate the patient's nostrils frequently to prevent tube-caused pressure areas.

- Irrigate the nasogastric port every 2 h to ensure patency and to keep the stomach empty.
- Teach the patient to avoid coughing or straining, which increases intra-abdominal pressure and predisposes to further bleeding.
- Have a second nasogastric tube, suction, and scissors available at the bedside.
- If the gastric balloon ruptures, the tube can rise into the nasopharynx, obstructing the airway. If this occurs, cut the tube immediately to deflate the balloon rapidly.
- Cut and remove the tube whenever there is a question of respiratory insufficiency or aspiration.
- Restrain the patient's arms if the patient is at risk for pulling out the tube. Agitation, confusion, and restlessness are risk factors.
- Assess for complications, including rupture or deflation of the balloon, pulmonary aspiration, and esophageal rupture.

tial resuscitation, massive bleeding that is immediately life-threatening, unavailable or failed endoscopic therapy, perforation, obstruction, suspicion of malignancy, or continued bleeding despite aggressive medical therapies.[15]

Surgical options for a bleeding peptic ulcer depend on the age and the condition of the patient, as well as on the location, size, and anatomy of the bleeding source. Emergency surgery of a bleeding duodenal ulcer may be a simple suturing (e.g., oversew) of the ulcer. Bleeding duodenal ulcers can also be treated using one of the following procedures:

- Truncal vagotomy and pyloroplasty with suture ligation of the ulcer
- Truncal vagotomy and antrectomy with resection or suture ligation of the ulcer
- Proximal gastric vagotomy with duodenotomy and suture ligation of the ulcer[15]

Bleeding gastric ulcers are commonly treated with one of the following procedures:

- Truncal vagotomy and pyloroplasty with wedge resection of the ulcer
- Antrectomy with wedge excision of the proximal ulcer
- Distal gastrectomy with or without truncal vagotomy
- Wedge resection of the ulcer[15]

A vagotomy involves severing the vagus nerve, which innervates the gastric cells. This results in decreased gastric acid secretion. A truncal (gastric) vagotomy selectively cuts the vagus distribution to the stomach. A pyloroplasty is necessary in conjunction with the vagotomy because denervation of the vagus nerve affects gastric motility. A pyloroplasty allows for continued gastric emptying. An antrectomy removes acid-producing cells in the stomach. A Billroth I procedure includes a vagotomy and antrectomy with anastomosis of the stomach to the duodenum. A Billroth II procedure involves a vagotomy, resection of the antrum, and anastomosis of the stomach to the jejunum (Fig. 41-2). A gastric perforation

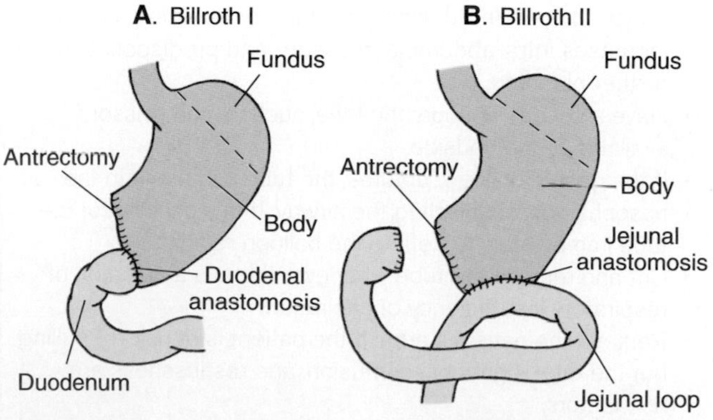

Figure 41-2 • A: The Billroth I procedure includes a vagotomy and antrectomy with anastomosis of the stomach to the duodenum. B: The Billroth II procedure includes a vagotomy, antrectomy, and anastomosis of the stomach to the jejunum.

can be surgically treated by simple closure or use of a patch to cover the mucosal hole.

Surgical decompression of portal hypertension can be used in patients with esophageal or gastric varices that are unresponsive to medical and endoscopic therapy. In this surgery, a portosystemic shunt is created, connecting the portal vein and the inferior vena cava to divert blood flow into the vena cava to decrease pressure.

Medical Management Once bleeding is controlled, management focuses on treating the underlying cause of the acute upper GIB. For patients with peptic ulcer disease, eradication of *H. pylori* and elimination of NSAID use increases the healing rate and markedly reduces the recurrence of a rebleed. Esophageal varices can be obliterated in subsequent endoscopy sessions, and β-blockade with propranolol (Inderal) or nadolol (Corgard) can be instituted to decrease the rebleeding rate. The dose should be titrated to achieve a 25% decrease in resting heart rate or a heart rate about 60 beats/minute as the desired end point.[14,16] The addition of isosorbide mononitrate may further decrease the risk for rebleeding. Cessation of alcohol ingestion is imperative. See Box 41-5 for nursing interventions in the care of the patient with acute GIB.

LOWER GASTROINTESTINAL BLEEDING

Etiology

Common causes of lower GIB are listed in Box 41-1. Most cases of acute lower GIB that require ICU admission result from diverticulosis or angiodysplasia, although bleeding from neoplasm, colitis, inflammatory bowel disease, and hemorrhoids is also seen.

Diverticulosis
Diverticula are saclike protrusions in the colon wall that usually develop at the point where arteries penetrate the colon wall. These vessels are separated from the bowel lumen only by the mucosa and are subsequently prone to injury. Diverticular bleeding accounts for 30% to 50% of all cases of acute lower GIB.[17] In the elderly, colonic diverticula account for up to 60% of all such cases.[18] Most patients with diverticular bleeding will stop bleeding spontaneously, but up to 25% of bleeding may be massive, resulting in hemorrhage and the need for surgery.[18,19] Risk factors for diverticular bleeding include a diet low in fiber, aspirin and NSAID use, advanced age, and constipation.

Angiodysplasia
Angiodysplasia, also called arteriovenous malformation or angioma, is the term used to describe dilated, tortuous submucosal veins, small arteriovenous communications, or enlarged arteries. The walls of the vessels lack smooth muscle and are composed of endothelial cells. The incidence of angiodysplasia increases with age owing to degeneration of the vessel walls; most cases occur in people older than 50 years, and two thirds occur in those older than

70 years. Acute lower GIB from angiodysplasia accounts for up to 39% of cases.[18] Angiodysplasia can occur anywhere in the colon, although it most often occurs in the cecum or ascending colon. As opposed to bleeding from diverticula, bleeding from angiodysplasia may be venous or arteriovenous in nature and is therefore usually less severe than bleeding from diverticular disease, which is arterial. Angiodysplasia is a common cause of lower GIB in patients with renal disease.

Clinical Presentation

Acute lower GIB is defined by the presence of hemodynamic instability and the passage of hematochezia. Patients with diverticular bleeding usually describe the sudden onset of painless maroon or bright red hematochezia, although melena can rarely occur. Diverticular bleeding is often painless, although patients may complain of cramping (which results from colonic spasm secondary to intraluminal exposure to blood). Blood loss from angiodysplasia usually presents as painless hematochezia.

If lower GIB is chronic, patients may present with iron-deficiency anemia and symptoms related to the anemia, such as weakness, fatigue, or dyspnea on exertion. Massive bleeding from hemorrhoids is rare but can occur in patients with rectal varices from portal hypertension.

Assessment

History

Relevant findings in the past medical history include abdominal surgery; a previous bleeding episode; peptic ulcer disease; inflammatory bowel disease; radia-tion to the abdomen or pelvis; or cardiopulmonary, renal, or liver disease. Knowledge of the patient's current medications and the existence of any allergies can also assist in diagnosis. A history of associated symptoms, including abdominal pain, fever, rectal urgency, tenesmus, weight loss, or a change in bowel habits or stool should be elicited. The color and consistency of stool should be determined; in a brisk bleed, frequent red or maroon stools are more likely, and brown or infrequent stools are unlikely.[19] The age of the patient may give a clue to diagnosis, because the risk for bleeding from diverticula and angiodysplasia increases with age.

Physical Examination

The physical examination is often unremarkable. Vital signs are closely monitored to assess for hemodynamic instability. A palpable mass may reveal a neoplasm. A rectal examination is essential to assess for hematochezia and melena and exclude the possibility of bleeding hemorrhoids, which can occasionally present as a hemorrhage.

Laboratory Studies

The initial laboratory studies include a complete blood count, serum electrolytes, BUN and creatinine levels, and PT and partial thromboplastin time (PTT). As in acute upper GIB, type and cross-match is mandatory before RBC transfusion.

Management

Resuscitation

The management of acute lower GIB requires aggressive fluid resuscitation, as described for acute upper GIB. Patients with hematochezia should have a nasogastric tube inserted to exclude an upper GI source of bleeding because 10% of suspected lower GIB occurs from upper GI sources.[9,20] The presence of bloody aspirate confirms an upper GI source of bleeding. However, the absence of blood does not exclude an upper GI source because bleeding from a site in the duodenum may not reflux into the stomach. Nasogastric aspirate that reveals bile without blood is unlikely in bleeding from an upper GI source. Once it is determined that bleeding is coming from a lower GI source, colonoscopy is the procedure of choice for both diagnosis and treatment.

Definitive Diagnosis

Endoscopy Colonoscopy is the test of choice for the evaluation of lower GIB; it has a diagnostic accuracy of up to 95% in affected patients.[18,19] Other advantages of colonoscopy are the ability to locate the source of the bleeding precisely, the ability to perform biopsies, and the potential for therapeutic intervention. Before colonoscopy, the colon needs to be cleansed with 4 L of polyethylene glycol solution given orally or by nasogastric tube until the waste is clear. For those patients in whom bleeding has stopped, it is reasonable to perform colonoscopy on an elective rather than emergent basis. If a source of bleeding is identified during colonoscopy, therapeutic options include thermal coagulation or injection with epinephrine or other sclerosants, as discussed previously. Upper endoscopy should be performed if colonoscopy is unable to distinguish a lower GI source.

Radionucleotide Imaging When colonoscopy fails to identify a bleeding source, radionucleotide scanning can detect bleeding that occurs at rates as low as 0.04 to 0.05 mL/minute.[21,22] This is more sensitive than angiography but less specific than either colonoscopy or a positive angiogram. The two types of scanning available are the technetium (^{99m}Tc)–sulfur colloid and ^{99m}Tc pertechnetate–labeled autologous RBCs. Unfortunately, both of these techniques provide poor localization because of the peristaltic action of the bowel. However, these scans may be useful before angiography because a positive scan can aid in the localization of the bleed.

Angiography Angiography is reserved for patients with massive, ongoing bleeding when endoscopy is not an acceptable option or with recurrent or persistent bleeding from a source not identified on colonoscopy. Angiography requires the active blood loss of 0.5 to 1.0 mL/minute to localize a bleeding site because the contrast in the arterial system is present for only a short time.[13,19] A positive angiogram is associated with a high likelihood for surgical intervention. When an active source is identified, arteriographic intervention with intra-arterial vasopressin or embolization may be used. However, embolization with gelatin sponges, microcoils, or polyvinyl alcohol particles is replacing vasopressin because of the high incidence of complication and rebleeding after stopping the infusion.[19,22] The nurse must be aware of the potential complications associated with arteriography, which include allergy to contrast, contrast-induced renal failure, bleeding from the arterial puncture site, and even embolism from thrombus.

Surgical Intervention

Surgical management of lower GIB is indicated for massive or recurrent bleeding and in those patients with high transfusion requirements. An exploratory laparotomy to identify the source of the bleeding is often performed. A segmental bowel resection with a primary anastomosis is often necessary for definitive treatment of lower GIB. In patients who are unstable, a stoma and mucus fistula may be created. In those patients with severe lower GIB without a localized source, a blind total colectomy may be the operative choice. Surgical management of diverticular bleeding is indicated if bleeding is not controlled with endoscopic or angiographic means or in patients with recurrent bleeding from the same segment.

• Intestinal Obstruction and Ileus

Intestinal obstruction occurs when the passage of intestinal contents through the lumen is impaired. This can result from either mechanical (anatomical) or nonmechanical causes. Ileus is the failure of passage of intestinal contents in the absence of mechanical obstruction. Intestinal obstruction is classified as either partial or complete, depending on the degree of obstruction. In a simple obstruction there is no ischemia, whereas in cases of strangulated obstruction, ischemia is present. A closed-loop obstruction describes a mechanical obstruction with a proximal and distal occlusion of the affected intestinal segment.

Bowel obstruction can occur in both the small and large bowel. The small bowel is most commonly affected, with the ileum as the most common site of obstruction. In large bowel obstruction, the sigmoid colon is the most common site of obstruction. The location of the obstruction, the degree of obstruction, and the presence of ischemia are important distinctions because treatment varies. Prompt recognition of bowel obstruction is important for the nurse because intestinal obstruction can progress to bowel strangulation, infarction, and perforation and result in potentially life-threatening peritoneal and systemic infection. The mortality rate associated with a strangulated obstruction is 30%.[23]

The causes of mechanical obstruction are varied and classified as extrinsic, intrinsic, and intraluminal (Box 41-6). Extrinsic lesions occur outside of the bowel. Examples of extrinsic lesions are adhesions, hernias, volvulus (twisting of a segment of the bowel on itself), and masses. Intrinsic lesions extend into the bowel wall. Diverticulitis, neoplasms, and radiation enteritis are examples of intrinsic lesions. Intraluminal causes of obstruction can result from the

Box 41-6 • Causes of Mechanical Obstruction

Extrinsic Lesions
Adhesions and congenital
 bands
Hernias
 External hernias
 Internal hernias
 Diaphragmatic hernias
 Pelvic hernias
Volvulus
 Gastric
 Midgut
 Cecal
 Sigmoid
Extrinsic masses
 Benign or malignant
  tumors
 Abscesses
 Aneurysms
 Hematomas
 Endometriosis

Intrinsic Lesions
Benign and malignant
 neoplasms
 Adenocarcinomas
 Lymphomas,
  lymphosarcomas
 Carcinoid tumors
Inflammatory conditions
 Tuberculous enteritis,
  Crohn's disease
 Strictures secondary to
  potassium chloride,
  nonsteroidal anti-
  inflammatory drugs,
  and ischemia

Radiation injury, caustic
 ingestants
Eosinophilic
 gastroenteritis,
 ameboma
Diverticulitis, pelvic
 inflammatory disease
Intussusception
Congenital defects
 Hypertrophic pyloric
  stenosis, annular
  pancreas
 Intestinal atresia/agenesis
 Malrotation/volvulus
 Intestinal duplication,
  mesenteric cysts
 Meckel's diverticulum
 Hirschsprung's disease
Hematoma
 Abdominal trauma
 Thrombocytopenia
 Henoch-Schönlein purpura

Intraluminal Causes
Meconium ileus
Barium impaction
Fecal impaction
Gallstone ileus
Gastric bezoars
Foreign bodies

From Yamada T, Alpers DH, Laine L, et al (eds): Textbook of Gastroenterology, 4th ed. Philadelphia: Lippincott Williams & Wilkins, 2003, p. 834.

ingestion of foreign bodies, intussusception, and neoplasms.

SMALL BOWEL OBSTRUCTION
Etiology

Adhesions are the most common cause of small bowel obstruction (SBO) in adults and account for 50% to 75% of obstructions.[24,25] Adhesions most commonly occur after laparotomy for colectomy, appendectomy, or gynecological procedures. Adhesions can also develop after abdominal radiation, ischemia, or infection, or as the result of foreign bodies. Adhesions may develop only days after surgery and as late as 10 to 20 years later. Adhesive bands can form and contract and, in time, may entrap a loop of bowel.

Hernias are the second most common cause of SBO and account for 25% of cases.[24,25] SBO secondary to hernia carries a high risk for complete

obstruction and strangulation. The herniation of a portion of the bowel after laparotomy is called a Richter's hernia. The occurrence of SBO in the absence of previous laparotomy should suggest hernia as the cause.

Tumors are uncommon in the small bowel, and primary neoplasms of the small bowel account for less than 5% to 10% of SBO.[24] Luminal compression of the small bowel or local invasion by gastric, pancreatic, colonic, and gynecological cancers can cause extrinsic compression, which accounts for most cases of SBO that result from malignancy.

Pathophysiology

In SBO, large amounts of fluid and swallowed air accumulate in the intestinal lumen proximal to the obstruction, causing distention (Fig. 41-3). Fluid accumulates from oral intake; swallowed saliva; and gastric, biliary, and pancreatic juices. Swallowed air has a high nitrogen content and is poorly absorbed from the lumen.[26]

As the obstruction continues, the bowel wall and lumen become edematous and distended. Increased intraluminal pressure leads to increased capillary permeability and movement of fluid and electrolytes into the abdominal cavity. This extravasation of fluid and electrolytes into the peritoneal cavity, combined with fluid lost through vomiting, can lead to hypovolemia, hypokalemia, and hyponatremia. Peristalsis decreases, and the normal functions of the intestine decrease or halt. In the absence of normal intestinal motility, bacterial overgrowth occurs. If oral intake continues, bacterial fermentation can contribute to gas accumulation. Within hours of acute obstruction, the contents of the lumen proximal to obstruction become malodorous and feculent because of this bacterial overgrowth.

Clinical Presentation

The severity of symptoms is related to the site and degree of obstruction and the presence and severity of ischemia (Table 41-1). Patients with SBO usually complain of the acute onset of intermittent, crampy abdominal pain. Bursts of peristalsis above the obstruction cause pain. The pain is often more severe the more proximal the obstruction. Patients with an incomplete obstruction often describe crampy abdominal pain after meals. The pain in incomplete obstruction may be exacerbated by the ingestion of high-fiber meals. In patients with proximal SBO, vomiting occurs frequently and early in the course of obstruction. The emesis is usually bilious, and vomiting often relieves the pain. Minimal abdominal distention usually accompanies proximal SBO.

In distal SBO, moderate abdominal distention and intermittent or constant pain are often present. Vomiting is intermittent. In ileal SBO, the emesis may be feculent secondary to bacterial overgrowth.

In strangulated SBO, the pain is more localized and may be steady and severe. When vomiting is protracted, dehydration and hypovolemia may occur.

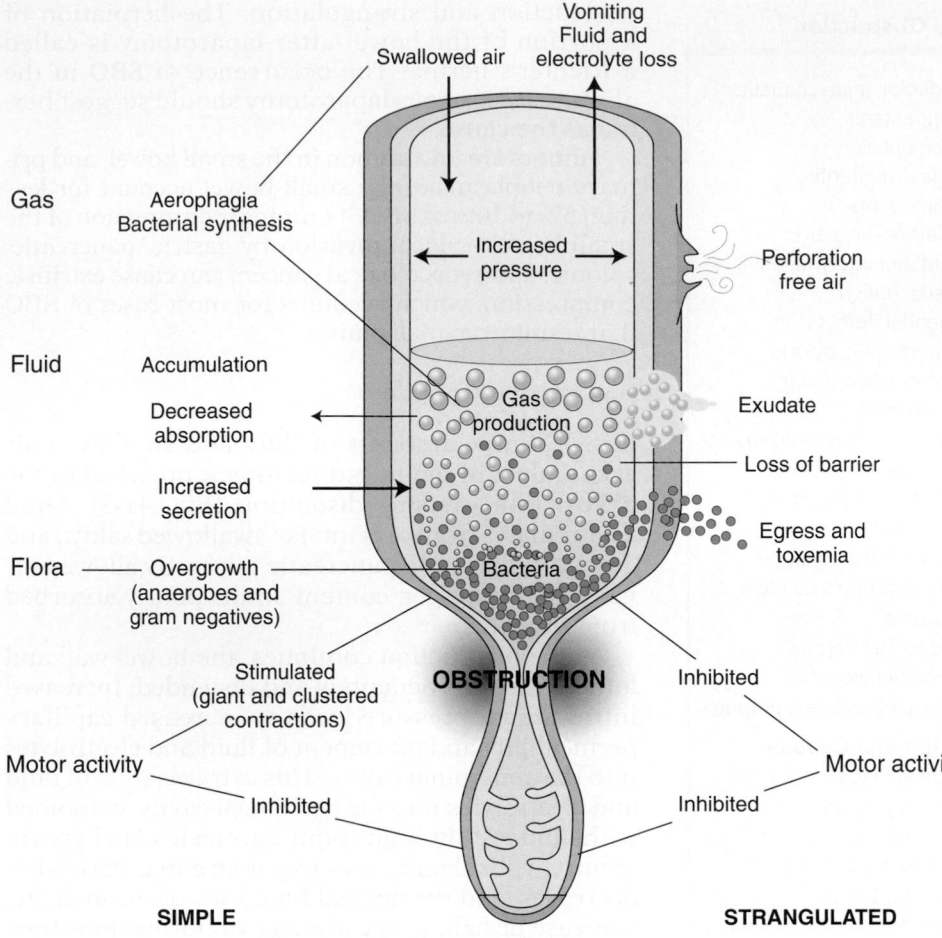

Figure 41-3 • The pathophysiology of simple obstruction (*left*) and strangulated obstruction (*right*) in the small intestine. (From Yamada T, Alpers DH, Laine L, et al [eds]: Textbook of Gastroenterology, 4th ed. Philadelphia: Lippincott Williams & Wilkins, 2003, p 830.)

Fever may be present secondary to an inflammatory process or in response to bowel ischemia or perforation. Constipation is also a common complaint, although patients may continue to pass gas and stool as the bowel distal to the obstruction empties. Obstipation, a reliable indicator of complete obstruction,[25] refers to extreme and persistent constipation caused by obstruction in the intestinal system. Depending on the duration and severity of the obstruction,

hemodynamic instability may develop as the result of massive fluid trapping in the lumen with leakage into the peritoneum.

Assessment

History

A careful history provides clues to etiology. A past medical history of previous abdominal surgery or

Table 41-1 • Clinical Features of Ileus and Obstruction Dependent on Anatomic Site

| | Ileus | Site of Obstruction | | | |
		Gastric Outlet	Distal Duodenum	Jejunoileal	Colon
Pain	Mild	Mild	Mild	Moderate	Severe
Distention	Moderate to severe	Mild	Mild	Moderate	Severe
Emesis					
Amount/frequency	Small, infrequent	Copious, frequent	Copious, frequent	Smaller/less frequent	Uncommon
Nature	Sour, bilious	Clear, sour, HCl, KCl	Bile-stained, bitter, NaCl, NaHCO₃	Malodorous, feculent	Variable
Acid–base imbalance	Variable	Metabolic alkalosis	Metabolic acidosis	Dehydration, hypotension	Usually not severe

HCl, hydrogen chloride; KCl, potassium chloride; NaHCO₃, sodium bicarbonate; NaCl, sodium chloride.
From Yamada T, Alpers DH, Laine L, et al (eds): Textbook of Gastroenterology, 4th ed. Philadelphia: Lippincott Williams & Wilkins, 2003, p 833.

trauma increases the risk for adhesions. Other pertinent past medical history findings include inflammatory bowel disease, diverticulitis, abdominal or pelvic radiation, peptic ulcer disease, pancreatitis, and previous obstruction or cancer. Correlation to menses suggests endometriosis. A complete medication history is also essential. Patients with a psychiatric history should be questioned about ingestion of foreign objects.

Physical Examination
Inspection of the abdomen often reveals visible peristalsis and distention. Patients with a proximal SBO may have epigastric or periumbilical tenderness, whereas those with distal SBO often have more diffuse tenderness. Bowel sounds are usually hyperactive in the early course of the obstruction, then high-pitched and tinkling with loud rushes as peristaltic waves attempt to push intestinal contents past the obstruction. Skin turgor and mucous membranes may show signs of dehydration. A palpable mass may represent a neoplasm or volvulus. It is necessary to perform a rectal examination to assess for blood. Inspection may reveal scars and external hernias. Hepatomegaly, liver masses, or other abdominal masses suggest malignancy. Abdominal tenderness and palpable masses may suggest abscess. Fever, rigors, and declining clinical status suggest bowel strangulation. Patients with a closed-loop obstruction may describe pain out of proportion to physical findings. Borborygmi are often audible and may correlate with abdominal cramping. Borborygmi are rumbling, gurgling, and tinkling noises produced by hyperactive intestinal peristalsis. If rebound tenderness is present, observe for signs and symptoms of shock because perforation is a possibility. Percussion of the abdomen may reveal resonance or tympany from fluid trapped in the intestine. Shifting dullness to percussion indicates ascites. Palpate for inguinal, femoral, and umbilical hernias. A tender mass at the site of a hernia suggests the etiology. Erythema overlying the skin may result from strangulation.[24] Tachycardia, tachypnea, altered mental status, oliguria, and hypotension may all be present in hypovolemia.

Laboratory Studies
Although there is no single laboratory value that is diagnostic for SBO, laboratory values are important in the management of SBO. Mild leukocytosis is present with simple obstructions, whereas white blood cell (WBC) elevations from 15,000 to 25,000/µL accompany strangulation. Mesenteric occlusion and perforation result in WBC elevations of 25,000/µL or more.[27] In proximal obstruction, potassium, sodium, hydrogen, and chloride may be lost in emesis, resulting in metabolic alkalosis.[25,27] BUN, creatinine, sodium, and osmolality levels reflect the fluid and electrolyte shifts that occur as fluid leaks out of the intestine and electrolytes are either reabsorbed or lost. As dehydration increases, the hemoglobin and hematocrit levels are elevated, reflecting hemoconcentration. In ischemia or strangulation, amylase, lipase, alkaline phosphatase, creatine phosphokinase, aspar-

tate aminotransferase (AST), alanine aminotransferase (ALT), and lactate dehydrogenase levels may rise.[24] Heme-positive stools are often present in ischemia or carcinoma. Metabolic acidosis suggests severe hypoxemia due to hypoperfusion, and metabolic acidosis refractory to fluid resuscitation suggests strangulation.[24]

Imaging Studies
Radiography When SBO is suspected, abdominal radiographs with the patient in upright, flat, and side-lying positions can confirm the diagnosis of obstruction, localize the site of obstruction, and assist in determining whether the obstruction is complete or partial. Normally there is little air in the small bowel. In complete SBO, gas and fluid accumulate proximal to the obstruction. Multiple air–fluid levels may be visible, with a stepladder pattern that demonstrates multiple loops of bowel with different air levels. Distal to the obstruction, the bowel lumen empties and collapses within 12 to 24 hours. Successive films may also confirm the diagnosis.

Barium studies may be helpful in the diagnosis of obstruction if plain films are nondiagnostic. Contrast studies can differentiate between a complete or partial obstruction. Barium is the agent of choice if SBO is suspected because it provides a better contrast than water-soluble material. In SBO, the large amount of water present proximal to the obstruction dilutes water-soluble contrast. However, if there is any question about bowel perforation, barium should be avoided because free barium in the peritoneum can cause significant inflammation. If colonic obstruction is suspected, a limited barium enema is used for diagnosis before barium is given by mouth.

Computed Tomography Abdominal computed tomography (CT) can help identify obstructive lesions, neoplasms, hernias, and signs of ischemia. Abdominal CT with oral or IV contrast can help differentiate mechanical obstruction from pseudo-obstruction. The CT diagnosis of a complete SBO requires a transition zone between dilated and collapsed loops of bowel, suggesting the point of obstruction. CT is less sensitive in the diagnosis of a partial SBO. CT can also assess the entire abdomen, which can suggest alternative diagnoses and identify any complications associated with obstruction. CT is also accurate in determining the presence of strangulation or a closed-loop obstruction.

Endoscopy Direct visualization with endoscopy may confirm the obstruction in the colon or proximal small bowel and aid in determining the type.

Management

Medical Management
When possible, obstructions, especially incomplete obstructions, are treated medically rather than surgically. Oral food and fluid are withheld (i.e., the patient is put on NPO status), and a nasogastric tube is placed to decompress the stomach or duodenum.

Fluid and electrolytes are repleted intravenously with Ringer's lactate or saline solution based on central venous pressure (CVP) readings and electrolyte results. When possible, the underlying causes are treated. Total parenteral nutrition (TPN) may be required to provide nutritional support. A Foley catheter is inserted to allow continual assessment of the fluid replacement. In patients with renal or cardiac disease, a CVP or pulmonary artery catheter may guide fluid replacement.

If patients continue to pass gas and stool, supportive management is continued. If patients show no improvement within 24 to 48 hours, or if fever or rebound tenderness occurs, a surgical evaluation is indicated. All patients with intestinal obstruction should be watched closely for signs and symptoms that reflect sepsis, perforation, ischemia, necrosis, or gangrene. Broad-spectrum antibiotics are started immediately when strangulation or sepsis is suspected. The mortality rate associated with bowel ischemia resulting from obstruction is high.

Surgical Management

Acute complete SBO is a surgical emergency. Acute complete SBO is suspected when the patient fails to pass gas and stool and gas is not evident in the distal intestine on radiography. An acute complete SBO is accompanied by the risk for bowel strangulation. Patients with strangulated bowel, volvulus, and incarceration of bowel loop in a hernia or a closed-loop obstruction require immediate surgery. In addition, those patients who fail conservative therapy or experience a decline in clinical status warrant surgical intervention.

Surgical procedures include laparoscopic lysis of adhesions, reduction of volvulus, resection of the involved and surrounding area of bowel with impaired blood supply, bowel decompression, and possible ostomy. These patients may require a second surgery to assess bowel viability.

COLONIC OBSTRUCTION

Etiology

Carcinoma, sigmoid diverticulitis, and volvulus are the three most common causes of colonic obstruction and together account for 90% of colonic obstructions.[24] Malignancy is the most common cause of colonic obstruction in the United States, accounting for approximately 50% of cases.[24,25] Patients with colorectal cancer present with a colonic obstruction 20% of the time.[24] Diverticulitis can cause strictures in the colon that can lead to mechanical obstruction, resulting in approximately 10% of cases of colonic obstruction.[24] Volvulus, which occurs most commonly in the sigmoid colon and the cecum, causes 10% to 15% of colonic obstructions in the United States.[24] A closed-loop obstruction is usually produced with volvulus and carries a high incidence of strangulation.[24] A history of laxative use and constipation is common in patients with volvulus.

Pathophysiology

When the ileocecal valve is competent, a closed-loop obstruction can occur because the cecum does not allow decompression of fluid and gas into the small bowel. As fluid and gas accumulate, the intraluminal pressure increases, and the colonic wall can become ischemic if this pressure exceeds the capillary pressure. In some cases, the cecum may become so severely distended that it inhibits intramural blood flow, which can result in necrosis and gangrene.[24] In colonic obstruction, the normal colonic flora produces methane and ammonia, which contribute to the distention. Dehydration results when secretions are sequestered in the colon.

Patients with colonic obstruction have changes in intestinal flora and translocation of bacteria in mesenteric lymph nodes. This is the most likely cause of septic complications of colonic obstruction.

Clinical Presentation

The clinical presentation of patients with colonic obstruction depends on the degree of obstruction, the cause, the presence of comorbidity, the presence of closed-loop obstruction, and the competency of the ileocecal valve. Patients with colonic obstruction typically present with abdominal pain and distention. The pain may be colicky or severe and unremitting if peritonitis is present. Severe, constant pain suggests gangrenous bowel. If vomiting occurs, it tends to be late in the course of obstruction, especially in patients with a competent ileocecal valve. Patients with volvulus may present with a sudden onset of marked abdominal distention. Patients with obstruction from colon cancer may describe altered bowel habits or a change in stool caliber. Dehydration results when secretions become sequestered in the colon. Patients with a competent ileocecal valve may have greater distention, which increases the risk for ischemia and perforation because an incompetent ileocecal valve allows decompression into the small intestine. Most patients with colonic obstruction complain of constipation; however, diarrhea may be present if stool is leaking past an obstruction. Patients may complain of dyspnea if diaphragmatic excursion is compromised by abdominal distention.

Assessment

History

A history of altered bowel movements, blood in the stool, or iron deficiency anemia is suggestive of carcinoma, as are weight loss and anorexia. Diverticulitis typically presents with left lower quadrant pain and associated fever. There may be a change in bowel habits as well. Bleeding is not usually associated with diverticulitis.

Physical Examination

Abdominal distention is common. Signs of dehydration may be seen. Abdominal masses and signs of peritoneal irritation may be elicited. Bowel sounds may be altered. Ascites and hepatomegaly may be present in patients with colon cancer with liver metastasis. A rectal examination may be helpful in identification of rectal cancer. High fever and tachycardia, regardless of rehydration or the presence of peritoneal signs, suggest strangulation and warrant urgent surgical evaluation.

Laboratory Studies
Iron-deficiency anemia may be present if obstruction results from neoplasm. Marked leukocytosis suggests diverticulitis, ischemia, or perforation.

Imaging Studies
Plain abdominal films in the supine and upright positions can reveal findings suspect for the diagnosis of colonic obstruction but may not be able to identify the site or its cause. Obstruction in patients with a competent ileocecal valve causes dilation confined to the colon. Small bowel distention may be visible on abdominal films in patients with acute colonic obstruction in patients with intact ileocecal valves.

Barium should never be given orally unless a barium enema, CT scan, or colonoscopy has ruled out colonic obstruction. Oral barium accumulates proximal to the colonic obstruction, and water will continually be extracted, causing a barium impaction.

CT may be valuable in distinguishing between an anatomic obstruction and a pseudo-obstruction.[28] CT can also diagnose other causes of colonic obstruction, such as inflammation as a result of colitis or diverticulitis and perforation as a result of colorectal cancer.[28]

Management

Medical Management
The medical management of the patient with acute colonic obstruction is similar to that of the patient with SBO. Medical management focuses on fluid and electrolyte replacement. Oral intake is limited, or the patient is placed on NPO status. Nasogastric suction may assist in decompression of abdominal distention. Colonic decompression in the setting of a volvulus can be attempted by colonoscopy.

Surgical Management
Colonic obstruction usually requires surgery. The goals of surgery are to decompress the colon and to treat the obstructive lesion. Surgical management of the colonic obstruction is warranted if the patient fails to improve with medical management, the patient's clinical status deteriorates, or the patient has a complete colonic obstruction with a competent ileocecal valve. For obstruction of the left colon, operative decompression followed by primary anastomosis after intraoperative lavage is the treatment of choice. For obstruction in the transverse and right colon, primary resection and anastomosis can also be performed safely. Stents that are placed endoscopically can be used as a temporary measure before surgical resection of obstruction from malignancy or as a palliative measure in nonoperative colorectal cancer.[23,25]

ILEUS

Ileus, often called paralytic ileus or adynamic ileus, is the failure of intestinal contents to pass in the absence of mechanical obstruction. Ileus can have intra-abdominal or extra-abdominal causes (Box 41-7), many of which are likely to be seen in the ICU setting. Acute colonic pseudo-obstruction, also called Ogilvie's syndrome, implies nonmechanical obstruction of the colon that is temporary and reversible.

Etiology

Postoperative ileus (a transient inhibition of normal GI motility that usually lasts for 3 to 5 days after surgery) is the most common cause of a delayed discharge after surgery, abdominal[29] or otherwise. Other causes of acute ileus include metabolic abnormalities (electrolyte disturbances, uremia, heavy metal poisoning), drugs (narcotics, catecholamines, adrenocorticotropic

---

Box 41-7 • Causes of Adynamic Ileus and Acute Colonic Pseudo-obstruction

Intra-abdominal Causes	Extra-abdominal Causes
Reflex inhibition	Reflex inhibition
Laparotomy	Craniotomy
Abdominal trauma	Rib, spine, or pelvic
Renal transplantation	fractures
Inflammatory conditions	Myocardial infarction
Perforated viscus or	Coronary bypass
penetrating wounds	Open heart surgery
Bile peritonitis	Pneumonia,
Chemical peritonitis	pulmonary embolus
Intraperitoneal hemorrhage	Burns
Toxic megacolon	Black widow spider
Familial Mediterranean fever	bites
Acute pancreatitis	Drug-induced
Acute cholecystitis	Anticholinergic/
Celiac disease	ganglionic
Inflammatory bowel disease	antagonists
Acute irradiation injury	Opiates
Abdominal irradiation	Chemotherapeutic
Infectious processes	agents
Bacterial peritonitis	Tricyclic anti-
Appendicitis	depressants
Diverticulitis	Phenothiazines
Herpes zoster virus	Metabolic abnormalities
Anorectal herpes simplex	Septicemia
virus	Electrolyte imbalance
Ischemic processes	Heavy metal poison-
Arterial insufficiency	ing (lead, mercury)
Venous thrombosis	Porphyria
Mesenteric arteritis	Uremia
Strangulation obstruction	Diabetic ketoacidosis
Retroperitoneal processes	Sickle cell disease
Ureteropelvic stones	Pulmonary failure
Pyelonephritis	
Retroperitoneal hemorrhage	
Pheochromocytoma	
Malignancy	
(Ogilvie's syndrome)	

From Yamada T, Alpers DH, Laine L, et al (eds): *Textbook of Gastroenterology*, 4th ed. Philadelphia: Lippincott Williams & Wilkins, 2003, p. 836.

hormones, anticholinergics), and local or systemic inflammation (peritonitis, ischemia, pancreatitis). Ileus may also be present after spinal cord injury. Blood-borne toxins, abnormalities in acid–base balance, electrolyte disturbances, and decreased oxygen supply are all possible causes of ileus.[25]

Pathophysiology

Although the etiology of ileus can be defined, the pathophysiology of ileus is poorly understood. Postoperative ileus has been widely studied, and multiple mechanisms are thought to play a role, including sympathetic neural reflexes, local and systemic inflammatory mediators, and changes in neural and hormonal transmitters.[29–31] The effects of anesthesia, combined with inflammation or ischemia in the operative area, may also interfere with nerve conduction. Opioid narcotics may also contribute to postoperative ileus because they decrease propulsive motility of the intestine.

In ileus, peristalsis ceases and distention of the intestine occurs as fluid and electrolytes accumulate in a process similar to that seen in mechanical obstruction.

Clinical Presentation

Patients may complain of diffuse abdominal discomfort and distention (see Table 41-1). Nausea and vomiting are often predominant in patients with postoperative ileus. Vomiting is frequent, and the emesis usually contains gastric contents and bile. The vomiting of feculent material is rare. The pain is usually less intense than in small bowel or colonic obstruction. The patient with ileus also complains of constipation and usually denies the passage of flatus. Other common symptoms are nausea, anorexia, hiccups, and bloating.

Assessment

History
A history of thyroid or parathyroid disease, heavy metal exposure, diabetes mellitus, and scleroderma should be elicited to identify underlying causes.[23]

Physical Examination
Abdominal distention is often prominent in ileus. Auscultation of the abdomen usually reveals infrequent or absent bowel sounds. The abdomen is usually resonant to percussion secondary to air in the dilated loops of intestine. Abdominal girth is assessed at frequent intervals. Signs of peritoneal irritation or sepsis are also sought during the abdominal examination.

Laboratory Studies
Electrolyte abnormalities commonly associated with ileus are similar to those seen in patients with mechanical obstruction.

Imaging Studies
Abdominal radiographs that show massive colonic dilation confirm the diagnosis of ileus.[25] In ileus, gas and fluid accumulate in loops of mildly dilated bowel proximal or adjacent to the site of an acute inflammatory process such as appendicitis or pancreatitis. These loops are involved in localized ileus and are called sentinel loops.[23] In acute colonic pseudo-obstruction, the entire colon becomes dilated, with the cecal diameter the greatest. Chest radiographs may help identify pneumonia or other causes of ileus. Contrast enema studies can be used to differentiate complete obstruction from partial obstruction and ileus. CT of the abdomen may identify causes that can contribute to ileus. Ultrasonography has no role in the diagnosis of ileus because the dilated loops of bowel prevent imaging.

Management

Treatment of ileus focuses on management of underlying causes. Because ileus may present in much the same way as mechanical obstruction, exclusion of mechanical causes is necessary. Treatment usually consists of supportive care. Patients with ileus are usually placed on NPO status. Fluid and electrolyte replacement is directed by clinical status and laboratory values as needed. Nasogastric suction limits the collection of swallowed air that can contribute to abdominal distention. Medications that can adversely affect colonic motility are halted when possible. Laxative use is avoided because these agents can provide a substrate for bacterial fermentation, which results in further gas accumulation. In addition, patients should be mobilized and encouraged to get out of bed if they are ambulatory.

If patients show no improvement in 3 to 5 days, a further search for underlying causes is initiated. Neostigmine has been effective in the treatment of colonic ileus not responsive to conservative therapy. Neostigmine is a parasympathomimetic that can correct the autonomic imbalance thought to contribute to ileus.[23,25,31] Prokinetic medications, such as metoclopramide (Reglan) and erythromycin, have not been found to be effective in the treatment of ileus.[30]

Therapeutic interventions for the decompression of the colon include colonoscopy, open or percutaneous cecostomy, and a decompression colostomy. Colonoscopy is the procedure of choice for decompression in patients who do not respond to conservative or medical therapy. Surgery is indicated if patients develop a perforation or evidence of ischemia.

• Acute Pancreatitis

Acute pancreatitis is an acute inflammation of the pancreas that can also involve surrounding tissues, remote organs, or both. Acute pancreatitis can be mild or severe. In mild acute pancreatitis, there are areas of fat necrosis in and around pancreatic cells, along with interstitial edema. Mild pancreatitis is not associated with organ dysfunction or complications, and recovery is usually uneventful. Approximately 10% to 20% of patients with acute pancreatitis develop severe acute pancreatitis, also called necrotic or hemorrhagic pancreatitis.[32,33] In severe acute pancreatitis, there is extensive fat necrosis in and around the pancreas, pancreatic cellular necrosis, and hemorrhage in the pancreas. Severe acute pancreatitis is associated with local and systemic complications. The incidence of acute pancreatitis varies among populations based on the prevalence of precipitating factors such as alcohol use and gallstone disease. The incidence of acute pancreatitis is 1 to 5 per 10,000 people in the United States.[34] The mortality rate associated with acute pancreatitis is approximately 10%.[33,35]

ETIOLOGY

There are multiple causes of acute pancreatitis (Box 41-8). Gallstones and excessive alcohol use together account for 70% to 80% of cases.[36] Gallstone pancreatitis is more common in women, and alcoholic pancreatitis is more common in men. Acute pancreatitis often follows the ingestion of a large meal or drinking episode. Biliary stones and biliary sludge may also precipitate acute pancreatitis as they pass through the ampulla of Vater. Many drugs, including diuretics, sulfonamides, metronidazole, aminosalicylates, and estrogen, can precipitate acute pancreatitis as a result of toxic metabolites or a drug reaction. Hypercalcemia and hypertriglyceridemia are metabolic causes of acute pancreatitis. Idiopathic pancreatitis is associated with pregnancy, the administration of TPN, or major surgery. Pancreatitis has also occurred after blunt or penetrating abdominal trauma or after endoscopic manipulation of the ampulla of Vater. Other possible precipitating factors include infectious processes, such as mumps, staphylococcal infection, scarlet fever, and viral infections, as well as the congenital variant of pancreas divisum. Pancreatitis may occur as an isolated event, or the patient may suffer repeated attacks.

PATHOPHYSIOLOGY

The acinar cells of the pancreas synthesize and secrete digestive enzymes to assist in the breakdown of starch, fat, and proteins. Under normal circumstances, these enzymes remain inactive until they enter the duodenum. As pancreatic juice enters the duodenum, trypsinogen is activated by enterokinase into its active form, trypsin.

In acute pancreatitis, pancreatic enzymes become prematurely activated in the pancreas. This premature activation results in autodigestion of the pancreas and the peripancreatic tissue. The exact mechanism by which pancreatic enzymes become activated and initiate autodigestion is not fully understood. However, the activation of trypsinogen is thought to be the critical event that promotes the activation of other injurious enzymes, including elastase, kinases, and phospholipase A. Elastase can cause dissolution of elastic fibers in blood vessels, which can lead to hemorrhage. Activated kinins cause systemic vasodilation and increased vascular permeability, which promotes edema.[34] Phospholipase A causes necrosis of the pancreas and the surrounding fatty tissue.

Pancreatic enzymes, vasoactive substances, hormones, and cytokines released from the injured pancreas cause a cascade of events that can lead to edema, vascular damage, hemorrhage, and necrosis. Systemic effects mediated by the immune system can lead to a systemic inflammatory response syndrome (SIRS), which can result in distant organ damage and multisystem organ failure. This immune response is independent of the event that causes acute pancreatitis but is responsible for the majority of the morbidity and mortality associated with it.

CLINICAL PRESENTATION

Abdominal pain is the hallmark of acute pancreatitis. The severity of the pain correlates to the degree of pancreatic involvement. The pain is usually mid-epigastric or periumbilical, with radiation to the back, but it may radiate to the spine, flank, or left shoulder. The pain usually begins abruptly, often after a large meal or large intake of alcohol. It may be steady and severe, or it may increase in intensity over several hours. The pain is usually exacerbated when the patient lies supine and is usually relieved when the patient sits and leans forward or lies in a fetal position. Nausea, vomiting without pain relief, tachycardia, abdominal distention, and hypotension are other common symptoms. A low-grade fever may or may not be present. A persistent fever may indicate complications, such as peritonitis, cholecystitis, or intra-abdominal abscess.

The diagnosis of acute pancreatitis is often challenging because acute pancreatitis can mimic many other conditions. The differential diagnosis includes gastritis, perforated duodenal or gastric ulcers, acute SBO, ruptured ectopic pregnancy, sickle cell crisis, acute cholecystitis, mesenteric artery occlusion, and ruptured aortic aneurysm. Diagnosis is made on the basis of the patient's clinical presentation, history, and physical examination findings, and the results of laboratory and radiographic studies (Box 41-9). The diagnosis of acute pancreatitis requires two of the following three features: abdominal pain characteristic of acute pancreatitis, serum amylase or lipase

---

Box 41-8 • Major Causes of Acute Pancreatitis

- Biliary disease: gallstones or microlithiasis, common bile duct obstruction, biliary sludge
- Pancreas divisum
- Alcohol abuse
- Drugs: thiazide diuretics, furosemide, procainamide, tetracycline, sulfonamides, azathioprine, 6-mercaptopurine, angiotensin-converting enzyme inhibitors, valproic acid
- Hypertriglyceridemia
- Hypercalcemia
- Idiopathic
- Miscellaneous (postoperative, ectopic pregnancy, ovarian cyst, total parenteral nutrition)
- Abdominal trauma
- Endoscopic retrograde cholangiopancreatography
- Infectious processes

Box 41-9 • Clinical Manifestations of Acute Pancreatitis

Physical Examination Findings
- Abdominal pain
- Low-grade fever
- +/− Jaundice
- Abdominal guarding or distention
- Paralytic ileus
- Grey Turner's sign
- Cullen's sign
- Nausea or vomiting without relief

Laboratory Findings
- Elevated serum and urine amylase
- Elevated serum lipase
- Elevated white blood cell count
- Hypokalemia
- Hypocalcemia
- Elevated bilirubin, aspartate aminotransferase, and prothrombin time (with liver disease)
- Elevated alkaline phosphatase level (with biliary disease)
- Hypertriglyceridemia
- Hyperglycemia
- Hypoxemia

---

greater than or equal to the upper limits of normal, and characteristic findings on CT.[32]

ASSESSMENT

History

A careful history can provide important clues to diagnosis. A history of biliary tract disease, alcohol intake, and medication use should be elicited to identify precipitating causes. A family history of acute pancreatitis may suggest hereditary causes. The patient may report anorexia, weight loss, nausea, vomiting, or abdominal distention. Assessment of the location, duration, quality, quantity, and precipitating factors of pain is important to help identify potential causes.

Physical Examination

Diffuse abdominal tenderness and guarding may be present during abdominal palpation. The upper abdomen may be distended and tympanic to percussion. Bowel sounds may be hypoactive or absent owing to decreased intestinal mobility or paralytic ileus. Jaundice may be present in gallstone disease or from obstruction of the biliary tree from pancreatic edema. Ascites or palpable abdominal masses may be present. Patients with severe acute hemorrhagic pancreatitis may have signs of dehydration and hypovolemic shock. These signs may worsen when fluid is lost into the bowel lumen because of a paralytic ileus. The presence of a bluish discoloration of the lower abdominal flanks (Grey Turner's sign) or around the umbilical area (Cullen's sign) indicates hemorrhagic pancreatitis and an accumulation of blood in these areas. These findings are rare, but if they occur, the findings usually do not appear until 48 hours or more after onset of symptoms.[37]

Laboratory Studies

No single laboratory study is diagnostic of acute pancreatitis; however, elevations of serum amylase and lipase enzymes are often seen in acute pancreatitis. These enzymes are released as the pancreatic cells and ducts are destroyed. Serum amylase levels rise within 2 to 12 hours of the onset of symptoms and gradually return to baseline within 3 to 5 days in acute pancreatitis.[38] In mild pancreatitis, amylase levels can be close to normal. If a few days have elapsed since symptoms began, amylase values can also be normal even with an active inflammatory process in the pancreas. The sensitivity of serum amylase is limited in patients with elevated serum triglycerides and in acute pancreatitis related to alcohol.[38] The specificity of serum amylase is decreased in biliary tract disease, tumors, salivary gland lesions, cerebral trauma, gynecological disorders, and renal failure. However, the specificity for serum amylase in the diagnosis of acute pancreatitis is increased if levels are more than 2 to 3 times the upper limits of normal.[38]

Compared with serum amylase levels, serum lipase levels rise later and remain elevated. Serum lipase levels usually rise within 4 to 8 hours of the onset of symptoms, peak at 24 hours, and return to normal after 8 to 14 days.[38] Because serum lipase stays elevated longer, it is a useful test in diagnosis if there is a delay in examination. Like amylase, serum lipase levels may be elevated in patients who have intra-abdominal inflammation or renal insufficiency.

Elevations of isoenzymes, urinary amylase, and the amylase values of pleural fluid and paracentesis drainage support the presence of acute pancreatitis. Leukocytosis, hypokalemia, hypocalcemia, and hypertriglyceridemia may be present but are not specific to acute pancreatitis. Leukocytosis with WBCs of more than 15,000/µL frequently results from infection, stress, or dehydration.[35] Persistent vomiting may result in hypokalemia. Hypocalcemia may indicate the presence of pancreatic fat necrosis because calcium binds with fatty acids during tissue necrosis. In addition, trypsin inactivates parathyroid hormone, which is needed for calcium absorption. Hyperglycemia may result from decreased insulin release from damaged β cells, increased glucagon release, and the stress response. Hemoconcentration may occur as fluid is lost into the peritoneal space. Elevations in serum bilirubin, AST, and PT are common in the presence of concurrent liver disease. A greater than threefold elevation in ALT suggests biliary pancreatitis.[24] Alkaline phosphatase is elevated with biliary tract disease. Triglyceride levels associated with acute pancreatitis are usually greater than 800 to 1,000 mg/dL.[38]

Imaging Studies

Radiographs of the chest and abdomen are useful to exclude other causes of abdominal pain, including intestinal ileus, perforation, pericardial effusion, and pulmonary disease.

Abdominal ultrasound is of limited use in visualization of the pancreas due to intestinal gas and adipose tissue. Abdominal ultrasound is used to evaluate the biliary tree for gallstones, sludge, or ductal dilation as the etiology of pancreatitis.[32]

CT is the best imaging study to confirm the diagnosis and determine the severity of acute pancreatitis. CT can visualize the size of the pancreas and identify the presence of peripancreatic fluid, pancreatic pseudocysts, and abscesses. Dynamic CT done with contrast can help identify areas of necrosis in the pancreas. CT findings of extensive necrosis have correlated with a high risk for pancreatitis-related infection and death. Sequential CT allows for assessment of progressive disease or resolution. CT can also demonstrate fluid collection and areas of necrosis and can be used to guide percutaneous needle aspiration for culture.

Magnetic resonance cholangiopancreatography may have a sensitivity of more than 90% for bile duct stones. Endoscopic retrograde cholangiopancreatography plays a role in locating and removing stones in the common bile duct if gallstone pancreatitis is present.

Tools for Predicting Severity

Acute pancreatitis is self-limiting and mild in 80% to 90% of patients, resolving spontaneously within 5 to 7 days.[37] These patients usually require conservative care. However, in 10% to 20% of patients with acute pancreatitis, increased intrapancreatitis and extrapancreatic inflammation result in systemic inflammatory responses. Although the mortality rate for severe acute pancreatitis is 10%, this value rises to 50% or more when there are complications.[33,39] Multiple assessment tools have been developed in attempts to identify patients who are likely to develop severe acute pancreatitis so that aggressive treatment and surveillance can decrease complications and mortality.

Ranson's criteria have been widely used to assess the severity of acute pancreatitis (Box 41-10). Ranson's criteria consist of multiple clinical criteria used to identify those patients at risk for increased morbidity and mortality. The criteria assessed at admission indicate the severity of the acute inflammatory response, and the criteria assessed at 48 hours evaluate systemic effects. Three or more signs identified at the time of admission or during the initial 48 hours are predictive of severe acute pancreatitis, with an associated mortality rate of 10% to 20%.[32,33,40] Six or more have a corresponding mortality rate of 39%.[32,33] Ranson's criteria have a greater than 90% accuracy rate and are useful clinically in identifying high-risk patients. The primary disadvantage to Ranson's criteria is the 48-hour delay before the assessment is completed.

The Acute Physiology and Chronic Health Evaluation II (APACHE II) score has also been studied and found to be useful in predicting severity of acute pancreatitis (Table 41-2). The APACHE II uses the worst values of physiological measures, age, and previous health status at admission, at 24 hours, and at 48 hours to predict severity of acute pancreatitis. An APACHE II score on admission of 8 or more predicted 68% of severe attacks.[37] An advantage of the APACHE II score is that it can be used daily. An APACHE II score that increases during the first 48 hours strongly suggests severe pancreatitis.[32] Both Ranson's criteria results and APACHE II scores are comparable at 48 hours.

Extravasation and third-spacing seen in severe acute pancreatitis can cause significant intravascular volume depletion. This depletion can lead to decreased perfusion of the pancreas and cause pancreatic necrosis. Some experts have proposed that hemoconcentration, as detected by an elevated serum hematocrit, is a reliable predictor of necrotizing pancreatitis; however, there is no consensus. Experts do agree that necrotizing pancreatitis is unlikely in the absence of hemoconcentration at admission.[32]

The presence of peripancreatic inflammation, peripancreatic fluid collection, and extent of pancreatic necrosis found on CT have been shown to predict severity of acute pancreatitis. The CT severity index uses CT findings to grade pancreatic severity.

The use of serum markers to prognosticate severity has been tested. The most promising have been quantification of C-reactive protein (CRP) and trypsinogen active peptide (TAP). CRP levels greater than 130 mg/L within the first 72 hours of acute pancreatitis have correlated with the presence of necrosis with sensitivity and sensitively of greater than 80%.[32,36] CRP rises in relation to severity, is inexpensive, and readily available. Unfortunately, CRP does not become significantly elevated until 48 hours after inflammation, which limits its use in diagnosis of acute pancreatitis.[37] TAP is released when trypsinogen is activated into trypsin, which makes this an attractive marker for acute pancreatitis; however, false-negative and false-positive responses remain a concern.[37,39] Unfortunately, TAP is not available commercially.

COMPLICATIONS

The local and systemic complications of acute pancreatitis are summarized in Box 41-11.

Box 41-10 • Ranson's Criteria for Acute Pancreatitis

Evaluate on admission or on diagnosis:

- Age >55 y
- Leukocyte count >16,000/mL
- Serum glucose >200 mg/dL
- Serum lactate dehydrogenase >350 IU/mL
- Serum aspartate aminotransferase >250 IU/dL

Evaluate during initial 48 h:

- Fall in hematocrit >10%
- Blood urea nitrogen level rise >5 mg/dL
- Serum calcium <8 mg/dL
- Base deficit >4 mEq/L
- Estimated fluid sequestration >6 L
- Arterial PaO_2 <60 mm Hg

Table 41-2 • The Acute Physiology and Chronic Health Evaluation II (APACHE II) Classification System

Physiologic Variable	High Abnormal Range				0	Low Abnormal Range			
	+4	+3	+2	+1		+1	+2	+3	+4
Temperature rectal (°C)	≥41	39–40.9		38.5–38.9	36.0–38.4	34–35.9	32–33.9	30–31.9	≤29.9
Mean arterial pressure = (2 × diastolic + systolic)/3	≥160	130–159	110–129		70–109		50–69		≤49
Heart rate (ventricular response)	≥180	140–179	110–139		70–109		55–69	40–54	≤39
Respiratory rate (nonventilated or ventilated)	≥50	35–49		25–34	12–24	10–11	6–9		<5
Oxygenation A-aDo$_2$ or Pao$_2$ (mm Hg); Fio$_2$ >0.5; record A–aDo$_2$;	≥500	350–499	200–349		<200				
Fio$_2$ <0.5, record only Pao$_2$					>70	61–70		55–60	<55
Arterial pH (if no arterial blood gases [ABGs] record serum HCO$_3$ below)*	≥7.7	7.6–7.69		7.5–7.59	7.33–7.49		7.25–7.32	7.15–7.24	<7.15
Serum sodium	≥180	160–179	155–159	150–154	130–139		120–129	111–119	≤110
Serum potassium	≥7	6–6.9		5.6–5.9	3.5–5.4	3–3.4	2.5–2.9		<2.5
Serum creatinine (mg/dL) (double point for acute renal failure)	≥3.5	2–3.4	1.5–1.9		0.6–1.4		<0.6		
Hematocrit (%)	≥60		50–59.9	46–49.9	30–45.9		20–29.9		<20
White blood count	≥40		20–39.9	15–19.9	3–14.9		1–2.9		<1
Glasgow coma scale (GCS) (score = 15 minus actual GCS)†	15 – GCS =								
A Total acute physiology score (APS)	Sum of the 12 individual variable points =								
*Serum HCO$_3$ (venous mmol/L) (not preferred, use if no ABGs)	<52	41–51.9		32–40.9	22–31.9		18–21.9	15–17.9	<15

†Glasgow Coma Scale	(Circle Appropriate Response)	B (Age and Points)		C (Chronic Health Points)	
Eyes open	*Verbal—nonintubated*	Age	Points	If any of the 5 CHE categories is answered with yes give +5 points for nonoperative or emergency post-operative patients	
4 - spontaneously	5 - oriented and converses	<44 y	0		
3 - to verbal command	4 - disoriented and talks	45–54 y	2		
2 - to painful stimuli	3 - inappropriate words	55–64 y	3	Liver	Cirrhosis with portal hypertension or encephalopathy
1 - no response	2 - incomprehensible sounds	65–74 y	5		
	1 - no response	>75 y	6	Cardiovascular	Class IV angina at rest or with minimal self-care activities
Motor response	*Verbal—intubated*				
6 - to verbal command	5 - seems able to talk			Pulmonary	Chronic hypoxemia or hypercapnia or polycythemia or pulmonary hypertension >40 mm Hg
5 - localizes to pain	3 - questionable ability to talk				
4 - withdraws to pain	1 - generally unresponsive				
3 - decorticate				Kidney	Chronic peritoneal or hemodialysis
2 - decerebrate				Immune	Immune-compromised host
1 - no response					
		Age points =		Chronic health points =	

Credit given to Nick Mendel, Kiev, Ukraine, for producing this document.
APACHE II score **(sum of A + B + C): A** APS points + **B** age points + **C** chronic health points = total APACHE II.
From Triester SL, Kowdley KV: Prognostic factors in acute pancreatitis. J Clin Gastroenterol 34(2):167–176, 2002.

Box 41-11 • Major Complications of Acute Pancreatitis

Local
- Pancreatic necrosis
- Pancreatic pseudocyst
- Pancreatic abscess

Pulmonary
- Atelectasis
- Acute respiratory distress syndrome
- Pleural effusions

Cardiovascular
- Hypotensive shock
- Septic shock
- Hemorrhagic shock

Renal
- Acute renal failure

Hematological
- Disseminated intravascular coagulation

Metabolic
- Hyperglycemia
- Hypertriglyceridemia
- Hypocalcemia
- Metabolic acidosis

Gastrointestinal
- Gastrointestinal bleed

Local Complications

The local effects of pancreatitis include inflammation of the peritoneum around the pancreas and fluid accumulation in the peritoneal cavity. These changes can lead to pancreatic pseudocyst, pancreatic abscess, and acute GI hemorrhage.

Pancreatic pseudocysts occur in up to 15% of all cases of acute pancreatitis.[33] A pseudocyst is a collection of inflammatory debris and pancreatic secretions enclosed by a lined epithelial tissue and free of solid debris that must be present for 4 weeks or more.[33] The pseudocyst can rupture and hemorrhage or become infected, causing bacterial translocation and sepsis. A pseudocyst is suspected in any patient who has persistent abdominal pain with nausea and vomiting, a prolonged fever, and elevated serum amylase. Surgery may also be indicated for pseudocysts; however, it is usually delayed because most pseudocysts resolve spontaneously. Surgical treatment of the pseudocyst can be done through internal or external drainage or needle aspiration. Acute surgical intervention may be required if the pseudocyst becomes infected or perforates.

A pancreatic abscess is a walled-off collection of purulent material in or around the pancreas that usually occurs 6 weeks or more after the onset of acute pancreatitis.[33] Signs and symptoms of an abdominal abscess or infected pancreatic necrosis include increased WBC count, fever, abdominal pain, and vomiting. Pancreatic infection from an abscess, pseudocyst, or necrotic tissue may be present when-

ever a patient has a temperature greater than 39°C (102.2°F), tachycardia, or leukocytosis greater than 20,000/μL, or shows other signs of clinical deterioration. Infections after the onset of pancreatitis, if untreated, are often fatal. Broad-spectrum antibiotics are given to those patients with suspected infection.

GI complications of acute pancreatitis include GIB and bacterial translocation. GIB, the most common GI complication of acute pancreatitis, includes bleeding from peptic ulcers, hemorrhagic gastroduodenitis, stress ulcers, and Mallory-Weiss syndrome. Decreased peristalsis can lead to bacterial translocation.

Pulmonary Complications

Enzymes and inflammatory cytokines that reach the pulmonary circulation are thought to cause the many pulmonary complications associated with acute pancreatitis. Leukocytes that reach the pulmonary microcirculation migrate into the interstitium, which results in endothelial permeability and tissue edema. This causes lung congestion and alveolar collapse, and it can lead to adult respiratory distress syndrome.[39] Arterial hypoxemia can occur in patients with mild disease without clinical or radiographic findings to support the pulmonary dysfunction. In severe acute pancreatitis, arterial blood gases should be drawn every 8 hours for the first few days to detect this complication. Treatment of hypoxemia includes vigorous pulmonary care (e.g., deep breathing and coughing) and frequent position changes. Oxygen therapy can also be used to improve overall oxygenation status. Careful fluid administration is also necessary to prevent fluid overload and pulmonary congestion. Patients with acute respiratory compromise may require mechanical ventilatory support. Abdominal distention and diminished diaphragmatic excursion may also contribute to atelectasis seen in acute pancreatitis.

Cardiovascular Complications

Hemodynamically significant fluid sequestration is characteristic of fulminant pancreatitis. Another major systemic effect of enzyme release into the circulatory system is peripheral vasodilation, which in turn can cause hypotension and shock.

Decreased perfusion to the pancreas itself can result in the release of myocardial depressant factor (MDF). MDF decreases heart contractility and affects cardiac output. Perfusion of all body organs can then become compromised. Early and aggressive fluid resuscitation is thought to prevent the release of MDF. Trypsin activation causes abnormalities in blood coagulation and clot lysis. This promotes the development of disseminated intravascular coagulation (DIC) with its associated bleeding (see Chapter 49).

Renal Complications

Acute renal failure is thought to be a consequence of hypovolemia and decreased renal perfusion. Death during the first 2 weeks of acute pancreatitis usually results from pulmonary or renal complications.

Metabolic Complications

Metabolic complications of acute pancreatitis include hypocalcemia and hyperlipidemia, which are thought to be related to areas of fat necrosis around the inflamed pancreas. Hyperglycemia may occur as a result of damage to the cells of the islets of Langerhans; metabolic acidosis can result from hypoperfusion and activation of anaerobic metabolism.

MANAGEMENT

Medical Management

Conventional care of the patient with acute pancreatitis focuses on fluid and electrolyte replacement to maintain or replenish vascular volume and electrolyte balance, pain management, resting the pancreas in an effort to prevent the release of pancreatic secretions, and maintaining the patient's nutritional status (Box 41-12). Close observation and clinical judgment are the basis for therapy and management.

Fluid and Electrolyte Replacement

Most patients with acute pancreatitis require the infusion of IV fluids to replace fluid lost through third-spacing into the retroperitoneal space or peritoneal cavity, and intravascular volume depletion as a result of inflammatory mediators and local inflammation caused by pancreatic enzyme exudates.[32] Patients with severe acute pancreatitis may need up to 5 to 10 L of fluid replacement within 24 hours during their initial days of hospitalization.[36] The goal is to administer enough fluid to obtain a circulating volume sufficient to maintain organ and tissue perfusion and prevent end-stage shock. Hypovolemia and shock are major causes of death early in the disease process when aggressive fluid resuscitation fails to reverse the shock process.

Colloid and crystalloid solutions, such as albumin and Ringer's lactate solution, are used for volume replacement. Patients with acute hemorrhagic pancreatitis may also need PRBCs to restore blood volume. Fluid replacement is evaluated by monitoring intake and output and daily weights. Patients with more severe disease may require hemodynamic monitoring with measurement of pulmonary artery wedge pressure or CVP. CVP should be within 8 to 12 mm Hg.[36]

Patients with severe disease whose hypotension fails to respond to fluid therapy may need medications to support blood pressure. The drug of choice is dopamine at low doses to maintain renal perfusion while supporting blood pressure.

Urinary output is a sensitive measure of the adequacy of fluid replacement, and it should be maintained at greater then 30 mL/hour or 0.6 mL/kg/hour. Blood pressure and heart rate are also sensitive measures of volume status.

Patients with severe hypocalcemia are placed on seizure precautions with respiratory support equipment on hand. The nurse is responsible for monitoring calcium levels, administering replacement solutions, and evaluating the patient's response to any calcium supplementation. Calcium replacements should be infused through a central line because peripheral infiltration can cause tissue necrosis. The patient also needs to be monitored for calcium toxicity; symptoms include lethargy, nausea, shortening of the QT interval, and decreased excitability of nerves and muscles. Hypomagnesemia may also be present, so magnesium may need to be replaced as well. Serum magnesium levels usually need to be corrected before calcium levels can return to normal. Potassium may need to be replaced early in the treatment regimen because it is lost through vomiting and sequestration of potassium-rich pancreatic juices.

Hyperglycemia is related to impaired secretion of insulin, an increased release of glucagon, or increased stress response. In some cases, hyperglycemia can be associated with dehydration or other electrolyte imbalances. Sliding-scale regular insulin may be ordered; it needs to be administered very cautiously because glucagon levels are only transiently elevated in acute pancreatitis. Successful fluid replacement is marked by return of alert mental status, urine output, cardiac output, stable hemodynamic values, and a normal serum lactate level.

Pain Management

Pain control is a nursing priority for patients with acute pancreatitis, not only because of the extreme discomfort, but also because pain increases pancreatic enzyme secretion. Pain is related to the degree of pancreatic inflammation, can be severe and constant, and can last for many days.

Adequate pain control with the use of IV narcotics, preferably delivered by patient-controlled analgesia, is essential in the treatment of acute pancreatitis. Meperidine (Demerol) has traditionally been the analgesic of choice because of the potential for sphincter of Oddi spasm that can accompany opioid use. However, meperidine is not always effective, and other analgesics (including opioids) should not be withheld. Fentanyl citrate (Sublimaze), although an opiate, has been used successfully to control the pain of acute pancreatitis.

Analgesia should be routinely administered at least every 3 to 4 hours to prevent uncontrollable abdominal pain. Use of a pain rating scale is recommended for evaluating the patient's response to medication. Be alert to the patient's respiratory status because narcotics can induce respiratory depression. A nasogastric tube attached to low intermittent suction can help ease pain considerably, although the use of a nasogastric tube is controversial in patients without vomiting. Patient positioning can also relieve some of the discomfort.

Resting the Pancreas

In some patients with acute pancreatitis, nasogastric suction is used to decompress the stomach and decrease stimulation of secretin. Secretin, which stimulates production of pancreatic secretions, is released in response to acid in the duodenum. Nausea, vomiting, and abdominal pain may decrease when a nasogastric tube is placed and connected to suction early in treatment. A nasogastric tube is also

Box 41-12 • COLLABORATIVE CARE GUIDE for the Patient With Pancreatitis

OUTCOMES	INTERVENTIONS
Oxygenation/Ventilation Arterial blood gases are maintained within normal limits. The patient's lungs are clear. The patient has no evidence of atelectasis, pneumonia, or acute respiratory distress syndrome.	• Assist patient to turn, deep-breathe, cough, and use incentive spirometer q4h and PRN. Provide chest physiotherapy. • Assess for hypoventilation, rapid and shallow breathing, and respiratory distress. • Monitor pulse oximetry, end-tidal CO_2, and arterial blood gases. • Administer analgesics if splinting is reducing effective ventilation. • Provide supplemental oxygen as needed. • Auscultate breath sounds q2–4h and PRN. • Suction only when rhonchi are present or secretions are visible in endotracheal tube. • Hyperoxygenate and hyperventilate before and after each suction pass.
Circulation/Perfusion Blood pressure, heart rate, and hemodynamic parameters are within normal limits. Serum lactate will be within normal limits. Patient will not experience bleeding related to acute gastro-intestinal hemorrhage, coagulopathies, or disseminated intravascular coagulation.	• Monitor vital signs q1–2h. • Monitor pulmonary artery pressures and right atrial pressure q1h and cardiac output, systemic vascular resistance, and peripheral vascular resistance q6–12h if pulmonary artery catheter is in place. • Maintain patent IV access. • Administer intravascular volume as indicated by real or relative hypovolemia, and evaluate response. • Monitor lactate qd until it is within normal limits. • Administer red blood cells, positive inotropic agents, colloid infusion as ordered to increase oxygen delivery. • Monitor prothrombin time, partial thromboplastin time, complete blood count daily or PRN. • Assess for signs of bleeding. Observe for Cullen's or Grey Turner's signs. • Administer blood products as indicated.
Fluids/Electrolytes Patient is euvolemic. No evidence of electrolyte imbalance or renal dysfunction.	• Maintain patent IV access. • Monitor daily weights. • Monitor intake and output. • Measure abdominal girth q8h at the same location on the abdomen. • Monitor electrolytes daily and PRN. • Assess for signs of lethargy, tremors, tetany, and dysrhythmias. • Replace electrolytes as ordered. • Monitor blood urea nitrogen, creatinine, serum osmolality, and urine electrolytes daily.
Mobility/Safety No evidence of complications related to bed rest and immobility. Patient achieves or maintains ability to conduct activities of daily living and mobilize self.	• Initiate deep venous thrombosis prophylaxis. • Reposition frequently. • Ambulate to chair when acute phase is past, hemodynamic stability and hemostasis achieved. • Consult physical therapist. • Conduct range-of-motion and strengthening exercises.

(continued)

Box 41-12 • COLLABORATIVE CARE GUIDE for the Patient With Pancreatitis **(Continued)**

OUTCOMES	INTERVENTIONS
No evidence of infection, WBC within normal limits.	• Monitor for systemic inflammatory response syndrome. Criteria: increased WBC count, increased temperature, tachypnea, tachycardia. • Use strict aseptic technique during procedures. • Maintain invasive catheter tube sterility. • Change invasive catheters, culture blood, line tips, or fluids, etc., according to hospital protocol.
Skin Integrity Skin will remain intact.	• Assess skin q8h and each time patient is repositioned. • Turn q2h. • Consider pressure relief/reduction mattress.
Nutrition Caloric and nutrient intake meet metabolic requirements per calculation (e.g., basal energy expenditure). Evidence of metabolic dysfunction is minimal.	• Provide parenteral feeding. • Maintain NPO. • Consult dietitian or nutritional support service. • Fat or lipid restriction. • Provide small, frequent feedings. • Monitor albumin, prealbumin, transferrin, cholesterol, triglycerides, glucose.
Comfort/Pain Control Patient will have minimal pain, < 5 on pain scale. Patient will have minimal nausea.	• Assess pain and discomfort using objective pain scale q4h PRN and after administration of pain medication. • Administer analgesics and monitor patient response. • Use nonpharmacological pain management techniques (e.g., music, distraction, touch) as adjunct to analgesics. • Maintain nasogastric tube patency. • Monitor nausea and vomiting. • Administer antiemetic as ordered.
Psychosocial Patient demonstrates decreased anxiety.	• Listen to patient's worries and fears. • Assess patient's response to anxiety. • Support effective coping behaviors. • Teach alternative behaviors for those that are not helpful. • Help patient increase sense of control by providing information and explanation. • Allow choices when possible. • Provide as much predictability in routine as possible.
Teaching/Discharge Planning Patient/significant others understand procedures and tests needed for treatment. Significant others understand the severity of the illness, ask appropriate questions, anticipate potential complications.	• Prepare patient/significant others for procedures such as paracentesis, pulmonary artery catheter insertion, or laboratory studies. • Explain the widespread effects of pancreatitis and the potential for complications such as sepsis or acute respiratory distress syndrome. • Encourage significant others to ask questions related to pathophysiology, monitoring, treatments, etc. • Instruct patient and family in discharge regimen that may include wound care, medications, and dietary limitations.

necessary in patients with severe gastric distention or a paralytic ileus. Patients with acute pancreatitis should be placed on NPO status until the abdominal pain subsides and serum amylase levels have returned to normal. Starting oral intake sooner can cause the abdominal pain to return and can induce further inflammation of the pancreas by stimulating the autodigestive disease process.

Nutritional Support
For those patients with acute pancreatitis who are being kept on prolonged NPO status with nasogastric

suction because of paralytic ileus, persistent abdominal pain, or pancreatic complications, nutritional support is recommended. TPN has been traditionally used because it was believed that stimulation of the pancreas by solid or liquid nutrients caused pancreatic stimulation and adversely affected the course of acute pancreatitis. Increasing evidence suggests that the use of enteral nutrition delivered past the ligament of Treitz to the distal duodenum or jejunum is safe. In addition, enteral nutrition may reduce infectious complications by maintaining intestinal barrier function and avoiding some of the complications of parental nutrition. Lipid administration is avoided to prevent increasing triglyceride levels, which can exacerbate the inflammatory process. In the patient with mild acute pancreatitis, oral fluids can usually be restarted within 3 to 7 days, with solid food introduced slowly and as tolerated. Supplementation with TPN is appropriate if oral and enteral nutrition cannot provide enough calories to prevent catabolism

Prolonged NPO status is often difficult for patients. Frequent mouth care and proper positioning of the nasogastric tube are important to maintain skin integrity and maximize patient comfort. Bed rest is prescribed to decrease the patient's basal metabolic rate; this, in turn, decreases the stimulation of pancreatic secretions.

Surgical Management

Surgery for acute pancreatitis is indicated if massive pancreatic necrosis is present in a patient with a worsening clinical status. A pancreatic resection for acute necrotizing pancreatitis can be performed to prevent systemic complications of the disease process. In this procedure, dead or infected pancreatic tissue is surgically removed. In some cases, the entire pancreas is removed. Broad-spectrum antibiotics are given to patients who require surgical débridement of necrotic tissue.

• Hepatitis

ETIOLOGY

Diffuse inflammation of the liver, otherwise known as hepatitis, can be noninfectious or infectious in origin (Box 41-13). Acute hepatitis lasts less than 6 months; it either resolves completely with return of normal liver function or progresses to chronic hepatitis, then cirrhosis, and possibly liver failure. Chronic hepatitis is an inflammatory process that lasts longer than 6 months and may also progress to cirrhosis and possibly liver failure.

Noninfectious Hepatitis

Noninfectious hepatitis can be caused by excessive alcohol consumption, autoimmune disorders, metabolic or vascular disorders (including right-sided heart failure), acute biliary obstruction, and many individual drugs and drug classes (depending on the amount

---

Box 41-13 • Selected Causes of Hepatic Inflammation

Infectious Diseases
- Viral hepatitis (A, B, C, D, E)
- Epstein-Barr virus
- Cytomegalovirus
- Herpes simplex virus
- Coxsackievirus B
- Toxoplasmosis
- Adenovirus
- Varicella-zoster virus

Drugs and Toxins
- Alcohol
- Acetaminophen
- Isoniazid
- Salicylates
- Anticonvulsants
- Antimicrobials
- HMG-CoA reductase inhibitors
- α-Methyldopa
- Amiodarone
- Estrogens
- *Amanita phalloides* mushrooms
- Ecstasy (methylenedioxymethamphetamine)
- Herbal medicines (ginseng, comfrey tea, pennyroyal oil, *Teucrium polium*)

Autoimmune Diseases
- Autoimmune hepatitis
- Primary biliary cirrhosis
- Primary sclerosing cholangitis

Congenital Diseases
- Hemochromatosis (iron overload)
- Wilson's disease (copper deposition)
- α₁-Antitrypsin deficiency

Miscellaneous Causes
- Nonalcoholic fatty liver
- Fatty liver of pregnancy
- Severe right-sided congestive heart failure
- Budd-Chiari syndrome (vascular obstruction)

---

ingested and length of exposure). Examples include but are not limited to acetaminophen (both intentional and unintentional overdosing), isoniazid, HMG-CoA reductase inhibitors, anticonvulsants, antimicrobials, α-methyldopa, amiodarone, and estrogens.[41] Although only a minority of chronic alcohol abusers develop the syndrome of alcoholic hepatitis, severe cases carry a significant mortality rate of 60% within the first 4 weeks of diagnosis.[42]

Other liver toxins include poisonous mushrooms (*Amanita phalloides*), Ecstasy (methylenedioxymethamphetamine), and some herbal medicines (ginseng, comfrey tea, pennyroyal oil, and *Teucrium polium*).[43] Autoimmune hepatitis, a condition in which the patient's own immune system attacks the liver, causes inflammation and hepatocyte injury or death. Autoimmune hepatitis can be mistaken for an acute viral hepatitis if the patient presents with severe symptoms.

Infectious Hepatitis

Viral hepatitis is a highly contagious inflammatory condition. Just like noninfectious hepatitis, infectious hepatitis can be acute, or it can be chronic if infection lasts longer than 6 months. Viral infections of the liver parenchyma have been classified according to their specific infecting agent and corresponding serology markers. Hepatitis A, B, C, D, and E are summarized in Table 41-3. Other viral causes of hepatitis include herpes simplex virus (HSV), Epstein-Barr virus (EBV), cytomegalovirus (CMV), adenovirus, coxsackievirus B, and varicella-zoster virus (VZV). Typically patients with viral hepatitis present with nonspecific, flu-like symptoms such as malaise, nausea, vomiting, diarrhea, loss of appetite, mid-epigastric abdominal discomfort, and low-grade fever. In patients with hepatitis B virus (HBV), symptoms may be more severe.

Hepatitis A

In the United States, the Centers for Disease Control and Prevention (CDC) have reported a significant decline in the incidence of acute hepatitis A (HAV); the incidence of acute liver failure from HAV is considered low at an estimated 2,000 to 3,000 total cases per year, with a higher mortality rate in patients either older than 50 or younger than 5 years of age.[44-46] However, sporadic outbreaks continue to be reported due to consumption of contaminated food or direct person-to-person contact.[47] HAV is caused by an RNA enterovirus transmitted through the oral–fecal route, predominantly by ingestion of contaminated water or raw or partially cooked shellfish. In most patients, symptoms of HAV infection are either relatively mild or nonexistent, although older patients are at greater risk for more severe symptoms. The incubation period ranges from 15 to 45 days after exposure. HAV infection causes only acute liver disease; recovery is usually complete and does not lead to chronic hepatitis or cirrhosis. Blood tests usually reveal elevations in the aminotransferases (ALT and AST), bilirubin concentrations, and alkaline phosphatase level. In severe cases, the PT may be prolonged. Diagnosis can be made with serology antibody testing. Anti-HAV immunoglobulin G (IgG) antibodies provide immunity and can be found in people who have had a previous HAV infection, but these are not helpful in diagnosing an acute infection. Instead, a positive anti-HAV IgM serology marker indicates HAV infection within the preceding 6 months. HAV infection does not induce a carrier state.

Early in the course of the disease, there is an incubation period during which the patient is asymptomatic but highly contagious, particularly with high HAV levels in the stool. After symptoms are apparent, the hepatitis infection can be misdiagnosed because many of the symptoms are similar to those of the flu. Some patients seek medical attention because they become jaundiced. The two most common physical examination findings are jaundice and hepatomegaly. Acute symptoms can progress or disappear once jaundice is present. By the time symptoms occur, the virus is no longer shed in the stool, and the patient is usually not infectious. Recovery is signaled by liver function test results returning to normal.

After exposure to HAV, passive immunization can be achieved through the use of immune serum globulin. Most preparations of immune serum globulin

Table 41-3 • Summary of Types of Hepatitis

	Hepatitis A	Hepatitis B	Hepatitis C	Hepatitis D	Hepatitis E
Incubation (days)	15–45	30–180	15–160	30–180	14–60
Onset	Acute	Insidious	Insidious	Acute or insidious	Acute
Transmission	Fecal/oral Contaminated food, water	Blood Sexual Perinatal Percutaneous	Blood May be sexual	Blood Sexual (comorbid infection with HBV)	Fecal/oral Contaminated food, water
Severity	Mild	Often severe	Moderate	May be very severe	Virulent, especially in pregnant women
Prognosis	Generally good	Worse with age, debility	Moderate	Fair, worse with chronic disease	Good, unless pregnant
Diagnosis					
Acute	Anti-HAV IgM	HBsAG Anti-HBc (IgM) HBeAg	HCV ELISA Anti-HCV recombinant strip immunoblot assay (RIBA) HCV RNA	HDV Ag	Clinical
Chronic	—	Anti-HBc (IgG)	Anti-HCV	Anti-HDV	—
Prophylaxis (adults)	Immune globulin	Hepatitis B vaccine Immune globulin	?Immune globulin	None available	None available
Carrier	No	Yes	?	Yes	No

contain adequate quantities of anti-HAV and should be given within 2 weeks of exposure. The immune serum globulin may not entirely abort an infection, but it significantly ameliorates the symptoms. It is usually given to intimate contacts of patients with HAV. There are also two U.S. Food and Drug Administration (FDA)–approved vaccines, Havrix and Vaqta, for people 2 years of age and older. Vaccination is encouraged for all high-risk people, particularly children who live in states where the incidence of HAV between the years 1987 and 1997 was twice the national average (e.g., Arizona, Alaska, California, Idaho, Nevada, New Mexico, Oklahoma, Oregon, South Dakota, Utah, and Washington).[44] The intramuscular dosage is variable.

Hepatitis B

Hepatitis B virus (HBV) is a DNA virus of the Hepadnaviridae family that replicates by reverse transcription. Infection causes both acute and chronic hepatitis, and the incubation period is 30 to 180 days, with the average at 12 weeks. HBV is spread by contact with blood or blood products. The antigen has been identified in body secretions, such as semen, mucus, and saliva; sexual exposure to a person with HBV is the most common mode of transmission.[44] It appears that a break in the skin or the mucous membrane is necessary for the transmission to occur. HBV is also transmitted parenterally through blood transfusions, occupational needlestick injuries, and the use of contaminated needles (e.g., illicit drug use). Maternal perinatal transmission can also occur.

Incorrect interpretation of HBV serologic markers is common. Familiarity with the serology testing is important for the nurse who is assisting in the diagnostic evaluation of a suspected case of viral hepatitis to prevent inappropriate laboratory testing and patient discomfort. Hepatitis B surface antigen (HBsAg) is a protein that coats the outer surface of the HBV and is produced in great excess during viral replication. HBsAg is the single most important test to detect infection with HBV. A positive result indicates that a patient is infected with HBV. If the presence of HBsAg is associated with an acute illness and a marked rise in the aminotransferases as well as the presence of hepatitis B core IgM antibody (IgM anti-HBc), the patient has acute HBV. If HBsAg disappears from the blood within 6 months, there is resolution of infection, and the patient does not advance to chronic disease. Patients with acute HBV infection who overcome their infection and eradicate the virus develop antibodies against hepatitis B surface antigen (anti-HBs). In some laboratories, these results may be reported as hepatitis B surface antibody (HBsAb) instead of anti-HBs. Regardless of the nomenclature, these people are protected against future HBV infection. A person who receives the HBV vaccine also develops HBsAb. An acute HBV infection is also associated with elevated serum aminotransferase levels of 1,000 to 2,000 U/L, with ALT typically greater than AST, although peak ALT levels do not correlate with prognosis. Instead, the prolongation of the PT is the best indicator of prognosis.[48]

Acute HBV infection can lead to fulminant liver failure in less than 1% of cases, and this occurs within 4 weeks of the onset of symptoms. It is associated with encephalopathy, multiorgan failure, and a mortality rate of 80% if not treated with liver transplantation.[48] The likelihood of chronicity is inversely proportional to age; chronic active HBV is seen in 5% to 10% of the patients.[44] These patients continue to have high levels of HBsAg and can be infectious to others. Anti-hepatitis B core (anti-HBc), also called hepatitis B core antibody (HBcAb), also appears early in the course of infection and may persist for many years, but it is helpful in evaluating an acute versus chronic infection because anti-HBc can be further divided into two subtypes. Anti-HBc (IgM) is the initial response to infection and lasts for 6 to 18 months after recovery from infection. Therefore, high titers of anti-HBc (IgM) indicate the presence of acute infection, and low titers indicate chronic liver infection. Anti-HBc (IgG) is the second subtype and is positive in patients who are either chronically infected or previously infected, persisting in the bloodstream for a lifetime. Once an infection by HBV is established with HBsAg and anti-HBc, further serological testing can be ordered. For instance, the presence of the hepatitis Be antigen (HBeAg) indicates active viral replication and helps in diagnosing disease severity, prognosis, and treatment options. Those patients who have a positive HBeAg are considered highly infectious. The degree of liver impairment in chronic active hepatitis is variable from mild to serious and can progress to cirrhosis and hepatocellular carcinoma.[49] Cirrhosis should be suspected if the patient develops hypersplenism, hypoalbuminemia (in the absence of nephropathy), or prolongation of the PT. In advanced cirrhosis, serum AST level is typically higher than ALT levels.[48]

Clinical signs and symptoms of HBV infection during the acute phase are the same as those of HAV infection. Arthralgia, high fever, and rash are hallmark signs of HBV infection. However, there is a greater risk for the development of fulminant hepatic failure in patients with HBV infection, which is characterized by jaundice, hepatic encephalopathy, and rapidly deteriorating hepatic synthetic function.

HBV exposure is associated with high risk. After accidental exposure, such as an inadvertent needlestick, passive immunoprophylaxis can be achieved by using high anti-HBs titer hepatitis B immune globulin (HBIG). This is a pooled serum containing high titers of the anti-hepatitis B immune globulin. It is recommended that HBIG be given within 48 hours of postexposure as inoculations to high-risk patients, to close contacts of patients with active HBV (within 2 weeks after sexual or personal contact with infected body fluids), and to those traveling to endemic areas who do not have time to go through the normal three-dose vaccination series.[44]

Many new HBV nucleoside analog treatments are under review. The following six medications are currently approved by the FDA for the treatment of chronic HBV: interferon-α 2b (INF-α 2b), pegylated INF-α 2a, lamivudine, adefovir dipivoxil, entecavir, and recently, telbivudine.[50] Fortunately, a vaccine exists for active immunization against HBV (Recombivax-HB, Engerix-B). This vaccine, administered prophylactically over a 6-month period, provides active immunization against HBV. It is highly recommended for health care personnel at risk for infection with HBV. It is also recommended for people who have had intimate contacts with people already infected with HBV. Precautions to protect against exposure to blood-borne pathogens must be followed. In the United States, children are universally vaccinated against HBV.

Hepatitis C

Hepatitis C virus (HCV) has surpassed alcoholism to become the leading cause of liver cirrhosis and the leading cause of liver transplantation in the United States.[44] As diagnostic tests improved, HCV, formerly called non-A, non-B hepatitis, was identified in 1989. It is a single-stranded RNA virus related to the Flaviviridae family. In the one HCV serotype, there are at least six different genotypes (or expressions). These variations in genotype have led to variations in clinical course, problems with vaccine development, treatment response, and in many cases, duration of treatment.[51] In the United States, genotypes 1 and 4 make up 70% to 75% of people infected with HCV; genotypes 2 and 3 account for the remaining 25% to 30% of cases.[52] Although genotype does not predict outcome of infection, it does predict the likelihood of treatment response and, in many cases, determines the duration of treatment.[51]

HCV, a blood-borne virus, can cause both acute and chronic hepatitis. Of those people who develop acute HCV, chronicity can occur in as many 55% to 85%, and 5% to 20% reportedly develop cirrhosis over approximately 20 to 25 years.[51] People with HCV-related cirrhosis are at risk for developing end-stage liver disease (a risk of approximately 30% over 10 years) as well as hepatocellular carcinoma (a risk of approximately 1% to 2% per year).[51]

Before 1992, when testing for HCV was mandated, many people acquired HCV through blood transfusions. The main risk factors in the United States include shared contaminated needles from illicit drug use and occupational needlestick exposure. There are indications that the virus might also be transmitted through perinatal, sexual, and household contacts (e.g., sharing of razors and toothbrushes), although these modes of transmission are not as common. It has also been suggested that acupuncture, body piercing, tattooing, and even commercial barbering carry a risk for HCV transmission.[51] Incubation of HCV is 15 to 160 days, with an average of 7 weeks. Within 6 months of infection, patients may produce anti–hepatitis C antibodies, but these do not confer immunity.

Although most patients are asymptomatic, the most commonly reported symptoms of HCV infection include fatigue, anorexia, weight loss, and abdominal pain. Diagnostic evaluation for HCV infection includes an HCV enzyme-linked immunosorbent assay (ELISA; ordered when the aminotransferase levels are elevated and for screening patients on hemodialysis), an anti-HCV recombinant strip immunoblot assay (RIBA; ordered to confirm a positive HCV test or if a patient presents with symptoms of hepatitis), or an HCV RNA test (ordered when HCV RIBA findings are indeterminate, but there remains a high index of suspicion for HCV). HCV RNA, which tests for the presence of the virus RNA in the blood (rather than antibodies against the virus), is the gold standard for detecting HCV. HCV RNA levels are used to gauge response to treatment, but they are not serially checked because viral load has no correlation to the degree or rate of liver injury progression.[53]

HCV is the leading cause of death from liver disease in the United States, but it is rarely diagnosed as the acute infection.[51] The goal of treatment is virus eradication and prevention or delay of cirrhosis and end-stage liver disease. Patients who develop end-stage liver disease may be candidates for liver transplantation.[53,54]

Currently, no vaccine is available to prevent HCV, and immune globulin does not afford protection to people who have been exposed. Current combination therapy consists of pegylated INF-α 2a or 2b plus ribavirin. Infection is considered eradicated when there is a sustained viral response (SVR), which is defined as the absence of HCV RNA (aviremia) at the end of treatment and then 6 months after treatment. Genotypes 1 and 4 are considered the most difficult strains to treat; they require a longer duration of treatment (48 weeks) and have a lower post-treatment SVR rate (40%) compared with genotypes 2 and 3. Genotypes 2 and 3 require a shorter duration of treatment (24 weeks) and have a higher SVR rate of 79% to 82%.[44,49,53,55,56] These treatment variations highlight the importance of genotyping to determine who may benefit from combination therapy and optimal treatment duration.

Hepatitis D

Hepatitis D (delta virus or HDV) is an incomplete RNA virus that depends on HBV envelope proteins to reproduce. HDV infection may occur as a superinfection in the patient who has chronic HBV, or it may occur simultaneously with an acute HBV infection. HDV can progress to fulminant hepatitis and chronic disease. In the United States, HDV infection occurs primarily among people receiving multiple transfusions and those abusing illicit IV drugs. Early in the disease, the hepatitis D antigen (HDV Ag) is present in the blood. Later in the disease, antibodies to the HDV are present (anti-HDV).

Because this disease coexists with HBV, patients with HDV have symptoms similar to those of acute or chronic HBV, but symptoms may be more pronounced. Quantitative real-time polymerase chain reactions (PCR) assays for HDV RNA are monitored at 3 and 6 months. Current treatment includes standard INF, and recent research suggests that pegylated INF-α 2b may improve SVR. The addition of ribavirin has not shown to provide any additional benefit.[49,57] Vaccination against HBV also protects against HDV infection.[44]

Hepatitis E

Hepatitis E virus (HEV) is a single-stranded RNA virus similar to HAV. It is transmitted by the oral–fecal route from contaminated water and food. In some cases, the source of infection has been traced to contact with infected animals or animal products, notably swine.[49] The incubation period is 14 to 60 days, and it has an overall low mortality rate among the general population.[58] HEV has been implicated in epidemics in Asia (Afghanistan, Bangladesh, Burma [Myanmar], China, India, Indonesia, Kazakhstan, Kyrgyzstan, Malaysia, Mongolia, Nepal, Pakistan, Tajikistan, Turkmenistan, and Uzbekistan), Mexico, the Middle East, Northern Africa, and sub-Saharan Africa. No outbreaks have occurred in Europe, the United States, Australia, or South America.[58] For reasons that are still unclear, pregnant women with HEV infection have died more often and had more obstetric complications and worse fetal outcomes than women with other forms of viral hepatitis.[59] Because the incidence of HEV infection is less than 1% in the United States, the nurse should pay careful attention if a patient presents with symptoms of hepatitis and has recently traveled or lived in endemic areas. Unfortunately, previous HEV infection is not necessarily protective.

Hepatitis F and Hepatitis G

It was formerly believed that a virus isolated from rare blood samples was a newly identified virus, labeled hepatitis F. However, further investigation has found this virus to be a variant of HCV, and additional research has failed to demonstrate the existence of a new virus. Little is known about the most recently identified virus, hepatitis G (HGV), which has been identified with PCR testing. It is a single-stranded enveloped RNA virus similar to HCV. As with HBV and HCV, HGV is transmitted by blood and body fluids; infection is diagnosed by seroconversion of HGV RNA in blood or liver tissue. No vaccine has been developed against HGV, and current treatment is supportive and focused on symptom management. Infection is considered benign and is rarely associated with elevated liver function tests.[44]

PATHOPHYSIOLOGY

To improve patient outcomes, nurses must have a solid knowledge base regarding the underlying pathophysiology, assessment, and management of acute and chronic liver disease. Hepatocytes, the functional cells of the liver, perform many essential functions, including the metabolism of nutrients (e.g., glucose, proteins, lipids, vitamins) and the detoxification of medications, alcohol, ammonia, toxins, and hormones. In addition, hepatocytes are responsible for synthesis of clotting factors, conjugation and secretion of bilirubin, and synthesis of bile salts. Abnormal liver function is usually not apparent unless a significant acute insult occurs or chronic liver disease is fairly advanced. Liver failure occurs when there is a loss of 60% of the hepatocytes, and symptoms are usually detectable after 75% or more of the hepatocytes are injured or killed. Liver function testing and evaluation begin with a complete history and physical examination. Interpretation of liver serum enzymes, synthetic function, and cholestasis (or excretory function) tests are important for the nurse to understand and are discussed later in this chapter.

Acute liver disease, typically caused by viral or chemical insults, occurs suddenly and resolves, becomes chronic, or results in a patient's death. Chronic liver disease leading to cirrhosis, typically more insidious in nature, is the 12th leading cause of death in the United States.[60] Disease processes in the liver can affect the hepatocytes, the blood vessels, and the Kupffer cells, which are responsible for uptake and subsequent degradation of foreign and potentially harmful substances in the body. If the injury is mild and reversible, hepatocytes may regenerate, and liver function may return to normal. However, if the injury is more severe or sustained, regeneration may be incomplete, or the healing process may cause fibrosis. Fibrotic changes alter the liver architecture and can lead to cirrhosis and impediment of blood flow through the liver. An acute insult to the liver can progress to fulminant liver failure, which is defined as hepatic encephalopathy occurring within 8 weeks of jaundice. Hepatic encephalopathy is a state of abnormal mental functioning as a result of the inability of the liver to remove ammonia and other toxins from the blood. If liver function does not return and liver transplantation is unavailable, fulminant liver failure can progress to cerebral edema, coma, and death from brain herniation.

ASSESSMENT

History

Questions regarding the patient's alcohol consumption and illicit drug use, use of prescription and over-the-counter medications, use of herbal supplements, surgical and transfusion history, occupational or travel exposure history, and sexual history may be helpful in determining the diagnosis, nursing plan of care, and teaching needs of the patient. In chronic hepatitis, most patients are asymptomatic except for mildly elevated liver enzymes. Constitutional symptoms vary widely but typically include malaise, fatigue, low-grade fever, nausea, vomiting, and sometimes diarrhea.

Physical Examination

When cirrhosis and portal hypertension resulting from chronic hepatitis are present, jaundice (yellow staining of the skin and mucous membranes as a result of bilirubin pigments) may be noted. Hepatomegaly (enlargement of the liver) may result in right upper quadrant tenderness and is a result of portal hypertension or congestion in the liver from altered blood flow due to cirrhosis. The liver edge is often firm and nodular. In advanced cirrhosis, although the left lobe may be enlarged, overall liver size is often decreased and difficult to palpate. Dullness of percussion over the liver span can provide serial observations of resolution of hepatitis or progression of cirrhosis. Splenomegaly as a result of portal hypertension and sequestration of fluid in the spleen may result in left upper quadrant tenderness. Muscle wasting and abdominal ascites may develop as a result of malnutrition, portal hypertension, and hypoalbuminemia due to the liver's impaired ability to synthesize proteins. Peripheral edema may result from hypoalbuminemia, sodium retention, and ascites obstructing blood return from the lower extremities. Vitamin deficiencies may result in glossitis of the tongue and cheilosis of the lips. Bruising and bleeding tendencies may develop as a result of impaired production of clotting factors and sequestration of platelets in the spleen. Other manifestations include telangiectasis or spider nevi (usually of the upper half of the body). These lesions consist of a pulsating arteriole from which smaller vessels radiate. Palmar erythema, or redness of the palms, is a result of increased blood flow from hyperdynamic cardiac dysfunction associated with hepatitis (with ascites). In men, there may be a loss of body hair, testicular atrophy, and gynecomastia. These changes are thought to be related to altered hormone metabolism and estrogen excess in the liver.

Physical examination may also reveal abdominal wall vein dilation around the umbilicus, known as caput medusae. This is the result of portal hypertension and congestion and collateral vessel development (Fig. 41-4). This congestion may be auscultated

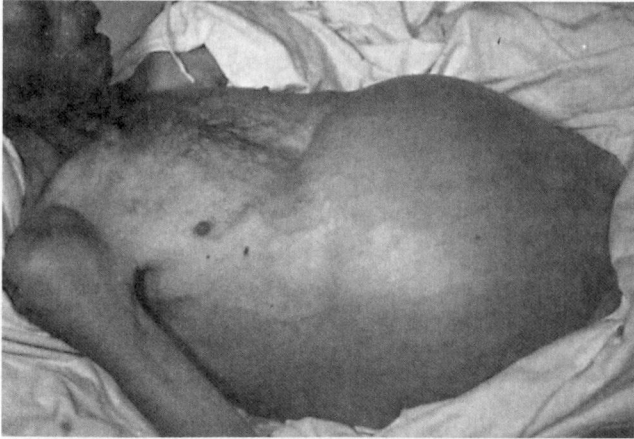
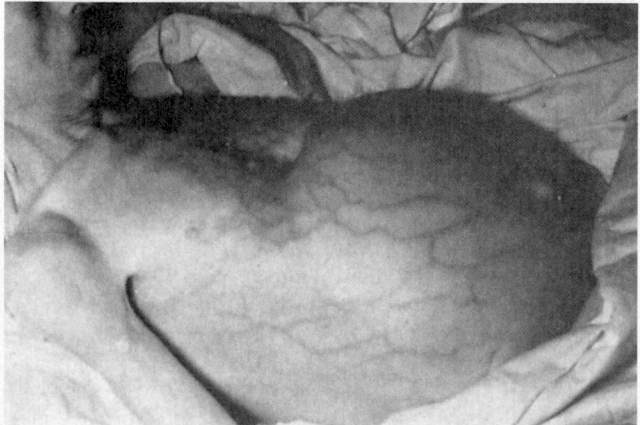

Figure 41-4 • Collateral abdominal veins on the anterior abdominal wall in a patient with alcoholic liver disease as recorded by black and white photography (*top*) and infrared photography (*bottom*). (From Schiff L: Diseases of the Liver. Philadelphia: JB Lippincott, 1982).

as an arterial bruit (systolic phase) or a venous hum (both systolic and diastolic phases) over the liver and epigastrium. Encephalopathy, ascites, and peripheral edema, reflective of advanced disease, may be present. Other observable assessment findings include frothy, dark amber urine and clay-colored stools as a result of alterations in bilirubin excretion. Common signs and symptoms of noninfectious and infectious hepatitis are summarized in Table 41-4. Patients with signs and symptoms of hepatic decompensation (e.g., portal hypertension, ascites, encephalopathy, and coagulopathy) should be hospitalized, evaluated, and treated more expeditiously than those patients who demonstrate adequate hepatic compensation and stability.

Laboratory Studies

Tests for Evaluating Hepatocellular Injury
The clinical significance of any liver chemistry must be evaluated in the context of the patient's history and clinical situation. Liver function tests (LFTs) is a commonly used but inaccurate term. Some laboratory tests do measure liver synthetic function, and these include albumin, PT, and total bilirubin. However, other laboratory tests are markers of hepatocellular injury and include AST (aspartate aminotransferase), previously known as SGOT (serum glutamic oxaloacetic transaminase), and ALT (alanine aminotransferase), previously known as SGPT (serum glutamic pyruvic transaminase).

ALT and AST are enzymes present inside the hepatocytes. When hepatocytes are injured or die, they release AST and ALT into the serum. Therefore, the presence of these enzymes in the blood signals the presence of hepatocyte injury. However, AST and ALT lack sensitivity (for a particular diagnosis) in evaluating chronic liver injury for two reasons. First, AST and ALT are also found (to a lesser degree) in the skeletal muscle, and as such, elevations may be related to a skeletal muscle injury or overexertion. This is particularly true for AST because ALT is almost exclusively present in hepatocytes and is the most specific test for hepatocellular damage. Second, it is thought that dying hepatocytes synthesize less AST and ALT enzymes than healthy ones. Therefore, despite inflammation detected on a liver biopsy, patients with chronic hepatitis may have relatively normal levels of AST and ALT.

Despite these difficulties in laboratory interpretation, elevations of AST and ALT are often helpful in evaluating acute liver injury, response to treatment, and monitoring those at risk for liver disease because of medical interventions. Elevations of these enzymes suggest hepatocyte death and the degree of elevation roughly approximates the amount of liver cell death. AST and ALT elevate at relatively equal levels, but an exception occurs in alcoholic hepatitis, in which AST levels tend to be higher than ALT levels. Although the AST/ALT ratio is not diagnostic, a ratio greater than 2:1 is suggestive of alcohol-induced injury, and a ratio of 3:1 increases the likelihood even more.[61–63] This is thought to be due to the depletion of vitamin B_6 (pyridoxine) in patients with chronic alcoholism;

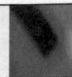

Table 41-4 • Common Signs and Symptoms of Hepatitis

Signs and Symptoms	Cause
Constitutional	
Fever, chills	Immune response to viral infection
Generalized weakness, malnutrition	Inability to metabolize nutrients
Gastrointestinal	
Right upper quadrant pain	Hepatomegaly
Left upper quadrant pain	Splenomegaly
Loss of appetite	Ascites, fatigue
Abdominal distention	Ascites
Nausea, vomiting/hematemesis	Portal hypertension
Clay-colored feces	Inability to excrete conjugated bilirubin
Diarrhea	Impaired fat metabolism
Melena, hematochezia	Portal hypertension
Pulmonary	
Shortness of breath	Ascites, decreased lung and diaphragmatic expansion
Increased work of breathing	
Decreased oxygen saturation	
Decreased partial pressure of oxygen	
Cardiac	
Increased heart rate	Hypotension, sequestration of fluid in the liver and spleen, third-spacing in the peripheral
Decreased blood pressure	extremities from decreased protein metabolism/low albumin levels
Dysrhythmias	Electrolyte disturbances
Peripheral edema	Impaired protein metabolism
Neurological	
Headache	Impaired metabolism of ammonia and other circulating toxins
Depression/irritability	
Asterixis	
Genitourinary	
Decreased urinary output	Decreased circulating volume and impaired glomerular filtration rate
Frothy, dark amber urine	Excretion of conjugated bilirubin (water-soluble bile)
Integumentary	
Jaundice	Impaired excretion of bile
Pruritus, dry skin	Impaired excretion of bile
Bruising, ecchymosis	Impaired ability to synthesize clotting factors
Spider nevi, caput medusae	Portal hypertension
Palmar erythema	Portal hypertension
Hair loss	Impaired metabolism of circulating hormones
Endocrine	
Hypoglycemia	Impaired glucose metabolism and storage
Increased weight	Ascites, third-spacing of fluid
Gynecomastia, testicular atrophy (in men)	Inability to metabolize hormones (e.g., estrogens)
Immune	
Infection, spontaneous bacterial peritonitis	Impaired Kupffer cell function, splenomegaly

ALT synthesis is more strongly inhibited by pyridoxine deficiency than AST synthesis. In chronic hepatitis, AST and ALT levels are usually less than 10 times normal. However, in acute viral, toxin-induced, or ischemic hepatitis, these elevations may be greater than 1,000 U/L. In addition, alcoholic hepatitis causes smaller elevations (<300 U/L). Unfortunately, AST and ALT levels have low prognostic value.

Tests for Evaluating Liver Synthetic Function

As mentioned earlier, albumin, total protein, and PT are measures of actual liver synthetic function. Because proteins are synthesized by the liver, albumin and other proteins are an index of liver function. Albumin is the predominant protein in the serum; patients with advanced liver disease and cirrhosis tend to

have low serum concentrations (hypoalbuminemia). Because albumin is responsible for colloid osmotic pressure, low concentrations lead to leakage of intravascular fluids into interstitial spaces and peripheral edema. Because albumin levels are also influenced by poor nutrition and renal disease, care must be taken when interpreting laboratory test results.

The PT is a measure of the liver's capacity to synthesize clotting factors. The liver synthesizes blood clotting factors II, V, VII, IX, and X. An elevation in PT values is not seen until more than 80% of hepatocyte function is lost. However, because of the short half-life of factor VII, a PT is helpful in evaluating acute liver failure. Evaluation for vitamin K deficiency is performed because malabsorption or poor nutritional intake must be excluded in a patient who is hypoprothrombinemic. Failure of improvement in a PT level after vitamin K supplementation (5 to 10 mg orally for 3 days) may indicate intrinsic liver disease.

Tests for Evaluating Cholestasis (Excretory Function)

Tests for cholestasis (lack of bile flow) help determine what is happening in the bile ducts. Obstruction of bile flow may be extrahepatic (e.g., gallstones, post-surgical stricture, or malignancy) or intrahepatic (e.g., poor hepatocyte function or damage to the small septal or intralobular bile ducts). Present in the biliary epithelium, elevated alkaline phosphatase and γ-glutamyltransferase (GGT) levels reflect damage to the bile ducts or obstruction of bile flow.

An elevated serum bilirubin level is roughly proportional to the amount of liver dysfunction or disease severity. Bilirubin is the major source of hemoglobin metabolism from the destruction of adult RBCs. The unconjugated (indirect) form of bilirubin is not water soluble and is bound to albumin as a means of transport to the liver for conjugation and subsequent excretion in the bile. In the hepatocytes, unconjugated bilirubin is combined with glucuronic acid to make it water soluble (or conjugated) for excretion into the bile and feces. Cholestasis causes reflux of conjugated bilirubin into the blood (a condition called conjugated hyperbilirubinemia), so the conjugated bilirubin is instead excreted through the kidneys. The urine becomes frothy and very dark amber in color from bilirubin pigments. The nurse may be asked to perform a dipstick test on the urine for bilirubin to confirm this clinical suspicion. Unconjugated hyperbilirubinemia results from a poor nutritional state (e.g., decreased albumin available for transport of bilirubin to the liver) or hepatocyte dysfunction in the conjugation process. Jaundice is usually present when the serum bilirubin level is greater than 2 to 3 mg/dL.

MANAGEMENT

The primary treatment of acute hepatitis of any type is primarily supportive. Measures include providing rest and adequate nutrition and preventing further liver injury by the avoidance of hepatotoxic medications and substances. Hospitalization is rarely required but is needed in cases of disease complicated by hemodynamic instability, failure to maintain adequate nutrition and fluid intake, encephalopathy, blood coagulopathies, and renal failure.

In situations of hemodynamic instability, monitoring of blood pressure, heart rate, cardiac dysrhythmias, and urine output is essential. IV fluids will most likely need to be provided. It is important to avoid lactated Ringer's solutions because of the inability of the impaired liver to metabolize lactate, which could induce or exacerbate a metabolic acidosis. Frequent monitoring of hepatic enzymes and synthetic function is requested to evaluate disease progression and response to treatment interventions. Electrolyte, nutrient, and vitamin abnormalities from disease progression, malnutrition, and nausea

and vomiting require repletion. The nurse may have to assist in invasive treatments or procedures, such as placement of a Sengstaken-Blakemore tube for control of bleeding esophageal varices, paracentesis for ascites, and liver biopsy. In the event of fluid volume overload, diuretics, albumin, and protein supplements may be prescribed. Accurate intake and output, daily weight, and abdominal girth measurements may alert the nurse to significant volume shifts and potential hemodynamic or respiratory issues.

Maintaining adequate nutrition is a priority. Small, frequent meals and antiemetics are administered as needed. A high-calorie, low-protein diet is recommended to prevent complications associated with impaired protein and ammonia metabolism associated with acute hepatic encephalopathy. However, a low-protein diet is used only in the short term because seriously ill patients actually have increased protein requirements to build and maintain muscle mass and to assist in healing and repair. Parenteral nutrition is needed only if oral intake is impaired by intractable nausea and vomiting. Patients with severe fatigue require frequent rest and spacing of activities.

Because of the risk for coagulopathy, the nurse must monitor for bleeding gums, epistaxis, ecchymosis, petechiae, hematemesis, hematuria, and melena. Vitamin K may be prescribed to help reduce the effects of bleeding tendencies, and a PT may be ordered to monitor the efficacy of treatment.

Avoidance of alcohol, narcotics, barbiturates, and medications that are metabolized by the liver is recommended. Careful observation and documentation of patient responses (e.g., mental status, level of consciousness) to medications and treatment regimens is recommended. Because of the liver's inability to metabolize or detoxify many foods, drugs, and toxins, the nurse may be asked to administer frequent medications such as lactulose, neomycin sulfate, and metronidazole to treat hepatic encephalopathy. Lactulose is a laxative that acidifies the colon to prevent the absorption of ammonia. The dose of lactulose is titrated so that the patient has two to three soft stools per day without diarrhea. Neomycin and metronidazole act as antibiotics to clear the colon of bacteria that produce ammonia.

If severe pruritus from jaundice is present, a bile salt sequestering agent (e.g., cholestyramine), a topical emollient, or both can be used to help alleviate this symptom. Mittens may need to be used to prevent excessive scratching and subsequent skin breakdown in a confused patient.

Patient teaching for the patient with hepatitis includes measures to prevent infection and transmission, dietary limitations and alcohol avoidance, and the necessity for follow-up care. The patient is advised to monitor activity tolerance and fatigue. If signs and symptoms persist and liver enzymes remain elevated for greater than 6 months, the patient will progress to chronic disease. This is more common in HBV and HCV infection and is confirmed by liver biopsy.

• Complications of Liver Disease

Complications of advanced liver disease include cirrhosis, hepatic encephalopathy, hepatorenal syndrome, spontaneous bacterial peritonitis, and hepatocellular carcinoma.

CONCEPTS in action ANIMATION CIRRHOSIS

Etiology

In the United States, chronic HCV infection and alcohol abuse are the most common causes of liver cirrhosis.[44] However, cirrhosis of the liver can result from a number of other diseases, which include but are not limited to nonalcoholic steatohepatitis, hereditary hemochromatosis, Wilson's disease, and α_1-antitrypsin deficiency.

Pathophysiology

Cirrhosis, which develops over time, can cause severe alterations in the structural architecture of the liver and function of the hepatocytes. These changes are characterized by inflammation and liver cell necrosis, which can be focal or diffuse. Necrosis is followed by regeneration of liver tissue but not in a normal fashion. Fibrous tissue and regenerative nodules develop over time, which distorts the normal architecture of the liver lobule and alters blood flow. These fibrotic changes are irreversible, resulting in chronic liver dysfunction and eventual liver failure. Fatty deposits in the parenchymal cells may be seen initially. The cause of the fatty changes is unclear, but it may be a response to alterations in enzymatic function responsible for normal fat metabolism. Eventually, all of the liver's metabolic processes are altered.

Inflammation, fibrotic changes, and increased intrahepatic vascular resistance cause compression of the liver lobule, leading to increased resistance or obstruction of normal blood flow through the liver, which is normally a low-pressure system. This portal hypertension results in significant venous congestion and dilation (Fig. 41-5). Subsequently, nutrient-rich blood from the GI tract is shunted away from the liver, the first site of metabolism for many nutrients, drugs, and toxins. Pressure builds up in the systemic venous circulation, causing congestion where the portal and systemic venous systems connect: the esophagus, stomach, and rectum. These vascular changes result in varicose veins, or varices. Esophageal varices and gastric varices are of particular concern in the care of these patients because they are extremely friable. Rupture from these varices can result in massive internal bleeding that may be life-threatening. Portal hypertension also promotes increased collateral circulation and allows blood to flow from the intestines directly to the vena cava. This congestion

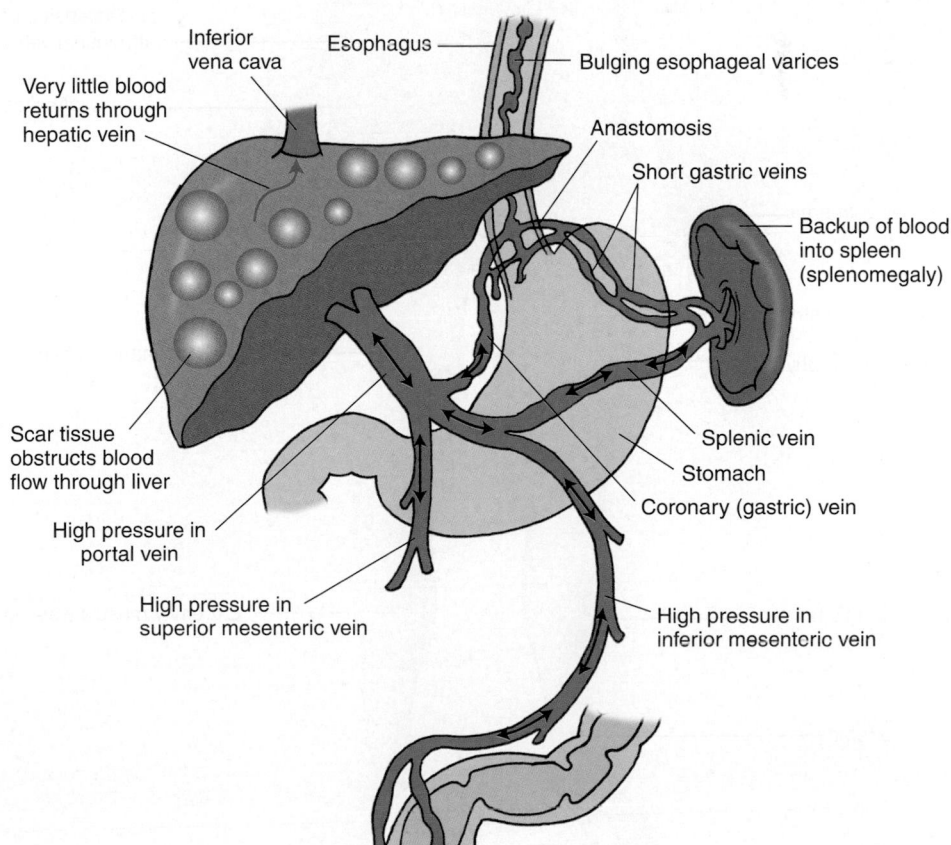

Figure 41-5 • Esophageal varices develop from increased portal pressure. In an attempt to return blood to the systemic circulation, collateral veins develop to bypass increased portal resistance. These collateral vessels become tortuous and distended and are called varices.

is often seen as a collection of prominent vessels on the surface of the abdomen and is known as caput medusae. Splenomegaly results from the sequestration of trapped blood from portal hypertension. Of particular concern is the trapping of platelets, which can be seen clinically by bleeding tendencies and a thrombocytopenia on laboratory evaluation. Frank hematemesis or bleeding from esophageal and gastric varices can cause melena. Hemorrhoidal varices, or hemorrhoids, can also result from portal hypertension. Finally, portal hypertension may result in

abdominal fluid accumulation, known as ascites. As liver disease progresses and cirrhosis develops, mild to moderate high-output cardiac dysfunction may occur. This hyperdynamic dysfunction is characterized by splanchnic and systemic vasodilation, an afterload effect that decreases cardiac work and elevates cardiac output. Clinically, it is seen as hypotension, tachycardia, and cardiac flow murmurs. As hepatic cirrhosis progresses, these clinical findings become more pronounced. Figure 41-6 illustrates clinical effects of cirrhosis.

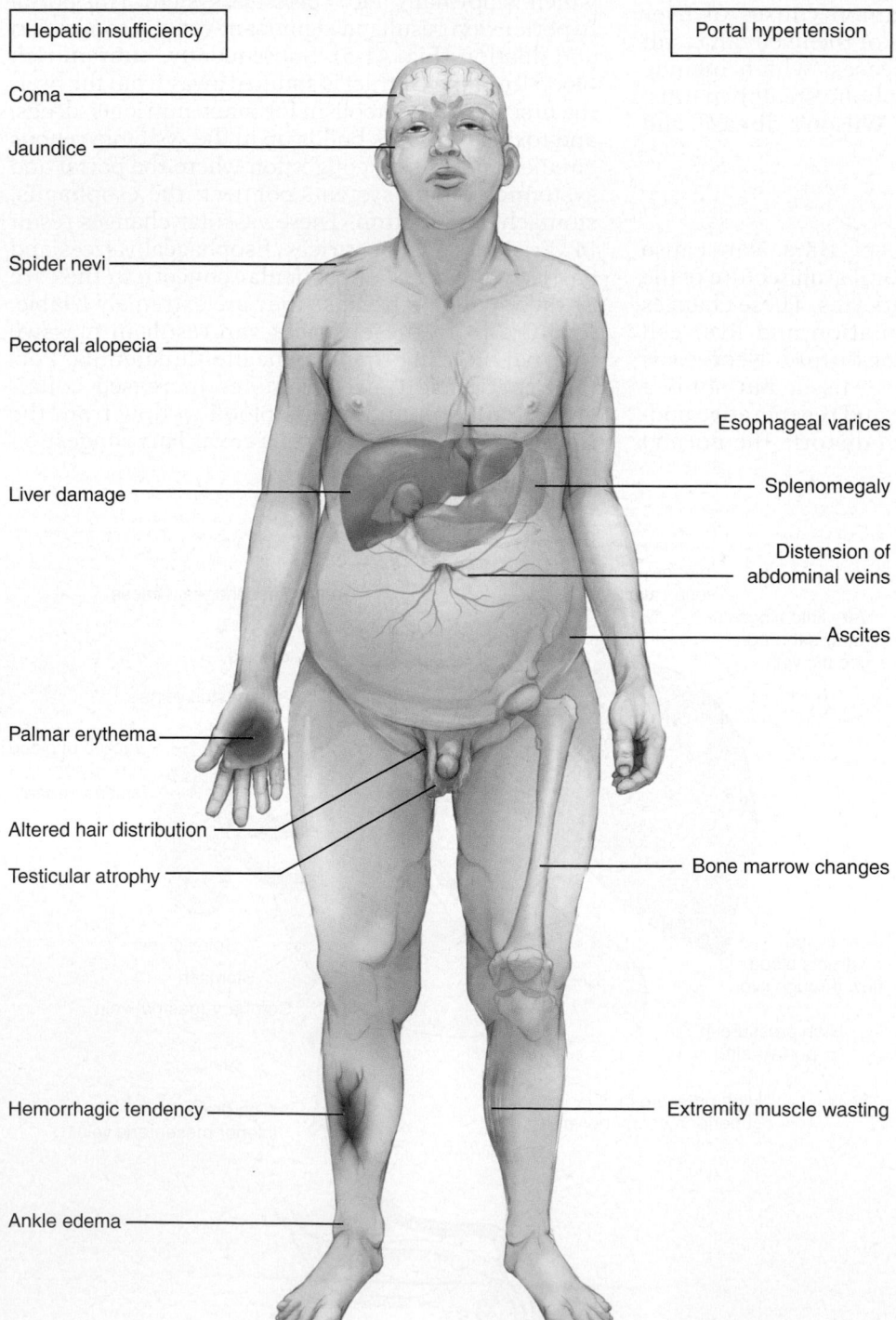

Hepatic insufficiency

- Coma
- Jaundice
- Spider nevi
- Pectoral alopecia
- Liver damage
- Palmar erythema
- Altered hair distribution
- Testicular atrophy
- Hemorrhagic tendency
- Ankle edema

Portal hypertension

- Esophageal varices
- Splenomegaly
- Distension of abdominal veins
- Ascites
- Bone marrow changes
- Extremity muscle wasting

Figure 41-6 • Clinical effects of cirrhosis of the liver. (From Bullock BL: Pathophysiology: Adaptations and Alterations in Function, 4th ed. Philadelphia: Lippincott-Raven, 1996.)

Assessment

In some patients, cirrhosis may be subclinical. However, history and physical examination findings may reveal clues to altered liver function. For example, altered carbohydrate metabolism can result in unstable blood sugars. Altered fat metabolism can cause fatigue and decreased activity tolerance. Altered protein metabolism results in a decreased synthesis of albumin. Albumin is necessary for colloid osmotic pressure, which holds fluid in the intravascular space. A decrease leads to interstitial tissue edema and decreased plasma volume. Globulin, another protein, is essential for normal blood clotting. This, coupled with a decreased synthesis of many blood clotting factors and decreased metabolism of vitamins and iron, predisposes the patient to hematological complications that range from bruising to hemorrhage. A low-grade DIC also may develop. Portal hypertension, ascites, and lower extremity edema cause hypotension. Initially, the patient may have flushed skin and bounding pulses from the vasodilation in the portal venous system, which leads to a hyperdynamic state with peripheral circulation vasodilation and hypotension. Table 41-5 summarizes laboratory findings in patients with cirrhosis and impending liver failure.

Management

Management goals include the prevention of additional stress on liver function and early recognition and treatment of complications. Liver functions under stress include nutritional metabolism, clearing medication and metabolic waste products, and formation of clotting factors. Interventions include monitoring nutritional markers and providing nutrition; moni-

toring fluid balance, urinary output, electrolyte and chemistry studies, drug type, and dose requirements; monitoring bleeding times, platelet function, and hematocrit; and detecting signs of bleeding (Box 41-14). Bowel cleansing regimens may be ordered. The early recognition of complications includes detecting signs of impending liver failure: changes in neurological and mental status, increasing ascites, and hepatorenal syndrome.

The critically ill patient in liver failure is often in some state of unconsciousness, with jaundiced skin and sclera. Coagulation times are prolonged, so bleeding is apt to occur from many sources. There is a risk for sores and skin breakdown because of the patient's debilitated state.

Maintaining fluid and electrolyte balance requires ongoing nursing assessment. Imbalance can result from replacement therapy, malnutrition, gastric suction, diuretics, vomiting, diaphoresis, ascites, diarrhea, inadequate fluid intake, and elevated aldosterone levels. The patient may complain of headache, weakness, numbness and tingling of extremities, muscle twitching, thirst, nausea, or muscle cramps and may become confused. The nurse is asked to monitor weight and CVP trends to help determine fluid retention and vascular loading. Other assessment clues to monitor include any increase or decrease in urinary output, cardiac dysrhythmias, changes in mental status or level of consciousness, prolonged vomiting or frequent liquid stools, muscle tremors, spasms, edema, or poor skin turgor.

Impaired handling of salt and water by the kidney and other abnormalities in fluid homeostasis predispose the patient to ascites, an accumulation of fluid in the peritoneum. This complication can be problematic because it can restrict movement of the diaphragm,

Table 41-5 • Laboratory Studies for Hepatic Injury and Function

Parameter	Normal	Increased	Decreased
Hepatocellular Injury			
ALT	5–35 IU/L	Acute viral hepatitis (ALT > AST)	Vitamin B deficiency
AST	5–40 IU/L	Biliary tract obstruction	
		Alcoholic hepatitis (AST > ALT)	
		Ischemia or hypoxia ("shock liver")	
		Drug toxicity	
		Right-sided heart failure	
		Liver cancer	
Liver Synthetic Function			
Albumin	3.4–4.7 g/dL	Dehydration, shock	Chronic liver disease, malnutrition, malabsorption
Total protein	6.0–8.0 g/dL		
PT	11–15 sec	Liver disease	N/A
International normalized ratio (INR)	0.8–1.2 sec	Vitamin K deficiency	
		Anticoagulants	
Cholestasis or Excretory Function			
Total bilirubin	0.2–1.3 mg/dL	Viral hepatitis	N/A
Conjugated (direct)	0.1–0.3 mg/dL	Alcoholic hepatitis	
Unconjugated (indirect)	0.2–0.7 mg/dL	Obstructive jaundice	
Alkaline phosphatase	30–115 IU/L	Primary biliary cirrhosis	
GGT	9–85 U/L		

N/A, not applicable.

Box 41-14 • COLLABORATIVE CARE GUIDE for the Patient With Cirrhosis and Impending Liver Failure

OUTCOMES	INTERVENTIONS
Oxygenation/Ventilation The patient's arterial blood gases will be within normal limits. The patient has no evidence of pulmonary edema or atelectasis. Breath sounds are clear bilaterally.	• Monitor pulse oximetry and arterial blood gases, respiratory rate and pattern, and ability to clear secretions. • Validate significant changes in pulse oximetry with co-oximetry arterial saturation measurement. • Assist patient to turn, cough, deep breathe, and use incentive spirometer q2h. • Provide chest percussion with postural drainage if indicated q4h. • Monitor effect of ascites on respiratory effort and lung compliance. • Position on side and with head of bed elevated to improve diaphragmatic movement.
Circulation/Perfusion Patient will achieve or maintain stable blood pressure and oxygen delivery. Serum lactate will be within normal limits. Patient will not experience bleeding related to coagulopathies, varices, hepatorenal syndrome.	• Monitor vital signs, including cardiac output, systemic vascular resistance, oxygen delivery, and oxygen consumption. • Monitor lactate daily until it is within normal limits. • Administer red blood cells, positive inotropic agents, colloid infusion as ordered to increase oxygen delivery. • Monitor prothrombin time, partial thromboplastin time, complete blood count daily. • Assess for signs of bleeding (e.g., blood in gastric contents, stools or urine); observe for petechiae, bruising. • Administer blood products as indicated. • Assist with insertion and manage the esophageal tamponade balloon tube. • Perform gastric lavage as needed.

Fluids/Electrolytes
Patient is euvolemic.
Patient will not gain weight due to fluid retention.
	• Daily weights.
	• Monitor intake and output.
	• Monitor electrolyte values.
	• Measure abdominal girth daily at the same location on the abdomen.
	• Monitor signs of volume overload:
	    Cardiac gallop
	    Pulmonary crackles
	    Shortness of breath
	    Jugular vein distention
	    Peripheral edema
	• Administer diuretics as ordered.

Mobility/Safety Patient is alert and oriented. Ammonia level is within normal limits. Patient achieves or maintains ability to conduct activities of daily living and mobilize self. No evidence of infection, WBC within normal limits.	• Assess serum ammonia level. • Administer lactulose as ordered. • Monitor level of consciousness, orientation, thought processing. • Assess asterixis. • Take precautions to prevent falls. • Consult physical therapist. • Conduct range-of-motion and strengthening exercises. • Monitor systemic inflammatory response syndrome criteria: increased WBC, increased temperature, tachypnea, tachycardia. • Use aseptic technique during procedures and monitor others.

(continued)

Box 41-14 • COLLABORATIVE CARE GUIDE for the Patient With Cirrhosis and Impending Liver Failure (Continued)

OUTCOMES	INTERVENTIONS
	• Maintain invasive catheter tube sterility.
	• Change invasive catheters, culture blood, line tips, or fluids, provide site care, etc., according to hospital protocol.
Skin Integrity Skin will remain intact.	• Assess skin q8h and each time patient is repositioned. • Turn q2h. Assist or teach patient to shift weight or reposition. • Consider pressure relief/reduction mattress.
Nutrition Caloric and nutrient intake meet metabolic requirements per calculation (e.g., basal energy expenditure).	• Provide nutrition by oral, enteral, or parenteral feeding. • Sodium, protein, fat, or fluid restriction may be necessary. • Consult dietitian or nutritional support service to evaluate nutritional needs and restrictions. • Provide small, frequent feedings.
Evidence of metabolic dysfunction is minimal.	• Monitor albumin, prealbumin, transferrin, blood urea nitrogen, cholesterol, triglycerides, bilirubin, aspartate transaminase, alanine transaminase • Administer cleansing enemas and cathartics if ordered.
Comfort/Pain Control Patient will have minimal pain. Patient will have minimal pruritus.	• Assess pain and discomfort from ascites, bleeding, pruritus. • Administer analgesics cautiously and monitor patient response. • Bathe with cool water, blot dry. • Lubricate skin. • Administer antipruritic medication; apply to skin PRN as ordered.
Psychosocial Patient demonstrates decreased anxiety.	• Assess patient's response to illness. Provide time to listen. • Assess effect of critical care environment on the patient. • Minimize sensory overload. • Provide adequate time for uninterrupted sleep. • Encourage flexible visiting hours for family. • Plan for consistent caregiver.
Teaching/Discharge Planning Patient/significant others understand procedures and tests needed for treatment of hepatic dysfunction.	• Prepare patient/significant others for procedures such as paracentesis or laboratory studies. • Teach patient and family information regarding sodium, protein, and fluid restrictions. Give written materials.
Patient/significant others are prepared for home care.	• Teach signs and symptoms of progressing hepatic failure (e.g., change in mentation, skin coloration, ascites). • Teach signs and symptoms of occult bleeding and respiratory infection. • Teach home medication regimen. • Teach comfort measures.

causing impairment of the patient's breathing pattern. Therefore, monitoring respiratory status by the nurse is crucial. Ascites is managed through bed rest, a low-sodium diet of no more than 2,000 mg/day, fluid restriction, and diuretic therapy.[64] It has been demonstrated that ascites absorption has an upper limit of 700 to 900 mL/day during diuresis therapy. If diuresis exceeds this limit, it may be at the expense of the intravascular volume and may potentiate hemodynamic instability. Diuresis with spironolactone, an aldosterone antagonist, is first-line diuretic therapy for ascites, although combination therapy with furosemide is more effective.[65] Monitoring for electrolyte imbalance, particularly hypokalemia, is essential. In addition to strict intake and output balance and daily weights, abdominal girth should be measured daily.

Paracentesis is also used to treat ascites in patients unresponsive to salt restriction and maximal diuretic therapy.[65] In this procedure, ascitic fluid is withdrawn from the abdomen through percutaneous needle aspiration. As much as 4 to 6 L/day of ascitic fluid can be withdrawn, and close monitoring of vital signs is important during this procedure because a sudden loss of intravascular pressure may precipitate hypotension, decreased renal perfusion, and tachycardia. Volume expanders are recommended if 5 L or more of ascitic fluid is withdrawn during a single paracentesis procedure (e.g., replacement of 5 g of albumin per liter of removed ascites fluid).[65] As with any invasive procedure, there is an increased risk for infection, particularly with repeated large-volume paracentesis procedures (e.g., refractory ascites). Refractory ascites results from continued deterioration of liver function and increased portal pressure, increased circulating vasoconstrictors, and decrease in renal blood flow. Refractory ascites marks a sentinel deterioration in the patient's disease trajectory with an estimated two year mortality of 50%.[65] Refractory ascites requires repeated paracentesis, with decreasing intervals of time between procedures. Unfortunately, paracentesis does not improve the overall poor prognosis, and all patients with refractory ascites should be referred for consideration for a liver transplantation.

A venous-peritoneal (VP) shunt is used to relieve ascites that is resistant to other therapies. The LeVeen shunt (Fig. 41-7) is inserted by placing the distal end of a tube in the abdominal cavity and tunneling the other end into a central vein (e.g., the superior vena cava). This perforated intra-abdominal tube allows for ascitic fluid to flow into the central vein. Complications related to placement and use include sepsis, peritonitis, DIC, thrombi formation, and variceal hemorrhage. It is not recommended for patients with infected ascites, encephalopathy, or renal failure. Although the VP shunt controls ascites better than paracentesis, occlusion rates within the first year of placement are high. Because of the aforementioned complications, these shunts are rarely placed in current hepatology practice.

A nonsurgical approach to managing ascites and acute variceal hemorrhage is the transjugular intrahepatic portosystemic shunt (TIPS), illustrated in Figure 41-8. The purpose of a TIPS is to decompress the portal venous system and therefore prevent rebleeding from varices or stop or reduce the formation of ascites.[66] Absolute contraindications to a TIPS procedure include congestive heart failure, severe tricuspid regurgitation, multiple hepatic cysts, uncontrolled systemic infection or sepsis, unrelieved biliary obstruction, and severe pulmonary hypertension (mean pressures > 45 mm Hg; these patients are not candidates for liver transplantation).[66,67] Rebleeding rates ranged from 1% to 18% after various inverse rates of reduction in portal pressure.[68] Using an angiographic catheter, a guide wire with a dilating balloon is inserted into the internal jugular vein and is advanced through the liver parenchyma, to connect the portal vein, where most of the blood flowing to the liver enters, to the hepatic vein, which empties blood into the inferior vena cava. A stent is then placed to create a conduit between the hepatic and portal vein, which decreases portal pressure. Complications include shunt occlusion, shunt stenosis, and hepatic encephalopathy.[69] Hepatic encephalopathy increases after a TIPS procedure because this portacaval shunt diverts portal blood flow away from the liver parenchyma. Although TIPS is fairly successful in the treatment of ascites, recent meta-analyses concluded that it can also be associated with the development of increased encephalopathy and offers no survival benefit.[64,70]

HEPATIC ENCEPHALOPATHY

Patients with severe liver disease can progress to hepatic encephalopathy (HE), a reversible decrease in neurologic function caused by liver disease. In general, clinical manifestations of HE can be subtle, with changes in memory, personality, concentration, and

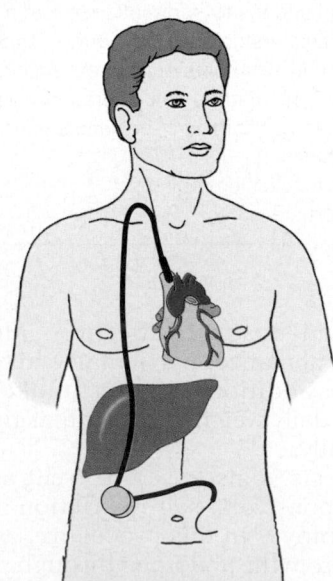

Figure 41-7 • The distal end of the LeVeen shunt is tunneled into a central vein. The shunt allows ascites fluid to drain from the abdominal cavity.

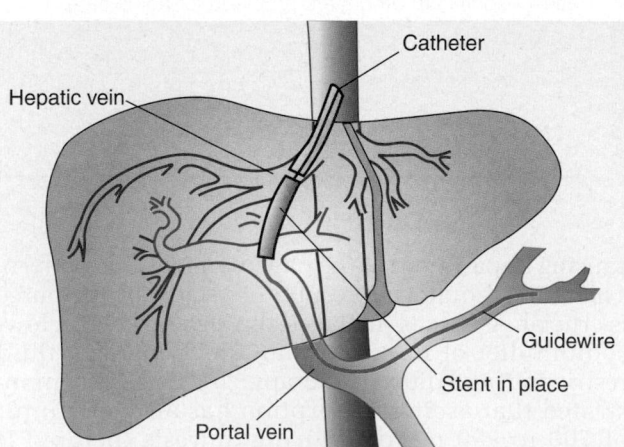

Figure 41-8 • Transjugular intrahepatic portosystemic shunt (TIPS). A stent is inserted through a catheter to the portal vein to divert blood flow and reduce portal hypertension. (From Smeltzer SC, Bare BG, Hinkle JL, Cheever KH: Brunner and Suddarth's Textbook of Medical–Surgical Nursing, 11th ed. Philadelphia: Lippincott Williams & Wilkins, 2008, p 1297.)

reaction times. HE can progress to more apparent neurologic cognitive changes, irritability or agitation, reversal of day and night schedules, somnolence, and eventually terminal coma if left untreated. These changes can be graded into stages (subclinical to stupor or coma) by evaluating both intellectual and neuromuscular function. In addition, they may fit into one of three clinical patterns. Type A is related to acute liver failure. Type B occurs in the setting of normal liver histology and the presence of a hepatic vascular bypass (e.g., TIPS). Type C is due to cirrhosis and represents most cases in the ICU; it can be divided further into acute and chronic subcategories.[64] Asterixis (a flapping tremor, usually of the hands) is a very early sign of HE. To test for this, the nurse should ask the patient to hold an arm and hand out, with fingers spread, as if stopping traffic and look for involuntary hand "flapping." Other signs are hyperreflexia and muscle rigidity.

The cause of the HE is thought to be related to the accumulation of toxic agents absorbed from the intestinal tract. These substances accumulate because the liver has lost the ability to metabolize and detoxify these substances. Elevated serum ammonia, a byproduct of protein and amino acid metabolism, is one of the suspected neurotoxins. Normally, ammonia is metabolized into urea before entering the systemic circulation, and the urea is then excreted. If the liver is unable to perform this detoxification or if a good portion of the portal blood is shunted around the liver from portal hypertension, the circulating level of ammonia rises. If ammonia and the other toxic agents can be reduced through effective therapy, the encephalopathy gradually clears. Although arterial ammonia levels are more reliable than venous samples, they are often more difficult to obtain and more painful for the patient. In addition, symptoms of HE may lag behind ammonia level elevations, and improvements in HE symptoms may occur before any improvement in ammonia levels.

Unfortunately, bypassing the liver with a shunt may result in decreased clearance and increased accumulation of toxins. HE can develop quite rapidly in patients with portosystemic shunts. People with portal hypertension can hemorrhage from esophageal varices or other sites in the GI tract. The hemorrhage produces a significant nitrogenous load to the intestinal tract in the form of blood, from which bacterial deamination produces the ammonia. Protein intake is limited to 20 to 40 g/day for the treatment of acute hepatic encephalopathy. Lactulose is used to facilitate bowel movements and clearance of nitrogenous products. Neomycin or metronidazole may be given to clear the gut of bacteria that promote nitrogenous production. Lactulose decreases the colonic pH to prevent the absorption of ammonia. Nursing measures to protect the patient with mental status changes from harm are a priority.

HEPATORENAL SYNDROME

Hepatorenal syndrome (HRS) is defined as the development of renal failure in patients with severe liver disease (acute or chronic) in the absence of any other identifiable cause of renal pathology.[71] Two patterns of HRS have been defined. Type 1 is often observed in acute liver failure or alcoholic hepatitis, or following acute decompensation of a patient with a history of cirrhosis. The most frequent cause of renal failure in cirrhosis is spontaneous bacterial peritonitis (SBP).[71] The onset of type 1 HRS is rapid, with a creatinine of more than 2.5 mg/dL or a 50% reduction in initial 24-hour creatinine clearance to less than 20 mL/min within 2 weeks. Patients often appear jaundiced and have a significant coagulopathy. Mortality from type 1 HRS is 80% (at 2 weeks) and usually results from a combination of liver and renal failure or variceal bleeding.[71] Type 2 HRS usually occurs in patients with diuretic-resistant ascites. Onset is more insidious, with deterioration in renal failure over months, but it is also associated with a poor prognosis.[71] In both types of HRS, failure of the kidneys is the result of the extreme systemic vasodilation (from the portal hypertension of liver failure), which decreases the effective circulating blood volume. This leads to a compensatory increase in cardiac output and maximal renal vasoconstriction, which reduces renal perfusion and subsequent renal failure.

Ascites, jaundice, hypotension, and oliguria are clinical findings in HRS; laboratory findings typically include azotemia, elevated serum creatinine, urine sodium less than 10 mEq/L, and hyponatremia. Management goals include therapies to support liver and kidney functions. Historically, liver transplantation had been the treatment of choice. However, because elevated pretransplantation serum creatinine levels have been demonstrated as a poor post-transplantation prognostic factor, it is now being suggested that both a liver and kidney transplantation would improve patient survival.[65,72,73]

SPONTANEOUS BACTERIAL PERITONITIS

Patients with liver disease may be more susceptible to infection because the hepatic Kupffer cells, which are responsible for uptake and subsequent degradation of foreign and potentially harmful substances in the body, do not function as efficiently. SBP occurs when there is a large accumulation of ascites without an identifiable intra-abdominal source of infection (e.g., absence of recognizable intestinal perforation). Ascitic fluid contains low concentrations of albumin, which is thought to normally provide some protection against bacteria. Subsequent leakage of bacteria through the abdominal wall or from invasive procedures (e.g., endoscopy, nasogastric tube, IV line, or indwelling bladder catheter placement) is thought to precipitate SBP.

Patients with SBP may complain of fever, chills, generalized abdominal pain, or tenderness with palpation (but rarely with rebound tenderness). However, symptoms may be minimal, with only subtle worsening of jaundice or encephalopathic trends.

Approximately 30% of patients with SBP develop renal failure, so if SBP is suspected, the ascitic fluid should be evaluated for cell count, differential, and culture.[71] While ascitic fluid bacterial cultures are pending, the diagnosis of SBP is highly likely if ascitic fluid leukocyte count is elevated at more than 500 cells/L (with a proportion of polymorphonuclear leukocytes of more than 50%).[71] The patient should be treated with broad-spectrum antibiotic coverage until the results of these tests are returned. SBP must be differentiated from peritonitis secondary to an abscess or perforation because the latter needs immediate surgical treatment.

Common nursing diagnoses for the patient with a GI disorder are listed in Box 41-15. A discharge planning guide for the patient with a GI disorder is given in Box 41-16.

• Clinical Applicability Challenges

Case Study

Mrs. K., a 42-year-old woman, has a 20-year history of ileocolonic Crohn's disease. She is status post (S/P) four small bowel resections and dilation of an ileoanastomotic stricture and had been

> **Box 41-15 · Examples of Nursing Diagnoses for the Patient With a Gastrointestinal Disorder**
>
> - Impaired Nutrition: Less Than Body Requirements related to altered pancreatic or liver function, impaired digestion from inadequate bile or pancreatic enzyme production, poor eating habits, excessive alcohol intake, nausea, vomiting, or anorexia
> - Excess Fluid Volume related to extravascular ascites, portal hypertension, and hypoalbuminemia
> - Risk for Deficient Fluid Volume related to overly aggressive diuresis, gastrointestinal bleeding and coagulopathies, and peritoneal sequestration of intra-abdominal fluids
> - Risk for Electrolyte Imbalance related to anorexia, nausea, and vomiting
> - Risk for Aspiration related to delayed gastric emptying, intestinal obstruction, ileus, or gastrointestinal bleeding
> - Risk for Impaired Gas Exchange related to decreased diaphragmatic excursion secondary to abdominal distention and potential for aspiration
> - Risk for Decreased Cardiac Output related to hepatic portal hypertension or blood loss from gastrointestinal bleeding
> - Acute Pain or Discomfort related to nasogastric tube irritation, pruritus related to accumulation of bilirubin pigment and salts, inflammation of the pancreas and surrounding tissues, and local peritonitis
> - Risk for Disturbed Sensory Perception related to hepatic encephalopathy and delirium tremens (in cases of alcohol abuse)
> - Risk for Ineffective Therapeutic Regimen Management related to insufficient knowledge of disease process, treatments, contraindications, dietary management, and follow-up care

> **Box 41-16 · DISCHARGE PLANNING GUIDE: Common Gastrointestinal Disorders**
>
> - Explain signs and symptoms of gastrointestinal bleeding: hematemesis, tarry stools, melena.
> - Explain signs and symptoms of recurrent ileus: nausea or vomiting, abdominal distention.
> - Explain signs and symptoms of acute or recurrent pancreatitis: severe left upper quadrant pain, especially after a large meal or alcohol intake. The pain may be intermittent or constant in the epigastric area and accompanied by nausea and anorexia.
> - Explain signs and symptoms of acute or worsening chronic hepatitis: generalized fatigue or malaise, right upper quadrant abdominal pain and distention, clay-colored stools or diarrhea, change in mental status, and jaundice.
> - Explain the importance of monitoring for fever, chills.
> - Explain how to check weight daily (same time of day) to monitor for increased ascites.
> - Review and provide written instructions for medications and treatments.
> - Discuss potential side effects of medications and treatments.
> - Encourage follow-up care.
> - Provide the patient and family with information regarding smoking cessation and alcohol and drug treatment programs as necessary.

admitted to the intensive care unit (ICU) from an outside hospital with a 3-day history of abdominal pain, nausea, and vomiting. Mrs. K. was in her usual state of health until 3 days before admission when she awoke from sleep at 4:00 a.m. with severe, crampy abdominal pain. The pain, located in the right upper quadrant, resolved after several minutes, and the patient returned to bed. The following day she experienced intermittent, crampy abdominal pain, accompanied by nausea and several episodes of the "dry heaves." She stayed in bed convinced she had a stomach virus, drank fluids, and ate no solids. She had several small solid bowel movements without relief of the abdominal pain and passed small amounts of flatus throughout the day. She awoke from sleep that night with increased pain, and she vomited a small amount of brownish emesis with partial relief of the abdominal pain. The following day the abdominal pain increased in intensity and frequency, the nausea persisted, and she vomited feculent emesis multiple times. That evening her husband persuaded her to go to the emergency department.

Physical examination reveals an alert, oriented, well-groomed, thin female in moderate distress. Vital signs are blood pressure, 171/95 mm Hg; heart rate, 112 beats/minute; respiratory rate, 20 breaths/minute; and temperature, 37.9°C (100.2°F). Examination of the oral cavity reveals no exudates or lesions and pink, dry mucous membranes. Cardiovascular examination reveals S1, S2, without audible murmur, rub, or gallop, with a regular rate and rhythm. No ectopy is apparent on cardiac monitor. The lungs were clear to auscultation, and chest expansion is equal. The patient's abdomen is round and mildly distended, without visible peristalsis. Well-healed midline incisional scars are evident, consistent with the patient's previous bowel resections. Bowel sounds are hyperactive, high-pitched, and tinkling in all four quadrants, with audible borborygmi. The patient's abdomen is diffusely tympanitic to percussion with tenderness to palpation in the epigastrium and right upper quadrant. There was no guarding or rebound. There are no palpable masses or bruits, and no hepatosplenomegaly. Rectal examination revealed normal sphincter tone, without palpable masses or lesions. Heme-negative brown stool was detected in the rectal vault.

Laboratory studies reveal sodium (Na^+), 132 mEq/L; potassium (K^+), 3.2 mEq/L; chloride (Cl^-), 93 mmol/L; blood urea nitrogen, 24 mg/dL; glucose, 172 mg/dL; alkaline phosphatase, 81 μg/L; aspartate transaminase, 40 μg/L; alanine transaminase, 37 μg/L; amylase, 72 U/L; lipase, 39 U/L; white blood cell count, 17.2 K/μL; hemoglobin, 16.1 g/dL; and hematocrit, 46.8%. An abdominal computed tomography scan shows new distention of the small bowel at 4.2 cm, with bowel dilation at the level of the distal ileum, focal wall thickening, and a transition zone. The patient receives a diagnosis of small bowel obstruction (SBO), and she is admitted to critical care for further evaluation and management.

On arrival in the ICU, the patient is made NPO, and a nasogastric tube is placed. Maintenance IV fluids and total parenteral nutrition are initiated after successful line placement. Medications prescribed included antiemetics. Frequent abdominal assessments were performed and included inspection, auscultation, percussion, and palpation. Serial radiographs (flat and upright) are taken daily without resolution of the SBO. On hospital day 4, the patient is taken to surgery for an exploratory laparotomy with extensive lysis of adhesions and resection of the terminal ileum and colon. On postoperative day 2, the patient is nausea free and was tolerating ice chips. On postoperative day 3, the nasogastric tube is removed. On postoperative day 4, a clear liquid diet is permitted, which is advanced as tolerated. The patient is hemodynamically stable and discharged to the floor with no further complications. She is subsequently discharged to home and is given discharge instructions to follow up with her primary gastroenterologist and surgeon in 1 month.

1. What is the most likely etiology of an SBO?
2. Describe the potential complications of an SBO.

Review Questions

1. A patient with a diagnosis of acute pancreatitis is receiving total parenteral nutrition (without lipids) and is eventually transitioned to a regular diet as tolerated. During discharge teaching, the nurse provides the patient with dietary modification information to help prevent future episodes of pancreatitis. Which of the following items should the patient limit in his diet?
   a. Carbohydrate intake
   b. Fat intake
   c. Protein intake
   d. Water intake

2. A patient has been admitted to the hospital with a diagnosis of acute pancreatitis. As the nurse assessing the patient's abdominal pain, which type of pain is most consistent with this diagnosis?
   a. Burning and aching, located in the left lower abdominal quadrant
   b. Burning and aching, located in the right lower abdominal quadrant
   c. Severe and unrelenting, located in the epigastrium and radiating to the back
   d. Severe and unrelenting, located in the right upper quadrant and radiating to the right shoulder

3. Mr. S. is admitted with intermittent left lower quadrant pain and rectal bleeding, which has increased in frequency over the past few days. As the nurse admitting this patient, you know that the most common cause of acute lower GI bleeding is
   a. hemorrhoids.
   b. diverticulosis.
   c. colon carcinoma.
   d. Mallory-Weiss tear.

4. As the nurse collecting a patient's current and past medical history, you have a strong clinical suspicion that he has an acute hepatitis B viral infection (HBV). Which of the laboratory tests would confirm an acute HBV infection?
   a. Acute infection diagnosed by a positive HBsAg, HBcAb, and IgM
   b. Acute infection diagnosed by a positive HBcAb and IgG
   c. Acute infection diagnosed by an AST > ALT, typically 1,000 to 2,000 IU/mL
   d. Acute infection diagnosed when HBsAb becomes detectable

5. A patient is being admitted to your unit with a diagnosis of chronic hepatitis C virus (HCV). Which of the laboratory tests would confirm an HCV infection?
   a. HCV enzyme-linked immunosorbent assay
   b. HCV RNA
   c. Anti-HCV recombinant strip immunoblot assay
   d. HCsAg total

References

1. Conrad SA: Acute upper gastrointestinal bleeding in critically ill patients: Causes and treatment modalities. Crit Care Med 30(Suppl 6):S365–368, 2002

2. Eisen GM, Dominitz JA, Faigel DO, et al: An annotated algorithmic approach to upper gastrointestinal bleeding. Gastrointest Endosc 53(7):864–866, 2001

3. Yavorski RT, Wong RKH, Maydonovitch C, et al: Analysis of 3,294 cases of upper gastrointestinal bleeding in military medical facilities. Am J Gastroenterol 90(4):568–573, 1995

4. Rivkin K, Lyakhovetskiy A: Treatment of nonvariceal upper gastrointestinal bleeding. Am J Health-System Pharmacists 62(11):1159–1170, 2005

5. D'Amico G, Pagliaro LLP, Pietrosi GGPI, Tarantino IITA: Emergency sclerotherapy versus medical interventions for bleeding oesophageal varices in cirrhotic patients. Cochrane Database Syst Rev 2, 2007

6. Chalasani N, Kahi C, Francois F, et al: Improved patient survival after acute variceal bleeding: A multicenter, cohort study. Am J Gastroenterol 98(3):653–659, 2003

7. Psilopoulos D, Galanis P, Goulas S, et al: Endoscopic variceal ligation vs. propranolol for prevention of first variceal bleeding: A randomized controlled trial. Eur J Gastroenterol Hepatol 17(10):1111–1117, 2005

8. Schmulewitz N, Baillie J: Dieulafoy lesions: A review of 6 years of experience at a tertiary referral center. Am J Gastroenterol 96(6):1688–1694, 2001

9. Rockey DC: Gastrointestinal bleeding. Gastroenterol Clin North Am 34:581–588, 2005

10. Kelley DM: Hypovolemic shock: An overview. Crit Care Nurs Q 28(1):2–19, 2005

11. Rockey DC: Gastrointestinal bleeding. In Feldman M, Friedman LS, Sleisenger MH (eds): Sleisenger & Fordtran's Gastrointestinal and Liver Disease, 8th ed. Philadelphia, WB Saunders, 2006, pp 255–300

12. Kupfer Y, Cappell MS, Tessler S: Acute gastrointestinal bleeding in the intensive care unit: The intensivist's perspective. Gastroenterol Clin North Am 29(2):275–307, 2000

13. Miller M, Smith TP: Angiographic diagnosis and endovascular management of nonvariceal gastrointestinal hemorrhage. Gastroenterol Clin North Am 34:735–752, 2005

14. Zaman A, Chalasani N: Bleeding caused by portal hypertension. Gastroenterol Clin North Am 34:623–642, 2005

15. Stabile BE, Stamos MJ: Surgical management of gastrointestinal bleeding. Gastroenterol Clin North Am 29(1):189–222, 2000

16. Shah VH, Kamath PS: New developments in portal hypertensive bleeding. Clin Perspect Gastroenterol 5(1),17–22, 2002

17. Bloomfield RS, Rockey DC, Shetzline MA: Endoscopic therapy of acute diverticular hemorrhage. Am J Gastroenterol 96(8):2367–2372, 2001

18. Strate LL: Lower GI bleeding: Epidemiology and diagnosis. Gastroenterol Clin North Am 34:643–664, 2005

19. Green BT, Rockey DC: Lower gastrointestinal bleeding management. Gastroenterology Clinics of North America, 34:665–678, 2005

20. Byers SE, Chudnofsky CR, Sorondo B, et al: Incidence of occult upper gastrointestinal bleeding in patients presenting to the ED with hematochezia. Am J Emerg Med 25:340–344, 2007

21. Hammond KL, Beck DE, Hicks TC, et al: Implications of negative technetium 99m-labeled red blood cell scintigraphy in patients presenting with lower gastrointestinal bleeding. Am J Surg 193(3):404–408, 2007

22. Elta GH: Urgent colonoscopy for acute lower-GI bleeding. Gastrointest Endosc 59(3):402–408, 2004

23. Summers RW: Approach to the patient with ileus and obstruction. In Yamada T, Alpers DH, Kaplowitz N, et al (eds): Textbook of Gastroenterology, vol I, 4th ed. Philadelphia: Lippincott Williams & Wilkins, 2003, pp 829–843.

24. Turnage RH, Heldmann M, Cole P: Intestinal obstruction and ileus. In Feldman M, Friedman LS, Brandt LJ (eds): Sleisenger & Fortran's Gastrointestinal and Liver Disease: Pathophysiology, Diagnosis and Management, 8th ed. Philadelphia: WB Saunders, 2006, pp 2653–2679

25. Kahi CJ, Rex DK: Bowel obstruction and pseudo-obstruction. Gastroenterol Clin North Am 32:1229–1247, 2003

26. Silen W: Acute intestinal obstruction. In Braunwald E, Fauci AS, Kasper DL, et al (eds): Harrison's Principles of Internal Medicine, 15th ed. New York: McGraw-Hill, 2001, pp 1703–1705

27. Shelton BK: Intestinal obstruction. AACN Clin Issues 10(4): 478–491, 1999

28. Frager D: Intestinal obstruction: Role of CT. Gastroenterol Clin North Am 31:777–799, 2002

29. Luckey A, Livingston E, Tache Y: Mechanisms and treatment of postoperative ileus. Arch Surgery 138(2):206–214, 2003

30. Behm B, Stollman N: Postoperative ileus: Etiologies and interventions. Practical Gastroenterol Hepatol 1(2):71–80, 2003

31. Bauer AJ, Schwarz NT, Moore BA, et al: Ileus in critical illness: Mechanisms and management. Curr Opin Crit Care 8:152–157, 2002

32. Bank PA, Freeman ML, for the Practice Parameters Committee of the American College of Gastroenterology: Practice guidelines in acute pancreatitis. Am J Gastroenterol 101:2379–2400, 2006

33. Law NM, Freeman ML: Emergency complications of acute and chronic pancreatitis. Gastroenterol Clin North Am 32(4): 1169–1194, 2003

34. Topazian M, Gorelick FS: AP. In Yamada T, Alpers DH, Kaplowitz N, et al (eds): Textbook of Gastroenterology, vol II, 4th ed. Philadelphia: Lippincott Williams & Wilkins, 2003, pp 2026–2060

35. Granger J, Remick D: Acute pancreatitis: Models, markers, and mediators. Shock 24(Suppl):45–51, 2005

36. Mayerle J, Simon P, Lerch MM: Medical treatment of acute pancreatitis. Gastroenterol Clin North Am 33:855–869, 2004

37. Triester SL, Kowdley KV: Prognostic factors in acute pancreatitis. J Clin Gastroenterol 34(2):167–176, 2002

38. Smotkin J, Tenner S: Laboratory diagnostic tests in acute pancreatitis. J Clin Gastroenterol 34(4):459–462, 2002

39. Papachristou GI, Whitcomb DC: Predictors of severity and necrosis in acute pancreatitis. Gastroenterol Clin North Am 33:871–890, 2004

40. Despins LA, Kivlahan C, Cox KR: Acute pancreatitis: Diagnosis and treatment of a potentially fatal condition. Am J Nurs 105(11):54–57, 2005

41. Larson AM, Polson J, Fontana RJ, et al: Acetaminophen-induced acute liver failure: Results of a U.S. multicenter, prospective study. Hepatology 42(6):1364–1372, 2005

42. Madhortra R, Gilmore IT: Recent developments in the treatment of alcoholic hepatitis. Q J Med 96:391–400, 2003

43. Vargus HI: (2002). Hepatobiliary disease. In Bongard FS, Sue DY (eds): Current Critical Diagnosis and Treatment, 2nd ed. New York: McGraw Hill, 2002, pp 768–776

44. Holcomb SS: An update on hepatitis. Dimens Crit Care Nurs 21(5):170–177, 2002

45. Kim WR, Brown RS, Terrault NA, El-Serag H: Burden of liver disease in the United States: Summary of a workshop. Hepatology 36:227–242, 2002

46. Taylor RM, Davern T, Munoz S, et al: Fulminant hepatitis A virus infection in the United States: Incidence, prognosis, and outcomes. Hepatology 44(6):1589–1597, 2006

47. Wheeler C, Vogt TM, Armstrong GL, et al: An outbreak of hepatitis A associated with green onions. N Engl J Med 353:890–897, 2005

48. Perrillo R, Nair S: Hepatitis B and D. In Feldman M, Friedman LS, Sleisenger MH (eds): Sleisenger & Fordtran's Gastrointestinal and Liver Disease, 8th ed. Philadelphia, WB Saunders, 2006, pp 1647–1681

49. Tan J, Lok ASF: Update on viral hepatitis: 2006. Curr Opin Gastroenterol 23:263–267, 2007

50. Rivkin A: Entecavir: A new nucleoside analogue for the treatment of chronic hepatitis B. Drugs Today (BARC) 43(4): 201–220, 2007

51. Strader DB, Wright T, Thomas DL, Seeff LB: AASLD Guidelines: Diagnosis, management, and treatment of hepatitis C. Hepatology 39:1147, 2004

52. Larson A, Carithers R: Hepatitis C in clinical practice. J Intern Med 249(2):111–120, 2001

53. Gardenier D, Alfandre D: Primary care of the patient with chronic hepatitis C. J Nurse Pract 2(8):517–524, 2006

54. Muir A: The natural history of hepatitis C viral infection. Semin Gastroenterol Dis 11(2):53–61, 2000

55. Liang T, Rehermann B, Seeff L, Hoofnagle J: Pathogenesis, natural history, treatment, and prevention of hepatitis C. Ann Intern Med 132(4):296–305, 2000

56. Manns M, McHutchison J, Gordon S, et al: Peginterferon alfa-2b plus ribavirin compared to interferon alpha-2b plus ribavirin for initial treatment of chronic hepatitis C: A randomised trial. Lancet 358(9286):958–965, 2001

57. Castelnau C, LeGal F, Ripault MP, et al: Efficacy of peginterferon alpha-2b in chronic hepatitis delta: Relevance of quantitative RT-PCR for follow-up. Hepatology 44:728–735, 2006

58. Labrique AB, Thomas DL, Stoszek SK, Nelson KE: Hepatitis E: An emerging infectious disease. Epidemiol Rev 21:162–179, 1999

59. Patra S, Kumar A, Trivedi SS, et al: Maternal and fetal outcomes in pregnant women with acute hepatitis E virus infection. Ann Intern Med 147(1):28–33, 2007

60. Miniño AM, Heron M, Murphy SL, Kochanek KD: National Vital Statistics Report, deaths: Final data for 2004. Retrieved June 15, 2007, from http://www.cdc.gov/nchs/products/pubs/pubd/hestats/finaldeaths04/finaldeaths04

61. Pratt DS, Kaplan MM: Evaluation of abnormal liver-enzyme results in asymptomatic patients. N Engl J Med 342:1266–1271, 2000

62. Rochling FA: Evaluation of abnormal liver tests. Clin Cornerstone 3:1–12, 2001

63. Stonesifer E: Common laboratory and diagnostic testing in patients with gastrointestinal disease. AACN Clin Issues 15(4):582–594, 2004

64. Han MK, Hyzy R: Advances in critical care management of hepatic failure and insufficiency. Crit Care Med 34(9):S225–S231, 2006

65. Blendis L, Wong F: The natural history and management of hepatorenal disorders: From pre-ascites to hepatorenal syndrome. Royal Coll Physicians 3(2):154–159, 2003

66. Boyer TD, Haskal ZJ: The role of TIPS in management of portal hypertension. Hepatology 41:386, 2005

67. Hoeper MM, Krowka MJ, Strassburg CP: Portopulmonary hypertension and hepatopulmonary syndrome. Lancet 363:1461–1468, 2004

68. Rossle M, Siegersterrer V, Olschewski M, et al: (2001). How much reduction in portal pressure is necessary to prevent variceal rebleeding? A longitudinal study in 225 patients with transjugular intrahepatic portosystemic shunts. Am J Gastroenterol 96:3379–3383, 2001

69. Peron JM, Barange K, Otal P, et al: Transjugular intrahepatic portosystemic shunts in the treatment of refractory ascites: Results in 48 consecutive patients. J Vasc Intervent Radiol 11:1211–1216, 2000

70. Deltenre P, Mathurin P, Dharancy S, et al: Transjugular intrahepatic portosystemic shunt in refractory ascites: A meta-analysis. Liver Int 25:349–356, 2005

71. Dagher L, Moore K: The hepatorenal syndrome. Gut 49:729–737, 2001

72. Nahr S, Verma S, Thuluvath PJ: Pretransplant renal function predicts survival in patients undergoing orthotopic liver transplantation. Hepatology 35:1179–1185, 2002

73. Jeyarah DR, Gonwa TA, McBride M, et al: Hepatorenal syndrome: Combined liver kidney transplant versus isolated liver transplant. Transplantation 64:1760–1765, 1997

Other Selected Readings

Martin B: Prevention of gastrointestinal complications in the critically ill patient. AACN Clin Issues 18(2):158–166, 2007

Milanchi S, Allins A: Early pneumoperitoneum after percutaneous endoscopic gastrostomy in intensive care patients: Sign of possible bowel injury. Am J Crit Care 16(2):132–136, 2007

Spirt MJ, Stanley S: Update on stress ulcer prophylaxis in critically ill patients. Crit Care Nurse 26(1):18–28, 2006

White KA: Ogilvic's syndrome: No ordinary constipation. Am Nurse Today (2)8:12–12, 2007

Endocrine System

PART 10

INTERNET RESOURCES

Topic	Web Page Address
American Association of Clinical Endocrinologists	www.aace.com
American Association of Diabetes Educators	www.aadenet.org
American Diabetes Association	www.diabetes.org
American Dietetic Association	www.eatright.org
American Thyroid Association	www.thyroid.org
Canadian Diabetes Association	www.diabetes.ca
Centers for Disease Control and Prevention	www.cdc.gov/diabetes
Diabetes Action Research and Education Foundation	www.diabetesaction.org
Diabetes Exercise and Sports Association	www.diabetes-exercise.org
Endocrine Disorders and Endocrine Surgery	www.endocrineweb.com
Endocrine Nurses' Society	www.endo-nurses.org
Endocrine Online	www.endocrineonline.org
The Endocrine Society	www.endo-society.org
Endocrine Surgery Website by Johns Hopkins Hospital	http://www.path.jhu.edu/endocrine/
European Federation of Endocrine Societies	www.euro-endo.org
Federation of European Nurses in Diabetes	www.fend.org
International Association of Endocrine Surgeons	www.iaes-endocrine-surgeons.com
International Diabetes Federation	www.idf.org
Joslin Diabetes Center	www.joslin.org
Juvenile Diabetes Research Foundation International	www.jdrf.org
National Adrenal Diseases Foundation	www.medhelp.org/nadf/
National Institute of Diabetes and Digestive and Kidney Disorders	www.niddk.nih.gov
National Kidney Foundation	www.kidney.org
Thyroid Federation International	www.thyroid-fed.org
Thyroid Foundation of America	www.allthyroid.org

Anatomy and Physiology of the Endocrine System

Jane Kapustin

42

The Hypothalamus and Pituitary Gland
    Posterior Pituitary (Neurohypophysis) Hormones
    Anterior Pituitary (Adenohypophysis) Hormones
The Thyroid and Parathyroid Glands
    Thyroid Hormones
    Calcitonin and Parathyroid Hormone
The Endocrine Pancreas
    Insulin
    Glucagon
    Somatostatin
    Pancreatic Polypeptide
The Adrenal Glands
    Medullary Hormones
    Cortical Hormones
Atrial Natriuretic Peptide (Natriuretic Hormone)

Objectives

Based on the content in this chapter, the reader should be able to:

❶ Describe the production, action, and regulation of antidiuretic hormone, growth hormone, and the thyroid hormones.

❷ Describe how activated vitamin D, parathyroid hormone, and calcitonin each influence calcium concentrations in the blood.

❸ Describe the production, action, and regulation of insulin.

❹ Compare and contrast the pathophysiology of types 1 and 2 diabetes.

❺ Describe the production, action, and regulation of glucagon.

❻ Explain how glucocorticoids are secreted.

❼ Discuss the significant effects of glucocorticoid medications.

❽ Summarize the renin–angiotensin mechanism for regulating mineralocorticoid secretion.

Communication between systems in the body is accomplished in three ways. One method of communication is the nervous system. A second method is the cellular secretion of chemicals that are released into the interstitial fluid. Examples of this method of communication include the chemicals that trigger a local inflammatory response, such as histamine, complement, and prostaglandins. The third method of communication is the cellular secretion of chemicals that are circulated through the bloodstream. This communication is known more commonly as the endocrine system (Fig. 42-1, Table 42-1). The secretions of endocrine cells are termed hormones. Hormones are molecules synthesized and secreted by specialized cells and released into blood vessels to exert biochemical effects on target cells distant from the site of origin. They control metabolism, transport of substances across the cell membrane, fluid and electrolyte balance, growth and development, adaptation, and reproduction.

Hormone action is specific and depends on linkage with a specialized hormone receptor on the target cell. This hormone–receptor complex is responsible for a series of biological responses. Hormones are either stimulatory or inhibitory. Either their actions are very organ specific, such as prolactin (which only affects the mammary glands), or their effects are generalized, such as insulin (which affects most cellular functions of the body).

Hormone production is maintained by a feedback loop mechanism involving the hypothalamic–pituitary axis system (Fig. 42-2). Release of a specific hormone is made possible when the circulating level of that hormone is low (positive feedback). Conversely, when the circulating level of a hormone is high, the release of more hormone is inhibited (negative feedback) until a lower level is reached. This system is regulated by specialized sensors in the hypothalamus that continuously monitor hormone assays to maintain self-regulated homeostasis.

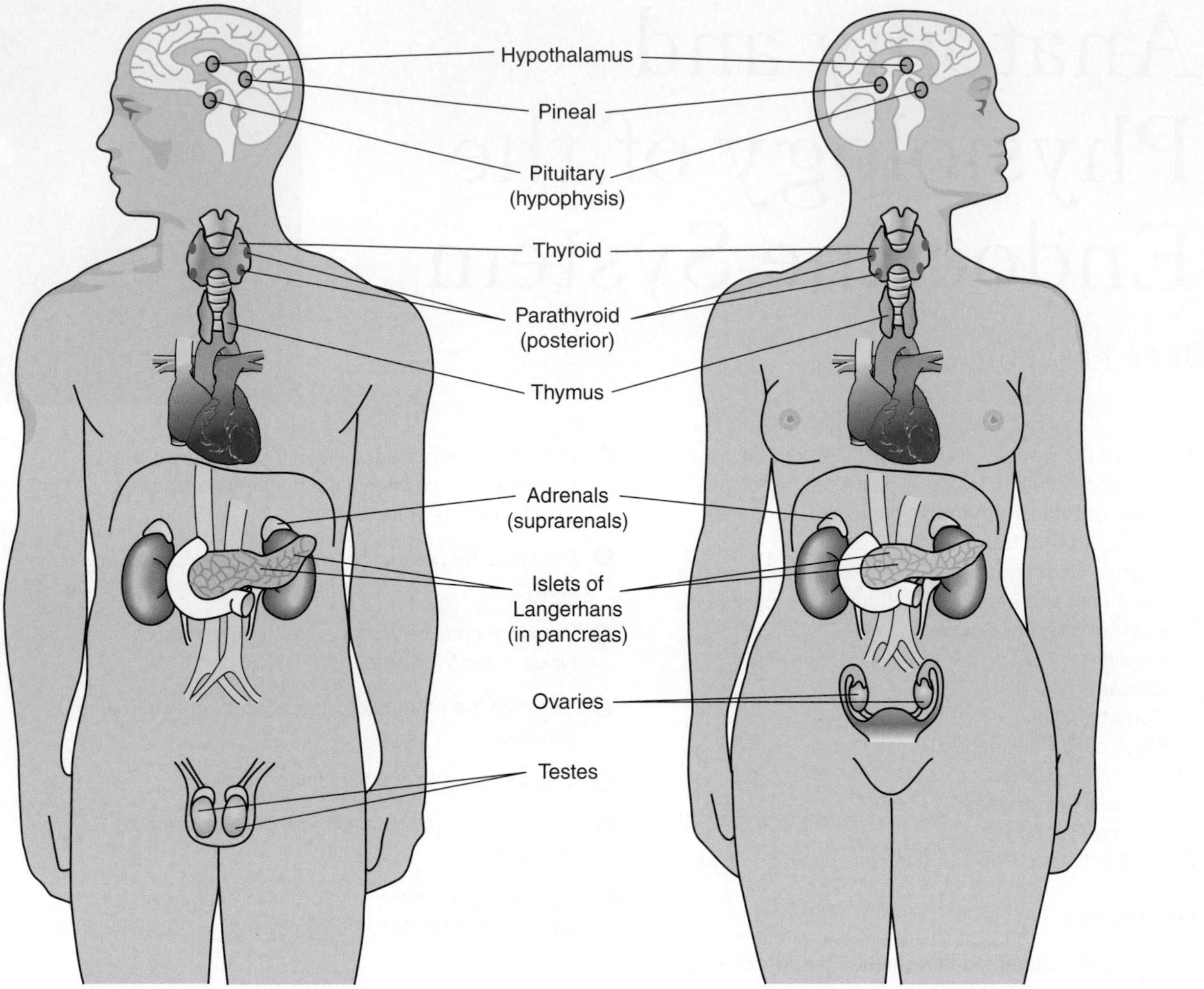

Figure 42-1 • The endocrine system. (From Smeltzer SC, Bare BG, Hinkle JL, Cheever KH: Brunner & Suddarth's Textbook of Medical–Surgical Nursing, 11th ed. Philadelphia: Lippincott Williams & Wilkins, 2008, p 1142.)

Theoretically, when functioning properly, this system prevents the overproduction of hormones.

The effects of aging can influence the endocrine system as well (Box 42-1). As humans age, target organ sensitivity decreases. The target organs demonstrate the effects of aging by either increasing in pigmentation or shrinking in size. This, in effect, decreases hormone receptor binding. This phenomenon explains why older patients are at higher risk for development of hypothyroidism: aging can decrease production of triiodothyronine (T_3) and thyroxine (T_4) and can lead to thyroid gland atrophy. Women are 4 to 5 times more likely to develop hypothyroidism than men.

Endocrine dysfunction can be identified as belonging to one of five major categories:

▶ Subnormal hormone production as a result of gland destruction or malformation

▶ Hormone excess

▶ Production of abnormal hormone resulting from gene mutation

▶ Hormone receptor disorders resulting from autoimmune processes

▶ Disorders of hormone transport or metabolism, resulting in increased levels of "free" hormones in the blood

• The Hypothalamus and Pituitary Gland

The key to understanding the physiology of the hormones of the pituitary gland lies in visualizing the anatomy of the gland and its blood supply. The hypothalamus and pituitary share two connecting pathways: a rich vascular network, which connects the hypothalamus with the anterior pituitary; and nerve fibers, which link the hypothalamus with the posterior pituitary. Together, these two glands form a unit that controls the thyroid gland, the adrenal glands, and the gonads, and exerts control over the growth and metabolism of the organism.

Because of the control the pituitary gland exerts over all body functions, it is often referred to as the master gland. It has two distinct regions: the anterior (front) lobe and the posterior (back) lobe. Located at

Table 42-1 • Endocrine System in Summary

Endocrine Gland and Hormone	Principal Site of Action	Principal Processes Affected
Pituitary Gland		
Anterior Lobe		
Growth hormone (GH, somatotropin)	General	Growth of bones, muscles, and other organs
Thyroid-stimulating hormone (TSH)	Thyroid	Growth and secretory activity of thyroid gland
Adrenocorticotropic hormone (ACTH)	Adrenal cortex	Growth and secretory activity of adrenal cortex
Follicle-stimulating hormone (FSH)	Ovaries	Development of follicles and secretion of estrogen
	Testes	Development of seminiferous tubules, spermatogenesis
Luteinizing hormone (LH) or interstitial cell-stimulating hormone (ICSH)	Ovaries	Ovulation, formation of corpus luteum, secretion of progesterone
Prolactin (luteotropic hormone, LTH)	Testes	Secretion of testosterone
Melanocyte-stimulating hormone (MSH)	Mammary glands and ovaries	Secretion of milk; maintenance of corpus luteum
β-lipotropin	Skin	Pigmentation
Posterior Lobe		
Antidiuretic hormone (ADH, vasopressin)	Kidney	Reabsorption of water; water balance
	Arterioles	Blood pressure
Oxytocin	Uterus	Contraction
	Breast	Expression of milk
Pineal Gland		
Melatonin	Gonads	Sexual maturation
Thyroid Gland		
Thyroxine (T_4) and triiodothyronine (T_3)	General	Metabolic rate; growth and development; intermediate metabolism
Calcitonin	Bone	Inhibits bone resorption; lowers blood level of calcium
Parathyroid Glands		
Parathyroid hormone (PTH)	Bone, kidney, intestine	Promotes bone resorption; increases absorption of calcium; raises blood calcium level
Adrenal Glands		
Cortex		
Mineralocorticoids (eg, aldosterone)	Kidney	Reabsorption of sodium; elimination of potassium
Glucocorticoids (eg, cortisol)	General	Metabolism of carbohydrate, protein, and fat; response to stress; anti-inflammatory
Sex hormones	General	Preadolescent growth spurt
Medulla		
Epinephrine	Cardiac muscle, smooth muscle, glands	Emergency functions: same as stimulation of sympathetic nervous system
Norepinephrine	Organs innervated by sympathetic nervous system	Chemical transmitter substance; increases peripheral resistance
Islet Cells of Pancreas		
Insulin	General	Lowers blood sugar; utilization and storage of carbohydrate; decreases gluconeogenesis
Glucagon	Liver	Raises blood glucose; glycogenolysis
Somatostatin	General	Lowers blood glucose by interfering with release of growth hormone and glucagon
Testes		
Testosterone	General	Development of secondary sex characteristics
	Reproductive organs	Development and maintenance; normal function
Ovaries		
Estrogens	General	Development of secondary sex characteristics
	Mammary glands	Development of duct system
	Reproductive organs	Maturation and normal cyclic function
Progesterone	Mammary glands	Development of secretory tissue
	Uterus	Preparation for implantation; maintenance of pregnancy
Gastrointestinal Tract		
Gastrin	Stomach	Production of gastric juice
Enterogastrone	Stomach	Inhibits secretion and motility
Secretin	Liver and pancreas	Production of bile; production of watery pancreatic juice (rich in $NaHCO_3$)
Pancreozymin	Pancreas	Production of pancreatic juice rich in enzymes
Cholecystokinin	Gallbladder	Contraction and emptying

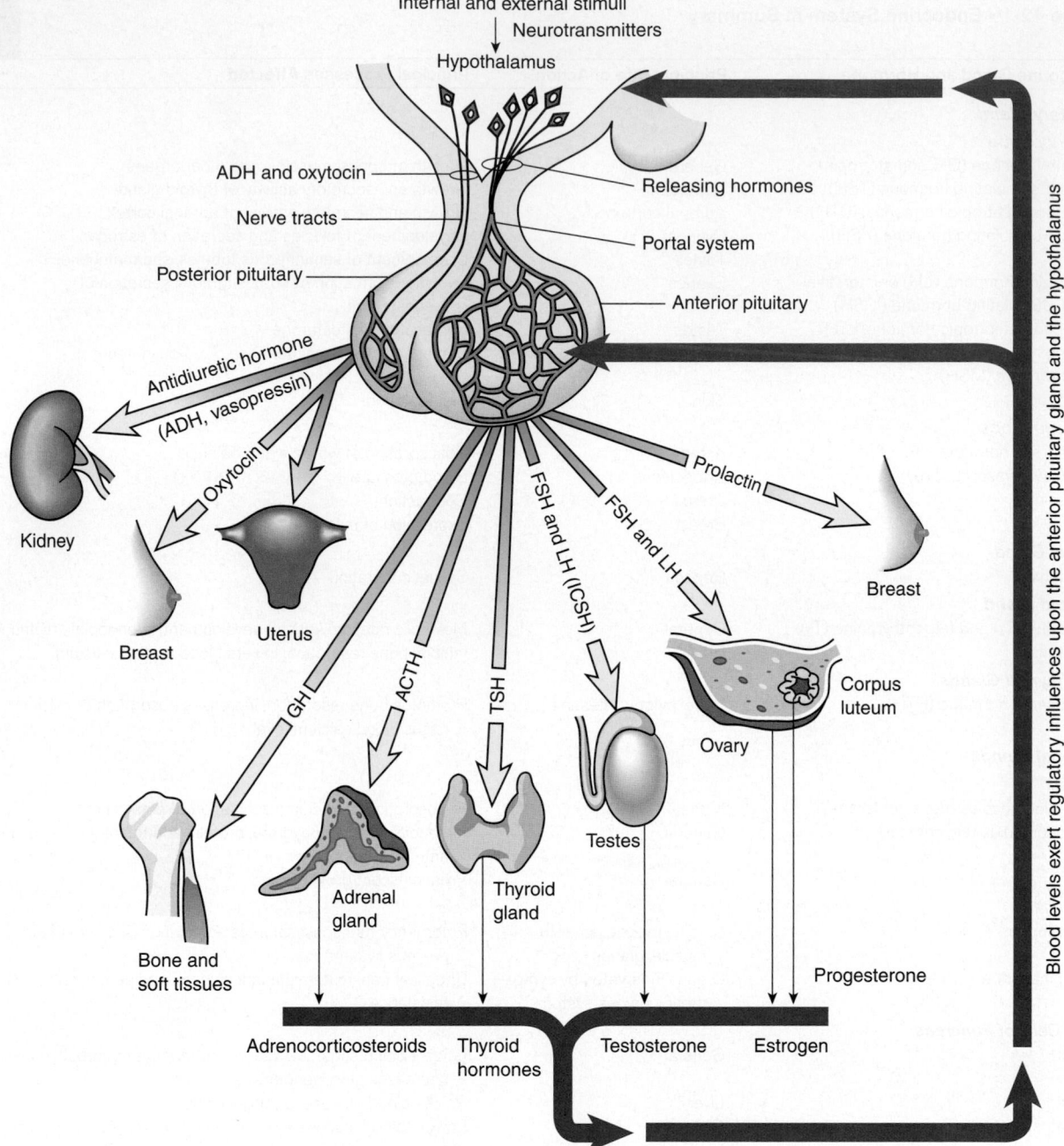

Figure 42-2 • The feedback loop mechanism that controls hormone production. Sensors in the hypothalamus monitor hormone levels and initiate or suppress production accordingly. ACTH, adrenocorticotropic hormone; ADH, antidiuretic hormone; CNS, central nervous system; FSH, follicle-stimulating hormone; LH, luteinizing hormone; TSH, thyroid-stimulating hormone. (From Smeltzer SC, Bare BG, Hinkle JL, Cheever KH: Brunner & Suddarth's Textbook of Medical–Surgical Nursing, 11th ed. Philadelphia: Lippincott Williams & Wilkins, 2008, p 1445.)

the base of the skull in the sphenoid bone at a site referred to as the sella turcica, this well-protected gland is difficult to reach surgically because it is so deeply embedded in the skull. Despite being well protected, the pituitary is still susceptible to injury as a result of head or facial trauma, edema, or surgical complications. Because it is so vascular, the pituitary is extremely vulnerable to injury from ischemia and infarction.

The hypothalamus is a small area at the base of the brain connected to the posterior pituitary (also

known as the neurohypophysis) by the pituitary stalk. This stalk is a direct outgrowth of the neuroectoderm of the base of the brain that drops during development of the gland into the bony sella turcica. This is in direct contrast to the anterior pituitary (adenohypophysis), which arises from the buccal endothelium and develops separately in the same bony structure. Besides being embryogenically separate, the blood supplies of the anterior and posterior pituitary differ. The hypothalamus has specialized nerve cells that are in constant communication with the third ventri-

> **Box 42-1 • CONSIDERATIONS FOR THE OLDER PATIENT: Physiological Changes in the Endocrine System That Occur With Aging**
>
> - Production of thyroid hormone, cortisol, and aldosterone decreases with age.
> - Levels of somatostatin, triiodothyronine (T_3), thyroxine (T_4), aldosterone, renin, calcitonin, and vasopressin decrease with age, as does glucose tolerance.
> - Levels of norepinephrine, parathyroid hormone (PTH), atrial natriuretic peptide (ANP), insulin, and glucagon increase with age.

cle of the brain where continuous sampling of serum osmolality can occur. Information about the osmolality influences the release or inhibition of hormones. It is through this relationship that the hypothalamus influences the release of chemical and neural signals to maintain homeostasis. Because the hypothalamus controls the releasing or inhibiting hormones that influence the pituitary, it assumes the function of the coordinating center of the brain for endocrine, behavioral, and autonomic nervous system function. The hypothalamus is responsible for communicating emotion, pain, body temperature, and other neural input to the endocrine system.

The anterior pituitary hormones are controlled by releasing factors that are secreted from the hypothalamus and are called hypophysiotropic hormones. The hypophysiotropic hormones are secreted into the primary capillary plexus near the median eminence that supplies blood to the anterior pituitary (Fig. 42-3). This blood may also travel in a retrograde fashion and may be responsible for one level of feedback control of the anterior pituitary and hypophysiotropic hormones. A given hypophysiotropic hormone regulates the secretion of one or two anterior pituitary hormones. Both growth hormone (GH, somatotropin) and prolactin are dually controlled by a stimulatory and an inhibitory hypophysiotropic hormone. The posterior pituitary is a direct neural extension of the hypothalamus, and the controlling factors reside in

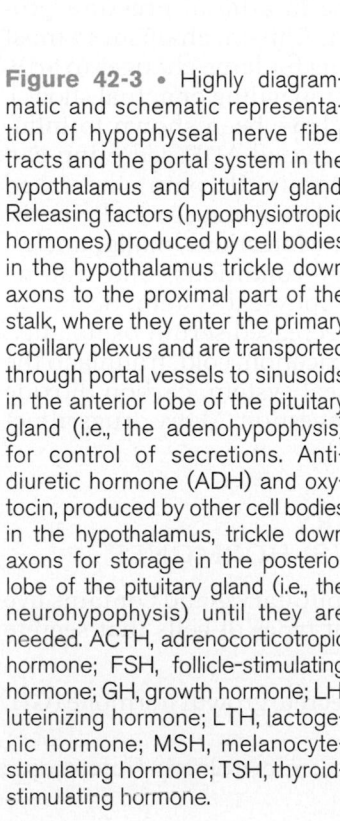

Figure 42-3 • Highly diagrammatic and schematic representation of hypophyseal nerve fiber tracts and the portal system in the hypothalamus and pituitary gland. Releasing factors (hypophysiotropic hormones) produced by cell bodies in the hypothalamus trickle down axons to the proximal part of the stalk, where they enter the primary capillary plexus and are transported through portal vessels to sinusoids in the anterior lobe of the pituitary gland (i.e., the adenohypophysis) for control of secretions. Antidiuretic hormone (ADH) and oxytocin, produced by other cell bodies in the hypothalamus, trickle down axons for storage in the posterior lobe of the pituitary gland (i.e., the neurohypophysis) until they are needed. ACTH, adrenocorticotropic hormone; FSH, follicle-stimulating hormone; GH, growth hormone; LH, luteinizing hormone; LTH, lactogenic hormone; MSH, melanocyte-stimulating hormone; TSH, thyroid-stimulating hormone.

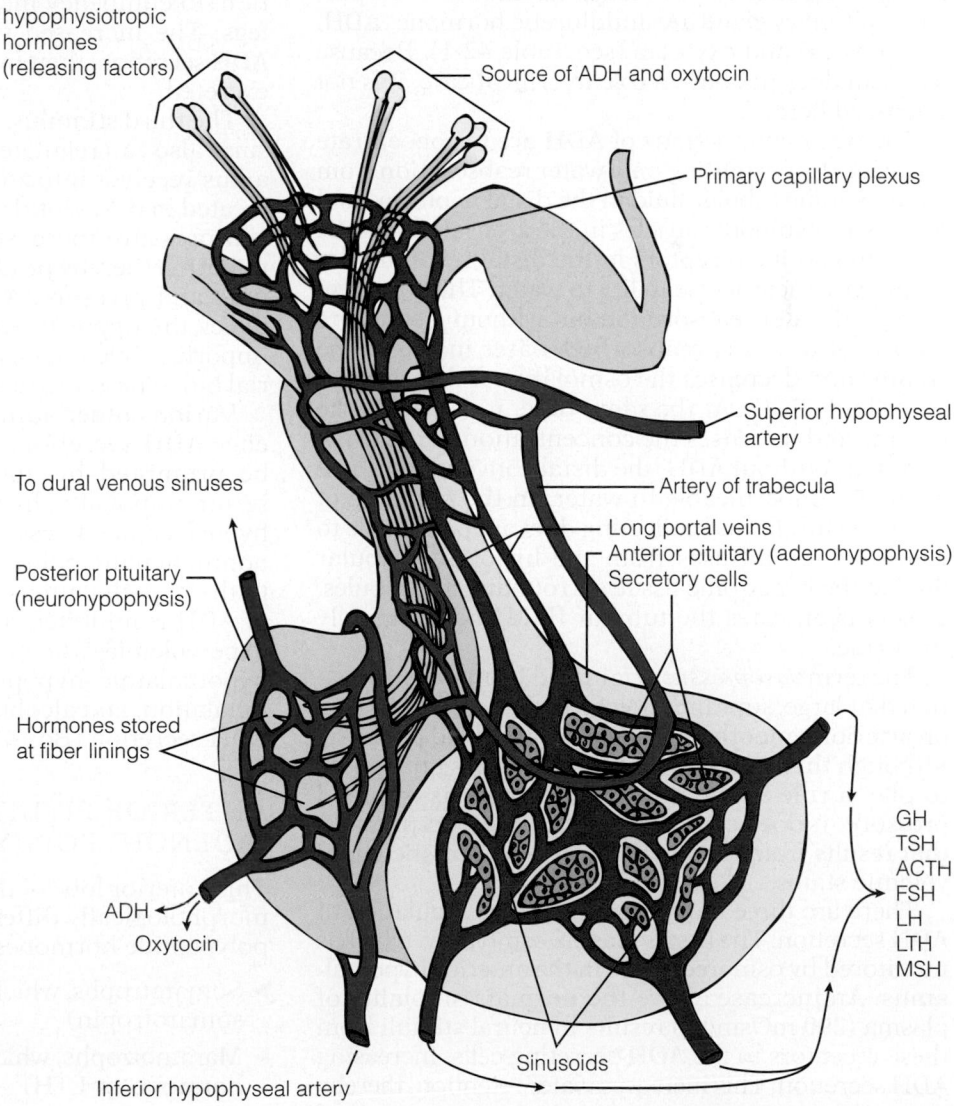

the neural chiasma of the hypothalamus; they are secreted by those cells into the posterior pituitary (see Fig. 42-3). In addition to controlling the pituitary gland through releasing factors, the hypothalamus controls other endocrine roles through releasing factors that control appetite, thirst, emotions, sleep–wake cycles, and cognition.

Such hypothalamic regulation of pituitary functioning can be disrupted by hypothalamic lesions. This can lead to oversecretion or undersecretion of one or more hormones released from the anterior or posterior pituitary. The hypothalamus also receives input from various higher and lower brain centers. These neural connections, together with the influence of the hypothalamus on the pituitary, provide the biological basis for the construction of conceptual models that describe how stress, emotions, environmental stimuli, and perceptions affect endocrine functions.

POSTERIOR PITUITARY (NEUROHYPOPHYSIS) HORMONES

The posterior pituitary (neurohypophysis) makes up 20% of the gland. The two major hormones of the posterior pituitary gland are antidiuretic hormone (ADH, vasopressin) and oxytocin (see Table 42-1). Because oxytocin does not have a role in critical care, it is not discussed here.

The two major actions of ADH are to concentrate the urine (by permitting only water reabsorption from the hypotonic tubular fluid in the distal nephron) and to constrict smooth muscles in the arterial wall. ADH binds to specific receptors in the distal renal tubules to increase their permeability to water. This results in increased water reabsorption but without electrolyte reabsorption. This reabsorbed water increases the volume and decreases the osmolality of the extracellular fluid (ECF). At the same time, it decreases the volume and increases the concentration of the urine excreted. Without ADH, the distal convoluted tubule would be impermeable to water. In the presence of ADH, the tubule and collecting duct are permeable to water, which diffuses from the hypotonic tubular fluid to the hypertonic tissue surrounding the tubules. This concentrates the tubular fluid and ultimately the urine.

The term *vasopressin* originated from the observation that large, supraphysiological dosages of ADH act on arteriole smooth muscle to elevate blood pressure. Although this pressor action of ADH does not appear to play a role in the normal homeostasis of blood pressure, it does counteract a fall in blood pressure that results from hemorrhagic or other drastic hypovolemic states.

There are three major stimuli for the regulation of ADH secretion. The first is plasma osmolality, which is monitored by osmoreceptors in the anterior hypothalamus. An increase above the normal osmolality of plasma (290 mOsm/kg) results in neural stimuli from these receptors to the ADH-secreting cells, increasing ADH secretion. This increases water retention, thereby diluting the ECF and lowering the plasma osmolality back to normal. Similarly, a fall in plasma osmolality triggers a decrease or cessation in ADH secretion. This allows more water excretion, thereby raising the ECF osmolality. ADH secretion can be altered by changes in osmolality of less than 1%. This osmoreceptor-mediated reflex arc functions to maintain osmotic homeostasis of the ECF.

The second stimulus consists of changes in ECF volume. Stretch receptors in the low-pressure portion of the cardiovascular system (e.g., the vena cava, the right side of the heart, and the pulmonary vessels) monitor blood volume. Stimuli from these receptors are conducted by afferent fibers to the hypothalamus (by way of the brainstem). A decrease in blood volume stimulates ADH secretion. The resultant increase in water retention elevates the blood volume. An increase in blood volume stops ADH secretion. This halts water retention, thereby restoring the normal volume of the ECF compartment. This mechanism alters ADH secretion in response to changes in body position. Movement from the recumbent to the upright position causes a temporary decrease in the stimulation of volume receptors because blood pools in the legs. This results in an increase in ADH secretion. Recumbency increases venous return from the legs. The increased volume triggers a decrease in ADH secretion, thereby increasing the volume of urine excreted.

The third stimulus, changes in arterial blood pressure, also can regulate ADH secretion. The hypothalamus receives information from pressure receptors located in the carotid sinuses and aorta. A fall in arterial pressure increases ADH secretion. The water retention thereby produced increases the plasma volume and pressure. A rise in arterial pressure produces the opposite effect. This mechanism is most important in compensating for large changes in arterial blood pressure (e.g., impending or actual shock).

Various other stimuli have been shown to influence ADH secretion. Increased ADH secretion can be prompted by angiotensin II, pain, increased serum osmolality, hypovolemia, nausea and emesis, hypoglycemia, stress, acute infections, malignancies, nonmalignant pulmonary conditions, and trauma to the hypothalamic–hypophyseal system. Secretion of ADH is inhibited by decreased serum osmolality, hypervolemia, water intoxication, cold, trauma to the hypothalamic–hypophyseal system, carbon dioxide inhalation, and alcohol ingestion. Many drugs affect ADH secretion (Box 42-2).

ANTERIOR PITUITARY (ADENOHYPOPHYSIS) HORMONES

This anterior lobe of the pituitary gland contains five morphologically different types of cells that secrete polypeptide hormones:

▶ Somatotrophs, which secrete growth hormone (GH, somatotropin)

▶ Mammotrophs, which secrete prolactin (luteotropic hormone, or LTH)

The production and secretion of GH occurs in the anterior pituitary in response to growth hormone–releasing hormone (GHRH) produced in the hypothalamus. Growth-inhibiting hormone (GIH) inhibits the secretion of GH. GH acts both directly on target cells and indirectly by stimulating the liver and other as-yet-unidentified tissues to secrete various growth factors termed somatomedins. These growth factors are structurally similar to insulin. Direct actions of GH include increasing the breakdown of fats (lipolysis) in adipose cells and releasing the fatty acids produced by lipolysis into the bloodstream (this is termed its ketogenic effect); increasing hepatic glycolysis and thereby increasing plasma glucose levels; increasing the sensitivity of insulin-producing cells to certain stimuli; increasing the cellular uptake of amino acids; and stimulating erythropoiesis.

▶ Thyrotrophs, which secrete thyroid-stimulating hormone (TSH)

▶ Corticotrophs, which secrete adrenocorticotropic hormone (ACTH), β-lipotropin, β-endorphin, and melanophore-stimulating hormone (MSH)

▶ Gonadotrophs, which secrete luteinizing hormone (LH) and follicle-stimulating hormone (FSH)

Each type of cell is separately regulated by hypophysiotropic hormones (Fig. 42-4).

LTH, LH, and FSH are not significant in the critical care arena and are not discussed in this chapter. TSH, which stimulates cells of the thyroid gland to produce and secrete the two thyroid hormones, is discussed later in this chapter, and GH is described in the following paragraph.

• The Thyroid and Parathyroid Glands

The thyroid gland is a bilobed, richly vascularized structure. The lobes lie lateral to the trachea just beneath the larynx and are connected by a bridge of thyroid tissue, the isthmus, that runs across the anterior surface of the trachea (Fig. 42-5). Microscopically, the thyroid is composed primarily of spheroid follicles, each of which stores a colloid material in its center. The follicles produce, store, and secrete the two major thyroid hormones: T_3 and T_4. If the gland is actively secreting, the follicles are small and contain little colloid. Inactive thyroid tissue contains large follicles, each of which possesses a large quantity of stored colloid. Parafollicular cells (C cells), which produce the hormone calcitonin, are scattered between the follicles of the thyroid gland.

Each lobe of the thyroid gland typically contains two parathyroid glands: one in its superior pole and one in its inferior pole. Individual variation exists with

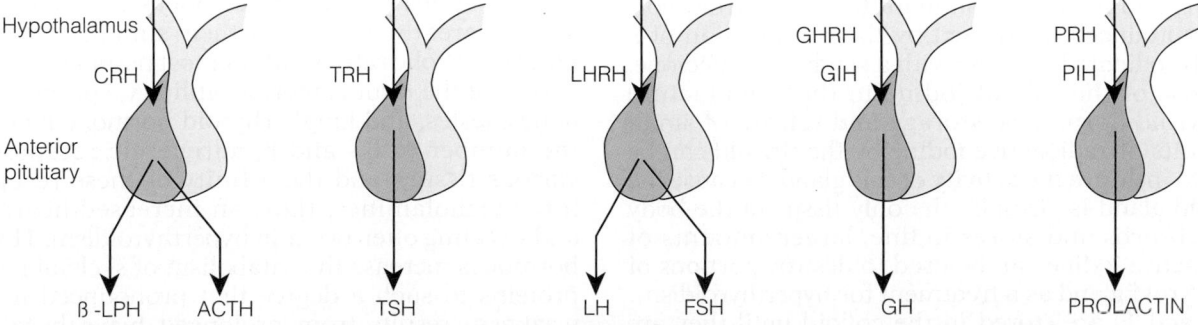

Figure 42-4 • Effects of the hypophysiotropic hormones on the secretion of anterior pituitary hormones. The hypophysiotropic hormones are corticotropin-releasing hormone (CRH), thyrotropin-releasing hormone (TRH), luteinizing hormone–releasing hormone (LHRH), growth hormone–releasing hormone (GHRH), growth-inhibiting hormone (GIH), prolactin-inhibiting hormone (PIH); and prolactin-releasing hormone (PRH). CRH prompts the release of β-lipotropin (β-LPH) and adrenocorticotropic hormone (ACTH). TRH prompts the release of thyroid-stimulating hormone (TSH). LHRH prompts the release of luteinizing hormone (LH) and follicle-stimulating hormone (FSH). GHRH and GIH promote and inhibit the secretion of growth hormone (GH), respectively. PRH and PIH promote and inhibit the secretion of prolactin, respectively.

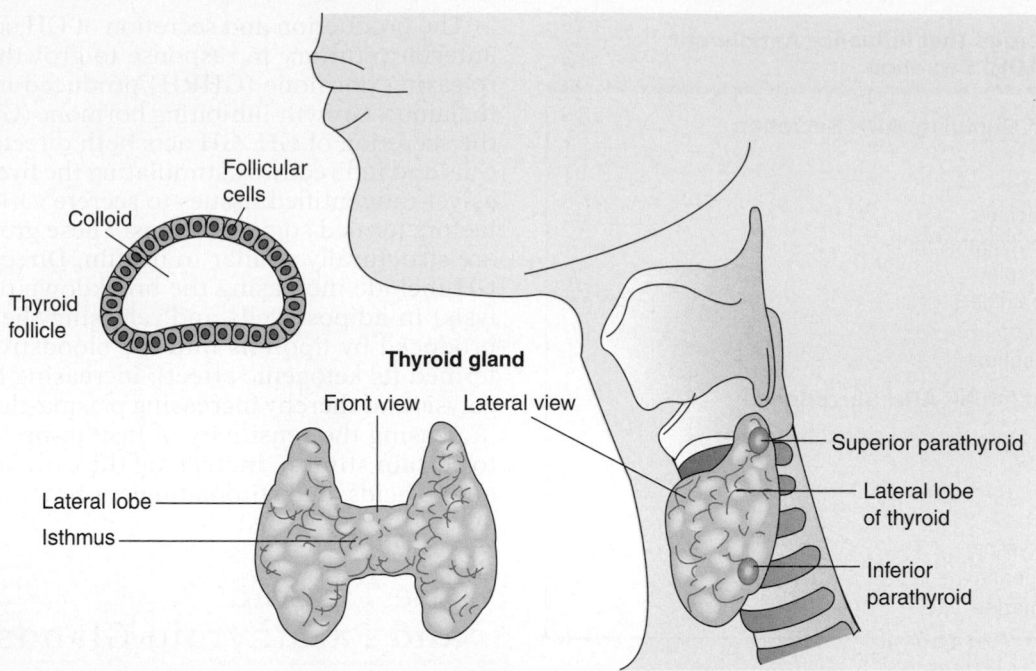

Figure 42-5 • The thyroid gland. (From Porth CM: Pathophysiology: Concepts of Altered Health States, 7th ed. Philadelphia: Lippincott Williams & Wilkins, 2005, p 970.)

respect to the number and distribution of parathyroid glands. Some people have more or fewer than four. Others have parathyroid tissue in the mediastinum. The parathyroid glands produce parathyroid hormone (PTH).

THYROID HORMONES

The follicular cells absorb tyrosine (an amino acid) and iodide from the plasma and secrete them into the central colloid portion of the follicle, where they are used in the synthesis of T_3 and T_4. (The subscript refers to the number of iodide molecules that each substance contains.) Two iodide molecules are attached, first one and then the other, to each tyrosine molecule. Two such doubly iodinated tyrosines are combined to form T_4. T_3, which is much more biologically active than T_4 and is the predominant form of thyroid hormone produced, is formed by the combination of a doubly iodinated tyrosine with a singly iodinated one. Because of the role of iodine in the manufacture of thyroid hormones, storage and release of small amounts of radioactive iodine by the thyroid can be used to measure the activity of this gland. Because the thyroid gland is virtually the only tissue of the body that absorbs and stores iodine, larger amounts of radioactive iodine can be used to destroy portions of the thyroid gland as a treatment for hyperthyroidism.

T_3 and T_4 are stored in the colloid until they are needed. When they are to be secreted, the follicular cells transport them from the colloid to the plasma. Less than 1% of the secreted T_3 and T_4 remains free and physiologically active in the plasma. The remainder is bound to plasma proteins. The plasma proteins involved in transporting T_3 and T_4 are manufactured in the liver. Consequently, liver damage that decreases

the plasma levels of these proteins can produce a condition resembling thyroid hormone excess (i.e., hyperthyroidism). Plasma levels of these proteins can also be depressed by glucocorticoids, androgens, and L-asparaginase (an antineoplastic drug). They are elevated during pregnancy, and by estrogens, opiates, clofibrate, and major tranquilizers. Thyroid hormones are deiodinated and catabolized by the liver, kidneys, and various other tissues. A small amount of degraded hormone is added to the bile secreted by the liver and is excreted in the stool.

T_3 directly crosses target cell membranes, whereas T_4 is changed into T_3 by target cell membranes before crossing. The conversion of T_4 to T_3 occurs in the peripheral tissues of the liver and kidneys and accounts for 80% of the T_3 available for metabolic activity. T_4 is 100% produced in the thyroid.

The actions of thyroid hormones are widespread and apparently arise from their stimulation of the basal metabolic rate (BMR) of most tissues (excluding tissues of the brain, anterior pituitary, spleen, lymph nodes, testes, and lung). Thyroid hormone increases the number of β_1- and β_2-adrenergic receptors in various tissues and the affinity of these receptors for catecholamines; thus, an increased heart rate and sweating often occur in hyperthyroidism. Thyroid hormones increase the catabolism of skeletal muscle proteins to such a degree that pronounced muscle weakness results from prolonged hyperthyroidism (thyrotoxic myopathy). Thyroid hormones increase the rate of carbohydrate absorption from the small intestine and decrease circulating levels of cholesterol.

Thyroid hormones are essential for the normal growth and development of many body systems, notably the skeletal and nervous systems. These hormones stimulate the secretion of GH and potentiate its effect on various tissues. Thyroid hormones are also necessary for normal levels of neuronal functioning. Thyroid insufficiency leads to slowed reflexes, slowed mentation, and decreased level of consciousness (through decreased levels of reticular activating system activity). Hyperthyroidism lowers synaptic thresholds in the central nervous system (CNS), causing hyperreflexia and a fine muscle tremor. The pervasive effects of thyroid hormones on the nervous system are best illustrated by cretinism, a condition resulting from congenital thyroid insufficiency.

The secretion of T_3 and T_4 by the thyroid gland is primarily regulated by the secretion of TSH from the anterior pituitary. In turn, TSH secretion is regulated by a hypothalamic neurosecretory material termed thyrotropin-releasing hormone (TRH). After receiving stimuli from TRH from the hypothalamus, the thyroid secretes TSH to stimulate the manufacture and secretion of T_3 and T_4. A negative feedback regulatory loop exists whereby increased levels of free (unbound) T_3 and T_4 suppress TSH secretion. Decreased plasma TSH results in decreased thyroid function, which causes a fall in free plasma T_3 and T_4. Low T_3 and T_4 levels stimulate TSH secretion. If a TSH-induced increase in thyroid activity does not raise the plasma levels of free T_3 and T_4, the continued high levels of TSH eventually cause an increase in the size of the thyroid gland (nontoxic goiter). In this case, an enlarged thyroid is not associated with overproduction of hormone. This feedback loop maintains homeostasis of the daily secretion of TSH and thyroid hormones.

CALCITONIN AND PARATHYROID HORMONE

Calcitonin, which is secreted by the parafollicular cells of the thyroid gland, and PTH, which is produced and secreted by the parathyroid glands, exert a major influence on calcium metabolism in conjunction with 1,25-dihydroxycholecalciferol, which is produced by the action of the liver and the kidneys on vitamin D. Ultraviolet light changes 7-dehydrocholesterol provitamins in the skin to a group of compounds, collectively called vitamin D. One of these, D_3, can also be obtained from vitamin D–enriched and other foods. The liver converts D_3 to 25-hydroxycholecalciferol, which is then altered by kidney cells to a more active form, 1,25-dihydroxycholecalciferol. (The hypocalcemia seen in chronic renal disease results from an activated vitamin D deficiency.) Activated vitamin D acts on intracellular enzymes of the intestinal mucosal cells to increase calcium absorption. To a lesser extent, it also increases the active transport of calcium out of osteoblasts into the bloodstream. Both of these actions elevate plasma calcium levels. In vitamin deficiency states, the effect of decreased intestinal absorption outweighs any decrease in the mobilization of calcium from bone to produce an overall hypocalcia and poor mineralization of bone.

Vitamin D is synthesized in the skin, absorbed in the small intestine, and transported into the plasma bound to vitamin D–binding proteins. The metabolism of vitamin D is strictly regulated by phosphate concentration in the kidney and by PTH. Thus, the effect of a decrease in dietary phosphate or serum phosphate is to increase levels of 1,25-dihydroxycholecalciferol.

Parathyroid Hormone

PTH is a polypeptide produced and secreted by the chief cells of the parathyroid glands. This hormone is stored in secretory granules and released in response to a decrease in ionized calcium concentrations. It is cleaved into active form in the kidneys and liver. Plasma calcium and phosphate levels operate in a negative feedback loop to influence the activity of the renal enzyme system, which catalyzes the conversion of metabolically inactive vitamin D to the metabolically active form. High plasma calcium levels decrease this activation process, whereas low levels increase it. The formation of activated vitamin D is also facilitated by PTH and decreased by metabolic acidosis and hypoinsulinemia (diabetes mellitus).

PTH is transported free (unbound) in the plasma, has a half-life of less than 20 minutes, and is metabolically degraded by cells in the liver. A decrease in calcium concentration increases PTH secretion. PTH acts on two target tissues: bone cells and kidney tubules. In bone, it stimulates osteoclast activity and inhibits osteoblast activity. This results in bone reabsorption with consequent mobilization of calcium and phosphate from the bony matrix into the bloodstream. In the kidney, PTH increases the reabsorption of calcium by distal tubule cells and decreases the reabsorption of phosphate by proximal tubule cells. The effect of these multiple actions is elevation of plasma calcium levels and lowering of plasma phosphate levels.

Plasma calcium levels alter PTH secretion through a negative feedback loop. Secretion is inhibited by high plasma calcium levels and stimulated by low blood levels of calcium. The activated vitamin D deficiency–induced hypocalcemia, which occurs in chronic renal failure, typically produces a secondary hyperparathyroidism. Secretion of PTH by the parathyroid gland is also stimulated by hypomagnesemia, adrenergic agonists, and prostaglandins.

Calcitonin

This polypeptide hormone is produced by the parafollicular cells (C cells) of the thyroid gland. It can also be secreted by nonthyroidal tissue (e.g., tissue of the lung, intestine, pituitary, and bladder). Calcitonin is transported unbound in the plasma. It has a half-life of 5 minutes and is predominantly metabolized in the kidney. Calcitonin lowers plasma calcium and phosphate levels by inhibiting osteoclastic bone reabsorption and increasing urinary phosphate and calcium excretion. Calcitonin levels are elevated during pregnancy and lactation, suggesting that calcitonin may help to protect the mother's skeleton from excess calcium loss during these periods of calcium drain.

Calcitonin does not function in the normal daily homeostasis of plasma calcium levels. It appears to serve more of an emergency function in that it is

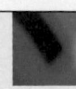

Table 42-2 • Hormones of the Thyroid and Parathyroid Glands and Their Actions

Gland	Hormone	Action
Thyroid gland	Thyroxine (T_4)	Controls basic metabolic rate
	Triiodothyronine (T_3)	Induces growth and development
		Inhibits bone resorption
	Calcitonin	Inhibits calcium reabsorption in gastrointestinal tract
		Increases calcium excretion from kidney
Parathyroid gland	Parathyroid hormone	Promotes bone resorption
		Increases calcium reabsorption
		Increases calcium blood levels

secreted only if the plasma calcium level exceeds 9.3 mg/dL. At high blood calcium levels, calcitonin secretion is stimulated by increased levels of plasma calcium. Calcitonin is also released by the action of gastrin, glucagon, and secretion of gastrointestinal hormones.

Table 42-2 summarizes the hormones secreted by the thyroid and parathyroid glands.

• The Endocrine Pancreas

The pancreas lies transversely under the stomach between the duodenum and spleen. Because of its posterior position, it is essentially hidden and is not palpable. The pancreas has both endocrine and exocrine functions, which are under the control of different groups of cells. The organ is made up of two tissue types: the acini, the exocrine portion; and the islets of Langerhans, the endocrine portion. The acini secrete digestive enzymes into the duodenum, whereas the islets of Langerhans secrete hormones into the blood.

The islets of Langerhans secrete the peptide hormones involved in blood glucose regulation. The name "islets of Langerhans" refers to the more than 1 million ovoid islands (clusters) of cells that are scattered throughout the pancreas, predominantly in the tail. Because of this distribution of islet cells, acute attacks of pancreatitis, which usually spare the tail, tend to spare the islets. Episodes of chronic recurrent pancreatitis typically involve the entire pancreas. Consequently, these episodes cause islet cell destruction and diabetes mellitus.

Each cell cluster is richly supplied with capillaries, into which its hormones are secreted. The islets are composed of four types of cells: α cells, which secrete glucagon; β cells, which secrete insulin; δ cells, which secrete somatostatin; and F cells, which secrete pancreatic polypeptide. The hormones secreted by the pancreas are summarized in Table 42-3.

INSULIN

Insulin, an anabolic hormone, is regulated by a number of stimulatory and inhibitory factors. It is responsible for the control of blood glucose concentrations and storage of carbohydrate, proteins, and fats. Insulin facilitates the use of glucose as the main source of energy for most body tissues. Insulin is the only hormone with the ability to directly lower the blood glucose level. Also, insulin facilitates an increase in the cellular transport of glucose, amino acids, and fatty acids across cell membranes and modulates intracellular metabolic synthesis of nucleic acids.

The precursor of insulin, proinsulin, is manufactured in the β cells of the islets of Langerhans. Proinsulin can be thought of as a "necklace" of amino acid

Table 42-3 • Hormones of the Pancreas and Their Actions

Hormone	Cell	Stimulant	Response
Insulin	β	Glucose	Decreased glucose level
			Increased fat storage
			Increased protein synthesis
			Increased glucogenesis
Glucagon	α	Decreased glucose level, exercise	Increased glucose level
			Increased gluconeogenesis
			Increased glycogenolysis
Somatostatin	δ	Hyperglycemia	Increased glucose
			Increased glycogen
Pancreatic polypeptide	F	Acute hypoglycemia	Increased gallbladder contraction
			Increased pancreatic enzymes

beads and is stored as secretory granules in another cell structure. Proinsulin can be found in the plasma as a result of certain islet tumors (insulinoma) or overstimulation of the β cells. Connecting peptide (C-peptide) is a biologically inactive chain and is secreted into the bloodstream along with insulin. Because there is a 1:1 ratio between C-peptide and insulin, plasma C-peptide levels can be used to measure endogenous insulin secretion or degree of β cell activity. Clinically, C-peptide levels can assist with distinguishing between types 1 and 2 diabetes (C-peptide is low in type 1 diabetes, reflecting autodestruction of β cells and no further production of insulin).[1]

The actions of insulin are summarized in Box 42-3. In addition to facilitating glucose uptake by muscle and adipose cells, insulin facilitates glucose uptake by connective tissue, leukocytes, mammary glands, the lens of the eye, the aorta, the pituitary gland, and α islet cells. In general, insulin enables glucose to be readily available for aerobic oxidation in muscle, adipose, and connective tissue cells. Facilitation of the preferential use of glucose as cellular fuel means that the cells do not need to oxidize fatty or amino acids. Instead, these can be conserved. Protein synthesis and fat storage are increased in liver, muscle, and adipose tissue. Breakdown of fats and proteins is decreased. Hepatic gluconeogenesis also is decreased or halted, and glycogen synthesis is increased.

Insulin acts only on a few types of tissues. However, the membranes of nearly all types of body cells possess insulin receptors. Binding of insulin to the insulin receptors initiates the physiological action of insulin on the cell. Plasma insulin has a half-life of approximately 5 minutes. About 80% of all circulating insulin is catabolized by liver and kidney cells.

Insulin secretion is influenced by a variety of factors as listed in Box 42-4. Monosaccharides are the primary regulatory mechanism for insulin secretion. Elevated plasma levels of glucose act in a negative feedback loop to increase the secretion of insulin. Lower levels of glucose decrease insulin output. Glucagon, β-adrenergic agonists, and theophylline increase insulin secretion. B cells are also stimulated to secrete insulin by tolbutamide and other sulfonylurea derivatives; acetylcholine; impulses from vagal nerve branches to the

islets; selected amino acids, such as arginine; and β-ketoacids. The mechanisms of action of these stimuli are as yet unclear. Insulin production is inhibited by α-adrenergic agonists, β-adrenergic blocking agents, diazoxide (Proglycem), thiazide diuretics, phenytoin (Dilantin), alloxan, agents that prevent glucose metabolism (e.g., 2-deoxyglucose and mannoheptulose), somatostatin, and insulin itself.

Chronic stimulation of β cells, such as by a high-carbohydrate diet for several weeks, can cause a limited amount of hypertrophy and subsequent increase in the insulin-producing capacity. However, overstimulation produces β-cell exhaustion. Stimulation of these exhausted cells produces β-cell death and depletes the β-cell reserve. β-Cell activity is also decreased by the administration of exogenous insulin. Such decreased activity enables the cells to rest and results in temporary hyperproduction after the withdrawal of exogenous insulin.

INSULIN RESISTANCE

Insulin resistance, which may be characteristic of type 2 diabetes, is the main defect seen with the development of hyperglycemia, hyperinsulinemia, and consequent β-cell exhaustion. Insulin resistance is a physiological condition in which a person needs more insulin to lower serum glucose effectively than would normally be required. To compensate for insulin resistance, the pancreas secretes more insulin in an attempt to maintain normal glucose levels. The degree of obesity directly affects the resistance to insulin in most patients with type 2 diabetes. One principal mechanism may be a defect in insulin receptor function due to a genetic mutation of the insulin receptor gene. The quantity and activity of insulin receptors

---

Box 42-4 • Factors Affecting Insulin Secretion

Stimulators	Inhibitors
Glucose	Somatostatin
Mannose	2-Deoxyglucose
Amino acids (leucine, arginine, others)	Mannoheptulose
Intestinal hormones (gastric inhibitory peptide [GIP], gastrin, secretin, cholecystokinin [CCK], glucagon, others?)	α-Adrenergic-stimulating agents (norepinephrine, epinephrine)
β-Keto acids	β-Adrenergic-blocking agents (propranolol)
Acetylcholine	Diazoxide
Glucagon	Thiazide diuretics
Cyclic adenosine monophosphate (AMP) and various cyclic AMP–generating substances	Phenytoin
	Alloxan
β-Adrenergic-stimulating agents	Microtubule inhibitors
Theophylline	Insulin
Sulfonylureas	

Box 42-3 • Major Actions of Insulin on Adipose and Muscle Cells

Muscle Cells	Adipose Cells
Increased glucose entry	Increased glucose entry
Increased K+ uptake	Increased K+ uptake
Increased glycogen synthesis	Increased fatty acid entry and synthesis
Increased amino acid entry	Increased fat deposition
Increased protein synthesis	Increased conversion of glucose to fatty acids
Decreased protein catabolism	Inhibition of lipolysis
Increased ketone entry into cells	

also can be regulated by various factors. Increased amounts of insulin, obesity, acromegaly, excess gluco-corticoids, and human immunodeficiency virus (HIV) therapies can exacerbate insulin resistance by decreasing the receptors' number or activity, or both. Exercise and decreased circulating levels of insulin increase the activity of insulin receptors[2]; therefore, leading a sedentary lifestyle may contribute to insulin resistance.

Additional conditions play a role in the pathogenesis of type 2 diabetes mellitus: β-cell dysfunction and excess hepatic glucose production that contributes to hyperglycemia. β-Cell dysfunction results when the pancreas is unable to meet the high demands for insulin due to insulin resistance. When type 2 diabetes mellitus is diagnosed, approximately 50% of β-cell function is already lost.

Several theories explain the development of β-cell dysfunction:

▶ Cell exhaustion results when the pancreas must keep up with the higher demands for insulin. Some functional and morphological changes occur to compensate for the increased demand, but eventually β-cell exhaustion occurs.

▶ Chronic hyperglycemia leads to the development of glucotoxicity—direct toxicity to the β cells.

▶ Chronic exposure of β cells to excess free fatty acids damages them, leading to lipotoxicity.

▶ Apoptosis, or programmed cell death, occurs secondary to chronic glucotoxicity and lipotoxicity. This leads to progressive β–islet cell loss.

▶ Abnormal deposition of amyloid matter leads to islet cell destruction.[3]

Insulin resistance interferes with normal cellular interactions between insulin, skeletal muscles, and adipose tissues. Insulin binds with cell surface receptors, causing a cascade of intracellular signals; this results in the translocation of glucose transporter cells to cell surfaces and allows entry of glucose into the cell. In addition, insulin may bind normally to receptors but has to work with disrupted signals, resulting in insufficient translocation of glucose transporter molecules. This ultimately leads to excess glucose accumulation.[2]

Insulin resistance triggers β cells to produce more insulin as a compensatory mechanism. Hyperinsulinemia initially meets the additional needs created by excess glucose. However, when β-cell function fails to satisfy these demands, hyperglycemia and type 2 diabetes mellitus ensue. This is termed the dual phenomenon or dual abnormality: insulin resistance and β-cell dysfunction.[3] Data from a landmark trial, the United Kingdom Prospective Diabetes Study (UKPDS), suggest that the process of declining β-cell function occurs for approximately 10 years before the diagnosis of type 2 diabetes is made.[4]

GLUCAGON

This polypeptide hormone is manufactured and secreted by the α cells of the islets of Langerhans and is stimulated by pure protein meal ingestion that produces an aminoacidemia. The half-life of plasma glucagon is 5 to 10 minutes. Glucagon influences enzyme systems in liver, fat, and muscle cells and is degraded mainly by the liver.

The major function of glucagon, which stimulates the synthesis of the gluconeogenic enzyme fructose-1,6-biphosphate, is to elevate blood glucose levels and then to enable this plasma glucose to enter and be used by the cells of the body (e.g., the muscle cells) by stimulating the secretion of insulin. In this manner, glucagon prevents hypoglycemia between meals, during exercise, during the first few days of fasting, and after a high-protein meal. Dietary protein stimulates an increase in plasma insulin, which causes a rapid cellular uptake of absorbed dietary carbohydrates.

To elevate blood glucose levels, glucagon stimulates liver cells to perform glycogenolysis and gluconeogenesis. This increases the glucose concentration in liver cells, and because these cells can dephosphorylate intracellular glucose, this glucose can be released from the liver into the bloodstream. The fatty acids and amino acids needed for gluconeogenesis are supplied by the glucagon-stimulated breakdown of fats in adipose cells and the release of fatty acids into the bloodstream. If the supply of fatty acids is not sufficient, glucagon also stimulates the breakdown of proteins into amino acids in muscle cells and the release of amino acids into the plasma. These fatty acids and amino acids are then taken up by hepatocytes and used as raw materials in gluconeogenesis. Glucagon also elevates plasma ketone levels by increasing hepatic ketone production, and promotes the secretion of somatostatin and GH.

Although glucagon opposes the effects of insulin on blood sugar levels, it also stimulates the secretion of insulin. This apparent contradiction is actually a logical second step in the biological function of this hormone. It enables the increased plasma glucose to enter and be used by various tissues. An elevated plasma glucose level stimulates insulin secretion, but this takes a while. The direct action of glucagon on β cells simply is faster.

As is the case with β cells, α cells are stimulated by β-adrenergic agonists, theophylline, elevated plasma levels of dietary amino acids (primarily those used in gluconeogenesis), and vagal (cholinergic) stimulation. Glucagon secretion is also prompted by glucocorticoids (e.g., cortisol), catecholamines, growth hormone, cholecystokinin (CCK), and gastrin. Exercise, physical stress, and infections also increase α-cell activity. Whereas the effects of exercise on glucagon secretion appear to be mediated by increased β-adrenergic activity, stress and infection probably operate by increasing plasma glucocorticoid levels. Dietary amino acids are believed to enhance glucagon secretion by their effects on CCK or gastrin, or both, because intravenous amino acids exert little or no effect on α cells.

Elevated plasma glucose levels enact a negative feedback loop to retard or halt the output of glucagon; however, plasma insulin must be present for this mechanism to operate. Like β-cell secretion, α-cell secretion is inhibited by adrenergic agonists, phenytoin, and somatostatin. Fatty acids and ketone bodies in the plasma can inhibit glucagon secretion, but this inhibition must be weak because plasma glucagon levels can be quite elevated during diabetic ketoacidosis.

In addition to glucagon, other hormones—cortisol, epinephrine, and GH—have great influence on the regulation of glucose and insulin. These counter-regulatory hormones have a synergistic effect on glucose production as a mechanism to protect the body during stress. They act to inhibit insulin while increasing glucagon, producing an insulin-resistant state, and increasing overall serum glucose levels to produce sufficient energy levels during "fight-or-flight" responses. These hormones elevate serum glucose levels to protect against hypoglycemia and to prepare the body for stress. However, they can also further aggravate a state of hyperglycemia and can lead to dangerous levels of glucose, as seen in diabetic emergencies.[5]

SOMATOSTATIN

This tetradecapeptide is produced not only by the δ cells of the pancreas but also by the hypothalamus, where it functions as an inhibitor of anterior pituitary GH secretion; neurons of the CNS, where it probably functions as a synaptic neurotransmitter agent; and δ cells in the gastric mucosa, where it inhibits the secretion of gastrin and other, lesser known gastrointestinal hormones. Islet cell somatostatin is secreted into the bloodstream and therefore functions as a hormone. Little is known of the metabolism of somatostatin because it is so tightly bound with the actions of GH.

Somatostatin inhibits the release of insulin and glucagons from the pancreas. Pancreatic somatostatin inhibits the activity of all other islet cells. The biological significance of this action is not yet known. The only clinical data of relevance concern δ-cell tumors. These produce a clinical picture that resembles diabetes mellitus but that is reversible with tumor ablation. The secretion of somatostatin from islet cells is increased by glucose, certain amino acids, and CCK. Factors that inhibit islet somatostatin secretion are unknown.

PANCREATIC POLYPEPTIDE

Not much is known about this islet hormone in humans. It is produced by the endocrine cells found in small clusters of cells located between the cells of the islets of Langerhans and the acinar cells of the pancreas. Its secretion in humans is enhanced by dietary protein, exercise, acute hypoglycemia, and fasting. Somatostatin and elevated plasma glucose levels decrease the secretion of this polypeptide. No definite actions of this hormone have been established for humans, but it appears to have a role in smooth muscle relaxation of the gallbladder.

• The Adrenal Glands

The adrenal glands lie at the superior pole of each kidney retroperitoneally. Each gland is composed of an inner core, the medulla, surrounded by an outer layer, the cortex (Fig. 42-6). Although they are structurally related, the medulla and cortex are derived from different embryological tissues and function as separate entities. The hormones produced by the adrenal glands are summarized in Table 42-4.

MEDULLARY HORMONES

The adrenal medulla is basically a modified sympathetic ganglion. The axons of preganglionic sympathetic neurons arrive from the thoracic cord by way of splanchnic nerves. They synapse in the adrenal medulla with modified postganglionic cells that have

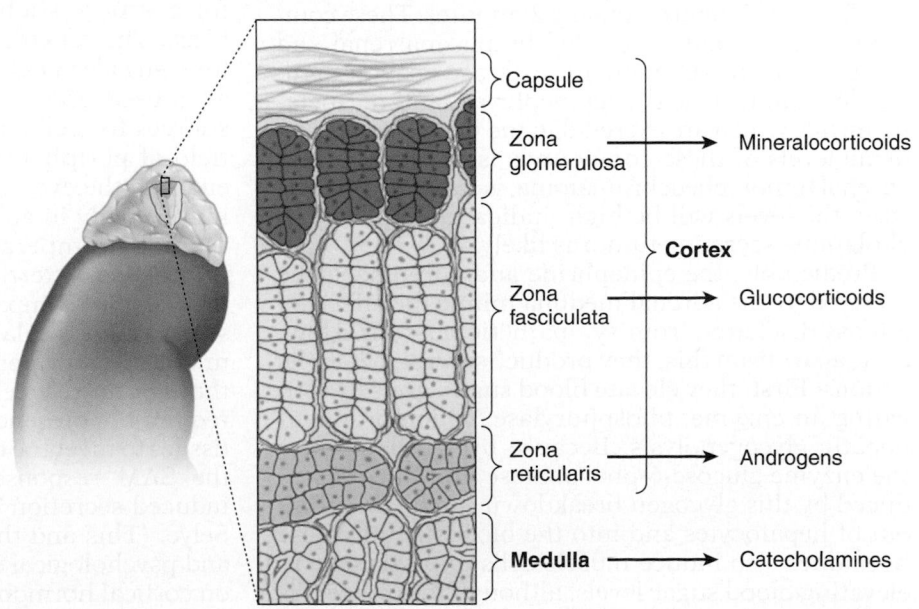

Figure 42-6 • The adrenal gland has a cortex and a medulla. (From Seifter J, Ratner A, Sloane D: Concepts in Medical Physiology. Philadelphia: Lippincott Williams & Wilkins, 2005, p 541.)

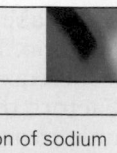

Table 42-4 • Hormones of the Adrenal Gland and Their Actions

Gland	Hormone	Action
Adrenal gland cortex	Mineralocorticoids	Reabsorption of sodium Elimination of potassium
	Glucocorticoids	Responds to stress Decreases inflammation Alters metabolism of protein and fat
Medulla	Epinephrine	Stimulates sympathetic system
	Norepinephrine	Increases peripheral resistance

lost their axons and secrete chemicals directly into the bloodstream. Therefore, the adrenal medulla may appropriately be viewed as an endocrine extension of the autonomic nervous system.

Four chemicals are produced and secreted in the adrenal medulla by two morphologically different cell types:

▶ Dopamine, a precursor of norepinephrine

▶ Norepinephrine, the typical product of postganglionic sympathetic neurons

▶ Epinephrine, a methylated version of norepinephrine

▶ Opioid peptides (enkephalins)

Not much is known about the opioid peptides. The specific stimulus for their secretion has yet to be identified, and their physiological actions are unknown, as are their metabolism and fate. Dopamine, norepinephrine, and epinephrine are collectively termed catecholamines. They are stored in granules in the medullary cells. The secretion of these chemicals is triggered by stimulation of the preganglionic neurons that innervate the medulla. This causes the neurons to release acetylcholine, which in turn prompts the medullary cells to secrete. The half-life of plasma catecholamines is approximately 2 minutes. These compounds are rapidly degraded by plasma renal and hepatic catechol-O-methyltransferase enzymes into vanillylmandelic acid, metanephrine, and normetanephrine, which are excreted in the urine. Measuring urine levels of these compounds is significant if an adrenal tumor, pheochromatoma, is suspected. In this case, the levels will be high, indicating that a catecholamine secreting tumor is likely.

Predictably, the epinephrine and norepinephrine secreted by the adrenal medulla mimic the effects of a mass discharge from sympathetic neurons. However, apart from this, they produce several metabolic actions. First, they elevate blood sugar levels by activating an enzyme, phosphorylase, which promotes hepatic glycogenolysis. Because liver cells possess the enzyme glucose-6-phosphatase, the glucose produced by this glycogen breakdown is able to diffuse out of hepatocytes and into the bloodstream. These hormones also induce muscle cells to participate in elevating blood sugar levels, although this process is

less direct. These hormones can also elevate plasma glucose levels by stimulating the secretion of glucagon and can increase the uptake of glucose into body tissues by stimulating the secretion of insulin. Epinephrine and norepinephrine can also produce the opposite effects by stimulating α-adrenergic receptors on islet cells. Because of differential effects of both hormones on α- and β-adrenergic receptors, the result is that epinephrine elevates plasma glucose levels much more than does norepinephrine.

A second metabolic effect of catecholamines is promotion of lipolysis in adipose tissue. This elevates plasma free fatty acid levels and provides an alternative energy source for many body cells. Circulating catecholamines also increase alertness by stimulating the reticular activating system. Last, these hormones produce an increase in the metabolic rate of the body and a cutaneous vasoconstriction, both of which result in an elevation in body temperature. However, the accelerated metabolism requires the presence of the thyroid and adrenal cortex hormones.

Although the physiological action of adrenal medullary dopamine is unknown, exogenous dopamine is useful in combating certain shocks because it has a positive inotropic effect on the heart (by way of β receptors) and produces renal vasodilation and peripheral vasoconstriction. The overall effect of moderate dosages is elevation of systolic blood pressure (without an appreciable increase in diastolic blood pressure) together with retention or restoration of renal output.

Stimulation of the adrenal medulla glands is part of a general sympathetic–adrenal medulla (SAM) response to exercise and to perceived threats to biopsychological integrity and survival. (Cannon called the latter the "fight-or-flight" response.) Hypoglycemia also stimulates increased adrenal medullary secretion. The results of the SAM response enable the body to perform vigorous physical exertion optimally. The heart rate and blood pressure are increased (increasing perfusion), and blood flow is shunted away from the skin and gastrointestinal tract to more vital organs for exertion, such as skeletal muscles, brain, and heart. The reticular activating system is stimulated, fostering alertness. Blood glucose and fatty acid levels are raised, thereby increasing the available energy sources for cells. Pupils are dilated, increasing the field of peripheral vision and the amount of light entering the eyes. Sweat glands are stimulated, cooling the body in advance of and during the time that the body temperature is elevated as the result of the physical exertion. Most of this SAM response is mediated by sympathetic nerve fibers to various body structures; circulating catecholamines play only a minor role. Furthermore, many tissue responses (e.g., those of muscle cells) to such sympathetic demands require the presence of glucocorticoids to enable the tissues to meet the demands of the SAM response, and the SAM response often accompanies the stress-induced secretion of adrenal steroids discovered by Selye. (This and the endocrine response to physical and psychological stress are discussed in the section on cortical hormones.)

CORTICAL HORMONES

The adrenal cortex is composed of three histologically different layers (see Fig. 42-6). Its exterior is covered by a capsule. The outermost layer, the zona glomerulosa, lies just beneath the capsule. It produces and secretes primarily mineralocorticoids, such as aldosterone. The inner two layers, the zona fasciculata and zona reticularis, manufacture and secrete glucocorticoids (cortisol and corticosterone) and adrenal androgens and estrogens. If these inner cortical layers are destroyed, they can be regenerated from zona glomerulosa cells.

Figure 42-7 depicts the metabolic pathways for synthesis of all adrenocortical hormones. Each of these metabolic steps is governed by a specific enzyme. Genetic deficiencies in one or more of these enzymes produce syndromes involving the underproduction or overproduction of various cortical hormones. Drugs that inhibit specific enzymes are used clinically to assess cortical function. One such drug is metyrapone, which inhibits cortisol synthesis.

After secretion, plasma cortisol and, to a lesser extent, corticosterones are bound to a plasma globulin called corticosteroid-binding globulin (CBG), or transcortin. Only the unbound hormones are physiologically active. The bound glucocorticoids serve as a hormone reservoir that is used to replace degraded unbound hormone. The half-lives of plasma corticosterone and cortisol are approximately 50 and 80 minutes, respectively. CBG is manufactured by liver cells. Therefore, decreased hepatic function (e.g., cirrhosis) can lead to subnormal quantities of plasma CBG, resulting in excess quantities of circulating unbound, active glucocorticoids. Only a small amount of aldosterone is bound to plasma proteins. Its half-life is approximately 20 minutes.

Adrenal steroids are degraded by the liver. Depressed hepatic function can retard the degradation of adrenal steroids, thereby producing a clinical picture of hormone excess. The soluble degraded steroid metabolites are excreted by the kidneys.

Glucocorticoids

As the name glucocorticoid suggests, cortisol and corticosterone influence glucose metabolism. They elevate plasma glucose levels by promoting hepatic gluconeogenesis and glycogenolysis. To facilitate gluconeogenesis, these hormones cause the breakdown of fat and proteins and the release of fatty and amino acids into the bloodstream, which carries them to the liver. Excessive gluconeogenesis can lead to severe hyperglycemia often seen in diabetic patients receiving glucocorticoids.

Glucocorticoids enable tissues to respond to glucagon and catecholamines; they also prevent rapid fatigue of skeletal muscle. Cortisol and corticosterone also act on the kidneys to permit the excretion of a normal water load in one of three ways: glucocorticoids make distal or collecting tubules more permeable to the reabsorption of water independently of sodium reabsorption, they increase the glomerular filtration rate (GFR), or they reduce the output of ADH.

The effects of glucocorticoids on plasma components are mixed. They decrease the number of plasma eosinophils and basophils but increase the number of circulating neutrophils, platelets, and erythrocytes. By

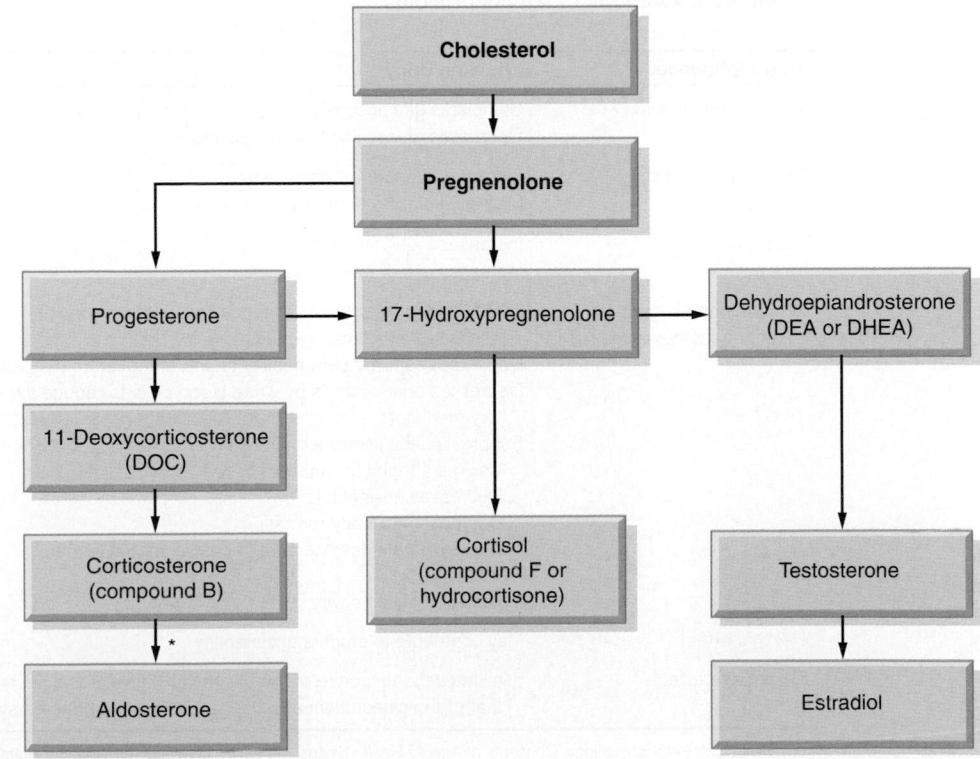

Figure 42-7 • Biosynthetic pathways for adrenal cortical hormones. Only cells of the zona glomerulosa can convert corticosterone to aldosterone (*). All the other pathways can be carried out by cells in all three layers of the adrenal cortex.

suppressing production and increasing destruction, glucocorticoids decrease the number of lymphocytes. They also decrease the size of lymph nodes. A major function of lymphocytes is to provide either humoral immunity (with antibodies) or cell-mediated immunity. Stress-induced elevations in glucocorticoid secretion and the resulting decrease in lymphocytes may explain the decrease in immunocompetence that often occurs in people who are under psychological or physical stress.

Other effects of physiological levels of glucocorticoids include decreasing olfactory and gustatory sensitivity. People with adrenal insufficiency can detect various chemicals (e.g., sugar, salt, urea, and potassium chloride) by either taste or smell with a sensitivity that is 40 to 120 times greater than normal.

The effects of pharmacological dosages of glucocorticoids are considered separately from those of normal physiological levels. In pharmacological dosages, glucocorticoids possess immunosuppressive anti-inflammatory and antihistaminic activity. Glucocorticoids suppress the immune system by inhibiting the production of interleukin-2 by T4 (helper) lymphocytes. Decreases in interleukin-2 reduce the proliferation of T8 (suppressor, cytotoxic) T cells and B lymphocytes. Glucocorticoids act in several ways to suppress the inflammatory response, including the influx of phagocytes and the activation of complement and kinins.

Conversely, glucocorticoids can be of great benefit in the treatment of certain noninfective inflammatory conditions (e.g., rheumatoid arthritis and systemic lupus erythematosus). Glucocorticoids can also be beneficial in the treatment of certain allergies (e.g., asthma, hives, and minimal-change glomerular disease) because they prevent the release of histamines from mast cells. Their use as immunosuppressives enables patients to receive organ transplants. In any case, the potentially deleterious side effects of glucocorticoids usually require that they be used only after other treatments (e.g., nonsteroidal anti-inflammatory drugs [NSAIDs] or antihistamines) have failed or if the benefits clearly outweigh the risks (e.g., in renal disease or with organ transplants). In addition to immunosuppression, glucocorticoids trigger the development of all or part of Cushing's syndrome (e.g., diabetes, hypertension, protein wasting, and osteoporosis) and inhibit growth in infants and children. The pharmacological and physiological actions of glucocorticoids are summarized in Table 42-5.

Regulation of glucocorticoid secretion is outlined in Figure 42-8. The secretion of glucocorticoids is triggered by the release of corticotropin-releasing hormone (CRH), a neurosecretory material released by the hypothalamus. CRH stimulates the cells of the anterior pituitary to secrete ACTH. Without the stimulus of ACTH, the cells of the zona fasciculata and zona reticularis do not secrete glucocorticoids. Elevated plasma glucocorticoid levels function in a negative feedback loop to decrease or halt the secretion of CRH and thereby indirectly inhibit the secretion of ACTH as well.

There is a diurnal rhythm to the secretion of CRH that causes a similar rhythm in the output of ACTH and glucocorticoids. The result is that maximal glucocorticoid secretion occurs between 6:00 a.m. and

Table 42-5 • Actions of Glucocorticoids

Major Influence	Effect on Body
Glucose metabolism	Stimulates gluconeogenesis Decreases glucose use by the tissues
Protein metabolism	Increases breakdown of proteins Increases plasma protein levels
Fat metabolism	Increases mobilization of fatty acids Increases use of fatty acids

Anti-inflammatory action (pharmacological levels)	Stabilizes lysosomal membranes of the inflammatory cells, preventing the release of inflammatory mediators
	Decreases capillary permeability to prevent inflammatory edema
	Depresses phagocytosis by white blood cells to reduce the release of inflammatory mediators
	Suppresses the immune response
	   Causes atrophy of lymphoid tissue
	   Decreases eosinophils
	   Decreases antibody formation
	   Decreases the development of cell-mediated immunity
	Reduces fever
	Inhibits fibroblast activity

Psychic effect	May contribute to emotional instability
Permissive effect	Facilitates the response of the tissues to humoral and neural influences, such as that of the catecholamines, during trauma and extreme stress

From: Porth CM: Pathophysiology: Concepts of Altered Health States, 7th ed. Philadelphia: Lippincott Williams & Wilkins, 2005, p. 930.

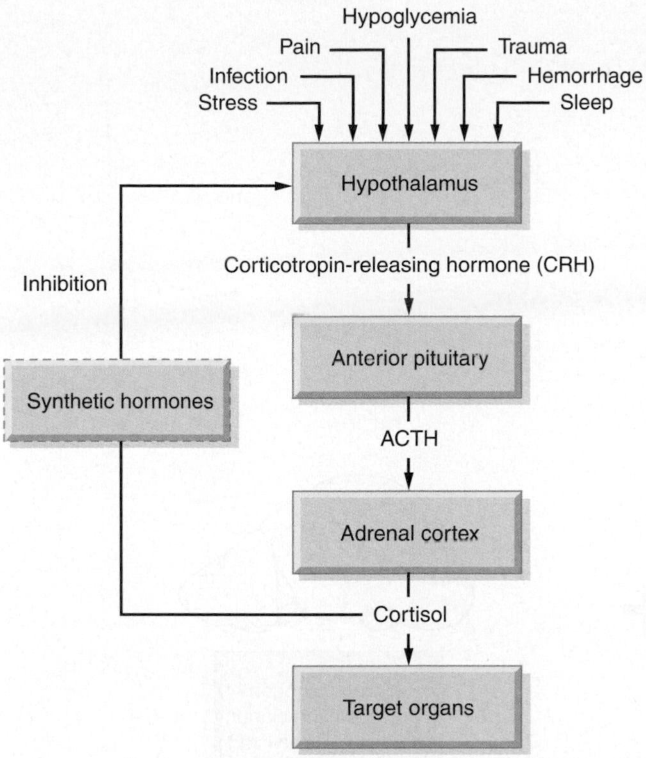

Figure 42-8 • The hypothalamic–pituitary–adrenal (HPA) feedback system that regulates glucocorticoid (cortisol) levels. Cortisol release is regulated by adrenocorticotropic hormone (ACTH). Stress exerts its effects on cortisol release through the HPA system and corticotropin-releasing hormone (CRH), which controls the release of ACTH from the anterior pituitary gland. Increased cortisol levels incite negative feedback inhibition of ACTH release. Pharmacological doses of synthetic steroids inhibit ACTH release by way of the hypothalamic CRH.

8:00 a.m. in people sleeping from midnight to 8:00 a.m. in a 24-hour day. Tumors that secrete CRH, ACTH, or glucocorticoids do not demonstrate such a rhythm, a fact that is useful in their diagnosis. The biological clock that regulates this and other diurnal, or circadian, rhythms is located in the hypothalamus, just above the area where the optic nerves cross (optic chiasma).

The beneficial functions of normal levels of glucocorticoids in enabling tissues to respond to glucagon and catecholamines are more than adequate to meet the needs of the SAM mechanism for a short time. If these needs continue, additional stress-induced glucocorticoid secretion is required. Eventually, if the stress continues unameliorated, exhaustion of the adrenal cortex occurs, glucocorticoid levels drop, tissues are no longer able to meet the demands of the SAM mechanism, muscle fatigue occurs, readily available cell energy sources (e.g., plasma glucose and fatty acid) are depleted, and vascular collapse and death result.

Mineralocorticoids

Aldosterone and glucocorticoids that have some mineralocorticoid function (e.g., 11-deoxycorticosterone) increase sodium reabsorption by the cells of the collecting ducts and distal tubules of the nephrons. Because of the cation exchange system in the distal tubule cells, such sodium reabsorption can increase potassium secretion and thereby foster potential hypokalemia. The reabsorption of sodium osmotically causes water reabsorption. This expands the volume of ECF. The increase in blood volume causes an elevation in blood pressure. However, edema does not usually result. Above a certain level of aldosterone-induced sodium reabsorption, the expansion of the ECF compartment can trigger secretion of natriuretic hormone or decreased sodium reabsorption in the proximal tubule. Either of these effects opposes the action of aldosterone and sodium excretion.

The primary mechanism for regulating aldosterone secretion is the renin–angiotensin system (Fig. 42-9). Pituitary ACTH does not stimulate zona glomerulosa cells under normal conditions. Cells of the juxtaglomerular apparatus are wedged between the renal afferent arteriole as it enters the glomerulus and the distal tubule as it passes by this area. The juxtaglomerular apparatus contains baroreceptor cells that monitor the afferent arteriole blood pressure and other cells that monitor the sodium and chloride concentration in the urine in the distal tubule (the lower the concentration, the slower the formation of filtrate, if all other factors are equal). A decrease either in blood pressure or in the concentration of electrolytes stimulates the juxtaglomerular apparatus to secrete the glycoprotein hormone renin. The major classes of stimuli that trigger renin secretion are decreased renal perfusion (e.g., cardiac failure, dehydration, and hemorrhage) and low ECF salt concentrations (e.g., from excessive use of diuretics).

Renin converts a circulating plasma globulin into angiotensin I. As the blood passes through the lungs (and to a lesser extent in other parts of the circulatory system), angiotensin I is converted to angiotensin II. This physiologically active chemical acts on the zona glomerulosa to promote aldosterone secretion, which leads to retention of salt and water, and contraction of vascular smooth muscle, thereby stimulating profound vasoconstriction. The result of both actions of angiotensin II is elevation of systemic blood pressure, which, among other things, improves renal perfusion.

The juxtaglomerular apparatus contains β_1 receptors and can be stimulated by sympathetic fibers. Prostaglandins also stimulate the juxtaglomerular apparatus. Sympathetic stimulation through β_1 receptors, renal artery hypotension, and decreased sodium delivery to distal tubules stimulate the secretion of renin. Therefore, the secretion of renin can be pharmacologically decreased by β-blockers (e.g., propranolol or atenolol). Prostaglandin inhibitors (aspirin and NSAIDs) can exert a similar action. Angiotensin-converting enzyme (ACE) inhibitors (e.g., lisinopril) prevent the conversion of angiotensin I to angiotensin II. These effects have made ACE inhibitors and β-blockers useful as antihypertensive agents.

Aldosterone secretion is also stimulated by an increase in plasma potassium levels, but not by increased sodium levels. Another regulating factor for

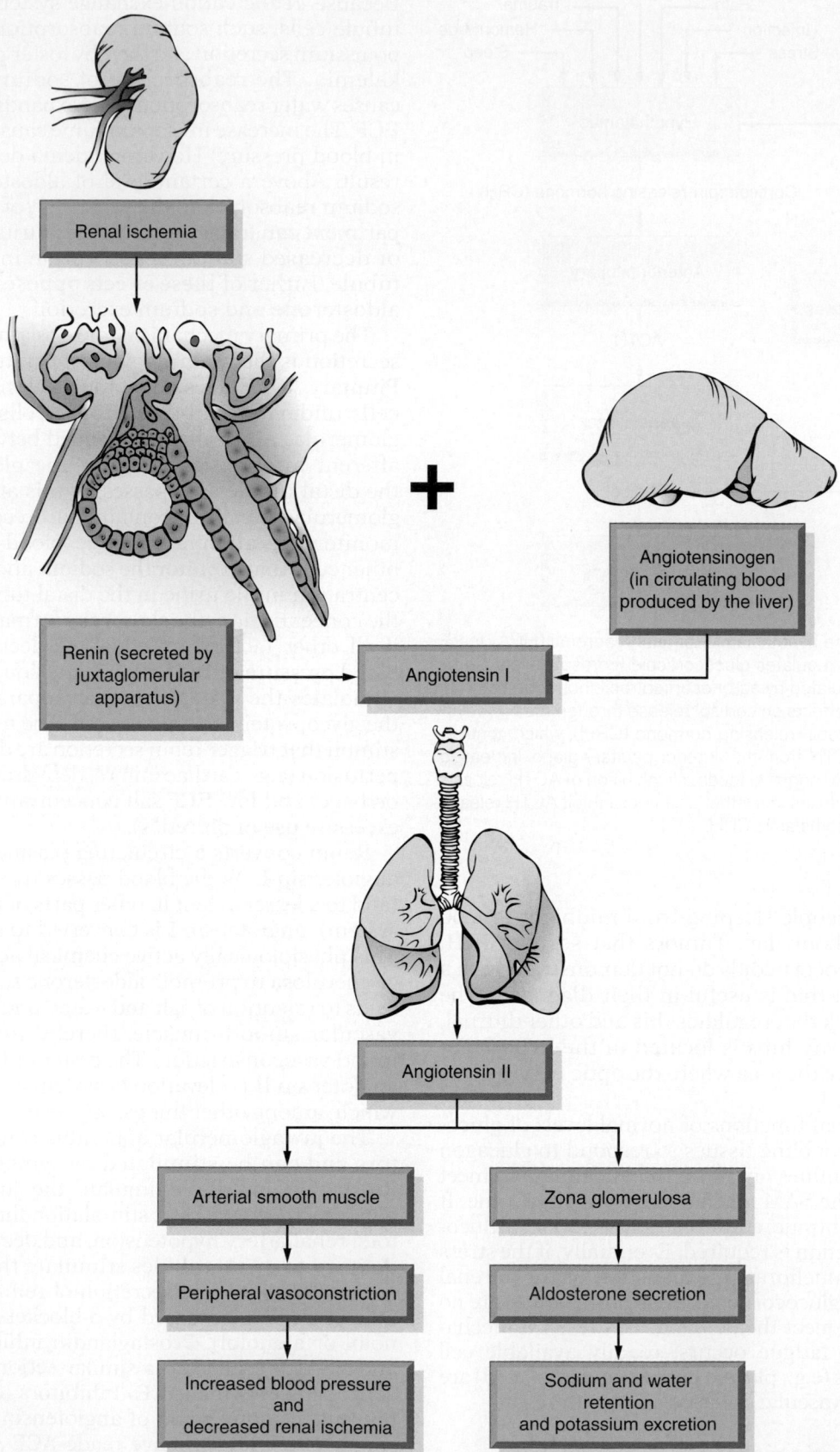

Figure 42-9 • The renin–angiotensin system induces aldosterone secretion and vasoconstriction, which in turn elevates the systemic blood pressure.

aldosterone secretion is posture. An upright body position increases aldosterone levels by increasing production and decreasing degradation. How this works is unclear, but because of this, aldosterone levels of bedridden patients are slightly subnormal. There also is a poorly understood diurnal rhythm of aldosterone secretion, with highest levels occurring in the early morning hours just before the person's awakening.

• Atrial Natriuretic Peptide (Natriuretic Hormone)

Atrial natriuretic peptide (ANP) is manufactured by cells in the walls of the atria of the heart. The main stimulus for ANP secretion is atrial stretch. ANP increases renal excretion of salt and water. Some evidence suggests that ANP acts by increasing glomerular filtration. Other evidence indicates that ANP inhibits the membrane active transport mechanism responsible for the reabsorption of sodium by renal tubule cells. Decreased sodium reabsorption decreases the movement of water from the urine in the nephron back into the blood of the peritubular capillaries, thereby increasing the elimination of water and salt from the body. ANP also inhibits the secretion of renin by the juxtaglomerular apparatus, thereby lowering plasma angiotensin levels. In addition, ANP inhibits the membrane active transport mechanism responsible for pumping sodium out of vascular smooth muscle cells. The consequent rise in intracellular sodium inhibits the entry of calcium ions, thereby lowering the intracellular concentration of calcium ions. The decrease in the intracellular free calcium promotes vasodilation and a lowering of the systemic blood pressure.

ANP is secreted in response to an increase in ECF volume caused by the ingestion of salt and water. The exact stimulus appears to be a stretch of the muscle fibers in the atrial walls, which results from the increased venous return that is caused by the rise in ECF volume. As the natriuresis causes the ECF volume to fall back to normal, the secretion of ANP stops. The capability of ANP to increase the GFR, together with its direct effects on the collecting tubules, results in a profound natriuresis and diuresis.

The metabolic fate of ANP is unknown, but circulating levels of this hormone are elevated in patients with congestive heart failure, cirrhosis, or renal insufficiency and are low in those with nephrotic syndrome or volume depletion. These results suggest liver and kidney regulation.

• Clinical Applicability Challenges

Short-Answer Questions

1. Explore physiological implications when there is faulty regulation of antidiuretic hormone (ADH) by the posterior pituitary.

2. Compare and contrast the feedback mechanisms that affect the synthesis and production of thyroxine (T_4) by the thyroid and cortisol by the adrenal cortex.

3. Compare and contrast the pathogenesis of types 1 and 2 diabetes mellitus.

Review Questions

1. Actions of glucocorticoids include
   a. glucose elevation by gluconeogenesis.
   b. suppression of the anti-inflammatory response.
   c. stimulation of histamine triggers.
   d. stimulation of water excretion in the kidney.

2. Blood glucose regulation is affected by which of the following hormones?
   a. Aldosterone
   b. Calcitonin
   c. Glucagon
   d. Antidiuretic hormone

3. The renin–angiotensin–aldosterone system is stimulated in which of the following conditions?
   a. Hemorrhage
   b. Hypervolemia
   c. Hypertension
   d. Hyperventilation

4. Antidiuretic hormone (ADH) is suppressed by which of the following stimuli?
   a. High serum osmolality
   b. Positive pressure ventilation
   c. Hypovolemia
   d. Ethanol

5. Higher levels of thyroid-stimulating hormone (TSH) are associated with which of the following?
   a. Hyperthyroidism
   b. Hyperadrenalism
   c. Hypothyroidism
   d. Hypoadrenalism

6. Aldosterone is secreted from which of the following cells of the adrenal gland?
   a. Medulla
   b. Zona reticularis
   c. Zona fasciculata
   d. Zona glomerulosa

7. Which of the following stimuli regulate antidiuretic hormone (ADH) secretion?
   a. Ectopic foci of ADH-secreting tissue
   b. Changes in serum osmolality as detected by the hypothalamus
   c. An active thirst center
   d. Detectable levels of aldosterone hormone

8. Which of the following mechanisms describes the role of counter-regulatory hormones on the regulation of glucose metabolism?
   a. Catecholamines block gluconeogenesis, lowering glucose
   b. Growth hormone (GH) exacerbates a hyperglycemic state
   c. Cortisol suppresses the immune response to glucagons
   d. Catecholamines synergize insulin to increase glucose levels

9. Which of the following statements about hyperglycemia and type 2 diabetes mellitus are true?
   a. Both conditions result from undersecretion of insulin
   b. Both conditions result from inability to use available insulin
   c. Both conditions result from autoimmune destruction of islet cells
   d. Both conditions result from high levels of circulating insulin

10. Which of the following statements best explains the β-cell dysfunction seen in type 2 diabetes mellitus?
   a. Chronic exposure to high levels of insulin damages β cells.
   b. High levels of potassium trigger apoptosis.
   c. An autoimmune process damages β cells.
   d. High demands for insulin lead to β cell exhaustion.

References

1. Newton CA, Raskin P: Diabetic ketoacidosis in type 1 and 2 diabetes mellitus. Arch Intern Med 164:1925–1931, 2004
2. Robinson LE, van Soeren MH: Insulin resistance and hyperglycemia in critical illness: Role of insulin in glycemic control. AACN Clin Issues 15(1):45–62, 2004
3. Osei K, Rhinesmith S, Gallard T, Schuster D: Impaired insulin sensitivity, insulin secretion, and glucose effectiveness predict future development of impaired glucose tolerance and type 2 diabetes in pre-diabetic African Americans. Diabetes Care 27(6):1439–1446, 2004
4. United Kingdom Prospective Diabetes Study (UKPDS) VIII: Study design, progress, and performance. Diabetologia 34: 877–890, 1991
5. Umpeirrez GE, Murphy MB, Kitabchi AE: Diabetic ketoacidosis and hyperglycemic hyperosmolar syndrome. Diabetes Spectrum 15(1):28–36, 2002

Other Selected Readings

American Diabetes Association: Standards of Medical Care in Diabetes—2007. Diabetes Care 30(Suppl 1):S4–S47, 2007

Beaser RS, Caballero E, Leahy JL: Diabetes and insulin: Indications, initiation, and innovations. CMI-accredited symposium developed by Medscape, September 2005. Retrieved July 14, 2006, from http://www.medscape.com/viewprogram/5500_pnt.

Becker KL (ed): Principles and Practice of Endocrinology and Metabolism, 3rd ed. Philadelphia: Lippincott Williams & Wilkins, 2001.

Camacho PM, Gharib H, Sizemore GW: Evidence-Based Endocrinology, 2nd ed. Philadelphia: Lippincott Williams & Wilkins, 2007

Harris PE, Bouloux PM: Endocrinology in Clinical Practice. London: Martin Dunitz Ltd, 2003

Harmel AP, Mathur R: Davidson's Diabetes Mellitus: Diagnosis and Treatment, 5th ed. Philadelphia: Saunders Elsevier, 2004

Lebovitz HE: Clinician's Manual on Insulin Resistance. London: Science Press, 2002

McCance KL, Huether SE: Pathophysiology: The Biologic Basis for Disease in Adults and Children, 5th ed. St. Louis: Mosby–Year Book, 2005

Melmed S, Conn PM: Endocrinology, 2nd ed. Totowa, NJ: Humana Press, 2005

Porth CM: Pathophysiology: Concepts of Altered Health States, 7th ed. Philadelphia: Lippincott Williams & Wilkins, 2005

Seifter J, Ratner A, Sloane D: Concepts in Medical Physiology. Philadelphia: Lippincott Williams & Wilkins, 2005

Smeltzer SC, Bare BG, Hinkle JL, Cheever KH: Brunner & Suddarth's Textbook of Medical–Surgical Nursing, 11th ed. Philadelphia: Lippincott Williams & Wilkins, 2008, p 1441

U.S. Preventive Services Task Force: Screening for type 2 diabetes mellitus in adults: Recommendations and rationale. Ann Intern Med 138:212–214, 2003

Patient Assessment: Endocrine System

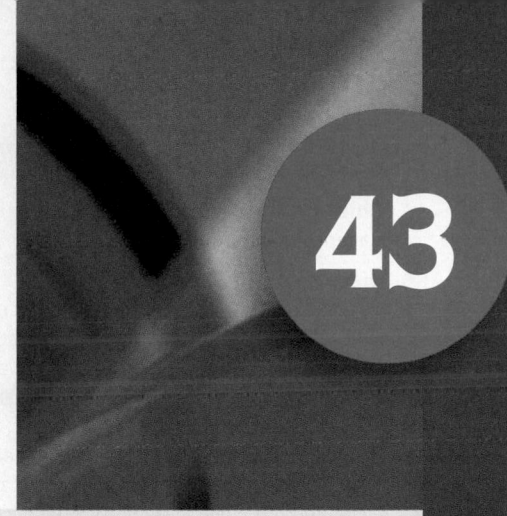

43

Jane Kapustin

Objectives

Based on the content in this chapter, the reader should be able to:

1. Analyze the relationship between dysfunction of the hypothalamus and the pituitary gland and the signs and symptoms of the resultant disorder.

2. Consider the signs and symptoms of hypothyroidism and hyperthyroidism as they reflect thyroid gland dysfunction.

3. Formulate a plan for collecting history and physical examination data when the patient may have an acute pancreatic illness such as diabetic ketoacidosis or hyperglycemic hyperosmolar syndrome.

4. Differentiate between normal and abnormal findings for an adrenal gland disturbance.

5. Explain laboratory tests used to diagnose acute endocrine disorders.

Endocrine disorders can affect all body systems and are usually caused by the overproduction or underproduction of hormones. This chapter presents an overview of the history, physical examination, and diagnostic studies that help diagnose the following specific endocrine disorders: thyroid crisis; myxedema coma; adrenal crisis; syndrome of inappropriate antidiuretic hormone (SIADH); diabetes insipidus; diabetic ketoacidosis (DKA); hyperglycemic hyperosmolar syndrome (HHS); and hypoglycemia. It builds on the content presented in Chapter 42, which explored the far-reaching effects of the endocrine system on body functions. This chapter also provides a foundation for understanding specific applications described in Chapter 44.

Because the endocrine system affects so many general areas of the body, assessment must include a variety of signs and symptoms. General manifestations of disorders are evident through vital signs, energy level, fluid and electrolyte imbalances, and ability to carry out activities of daily living. Other parameters to be observed include heat or cold intolerance, changes in weight, fat redistribution, changes in sexual functioning, and altered sleep patterns. Box 43-1 summarizes the approach used to assess a patient suspected of having an acute endocrine disorder.

Because the endocrine system exerts control over the entire body, many laboratory tests that have been discussed in other chapters are applicable to the assessment of an acute endocrine disorder. For example, fluid and electrolyte problems accompany many acute endocrine disorders. Therefore, serum sodium, potassium, magnesium, and osmolality are assessed. Blood urea nitrogen (BUN) and creatinine levels may also help assess renal involvement (see Chapter 29). Arterial blood gases (ABGs), bicarbonate levels, and anion gap calculation may be necessary to diagnose acidosis. Laboratory studies specific to endocrine gland dysfunction are described in the following sections and summarized in Table 43-1.

Box 43-1 • Endocrine Health History

Chief Complaint

Patient's description of the problem

History of the Present Illness

Hypothalamus and pituitary disorders: excessive or inadequate urinary output, excessive thirst, poor skin turgor, cognitive changes, dehydration or water intoxication

Thyroid disorders: Cold or heat intolerance; edema; cognitive changes, such as slowed mentation, agitation, memory impairment, and stupor; tremulousness; insomnia; fatigue; tachycardia, atrial fibrillation; bradycardia; hypoventilation; constipation; diarrhea; menstrual cycle irregularities; skin problems; husky voice; diplopia, exophthalmos; eye pain, change in vision; depression; hematuria

Parathyroid disorders: apathy, fatigue, weakness, tetany, joint pain

Diabetes mellitus: weight gain or loss, excessive urination, excessive thirst, excessive appetite, blurred vision, dental caries, poor wound healing, chronic vaginitis, neuropathy, dehydration, cognitive changes

Adrenal disorders: nausea, vomiting; striae; central obesity with peripheral wasting; moon facies; hirsutism; petechiae, easy bruising; dehydration; fatigue, lethargy

Past Health History

Relevant childhood illnesses and immunizations: history of adenoid or neck/chest radiation, mental retardation, iodine deficiency

Past acute and chronic medical problems: diabetic emergencies, hypertension, high cholesterol, tachydysrhythmias, congestive heart failure, myocardial infarction, Graves' disease, Hashimoto's thyroiditis, head injury, cerebral vascular accident, pancreatitis, unexplained infections

Risk factors: age, heredity, gender, race, tobacco use, alcohol use, elevated cholesterol, obesity, sedentary lifestyle, growth spurt cycles, pregnancy, gestational diabetes, delivery of an infant weighing more than 9 lb, anemia

Past surgeries: neurosurgical procedures, thyroidectomy, parathyroidectomy, adrenalectomy

Medications: amiodarone, phenytoin, carbamazepine, chlorpropamide, corticosteroids, opioids, lithium, aspirin, iodides, heparin, levothyroxine (Synthroid), neoplastic drugs, estrogen, methadone, androgens, β-blockers, nonsteroidal anti-inflammatory drugs, potassium, diuretics

Allergies and reactions to medication, foods, contrast dye, latex, or other materials

Transfusion history

Family history: thyroid disease, diabetes, lipid disorders, cerebral aneurysms, cancers, autoimmune disorders

Personal and social history: tobacco, alcohol, substance abuse; occupation; living environment; diet, exercise; sleep patterns; cultural beliefs; spiritual/religious beliefs; leisure activities

Review of Other Systems

HEENT: headaches, dizziness, weakness, visual changes

Lymphatics: edema, lymphadenopathy

Genitourinary: sexual dysfunction, infertility, abnormal vaginal bleeding

Table 43-1 • Sampling of Laboratory Studies Used to Assess Acute Endocrine Disorders

Test	Normal Adult Values	Abnormal Values
Total T_4	4–12 µg/dL	High in hyperthyroidism Low in hypothyroidism
Free T_4	0.8–2.7 ng/mL	High in hyperthyroidism Low in hypothyroidism
Free T_4 index	4.6–12 ng/mL	High in hyperthyroidism Low in hypothyroidism
Free T_3	260–480 pg/dL	Low in hypothyroidism
Thyroid-stimulating hormone (TSH)	260–480 pg/dL	High in hypothyroidism (primary) Low in hypofunction of anterior pituitary (secondary hypothyroidism)
Cortisol	8 a.m. 5–23 µg/dL 4 p.m. 3–16 µg/dL	High in Cushing's disease (increased ACTH secretion by pituitary) High in stress, trauma, and surgery Low in hyposecretion of ACTH by pituitary and adrenal insufficiency
Cortisol stimulation	Should increase to 18 µg/dL	Low or absent in adrenal insufficiency and hypopituitarism
Urine vanillylmandelic acid and catecholamines	VMA up to 2–7 mg/24 h Catecholamines: 270 µg/24 h	High in pheochromocytoma High in hypothyroidism and diabetic acidosis
Urine specific gravity	1.010–1.025 with normal hydration and volume	Low in diabetes insipidus High in diabetes mellitus with dehydration High in SIADH
Urine ketones	Negative	Positive in diabetic ketoacidosis

SIADH, syndrome of inappropriate antidiuretic hormone; T_3, triiodothyronine; T_4, thyroxine.

Similarly, in the evaluation of endocrine disorders, it is often necessary to evaluate body systems other than the endocrine system using diagnostic studies. For example, electrocardiography and cardiac monitoring may be needed to diagnose cardiac problems, whereas a chest radiograph may be necessary to detect pulmonary problems, such as the pleural effusion that can occur in myxedema coma. Computed tomography (CT), magnetic resonance imaging (MRI), and ultrasound may be used to localize tumors.

• The Hypothalamus and Pituitary Gland

Some of the hormones of the hypothalamus and the pituitary have a profound impact on the critically ill patient and are described in detail in this section (antidiuretic hormone [ADH], adrenocorticotropic hormone [ACTH], thyroid-stimulating hormone [TSH]). Those hormones that are mainly responsible for normal physiological functioning of the reproductive system are not significant in the care of the critically ill adult and therefore are not covered in this section (oxytocin, follicle-stimulating hormone [FSH], luteinizing hormone [LH], growth hormone [GH], melanophore-stimulating hormone [MSH]).

The pituitary gland hormones are under the control of the hypothalamus. The posterior lobe of the pituitary stores and secretes ADH (vasopressin) in response to serum osmolality. Because the primary function of ADH is to control water excretion by the kidney, attention must be focused on the patient's hydration status and serum and urine osmolality to acquire information about the general functioning of this part of the pituitary.

HISTORY AND PHYSICAL EXAMINATION

The nurse obtains important information about the nature of endocrine disorders by conducting a thorough history. Because disorders of the pituitary that could result in critical care admission affect fluid and electrolyte balance, the nurse inquires about general hydration status. Specific parameters are included in the endocrine health history (see Box 43-1).

Physical examination of the patient includes assessment of hydration status. Skin turgor, buccal membrane moisture, vital signs, and weight are assessed. A patient with hypovolemia (as seen in diabetes insipidus) would experience weight loss from excretion of large volumes of dilute urine. Eventually, the patient would experience tachycardia, hypotension, poor skin turgor, dry buccal membranes, and cognitive changes associated with dehydration and hypernatremia. Conversely, a patient with hypervolemia (as seen in SIADH) would display signs of water intoxication, such as edema, scant urinary output, weight gain, hypertension, moist buccal membranes, good skin turgor, and cognitive changes associated with hyponatremia.

For patients experiencing fluid balance alterations, the nurse needs to maintain strict measuring of intake and output. Urine specific gravity is measured routinely, noting the nature of the urine (color, concentration, and volume). In addition, critically ill patients with fluid imbalance often have advanced monitoring techniques in place such as central venous pressure or hemodynamic monitoring with a pulmonary artery catheter. Vigilant monitoring of the patient's fluid status needs to be maintained.

LABORATORY STUDIES

Serum Antidiuretic Hormone

The normal serum ADH level is 1 to 13.3 pg/mL. This radioimmunoassay level distinguishes between central diabetes insipidus and SIADH. Elevated serum ADH compared with low serum osmolality and elevated urine osmolality confirms the diagnosis of SIADH. Conversely, reduced levels of ADH with a correspondingly high serum osmolality, hypernatremia, and reduced urine concentration indicate central diabetes insipidus. Table 43-2 compares and contrasts laboratory values for diabetes insipidus and SIADH.

Urine Specific Gravity

Specific gravity reflects the kidneys' ability to dilute and concentrate urine. The range depends on hydration, urine volume, and the amount of solids in the urine. The specific gravity can be measured by using a multiple-test dipstick that has a reagent for specific gravity or by using a refractometer. Low specific gravity (1.001 to 1.010) is seen in diabetes insipidus and is accompanied by copious, dilute urine. Increased specific gravity (1.025 to 1.030) is seen in diabetes mellitus with dehydration; the urine in general is more concentrated with smaller volumes.

Serum Osmolality

Serum osmolality ranges from 270 to 300 mOsm/kg and measures the concentration of diluted particles in the bloodstream. Elevated serum osmolality (hemoconcentration) stimulates the release of ADH, which enhances the reabsorption of fluid and sodium at the nephron level. Through this process, extracellular fluid (ECF) volume is restored, and the plasma becomes less concentrated.

Table 43-2 • Comparison of Laboratory Values in Diabetes Insipidus and Syndrome of Inappropriate Antidiuretic Hormone (SIADH)		
Laboratory Test	**Diabetes Insipidus**	**SIADH**
Antidiuretic hormone (ADH)	Decreased	Increased
Serum osmolality	Increased	Decreased
Sodium	Increased	Decreased
Urinary output	Increased	Decreased
Urine specific gravity	Decreased	Increased
Urine osmolality	Decreased	Increased

Conversely, hemodilution or decreased serum osmolality inhibits ADH, causing excess fluid to be eliminated by the kidneys to maintain homeostasis. Concentration of the plasma is restored.

Urine Osmolality

This test is a more exact measure of urine concentration. It is also a more useful test when performed in conjunction with serum osmolality. It can be used to diagnose kidney function, diabetes insipidus, and psychogenic water drinking. The urine osmolality is increased in Addison's disease, SIADH, dehydration, and renal disease. It is decreased in diabetes insipidus and psychogenic water drinking. The normal range is 300 to 900 mOsm/kg per 24 hours and 50 to 1,200 mOsm/kg in a random sample.

Water Deprivation Test

Water restriction is a useful test because healthy people respond with a rapid decrease in urine volume when water intake is withheld. However, people with diabetes insipidus have no decrease in urine volume in response to severe water restriction. This signifies that the normal mechanism of ADH release in the face of water restriction and dehydration is dysfunctional. This test is rarely performed in a critical care unit because the patient is too ill and fragile to withstand the rigors of severe dehydration. The preferred test is measurement of serum ADH to diagnose diabetes insipidus.

Antidiuretic Hormone Administration

One final laboratory test used to diagnose diabetes insipidus is ADH administration. Exogenous ADH (vasopressin or Pitressin) given subcutaneously to the person suspected of having diabetes insipidus causes a temporary increase in urine osmolality. For a brief time, the person displays the appropriate response to ADH by conserving water at the kidney level, and urine output slows down in an attempt to restore ECF. This test also helps distinguish between the two types of diabetes insipidus, nephrogenic and central. In nephrogenic diabetes insipidus, the person does not demonstrate a reaction to exogenous ADH because the kidney receptors in the collecting duct are unresponsive to ADH. People with central diabetes insipidus respond readily to the exogenous ADH.

DIAGNOSTIC STUDIES

Diagnostic imaging studies are frequently used for patients suspected of having pituitary or hypothalamic disorders. CT and MRI are essential in diagnosing primary diseases affecting this area of the brain. Examples of disorders that affect the pituitary–hypothalamic axis are brain tumors, aneurysms, edema from surgical exploration or traumatic injuries, and necrotic lesions. Imaging techniques are used to view the sella turcica and the surrounding structures, including the pituitary within the bony encasement of the middle cranial fossa. Angiography assists with precise viewing of the vascular supply in the area. Figure 43-1 provides examples of MRI and CT scans of a pituitary tumor.

The critically ill patient requires monitoring at all times during these procedures. Quite often, the patient requires sedation to eliminate all patient motion in an effort to ensure clear images. Institutional policies and procedures need to be followed during diagnostic testing.

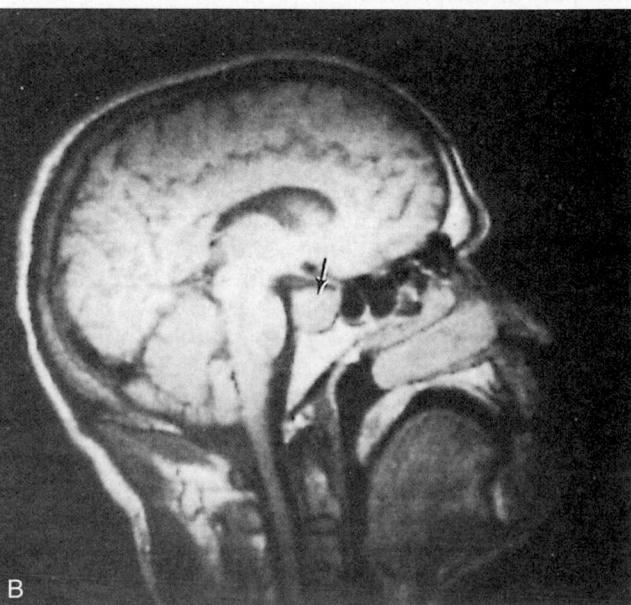

Figure 43-1 • A: Computed tomography scan showing a suprasellar pituitary tumor (*arrow*) in a thyroid-toxic patient with a thyroid-stimulating hormone (TSH)–secreting pituitary tumor. **B:** T1-weighted magnetic resonance image in the same patient showing a 2- × 2-cm pituitary tumor (*arrow*). T1-weighted images are favorable for demonstrating anatomical detail. (Adapted from Smallridge RC: Thyrotropin-secreting pituitary tumors. Endocrinol Metab Clin North Am 16:3, 1987.)

• The Thyroid Gland

The thyroid hormones are regulated by the hypothalamus and the pituitary gland in a negative feedback system as previously described. Low levels of triiodothyronine (T_3) and thyroxine (T_4) cause the hypothalamus to secrete thyrotropin-releasing hormone (TRH), which then stimulates the anterior pituitary gland to release TSH. TSH stimulates the production and release of the thyroid hormones (Fig. 43-2).

Increased thyroid hormone production results in hyperthyroidism, which can lead to an extreme form of thyrotoxicosis. This is a rare, life-threatening illness necessitating critical care admission for management of the patient. Conversely, hypothyroidism can occur, resulting in a severe hypometabolic state. If hypothyroidism is untreated, myxedema coma can develop in the patient, which is most likely to be managed and treated in a critical care unit.

HISTORY AND PHYSICAL EXAMINATION

Thyroid hormones affect nearly every cell and tissue in the body. Therefore, manifestations of these disorders are widespread. The typical course of disease progression is insidious, and the nurse needs to take a detailed history to uncover signs and symptoms of either hypothyroidism or hyperthyroidism. History taking focuses on the variety of expected signs and symptoms associated with hypothyroidism and hyperthyroidism. Table 43-3 compares and contrasts the two disorders. Box 43-2 explores the incidence of thyroid disorders in the older patient.

Because of their deep, protected locations in the body, the endocrine glands are in general inaccessible to palpation, percussion, and auscultation. The exception is the thyroid gland, which can be examined physically when it is enlarged. Assess-

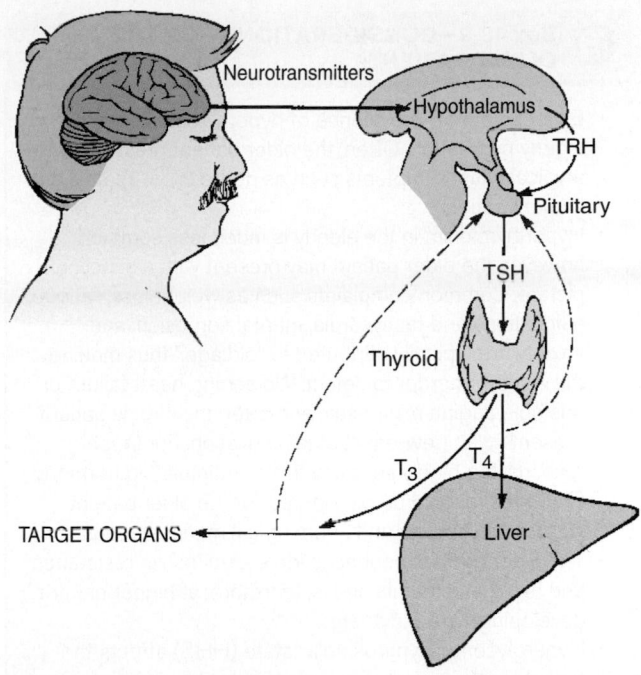

Figure 43-2 • The hypothalamic–pituitary–thyroid axis. Thyrotropin-releasing hormone (TRH) from the hypothalamus stimulates the pituitary gland to secrete thyroid-stimulating hormone (TSH). TSH stimulates the thyroid to produce thyroid hormone (T_3 and T_4). High circulating levels of T_3 and T_4 inhibit further TSH secretion and thyroid hormone production through a negative feedback mechanism (*dashed lines*). (From Smeltzer SC, Bare BG, Hinkle JL, Cheever KH: Brunner & Suddarth's Textbook of Medical–Surgical Nursing, 11th ed. Philadelphia: Lippincott Williams & Wilkins, 2008, p 1449.)

ment begins with inspection of the neck area for enlargement, nodules, and symmetry of the gland. The patient is then asked to swallow while the nurse observes the thyroid rising. Next, the thyroid is palpated for size, shape, symmetry, and presence of tenderness (Fig. 43-3). See Box 43-3 for a more

Table 43-3 • Manifestations of Hypothyroid and Hyperthyroid States

Symptoms of Thyroid Dysfunction		Signs of Thyroid Dysfunction	
Hyperthyroidism	*Hypothyroidism*	*Hyperthyroidism*	*Hypothyroidism*
Nervousness	Fatigue, lethargy	Tachycardia or atrial fibrillation	Bradycardia and, in late stages, hypothermia
Weight loss despite an increased appetite	Modest weight gain with anorexia	Increased systolic and decreased diastolic blood pressures	Decreased systolic and increased diastolic blood pressures
Excessive sweating and heat intolerance	Dry, coarse skin and cold intolerance	Hyperdynamic cardiac pulsations with an accentuated S_1 sound	Intensity of heart sounds sometimes decreased
Palpitations	Swelling of face, hands, and legs	Warm, smooth, moist skin	Dry, coarse, cool skin, sometimes yellowish from carotene, with nonpitting edema and loss of hair
Frequent bowel movements	Constipation	Tremor and proximal muscle weakness	Impaired memory, mixed hearing loss, somnolence, peripheral neuropathy, carpal tunnel syndrome
Muscular weakness of the proximal type and tremor	Weakness, muscle cramps, arthralgias, paresthesias, impaired memory and hearing	With Graves' disease, eye signs such as stare, lid lag, and exophthalmos	Periorbital puffiness

Box 43-2 • CONSIDERATIONS FOR THE OLDER PATIENT: Endocrine Disorders

- Expect a higher prevalence of hypothyroidism in the elderly population. Often, the older patient presents with atypical initial symptoms such as depression, apathy, and immobilization.
- Hyperthyroidism in the elderly is much less common; however, the older patient may present with a subclinical picture. Common complaints such as weight loss, fatigue, palpitations and tachycardia, mental confusion, and anxiety are typically attributed to "old age," thus making the disorder harder to detect. Worsening heart failure or unstable angina may result, and often the elderly patient presents with new-onset atrial fibrillation. For these reasons, the highly sensitive thyroid-stimulating hormone (TSH) test should be considered for the older patient with cardiovascular and neurological manifestations.
- The older adult experiences increased insulin resistance and hyperinsulinemia and is, therefore, at higher risk for developing type 2 diabetes.
- Hyperglycemic hyperosmolar state (HHS) affects the frail elderly population, with the acutely ill older patient at higher risk. Be suspicious of the older patient with diabetes and the new onset of acute illness, such as myocardial infarction, pancreatitis, pneumonia, or other serious infections or illnesses.
- Another expected result of aging is the decrease in secretion of aldosterone and cortisol. This can result in a diminished response to acute illness or trauma. The older patient may have a decreased ability to maintain appropriate fluid and electrolyte balance. In general, older adults display diminished responses to stressors such as critical illness or trauma.

Box 43-3 • Steps for Palpating the Thyroid Gland

- Ask the patient to flex the neck slightly forward to relax the sternomastoid muscles.
- Place the fingers of both hands on the patient's neck so that your index fingers are just below the cricoid cartilage.
- Ask the patient to sip and swallow water as before. Feel for the thyroid isthmus rising up under your finger pads. It is often but not always palpable.
- Displace the trachea to the right with the fingers of the left hand; with the right-hand fingers, palpate laterally for the right lobe of the thyroid in the space between the displaced trachea and the relaxed sternomastoid. Find the lateral margin. In similar fashion, examine the left lobe.

  The lobes are somewhat harder to feel than the isthmus, so practice is needed.

  The anterior surface of a lateral lobe is approximately the size of the distal phalanx of the thumb and feels somewhat rubbery.
- Note the *size, shape,* and *consistency* of the gland and identify any *nodules* or *tenderness.*

If the thyroid gland is enlarged, listen over the lateral lobes with a stethoscope to detect a bruit, a sound similar to a cardiac murmur but of noncardiac origin.

From Bickley LS: Bates' Guide to Physical Examination and History Taking, 8th ed. Philadelphia: Lippincott Williams & Wilkins, 2002, p 167.

detailed description of the steps for palpating the thyroid gland. Thyromegaly (goiter) or thyroid nodules can be detected by palpation. Both lobes of the gland and the isthmus are palpated.

Occasionally, a thyroid bruit can be detected by listening over the gland with the bell of the stetho-scope (Fig 43-4). A bruit is caused by excessive or turbulent blood flow associated with hyperthyroidism and the resultant hypermetabolic state.

Other assessment parameters include noting vital sign changes, skin changes (including edema), neurological changes, and weight changes associated with either disorder. Hypothyroidism is frequently associated with hypotension, bradycardia, hypoventilation, and subnormal temperature. The patient often has dry, flaky skin; edema over the pretibial area; and a deep or husky voice. The patient displays slowed cognitive functioning with slower-than-normal verbal

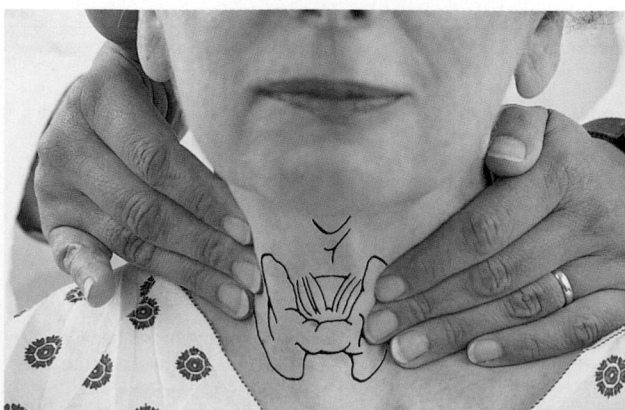

Figure 43-3 • The thyroid is examined from behind, with the patient in a sitting position, avoiding hyperextension of the neck. (© B. Proud.)

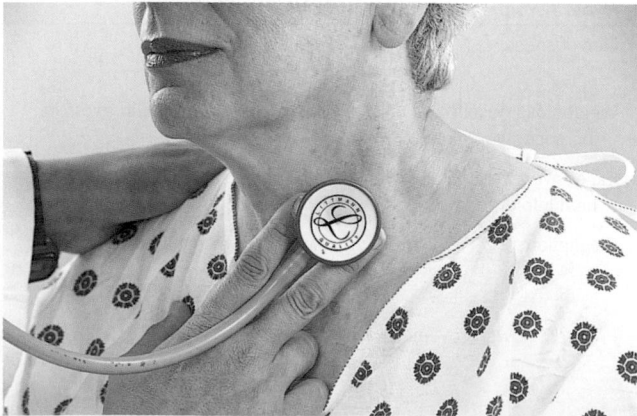

Figure 43-4 • Auscultating for bruits over the thyroid gland. (From Weber J, Kelley J: Health assessment in nursing, 3rd ed. Philadelphia: Lippincott Williams & Wilkins, 2007, p 205. © B. Proud.)

responses, slowed rapid alternating movements, and decreased deep tendon reflexes.

Patients with hyperthyroidism have more neurological manifestations such as tremor, nervousness, insomnia and restless movements, and hyperactive reflexes. Vital signs are characteristic: hypertension, tachycardia, tachypnea, and hyperthermia. The patient may have a goiter with detectible bruit. Also, the patient may have exophthalmos or proptosis of the eyes. The eyes may unilaterally or bilaterally protrude from the eye sockets, rendering the patient unable to close one or both eyes (Fig. 43-5).

LABORATORY STUDIES

Thyroid-Stimulating Hormone Test (Thyrotropin Assay)

The TSH test is a highly sensitive test used to diagnose hypothyroidism and hyperthyroidism. The third-generation immunometric assay tests of TSH are 100 times more sensitive than the earlier methods for measuring TSH, and this test is the preferred method for diagnosing and monitoring progression of thyroid disease. Box 43-4 provides a review of common thyroid tests. Table 43-4 lists medications that may interfere with thyroid tests.

The TSH test measures circulating TSH from the anterior pituitary. TSH stimulates the release and distribution of the T_3 and T_4 stored in large amounts in the thyroid gland. Measuring TSH helps determine whether the hypothyroidism is primary (i.e., caused by dysfunction of the thyroid gland) or secondary (i.e., caused by hypofunction of the anterior pituitary gland). A high TSH level helps diagnose primary hypothyroidism. Measuring the TSH level also helps guide medication titrations for patients requiring exogenous thyroid hormone.

However, the levels of TSH and free T_4 are highly influenced by stress in critically ill patients because of problems with protein levels that are often seen in critical care. Malnutrition, hepatic dysfunction, pregnancy, and drugs affect the TSH and free T_4 levels.

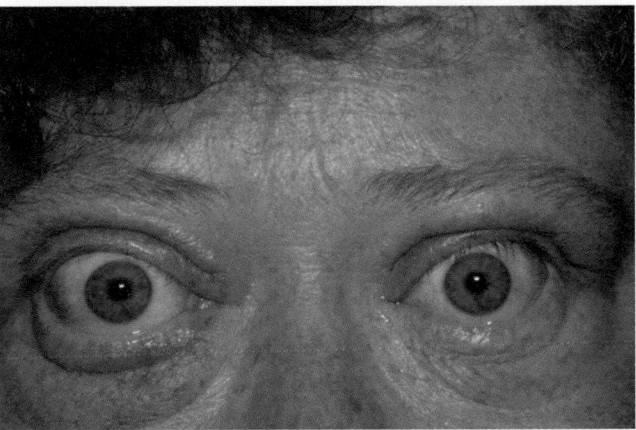

Figure 43-5 • A woman with Graves' disease (hyperthyroidism). Note the exophthalmos. (From Goodheart HP: Goodheart's Photoguide of Common Skin Disorders: Diagnosis and Management, 2nd ed. Philadelphia: Lippincott Williams & Wilkins, 2003, p 391.)

Box 43-4 • Laboratory Evaluation of the Thyroid

Tests That Assess Thyroid Function
• Radioactive iodine uptake

Tests That Assess the Hypothalamic–Pituitary Axis
• Sensitive thyroid-stimulating hormone (TSH)
• TSH-releasing hormone stimulation test

Tests That Assess Thyroid Hormone Binding Peripherally
• Total thyroxine (T_4) and total triiodothyronine (T_3)
• Free T_4 and free T_3
• In vitro uptake tests (T_3 resin uptake)
• Thyroid hormone–binding ratios (free T_4 index)
• T_4-binding globulin

Diagnostic Studies
• Iodine-131, technetium-99m scans
• Ultrasound
• Computed tomography (CT)
• Magnetic resonance imaging (MRI)
• Computerized rectilinear thyroid (CRT)

Miscellaneous Tests
• Thyroid antibodies (thyroid peroxidase, thyroid-stimulating immunoglobulin)
• Thyroglobulin
• Calcitonin
• Basal metabolic rate (BMR)

Therefore, the results of the TSH test need to be analyzed carefully in the critically ill patient. The normal adult value for TSH is 0.4 to 5.4 mU/L.

Total Thyroxine

Total T_4 measures both the free T_4 and the portion carried by thyroxine-binding globulin (TBG). T_4 is increased in hyperthyroidism and decreased in hypothyroidism. Any factor that affects protein binding affects the results of the total T_4. These factors include pregnancy; estrogen or androgen therapy; and taking oral contraceptives, salicylates, or phenytoin. Normal values depend on the laboratory method used. The normal value is 16.5 fg/dL in infants; childhood norms are up to 15 fg/dL. Normal adult values range from 4 to 12 fg/dL and are higher during pregnancy. Older adults have lower values because plasma proteins decrease as people age.

Free Thyroxine and Free Thyroxine Index

Free T_4 and free T_4 index measure the free part of T_4, the part that is not bound to protein. Free T_4 is the metabolically active form of the hormone that can be used by tissues. It makes up a small part of the total T_4. The free T_4 test is more useful than the total T_4 test in diagnosing hypofunction and hyperfunction of the thyroid gland because it helps diagnose thyroid function when people have abnormal TBG levels. This

⋯⋮⋮⋮⋮⋮⋯ Table 43-4 • Medications That May Interfere With Thyroid Tests		
Substance Determined	**Drugs Causing Increased Values or False-Positive Values**	**Drugs Causing Decreased Values or False-Negative Values**
Calcitonin (Plasma)	Estrogen/progestin, calcium, cholecystokinin, epinephrine, glucagon	Octreotide, phenytoin
Thyroxine (T₄) Free (Serum)	Amiodarine, aspirin, carbamazepine, danazol, furosemide, levothyroxine, phenytoin, probenecid, propranolol, radiographic agents, tamoxifen, thyroxine, valproic acid	Amiodarone, anabolic steroids, anticonvulsants (e.g., carbamazepine), asparaginase, clofibrate, corticosteroids, furosemide, isotretinoin, levothyroxine, methadone, methimazole, octreotide, oral contraceptives, phenobarbital, phenytoin, ranitidine
Free Triiodothyronine (T₃) (Serum)	Amiodarone, aspirin, carbamazepine, fenoprofen, levothyroxine, phenytoin, ranitidine, thyroxine	Amiodarone, carbamazepine, corticosteroids, methimazole, phenytoin, propranolol, radiographic agents, somatostatin
Free Thyroxine Index (Serum)	Amiodarone, amphetamine, furosemide, oral contraceptives, propranolol	Aspirin, carbamazepine, clomiphene, corticosteroids, co-trimoxazole, ferrous sulfate, iodides, isotretinoin, lovastatin, methimazole, phenobarbital, phenytoin, primidone
Thyroglobulin (Serum)		Carbamazepine, neomycin, thyroxine
Thyroid Stimulating Hormone (Serum)	Aminoglutethimide, amphetamine, calcitonin, carbamazepine, chlorpromazine, clomiphene, ethionamide, ferrous sulfates, furosemide, iodides, lithium, lovastatin, mercaptopurine, metoprolol, morphine, nitroprusside, phenytoin, potassium iodide, prazosin, prednisone, propranolol, radiographic agents, rifampin, sulfonamides, thyrotropin-releasing hormone	Amiodarone, anabolic steroids, antithyroid drugs, aspirin, carbamazepine, clofibrate, corticosteroids, danazol, dobutamide, dopamine, fenoldopam, growth hormone-releasing hormone, hydrocortisone, interferon, levodopa, levothyroxine, nifedipine, octreotide, phenytoin, pimozide, pyridoxine, somatostatin, thyroxine, troleandomycin
Thyroxine-Binding Globulin (Serum)	Carbamazepine, clofibrate, diethylstilbestrol, estrogens, mestranol, oral contraceptives, perphenazine, phenothiazines, progesterone, tamoxifen, thyroid agents, warfarin	Anabolic steroids, asparaginase, aspirin, chlorpropamide, colestipol, corticosteroids, cortisone, cytostatic therapy, phenytoin, propranolol, sulfonamides
Triiodothyronine (T₃) Total (Serum)	Amiodarone, amphetamine, clofibrate, estrogens, fenoprofen, fluorouracil, insulin, levothyroxine, mestranol, methadone, opiates, phenothiazines, phenytoin, propylthiouracil, prostaglandins, ranitidine, rifampin, somatotropin, tamoxifen, terbutaline, thyrotropin-releasing hormone, valproic acid	Amiodarone, anabolic steroids, androgens, anticonvulsants (eg, phenytoin), asparaginase, aspirin, arenolol, cholestyramine, cimetidine, clomiphene, clomipramine, colestipol, corticosteroids, co-trimoxazole, furosemide, interferon, iodides, isotretinoin, lithium, methimazole, metoprolol, neomycin, netilmicin, oral contraceptives, penicillamine, phenobarbital, phenytoin, potassium iodide, propranolol, propylthiouracil, radiographic agents, reserpine, salicylates (eg, aspirin), somatostatin, sulfonylureas
Triiodothyronine Uptake (Blood)	Anabolic steroids, androgens, aspirin, colestipol, corticosteroids, cytostatic therapy, dicoumarol, heparin, phenytoin, propranolol, salicylates, sulfonamides, thyroid agents, warfarin	Antiovulatory drugs, antithyroid drugs, carbamazepine, clofibrate, diethylstilbestrol, estrogens, heparin, heroin, mestranol, methadone, oral contraceptives, perphenazine, phenothiazines, progesterones, tamoxifen, thiazide diuretics (eg, hydrochlorothiazide), thyroid agents, warfarin

From Fischbach FT: A Manual of Laboratory and Diagnostic Tests, 6th ed. Philadelphia: Lippincott Williams & Wilkins, 1999, pp 1232–1234.

test can also evaluate thyroid replacement therapy. Radioisotopes can interfere with test results, and heparin can give false high readings. This test can be performed by direct assay or by indirect measurement. The direct assay normal value is 0.8 to 2.7 ng/mL, whereas the free T₄ index is 4.6 to 12 ng/mL.

Free Triiodothyronine

Free T₃ measures the circulating T₃ that exists in the free state in the blood, unbound to protein. This is one

measure to evaluate thyroid function. T₃ is about 5 times more potent than T₄ and is more metabolically active. Decreased values indicate hypothyroidism. Radioisotopes also affect results. Normal adult values are 260 to 480 pg/dL.

Triiodothyronine Resin Uptake Test

The T₃ resin uptake test is an indirect measure of TBG available to bind T₃ and T₄. It is increased with thyrotoxicosis.

Calcitonin

Calcitonin, or thyrocalcitonin, is a hormone secreted by the thyroid. It is secreted in response to high levels of calcium and reduces the calcium level by increasing its deposition in bone.

Thyroid Antibodies

Several autoimmune thyroid diseases produce detectable antibodies. Specifically, Graves' disease, Hashimoto's thyroiditis, and chronic autoimmune thyroid disease cause elevations in antithyroid antibodies, detectable by immunoassay techniques. These conditions can lead to severe hypothyroidism or hyperthyroidism if not treated.

Thyroglobulin

Thyroglobulin can be measured by radioimmunoassay and is elevated in most thyroid disorders. This test has limited diagnostic value because it is nonspecific. It is used clinically to follow the progression of disease in a patient being treated for thyroid cancer.

DIAGNOSTIC STUDIES

Thyroid Scan and Radioactive Iodine Uptake

The radioactive iodine uptake test measures the rate of iodine uptake by the thyroid gland after the administration of iodine-123 tracer (by capsule, solution, or intravenous injection). A scintillation counter then measures gamma rays released from the breakdown of the tracer in the thyroid. This produces a visual representation of the radioactivity in the thyroid gland, neck, and mediastinum. Scan time is about 20 minutes. Normally, the radioactive iodine is evenly distributed in the thyroid gland, and the scan shows a normal size, position, and shape.

The thyroid scan may be performed in conjunction with a radioactive iodine uptake study. After the patient takes the radioactive iodine, a count is made over the thyroid gland with a scintillation counter at specific times. These nuclear tests can indicate areas of increased and decreased function and provide data to diagnose hyperthyroidism, hypothyroidism, nodules, ectopic thyroid tissue, and cancer of the thyroid.

Fine-Needle Biopsy

Fine-needle biopsy is the diagnostic tool of choice for detecting malignancy for a thyroid nodule. It is often the initial test for evaluation of any thyroid mass. The test is safe, quick, and accurate, and results are usually available within hours to several days.

Ultrasound

Ultrasound of the thyroid gland uses high-frequency sound waves to produce an image of the gland. Ultrasound is an easy, noninvasive procedure that has no radiation risks and can be performed at the bedside. The test produces good images of structures and can detect masses, cysts, and enlargements of the gland.

• The Parathyroid Gland

The parathyroid gland produces parathyroid hormone (PTH), which maintains blood calcium and phosphorus levels, neuromuscular activity, blood clotting function, and cell membrane permeability. The four parathyroid glands are located just posterior to the thyroid gland and are sometimes damaged during thyroid surgery.

The output of PTH is regulated by the serum level of calcium under a negative feedback system. Overproduction of PTH results in hyperparathyroidism and is characterized by bone decalcification and the development of renal stones containing calcium.

Hypocalcemia as a result of hypoparathyroidism manifests neurologically. The patient manifests tetany (general muscular hypertonia, tremor, and spasmodic movements) as calcium levels dip below 5 to 6 mg/dL. The patient may complain of numbness, tingling, and cramps in the extremities. As the hypocalcemia worsens, the patient experiences bronchospasm, laryngeal spasm, carpopedal spasm (flexion of the elbows and wrists with extension of the carpophalangeal joints), dysphagia, photophobia, cardiac dysrhythmias, and seizures.

HISTORY AND PHYSICAL EXAMINATION

The nurse ascertains a history of electrolyte imbalance, specifically calcium and phosphorus. Additional information includes a history of a variety of other symptoms listed in the endocrine health assessment (see Box 43-1). The patient may present with kidney stone symptoms such as severe flank pain, groin pain, frequent urination, hematuria, and nausea and vomiting. The patient may experience joint and bone pains and may sustain pathological fractures, especially of the spine. The nurse remains vigilant for signs of tetany (Fig. 43-6) and related complications.

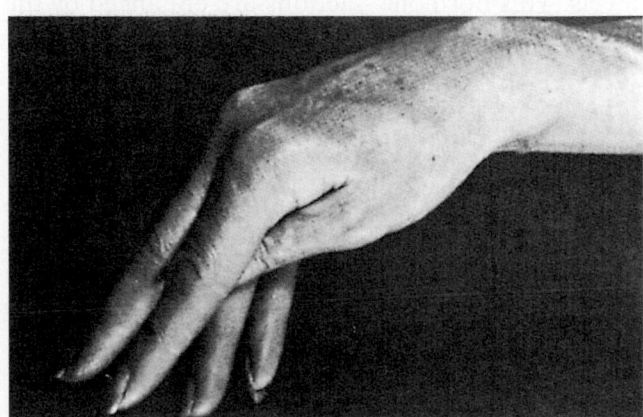

Figure 43-6 • Tetany is caused by tonic spasm of the intrinsic hand muscles. (From Spillane R: An Atlas of Clinical Neurology, 3rd ed. London: Oxford University Press, 1982, p 295.)

Tetany can be assessed by evaluating the patient for Trousseau's sign or Chvostek's sign. Trousseau's sign is positive when carpopedal spasm is induced by occluding the blood flow to the arm for 3 minutes with the use of a blood pressure cuff. If tapping over the facial nerve just in front of the parotid gland causes twitching of the mouth or eye, the patient has a positive Chvostek's sign.

LABORATORY STUDIES

Serum Calcium Level

Normal calcium levels range from 8.6 to 10.3 mg/dL. Most (99%) of body calcium is in the bone. The remaining 1% is in the ECF. Nearly 50% of serum calcium is ionized or free, whereas the remainder is bound to albumin. Changes in serum albumin alter total serum calcium concentration. Therefore, if albumin levels are also abnormal, clinical decisions regarding calcium should be based on the free calcium levels.

Marked serum calcium elevations are the most obvious manifestation of hyperparathyroidism. Calcium levels greater than 10.3 mg/dL are considered abnormally elevated. The common causes of hypercalcemia include primary hyperparathyroidism, malignancy, sarcoidosis, vitamin D toxicity, hyperthyroidism, and some medications such as thiazide diuretics and lithium.

Low serum calcium levels are the marker for hypoparathyroidism. Tetany develops at calcium levels of 5 to 6 mg/dL or lower. Common causes of hypocalcemia include hypoalbuminemia, renal failure, hypoparathyroidism, acute pancreatitis, tumor lysis syndrome, severe hypomagnesemia, and multiple citrated blood transfusions.

Parathyroid Hormone Level

Radioimmunoassay reveals elevated PTH levels in hyperparathyroidism and decreased PTH levels in hypoparathyroidism. PTH regulates calcium and phosphorus metabolism. Increased secretion of PTH results in increased calcium absorption from the kidneys, intestines, and bones, thereby raising calcium levels. This hormone's actions are enhanced by the presence of vitamin D.

DIAGNOSTIC STUDIES

Radiographic Studies

Plain films, bone scans, MRI, ultrasound, or a combination of these modalities may be used to examine the parathyroid glands and evaluate the bone changes that have occurred as a result of the disease.

• The Endocrine Pancreas

Disorders of the endocrine pancreas are characterized by chronic hyperglycemia and result in major shifts of fluids and electrolytes as well as in blood glucose lev-els. The risk for developing diabetes increases with age. The two main types of diabetes are type 1 and type 2, and both forms of diabetes can lead to serious illnesses requiring critical care.

HISTORY AND PHYSICAL EXAMINATION

A complete history is multisystem focused because glucose dysfunction affects every system of the body. A good family history is obtained to document the role of familial patterns often seen in type 2 diabetes. The characteristics of patients at risk for developing type 2 diabetes are reviewed in Box 43-5.

For the patient with known diabetes who enters the critical care arena, the nurse focuses on gathering information about the extent of the disease and its duration, the onset of complications, the medications taken for the disease, and other past medical and surgical history. Chronic complications such as neuropathy, retinopathy, and nephropathy are explored, as well as the existence of other medical conditions such as hypertension, hyperlipidemia, obesity, and peripheral vascular disease. Refer to Box 43-1 for a health history review of the endocrine system.

Physical examination focuses on the severe fluid and electrolyte and neurological dysfunction seen with acute diabetes complications such as DKA, HHS, and hypoglycemia. Observation of fluid status and hydration is mandatory. Skin turgor, buccal membranes, weight, urine specific gravity, and vital signs are assessed. The nurse monitors the patient's neurological status frequently as well as central venous pressures and other advanced monitoring if available. The presence of a fruity odor on the breath (associated with ketonemia) should be noted. In addition, the patient may display Kussmaul's respirations as an attempt to rapidly exhale excess carbon dioxide. This respiratory pattern is characterized by deep, rapid breathing. Figure 43-7 summarizes the physical features seen in the patient with diabetes mellitus.

Box 43-5 • RED FLAG: Risk Factors Associated With Developing Type 2 Diabetes

- Family history of diabetes (parents, grandparents, siblings)
- Obesity (body mass index [BMI] greater than 27 kg/m²)
- Race and ethnicity (African American, Native American, Hispanic American, Asian American, Pacific Islander)
- Age greater than 45 years
- History of impaired fasting glucose or impaired glucose tolerance
- Hypertension
- High-density lipoprotein (HDL) cholesterol less than 35 mg/dL
- Triglyceride level greater than 250 mg/dL
- History of gestational diabetes, the delivery of a baby greater than 9 pounds, or both

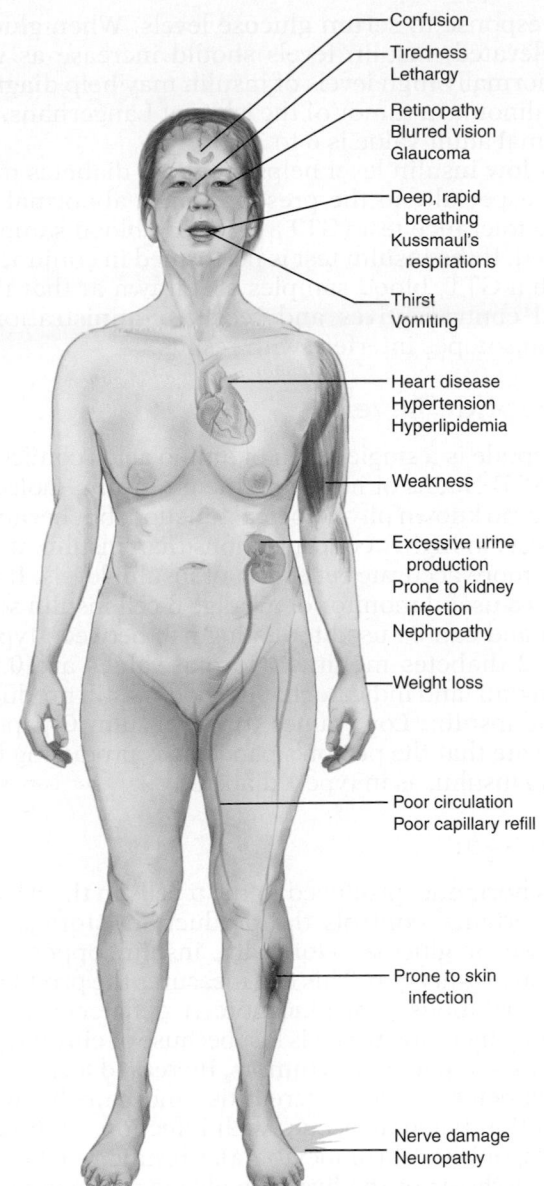

- Confusion
- Tiredness
- Lethargy
- Retinopathy
- Blurred vision
- Glaucoma
- Deep, rapid breathing
- Kussmaul's respirations
- Thirst
- Vomiting
- Heart disease
- Hypertension
- Hyperlipidemia
- Weakness
- Excessive urine production
- Prone to kidney infection
- Nephropathy
- Weight loss
- Poor circulation
- Poor capillary refill
- Prone to skin infection
- Nerve damage
- Neuropathy

Figure 43-7 • Clinical features of diabetes mellitus.

Box 43-6 • Criteria for the Diagnosis of Diabetes Mellitus

1. Symptoms of diabetes plus casual plasma glucose concentration ≥200 mg/dL (11.1 mmol/L). Casual is defined as any time of day without regard to time since last meal. The classic symptoms of diabetes include polyuria, polydipsia, and unexplained weight loss.

   OR

2. FPG ≥126 mg/dL (7.0 mmol/L). Fasting is defined as no caloric intake for at least 8 h.

   OR

3. 2-h postload glucose ≥200 mg/dL (11.1 mmol/L) during an OGTT. The test should be performed as described by WHO, using a glucose load containing the equivalent of 75 g anhydrous glucose dissolved in water.

In the absence of unequivocal hyperglycemia, these criteria should be confirmed by repeat testing on a different day. The third measure (oral glucose tolerance test, OGTT) is not recommended for routine clinical use.
From American Diabetes Association. Position statement: Diagnosis and Classification of Diabetes Mellitus. Diabetes Care 31 (1):S55–S60, 2008.

LABORATORY STUDIES

Fasting Blood Glucose Level and Fingerstick Glucose Analysis

The fasting blood glucose level provides a foundation for managing diabetes mellitus. Very high blood glucose levels can occur in DKA and HHS. In addition, elevated glucose levels can occur in Cushing's syndrome, high-stress states, pancreatitis, and chronic renal and liver disease. Hypoglycemia can occur in Addison's disease, pancreatic tumors, starvation, and hypopituitary problems. The normal value for adults is 65 to 110 mg/dL. Two-hour postprandial blood glucose testing helps further evaluate carbohydrate metabolism, especially in people with diabetes mellitus. The normal value is 65 to 126 mg/dL. The American Diabetes Association (ADA) criteria for the diagnosis of diabetes are given in Box 43-6.

In addition, the ADA recognizes an intermediate group of people who have glucose levels less than 126 mg/dL but nonetheless have glucose levels too high to be considered normal. If their fasting glucose is greater than 100 mg/dL but less than 126 mg/dL, they have the abnormality known as impaired fasting glucose (IFG). If the oral glucose tolerance test is performed to diagnose glucose abnormalities, the 2-hour postload level of less than 140 mg/dL is considered normal, a level of 140–199 mg/dL is considered impaired glucose tolerance (IGT), and a level of greater than 200 mg/dL is provisionally diagnostic of diabetes. Patients with IFG or IGT are now diagnosed with "prediabetes"; they are considered to have a very high risk for developing diabetes as well as cardiovascular disease. IFG and IGT are associated with metabolic syndrome, which is manifested by increased abdominal obesity, high triglyceride levels, low high-density lipoprotein cholesterol levels, and hypertension.[1]

Numerous drugs can interfere with glucose regulation, including corticosteroids, diuretics, lithium, phenytoin, β-blockers, and estrogen. Hypoglycemic reactions can result from sulfonylureas, insulin, alcohol, β-blockers, angiotensin-converting enzyme inhibitors, and aspirin.

Fingerstick glucose testing can be used at the bedside for immediate feedback regarding the patient's glucose status. In addition, patients can be taught to use fingerstick devices at home to monitor their glucose levels and responses to medication. Standardization of the equipment must be ensured when these devices are used for patient monitoring.

In general, point-of-service testing such as this may not be appropriate for the critically ill patient because fingerstick testing requires adequate tissue perfusion for accuracy, and many critically ill patients do not have this required level of perfusion. Testing glucose from more direct sources of blood (i.e., veins, venous lines, central lines, arterial lines) may enhance accuracy.

Glycosylated Hemoglobin

Glycosylated hemoglobin (HbA$_{1c}$) testing offers information about the average amount of glucose present in the patient's bloodstream for the 100- to 120-day life span of erythrocytes. This information is useful to assess data trends for a person who has been previously diagnosed with diabetes. The percentage result (normal: 4% to 7%) that reflects an average of 3 months enhances accuracy because it controls for many variables such as stress, exercise, fasting state, interfering medications, and recent changes in patient compliance. In comparison with the highly variable, "snapshot view" that is provided by a fasting glucose level, HbA$_{1c}$ testing provides insight into the patient's overall status over the previous months.[1] Figure 43-8 compares the HbA$_{1C}$ value to the average blood glucose value.

Fructosamine

Serum fructosamine level measures glycosylation of serum protein albumin. Albumin has a half-life of approximately 2 weeks, as opposed to the half-life of hemoglobin. It is a useful index that reflects chronic glycemia control in patients with diabetes for whom HbA$_{1C}$ may be inaccurate such as those with anemia or hemoglobin abnormalities (e.g., sickle cell disease).[2]

Insulin

This test helps measure abnormal carbohydrate metabolism by measuring the amount of circulating serum insulin in the fasting state. Insulin is released in response to serum glucose levels. When glucose is elevated, insulin levels should increase as well. Abnormally high levels of insulin may help diagnose insulinoma, a tumor of the islets of Langerhans. The normal adult value is 6 to 24 fU/mL.

A low insulin level helps diagnose diabetes mellitus, especially in the presence of an abnormal glucose tolerance test (GTT). A fasting blood sample is tested. If the insulin test is performed in conjunction with a GTT, blood samples are drawn at that time. Oral contraceptives and recent administration of radioisotopes interfere with results.

C-Peptide Level

C-peptide is a single chain of amino acids connecting A and B chains of insulin in the proinsulin molecule. It has no known physiological function, but because it persists in higher concentrations than insulin, it may be a more accurate reflection of insulin levels. It provides a useful monitor of average β-cell insulin secretion and can be used to distinguish between types 1 and 2 diabetes mellitus. Normal values are 0.5 to 2.0 ng/mL and indicate that the body is still producing some insulin. Low values (or no insulin C-peptide) indicate that the person's pancreas is producing little or no insulin, as in type 1 diabetes.[1]

Glucagon

This hormone, produced in the α cells in the islets of Langerhans, controls the production, storage, and release of glucose. Normally, insulin opposes the action of glucagon. This test measures the production and metabolism of glucagon. A deficiency occurs when pancreatic tissue is lost because of chronic pancreatitis or pancreatic tumors. Increased levels occur in diabetes, acute pancreatitis, and catecholamine secretion (such as occurs with infection, high stress levels, or pheochromocytoma). Chronic renal failure and cirrhosis of the liver can also increase glucagon levels. Normal fasting values are 50 to 200 pg/mL.

Serum Ketones

Measuring serum ketones reveals information about the use of fat metabolism in lieu of carbohydrates as seen in the critically ill person with diabetes. The normal serum ketone level is 2 to 4 mg/dL. Ketonemia (ketone bodies in the bloodstream) is manifested by Kussmaul's respirations and a fruity, sweet-smelling odor on the exhaled breath. These signs are the result of the patient's attempt to maintain a normal pH during extreme metabolic acidosis.[1] In DKA, metabolic acidosis is primarily the result of the accumulation of acetoacetic acid and β-hydroxybutyric acid.[3]

Urine Ketones

Ketones are not normally found in the urine. Ketones in the urine are associated with diabetes and other diseases of altered carbohydrate metabolism. People with diabetes should test for ketones whenever their urine or blood sugar is high. Because ketones appear in the urine before they can be detected in the blood,

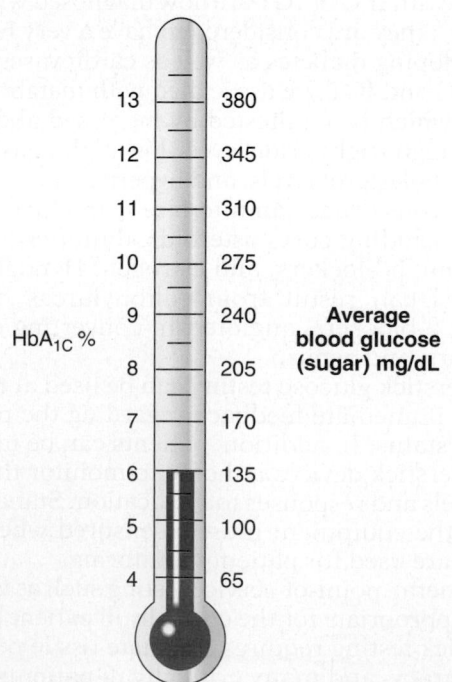

Figure 43-8 • Comparison of glycosylated hemoglobin (HbA$_{1c}$) to average blood glucose level. The normal range is shown in *red*.

this test is often used in the emergency department when screening for acidosis. The test is performed by dipping a ketone reagent strip in a fresh urine sample. The presence of ketones in the urine results from lipolysis or fat breakdown in the absence of adequate insulin.

• The Adrenal Gland

The adrenal gland is anatomically and functionally divided into two distinct parts—the outer cortex and the inner medulla (see Chapter 42, Fig. 42-6). The two regions secrete different hormones. The cortex produces mineralocorticoids (e.g., aldosterone), glucocorticoids (e.g., cortisol), and androgens. The medulla secretes catecholamines such as epinephrine, norepinephrine, and dopamine. Disorders of the adrenal gland have widespread effects on the human body because these hormones regulate major body functions such as fluid and electrolyte balance, sympathetic nervous system responses, inflammation, and metabolism.

The secretion of hormones by the adrenal gland is regulated in a negative feedback system through the hypothalamic–pituitary axis. The hypothalamus releases corticotropin-releasing hormone (CRH), which in turn stimulates the release of ACTH from the anterior pituitary. ACTH then stimulates the adrenal cortex to secrete cortisol.

HISTORY AND PHYSICAL EXAMINATION

Refer to Box 43-1 for a review of relevant health history questions related to adrenal disorders.

Clinical manifestations of adrenal gland dysfunction depend on the nature of the lesion and which hormone is adversely affected. Adrenal cortex lesions may affect the release of catecholamines and cause sudden, severe headache, diaphoresis, palpitations, and other symptoms associated with paroxysmal hypertension. One such lesion is pheochromocytoma, a benign adrenal cortex tumor that mediates this severe outpouring of catecholamines.

Another common pathology affecting the adrenal gland is a pituitary tumor that leads to hypersecretion of ACTH. The resulting disease, Cushing's syndrome, manifests as central obesity, unusual fat deposits, thin extremities, fragile skin, skin discoloration (striae), sleep disturbances, and catabolism (Fig. 43-9). The same clinical picture can result from chronic exogenous steroid use.

Adrenal insufficiency from autoimmune Addison's disease can lead to an adrenal crisis. The patient lacks adequate stimulation of the adrenal gland, or the adrenal gland is rendered ineffective and stops secreting adequate levels of hormone. Consequently, the patient becomes lethargic, dehydrated, and unable to mount any stress response to handle acute illness or trauma. The critically ill patient often suffers from mild forms of adrenal insufficiency because the patient's normal stores of hormones are used quickly in response to the illness. Many require exogenous

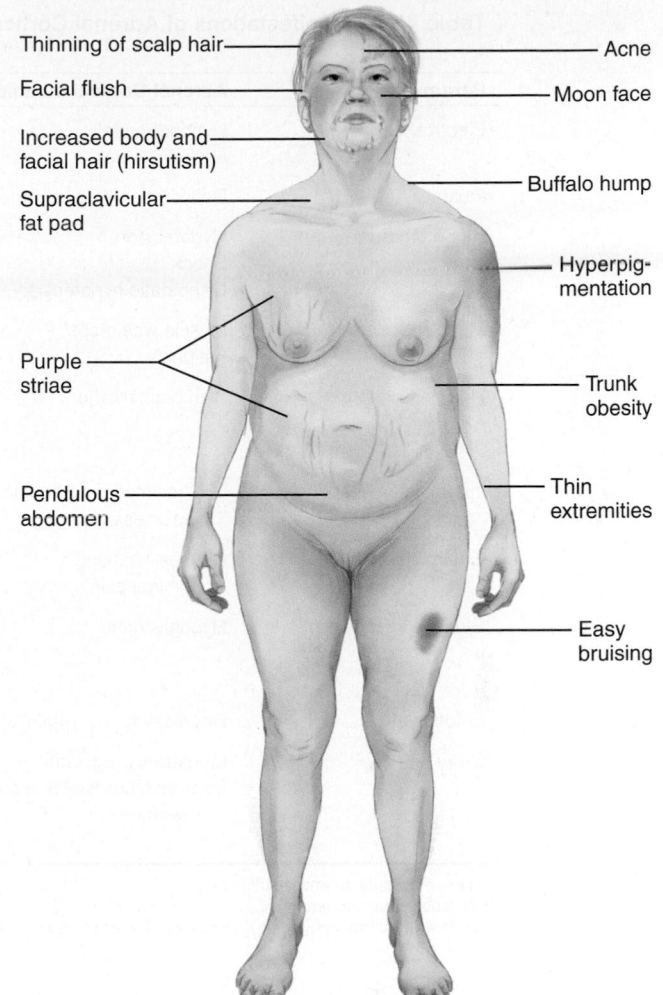

Thinning of scalp hair
Facial flush
Increased body and facial hair (hirsutism)
Supraclavicular fat pad
Purple striae
Pendulous abdomen

Acne
Moon face
Buffalo hump
Hyperpigmentation
Trunk obesity
Thin extremities
Easy bruising

Figure 43-9 • Clinical manifestations of Cushing's syndrome.

steroids to assist with recovery. A summary of the clinical manifestations of adrenal cortical insufficiency and glucocorticoid excess is given in Table 43-5.

LABORATORY STUDIES

Cortisol (Hydrocortisone)

This test evaluates the ability of the adrenal cortex to produce the glucocorticoid hormone cortisol. Cortisol is elevated in adrenal hyperfunction and decreased in adrenal hypofunction. Adrenal hyperfunction may be caused by excess secretion of ACTH by the pituitary gland (Cushing's syndrome), high stress, trauma, and surgery. Adrenal hypofunction may be the result of anterior pituitary hyposecretion, hepatitis, and cirrhosis.

Cortisol secretion is diurnal; it is normally higher in the early morning (6:00 a.m. to 8:00 a.m.) and lower in the evening (4:00 p.m. to 6:00 p.m.). This variation is lost in patients with adrenal hyperfunction and in people under stress. Serum samples are drawn between 6:00 a.m. and 8:00 a.m. and between 4:00 p.m. and 6:00 p.m. Normal 8:00 a.m. values are 5 to 23 fg/dL or 138 to 635 mmol/L. Normal 4:00 p.m. values are 3 to 16 fg/dL or 83 to 441 mmol/L.

Table 43-5 • Manifestations of Adrenal Cortical Insufficiency and Excess

Parameter	Adrenal Cortical Insufficiency	Glucorticoid Excess
Electrolytes	Hyponatremia* Hyperkalemia*	Hypokalemia
Fluids	Dehydration* (e.g., elevated BUN)	Edema
Blood pressure	Hypotension Shock* Orthostatic hypotension	Hypertension
Musculoskeletal	Muscle weakness* Fatigue*	Muscle wasting Fatigue
Hair and skin	Skin pigmentation	Easy bruisability Hirsutism, acne, and striae (abdomen and thighs)

Inflammatory response	Low resistance to trauma, infection
	    and stress
		Decrease in eosinophils,
		    lymphocytopenia

Gastrointestinal	Nausea, vomiting* Abdominal pain*	Possible gastrointestinal bleeding
Glucose metabolism	Hypoglycemia*	Impaired glucose tolerance Glycosuria Elevated blood sugar
Emotional	Depression and irritability	Emotional lability to psychosis

Other	Menstrual irregularity
	Decreased axillary and pubic hair
	    in women
		Oligomenorrhea
		Impotence in the male
		Centripetal obesity (moon face and
		    buffalo hump)

*Occurs with acute adrenal insufficiency.
BUN, blood urea nitrogen.
From Porth CM: Pathophysiology: Concepts of Altered Health States, 5th ed. Philadelphia: Lippincott Williams & Wilkins, 1998, p 80.

Cortisol (Dexamethasone) Suppression

When healthy people receive a low dose of dexamethasone (chemically similar to cortisol), ACTH production is suppressed. However, people with adrenal hyperfunction and some with endogenous depression continue to produce ACTH and do not have a diurnal variation of cortisol.

For this test, dexamethasone is given at bedtime. Blood samples are taken the next day at 8:00 a.m. and 4:00 p.m. Medications are discontinued for 24 to 48 hours before this test is started, especially estrogens, phenytoin, and cortisol-related preparations. Radioisotopes should not be given within 1 week of this test. This test is the test of choice to diagnose Cushing's syndrome.[4]

Cortisol Stimulation

This test measures the response of the adrenal glands to an injection of cosyntropin (Cortrosyn, a synthetic ACTH preparation). A fasting 8:00 a.m. cortisol level is drawn before cosyntropin is administered, and then blood samples are taken 30 and 60 minutes after it is administered. The adrenal glands normally respond to the cosyntropin by synthesizing and secreting adrenocorticoids. The plasma cortisol level should increase to at least 18 fg/dL. The response to cosyn-

tropin is decreased or absent in people with adrenal insufficiency or hypopituitarism. Long-term steroid therapy affects results. This test may be contraindicated in the presence of infections, inflammatory diseases, and cardiac disease. Cortisol stimulation is the preferred test to diagnose Addison's disease.

Urine Vanillylmandelic Acid and Catecholamine Levels

Urine vanillylmandelic acid is a metabolite of catecholamines. It has a high concentration in the urine and is easy to detect. Therefore, this 24-hour urine test is performed when a person is suspected of having hypertension due to pheochromocytoma. Catecholamines can also be detected in the urine. Elevated levels of catecholamines can be found in patients with hypothyroidism, DKA, neuroblastomas, and ganglioneuromas.

Urine should not be collected when the patient is NPO. Test results are also affected by many drugs and foods, such as tea, coffee, vanilla, and fruit juice. Therefore, some laboratories restrict certain foods for 2 days before testing and on the day of testing. Certain drugs may also be discontinued for 4 to 7 days before testing. Normal adult values for urine vanillylmandelic acid are 2 to 7 mg/24 hours, and for catecholamines, 270 fg/24 hours.

Urine 17-Ketosteroids and 17-Hydroxycorticosteroids

These 24-hour urine collection tests reflect adrenal function by measuring the urinary excretion of steroids. They are used infrequently because they have been replaced by serum immunoassays.

DIAGNOSTIC STUDIES

Adrenal Scan

This scan is used to identify the site of certain tumors or sites that produce excessive amounts of catecholamines. The radionuclide iobenguane (^{131}I) is injected intravenously, and scans are performed on days 2, 3, and 4. Sometimes only 1 day is needed, and other times imaging is needed on days 6 and 7. Normally tumors and sites of hypersecretion are absent. If ACTH levels are elevated, MRI of the pituitary should be done to seek the source.[4]

• Clinical Applicability Challenges

Case Study: Diabetes Mellitus

Mr. J., a 58-year-old African American, arrives in the emergency department after his wife discovers him unarousable at their home. She tells the nurse that he has been very fatigued and lethargic for the past several days, and she has noticed that he had been drinking a lot of juice lately. In addition, she reports that he has been getting up frequently at night to urinate and has complained of blurred vision. He takes medication for high blood pressure and high cholesterol, but his wife is not sure of the exact names. The patient is a nonsmoker, and he drinks a glass of wine every other week at home. He is not allergic to any medications. Both of his parents had diabetes, and two of his brothers have diabetes as well. Currently, he works at a computer firm and is relatively sedentary.

The nurse notes that Mr. J. is a lethargic but fully oriented, overweight male with flushed, slightly diaphoretic skin. His skin turgor is poor, with a sluggish capillary refill time. His vital signs are blood pressure, 95/50 mm Hg; heart rate, 118 beats/minute; and respiratory rate, 24 breaths/minute. He is afebrile.

Mr. J.'s lab results show a glucose level of 610 mg/dL, serum ketones are mildly positive, and white blood cells are normal. Mr. J.'s electrocardiogram shows sinus tachycardia (rate, 115 to 120 beats/minute), he has postural hypotension, and he is slightly tachypneic. He repeatedly asks for something to drink as the staff prepares to start an intravenous line for fluids and to initiate an insulin infusion.

1. What is the constellation of symptoms that Mr. J. displayed at home that are associated with the insidious development of diabetes mellitus?

2. What specific risk factors for type 2 diabetes mellitus are illustrated in this case study?

3. In the emergency department, Mr. J. demonstrates typical signs and symptoms associated with diabetes mellitus. Explain the pathogenesis of these abnormalities.

Review Questions

1. Ms. K has been diagnosed with syndrome of inappropriate antidiuretic hormone (SIADH). The expected serum osmolality for Ms. K is
   a. decreased.
   b. increased.
   c. completely normal.
   d. same as the urine osmolality.

2. Which group of signs/symptoms is associated with hyperthyroidism?
   a. Bradycardia, dysrhythmias, hypertension, hyporeflexia
   b. Tachycardia, dysrhythmias, hypotension, hyperreflexia
   c. Heat intolerance, hypertension, tachycardia, hyperreflexia
   d. Cold intolerance, hypertension, tachycardia, hyperreflexia

3. A male patient's laboratory values indicate that he continues to have hypocalcemia and is at risk for development of tetany. Tetany is assessed by which one of the following parameters?
   a. Positive Hoffmann's sign
   b. Positive Turner's sign
   c. Positive Trousseau's sign
   d. Positive Rovsing's sign

4. The glycosylated hemoglobin (HbA$_{1c}$) is reflective of glucose saturation on the hemoglobin molecule for what length of time?
   a. 1 month
   b. 2 months
   c. 3 months
   d. 6 months

5. A female patient has been diagnosed with hypersecretion of adrenocorticotropic hormone (ACTH) and adrenal cortical excess. What signs and symptoms is she most likely to have?
   a. Lethargy and striae
   b. Central obesity and unusual fat deposits
   c. Dehydration and diabetes mellitus
   d. Skin pigmentation and hypoglycemia

References

1. American Diabetes Association: Position statement: Diagnosis and classification of diabetes mellitus. Diabetes Care 30(1): S42–S47, 2007
2. Ko GT, Chan JC, Yeung VF, et al: Combined use of a fasting plasma glucose concentration and HBA$_{1}$c or fructosamine predicts the likelihood of having diabetes in high-risk subjects. Diabetes Care 21(8):1221–1225, 1998

3. Newton CA, Raskin P: Diabetic ketoacidosis in type 1 and type 2 diabetes mellitus. Arch Intern Med 164:1925–1931, 2004
4. Holcomb SS: Confronting Cushing's syndrome. 35 (9):32hn1–32hn6, 2006

Other Suggested Readings

American Diabetes Association: Position statement: Hyperglycemic crises in patients with diabetes mellitus. Diabetes Care 27(Suppl l):S94–S102, 2004

American Diabetes Association: Position statement: Diagnosis and classification of diabetes mellitus. Diabetes Care 31(1): S55–S60, 2008

American Diabetes Association: Clinical practice recommendations 2008. Diabetes Care 31(Suppl 1):S51–S108, 2008

Bazakis AM, Kunzler C: Altered mental status due to metabolic or endocrine disorders. Emerg Med Clin North Am 23(3): 901–908, 2005

Bloomgarden ZT: Aspects of type 2 diabetes and related insulin-resistant states. Diabetes Care 29(3):732–740, 2006

Brackenridge A, Wallbank H, Lawrenson RA, Russell-Jones D: Emergency management of diabetes and hypoglycaemia. Emerg Med J 23(3):183–185, 2006

Brenner ZR: Management of hyperglycemic emergencies. AACN Clin Issues 17(1):56–65, 2006

Fonseca VA: Clinical Diabetes: Translating Research into Practice. Philadelphia: Saunders, Elsevier, 2006

Harmel AP, Mathur R: Davidson's Diabetes Mellitus: Diagnosis and Treatment, 5th dd. Philadelphia: Saunders, Elsevier, 2004

Harris PE, Bouloux PM: Endocrinology in Clinical Practice. London, UK: Martin Dunitz Ltd, 2003

Holcomb SS: Detecting thyroid disease. Nursing 2006 35(10):4–8, 2006

Holcomb SS: Detecting thyroid disease, Part 1. Nursing 2003 33(8):32cc1–32cc4, 2006

Krentz AJ: Emergencies in Diabetes: Diagnosis, Management and Prevention. Southhampton University, UK: John Wiley & Sons, 2004

Lacara T, Domagtoy C, Lickliter D, et al: Comparison of point-of-care and laboratory glucose analysis in critically ill patients. Am J Crit Care 16(4):336–346, 2007

Mauk KL: Rooting out hypothyroidism in the elderly. Nursing 2005 35(12):65–66, 2005

Melmed S, Conn PM: Endocrinology, 2nd ed. Totowa, NJ: Humana Press, 2005

Mesa J, Salcedo D, de la Calle H, et al: Detection of ketonemia and its relationship with hyperglycemia in type 1 diabetic patients. Diabetes Res Clin Pract 72(3):292–297, 2006

Moore T: Diabetic emergencies in adults. Nurs Stand 18(46): 45–54, 2004

Newton CA, Raskin P: Diabetic ketoacidosis in type 1 and type 2 diabetes mellitus. Arch Intern Med 164:1925–1931, 2004

Palmer R: An overview of diabetic ketoacidosis. Nurs Stand 19(10):42–44, 2004

Pfadt E, Carlson DS: Acute adrenal crisis. Nursing 2006 36(8): 80–81, 2006

Porth CM: Pathophysiology: Concepts of Altered Health States, 7th ed. Philadelphia: Lippincott Williams & Wilkins, 2005

Reid JR, Wheeler SF: Hyperthyroidism: Diagnosis and treatment. Am Fam Physician 72(4):623–631, 2005

Rhoades J: Advanced health assessment and diagnostic reasoning. Philadelphia: Lippincott Williams & Wilkins, 2006

Robinson LE, van Soeren MH: Insulin resistance and hyperglycemia in critical illness: Role of insulin in glycemic control. AACN Clin Issues 15(1):45–62, 2004

Smeltzer SC, Bare BG, Hinkle JL, Cheever KH: Brunner & Suddarth's Textbook of Medical–Surgical Nursing, 11th ed. Philadelphia, Lippincott Williams & Wilkins, 2008

Umpeirrez GE, Smily D, Kitabchi AE: Narrative review: Ketosis-prone diabetes mellitus. Ann Intern Med 144(5):350–357, 2006

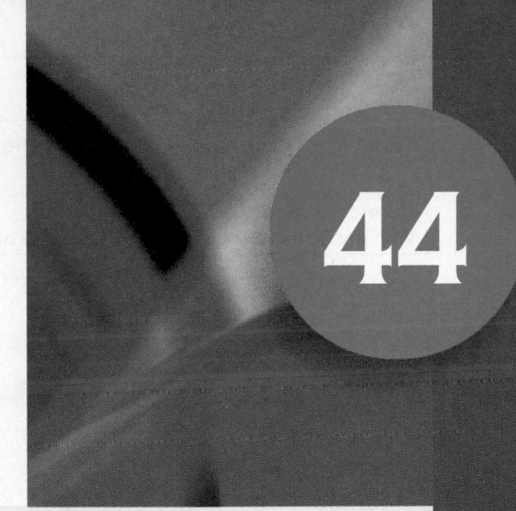

Common Endocrine Disorders

Jane Kapustin

Objectives

Based on the content in this chapter, the reader should be able to:

❶ Examine the pathophysiological principles that help explain thyrotoxic crises, myxedema coma, adrenal crises, syndrome of inappropriate antidiuretic hormone secretion, diabetes insipidus, diabetic ketoacidosis, hyperglycemic hyperosmolar syndrome, and hypoglycemia.

❷ Distinguish key precipitating factors, history, and clinical manifestations of endocrine disorders.

❸ Discuss five laboratory studies that are useful in diagnosing acute endocrine disorders.

❹ Analyze the similarities and differences in caring for patients with endocrine disorders.

❺ Explore the nursing role in assessing, managing, and evaluating a plan of care for patients with endocrine disorders.

Endocrine disorders have multisystem effects. At the same time, acute illness may lead to hypofunction and, less commonly, hyperfunction of the neuroendocrine system. Patients with acute illness who are at risk for endocrine dysfunction may have a preexisting endocrine disorder. Although that disorder may have already been diagnosed, many endocrine dysfunctions are not recognized before acute illness. For this reason, endocrine dysfunction should be considered in the assessment and management of all critically ill patients.

• Hypothalamic–Pituitary–Adrenal Function During Critical Illness

Severe illness and stress activate the HPA, resulting in the release of cortisol from the adrenal cortex. This mechanism is key to providing for positive adaptation to severe stressors and for general cellular and organ homeostasis. The nervous and endocrine systems are both influenced by the responses to stress, and the actions of these systems are intertwined and interdependent. For example, the neurosensory pathways and chemical mediators in the vascular system will detect a potential stressor, and the endocrine and immune systems will be stimulated to provide both an interaction and reaction to deal effectively with it. Table 44-1 defines the hormones that are intricately involved in the response to stress. The stress response is first activated at the level of the central nervous system (CNS). Communication occurs along the many neuronal pathways in the cerebral cortex, limbic system, thalamus, hypothalamus, pituitary gland, and reticular activating system (Fig. 44-1). One area of the brainstem, the locus ceruleus, is responsible for the autonomic nervous system release of norepinephrine, one of the most basic survival responses to stress. This release causes a chain of events that prepares humans for mounting an appropriate reaction to the stressor. In turn, corticotropin-releasing factor induces the

Table 44-1 • Hormones Involved in the Neuroendocrine Response to Stress

Hormones Associated With the Stress Response	Source of the Hormone	Physiologic Effects
Catecholamines (norepinephrine, epinephrine)	Locus ceruleus, adrenal medulla	Produces a decrease in insulin release and an increase in glucagon release resulting in increased glycogenolysis, gluconeogenesis, lipolysis, proteolysis, and decreased glucose uptake by the peripheral tissues; an increase in heart rate, cardiac contractility, and vascular smooth muscle contraction; and relaxation of bronchial smooth muscle
Corticotropin-releasing factor (CRF	Hypothalamus	Stimulates ACTH release from anterior pituitary and increased activity of neurons in locus ceruleus
Adrenocorticotropic hormone (ACTH)	Anterior pituitary	Stimulates the synthesis and release of cortisol
Glucocorticoid hormones (e.g., cortisol)	Adrenal cortex	Potentiates the actions of epinephrine and glucagon; inhibits the release and/or actions of the reproductive hormones and thyroid-stimulating hormone; and produces a decrease in immune cells and inflammatory mediators
Mineralocorticoid hormones (e.g., aldosterone)	Adrenal cortex	Increases sodium absorption by the kidney
Antidiuretic hormone (ADH, vasopressin)	Hypothalamus, posterior pituitary	Increases water absorption by the kidney; produces vasoconstriction of blood vessels; and stimulates the release of ACTH

From Porth CM: Concepts of Altered Health States, 7th ed. Philadelphia: Lippincott Williams & Wilkins, 2005, p 190.

secretion of adrenocorticotropic hormone (ACTH), which triggers the synthesis and release of cortisol from the adrenal gland.[1]

Acute and chronic stressful events can initiate a significant physiological response in an effort to maintain homeostasis. The "fight-or-flight" response is the initial reaction to a severe stressor, and release of norepinephrine and epinephrine follows. Activation of the hypothalamic–pituitary–adrenal (HPA) axis occurs in response to stress and critical illness, and secretion of cortisol, the primary glucocorticoid hormone, results. Cellular actions of cortisol include

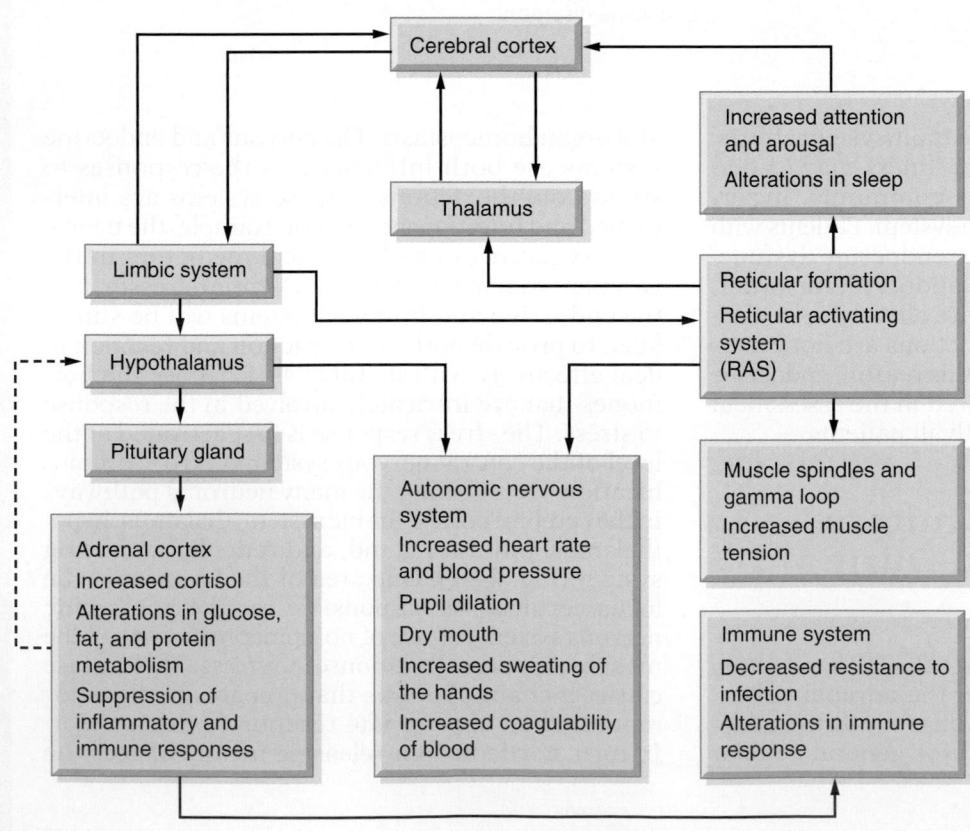

Figure 44-1 • Stress pathways. The broken line represents negative feedback. (From Porth CM: Pathophysiology: Concepts of Altered Health States, 7th ed. Philadelphia: Lippincott Williams & Wilkins, 2005.)

stimulation of gluconeogenesis, anti-inflammatory effects of the immune system, maintenance of vascular tone and endothelial integrity, increased sensitivity to pressors, reduction of nitric oxide–mediated vasodilation, and modulation of angiotensinogen synthesis. This hormone plays an important role in survival from major stressful events. Cortisol stimulates the HPA axis during acute and chronic events such as surgery, sepsis, trauma, burns, and other severe critical illnesses. Initially, elevated cortisol levels are often detected in the critically ill. If the stressor is prolonged, cortisol levels become depleted. Refer to Table 44-1 and to Chapter 42 for a review of the hormones activated in the neuroendocrine response to stress.

This chapter now presents an overview of the pathophysiology, assessment, management, and complications of patients with acute endocrine disorders. These disorders are thyroid dysfunctions, adrenal gland dysfunctions, antidiuretic hormone (ADH) dysfunctions, and emergencies in patients with diabetes.

• Thyroid Dysfunction

Thyroid dysfunction is a common clinical problem in the United States. Women are 5 to 10 times more likely than men to present with thyroid disease. The most common thyroid conditions are hyperthyroidism, hypothyroidism, and thyroid nodule. Clinical presentations may be quite subtle; therefore, patients with endocrine manifestations must be regarded with a high index of suspicion. Extremes of these two conditions are discussed in greater detail in this chapter. Figure 44-2 compares the signs and symptoms of hyperthyroidism and hypothyroidism.

THYROTOXIC CRISIS

Thyrotoxic crisis is a severe form of hyperthyroidism often associated with physiological or psychological stress. When the thyroid state worsens critically, it is called thyrotoxic crisis. Rapid deterioration and death can occur if the condition is untreated. These patients must be admitted to the intensive care unit for supportive measures, antithyroid medications, steroids, and continuous nursing care. Consultation with an endocrinologist and cardiologist is essential. Even without preexisting coronary artery disease (CAD), untreated thyrotoxic crisis can cause angina pectoris and myocardial infarction, heart failure, cardiovascular collapse, coma, and death. The condition may develop spontaneously, but it occurs most frequently in people who have undiagnosed or partially treated severe hyperthyroidism.

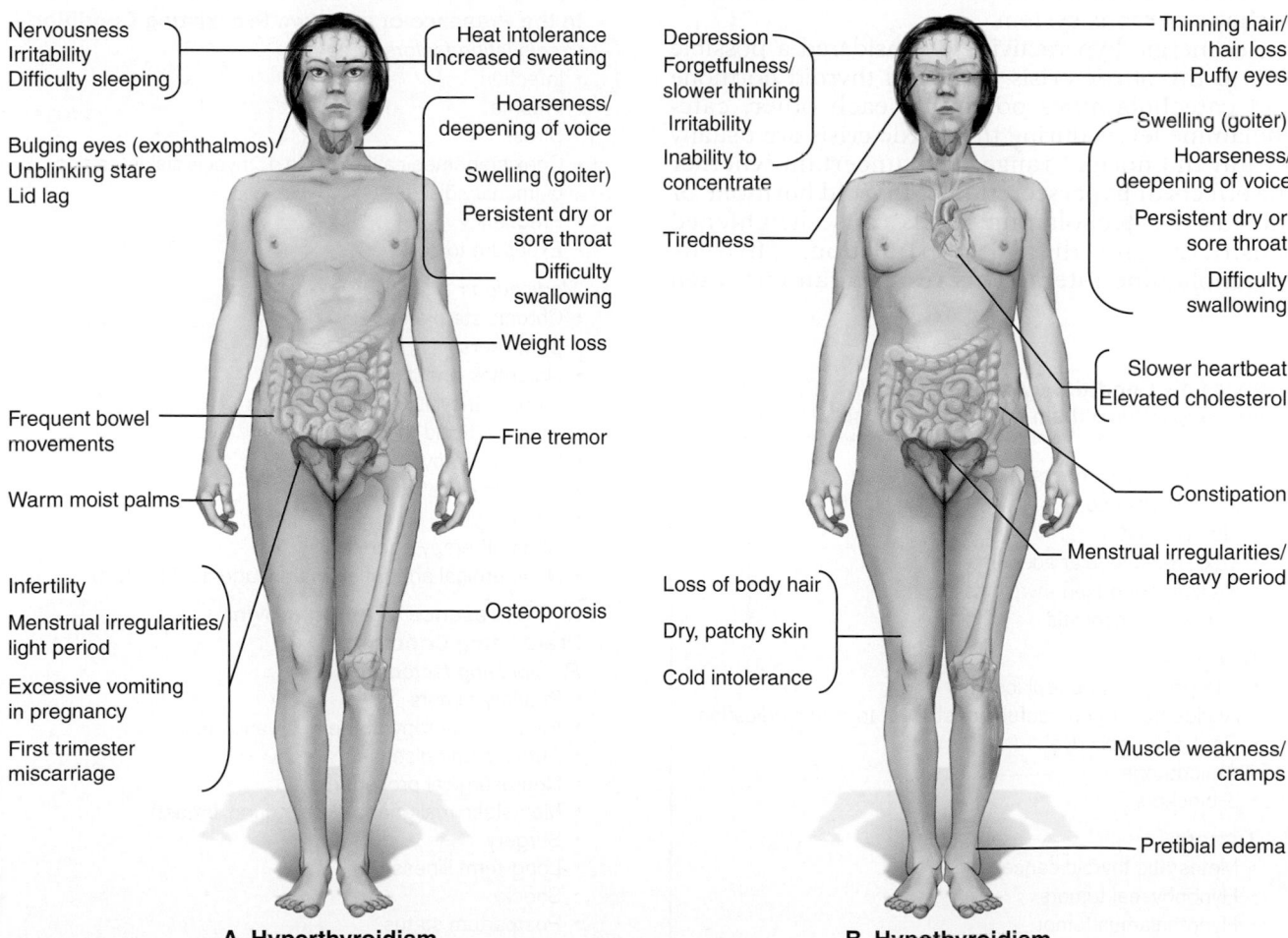

A. Hyperthyroidism

Nervousness
Irritability
Difficulty sleeping

Heat intolerance
Increased sweating

Bulging eyes (exophthalmos)
Unblinking stare
Lid lag

Hoarseness/
deepening of voice

Swelling (goiter)

Persistent dry or
sore throat

Difficulty
swallowing

Weight loss

Frequent bowel
movements

Fine tremor

Warm moist palms

Infertility

Menstrual irregularities/
light period

Osteoporosis

Excessive vomiting
in pregnancy

First trimester
miscarriage

B. Hypothyroidism

Depression
Forgetfulness/
slower thinking
Irritability
Inability to
concentrate

Thinning hair/
hair loss
Puffy eyes

Swelling (goiter)

Hoarseness/
deepening of voice

Persistent dry or
sore throat

Tiredness

Difficulty
swallowing

Slower heartbeat
Elevated cholesterol

Constipation

Menstrual irregularities/
heavy period

Loss of body hair

Dry, patchy skin

Cold intolerance

Muscle weakness/
cramps

Pretibial edema

Figure 44-2 • Clinical manifestations of hyperthyroidism (**A**) and hypothyroidism (**B**).

By definition, hyperthyroidism is a condition in which the actions of the thyroid hormones result in greater-than-normal responses. Specific diseases that can cause hyperthyroidism include Graves' disease, exogenous hyperthyroidism, thyroiditis, toxic nodular goiter, toxic multinodular goiter, and thyroid cancer. Certain drugs, such as contrast material for radiographic procedures or amiodarone (an antidysrhythmic drug), may precipitate the thyrotoxic state because of their high iodine content. The conditions associated with hyperthyroidism are summarized in Box 44-1.

Pathophysiology

The cause of thyrotoxic crisis, often referred to as thyroid storm, is poorly understood. Physiological mechanisms that are thought to induce thyrotoxic crises include the sudden release of large quantities of thyroid hormone, low tissue tolerance to triiodothyronine (T_3) and thyroxine (T_4), adrenergic hyperactivity, and excessive lipolysis and fatty acid production. The abrupt release of large quantities of thyroid hormone is thought to produce the hypermetabolic manifestations seen during thyrotoxic crises. The many different endocrine, reproductive, gastrointestinal, integumentary, and ocular manifestations are caused by increased circulating levels of thyroid hormone and by stimulation of the sympathetic nervous system.

Adrenergic hyperactivity is considered a possible link to thyrotoxic crisis. Although thyroid hormone and catecholamines potentiate each other, catecholamine levels during thyrotoxic crisis are usually within the normal range. It is uncertain whether the effects of hypersecretion of thyroid hormone or increased catecholamine levels cause heightened sensitivity and thyroid overfunction. Thyroid–catecholamine interactions result in an increased rate of chemical reactions, increased nutrient and oxygen consumption, increased heat production, alterations in fluid and electrolyte balance, and a catabolic state.

Another mechanism that may contribute to thyrotoxic crisis is excessive lipolysis and fatty acid production. With excessive lipolysis, increased fatty acids are oxidized and produce an overabundance of thermal energy that is difficult to dissipate through vasodilation.

Assessment

History and Physical Examination
Accurate identification of the precipitating factor for thyrotoxic crisis allows for proper treatment to be initiated. Precipitating factors for people with recognized and unrecognized existing thyroid disease are listed in Box 44-2. Hyperthyroidism's most common form, Graves' disease, is an autoimmune condition caused by thyroid-stimulating immunoglobulins. It is not always apparent that the patient is suffering from this particular disease. Therefore, subtle clues need to be explored, such as the patient's exposure to

---

Box 44-2 • RED FLAG: Risk Factors for Development of Thyroid Crisis

In the Presence of a Known Preexisting Condition
Precipitating factors
• Infection
• Trauma
• Stress
• Coexistent medical illness (e.g., myocardial infarction, pulmonary disease)
• Pregnancy
• Exposure to cold

Medications
• Chronic steroid therapy
• β-blockers
• Narcotics, anesthetics
• Alcohol, tricyclic antidepressants
• Glucocorticoid therapy
• Insulin therapy
• Thiazide diuretics
• Phenytoin
• Chemotherapy agents
• Nonsteroidal anti-inflammatory agents (NSAIDs)

In the Presence of an Unknown Preexisting Condition
Precipitating factors
• Pituitary tumors
• Radiation therapy of the head and neck
• Autoimmune disease
• Neurosurgical procedures
• Metastatic malignancies (e.g., lung, breast)
• Surgery
• Long-term illness
• Shock
• Postpartum status
• Trauma

Box 44-1 • Conditions Associated With Hyperthyroidism or Thyrotoxicosis

Endocrine Disorders
• Graves' disease
• Nodular goiter
• Toxic multinodular adenoma
• Radiation-induced thyroiditis
• Subacute thyroiditis

Drugs
• Iatrogenic thyroid replacement
• Accidental or purposeful ingestion of thyroid medication
• Contrast media dye
• Amiodarone
• β-blockers

Tumors
• Metastatic thyroid cancer
• Hypophyseal tumors
• Hypothalamus tumor
• Hydatidiform mole

iodine, prior or current use of thyroid hormone, anterior neck pain, thyroid enlargement, exophthalmos (i.e., protrusion of one or both eyes) or other eye symptoms, pregnancy, a history of goiter, and a family history of thyroid disease.

Signs and symptoms of hyperthyroidism affect all body systems and include sweating, heat intolerance, nervousness, tremors, palpitations, tachycardia, hyperkinesis, and increased bowel sounds. Extremes of these manifestations, specifically a temperature greater than 104°F (40°C) in the absence of an infection, tachycardia, and CNS dysfunction, may be present in hyperthyroidism. CNS abnormalities include agitation, restlessness, delirium, seizures, or coma. Signs of thyroid emergencies are listed in Box 44-3.

As discussed in Box 44-4, older patients may not have the classic signs and symptoms of thyrotoxic crisis, causing this condition to be overlooked. However, they frequently have suggestive signs and symptoms. In these circumstances, the nurse asks older patients if they have heart disease and what medications they take. This can be important in determining whether there is underlying thyroid disease because β-blocker medication may mask cardiovascular clues.

Laboratory Studies

Laboratory studies may show elevated total T_4, free T_3, and free T_4 levels. The thyroid-stimulating hormone (TSH) level is extremely low in hyperthyroidism. TSH is suppressed because the levels of circulating hormones, T_3 and T_4, are so elevated. Recall that TSH is secreted when thyroid hormone levels are low.

Serum electrolytes, liver function tests, and complete blood counts, although not diagnostic, may help uncover abnormalities that require treatment. They may also help identify the precipitating cause. Electrolyte imbalances due to dehydration, excessive bone resorption, and increased insulin degradation often

occur. The serum calcium is often elevated, whereas potassium and magnesium are decreased, and liver function test values are increased. Hyperglycemia due to insulin resistance and breakdown of stored glucose often occurs.

Diagnostic Studies

Diagnostic tests include the radioactive iodine uptake test, which is usually increased. Electrocardiography (ECG) and cardiac monitoring may show atrial fibrillation, supraventricular tachycardia, sinus bradycardia, heart block, conduction disturbances, and ventricular dysrhythmias, all reflective of the hypermetabolic state and the synergized catecholamines.

Management

Management goals for thyrotoxic crises are fourfold: (1) treating the precipitating factor or factors, (2) controlling excessive thyroid hormone release, (3) inhibiting the thyroid hormone biosynthesis, and (4) treating the peripheral effects of thyroid hormone.[2]

Antithyroid drugs (Table 44-2) are used to control thyroid release or biosynthesis. Propylthiouracil is the preferred agent, although it can be given only orally. Propylthiouracil is preferred because it blocks the conversion of T_4 to T_3 in peripheral tissues and binds iodine to prevent synthesis of the hormone. If the oral route is not possible, methimazole can be given rectally.

Iodine solutions, such as sodium iodide intravenously or potassium iodide (SSKI) or Lugol's solution orally, are given to block the release of thyroid hormone. These agents should not be given until 1 hour after the administration of antithyroid medications. Lithium is the choice for patients who are iodine sensitive. Glucocorticoids may be ordered because they also inhibit thyroid hormone release.

Emergency removal of excess circulating hormone replacement therapy can be accomplished by instituting plasmapheresis, dialysis, or hemoperfusion adsorption. Cholestyramine may be used to assist with oral absorption of excess hormone.

Blocking the catecholamine effects that may result in cardiovascular decompensation secondary to decreased stroke volume and reduced cardiac output may be instituted. β-Blockers, specifically propranolol, are used to treat the symptoms of the hyperthyroidism

Box 44-4 • CONSIDERATIONS FOR THE OLDER PATIENT: Hyperthyroidism

Elderly patients with hyperthyroidism often present with atypical signs and symptoms of the disorder. Apathetic hyperthyroidism, as seen in the older patient, manifests with a single symptom such as depression or muscle weakness. Thus, the elderly patient may present with palpitations, shortness of breath, tremor, and nervousness, but many other symptoms, as seen in younger patients, are masked. Much time can transpire until the patient deteriorates into full-blown thyroid storm.

Box 44-3 • RED FLAG: Possible Indications of Thyroid Emergencies

THYROID STORM	MYXEDEMA COMA
Tachycardia	Bradycardia
Hyperthermia	Hypothermia
Tachypnea	Hypoventilation
Diaphoresis	
Hypercalcemia	Hyponatremia
Hyperglycemia	Hypoglycemia
Metabolic acidosis	Respiratory and metabolic acidosis
Diarrhea	
Cardiovascular collapse	Cardiovascular collapse
Cardiogenic shock	Decreased vascular tone
Hypovolemia	
Cardiac arrhythmias	
Irritability	
Depressed level of consciousness	Depressed level of consciousness
Emotional lability	Seizures, coma
Psychosis	
Tremors, restlessness	Hyporeflexia
Weight loss	Weight gain

Table 44-2 • Pharmacologic Agents Used to Treat Hyperthyroidism			
Drug	**Dose**	**Action**	**Nursing Considerations**

Propylthiouracil (PTU)	Loading: 800–1,200 mg
	Maintenance: 100–400 mg
	  every 4–6 h orally (PO)
		Blocks synthesis of hormones
		(conversion of T_3 to T_4)
			Monitor cardiac parameters.
			Observe for conversion to hypothyroidism.
			Must be given by mouth.
			Watch for rash, nausea, vomiting, agranulocytosis,
			  lupus syndrome.

Methimazole	10–20 mg every 6–8 h PO	Blocks synthesis of thyroid hormone	More toxic than PTU. Watch for rash and other symptoms as for PTU.
Sodium iodide	1 g every 12 h intravenously (IV)	Suppresses release of thyroid hormone	Given 1 h after PTU or methimazole. Watch for edema, hemorrhage, gastrointestinal upset.
Potassium iodide	2–5 gtt every 8 h PO	Suppresses release of thyroid hormone	Discontinue for rash. Watch for signs of toxic iodinism.
SSKI	5–10 drops every 8 h PO	Suppresses release of thyroid hormone	Mix with juice or milk. Give by straw to prevent staining of teeth.
Dexamethasone	2 mg every 6 h IV	Suppresses thyroid hormone release	Monitor intake and output. Monitor glucose. May cause hypertension, nausea, vomiting, anorexia, infection.
β-blocker (e.g., propranolol)	13 mg every 1–4 h IV	β-adrenergic blocking agent	Monitor cardiac status. Hold for bradycardia or decreased cardiac output. Use with caution in patients with heart failure.

rather than the primary thyroid disease. This therapy may be ordered to restore cardiac function by decreasing the catecholamine-mediated symptoms. The response to β-blockers is carefully monitored because intrinsic cardiac disease may worsen as a result of the negative inotropic effects.[3] Digoxin, diltiazem (Cardizem), diuretics, or a combination of these agents may also be used to treat congestive heart failure or supraventricular tachydysrhythmias. Oxygen is delivered to address the additional metabolic requirements. The goal of therapy is to decrease myocardial oxygen consumption, decrease the heart rate (ideally to below 100 beats/minute), and increase cardiac output.

Corticosteroids may be used to help treat coexisting adrenal insufficiency and thyroid storm. Intravenous dexamethasone or hydrocortisone can be given to assist with blunting excess thyroid hormone release in this emergency state.

Management also focuses on monitoring multisystem effects from the hypermetabolism of thyrotoxic crisis and the response to treatment. Cardiovascular function, fluid and electrolyte balance, and neurological status require close attention. It is necessary to assess blood pressure, heart rate and rhythm, respiratory rate, and extra heart sounds every hour.

The nurse evaluates fluid status and laboratory values. Hourly monitoring of body temperature is warranted because the patient is at risk for hyperthermia. Antipyretic agents, particularly acetaminophen, are recommended for fever control; aspirin is not appropriate because it increases free T_3 and T_4 levels. Tepid baths or a cooling blanket may be necessary. It is important to avoid cooling to the point of shivering and piloerection because this may have a rebound effect of raising body temperature. Intravenous fluids are necessary to replace the fluids lost due to excessive hyperthermia, tachypnea, diaphoresis, and diarrhea that often accompany thyrotoxic crisis.

The nurse assesses neurological status at least hourly. Seizure precautions and safety measures prevent injury. If the patient's level of consciousness decreases, it is important to assess airway patency and safety issues. Maintaining a calm environment is necessary to help manage the extreme agitation and restlessness seen in the patient with thyrotoxic crisis.

Energy and nutritional needs are heightened because of the hypermetabolism. Interventions include administering glucose-containing solutions, nutritional support, vitamin supplementation, and sedation if needed. The nurse monitors the patient's glycemic status because the administration of corticosteroids and excess glucose rich nutrients may lead to hyperglycemia in some patients. Box 44-5 lists examples of nursing diagnoses for the patient in thyrotoxic crisis.

> **Box 44-5 Examples of Nursing Diagnoses and Collaborative Problems for the Patient in Thyroid Crisis**
>
> - Deficient Fluid Volume related to hypermetabolic state
> - Hyperthermia related to hypermetabolic state
> - Decreased Cardiac Output related to hypermetabolic state and heart failure
> - Impaired Cerebral Tissue Perfusion related to hypermetabolic state and heart failure
> - Potential for Injury related to altered mental status

Effective therapy can be expected to result in clinical improvement within 24 to 48 hours. The nurse monitors the patient's mental status carefully and also checks for stabilization of vital signs and normalization of body temperature. Patient follow-up to prevent another episode is necessary and may involve lifelong medication or suppressive therapy with thyroid ablation.

MYXEDEMA COMA

Hypothyroidism is a common disorder with a broad clinical spectrum—patients may be asymptomatic, or they may be severely ill with myxedema coma. Hypothyroidism is more common among women, and the incidence increases with age. Approximately 10% to 15% of elderly patients have elevated TSH associated with hypothyroidism, and routine screening of high-risk populations is often done in primary care settings.[3]

Myxedema coma is a rare, life-threatening emergency brought on by extreme hypothyroidism. It usually is seen in older patients during winter months after certain precipitating factors such as stress, exposure to extreme cold temperatures, or trauma. In addition to coma, complications of myxedema coma include pericardial and pleural effusions, megacolon with paralytic ileus, and seizures. Death can result if severe hypoxia and hypercapnia are not reversed.

Pathophysiology

Deficient production of thyroid hormone results in the clinical state termed hypothyroidism. Hypothyroidism, a chronic disease, is 10 times more common in women than in men. It occurs in all age groups but most commonly in those older than 50 years. It is more common than hyperthyroidism.

Hypothyroidism can be primary or secondary. Primary causes include congenital defects, loss of thyroid tissue after treatment for hyperthyroidism, defective hormone synthesis due to an autoimmune process, and antithyroid drug administration or iodine deficiency. Secondary causes include peripheral resistance to thyroid hormone, pituitary infarction, and hypothalamic disorders. Transient hypothyroidism can occur after withdrawal of prolonged T_4 or T_3 treatment. The common causes of hypothyroidism are summarized in Box 44-6.

Hypothyroidism usually affects all body systems. A low basal metabolic rate (BMR) and decreased energy metabolism and heat production are characteristic. The patient with chronic hypothyroidism may have myxedema, an alteration in the composition of the dermis and other tissues. The connective fibers are separated by an increased amount of protein and mucopolysaccharides. This binds water, producing nonpitting, boggy edema, especially around the eyes, hands, and feet; it is also responsible for thickening of the tongue and the laryngeal and pharyngeal mucous membranes, resulting in slurred speech and hoarseness.

Box 44-6 • Causes of Hypothyroidism

- Destruction of the thyroid gland (e.g., surgery, radioactive iodine, external radiation to the neck)
- Infiltrative disease (e.g., sarcoidosis, amyloidosis, lymphoma)
- Autoimmune disease (e.g., Hashimoto's disease, post-Graves' disease)
- Thyroiditis (e.g., viral, silent, postpartum)
- Drug induced (e.g., iodides, lithium, amiodarone)
- Hereditary hypothyroidism
- Thyrotropin-releasing hormone (TRH) deficiency
- Thyroid-stimulating hormone (TSH) deficiency

Assessment

History and Physical Examination

Signs and symptoms of hypothyroidism include fatigue, weakness, decreased bowel sounds, decreased appetite, weight gain, and ECG changes. Myxedema coma is a rare manifestation of hypothyroidism, characterized by severe depression of the sensorium, hypothermia, hypoventilation, hypoxemia, hyponatremia, hypoglycemia, hyporeflexia, hypotension, and bradycardia. Patients with myxedema coma do not shiver, although body temperatures below 80°F (26.6°C) have been reported. The diagnosis of myxedema coma depends on recognizing the clinical symptoms and identifying the underlying precipitating factor. The most common precipitating factor is pulmonary infection; other factors include trauma, stress, infections, drugs (e.g., narcotics or barbiturates), surgery, and metabolic disturbances (see Box 44-3).

Laboratory Studies

A decrease in T_4 and free T_4 is most common, whereas sodium is usually decreased, and potassium is increased. TSH is markedly elevated in severe hypothyroidism. Arterial blood gases (ABGs) usually show a severe hypercapnia with a decreased arterial oxygen tension (PaO_2) and increased arterial carbon dioxide tension ($PaCO_2$).

Diagnostic Studies

A chest radiograph detects pleural effusion. ECG changes include bradycardia, a prolonged PR interval, and decreased amplitude of the P wave and QRS complex. Heart block may develop.

Management

The most serious complication of hypothyroidism is progression to myxedema coma and death, if the condition is untreated. A multisystem approach must be used in treating this emergency. Mechanical ventilation is used to control hypoventilation, hypercapnia, and respiratory arrest. Intravenous hypertonic normal saline and glucose correct the dilutional hyponatremia and hypoglycemia. Fluid administration plus vasopressor therapy may be necessary to correct hypotension.

Pharmacological therapy includes the administration of thyroid hormone and corticosteroids. There are several approaches to this aspect of medical management. Initial drug therapy includes 300 to 500 µg T_4 intravenously to saturate all protein-binding sites and establish a relatively normal T_4 level. Subsequent doses may include 75 to 100 µg daily. Intravenous or oral T_3 is an alternative order. Guidelines to T_3 replacement are 25 µg intravenously every 8 hours for the first 24 to 48 hours. Oral T_3 doses every 8 hours are also ordered. Hormone replacement should occur slowly, with continuous monitoring of the patient during treatment to avoid sudden increased metabolic demand and resultant myocardial infarction. Methodical fluid replacement and rewarming of the patient also help to avoid complications.

Additional interventions include treating abdominal distention and fecal impaction and managing hypothermia by gradually rewarming the patient using blankets and socks. Mechanical devices are not used. The nurse monitors the patient for neurological status and changes in level of consciousness and implements seizure precautions. Care of the comatose patient includes preventing complications related to aspiration, immobility, skin breakdown, and infection. Monitoring of cardiovascular and respiratory function is necessary. Fluid administration must also be monitored because of a risk for fluid overload. An important aspect of care is to detect early signs of complications. As the patient recovers, interventions focus on patient self-care and education.

Patient follow-up includes a thorough investigation of how the severe hypothyroidism occurred and how it can best be avoided in the future. Patient teaching, family follow-up, medical alert activation, and involvement of community supports may be necessary for this complex patient.

• Adrenal Gland Dysfunction

ADRENAL CRISIS

Pathophysiology

Adrenal insufficiency, also known as hypoadrenalism or hypocorticism, is a rare but life-threatening dysfunction of the adrenal cortex. Adrenal hormone insufficiency may be either primary (i.e., directly involving the adrenal gland) or secondary (i.e., due to hypothalamic–pituitary disease).

Primary adrenal insufficiency is termed Addison's disease. The most common cause of primary hypoadrenalism in the industrialized West is autoimmune adrenalitis. Autoimmune antibody formation leads to the gradual destruction of the adrenal gland, resulting in adrenal insufficiency. The second leading cause of primary adrenal insufficiency is destruction of the gland secondary to *Mycobacterium tuberculosis* infection. Worldwide, tuberculosis remains the most common cause of primary adrenal insufficiency. Other causes include bilateral hemorrhage of the glands secondary to bacterial infection with sepsis and shock, metastatic malignancies, acquired immunodeficiency syndrome (AIDS), fungal infections, surgical adrenalectomy, and sarcoidosis.

The most common cause of secondary adrenal insufficiency is iatrogenic, resulting from abrupt withdrawal of exogenous ACTH or as a complication of cortisol therapy. Suppressed ACTH secretion as a result of exogenous cortisol therapy disrupts the body's natural feedback loop that controls cortisol secretion, rendering the patient in an acute state of adrenal insufficiency. Other causes of secondary adrenal insufficiency include metastatic carcinomas of the lung or breast, pituitary infarction, surgery or irradiation, and CNS disturbances, such as basilar skull fractures or infections.

Acute adrenal insufficiency or adrenal crisis occurs when there is a change in the chronic condition or massive adrenal hemorrhage. In addition to the chronic disease, severe infection, septic shock, trauma, surgical procedure, or some extra stress occurs, precipitating acute adrenal crisis in the patient. The patient is therefore unable to meet the requirements for normal metabolic function or increased metabolic needs as necessary for stress or illness. Any stressed, critically ill patient can develop adrenal insufficiency as a result of suddenly imposed extraneous stressors. As the patient struggles to survive, he or she quickly depletes cortisol stores and may require exogenous replacement.[1]

Assessment

History and Physical Examination
Symptoms of adrenal insufficiency are the same for primary and secondary disease. Because adrenal insufficiency affects both glucocorticoids and mineralocorticoids, many body functions are affected, including glucose metabolism, fluid and electrolyte balance, cognitive state, and cardiopulmonary status. Weakness, fatigue, anorexia, nausea, vomiting, diarrhea, and abdominal pain may be initial clues to adrenal crisis. These findings are nonspecific until linked with the history of a chronic condition requiring past or present corticosteroid use.[4] Specifically, use of more than 20 mg of hydrocortisone or its equivalent, taken for longer than 7 to 10 days, has the potential for suppressing the HPA axis.

Hyperpigmentation on areas of the elbows, knees, hands, or buccal mucosa is seen in primary adrenal insufficiency. The presence of hyperpigmentation, secondary to the deposition of melanin in the skin, strengthens the clinical picture of adrenal crisis. The most common physical changes include signs of severe dehydration, such as weight loss and orthostatic hypotension. Dehydration occurs secondary to the nephrons' insufficient ability to reabsorb sodium and water. Signs and symptoms of an impending adrenal crisis are summarized in Box 44-7.

Laboratory Studies
Laboratory values in acute conditions of glucocorticoid and mineralocorticoid deficiency show hyponatremia, hyperkalemia, decreased serum bicarbonate

Associated medical or surgical problems may indicate the need for invasive blood pressure and hemodynamic monitoring.

Another management goal is to prevent complications. This includes monitoring signs and symptoms of electrolyte imbalance (hyponatremia and hypercalcemia) and respiratory and cardiovascular function. The nurse looks for changes in blood pressure, heart rate and rhythm, skin color and temperature, capillary refill time, and central venous pressure (CVP). There is a risk for orthostatic hypotension, bradycardia, and dysrhythmias. The nurse also monitors neuromuscular signs, such as weakness, twitching, hyperreflexia, and paresthesia.

Emotional support, a simple explanation, and a quiet environment are effective in assisting the patient emotionally through the physiological crisis. Once the acute crisis is over, patient education is a goal of care. Patient education is necessary because the ultimate prognosis depends on the patient's ability to understand and follow through with self-care. Self-care includes knowing the medication regimen, stress factors and their effect on the disease, and the signs of impending crisis; wearing a medical alert tag or bracelet, or carrying a wallet card; and taking medication as prescribed.

levels, and elevated blood urea nitrogen (BUN). Metabolic acidosis may occur because of dehydration. Hypoglycemia is usually present. Other abnormal laboratory findings include anemia and lymphocytosis with eosinophilia. In primary adrenal insufficiency, the patient presents with chronically elevated ACTH levels. ACTH levels are normal or decreased in the patient with secondary adrenal insufficiency.

Serum cortisol levels and cortisol stimulation (ACTH stimulation) tests are also used to confirm the diagnosis. Cortisol levels below 15 µg/dL are indicative of adrenal dysfunction. In primary adrenal insufficiency, repeated injections of ACTH (or Cortrosyn) do not cause a rise in cortisol levels because the adrenal gland is dysfunctional. In secondary adrenal insufficiency, ACTH injections cause a normal but delayed response.

Diagnostic Studies

A computed tomography (CT) scan of the adrenal glands and the head may be done to detect tumors or other pathology of the adrenal and pituitary gland.

Management

The immediate goal of therapy is to administer the needed hormones and restore fluid and electrolyte balance. Hydrocortisone, 100 mg intravenously, is administered immediately, followed by 100 mg every 6 to 8 hours. Fluid resuscitation is also started immediately with normal saline and 5% dextrose solutions. The rate of fluid and electrolyte replacement is dictated by the degree of volume depletion, serum electrolyte levels, and clinical response to therapy.

PHEOCHROMOCYTOMA

Pheochromocytoma is a very rare catecholamine-secreting tumor that arises from chromaffin cells in the adrenal gland. Because of the excessive catecholamine secretion, pheochromocytoma may precipitate life-threatening hypertension or cardiac dysrhythmias when norepinephrine or epinephrine are released in larger quantities. The trigger for the release of catecholamines is unknown, but the high levels can lead to severe hypertension, atrial fibrillation, ventricular fibrillation, myocardial infarction, or cerebral infarction.

Pheochromocytomas can occur in people of all ages and ethnicities, and the peak incidence is between the third and fifth decades of life. Classic symptoms include headaches, palpitation, and diaphoresis in association with severe, paroxysmal hypertension. Typically the symptoms worsen with time and become more severe as the tumor grows.

Diagnosis is based on the suspicion of pheochromocytoma for the patient who presents with paroxysmal hypertension and other associated symptoms. Choice laboratory studies include measurement of plasma metanephrines and urinary catecholamines, metanephrines, and vanillymandelic acid. Diagnosis is confirmed with imaging studies such as abdominal magnetic resonance imaging (MRI) or CT scanning. Medical care includes surgical resection of the tumor and careful control of the hypertension. α-Blockers and β-blockers are required preoperatively to control blood pressure and to prevent hypertensive crisis. Usually, the hypertension is no longer a problem postoperatively.

neurological symptoms, including disorientation and decreasing consciousness. Seizure precautions may be necessary. Complications of SIADH include neurological deterioration leading to seizures, coma, and death.

Patients may find it difficult to limit their fluid intake. Mealtimes may also be difficult because menus are aimed at meeting nutritional needs without increasing fluid intake. Providing good oral care and offering substitutions for fluids (e.g., Toothettes, lemon-glycerin swabs) may be helpful for the persistently thirsty patient. Providing information and emotional support and acknowledging the deprivation may help patients through this period.

DIABETES INSIPIDUS

Pathophysiology

Diabetes insipidus is a disease characterized by water imbalance resulting from inadequate ADH or resistance to ADH, leading to water diuresis and dehydration. In diabetes insipidus, the kidneys excrete great quantities of dilute urine, at times up to 20 L/day. Normally, the posterior pituitary releases ADH, which then acts on the distal renal tubules to promote reabsorption of water. When there is an absence of or deficit in ADH, the kidneys lose their ability to reabsorb water and control fluid output (see Chapter 42).

Diabetes insipidus may manifest in two forms: central or nephrogenic. Central diabetes insipidus is the more common condition that results in ADH deficiency and responds favorably to exogenous vasopressin administration. This type of diabetes insipidus is the disease most often encountered in the critical care environment. Nephrogenic diabetes insipidus is a very rare genetic disorder that results from the failure of the kidney to respond to ADH. Only central diabetes insipidus is discussed in this chapter.

Diabetes insipidus can be transient, temporary, partial, or permanent, depending on the initial cause and circumstances surrounding the patient illness or injury. The osmolality sensors of the hypothalamus control ADH release from the posterior pituitary. As the osmolality increases, the osmoreceptors are stimulated, releasing more ADH. In the kidneys, ADH causes more water and sodium to be absorbed, restoring adequate fluid balance. In the absence of ADH, the renal tubules and collecting ducts are impermeable to water. Consequently, large volumes of dilute urine are excreted. Serum osmolality and sodium rise, and the patient continues to become progressively more dehydrated. The thirst sensation may or may not be affected, depending on the patient's level of consciousness. For patients with an impaired thirst mechanism, dehydration and hypovolemic shock will result more quickly if the condition is not corrected.

Diabetes insipidus can develop after any event that causes edema or direct damage to the neurohypophysis. After surgery, diabetes insipidus may occur when regions of the brain around the hypothalamus and pituitary are affected. It can occur after head injuries, gunshot wounds, and lesions that disrupt blood supply to the area. Damage to the sphenoid bone, max-

illofacial injuries, hypothalamic tumors, and nasopharyngeal tumors that invade the base of the skull may also lead to the development of diabetes insipidus. Direct trauma or ischemic events involving the hypothalamus, such as hemorrhage, infection, or neoplasm, may result in diabetes insipidus. Also, diseases or drugs that affect the renal collecting tubules may lead to diabetes insipidus. There is also a psychogenic polydipsia, in which excessive water is consumed, resulting in excess output.

After trauma or surgery, diabetes insipidus can be transient until initial edema subsides. The neurohypophysis is very sensitive to extraneous pressure; consequently, these structures may be unable to produce, secrete, or release ADH as needed. The patient displays temporary signs of diabetes insipidus. As the edema abates, ADH secretion resumes its normal course, and the diabetes insipidus eventually is corrected. In some cases of severe trauma or hemorrhage, the structures may be completely damaged, and the patient may permanently develop diabetes insipidus.

The classic example of the transient type of disorder is illustrated by the patient undergoing a transsphenoidal approach for a hypophysectomy to remove a pituitary tumor. In most cases, the patient experiences temporary problems related to an inability to synthesize, store, or release ADH due to edema of the hypothalamus and pituitary. This patient requires close monitoring for the development of diabetes insipidus and may need treatment. Figure 44-3 illustrates a transsphenoidal approach to a pituitary tumor.

Assessment

Polyuria, polydipsia, and dehydration are the hallmarks of diabetes insipidus. Patients can excrete

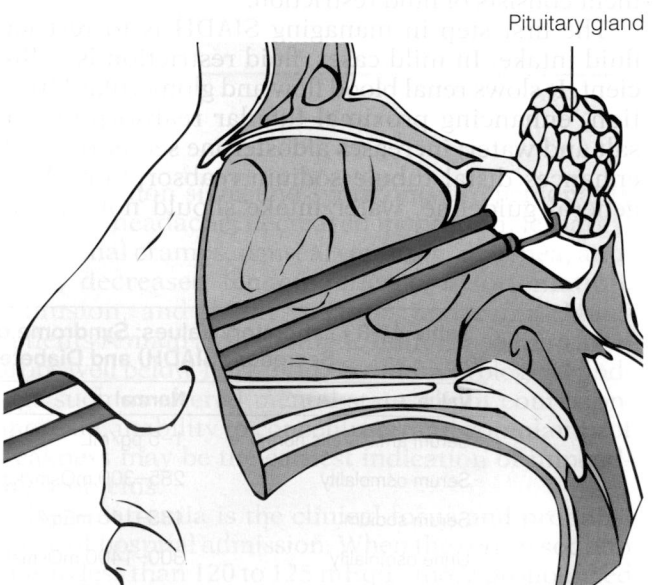

Pituitary gland

Figure 44-3 • The transsphenoidal approach to a pituitary tumor can lead to transient diabetes insipidus. The neurohypophysis is very sensitive to extraneous pressure; consequently, these structures may be unable to produce, secrete, or release antidiuretic hormone (ADH) as needed. The resultant diabetes insipidus resolves as the edema (from the surgery) resolves.

from 3 to 20 L of urine per day. When patients are alert, they experience excessive thirst and excessive urinary output. They try to increase their fluid intake, but this can cause exhaustion and eventually result in dehydration. On the other hand, when people are not alert enough to detect thirst and increase their fluid intake, they can quickly become hypovolemic because of the fluid loss. If left untreated, this can lead to death.

Signs of dehydration include dry skin, dry mucous membranes, confusion, sunken eyeballs, constipation, poor skin turgor, lethargy, muscle weakness, muscle pain, and pallor. Vital signs are adversely affected, with severe tachycardia, hypotension, low CVP, and a possible rise in body temperature. Weight loss may be apparent.

Recognizing diabetes insipidus may be more difficult when patients are recovering from surgery because steroids and cerebral dehydrating agents used before and during surgery promote diuresis for the first postoperative day or so. If awake, the patient complains of progressive thirst if diabetes insipidus is present. Urine output increases and persists regardless of the amount of fluid intake. Urine specific gravity falls or remains at about 1.001 to 1.005. Urine is copious, clear, and almost colorless. Plasma osmolality increases, often to levels greater than 300 mOsm/kg. Urine osmolality decreases to 50 to 100 mOsm/kg. The urine sodium is below normal, whereas the serum sodium is elevated (see Chapter 43, Table 43-2). The water deprivation test is also helpful to diagnose diabetes insipidus. These tests, combined with the constellation of signs and symptoms, lead to the diagnosis. Table 44-3 presents laboratory values for patients with diabetes insipidus.

Management

The objective of therapy is to prevent dehydration and electrolyte imbalance, while treating the underlying cause and preventing complications. Hypotonic intravenous solutions, such 0.45% sodium chloride, are administered to match the urine output. The volume of replacement fluids depends on the degree of dehydration and the amount needed to reverse hypovolemic shock.

A variety of replacement ADH (vasopressin) therapies are available. Desmopressin acetate (DDAVP) is synthetic ADH that can be administered intravenously or as a nasal spray. Aqueous vasopressin (Pitressin) may be given as an intravenous bolus, continuous infusion, or subcutaneously. The medications can be used for temporary or permanent ADH replacement. Permanent hormone replacement requires more patient and family education. In addition, the patient should obtain medical alert identification to wear at all times. Table 44-4 reviews the commonly administered medications for diabetes insipidus.

Management also focuses on monitoring fluid and electrolyte balance. The nurse detects fluid excesses or deficits by evaluating hourly intake and output, serum and urine electrolytes and osmolality results, and urine specific gravity. In addition, he or she notes changes in blood pressure, pulse, and respirations, as well as the onset of pulmonary crackles, neck vein distention, peripheral edema, and increasing CVP and pulmonary artery wedge pressure. The nurse observes skin turgor and mucous membranes and changes in alertness and cognition. Drowsiness, confusion, and headache may indicate water intoxication. Weight is another indicator of fluid status.

Complications

Major complications of diabetes insipidus are cardiovascular collapse and tissue hypoxia. Seizures and encephalopathy can also result from fluid and electrolyte imbalance. Prognosis is excellent as long as the patient receives prompt and aggressive treatment.

• Emergencies for Patients With Diabetes Mellitus

Diabetes mellitus is a complex and chronic metabolic disorder characterized by hyperglycemia and defects in insulin secretion. Figure 44-4 illustrates

Table 44-4 • Common Administered Medications for Diabetes Insipidus				
Drug	Dosage	Route of Administration	Duration of Drug	Adverse Effects
Desmopressin (DDAVP)	5–20 µg each day	Nasal spray (cannot be given if nasal passages blocked)	8–24 h	Headache, chest pain, nausea, diarrhea, edema
Aqueous pitressin	2–4 units every 4–6 h	Intramuscularly, subcutaneously, intranasally	1–8 h	Headache, chest pain, nausea, diarrhea, edema
Pitressin tannate in oil	2.5–5 units	Intramuscularly	36–48 h	Headache, chest pain, nausea, diarrhea, edema
Lysine vasopressin nasal spray	5–20 units three to seven times daily; titrate to output	Intranasally	2–6 h	—
Chlorpropamide (Diabinese)	100–250 mg/day	By mouth	60–72 h	Hypoglycemia, headache, tinnitus, alcohol intolerance, gastrointestinal disturbances, diarrhea
Clofibrate	250–500 mg	By mouth	6–8 h	Gastrointestinal disturbances

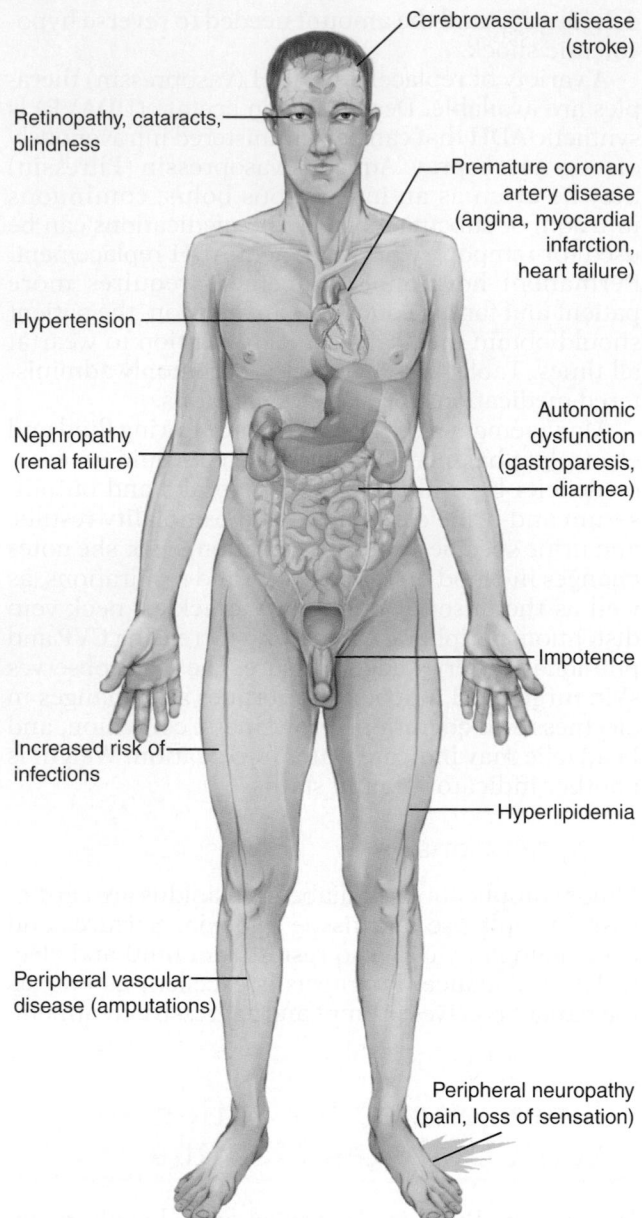

Cerebrovascular disease (stroke)

Retinopathy, cataracts, blindness

Premature coronary artery disease (angina, myocardial infarction, heart failure)

Hypertension

Nephropathy (renal failure)

Autonomic dysfunction (gastroparesis, diarrhea)

Impotence

Increased risk of infections

Hyperlipidemia

Peripheral vascular disease (amputations)

Peripheral neuropathy (pain, loss of sensation)

Figure 44-4 • The complications of diabetes can be widespread.

how chronic hyperglycemia is associated with long-term organ dysfunction, particularly of the eyes, kidneys, nerves, heart, and blood vessels. These long-term microvascular and macrovascular complications of retinopathy, neuropathy, nephropathy, and cardiovascular disease are the primary causes of morbidity and mortality in people affected with diabetes.

The incidence of diabetes in the United States has risen dramatically, and diabetes morbidity and mortality are also increasing. Diabetes is one of the most common diseases in the United States, with an estimated 16.7 million adults afflicted; it is the seventh leading cause of death in the United States.[5] Prevalence rates approach 50% in certain population subgroups (Native American, Hispanic American, African American). This rate is strongly related to the epidemic of obesity and the socioeconomic inequalities that plague the United States.

The pathogenic processes associated with diabetes mellitus range from autoimmune destruction of the islet β cells of the pancreas (type 1 diabetes mellitus) to insulin resistance (type 2 diabetes mellitus). The derangements of carbohydrate, protein, and fat metabolism all result from deficient action of insulin on target tissues. The main effect is hyperglycemia. Hyperglycemia is manifested as polyuria, polydipsia, polyphagia, weight loss, and blurred vision. Acute, critical illnesses associated with diabetes are hyperglycemia with ketoacidosis and nonketotic hyper-osmolar syndrome.

Often almost half of patients with type 2 diabetes mellitus are not diagnosed until complications have already developed, and many suffer acute syndromes requiring emergency department evaluation, intensive care management, or both. The critical care nurse must be vigilant in identifying high-risk patients. Box 43-6 in Chapter 43 contains the American Diabetes Association's Position Statement on the diagnostic parameters for diabetes.

Most patients with diabetes can be classified into two main groups, those with type 1 diabetes mellitus and those with type 2 diabetes mellitus (Table 44-5). The cause of type 1 diabetes is an absolute deficiency of insulin secretion. This insulin secretion impairment results from autoimmune destruction of the β cells of the pancreas. Markers of immune destruction include islet cell autoantibodies (ICAs). These autoantibodies include glutamic acid decarboxylase antibodies (GAD-65), islet cell antibodies (ICA512-1A-2), and insulin antibodies (IAAs). The best predictor for future development of type 1 diabetes is the expression of multiple autoantibodies.[6] The rate of islet cell destruction is variable, and it occurs more rapidly in younger patients and more slowly in older patients. Some children and adolescents present with ketoacidosis as the first manifestation of the disease. As the islet cell destruction occurs, the patient is rendered insulin dependent for survival.

Type 1 diabetes is a disease of the young, with a peak incidence at ages 10 to 12 years for females and 12 to 14 years for males. Although onset occurs mainly during childhood or at puberty and most patients receive a diagnosis before age 20 years, the disease can occur at any age. Type 1 diabetes accounts for approximately 10% to 20% of all cases of diabetes. A genetic predisposition for type 1 diabetes may exist because it appears that genetically predisposed patients contract the disorder after an environmental factor (viruses, congenital rubella, enteroviruses) triggers the autoimmune destruction of the islet cells, leading to insulin deficiency.[7] These patients are rarely obese. Type 1 diabetes is associated with other autoimmune diseases such as Graves' disease, Addison's disease, and autoimmune polyendocrine syndromes.

Type 2 diabetes mellitus manifests as insulin resistance with relative, rather than absolute, insulin deficiency. Most of the patients with this form of diabetes do not require insulin, at least initially. The specific cause of insulin resistance is multifactorial; however, these patients do not suffer from autoimmune destruction of the islet cells of the pancreas. Most patients

Table 44-5 • Comparison of Type I and Type 2 Diabetes Mellitus

	Type 1 Diabetes	Type 2 Diabetes
Etiology	Autoimmune destruction of islet cells	Insulin resistance
Incidence	10%	90%
Age of onset	Usually before 35 years	Usually after 35 years
Speed of onset	Usually rapid	Usually gradual
Nutritional state	Usually thin	Usually overweight, obese
Endogenous insulin	Absent	Low or high, rarely absent
Symptoms	Polyuria, polydipsia, polyphagia, weight loss	Same, plus blurred vision, fatigue
Ketosis	Frequently present with poor control	Infrequent
Treatment goal	Exogenous insulin management	Weight loss, exercise, improved insulin resistance
Treatment	Exogenous insulin, diet control, exercise, weight maintenance	Oral agents, diet control, exercise, weight loss

are overweight or obese, and excess adiposity itself can lead to insulin resistance.[8] Ketoacidosis seldom occurs in this form of diabetes because the patient still secretes just enough insulin to avoid critical illness. When the patient does sustain severe complications associated with hyperglycemia, usually he or she has concomitant illness such as myocardial infarction, infection, or trauma. Because of the high incidence of insulin resistance and relative insulin deficiency, hyperglycemic hyperosmolar syndrome (HHS) usually develops in patients with type 2 diabetes when they become critically ill.

Type 2 diabetes can go undiagnosed for many years because this disease progresses slowly. However, the patient is at high risk for developing macrovascular and microvascular complications. Quite often, these patients have normal to higher-than-normal insulin levels because of the ensuing insulin resistance that they develop. Insulin resistance develops, and their circulating insulin is insufficient to prevent hyperglycemia. Insulin resistance is best treated with weight loss, exercise, and pharmacological management.[9] The medications to treat type 2 diabetes range from insulin secretagogues and medications that affect insulin sensitivity to insulin. Refer to Table 44-6 and Figure 44-5 for a review of the commonly used oral medications for type 2 diabetes and their mechanisms of action.

Eventually, many people with diabetes require insulin as their disease progresses. The risk for developing type 2 diabetes increases with age, obesity, sedentary lifestyle, and family history of type 2 diabetes. Its incidence varies with ethnicity but is increasingly more common in African Americans, Hispanics, Native Americans, South Pacific Islanders, and Asian Americans. Epidemiological and genetic studies suggest a strong genetic basis for developing type 2 diabetes; however, candidate genes that account for the majority of cases have not been identified. Type 2 diabetes is a multifactorial disorder with genetic and environmental implications.[5]

Results from two landmark trials involving people with types 1 and 2 diabetes mellitus, the Diabetes Control and Complications Trial[10] and the United Kingdom Prospective Diabetes Study,[11] have profoundly affected the current management of diabetes. These two trials have demonstrated that very tight glycemic control is necessary to avoid the costly and life-threatening complications resulting from poorly controlled diabetes. This approach extends to the management of diabetic emergencies in the critical care arena as well. It has created a need for continuous intravenous insulin infusions to control the patient's glucose at all times.[12] The critical care nurse needs to monitor the patient very closely to avoid serious complications associated with insulin infusions.

DIABETIC KETOACIDOSIS
Pathophysiology

Diabetic ketoacidosis (DKA) is a critical illness that manifests with severe hyperglycemia, metabolic acidosis, and fluid and electrolyte imbalances. DKA results from severe insulin deficiency that leads to the disordered metabolism of proteins, carbohydrates, and fats. The concomitant elevation of counter-regulatory hormones such as growth hormone (GH), cortisol, epinephrine, and glucagon exacerbates the condition, leading to further hyperglycemia and hyperosmolality, ketoacidosis, and volume depletion. Figure 44-6 outlines these mechanisms and their interrelationships.

DKA continues to be an important cause of morbidity and mortality among people with diabetes. DKA is responsible for more than 100,000 hospital admissions per year in the United States. Most patients with DKA have type 1 diabetes mellitus; however, it is possible for patients with type 2 diabetes to manifest DKA during catabolic stress associated with severe critical illness. DKA is associated with a 2% to 5% mortality rate and is a common cause of death among children and adolescents with type 1 diabetes mellitus.[13] Treatment

Table 44-6 • Oral Pharmacologic Agents to Treat Diabetes Mellitus

Drug	Example	Action	Duration of Action	Nursing Considerations
First-generation sulfonylureas	Tolinase, Diabinese	Stimulates pancreatic insulin secretion	12–60 h	Side effects include hypoglycemia, gastrointestinal disturbances, and rash Contraindicated in pregnancy Seldom used
Second-generation sulfonylureas	Glyburide, Glucotrol, Micronase, Amaryl	Stimulates pancreatic insulin secretion	10–24 h	Side effects include hypoglycemia, gastrointestinal disturbances, and rash Safer in elderly patients
Biguanides	Metformin (Glucophage)	Reduces hepatic glucose production, increases insulin sensitivity	8 h	Lactic acidosis is a serious side effect (stop when using contrast medium for x-rays); other side effects include gastrointestinal disturbances (e.g., flatulence, diarrhea, nausea) Use with caution in patients with renal disease Improves insulin resistance Promotes weight loss
Thiazolidinediones	Actos, Avandia	Enhances insulin's effects at receptor sites	12–24 h	Will not increase level of circulating insulin Side effects include edema, weight gain, and anemia Monitor liver function tests Improves lipid profile Extreme caution with heart failure
α-glucosidase inhibitors	Precose, Miglitol	Inhibits metabolism of carbohydrates in intestines	8 h	Take with meals Side effects include gastrointestinal symptoms (e.g., flatulence, abdominal pain, diarrhea, nausea) Use with caution in patients with renal disease
Meglitinides	Prandin	Stimulates β-cell insulin release		Side effects include hypoglycemia, upper respiratory infection, headache, and diarrhea Use with caution in patients with hepatic or renal disease
Amino acid derivatives (insulin secretagogue)	Starlix	Stimulates β-cell insulin release		Side effects include hypoglycemia, gastrointestinal disturbances (e.g., nausea), upper respiratory tract symptoms, and dizziness Use with caution in patients with hepatic disease
Combination therapy (Glucovance)	Glyburide and metformin	As above with each drug	As above with each drug	As above with each drug
Avandamet metaglip	Avandia and metformin	As above with each drug	As above with each drug	As above with each drug
	Metformin and glipizide	As above with each drug	As above with each drug	As above with each drug
Incretion mimetics	Byetta, symlin	Decreases post-prandial glucose rise and slows gastric emptying, promotes satiety	8–12 hours	Given subcutaneously 1°AC May produce weight loss

can cost more than one of every four health care dollars spent on direct medical care for adults with type 1 diabetes mellitus. The cause of death is rarely a direct result of the metabolic acidosis or from hyperglycemia; instead, death is more often related to the underlying illness that precipitated the metabolic decompensation. Therefore, successful treatment requires prompt attention to the precipitating causes of the hyperglycemic event.

Three major physiological disturbances exist in DKA: (1) hyperosmolality due to hyperglycemia, (2) metabolic acidosis due to accumulation of ketoacids, and (3) volume depletion due to osmotic diuresis. Each of these three disturbances may be more

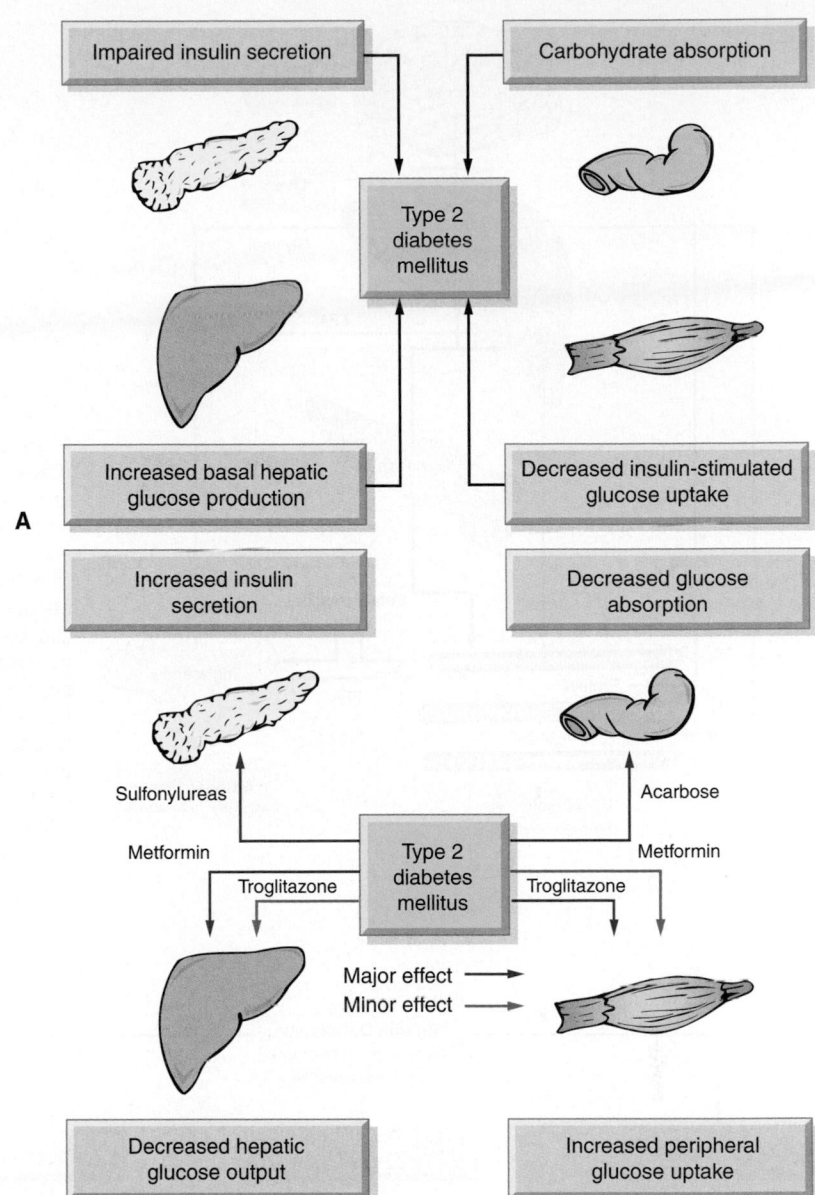

Figure 44-5 • A: Factors leading to elevated blood glucose levels in type 2 diabetes mellitus. **B:** Mechanisms of action of the oral hypoglycemic agents used in the treatment of type 2 diabetes mellitus. (From Porth CM: Pathophysiology: Concepts of Altered Health States, 7th ed. Philadelphia: Lippincott Williams & Wilkins, 2005.)

or less severe in any patient. Furthermore, interactions among these disturbances may occur, aggravating (or possibly partially compensating for) one another.

Hyperglycemia and Hyperosmolality

The first major consequence of DKA is hyperosmolality due to hyperglycemia. The hyperglycemia seen in DKA is the result of insulin deficiency and excessive hepatic (gluconeogenesis) and renal (glycogenolysis) glucose production and reduced glucose utilization in peripheral tissues. With insulin deficiency, the plasma glucose level rises. As illustrated in Figure 44-7, the concomitant effects of the counter-regulatory hormones, particularly cortisol and catecholamines, further aggravate hyperglycemia by enhancing gluconeogenesis, insulin resistance, and lipolysis.

The central mechanism that protects against hyperosmolality is excretion of glucose by the kidneys. Glucose is filtered at the kidney glomerulus. With normal circulating blood volume and a normal glucose load, all this glucose is reabsorbed into the bloodstream. However, when the blood sugar exceeds the normal threshold of about 180 mg/dL, glucose begins to escape into the urine because the reabsorption capacity of the tubules is exceeded. As the glucose load to be filtered increases, glucose is lost rapidly in the urine. Eventually, nearly all of the additional glucose put into the circulation is lost into the urine. The renal "escape valve" serves as a protective device to prevent extreme accumulation of glucose in blood. Indeed, in people with diabetes whose circulating blood volume is well maintained, it is extremely unusual to find blood sugar levels in excess of 500 mg/dL because of the intense glucose diuresis. Conversely, any patient whose blood sugar is higher than this level has either a severely reduced circulating blood volume, renal damage, or both.

Glycosuria is largely responsible for volume depletion. Additionally, high ketone levels cause osmotic

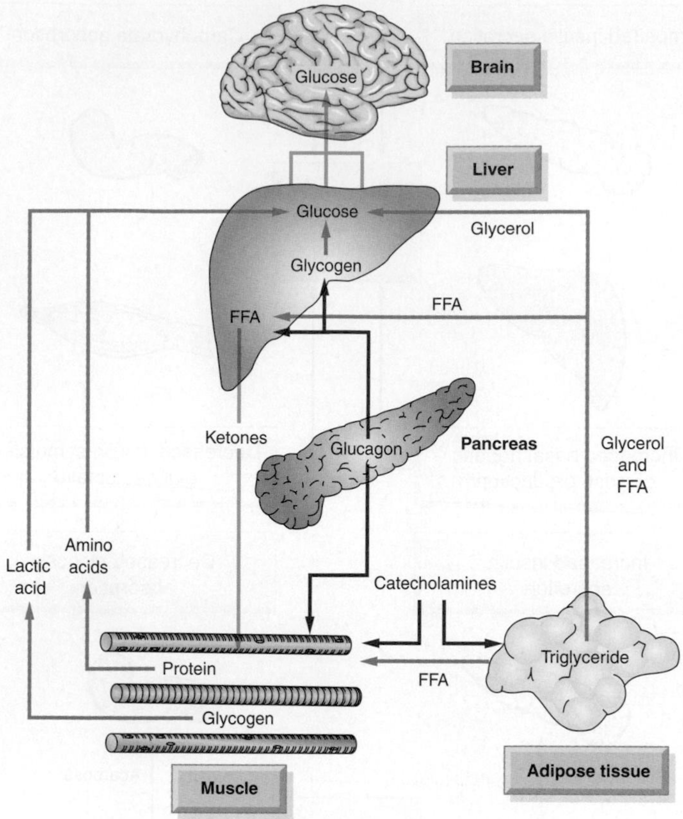

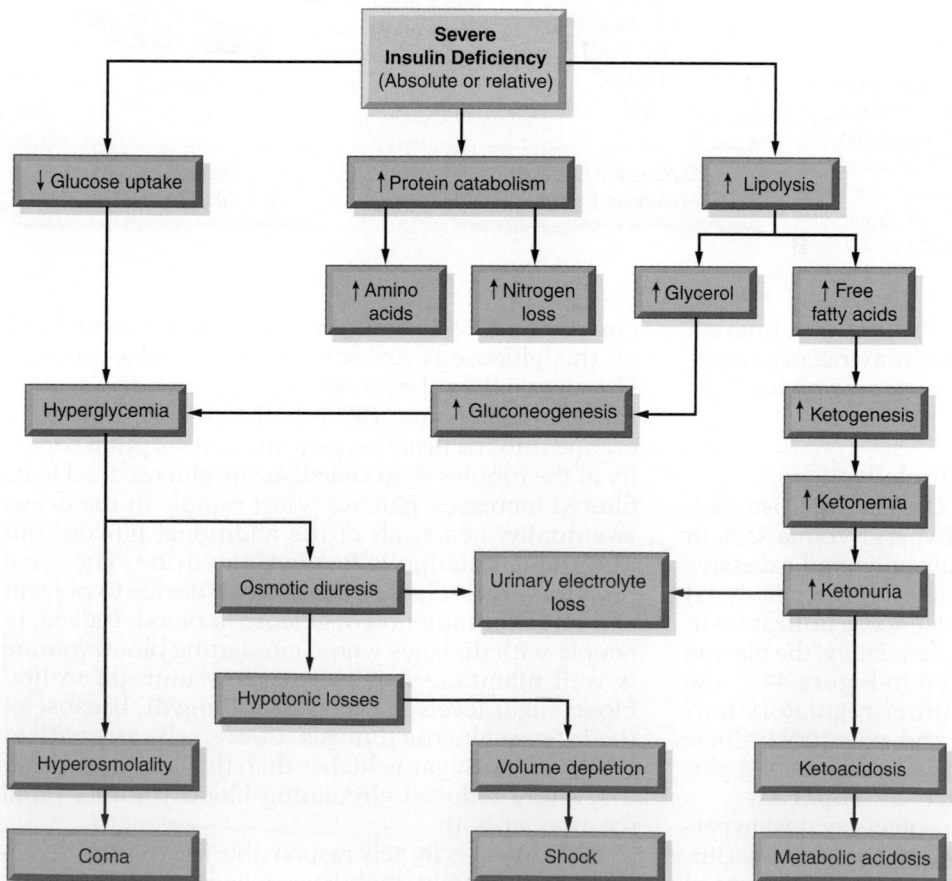

Figure 44-6 • Mechanisms of diabetic ketoacidosis (DKA). DKA is associated with very low insulin levels and extremely high levels of glucagon, catecholamines, and other counter-regulatory hormones. Increased levels of glucagon and catecholamines (*red arrows*) lead to mobilization of substrates (*blue arrows*) for gluconeogenesis and ketogenesis by the liver (*green arrows*). Gluconeogenesis in excess of that needed to supply glucose to the brain and other glucose-dependent tissues produces a rise in blood glucose levels. Mobilization of free fatty acids (FFAs) from triglyceride stores in adipose tissue leads to accelerated ketone production and ketosis. (From Porth CM: Pathophysiology: Concepts of Altered Health States, 7th ed. Philadelphia: Lippincott Williams & Wilkins, 2005, p 943.)

Figure 44-7 • The metabolic consequences of severe insulin deficiency and the interrelations of these consequences lead to diabetic ketoacidosis (DKA).

diuresis that leads to hypovolemia and decreased glomerular filtration rate. A vicious cycle occurs in a patient whose diabetes is badly out of control and who cannot take in enough sodium and water to compensate for urinary losses. Hyperglycemia leads to volume depletion, which in turn reduces urinary glucose losses and permits the blood sugar to rise even higher.

This hyperosmolality of body fluids and dehydration probably accounts for the lethargy, stupor, and ultimately, coma that occurs as DKA worsens. Diabetic patients who have ketoacidosis without hyperosmolality are less likely to have changes in consciousness.

Ketosis and Acidosis

The second major consequence of severe insulin deficiency is uncontrolled ketogenesis (see Fig. 44-7). The combination of insulin deficiency and enhanced effects of the counter-regulatory hormones causes the activation of lipase in adipose tissue. Lipase causes the breakdown of triglycerides into glycerol and free fatty acids; massive amounts of free fatty acids are released as precursors of ketoacids. In the liver, they are oxidized to ketone bodies.

As ketoacids enter the ECF, the hydrogen ion is stripped from the molecule and neutralized by combining with bicarbonate ion buffer, thereby protecting the pH of the ECF and leaving behind ketoacid anion residues. The resulting carbonic acid breaks down into water and carbon dioxide gas, which is exhaled. As ketoacid anions accumulate, they progressively displace bicarbonate from the ECF. The usual laboratory determination of electrolytes does not measure ketoacid concentration directly. However, an excess of total measured cations (sodium plus potassium) over total measured anions (chloride plus bicarbonate) provides a clue to the presence of these so-called unmeasured anions. This excess, referred to as the anion gap, can serve as an indirect measure of the quantity of ketoacids present.

The following formula is used to calculate the anion gap:

$$(Sodium) - (chloride + HCO_3)$$

The normal value is less than 15 mEq/L. An abnormal result indicates metabolic acidosis. For example, if sodium = 144 mEq/L, chloride = 92 mEq/L, and bicarbonate = 26 mEq/L, then the anion gap is 26 mEq/L, a value that indicates severe metabolic acidosis. As the ketoacids continue to accumulate, the serum bicarbonate falls and the anion gap increases. If this continues, the pH falls, and the acidosis becomes life-threatening.

Another cause of metabolic acidosis in DKA is the formation of lactic acidosis resulting from poor tissue perfusion and hypovolemia. This further exacerbates the anion gap, decreasing the serum bicarbonate level. Neutrality of body fluids is protected primarily by the bicarbonate buffering system, which determines the pH at all times by the ratio of bicarbonate anion to carbon dioxide in plasma. If bicarbonate anion is lost because of its displacement by ketoacid anions, excess carbon dioxide gas must be driven off at the

level of the lung by hyperventilation. This process keeps the ratio at or close to its usual value of 20:1 and maintains the pH close to its physiological value of 7.4. Hyperventilation, which is gradual at first and then rapidly becomes more vigorous and more obvious as the arterial pH drops below 7.2, is a characteristic physical finding in DKA.

This dramatic increase in ventilation, which occurs more by an increase in the depth than in the frequency of breathing, is known as Kussmaul's respirations. It is associated with the classic "fruity" odor of the breath in DKA. The presence of clearcut Kussmaul's respirations is a signal that the ECF pH is at or below 7.2, a relatively severe degree of acidosis.

Volume Depletion

Ketoacids are excreted in the urine largely as sodium, potassium, and ammonium salts. This contributes to the third pathophysiological problem of DKA: volume depletion and fluid and electrolyte loss as a result of osmotic diuresis. The fluid loss associated with DKA is approximately 6 liters.

Although loss of glucose through the kidneys helps protect against the ravages of extreme hyperosmolality, the diabetic patient who develops ketoacidosis pays a price for this glycosuria. Glucose remaining in the glomerular filtrate, after the renal tubules have reabsorbed all they can, forces water to remain in the tubules. This glucose-rich filtrate then flows out of the body, carrying with it water, sodium, potassium, ammonium, phosphate, and other salts. This rapid urine flow and obligate loss of water and electrolytes is known as an osmotic diuresis. Salts of ketone bodies and the urea resulting from rapid protein breakdown and accelerated gluconeogenesis also contribute to the solute load in the renal tubule, further aggravating the diuresis. The average amounts of salts and water lost to the body through osmotic diuresis during the development of DKA have been measured. Overall water loss in a 70-kg adult patient with DKA can be 5 to 8 L, or 15% of total-body water.

The fluid lost to the body is slightly hypotonic; it contains a slight excess of water compared with the volume of salts. This is expected from an osmotic diuresis due to glucose and urea. The fluid losses result from the combination of many different factors, including the intensity and duration of the hyperglycemia and osmotic diuresis; the amount of water and electrolyte replaced orally during this time; the presence of other fluid and electrolyte losses, such as vomiting, diarrhea, or sweating; and the integrity of renal function.

Sodium and water make up the central structure of the ECF, including the vascular volume. When large quantities of sodium and water are lost in the urine, the body perceives it as a serious threat to the maintenance of the circulation. A variety of compensatory mechanisms are called into play to prevent vascular collapse and shock. For example, an increase in pulse rate usually occurs, which helps maintain cardiac output in the face of shrinking intravascular volume.

At least as important, however, is a protective shift in body fluid brought about by the hyperglycemia.

Because free glucose is limited almost entirely to the extracellular water, an osmotic pressure gradient is set up across the cell membrane, between the extracellular compartment and the interior of the cells. Therefore, the higher the blood sugar, the more water is drawn out of cells and into the extracellular space. Therefore, as sodium and water are lost into the urine, shrinking the ECF, they are "replaced" (at least as to their osmotic effect) by glucose entering from the liver and by water entering from all cells. This re-expands the ECF.

Although hyperosmolality produces damaging CNS effects and osmotic diuresis, it provides a temporary mechanism for preventing vascular collapse. Despite these compensatory mechanisms, circulatory volume falls as DKA progresses. This leads to decreased glomerular filtration, decreased tissue perfusion, metabolic acidosis, and shock.

As the vascular volume falls, glomerular filtration also falls. This decreasing renal function leads to increasing blood levels of glucose, potassium, urea nitrogen, and creatinine. The excretion of potassium by the kidney occurs through the exchange of potassium for sodium. Therefore, adequate sodium must be present at the exchange site in the kidney for the rate of potassium excretion to keep pace with the need for excretion. If renal perfusion falls, enough sodium may not be available for this exchange. As a result, despite a total-body depletion of potassium, the serum potassium level may rise above normal, even to dangerously high levels.

A second major consequence of diminished vascular volume is a generalized decrease in tissue perfusion. Well before the drop in volume has reached the point at which blood pressure actually falls and full-blown shock occurs, blood is shunted away from many tissues, and the perfusion of nearly all tissues suffers. The resulting decrease in oxygen causes those tissues to shift to some degree of anaerobic glucose metabolism. This results in the increased production of lactic acid. The release of lactic acid into the circulation lowers the bicarbonate further, aggravating the already existing metabolic acidosis. Therefore, in patients with DKA, combined lactic acidosis and ketoacidosis is a common finding.

The loss of phosphate in the urine worsens tissue hypoxia. As body phosphate stores are depleted, circulating plasma phosphate levels fall quite low, depriving the red blood cells of organic phosphate compounds. Under these circumstances, the red blood cells become depleted of certain key phosphate derivatives, which in turn increases the tightness of oxygen binding to the hemoglobin in these cells. As these cells pass through poorly perfused tissues, less oxygen is given up, and tissue hypoxia worsens.

Finally, if vascular volume falls low enough, compensation mechanisms fail, blood pressure drops, and true shock supervenes. A rapidly worsening cycle of acidosis, tissue damage, and deepening shock may then occur, leading ultimately to irreversible vascular collapse and death. The full-blown syndrome of DKA is characterized by major contributions from all three major pathophysiological disruptions, each of which is primarily responsible for one of the major clinical features: coma, shock, and metabolic acidosis.

Causes

The most common cause of DKA is infection, occurring in 30% to 50% of cases. Urinary tract infection and pneumonia account for the majority of infections.[14] Other precipitating factors include severe illness (cerebrovascular accident [CVA], myocardial infarction, pancreatitis), alcohol abuse, trauma, and drugs. In addition, many people with type 1 diabetes present with DKA on initial diagnosis. Also, many patients with type 1 diabetes suddenly discontinue their insulin and deteriorate; reasons for insulin omission in younger patients include fear of weight gain, fear of hypoglycemia, rebellion against authority, and the stress of chronic disease. In one study of 341 females with type 1 diabetes, psychological problems complicated by eating disorders were a contributing factor in 20% of cases.[14] Other reasons given for sudden discontinuation of insulin or oral medications include lack of knowledge and poor compliance related to lack of financial resources. Noncompliance with therapy has been implicated as a major precipitating cause of DKA in urban African American and medically indigent patients.[14]

Assessment

Initial laboratory analysis should include an immediate glucose level using a venous sample and glucose meter measurement at the bedside to confirm the diagnosis. While these preliminary data are collected, the nurse inserts an intravenous line and starts volume replacement. A more considered assessment follows, which begins with details of the history and physical examination, a search for precipitating causes, and more complete laboratory tests. Physical examination and laboratory findings in DKA are summarized in Box 44-9.

History and Physical Examination

If ketoacidosis is strongly suspected, an effort is made to establish the diagnosis quickly so that life-preserving therapy can be started. Initial data collection includes an abbreviated history from the family or friends of an unconscious patient, a search for a dia-

---

Box 44-9 • Signs of Diabetic Ketoacidosis (DKA)

- Hyperventilation
- Kussmaul's respirations and "fruity" breath
- Lethargy, stupor, coma
- Hyperglycemia
- Glycosuria
- Volume depletion
- Hyperosmolality
- Increased anion gap (>7 mEq/L)
- Decreased bicarbonate (<10 mEq/L)
- Decreased pH (<7.4)

betic identification card, and rapid assessment for clinical clues of volume depletion. After asking about the diabetic regimen, medications, and recent changes in health, the clinician should perform a review of systems. Questions concern appetite, weight change, food and fluid intake, thirst, abdominal bloating and discomfort, bowel function, and urinary frequency and amount. During the interview, he or she should observe the patient's cognition and responsiveness.

DKA develops rapidly, and patients may display polydipsia, polyuria, and weight loss several days before ketoacidosis is established. Frequently, abdominal pain and vomiting are presenting symptoms. Approximately 40% to 75% of patients experience abdominal pain that mimics an acute abdomen; the severity of abdominal pain often correlates with more severe metabolic acidosis. Other possible findings include thirst, frequent urination, poor appetite, nausea and vomiting, fatigue, weakness, and drowsiness. The patient may also have symptoms related to urinary tract infection, upper respiratory infection, and chest symptoms because infection is often a precipitating factor.

The physical examination includes blood pressure, heart and respiratory rate, breathing pattern, heart sounds and rhythm, breath sounds, capillary refill, color and warmth of extremities, temperature, signs of hydration (e.g., skin turgor, mucus pool under tongue), deep tendon reflexes, level of consciousness, and an abdominal examination. Possible findings include hyperventilation, Kussmaul's respirations and fruity breath, dehydration, abdominal distention, dry mucous membranes, flushed skin, poor skin turgor and perfusion, hypotension, tachycardia, and varying degrees of responsiveness from lethargy to coma.

Laboratory Studies
Laboratory studies include blood glucose, chemistries, osmolality, anion gap, pH, ABGs, urine acetone, and glucose. Possible findings include hyperosmolality, increased anion gap (>7 mEq/L), decreased bicarbonate (<10 mEq/L), and decreased pH (<7.4). The serum glucose may range from 300 mg/dL to 800 mg/dL or higher. Sodium, potassium, creatinine, and BUN are all elevated. Magnesium and phosphate may also be high. Patients with DKA often present with leukocytosis and the presence of greater than 10% neutrophil bands.

Diagnostic Studies
Throat, urine, or blood cultures may also be performed to determine the presence of infection. A chest radiograph should be obtained to rule out acute infection, and an ECG should be obtained.

Management

Treatment goals for the patient with DKA include the following:

▶ Improve circulatory volume and tissue perfusion
▶ Correct electrolyte imbalances
▶ Decrease serum glucose
▶ Correct ketoacidosis
▶ Determine precipitating events

Treatment protocols for the adult with DKA are given in Figure 44-8, and a Collaborative Care Guide is given in Box 44-10.

Fluid Replacement
The immediate threat to life in a critically ill ketoacidotic patient is volume depletion. After establishing an intravenous line, the nurse rapidly infuses 0.9% (normal) saline. The goal is to reverse the severity of the extracellular volume depletion and restore renal perfusion as soon as possible. The first liter may be infused in 1 hour in patients with normal cardiac function. This replaces only a fraction of the extracellular loss in the average patient, which can range from 6 to 10 L.

Fluid replacement continues at roughly 1 L/hour until the heart rate, blood pressure, and urine flow indicate that hemodynamic stability is attained. Hypotonic solutions, such as 0.45% normal saline, can be administered at a rate of 150 to 250 mL/hour after the intravascular volume has been restored, or if the serum sodium level is greater than 155 mg/dL. Other plasma expanders, such as albumin and plasma concentrates, may be necessary if low blood pressure and other clinical signs of vascular collapse do not respond to saline alone.

Rapid infusion of saline in DKA has possible complications. It can dilute plasma proteins and lower the osmotic pressure of the plasma. This allows fluid to leak out of the vascular space through the capillary walls and contributes to the development of pulmonary edema or cerebral edema, particularly in children and older adults. Therefore, patients must be observed carefully during the first 24 to 36 hours for signs of pulmonary or cerebral edema.

Volume losses continue throughout the first hours of treatment until the glycosuria and osmotic diuresis are controlled. The next step of fluid replacement can be based on an estimate of the patient's total-body fluid loss. About 80% of the fall in blood sugar during treatment of DKA is due to glucose loss into the urine, rather than the result of insulin-induced changes in glucose production and consumption. Therefore, in the earliest phases of treatment, insulin therapy complements fluid and electrolyte replacement.

Insulin Therapy
Insulin is the cornerstone of management of ketoacidosis for several reasons. It decreases the production of ketones by shutting off the supply of free fatty acids emerging from adipose tissue. It inhibits hepatic gluconeogenesis, thus preventing further glucose from being added to the ECF. Simultaneously, hepatic ketogenesis is further reduced. Insulin also restores cellular protein synthesis. This effect occurs more slowly and permits the restoration of normal potassium, magnesium, and phosphate stores in tissues. Insulin also increases peripheral glucose utilization.

Tight glycemic control is the goal for managing patients with diabetes in the acute care setting. However, blood sugar should not fall too fast or too far.

Confusion and lethargy ensue quickly. Hemoconcentration of the blood increases the risk for clot formation, thromboemboli, and infarcts in major organs.

Causes

Infection is a major cause of HHS, occurring in 30% to 60% of patients. Urinary tract infections and pneumonia are the most common associated infections. In some cases, acute illness such as CVA, myocardial infarction, or pancreatitis provokes the release of counter-regulatory hormones resulting in hyperglycemia. HHS may also occur secondary to extreme stress associated with severe medical illness such as stroke, myocardial infarction, pancreatitis, trauma, sepsis, burns, or pneumonia. Often, HHS results from excessive carbohydrate intake or exposure such as dietary supplements, total enteral support with tube feedings, or peritoneal dialysis. Elderly people are at particularly high risk, especially those who have impaired cognition and who are in long-term chronic care facilities. Drugs such as corticosteroids, thiazide diuretics, sedatives, and sympathomimetics affect carbohydrate metabolism adversely and may lead to glucose impairment.

Assessment

History and Physical Examination

The nurse assesses the patient for precipitating or associated events. This syndrome can be iatrogenic (e.g., induced by certain medications such as steroids, hemodialysis against hyperosmolar glucose solutions, or prolonged intravenous hypertonic glucose infusions such as those given for total parenteral nutrition). It can also be precipitated by serious medical illnesses such as pneumonia or pancreatitis.

Often family members or long-term care personnel report that the patient has become a bit drowsy, taken in less food and fluid over several days, and slept more until he or she became difficult to awaken. The patient often arrives at the hospital with serious volume depletion and in a stupor or coma. The signs and symptoms of HHS are given in Table 44-8.

The clinical manifestations may take days to weeks to develop, and the patient often displays weakness, polyuria, polydipsia, and impaired mental state ranging from confusion to coma. Dehydration is manifested by tachycardia, hypotension, low cardiac output, poor skin turgor, rapid respirations without Kussmaul's breathing, and warm, flushed skin. The presence of hypothermia is a poor prognostic sign in HHS.

Laboratory Studies

Laboratory values for HHS are similar or those with DKA with four main exceptions:

1. The hyperglycemia in HHS is, by definition, a blood glucose level greater than 600 mg/dL, and this is significantly higher than DKA. Glucose can be in excess of 2,000 mg/dL.

2. Plasma osmolality is higher than DKA and is reflective of more severe dehydration. In addition to extracellular sodium and water losses, a large additional "free water" deficit exists, probably because patients do not become thirsty, causing them to take in decreasing amounts of fluid. As a result, patients have very high serum levels of sodium and glucose. Serum osmolality is extremely high (>310 to 320 mOsm/kg).

3. Patients may have some degree of ketosis as well but usually are nonketotic. In DKA, the degree of ketosis is much more severe.

4. In HHS, acidosis is not present or is very mild. In HHS, the anion gap attributable to ketoacids usually is less than 7 mEq/L. The patient may present with azotemia, hyperkalemia, and lactic acidosis.

Management

Therapy for HHS is directed at correcting the volume depletion, controlling hyperglycemia, and identifying the underlying cause of HHS and treating it. The volume depletion is usually greater in HHS than in DKA. Rapid rehydration is more cautiously carried out because of the fragile state of the patient, who often has comorbidities. Isotonic saline or hypotonic saline is administered initially to correct the fluid imbalance, and some patients may require as many as 9 to 12 L of fluid overall. The nurse should be vigilant for the signs of fluid overload during rehydration. Figure 44-9 presents an algorithm for caring for people with HHS who are older than 20 years of age.

Critically ill patients require hemodynamic monitoring during fluid resuscitation, especially elderly patients with cardiac or renal disease. Careful monitoring of fluid intake, urine output, blood pressure, central pressures, pulse, breath sounds, and neurological status is one of the nurse's primary responsibilities. In addition, the patient requires frequent laboratory monitoring.

Patients receive low doses of insulin along with the fluid replacement. It is necessary to give low-dose insulin by continuous infusion (0.1 mg/kg/hour) because these patients are vulnerable to the sudden loss of circulating blood volume that occurs with higher doses of insulin and a rapid blood sugar reduction. As the glucose level returns close to normal (250 to 300 mg/dL), it is appropriate to stop the insulin infusion and add dextrose to the intravenous fluids to prevent a sudden drop in the blood glucose level. At this point, subcutaneous administration of insulin can proceed.

Investigation of the underlying cause of HHS is warranted, and treatment, if possible, is necessary. For example, management of underlying infection from pneumonia involves aggressive use of antibiotics, chest physiotherapy, turning, and coughing and deep breathing or suctioning as needed to clear the infiltrate. Removal of exogenous sources of glucose (tube feedings, peritoneal dialysis, medications) is appropriate while treating the hyperglycemic state.

Older patients who develop HHS have frequent complications and high mortality rates. They often have difficulty handling the fluid volume shifts that occur during the development and treatment of this

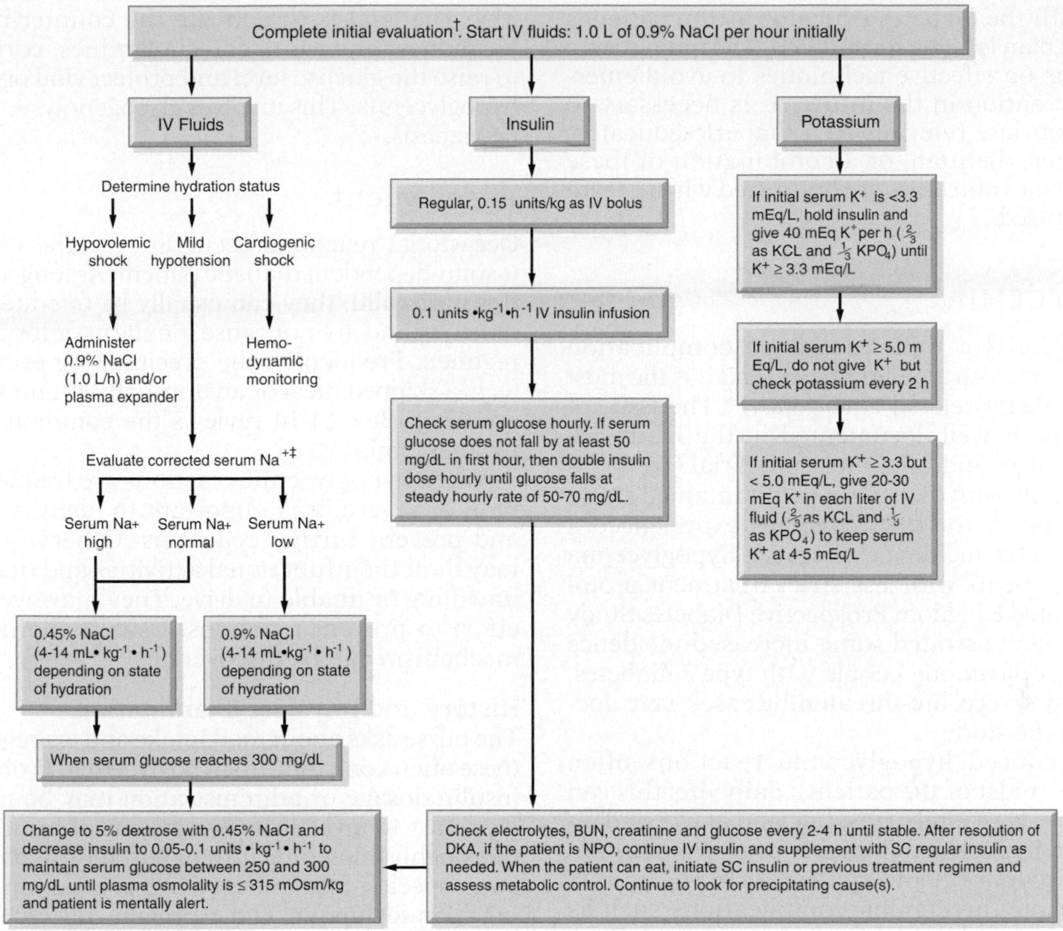

Complete initial evaluation†. Start IV fluids: 1.0 L of 0.9% NaCl per hour initially

IV Fluids

Determine hydration status

Hypovolemic shock   Mild hypotension   Cardiogenic shock

Administer 0.9% NaCl (1.0 L/h) and/or plasma expander

Hemodynamic monitoring

Evaluate corrected serum Na$^{+‡}$

Serum Na+ high   Serum Na+ normal   Serum Na+ low

0.45% NaCl (4-14 mL• kg^{-1} • h^{-1}) depending on state of hydration

0.9% NaCl (4-14 mL•kg^{-1} • h^{-1}) depending on state of hydration

When serum glucose reaches 300 mg/dL

Change to 5% dextrose with 0.45% NaCl and decrease insulin to 0.05-0.1 units • kg^{-1} • h^{-1} to maintain serum glucose between 250 and 300 mg/dL until plasma osmolality is ≤ 315 mOsm/kg and patient is mentally alert.

Insulin

Regular, 0.15 units/kg as IV bolus

0.1 units •kg^{-1}•h^{-1} IV insulin infusion

Check serum glucose hourly. If serum glucose does not fall by at least 50 mg/dL in first hour, then double insulin dose hourly until glucose falls at steady hourly rate of 50-70 mg/dL.

Check electrolytes, BUN, creatinine and glucose every 2-4 h until stable. After resolution of DKA, if the patient is NPO, continue IV insulin and supplement with SC regular insulin as needed. When the patient can eat, initiate SC insulin or previous treatment regimen and assess metabolic control. Continue to look for precipitating cause(s).

Potassium

If initial serum K$^+$ is <3.3 mEq/L, hold insulin and give 40 mEq K$^+$ per h ($\frac{2}{3}$ as KCL and $\frac{1}{3}$ KPO$_4$) until K$^+$ ≥ 3.3 mEq/L

If initial serum K$^+$ ≥ 5.0 m Eq/L, do not give K$^+$ but check potassium every 2 h

If initial serum K$^+$ ≥ 3.3 but < 5.0 mEq/L, give 20-30 mEq K$^+$ in each liter of IV fluid ($\frac{2}{3}$ as KCL and $\frac{1}{3}$ as KPO$_4$) to keep serum K$^+$ at 4-5 mEq/L

Figure 44-9 • Management of adults with hyperglycemic hyperosmolar syndrome (HHS). *Diagnostic criteria: blood glucose >600 mg/dL, arterial pH >7.3, bicarbonate >15 mEq/L, mild ketonuria or ketonemia, and effective serum osmolality >320 mOsm/kg H2O. This protocol is for patients admitted with mental status change or severe dehydration who require admission to an intensive care unit. Effective serum osmolality calculation: 2 [measured Na (mEq/L)] + glucose (mg/dL)/18. †After history and physical examination, obtain arterial blood gases, complete blood count with differential, urinalysis, plasma glucose, blood urea nitrogen (BUN), electrolytes, chemistry profile, and creatinine levels STAT as well as an electrocardiogram. Obtain chest x-ray and cultures as needed. ‡Serum Na should be corrected for hyperglycemia (for each 100 mg/dL glucose >100 mg/dL, add 1.6 mEq to sodium value for corrected serum value). IV, intravenous; SC, subcutaneous. (Copyright © 2004 American Diabetes Association. From Diabetes Care®, Vol. 27, S94–S102. Reprinted with permission from The American Diabetes Association.)

syndrome. The nurse gives fluid slowly to avoid complications associated with cerebral edema such as seizures and an altered neurological state. These patients are also at risk for intravascular thrombosis and focal seizures because of the hemoconcentration of the blood and the hyperosmolar state. Use of seizure precautions is necessary at all times. Treatment of acute cerebral edema usually involves infusion of osmotic diuretic such as 20% mannitol. Because these patients usually have a preexisting cardiac or renal history that predisposes them to complications, fluid resuscitation should proceed slowly and carefully.

Critical care management continues until the patient's hyperglycemic state has stabilized, his or her neurological condition and vital signs return to normal, and the precipitating cause has resolved. Discharge criteria also include having an adequate plan in place for the patient to maintain glycemic control and avoid future hyperglycemic emergencies.

Patient Education

As with patients with DKA, the patient and family experiencing HHS need education. The prevention of many cases of HHS and DKA entails better access to medical care, proper education, and effective communication with a health care provider during an intercurrent illness. Many uninsured or underinsured patients stop insulin for economic reasons. The nurse must assess for this possibility.

For the person with newly diagnosed diabetes, the nurse needs to provide information about the pathophysiology of the disease, the signs and symptoms of complications, and methods of treatment, including medications, diet, and exercise. Information about how to manage "sick days" and other tips to avoid acute complications such as HHS must be part of the educational plan.

The patient may need instruction on home management and glucose testing. Often the critical care staff consults with the diabetes educator as the patient's educational plan is being formulated. The main theme should focus on effective techniques to avoid emergency intervention in the future. It is necessary to make appropriate referrals to a diabetic educator, social worker, dietitian, or a combination of these because diabetes outcomes are optimized when a team approach is used.

HYPOGLYCEMIA

Hypoglycemia is a well-recognized complication among patients with type 1 diabetes, and it is the most common diabetes-related emergency.[15] The issue of hypoglycemia is well documented in the landmark Diabetes Control and Complications Trial (DCCT),[10] in which people with diabetes who maintained strict, intensive therapy for their diabetes experienced a threefold greater incidence of severe hypoglycemia than those patients with less strict treatment protocols. The United Kingdom Prospective Diabetes Study (UKPDS)[11] demonstrated some increased incidence of hypoglycemia among people with type 2 diabetes, although few severe, life-threatening cases were documented in the study.

Insulin-induced hypoglycemia reactions often occur in the midst of the patient's daily life; this can be, at the very least, embarrassing, and at worst, dangerous. Mild hypoglycemia causes unpleasant symptoms and discomfort; however, severe hypoglycemia can lead to life-threatening complications such as seizures, coma, and even death if not reversed. Even though measurable recovery from hypoglycemia is rapid and complete within minutes after proper treatment, many patients remain emotionally (and possibly physiologically) shaken for hours or even days after insulin reactions. In extreme situations, prolonged or recurrent hypoglycemia, although uncommon, has the potential to cause permanent brain damage and can even be fatal.

Pathophysiology

Minute-to-minute dependence of the brain on glucose supplied by the circulation results from the inability of the brain to burn long-chain free fatty acids, the lack of glucose stored as glycogen in the adult brain, and the unavailability of ketones. The brain recognizes its energy deficiency when the serum glucose level falls abruptly to about 45 mg/dL. The term neuroglycopenia refers to the degree of hypoglycemia sufficient to cause brain dysfunction resulting in personality changes and intellectual deterioration. The exact level at which symptoms occur varies widely from person to person, however, and it is not uncommon for levels as low as 30 to 35 mg/dL to occur (e.g., during glucose tolerance tests) with no symptoms whatsoever among the long-term diabetic population.

Symptoms result from either the sympathetic nervous system response to hypoglycemia or the neuroglycopenic response. The hypothalamus reacts to the lower glucose levels to mount the adrenergic response, including tachycardia, palpitations, tremors, and anxiety. The goal is to activate the counter-regulatory hormones (glucagon, catecholamines, cortisol, GH) to raise the glucose level and protect vital organs from hypoglycemia. This involves glycogenolysis and gluconeogenesis.

Assessment

Occasional reactions occur in even the most stable insulin-dependent diabetic patient. As long as the reactions are mild, they can usually be tolerated without difficulty and are not cause for alarm or for changes in regimen. Frequently, the precipitating event is clear (e.g., a skipped meal or an unusually strenuous bout of exercise). Box 44-14 reviews the common causes of hypoglycemia.

When hypoglycemic reactions are frequent, recurrent, or severe, it is important to identify the cause and prevent further reactions. Otherwise patients may limit their functional activities and may become unwilling or unable to drive. They may overeat in an effort to prevent reactions. Usually the underlying mechanism can be discovered.

History and Physical Examination

The nurse asks about food intake and exercise because these often contribute to hypoglycemia. Problems with insulin dosage or administration may be noted. It is necessary to investigate every detail of insulin therapy thoroughly, including insulin purchase and its appearance, species, and units; syringes, injection sites, and injection technique; and especially any recent change in any part of the regimen. The nurse explores for flaws and inconsistencies in reporting. Prescription errors,

---

Box 44-14 • Common Causes of Hypoglycemia

- Insulin shock
- Insulinoma
- Inborn errors of metabolism
- Stress
- Weight loss
- Postgastrectomy
- Alcohol-related
- Glucocorticoid deficiency
- Fasting hypoglycemia
- Profound malnutrition
- Prolonged exercise
- Severe liver disease
- Severe sepsis
- Drug effects
    - Ethanol
    - Salicylates
    - Quinine
    - Haloperidol
    - Insulin
    - Sulfonylureas
    - Sulfonamides
    - Allopurinol
    - Clofibrate
    - β-adrenergic agents

mismatched syringe and insulin units, use of new injection sites, and other errors may emerge.

The administration or withdrawal of other drugs may be the precipitating event for recurrent insulin reactions. For example, salicylates in large doses can reduce blood sugar and, in combination with insulin, can produce hypoglycemia. Also, the nurse asks about the use of glucocorticoid medications. Because these medications cause insulin resistance, insulin doses are often raised to meet the increased insulin demand. If the steroids are then tapered without reducing the insulin dose, hypoglycemic reactions can occur. Alcohol often causes hypoglycemia. Not only do patients often eat less when they have a few drinks, but also alcohol shuts off gluconeogenesis by interfering with intermediate biochemical steps in the liver. When combined with injected insulin, this frequently leads to hypoglycemia. Oral hypoglycemic agents can also produce severe and long-lasting hypoglycemia. Patients who experience such episodes tend to be older and undernourished with impaired renal or hepatic function. Nevertheless, any patient on oral agents can become hypoglycemic, especially when substances such as salicylates and alcohol potentiate the effects of the oral agents.

Another common mechanism that can cause hypoglycemia is an atypical (e.g., early or late) response to insulin therapy. Once the response pattern is defined, it is possible to adjust the insulin regimen and eliminate the insulin reactions. Occasionally, when a stable, reaction-free patient begins to experience hypoglycemic episodes, the clinician should explore the likelihood of insulin sensitivity due to weight loss or the onset of azotemia.

As the blood sugar level falls below normal, the CNS responds in two distinct ways: first, with impairment of higher cerebral functions, and second, soon thereafter with an "alarm" response in vegetative functions. Patients most commonly describe the symptoms of mild or early insulin reactions as fuzziness in the head, trouble thinking or concentrating, shakiness, light-headedness, or giddiness. These changes occur when the cerebral cortex is deprived of its main energy supply, usually when the blood glucose has fallen to 50 mg/dL or less or is rapidly declining. This part of the brain is apparently the most sensitive to the loss of glucose.

Changes in personality and behavior vary with the person and may not be apparent to them during an insulin reaction. Changes range from silly, manic, inappropriate behavior to withdrawn, sullen, grumpy, irritable, suspicious behavior. There may be difficulties in motor function, such as trouble walking and slurred speech, and patients who are well into insulin reactions may closely resemble people who have been drinking alcohol.

Some patients experience aphasia, vertigo, localized weakness, and even focal seizures with their insulin reactions. Such focal changes usually occur when there is prior damage to a specific area of the cortex, such as a head injury or CVA.

Closely following the cortical changes is a series of autonomic neurological responses. The primary response is discharge from the centers that control adrenergic autonomic impulses. This results in the release of norepinephrine throughout the body and epinephrine from the adrenals. Tachycardia, pallor, sweating, anxiety, and tremor are characteristic signs of hypoglycemia and are important early warning signs for patients who recognize a reaction. Headache can occur, and the stress response can occasionally trigger secondary sequences of symptoms, including angina or pulmonary edema in patients with fragile cardiovascular disease.

As hypoglycemia persists and worsens, consciousness is progressively impaired, leading to stupor, seizure, or coma. This is characteristic of severe hypoglycemia. The autonomic centers controlling fundamental systems, such as respiration and blood pressure, are the most resistant to hypoglycemia and continue to function even when most other cerebral functions are lost.

The more profound the hypoglycemia and the longer it lasts, the greater the chance of transient or even permanent cerebral damage after blood glucose is restored. There does not seem to be a clear duration threshold for such damage, but severe hypoglycemia lasting more than 15 to 30 minutes can result in some symptoms that persist for a time after glucose is given. Blood sugar measurement, before the administration of glucose if possible, verifies the diagnosis.

Management

Treatment of insulin reactions is always glucose. If the patient can swallow, the most convenient form is a glucose- or sucrose-containing drink because it probably gets through the stomach and into the absorbing intestine in this form in the shortest possible time. If the patient is too groggy, stuporous, or uncooperative to drink, the glucose is in the form of an intravenous bolus of 25 g of 50% dextrose given over several minutes. If this route or dosage is unavailable, 1 mg of glucagon given subcutaneously or intramuscularly reverses the symptoms by inducing a rapid breakdown and release of glucose into the bloodstream from hepatic glycogen stores.

The amount of glucose needed to reverse an insulin reaction acutely is not large. In an average-sized adult, less than 15 g (3 tsp) of glucose can raise the blood sugar from 20 to 120 mg/dL. Glucose in almost any oral form will serve. Typical treatments for hypoglycemia include 3 glucose tablets, 6 ounces of regular cola, 6 ounces of orange juice, 4 ounces of 2% or skim milk, or 6 to 8 Lifesaver candies. Starch, found in crackers and cookies, is broken down to free glucose after passing through the stomach and is absorbed so rapidly that blood sugar rises virtually as fast as with free glucose or sucrose.

Patients frequently express concern about what to do if they do not respond to the initial therapy, and they fear that they might "never wake up" from a nocturnal insulin reaction. The nurse must reassure them that if the first bolus of glucose consumed does not seem to work, the sensible thing to do is to take in more. Insulin reactions are always reversible with enough glucose. The response to oral glucose, of course, takes time, perhaps 5 to 15 minutes, whereas the response to intravenous glucose should occur within 1 or 2 minutes at most. Failure to respond fully in the appropriate time indicates that not enough glucose has been given, that the diagnosis is incorrect, or that the hypoglycemia has been long and severe enough to produce persistent, although not necessarily permanent, cerebral dysfunction.

Patient Education

The nurse should teach all people with diabetes to report hypoglycemic reactions to their health care provider for adjustments in their medical regimen. If they are taking insulin, they should know when to expect peak effects of the drug so that they can predict high-risk times for hypoglycemia. They should always carry a high-glucose snack with them for emergency use. The nurse should encourage them to carry medical alert information at all times.

• Clinical Applicability Challenges

Case Study: Complications of Diabetes Mellitus

Mr. B., a 19-year-old man, was admitted to the hospital with the chief complaints of fatigue, weakness, nausea, and vomiting for 4 days. His college roommates brought him to the emergency department. He had been diagnosed with diabetes mellitus at 8 years of age. Since that time, he had been taking a maintenance insulin regimen of 22 units of longer-acting insulin glargine at bedtime and a sliding scale of NovoLog pre-meals. Four days before admission, he became ill with flu-like symptoms such as cough, fatigue, fever and chills, and nausea and intermittent vomiting. During this period, he omitted his evening insulin and then took no further insulin for several days because he was not eating anything.

On admission, the patient's vital signs are temperature (rectal), 100.6°F (38.1°C); pulse, 128 beats/minute; respirations, 32 breaths/minute and deep; and blood pressure, 90/52 mm Hg. He is oriented but lethargic, with coarse rales at both lung bases. Admission laboratory work reveals hematocrit, 48.6%; white blood cells, 36,400/mm^3; glucose, 710 mg/dL; sodium, 128 mEq/L; potassium, 5.7 mEq/L; chloride, 90 mEq/L; bicarbonate, 4 mEq/L; blood urea nitrogen, 43 mg/100 mL; creatinine, 2.3 mg/dL; serum ketones, 4+; and urine glucose and ketones 4+. Arterial blood gas values are arterial blood pH, 7.06; PaO$_2$, 112 mm Hg; PaCO$_2$, 13 mm Hg; and bicarbonate, 2.5 mEq/L. The admission chest film is negative for pneumonia.

Emergency department physicians diagnose Mr. B. with DKA, and the initial therapy consists of several liters of intravenous infusion of normal saline and 20 units regular insulin by intravenous push, followed by an infusion of insulin at 5 units per hour during the first 9 hours. Mr. B.'s mental status improves rapidly. The flow sheet below summarizes the biochemical changes over the first 15 hours.

By the time of discharge 4 days later, Mr. B. is eating well, and it is evident that his blood glucose is controlled on his usual doses of insulin glargine.

1. Mr. B. receives diagnoses of ketosis and acidosis. What are the indicators of ketosis and acidosis?
2. Mr. B. experiences volume depletion and electrolyte imbalances. Why does this occur and what are the clues?
3. How could Mr. B.'s complication of diabetes been prevented?

Review Questions

1. A 58-year-old man was admitted with hyponatremia following an aneurysm rupture. His sodium level is now 128. In addition to fluid restriction, which one of the following pharmacological agents is indicated for the treatment of mild syndrome of inappropriate antidiuretic hormone secretion (SIADH)?
   a. Aspirin
   b. Synthroid
   c. Demeclocycline
   d. Propylthiouracil

Biochemical Flow Sheet Indicating Diabetic Ketoacidosis in Mr. B.

Time	Sugar	pH	Na	K	Cl	HCO$_3$	BUN/Creatinine
1:00 pm	710	7.06	128	5.7	90	4	43/2.3
3:00 pm	492		132	4.8	101	6	41/1.7
5:15 pm	375	7.25	137	4.1	106	8	45/1.4
10:00 pm	303		139	4.7	114	15	27/1.2
4:00 am	304		143	4.3	113	22	22/1.1

2. A 23-year-old woman who suffered a severe closed head injury displays signs of polyuria and dehydration, and her intracranial pressure is elevated. Which laboratory value is most consistent with diabetes insipidus?
   a. Blood glucose greater than 200 mg/dL
   b. Hematocrit less than 30%
   c. Serum osmolality greater than 295 mOsm/L
   d. Urine osmolality greater than 150 mOsm/L

3. An elderly resident of a nursing home is transferred to a local hospital when she is found less cognitively responsive and more sluggish in her reactions. She has a long history of hypothyroidism and has been mistakenly off her thyroid medication for more than 3 months. Myxedema coma is characterized by which one of the following sets of symptoms?
   a. Hypotension, bradycardia, hypothermia
   b. Tachycardia, hypotension, hypothermia
   c. Hypothermia, tachycardia, hypertension
   d. Hypoventilation, bradycardia, hyperthermia

4. A severely ill female patient who has been in the intensive care unit for more than 2 weeks is found to have a low cortisol level associated with adrenal insufficiency. One of the most common underlying problems for this condition is
   a. myocardial infarction.
   b. septic shock.
   c. syndrome of inappropriate antidiuretic hormone secretion (SIADH).
   d. hypothyroidism.

5. A 19-year-old college student with type 1 diabetes mellitus is brought to the emergency room after her roommate noticed that she was becoming increasingly ill. The nurse suspects diabetic ketoacidosis and knows that diabetic ketoacidosis is often precipitated by which one of the following conditions?
   a. Overuse of insulin
   b. Urinary tract infection
   c. Compliance with oral medications
   d. Taking insulin when acutely ill

6. An elderly man is admitted to the intensive care unit with the diagnosis of hyperosmolar hyperglycemic syndrome (HHS). In addition to searching for the cause of the event, traditional therapy for HHS consists of which one of the following?
   a. Fluid replacement with isotonic saline, intravenous insulin infusion, possible potassium replacement
   b. Fluid replacement with hypertonic saline, intravenous insulin infusion, sodium bicarbonate replacement
   c. Fluid replacement with dextrose in 5% lactated Ringer's solution (D5LR) initially, intravenous insulin infusion, chloride bolus
   d. Hemodialysis to correct underlying fluid and electrolyte disturbances, intravenous insulin infusion, oxygen

7. A patient with hyperosmolar hyperglycemic syndrome (HHS) will present with lab work that is often in contrast to the lab work associated with a patient with diabetic ketoacidosis. Which of the following results is considered typical of HHS?
   a. The anion gap is usually 15 mEq/L or greater.
   b. Ketonemia is present.
   c. Serum glucose levels may be 600 to 2400 mg/dL.
   d. The serum bicarbonate level is less than 10 mEq/L.

8. One initial treatment goal of hyperglycemic hyperosmolar syndrome (HHS) is to
   a. bring the blood glucose level to a normal range quickly.
   b. alleviate ketosis.
   c. diurese the patient aggressively.
   d. rehydrate the patient slowly.

9. A 27-year-old man is admitted to the emergency room following a minor motor vehicle crash. He is initially unresponsive. The emergency room nurse discovers his diabetes alert necklace, and the physician orders an intravenous bolus of 50% dextrose. Severe hypoglycemia is usually caused by which one of the following?
   a. Missed meals or too much exercise
   b. Counter-regulatory hormones such as cortisol or epinephrine
   c. Skipping oral hypoglycemic medications
   d. Severe, critical illness in a patient with diabetes

10. Hypoglycemia for the fully conscious patient is best treated by which of the following initial interventions?
    a. Glipizide orally
    b. Three or four crackers orally
    c. Cake icing sublingually
    d. Orange juice orally

References

1. Arafah BM: Hypothalamic pituitary adrenal function during critical illness: Limitations of current assessment methods. J Clin Endocrinol Metab 91(10):3725–3745, 2006
2. Reid JR, Wheeler SF: Hyperthyroidism: Diagnosis and treatment. Am Fam Physician, 72(4):623–631, 2005
3. Mauck KL: Rooting out hypothyroidism in the elderly. Nursing 2005 35(12):65–66, 2005
4. Pfadt E, Carlson RS: Acute adrenal crisis. Nursing 2006 36(8):80–81, 2006
5. American Diabetes Association: All about diabetes, 2006. Retrieved September 27, 2007, from http://www.diabetes.org/about-diabetes.jsp
6. Newton CA, Raskin P: Diabetic ketoacidosis in type 1 and 2 diabetes mellitus. Arch Intern Med 164:1925–1931, 2004
7. Fonseca VA: Clinical Diabetes: Translating Research into Practice. Philadelphia: Saunders, Elsevier, 2006
8. Bloomgarden ZT: Aspects of type 2 diabetes and related insulin-resistant states. Diabetes Care 29(3):732–740, 2006
9. Umpeirrez GE, Smily D, Kitabchi AE: Narrative review: Ketosis-prone diabetes mellitus. Ann Intern Med 144(5):350–357, 2006
10. Diabetes Control and Complications Trial (DCCT) Research Group: The effect of intensive treatment of diabetes on the development and progression of long-term complications in insulin-dependent diabetes mellitus. N Engl J Med 329:977–986, 1993
11. United Kingdom Prospective Diabetes Study Group: Tight blood pressure control and risk of macrovascular and microvascular complications in type 2 diabetes (UKPDS 38). BMJ 317:703–713, 1998
12. Brenner ZR: Management of hyperglycemic emergencies. AACN Clin Issues 17(1):56–65, 2006

13. Krentz AJ: Emergencies in Diabetes: Diagnosis, Management and Prevention. Southhampton University, UK: John Wiley & Sons, 2004

14. Umpeirrez GE, Murphy MB, Kitabchi AE: Diabetic ketoacidosis and hyperglycemic hyperosmolar syndrome. Diabetes Spectrum 15(1):28–36, 2002

15. Brackenridge A, Wallbank H, Lawrenson RA, Russell-Jones D: Emergency management of diabetes and hypoglycemia. Emerg Med J 23(3):183–185, 2006

Other Suggested Readings

Aguilar, BR: The diabetes epidemic: Special populations, special considerations. 2006. Available at: http://www.medscape.com

American Diabetes Association: Position statement: Hyperglycemic crises in patients with diabetes mellitus. Diabetes Care 27(Supp. l):S94–S102, 2004

American Diabetes Association: Standards of medical care in diabetes 2008. Diabetes Care 31(Suppl 1):S4–S108, 2008

Arafah BM: Hypothalamic pituitary adrenal function during critical illness: Limitations of current assessment methods. J Clin Endocrinol Metab 91(10):3725–3745, 2006

Aragon D: Evaluation of nursing work effort and perceptions about blood glucose testing in tight glycemic control. Am J Crit Care 15(4):378–388, 2006

Arcangelo VP, Peterson AM: Pharmacotherapeutics for Advanced Practice, 2nd ed. Baltimore: Lippincott Williams & Wilkins, 2006

Bloomgarden ZT: Aspects of type 2 diabetes and related insulin-resistant states. Diabetes Care 29(3):732–740, 2006

Brenner Z: Management of hyperglycemic emergencies. AACN Clin Issues 17(1):56–65, 2006

Clement S: Better glycemic control in the hospital: Beneficial and feasible. Cleve Clin J Med 74(2):111–120, 2006

Eigsti J, Henke K: Innovative solutions: Development and implementation of a tight blood glucose management protocol: One community hospital's experience. Dimens Crit Care Nurs 25(2): 62–65, 2006

Fatourechi V: Pretibial myxedema: Pathophysiology and treatment options. Am J Clin Dermatol 6(5):295–309, 2005

Fonseca VA: Clinical Diabetes: Translating Research into Practice. Philadelphia: Saunders, Elsevier, 2006

Gearhart M, Parbhoo S: Hypoglycemia in the critically ill patient. AACN Clin Issues 17(1):50–55, 2006

Gerard SO, Neary V, Apuzzo D, et al: Implementing an intensive glucose management initiative: Strategies for success. Crit Care Nurs Clin North Am 18(4):331–344, 2006

Goldberg P, Siegel M, Sherwin R, et al: Implementation of a safe and effective insulin infusion protocol in a medical intensive care unit. Diabetes Care 27(2):461–467, 2004

Harmel AP, Mathur R: Davidson's Diabetes Mellitus: Diagnosis and Treatment, 5th ed. Philadelphia: Saunders, Elsevier, 2004

Harris PE, Bouloux PM: Endocrinology in Clinical Practice. London: Martin Dunitz Ltd, 2003

Haskal R: Current issues for nurse practitioners: Hyponatremia. J Am Acad Nurse Practitioners 19(11):563–579, 2007

Hirsch IB, Bergenstal RM, Parkin CG, et al: A real-world approach to insulin therapy in primary care practice. Clin Diabetes 23(2):78–86, 2005

Holcomb SS: Detecting thyroid disease. Nursing 2006 35(10):4–8, 2006

Johnson K, Renn C: The hypothalamic-pituitary-adrenal axis in critical illness. AACN Clin Issues 17(1):39–49, 2006

Krentz AJ: Emergencies in Diabetes: Diagnosis, Management and Prevention. Southhampton University, UK: John Wiley & Sons, 2004

Kreshak A, Chen EH: Arterial blood gas analysis: Are its values needed for the management of diabetic ketoacidosis? Ann Emerg Med 45(5):550–551, 2005

Kudva YC, Sawka AM, Young WF: Clinical review 164. The laboratory diagnosis of adrenal pheochromocytoma; the Mayo Clinic experience. J Clin Endocrinol Metab 88(10):4533–4539, 2003

LaSalle JR: New insulin analogs: Insulin detemir and insulin glulisine. Pract Diabetol 25(3):34–44, 2006

Melmed S, Conn PM: Endocrinology, 2nd ed. Totowa, NJ: Humana Press, 2005

Moore T: Diabetic emergencies in adults. Nurs Stand 18(46):45–54, 2004

Muir AB, Quisling RG, Yang MC: Cerebral edema in childhood diabetic ketoacidosis: Natural history, radiographic findings, and early identification. Diabetes Care 27(7);1541–1546, 2004

Newton CA, Raskin P: Diabetic ketoacidosis in type 1 and 2 diabetes mellitus. Arch Intern Med 164:1925–1931, 2004

Palmer R: An overview of diabetic ketoacidosis. Nurs Stand 19(10):42–44, 2004

Porsche R, Brenner ZR: Amiodarone-induced thyroid dysfunction. Crit Care Nurse 26(3):34–41, 2006

Porth CM: Pathophysiology: Concepts of Altered Health States, 7th ed. Philadelphia: Lippincott Williams & Wilkins, 2005

Read J, Cheng E: Intensive insulin therapy for acute hyperglycemia. AACN Adv Crit Care 18(2):200–212, 2007

Reid JR, Wheeler SF: Hyperthyroidism: Diagnosis and treatment. Am Fam Physician 72(4):623–631, 2005

Rodriguez I, Fluiters E, Perez-Mendez LF, et al: Factors associated with mortality of patients with myxoedema coma: Prospective study in 11 cases treated in a single institution. J Endocrinol 180(2):347–350, 2004

Rottmann CN: SSRIs and the syndrome of inappropriate antidiuretic hormone secretion. Am J Nurs 107(1):51–58, 2007

Selig P: Metabolic syndrome in the acute care setting. AACN Clin Issues 17(1):79–85, 2006

Siu CW, Yeung CY, Lau CP, Tse HF: Incidence, clinical characteristics, and outcome of congestive heart failure as the initial presentation in patients with primary hyperthyroidism. Heart 93:483–487, 2007

Smeltzer SC, Bare BG, Hinkle JL, Cheever KH: Brunner & Suddarth's Textbook of Medical–Surgical Nursing, 11th ed. Philadelphia: Lippincott Williams & Wilkins, 2008

Susia G: Implementing glucose control protocols in critically ill patients. AACN Adv Crit Care 18(1):5–9, 2007

Turina M, Christ-Crain M, Polk HC: Diabetes and Hyperglycemia: Strict glycemic control. Crit Care Med Suppl 34(9):S291–S300, 2006

Umpeirrez GE, Smily D, Kitabchi AE: Narrative review: Ketosis-prone diabetes mellitus. Ann Intern Med 144(5):350–357, 2006

Van den Berghe G, Wouter P, Weekers F, et al: Intensive insulin therapy in the critically ill patients. N Engl J Med 345:1359–1367, 2001

Hematological and Immune Systems

PART 11

INTERNET RESOURCES

Topic	Web Page Address
AIDS.Org	www.immunet.org
American Cancer Society	www.cancer.org
American Organ Transplant Association	www.a-o-t-a.org
America Society of Clinical Oncology	www.oncology.com
American Society of Hematology	www.hematology.org
American Society of Pediatric Hematology	www.aspho.org
Association of Nurses in AIDS Care	www.anacnet.org
The Body: An AIDS and HIV Information Resource	www.thebody.com
Canadian Cancer Society	www.cancer.ca
Community AIDS Treatment Information Exchange	www.catie.ca
HIV/AIDS Treatment Information Service	www.hivatis.org
HIV InSite	http://hivinsite.ucsf.edu
International Transplant Nurses Society	www.itns.org
Johns Hopkins AIDS Service	www.hopkins-aids.edu
Leukemia and Lymphoma Society	www.leukemia.org
National AIDS Treatment Advocacy Project	www.natap.org
National Cancer Institute	www.cancer.gov
Neutropenia Support Association, Inc.	www.neutropenia.ca
North American Transplant Coordinators Organization	www.Natco1.org
Oncolink: U of Penn Cancer Center Resource	www.oncolink.upenn.edu
Oncology Nursing Society	www.ons.org
Scientific Registry of Transplant Recipients	www.ustransplant.org
Tumor Cell and Tissue Banking	www.cryoma.com
United Network for Organ Sharing	www.unos.org
United States Website for Organ Donation	www.organdonor.gov

Anatomy and Physiology of the Hematological and Immune Systems

45

Thomasine Guberski

Hematological System
   Blood and Its Functions
   Components of Blood
   Blood Coagulation
Immune System
   Immune Response
   Impaired Host Resistance

Objectives

Based on the content in this chapter, the reader should
be able to:

❶ Describe the blood and its components and the
function of each component.

❷ Delineate the clotting factors and the role each
plays in coagulation.

❸ Describe the anatomy and physiology of the
immune system.

❹ Differentiate between humoral and cell-mediated
immunity.

Because cells for both the hematological and the immune systems originate in bone marrow, the systems are interrelated. As a result, a change in one system can manifest itself in the other system. For example, a decrease in the number of white blood cells results in an immune system that is less able to resist infection. The anatomy and physiology of these two systems are discussed separately in this chapter, but the reader should keep in mind their close relationship.

• Hematological System

Veins, venules, capillaries, arterioles, and arteries constitute an intricate network of conduits for the transportation of blood, which carries respiratory gases, nutrients, and waste products to and from body tissue. Patency of the conduits and containment of blood within the vasculature depend on the integrity of the transporting conduits. A delicate balance must be maintained in the vasculature to ensure both its patency and a liquid state of blood so that neither thrombosis nor hemorrhage occurs. This delicate balance is provided by the hemostatic and fibrinolytic systems working in concert.

BLOOD AND ITS FUNCTIONS

Blood is an aqueous solution of colloid and electrolytes that serves as a medium of exchange between body cells (interior environment) and the exterior, or external, environment. It has distinct characteristics, including variable color (arterial blood is bright red; venous blood is dark red), viscosity (blood is 3 to 4 times thicker than water), a pH of 7.35 to 7.4, and a volume of approximately 70 to 75 mL/kg of body weight (5 to 6 L). Plasma constitutes approximately 55% of blood volume, whereas cellular elements suspended in the plasma constitute the remaining 45%.

The vital functions of blood are as follows:

▶ Transport of oxygen and absorbed nutrients to cells

▶ Transport of carbon dioxide and other waste products to the lungs, kidneys, gastrointestinal system, and skin

▶ Transport of hormones from endocrine glands to target organs and tissues

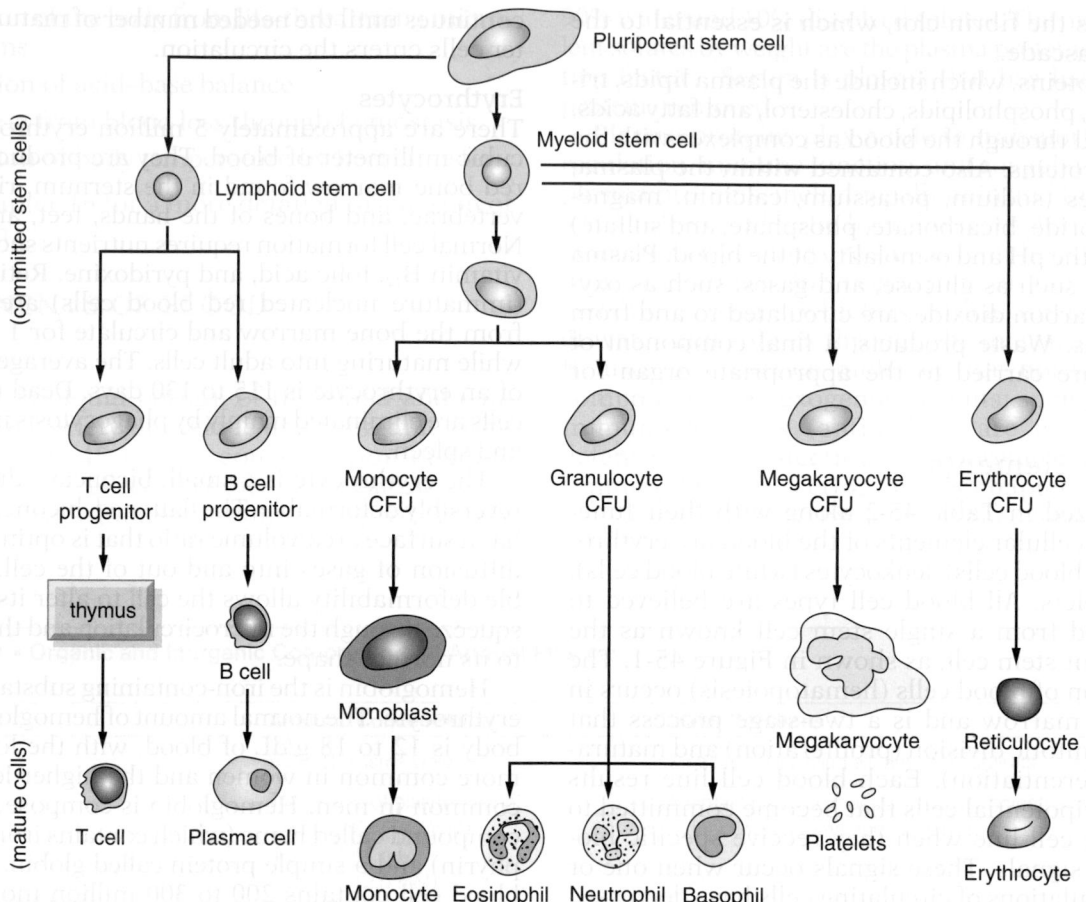

Figure 45-1 • Major maturational stages of blood cells. (From Porth CM: Pathophysiology: Concepts of Altered Health States, 7th ed. Philadelphia: Lippincott Williams & Wilkins, 2005, p 283.)

oxyhemoglobin. Hemoglobin also combines with carbon dioxide. Thus, the blood can carry oxygen to the tissues and carbon dioxide from the tissues to the alveoli of the lungs, where it is expelled into the atmosphere. Hemoglobin can also combine preferentially with carbon monoxide, which displaces oxygen.

One iron atom is present for each heme molecule. Total body iron ranges from 2 to 6 g. Two thirds of this is in hemoglobin, whereas the rest is stored in the bone marrow, spleen, and liver. When red blood cells break down, hemoglobin splits into heme and globin factors. The liver stores the iron portion of heme for production of new hemoglobin, and the remainder is converted into bilirubin, which is excreted in feces and urine after conjugation by the liver. This conjugation process is important to the excretion of bilirubin, which causes jaundice when it accumulates in the tissues (see Chapter 38).

Respiration is a major function of erythrocytes. Hemoglobin combines with oxygen in the lungs. The saturation of hemoglobin with oxygen is influenced by the partial pressure of oxygen available in the lungs, the temperature of the blood, the pH of the blood, and the amount of intracellular 2,3-biphosophyglycerate. For example, people who live at sea level and vacation in high altitudes, where the partial pressure of oxygen in the lungs is lower, may experience shortness of breath with activity because less oxygen is available to combine with hemoglobin.

Leukocytes

Leukocytes, or white blood cells, are transported in the circulation but act primarily in the body tissues, defending the body against microorganisms and foreign antigens and removing debris such as dead or injured host cells. There are approximately 5,000 to 10,000 white blood cells per cubic millimeter of blood. The two major categories of leukocytes are granulocytes and agranulocytes.

Granulocytes make up approximately 70% of all white blood cells and include neutrophils, eosinophils, and basophils. They are produced by the bone marrow from myeloid stem cells, and their function depends on the type of enclosed granule. Polymorphonuclear leukocytes, or neutrophils, fight bacterial and fungal infections and digest foreign particulate matter or break down products from cells through phagocytosis. Neutrophils are present during the early acute phase of an inflammatory reaction. After bacterial invasion or tissue injury, they migrate from the capillaries into the inflamed area, reaching their peak activity in 6 to 12 hours. In the inflamed area, they destroy and ingest microorganisms and other debris. They die in 1 or 2 days, releasing digestive enzymes that dissolve cellular debris and prepare the inflamed site for healing.

Eosinophils are particularly important in detoxifying foreign protein. They ingest antigen–antibody complexes, attack parasites, and are elevated during allergic reactions. Eosinophils have surface receptors for immunoglobulins and histamine.

Basophils contain cytoplasmic granules with vasoactive amines (histamine, bradykinin, and serotonin), which are thought to play a role in the symptoms of acute systemic allergic reactions. Basophils also contain the anticoagulant heparin, histamine, and other vasoactive substances.

Agranulocytes (monocytes, macrophages, and lymphocytes) are leukocytes that do not contain lysosomal granules in their cytoplasm. Agranulocytes also come from the myeloid stem cell. Monocytes (immature macrophages) and macrophages comprise the mononuclear phagocyte system (formerly called the reticuloendothelial system). They are responsible for the phagocytosis of dead leukocytes and erythrocytes in the blood and for the processing of antigenic material as the neutrophils start to decrease in number. Some of the circulating macrophages migrate out of the blood vessels in response to inflammation or infection, whereas others migrate to fixed sites in lymphoid tissues of the liver, spleen, lymph nodes, peritoneum, or gastrointestinal tract, where they may remain active for months or years. Lymphocytes are immunocompetent cells that are involved in producing antibodies and maintaining the immune response. The most important classifications are B and T lymphocytes, which are discussed later in the chapter.

Platelets

Platelets are disk-shaped cytoplasmic fragments formed from stem cells in the bone marrow, specifically, a giant cell called the megakaryocyte. Platelets maintain capillary integrity, accelerate coagulation, and retract clots. There are approximately 250,000 to 500,000 platelets per cubic millimeter of blood; one third of them reside in a reserve pool in the spleen. Platelets live about 10 days; when they die, they are removed from the circulation by macrophages, mostly in the spleen.

BLOOD COAGULATION

Hemostatic homeostasis is maintained through three interdependent components: blood vessels, platelets, and blood coagulation factors. In the course of normal wear and tear, the endothelial lining of blood vessels is subject to damage that requires local repair to prevent blood leakage. The body repairs the vessels through a process called coagulation. In this process, damage to, or sloughing of, the endothelium exposes the underlying collagen. This exposed collagen attracts and activates platelets to adhere to it, which begins the formation of platelet plugging. With the attraction of platelets to the exposed collagen, an initial barrier of platelets is formed. These platelets release small amounts of adenosine diphosphate, which causes additional platelets to be attracted and stick to each other. Following this process, there is a release of platelet factor 3 from the platelet membrane, which interacts with various blood coagulation proteins and accelerates clotting.

Platelets play two major roles in the clotting process. First, the platelet plug temporarily plugs the leak in the blood vessel. This plug provides the architectural foundation for the building of the fibrin clot. Second, platelets initiate clotting by way of the intrinsic pathway through the release of platelet factor 3.

Coagulation Factors

CONCEPTS in action **ANIMATION**

Coagulation factors are designated by Roman numerals and numbered according to the order in which they were first identified. When the factors are in active form, they are designated by a lowercase "a" (e.g., factor XIIa). Box 45-1 lists the factors by Roman numeral and common name.

Coagulation Pathways

Blood coagulation proteins, or coagulation factors, are found in the extrinsic and intrinsic pathways to coagulation. The trigger for coagulation activates either the extrinsic or intrinsic pathway. Recent information about the coagulation cascade indicates some interplay between the extrinsic and intrinsic pathways. Specifically, factor VII, found in the extrinsic pathway, can activate intrinsic pathway factor XI. Likewise, several factors in the intrinsic pathway activate factor VII.[1]

Extrinsic Pathway

The extrinsic pathway is a series of chemical reactions that originate outside the injured structure (Fig. 45-2). Injury to tissues and blood vessels triggers coagulation and results in the release of factor III (thromboplastin) into the circulation. Factor III, catalyzed by factor VII (proconvertin), activates factor X (Stuart-Prower factor). In the presence of calcium ions, factor V (proaccelerin), and platelet factor 3, factor Xa catalyzes the conversion of factor II (prothrombin) to IIa (thrombin) and factor I (fibrinogen) to the fibrin clot.

Box 45-1 • Coagulation Factors

   I. Fibrinogen
  II. Prothrombin (thrombin in active form—IIa)
 III. Thromboplastin
 IV. Calcium
  V. Proaccelerin
 VI. Unassigned
 VII. Proconvertin; prothrombinogen; convertin
VIII. Antihemophiliac factor A (factor VIIIR–von Willebrand)
 IX. Antihemophiliac factor B; Christmas factor; platelet cofactor II
  X. Stuart-Prower factor; prothrombinase
 XI. Plasma thromboplastin antecedent
 XII. Hageman factor; glass factor
XIII. Fibrin-stabilizing factor; Laki-Lorand factor

IMMUNE RESPONSE

CONCEPTS in action ANIMATION

The immune system is the body's internal response to substances recognized as foreign. People have two types of immunity: general (innate) immunity and specific (acquired) immunity. Innate immunity is the body's capacity to resist invasion by foreign agents. Collectins are glycoproteins that facilitate recognition of pathogenic microorganisms in innate immunity.[2] In addition, innate immunity makes use of phagocytes and natural killer cells (NKCs) in its inflammatory response to microorganisms. Innate immunity is nonspecific and has no memory.

Acquired immunity is the specific capacity of a person's immune system to identify a substance as foreign. It occurs when a person develops his or her own antibodies in response to exposure to an antigen. Antibodies function as memory cells, so that subsequent exposures to specific antigens cause a quicker response. Acquired immunity also occurs when another source supplies a person with antibodies. The maternal-to-fetal transfer of antibodies is an example of one person supplying antibodies to another. Because it may take several days for acquired immunity to generate sufficient activity to protect a person, a major role of the innate immune system is to limit microbial replication until the specific immune response is mobilized.[3]

Basically, the immune system protects the body, or "self," from invasion by "nonself." The concept of immune tolerance infers a nonactive immune system with self while producing immunity to foreign substances.[3] Any foreign substance capable of eliciting a specific immune response is referred to as an antigen. Antigens are most often composed of proteins, but polysaccharides, complex lipids, and nucleic acids also can act as antigenic materials; bacteria, viruses, fungi, parasites, and foreign tissue are all antigens. For instance, transplant rejection occurs when the body recognizes transplanted tissues or organs as foreign. Discrete, immunologically active sites on antigens enable immunoglobulins, lymphocytes, or antibodies to identify target cells, against which destructive forces are directed. Immune responses are not equally potent. The intensity of the system's response is affected by the route of invasion, the dosage of the antigen, and the antigen's degree of foreignness.

Immunological competence refers to the immune system's capacity to identify and reject foreign materials. The system's failure to recognize antigens and mobilize effective defenses results in infection or malignancy. Failure to recognize markers of self can result in autoimmune diseases, such as multiple sclerosis, rheumatoid arthritis, or systemic lupus erythematosus. The system's "battle against imaginary enemies," such as pollen or dust, may result in allergies.

The major histocompatibility complex, essential for recognizing self from nonself, is a group of genes contained in a section of chromosome 6 that encode molecules that mark a cell as self. These genes vary widely in structure from one person to another. Their presence is a major factor in transplant rejection because they determine to which antigens one responds and how strongly. They also allow immune cells to recognize and communicate with one another.

General Immunity

General immunity is present in all healthy people and forms the first line of defense against illness. Previous exposure to an organism or toxin is not required. Also, mechanisms of general immunity do not distinguish among microorganisms of different species and do not alter in intensity on re-exposure. General immune defenses include physical, chemical, and mechanical barriers; biological defenses; phagocytosis; inflammatory processes; and cytokines.

Physical, Chemical, and Mechanical Barriers

Physical barriers prevent harmful organisms and other substances from gaining entrance into the body or body cavities. These barriers include skin, mucous membranes, the epiglottis, respiratory tract cilia, and sphincters. Chemical barriers such as antibacterial agents, antibodies, and acid solutions create an environment hostile to many pathogens. Lysozymes in tears, lactic acid in vaginal secretions, and hydrochloric acid in gastric secretions all act as chemical barriers. Mechanical barriers help rid the body of potentially harmful substances through some action (e.g., lacrimation, intestinal peristalsis, urinary flow).

Biological Defenses

Under normal conditions, large areas of the human body are colonized with microorganisms of low pathogenicity. The skin and mucous membranes of the oropharynx, nasopharynx, intestinal tract, and parts of the genital tract each have their own microflora, referred to as normal flora. These microorganisms influence patterns of colonization by competing with more harmful organisms for essential nutrients and by producing substances that inhibit the growth of other microorganisms.

Phagocytes and Phagocytosis

Phagocytosis is a process by which injured cells and foreign invaders are ingested by leukocytes, specifically, neutrophils and mononuclear phagocytes (monocytes and macrophages). Both cell types originate from stem cells in the bone marrow and, although structurally different, approach phagocytosis in a similar manner.

Surface receptors on their cell membranes allow them to attach to foreign substances and then engulf, internalize, and destroy these substances using enzymes present in their cellular interior. Both neutrophils and macrophages are attracted to the site of microorganism invasion by chemokines. Neutrophils provide the "first-wave" cellular attack on invading organisms during the acute inflammatory process. The number of neutrophils at the site peaks in 6 to 12 hours after inflammation begins. The second wave of cells is primarily monocytes. Monocytes spend only a short time in the bloodstream before escaping through the capillary membranes into the tissue.

Once in the tissue, they swell to much larger sizes to become macrophages, which either attach to certain tissues and destroy bacteria, or wander through the tissue phagocytizing foreign matter. These cells are strategically placed throughout the body tissues, where they can exist for months and even years. Macrophages in different tissues differ in appearance because of environmental variations and are known by different names (i.e., Kupffer's cells in the liver, alveolar macrophages in the lungs, histiocytes in the skin and subcutaneous tissue, and microglia in the brain).

Inflammatory Responses

CONCEPTSin action ANIMATI●●N

Inflammation is an acute physiological nonspecific response of the body to tissue injury caused by factors such as chemicals, heat, trauma, or microbial invasion. It is the primary process through which the body repairs tissue damage and defends itself against infection. The initial inflammatory response is localized but may lead to systemic consequences such as fever, malaise, and neutrophilia. The inflammatory response contains three stages:

1. The vascular stage involves an immediate but short-term vasoconstriction, followed by vasodilation of arterioles and venules and hyperemia and swelling resulting from the secretion of histamine, prostaglandins, serotonin, and kinins.

2. The cellular exudate stage is characterized by neutrophilia, secretion of colony-stimulating factors into the interstitial fluid, and formation of exudate, a clear serous fluid with a high protein count. The functions of exudate are to transport leukocytes and antibodies to the inflammatory site, dilute toxins and irritating substances, and transport materials necessary for tissue repair. As the inflammatory process continues, the serous exudate changes to a creamy white fluid containing cellular debris.

3. The tissue repair and replacement stage, in which inflammatory material is removed and connective tissue cells proliferate. Collagen synthesis occurs, resulting in tissue replacement.

The most important result of these processes is accumulation at the site of injury of large numbers of neutrophils and macrophages, which inactivate or destroy invaders, remove debris, and begin the initial tissue repair.

Cytokines

Cytokines are chemical messengers that function as immune system hormones and play a role in acquired immunity and in mediating the inflammatory response. They enhance cell growth, promote cell activation, direct cellular traffic, stimulate macrophage function, and destroy antigens. They are also called interleukins (ILs) because they serve as messengers between leukocytes. Interferons and tumor necrosis factor are also cytokines.

Interleukin-1 (IL-1) augments the synthesis of IL-2, IL-3, IL-4, interferon-γ, and IL-2 receptors. It can also activate lymphokine-activated killer cells. IL-2 binds to specific receptors on activated T cells and markedly enhances the cytolytic activity of NKCs, which are a specialized group of lymphoid cells that act directly, without prior sensitization, to lyse a variety of malignant and virus-infected cells. IL-3 and B-cell differentiation factor provide critical signals for the growth and maturation of antigen-primed B cells.

Cytokines can be classified as either lymphokines (secreted by lymphocytes) or monokines (secreted by monocytes or macrophages). Interferons (a type of lymphokine) provide some protection to the body against invasion by viruses until more slowly reacting specific immune responses take over. Interferons are produced when a virus infects a host cell; they affect the transcription and translation of viral genes. In addition, interferons appear to be involved in protecting the body against some forms of cancer. Specifically, these substances have been demonstrated to interfere with cellular division and proliferation of abnormal cells. They also enhance the activity of NKCs.

Specific Immunity

If a foreign agent persists despite general immune responses, the activation of specific immune responses occurs. To be most effective, these responses require previous exposure to a foreign agent or organism. The cellular components of these types of responses are capable of distinguishing among microorganisms and can alter their intensity and response time significantly on re-exposure.

Two types of specific immune responses have been identified: cell-mediated immunity and humoral immunity. Most foreign substances stimulate both cellular and humoral immune responses; this results in an overlapping of their reactions and maximal protection against damage from the invading substances.

B and T Lymphocytes
B and T lymphocytes originate from stem cells produced in the bone marrow. During fetal development and shortly after birth, primary lymphoid organs are the sites where these cells differentiate and mature into the competent cells responsible for cell-mediated and humoral immune responses. For B lymphocytes, this preprocessing is believed to occur in the bone marrow and, possibly, the fetal liver; for T lymphocytes, it occurs in the thymus gland.

As they develop, both B and T lymphocytes acquire receptors for specific antigens that commit them to a single antigenic specificity for their lifetime. Subsequently, each of these "preprogrammed" B or T lymphocytes (on activation by its specific antigen) is capable of producing tremendous numbers of clones or duplicate lymphocytes. The different types of T cells produced are categorized according to their function, as shown in Table 45-3.

Lymphoid System
After preprocessing in the primary lymphoid organs, B and T lymphocytes migrate to secondary lymphoid tissues, where the interaction with antigens and immune responses actually occurs. Secondary lymphatic tissue is located extensively in the lymph nodes. It is also found in special lymphoid tissue, such as that

Table 45-3 • Types of T Cells and Their Functions

Cell Type	Function
Cytotoxic T cells (T8)	Direct-attack cells capable of killing many microorganisms; predominant effector cell Virus-infected cells, cancer cells, and transplanted cells especially susceptible
Helper-inducer T cells (T4)	Most numerous Play pivotal role in overall regulation of immune response Often called "master conductor" Secrete lymphokines
Suppressor T cells (T8)	Act as negative feedback controllers of T4 cells May also limit ability of immune system to attack body tissues
Memory T cells	Sensitized to antigens during specific immune responses Remain stored in body Capable of initiating far more rapid response by T cells on re-exposure to same antigen

of the spleen, tonsils, adenoids, appendix, bone marrow, and gastrointestinal tract. This lymphoid tissue is placed advantageously throughout the body to intercept invading organisms or toxins before they can enter the bloodstream and disseminate widely.

Cell-Mediated Immune Response

Cell-mediated immunity provides a response to fungi, parasites, and intracellular bacteria. It also plays a major role in the rejection or acceptance of certain tissue grafts, the stimulation and regulation of antibody production, and defense against various malignant changes. As noted, T lymphocytes contain an antigen receptor that allows for the binding of a specific type of antigen.

Each T cell, when activated by its specific antigen, is capable of producing large numbers of clones. After preprocessing, T cells migrate to lymphoid tissue, where they act as effector cells (directly attacking antigens and malignant cells) and regulators of both the cellular and humoral immune response.

Antigenic stimulation of T lymphocytes initiates the cell-mediated response. This step of the response may be mediated by macrophages that bind to the antigen, facilitating its recognition. The macrophages then produce cytokines, which stimulate T lymphocytes, increase B-lymphocyte proliferation, and activate phagocytes. People with impaired cell-mediated immunity are at high risk for infections with pathogens that replicate within cells such as viruses or parasites.[3]

Humoral Immune Response

The humoral immune response is extracellular; that is, it occurs in blood and tissue fluid. It begins in response to most bacteria, bacterial toxins, and the extracellular phase of viral invasion. Humoral immunity involves two types of serum proteins: immunoglobulins (Igs) and complement.

Igs are antibody molecules made by B lymphocytes that differentiate to plasma cells and memory cells. The plasma cells then secrete antibodies that bind to antigens; the resulting antigen–antibody complexes are ingested by phagocytes. After the complexes are eliminated, the memory cells remain in circulation and in lymphoid tissue to mature into plasma cells when the antigen is encountered again. Immunoglobulins are specific to antigens and are of several types:

▶ IgA (two types) concentrates in body fluids, such as tears, saliva, and secretions of respiratory and gastrointestinal tracts; it guards entrances to the body.

▶ IgM tends to remain in the bloodstream, where it is effective in killing bacteria.

▶ IgG (four types) is able to enter tissue spaces and works efficiently to coat microorganisms before phagocytosis occurs.

▶ IgD is found mostly in the membrane of B cells, where it is believed to regulate the cells' activation.

▶ IgE is normally present in only trace amounts; it is responsible for symptoms of allergy by activating mast cells.

Complement is a nonspecific series of 15 proteins that circulate in an inactive form in the bloodstream. These proteins activate one another in a cascading sequence when the first complement molecule C1 encounters an antigen–antibody complex. The end product of the cascade is a cylinder that lyses the cell membrane of the target cell, allowing fluids and molecules to flow in and out, which kills the target cell.

Complement can be activated in three ways. Classic activation is initiated by the antibody–antigen complex. The alternate pathway and lectin pathways are not initiated by antibodies but start in response to polysaccharides found on the surfaces of some bacteria (Fig. 45-4).[2] In addition, complement facilitates the interaction of antigens and antibodies and enhances all aspects of the inflammatory process, especially increasing vascular permeability and phagocytosis.

Combined Immune Responses

The specific immune response is complex and involves the interaction of macrophages, complement proteins, and the cellular components of both the cellular and humoral systems (Fig. 45-5). Macrophages initially function to recognize, process, and present the antigen

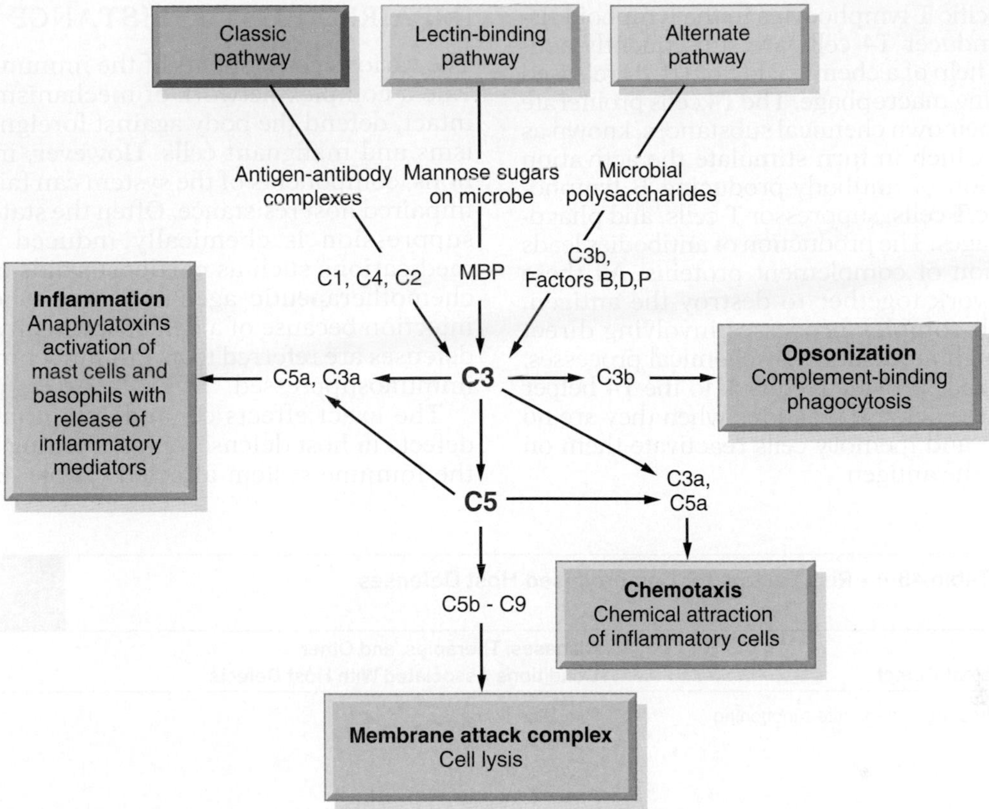

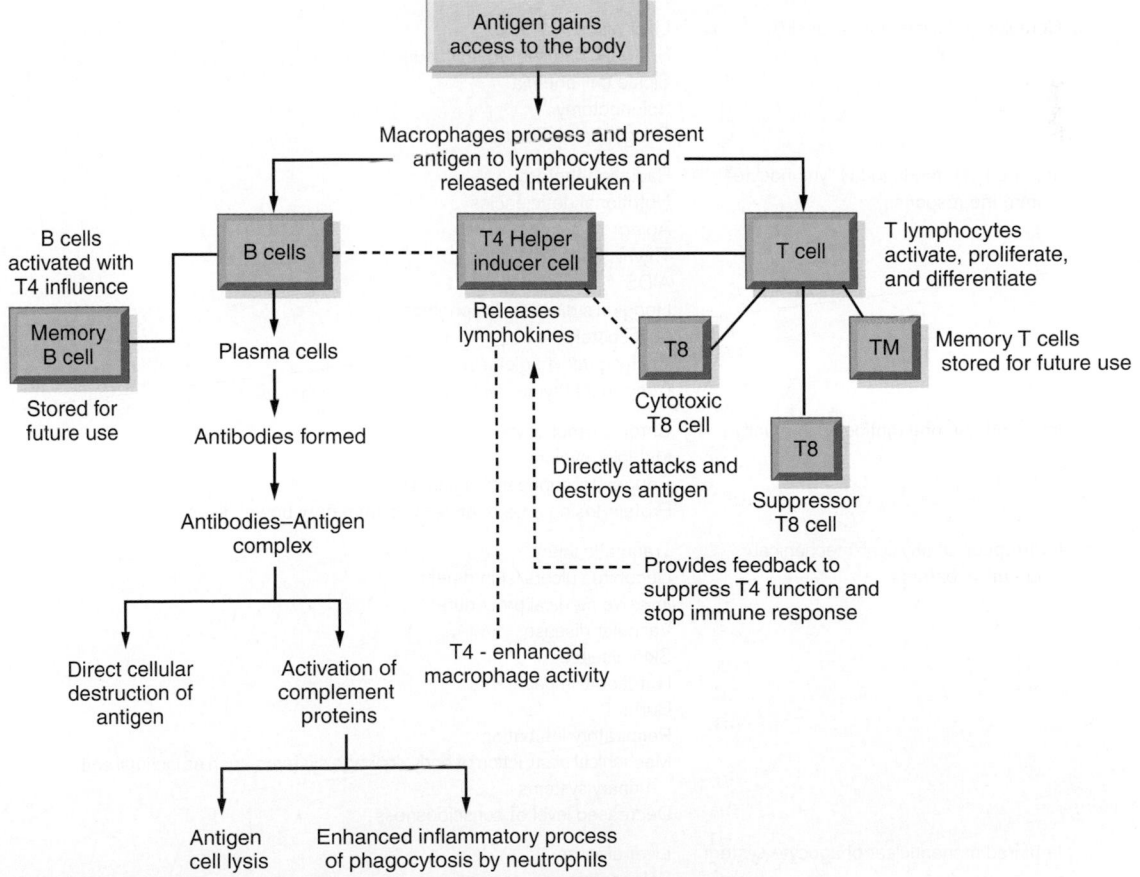

Figure 45-4 • Classic, lectin, and alternative complement pathways. (From Porth CM: Pathophysiology: Concepts of Altered Health States, 7th ed. Philadelphia: Lippincott Williams & Wilkins, 2005, p 381.)

Figure 45-5 • A schematic representation of the combined immune responses.

to antigen-specific T lymphocytes in the lymphoid tissues. Helper-inducer T4 cells are subsequently activated with the help of a chemical factor (IL-1) released by the presenting macrophage. The T4 cells proliferate and produce their own chemical substances, known as lymphokines, which in turn stimulate the activation and proliferation of antibody-producing B lymphocytes, cytotoxic T cells, suppressor T cells, and phagocytic macrophages. The production of antibodies leads to the activation of complement proteins. All these components work together to destroy the antigen, either through complex processes involving direct attack or through modulation by chemical processes. Suppressor T cells provide feedback to the T4 helper cells to halt these defense reactions when they are no longer needed, and memory cells reactivate them on re-exposure to the antigen.

IMPAIRED HOST RESISTANCE

The various components of the immune system provide a complex network of mechanisms that, when intact, defend the body against foreign microorganisms and malignant cells. However, in some situations, components of the system can fail, resulting in impaired host resistance. Often the state of immunosuppression is chemically induced by drugs or medications such as corticosteroids and cytotoxic chemotherapeutic agents. People who acquire an infection because of a deficiency in any of their host defenses are referred to as immunocompromised, or immunosuppressed.

The exact effects of, and symptoms related to, defects in host defense vary according to the part of the immune system affected (Table 45-4). General

Table 45-4 • Risk Factors for Compromised Host Defenses

Host Defect	Diseases, Therapies, and Other Conditions Associated With Host Defects
Impaired phagocyte functioning	Radiation therapy Nutritional deficiencies Diabetes mellitus Acute leukemias Corticosteroids Cytotoxic chemotherapeutic drugs Aplastic anemia Congenital hematological disorders Alcoholism
Complement system deficiencies	Liver disease Systemic lupus erythematosus Sickle cell anemia Splenectomy Congenital deficiencies
Impaired cell-mediated (T lymphocyte) immune response	Radiation therapy Nutritional deficiencies Aging Thymic aplasia AIDS Hodgkin's disease/lymphomas Corticosteroids Antilymphocyte globulin Congenital thymic dysfunctions
Impaired humoral (antibody) immunity	Chronic lymphocytic leukemia Multiple myeloma Congenital hypogammaglobulinemia Protein-losing enteropathies (inflammatory bowel disease)
Interruption of physical/mechanical/ chemical barriers	Traumatic injury Decubitus ulcers/skin defect Invasive medical procedures Vascular disease Skin diseases Nutritional impairments Burns Respiratory intubation Mechanical obstruction of body drainage systems, such as lacrimal and urinary systems Decreased level of consciousness
Impaired mononuclear phagocyte system	Liver disease Splenectomy

features associated with compromised host resistance include recurrent infections, infections caused by usually harmless agents (opportunistic organisms), chronic infections, skin rashes, diarrhea, growth impairment, and increased susceptibility to certain cancers.

• Clinical Applicability Challenges

Short-Answer Questions

1. People infected with the human immunodeficiency virus (HIV) often develop opportunistic infections. How does this happen immunologically?

2. A patient is diagnosed with aplastic anemia. Discuss how the loss of bone marrow function would affect the hematologic and immune systems.

3. Explain the mechanism that causes a blunted fever response in a patient who has had a transplant.

Review Questions

1. A patient has a viral infection. Which of the following elements of the immune response would be involved?
   a. T lymphocytes
   b. Null cells
   c. Complement
   d. B lymphocytes

2. A patient is admitted to the hospital because of an allergic reaction to penicillin. Which of the following immunoglobulins (Igs) would you expect to be present in larger than normal amounts?
   a. IgA
   b. IgD
   c. IgE
   d. IgG

3. You are reviewing a patient's laboratory results. The absolute neutrophil count is 900 cells/mm^3. This is an indication of the patient's
   a. decreased ability to respond to infections.
   b. increased risk for allergic reactions to therapy.
   c. risk for neoplastic leukocytes.
   d. probable need for prolonged convalescence.

4. You are working in the emergency department and a patient presents with carbon monoxide poisoning. Which of the following would you expect in the blood gas analysis?
   a. Decreased PCO_2
   b. Decreased PO_2
   c. Increased hemoglobin
   d. Increased porphyrin

5. The component of the immune system responsible for transplant rejection is
   a. activation of complement.
   b. leukocyte phagocytosis.
   c. major histocompatibility complex.
   d. transforming growth factor.

References

1. Hoffman R: Hematology: Basic Principles and Practice, 4th ed. New York: Churchill Livingstone, 2005
2. Porth C: Pathophysiology, Concepts of Altered Health Status, 7th ed. Philadelphia: Lippincott Williams & Wilkins, 2005
3. Andreoli TE, Carpenter CC, Bennett JC, Plum F: Cecil Essentials of Medicine. Philadelphia: Saunders, 2004

Other Selected Readings

Corwin EJ: Handbook of Pathophysiology, 3rd ed. Philadelphia: Lippincott, Williams & Wilkins, 2007
Lichtman MA, Beutler E, Kaushansky K, Kipps TJ: Williams Hematology, 7th ed. New York: McGraw-Hill, 2005
Pieracci FM, Barie PS: Diagnosis and management of iron-related anemias in critical illness. Crit Care Med 34(7):1898–1906, 2006
Smith JW, Gamelli RL, Jones SB, Shankar R: Immunologic responses to critical injury and sepsis. J Intens Care Med 21(3): 160–172, 2006

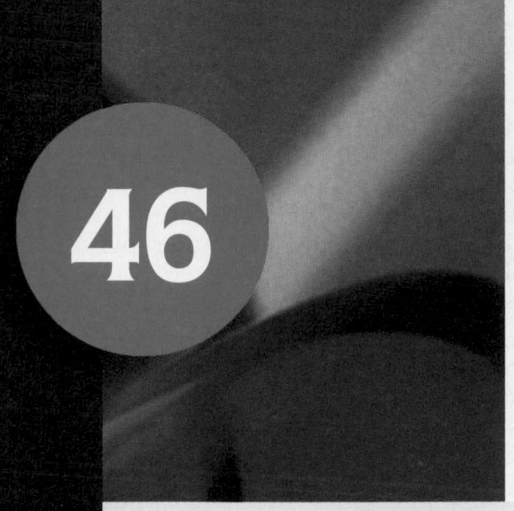

46

Patient Assessment: Hematological and Immune Systems

Kenneth Rempher • Patricia Morton

Assessment
History
Physical Examination
Diagnostic Studies and Results Interpretation
Tests to Evaluate Red Blood Cells
Tests to Evaluate White Blood Cells
Tests to Evaluate Disorders of Primary Hemostasis
Tests to Evaluate Disorders of Secondary
Hemostasis
Tests to Evaluate Hematological and Immune
Disorders
Assessment of the Immunocompromised Patient
History
Risk Factors for Immunocompromise

Objectives

Based on the content in this chapter, the reader should be able to:

❶ Identify areas of a patient's history and physical assessment pertinent to assessing hematological and immune disorders.

❷ Differentiate diagnostic tests used to assess hematological and immune disorders.

❸ Synthesize the results of a patient's history, physical examination, and diagnostic tests to identify hematological and immune disorders.

❹ Describe key aspects of the assessment of the immunocompromised patient.

Hematological and immune disorders encompass numerous ailments, many of which are life-threatening. In general, hematological disorders can be classified as overproduction or underproduction of hematological components or dysfunction of these components. Immune disorders usually are caused by underactivity or overactivity of immune system elements. Immune disorders can be inherited, or they can be acquired through disease or treatments such as chemotherapy and transplant immunosuppression. The hematological and immune systems are complex and closely interrelated; therefore, disorders or dysfunctions of one system often alter the effectiveness of the other.

• Assessment

HISTORY

The patient history is essential when evaluating potential hematological or immune disorders. While discussing the chief complaint, a patient may state symptoms that seem vague and unrelated, so a detailed history is critical. It is important to keep in mind the complex physiology of these systems when assessing a patient's health history (see Chapter 45).

After obtaining information about the chief complaint and history of the present illness, the nurse inquires about the patient's past health history, family history, and personal and social history[1-3] (Box 46-1). The patient's immunization history and occupation may provide helpful clues. A review of relevant systems concludes the history. Table 46-1 summarizes conditions and treatments that may predispose patients to hematological and immune disorders (see Chapters 48 and 49). Box 46-2 summarizes special considerations for older patients.

PHYSICAL EXAMINATION

A thorough physical examination is necessary to identify physical signs that may indicate a hematological or immune system disorder. Table 46-2 summarizes physical findings that may suggest various disorders of these systems. (Many of these disorders are further described in Chapter 49.)

The physical examination of the hematologically or immunocompromised patient focuses on four major areas: skin, liver, spleen, and lymph nodes. The entire examination must be thorough to help identify the exact source of the problem. The nurse examines the patient's skin for pallor or jaundice as well as for signs of abnormal bleeding. He or she

Box 46-1 • Hematological and Immune Health History

Chief Complaint
- Patient's description of the problem

History of the Present Illness
- Complete analysis of the following signs and symptoms (using the NOPQRST format; see Box 17-1)
- Unusual bruising or bleeding, frequent infections, fatigue/malaise, headache, dizziness/gait disturbance, pain, enlarged lymph nodes, fevers, night sweats, weakness, limb pain/limp, seizure, weight loss, abdominal pain, vomiting, heat intolerance, poor wound healing, nevi

Past Health History
- Relevant childhood illnesses and immunizations—mononucleosis, malabsorption, hepatitis, pernicious anemia
- Past acute and chronic medical problems, including treatments and hospitalizations—anemia, cancer, infections, autoimmune hemolytic anemia/Evans syndrome, hemochromatosis, hereditary spherocytosis, iron deficiency anemia, polycythemia, hemophilia, sickle cell disease, thalassemia, idiopathic thrombocytopenia, glucose-6-phosphate dehydrogenase (G6PD) deficiency, aplastic anemia, myelodysplastic syndrome, cirrhosis, HIV, major trauma, sepsis
- Risk factors—recent exposure to benzenes, pesticides, mustard gas, antineoplastic agents
- Past surgeries—splenectomy, cardiothoracic surgery, total gastrectomy
- Past diagnostic tests and interventions—bone marrow aspiration, radiation therapy, chemotherapy, multiple blood transfusions, administration of blood products (cryoprecipitate)
- Medications—chemotherapeutic agents, antibiotics, antihypertensives, diuretics, glucocorticoids, nonsteroidal anti-inflammatory drugs, aspirin, heparin, warfarin, antiplatelet agents
- Allergies and reactions
- Transfusions

Family History
- Health status or cause of death of parents and siblings—cancer, anemia, hereditary spherocytosis, G6PD deficiency, sickle cell anemia, methemoglobinemia, thalassemia, Glanzmann's thrombasthenia, von Willebrand's disease, polycythemia

Personal and Social History
- Tobacco, alcohol, and substance use
- Family composition
- Occupation and work environment—exposure to chemicals: benzenes, mustard gas, cigarette smoke, butadiene, dioxins (pesticides), hexachlorobenzene, ozone, polybrominated biphenyls, polychlorinated biphenyls (PCBs), phenols, toluene-di-isocyanate vinyl chloride, lead, naphthalene
- Living environment; see above
- Diet (insufficient intake of foods rich in iron and folic acid, including liver, eggs, whole grains, breads, cereals, potatoes, leafy green vegetables, fruits, and legumes). Assess for poor intake of foods rich in vitamin B_{12}, including liver, fish, and fortified cereals.
- Sleep patterns—disruptive sleep patterns modulate changes in immune system activity[1]
- Exercise—regular exercise is associated with optimizing immunity[2]
- Cultural beliefs
- Spiritual or religious beliefs—refusal of blood products, including transfusions is a core belief for some patients, including some Jehovah's Witnesses[3]
- Coping patterns and social support systems
- Leisure activities
- Sexual activity
- Recent travel

Review of Systems
- HEENT: oral infections, gum bleeding, epistaxis, mouth sores, sore throat, smooth tongue texture, jaundiced sclera, conjunctival pallor, retinal hemorrhages
- Cardiac: tachycardia, S_4 sounds
- Respiratory: recent upper or lower respiratory infections, hemoptysis
- Gastrointestinal: blood in emesis, blood in stools, dark tarry stools, unintentional weight loss, splenomegaly, hepatomegaly, splenic bruits and rubs
- Musculoskeletal: weakness, bone pain, back pain, arthralgia
- Neurological: mental status changes, pain to touch, position and vibratory sensation, tendon reflexes
- Genitourinary: blood in urine, urinary tract infections
- Reproductive: heavy menstruation, vaginal bleeding

---

also evaluates the patient's joints for pain, swelling, and limited range of motion, which may suggest hemarthrosis from coagulopathy or sickle cell anemia. Superficial mucocutaneous bleeding and a dependent distribution of petechiae can indicate thrombocytopenia, whereas clusters of palpable, pruritic petechiae can suggest vasculitis. Extensive superficial purpura, deep hematomas, or hemarthroses may indicate a coagulation disorder. The nurse also notes skin rashes, pruritus, and excoriations. It is necessary to assess the extremities for areas of redness, tenderness, warmth, or swelling, which can indicate thrombophlebitis. Leg and ankle ulcers may be present in patients with sickle cell anemia. The nurse assesses the lips and nail beds for cyanosis; digital clubbing may be present in patients with chronic hypoxemia.

The nurse also examines the patient's eyes and mouth. Visual changes can indicate hyperviscosity from polycythemia or retinal infarcts from sickle cell anemia. It is important to assess the nares, gums, and mucous membranes of the mouth for signs of bleeding. The oral examination is a good time to ask about bleeding gums while brushing. Pallor of the oral mucosa can be a significant indicator of anemia. Tongue changes can occur in patients with an iron deficiency and megaloblastic anemias. Inspection of the throat and palpation of lymph nodes to assess for infection or malignancy is warranted. Figure 46-1 shows palpation of the lymph nodes in the neck.

1174

Table 46-1 • Hematological and Immune Disorders Based on Patient History

Patient History	Potential Disorder
Chronic disease (inflammation, infection)	Anemia
Nutritional deficiencies (iron, folate, vitamin B$_{12}$)	Anemia
Nutritional deficiencies (vitamin K, malabsorption)	Coagulopathy
Endocrine (thyroid, pituitary) dysfunction	Anemia
Hypersplenism	Anemia, thrombocytopenia
Acquired immunodeficiency syndrome	Anemia, neutropenia
Malignancy	Pancytopenia
Chemical exposure	Neutropenia, hemolytic anemia
Prosthetic heart valve or vascular graft	Hemolytic anemia
Collagen vascular disorder	TTP
Hypersensitivity reaction	TTP
Viral, bacterial, or fungal infection	TTP
Uremia	Coagulopathy
Chronic alcoholism	Coagulopathy
Liver disease	Coagulopathy, thrombosis
Vasculitis	Thrombosis
Atherosclerosis	Thrombosis
Chronic obstructive pulmonary disease	Polycythemia
Smoking	Polycythemia
Congenital cardiac disease	Polycythemia
Previous Therapies/Medications	
Heparin	Thrombocytopenia
Antibiotics	Agranulocytosis
Carbamazepine	Agranulocytosis
Alkylating agents	Leukemia, lymphoma, pancytopenia
Blood transfusion	Anemia
Aspirin, nonsteroidal anti-inflammatory drugs	Coagulopathy
Warfarin	Coagulopathy
Steroids	Leukocytosis
Various drugs, chemicals, and toxins (see Box 49-1)	Hemolytic anemia
Family History	
Sickle cell anemia	Anemia
Thalassemia	Anemia
Congenital hemolytic anemia	Anemia
Polycythemic disorders	Polycythemia vera
von Willebrand's disease	Bleeding disorder
Hemophilia	Bleeding disorder

TTP, thrombotic thrombocytopenic purpura.

Box 46-2 • CONSIDERATIONS FOR THE OLDER PATIENT: Risk Factors for Hematological Disorders

- Decreased iron intake, resulting from poor dentition (difficulty chewing meat) or a fixed income (making sources of iron such as meat or supplements unaffordable), can place the older adult at risk for iron-deficiency anemia. Older adults may also experience low-grade gastrointestinal bleeding as a result of nonsteroidal anti-inflammatory drug use for the treatment of arthritis, from hemorrhoids and polyps, or from undiagnosed colon cancer. This blood loss may also place them at risk for iron deficiency anemia.
- Poor absorption of vitamin B$_{12}$ (as a result of atrophic gastritis) places the older adult at risk for megaloblastic anemia.
- Declining immune function places the older adult at risk for leukemia, lymphoma, and multiple myeloma.
- Anticoagulation therapy (e.g., to treat atrial fibrillation) can result in platelet dysfunction and places the older adult at risk for hemorrhage. This is a particularly significant risk in older adults who are disoriented or have decreased mobility.

tion and hemoptysis. Symptoms of intermittent claudication (see Chapter 19) and angina pectoris (see Chapter 21) indicate problems with oxygen delivery in patients with polycythemia. Polycythemia is an unusual myeloproliferative disease in which there is excessive production of erythrocytes. The increased number of erythrocytes results in increased blood volume, increased viscosity of blood, and clogging of microcirculatory blood vessels, which leads to decreased tissue perfusion.[4] Subsequently, patients with polycythemia commonly experience hypertension as part of the sympathetic response to decreased tissue perfusion.

Pertinent physical assessment findings of the abdominal and pelvic region include lymphadenopathy, splenomegaly, and hepatomegaly, which can indicate a number of hematological or immune conditions. Figure 46-2 shows the technique for palpating the spleen in the supine and side-lying positions. Figure 46-3 shows the degrees of splenomegaly. The nurse also thoroughly assesses for urinary tract infections, vaginal infections (including those with yeast), and perirectal inflammation. In addition, the nurse checks all body secretions and fluids (stool, urine, emesis, or gastric secretions) for the presence of blood.

Neurological abnormalities may be present in patients with hematological conditions. Altered mental status, paresis, aphasia, dysphasia, coma, seizures, paresthesia, and visual problems may be caused by thrombotic thrombocytopenic purpura (TTP; see Chapter 49). An altered level of consciousness, papilledema, vomiting, and bradycardia with widening pulse pressure are signs of increased intracranial

Tachycardia and tachypnea may be present in patients with anemia or infection. An S$_4$ heart sound may be heard in persons with severe anemia. Dyspnea on exertion and orthostatic changes in blood pressure can be other symptoms of anemia and not just volume insufficiency. Many patients present with new-onset chest pain made worse by anemia. As the body loses oxygen carrying capacity resulting from loss of hemoglobin, the myocardium becomes stressed and can trigger angina. It is necessary to perform thorough lung auscultation and inspection of sputum, if present, to rule out respiratory infec-

Table 46-2 • Findings Indicating Possible Hematological or Immune Disorders

Physical Findings*	Related Information From Patient History	Possible Disorder
Pallor, dyspnea, dizziness, tachycardia, glossitis	Fatigue Headache Pica (compulsive craving for clay, laundry starch, earth, or ice)	Iron-deficiency anemia
As above, also smooth tongue, stomatitis, icterus, paresthesias, gait ataxia, mental status changes	Fatigue Headache Premature graying of hair	Megaloblastic anemia
Bleeding (ecchymosis, petechiae, epistaxis, hemorrhage), pallor, dizziness, tachycardia	Fatigue Headache History of frequent infections (e.g., upper respiratory, cellulitis, perirectal) Previous viral infection (hepatitis, infectious mononucleosis, HIV, cytomegalovirus) Family history of aplastic anemia	Aplastic anemia
Pallor of conjunctiva, mucous membranes, palms and soles of feet; dyspnea; dizziness; tachycardia; bone pain; pain in chest or abdomen; splenomegaly; fever; leg and ankle ulcers; painless hematuria	African American descent Family history of sickle cell anemia Frequent infections Impaired vision Damage to joints Chronic renal failure History of stroke	Sickle cell anemia
Pallor, dyspnea, dizziness, jaundice, splenomegaly, cholelithiasis	Mediterranean descent, also Middle Eastern, South and Southeast Asian, and African	Thalassemia
Splenomegaly, hepatomegaly, facial and conjunctival plethora, hypertension, pruritus, dizziness, headache, thrombosis, thrombophlebitis	Visual disturbances Epigastric distress Cardiovascular insufficiency Bleeding tendency Numbness and burning of toes (from peripheral vascular insufficiency)	Polycythemia
Mouth sores, sore throat, lymphadenopathy, splenomegaly, hepatomegaly, infection (signs of infection may be minimal)	History of recurrent, severe infections Fatigue Recent radiation or chemotherapy treatment	Leukopenia
Infection, bleeding, bone pain, splenomegaly, skin and gum lesions, leukostasis if WBC count is extremely high (headache, confusion, CNS infarcts, acute respiratory insufficiency, pulmonary infarcts)	History of recurrent infections Fatigue Anorexia Weight loss	Acute or chronic leukemia
Bone pain, pallor, weakness, fatigue	History of recurrent infections Renal insufficiency Hypercalcemia (thirst, lethargy, confusion, polyuria, constipation)	Multiple myeloma
Weight loss, fever, night sweats, painless lymphadenopathy, splenomegaly, abdominal pain	Fatigue Anorexia History of infections	Hodgkin's disease or non-Hodgkin's lymphoma
Superficial mucocutaneous bleeding, petechiae on dependent areas of the body, epistaxis, hemoptysis, hematemesis, hematuria, rectal bleeding, vaginal bleeding, intra-abdominal hemorrhage (diffuse abdominal pain, restlessness, anxiety, pallor, rigidity, dusky coloration of abdominal skin, tachycardia, tachypnea, and hypotension), intracranial bleeding (headache, vomiting, decreasing level of consciousness, papilledema, bradycardia)	History of viral or bacterial infection Hypersplenism Malignancies affecting the bone marrow History of immune disorders Alcoholism Pregnancy	Thrombocytopenia
Confusion, headache, altered mental status, paresis, aphasia, dysphagia, coma, seizures	Paresthesias Visual disturbances	TTP

(continued)

Table 46-2 • Findings Indicating Possible Hematological or Immune Disorders (Continued)

Physical Findings*	Related Information From Patient History	Possible Disorder
Superficial purpura, mucocutaneous bleeding, hemorrhage, joint pain and swelling (from bleeding into joints), deep hematomas	History of excessive or recurrent bleeding in patient or family members Alcoholism Hepatitis Liver disease Malnutrition Malabsorption syndromes (affects absorption of vitamin K from gastrointestinal tract)	Coagulation disorder

CNS, central nervous system; TTP, thrombotic thrombocytopenic purpura; WBC, white blood cell.
*Findings listed may not always be present.

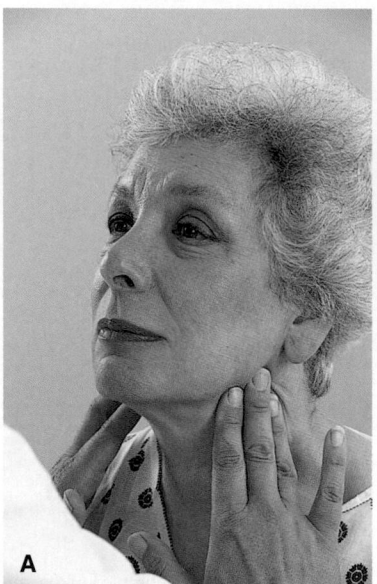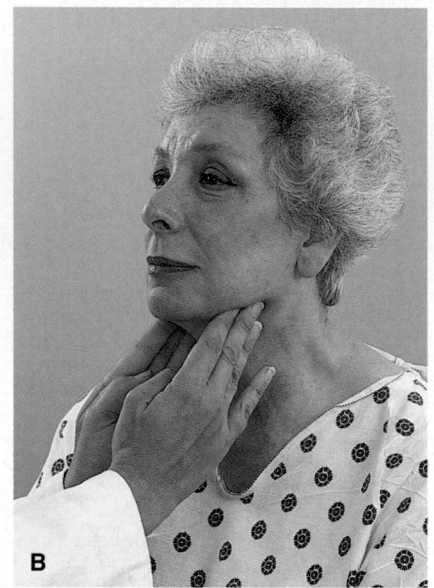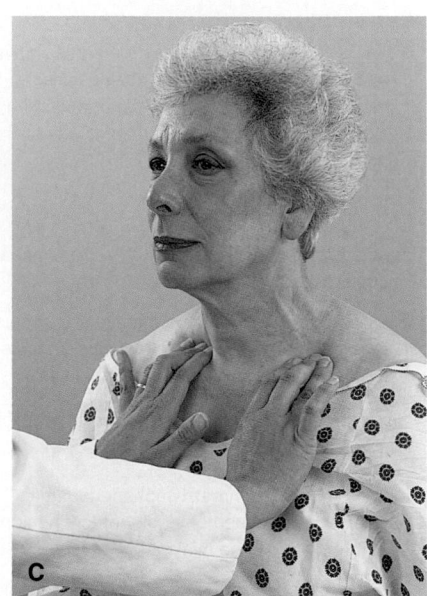

Figure 46-1 • A: Palpating the tonsillar nodes. **B:** Palpating the submandibular nodes. **C:** Palpating the supraclavicular nodes. (From Weber J, Kelley J: Health Assessment in Nursing, 3rd ed. Philadelphia: Lippincott Williams & Wilkins, 2007, pp 205, 207. Copyright B. Proud.)

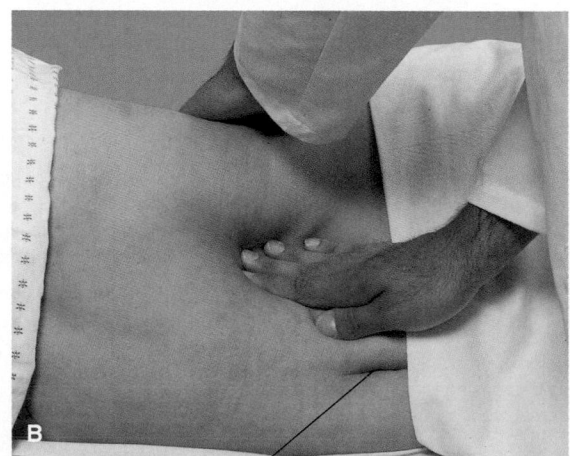

Umbilicus

Figure 46-2 • A: Palpating the spleen in the supine position. **B:** Palpating the spleen in the side-lying position. (From Weber J, Kelley J: Health Assessment in Nursing, 3rd ed. Philadelphia: Lippincott Williams & Wilkins, 2007, p 452.)

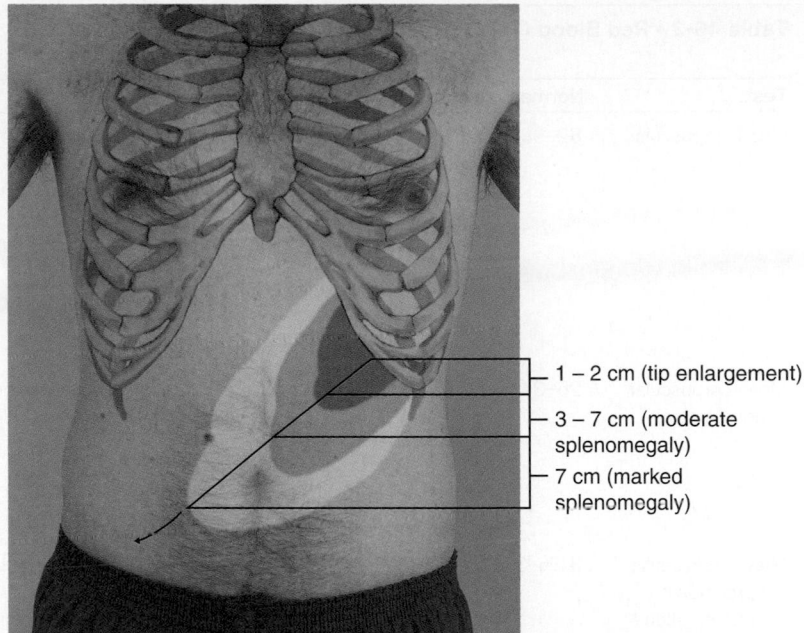

— 1 – 2 cm (tip enlargement)

— 3 – 7 cm (moderate splenomegaly)

— 7 cm (marked splenomegaly)

Figure 46-3 • Degrees of splenomegaly. (From Rhoads J: Advanced Health Assessment and Diagnostic Reasoning. Philadelphia: Lippincott Williams & Wilkins, 2006, p 283.)

pressure, which may be caused by intracranial bleeding in patients with coagulopathy.

• Diagnostic Studies and Results Interpretation

Laboratory test results are usually the most sensitive and specific determinants of hematological and immune problems. Specialized testing may be required to ascertain whether the components are functioning properly. Because patients with severe presentations of hematological and immune conditions may be seen in the intensive care unit (ICU), tests to differentiate the conditions and their causes are presented here.

TESTS TO EVALUATE RED BLOOD CELLS

Red blood cells (RBCs) are essential for oxygenating tissues. An overproduction of RBCs results in polycythemia, which is indicated by a high hematocrit level and an increased RBC mass (see Chapter 49). Anemia is a condition marked by a decrease in the RBC mass caused by decreased production of RBCs, increased RBC destruction, a combination of these two conditions, or acute blood loss. All patients being evaluated for anemia should have a complete blood count (CBC) with RBC indices, a reticulocyte count, iron studies, and a peripheral smear analysis. Abnormalities in these test results indicate the need for subsequent testing.

Complete Blood Count

The CBC provides an overall indication of bone marrow production of RBCs, white blood cells (WBCs), and platelets. It also indicates the patient's hemoglobin level, hematocrit level, RBC indices, and WBC differential. (See Chapter 17, Table 17-2 for normal hemoglobin and hematocrit values.) Patients usually extract about 25% of the oxygen from saturated hemoglobin. An increase in oxygen extraction can occur in patients with extreme anemia. As the patient's extraction increases, so does his or her oxygen debt and shock state. Anemia from any cause is a major determinant in tissue hypoxia.

Red Blood Cell Indices

RBC indices are laboratory values that describe RBC structure or function. Table 46-3 presents RBC indices and some of the conditions that can cause abnormal laboratory results.

Peripheral Smear

The peripheral smear can indicate disorders of the structure of RBCs. Table 46-4 lists various abnormalities detected by examining the peripheral smear, along with further testing that may be appropriate.

Mature RBCs do not contain a nucleus. Nucleated RBCs mature in the bone marrow and are not normally present in peripheral blood. They appear in the peripheral smear after profound stimulation, such as that from acute hemorrhage, hypoxemia, hemolytic anemia, or megaloblastic anemia.[5] If these causes are ruled out, the appearance of nucleated RBCs may be caused by infiltrative processes in the bone marrow from malignancy, myelofibrosis, or granuloma. Nucleated RBCs may also be seen in asplenic patients because the spleen normally recognizes and removes these abnormal cells.

Spherocytes and elliptocytes are abnormally shaped RBCs. They usually appear in patients with a hereditary disorder that causes RBC membrane defects. These irregular cells are trapped and destroyed in the

Table 46-3 • Red Blood Cell Indices: Laboratory Abnormalities

Test	Normal Value	Significance	Possible Causes for Abnormal Results
Mean corpuscular volume	82–98 m³	Indicates the average volume of an RBC in the blood sample. Low value indicates RBCs are smaller than normal (microcytic). High value indicates RBCs are larger than normal (macrocytic).	Decreased: Anemia (iron-deficiency, sickle cell, hemolytic), α- or β-thalassemia, chronic disease, radiation therapy, endocarditis, diverticulitis, warm autoantibodies Increased: Alcoholism, cirrhosis, folate deficiency, vitamin B_{12} deficiency, pancreatitis, chronic lymphocytic leukemia, aplastic anemia
Mean corpuscular hemoglobin	26–34 pg	Indicates the average weight of hemoglobin in each RBC.	Decreased: Anemia (iron-deficiency, microcytic, normocytic) Increased: Anemia (macrocytic, pernicious), cold agglutinin conditions, presence of monoclonal blood proteins, heparin sodium, heparin calcium
Mean corpuscular hemoglobin concentration	31%–38%	Indicates the amount of hemoglobin in the RBC compared with its size. Results expressed as hypochromic or normochromic, referring to the concentration of hemoglobin and color of RBCs.	Decreased: Anemia (iron-deficiency, chronic, megaloblastic, microcytic, sideroblastic) Increased: Cold agglutinins, hereditary spherocytosis, intravascular hemolysis, heparin calcium, heparin sodium
Red cell distribution width	13.4%–14.6%	Measures the amount of homogeneity in the RBC width in the blood sample. Much variation in RBC width indicates the red cell distribution width is elevated. RBCs of similar size indicates red cell distribution width is low.	Decreased: Defects in iron reutilization Increased: Iron-deficiency states
Reticulocyte count	1%–2%	Indicates the amount of immature RBCs that have been recently released from the bone marrow, expressed as a percentage of the total RBCs. Low reticulocyte count in presence of decreased RBCs indicates possible bone marrow dysfunction.	Decreased: Alcoholism, anemia (aplastic, iron deficiency, megaloblastic, pernicious), chronic infection, myxedema, radiation therapy Increased: Hemolytic anemia, hemorrhage, leukemia, malaria, polycythemia, pregnancy, sickle cell anemia, thalassemia, thrombotic thrombocytopenic purpura
Serum iron	Adult men 50–160 µg/dL Adult women 40–150 µg/dL	Indicates the amount of iron in the serum. Low serum iron needs to be correlated with other testing (i.e., ferritin, transferrin, and total iron binding capacity) to determine if iron deficiency anemia is present.	Decreased: Acute blood loss, iron deficiency anemia, gastrectomy, malabsorption, malignancy, rheumatoid arthritis, uremia Increased: Acute hepatitis, aplastic anemia, blood transfusion, hemochromatosis, lead poisoning, pernicious anemia, thalassemia, vitamin B_6 deficiency
Serum ferritin	Adult men 15–200 ng/mL Adult women ≤40 y 11–122 ng/mL Adult women >40 y 12–263 ng/mL	Correlates well to the size of iron stores in the body. Ferritin is stored in the liver and reticuloendothelial system and released into the serum to meet the body's demand for iron.	Decreased: Hemodialysis, inflammatory bowel disease, iron-deficiency anemia, gastrointestinal surgery, pregnancy Increased: Anemia (chronic, hemolytic, megaloblastic, pernicious, sideroblastic), chronic infection, chronic inflammation, chronic renal disease, excess ingestion of iron, hepatic disease, liver disease, malignancy, multiple blood transfusions, rheumatoid arthritis, thalassemia
Total iron-binding capacity	250–400 mg/dL	Indicates the maximum amount of iron that can be bound to transferrin. Useful for differentiating anemia from chronic inflammatory disorders.	Normal: Chronic inflammatory disorders Increased: Iron-deficiency anemia
Serum transferrin	200–400 mg/dL	Plasma protein that transports iron by binding iron to serum transferrin receptors. Emerging as more sensitive indicator of iron deficiency and may replace more conventional indices (serum iron and ferritin).	Decreased: Cirrhosis, hemochromatosis, inflammatory states, renal disease, hemorrhage, hepatitis, hypothyroidism, microcytic anemia, pernicious anemia, thalassemia Increased: Iron-deficiency states

From Chernecky CC, Berger BJ: Laboratory Tests and Diagnostic Procedures, 2nd ed. Philadelphia: WB Saunders, 1997.

Table 46-4 • Peripheral Smear Red Blood Cell Abnormalities

Abnormality	Potential Diagnoses	Further Testing
Nucleated RBCs	Acute hemorrhage, hypoxia, megaloblastic anemia	Vitamin B_{12} and folate levels; assess for bleeding; O_2 saturation, arterial blood gases for hypoxia
Spherocytes, elliptocytes	Hemolytic anemia from hereditary spherocytosis, hereditary elliptocytosis	Reticulocyte count, serum bilirubin, serum lactate dehydrogenase, direct Coombs', osmotic fragility
Rouleaux formations	Multiple myeloma	Serum protein electrophoresis, urine for Bence Jones proteins
Target cells, sickle cells, red cell cytoplasmic inclusions	Sickle cell anemia, thalassemia	Hemoglobin studies (hemoglobin electrophoresis, hemoglobin F and A_2)
Schistocytes	Thrombotic thrombocytopenic purpura, mechanical hemolysis	Reticulocyte count, serum lactate dehydrogenase, serum bilirubin, coagulation studies, cardiac auscultation

spleen, causing hemolytic anemia. Testing for RBC osmotic fragility demonstrates that these cells are more likely to lyse than normal RBCs. Serum lactate dehydrogenase and serum bilirubin levels should be ordered if hemolysis is suspected.

The presence of Rouleaux formations (the RBCs on the peripheral smear resemble a stack of coins) can indicate multiple myeloma.[6] If clinical findings support this suspicion, serum protein electrophoresis and urine analysis for Bence Jones protein are the next steps in determining a diagnosis.

Target cells, sickled cells, and RBC cytoplasmic inclusions on the peripheral smear suggest the need for hemoglobin electrophoresis and hemoglobin F and A_2 levels. The most common anemias diagnosed in this manner are β-thalassemia and sickle cell anemia.

The presence of schistocytes in a patient with a prosthetic heart valve may indicate mechanical hemolysis.[7] Schistocytes in a patient with fever, thrombocytopenia, renal dysfunction, and neurolog-

ical abnormalities require immediate interventions for suspected TTP (see Chapter 49).

TESTS TO EVALUATE WHITE BLOOD CELLS

Because WBCs detect and destroy pathogens, an elevated WBC count usually indicates infection and tends to correlate with the severity of the infection.

White Blood Cell Count

The WBC count measures circulating leukocytes and should always be assessed in conjunction with the WBC differential and the patient's clinical condition. The WBC differential is relative and describes the percentages of the WBC subtypes (neutrophils, eosinophils, basophils, monocytes, and lymphocytes). WBC subtypes can also be measured using absolute numbers. It is important to consider both the absolute and relative values of the WBC subtypes when assessing the differential. For example, 60% segmented neutrophils may seem within normal limits, but if the total WBCs are 18,000 cells/mm³, the absolute value (18,000 × 0.60) is 10,800 cells/mm³, which is well above normal. Table 46-5 indicates normal absolute and differential values for the WBC count.

Conditions other than infection that may elevate the WBC count include use of steroids, trauma, stress, leukemia, hemorrhage, tissue necrosis, and dehydration. Table 46-5 summarizes abnormalities of WBC overproduction and potential physiological causes. In some cases, patients with leukemia have WBC counts greater than 100,000 cells/mm³ because of excessive bone marrow production of blast cells (immature granulocytes). These patients are at risk for leukostasis, in which blasts aggregate in the capillaries of the brain and lungs. Clinical findings of leukostasis include headache, confusion, central nervous system infarcts, acute respiratory insufficiency, and pulmonary infiltrates.

A low WBC count usually indicates decreased production caused by immunosuppressive therapy or a disorder of bone marrow production due to infiltrative processes or bone marrow failure. Decreases in circulating neutrophils may be caused by decreased production from bone marrow injury, bone marrow infiltration, nutritional deficiencies, or congenital defects of the stem cells in the bone marrow. Other causes of neutropenia are splenic sequestration and destruction, immune-mediated granulocyte destruction, or overwhelming infection. Lymphocytopenia is most commonly caused by malignancy, followed by collagen vascular disease. Acquired immunodeficiency syndrome (AIDS) and AIDS-related complex are other notable causes of lymphocytopenia (see Chapter 48).

There are numerous potential abnormalities in the WBC differential. A left shift refers to an increase in the number of bands (neutrophil precursors), which usually indicates an infectious process. The presence of blasts in the peripheral blood is always an aberrant finding and suggests the presence of leukemia or a myeloproliferative disorder.

T and B Lymphocyte Tests

As discussed in Chapter 45, lymphocytes are classified as T cells and B cells. T cells are important in the body's ability to distinguish between self and nonself. Monoclonal antibodies against specific lymphocyte surface proteins are used to identify types of circulating lymphocytes and their subset populations, which can be useful in characterizing hematological malignancies and identifying immunological and autoimmune diseases. A specific example of this is assessment of the CD4⁺ subpopulation of T cells in patients with AIDS; a CD4⁺ count of less than 400/mm³ is associated with a poorer prognosis. Table 46-6 lists possible causes of lymphocytosis and lymphopenia.

When an antigen stimulates B cells, they differentiate into plasma cells and produce antibodies. Although plasma cells reside in lymphoid tissue, their antibody production can be evaluated through serum and urine protein electrophoresis. Autoimmune diseases occur when the body produces antibodies directed against its own tissues. These diseases can be organ specific (e.g., Graves' disease in the thyroid) or widely disseminated and involve multiple organs, such as systemic lupus erythematosus (SLE), which can attack almost every body system. Laboratory testing is aimed at the detection of serum antibodies against various tissues. C-reactive protein, antinuclear antibody, rheumatoid factor, and erythrocyte sedimentation rate are additional tests used in diagnosing autoimmune disorders.

TESTS TO EVALUATE DISORDERS OF PRIMARY HEMOSTASIS

Laboratory testing that evaluates hematological dysfunction should be guided by the information gathered in the history and physical examination. Family history, underlying clinical conditions, and the duration and type of abnormal bleeding can indicate appropriate testing and diagnostic workup. Because hematological and immune disorders are so pervasive in the human body, the nurse must be careful not to disregard innocuous symptoms. The patient's history must be thorough.

Primary bleeding disorders are caused by problems with platelets and small blood vessels that can result in subtle bleeding. For instance, mucocutaneous bleeding, petechiae, and superficial purpura may be early signs of impending critical illness. Decreased platelets or increased capillary fragility can cause the sudden appearance of petechiae, especially in dependent areas, such as the lower extremities.

Platelet Count

The primary phase of hemostasis involves aggregation of platelets at the site of vessel injury. These platelets initiate the coagulation cascade, which results in the deposit of fibrin at the site of injury to stabilize the clot (secondary hemostasis). See Chapter 45, Figure 45-2 for an illustration of the processes that occur during hemostasis.

When evaluating primary hemostasis, one first obtains a platelet count from the CBC. A platelet count of less than 150,000/mm³ is abnormal, but bleeding from thrombocytopenia alone usually does not happen unless the platelet count falls below 20,000/mm³. However, prolonged bleeding from surgery or trauma may occur with platelet counts of 40,000 to 50,000/mm³. Severe, spontaneous hemorrhage may result when platelet counts reach 5,000 to 10,000/mm³. Causes of thrombocytopenia include decreased bone marrow production, splenic sequestration due to splenomegaly, or peripheral destruction of platelets by the body's own immune system. Disseminated intravascular coagulation (DIC) and TTP (see Chapter 49) are other serious disorders that involve low platelet counts. Drugs are the first suspect

Table 46-5 • White Blood Cell (WBC) Count and Differential: Laboratory Abnormalities

Test	Normal Value: Relative	Normal Value: Absolute (cells/mm³)	Significance	Possible Causes of Abnormal Results
White blood cell (WBC) count		4,500–10,000	Measures number of WBCs	Infection, inflammation, leukemia, trauma, stress
Differential	All percentages for various types of WBCs must add up to 100%		Describes the percentage of each WBC found in blood	See examples of specific cell type below
Granulocytes			Type of WBC categorized by presence of granules in cytoplasm	See specific granulocyte subtypes below
Segmented neutrophils	50%–70%	2,500–7,000	Mature neutrophil with nuclei segmented into lobes	*Increased:* bacterial infection, inflammatory disorder, tissue destruction, malignancy, drug-induced hemolysis, diabetic ketoacidosis, myeloproliferative disorders, idiopathic, smoking, obesity *Decreased:* compromised immune system, depressed bone marrow, heart-lung bypass, hemodialysis, overwhelming infection, tuberculosis, typhoid
Band neutrophils	3%–5%	135–500	Immature neutrophil with nuclei that have smooth edges, unsegmented	*Increased:* acute stress, active bacterial infection *Decreased:* compromised immune system
Eosinophils	1%–3%	100–300	Also known as acidophils (acid loving); combat infections caused by parasites; play a role in allergic reactions; cause bronchoconstriction in asthma	*Increased:* parasitic infection, asthma, allergies, dermatoses (hives and eczema), adrenal insufficiency *Decreased* (note: a low eosinophil count is not a cause for concern); Cushing's disease; administration of glucocorticosteroids; various pharmaceuticals
Basophils	0.4%–1%	40–100	Similar mechanism to mast cells in allergic response; triggered by immunoglobulin E binding to antigens; releases pro-inflammatory mediators	*Increased:* hyperlipidemia, viral infections (smallpox, chickenpox), inflammatory conditions (ulcerative colitis, chronic sinusitis, asthma), Hodgkin's lymphoma, increased estrogen, hypothyroidism, myeloproliferative disorders, *Decreased:* stress, hyperthyroidism, pregnancy
Monocytes	4%–6%	200–600	Monocytes become macrophages after migration into tissue; macrophages perform phagocytosis	*Increased:* viral infection, parasitic infection, myeloproliferative disorders, inflammatory bowel disease, sarcoidosis, cirrhosis, drug reactions *Decreased:* administration of glucocorticoids, aplastic anemia, lymphocytic anemia
Lymphocytes	25%–35%	1,700–3,500	Primary source of viral defense and antibody production	*Increased:* viral infections, pertussis, tuberculosis, acute lymphoblastic leukemia, cytomegalovirus infection, mononucleosis, post transfusion, splenomegaly, hyperthyroidism, connective tissue disorder *Decreased:* AIDS, bone marrow suppression, aplastic anemia, steroid use, neurological disorders (multiple sclerosis, myasthenia gravis, Guillain-Barré syndrome)

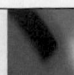

Table 46-6 • Possible Causes of Lymphocytosis and Lymphopenia

Finding	Possible Causes
Lymphocytosis	Cytomegalovirus infection, hepatitis, infectious mononucleosis, lymphocytic leukemia, syphilis, diverticulitis, endocarditis, pertussis, toxoplasmosis Drugs and chemicals include aspirin, haloperidol, lead intoxication, levodopa, phenytoin, carbon disulfate poisoning, tetrahydrochloride poisoning
Lymphopenia	Aplastic anemia, Cushing's syndrome, malignancy, chronic myelogenous leukemia, systemic lupus erythematosus, radiation therapy to the lymphatics, immunoglobulin deficiencies, uremia Drugs include chemotherapeutic agents, glucocorticoids, lithium, niacin, epinephrine

From Chernecky CC, Berger BJ: Laboratory Tests and Diagnostic Procedures, 2nd ed. Philadelphia: WB Saunders, 1997.

Box 46-4 • Causes of Platelet Disorders in the Intensive Care Unit

Thrombocytopenia
Heparin (1%−−3%)
Sepsis (>50%)
AIDS (40%–60%)
Disseminated intravascular coagulation (DIC)
Thrombotic thrombocytopenic purpura (TTP)

Abnormal Platelet Function
Renal insufficiency
Cardiopulmonary bypass
Aspirin
Dextran

The incidence of platelet disorders is indicated in parentheses.
From Marino PL: The ICU Book, 2nd ed. Philadelphia: Lippincott Williams & Wilkins, 1998, p 710.

in thrombocytopenia (Box 46-3); once the nurse has ruled them out, he or she moves to nonpharmacological causes (Box 46-4). Finally, one must consider that some people may produce adequate numbers of platelets but ones that function abnormally.

An elevated platelet count greater than 400,000/mm³ indicates increased platelet production or decreased platelet destruction. These platelets may function abnormally, causing aberrant bleeding and clotting. A cause of primary thrombocytosis is bone marrow disease. Causes of reactive thrombocytosis include chronic inflammation, infection, malnutrition, acute stress, malignancy, splenectomy, or the postoperative state.

Peripheral Smear

A peripheral blood smear may reveal megathrombocytes (large platelets), which may be present during premature platelet destruction. Also, note that some patients' platelets clump when exposed to EDTA (the anticoagulant used in the "purple top" or CBC tube). Examination of the peripheral smear shows this clumping, and a repeat CBC in a heparinized "green top" blood collection tube reveals an accurate platelet count.

Platelet Function Assay

The platelet function assay (PFA) is a screening method that tests platelet function in adhesion and aggregation quality. This test is helpful in the evaluation of platelet function in patients with menorrhagia, drug-induced platelet dysfunction, and high-risk pregnancy.

Bleeding Time

The bleeding time test assesses the length of time required for a clot to form at the site of vessel injury. A prolonged bleeding time in a patient with a normal platelet count may indicate a disorder of platelet function that requires further testing. Remember that patients can bleed to hemorrhage with a normal platelet count if the platelets are not functioning. A deficiency in factor VIIIR (von Willebrand's disease) results in decreased ability of the platelets to adhere to the injured vessel wall. Uremia from renal failure, drugs (especially aspirin), foods, and spices can also cause abnormal platelet function. Box 46-3 lists some drugs known to decrease platelet production or function. Platelet aggregation studies are performed to detect inherited or acquired disorders in platelet function.

Box 46-3 • RED FLAG: Drugs That Decrease Platelet Production or Function

- Aspirin
- Benzene and benzene derivatives
- Cimetidine
- Chemotherapeutic agents
- Chloramphenicol
- Chlorothiazides
- Digitalis
- Digoxin
- Estrogen
- Furosemide
- Gold
- Heparin
- Penicillin
- Phenytoin
- Quinidine
- Streptomycin
- Sulfonamides
- Tetracycline
- Vitamin E

From Doyle B, Porter DL: Thrombocytopenia. AACN Clin Issues 8:469–480, 1997.

Prothrombin Time and Activated Partial Thromboplastin Time

Screening for coagulation abnormalities includes evaluating the prothrombin time (PT) and the activated partial thromboplastin time (aPTT). Prolongation of either of these tests indicates coagulation factor deficiencies or inhibition. The PT test screens for dysfunction in both the extrinsic portion that includes tissue thromboplastin and factor VII and in the common pathway that includes factors X, V, and II and fibrinogen. Prolongation of PT can result from disorders such as liver disease, vitamin K deficiency, clotting factor deficiencies, or DIC. Numerous medications, including allopurinol, aspirin, β-lactam antibiotics, chlorpropamide, digoxin, diphenhydramine, and phenytoin sodium, can also cause a prolonged PT. PT is also used to monitor patient response to anticoagulation therapy with warfarin.

In 1983, the World Health Organization introduced the international normalized ratio (INR) to provide a common standard for interpretation of PT. The INR value depends on the sensitivity ratio of the thromboplastin reagent used in the laboratory to the International Reference Preparation. It is now widely accepted practice to assess the level of anticoagulation and warfarin dosing based on the INR ratio.

The aPTT measures how well the coagulation sequences of the intrinsic pathway (factors XII, XI, IX, VIII) and the common pathway (factors X, V, II, and fibrinogen) are functioning. An elevated aPTT could indicate disorders of any coagulation factors except VII and XIII. Clinical conditions associated with an elevated aPTT include DIC, von Willebrand's disease, and liver disease. Drugs that may affect aPTT include chlorpromazine, codeine, phenothiazines, salicylates, and warfarin. The aPTT test is also used to monitor patient response to heparin therapy.

▶ **Thrombin time:** Thrombin time is a test that measures the clotting time of a sample of plasma to which thrombin has been added. Thrombin is important in converting fibrinogen to fibrin in the final phase of the coagulation cascade. Thrombin time is increased in conditions such as DIC, liver disease, clotting factor deficiencies, shock, and hematological malignancies. Decreased thrombin time occurs with thrombocytosis.

▶ **Fibrinogen level:** Fibrinogen is converted by thrombin to fibrin, which then combines with platelets to form a stable clot. Patients with DIC, severe liver disease, sepsis, TTP, or trauma have a low fibrinogen level. Elevated fibrinogen levels occur in conditions involving tissue damage and inflammation.

▶ **Fibrin degradation product level:** Fibrin degradation products (FDPs) accumulate when a large amount of clotting has occurred and has then been broken down. Increased FDPs, along with an elevated PT/aPTT, decreasing platelets, and a low fibrinogen level, indicate possible DIC (see Chapter 49).

▶ **D-Dimer:** D-Dimer is a more specific test than FDP measurement for detecting an event in which fibrin is being broken down. Its indications include ruling out and monitoring DIC, deep venous thrombosis, pulmonary embolism, and venous and arterial thrombotic conditions, and the monitoring of thrombolytic therapy.

TESTS TO EVALUATE DISORDERS OF SECONDARY HEMOSTASIS

Disorders of secondary hemostasis involve clotting factor deficiencies and are characterized by recurrent oozing of blood and hematoma formation. The onset of these symptoms may be delayed because of the initial plugging of the vessel injury; however, defective clotting mechanisms fail to provide a stable fibrin clot.

When assessing disorders of secondary hemostasis, one must determine whether the disorder is congenital or acquired. A history of excessive or recurrent bleeding in the individual or family members suggests a congenital disorder as the more likely cause. Table 46-7 describes potential complications experienced by people with congenital bleeding disorders. The most common congenital bleeding disorders are von Willebrand's disease, hemophilia A, and hemophilia B. PT and aPTT are ordered for patients with suspected congenital disorders, along with factor VIIIR, VIII, and IX assays. A deficiency in von Willebrand's factor (VIIIR) results in the decreased ability of platelets to adhere to the injured vessel wall and a deficiency of factor VIII. A deficiency of factor VIII causes hemophilia A; a deficiency of factor IX causes hemophilia B. Table 46-8 summarizes laboratory abnormalities that indicate these congenital disorders.

An acute bleeding problem without a prior history of chronic bleeding suggests an acquired disorder. Acquired disorders of hemostasis occur with vitamin K deficiency, severe trauma, hemorrhage, massive transfusion, overwhelming infection, severe liver disease, and DIC. A deficiency of vitamin K decreases synthesis of prothrombin, factor VII,

Table 46-7 • Potential Complications in Congenital Bleeding Disorders	
Site	**Potential Complication**
Abdomen (e.g., retroperitoneal)	Hypotension, hypovolemic shock
Muscle	Compartment syndrome
Joint	Hemarthrosis with destruction of bone and cartilage in joint capsule
Intracranial	Increased intracranial pressure
Retropharyngeal	Airway obstruction
Gastrointestinal	Anemia, melena
Urinary tract	Hematuria; clots in ureters may occur after factor administration

From Stabler SP: Hemophilia. In Wood ME (ed): Hematology/Oncology Secrets. Philadelphia: Hanley & Belfus, 1999.

Table 46-10 • Common Laboratory Tests of the Immune System

Laboratory Test	Reference Range	Use
C-reactive protein	Not available; levels < 10 mg/L indicate patient no longer has clinically active inflammation; high or increasing levels are consistent with infection and/or inflammation	Evaluation of various inflammatory conditions, including rheumatoid arthritis and systemic lupus erythematosus
Antinuclear antibody (ANA)	Low titers are negative; elevated titers demonstrate an elevated concentration of antinuclear antibodies	Screening and diagnosis of autoimmune disorders
Human leukocyte antigen (HLA) typing	Reported as phenotype for each of the six HLA loci tested. HLA (protein marker found on most of the body's cells) typing involves either serologic or DNA methods. Antibody screen test is reported as the percentage of panel reactive antibodies (PRAs); percent PRA is number of wells reactive with patient's serum expressed in percent. Cross-match is reported as compatible or incompatible.	Determination of tissue compatibility for organ transplantation; also used to determine paternity and to diagnose HLA-related disorders
Erythrocyte sedimentation rate (ESR)	1–13 mm/h for males; 1–20 mm/h for females	Evaluation of inflammatory state; females tend to have a higher ESR; ESR increases with age
Immunoglobulins (Igs)	IgA: 160–260 mg/dL IgG: 950–1550 mg/dL IgM: 50–300 mg/dL IgD: 0–9 mg/dL IgE: 0.002–0.2 mg/dL	Assessment of immunodeficiency state and certain cancers, including multiple myeloma and macroglobulinemia; also used to assess response to immunizations
Complement system	C3: 75–150 mg/dL C4: 13–40 mg/dL	Diagnosis of systemic lupus erythematosus and other immunological disorders

Chronic Disease

Many chronic diseases are associated with compromised immune functioning. Diabetes, hepatic disorders, cancer, and aplastic anemia are just a few examples of diseases in which immune deficiencies occur. Because many critically ill patients have an underlying chronic disease, the existence and severity of such diseases should be considered contributing factors to immunocompromise when these patients are assessed.

Immunosuppressed States

Patients with leukemia, lymphoma, multiple myeloma, and other hematological conditions can experience impaired immunity and recurrent infections. Immunodeficiency states can be congenital or acquired. People with congenital immunodeficiencies frequently do not survive childhood. Immunodeficiency syndromes in adults may occur through a spontaneous defect in the immune system or through HIV infection (see Chapter 48).

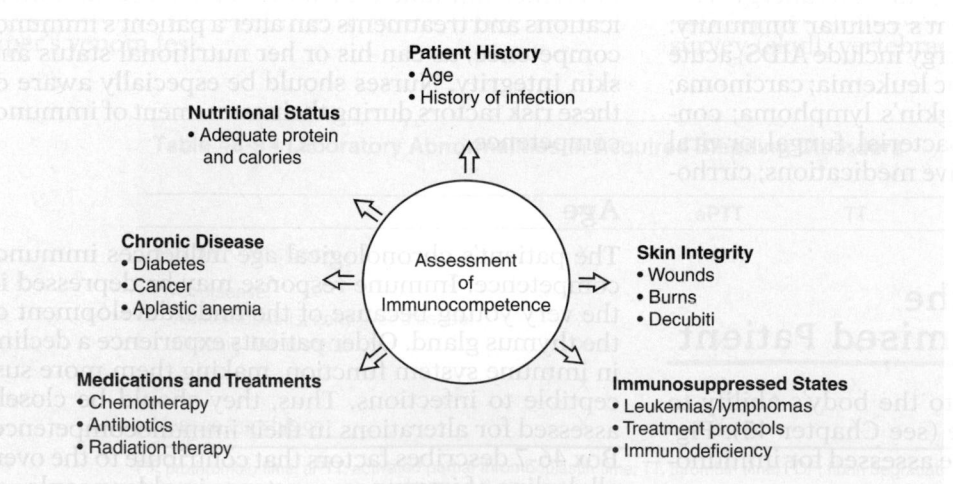

Patient History
• Age
• History of infection

Nutritional Status
• Adequate protein and calories

Chronic Disease
• Diabetes
• Cancer
• Aplastic anemia

Medications and Treatments
• Chemotherapy
• Antibiotics
• Radiation therapy

Assessment of Immunocompetence

Skin Integrity
• Wounds
• Burns
• Decubiti

Immunosuppressed States
• Leukemias/lymphomas
• Treatment protocols
• Immunodeficiency

Figure 46-4 • In addition to obtaining his or her history, assessment of the immunocompromised patient should cover six major areas.

Box 46-6 • RED FLAG: Signs of Early Septic Shock

- Fever
- Chills
- Confusion
- Irritability
- Tachycardia
- Tachypnea
- Decreased peripheral pulses
- Hypotension
- Warm, dry skin

Patients who are severely immunosuppressed have impaired responses to infectious agents and may not display the typical signs of infection. Fever and redness or pus at infection sites may be diminished because of the decreased numbers of WBCs required to promote these physical signs. Nurses should thus be extremely vigilant about monitoring for potential infection.

Medications and Treatments

Many medications affect immunocompetence. Antibiotics such as tetracycline and chloramphenicol impair bone marrow function.[8] Steroids display many immunological effects, including decreased lymphocyte and antibody concentration. Patients who have received organ or bone marrow transplants (see Chapter 47) often must remain on medications (e.g., cyclosporine) that severely suppress the immune system. Patients placed on treatment regimens with any immunosuppressive medications are monitored for early symptoms of infection that would indicate compromise in immune functioning.

Various treatments also impair immunocompetence. Treatment protocols for patients with cancer can lead to life-threatening complications, such as infection and sepsis. Biological therapy with inter-

feron-α and interleukin-2 can cause leukopenia. Patients who receive multiple transfusions with RBCs can demonstrate suppressed immunity. Most chemotherapeutic agents and radiation to the pelvis, spine, ribs, sternum, skull, and metaphyses of the long bones can adversely affect the bone marrow's ability to produce WBCs. The lowest point in WBC levels, or the nadir, may not be seen until several days or weeks after the initiation of treatment. The absolute neutrophil count (ANC) is calculated in neutropenic patients to determine the degree of immunosuppression. The ANC is calculated as follows:

1. Add segmented neutrophils and band neutrophils (from the WBC differential).
2. Multiply the total WBC count by the total obtained in step 1.

> Example:
>
> Segs = 42%
>
> Bands = 10%
>
> Total WBC count = 4,100 cells/mm³
>
> 42 + 10 = 52%
>
> 4,100 × 0.52 = 2,132 cells/mm³ (ANC)

Usually, protective measures, such as those summarized in Box 46-8, are instituted for patients with an ANC of less than 1,000 cells/mm³. However, all patients in the ICU are considered at risk for immunocompromise and should have the benefit of scrupulous handwashing, rigorous monitoring, and protective interventions.

Nutritional Status

The patient's nutritional status has a major impact on immune function. Inadequate intake of protein and calories can alter immune responses and resistance to infection by decreasing lymphocyte and antibody production as well as impairing wound healing. A multidisciplinary approach using a nutritionist can assist the nurse in assessing dietary intake and nutritional requirements for the critically ill immunocompromised person. Supplemental intravenous or enteral feedings may be necessary to prevent further deterioration of the body's nutritional status and ability to fight infection.

Skin Integrity

The integumentary system, including the skin and mucous membranes, provides a physical barrier to infection. Surgical or traumatic wounds, burn injuries, or pressure sores breach these physical defenses and predispose the critically ill patient to infection. Also, in a critical care setting in which intravenous and intra-arterial catheters, urethral catheters, or endotracheal tubes are used, multiple portals of entry for pathogens can provide simultaneous sites for potential infection. Therefore, all wounds and portals of entry should be carefully monitored for signs and symptoms of infection.

Box 46-7 • CONSIDERATIONS FOR THE OLDER PATIENT: Factors Contributing to Diminished Immunocompetence

- Decline in immune system functioning
- Decreased nutritional intake (decreased taste, poor teeth, declining appetite)
- Chronic illnesses (diabetes, chronic obstructive pulmonary disease, renal disease)
- Increased risk for malignancy
- Possible urinary incontinence
- Prostatic hypertrophy and urinary retention
- Skin breakdown and impaired wound healing
- Decreased ability to care for self
- Impaired communication
- Decreased mobility

47

Organ and Hematopoietic Stem Cell Transplantation

Sandra A. Mitchell • JoAnn Sikora

Objectives

Based on the content in this chapter, the reader should be able to:

❶ Analyze the criteria used to evaluate and prepare patients for transplantation.

❷ Evaluate the principles of organ and hematopoietic stem cell compatibility and immunosuppression.

❸ Discuss nursing assessment and management for patients undergoing solid organ transplantation (kidney, liver, heart, pancreas, lung) or hematopoietic stem cell transplantation.

❹ Describe the early- and late-phase complications of organ and hematopoietic stem cell transplantation.

Transplant research began in the early 1900s, but kidney transplantation did not become a realistic treatment for chronic renal failure in humans until the early 1950s. Heart and liver transplantations followed in the 1960s and have steadily increased in frequency as a treatment for end-stage organ failure since the 1980s. Pancreas transplantation also began in the mid-1960s and achieved good graft survival rates in the 1980s. The number of lung transplantations is small, primarily because of a lack of medically suitable donors. Table 47-1 gives survival rates for solid organ transplantations.

During the past 30 years, hematopoietic stem cell transplantation (HSCT) has evolved from an experimental treatment for patients with advanced acute leukemia into a therapeutically effective modality that is now standard therapy for selected diseases. HSCT, which is known to be curative in several malignant and nonmalignant disorders, is a transplantation using hematopoietic stem cells at various stages of differentiation and maturation. Decreased treatment-associated mortality and improved supportive care have helped make this possible.

Astute nursing care is essential to prevent treatment-related complications and death. Other factors that may affect the outcomes of HSCT include the type and stage of disease at the time of transplantation, the type of transplant (allogeneic versus autologous), the degree of human leukocyte antigen (HLA) matching in allogeneic transplants, the stem cell source, the intensity of the conditioning regimen, the ages of both the donor and the recipient,

Table 47-1 • Graft and Patient One-Year Survival Rates for Adult Solid Organ Transplants Performed in 2003–2004

Organ	Graft Survival Rate (%)	Patient Survival Rate (%)
Kidney—living donor	95	98
Kidney—deceased donor	90	95
Heart	88	88
Lung	83	85
Liver—living donor	84	91
Liver—deceased donor	82	87
Pancreas	73	95
Kidney-pancreas	92 (kidney); 85 (pancreas)	95
Intestine	79	88

Data from the 2006 Annual Report of the U.S. Organ Procurement and Transplantation Network and the Scientific Registry of Transplant Recipients: Transplant Data 1996–2005. Health Resources and Services Administration, Healthcare Systems Bureau, Division of Transplantation, Rockville, MD.

and the experience of the transplantation center. In general, the transplant-related mortality risk in allogeneic HSCT is about 20% to 30% higher than in autologous HSCT. The transplant-related mortality rate in autologous HSCT is less than 5% at most centers.

Even when a patient is cured of the original disease, he or she may experience delayed and long-term complications that can shorten or negatively affect the quality of his or her remaining life. These complications include infections, chronic graft-versus-host disease (GVHD; seen in allogeneic HSCT), thyroid dysfunction, pulmonary complications, cataracts, and the development of second malignancies. In general, autologous transplantation has fewer long-term complications, largely because no GVHD is associated with autologous transplantation. Disease-free survival

5 years after HSCT varies substantially, depending on the age of the recipient, the underlying disease, prognostic risk factors, disease status at the time of transplantation, the type of HSCT procedure, and the extent of prior treatment. Depending on these factors, disease-free survival rates vary from 10% to 75%[1-7] (Table 47-2). Advances in histocompatibility matching, immunosuppression, stem cell collection, and cryopreservation techniques, as well as the development of safer and less toxic conditioning regimens along with more effective drugs to manage posttransplantation infections and stimulate hematopoiesis, have helped increase the success of HSCT.[8]

This chapter describes the major aspects of care for patients receiving kidney, liver, heart, pancreas, and lung transplantations and HSCT. It covers principles

Table 47-2 • Disease-Free Survival 5 Years After Hematopoietic Stem Cell Transplantation

Disease and Stage	Allogeneic (% Survival)	Autologous (% Survival)
Acute myeloid leukemia		
First remission	45–70	40
First relapse, second or later remission	23–45	20–30
Refractory, multiply relapsed	10–15	<10
Acute lymphocytic leukemia		
First or second remission	30–60	40
Relapse	10	–
Chronic myelogenous leukemia		
Chronic phase	50–70	–
Accelerated or blastic phase	10–30	–
Aplastic anemia		
Untranfused	80–90	–
Transfused	50–70	–
Myelodysplastic syndrome	10–25	–
Hodgkin's lymphoma	–	50–80
Non-Hodgkin's lymphoma	40–50	30–60
Multiple myeloma	20–40	<10*

*15%–25% with tandem autologous transplantation
Data from Tabara et al: 2002; Barrett, Chao, Bishop: 2007; Pant, Copelan: 2007; and the National Marrow Donor Program. Available at: http://www.marrow.org.

that apply to all types of transplantation and discusses content unique to specific types of transplants.

• Indications for Transplantation

Many factors influence the indications and patient eligibility for transplantation. Currently, end-stage disease is the primary reason for most organ transplantations. HSCT is now used when bone marrow is defective or destroyed by a disease process or as a result of treating an underlying disease.[9] New information concerning patient outcomes, complications, surgical techniques, immunosuppressive drugs, and availability of organs and hematopoietic stem cells is also considered. Table 47-3 presents indications for transplantation.

• Patient Evaluation and Contraindications to Transplantation

Selecting the ideal candidate for transplantation is an intricate process. To evaluate a patient's suitability for transplantation, a comprehensive multisystem analysis is performed. This includes both physiological and psychosocial factors that affect the patient's chance for a successful transplantation. During this evaluation phase, treatment of newly diagnosed conditions occurs, and clinicians make plans to ensure adequate nutrition, mobility, and muscle strength. The goal is to have the patient in the best possible physical condition for transplantation. When transplantations are performed earlier rather than later in the disease process, there are fewer disabilities and a greater chance for survival.

Financial guidance is provided so that patients and families know what their insurance will cover and the nature and amount of their expected out-of-pocket expenses. Costs for transplantations range from $80,000 to $250,000. Medications after transplantation can cost $10,000 to $16,000 a year.[10–12] Transplantation centers may require proof of the patient's ability to cover their medication expenses before accepting a patient for transplantation.

The following general criteria guide the selection for transplantation:

▶ Age is evaluated individually. Ages may range from newborn (patients who may have heart transplantation for hypoplastic left heart syndrome) to 70 years. People older than 55 years of age may be at increased risk for complications.

▶ Acute or chronic infection is absent or has been treated. Localized liver infection may be an exception. Inflammatory diseases, such as systemic lupus erythematosus, do not rule out transplantation but should be quiescent at the time of the procedure.

▶ For the patient undergoing HSCT for a malignancy, care is taken to distinguish patients who can be

Table 47-3 • Indications for Transplantation

Organ	Indications for Transplantation	Common Causes
Kidney	End-stage renal disease	Hypertension, diabetes mellitus, glomerular nephritis, urological disorders, cancer, nephrotoxins, trauma, hemolytic disorders, congenital anomalies
Liver	Adults: irreversible liver disease, malignancy, and hepatic failure resulting in synthetic liver dysfunction Children: biliary atresia, α1-antitrypsin deficiency	Acute or chronic hepatitis, primary sclerosing cholangitis, primary biliary cirrhosis, hepatocellular carcinoma, Budd-Chiari syndrome, alcoholic cirrhosis
Heart	End-stage heart failure	Ischemic cardiomyopathy, idiopathic cardiomyopathy, valvular heart disease, congenital anomalies
Pancreas	Type 1 diabetes mellitus with end-stage renal disease either alone or in combination with a kidney transplant	Diabetes mellitus
Lung	Chronic obstructive pulmonary disease (COPD)	Emphysema and bronchiectasis, idiopathic pulmonary fibrosis, emphysema due to a1-antitrypsin deficiency, primary pulmonary hypertension
Heart–lung	Eisenmenger's syndrome	Pulmonary hypertension with irreversible right-sided heart failure not amenable to heart transplantation alone
Hematopoietic stem cell	Malignant disorders	Leukemias, myelodysplastic syndrome, Hodgkin's lymphoma, non-Hodgkin's lymphoma, multiple myeloma, and selected solid tumors (e.g., renal cell tumors, germ cell tumors, neuroblastoma, pinealoblastoma)[1]
	Nonmalignant disorders	Aplastic, sickle cell, and Fanconi's anemias; selected metabolic disorders; thalassemia; and immunodeficiency syndromes[1]

saved by transplantation from those who may relapse or succumb to the rigors and toxicities of treatment.

Table 47-4 lists organ-specific criteria for transplantation.

In general, evaluation common to all transplantations includes the following:

▶ ABO typing
▶ Tissue typing, HLA matching, mixed lymphocyte culture (MLC) matching
▶ Transfusion history
▶ Infectious disease screening (tuberculin skin test, human immunodeficiency virus [HIV], hepatitis B surface antigen, hepatitis C virus, Epstein-Barr virus, cytomegalovirus [CMV], toxoplasmosis titers, herpes simplex, varicella virus, venereal disease)
▶ Liver function studies
▶ Renal function studies
▶ Complete blood count (CBC)
▶ Coagulation studies
▶ Gastrointestinal evaluation (depending on age and history)
▶ Gynecological examination
▶ Electrocardiogram (ECG)
▶ Chest radiograph
▶ Dental examination to rule out infection
▶ Social history, review of patient motivation, ability to follow postoperative regimen, and psychiatric evaluation

Contraindications are based on conditions and behaviors that decrease the chance of survival. For solid organ transplantation, these include serious active infection or sepsis, recent cancer (unless that is the reason for transplantation), current substance abuse, HIV infection, severe cachexia, active peptic ulcer disease, psychiatric disorders that impair the ability to give informed consent or adhere to the treatment regimen, and repeated noncompliance. Table 47-4 lists these contraindications.

• Donor Selection

After a person is determined to be a candidate for transplantation, a donor source must be selected.

DETERMINING COMPATIBILITY
Organ Transplantation

Determination of compatibility in transplantation involves the evaluation of two major antigen systems. The primary determinant for solid organ transplantation is ABO grouping. A mismatch in compatibility may cause an immediate reaction leading to organ loss. The rules of compatibility that apply to the administration of blood products also apply to solid

organ transplantation: type A blood has the A antigen, type B blood has the B antigen, type AB blood has both A and B antigens, and type O blood has neither antigen.

Histocompatibility testing (tissue typing) is the identification of donor and recipient antigens and the evaluation of donor antigens against recipient antibodies. This evaluation determines the compatibility between donor and recipient, which predicts the chances of graft acceptance. In the HLA antigen system, genes of the major histocompatibility complex code for the antigens that compose a person's tissue type. These genes contain information for antigens present on the surface of the nucleated cells and serve to signal the immune system in differentiating self from nonself. The major histocompatibility complex involved in the immune response includes class I antigens (A, B) and class II (DR) antigens. Class I antigens (HLAs) are present on the surface of all nucleated cells and platelets, whereas class II antigens are found on the surface of lymphocytes. Each person has six A-, B-, and DR-locus antigens that are inherited as a haplotype (i.e., a single unit), receiving one HLA haplotype from each parent. Individuals have two HLA haplotypes, one for each chromosome. Offspring then share one haplotype with each parent, and on average, there is a one in four chance that they will share both haplotypes with at least one of their siblings. There is also a one in four chance that they will share neither haplotype with their siblings. Many possible alleles occur at each locus, resulting in a large number of HLA combinations. Therefore, it is rare that unrelated people have identical antigens.

The higher the number of antigens that match, the higher the likelihood of compatibility, and the lower the risk for rejection. A six-antigen match is associated with the greatest potential for successful transplantation. HLA matching is performed for both solid organ and hematopoietic stem cell transplants. It is most important in kidney and stem cell transplantation. Transplantation requires the suppression of the normal immune response with the postoperative administration of antirejection medications to prevent graft rejection. The greater the similarity of the donor and recipient tissue type, the less likely the occurrence of rejection.

In the case of living related donors, a direct white blood cell (WBC) cross-match may be performed. The sera of the donor and the recipient are tested and evaluated for cell death. For those patients not receiving living related donation, screening is routinely performed against a pool of lymphocyte samples from multiple random donors against the sera of the recipient. The percentage of samples to which the recipient reacts is referred to as the panel reactive antibody percentage (PRA). A high PRA is predictive of a high risk for rejection, and a prospective cross-match, such as is used in living donors, would be advised. PRA should be repeated monthly because the titer may change from time to time.

Blood transfusions are avoided if possible in patients awaiting organ transplantation because of the risk for antibody production and a resultant high

Table 47-4 • Criteria, Contraindications, and Evaluations in Transplantation

Organ	Specific Criteria	Contraindications	Specific Evaluation
Kidney	• End-stage or near end-stage renal failure (defined as a glomerular filtration rate of <10 mL/min) • Pre–end stage preferable for some patients (i.e., children, patients with diabetes mellitus, and those for whom there is a living donor)	• Severe or uncorrectable coronary artery disease, peripheral vascular disease, or pulmonary disease • Severe cardiomyopathy	• Voiding cystourethrogram to evaluate for obstruction or reflux (medical history dependent) • Cardiac evaluation (age and medical history dependent)
Liver	• Malnutrition • Severe blood clotting abnormalities • Variceal bleeding • Hepatic encephalopathy • Severe, intractable ascites • Severe, intractable pruritus	• Multiple uncorrected congenital anomalies • Advanced cardiopulmonary disease • Severe pulmonary hypertension	• Abdominal computed tomography (CT) scan (to detect hepatoma) • Doppler ultrasound (to identify patency of portal vein) • Liver disease studies and auto-immune markers, such as cerulo-plasmin, carcinoembryonic antigen (CEA), alpha-fetoprotein (AFP), antimitochondrial and antinuclear antibody • Endoscopic retrograde cholangio-pancreatography (ERCP)/cholangiogram (if indicated, usually for patients with cholestasis) • Liver biopsy (if indicated) • Upper and lower endoscopy (if indicated)
Pancreas	• End-stage renal failure (combine kidney and pancreas transplant) • Absence of (or corrected) coronary artery disease	• Severe or uncorrectable coronary artery disease, peripheral vascular disease, or pulmonary disease • Previous major amputation • Blindness (not absolute contraindication) • Severe cardiomyopathy	• Thallium stress test or coronary angiogram • Cardiology consult • Gastric emptying study • Ophthalmology evaluation • Endocrine studies: glycosylated hemo-globin, serum amylase and lipase, islet cell antibody, urine and serum peptide measurements
Heart	• Cardiac disease, New York Heart Association Class IV (or advanced III) • Condition not amenable to other forms of medical or surgical therapy • End-stage cardiac disease with less than a 25% likelihood of survival at 1 year without a transplant • Patients with potentially fatal arrhythmia not amenable to other therapies	• Fixed pulmonary hypertension with pulmonary vascular resistance: >6–8 Wood units (>480–640 dynse/sec/cm^{-5} or pulmonary arteriolar gradient >15 mm) • Recent unresolved pulmonary infarct (increased post-transplant risk for pulmonary infection) • Advanced or poorly controlled diabetes mellitus	• Right heart catheterization; full cardiac catheterization if indicated • Cardiopulmonary exercise testing (MVO$_2$) • Pulmonary function tests, including diffusion capacity (DLCO) • Cardiac rehabilitation consultation • Multigated acquisition analysis (MUGA) or echocardiogram
Lung	• Untreatable end-stage pulmonary disease (parenchymal or vascular) • Medical therapy ineffective • Estimated survival (without lung trans-plant) less than probability of survival with lung transplant	• Significant coronary artery disease • Poor nutritional status (i.e., <10%–15% of ideal body weight) • Previous cardiothoracic surgery • Corticosteroid use >15 mg/d • Ventilation dependency	• Quantitative ventilation/perfusion scan • Cardiac evaluation • Full pulmonary function testing, including DLCO, arterial blood gases, lung volume • 6-min walk test (rehabilitation assessment) • Nutritional assessment
Hematopoietic stem cells	• **Malignant disorders:** replacement of hematopoietic and immune system destroyed by high-dose chemother-apy or radiation with new immune sys-tem that can recognize malignant cells as foreign and mount immuno-logic response against tumor	• Poor or no response to conventional-dose chemotherapy for malignant disorders (exception is acute leukemia that fails to respond to induction therapy [primary induction failure]; high-dose chemotherapy and allogeneic transplant is an accepted indication)	• Disease restaging, including CT scans, nuclear medicine scans, bone marrow aspirate and biopsy, lumbar puncture, immunoglobulin levels, cytogenetics, molecular diagnostics, and measures of minimal residual disease • DNA procurement for future engraft-ment studies

(continued)

Table 47-4 • Criteria, Contraindications, and Evaluations in Transplantation (Continued)

Organ	Specific Criteria	Contraindications	Specific Evaluation
	• **Nonmalignant disorders:** replacement of an immune or hematopoietic system that is either defective or has failed	• Poor performance status (using Karnofsky Performance Status scale to assess physical functioning) • Advanced cardiopulmonary or renal disease (left ventricular ejection fraction [LVEF] <50%; DLco <70; creatinine clearance, 60 mL/min [exception may be multiple myeloma patients]) • Brain metastasis • Age >70 years	• ABO and Rh typing • HLA typing and HLA-matched platelet transfusion support (allogeneic transplant patients only) • Chest x-ray, ECG and MUGA scan, pulmonary function tests, including DLCO, 24-hour urine for creatinine clearance • Baseline CT scans of chest and sinuses, particularly if there are symptoms or a history of repeated infections • Dental evaluation, including full mouth x-rays and cleaning • Sperm/fertilized embryo banking • Autologous stem cell backup if patient is undergoing unrelated or mismatched transplantation • Consultations with radiation therapy and infectious disease

PRA or positive cross-match between donor and recipient. If blood transfusions are necessary, leukocyte-filtered blood should be administered.

Hematopoietic Stem Cell Transplantation

Selection of a donor for HSCT is based on the type and stage of the underlying disease, age, comorbidities, and availability of an appropriate HLA- and MLC-matched donor. MLC matching is performed to observe for interaction between the potential donor's cells and recipient cells. Low reactivity indicates greater compatibility.

There are many sources of hematopoietic stem cells. The types of HSCT may be differentiated in terms of the hematopoietic stem cell donor, the method used to collect the cells, and the intensity of the conditioning regimen (Box 47-1).

For patients who receive hematopoietic stem cells from another person (i.e., allogeneic transplant), donor selection is based on the availability of HLA- and MLC-matched donors, who may or may not be related. A related donor is usually a sibling (siblings have the greatest chance of matching on both HLA and on other minor and as yet unrecognized antigens). If more than one donor is HLA-identical to the patient, donor selection is based on sex compatibility with the patient, ABO compatibility with the patient, negative viral titers, overall health, younger donor age, minimal donor exposure to blood products, and donor nulliparity, because all these factors are associated with an improved outcome of HSCT.

If the patient does not have a suitable family donor, a search for an unrelated donor may be undertaken. The National Marrow Donor Program (NMDP), a donor registry developed in 1986, allows patients without a related donor to find an HLA-matched unrelated donor (Box 47-2). Umbilical cord blood is another

potential stem cell source, particularly in pediatric allogeneic transplantation.

A difference in ABO blood groups between patient and donor does not interfere with donor selection; however, it does present unique clinical problems. The hematopoietic stem cell product may have to be

---

Box 47-1 • Types of Hematopoietic Stem Cell Transplantation

Differentiated based on *donor* source for stem cells
- *Autologous*—self
- *Syngeneic*—identical twin
- *Allogeneic*—non-self
  - Related
  - Unrelated (National Marrow Donor Program)
- *Cord blood*
  - Related
  - Unrelated (cord blood bank)

Differentiated based on *method* of collecting stem cell
- Bone marrow harvest
- Peripheral blood stem cell collection by apheresis

Differentiated based on *intensity* of conditioning regimen
- Myeloablative: high doses of chemotherapy and sometimes radiation therapy given to destroy hematopoietic and immune systems of recipient. Transplantation of new stem cells allows hematopoietic and immune reconstitution. High morbidity and mortality rates restrict this treatment to younger patients and those in good medical condition.
- Reduced intensity: lower chemotherapy doses (those that do not fully destroy patient's own hematopoietic and immune systems) are given along with immunosuppression to facilitate engraftment of donor hematopoietic cells. Significant long-term risks for infection and chronic graft-versus-host disease persist.

determine appropriate intervention. An ECG and echocardiogram are required for heart donation, and serial chest radiographs, sputum for Gram stain, bronchoscopy, and visual inspection at the time of organ procurement are required for lung donation.

Role of the Donor Coordinator

The role of the donor coordinator has developed as a result of the disparity between potential donors and the numbers of patients awaiting organ donation. The donor coordinator allows for the introduction of the concept of organ donation by a nurse not associated with transplantation. This approach results in the highest rates of consent.[15] Kidneys are the most commonly transplanted organ, and heart, lung, liver, pancreas, intestine, cornea, skin, bone, and other organs or tissue may also be donated. The donor coordinator is involved in the coordination and procurement of all transplantable organs. In addition, the donor coordinator usually ensures that the family has the information necessary to give informed consent and provides them with access to bereavement support. The donor coordinator also serves as a resource for the health care team and as a liaison between the transplantation program and the critical care area. Cooperation between the critical care staff and the transplantation program helps ensure that the option of donation is offered to families of all potential donors.

It is important that all potential organ donors be identified. Potential donors often are victims of trauma or cerebral aneurysm or a variety of other circumstances. Criteria for organ donation vary widely. Therefore, it is recommended that any patient for whom the possibility of donation is considered be referred to the local OPO (to find a local OPO visit www.transweb.org/reference/maps/opo).

Preservation Time

There is a broad range of acceptable preservation times for organs. However, the goal is to transplant organs as soon as possible. Kidneys can be stored for up to 48 hours using pulsatile perfusion preservation and for 24 to 36 hours using cold storage. Livers can be stored for up to 20 hours, pancreata up to 12 hours, and hearts and lungs for 4 to 6 hours. To decrease cellular injury, organs are stored in a solution and kept in ice. The preservative solutions used are different for each organ and are based on the metabolic needs of the organ, with center-specific variability. The focus of preservation is to protect the organ from ischemic injury.[18]

• Assessment and Management in Organ Transplantation

The role of the transplant coordinator extends across the continuum of care from pre-evaluation of potential recipients through transplantation and follow-up. This person is responsible for coordinating the

evaluation and teaching the recipient and family about the evaluation testing process, the listing process, and organ allocation. A major contribution is reviewing preoperative through postoperative procedures, the immunosuppressive regimen, and follow-up care. In many institutions, a nurse practitioner, who also provides medical care and follow-up for the patients, fulfills this role.

PREOPERATIVE PHASE

The immediate preoperative phase, which is usually only a matter of hours, includes comprehensive laboratory studies, chest radiograph, ECG, and, for kidney transplant recipients, dialysis within 24 hours of transplantation. Laboratory studies usually include CBC, prothrombin time (PT), partial thromboplastin time (PTT), electrolytes, blood sugar, blood urea nitrogen (BUN), creatinine, liver function tests, type and cross-match, and urinalysis.

SURGICAL PROCEDURE

Kidney

Typically, the kidney is placed retroperitoneally in the iliac fossa. The hypogastric or internal artery and the external iliac vein are usually used for vascular anastomosis. When it is mechanically difficult to access these vessels, as with children, it may be necessary to anastomose the renal vessels to the inferior vena cava and aorta.

Two common types of ureteral anastomoses can be performed. In the first procedure, the donor ureter is implanted into the recipient's bladder by a vertical cystotomy and a submucosal antireflux tunnel because the ureter lacks innervation and normal peristalsis. In the second type, used less frequently, the donor kidney is anastomosed at the ureteropelvic junction to the recipient ureter. An indwelling catheter is used for both types of anastomoses, and occasionally a ureteral stent may be used. In either case, hematuria is present for several days. In the first, more common procedure, clots may be seen in the urine because of the vascular nature of the bladder. In the second, less common, procedure, the urine changes to pink within the first postoperative day because there are no sutures in the bladder.

Liver

The liver is transplanted orthotopically, that is, in its normal position after the native liver is removed. Four vascular anastomoses must be performed: the suprahepatic vena cava, the infrahepatic vena cava, the portal vein, and the hepatic artery (Fig. 47-1). Then the liver is reperfused, and the bile duct is anastomosed, usually to the recipient bile duct.[19] A T tube is usually inserted. During liver transplantation, a rapid infusion system is used for administering blood and blood products, a cell saver is often used to limit the amount of banked blood required, and a pump for venovenous bypass is often used in adults to return blood to the heart. This is performed by inserting

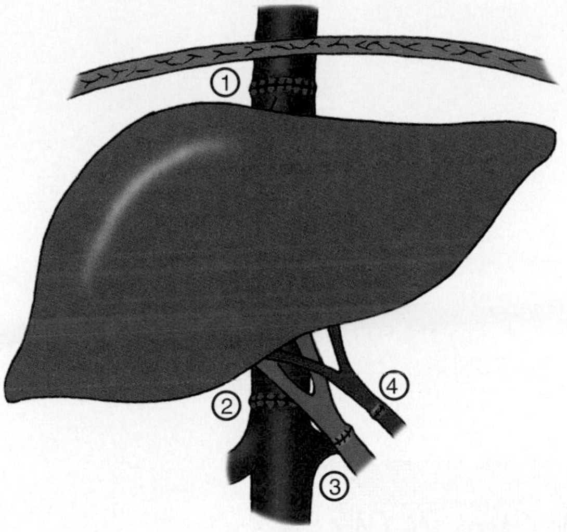

Figure 47-1 • Diagram of vascular anastomoses in liver transplantation: (1) suprahepatic vena cava; (2) infrahepatic vena cava; (3) portal vein; and (4) hepatic artery.

a catheter into the saphenous or femoral vein and another into the axillary vein (usually on the left side), which allows blood to circulate from the lower extremities back to the heart. Surgery usually takes between 8 and 16 hours.

Heart

Orthotopic Transplantation

Orthotopic heart transplantation (OHT) is the most common heart transplantation performed. The recipient's heart is excised, and the donor heart is implanted in its place. A median sternotomy incision is made, cardiopulmonary bypass is initiated, and the recipient's heart is removed by incising the left and right atria, pulmonary artery, and aorta. The Lower and Shumway technique has been the gold standard for OHT. The atrial septum and posterior and lateral walls of the recipient's atria are left intact, including the areas of the sinoatrial node, inferior and superior venac cavae to the right atrium, and pulmonary veins to the left atrium. The remnant atria serve as anchors for the donor heart.

The donor atria are trimmed to preserve the anterior arterial walls, sinoatrial node, and internodal conduction pathways. Then anastomoses are made between the recipient and donor left and right atria, the pulmonary arteries, and the aortas. Atrial and ventricular pacing wires are placed at the time of surgery so that temporary pacing can easily be initiated. Cardiopulmonary bypass is weaned off, and the donor heart assumes the role of providing the cardiac output (Fig. 47-2A).

An alternative to the atrial-to-atrial cuff technique is the bicaval technique (see Fig. 47-2B), which preserves atrial anatomy disrupted by the Lower and Shumway technique. The donor atria are intact, and the anastomoses are between the donor and recipient inferior and superior venae cavae rather than the atria. This avoids the loss of atrial anatomy, which

has been demonstrated to be responsible for the development of post-transplantation complications such as mitral and tricuspid regurgitation, atrial thrombus formation, and tachydysrhythmia.[20]

Heterotopic Transplantation

Heterotopic transplantation, or piggyback procedure, is an infrequently used technique. The recipient's heart is left in place, and the donor heart is placed next to it in the right chest. The two hearts are connected in parallel by anastomoses made between the donor and recipient left and right atria, aortas, and pulmonary arteries using a synthetic tube graft. By allowing blood to flow through either or both hearts, two functional hearts work together to provide the cardiac output (Fig. 47-3).

Heterotopic transplantation may be used in patients with pulmonary hypertension in whom the donor heart alone would not have a strong enough right ventricle to pump against the increased pulmonary vascular resistance. It can also be used as a life-saving procedure in urgent cases if the only available donor heart is too small for the size of the recipient. Limitations of heterotopic transplantation include thromboembolism from the native heart with need for anticoagulation, limited space in the chest cavity, and, in ischemic heart disease, ongoing angina and the possibility of ischemia-induced dysrhythmias in the native heart. The survival rates are less favorable for heterotopic transplantation than for orthotopic transplantation.

Pancreas

Transplantation of the entire pancreas is performed most commonly. Pancreas transplantation may be performed in combination with kidney transplantation for recipients with end-stage renal disease secondary to diabetes mellitus. The pancreas and kidney may be transplanted at the same time or months apart. Clinical trials are ongoing to determine the feasibility and outcomes of islet cell transplantation for patients with type 1 diabetes not controlled with insulin. With this experimental procedure, only the insulin-producing islet cells are transplanted. The recipient still requires immunosuppressive medications to prevent rejection.

The pancreas is placed into a heterotopic position, usually the right iliac area. Techniques vary for vascular and exocrine anastomoses. The most controversial aspect of the surgical technique is the approach for draining exocrine secretions. The exocrine duct may be occluded, or exocrine secretions may drain either into the small bowel or bladder. There is no consensus about the best approach, and all have advantages and disadvantages.

Lung

Both single- and double-lung transplantations are performed. In single-lung transplantations, the left lung mainstem bronchus is longer, which makes the procedure easier technically. The preferred lung is based on perfusion abnormalities (as determined by

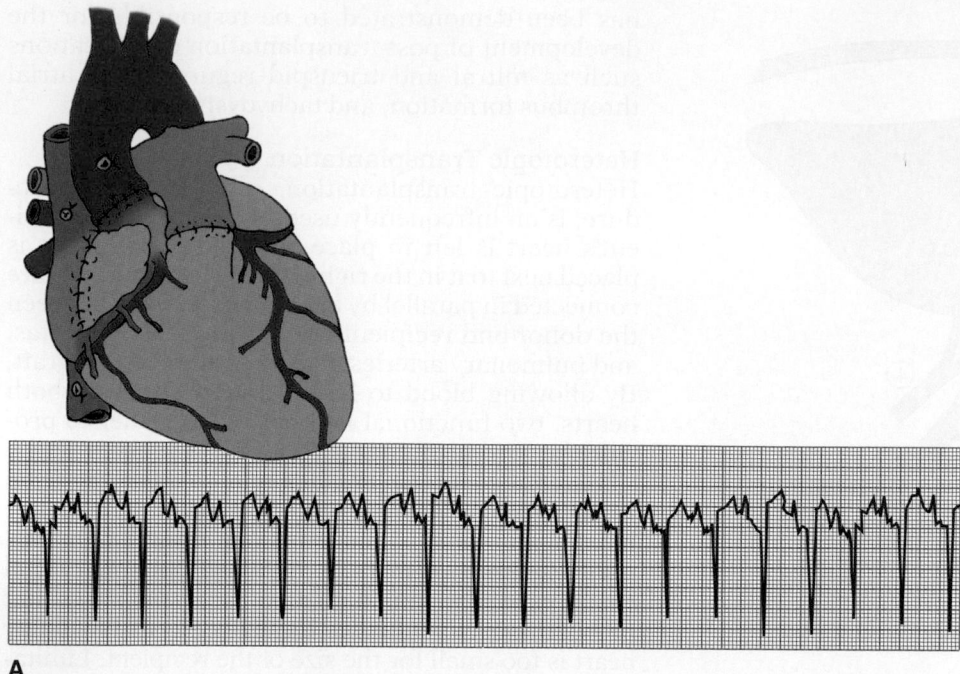

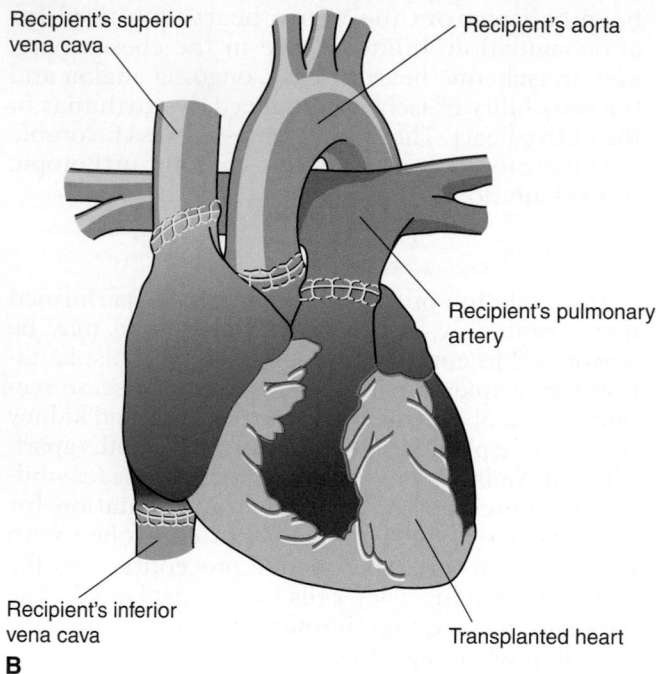

Recipient's superior vena cava

Recipient's aorta

Recipient's pulmonary artery

Recipient's inferior vena cava

Transplanted heart

B

Figure 47-2 • Orthotopic method of transplantation. **A:** Lower and Shumway technique. Both the donor and the recipient sino-atrial nodes are intact (X), resulting in the electrocardiogram tracing. Note the double P wave at the independent rates. **B:** Bicaval technique. The anastomoses are made between the inferior and superior venae cavae rather than the atria. (**B** from Smeltzer SC, Bare BG, Hinkle JL, Cheever KH: Brunner and Suddarth's Textbook of Medical-Surgical Nursing, 11th ed. Philadelphia: Lippincott Williams & Wilkins, 2008, p 929.)

ventilation–perfusion scan) and functional abnormalities. Anastomoses are made at the mainstem bronchus, pulmonary artery, and cuff of atrium containing pulmonary veins. Cardiopulmonary bypass is not always necessary and depends on the patient's pulmonary artery pressure, blood pressure, and gas exchange. Incision is made at the fifth intracostal space using a posterior lateral thoracotomy for single-lung transplantations, whereas a median sternotomy incision or a clamshell incision is made for double-lung transplantations. Surgeons telescope the recipient's bronchus into the donor lung or vice versa, or perform an end-to-end anastomosis with omentopexy in which an omental flap is wrapped around

the tracheal anastomosis to increase blood supply to the area.

POSTOPERATIVE PHASE

Immediately after surgery, transplant recipients require care in a closely monitored area until stable. Kidney transplant recipients often go to a postanesthesia care unit and then directly to a transplant unit. Other organ recipients go to an intensive care unit (ICU) from the operating room. When a patient arrives in the postanesthesia or intensive care area, the nurse makes the following assessments:

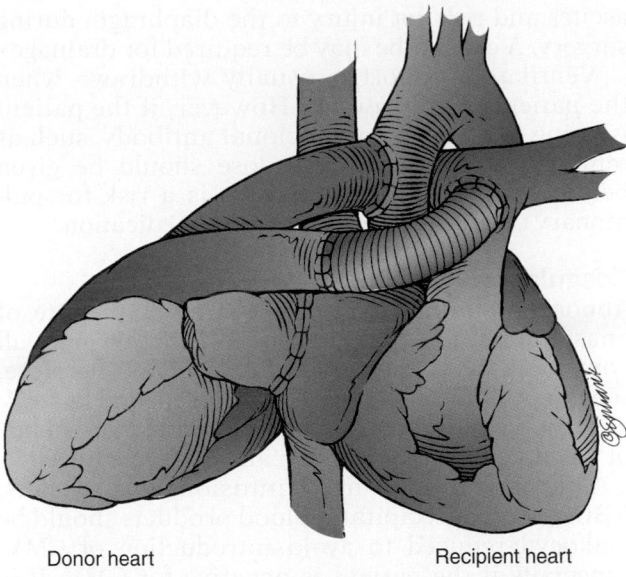

Donor heart   Recipient heart

Figure 47-3 • Heterotopic method of heart transplantation. The donor heart is anastomosed with a Dacron graft to the recipient's heart, resulting in this electrocardiogram tracing. Note the "extra" QRS at an independent rate. (From Smeltzer SC, Bare BG: Brunner and Suddarth's Textbook of Medical-Surgical Nursing, 10th ed. Philadelphia: Lippincott Williams & Wilkins, 2004, p 775.)

▶ Blood pressure, heart rate, respirations, oxygenation and ventilator settings, temperature, central venous pressure, and cardiopulmonary hemodynamics. In renal transplant recipients, it is necessary to take blood pressure on an extremity that does not have a functioning vascular access site because even momentary interference with arterial blood flow may lead to access malfunction.

▶ Patient's level of consciousness and degree of pain

▶ Number of intravenous and arterial lines, noting the site, type of solution, and flow rate

▶ Abdominal or chest dressing for drainage, noting the presence of drains and amount and type of drainage

▶ Presence of bladder and possible ureteral catheters and patency and urinary drainage

▶ Attachment of nasogastric tube to appropriate drainage system and amount and character of drainage

▶ Most recent hemodynamic and intraoperative laboratory results

Kidney

Care of the kidney transplant recipient emphasizes assessing renal function and administering immunosuppressive therapy. Therefore, answers to the following questions help guide care:

▶ Are the patient's own kidneys present in addition to the graft, and if so, how much urine do they produce daily? This information helps determine how much urine is from the transplanted kidney.

▶ What are the preoperative results of laboratory tests (BUN, creatinine, hematocrit)?

▶ How much and what kind of intravenous fluid has the patient received?

▶ What immunosuppressive drugs were given before or during surgery? What immunosuppressive therapy should be given after surgery?

Nursing responsibilities also involve the following:

▶ Observing the function of the transplanted kidney

▶ Monitoring fluid and electrolyte balance

▶ Helping avoid sources of infection

▶ Detecting early signs of complications

▶ Supporting the patient and family through the recovery phase

In addition, at regular intervals, the nurse evaluates the patency and the vascular access used for dialysis. This is done by placing either fingers or a stethoscope directly over the access site and feeling or listening for a characteristically loud, pulsating noise called a *bruit*. If the patient has been maintained on peritoneal dialysis and the catheter is in place, it is essential that the catheter system is sterile and capped.

Renal Graft Function

The amount of urine produced by the transplanted kidney varies from a large amount (200 to 1,000 mL/hour) to small amounts (<20 mL/hour). The degree of renal function is related to ischemic injury in the donor kidney, usually from either hypotensive periods in a cadaveric donor or from the time the kidney is stored outside the body (preservation time). Renal function is better when kidney preservation time is less than 24 hours. Most post-transplantation dysfunction is reversible but may take up to 4 weeks to return to normal.

Assessments of renal function include periodic blood urea nitrogen and creatinine levels and, in some centers, a β_2-microglobulin level. The glomerular basement membrane readily filters this low–molecular-weight globulin, which the proximal renal tubules reabsorb and metabolize almost completely.

A renal scan is a radionuclide test used to determine renal perfusion, filtration, and excretion. It is usually performed in the first 24 hours to obtain baseline data and then periodically thereafter when laboratory values or clinical changes suggest an alteration in renal function.

Urinary Drainage Problems

When a change in urinary output occurs, such as a large volume one hour and a diminished amount the next, mechanical factors that interfere with urinary drainage should be suspected. Clotted, kinked, or compressed tubing in the urinary drainage system may be the cause of the decreased output. When the catheter is occluded by a clot, the patient may complain of pain, feel an urgency to void, or have bloody leakage around the catheter. Milking is the preferred way to dislodge clots because irrigation, even under aseptic conditions, increases the risk for infection. However, gentle irrigation with strict aseptic technique may be necessary. Small amounts of irrigant (≤30 mL) are recommended because patients commonly have small bladders. Vigorous irrigation also could cause extravasation at the ureteral anastomosis site.

Urinary Leakage

Urinary leakage on the abdominal dressing and severe abdominal discomfort or distention may indicate retroperitoneal leakage from the ureteral anastomosis site. It is important to report decreased urinary output or severe abdominal pain in the presence of good renal function and adequate pain medication because technical and surgical complications can result in loss of graft function.

Hyperkalemia

The most frequent electrolyte disturbance in the acute postoperative phase is hyperkalemia. If the graft functions and excretes a high volume of urine, it is usually also able to excrete the excessive serum potassium created by surgical tissue damage. If the patient is oliguric or anuric after surgery, the serum potassium may increase to unacceptable levels. Interventions include administration of glucose and insulin to transport potassium into the cell and administration of oral polystyrene sulfonate.

Liver

Immediate postoperative care is focused on hemodynamic stability, adequate oxygenation, fluid and electrolyte balance, adequate hemostasis, and graft function. An arterial line and pulmonary artery catheter are in place. The pulmonary artery catheter readings help monitor cardiac function and fluid status because high cardiac output and low systemic vascular resistance related to the effects of end-stage liver disease continue immediately after surgery.

Vasopressors and additional fluid boluses may be required in the first 24 to 36 hours. Central venous pressure should be maintained at greater than 10 cm H_2O to balance the importance of good cardiac function against the risk for passive congestion of the liver. Hypotension is most often caused by intra-abdominal bleeding. An increase in abdominal girth or excess bloody drainage from Jackson-Pratt drains is indicative of a severe problem.

Oxygenation

Adequate ventilation is crucial for graft perfusion and helps reduce the risk for pulmonary complications. The critical care team determines ventilator settings, and the nurse monitors the arterial (SaO_2) and mixed venous (SvO_2) oxygen saturations. Pulse oximetry may be used, but severe jaundice may interfere with saturation measurements. Postoperative pleural effusion is common owing to the presence of

ascites and risk got injury to the diaphragm during surgery. A chest tube may be required for drainage.

Ventilator support is usually withdrawn when the patient is fully awake. However, if the patient is going to receive a monoclonal antibody, such as muromonab-CD3, the first dose should be given before extubation because there is a risk for pulmonary edema as a reaction to the medication.

Coagulation

Abnormal clotting factors, bleeding at the site of anastomosis, and impaired graft function may all contribute to problems with hemostasis. Therefore, the nurse monitors PT, PTT, fibrinogen, and factor V level along with the amount, color, and consistency of bleeding from the incision and drainage tubes.

The patient may need infusions of platelets, RBCs, or cryoprecipitate. Blood products should be leukocyte-reduced to avoid introduction of CMV, especially if the patient is negative for CMV. It is necessary to take care to avoid overcorrecting coagulation deficiencies, which could lead to vascular thrombosis of the extremities or the graft. As a result of the venovenous bypass system, there is also a risk for phlebitis or thrombosis in the femoral and axillary access site. This may be indicated by ipsilateral swelling in these extremities. Anticoagulation or an inferior vena cava filter may be necessary if deep venous thrombosis develops.

Electrolyte Balance

Hyperglycemia; hyperkalemia; metabolic alkalosis; and calcium, phosphorus, and magnesium disorders may occur. Hyperglycemia is an indication that the liver is able to store glycogen and convert it to glucose. Hyperkalemia can indicate nonfunctional hepatocytes and, in turn, a nonfunctional graft. Metabolic alkalosis is related to the citrate in stored blood (metabolized to bicarbonate), hypokalemia, diuretic therapy, and the administration of large volumes of fresh frozen plasma. This usually resolves spontaneously, but hypoventilation in response to the alkalosis may slow weaning from mechanical ventilation. Calcium, phosphorus, and magnesium disturbances are primarily due to the administration of fluid and blood products.

Some degree of postoperative renal dysfunction is also common due either to hepatorenal syndrome or hypotension during surgery. In addition, some immunosuppressive medications are nephrotoxic. This can affect fluid and electrolyte balance. On occasion, when dialysis is needed, continuous arteriovenous or venovenous hemofiltration is used because it interferes least with hemodynamic stability.

Liver Function

Function of the transplanted liver can range from excellent to primary nonfunction. Although the cause of primary nonfunction is not known, it is believed to be related to preservation injury, and retransplantation is necessary. Liver function is initially assessed by bile production, coagulation factors, and later by liver function tests. Measuring bile production from the biliary drainage tube helps assess the excretory function of the liver and is a good early indicator of graft function. PT and the international normalized ratio (INR) provide a measure of the synthetic function of the liver. Aminotransferases (alanine aminotransferase and aspartate aminotransferase) provide information about the degree of hepatic injury related to preservation. In addition, improvement in the clearance of lactate, encephalopathy, and glucose metabolism are also assessments of liver function. All liver function test results are elevated initially and gradually decrease.

Heart

Postoperative care of the heart transplant recipient is similar to that for any person undergoing cardiac surgery. However, there are several major differences, including changes in cardiac rhythm and function caused by denervation of the donor heart and the potential for right ventricular failure. Only the more common orthotopic transplantation is discussed here.

Remnant P Waves

In the standard atrial cuff technique, the recipient sinoatrial node and portions of the recipient atria are left intact at the time of surgery. Therefore, two P waves are usually seen on the ECG. The recipient sinoatrial node initiates an impulse that depolarizes the remnant recipient atria; however, this depolarization wave usually does not cross the atrial suture line. The donor sinoatrial node initiates the impulse that causes depolarization of the entire donor heart and elicits the QRS complex. Because the two sets of atria beat independently of each other, two different P waves may appear on the ECG. Remnant P waves may be identified by their dissociation or lack of relationship to the QRS complexes. They usually occur at a slower rate than the donor P waves, and their rate may speed up or slow down because the remnant P waves are still under autonomic nervous system influence, whereas the donor P waves are denervated. The two sets of atria may also be in different rhythms. For example, the recipient atrial remnants may be in atrial fibrillation while the donor heart is in normal sinus rhythm.

Effects of Denervation

During removal of the donor heart, the nerve supply is severed, resulting in a lack of autonomic nervous system innervation of the transplanted heart. Because of the loss of vagal influence, the resting sinus rate is higher than normal—usually between 90 and 110 beats/minute—and heart rate variations due to respiration do not occur.

Decreased donor sinoatrial node automaticity can also occur after transplantation as a result of injury to the node during procurement, transport, surgical procedure, or postoperative edema of the atrial suture line. Usually, these problems resolve within 1 to 2 weeks after transplantation, but temporary pacing may be needed to maintain an adequate heart rate. Atropine, which blocks vagal stimulation, is ineffective in treating bradydysrhythmias in the transplanted heart because there is no parasympathetic innerva-tion. If the sinus rate is reduced, junctional rhythms can occur earlier than normal because of the loss of vagal tone.

Normal cardiovascular reflexes are also removed by denervation. In the normal heart, increased body metabolic demands cause direct compensatory stimulation of the heart by the sympathetic nervous system, which immediately increases heart rate, contractility, and cardiac output. Because direct sympathetic nervous system stimulation of the transplanted heart is absent, this response is mediated through release of circulating catecholamines from the adrenal medulla. Therefore, increases in heart rate, contractility, and cardiac output occur much more slowly than normal. With exercise, heart rate and cardiac output increase gradually over 3 to 5 minutes and remain elevated longer after exercise. Prolonged warm-up before and cool-down after exercise help compensate for these changes.

Orthostatic hypotension can occur because the normal, immediate reflex tachycardia, which compensates for venous pooling with position change, does not occur. When patients begin ambulating, they should be cautioned to change position gradually to prevent orthostatic hypotension.

Because of denervation, the cardiac effects of medications normally mediated by the autonomic nervous system are abnormal. Atropine, which increases heart rate by blocking parasympathetic influence, is ineffective. Isoproterenol, a positive chronotropic agent, has been widely used because it stimulates myocardial receptors directly for pharmacological management of symptomatic bradydysrhythmias. However, isoproterenol is not widely available. Instead, dobutamine and epinephrine, along with temporary epicardial pacing, are frequently used.

Digitalis preparations are ineffective in decreasing the heart rate or increasing the atrioventricular nodal refractory period because these effects are mediated primarily by the parasympathetic nervous system. Digitalis does increase myocardial contractility by its direct action on myocardial cells. β-Blocking drugs or calcium channel blockers (e.g., verapamil) can be used to control supraventricular tachydysrhythmias in the transplanted heart; carotid sinus pressure, the Valsalva maneuver, and digitalis are ineffective.

Finally, denervation prevents transmission of pain impulses from ischemic myocardium to the brain, so the patient does not experience angina. Severe myocardial ischemia or infarction may go unnoticed. For this reason, ECG stress testing and annual coronary angiography or coronary vascular ultrasonography are usually performed.

Potential for Ventricular Failure

Post-transplantation ventricular failure, causing decreased cardiac output, occurs for the same reasons as in other cardiac surgical procedures. In addition, a prolonged ischemia time, inotropic support of the donor, or rejection can cause myocardial depression in a transplant recipient.

Right ventricular failure is the most common cause of primary graft failure after transplantation. Reasons for right-sided heart dysfunction are not entirely clear but are related to acute changes in pulmonary vascular resistance. The newly transplanted heart is required to work against elevated pulmonary pressures secondary to long-standing heart failure in the recipient.[21] Postoperative changes in pH or ABGs can cause pulmonary vascular spasm. Both pulmonary hypertension and spasm increase the pulmonary vascular resistance or resistance to ejection of blood by the right ventricle. The normal right ventricle of the donor heart may be unable to increase its output acutely to overcome a high preexisting pulmonary vascular resistance. Signs of acute right ventricular failure include elevated central venous pressure and jugular venous distention. Left ventricular cardiac output decreases because the right ventricle is unable to pump enough blood through the lungs.

Treatment of post-transplantation right-sided heart failure involves the use of drugs to decrease right heart afterload (dobutamine, milrinone, inhaled nitric oxide). Inhaled nitric oxide, a direct pulmonary vasodilator, may be administered through the ventilator circuit, thereby avoiding the systemic affects of the drugs that are administered intravenously. Conditions that increase right heart afterload (e.g., hypoxia, acidosis, excessive blood transfusions) should be avoided.

Pancreas

The critical care of a pancreas transplant recipient is comparable to the critical care of any patient who has had major abdominal surgery. The differences relate to pancreatic function, the type of surgical procedure, and secondary effects of diabetes mellitus.

Blood glucose response usually returns within the first few postoperative hours; however, an insulin drip may be required until blood glucose is normal. Pancreatic function is monitored by glucose levels before and after meals, by the results of glycosylated hemoglobin, and sometimes by glucose tolerance testing. Even minor abnormalities may indicate rejection or vascular thrombosis of the graft.

When a section of duodenum is used for exocrine drainage, the prevention of infection is particularly challenging. Antibiotics are usually administered until the intraoperative culture of the duodenum is reported. When the bladder is used for exocrine drainage, bicarbonate wasting in the urine may occur. The standard method for pancreatic transplantation involves drainage of exocrine secretions into the urinary bladder with venous outflow into the systemic circulation. Despite the high success rate associated with this approach, it often leads to complications, which can include urinary tract infections, reflux pancreatitis, metabolic acidosis, and hyperinsulinemia. Depending on the patient's ability to void, the catheter may be needed for several days or possibly weeks if there is long-standing neurogenic bladder dysfunction secondary to diabetes mellitus. The surgical approach remains center and surgeon specific.

It is necessary to keep a nasogastric tube in place until bowel activity returns. This may take 3 to 5 days if there is diabetic gastroparesis. If the nasogastric tube remains in place, enteral or parenteral feedings may be necessary.

Lung

On arrival to the ICU, the lung transplant recipient is anesthetized, intubated, and mechanically ventilated. Usually, extubation occurs 24 to 36 hours after surgery when the patient's oxygenation is optimized and secretions are minimal. Extubation usually proceeds more quickly in patients with emphysema and a single-lung transplant than in patients with pulmonary hypertension, who may need a longer intubation period.

The lung transplant recipient does not have a cough reflex because of denervation. Therefore, when suctioning, the nurse avoids inserting the catheter where it can cause damage. The surgical team performs frequent bronchoscopy to ensure intact anastomoses and pulmonary toileting. A common problem in the immediate post-transplantation period is pulmonary edema due to a phenomenon known as "reperfusion" injury. As a result, it is best to maintain the patient in a relatively hypovolemic state for the first few days. Diuresis begins when the patient is hemodynamically stable.

The lungs are constantly exposed to the outside world, and therefore prevention of infection is especially important after lung transplantation. Antibiotics are given prophylactically and are determined by donor cultures, preoperative serology results, and sputum samples. Patient care measures to prevent infection include giving oral care, encouraging physical activity early in the postoperative course, and performing daily respiratory and chest physiotherapy. Continuous pulse oximetry is used to monitor oxygen saturation, and daily chest radiographs help monitor progress. Infection control measures by staff include washing hands and using aseptic suctioning technique. Staff and visitors with active infections should avoid caring for or visiting the patients.

● Assessment and Management in Hematopoietic Stem Cell Transplantation

HSCT involves replacing diseased, destroyed, or nonfunctioning hematopoietic cells with healthy progenitor cells, also called stem cells. Stem cells are primitive hematopoietic cells capable of self-renewal, and they are pluripotent, meaning that they are capable of maturation into an RBC, WBC, or platelet. These stem cells may be collected directly from the bone marrow spaces by a bone marrow harvest procedure, or from the peripheral blood, by apheresis. HSCT is an important advance in restoring hematopoietic function in patients whose bone marrow has been destroyed by high-dose chemotherapy and radiation therapy (see Table 47-1).

In both autologous and allogeneic HSCT, peripheral blood stem cells have become the preferred source of hematopoietic stem cells for grafting, although for selected allogeneic HSCT recipients, bone marrow grafting may offer specific advantages over peripheral blood stem cells. Collection of cells through apheresis is easier and less costly and may also result in a more rapid recovery of neutrophil and platelet counts. In unrelated allogeneic transplantation, the source of stem cells may be either a bone marrow harvest procedure or a peripheral blood stem cell collection. Table 47-5 presents a detailed comparison of autologous and allogeneic stem cell transplantation. Box 47-3 outlines the benefits and limitations of the various sources of stem cells for transplantation.

STEM CELL HARVESTING, MOBILIZATION, AND COLLECTION

Stem cells are most numerous in the bone marrow spaces, and some circulate in the peripheral blood. The process of harvesting and collecting hematopoietic stem cells differs depending on whether progenitor cells will be obtained through a bone marrow harvest or collected from the peripheral bloodstream.

When stem cells are obtained from the bone marrow, the harvesting procedure is performed in the operating room with the patient anesthetized. Multiple aspirations are obtained from each posterior iliac crest using large-bore needles until a total of 2 to 3 × 10^8 nucleated cells per kilogram of recipient body weight is obtained. The total volume of aspirate is 1 to 2 L. The marrow is placed in a heparinized tissue culture medium and filtered for the removal of fat and bone particles, and the cells are taken directly to the recipient's room for infusion. The bone marrow harvest procedure usually takes 1 to 2 hours. Pressure dressings are applied to the aspirate sites, and the donor is usually admitted for overnight observation. The harvest sites may be mildly uncomfortable for 2 to 7 days after the procedure.

Hematopoietic stem cells may also be collected from the peripheral blood. However, because stem cells are not abundant in the peripheral blood, chemotherapy or colony-stimulating factors (granulocyte colony-stimulating factor [G-CSF] or granulocyte–macrophage colony-stimulating factor [GM-CSF]) must be given before collection to drive progenitor cells into the peripheral circulation. This process is termed *mobilization* or *priming*. The chemotherapy that patients receive for stem cell mobilization is also useful for tumor reduction. For related and unrelated donors, colony-stimulating factors alone are used to increase the number of stem cells in the peripheral blood. Protocols vary, but G-CSF or GM-CSF is given by a subcutaneous injection daily. Stem cell collections begin after 4 or 5 days of cytokine injections.

Hematopoietic progenitor cells are collected from the peripheral blood by a method called *leukapheresis*. A commercial cell separator machine collects the progenitor cells and returns the remainder of the plasma and cellular components to the bloodstream. This is performed either through wide-bore double-lumen central catheters or large-bore antecubital intravenous catheters. The procedure takes approximately 3 to 4 hours, and the number of leukapheresis procedures required is determined by the number

---

Table 47-5 • Comparison of Autologous and Allogeneic Stem Cell Transplantation

	Autologous	Allogeneic
Indications	Hematological malignancies and solid tumors Possible role in treatment of autoimmune disorders Future role in combination with gene therapy to treat genetic disorders and HIV infection	Hematological malignancies, aplastic anemia, congenital bone marrow disorders, immune deficiency states, some inborn errors of metabolism
Source of stem cells	Stem cells collected from bone marrow or peripheral blood of the patient and then reinfused after high-dose conditioning regimen Stem cells given to rescue the patient from hematological toxicity of conditioning regimen	Marrow, peripheral blood, cord blood, family donors, unrelated donors, HLA-matched or partially matched
Preparative regimen	High-dose chemotherapy to eradicate malignant disease	High-dose chemotherapy and sometimes total-body radiation as intensive therapy for malignant disease and to provide immunosuppression to allow engraftment (makes "space" for incoming stem cells)
Post-transplantation treatment	Supportive care, transfusions, growth factors, immune manipulation	Supportive care, transfusions, growth factors, immune manipulation, prophylaxis and treatment of GVHD
Risk for infectious complications	Lower risk; infections occur mainly in early post-transplantation period	Higher risk; sustained risk for infection for months or years
Major complications	Preparative regimen toxicity, disease recurrence or progression	Preparative regimen toxicity, disease recurrence or progression, GVHD, immunodeficiency
Treatment-related mortality rate	Usually <5%	5%–30% depending on many patient-, donor-, and disease-related factors

Adapted from Barrett J, Warwick R: In Barrett J, Treleaven J (eds): The Clinical Practice of Stem Cell Transplantation. Oxford: Isis Medical Media, 1998.

of stem cells harvested at each session. The goal is to collect 5×10^6 CD34-positive cells per kilogram of recipient body weight. The CD34-positive antigen is an antigen expressed on the surface of early progenitor cells. With autologous hematopoietic progenitor cells, the cells are immediately cryopreserved and stored in liquid nitrogen until the recipient is ready for reinfusion. The donor may experience a transient hypocalcemia reaction with chills, fatigue, tingling in the lips and extremities, and vertigo resulting from the citrate infusion, which is used to prevent clotting of the blood during the procedure. The symptoms can be prevented or treated by taking a calcium supplement.

CONDITIONING REGIMEN

After the progenitor cells have been obtained, the recipient begins the conditioning regimen designed to prepare him or her to receive transplanted stem cells. The goal of the conditioning regimen depends in part on whether the transplant is autologous or allogeneic and on the nature of the recipient's underlying disease. In allogeneic transplantation, the purpose of conditioning is to eradicate any malignant disease, eliminate the bone marrow to create a space for the new donor stem cells, and provide sufficient immunosuppression to allow engraftment of the transplanted stem cells. In autologous transplantation, immunosuppression is not required because the recipient of the hematopoietic stem cells is also the donor and there is therefore no tissue incompatibility. However, the high-dose therapy is still needed to eradicate malignant disease.

High-dose chemotherapy treatment is based on the hypothesis that increasing the total dose or dose rate will kill more tumor cells, resulting in improved response and survival rates. Drugs with different (i.e., non-overlapping) nonhematologic dose-limiting toxicities are combined in maximal doses.[22,23] Alkylating agents (cyclophosphamide, carboplatin, busulfan, thiotepa, cisplatin, melphalan, carmustine), etoposide, cytarabine, and sometimes total-body irradiation are used to destroy the bone marrow and eradicate disease. The regimen is administered over 2 to 8 days. The individual drugs that may be used in combination as part of the transplant conditioning regimen may have several adverse effects (Table 47-6).

The stem cell recipient is then allowed 1 to 2 rest days to clear the chemotherapy from the system before the infusion of stem cells. Bone marrow aplasia occurs within days after the conditioning regimen is completed. The acute toxicity from the regimen can last for a few weeks or until engraftment occurs.

Research is underway to study whether a reduced intensity conditioning regimen (sometimes called nonmyeloablative) followed by allogeneic HSCT provides improved transplantation outcomes for selected candidates. Reduced intensity transplantation may provide a treatment option for patients who, because of advanced age or preexisting lung, kidney, or liver damage, cannot tolerate the toxicities of a traditional allogeneic transplant.[24] The theory behind a reduced-intensity transplantation is that the immune-mediated graft-versus-tumor effect provided by the new immune system, rather than the conditioning regimen itself, cures the disease. Specific regimens under investigation include fludarabine, single-dose total-body irradiation, and a combination of potent immunosuppressive medications. These regimens are not without risk, and patients undergoing reduced intensity transplantation still experience many of the expected complications of myeloablative allogeneic transplantation. The problems encountered in the early post-transplantation period, such as infection, bleeding, and regimen-related toxicities, may be reduced compared with myeloablative transplantation, but the risk for GVHD and the long-term risks for infection continue to be important.

TRANSPLANTATION/HEMATOPOIETIC STEM CELL INFUSION

In allogeneic HSCT, the stem cells are usually infused immediately after they are collected. Autologous stem cells are cryopreserved with dimethylsulfoxide (DMSO) and must be thawed in a warm normal saline bath at the bedside immediately before reinfusion.

The actual infusion of stem cells is a relatively simple procedure, much like a blood transfusion. The cells are infused into a central venous catheter over 30 to 60 minutes, depending on the total volume of the product. Patients usually are premedicated with acetaminophen, hydrocortisone, and diphenhydramine, and they are prehydrated to maintain renal perfusion. Diuretics, mannitol, and antihypertensives may be required to prevent volume overload and manage hemodynamic changes during infusion. Vital signs are monitored, and oxygen and cardiac monitoring are readily available.

⋯ Table 47-6 • Nonhematological Adverse Effects of High-Dose Therapy Regimens

Drug or Therapy	Adverse Effects
Busulfan	Interstitial pulmonary fibrosis, hepatic dysfunction (including veno-occlusive disease of the liver), acute cholecystitis, generalized seizures, mucositis, skin adverse effects (hyperpigmentation, desquamation, acral erythema), nausea and vomiting
Carmustine (BCNU)	Hepatic, pulmonary, and central nervous system adverse effects, cardiac adverse effects (dysrhythmias and hypotension), nausea and vomiting
Cytosine arabinoside (Ara-C)	Cerebellar toxicity, encephalopathy, seizures, conjunctivitis, skin adverse effects (rash, acral erythema), nausea and vomiting, diarrhea, renal insufficiency, liver function abnormalities, pancreatitis, noncardiogenic pulmonary edema, fever, arthralgias
Cyclophosphamide	Cardiac adverse effects (cardiomyopathy, congestive heart failure, hemorrhagic cardiac necrosis, pericardial effusion, ECG abnormalities), interstitial pulmonary fibrosis, hemorrhagic cystitis, elevation in liver enzymes, nausea and vomiting, metabolic adverse effects (syndrome of inappropriate anti-diuretic hormone secretion [SIADH])
Carboplatinum	Nausea and vomiting, nephrotoxicity, liver function abnormalities (including veno-occlusive disease of the liver), ototoxicity
Cisplatinum	Nausea and vomiting, neurotoxicity (peripheral neuropathy, ataxia, visual disturbances), ototoxicity, renal adverse effects
Etoposide	Hypersensitivity reactions, hypotension, liver function abnormalities and chemical hepatitis, renal dysfunction, nausea and vomiting, metabolic adverse effects (metabolic acidosis), mucositis, stomatitis, painful skin rash (on the palms, soles, and periorbital area)
Ifosfamide	Hemorrhagic cystitis, nausea, vomiting
Melphalan	Acute hypersensitivity reaction, renal adverse effects, mucositis, nausea and vomiting, hepatic toxicity (including veno-occlusive disease of the liver)
Thiotepa	Hyperpigmentation, acute erythroderma, dry desquamation, liver function abnormalities (including veno-occlusive disease of the liver), mucositis, esophagitis, dysuria, hypersensitivity reactions
Total-body irradiation	Nausea and vomiting, diarrhea, parotitis, xerostomia, stomatitis, erythema, pneumonitis, veno-occlusive disease of the liver

Complications of allogeneic HSCT may include pulmonary edema, hemolysis, infection, and anaphylaxis; however, these are rare. A garlicky odor or taste may occur; excretion of DMSO causes this. DMSO-associated RBC hemolysis may also occur, and patients require vigorous hydration to prevent renal toxicity. An infusion reaction that may include bradycardia (rarely heart block), hypertension, and an acute hypersensitivity reaction is another potential adverse effect of DMSO during the administration of cryopreserved autologous HSCT. During HSCT, monitoring for volume overload and for complaints suggestive of embolism such as chest pain, dyspnea, and cough is necessary. Patients may also experience an acute hemolytic transfusion reaction if they are receiving hematopoietic stem cells from an ABO-mismatched donor.

ENGRAFTMENT

After intravenous infusion, the hematopoietic stem cells migrate to the bone marrow spaces, where they are attracted by chemotactic factors. Engraftment occurs when the transplanted progenitor cells begin to grow and manufacture new hematopoietic cells in the bone marrow. Engraftment is generally defined as an absolute neutrophil count greater than 0.5×10^9/L for 3 consecutive days, and a platelet count greater than 20×10^9/L achieved without transfusion support. The rate of engraftment depends on the source of the progenitor cells, the total progenitor cell dose, the use of colony-stimulating factors, the complications the patient experiences in the pre-engraftment period, and the choice of prophylaxis against GVHD. Time to engraftment in HSCT varies according to the origin of the hematopoietic stem cells: for bone marrow–derived stem cells, 2 to 3 weeks; for peripheral blood stem cells, 11 to 16 days; and for cord blood–derived stem cells, 26 days (average; as long as 42 days).

Patients usually receive their conditioning treatment and immediate post-transplantation care in an inpatient unit. However, improved symptom management and technological advances, including the use of hematopoietic growth factors, have allowed earlier discharge from the hospital. Box 47-4 presents the criteria for hospital discharge after HSCT. Many institutions now have outpatient care facilities available for transplant recipients that permit outpatient treatment and evaluation 7 days per week.[25]

Box 47-4 • Criteria for Hospital Discharge After Hematopoietic Stem Cell Transplantation

Discharge from hospital is usually permitted when:
- The patient has been afebrile for at least 24 hours
- A 24-hour outpatient medical facility is available
- Family caregiver support is available
- The patient is independent in basic activities of daily living
- Acute post-transplantation complications have been resolved or controlled
- The patient is achieving oral intake of at least 1,500 mL per day, or a plan to meet the patient's fluid needs through self-administration of intravenous fluids or daily intravenous fluid administration in clinic is in place
- Nausea and vomiting are controlled
- The patient is able to tolerate oral medications
- Availability of appropriate transfusion support in a clinic environment and access to irradiated blood products have been determined
- The patient's platelet count is supportable with no more frequent than daily platelet product
- The patient's white blood cell count is greater than 1×10^9/L
- A hematocrit of 25% is supportable with no more than daily transfusion of one unit of packed red blood cells

After the transplantation but before complete hematopoietic cell engraftment, patients experience severe pancytopenia and immunosuppression, and the resulting complications may include infection and bleeding. Patients take hematopoietic growth factors (e.g., G-CSF, GM-CSF) to accelerate neutrophil recovery, thereby reducing the period of pancytopenia and the highest risk for infection. While patients have pancytopenia, until their blood counts begin to recover, they typically receive broad-spectrum antimicrobial drugs directed at bacteria, viruses, and fungi, as well as blood components such as platelets and packed red blood cells.

All blood products given to HSCT recipients require filtration to remove WBCs that may transmit CMV and irradiation to prevent transfusion-associated GVHD. Studies have determined that leukodepletion by either bedside filtration during transfusion or by prestorage leukocyte depletion of blood products is an effective method of preventing transfusion-associated CMV infection in HSCT because leukocytes transmit CMV.[26] In addition, filtered blood products may also prevent febrile transfusion reactions and delay alloimmunization.[27–28] However, use of a leukocyte depletion filter does not affect the risk for transmission of viral hepatitis.

Transfusion-associated GVHD is a rare but almost uniformly fatal complication of transfusion, resulting from the infusion of immunocompetent lymphocytes capable of proliferation into an immunocompromised recipient who is unable to destroy them.[26] The infused lymphocytes recognize host tissues as foreign and mount a reaction.

To prevent transfusion-associated GVHD, all cellular blood products, except for stem cell grafts and donor lymphocytes given for graft-versus-tumor effect, irradiation to 2,500 cGy is necessary.[26] The blood component should be labeled as irradiated. It is not radioactive, and no additional precautions for handling the blood product are required. Other patients can use irradiated blood products; the irradiating process does not alter the efficacy or cellular content of the product and does not harm the recipient in any way. Patients who have undergone allogeneic or autologous HSCT should receive irradiated cellular components, both before and after stem cell transplantation.[25] Most centers recommend that allogeneic stem cell recipients receive irradiated blood products for the rest of their lives. Box 47-5 shows a Collaborative Care Guide for the patient with allogeneic HSCT.

• Immunosuppressive Therapy

In solid organ transplantation, the transplanted organ is foreign to the recipient, whose immune system eventually will recognize this and mobilize to reject

(text continues on page 1213)

Box 47-5 • COLLABORATIVE CARE GUIDE for the Allogeneic Hematopoietic Stem Cell Transplantation

OUTCOMES	INTERVENTIONS
Oxygenation/Ventilation The patient will demonstrate pulmonary hygiene techniques, including coughing, deep breathing, incentive spirometry, and daily exercise as tolerated. The patient will demonstrate improvement in respiratory pattern and lung sounds, with subjective reduction in complaints of dyspnea, cough, pleuritic chest pain, and weakness. The patient's risk for aspiration will be eliminated or minimized.	• Auscultate lung sounds and vital signs and pulse oximetry q4h and PRN. • Note skin color capillary refill and presence of central or peripheral cyanosis. • Assess the quality of respirations including use of accessory muscles, nasal flaring, and grunting. • Note cough and complaints of shortness of breath, orthopnea, or pleuritic pain. • Determine effects of medications that may affect respiratory status, including narcotics and sedatives.

(continued)

Box 47-5 • COLLABORATIVE CARE GUIDE for the Allogeneic Hematopoietic Stem Cell Transplantation (Continued)

OUTCOMES	INTERVENTIONS
	• Suction oropharynx or nasotrachea to remove secretions.
	• Encourage deep-breathing and coughing exercises, and teach patient proper use of incentive spirometry.
	• Encourage patient to maintain optimal level of activity, including walking, exercise bicycle, and working daily with physical therapist.
	• Instruct patient on methods of preventing respiratory complications related to mucositis or aspiration, such as avoiding drinking liquids after using topical local anesthetics, keeping head of bed elevated and having oral suction in a convenient location.
	• Implement measures to manage anemia and control bleeding, if present.
	• Administer supplemental oxygen as indicated.
	• Administer diuretics as ordered.
Circulation/Perfusion	
The patient will exhibit the absence or control of signs and symptoms of potential physiological problems:	• Develop a nursing plan to manage individual cardiovascular problems. Cardiovascular problems may include hypertension, orthostatic hypotension, sepsis-induced hypotension, dysrhythmias, pericarditis, superior vena cava syndrome, thrombus formation, and myocardial infarction.
Bleeding/hemorrhage	
Hypotension secondary to sepsis, hemorrhage, medication side effects, or dehydration	
Hypertension secondary to medication side effects	• Replace fluid losses with packed red blood cells or hydration.
Dehydration secondary to decreased oral fluid intake as a result of nausea, vomiting, or mucositis, or increased fluid losses through fever, diarrhea, or insensible fluid losses through the skin	• Use appropriate measures to decrease fluid losses secondary to fever, diarrhea, vomiting, or hemorrhage.
	• Administer antihypertensives, diuretics, antidysrhythmics, or vasoactive drugs as ordered and monitor their effectiveness.
	• Provide information to patient and family regarding cardiac status, and rationale for specific nursing interventions.
	• Monitor platelet count and coagulation profile carefully, especially in patients experiencing hypertension.
	• Instruct patient about appropriate safety measures during period of altered cardiac status. Patients who are orthostatic may become dizzy when standing. Provide assistance as needed.
	• Although hypotension and hypertension may occur without symptoms, alert patient to these signs and symptoms, and encourage prompt reporting to the health care team. Common signs of hypertension include headache and visual disturbance. Hypotension may be associated with dizziness, visual disturbances, tachycardia, and cool or diaphoretic skin.
	• Emphasize the importance of taking oral antihypertensive medications when scheduled.
Fluids/Electrolytes	
The patient will exhibit the absence of or control of signs and symptoms of potential physiological problems:	• Strictly monitor intake, output, and fluid balance q4–8h.
	• Check weight twice daily.
Veno-occlusive disease of the liver, as manifested by sudden weight gain, increase in bilirubin, aspartate aminotransferase, and alkaline phosphatase levels, hepatomegaly, ascites, and encephalopathy	• Measure abdominal girth daily in patients with veno-occlusive disease.
	• Perform pulmonary assessment, including pulse oximetry, respiratory rate, quality, and presence of adventitious breath sounds.
Renal insufficiency/failure, as manifested by a decreased urine output or rising serum creatinine	• Perform cardiac assessment, noting presence of orthostatic hypotension, extra heart sounds, or neck vein distention.
Dehydration secondary to decreased oral fluid intake as a result of nausea, vomiting, or mucositis, or increased	• Assess for peripheral and sacral edema.

(continued)

Box 47-5 • COLLABORATIVE CARE GUIDE for the Allogeneic Hematopoietic Stem Cell Transplantation (Continued)

OUTCOMES	INTERVENTIONS
fluid losses through fever, diarrhea, or insensible fluid losses through the skin. **Electrolyte disorders** secondary to steroid-induced hyperglycemia, syndrome of inappropriate antidiuretic hormone secretion (SIADH), tumor lysis syndrome, or medication-induced electrolyte shifts	• Monitor serum electrolytes, liver function tests, and urine specific gravity once or twice daily as ordered. • Monitor for and treat steroid-induced hyperglycemia. • Adjust dose or eliminate nephrotoxic drugs in patients with renal insufficiency or renal failure. • Administer intravenous fluids as ordered to replace gastrointestinal losses and to supplement inability to consume sufficient oral fluids. • Administer electrolyte replacements as ordered. • Administer antiemetics and antidiarrheal agents as ordered. • Monitor stools for volume, consistency, color, and odor. • Monitor for fluid losses through sloughing of the skin.
Mobility/Safety The patient will: Maintain baseline strength and endurance and minimize focal muscle weakness, fatigue, and dyspnea Participate in measures to prevent a decrease in strength and endurance Experience minimal complications from decreased mobility Use safety measures to prevent injury	• Encourage patient to continue daily activities throughout the transplantation course. Provide rationale and explain the complications of inactivity to both patient and family. • Develop an individualized plan to address factors contributing to limited mobility, including pain, nonadherence, depression, medication side effects, nausea, generalized weakness and malaise, and altered level of consciousness. • Refer to physical and occupational therapy for assessment and treatment. • Encourage focused exercises that provide proximal muscle strengthening in patients on corticosteroids. • Encourage patient to maintain maximal independence in ADLs and self-care. • Develop a schedule that allows adequate rest by coordinating all activity and treatments (ADLs, medications, health team rounds). • Identify signs of impaired activity tolerance and set specific goals for improving tolerance/endurance in activities.
Skin Integrity The patient will: Maintain skin integrity Demonstrate techniques of skin care Demonstrate basic understanding of skin GVHD Exhibit control of symptoms associated with skin GVHD	• Assess skin daily for maculopapular rash, erythema, sloughing, or open lesions. • Monitor skin for the development of signs of infection such as warmth, erythema, swelling, or tenderness. • Apply skin emollients and other topical agents, including topical antimicrobial agents, as ordered. • Consider use of antipruritic or steroid topical agents to manage symptoms of itching and inflammation. • If skin breakdown occurs, consult enterostomal therapist or wound management specialist concerning nonadherent, absorptive dressings and the role of special beds/mattresses. • Monitor patient for dehydration if there are increased insensible losses of fluid through the skin. • Teach patient and family the importance of avoiding direct sun exposure and the importance of using sun block and protective clothing when outdoors because sun exposure can initiate a flare of GVHD of skin.
Nutrition The patient will: Have nutritional balance maintained through diet and parenteral nutrition Demonstrate understanding of dietary restrictions related to a specific gastrointestinal problem	• Evaluate oral mucosal integrity and note presence of oral problems. • Note subjective data, including complaints of nausea, loss of appetite, taste changes, early satiety, pain or abdominal cramping, and any precipitating factors.

(continued)

Box 47-5 • COLLABORATIVE CARE GUIDE for the Allogeneic Hematopoietic Stem Cell Transplantation (Continued)

OUTCOMES	INTERVENTIONS
Demonstrate methods for maintaining nutritional requirements as an outpatient	• Monitor calorie counts, intake and output totals, and weights to determine adequacy of nutritional intake. • Develop a multidisciplinary plan for nutritional management. Discuss approaches to use when experiencing taste changes; thick, viscous saliva and mucus; xerostomia; early satiety; nausea/vomiting; mucositis or esophagitis; and other troubling symptoms. • If patient is receiving high-dose steroids, ensure increased protein intake and calcium and vitamin D supplementation. Consider restricted concentrated carbohydrate intake if hyperglycemia is present. Consider restricted sodium intake if fluid retention is especially problematic. • Increase protein intake in patients with extensive skin or gastrointestinal GVHD. • Consider multiple vitamin without iron (to prevent iron overload), and folic acid supplementation 1 mg orally qd. • Maintain nutritional requirements through use of hyperalimentation as required. • Encourage patient to try different foods as tolerated. • Advance diet as tolerated and note response to advancement. • Encourage small, frequent meals and a bedtime snack. • Medicate for nausea or pain as needed. • Encourage family members to be supportive and patient. Pressure from family or staff can produce anxiety that will have a negative effect on eating habits.

Comfort/Pain Control
Patient will be able to:
  Identify activities that increase or decrease pain
  Relate location and characteristics of pain as well as degree of pain relief to the health care team
  Participate in daily care without interference from pain or side effects of pain control measures
  Achieve acceptable level of pain control
	• Monitor for the potential sources of pain/discomfort in the hematopoietic stem cell transplant recipient, including:
	  Pain associated with diagnostic or therapeutic procedures
	  Neuropathic pain secondary to immunosuppressive medications
	  Mucositis/esophagitis
	  Rectal pain/hemorrhoids
	  Painful urination from hemorrhagic cystitis
	  Abdominal pain secondary to infections, severe diarrhea/enteritis, or liver distention
	  Cutaneous discomfort secondary to GVHD of skin
	• Teach patient importance of reporting pain and the effectiveness of pain relief measures to health care team.
	• Assess location, onset, frequency, intensity, and quality of pain. Use a 0–10 pain scale to assess patient's perception of pain and to assist in evaluating effectiveness of treatment. For patients unable to communicate, monitor changes in vital signs and observe for increased restlessness, which could indicate inadequate pain control.
	• Premedicate patient before potentially painful procedures.
	• Teach proper and safe use of patient-controlled analgesia if ordered.
	• For patients receiving continuous infusion, consider the need for a bolus of analgesic before disconnecting patient from continuous infusion, while disconnected, and after resuming continuous infusion.
	• Suggest consultation with pain management team if indicated.

(continued)

Box 47-5 • COLLABORATIVE CARE GUIDE for the Allogeneic Hematopoietic Stem Cell Transplantation (Continued)

OUTCOMES	INTERVENTIONS
	• Monitor narcotic dosages and patient response carefully in patients with hepatic dysfunction secondary to veno-occlusive disease or GVHD.
	• In the nonventilated patient, adjust analgesic dosages in the presence of markedly deceased respiratory rate or markedly altered level of consciousness.

Psychosocial–Individual and Family
Patient and family will be able to:
  Identify effective and ineffective coping patterns
  Identify personal strengths
  Verbalize their needs
  Actively participate in problem solving
  Use resources and support systems to strengthen their coping skills
	• Provide opportunities for patient and family to communicate with each other, as well as with psychosocial support professionals and other health care team members.
	• Reinforce successful coping skills (i.e., clearly verbalizing needs, using activities that reduce stress, and effective patient/family/team communication).
	• Provide reassurance and review support systems, options, and resources available to support effective coping.
	• Establish trust and congruence in goals and objectives.
	• Provide information in a timely and specific manner.
	• Allow patient as much choice and control as appropriate and feasible.
	• Avoid the use of approaches that foster dependency (coercion, persuasion, manipulation).
	• Demonstrate caring, respect, and concern for patient and family.
	• Use positive reinforcement.

Teaching/Discharge Planning
The patient and family will demonstrate knowledge of:
  The overall process of hematopoietic stem cell transplantation and the expected complications and self-care requirements, including preparative regimen and side effects, infusion of peripheral stem cells and side effects, engraftment, complications, discharge criteria, follow-up care, symptoms to report, protective precautions (neutropenic and thrombocytopenic precautions), dietary restrictions, and specific psychomotor skills, including central venous catheter care, medication administration, and vital sign monitoring
  The structure of the inpatient unit, unit routines, and the programs and resources available to make their inpatient stay more comfortable and facilitate their self-care
  The importance of the active involvement of patient and family in the daily care and decision making through-out the hematopoietic stem cell transplantation process
On discharge, patient and family will demonstrate knowledge of:
  Signs and symptoms that should be reported immediately to the health care team, including fever, chills, skin rash, bleeding, nausea, vomiting, diarrhea or abdominal pain, shortness of breath, cough, dyspnea, and an inability to take oral medication or consume sufficient fluids
  Names of medication, rationale for each medication, the required schedule for administration, and potential side effects
  Contact telephone numbers for day and after-hours care
  Psychomotor skills necessary for administration of oral and intravenous (IV) medications, self-care of central venous catheter, and any other self-care skills such as administration of total parenteral nutrition and home IV hydration
	• Orient patient to unit, room environment, ancillary services, and general routines. The patient and family may be initially overwhelmed by the amount of new information and may require reinforcement of information.
	• Allow patient and family to share concerns and request additional information about the transplantation process.
	• Encourage questions throughout the transplantation process, and provide clarification on all aspects of treatment.
	• Explain the need for active patient and family involvement in daily care and decision making throughout the hematopoietic stem cell transplantation process.
	• Teach the importance of daily hygiene, diligent oral care, daily exercise, nutrition, and other routines.
	• Encourage patient to maintain open communication with health care team.
	• Integrate discharge teaching while fostering patient family participation in daily care.
	• Provide patient with written instructions on outpatient self-care guidelines, medication schedule, and other self-care activities.
	• Refer to home health agency for continued education and support of patient at home, as indicated.
	• Provide teaching/instruction using methods adapted to patient's learning style. Discuss with patient how he or she learns best: by doing, by listening, or by watching.
	• Document teaching provided, areas requiring continued reinforcement and follow-up, and learning outcomes achieved in the patient's record.

the transplanted organ. Therefore, immunosuppressive therapy is necessary to suppress the immune response so the transplanted organ will be accepted. In allogeneic HSCT, because the immune system is generated from donor cells, immunosuppressive therapy is used to prevent GVHD, a response in which donor T lymphocytes attack the recipient's cells. The challenge of immunosuppressive therapy is to provide the recipient with adequate immunosuppression without undue toxicity, unfavorable reactions, and excess susceptibility to opportunistic infections. Therapeutic regimens may be individualized based on the needs of a particular patient.

To suppress the immune response in solid organ transplant recipients, several drugs may be necessary (Table 47-7). A single medication usually cannot do this effectively. Therefore, immunosuppressive regimens include medications that complement each other and increase the effectiveness of the immunosuppression. The foundation of most immunosuppressant regimens for solid organ transplantation is triple, or three-drug, therapy. The combination of drugs used for organ transplantation and HSCT may differ.

Triple therapy is a combination of low-dose prednisone, azathioprine or mycophenolate mofetil, and cyclosporine A or tacrolimus. By combining these three agents, the dose of each drug is lower so that patients experience fewer adverse effects than they would from one drug alone. For example, the risk for aseptic necrosis, diabetes mellitus, cataracts, and gastrointestinal complications attributed to chronic steroid therapy is greatly reduced with the combination therapy. Because the dosage of azathioprine is low, the potential for hepatotoxicity and leucopenia is decreased. Problems associated with higher doses of cyclosporine A, including lymphoma, hirsutism, hepatotoxicity, gingival hyperplasia, seizures, and gastrointestinal disturbances, occur at a lower frequency.

Quadruple, or sequential, therapy is a combination of the same three drugs that are used in triple therapy (prednisone, azathioprine or mycophenolate mofetil, and either cyclosporine A or tacrolimus) plus antithymocyte antibody preparations or monoclonal antibody, monomurab-CD3. The calcineurin inhibitors, cyclosporine A or tacrolimus, are withheld until renal function is present. All four drugs *(text continues on page 1216)*

Table 47-7 • Selected Immunosuppressive Drugs Used in Solid Organ Transplantation

Drug	Adverse Reactions	Dosing/Administration	Comments
Methylprednisolone (Solu-Medrol) (IV) Prednisone (PO)	Increased susceptibility to infection	Initial: 0.5–3 mg/kg of body weight, tapered to an adequate oral maintenance dose	
	Masks symptoms of infection Peptic ulcer, GI bleeding		An antacid and H$_2$ blockers or a proton pump inhibitor are given while patient is on steroids to reduce the risk for gastric irritation and ulceration.
	Increased appetite, weight gain Increased sodium and water retention, which exaggerate hypertension Delayed healing Negative nitrogen balance Adrenal gland suppression Behavior and personality changes Diabetogenic effect Muscle weakness Osteoporosis with long-term therapy Skin atrophy, striae Easy bruising Glaucoma, cataracts Hirsutism Acne Avascular/aseptic necrosis	During rejection: methylprednisolone may be given in IV boluses up to 1 g/dose	Cardiac arrest can occur if IV bolus of 1 g is given rapidly. Sodium restriction may be necessary when steroid dosage is high or when fluid retention increases.
Azathioprine (Imuran) (IV or PO)	Bone marrow suppression: leukopenia, thrombocytopenia, anemia, pancytopenia Rash Alopecia Liver damage, jaundice Increased susceptibility to infection	Regulated to keep WBC 5,000–10,000; drug usually stopped when WBC 3,000 or less Initial 2–5 mg/kg of body weight Maintenance: 2–3 mg/kg of body weight During rejection: maximum of 3 mg/kg of body weight, dose not usually increased with rejection	The dose is lowered when allopurinol is added to medication regimen because allopurinol delays metabolism of azathioprine (allopurinol and azathioprine are synergistic).

(continued)

Table 47-7 • Selected Immunosuppressive Drugs Used in Solid Organ Transplantation (Continued)

Drug	Adverse Reactions	Dosing/Administration	Comments
Cyclosporine (Sandimmune) (IV or PO) Neoral (PO, microemulsion)	Nephrotoxicity Hepatotoxicity	Initial: 4 mg/kg/day (IV) Maintenance: 5–15 mg/kg/day PO may be used as part of triple-therapy regimen (prednisone, azathioprine, cyclosporine), or quadruple-therapy regimen (same as triple therapy plus ALG or OKT3)	Initially, nephrotoxicity and hepato-toxicity seem to be dose related and respond to dose reduction.
	Hypertension Hirsutism Gum hyperplasia Malignancy Nausea, vomiting, diarrhea Tremors/seizures Diabetogenic effects Anaphylactic reactions have been seen with IV administration	The dose for Sandimmune and Neoral are not interchangeable owing to differences in bioavailability. When prepara-tions are changed, dose adjustments are based on blood levels. Dosage altered by monitoring drug levels at least during initial period	Long-term nephrotoxicity is a major concern. Nephrotoxicity is sometimes difficult to differentiate from rejection or acute tubular necrosis in renal patients. Metabolized by cytochrome P-450 enzymes. Drugs that are inducers or inhibitors for P-450 enzymes may increase or decrease cyclosporine concentrations. Trough levels done to monitor and titrate dosage. Drug interactions can raise or lower blood levels. Risk for anaphylaxis is reduced if slow continuous infusion is given.
Tacrolimus (Prograf)	Infection Nephrotoxicity Neurotoxicity Hypertension Diabetogenesis Tremors	Dosage varies 0.10 mg/kg/day IV 0.05–0.2 mg/kg/day PO (given in divided doses)	Dose based on trough levels. May be able to discontinue steroids. Monitor renal and liver function. Drug interactions and liver function can affect blood levels. Metabolized by cytochrome P-450 enzymes. Drugs that are inducers or inhibitors for P-450 enzymes may increase or decrease cyclosporine concentrations.
Muromonab-CD3 (Orthoclone OKT3)	Febrile reactions; fever, chills, tremor Respiratory: dyspnea, chest pain, wheezing, pulmonary edema GI: nausea, vomiting, diarrhea Anemia, thrombocytopenia	2.5–5 mg/day IV bolus over 30–60 s, for 10–14 days	Reactions are greatest with first dose and occur within 30–60 min. To minimize first dose reaction, pre-treat with methylprednisolone, acetaminophen, and diphen-hydramine hydrochloride. Monitor vital signs q15min for 2 h, then q30min first two doses. Have emergency equipment and cooling blanket available. Repeat administrations may cause seri-ous reactions if antibodies develop.
Antilymphocyte globulin (ALG)	Anaphylactic shock due to hyper-sensitivity to animal serum	Skin test for hypersensitivity to animal serum performed before initial dose	
Antithymocyte globulin (ATG) Antilymphocyte serum (ALS) Antithymocyte serum (ATS) (usually IV, IM, or deep SC)	Fever (up to 105°F or 40.6°C) and chills Increased susceptibility to infections due to decreased lymphocytes IM or deep SC injection site swollen, red, and painful, with abscess formation Difficulty walking if IM or SC injec-tion given in thigh	Dosage may vary	Lymphocyte and platelet counts may decrease sharply with drug admin-istration; therefore, a CBC with dif-ferential should be drawn before infusion is started. Usually given only for short period of time either to prevent or treat rejec-tion; not a long-term immunosup-pressant.

(continued)

Table 47-7 • Selected Immunosuppressive Drugs Used in Solid Organ Transplantation (Continued)

Drug	Adverse Reactions	Dosing/Administration	Comments
Cyclophosphamide (Cytoxan)	Leukopenia, thrombocytopenia Increased susceptibility to infections Metabolite of cyclophosphamide is a direct irritant to bladder mucosa and may cause hemorrhagic cystitis	1–2 mg/kg (or 1/2 to 2/3 of azathioprine dosage)	Given in place of azathioprine in patients with hepatotoxicity. Administer on awakening to avoid accumulation of metabolites in bladder while sleeping. Observe for hematuria. Urine output of at least 100 mL/h should be maintained for at least 72 h after Cytoxan is administered to dilute metabolites.
Mycophenolate mofetil (Cellcept)	Alopecia Nausea Vomiting Diarrhea Dyspepsia	Usual dosage 1 g bid (250-mg capsules)	GI symptoms may be dose related and may improve with decrease. Preferable to take on an empty stomach unless GI symptoms are intolerable.
Methotrexate (MTX)	Myelosuppression Mucositis Hepatotoxicity	15 mg/m2 day 1, then 10 mg/m2 day 3, 6, 11	The myelosuppressive effects of MTX exposure can be reversed by leukovorin. Most of the drug is excreted through the kidney, with a small fraction excreted through the bile. Standard doses in patients with good renal function, bilirubin less than 10 mg/dL and without effusions or ascites are not likely to produce serious toxicity
Sirolimus (Rapamune)	Hypercholesterolemia Elevated triglycerides Thrombocytopenia (dose related) Leukopenia	Loading dose 6–15 mg Maintenance dose 2–5 mg/day	Monitoring by trough levels Therapeutic levels: 5–20 ng/mL May impair wound healing.

Daclizumab	Common
	  Cough
	  Dizziness, fatigue, headache, tremor
	  Dysuria
	  GI effects, vomiting
	  Insomnia
	  Pain
	Serious
	  Anaphylaxis
	  Bleeding, thrombosis
	  Dyspnea
	  Edema, hypertension, hypotension, tachycardia
	  Fever
	  Infection
	  Lymphoproliferative disorders
		1 mg/kg IV beginning within 24 h before transplantation, then 1 mg/kg IV every 14 days for a total of five doses	Used for induction therapy to prevent acute rejection early in transplant.
			Not used for treatment of acute rejection.

Basiliximab	Common
	  Abdominal pain
	  Vomiting
	  Asthenia
	  Dizziness
	  Insomnia
	Serious
	  Acute hypersensitivity reaction
	  Anemia
	  Candidiasis (frequent)
	  Cytomegalovirus infection
		20 mg IV within 2 h before transplantation surgery; then another 20-mg IV dose day 4 after surgery	Used for induction therapy to prevent acute rejection early in transplant.
			Not used for treatment of acute rejection.

GI, gastrointestinal; IM, intramuscular; IV, intravenous; PO, oral; SC, subcutaneous.

are given for several days, after which the polyclonal or monoclonal antibody preparation is discontinued. A triple-drug regimen is then continued for maintenance therapy.

Because of the nephrotoxicity of calcineurin inhibitors and the risks for drug accumulation and resultant toxicity in the absence of renal function, not using the calcineurin inhibitors in the early posttransplantation period has advantages. Quadruple therapy permits both broad and specific immunosuppression while limiting toxicity until renal function has improved. However, it does have a disadvantage: the potential inability to use the polyclonal or monoclonal antibody preparation for treatment of rejection episodes or as "rescue" therapy.

• Complications of Transplantation

Complications after solid organ transplantation and HSCT are usually due to graft function, problems with immunosuppression, or the adverse effects of the transplantation preconditioning regimen. Other common complications after HSCT are GVHD and infection.

ORGAN TRANSPLANTATION

Organ Rejection

The early recognition and management of organ rejection and its associated problems are key priorities for the critical care nurse. The transplanted organ represents a continuous source of HLA alloantigens capable of inducing a rejection response. This immunologic response involves the recognition of HLA antigens of donor endothelial tissues cells by recipient lymphocytes or antibodies. The allograft continuously activates the immune response, resulting in lifelong overproduction of cytokines, constant cytotoxic activity, and sustained alteration in the graft vasculature. Transplantation of a vascular organ induces sensitization through direct stimulation of circulating host immune cells as they encounter donor antigens on allograft cell surfaces. Rejection leads to subsequent destruction of the antigen-bearing graft. The pathophysiologic mechanisms of graft rejection are depicted in Figure 47-4.

Both donor and host factors contribute to the immune response of rejection. The major donor factor is the expression of antigens on the donor tissue and the presence of antigen-presenting cells within the transplanted graft. The major host factor is prior sensitization against ABO and HLA antigens expressed in the graft.[29]

Because the transplanted organ is not immunologically identical to the recipient, it acts as an antigen or foreign substance and triggers the immune system to reject it. Rejection can vary in degree from mild to severe and may be irreversible. Rejection may occur at any time, but the risk is highest in the first 3 months after transplantation. The earlier and more severe the rejection episode, the worse the prognosis for graft survival. Biopsy of the transplanted organ is usually needed to diagnose rejection definitively. Four types of rejection are defined: hyperacute, accelerated, acute, and chronic, although all types do not occur in all transplanted organs.

Hyperacute Rejection

Hyperacute rejection occurs in the operating room immediately after transplantation. It is a humoral immune response in which the recipient has preformed antibodies that immediately react against antigens of the donor organ. Vascular damage occurs, resulting in severe thrombosis and graft necrosis. In kidney and heart transplantation, hyperacute rejection always results in graft failure and the need for retransplantation. Fortunately, hyperacute rejection is uncommon and can usually be prevented by pretransplantation cross-matching.

Accelerated Rejection

Accelerated rejection is defined only in kidney transplantation, and it occurs within 1 week after transplantation. Clinically, the patient may have anuria, increased BUN and creatinine, and pain at the graft site. Accelerated rejection is due either to preformed antibodies against the donor antigens in the recipient's blood or to lymphocytes in the recipient that are already sensitized to some of the donor antigens. Like hyperacute rejection, accelerated rejection is seen infrequently because of improved tissue typing and cross-matching. It is treated aggressively with immunosuppressants and usually results in loss of the transplanted kidney.

Acute Rejection

Acute rejection occurs within the first 3 months after transplantation. This is the most common type of rejection, and most patients experience at least one episode. Acute rejection occurs when antigens on the donor organ trigger lymphocytes to mature into helper T cells. The helper T cells increase the production of cytotoxic killer T cells, which bind to the transplanted organ and damage it by secreting lysosomal enzymes and lymphokines. Acute rejection is also the type of rejection that responds best to immunosuppressive therapy.

Chronic Rejection

The pathophysiology of chronic rejection is not completely understood. Most likely it is a combination of a cell-mediated response and a response to circulating antibodies. Second in frequency to acute rejection, chronic rejection usually occurs from 3 months to years after transplantation and is accompanied by deteriorating organ function.

Kidney Acute rejection occurs after the first postoperative week. It is the most frequently seen form of rejection and the type that responds best to therapy. Changes in laboratory values are the earliest and most reliable indicators that graft function is deteriorating. Clinical manifestations of rejection are more subtle and may not be seen. The patient may experience any, all, or none of the following during an acute rejection episode.

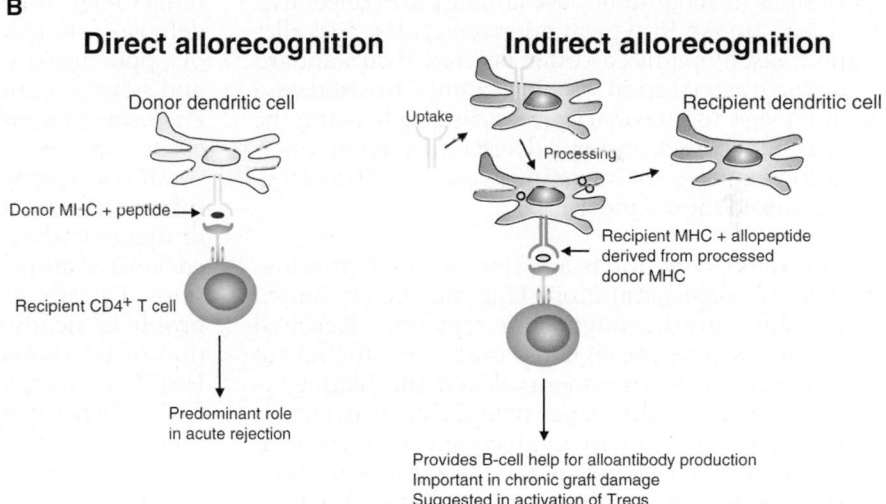

Figure 47-4 • Mechanisms of graft rejection. **A:** Within 24 to 48 hours after engraftment, dendritic cells that normally reside within the donor organ migrate to regional recipient lymphoid tissue. In the lymph node, they stimulate alloreactive CD4+ and CD8+ T cells. Activated T cells, particularly CD4+ cells, produce cytokines (e.g., interleukin-2, interleukin-4, interferon-γ), and both populations respond by proliferating and differentiating. Activated T lymphocytes can cause graft destruction by direct lysis (cytotoxic T lymphocytes, or CTLs) or by local production of cytokines, a delayed-type hypersensitivity (DTH) reaction. Cytokines also promote macrophage and eosinophil activation and recruitment, and these cells can also secrete soluble inflammatory mediators that kill their targets. Lastly, activated T cells provide help for alloantibody production by B cells. **B:** There are two types of allorecognition. Direct allorecognition occurs when T cells recognize intact foreign major histocompatibility complex (MHC) molecules (as depicted in part **A**). This is thought to be the dominant initiator of acute graft rejection. T cells may also recognize peptide fragments derived from processing of donor antigens presented on self-MHC molecules. This is termed *indirect allorecognition,* and it is believed to be important in chronic graft dysfunction, in part perhaps because of its role in providing T-cell help for alloantibody production by B cells. Indirect allorecognition is also implicated in activating regulatory T cells, which may act to limit graft damage and promote tolerance. (From Lechler RI, Sykes M, Thomson AW, Turka LA: Organ transplantation: How much of the promise has been realized? Nat Med 11[6]:605–613, 2005.)

Laboratory Findings

▶ Increased serum creatinine, BUN, serum β2-microglobulin
▶ Decreased creatinine clearance
▶ Decreased urine creatinine
▶ Possibly decreased urine sodium
▶ Decreased blood flow on renal scan

Clinical Manifestations

▶ Decreased urine output
▶ Weight gain
▶ Edema
▶ Temperature at least 100°F (37.8°C)

▶ Tenderness over the graft site, with possible swelling of the kidney
▶ General malaise
▶ Increased blood pressure

Chronic rejection is the result of repeated episodes of acute rejection in which the vessels become infarcted owing to the vasculitis, and the renal tissue becomes scarred. This gradually leads to deteriorating kidney function. The symptoms are similar to those of acute rejection except for fever and graft enlargement. Laboratory findings are similar to those of acute rejection but also include signs of chronic renal failure, such as a declining hematocrit and calcium–phosphorus imbalance. The rate of deterioration can vary from months to years. A transplant nephrectomy is not usually required unless the kidney becomes necrotic and life-threatening.

Liver Acute rejection in liver transplantation is suspected when liver function tests, specifically PT/INR (most sensitive), aminotransferases, alkaline phosphatase, and total bilirubin, are increased. Clinical signs, such as decreased bile production and perigraft tenderness, may or may not occur.[19] Chronic rejection is believed to be due to multiple acute rejection episodes or a positive cross-match. A definitive diagnosis is made when a biopsy shows portal and bile duct inflammation and the presence of inflammatory cells, such as T lymphocytes.[19]

Heart Although acute rejection is often asymptomatic, subtle signs and symptoms may include decreased cardiac output, atrial flutter or fibrillation, elevated WBC count, and low-grade fever. Endomyocardial biopsy is performed weekly for the first month and then less frequently to diagnose rejection. Acute rejection is a major cause of death in the first year after transplantation. Chronic rejection is the leading cause of death after the first year of cardiac transplantation. The prevalence within 5 years of transplantation is at least 60%. This cell-mediated rejection causes progressive myocardial fibrosis, leading to heart dysfunction. The lesions in allographic vasculopathy are concentric, not focal, unlike in typical atherosclerosis, and allographic vasculopathy can often be missed on standard cardiac catheterization. Angina cannot be used as a warning sign for coronary artery disease because the heart is denervated. Instead, decreased exercise tolerance during stress testing or intravascular ultrasonography is used for diagnosis.[30]

Pancreas Rejection is a major cause of graft loss in pancreas transplantation. This may be attributed to the difficulty in diagnosing rejection. Elevated blood glucose is a late sign and may occur too late to initiate successful treatment. When the bladder is used for exocrine drainage, urinary amylase levels reflect rejection before hyperglycemia becomes obvious. In combined kidney–pancreas transplantation, an elevated serum creatinine may indicate rejection, although rejection can occur in one organ and not the other. Some experts state that chronic pancreas rejection may not occur in combined kidney–pancreas transplantation. The best pancreas transplant survival rate occurs when the procedure is performed simultaneously with kidney transplantation[10] (see Table 47-1). Needle biopsy during cystoscopy is used for definitive diagnosis.

Lung The signs and symptoms of lung transplant rejection are difficult to distinguish from pulmonary infection. Decreased lung function (i.e., forced expiratory volume), dyspnea, cough, decreased breath sounds, fever, and tachypnea may occur in both rejection and infection. Immediately after surgery, rejection may also be confused with volume overload, reperfusion injury, or ischemic injury secondary to preservation. Chest radiographs showing interstitial and perihilar edema may be signs of rejection and signal the need for biopsy. Even so, biopsies must be carefully interpreted to rule out infectious complications, such as infection with CMV or *Pneumocystis carinii*, which can have histological findings similar to those of acute rejection.

Chronic rejection is known as obliterative bronchiolitis and occurs in approximately 15% to 25% of lung transplant recipients. Acute rejection and infection are believed to play a role in obliterative bronchiolitis.[30]

Infection

Infection is the most common post-transplantation complication. Alterations in the integrity of mucosal barriers and severe neutropenia from the pretransplantation conditioning regimen produce an environment conducive to serious bacterial and fungal infection.

The causative agents are often from the patient's own flora, particularly from the gastrointestinal tract and integumentary system. Pathogens may be bacteria, fungi, viruses, and even protozoa. The latter three groups of organisms are referred to as opportunistic pathogens. Normally harmless and found in humans and in the environment, they pose serious threats to patients with compromised immune systems. They take advantage of the decreased host defenses—hence the term "opportunistic." Examples of opportunistic infections include herpes simplex and herpes zoster viruses, CMV, *Candida albicans*, *Pneumocystis carinii*, *Aspergillus* species, and *Cryptococcus* species.

All transplant recipients are at risk for bacterial infections due to intravascular lines and urinary drainage catheters, but organ transplant recipients can also acquire postoperative wound and lung infections. Usually broad-spectrum antibiotics are given prophylactically for 48 hours after organ transplantation or until invasive lines and drains are removed. HSCT recipients receive antibiotics prophylactically for months after transplantation. Table 47-8 lists infections caused by bacteria and other organisms that commonly occur after allogeneic HSCT.

Recipients of organ transplants are at high risk for infection during the first 3 months after transplantation because they receive high dosages of immunosuppressants. Infections in the post–stem cell transplantation period usually follow a predictable pattern based on the recovery of the immune system. Therefore, recipients of HSCT are at high risk for infection during the first month, which is the pre-engraftment phase, because of neutropenia. HSCT recipients may receive colony-stimulating factors to reduce their risk for infection by accelerating WBC recovery. They remain at high risk for infection if they are receiving immunosuppressive medications to prevent or treat GVHD.

During the first month, the predominant fungal infections in recipients of HSCT are *Aspergillus* species and *Candida* species, for which amphotericin B or fluconazole may be used prophylactically. The most fre-

Table 47-8 • Infections After Allogeneic Hematopoietic Stem Cell Transplantation

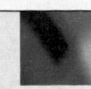

Period of Neutropenia (Days 0–30)	Period of Acute GVHD (Days 30–100)	Period of Chronic GVHD (Days 100+)
Gram-negative bacteria	Gram-negative bacteria	Encapsulated bacteria
Gram-positive bacteria	Gram-positive bacteria	Varicella-zoster virus
Herpes simplex	Cytomegalovirus	Cytomegalovirus
Candida species	Polyomavirus (BK virus)	*P. carinii*
Aspergillus species	Adenovirus	*Aspergillus* species
	Varicella-zoster virus	
	Candida species	
	Aspergillus species	
	Pneumocystis carinii	
	Toxoplasma gondii	

Adapted from Burt RK, Walsh T: Infection prophylaxis in bone marrow transplant recipients: Myths, legends and microbes. In Burt RK, Deeg HJ, Lothian S, et al (eds): Bone Marrow Transplantation. Austin, TX: Landes Bioscience, 1998, pp. 438–451.

quent viral infection is herpes simplex, and 80% of the patients who were seropositive before transplantation experience a reactivation of herpes simplex unless they receive acyclovir prophylactically.[31]

After the first month, the most common infection in all transplant recipients is CMV. To prevent CMV infection, patients who are CMV seronegative should receive only CMV-negative blood products. Many centers require that all blood transfusions be filtered. Ganciclovir may be appropriate for patients who are CMV seropositive and who are receiving increased immunosuppression for an episode of acute organ rejection. Close monitoring of HSCT recipients for CMV reactivation, as demonstrated by a rising level of CMV antigen by polymerase chain reaction in the blood, is imperative, with early preemption. Prevention is important in heart transplant recipients because there is a connection between CMV and coronary artery disease.[32,33] CMV may affect many organ systems; therefore, signs and symptoms of hepatitis, retinitis, enteritis, pneumonitis, fever, chills, and malaise may occur.

A small number of HSCT recipients contract severe and potentially fatal infections 3 months or more after transplantation, during the late recovery phase, because of cellular and humoral immune deficiencies. The most frequent causes of these infections are *Pneumococcus* species, *Staphylococcus aureus*, *Candida* species, and varicella-zoster virus.

If infection develops in immunosuppressed patients, the usual signs and symptoms may be absent. In these patients, even a small increase in temperature (99°F [37.2°C]) may be significant. Daily monitoring of the WBC count is necessary. After organ transplantation, the leukocyte count is usually slightly elevated because of surgery and steroid treatment. However, infection may be present if the elevation persists, a rapid elevation occurs after a decline,

or there is an increase in the percentage of immature WBCs (bands) noted on the differential.

It is essential to prevent infection in transplant recipients, who are immunosuppressed and may be neutropenic. Important nursing responsibilities include maintaining protective environments, practicing consistent and thorough provider handwashing and good oral and skin hygiene, monitoring vital signs frequently, and performing head-to-toe assessments. In some centers, additional protective measures include protective isolation systems, air filtration, gut and skin decontamination, and low-microbial diets. The benefit of these interventions has been debated, and their application is institution or protocol specific.[34–36]

In combined kidney–pancreas transplantation, immunosuppressive drugs may be discontinued in the presence of a severe infection to mobilize the patient's immune system. Consequently, the graft may be lost to save the patient. In heart, lung, and liver transplantation, immunosuppression may be decreased but must be continued.

Bleeding

Bleeding, oozing from the surface of the transplanted organ, or the presence of hematoma or lymphocele may occur after surgery. The heart transplant recipient is at risk for bleeding because the pericardial sac has stretched to accommodate an enlarged heart. When a smaller, healthy heart is implanted, the larger pericardial sac becomes a reservoir that can conceal postoperative bleeding. This may result in cardiac tamponade. Long-term coagulation therapy and liver congestion from pretransplantation heart failure also increase the risk for bleeding.

After liver transplantation, bleeding may occur as a result of coagulopathy because of liver dysfunction or from small vessels that continue to bleed after surgery. When the bladder drainage technique is used for exocrine drainage in pancreas transplantation, patients may have postoperative hematuria if the transplanted duodenal segment becomes ulcerated or if cystitis develops. Electrocautery using cystoscopy may be required for severe bleeding.

Gastrointestinal Complications Related to Steroid Therapy

Chronic steroid therapy increases the risk for peptic ulceration and erosive gastritis because it increases the secretion of hydrochloric acid and pepsinogen. Massive gastrointestinal bleeding may occur not only from steroid therapy but also from stress and decreased tissue viability caused by long-term protein restriction. For these reasons, patients usually are given histamine-2 (H$_2$) receptor antagonists (e.g., nizatidine or ranitidine) or proton pump inhibitors (e.g., omeprazole). The degree of renal function, together with concurrent medications, dictates which class of agent is selected for gastric cytoprotection.

Other serious gastrointestinal complications include acute pancreatitis, diverticulitis, *Candida* infection, esophagitis, obstruction from bowel adhesions, and ulcerative colitis. Infection becomes an added risk if the patient has an intestinal perforation. Ischemic bowel disease has been observed in the early post-transplantation period as a result of dehydration or ischemia due to low cardiac output.

More than one complication may occur simultaneously. In addition, signs and symptoms of gastrointestinal bleeding or perforation may be obscured by the anti-inflammatory effects of steroids. Therefore, complaints and changes in the patient's progress require thorough and prompt assessment.

The gastrointestinal tract of the patients who have had HSCT may also suffer the effects of the total-body irradiation and chemotherapy used in the preparatory regimen. Symptoms may include mucositis, nausea, vomiting, diarrhea, cramping, dyspepsia, anorexia, taste changes, and xerostomia.

HEMATOPOIETIC STEM CELL TRANSPLANTATION

Graft Failure

Graft failure is usually defined precisely by institutional protocols. However, all definitions include a complete absence of engraftment or a seemingly initial hematopoiesis after transplantation, with later decreasing blood cell counts and an absence of hematopoiesis.[37] The clinical features of graft failure include neutropenia, anemia, and thrombocytopenia occurring beyond the initial period expected as a result of high-dose chemotherapy or chemoradiation therapy.

The overall incidence of graft failure is less than 5%, and it occurs most often in patients with aplastic anemia or those receiving unrelated donor transplants. The etiology is multifactorial. An important component in the evaluation is differentiating graft failure from disease recurrence or drug-induced myelosuppression. Table 47-9 describes graft failure in terms of its risk factors, possible causes, and therapeutic and preventive measures.

The HSCT recipient may be more susceptible to the myelosuppressive effects of various drugs after the transplantation. Drugs with a potential to cause myelosuppression should be used very cautiously, if at all, to minimize the risk for drug-induced graft failure. In patients with delayed engraftment, it is prudent to review all medications and consider eliminating those that are not absolutely essential.

Veno-occlusive Disease of the Liver

Veno-occlusive disease of the liver (also called sinusoidal obstructive syndrome, or SOS) is a potentially fatal liver disease that occurs in 15% to 20% of recipients of HSCT. Veno-occlusive disease is a complication of the conditioning regimen and usually develops within 2 weeks of transplantation. The risk for veno-occlusive disease is increased in patients who have received total-body irradiation. Veno-occlusive disease may be severe; some studies report an incidence of 25% and a mortality rate close to 50%.[38–40]

Veno-occlusive disease occurs when fibrous material accumulates, resulting in obstruction of small venules in the liver. Subsequently, portal hypertension, acute liver congestion, and destruction of liver cells develop. Liver disease ranges from mild to severe, and severe liver failure may occur. In addition, veno-occlusive disease affects the kidneys; there is a decrease in renal blood flow, causing further water and sodium retention. Mild veno-occlusive disease persists until liver tissue heals and resumes normal function, usually 10 to 14 days after onset. Severe disease may result in multisystem failure.

Clinical manifestations of veno-occlusive disease usually begin during the first 3 weeks after transplantation and are characterized by hyperbilirubinemia, rapid weight gain, ascites, right upper quadrant pain, hepatomegaly, splenomegaly, and jaundice.[40] Treatment is supportive and focuses on maintaining intravascular volume and renal perfusion while minimizing fluid accumulation.[41] This may require central venous pressure monitoring and mechanical ventilation, as well as pulmonary artery pressure monitoring if excess fluids accumulate in the lungs. Sodium restriction is warranted, and spironolactone administration is necessary to decrease extravascular accumulation. Other supportive strategies may include renal-dose dopamine infusion, avoidance of diuretics that deplete intravascular volume, and chest physiotherapy to avoid pulmonary atelectasis.[40]

Strategies for prevention of veno-occlusive disease of the liver are currently undergoing investigation. These include anticoagulation with heparin, fibrinolytics such as tissue plasminogen activator or antithrombin III concentrates, defibrotide, prostaglandin E, and ursodeoxycholic acid (Actigall).[38–40,42,43]

Pulmonary Complications

Pulmonary complications develop in 30% to 60% of patients after HSCT.[44] Pulmonary complications may result from (1) infection, pulmonary edema, aspiration pneumonia, acute respiratory distress syndrome (ARDS), and septic shock; and (2) lung damage from total-body irradiation or pulmonary toxic chemotherapy agents.[41,44–48] Table 47-10 lists the pulmonary complications of HSCT.

Graft-Versus-Host Disease

GVHD, which is unique to allogeneic HSCT, results when the infused donor stem cells (graft) recognize the recipient (host) as foreign tissue. The graft then mounts an immunologic response attacking the host tissues, resulting in a T-cell–mediated reaction in the skin (rash), gastrointestinal tract (enteritis), and liver (elevated liver function test results). Figure 47-5 shows examples of the skin and gastrointestinal tract manifestations that may occur in acute GVHD.

The incidence of GVHD is 30% to 60% in cases involving histocompatible, sibling-matched allografts,

Table 47-9 • Graft Failure After Hematopoietic Stem Cell Transplantation: Risk Factors, Causes, and Preventive Measures

	Risk Factors	Causes	Preventive/Supportive Measures
Autologous stem cell transplants	• Patients with acute myelocytic leukemia, patients extensively pretreated • Low cell dose • Purged marrow • Marrow-suppressive drugs • Viral infection	• Defective marrow micro-environment with stromal cell damage • Collection of damaged stem cells due to extensive previous treatment • Drug-induced myelosuppression • Viral effects on stroma of bone marrow	• Harvest autologous stem cells early, before multiple cycles of potentially stem cell–toxic regimens have been given • Maximize number of infused cells (minimum number of autologous peripheral blood stem cells that results in consistent engraftment is at least 1×10^6 CD34+ cells/kg of body weight, below which engraftment may be incomplete or there may be failure of engraftment) • Avoid all myelosuppressive drugs after transplantation • Adjust doses of medications for renal dysfunction • Treat/prevent viral infections • Keep unmanipulated cells as backup in case or purged or manipulated grafts • Ensure that there is no folate or vitamin B_{12} deficiency • Administer G-CSF and rEPO as needed
Allogeneic stem cell transplants	• Diseases associated with a defective marrow micro-environment, including aplastic anemia and myelofibrosis • Stem cell source from HLA-mismatched, unrelated, or cord blood donor • Pretransplant transfusions, especially from a related donor • T-cell depletion, low cell dose, purging • Patients whose clinical condition precludes a sufficiently intensive conditioning regimen • Inadequate post-transplantation immunosuppression • Marrow-suppressive drugs • Viral infection, including infection with CMV	• Defective marrow microenvironment with stromal cell damage • Histocompatibility barriers • Allosensitization by transfusions • Damaged or inadequate number of stem cells infused • Persistence of host hematopoiesis • Persistence of immuno-competent host lymphocytes • GYHD-associated damage to bone marrow microenvironment • Drug-induced myelosuppression • Viral effects on stroma of bone marrow	• Avoid pretransplantation transfusions, especially from relatives • Select histocompatible donors • Ensure that the conditioning regimen is adequately immunosuppressive • Provide sufficient stem cell dose (minimum number of allogeneic peripheral blood stem cells that results in consistent engraftment is at least 2×10^6 CD34+ cells/kg of body weight, below which engraftment may be incomplete or there may be failure of engraftment) • Use post-transplantation immunosuppression with cyclosporine, tacrolimus, or methotrexate • Avoid all myelosuppressive drugs after transplantation • Adjust doses of medications for renal dysfunction • Treat/prevent viral infections • Ensure that there is no folate or vitamin B_{12} deficiency • Administer G-CSF, rEPO as needed • Consider cryopreserving autologous peripheral blood stem cells preallograft for possible use in the event of graft failure and overwhelming clinical problems such as hemorrhage or life-threatening infection

rEPO, recombinant erythropoietin.
Based on information from references 23, 77, and 83.

with more GVHD occurring when there is greater HLA mismatch between the donor and recipient.[49,50] The mortality rate due directly or indirectly to GVHD may reach 50%.[50] Risk factors other than histoincompatibility include sex mismatching; donor parity; older age; post-transplantation infectious complications, especially viral infections; the use of donor lymphocyte infusions after transplantation; and the type of GVHD prophylaxis used.[50]

GVHD is a serious complication, but it also has a beneficial effect in controlling the patient's malignancy in that immunocompetent donor cells are able to recognize the patient's malignant cells as foreign and eliminate them. This effect was originally identified in leukemia patients and was termed *graft-versus-leukemia effect*. Leukemia relapse was seen less often in patients with GVHD than in those without GVHD. The absence of GVHD in autologous transplant recipients is suspected to play a role in the higher disease relapse rates these patients experience. Recently, researchers are applying the graft-versus-malignancy effect to prevent disease recurrence after stem cell transplantation by the infusion of donor lymphocytes. This approach is called donor lymphocyte infusion. Research is also underway to devise strategies to induce GVHD in autologous recipients of HSCT.[51]

Table 47-10 • Pulmonary Complications of Hematopoietic Stem Cell Transplantation

Time Line	Complication
Acute (before day 30)	Pulmonary edema (secondary to fluid overload, cardiac dysfunction, or allergic reaction to medications/therapy) Oropharyngeal mucositis Aspiration pneumonia Pulmonary hemorrhage/diffuse alveolar hemorrhage Bacterial or fungal pneumonia Atelectasis Pleural effusion Recall radiation pneumonitis Allergic bronchospasm Transfusion-associated lung injury ARDS and septic shock
Early (before day 100)	Idiopathic interstitial pneumonitis Pulmonary embolism Viral pneumonia (CMV, herpes simplex virus, varicella-zoster virus, respiratory syncytial virus, adenovirus, parainfluenza, influenza) Protozoal pneumonia (*Pneumocystis carinii* pneumonia) Fungal pneumonia Bacterial pneumonia Transfusion-associated lung injury ARDS and septic shock
Late (after day 100)	Idiopathic interstitial pneumonitis Bacterial, fungal, or viral pneumonia Bronchiolitis obliterans/GVHD of lung

ARDS, acute respiratory distress syndrome.

Acute Graft-Versus-Host Disease

Acute GVHD may occur as early as 7 to 21 days after transplantation but peaks 30 to 40 days after transplantation. Acute GVHD targets the skin, liver, and gastrointestinal system. Skin reactions, which often occur first, include an itchy maculopapular, erythematous rash on the palms, soles, ears, face, and trunk. This may resolve or progress to generalized erythroderma and desquamation. Gastrointestinal symptoms include nausea, vomiting, anorexia, abdominal cramping, and large-volume diarrhea that is green and watery. Stool may be guaiac-positive as a result of intestinal mucosa sloughing. An enlarged liver, right upper quadrant pain, jaundice, and elevated bilirubin and alkaline phosphatase levels may occur. The severity and extent of acute GVHD are evaluated using a grading system (Table 47-11).

Chronic Graft-Versus-Host Disease

Chronic GVHD usually occurs in patients who have had acute GVHD, although it can occur in the absence of acute GVHD. Chronic GVHD typically occurs 100 to 400 days after transplantation. Among patients who survived 150 days after allogeneic stem cell transplantation, researchers observed chronic GVHD in 33% to 49% of HLA-identical related transplants and in 64% of matched unrelated donor transplants.[52]

Risk factors for chronic GVHD include previous acute GVHD, older recipient age, and sex mismatching (female donor and male recipient).[53] The incidence of chronic GVHD may also be higher in recipients of peripheral blood stem cells than in recipients of bone marrow–derived stem cells.[52] Another significant risk factor for the development of chronic GVHD is a continuing need for corticosteroids for control of GVHD by day 100 after transplantation.[54]

Clinical manifestations of chronic GVHD, which may be limited or extensive, are present in the skin, liver, eyes, oral cavity, lungs, gastrointestinal system, neuromuscular system, and a variety of other body systems. Although the onset of chronic GVHD typically occurs much later than acute GVHD, 100 to 400 days after transplantation there is a growing recognition that acute and chronic GVHD are best differentiated by their features, not their onset. Features of acute GVHD, including erythematous skin rash, liver function test abnormalities, nausea, vomiting, diarrhea, and abdominal pain, may occur after donor lymphocyte infusion. Similarly, pigmentary skin changes, sclerotic skin features, bronchiolitis obliterans, keratoconjunctivitis sicca, and oral dryness, all considered to be characteristics of chronic GVHD, may be observed in patients before day 100 after transplantation. A new paradigm for identifying acute and chronic GVHD and for diagnosing and staging chronic GVHD is evolving[55]; classification is based on the signs and symptoms of acute or chronic GVHD rather than on the number of days after transplantation. In addition, contemporary classification systems now identify an overlap syndrome in which diagnostic or distinctive features of chronic GVHD and acute GVHD appear together. Table 47-12 summarizes the clinical features, screening and evaluation, and interventions recommended for patients with chronic GVHD.[52,56-67]

Treatment and Prophylaxis of Graft-Versus-Host Disease

The first and most important way to limit GVHD is to find an HLA-matched donor. Despite such optimal matching of donor and recipient, further strategies to limit GVHD must be taken. The two major approaches to the prophylaxis of GVHD after HSCT are T-cell depletion of the graft and pharmacological therapy to prevent and treat GVHD.

T cells play a major role in the recognition of self from nonself proteins, and decreasing the number of T cells in the graft before transplantation may decrease the incidence and severity of GVHD. Methods of T-cell depletion involve physical, immunological, and pharmacological techniques. The desired outcome is a reduction or elimination of T cells capable of initiating life-threatening GVHD. However, T cells also play a role in engraftment, and T-cell depletion carries greater risks for infection, graft failure, and disease relapse.

A variety of immunosuppressive agents, alone or in combination, have been used prophylactically for acute GVHD.[50] Immunosuppressive medications

(text continues on page 1225)

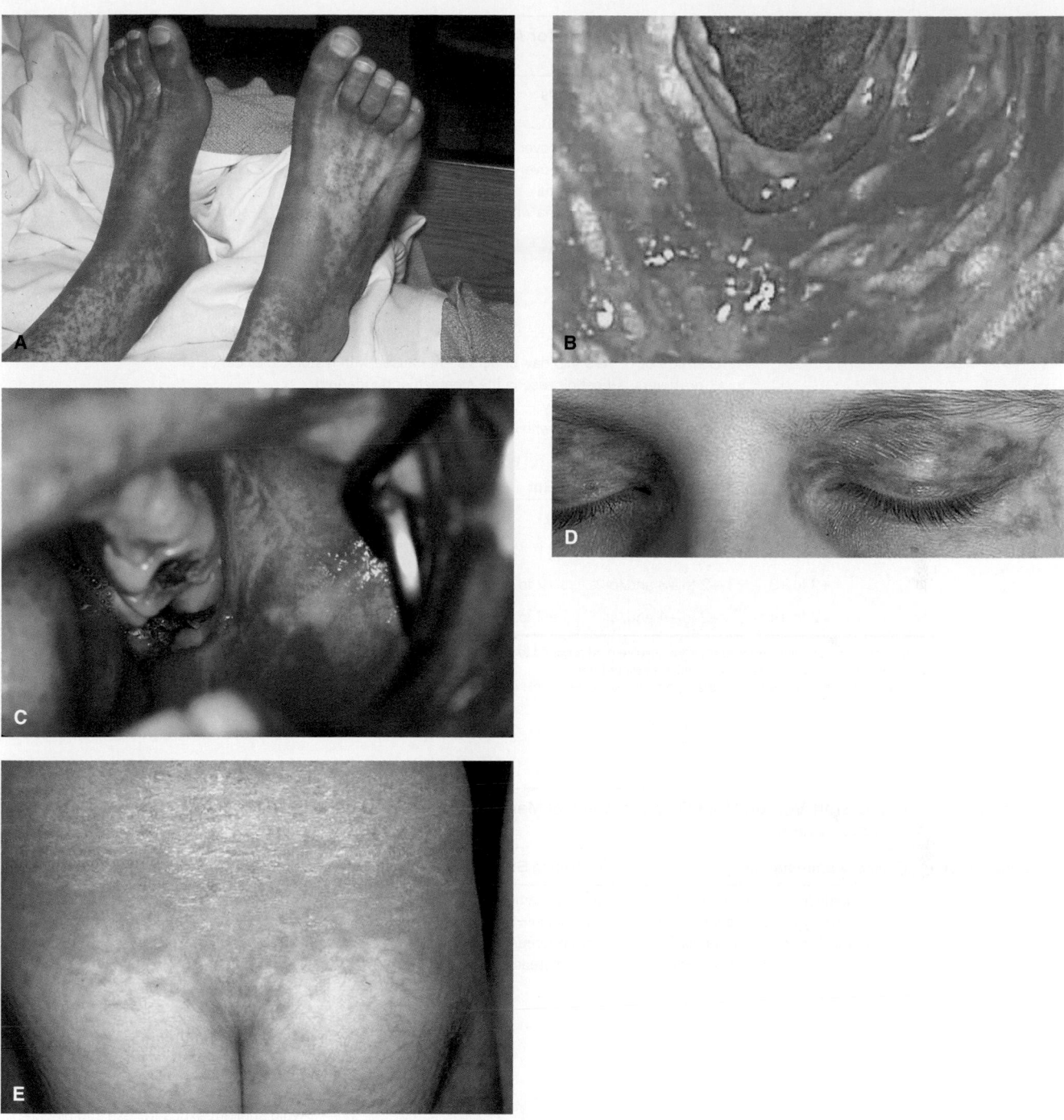

Figure 47-5 • Acute graft-versus-host disease (GVHD). **A:** GVHD of the skin is characterized by fine, discrete or confluent, erythematous macules and papules. Lesions may be pruritic or slightly tender with palpation. Earliest skin findings are usually seen on the face, palms and soles, and upper trunk. **B:** GVHD of the gastrointestinal tract. Images obtained during endoscopy demonstrate tissue edema, extensive erythema, and mucosal ulcerations. **C:** Oral lichen planus changes in a patient with GVHD more than 130 days after allogeneic peripheral blood stem cell transplantation. Note the confluent, smooth, white papules that create a lacy pattern on the buccal mucosa. **D:** Chronic GVHD of the skin with irregularly shaped, deeply hyperpigmented macular lesions. Note the atrophy of the dermal and subcutaneous tissues with paper-thin skin giving an easily wrinkled or shiny appearance. The term *poikiloderma* is used to describe the classic features of patchy hypopigmentation and hyperpigmentation, dermal atrophy, and telangiectasias (small-diameter linear blood vessels seen on the skins surface.) **E:** Lichenoid chronic GVHD of the skin of the lumbar region with flat-topped, violaceous papules; the surface is shiny and has a lacy white pattern. The eruption is confluent in some areas, and hypertrophic plaques have developed. Postinflammatory hyperpigmentation may develop. (**B,** photo courtesy of Bruce Greenwald, MD, University of Maryland Medical System, Baltimore Maryland; **C,** photo courtesy of Jane Fall-Dickson, RN, PhD, AOCN, National Institutes of Health, Bethesda Maryland; **D** and **E,** photos courtesy of T. L. Diepgen and G. Yihune, Dermatology Online Atlas [http://www.dermis.net/doia].)

Table 47-11 • Staging and Grading System for Acute Graft-Versus-Host Disease

Clinical Staging of Individual Organ Manifestations

Organ	Stage*	Description
Skin†	+1	Maculopapular eruption over <25% of body area
	+2	Maculopapular eruption over 25%–50% of body area
	+3	Generalized erythroderma
	+4	Generalized erythroderma with bullous formation and often with desquamation
Liver	+1	Bilirubin 2.0–3.0 mg/dL
	+2	Bilirubin 3.1–6.0 mg/dL
	+3	Bilirubin 6.1–15 mg/L
	+4	Bilirubin >15 mg/dL
Gut	+1	Diarrhea <500 mL/day
	+2	Diarrhea 500–999 mL/day, or persistent nausea with histologic evidence of graft-versus-host disease in the stomach or duodenum
	+3	Diarrhea ≥1,500 mL/day
	+4	Severe abdominal pain, with or without ileus

Overall Grade

Grade	Skin‡	Liver	Gut
I	+1 to +2	0	0
II	+1 to +3	+1 and/or	+1
III	+2 to +3	+2 to +3 and/or	+2 to +3
IV	+2 to +4	+2 to +4 and/or	+2 to +4

*Criteria for staging minimal degree of organ involvement required to confer that stage.
†Use rule of nines or burn chart to determine extent of rash.
‡If no skin disease is present, the overall grade is the highest single organ stage.

Table 47-12 • Chronic Graft-Versus-Host Disease: Clinical Manifestations, Screening/Evaluation, and Interventions

Organ/System	Clinical Manifestations	Screening Studies/Evaluation	Interventions
Dermal	Dyspigmentation, xerosis (dryness), erythema, hyperkeratosis, pruritus, sclerosis, lichenification, onycho-dystrophy (nail ridging/nail loss), alopecia	Clinical examination Skin biopsy—3-mm punch biopsy from forearm and posterior iliac crest areas	• Systemic Immunosuppressive therapy • PUVA; extracorporeal photopheresis • Topical tacrolimus ointment (Protopic) • Topical treatment with steroid creams, moisturizers/emollient, antibacterial ointments to prevent suprainfection; aggressive lubrication of the skin • Because the sweat glands are affected, avoid overheating because heat prostration and heat stroke can occur • Avoid sunlight exposure, use sun block lotion with a large hat that shades the face when outdoors
Oral	Lichen planus, xerostomia, ulceration	Oral biopsy from inner lower lip or buccal mucosa	• Steroid mouth rinses, oral PUVA, pilocarpine for xerostomia, fluoride gels/rinses to decrease caries • Careful attention to oral hygiene; regular dental evaluations
Ocular	Keratitis, sicca syndrome	Schirmer's test, ophthalmic evaluation	• Regular ophthalmological follow-up • Preservative-free tears • Temporary or permanent lacrimal duct occlusion • Fluid-ventilated, gas-permeable scleral lens prosthesis • Consider trial of cyclosporine ophthalmic emulsion (Restasis)

(continued)

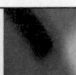

Table 47-12 • Chronic Graft-Versus-Host Disease: Clinical Manifestations, Screening/Evaluation, and Interventions (Continued)

Organ/System	Clinical Manifestations	Screening Studies/Evaluation	Interventions
Hepatic	Jaundice, abdominal pain	Liver function tests (alanine and aspartate aminotransferases, alkaline phosphatase, bilirubin)	• Consider bile acid displacement therapy with ursodeoxycholic acid (Actigall) 300 mg PO t.i.d.
Pulmonary	Obstructive/restrictive pulmonary disease, shortness of breath, cough, dyspnea, wheezing, fatigue, hypoxia, pleural effusion	Pulmonary function studies, peak flow, arterial blood gas, chest CT	• Prevent and treat pulmonary infections, including *Pneumocystis carinii and Streptococcus pneumoniae* • Aggressively investigate changes in pulmonary function because these may represent chronic GVHD of lung/bronchiolitis obliterans • Encourage smoking cessation
Gastrointestinal	Nausea, odynophagia, dysphagia, anorexia, early satiety, malabsorption, diarrhea, weight loss	Stool cultures, esophagogastroduodenoscopy, colonoscopy, nutritional assessment, fecal fat excretion studies, serum amylase, D-xylose absorption test, CT of the abdomen	• Referral to gastroenterologist; consultation with nutritionist and nutrition support • Consider empirical trial of pancreatic enzyme supplementation • Aggressive management of gastrointestinal symptoms such as nausea and vomiting • Consider the use of cholestyramine (Questran) in the management of diarrhea • Consider a trial of oral beclomethasone, budesonide, or both
Nutritional	Protein and calorie deficiency, malabsorption, dehydration, weight loss, muscle wasting	Weight, fat store measurement, prealbumin	• Nutritional monitoring, supplementation, symptom specific interventions • Trial of megestrol (Megace) or other approaches to appetite stimulation (e.g., mirtazapine [Remeron] or similar antidepressants; dronabinol [Marinol])
Genitourinary	Vaginal sicca, vaginal atrophy, stenosis, dyspareunia, vulvodynia	Pelvic examination; tissue biopsy	• Consider trial of mucosal application of corticosteroid ointment, cyclosporine ointment, or tacrolimus ointment • Vaginal dilators • Vaginal lubricants • Sexual counseling
Immunological	Hypogammaglobulinemia, autoimmune syndromes, development of autoantibodies	Quantitative immuno-globulin levels, CD4/CD8 lymphocyte subsets	• Intravenous immunoglobulin supplementation as indicated, and prophylactic antimicrobials (rotating antibiotics for recurrent sinopulmonary infections, PCP prophylaxis, topical antifungals) • Screening for CMV and other opportunistic infections with frequent surveillance cultures and antigen detection • Consider vaccination against influenza and pneumococcus
Musculoskeletal	Myositis fascritis, contractures, debility, muscle cramps/aches, carpal spasm	MRI measured range of motion, walk time, grip strength, CK, aldolase; performance status, formal quality-of-life evaluation (e.g., FACT-BMT), formal evaluation of rehabilitation needs (CARES)	• Physical therapy for stretching and endurance • Correct electrolyte imbalances • Consider clonazepam, magnesium supplementation treatment for muscle cramping or myalgias

CT, computed tomography; PCP, *Pneumocystis carinii* pneumonia; PUVA, psoralen and ultraviolet A.

minimize the ability of the newly developing donor immune system to recognize the host or patient as foreign and limit the immune response. Immunosuppressive drugs may need to be taken for months or years after an allogeneic HSCT. Immunosuppression may involve a single drug (often tacrolimus or cyclosporine A) or a combination of drugs (methotrexate, tacrolimus, cyclosporine A, steroids, mycophenolate mofetil, antithymocyte globulin), sometimes in combination with T-cell depletion.[50,68] Table 47-13 presents the immunosuppressive agents commonly used in

(text continues on page 1232)

Table 47-13 • Selected Immunosuppressive Drugs Used in Allogeneic [Hematopoietic] Stem Cell Transplantation

Agent/Drug	Mechanism of Action	Dosing/Administration	Adverse Reactions	Comments
Cyclosporine A (Sandimmune, Neoral)	Prevents IL-2 gene expression and thus impairs IL-2 synthesis and activation of T lymphocytes	Total daily dose: usually 1.5 mg/kg IV q12h, 0.75 mg/kg q6h or 3 mg/kg/d as a continuous infusion, with dosage adjusted to achieve therapeutic levels IV to PO conversion: approximately 1:3 Dosage dependent on achieving and sustaining therapeutic blood levels based on laboratory evaluation Therapeutic monitoring not required once drug is being tapered	Metabolic: hyperkalemia and hyperglycemia, hypomagnesemia, hyperlipidemia, hyperuricemia, diabetes mellitus Neurotoxicity: headache, tremor, insomnia, paresthesia, dizziness, seizures GI: diarrhea, nausea, constipation, anorexia, vomiting, abdominal pain, ascites, elevated liver function tests Renal: elevated creatinine, nephrotoxicity Cardiovascular: hypertension, chest pain Hematological: anemia Cutaneous: acneiform rash, striae Other: peripheral edema, infection, impaired wound healing, osteoporosis, gingival hyperplasia, flushing, sweating, hirsutism	• Bioavailability differs between oral solution and capsule formulation. Once regimen is established, patients should be instructed not to change formulation or brand. • Take with food. • Instruct patient on importance of strict adherence to administration schedule and to notify health care team immediately if unable to take due to GI side effects. • Monitor serum creatinine, BUN, potassium, magnesium, glucose, and triglyceride levels. • Avoid potassium-sparing diuretics. • Replete electrolytes as indicated. • Coadministration with grapefruit juice may increase cyclosporine levels and should be avoided. • Drug–drug interactions can lead to subtherapeutic or toxic cyclosporine levels. Drugs that inhibit or induce cytochrome P-450 are most responsible (see Table 47-14). • Cyclosporine trough levels to be drawn before administration of morning dose. Therefore, doses are usually timed for 10 a.m. and 10 p.m. to allow trough blood draw at morning clinic visit. Instruct patient to bring dose to clinic and to administer once trough level drawn. • Should not be used simultaneously with tacrolimus. • Tacrolimus should be discontinued 24 h before starting cyclosporine. In the presence of increased tacrolimus levels, initiation of cyclosporine should usually be further delayed. • Doses should be adjusted for renal dysfunction. • Monitor levels carefully in patients with renal or hepatic dysfunction.
Tacrolimus (Prograf)	Impaired synthesis of IL-2 and prevents T-lymphocyte proliferation; interferes with the gene transcription for a variety of cytokines including IFN-γ, TNF-α	Total daily dose: usually 1–2 mg PO q12h; 0.05–0.1 mg/kg/d as a continuous infusion, with dosage adjusted to achieve therapeutic levels	Metabolic: hyperkalemia and hypokalemia, hyperglycemia, hypomagnesemia, hyperlipidemia, hypophosphatemia, diabetes mellitus Neurotoxicity: headache, tremor, insomnia, paresthesia, dizziness, seizures GI: diarrhea, nausea, constipation, anorexia, vomiting, abdominal pain, ascites, elevated liver function tests	• Take on empty stomach. • Instruct patient on importance of strict adherence to administration schedule and to notify the health care team immediately if unable to take due to GI side effects. • Monitor serum creatinine, BUN, potassium, magnesium, phosphorus, glucose, and triglyceride levels. • Avoid potassium-sparing diuretics. • Replete electrolytes as indicated • Coadministration with grapefruit juice may increase tacrolimus levels and should be avoided.

	Action	Dosage	Adverse Effects	Nursing Considerations
		IV to PO conversion: approximately 1:4 Dosage dependent on achieving and sustaining therapeutic blood levels based on laboratory evaluation Therapeutic monitoring not required once drug is being tapered	Renal: elevated creatinine, nephrotoxicity Cardiovascular: hypertension, chest pain Hematological: anemia, leukocytosis, thrombocytopenia Cutaneous: pruritus, acneiform rash Pulmonary: pleural effusion, atelectasis, dyspnea Other: peripheral edema, infection, impaired wound healing, osteoporosis	• Drug–drug interactions can lead to subtherapeutic or toxic tacrolimus levels. Drugs that inhibit or induce cytochrome P-450 are most responsible (see Table 47-14). • Tacrolimus trough levels to be drawn before administration of morning dose. Therefore doses are usually timed for 10 a.m. and 10 p.m. to allow trough blood draw at morning clinic visit. Instruct patient to bring dose to clinic and to administer once trough level drawn. • Should not be used simultaneously with cyclosporine. • Cyclosporine should be discontinued 24 h before starting tacrolimus. In the presence of elevated cyclosporine levels, initiation of tacrolimus is delayed. • Doses should be adjusted for renal dysfunction. • Monitor levels carefully in patients with renal or hepatic dysfunction.
Corticosteroid	Decreases cytotoxic T-cell proliferation, inhibits production of IL-1 and IFN-g, prevents production of IL-2, inhibits neutrophils function by stabilizing leukocyte lysosomal membrane and inhibiting chemotaxis	Dosage varies according to institutional protocols Dosage: 0.5–2 mg/kg/d q12h, with tapering schedule determined based on starting dose and patient response	Metabolic: fluid and electrolyte imbalance, diabetes mellitus, hyperlipidemia Neurotoxicity: tremors, seizures, headache, difficulty concentrating, insomnia GI: GI irritation Cardiovascular: hypertension, dysrhythmias Cutaneous: bruising, fragile skin Neurotoxicity: tremors, seizures, headache Other: hunger, peripheral edema, infection, impaired wound healing, hirsutism, osteoporosis, weight gain, steroid myopathy, cataracts/ glaucoma, cushingoid changes, psychiatric disturbances (steroid psychosis, mood changes, confusion)	• Usually used in combination with cyclosporine or tacrolimus. • Consult physical therapy for proximal muscle strengthening exercise program. • Instruct patient in strategies to prevent or treat hyperglycemia, and in diabetic self-management. • Administer oral corticosteroids with food/milk to minimize GI upset. • Administer H-2 blockers as ordered. • May increase tacrolimus or cyclosporine levels. • Report complaints of visual changes and consult ophthalmology. • For patients on long-term steroids or otherwise at risk for or experiencing osteopenia (e.g., patients with acute lymphocytic leukemia, postmenopausal) ensure regular dual-energy x-ray absorptiometry scans, calcium and vitamin D supplementation and specific treatment for osteopenia with antiresorptive agents such as pamidronate, aledronate. • Tapering calendar specifying the dosage to be taken each day can help facilitate adherence in patients who are on tapering doses of steroids, or an alternate-day steroid regimen.

(continued)

Table 47-13 • Selected Immunosuppressive Drugs Used in Allogeneic [Hematopoietic] Stem Cell Transplantation (Continued)

Agent/Drug	Mechanism of Action	Dosing/Administration	Adverse Reactions	Comments
Mycophenolate mofetil (MMF) (Cellcept)	Antimetabolite that selectively inhibits the proliferation of T and B lymphocytes by interfering with purine nucleotide synthesis	Dosage: 1–1.5 g IV or PO q12h depending on institutional guidelines	Metabolic: hyperkalemia and hypokalemia, hyperlipidemia, hypophosphatemia, hyperglycemia Neurotoxicity: headache, insomnia, tremors, seizures GI: diarrhea, nausea, constipation, anorexia, vomiting, abdominal pain, hepatotoxicity Renal: elevated creatinine, nephrotoxicity Cardiovascular: hypertension, hypotension, dysrhythmias Hematological: anemia, leukocytosis, thrombocytopenia Cutaneous: acneiform rash Pulmonary: cough, dyspnea Other: fever, edema, pain, infection, muscle weakness, anxiety, depression	• MMF should be taken on an empty stomach. • Monitor complete blood count at regular intervals and adjust dosage for pancytopenia, as ordered. • Monitor liver function tests (bilirubin and serum aminotransferases) at regular intervals, adjust dosage for liver function abnormalities, as ordered. • Monitor serum levels of the MMF metabolic to guide treatment in patients with renal dysfunction. In the setting of renal impairment, or when coadministered with probenicid, acyclovir, or ganciclovir, the drug concentrations of MMF and of these drugs may increase. • There may be decreased MMF absorption when coadministered with magnesium oxide, aluminum- or magnesium-containing antacids, or cholestyramine.
Methotrexate	Antimetabolite that inhibits dihydrofolate reductase, thereby hindering DNA synthesis and cell reproduction, and thus inhibiting lymphocyte proliferation	Institutional protocols vary Usual dose: 5–15 mg/m² given IV on days 1, 3, 6, and 11 after transplantation	Myelosuppression, mucositis, photosensitivity, interstitial pneumonitis, hepatotoxicity, nephrotoxicity	• Dose and schedule for methotrexate prophylaxis for GVHD vary by institution. Common regimen is 5–15 mg/m2 on days 1, 3, 6 and 11 post-transplantation. • Doses may be adjusted or held for severe mucositis and renal or hepatic insufficiency. Doses may need to be adjusted for hypoalbuminemia. • Wait until at least 24 h after stem cell infusion to give day +1 dose.
Rituximab (Rituxan)	Rituximab binds specifically to the B-lymphocyte cell surface antigen CD20, inducing B-cell death. CD20 is a protein located on normal pre-B and mature B-lymphocytes	375 mg/m² by intravenous infusion given weekly for 4 wk. Administer slowly. The first infusion of rituximab should be initiated at a rate of 50 mg/h. If hypersensitivity or infusion-related events do not occur, the infusion rate should be increased by 50 mg/h increments every 30 min to a maximum of 400 mg/h. Subsequent infusions can be initiated at 100 mg/h, with increases of 100 mg/h every 30 min to a maximum of 400 mg/h. Protect from sunlight. Do not filter	Mild to moderate infusional toxicities consisting of fever and chills/rigors in the majority of patients during the first rituximab infusion. Other frequent infusion reaction symptoms include nausea, pruritus, angioedema, asthenia, hypotension, headache, bronchospasm, throat irritation, rhinitis, urticaria, rash, vomiting, myalgia, dizziness, and hypertension. These reactions generally occur within 30 to 120 min of beginning the first infusion and resolve with slowing or interruption of the rituximab infusion and with supportive care (diphenhy-	• Premedication consisting of acetaminophen and diphenhydramine should be considered before each infusion. • Medications and equipment necessary for the management of hypersensitivity/anaphylaxis should be readily available (e.g., epinephrine, antihistamines, corticosteroids, oxygen). • Assess baseline vital signs. Check complete blood count with differential and renal function. • Because of the potential for transient hypotension during infusion antihypertensive medication should not be taken 12 h prior to infusion. • The infusion should be interrupted if infusion-related reactions occur. Mild side effects usually resolve with temporary discontinuation of the infusion or administration of meperidine, diphenhydramine, or other supportive therapy such as bronchodilators or IV saline.

dramine, acetaminophen, IV saline, and vasopressors). The incidence of infusion reactions is highest during the first infusion (77%) and decreases with each subsequent infusion.

Other adverse effects include lymphopenia and decreased serum immunoglobulins, which can contribute to risk for serious infections, including hepatitis B reactivation with fulminant hepatitis, progressive multifocal leukoencephalopathy (PML), and other opportunistic infections.

Adverse effects also include cardiac dysrhythmias, renal toxicity, bowel obstruction and perforation; neutropenia, anemia; cough, rhinitis, bronchospasm, dyspnea, interstitial pneumonitis, bronchiolitis obliterans.

- Patients experiencing chills should be offered blankets and comfort measures until the reaction subsides. Administration of acetaminophen as often as every three hours as needed is recommended.
- Most patients who experience non–life-threatening reactions are able to complete the full course of therapy. Once the infusion-related side effect has completely resolved and the patient is comfortable (usually about 30 min), rituximab may be restarted at half the previous infusion rate. After restarting the infusion, recurrence of the side effect usually does not occur.
- Patients and family members should be advised concerning infusion-related side effects and informed that driving or operating equipment cannot be resumed until the effects of sedation are gone.
- Women of childbearing age should receive instructions to ensure that they are using effective contraceptive methods during therapy and for 12 mo after therapy is completed. Infant nursing should be discontinued until circulating levels are no longer detectable, which is usually 12 mo after therapy is completed.
- The safety of immunization with live viral vaccines following rituximab therapy has not been studied, and vaccination with live virus vaccines is not recommended.

Daclizumab (Zenapax)

Monoclonal antibody against the IL-2 receptor expressed on activated T cells.

Binds to the IL-2 receptor in a non-activating fashion, competing with IL-2 and thereby inhibiting IL-2 driven proliferation of the activated T lymphocyte

IL-2–induced proliferation of activated (antigen-stimulated) T lymphocytes is a critical step in proliferation and ultimately tissue destruction

Institutional protocols vary
Usual dose: 1 mg/kg by IV administration

Constipation, nausea, vomiting, diarrhea, abdominal pain, abdominal distention, edema, tremor, headache, dizziness, nephrotoxicity, chest pain, tachycardia, fever, pain, fatigue, hypertension, hypotension, dyspnea, pulmonary edema, coughing, musculoskeletal pain, back pain

- Anaphylactoid reactions after the administration of daclizumab have not been observed but can occur after the administration of proteins. Medications for the treatment of severe hypersensitivity reactions should be available for immediate use.
- The calculated volume of daclizumab should be mixed with 50 mL of sterile 0.9% sodium chloride solution and administered through a peripheral or central vein over a 15-min period. Once the infusion is prepared, it should be administered intravenously within 4 h. If it must be held longer, it should be refrigerated between 2°–8°C (36°–46°F) for up to 24 h. After 24 h, the prepared solution should be discarded.
- No incompatibility between daclizumab and PVC or polyethylene bags or infusion sets has been observed.
- No dosage adjustment is necessary for patients with severe renal impairment.

(continued)

Table 47-13 • Selected Immunosuppressive Drugs Used in Allogeneic [Hematopoietic] Stem Cell Transplantation (Continued)

Agent/Drug	Mechanism of Action	Dosing/Administration	Adverse Reactions	Comments
Infliximab (Remicade)	Monoclonal antibody against TNF-α Binds to soluble and membrane-bound TNF-α, producing reduction in serum IL-1 and reduced levels of nitric oxide synthase	Institutional protocols vary Usual dose: 10 mg/kg by IV administration Administer over at least 2 h Must be given with a low protein-binding filter of 1.2 μm or less	Headache, nausea, abdominal pain, fatigue, fever, and coughing Infusion reactions, including fever, chills, chest pain, hypotension, headache, and urticaria can occur during the infusion and for up to 2 h after the infusion is complete. There is no increase in the incidence of reactions after the initial infusion. Delayed, serum sickness–like reactions including myalgias, arthralgias, fever, rash, sore throat, dysphagia, and hand and facial edema can be seen 3–12 ds after infusion. Patients may develop human antichimeric antibody.	• Monitor patient for development of infusional toxicities. • Consider premedication with acetaminophen and diphenhydramine (Benadryl). • Initiate therapy at 10 mL/h × 15 min, increase to 20 mL/h × 15 min, and then increase to 40 mL/h × 15 min, then 80 mL/hr × 15 min, then 150 mL/h × 30 min, and then 250 mL/h × 30 min to complete infusion in 2 h. • Stop or slow infusion and give Benadryl, acetaminophen, or Solu-Cortef to treat mild to moderate infusion reaction. Resume infusion at 10 mL/h once reaction controlled or abated. • Medications for treating hypersensitivity reactions (e.g., acetaminophen, antihistamines, corticosteroids, or epinephrine) and supplemental oxygen should be available for immediate use in the event of a reaction. • Incompatible with PVC equipment or devices. Use glass infusion bottles and polyethylene–lined administration sets.
Alemtuzumab (Campath)	Monoclonal antibody directed against the cell surface antigen CD52, which is expressed on B and T lymphocytes	Institutional protocols vary Usual dose: 20 mg/d IV given over several hours for 5 ds, beginning before transplantation	Infusional toxicities may be severe, and include fever and rigors in more than 80% of patients. Other adverse effects include neutropenia, anemia, thrombocytopenia, nausea, vomiting, rash, fatigue, and hypotension.	• Premedicate patient with acetaminophen and Benadryl. • Medications for treating hypersensitivity reactions (e.g., acetaminophen, antihistamines, corticosteroids, or epinephrine) and supplemental oxygen should be available for immediate use in the event of a reaction. • Consider treatment with meperidine to control infusional rigors. • Administer fluid bolus as ordered to treat hypotension. • Produces profound and rapid lymphopenia; therefore, patients require broad antifungal, antibacterial, antiviral, and antiprotozoal prophylaxis for at least 4 mo after treatment.
Antithymocyte globulin (Atgam, equine) (Thymoglobulin, rabbit)	Polyclonal immunoglobulin composed of horse or rabbit antibodies capable of destroying human leukocytes	Institutional protocols vary Usual dose: 10–40 mg/kg/d for equine ATG, and 2.5 mg/kg/d for rabbit ATG	Seizures, laryngospasm, anaphylaxis, pulmonary edema, leukopenia, and thrombocytopenia. ATG is a foreign xenogeneic protein and an antibody, which may cause serum sickness, including myalgias, arthralgias, fever, rash, sore	• Monitor patient closely both during infusion and after infusion for signs of serum sickness and anaphylaxis. Consider premedication with corticosteroids, acetaminophen, and H_1 and H_2 blockers. • Medications for treating hypersensitivity reactions (e.g., acetaminophen, antihistamines, corticosteroids, or epinephrine) and supplemental oxygen should be available for immediate use in the event of a reaction.

throat, dysphagia and hand and facial edema.

Drug	Action	Dosing	Adverse effects
Sirolimus (Rapamune)	Structurally similar to tacrolimus and cyclosporine; however, it has a distinct immunosuppressant activity. Inhibits response of B and T lymphocytes to cytokine stimulation by IL-2 and inhibits antibody production by B cells	Long half-life permits once-daily dosing. Monitor trough blood levels	Hyperlipidemia, thrombocytopenia, leukopenia, headache, nausea, anorexia, dizziness
Methoxsoralen (Oxsoralen)	When photoactivated by ultraviolet light, drug inhibits mitosis by binding covalently to pyrimidine bases in DNA	400 µg/kg PO 1.5–2 h before exposure to ultraviolet light	

Nursing considerations:

- Because transient and at times severe thrombocytopenia may occur after ATG administration, in patients with platelet counts less than 100,000, monitor platelet count 1 h after ATG administration, and transfuse platelets as indicated.
- May suppress hematopoietic recovery if used in patients who have recently undergone high-dose therapy.
- Oral bioavailability is variable and is improved with high-fat meals.
- Like tacrolimus and cyclosporine, sirolimus is metabolized through the cytochrome P-450 3A system.
- Always administer doses in the evening to minimize impact of drowsiness on lifestyle and safety.
- Teach patient to use caution when taking thalidomide with other drugs that can cause drowsiness or neuropathy.
- Teach patient to rise slowly from a supine position to avoid lightheadedness.
- Teach patient to report immediately signs or symptoms suggestive of peripheral neuropathy, including numbness or tingling in the hands or feet or the development of skin rash or skin lesion. These may require immediate cessation of the drug until the patient can be evaluated for the neuropathy or skin rash.
- Teach patient to use protective measures (e.g., sunscreens and protective clothing) against exposure to ultraviolet light or sunlight.
- Control or manage constipation with a stool softener or mild laxative.
- May impair wound healing.
- Patients who have received cytotoxic chemotherapy or radiation and who are taking methoxsoralen are at increased risk for skin cancers, and long-term use may increase the risk of skin cancer.
- Toxicity increases with concurrent use of phenothiazines, thiazides, and sulfanilamides.
- Severe burns may occur from sunlight or ultraviolet A exposure if dose or treatment frequency is exceeded.
- Pretreatment eye examinations are indicated to evaluate for the presence of cataracts. Repeat eye examinations should be performed every 6 mo while patients are undergoing psoralen and ultraviolet A therapy.

ANC, absolute neutrophil count; GI, gastrointestinal; IFN, interferon; IL, interleukin; IV, intravenous; PO, oral; PVC, polyvinyl chloride; TNF, tumor necrosis factor.

patients undergoing HSCT and the associated nursing implications.[67,69–77]

For patients at higher risk for GVHD, especially those undergoing matched unrelated HSCT, more intensive strategies for GVHD prevention are necessary. Many drug–drug interactions are associated with cyclosporine A and tacrolimus. Table 47-14 lists drugs that may interact with cyclosporine A and tacrolimus.[69] It is important to instruct patients to take their immunosuppressive medication exactly as directed and to contact their physician before starting any new medication.

Prospective, randomized trials have demonstrated that combination therapy is superior to single-drug therapy in the prevention of acute GVHD. However, to date, research has not shown that any one prophylactic regimen is superior in preventing acute GVHD or improving overall outcome.[50,68] The most widely used pharmacological regimen for the prophylaxis of acute GVHD is a combination of methotrexate and either cyclosporine A or tacrolimus.[78] Other drugs included in some GVHD prophylaxis regimens are corticosteroids, antithymocyte globulin, daclizumab, and mycophenolate mofetil.[68,78–80] Table 47-15 presents several sample regimens for GVHD prophylaxis.

If grade II to IV acute GVHD develops, treatment is usually required.[56] Corticosteroids are the main component of therapy, along with continuing treatment with the immunosuppressive agent used for prophylaxis (tacrolimus or cyclosporine A). Corticosteroids are the main component of therapy, along with continuation of the immunosuppressive agents used for initial prophylaxis.[68,78–80] High doses of methylprednisolone (1 to 20 mg/kg/day) may be used. However, these high-dose regimens are associated with fatal infections and cannot be administered for more than a few days, and the dose of methylprednisolone is rapidly tapered to 2 mg/kg/day in divided doses. Once maximal improvement is achieved, the steroids are tapered over 8 to 20 weeks, based on patient response.

For patients with GVHD in whom initial therapy has failed, a variety of salvage or secondary regimens, including mycophenolate mofetil, infliximab, and daclizumab, are available. Once chronic GVHD develops, the usual therapy involves steroids, cyclosporine A, tacrolimus, and a variety of other immunosuppressive agents.[52,63,65,66,72,81] Gut rest, pain control, and antimicrobial prophylaxis coupled with hyperalimentation, if needed, are important aspects of the supportive care of patients with acute GVHD.[50] The outcome of treatment of acute GVHD is predicted by the overall grade of acute GVHD; higher overall grades are associated with poorer outcomes.[52,53] Response to treatment is another key determinant of outcome, and mortality is greatest in patients who do not achieve a complete response to the initial treatment strategy for acute GVHD.[54]

• Long-Term Considerations

Organ transplantation can lead to long-term survival. Increasing numbers of recipients lead healthier and longer lives. However, complications may occur long after transplantation.

Table 47-14 • Drugs That May Alter Levels of Cyclosporine and Tacrolimus

Effects	Known Interactions	Suspected Interactions
Increase serum levels	Erythromycin Clarithromycin Itraconazole Fluconazole Ketoconazole Corticosteroids	H₂ antagonists Cephalosporins Thiazide diuretics Furosemide Acyclovir Warfarin Calcium channel blockers (i.e., diltiazem, verapamil, nicardipine) Oral contraceptives Doxycycline Metoclopramide Coadministration with grapefruit juice
Decrease serum levels	Phenytoin or phenobarbital Rifampin or isoniazid Sulfadiazine + trimethoprim (intravenous)	Sulfinpyrazone Carbamazepine Anticonvulsants
Cause additive nephrotoxicity	Amphotericin B Aminoglycosides Melphalan Trimethoprim-sulfamethoxazole	Nonsteroidal anti-inflammatory drugs
Alter immunosuppressive effects		Propranolol Verapamil Etoposide

Based on information from Melocco T, Kerr S, McKenzie C: Drug toxicity and interactions posttransplant. In Atkinson K (ed): Clinical Bone Marrow Transplantation: A Clinical Textbook. Cambridge, UK: Cambridge University Press, 1994, pp 396–409.

·:::· **Table 47-15 • Examples of Commonly Used Drug Regimens for Prophylaxis of Acute GVHD**

Regimen	Dosing Schedule
Cyclosporine/steroids	Cyclosporine 3 mg/kg/day IV infusion from day −2, taper 10% weekly starting day +180* Methylprednisolone 0.25 mg/kg b.i.d. days +7 to +14, 0.5 mg/kg b.i.d. days +15 to +28, 0.4 mg/kg b.i.d. days +29 to +42, 0.3 mg/kg b.i.d. days +43 to +58, 0.25 mg/kg b.i.d. days +59 to +119, and 0.1 mg/kg daily days +120–180.
Cyclosporine/ methotrexate/ steroids	Cyclosporine 5 mg/kg/d IV infusion from day −2, taper 20% every 2 wk starting day +84* Methotrexate 15 mg/m2 on day +1, 10 mg/m2 on days +3 and +6 Methylprednisolone 0.25 mg/kg b.i.d. days +7 to +14, 0.5 mg/kg b.i.d. days +15 to +28, 0.4 mg/kg b.i.d. days +29 to +42, 0.3 mg/kg b.i.d. days +43 to +58, 0.25 mg/kg b.i.d. days +59 to +119, and 0.1 mg/kg daily days +120–180
Tacrolimus/ minimethotrexate	Tacrolimus 0.03 mg/kg/d infusion from day −2, taper 20% every 2 wk starting day +180* Methotrexate 5 mg/m2 on days +1, +3, +6, and +11
Antithymocyte globulin (ATG)/ cyclosporine/ methotrexate	ATG 20 mg/kg IV days −3, −2, and −1 Cyclosporine 5 mg/kg/d IV infusion from day −1, taper 10% weekly starting day +180* Methotrexate 10 mg/m² on days +1, +3, +6, and +11

*Either tacrolimus or cyclosporine has been used with this methotrexate or steroid dose schedule.

Long-term care focuses on monitoring the patient's progress and adherence to the health care regimen. In solid organ transplant recipients, a major cause of graft loss in the long term is failure of patients to adhere to the medication regimen. Patients must also be monitored for the development of late complications, including infections, hypertension and cardiovascular disease, chronic rejection, and recurrence of the original disease, such as hepatitis in liver transplantation and recurrent glomerulonephritis in kidney transplantation. There is also increased incidence of post-transplantation lymphoproliferative disease (PTLD) in solid organ transplant recipients who are receiving long-term immunosuppression.[82–83]

Weight gain can be a significant complication after transplantation as a result of steroid use or because of general improved well-being related to the organ transplantation. Osteoporosis secondary to high steroid use is also a long-term issue for organ transplant recipients, more often for heart, liver, and stem cell transplant recipients than for kidney transplant recipients.

The refinement and success of HSCT has resulted in a large population of patients who have achieved control of their underlying disease. However, these patients must often deal with long-term sequelae and late effects of HSCT. In addition to chronic GVHD and infectious risks, they may experience a wide range of complications (Box 47-6).[67,84–103] Most transplantation centers have unique requirements for continued follow-up care that depends on protocols. The nature of the patient's complications determines the frequency of clinic visits. Patients and clinicians can use the guidelines provided at http://www.cibmtr.org/PUBLICATIONS/guidelines.html to direct long-term follow-up care after hematopoietic stem cell transplantation. Table 47-16 presents guidelines for screening and management of late effects in HSCT recipients.[67,84.86,87,90-93,95–103]

Box 47-6 • Early and Late Complications of Autologous and Allogeneic Hematopoietic Stem Cell Transplantation

Early (Occurring Before Day 1100)

Regimen-related toxicity
- Hemorrhagic cystitis
- Veno-occlusive disease of the liver
- Pulmonary complications
- Renal complications
- Neurological complications
    Nutritional complications
    Idiopathic pneumonitis
    Graft failure
    Infection
- Viral
- Bacterial
- Fungal
    Graft-versus-host disease
    Relapse

Late (Occurring After Day +100)

Regimen-related toxicity
- Cataracts
- Neurological conditions (peripheral and autonomic neuropathies)
- Gonadal dysfunction
- Endocrine dysfunction
    Immunodeficiency
    Infection
    Musculoskeletal
- Osteoporosis
- Avascular necrosis
    Chronic graft-versus-host disease
    Relapse of malignancy
    Secondary malignancy

Table 47-16 • Evaluation and Screening of Late Effects of Hematopoietic Stem Cell Transplantation

System/Dimension	Possible Late Effects	Evaluation and Screening
Disease status	Relapse/recurrence	Determined based on site of original disease, but may include CT scans, bone marrow aspirate and biopsy, lumbar puncture, cytogenetics, and engraftment studies Evaluation for minimal residual disease (if available)
Engraftment	Graft failure/marrow dysfunction with cytopenia	CBC with differential Bone marrow aspirate and biopsy Engraftment studies: to detect differences between DNA of donor and recipient and thus establish engraftment: variable nucleotide tandem repeats or restriction fragment length polymorphisms; cytogenetic studies may also be used to establish engraftment if the donor and recipient are of opposite sexes
Immunological function/recovery	Disorders of B- and T-lymphocyte quantity and function Hypogammaglobulinemia	CD4/CD8 lymphocyte subsets Quantitative immunoglobulin levels Vaccination titers
Cardiopulmonary effects	Interstitial pneumonitis Bronchiolitis obliterans Hypertension, cardiomyopathy, pericardial damage, peripheral vascular disease, coronary artery disease	Chest x-ray Pulmonary function tests with diffusing capacity of lungs for carbon monoxide Electrocardiogram Echocardiogram History and physical examination
Neurological effects	Peripheral and autonomic neuropathies Cognitive changes, shortened attention span, difficulty with concentration Leukoencephalopathy Ototoxicity	Health history Neurological examination Neuropsychological testing Rehabilitation medicine Audiological testing
Gastrointestinal effects	Liver dysfunction Malabsorption syndromes	Liver function tests Hepatitis B serologies, hepatitis C polymerase chain reaction qualitative
Genitourinary effects	Renal dysfunction Radiation nephritis Hematuria, proteinuria Cancer of the bladder	BUN, creatinine Urinalysis with microscopy 24-h urine for creatinine clearance, total protein, if indicated
Endocrine **Thyroid function**	Hypothyroidism	TSH, T_3, T_4, free T_4
Gonadal function	Decreased production of gonadal hormones	LH, FSH, estradiol (women) Pelvic examination LH, FSH, testosterone (men)
Hypothalamic–pituitary	Abnormal pituitary gland function	Prolactin levels, FSH, LH, TSH
Ophthalmic	Cataracts	Ophthalmological examination to include slit-lamp examination and Schirmer's test
Dental/oral cavity	Sicca syndrome Caries Periodontal disease Xerostomia Oral malignancy	Regular dental evaluations Careful attention to oral hygiene Fluoride gels/rinses
Musculoskeletal	Osteoporosis Avascular necrosis Myopathy	Dual-energy x-ray absorptiometry scan MRI if pain in a joint, limited range of motion, or a limp MRI, neurological examination, electromyogram
Second malignancy	Nonmelanoma skin cancer Breast cancer	Complete physical examination with biopsy of suspect lesions; skin photographs may also help to monitor status Mammogram, self-examination

(continued)

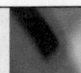

Table 47-16 • Evaluation and Screening of Late Effects of Hematopoietic Stem Cell Transplantation (Continued)

System/Dimension	Possible Late Effects	Evaluation and Screening
	Thyroid cancer	History and physical examination, ultrasound, ^{131}I scan
	Acute leukemia	CBC with differential
	Myelodysplastic syndrome	Bone marrow aspirate and biopsy (if CBC abnormal)
	PTLD	CT scans if PTLD suspected
	Cancer of the uterine cervix	Gynecological examination with Papanicolaou smear
	Cancer of the bladder	Urinalysis with micro to detect microhematuria, urine cytology, follow-up cystoscopy
Integumentary	Increased incidence of benign and malignant nevi	Complete physical examination Skin biopsy of suspect lesions
Psychological/ rehabilitation, quality of life	Changes in body image, roles, family relationships, lifestyle, occupation, discrimination, overcoming stigma, living with compromises, coping with symptoms	Assessment of individual adjustment, achievement of normal developmental tasks, marital stress, sexual function, body image, rehabilitation needs, symptom distress through systematic and structured evaluation

CBC, complete blood count; CT, computed tomography; FSH, follicle-stimulating hormone; LH, luteinizing hormone; MRI, magnetic resonance imaging; PTLD, post-transplantation lymphoproliferative disorder; T$_3$, triiodothyronine; T$_4$, thyroxine; TSH, thyroid-stimulating hormone.

• Clinical Applicability Challenges

Case Study

Ms. B., a 52-year-old woman, began experiencing shortness of breath in 2004. She initially took antibiotics for a presumed upper respiratory infection. The symptoms persisted, and she had a chest radiograph, which revealed an enlarged cardiac silhouette. An echocardiograph demonstrated an ejection fraction of 15%, with a dilated right ventricle, and a cardiac cathetcrization demonstrated clean coronary arteries. Other medical problems included type 2 diabetes mellitus, hyperlipidemia, and asthma. The patient received a referral for heart failure management. Despite maximal medical therapy, she experienced multiple admissions for heart failure exacerbation. She was evaluated for cardiac transplantation in 2006 and deemed a candidate for transplantation. The evaluation revealed an O-positive blood type and a panel reactive antibody of 2%. Her blood urea nitrogen was 23 mg/dL, with a creatinine of 1.0 mg/dL. Serologies were negative for cytomegalovirus (CMV) as well as hepatitis B and C antibodies. Serologies were positive for toxoplasmosis, Epstein-Barr virus, and herpes simplex virus type 1. She received a listing of status 2 (home, awaiting transplantation, not on inotropic therapy or mechanical support) as a blood group O.

Throughout early 2006, Ms. B. had several medical admissions for diuresis secondary to heart failure; in July, she experienced worsening shortness of breath with rest symptoms (New York Heart Association class IV failure) and was admitted for inotropic support. She was taken to the cardiac catheterization laboratory for placement of a Swan-Ganz catheter. Measurements of cardiac function were: right atrial (RA) pressure, 10 mm Hg; right ventricular (RV) pressure, 31/6 mm Hg; pulmonary artery (PA) pressure, 31/18 mm Hg, with a mean pressure of 24 mm Hg; pulmonary capillary wedge pressure (PCWP), 15 mm Hg; cardiac output, 3.0 L/min; and cardiac index (CI), 1.7 L/min/m², with a calculated pulmonary vascular resistance of 3 Woods units. Clinicians prescribed milrinone at 0.125 µg/kg/minute for her low cardiac indices.

Ms. B. remained in the critical care unit on inotropic support with a Swan-Ganz catheter in place. Her status for transplantation was upgraded to 1B. Clinicians considered placing a ventricular assist device to bridge her to transplantation. Fortunately, a suitable heart became available.

Ms. B. underwent an orthotopic heart transplantation. A standard biatrial approach was used. When she was separated from cardiopulmonary bypass, she was receiving dobutamine 8.0 µg/kg/minute, epinephrine 0.08 µg/kg/minute, vasopressin 0.07 units/minute, and isoproterenol 4 µg/minute. After bypass, nitric oxide was introduced through the ventilator for an elevated pulmonary pressure of 48/26 mm Hg. She remained intubated from the operative procedure. She was extubated on postoperative day 2.

Ms. B. had no bleeding complications in the intensive care unit. Weaning from the vasopressin and epinephrine occurred within the first 24 hours, but she remained on dobutamine for right ventricular heart support, and she continued on isoproterenol for chronotropic support. After stable pulmonary pressures and adequate oxygenation were achieved, weaning from the nitric oxide occurred over 24 hours. Stable pulmonary pressures were maintained. Immediately after the operation, she was started on Solu-Medrol, 125 mg intravenously for three doses, as well as mycophenolate mofetil (CellCept) for immunosuppression. After the intravenous therapy was completed, steroids were tapered to decreasing oral doses. Tacrolimus (Prograf) was held for the first 24 hours to ascertain that renal function was normalized. Tacrolimus was then initiated at low doses, with close attention to urinary output and renal indices. Blood urea nitrogen and creatinine remained within normal limits, and the tacrolimus was increased with a goal level of 12 to 15 ng/mL. Because of CMV mismatch (recipient negative/donor positive), she was started on prophylactic valganciclovir (900 mg twice daily). CMV by polymerase chain reaction was checked weekly to evaluate for early CMV reactivation. Dobutamine was slowly weaned completely over the week after transplantation.

Approximately 1 year later, the patient underwent endomyocardial biopsy and right heart catheterization. At this time, measurements of cardiac function were: RA pressure, 8 mm Hg; RV pressure, 31/14 mm Hg; PA, 27/17 mm Hg; PCWP, 14 mm Hg; and CI, 1.5 L/min/m². Despite relatively low intracardiac pressures, the CI was low. On the date of biopsy, the tacrolimus level was 6 ng/mL. The endomyocardial biopsy was a grade 3A rejection. The patient received Solu-Medrol, 1 gram intravenously for 3 days. The tacrolimus dose was aggressively titrated to maintain a level in the range of 12 to 15 ng/mL. One week later, the patient underwent repeat right heart catheterization and endomyocardial biopsy. On the date of biopsy, the tacrolimus level was 12.6 ng/mL. The pulmonary pressures were relatively unchanged; however, the CI was 2.8 L/min/m². The biopsy revealed a grade 0 rejection. The patient was discharged to home on prednisone 4 mg/day, mycophenolate mofetil 1,000 mg twice daily, and tacrolimus 10 mg twice daily.

1. Analyze the similarities and differences in the postoperative care of the transplantation patient compared with the routine surgical patient.
2. What was the major difference in immunosuppression between the first and the second biopsy?
3. What is this patient's major risk factor for post-transplantation coronary artery disease?

Review Questions

1. Mrs. Jones is a patient with a history of diabetes mellitus who is receiving high-dose conditioning therapy for 2 days consisting of total-body irradiation, 1,125 cGy; and cyclophosphamide (Cytoxan), 60 mg/kg. Her antiemetic regimen consists of dexamethasone, 40 mg orally (PO) each day; granisetron (Kytril), 1 mg intravenously (IV) each day; prochlorperazine (Compazine), 10 mg PO/IV every 4 hours as needed for nausea; and lorazepam (Ativan). Which of the following adverse effects would be anticipated during this period of high-dose therapy?

a. Parotitis, fever, electrocardiogram (ECG) abnormalities, and hypoglycemia
b. ECG abnormalities, syndrome of inappropriate antidiuretic hormone (SIADH), skin rash, and renal insufficiency
c. Fever, hyperglycemia, somnolence, mucositis, neutropenia
d. Fever, hyperglycemia, ECG abnormalities, and parotitis

2. Mrs. Jones is day 2 post–allogeneic transplantation after conditioning with total-body irradiation and cyclophosphamide (Cytoxan). Laboratory studies show white blood cells, 0.1 × 10⁹/L; hemoglobin, 8.2 g/dL; hematocrit, 24.6%; platelets, 17 × 10⁹/L; sodium, 120 mEq/L; potassium, 3.0 mEq/L; chloride, 98 mEq/L; carbon dioxide, 18 mEq/L; blood urea nitrogen, 11 mg/dL; and creatinine, 0.6 mg/dL. Vital signs are temperature, 98.1°F (36.7°C); pulse, 92 beats/minute; respirations, 22 breaths/minute; and blood pressure, 108/55 mm Hg. The patient's 24-hour fluid balance shows intake of 5,600 mL and output of 2,105 mL. She complains of nausea, vomiting, diarrhea, and abdominal pain. Based on these data, which of the following findings would be most likely on physical examination?

a. Rales, peripheral edema, jugular venous distention
b. Firm abdomen with absent bowel sounds and rebound tenderness, cardiac gallop (S₃), skin rash
c. Skin pallor, rales, peripheral edema, tenderness of the right upper quadrant
d. Erythema or shallow ulcerations of the oral cavity, weakness, erythema of the skin, conjunctival pallor, petechial skin rash

3. In addition to pancytopenia and gastrointestinal toxicity, Mrs. Jones demonstrates which of the following acute complications of high-dose therapy?
a. Syndrome of inappropriate antidiuretic hormone secretion
b. Veno-occlusive disease of the liver
c. Renal insufficiency
d. Sepsis

4. You are the nurse caring for a potential organ donor. The nurse from the organ procurement organization (OPO) is having difficulty controlling mean arterial pressure. The donor's mean arterial pressure is 100 mm Hg, and the goal is to achieve a mean arterial pressure of 60 to 80 mm Hg. Which of the following therapies is most likely to be ordered?
a. Fluid resuscitation with crystalloids or colloids
b. Norepinephrine
c. Dopamine
d. Sodium nitroprusside

5. Mr. Smith is a 55-year-old man who is 2 weeks postoperation from a lung transplantation. On previous walks with the physical therapist, Mr. Smith walked three laps around the ward. Today, he notes shortness of breath after only a half lap. The therapist reports it was necessary to place him on

3 liters/minutes of oxygen to maintain oxygen saturations above 90%. You call the nurse practitioner responsible for Mr. Smith to notify her of your findings. She orders a stat arterial blood gas and chest radiograph. She is suspicious for which of the following complications: (A) graft versus host disease, (B) reperfusion injury, (C) acute rejection, (D) infection?
a. B and D
b. C and D
c. None of these complications
d. A and C

6. Which of the following statements concerning irradiation of blood products in patients undergoing hematopoietic stem cell transplantation (HSCT) is correct?
  A. Irradiation inactivates immunologically competent T lymphocytes contained in the blood product.
  B. Transfusion-associated graft-versus-host disease (GVHD) develops when immunocompetent allogeneic lymphocytes are transfused into a severely immune compromised host.
  C. Gamma irradiation to 2,500 cGy is currently the most efficient and effective mode of irradiation.
  D. Blood products that have been irradiated cannot be used by other patients because the irradiating process alters the efficacy of the blood product.
    a. A, B, C
    b. A, C
    c. A, C, D
    d. All of the above

7. Which of the following would place a patient at a higher risk for the development of acute graft-versus-host disease (GVHD)?
  a. T-cell depletion
  b. Related, sex-matched donor as source of hematopoietic stem cells
  c. Younger patient or donor
  d. Post-transplantation cytomegalovirus (CMV) or other viral infections

8. Mrs. Jones is taking cyclosporine A to prevent acute graft-versus-host disease (GVHD). Which of the following statements would indicate inadequate knowledge of self-management principles in a patient receiving cyclosporine A?
  A. Mrs. Jones states that headache, tremor, or confusion may occur intermittently while taking cyclosporine A.
  B. To make up for a missed dose of cyclosporine A, Mrs. Jones takes 1.5 times the usual dose at the next regularly scheduled time.
  C. Mrs. Jones takes her usual cyclosporine A dose immediately before the clinic visit when drug levels are drawn.
  D. Mrs. Jones substitutes cyclosporine A capsules for cyclosporine elixir because the elixir has an oily, aversive taste and the capsules are easier to swallow.
    a. A, B, D
    b. B, C, D

  c. A, C, D
  d. A, B, C, D

9. Which of the following immunosuppressive drugs is dosed by levels and most likely to be nephrotoxic?
  a. Mycophenolate mofetil
  b. Tacrolimus
  c. Corticosteroids
  d. Azathioprine

10. Mr. Smith is 4 hours post–orthotopic heart transplantation. You note that his central venous pressure (CVP) has increased from 10 to 22 cm H_2O. His pulmonary artery pressures have gradually increased to 47/24 from 30/15 mm Hg. His systolic blood pressure is averaging 110 mm Hg. The physician suspects that Mr. Smith is experiencing right-sided heart dysfunction secondary to the acute change in pulmonary vascular resistance during transplantation of a healthy heart into the pulmonary bed of the previously failing heart. Which of the following medications is the physician most likely to prescribe?
  a. Epinephrine
  b. Dopamine
  c. Vasopressin
  d. Inhaled nitric oxide

11. Mr. Hitchcock is a 61-year-old man with end-stage heart failure and is awaiting heart transplantation. The patient's wife is worried that her husband's age and cardiac function will exclude him from consideration. Which of the following is a contraindication to transplantation?
  a. Age 60 years or older
  b. Fixed pulmonary hypertension with pulmonary vascular resistance of >6 Woods units
  c. Arrhythmias
  d. Chronically poor cardiac function requiring inotropic support

12. Which of the following nursing interventions are most likely to promote effective coping in organ transplant recipients and their families?
  A. Asking open-ended questions, which encourages the exploration of feelings
  B. Recommending that patients and family members keep their fears and concerns to themselves so that they do not add to each other's burdens
  C. Limiting the information provided so that patients and their families don't become overwhelmed
  D. Teaching problem-solving strategies
    a. A and D
    b. A, C and D
    c. B and D
    d. All of the above

References

1. Boyiadzis M, Pavletic S: Hematopoietic stem cell transplantation: Indications, clinical development and future directions. Expert Opin Pharmacotherapeutics 5(1):97–108, 2004.

2. Brunstein CG, Baker KS, Wagner JE: Umbilical cord blood transplantation for myeloid malignancies. Curr Opin Hematol 14:162–169, 2007

3. Chantry AD, Snowden JA, Craddock C, et al: Long-term outcomes of myeloablation and autologous transplantation of relapsed acute myeloid leukemia in second remission: A British Society of Blood and Marrow Transplantation registry study. Biol Blood Marrow Transplant 12:1310–1317, 2006

4. Koreth J, Cutler CS, Djulbegovic B, et al: High-dose therapy with single autologous transplantation versus chemotherapy for newly diagnosed multiple myeloma: A systematic review and meta-analysis of randomized controlled trials. Biol Blood Marrow Transplant 13:183–196, 2007

5. Nademanee A, Forman SJ: Role of hematopoietic stem cell transplantation for advanced-stage diffuse large cell B-cell lymphoma-B. Semin Hematol 43:240–250, 2006

6. Tabbara IA, Zimmerman K, Morgan C, Nahleh Z: Allogeneic hematopoietic stem cell transplantation: Complications and results. Arch Intern Med 162:1558–1566, 2002

7. Yakoub-Agha I, Mesnil F, Kuentz M, et al: Allogeneic marrow stem-cell transplantation from human leukocyte antigen-identical siblings versus human leukocyte antigen-allelic-matched unrelated donors (10/10) in patients with standard-risk hematologic malignancy: A prospective study from the French Society of Bone Marrow Transplantation and Cell Therapy. J Clin Oncol 24:5695–5702, 2006

8. Barrett JA, Chao NJA, Bishop MR: Are more patients being cured with allogeneic stem cell transplantation? American Society of Clinical Oncology, 2006 Educational Book. Alexandria, VA: American Society of Clinical Oncology, 2006

9. Williams LA, McCarthy PL: Diseases treated with peripheral stem cell transplantation. In Buchsel PC, Kapustay PM (eds): Stem Cell Transplantation: A Clinical Textbook. Pittsburgh: Oncology Nursing Press, 2000, pp 3.3–3.21

10. Scientific Registry of Transplant Recipients. 2005. Retrieved August, 2006, from http://www.ustransplant.org

11. United Network for Organ Sharing. Retrieved August, 2003, from http://www.unos.org

12. Medicare. Retrieved August, 2003, from http://www.medicare.org

13. Danovitch GM (ed): Handbook of Kidney Transplantation. Philadelphia: Lippincott Williams & Wilkins, 2001

14. Sheehy E, Conrad SL, Brigham LE, et al: Estimating the number of potential organ donors in the United States. N Engl J Med 349:667–674, 2003

15. Arbour R: Clinical management of the organ donor. AACN Clin Issues 16(4):551–580, 2005

16. Schneulle P, Berger S, DeBoer J, et al: Effects of catecholamine administration to brain-dead donors on graft survival in solid organ transplantation. Transplantation 72(3):455–463, 2001

17. Tuttle-Newhall JE, Collins BH, Kuo PC, Schroeder R: Organ donation and treatment of the multi-organ donor. Curr Probl Surg 40(5):253–310, 2003

18. Dubernard JM, Dawahra M, McMaster P (eds): Organ Preservation and Transplant Surgery. New York: Taylor & Francis, 2003

19. Penko ME: An overview of liver transplantation. AACN Clin Issues 10:176–184, 1999

20. Aziz TM, Burgess MI, El-Gamel A, et al: Orthotopic cardiac transplantation technique: A survey of current practice. Ann Thorac Surg 68:1242–1246, 1999

21. Poston RS, Griffith BP: Heart transplantation. J Intensive Care Med 19(1):3–12, 2004

22. Petros WP, Gilbert CJ: High-dose alkylating agent pharmacology/toxicity. In Burt RK, Deeg HJ, Lothian S, et al (eds): Bone Marrow Transplantation. Austin, TX: Landes Bioscience, 1998, pp 123–130

23. Rees C, Beale P, Judson I: Theoretical aspects of dose intensity and dose scheduling. In Barrett J, Treleaven J (eds): The Clinical Practice of Stem Cell Transplantation. Oxford, UK: Isis Medical Media, 1998, pp 17–29

24. Alousi A, de Lima M: Reduced-intensity conditioning allogeneic hematopoietic stem cell transplantation. Clin Adv Hematol Oncol 5(7):560–570, 2007

25. Schmit-Pokorny K, Franco T, Frappier B, et al: The cooperative care model: An innovative approach to deliver blood and marrow stem cell transplant care. Clin J Oncol Nurs 7(5):509–514, 556, 2003

26. Fox MC: Transfusions. In Burt RK, Deeg HJ, Lothian S, et al (eds): Bone Marrow Transplantation, pp 54–68. Austin, TX: Landes Bioscience, 1998

27. Davey DB, Crawford J: Hematologic support of the cancer patient. In Berger AM, Shuster JL, Von Roenn JH (eds): Principles and Practice of Supportive Oncology, 3rd ed. Philadelphia: Lippincott Williams & Wilkins, 2006, pp 727–740

28. Dodds A: ABO incompatibility and blood product support. In Atkinson K, Champlin R, Ritz J, Fibbe R, et al (eds): Clinical Bone Marrow and Blood Cell Transplantation, 3rd ed. Cambridge, UK: Cambridge University Press, 2004, pp 1077–1087

29. Smith S: 2002 Organ Transplant. Immunologic Aspects of Organ Transplantation. Available at: http://www.medscape.com/viewarticle/436533

30. Westall GP, Michaelides A, Williams TJ, et al: Bronchiolitis obliterans syndrome and early human CMV DNAemia dynamics after lung transplantation. Transplantation 75(12): 2064–2068, 2003

31. Burt RK, Walsh T: Infection prophylaxis in bone marrow transplant recipients: Myths, legends and microbes. In Burt RK, Deeg HJ, Lothian S, et al (eds): Bone Marrow Transplantation. Austin, TX: Landes Bioscience, 1998, pp 438–451

32. Potena L, Grigioni F, Ortolani P, et al: Relevance of cytomegalovirus infection and coronary-artery remodeling in the first year after heart transplantation: A prospective three-dimensional intravascular ultrasound study. Transplantation 75(6):839–843, 2003

33. Tu W, Potena L, Stepick-Biek P, et al: T-cell immunity to subclinical cytomegalovirus infection reduces cardiac allograft disease. Circulation 114(15):1608–1615, 2006

34. Shelton BK: Evidence-based care for the neutropenic patient with leukemia. Semin Oncol Nurs 19(2):133–141, 2003

35. Friese CR: Prevention of infection in patients with cancer. Semin Oncol Nurs 23(3):174–183, 2007

36. Zitella LJ, Friese CR, Hauser J, et al: Putting evidence into practice: Prevention of infection. Clin J Oncol Nurs 10(6): 739–750, 2006

37. Mielcarek M, Awaya N, Torok-Storb B: Mechanisms of failure of sustained engraftment. In Atkinson K, Champlin R, Ritz J, et al (eds): Clinical Bone Marrow and Blood Cell Transplantation, 3rd ed. Cambridge, UK: Cambridge University Press, 2004, pp 151–159

38. Ho VT, Linden E, Revta C, Richardson PG: Hepatic veno-occlusive disease after hematopoietic stem cell transplantation: Review and update on the use of defibrotide. Semin Thromb Hemost 33(4):373–388, 2007

39. Ho V, Momtaz P, Didas C, et al: Post-transplant hepatic veno-occlusive disease: Pathogenesis, diagnosis and treatment. Rev Clin Exp Hematol 8(1):E3, 2004

40. Wadleigh M, Ho V, Momtaz P, Richardson P: Hepatic veno-occlusive disease: Pathogenesis, diagnosis and treatment. Curr Opin Hematol 10(6):451–462, 2003

41. Saria MG, Gosselin-Acomb TK: Hematopoietic stem cell transplantation: Implications for critical care nurses. Clin J Oncol Nurs 11:53–63, 2007

42. Imran H, Tleyjeh IM, Zirakzadeh A, et al: Use of prophylactic anticoagulation and the risk of hepatic veno-occlusive disease in patients undergoing hematopoietic stem cell transplantation: A systematic review and meta-analysis. Bone Marrow Transplant 37(7):677–686, 2006

43. Tay J, Tinmouth A, Fergusson D, et al: Systematic review of controlled clinical trials on the use of ursodeoxycholic acid for the prevention of hepatic veno-occlusive disease in hematopoietic stem cell. Biol Blood Marrow Transplant 13(2):206–217, 2007

44. Afessa B, Litzow MR, Tefferi A: Bronchiolitis obliterans and other late onset non-infectious pulmonary complications in hematopoietic stem cell transplant. Bone Marrow Transplant 28:425–434, 2001

45. Watkins TR, Chien JW, Crawford SW: Graft versus host-associated pulmonary disease and other idiopathic pulmonary complications after hematopoietic stem cell transplant. Semin Respir Crit Care Med 26(5):482–489, 2005

46. Afessa B, Peters SG: Major complications following hematopoietic stem cell transplantation. Semin Respir Crit Care Med 27(3):297–309, 2006

47. Majhail NS, Parks K, Defor TE, Weisdorf DJ: Diffuse alveolar hemorrhage and infection-associated alveolar hemorrhage following hematopoietic stem cell transplantation: Related and high-risk clinical syndromes. Biol Blood Marrow Transplant 12(10):1038–1046, 2006

48. Soubani AO, Uberti JP: Bronchiolitis obliterans following haematopoietic stem cell transplantation. Eur Respir J 29(5):1007–1019, 2007

49. Goker H, Haznedaroglu I, Chao N: Acute graft-versus-host disease: Pathobiology and management. Exp Hematol 29:259–277, 2001

50. Jacobsohn DA, Vogelsang GB: Acute graft versus host disease. Orphanet J Rare Dis 2:35–39, 2007

51. Bolanos-Meade J, Garrett-Mayer E, Luznik L, et al: Induction of autologous graft-versus-host disease: Results of a randomized prospective clinical trial in patients with poor risk lymphoma. Biol Blood Marrow Transplant 13(10):1185–1191, 2007

52. Baird K, Pavletic SZ: Chronic graft versus host disease. Curr Opin Hematol 13:426–435, 2006

53. Holler E: Risk assessment in haematopoietic stem cell transplantation: GvHD prevention and treatment. Best Practice & Research. Clin Haematol 20:281–294, 2007

54. Lee SJ: New approaches for preventing and treating chronic graft-versus-host disease. Blood 105(11):4200–4206, 2006

55. Filipovich AH, Weisdorf D, Pavletic S, et al: National Institutes of Health consensus development project on criteria for clinical trials in chronic graft-versus-host disease. I. Diagnosis and staging working group report. Biol Blood Marrow Transplant 11:945–956, 2005

56. Abdelsayed RA, Sumner T, Allen C, et al: Oral precancerous and malignant lesions associated with graft-versus-host disease: Report of 2 cases. Oral Surg Oral Med Oral Pathol 93:75–80, 2002

57. Akpek G, Valladares JL, Lee L, et al: Pancreatic insufficiency in patients with chronic graft versus host disease. Bone Marrow Transplant 27:163–166, 2001

58. Aristei C, Allessandro M, Santucci A, et al: Cataracts in patients receiving stem cell transplantation after conditioning with total body irradiation. Bone Marrow Transplant 29:503–507, 2002

59. Baker KS, DeFor TE, Burns LJ, et al: New malignancies after blood or marrow stem-cell transplantation in children and adults: Incidence and risk factors. J Clin Oncol 21:1352–1358, 2003

60. Grigg AP, Angus PW, Hoyt R, et al: The incidence, pathogenesis, and natural history of steatorrhea after bone marrow transplantation. Bone Marrow Transplant 31:701–703, 2003

61. Lash AA: Sjögren's syndrome: Pathogenesis, diagnosis and treatment. Nurse Pract 26(8):50–58, 2001

62. Lee SJ, Vogelsang G, Flowers ME: Chronic graft versus host disease. Biol Blood Marrow Transplant 9(4):215–233, 2003

63. Vogelsang G: How I treat chronic graft-versus-host disease. Blood 97:1196–1201, 2001

64. Wagner JL, Flowers MED, Longton G, et al: Use of screening studies to predict survival among patients who do not have chronic graft-versus-host disease at day 100 after bone marrow transplantation. Biol Blood Marrow Transplant 7:239–240, 2001

65. Couriel D, Carpenter PA, Cutler C, et al: Ancillary therapy and supportive care of chronic graft-versus-host disease: National Institutes of Health consensus development project on criteria for clinical trials in chronic graft-versus-host disease. V: Ancillary Therapy and Supportive Care Working Group Report. Biol Blood Marrow Transplant 12:375–396, 2006

66. Higman MA, Vogelsang GB: Chronic graft versus host disease. Br J Haematol 125:435–454, 2004

67. Mitchell SA: Graft versus host disease. In Ezzone SA (ed): Peripheral blood stem cell transplant: Guidelines for oncology nursing practice. Pittsburg: Oncology Nursing Society Press, 2004

68. Deeg HJ: How I treat refractory acute graft versus host disease. Blood 109:4119–4126, 2007

69. Leather HL: Drug interactions in the hematopoietic stem cell transplant (HSCT) recipient: What every transplanter needs to know. Bone Marrow Transplant 33:137–152, 2004

70. Srinivas TR, Meier-Kriesche HU, Kaplan B: Pharmacokinetic principles of immunosuppressive drugs. Am J Transplant 5:207–217, 2005

71. Simpson D: New developments in the prophylaxis and treatment of graft versus host disease. Exp Opin Pharmacother 2:1109–1117, 2001

72. Simpson D: T-cell depleting antibodies: New hope for induction of allograft tolerance in bone marrow transplantation? BioDrugs 17:147–154, 2003

73. McPartland KJ, Pomposelli JJ: Update on immunosuppressive drugs used in solid-organ transplantation and their nutrition implications. Nutr Clin Pract 22(5):467–473, 2007

74. Chan B: The pharmacology of peripheral blood stem cell transplantation. In Buchsel PC, Kapustay PM (eds): Stem Cell Transplantation: A Clinical Textbook. Pittsburgh: Oncology Nursing Press, 2000, pp 8.3–8.24

75. Charuhas PM: Medical nutrition therapy in bone marrow transplantation. In McCallum PD, Polisena CG (eds): Clinical Guide to Oncology Nutrition. Chicago: American Dietetic Association, 2000, pp 90–98

76. Beauchesne PR, Chung NS, Wasan KM: Cyclosporine A: A review of current oral and intravenous delivery systems. Drug Dev Industr Pharm 33:211–220, 2007

77. Cronin DC, Faust TW, Brady L, et al: Modern immunosuppression. Clin Liver Dis 4:619–655, 2000

78. Bacigalupo A: Management of acute graft-versus-host disease. Br J Haematol 137(2):87–98, 2007

79. Kim SS: Treatment options in steroid-refractory acute graft-versus-host disease following hematopoietic stem cell transplantation. Ann Pharmacother 41(9):1436–1444, 2007

80. Bolanos-Meade J, Vogelsang GB: Acute graft-versus-host disease. Clin Adv Hematol Oncol 2(10):672–682, 2004

81. Seeley K, DeMeyer E: Nursing care of patients receiving Campath. Clin J Oncol Nurs 6(3):138–143, 2002

82. Frey NV, Tsai DE: The management of posttransplant lymphoproliferative disorder. Med Oncol 24(2):125–136, 2007

83. Lowe T, Bhatia S, Somlo G: Second malignancies after allogeneic hematopoietic cell transplantation. Biol Blood Marrow Transplant 13(10):1121–1134, 2007

84. Antin JH: Clinical practice: Long-term care after hematopoietic-cell transplantation in adults. N Engl J Med 347:36–42, 2002

85. Aziz NM: Cancer survivorship research: state of knowledge, challenges and opportunities. Acta Oncol (Stockholm, Sweden) 46:417–432, 2007

86. Baker KS, Gurney JG, Ness KK, et al: Late effects in survivors of chronic myeloid leukemia treated with hematopoietic cell transplantation: Results from the Bone Marrow Transplant Survivor Study. Blood 104:1898–1906, 2004

87. Bhatia S, Robison LL, Francisco L, et al: Late mortality in survivors of autologous hematopoietic-cell transplantation: Report from the Bone Marrow Transplant Survivor Study. Blood 105:4215–4222, 2005

88. Broers S, Kaptein AA, Le Cessie S, et al: Psychological functioning and quality of life following bone marrow transplantation: A 3-year follow-up study. J Psychosom Res 48:11–21, 2000

89. Chantry AD, Snowden JA, Craddock C, et al: Long-term outcomes of myeloablation and autologous transplantation of relapsed acute myeloid leukemia in second remission: A British Society of Blood and Marrow Transplantation registry study. Biol Blood Marrow Transplant 12:1310–1317, 2006

90. Cohen JM, Cooper N, Chakrabarti S, et al: EBV-related disease following haematopoietic stem cell transplantation with reduced intensity conditioning. Leuk Lymphoma 48:256–269, 2007

91. Doyle C, Kushi LH, Byers T, et al: Nutrition and physical activity during and after cancer treatment: An American Cancer Society guide for informed choices. CA Cancer J Clinicians 56:323–353, 2006

92. Gillis TA, Donovan ES: Rehabilitation following bone marrow transplantation. Cancer 92(4 Suppl):998–1007, 2001

93. Guise TA: Bone loss and fracture risk associated with cancer therapy. Oncologist 11:1121–1131, 2006

94. Harder H, Cornelissen JJ, Van Gool AR, et al: Cognitive functioning and quality of life in long-term adult survivors of bone marrow transplantation. Cancer 95:183–192, 2002

95. Kinch A, Oberg G, Arvidson J, et al: Post-transplant lymphoproliferative disease and other Epstein-Barr virus diseases in allogeneic haematopoietic stem cell transplantation after introduction of monitoring of viral load by polymerase chain reaction. Scand J Infect Dis 39:235–244, 2007

96. Lee SJ, Schover LR, Partridge AH, et al: American Society of Clinical Oncology recommendations on fertility preservation in cancer patients. J Clin Oncol 24:2917–2931, 2006

97. Lipkin AC, Lenssen P, Dickson BJ: Nutrition issues in hematopoietic stem cell transplantation: State of the art. Nutr Clin Pract 20:423–439, 2005

98. Ljungman P, Engelhard D, de la Camara R, et al: Vaccination of stem cell transplant recipients: Recommendations of the Infectious Diseases Working Party of the EBMT. Bone Marrow Transplant 35:737–746, 2005

99. Nuver J, Smit AJ, Postma A, et al: The metabolic syndrome in long-term cancer survivors, an important target for secondary preventive measures. Cancer Treat Rev 28:195–214, 2002

100. Rizzo JD, Wingard JR, Tichelli A, et al: Recommended screening and preventive practices for long-term survivors after hematopoietic cell transplantation: Joint recommendations of the European Group for Blood and Marrow Transplantation, the Center for International Blood and Marrow Transplant Research, and the American Society of Blood and Marrow Transplantation. Biol Blood Marrow Transplant 12:138–151, 2006

101. Sanders JE: Chronic graft-versus-host disease and late effects after hematopoietic stem cell transplantation. Int J Hematol 76(Suppl 2):15–28, 2002

102. Wingard JR, Vogelsang GB, Deeg HJ: Stem cell transplantation: Supportive care and long-term complications. Hematology (American Society of Hematology Education Program Book) 1:422–444, 2002

103. Baker KS, Ness KK, Steinberger J, et al: Diabetes, hypertension, and cardiovascular events in survivors of hematopoietic cell transplantation: A report from the bone marrow transplantation survivor study. Blood 109:1765–1772, 2007

Other Selected Readings

Abo-Zena RA, Horwitz ME: Immunomodulation in stem-cell transplantation. Curr Opin Pharmacol 2:452–457, 2002

Banner NR, Polak JM, Yacoub MH (ed): Lung Transplantation. Cambridge, UK: Cambridge University Press, 2003

Baumgartner WA, Reitz B, Kasper E, et al (eds): Heart and Lung Transplantation, 2nd ed. Philadelphia: WB Saunders, 2002

Burns JM, Tierney DK, Long GD, et al: Critical pathway for administering high-dose chemotherapy followed by peripheral blood stem cell rescue in the outpatient setting. Oncol Nurs Forum 22:1219–1224, 1995

Bush WW: Overview of transplantation immunology and the pharmacotherapy of adult solid organ transplant recipients: Focus on immunosuppression. AACN Clin Issues 10:253–269, 1999

Couples SA, Ohler L (eds): Transplantation Nursing Secrets. Philadelphia: Hanley & Belfus, 2003

Grant M, Cooke L, Bhatia S, Forman S: Discharge and unscheduled readmissions of adult patients undergoing hematopoietic stem cell transplantation: Implications for developing nursing interventions. Oncol Nurs Forum 32(1):E1–8, 2005.

Hakim N, Stratta R, Gray D (eds): Pancreas and Islet Transplantation. Oxford, UK: Oxford University Press, 2002

Kapustay PM, Buchsel PC: Process, complications, and management of peripheral stem cell transplantation. In Buchsel PC, Kapustay PM (eds): Stem Cell Transplantation: A Clinical Textbook. Pittsburgh: Oncology Nursing Press, 2000, pp 5.3–5.28

Kaufman DB, Shapiro R, Lucey MR, et al: 2003 SRTR report on the state of transplantation. Immuno Suppression: Practice and Trends. Am J Transplant 4(Suppl 9):38–53, 2004

Kirkland JK, Young JB, McGiffin DC (eds): Heart Transplantation. Philadelphia: Churchill Livingstone, 2002

Lanuza DM, McCabe MA: Care before and after lung transplant and quality of life research. AACN Clin Issues 12:186–201, 2001

Maddrey WC, Shiff ER, Sorrell MF (eds): Transplantation of the Liver. Philadelphia: Lippincott Williams & Wilkins, 2001

Marty FM, Rubin RH: The prevention of infection post-transplant: The role of prophylaxis, preemptive and empiric therapy. Transplant Int 19(10):2–11, 2006

Mattson MR: Graft-versus-host disease: review and nursing implications. Clin J Oncol Nurs 11(3):325–328, 2007.

Maurer JR, Frost AE, Estenne M, et al: International guidelines for the selection of lung transplant candidates. J Heart Lung Transplant 17:703–709, 1998

Mitchell SA: Hematopoietic stem cell transplantation. In Lin EM (ed): Advanced Practice in Oncology Nursing. Philadelphia: WB Saunders, 2001, pp 151–212

Saria MG, Gosselin-Acomb TK: Hematopoietic stem cell transplantation: Implications for critical care nurses. Clin J Oncol Nurs 11:53–63, 2007

Taylor DO: Cardiac transplantation: Drug regimens for the 21st century. Ann Thorac Surg 75:S72–S78, 2003

Wade CR, Reith KK, Sikora JH, Augustine SM: Postoperative nursing care of the cardiac transplant recipient. Crit Care Nurs Q 27(1):17–28, 2004

West F, Mitchell SA: Evidence-based guidelines for the management of neutropenia following outpatient hematopoietic stem cell transplantation. Clin J Oncol Nurs 8(6):601–613, 2004

Common Immunological Disorders

48

Kimmith Jones • Brenda Shelton

Objectives

Based on the content in this chapter, the reader should be able to:

❶ Describe the etiology and immunopathology associated with human immunodeficiency virus (HIV) infection and acquired immunodeficiency syndrome (AIDS).

❷ Explain standard precautions and transmission-based precautions and their implementation in the intensive care unit.

❸ Discuss the use of nucleoside reverse transcriptase inhibitors and protease inhibitors in the treatment of HIV infection and AIDS.

❹ Describe the pathophysiological processes of the oncological emergencies.

❺ Identify appropriate assessment data for each oncological emergency derived from patient history and physical examination, clinical manifestations, and diagnostic studies.

❻ Explain the anticipated medical management and rationale for the treatment of selected oncological emergencies.

❼ Describe relevant aspects of nursing management for each of the oncological emergencies.

Normally, an intact immune system provides protection from disease. When one or more components of this system is weakened or adversely altered, a person becomes susceptible to disease. An immunodeficiency that is congenital or inherited is classified as primary. Examples of primary immunodeficiencies include hypogammaglobulinemia, Bruton's disease, and Wiskott-Aldrich syndrome. An immunodeficiency is known as sec-ondary if it is acquired later in life. Examples of secondary immunodeficiency are human immunodeficiency virus (HIV) infection; acquired immunodeficiency syndrome (AIDS); any form of neoplastic disease; or immunosuppression as a result of drug therapy, such as cortisone or cyclophosphamide.

This chapter is divided into two parts that focus on two areas of secondary immunodeficiency: (1) HIV infection and AIDS, and (2) emergent situations precipitated by commonly occurring neoplastic disorders. The reader is encouraged to review Chapter 45, Anatomy and Physiology of the Hematological and Immune Systems. Especially important is the material relating to the immune mechanisms (humoral and cell-mediated immunity, complement system, and phagocytosis). This review will help the reader appreciate the pathophysiological changes occurring in the conditions discussed in this chapter.

Human Immunodeficiency Virus Infection

Impaired cellular immunity is the underlying pathophysiological condition of AIDS, which is caused by HIV. In 1981, AIDS was first recognized and reported to the Centers for Disease Control and Prevention (CDC).[1] In 1982, AIDS was defined by the CDC, and in 1993, the case definition for AIDS was updated and expanded. To be diagnosed with AIDS, a person with HIV infection must have one of the indicator conditions (Box 48-1).

HIV infection is a chronic illness. Currently, it is incurable. Initially, people believed that a person was exposed to HIV, converted to the HIV-positive status, developed one of the AIDS indicator conditions, and

died within a very short period. The long-term survival for patients infected with HIV has improved considerably because of advances in antiretroviral therapy (ART) and in the prophylaxis and treatment of opportunistic infections. Survival for patients receiving antiretroviral agents and therapy for opportunistic infections is now about 20 years.[1] The rate of progression to AIDS is significantly higher in people who are HIV positive and who are not receiving therapy. The higher the CD4 count and lower the viral load, the lower the risk for progression to AIDS (Table 48-1).

Many people with HIV infection require sophisticated medical and nursing care during the course of their illness. People with HIV may be admitted to the intensive care unit (ICU) because of complications of an opportunistic infection; for a completely unrelated problem, such as trauma; or for a surgical procedure. Their admission to the ICU may be the first indication of their HIV-positive status. As many as 40% of patients with HIV are unaware of their status when they are admitted to the ICU.[2] Recent recommendations, released from the CDC, advocate for routine screening of all people who visit any health care setting.[3] Knowledge of the patient's HIV status could affect the differential diagnosis and influence the diagnostic and treatment options. To achieve a positive patient outcome, it is essential to understand how HIV infection contributes to the reason for ICU admission. Critical care nurses must be knowledgeable about the disease process and the multisystem complications that may occur.

Box 48-1 • Case Definition of AIDS for Surveillance Purposes: Indicator Conditions

- Candidiasis of bronchi, trachea, or lungs
- Candidiasis, esophageal
- Cervical cancer, invasive*
- Coccidioidomycosis, disseminated or extrapulmonary
- Cryptococcosis, extrapulmonary
- Cryptosporidiosis, chronic intestinal (>1 mo duration)
- Cytomegalovirus disease (other than liver, spleen, or nodes)
- Cytomegalovirus retinitis (with loss of vision)
- Encephalopathy, HIV-related
- Herpes simplex: chronic ulcer(s) (>1 mo duration); or bronchitis, pneumonitis, or esophagitis
- Histoplasmosis, disseminated or extrapulmonary
- Isosporiasis, chronic intestinal (>1 mo duration)
- Kaposi's sarcoma
- Lymphoma, Burkitt's (or equivalent)
- Lymphoma, immunoblastic (or equivalent)
- Lymphoma, of brain, primary
- *Mycobacterium avium* complex or *Mycobacterium kansasii*, disseminated or extrapulmonary
- *Mycobacterium tuberculosis*, any site (pulmonary* or extrapulmonary)
- *Mycobacterium*, other species or unidentified species, disseminated or extrapulmonary
- *Pneumocystis jiroveci* pneumonia
- Pneumonia, recurrent bacterial*
- Progressive multifocal leukoencephalopathy
- *Salmonella* septicemia, recurrent
- Toxoplasmosis of brain
- Wasting syndrome due to HIV
- CD4+ count ≤200 cells/mL*

*Added in the 1993 expansion of the AIDS surveillance case definition.
From Centers for Disease Control and Prevention: 1993 Revised classification system for HIV infection and expanded surveillance case definition for AIDS among adolescents and adults. Morb Mortal Wkly Rep 41(RR-17), 1992.

• Epidemiology

At the end of 2003, an estimated 1,039,000 to 1,185,000 people in the United States were living with HIV/AIDS. An astounding 24% to 27% of these people were unaware of their HIV-positive status.[1] The majority of AIDS cases continue to occur in men between the ages of 30 and 44 years (Fig. 48-1). Most cases of AIDS in the United States are in urban areas. The U.S. states and territories with the highest cumulative totals of reported AIDS cases are (in descending order) New York, California, Florida, Texas, New Jersey, Illinois, Pennsylvania, Georgia, Puerto Rico, and Maryland.[4]

Throughout the AIDS epidemic, the largest proportion of AIDS cases has occurred as the result of male-to-male sexual contact (Fig. 48-2). About 46% of the total number of reported AIDS cases in the United States occur among men who have had sex with men.

Table 48-1 • Probability of Developing an AIDS-Defining Opportunistic Infection Within 3 Years in the Absence of Antiretroviral Therapy, Based on Baseline CD4 Count and Viral Load

	% AIDS-Defining Complication			
Viral Load (RT-PCR)*	N	3 y	6 y	9 y
CD4 <350 cells/mm³				
1,500–7,000*	30	0	18.8	30.6
7,000–20,000	51	8.0	42.2	65.6
20,000–55,000	73	40.1	72.9	86.2
>55,000	174	72.9	92.7	95.6
CD4 350–500 cells/mm³				
1,500–7,000	47	4.4	22.1	46.9
7,000–20,000	105	5.9	39.8	60.7
20,000–55,000	121	15.1	57.2	78.6
>55,000	121	47.9	77.7	94.4
CD4 >500 cells/mm³				
<1,500	110	1.0	5.0	10.7
1,500–7,000	180	2.3	14.9	33.2
7,000–20,000	237	7.2	25.9	50.3
20,000–55,000	202	14.6	47.7	70.6
>55,000	141	32.6	66.8	76.3

Data from Multicenter AIDS Cohort Study.
*Plasma HIV RNA levels in cells per milliliter using reverse transcriptase–polymerase chain reaction.
From Bartlett JG: The 2002 Abbreviated Guide to Medical Management of HIV Infection. Baltimore: Johns Hopkins University, Division of Infectious Diseases, 2002, p 23.

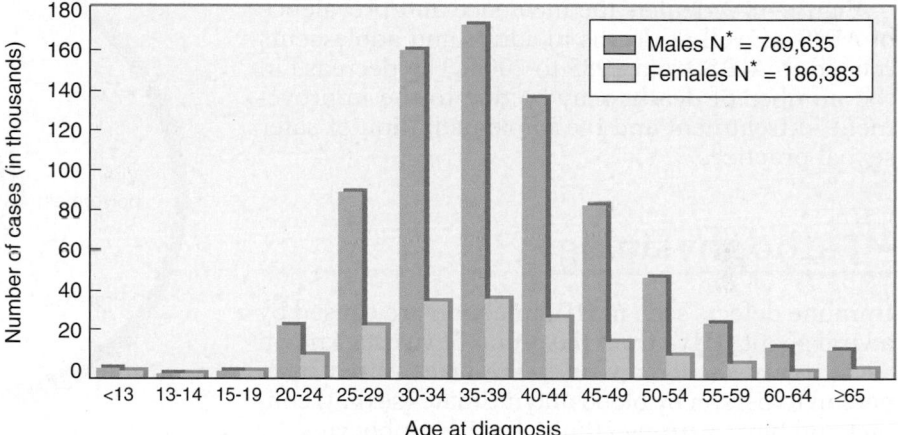

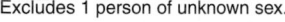

Figure 48-1 • Reported AIDS cases by age and sex in the United States, through 2005. (From the Centers for Disease Control and Prevention.)

*Excludes 1 person of unknown sex.

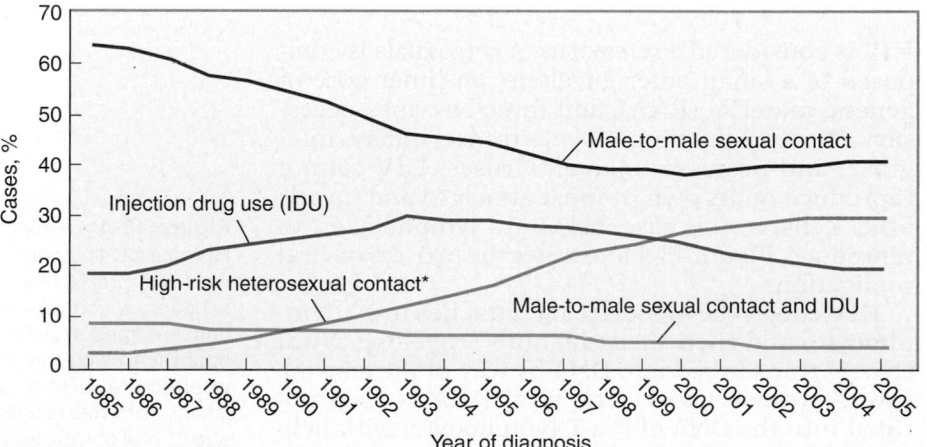

Figure 48-2 • Proportion of AIDS cases among adults and adolescents by transmission category and year of diagnosis in the United States, 1985 to 2005. (From Centers for Disease Control and Prevention.)

Note: Data have been adjusted for reporting delays and cases without risk factor information were proportionally redistributed.
*Heterosexual contact with a person known to have or to be at high risk for HIV infection.

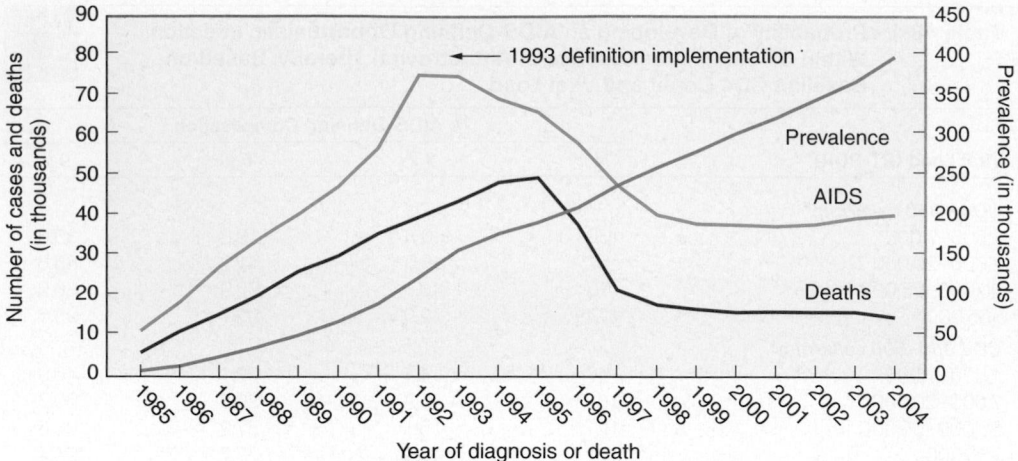

Figure 48-3 • Estimated incidence of AIDS, deaths of adults and adolescents with AIDS, and prevalence of AIDS, 1985 to 2004, in the United States (adjusted for reporting delays). (From Centers for Disease Control and Prevention.)

Even though the rate of new HIV infection in this transmission category has decreased considerably in the past decade, the number of AIDS cases increased between 2001 and 2005.[4] Women represent about 25% of all new cases of HIV.

Figure 48-3 depicts the incidence and prevalence of AIDS as well as deaths in adults and adolescents related to AIDS from 1985 to 2004. The decrease in the number of deaths may be due to the improvement in treatment and the implementation of safer sexual practices.

• Pathophysiology

Immune defects seen in HIV infection are caused by a viral agent (HIV) from the group of viruses known as retroviruses. Retroviruses are transmitted from person to person by blood and intimate (sexual) contact and have a strong affinity for T lymphocytes.

VIRAL REPLICATION

HIV is considered a retrovirus. A retrovirus is composed of a small outer envelope, an inner core of genetic material (RNA), and three enzymes necessary for reproduction: reverse transcriptase, integrase, and protease. Like all viruses, HIV cannot reproduce on its own. It must attach to and invade other cells, in this case, helper T4 lymphocytes, to reproduce. Figure 48-4 illustrates the process of viral replication.

HIV enters the bloodstream, attaches to a T lymphocyte, and then sheds its outer envelope. Viral RNA is transcribed into DNA by way of the enzyme reverse transcriptase. The viral DNA is incorporated into the DNA of the T lymphocyte, with help from the enzyme integrase. This process tricks the T lymphocyte into making components for more virus. The enzyme protease breaks the components down into functional pieces, which are assembled

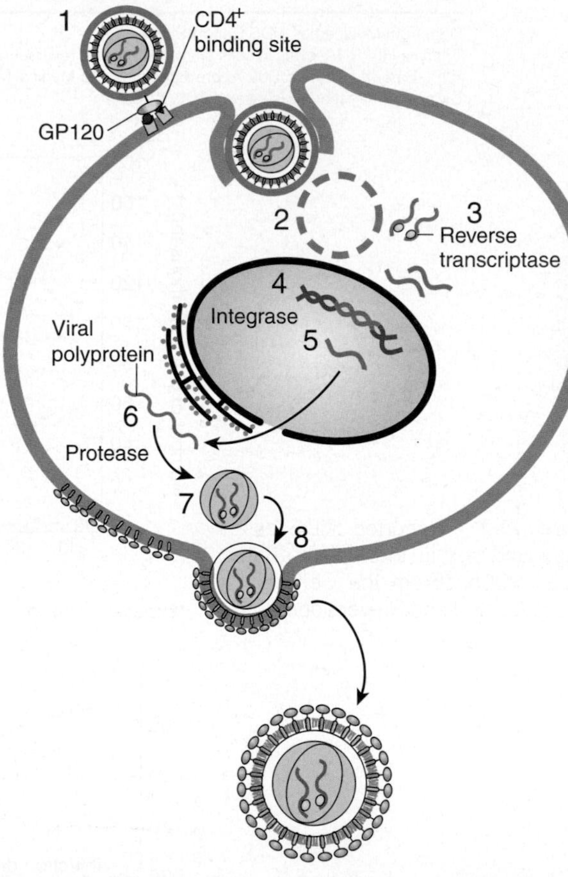

Figure 48-4 • Process of HIV replication. (1) Attachment of HIV to a CD4+ receptor. (2) Internalization and uncoating of the virus with viral RNA and reverse transcriptase. (3) Reverse transcription, which produces a mirror image of the viral RNA and double-stranded DNA molecule. (4) Integration of viral DNA into host DNA using the integrase enzyme. (5) Transcription of the inserted viral DNA to produce viral messenger RNA. (6) Translation of viral messenger RNA to create viral polyprotein. (7) Cleavage of viral polyprotein into individual viral proteins that make up the new virus. (8) Assembly and release of the new virus from the host cell. (From Porth C: Pathophysiology: Concepts of Altered Health States, 7th ed. Philadelphia: Lippincott Williams & Wilkins, 2005.)

into structurally intact and infectious units called virions.

Eventually, the new virions undergo a process of coating and are then expelled from the host cell by budding. During budding, the parent cell releases a daughter cell with its cytoplasmic material, which begins existence as a separate cell. These daughter cells disseminate through the bloodstream and infect other cells. Approximately 30% of the viral burden in a person who is HIV positive is regenerated daily. Extracellular virions have a half-life of about 6 hours.[5]

The T lymphocytes produce the viral components at varying rates depending on the person. It is unclear why the T lymphocytes of some patients produce the viral components slowly and others produce them more rapidly. Although new virions are being produced, there is a period of clinical latency during which the patient is asymptomatic. The asymptomatic period may last 8 to 11 years.[1]

IMMUNE DEFECTS

Patients with HIV infection exhibit impaired activation of both cellular and humoral immunity. HIV primarily infects the helper T4 cell of the immune system. As discussed in Chapter 45, the helper T4 cell plays a major role in the overall immune response. Infection of the helper T4 cell with HIV results in profound lymphopenia with decreased functional abilities, including decreased response to antigens and loss of stimulus for T- and B-cell activation. In addition, the cytotoxic activity of the T8 killer cell is impaired. Functional abilities of macrophages also are affected, with decreased phagocytosis and diminished chemotaxis. In humoral immunity, there is diminished antibody response to antigens, along with deregulation of antibody production. In essence, serum antibodies are increased, but their functional abilities are decreased. The total effect of these immune defects is increased susceptibility to opportunistic infections and neoplasms.

Figure 48-5 presents a summary of the immune defects associated with AIDS.

HIV TRANSMISSION

HIV is a fragile virus and cannot survive long outside the body. Survival time depends on the size of the liquid droplet in which it exists; the larger the droplet, the longer HIV can remain alive. As the droplet dries, HIV dies.

HIV has been isolated from all types of body fluids and tissues. However, not all body fluids have been implicated in the transmission of HIV. The four fluids from which large amounts of virus have been isolated and have been implicated in transmission include blood, semen, vaginal fluid, and breast milk.

The infectiousness of a fluid depends on the amount of virus present in the fluid and the ability of that fluid to reach the target cell, in this case the T lymphocyte. Although HIV has been isolated in all types of body fluids, the amount of virus present is very low (except in the four fluids associated with HIV transmission). In addition, for HIV to cause infection, it must leave the body of the infected person, travel to the body of another person, penetrate the skin barrier, enter the bloodstream, and attach itself to a T lymphocyte. The likelihood that this series of events will occur is low, especially because a certain amount of virus is required to cause an infection. Small tears in the anus or vagina provide a portal of entry for virus present in blood, semen, and vaginal fluid. The virus in breast milk can enter through cuts or irritation in the gastrointestinal tract of the infant.

There are three known modes of transmission of HIV:

▶ Unprotected vaginal or anal sexual contact with an infected person

▶ Inoculation with infected blood or blood products

▶ Pregnancy, delivery, or breast-feeding

A person does not become HIV positive immediately after the virus enters the body. Seroconversion is the development of antibodies from HIV exposure, which can be detected in the blood. In other words, seroconversion is the change from an HIV-negative result to an HIV-positive result. During the seroconversion process, the body recognizes HIV as an invader and develops antibodies to it, which are then

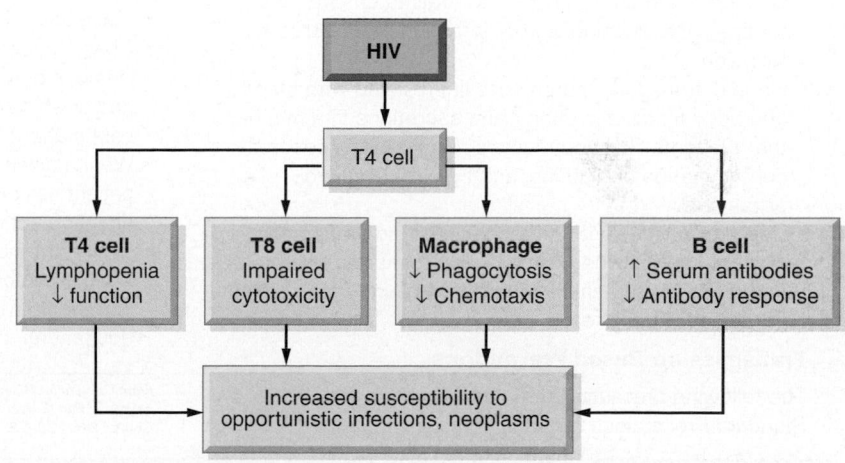

Figure 48-5 • Summary of immune defects in AIDS.

detectable by enzyme-linked immunosorbent assay (ELISA). In most people, seroconversion occurs 4 to 10 weeks after exposure to HIV.[6] During this time, a person can unknowingly transmit the virus because his or her ELISA may not be positive. In almost all people, seroconversion occurs within 6 months.[5] It is estimated that 252,000 to 312,000 people are not aware that they are HIV positive and therefore are not aware that they have the potential to transmit the virus to another person.[1]

The risk for HIV transmission to health care workers is low if Standard Precautions and Transmission-Based Precautions are followed[7] (Box 48-2). Occupational exposure can occur through a percutaneous injury (needlestick), contact with mucous membrane, or contact with nonintact skin (chapped, abraded, or affected by dermatitis).[8] The estimated average risk for HIV transmission after a percutaneous injury is

0.3%. The estimated average risk for HIV transmission after a mucous membrane exposure is 0.09%.[8] Factors that can influence HIV transmission in a health care setting include contact with a device that is visually contaminated with blood, exposure to a large quantity of blood, participating in a procedure in which a needle is placed in an artery or vein, and deep injuries.

Postexposure prophylaxis (PEP) should be started as soon as possible after exposure to HIV, preferably within 1 hour.[8] The decision about when to initiate PEP is based on the type of exposure, risk assessment of the incident, and risk assessment for HIV. Combination therapy using two or three medications is recommended in PEP; the number of medications depends on the type of exposure and the risk status of the source. Health care workers receiving PEP should continue the therapy for 4 weeks, which may

---

Box 48-2 • Summary of Recommended Practices for Standard and Transmission-Based Precautions

Standard Precautions

- Wash hands after touching blood, body fluids, secretions, excretions, and contaminated items, regardless of whether gloves are worn. Wash hands immediately after gloves are removed, between patient contacts, and whenever indicated to prevent transfer of microorganisms to other patients or environments. Use plain soap for routine handwashing and an antimicrobial or waterless antiseptic agent for specific circumstances.
- Wear clean, nonsterile gloves when touching blood, body fluids, excretions or secretions, contaminated items, mucous membranes, and nonintact skin. Change gloves between tasks on the same patient as necessary, and remove gloves promptly after use.
- Wear mask, eye protection, or face shield during procedures and care activities that are likely to generate splashes or sprays of blood or body fluids. Use gown to protect skin and prevent soiling of clothing.
- Ensure that used patient care equipment that is soiled with blood or identified body fluids, secretions, and excretions is handled carefully to prevent transfer of microorganisms, or cleaned and appropriately reprocessed if used for another patient.
- Use adequate environmental controls to ensure that routine care, cleaning, and disinfection procedures are followed.
- Handle, transport, and process linen soiled with blood and body fluids, excretions, and secretions in a manner that prevents skin and mucous membrane exposures, contamination of clothing, and transfer of microorganisms.
- Use previously identified techniques and equipment to prevent injuries when using needles, sharps, and scalpels, and place these items in appropriate puncture-resistant containers after use.

Transmission-Based Precautions

The following precautions are recommended in addition to Standard Precautions:

Airborne Precautions

- Place the patient in private room that has monitored negative air pressure in relation to surrounding areas, 6 to 12 air changes per hour, and appropriate discharge of air outside or monitored filtration if air is recirculated. Keep the door closed and the patient in the room.
- Use respiratory protection when entering room of patient with known or suspected tuberculosis. If patient has known or suspected rubeola (measles) or varicella (chickenpox), respiratory protection should be worn unless person entering room is immune to these diseases.
- Transport the patient out of the room only when necessary, and place a surgical mask on the patient if possible.
- Consult Centers for Disease Control and Prevention Guidelines for additional prevention strategies for tuberculosis.

Droplet Precautions

- Use a private room, if available. Door may remain open.
- Wear a mask when working within 3 ft of the patient.
- Transport the patient out of the room only when necessary, and place a surgical mask on the patient if possible.

Contact Precautions

- Place the patient in a private room if available.
- Change gloves after having contact with infective material. Remove gloves before leaving the patient environment, and wash hands with an antimicrobial or waterless antiseptic agent.
- Wear a gown if contact with infectious agent is likely or patient has diarrhea, an ileostomy, colostomy, or wound drainage not contained by a dressing.
- Limit movement of the patient out of the room.
- When possible, dedicate the use of noncritical patient care equipment to a single patient to avoid sharing equipment.

From Centers for Disease Control and Prevention: Guideline for isolation precautions in hospitals: Part II. Recommendations for isolation precautions in hospitals. Am J Infect Control 24(1):32–52, 1996.

be difficult if toxicities or side effects develop. Laboratory tests for toxicity should take place at the time of exposure and 2 weeks later and consist of a complete blood count (CBC) and renal and hepatic function tests. Health care workers exposed to HIV should have serological testing at the time of exposure and 6 weeks, 3 months, and 6 months after exposure.[8]

• Assessment

HISTORY AND PHYSICAL EXAMINATION

The spectrum of clinical findings ranges from asymptomatic infection with HIV, to a variety of infections and symptoms of decreasing immunocompetence, to unquestionable AIDS. Patients with HIV infection may become seriously ill, requiring frequent hospitalizations and care in the ICU. The critical care nurse more often encounters patients with AIDS when they have life-threatening opportunistic infections. Patients are often admitted to the ICU for an opportunistic illness and are diagnosed with AIDS at the same time.

Pneumocystis pneumonia (PCP), which is caused by *Pneumocystis jiroveci* (formerly known as *Pneumocystis carinii*), is the most common opportunistic infection requiring admission to the ICU. The organism is considered a fungus based on its genetic makeup. Even though the name has changed, the abbreviation PCP is still used to describe the pathogen. The most common presenting symptoms include fever, exertional dyspnea, nonproductive cough, and a normal chest radiograph.[9]

The major indication for critical care of patients with PCP is impending or actual respiratory failure. Symptoms of respiratory compromise often are more severe than diagnostic studies, such as chest radiographs and blood gas values, indicate. Therefore, early aggressive therapy for PCP using intravenous (IV) trimethoprim and sulfamethoxazole (Bactrim, Septra) and corticosteroids is the treatment of choice. Corticosteroids are given to reduce the inflammation caused by the death of *P. jiroveci* in the lungs. Even with urgent, aggressive treatment, many patients require mechanical ventilation for progressive alveolar hypoventilation. Adverse reactions to trimethoprim and sulfamethoxazole, including nausea and vomiting, maculopapular rash, bone marrow suppression, anorexia, headache, crystalluria, and fever, reportedly occur in more than 50% of patients.[10]

The research related to HIV was originally conducted in men. This body of knowledge could not be generalized to women because women did not participate in the studies. Many recent studies, which have included women, suggest that men and women do not differ in terms of the general characteristics of HIV disease.[6] The clinical course of infection, including time from HIV infection to AIDS, risk factors for HIV seroconversion, number and type of opportunistic illnesses, protection against infections, and the effectiveness of potent antiretroviral agents, all appear similar in both men and women.

No organ system escapes involvement in HIV infection. Single infections may develop in critically ill patients with AIDS, but patients often have multiple infections simultaneously that require a variety of treatment strategies. The decrease in immune system functioning causes the multisystem manifestations to develop, resulting in an increase in opportunistic infections. Figure 48-6 presents manifestations of HIV infection and AIDS. Box 48-3 lists examples of nursing diagnoses for patients with HIV infection.

In 1992, the CDC revised the classification system for AIDS; clinical categories and CD4 counts are used to determine where on the disease continuum a person fits. There are three clinical categories and three CD4 cell categories (Table 48-2). When a person has either one of the clinical conditions in category C or a CD4 lymphocyte count less than 200 cells/mm³, the diagnosis of AIDS is made. However, if the person falls within category A1, A2, B1, or B2, he or she is considered HIV positive.

The AIDS indicator conditions in category C are disorders caused by viruses, fungi, parasites, and bacteria, as well as cancers (see Box 48-1 for a detailed list of these conditions). All these agents are always present in the environment. In the immunocompetent person, the immune system keeps these opportunists under control, but in the immunosuppressed person, such as one who is HIV positive, the immune system loses this ability. Table 48-3 illustrates the correlation between CD4 counts and various infections and noninfectious complications seen in HIV infection.

LABORATORY AND DIAGNOSTIC STUDIES

Tests Used to Detect HIV

Several serological tests are used to determine whether a person has been exposed to HIV. Table 48-4 describes the U.S. Food and Drug Administration (FDA)–approved diagnostic tests for HIV. The most widely used test is the ELISA, which determines the presence of antibodies for HIV. The results of this rapid and inexpensive test are available in a few hours. ELISA is reported as reactive (positive) or nonreactive (negative) and has a sensitivity and specificity range from 96% to 99%.[11] Unfortunately, the presence of other antibodies may lead to a false-positive result, which means that the test result was HIV positive, but the person is actually HIV negative. With ELISA, the false-positive rate is 0.0004%, or 1 per 251,000.[12] A positive ELISA is always repeated, and if the second ELISA is positive, another confirmatory test is performed. Low production of antibodies at the time the test is performed may lead to a false-negative result. A false-negative result means that the test result was HIV negative but that the person is actually HIV positive.

The Western blot analysis is the most widely used confirmatory test and is as specific as the ELISA. The Western blot identifies the presence of antibodies to individual viral components. It should always be

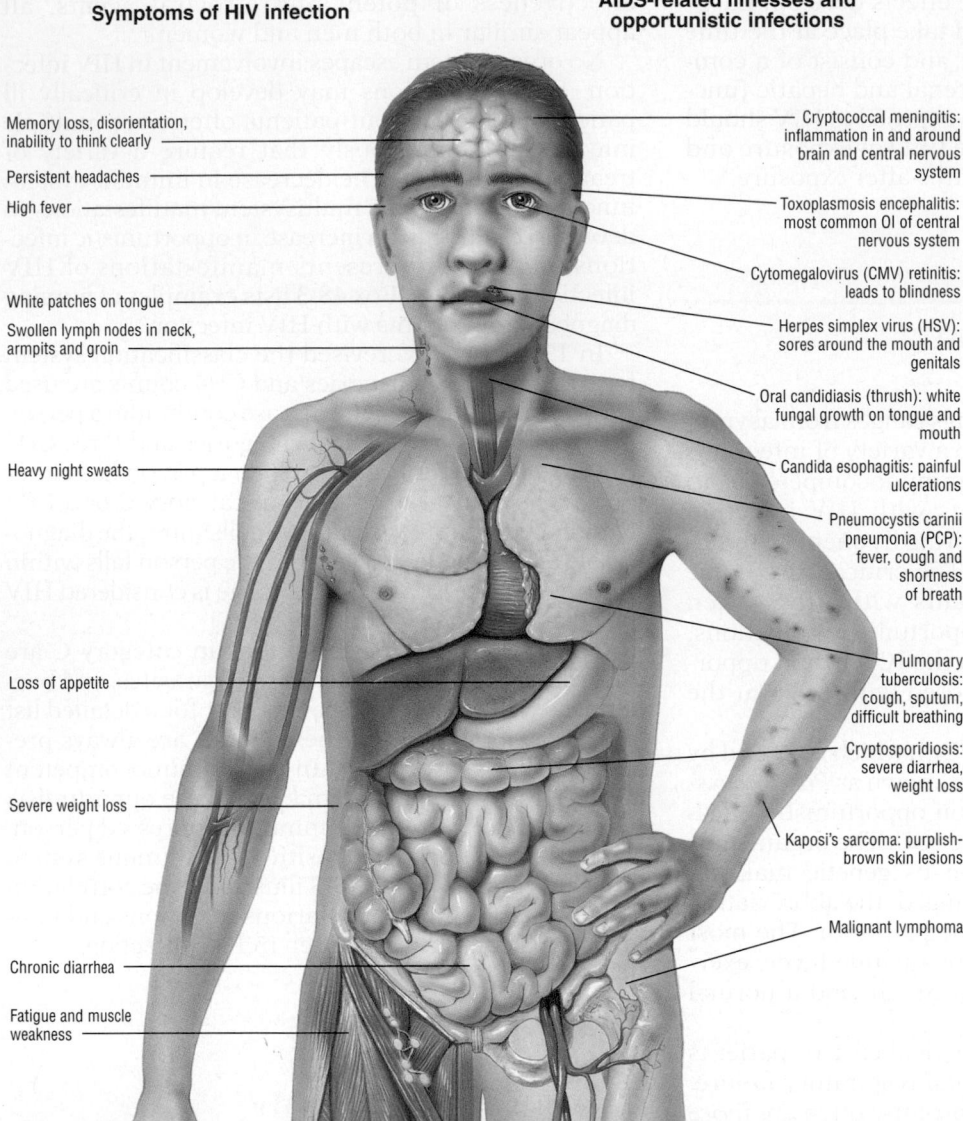

Symptoms of HIV infection

- Memory loss, disorientation, inability to think clearly
- Persistent headaches
- High fever
- White patches on tongue
- Swollen lymph nodes in neck, armpits and groin
- Heavy night sweats
- Loss of appetite
- Severe weight loss
- Chronic diarrhea
- Fatigue and muscle weakness

AIDS-related illnesses and opportunistic infections

- Cryptococcal meningitis: inflammation in and around brain and central nervous system
- Toxoplasmosis encephalitis: most common OI of central nervous system
- Cytomegalovirus (CMV) retinitis: leads to blindness
- Herpes simplex virus (HSV): sores around the mouth and genitals
- Oral candidiasis (thrush): white fungal growth on tongue and mouth
- Candida esophagitis: painful ulcerations
- Pneumocystis carinii pneumonia (PCP): fever, cough and shortness of breath
- Pulmonary tuberculosis: cough, sputum, difficult breathing
- Cryptosporidiosis: severe diarrhea, weight loss
- Kaposi's sarcoma: purplish-brown skin lesions
- Malignant lymphoma

Figure 48-6 • Manifestations of HIV infection and AIDS. (From Anatomical Chart Company: Atlas of Pathophysiology, 2nd ed. Springhouse, PA: Springhouse, 2006, p 261.)

Box 48-3 — Examples of Nursing Diagnoses and Collaborative Problems for the Patient With HIV Infections

- Risk for Infection related to HIV immunodeficiency
- Risk for Impaired Gas Exchange related to alveolar–capillary membrane changes with *Pneumocystis jiroveci* pneumonia infection
- Risk for Deficient Fluid Volume related to diarrhea, dysphagia
- Risk for Infection Transmission related to HIV
- Anxiety related to critical illness, fear of death
- Deficient Knowledge related to illness and impact on patient's future
- Risk for Disturbed Thought Processes related to HIV or opportunistic infection of central nervous system

---

used in combination with the ELISA because it has a 2% false-positive rate.[8] The Western blot is more expensive and requires more skill in interpretation than the ELISA.

Several alternative FDA-approved HIV detection methods are available, but usually they are not used as screening tests for adults. Most of them require traditional serological testing to confirm the presence of HIV.

The FDA approved a rapid test, the Single Use Diagnostic System (SUDS) test, in 1992. The SUDS test requires a trained laboratory technician to obtain the sample and perform the test. Results can be available in 10 to 15 minutes. Negative results may be definitive because of the high sensitivity and specificity; however, positive results require confirmation by standard serology. SUDS is used when rapid confirmation regarding a person's HIV status is required, such as after exposure to a pregnant

Table 48-2 • Assessment Parameters in Classification of HIV Disease

CD4 Cell Categories	Clinical Categories		
	A Asymptomatic, or PGL or Acute HIV Infection	B Symptomatic* (not A or C)	C† AIDS Indicator Condition (1987)
1. >500/mm³ (≥29%)	A1	B1	C1
2. 200–499/mm³ (14%–28%)	A2	B2	C2
3. <200/mm³ (<14%)	A3	B3	C3

*Symptomatic conditions not included in Category C that are (1) attributed to HIV infection or indicative of a defect in cell-mediated immunity, or (2) considered to have a clinical course or management that is complicated by HIV infection. Examples of B conditions include but are not limited to bacillary angiomatosis; thrush; vulvovaginal candidiasis that is persistent, frequent, or poorly responsive to therapy; cervical dysplasia (moderate or severe); cervical carcinoma in situ; constitutional symptoms such as fever (38.5°C) or diarrhea >1 mo; oral hairy leukoplakia; herpes zoster involving two episodes or >1 dermatome; idiopathic thrombocytopenic purpura; listeriosis; pelvic inflammatory disease (especially if complicated by a tubo-ovarian abscess); and peripheral neuropathy.
†All patients in categories A3, B3 and C1–3 (shown in gray) are reported as AIDS, based on the AIDS indicator conditions and/or a CD4 cell count <200/mm³.
PGL, persistent generalized lymphadenopathy
From Centers for Disease Control and Prevention: 1993 Revised classification system for HIV infection and expanded surveillance case definition for AIDS among adolescents and adults. MMWR Morb Mortal Wkly Rep 41(RR-17), 1992.

Table 48-3 • Correlation Between CD4 Count and HIV Complications

CD4 Count* (as cells/mm³)	Infectious Complications	Noninfectious† Complications
>500	Acute retroviral syndrome Candidal vaginitis	Persistent generalized lymphadenopathy Guillain-Barré syndrome Myopathy Aseptic meningitis
200–500	Pneumococcal and other bacterial pneumonia Pulmonary tuberculosis (TB) Herpes zoster Oropharyngeal candidiasis (thrush) Cryptosporidiosis, self-limited Kaposi's sarcoma Oral hairy leukoplakia	Cervical intraepithelial neoplasia Cervical cancer B-cell lymphoma Anemia Mononeuronal multiplex Idiopathic thrombocytopenic purpura Hodgkin's lymphoma Lymphocytic interstitial pneumonitis
<200	Pneumocystis jiroveci pneumonia Disseminated histoplasmosis and coccidioidomycosis Miliary/extrapulmonary TB Progressive multifocal leukoencephalopathy	Wasting Peripheral neuropathy HIV-associated dementia Cardiomyopathy Vacuolar myelopathy Progressive polyradiculopathy
<100	Disseminated herpes simplex Toxoplasmosis Cryptococcosis Cryptosporidiosis, chronic Microsporidiosis Candidal esophagitis	
<50	Disseminated cytomegalovirus Disseminated Mycobacterium avium complex	Central nervous system lymphoma

*Most complications occur with increasing frequency at lower CD4 counts.
†Some conditions categorized as noninfectious are often microbially mediated, such as lymphoma (Epstein-Barr virus) and cervical carcinoma (human papillomavirus).
From Bartlett JG: The 2002 Abbreviated Guide to Medical Management of HIV Infection. Baltimore: Johns Hopkins University, Department of Infectious Diseases, 2002, p 6.

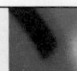

Table 48-4 • Diagnostic Tests for HIV Approved by the US Food and Drug Administration

Test Category/Test	Clinical Use	Comments
Antibody-based tests		
Enzyme-linked immunosorbent assay (ELISA)	Primary screening test	Sensitivity and specificity >99%. Patients recently infected with HIV have a "window period" between infection and reactivity.
Western blot	Most commonly used supplemental test to confirm the presence of HIV antibodies	Specificity of 97.8%. About 4% to 20% of sera that are repeatedly reactive by HIV-1 ELISA are interpreted as indeterminate by Western blot.
Indirect immunofluorescence assay	Confirms the presence of HIV antibodies	Sensitivity and specificity similar to Western blot.
Detection of viral antigens	Diagnostic aid	Used to evaluate acute symptomatic HIV disease and as a screening test in blood donors to reduce the "window period."
p24 antigen		
Viral nucleic acid detection	Monitor HIV progression and effectiveness of antiretroviral therapy	Useful in diagnosis of acute HIV infection in a high-risk patient with a negative or indeterminate Western blot test. A low-level positive viral load may be a false positive.
PCR and branched-chain DNA assays		
Viral culture	Diagnostic aid	Highly specific but relatively insensitive, due to varying degrees of viremia and technical difficulties.
HIV culture		
Alternative diagnostic modalities	Rapid test; notify patient in one visit	Sensitivity and specificity >99%. Positive results must be confirmed with a Western blot or indirect immuno-fluorescence assay.
Single-Use Diagnostic System		
OraSure oral test	Alternative to blood drawing	The patient places collection pad between cheek and gum. A health care professional then places pad in preservative solution and mails to a central laboratory. Initial studies reported a sensitivity and specificity >99%.
Calypte urine test	Alternative to blood drawing	Lower sensitivity and specificity than oral mucosal transudate testing.
Home Access Health Corporation	Home kit; patient reluctant to visit a health care facility	The blood-spot specimen is sent to a central laboratory. Results are available by phone within 3 to 7 days. Patients with positive results are referred to a physician.

Laboratory testing for infection with the human immunodeficiency virus: Established and novel approaches. Am J Med 109:571, 2000.

woman in labor or after possible exposure in a health care worker.

The FDA approved two home kits for HIV testing in 1994. To obtain the results, the user calls in about 7 days and listens to a prerecorded message. The test requires the person to use a lancet and filter strip with blotted blood, which is mailed to a laboratory using an anonymous code. People whose results are positive receive counseling and a referral to a health care provider.

The FDA approved an oral HIV test in 1994. The test involves collecting saliva and testing it for the presence of antibodies to HIV. The person places a specially treated pad between his or her lower cheek and gum for 2 minutes. Results are available by phone or fax within 3 days.

Lastly, the FDA approved a urine HIV test in 1996. The test uses the ELISA technology and is physician administered. Positive results must be confirmed by standard serology testing.

The p24 antigen test is used as a diagnostic tool. One of the core proteins of HIV is p24. Initially, p24 can be detected in the blood; however, during the latent phase of HIV, the protein drops to very low levels. As the virus becomes more active, p24 becomes detectable in the blood.[11] Some clinicians monitor p24 antigen to determine how rapidly the virus is multiplying.

Viral culture is used to grow HIV. It is mainly used in infants to detect HIV and in research. It is expensive and very labor intensive.

Periodic testing for HIV is recommended in people who practice high-risk behaviors, such as IV drug use and unprotected vaginal or anal sexual contact. Most authorities recommend testing at 6- to 12-month intervals; however, this time interval is arbitrary.[13]

Tests Used to Evaluate Progression of HIV Infection

HIV nucleic acid testing, also called viral load testing, in combination with the CD4 count is currently the best method available to determine progression on the HIV disease continuum. The viral load measures the amount of viral particles in 1 mL (mm³) of blood. The higher the viral load, the more rapid the progression to AIDS.[13] Three methods can be used to determine the viral load: polymerase chain reaction, branched-chain DNA (bDNA), and nucleic acid sequence–based amplification.[11] Polymerase chain reaction is the most common method. The test results are used to determine the best time to begin ART and when a change in therapy may be indicated.

The CD4 count is another important evaluation tool used to stage HIV disease and to make deci-

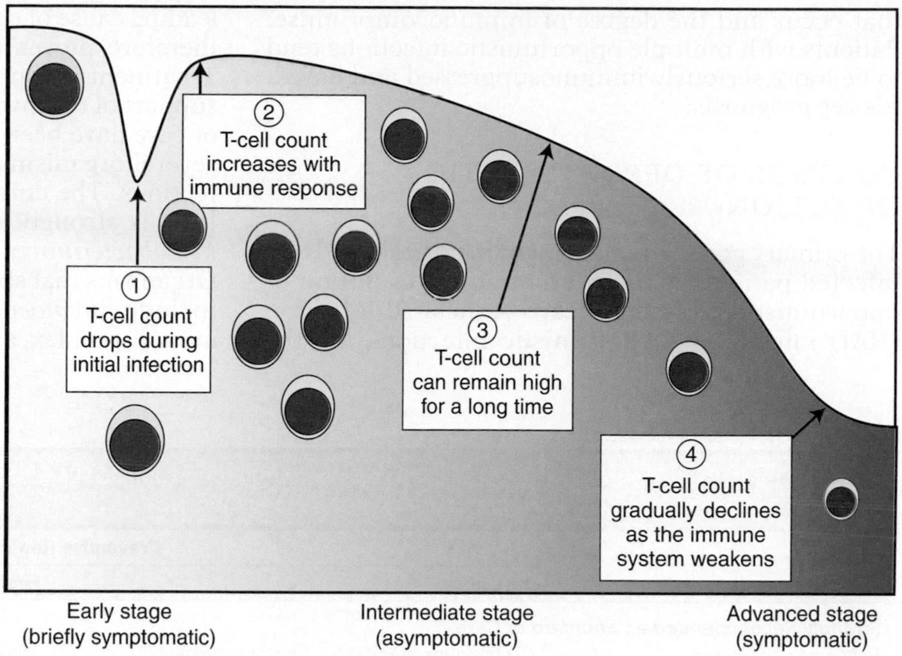

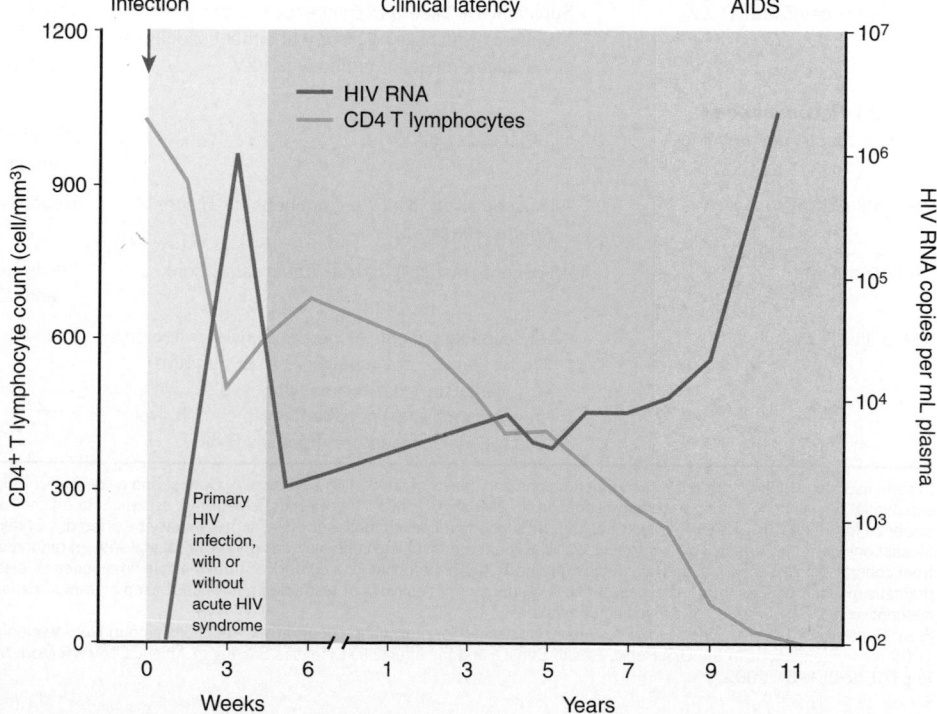

Figure 48-7 • Use of T-cell count (CD4) to stage HIV infection. (1) The T-cell count drops during initial infection because the virus is destroying the T cells. (2) Once the immune system starts to fight back, the T-cell count increases. T-cell counts can go up and down at different times during HIV disease, but they do not return to where they were before infection. (3) T-cell counts can remain fairly high for a long time—sometimes for years—but steadily lose ground. (Redrawn from Glaxo Wellcome: HIV: Understanding the Disease. Research Triangle Park, NC: Author, 1995.)

sions concerning the initiation of ART and prophylactic treatment for opportunistic organisms. The normal CD4 count is about 1,000 cells/mm³, and the count declines over time in the person with AIDS (Fig. 48-7). There is an inverse relationship between the viral load and CD4 count (Fig. 48-8). As HIV/AIDS progresses, the number of CD4 cells declines, and the amount of HIV in the blood increases.

Other tests used to evaluate HIV infection include CBC, rapid plasma reagin, chest radiograph, serum chemistries, Papanicolaou (Pap) tests in women, puri-

fied protein derivative skin test, hepatitis serology, toxoplasmosis serology, and cytomegalovirus antibody serology.

• Management

Management of patients with HIV disease involves a complex, multisystem assessment, including diagnostic tests that establish a baseline, to determine the appropriateness of therapy. Prognosis is based on the type and number of opportunistic infections

Figure 48-8 • Typical course of HIV infection. (From Understanding Disease and Management. Available at: http://www.Roche-hiv.com; modified from Fauci AS, Pantaleo G, Stanley S, Weissman D: Immunopathogenic mechanisms of HIV infection. 124[7]:654–663, 1996.)

that occur and the degree of immunocompromise. Patients with multiple opportunistic infections tend to be more seriously immunosuppressed and have a poorer prognosis.

CONTROL OF OPPORTUNISTIC INFECTION

The primary goal of management in critically ill HIV-infected patients is the prevention or resolution of opportunistic and health care–associated infection (HAI) infections. Opportunistic infections are the leading cause of death in patients with HIV infection; therefore, prevention is the cornerstone of treatment. Treatment of opportunistic infections is aimed at support of the involved system or systems. Standards of care have been developed for prophylaxis against several organisms associated with opportunistic infections. The current organisms for which prophylaxis is strongly recommended include *P. jiroveci, Mycobacterium tuberculosis,* and *Toxoplasma gondii.* Organisms that should be considered for prophylaxis include *Streptococcus pneumoniae, Mycobacterium avium* complex, and varicella-zoster. Table 48-5 lists

Table 48-5 • Prophylaxis to Prevent First Episode of Opportunistic Disease Among Adults and Adolescents Infected With Human Immunodeficiency Virus

Pathogen	Preventive Regimen	
	Indication	*First Choice*
Strongly Recommended as Standard of Care		
Pneumocystis jiroveci	CD4$^+$ counts of <200/μL or oropharyngeal candidiasis	Trimethoprim-sulfamethoxazole (TMP-SMZ), 1 double-strength tablet (DS) by mouth, daily (AI) or TMP-SMZ 1 single-strength tablet (SS) by mouth daily (AI)
Mycobacterium tuberculosis		
Isoniazid-sensitive	Tuberculin skin test (TST) reaction ≥5 mm or prior positive TST result without treatment or contact with person with active tuberculosis, regardless of TST result (BIII)	Isoniazid, 300 mg by mouth plus pyridoxine, 50 mg by mouth daily for 9 mo (AII) or isoniazid, 900 mg by mouth plus pyridoxine, 100 mg by mouth, twice weekly for 9 mo (BII)
Isoniazid-resistant	Same as previous pathogen; increased probability of exposure to isoniazid-resistant tuberculosis	Rifampin, 600 mg by mouth daily (AIII) or rifabutin, 300 mg by mouth (BIII) daily for 4 mo
Multidrug-resistant (isoniazid and rifampin)	Same as previous pathogen; increased probability of exposure to multidrug-resistant tuberculosis	Choice of drugs requires consultation with public health authorities; depends on susceptibility of isolate from source patient
Toxoplasma gondii	Immunoglobulin G antibody to Toxoplasma and CD4$^+$ count of <100/μL	TMP-SMZ, 1 DS by mouth daily (AII)
Mycobacterium avium complex	CD4$^+$ count of <50/μL	Azithromycin, 1,200 mg by mouth weekly (AI) or clarithromycin, 500 mg by mouth twice daily (AI)
Varicella-zoster virus (VZV)	Substantial exposure to chickenpox or shingles for patients who have no history of either condition or, if available, negative antibody to VZV	Varicella-zoster immune globulin (VZIG), 5 vials (1.25 mL each) intramuscularly, administered ≤96 h after exposure, ideally in ≤48 h (AIII)
Usually Recommended		
Streptococcus pneumoniae	CD4$^+$ count of ≥200/μL	23-valent polysaccharide vaccine, 0.5 mL intramuscularly (BII)
Hepatitis B virus	All susceptible patients (i.e., antihepatitis B core antigen–negative)	Hepatitis B vaccine: 3 doses (BII)
Influenza virus	All patients (annually, before influenza season)	Inactivated trivalent influenza virus vaccine: one annual dose (0.5 mL) intramuscularly (BII)
Hepatitis A virus	All susceptible patients at increased risk for hepatitis A infection (i.e., antihepatitis A virus–negative) (e.g., illegal drug users, men who have sex with men, hemophiliacs) or patients with chronic liver disease, including chronic hepatitis B or C	Hepatitis A vaccine: two doses (BIII)

System used to rate the strength of recommendations and quality of supporting evidence: A, Both strong evidence for efficacy and substantial clinical benefit support recommendation for use; should always be offered; B, Moderate evidence for efficacy or strong evidence for efficacy, but only limited clinical benefit, supports recommendation for use; should usually be offered; I, Evidence from at least one correctly randomized, controlled trial; II, Evidence from at least one well-designed clinical trial without randomization, from cohort or case-controlled analytic studies (preferably from more than one center), or from multiple time-series studies, or dramatic results from uncontrolled experiments; III, Evidence from opinions of respected authorities based on clinical experience, descriptive studies, or reports of consulting committees.
From Centers for Disease Control and Prevention: Guidelines for preventing opportunistic infections among HIV-infected persons: 2002 recommendations of the U.S. Public Health Service and the Infectious Diseases Society of America. MMWR Morb Mortal Wkly Rep 51(RR-8):1–51, 2002.

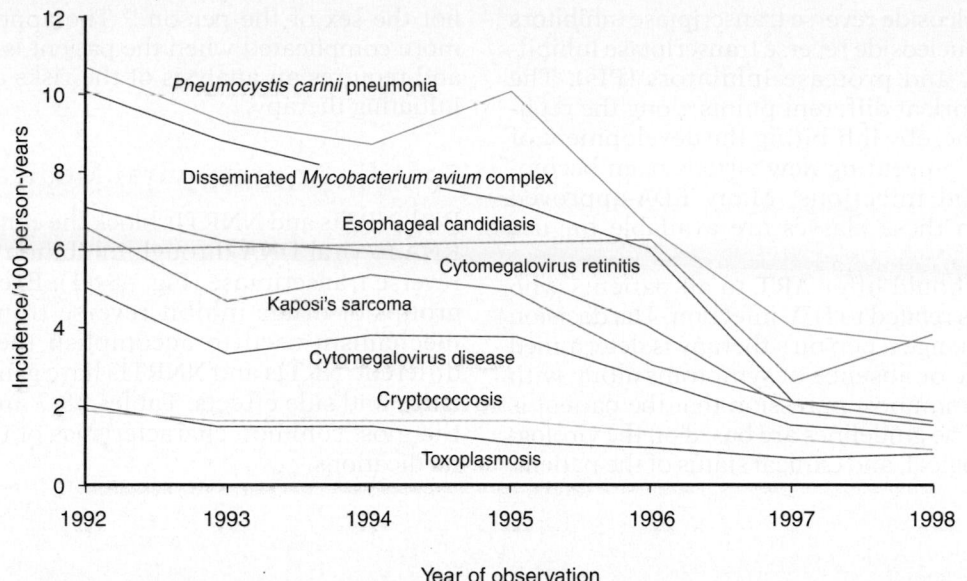

Figure 48-9 • Trends for opportunistic infections in HIV-infected adults and adolescents, ASD (Adult and Adolescent Spectrum of Disease) Project, 1992–1998. Data are standardized to the population of AIDS cases reported nationally in the same years by age, sex, race, HIV-exposure mode, country of origin, and CD4+ count. The median CD4+ count of reported patients with AIDS is 100 to 110/μL; therefore, rates indicate the incidence of opportunistic infections among persons with CD4+ counts in this range. The numbers of subjects included in the analysis are 10,441, 11,589, 11,276, 10,048, 9,250, 8,897, and 8,074, respectively, for the years 1992–1998. (From Kaplan JE, Hanson D, Dworkin MS, et al: Epidemiology of human immunodeficiency virus–associated opportunistic infections in the United States in the era of highly active antiretroviral therapy. Clin Infect Dis 30[Suppl 1]:S6, 2000.)

the organisms and the preferred choice for prophylaxis. Patients usually receive prophylaxis for the following organisms or infections: *S. pneumoniae,* hepatitis B, influenza, and hepatitis A. Maintenance of safe infection control measures to prevent bacterial contamination and complications in the ICU are essential when working with patients with AIDS.

The use of ART has had a significant impact on the treatment of opportunistic infections. The number of opportunistic infections has significantly decreased because of advances in ART[14] (Fig. 48-9). Prophylactic or suppressive treatment for PCP, toxoplasmosis, cytomegalovirus infection, *M. avium* complex infection, leishmaniasis, cryptococcosis, and candidal

thrush may be discontinued if the patient's CD4 count increases sufficiently.[5] Administration of ART also can rapidly reduce viral load, thereby decreasing the incidence of complications.

ANTIRETROVIRAL THERAPY

Originally, people believed that HIV-infected people progressed to AIDS and died within a short time, but we now know that HIV-positive people who receive ART can survive for many years after being infected with the virus and after receiving the diagnosis of AIDS (Fig. 48-10). The drug groups used to treat HIV

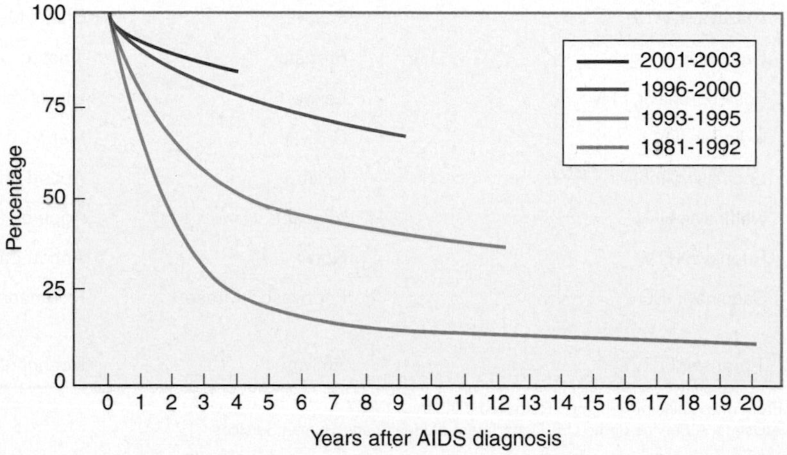

Figure 48-10 • Percentage of people surviving through June 2005, by years after AIDS diagnosis cohorts from 1981 to 2003 and by year of diagnosis, United States. The slope of the curve is dramatically reduced for people diagnosed after 1996. The flattened slope can be attributed to the implementation of antiretroviral therapy. (From Centers for Disease Control and Prevention: Epidemiology of HIV/AIDS— United States, 1981–2005. MMWR 55[21]:4, 2006.)

include the nucleoside reverse transcriptase inhibitors (NRTIs), non-nucleoside reverse transcriptase inhibitors (NNRTIs), and protease inhibitors (PIs). The drug groups work at different points along the replication cycle, thereby inhibiting the development of new virions or preventing new virions from becoming mature and infectious. Many FDA-approved medications in these classes are available for use (Table 48-6).[15]

Clinicians should offer ART to all patients who have symptoms related to HIV infection. The decision to initiate or change a person's therapy is determined by the presence or absence of symptoms along with the degree of immunosuppression that the patient is experiencing. The guidelines are based on the virological, immunological, and clinical status of the patient, not the sex of the person.[15] The approach becomes more complicated when the patient is asymptomatic and requires an analysis of the risks and benefits of initiating therapy.

Specific Antiretroviral Medications

Both NRTIs and NNRTIs block the conversion of viral RNA to viral DNA through inhibition of the enzyme reverse transcriptase (Fig. 48-11). Even though both groups of drugs inhibit reverse transcriptase, the mechanism used to accomplish the inhibition is different. NRTIs and NNRTIs have general characteristics and side effects. Tables 48-7 and 48-8 outline the most common characteristics of these groups of medications.

Table 48-6 • Food and Drug Administration–Approved Antiretroviral Agents			
Generic Name	Brand Name	Manufacturer Name	Approval Date
Non-nucleoside Reverse Transcriptase Inhibitors (NNRTIs)			
Delavirdine, DLV	Rescriptor	Pfizer	4-Apr-97
Efavirenz, EFV	Sustiva	Bristol Myers-Squibb	17-Sep-98
Nevirapine, NVP	Viramune	Boehringer Ingelheim	21-Jun-96
Nucleoside Reverse Transcriptase Inhibitors (NRTIs)			
Abacavir, ABC	Ziagen	GlaxoSmithKline	17-Dec-98
Abacavir, lamivudine	Epzicom	GlaxoSmithKline	2-Aug-04
Abacavir, zidovudine, and lamivudine	Trizivir	GlaxoSmithKline	14-Nov-00
Didanosine, ddI, dideoxyinosine	Videx, Videx EC	Bristol Myers-Squibb	9-Oct-91
Emtricitabine, FTC	Emtriva, Coviracil	Gilead Sciences, Inc.	2-Jul-03
Emtricitabine, tenofovir DF	Truvada	Gilead Sciences, Inc.	2-Aug-04
Lamivudine, 3TC	Epivir	GlaxoSmithKline	17-Nov-95
Lamivudine, zidovudine	Combivir	GlaxoSmithKline	27-Sep-97
Stavudine, d4T	Zerit	Bristol Myers-Squibb	24-Jun-94
Tenofovir DF, TDF	Viread	Gilead Sciences, Inc.	26-Oct-01
Zidovudine, AZT, ZDV	Retrovir	GlaxoSmithKline	19-Mar-87
Protease Inhibitors			
Amprenavir, APV	Agenerase	GlaxoSmithKline, Vertex Pharmaceuticals	15-Apr-99
Afazavavir, ATV	Reyataz	Bristol Myers-Squibb	20-Jun-03
Darunavir	Prezista	Tibotec	23-Jun-06
Fosamprenavir, FPV	Lexiva	GlaxoSmithKline, Vertex Pharmaceuticals	20-Oct-03
Indinavir, IDV	Crixivan	Merck	13-Mar-96
Lopinavir, ritonavir, LPV/r	Kaletra	Abbott Laboratories	15-Sep-00
Nelfinavir, NFV	Viracept	Agouron Pharmaceuticals	14-Mar-97
Ritonavir, RTV	Norvir	Abbott Laboratories	1-Mar-96
Saquinavir, SQV	Fortovase, Invirase	Hoffmann-La Roche	11/07/1997 12/06/1995
Tipranavir (TPV),	Aptivus	Boehringer Ingelheim	22-Jun-05

From http://aidsinfo.nih.gov/. Retrieved January 2, 2007.
AIDsinfo, A Service of the U.S. Department of Health and Human Services

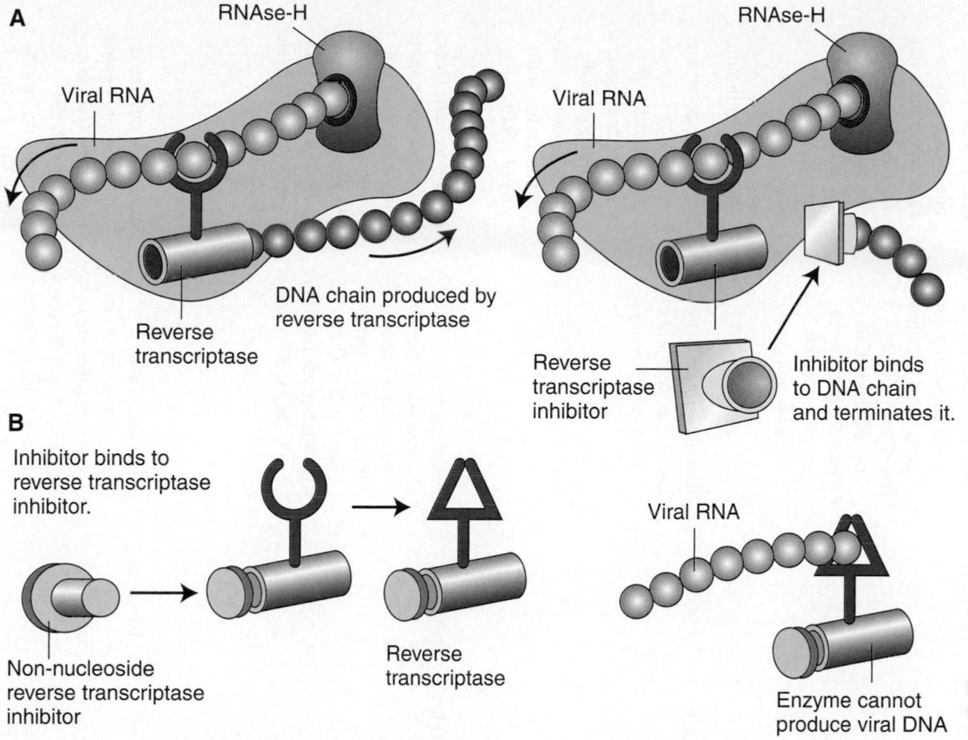

Figure 48-11 • Mechanism of action of nucleoside and non-nucleoside reverse transcriptase inhibitors. To enable HIV to be integrated into the host DNA, the single-stranded viral RNA must be converted to double-stranded DNA by the viral enzyme reverse transcriptase while the enzyme RNAse-H hydrolyses the RNA after it has been copied. Nucleoside and non-nucleoside reverse-transcriptase inhibitors are two classes of antiretroviral drugs that suppress HIV replication by attacking reverse transcriptase. **A:** Nucleoside reverse transcriptase inhibitors are similar in structure to the building blocks that make up DNA. By incorporating themselves into the DNA nucleoside chain being produced by reverse transcriptase, they stop attachment of further nucleosides and prevent ongoing viral DNA synthesis. **B:** Non-nucleoside reserve transcriptase inhibitors attach to the reverse transcriptase and affect the activity of the enzyme by restricting its mobility and making it unable to function. (From Richman DD: HIV chemotherapy. Nature 410:998, 2001.)

PIs, which began to be used in 1996, add to the arsenal against HIV. These agents are very beneficial in the treatment of HIV infection and were instrumental in the dramatic reduction in deaths related to AIDS (Fig. 48-12). When used in combination with NRTIs and NNRTIs, PIs provide even greater antiretroviral coverage. Protease is an enzyme necessary for breaking down large polyproteins into smaller viral proteins that are necessary for viral assembly, maturation, and budding. PIs bind with protease and block this process, resulting in viral particles that are immature and noninfectious (Fig. 48-13). These medications have limitations (including a low oral bioavailability and short half-life) that produce low trough concentrations (Table 48-9). This may require the administration of the medications at higher frequency and dose to achieve the desired effect, which may be difficult for some patients.[16] Other adverse effects include neurological, gastrointestinal, and urological complications; insulin intolerance; elevated cholesterol and triglycerides; and redistribution of body fat, with loss of fat from the face and limbs, along with central adiposity.[15] This latter side effect is known as lipodystrophy. Currently, 10 PI formulations are FDA approved (see Table 48-9).[15]

Potent Combination Antiretroviral Therapy

▶ Potent combination ART, also known as highly active antiretroviral therapy (HAART), became the standard of practice in 1996. Combination therapy is based on three different combination regimens: NNRTI based (one NNRTI and two NRTIs), PI based (one to two PIs and two NRTIs), and triple NRTI based (three NRTIs).

▶ Regardless of the combination selected, ART has four goals:[15]

  ▶ To suppress and maintain the viral load at nondetectable levels for as long as possible
  ▶ To restore and preserve immunological function
  ▶ To improve quality of life
  ▶ To reduce HIV-associated morbidity and mortality

The CD4 cell count is the most important marker in determining whether to start treatment.[15] The most recent guidelines recommend that ART be offered to all patients with a CD4 count of less than 200 cells/mm^3 and to those who have developed an

(*text continues on page 1258*)

Table 48-7 • Characteristics of Nucleoside Reverse Transcriptase Inhibitors (NRTIs)

Generic Name (Abbreviation)/ Trade Name	Formulation	Dosing Recommendations	Food Effect	Oral Bioavailability	Serum Half-Life	Intracellular Half-Life	Elimination	Adverse Events
Abacavir (ABC) Ziagen	Ziagen 300-mg tablets or 20-mg/mL oral solution	300 mg 2 times/ day; or 600 mg once daily; or as Trizivir—1 tablet 2 times/day	Take without regard to meals; alcohol increases abacavir levels 41%; abacavir has no effect on alcohol	83%	1.5 h	12–26 h	Metabolized by alcohol dehydrogenase and glucuronyl transferase. Renal excretion of metabolites 82% Trizivir & epzicom not for patients with CrCl < 50 mL/min	Hypersensitivity reaction, which can be fatal; symptoms may include fever, rash, nausea, vomiting, malaise or fatigue, loss of appetite, respiratory symptoms such as sore throat, cough, shortness of breath
Trizivir—w/ ZDV+3TC	Trizivir ABC 300 mg + ZDV 300 mg + 3TC 150 mg							
Epzicom—w/ 3TC	Epzicom ABC 600 mg + 3TC 300 mg	Epzicom—1 tablet once daily						
Didanosine (ddl) Videx EC, Generic didanosine enteric coated (dose same as Videx EC)	Videx EC 125, 200, 250, or 400 mg Buffered tablets (non-EC) are no longer available.	Body weight >60kg: 400 mg once daily EC capsule with TDF: 250 mg/day < 60 kg: 250 mg daily EC capsule with TDF: 200 mg/day	Levels decrease 55%; take ½ h before or 2 h after meal	30%–40%	1.5 h	> 20 h	Renal excretion 50% Dosage adjustment in renal insufficiency	Pancreatitis; peripheral neuropathy; nausea Lactic acidosis with hepatic steatosis is a rare but potentially life-threatening toxicity associated with use of NRTIs.
Emtricitabine (FTC) Emtriva Also available as: Atripla—w/ EFV & TDF Truvada—w/ TDF	Emtriva 200-mg hard gelatin capsule and 10-mg/mL oral solution Atripla—EFV 600 mg + FTC 200 mg + TDF 300 mg Truvada FTC 200 mg + TDF 300 mg	Emtriva 200-mg capsule once daily or 240 mg (24 mL) oral solution once daily Atripla 1 tablet once daily Truvada 1 tablet once daily	Take without regard to meals	93%	10 h	> 20 h	Renal excretion Dosage adjustment in renal insufficiency Atripla–not for patients with CrCl <50 mL/min Truvada not for patients with CrCl < 30 mL/min	Minimal toxicity; lactic acidosis with hepatic steatosis (rare but potentially life-threatening toxicity with use of NRTIs.) Hyperpigmentation/skin discoloration
Lamivudine (3TC) Epivir Combivir—w/ ZDV Epizicom—w/ ABC Trizivir—w/ ZDV+ABC:	Epivir 150-mg and 300-mg tablets or 10-mg/mL oral solution Combivir 3TC 150 mg + ZDV 300 mg Epizicom 3TC 300 mg + ABC 600 mg Trizivir 3TC 150 mg + ZDV 300 mg + ABC 300 mg	Epivir 150 mg 2 times/ day; or 300 mg daily Combivir 1 tablet 2 times/ day Epizicom 1 tablet once daily Trizivir 1 tablet 2 times/ day	Take without regard to meals	86%	5–7 h	18–22 h	Renal excretion Dosage adjustment in renal insufficiency Combivir, trizivir & epzicom not for patients with CrCl < 50 mL/min	Minimal toxicity; lactic acidosis with hepatic steatosis (rare but potentially life-threatening toxicity with use of NRTIs)

Drug	Formulation/Dose	Administration	Bioavailability	Half-life	Elimination/Dosage	Adverse Effects
Stavudine (d4T) **Zerit**	Zerit 15-, 20-, 30-, 40-mg capsules or 1 mg/mL for oral solution	Body weight >60 kg: 40-mg 2 times/day Body weight <60 kg: 30 mg 2 times/day	Take without regard to meals	86%	1.0 h	7.5 h	Renal excretion 50% Dosage adjustment in renal insufficiency	• Peripheral neuropathy; • Lipodystrophy • Pancreatitis • Lactic acidosis with hepatic steatosis—higher incidence than w/ other NRTIs • Hyperlipidemia • Rapidly progressive ascending neuromuscular weakness (rare)
Tenofovir Disoproxil Fumarate (TDF) **Viread** Also available as: **Atripla**—w/ EFV + FTC **Truvada**—w/ FTC	Viread 300 mg tablet Atripla—EFV 600 mg + FTV 200 mg + TDF 300 mg Truvada—TDF 300 mg + FTC 200 mg	Viread 1 tablet once daily Atripla 1 tablet once daily Truvada 1 tablet once daily	Take without regard to meals	25% in fasting state; 39% with high-fat meal	17 h	>60 h	Renal excretion Dosage adjustment in renal insufficiency Atripla—not for patients with CrCl <50 mL/min Truvada—not for patients with CrCl < 30 mL/min	• Asthenia, headache, diarrhea, nausea, vomiting, and flatulence; renal insufficiency • Lactic acidosis with hepatic steatosis (rare but potentially life-threatening toxicity with use of NRTIs)
Zidovudine (AZT, ZDV) **Retrovir** **Combivir**—w/ 3TC; **Trizivir**—w/ 3TC+ABC;	Retrovir 100-mg capsules, 300-mg tablets, 10-mg/mL intravenous solution, 10-mg/mL oral solution Combivir 3TC 150 mg + ZDV 300 mg Trizivir—3TC 150 mg + ZDV 300 mg + ABC 300 mg	Retrovir 300 mg 2 times/day or 200 mg 3 times/day Combivir or trizivir 1 tablet 2 times/day	Take without regard to meals	60%	1.1 h	7 h	Metabolized to AZT glucuronide (GAZT) Renal excretion of GAZT Dosage adjustment in renal insufficiency Combivir & trizivir—not for patients with CrCl <50 mL/min	• Bone marrow suppression: macrocytic anemia or neutropenia • Gastrointestinal intolerance, headache, insomnia, asthenia; • Lactic acidosis with hepatic steatosis (rare but potentially life-threatening toxicity associated with use of NRTIs)

Table 48-8 • Characteristics of Non-nucleoside Reverse Transcriptase Inhibitors (NNRTIs)

Generic Name (Abbreviation)/ Trade Name	Formulation	Dosing Recommendations	Food Effect	Oral Bioavailability	Serum Half-Life	Elimination	Adverse Events
Delavirdine (DLV)/ Rescriptor	100-mg tablets or 200-mg tablets	400 mg 3 times/ day; four 100-mg tablets can be dispersed in ≥3 oz of water to produce slurry; 200-mg tablets should be taken as intact tablets; separate dose from antacids by 1 h	Take without regard to meals	85%	5.8 h	Metabolized by cytochrome P-450 (3A inhibitor); 51% excreted in urine (<5% unchanged); 44% in feces	• Rash* • Increased transaminase levels • Headaches
Efavirenz (EFV)/ Sustiva Also available as **Atripla**— w/ FTC + TDF	50-, 100-, 200-mg capsules or 600-mg tablets Atripla™—EFV 600-mg + FTV 200-mg + TDF 300-mg	600 mg daily on an empty stomach, at or before bedtime	High-fat/ high-caloric meals increase peak plasma concentra- tion of capsules by 39% and tablets by 79%; take on an empty stomach	Data not available	40–55 h	Metabolized by cytochrome P-450 (3A mixed inducer/ inhibitor) No dosage adjustment in renal insuffi- ciency if EFV is used alone Atripla—not for patients with CrCl <50 mL/min	• Rash* • Central ner- vous system symptoms† • Increased transaminase levels • False-positive cannabinoid test • Teratogenic in monkeys‡
Nevirapine (NVP)/ Viramune	200-mg tablets or 50mg/ 5 mL oral suspension	200 mg daily for 14 days; there- after, 200 mg by mouth 2 times/ day	Take without regard to meals.	> 90%	25–30 h	Metabolized by cytochrome P-450 (3A inducer); 80% excreted in urine (glucu- ronidated metabolites; < 5% un- changed); 10% in feces	• Rash, includ- ing Stevens- Johnson syndrome* • Symptomatic hepatitis, including fatal hepatic necrosis, has been reported‡

*During clinical trials, NNRTI was discontinued because of rash among 7% of patients taking nevirapine, 4.3% of patients taking delavirdine, and 1.7% of patients taking efavirenz. Rare cases of Stevens-Johnson syndrome have been reported with the use of all three NNRTIs, the highest incidence seen with nevirapine use.

†Adverse events can include dizziness, somnolence, insomnia, abnormal dreams, confusion, abnormal thinking, impaired concentra- tion, amnesia, agitation, depersonalization, hallucinations, and euphoria. Overall frequency of any of these symptoms associated with use of efavirenz was 52%, as compared with 26% among controls subjects; 2.6% of those persons on efavirenz discontinued the drug because of these symptoms; symptoms usually subside spontaneously after 2–4 weeks.

‡Symptomatic, sometimes serious, and even fatal hepatic events (accompanied by rash in approximately 50% of cases) occur with significantly higher frequency in treatment-naive female patients with pre-nevirapine CD4+ T-cell counts >250 cells/mm³ or in treatment-naive male patients with pre-nevirapine CD4+ T-cell counts >400 cells/mm³. Nevirapine should not be initiated in these patients unless the benefit clearly outweighs the risk. This toxicity has not been observed when nevirapine is given as single doses to mothers or infants for prevention of mother-to-child HIV transmission.

AIDS-defining illness as well as those whose CD4 cell count is between 201 and 350 cells/mm³ (Table 48-10). If the CD4 cell count is greater than 350 cells/mm³ and the HIV RNA is greater than 100,000 copies/mL, clinicians commonly defer treatment; however, some experts initiate therapy. If the CD4 cell count is greater than 350 cells/mm³ and the HIV RNA is less than 100,000 copies/mL, treatment deferral is necessary to avoid virological failure.[15] The use of ART com- monly results in an increase in CD4 count of 100 to 150 cells/mm³ per year.[15] This increase may return the patient's number of CD4 cells to the normal range; this is known as immune reconstitution.[17]

NNRTI-based or PI-based regimens are the pre- ferred choice for patients who are just starting treat- ment (Table 48-11). Although the NNRTI-based regimens require the ingestion of fewer pills, viral strains that are resistant to these drugs are more

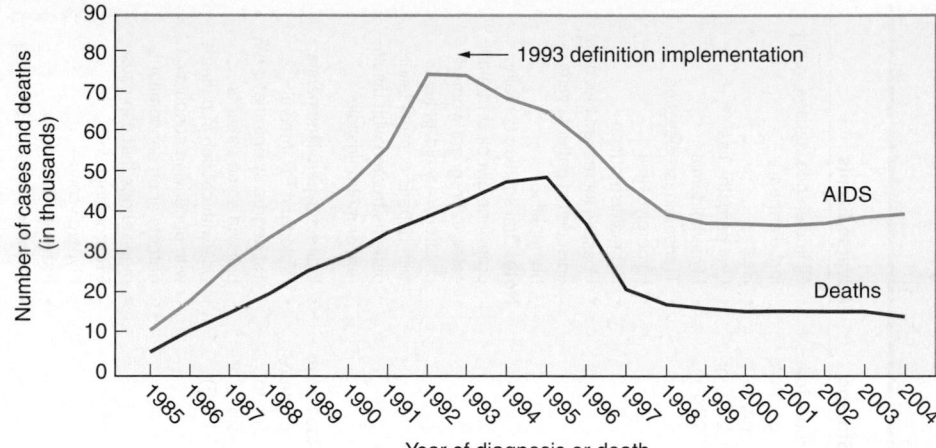

Figure 48-12 • AIDS cases and deaths among adolescents and adults with AIDS in the United States, 1985 to 2004. (From Centers for Disease Control and Prevention.)

prevalent. Triple NRTI-based regimens, which have not been able to achieve the desired virological response, are reserved for patients who cannot tolerate one of the preferred or alternate options. Each antiretroviral agent within a class has its own advantages and disadvantages (Table 48-12).

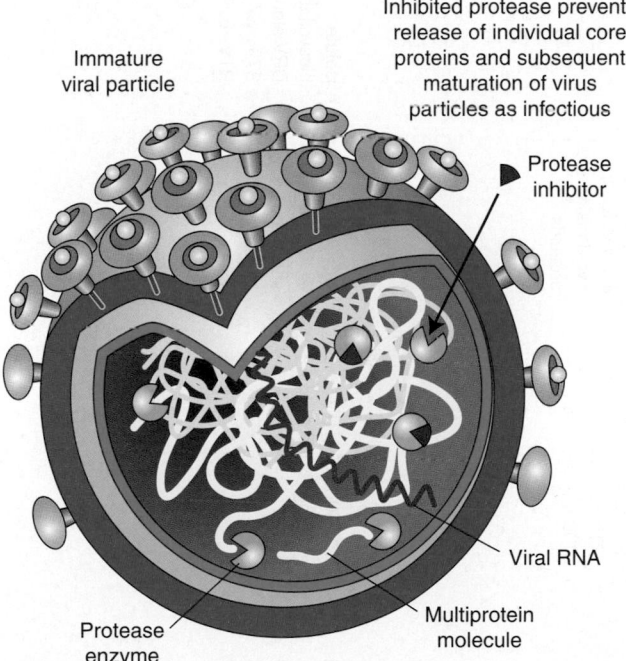

Figure 48-13 • Mechanism of action of protease inhibitors. After transcription in the nucleus, viral mRNA enters the cytoplasm and uses the host's cellular machinery to manufacture virus proteins. The viral components then gather at the cell membrane, and immature viruses bud off the cell. Core proteins are produced as part of long polypeptides, which must be cut into smaller fragments by the enzyme protease in order to form mature, functional proteins. Protease inhibitors bind to the site where protein cutting occurs and prevent the enzyme from releasing the individual core proteins. As a result of this, the new viral particles are unable to mature or become infectious. (From Richman DD: HIV chemotherapy. Nature 410:998, 2001.)

HIV-RNA levels are used to evaluate the effectiveness of ART. Once therapy has begun, a decrease in HIV-RNA should occur within 2 to 8 weeks. Within 4 to 6 months after starting ART, the patient's HIV-RNA level should be nondetectable (i.e., not measurable by current technology). The threshold for detectability of HIV-RNA varies by manufacturer but ranges from 50 to 80 copies/mL.[15] Viral load assessment should be repeated every 3 to 4 months to monitor effectiveness.[15] The frequency of monitoring HIV-RNA varies according to the patient's clinical status (Table 48-13).

There are times when the treatment does not achieve the desired effect. This is termed antiretroviral treatment failure. There are three types of treatment failure: virological failure, immunological failure, and clinical progression. Virological failure is defined as a viral load that decreases to nondetectable levels. Immunological failure is defined as a lack of the immune system to increase the CD4 cell count by 25 to 50 cells/mm³ over the patient's baseline within the first year of treatment or a drop in the CD4 count to below the patient's baseline. Clinical progression is defined as the occurrence or recurrence of an opportunistic illness after 3 months of receiving treatment with antiretroviral agents.[15]

When failure occurs, virological failure is most commonly the first to develop. Virological failure is typically followed by immunological failure and then clinical progression. The time interval between each is extremely varied and may be several years.[15]

Drug Resistance Testing

Genotypic resistance testing is used to determine whether the strain of HIV is resistant to current medications that a person is receiving. Results can be obtained within 1 to 2 weeks after obtaining a blood sample. Resistance testing helps to reduce the chance that antiretroviral treatment failure will occur.

Phenotypic resistance testing measures the ability of the virus to grow in different concentrations of a medication. This type of testing takes 2 to 3 weeks to complete and is more expensive than genotypic resistance testing (Table 48-14).[15]

(*text continues on page 1267*)

Table 48-9 • Characteristics of Protease Inhibitors (PIs)

Generic Name/ Trade Name	Formulation	Dosing Recommendations	Food Effect	Oral Bioavailability	Serum Half-Life	Route of Metabolism	Storage	Adverse Events
Amprenavir (APV)/ Agenerase	50-mg capsules, 15 mg/mL oral solution (capsules and solution NOT interchangeable on mg per mg basis) Note: APV 150-mg capsule is no longer available; consider using fosamprenavir in these patients.	1,400 mg 2 times/day (oral solution) Note: APV and RTV oral solution should not be coadministered because of competition of the metabolic pathway of the two vehicles.	High-fat meal decreases blood concentration 21%; can be taken with or without food, but high-fat meal should be avoided.	Not determined in humans	7.1–10.6 h	Cytochrome P-450 3A4 inhibitor, inducer, and substrate Dosage adjustment in hepatic insufficiency recommended	Room temperature (up to 25°C or 77°F)	• GI intolerance, nausea, vomiting, diarrhea • Rash • Oral paresthesias • Hyperlipidemia • Transaminase elevation • Hyperglycemia • Fat maldistribution • Possible increased bleeding episodes in patients with hemophilia **Note:** Oral solution contains propylene glycol; contraindicated in pregnant women, patients <4 y old, patients with hepatic or renal failure, patients treated with disulfiram or metronidazole
Atazanavir (ATV)/ Reyataz	100-, 150-, 200-mg capsules	400 mg once daily If taken with efavirenz or tenofovir: RTV 100 mg + ATV 300 mg once daily	Administration with food increases bioavailability Take with food; avoid taking with antacids	Not determined	7 h	Cytochrome P-450 3A4 inhibitor and substrate Dosage adjustment in hepatic insufficiency recommended	Room temperature (up to 25°C or 77°F)	• Indirect hyperbilirubinemia • Prolonged PR interval–1st degree symptomatic AV block in some patients • Use with caution in patients with underlying conduction defects or on concomitant medications that can cause PR prolongation • Hyperglycemia • Fat maldistribution • Possible increased bleeding episodes in pts with hemophilia
Darunavir (DRV) Prezista	300-mg tablet	(DRV 600mg + RTV 100mg) twice daily	Food ↑ Cmax & AUC by 30%—should be administered with food	Absolute bioavailability: DRV alone—37%; w/ RTV—82%	15 h (when combined with RTV)	Cytochrome P-450 3A4 inhibitor and substrate	Room temperature (up to 25°C or 77°F)	• Skin rash (7%)–DRV has a sulfonamide moiety; Stevens-Johnson Syndrome & erythema multiforme have been reported. • Diarrhea, nausea • Headache • Hyperlipidemia • Transaminase elevation • Hyperglycemia • Fat maldistribution • Possible increased bleeding episodes in pts with hemophilia

Drug	Formulation	Dosing	Food Effect	Bioavailability	Half-life	Metabolism	Storage	Adverse Effects
Fosamprenavir (fAPV)/Lexiva	700-mg tablet	ARV-naïve patients: • fAPV 1,400mg BID or • (fAPV 1,400 + RTV 200mg) QD or • (fAPV 700mg + RTV 100mg) BID; PI-experienced pts (QD not recommended): • (fAPV 700mg + RTV 100mg) BID; Coadministration w/ EFV (fAPV boosted only): • (fAPV 700mg + RTV 100mg) BID or • (fAPV 1,400mg + RTV 300mg) QD	No significant change in amprenavir pharmacokinetics in fed or fasting state	Not established	7.7 h (amprenavir)	Amprenavir is a cytochrome P-450 3A4 inhibitor, inducer, and substrate; Dosage adjustment in hepatic insufficiency recommended	Room temperature (up to 25°C or 77°F)	• Skin rash (19%) • Diarrhea, nausea, vomiting • Headache • Hyperlipidemia • Transaminase elevation • Hyperglycemia • Fat maldistribution • Possible increased bleeding episodes in patients with hemophilia
Indinavir/Crixivan	200-, 333-, 400-mg capsules	800 mg every 8 hours; With RTV: [IDV 800 mg + RTV 100 or 200 mg] every 12 hours	Unboosted IDV Levels decrease by 77% Take 1 h before or 2 h after meals; may take with skim milk or low-fat meal RTV-boosted IDV: Take with or without food	65%	1.5–2 h	Cytochrome P-450 3A4 inhibitor (less than ritonavir); Dosage adjustment in hepatic insufficiency recommended	Room temperature 15°C–30°C (59°F–86°F), protect from moisture	• Nephrolithiasis • GI intolerance, nausea • Indirect hyperbilirubinemia • Hyperlipidemia • Headache, asthenia, blurred vision, dizziness, rash, metallic taste, thrombocytopenia, alopecia, and hemolytic anemia • Hyperglycemia • Fat maldistribution • Possible increased bleeding episodes in pts with hemophilia
Lopinavir + ritonavir (LPV/r)/ Kaletra	Each tablet contains LPV 200 mg + RTV 50 mg; Oral solution: each 5 mL contains LPV 400 mg + RTV 100 mg; Note: Oral solution contains 42% alcohol	LPV 400 mg + RTV 100 mg (2 tablets or 5 mL) twice daily or LPV 800 mg + RTV 200 mg (4 tablets or 10 mL) once daily (Note: once-daily dosing only recommended for treatment-naïve patients; not for patients receiving EFV, NVP, fAPV, or NFV) With EFV or NVP: For treatment-experienced patients: LPV 600-mg + RTV	Oral tablet—No food effect; take with or without food; Oral solution— Moderately fatty meal ↑ LPV AUC & Cmin by 80% & 54%, respectively; take with food	Not determined in humans	5–6 h	Cytochrome P450 (3A4 inhibitor and substrate)	Oral tablet is stable at room temperature; Oral solution is stable at 2°–8°C until date on label; is stable when stored at room temperature (up to 25°C or 77°F) for 2 mo	• GI intolerance, nausea, vomiting, diarrhea (higher incidence with once-daily than twice-daily dosing) • Asthenia • Hyperlipidemia (esp. hypertriglyceridemia) • Elevated serum transaminases • Hyperglycemia • Fat maldistribution • Possible increased bleeding episodes in patients with hemophilia

(continued)

Table 48-9 • Characteristics of Protease Inhibitors (PIs) (Continued)

Generic Name/ Trade Name	Formulation	Dosing Recommendations	Food Effect	Oral Bioavailability	Serum Half-Life	Route of Metabolism	Storage	Adverse Events
		150 mg (3 oral tablets) twice daily or LPV 533 mg + RTV 133 mg (6.7 mL oral solution) twice daily with food						
Nelfinavir (NFV)/ Viracept	250-mg tablets or 625-mg tablets 50-mg/g oral powder	1,250 mg 2 times/day or 750 mg 3 times/day	Levels increase 2–3 fold Take with meal or snack	20%–80%	3.5–5 h	Cytochrome P450 3A4 inhibitor and substrate	Room temperature 15°–30°C (59°F–86°F)	• Diarrhea • Hyperlipidemia • Hyperglycemia • Fat maldistribution • Possible increased bleeding episodes among patients with hemophilia • Serum transaminase elevation
Ritonavir (RTV)/ Norvir	100-mg capsules or 600-mg/7.5-mL solution	600 mg every 12 h (when ritonavir is used as sole PI) As pharmacokinetic booster for other PIs—100–400 mg per day—in 1–2 divided doses	Levels increase 15% Take with food if possible; this may improve tolerability	Not determined	3–5 h	Cytochrome P450 (3A4 > 2D6; Potent 3A4 inhibitor)	Refrigerate capsules Capsules can be left at room temperature (up to 25°C or 77°F) for ≤30 d; Oral solution should NOT be refrigerated	• GI intolerance, nausea, vomiting, diarrhea • Paresthesias—circumoral and extremities • Hyperlipidemia, esp. hypertriglyceridemia • Hepatitis • Asthenia • Taste perversion • Hyperglycemia • Fat maldistribution • Possible increased bleeding episodes in patients with hemophilia

Drug	Formulation	Absorption	Administration	Tmax	Storage	Metabolism	Adverse effects
Saquinavir tablets and hard gel capsules (SQV)/ Invirase	200-mg hard gel capsules, 500-mg tablets	Unboosted SQV not recommended With RTV: • (RTV 100 mg + SQV 1,000 mg) 2 times/day	Take within 2 hours of a meal when taken with RTV	4% erratic (when taken as sole PI)	1–2 h	Room temperature 15°C–30°C (59°F–86°F)	Cytochrome P450 (3A4 inhibitor and substrate)	• GI intolerance, nausea and diarrhea • Headache • Elevated transaminase enzymes • Hyperlipidemia • Hyperglycemia • Fat maldistribution • Possible increased bleeding episodes in patients with hemophilia
Tipranavir (TPV)/ Aptivus	250-mg capsules	500 mg twice daily with ritonavir 200 mg twice daily Unboosted tipranavir is NOT recommended	Take both TPV & RTV with food. Bioavailability increased with high fat meal	Not determined	6 h after single dose of TPV/RTV	Refrigerated capsules are stable until date on label; if stored at room temperature (up to 25°C or 77°F)—must be used within 60 d	TPV— Cytochrome P-450 (3A4 inducer and substrate) Net effect when combined with RTV–CYP 3A4 inhibitor and CYP 2D6 inhibitor	• Hepatotoxicity—clinical hepatitis including hepatic decompensation has been reported, monitor closely, esp. in patients with underlying liver diseases • Skin rash—TPV has a sulfonamide moiety, use with caution in patients with known sulfonamide allergy • Rare cases of fatal and nonfatal intracranial hemorrhages have been reported. Most patients had underlying comorbidity such as brain lesion, head trauma, recent neurosurgery, coagulopathy, hypertension, alcoholism, or on medication with increase risk for bleeding • Hyperlipidemia (esp. hypertriglyceridemia) • Hyperglycemia • Fat maldistribution • Possible increased bleeding episodes in patients with hemophilia

*Dose escalation for ritonavir when used as sole PI: days 1 and 2: 300 mg 2 times; days 3–5: 400 mg 2 times; days 6–13: 500 mg 2 times; day 14: 600 mg 2 times/day.

Table 48-10 • Indications for Initiating Antiretroviral Therapy for the Chronically HIV-1–Infected Patient

The optimal time to initiate therapy is unknown among persons with asymptomatic disease and CD4+ T-cell count of >200 cells/mm³. This table provides general guidance rather than absolute recommendations for an individual patient. All decisions regarding initiating therapy should be made on the basis of prognosis as determined by the CD4+ T-cell count and level of plasma HIV RNA, the potential benefits and risks of therapy, and the willingness of the patient to accept therapy.

Clinical Category	CD4+ Cell Count	Plasma HIV RNA	Recommendation
AIDS-defining illness or severe symptoms* (AI)	Any value	Any value	Treat
Asymptomatic† (AI)	CD4+ T cells < 200/mm³	Any value	Treat
Asymptomatic (BII)	CD4+ T cells > 200/mm³ but ≤ 350/mm³	Any value	Treatment should be offered following full discussion of pros and cons with each patient (see text.)
Asymptomatic (CII)	CD4+ T cells > 350/mm³	≥ 100,000	Most clinicians recommend deferring therapy, but some clinicians will treat (see text.)
Asymptomatic (DII)	CD4+ T cells > 350/mm³	< 100,000	Defer therapy

*AIDS-defining illness per Centers for Disease Control, 1993. Severe symptoms include unexplained fever or diarrhea > 2–4 weeks, oral candidiasis, or > 10% unexplained weight loss.
†Clinical benefit has been demonstrated in controlled trials only for patients with CD4+ T cells < 200/mm³; however, the majority of clinicians would offer therapy at a CD4+ T-cell threshold < 350/mm³. A collaborative analysis of data from 13 cohort studies from Europe and North America found that lower CD4 count, higher HIV viral load, injection drug use, and age over 50 years were all predictors of progression to AIDS or death in antiretroviral-naive patients beginning combination antiretroviral therapy. These data indicate that the prognosis is better for patients who initiate therapy at >200 cells/mm³, but risk after initiation of therapy does not vary considerably at >200 cells/mm³ (for additional information, see **"When to Treat—Indications for Antiretroviral Therapy"**).

Table 48-11 • Antiretroviral Components Recommended for Treatment of HIV-1 Infection in Treatment-Naive Patients

A combination antiretroviral regimen in treatment-naive patients generally contains 1 NNRTI + 2 NRTIs or a single or ritonavir-boosted P1 + 2 NRTI. Selection of a regimen for an antiretroviral-naive patient should be individualized based on virologic efficacy, toxicities, pill burden, dosing frequency, drug–drug interaction potential, and comorbid conditions. Components listed below are designated as preferred when clinical trial data suggest optimal and durable efficacy with acceptable tolerability and ease of use. Alternative components are those for which clinical trial data show efficacy but that have disadvantages, such as antiviral activity or toxicities, compared with the preferred agent. In some cases, for an individual patient, a component listed as alternative may actually be the preferred component. Clinicians initiating antiretroviral regimens in the HIV-1–infected pregnant patient should refer to **"Recommendations for Use of Antiretroviral Drugs in Pregnant HIV-1-Infected Women for Maternal Health and Interventions to Reduce Perinatal HIV-1 Transmission in the United States"** at **http://aidsinfo.nih.gov/guidelines/.**

To Construct an Antiretroviral Regimen, Select 1 Component from Column A + 1 from Column B

	Column A (NNRTI or PI Options—in alphabetical order)			Column B (Dual-NRTI Options—in alphabetical order)
Preferred components	NNRTI— efavirenz (AII)	or PI- atazanavir + ritonavir (AIII) fosamprenavir + ritonavir (2 times/day) (AII) lopinavir/ritonavir² (2 times/day) (AII) (coformulated)	Preferred components	tenofovir/emtricitabine³ (coformulated) (AII); or zidovudine/lamivudine³ (coformulated) (AII)
Alternative to preferred components	NNRTI— nevirapine (BII)	or PI- atazanavir⁵ (BII) fosamprenavir (BII) fosamprenavir + ritonavir (1×/day) (BII) lopinavir/ritonavir (1×/day) (BII) (coformulated)	Alternative to preferred components	abacavir/lamivudine³ (coformulated) (BII) didanosine + (emtricitabine or lamivudine) (BII)

(+)

¹Efavirenz is not recommended for use in the 1st trimester of pregnancy or in sexually active women with child-bearing potential who are not using effective contraception
²The pivotal study that led to the recommendation of lopinavir/ritonavir as a preferred PI component was based on twice-daily dosing. A smaller study has shown similar efficacy with once-daily dosing but also showed a higher incidence of moderate to severe diarrhea with the once-daily regimen (16% vs. 5%).
³Emtricitabine may be used in place of lamivudine and vice versa.
⁴Nevirapine should not be initiated in women with CD4+ T-cell count >250 cells/mm³ or in men with CD4+ T-cell count >400 cells/mm³ because of increased risk for symptomatic hepatic events in these patients.
⁵Atazanavir must be boosted with ritonavir if used in combination with tenofovir.

Table 48-12 • Advantages and Disadvantages of Antiretroviral Components Recommended as Initial Antiretroviral Therapy

ARV Class	Antiretroviral Agent(s)	Advantages	Disadvantages
NNRTIs (in alphabetical order)		**NNRTI class advantages:** • Less fat maldistribution and dyslipidemia than PI-based regimens • Save PI options for future use	**NNRTI class disadvantages:** • Low genetic barrier to resistance (single mutation confers resistance) • Cross-resistance among approved NNRTIs • Skin rash • Potential for cytochrome P-450 drug interactions
	Efavirenz (EFV)	• Potent antiretroviral activity • Low pill burden; once-daily dosing • Fixed-dose combination with tenofovir + emtricitabine	• Neuropsychiatric side effects • Teratogenic in nonhuman primates, contraindicated in 1st trimester of pregnancy; avoid use in women with pregnancy potential
	Nevirapine (NVP)	• No food effect	• Higher incidence of rash than with other NNRTIs, including rare but serious hypersensitivity reactions (Stevens-Johnson syndrome or toxic epidermal necrolysis) • Higher incidence of hepatotoxicity than with other NNRTIs, including serious and even fatal cases of hepatic necrosis • Treatment-naive, female patients and treatment-naive patients with high pre-NVP $CD4^+$ counts (>250 cells/mm^3 females, >400 cells/mm^3 males) are at higher risk for symptomatic hepatic events. NVP not recommended in these patients unless benefit clearly outweighs risk.
PIs (in alphabetical order)		**PI class advantage:** • Save NNRTI for future use • Higher genetic barrier to resistance	**PI class disadvantages:** • Metabolic complications—fat maldistribution, dyslipidemia, insulin resistance • CYP3A4 inhibitors & substrates—potential for drug interactions (more pronounced w/ RTV-based regimens)
	Atazanavir (unboosted) (ATV)	• Less adverse effect on lipids than other PIs • Once-daily dosing • Low pill burden (2 pills per day)	• Indirect hyperbilirubinemia • PR interval prolongation—generally inconsequential unless combined with another drug with similar effect • Reduced drug exposure when used with TDF and EFV—need addition of RTV (ATV 300 mg qd + RTV 100 mg qd) • Absorption depends on food and low gastric pH—contraindicated with proton pump inhibitors; separate doses with antacid or H_2-blockers
	Atazanavir/ ritonavir (ATV/r)	• RTV-boosting: higher trough ATV conc. & greater antiviral effect • Once daily dosing	Potentially more adverse effect on lipids than unboosted atazanavir
	Fosamprenavir (unboosted) (fAPV)	• No food effect	• Skin rash
	Fosamprenavir/ ritonavir (fAPV/r)	• Twice daily dosing resulted in comparable efficacy as LPV/r • RTV-boosting: higher trough fAPV conc. & greater antiviral effect • Once daily can also be used • No food effect	• Skin rash • Once daily dosing less effective than twice daily dosing
	Lopinavir/ ritonavir (LPV/r)	• Co-formulated as Kaletra • Potential for once daily dosing in treatment-naïve patients • No food restriction with oral tablet formulation	• Gastrointestinal intolerance (higher incidence with once daily than twice daily dosing) • Hyperlipidemia • Preliminary data—lower drug exposure in pregnant women • Once-daily dosing—lower trough concentration than twice-daily dosing
	Nelfinavir (NFV)	• Favorable safety and pharmacokinetic profile for pregnant women when compared with other PIs	• Diarrhea • Higher rate of virologic failure when compared with other PIs (LPV/r & fAPV) and EFV in clinical trials • Food requirement
	Saquinavir + ritonavir (SQV/r)	• RTV boosting causes higher trough SQV conc. & greater antiviral effect	• Gastrointestinal intolerance • Need for use with RTV
Dual NRTIs		• Established backbone of combination antiretroviral therapy	• Rare but serious cases of lactic acidosis with hepatic steatosis reported (d4T>ddf = ZDV > TDF = ABC = 3TC = FTC)

(continued)

Table 48-12 • Advantages and Disadvantages of Antiretroviral Components Recommended as Initial Antiretroviral Therapy (Continued)

ARV Class	Antiretroviral Agent(s)	Advantages	Disadvantages
Dual-NRTI pairs (in alphabetical order)	Abacavir + lamivudine (ABC + 3TC)	• No food effect • Study showing noninferior to ZDV + 3TC as dual-NRTI backbone • Once-daily dosing • Coformulation (Epzicom)	• Potential for abacavir systemic hypersensitivity reaction
	Didanosine + lamivudine (ddI + 3TC)	• Once-daily dosing	• Peripheral neuropathy, pancreatitis—associated with didanosine • Food effect—needs to be taken on an empty stomach • Requires dosing separation from most PIs • Increase in toxicities when used with ribavirin, tenofovir, stavudine, or hydroxyurea
	Stavudine + lamivudine (d4T + 3TC)	• No food effect	• Peripheral neuropathy, lipoatrophy, hyperlactatemia, and lactic acidosis, reports of progressive ascending motor weakness, potential for hyperlipidemia with stavudine use • d4T—Higher incidence of mitochondrial toxicity than with other NRTIs

	Tenofovir/emtricitabine (or lamivudine) (TDF/FTC or 3TC)	• Good virologic response when used with efavirenz
		• Once-daily dosing
		• No food effect
		• Co-formulated as Truvada (TDF/FTC) and Atripla (EFV/TDF/FTC)
			• Tenofovir—some reports of renal impairment
			• Interactions with:
			  1. ATV—TDF reduces ATV levels need to add low dose RTV; and
			  2. ddI—TDF increases ddI level—need to reduce ddI dose

	Zidovudine + lamivudine (ZDV + 3TC)	• Extensive experience • Coformulated as Combivir • No food effect	• Bone marrow suppression with zidovudine • Gastrointestinal intolerance
	Emtricitabine (in place of lamivudine)	• Long half-life than lamivudine • Once daily dosing • Coformulation w/ TDF (Truvada) & w/ EFV/TDF (Atripla)	• Hyperpigmentation/skin discoloration
Triple-NRTI regimen	Abacavir (ABC) + zidovudine (ZDV) + lamivudine (3TC) only	• Coformulated as Trizivir • Minimal drug–drug interactions • Low pill burden • Saves PI & NNRTI for future use	• Inferior virologic responses when compared with efavirenz-based and indinavir-based regimens • Potential for abacavir hypersensitivity reaction

Table 48-13 • Indications for Plasma HIV RNA Testing*

Clinical Indication	Information	Use
Syndrome consistent with acute HIV infection	Establishes diagnosis when HIV antibody test is negative or indeterminate	Diagnosis[†]
Initial evaluation of newly diagnosed HIV infection	Baseline viral load setpoint	Use in conjunction with CD4+ T-cell count for decision to start or defer therapy
Every 3–4 mo in patients not on therapy	Changes in viral load	Use in conjunction with CD4+ T-cell count for decision to start therapy
2–8 wk after initiation of or change in antiretroviral therapy	Initial assessment of drug efficacy	Decision to continue or change therapy
3–4 mo after start of therapy	Assessment of virologic effect of therapy	Decision to continue or change therapy
Every 3–4 mo in patients on therapy	Durability of antiretroviral effect	Decision to continue or change therapy
Clinical event or significant decline in CD4+ T cells	Association with changing or stable viral load	Decision to continue, initiate, or change therapy

*Acute illness (e.g., bacterial pneumonia, tuberculosis, herpes simplex virus, *Pneumocystis jiroveci* pneumonia), and vaccinations can cause an increase in plasma HIV RNA for 2–4 weeks; viral load testing should not be performed during this time. Plasma HIV RNA results should usually be verified with a repeat determination before starting or making changes in therapy.
†Diagnosis of HIV infection made by HIV RNA testing should be confirmed by standard methods (i.e., ELISA and Western blot testing) performed 2–4 months after the initial indeterminate or negative test.

Table 48-14 • Recommendations for Using Drug Resistance Assays

Clinical Setting/Recommendation	Rationale
Drug Resistance Assay Recommended	
In acute HIV infection: *If the decision is made to initiate* therapy at this time, testing is recommended before initiation of treatment. A genotypic assay is generally preferred.	Drug resistance testing will determine whether drug-resistant virus was transmitted and will help to design initial or changed (if therapy was initiated before test results) regimens accordingly.
If treatment is deferred, resistance testing at this time should still be considered.	Earlier testing may be considered because of the potentially greater likelihood that transmitted resistance-associated mutations will be detected earlier in the course of HIV infection.
In chronic HIV infection: Drug resistance testing is recommended before initiation of therapy. A genotypic assay is generally preferred.	Transmitted HIV with baseline resistance to at least one drug may be seen in 6%–16% of patients. Suboptimal virologic responses may be seen in patients with baseline resistant mutations.
Resistance testing earlier in the course of HIV infection may be considered.	Earlier testing may be considered because of the potentially greater likelihood that transmitted resistance-associated mutations will be detected earlier in the course of HIV infection.
With virologic failure during combination antiretroviral therapy	Determine the role of resistance in drug failure and maximize the number of active drugs in the new regimen, if indicated.
With suboptimal suppression of viral load after antiretroviral therapy initiation	Determine the role of resistance and maximize the number of active drugs in the new regimen, if indicated.
Drug Resistance Assay Not Usually Recommended	
After discontinuation of drugs	Drug resistance mutations might become minor species in the absence of selective drug pressure, and available assays might not detect minor drug-resistant species. If testing is performed in this setting, the detection of drug resistance may be of value, but its absence does not rule out the presence of minor drug-resistant species.
When plasma viral load is <1,000 copies/mL	Resistance assays cannot be consistently performed because of low HIV RNA levels; patients/providers may incur charges and not receive results.

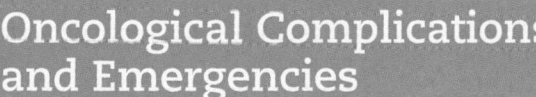

Oncological Complications and Emergencies

Oncological emergencies are potentially life-threatening complications that occur as a result of malignancy.[1] As many as 20% of people diagnosed with cancer have at least one oncological emergency during the course of their disease.[2] The incidence of these emergencies increases as patients with cancer live longer and develop complications that relate to progressive or advanced disease.[3] The nurse must recognize disease-related and patient-specific risk factors for the development of critical illness and plan appropriate assessment and intervention strategies for the most common oncological emergencies. These emergencies are classified by pathophysiological mechanism: hematological, anatomical–structural, and metabolic. Hematological complications involving bone marrow dysfunction, such as engraftment syndrome and leukostasis, commonly occur in neoplastic disorders. Anatomical–structural disorders such as cardiac tamponade, carotid artery rupture, hepatic veno-occlusive disease, obstruction of the superior vena cava, pleural effusion, spinal cord compression, and tracheobronchial obstruction are the result of tumor invasion or treatment-related destruction of normal anatomical structures. Metabolic disruptions from cancer or its treatment such as hypercalcemia, syndrome of inappropriate anti-diuretic hormone secretion (SIADH), and tumor lysis syndrome may involve hormone stimulation, procoagulant activity, and electrolyte imbalances.

• General Principles in the Critical Care of Patients With Cancer

Patients with cancer present unique concerns for the critical care nurse. A knowledge of preexisting illness, nature of the malignancy, treatment-related considerations, and prognostic implications must be incorporated into patient care. In addition, it is necessary to appreciate the psychosocial factors related to caring for patients with a chronic disease. Box 48-4 lists management factors in the evaluation and treatment of an oncological emergency.[4] Ideally, before any acute event, the oncologist or primary care physician has discussed end-of-life care and the oncological crises that should be treated and those that should not be treated with the patient and family members. However, this is not often the case, and the critical care nurse is an important liaison between the primary care physician and the intensivist. Each

Box 48-4 • NURSING INTERVENTIONS for Evaluation and Treatment of an Oncological Emergency

Symptoms and Signs
1. Are the symptoms and signs due to the tumor or to complications of treatment?
2. How quickly are the symptoms of the oncological emergency progressing?

Natural History of the Primary Tumor
1. Is there a previous diagnosis of malignancy?
2. What is the disease-free interval between the diagnosis of the primary tumor and onset of the emergency?
3. Has the emergency developed in the setting of terminal disease?

Efficacy of Available Treatment
1. Has there been no prior therapy or extensive pretreatment?
2. Should treatment be directed at the underlying malignancy or the urgent complications?
3. Will the patient's general medical condition influence the ability to administer effective treatment?

Treatment and Goals
1. What is the potential for cure?
2. Is prompt palliation required to prevent further debilitation?
3. What is the risk versus benefit ratio of treatment?
4. Should treatment be withheld if there is a minimal chance of response to available antitumor therapies?

Used with permission from Murphy GP, Lawrence W, Lenhard RE: Clinical Oncology. Atlanta: American Cancer Society, 1995, p. 597.

---

time a patient with cancer presents with critical illness, prognostic variables and information regarding treatment of the presenting condition should be used to advise the patient of the best course of action. Clearly there are times when the risk/benefit ratio of a lifesaving measure does not warrant its use; yet there are also many other situations in which a lifesaving intervention in a hopelessly ill patient may enhance the quality of life.[4,5] For example, a patient with advanced cancer may present with a potentially life-threatening pericardial effusion that can be effectively treated with insertion of a pericardial catheter. This patient may require a limited amount of intensive care after catheter insertion and fluid drainage, but the symptom relief may be advantageous in enhancing the quality of the last few weeks of the patient's life. Aggressive management of most oncological emergencies is indicated if a histological diagnosis of cancer has not been established, if the patient has a good prognosis or can achieve prolonged palliation with treatment, or if there is the possibility of restoring functional status.[5,6] The nursing intervention guidelines in Box 48-4 are presented as a list of clinical questions that should be considered when making a decision about whether to provide critical care interventions to the patient with cancer.

To provide high-quality, individualized care to patients with oncological emergencies, the critical care nurse should know a few facts regarding critical illness and the patient with cancer. Box 48-5 presents important conclusions drawn from multiple studies of critical illness in patients with cancer.[1,4] Box 48-6 lists nursing diagnoses and collaborative problems for patients with oncological emergencies.

• Hematological Complications

BONE MARROW SUPPRESSION

Cancer and its treatment often cause suppression of hematopoietic cell production or differentiation. Causes of bone marrow suppression are commonly associated with cancer invasion of the bone, chemotherapy and some radiation treatments, or blood and marrow transplantation. The clinical consequences are symptoms related to decreased red blood cell production (anemia), decreased platelet production (thrombocytopenia), and decreased white blood cell

Box 48-5 • Critical Care of Cancer Patients: Conclusions From the Literature

Incidence of Critical Illness
- Affects about 20% of patients
- More common in patients with hematological malignancy
- Most common critical illnesses:
    Respiratory distress
    Refractory hypotension
    Oncological emergencies

Prognostics of Critical Illness
- Survival is better in the newly diagnosed who have not yet received antineoplastic therapy.
- Survival from specific interventions:

Cardiac arrest:	<2% alive to discharge
Mechanical ventilation:	12%–45% alive to discharge (worst prognosis in patients receiving blood and marrow transplant, best prognosis in patients with a newly diagnosed solid tumor)
Dialysis:	21%–40% alive to discharge (prognosis has been improving with use of continuous renal replacement therapies)

- Most important predictor of survival: status of the underlying malignant disease
- Other poor prognostic variables:
    Age extremes
    Concomitant health problems
    Severity of cancer
    Aggressiveness/potency of treatment
    Reversibility of the specific crisis

production (leukopenia). Table 48-15 is a summary of the key clinical features and nursing implications of these three types of bone marrow suppression. These disorders are not uniquely oncological, but they are common in patients with cancer and influence the patient's response to other critical illnesses.

Other causes of bone marrow suppression must be considered if cancer-related etiological factors are not present. When serum tests are unclear in elucidating the etiology of bone marrow suppression, a bone marrow aspirate or biopsy may be performed to confirm the pathophysiological process. This test usually requires sedation and a local anesthetic before a large coring needle is used to remove the liquid red bone marrow from either the hip or sternum. Bone marrow biopsy determines whether the bone marrow defect is present during the cellular production phase, and it may be a basis for clinical management.[7]

Management of bone marrow suppression as a cluster involves determining whether the cause is time-limited and ascertaining the amount of supportive therapy required. Treatment may include administration of bone marrow growth factors specific to the deficient cellular component,[8] infusion of blood components, or prophylactic clotting enhancement and antimicrobial therapy to prevent life-threatening bleeding or infectious complications.

ENGRAFTMENT SYNDROME

Engraftment syndrome, also known as cytokine release syndrome, cytokine storm, and macrophage activation syndrome is a recently identified disorder that occurs infrequently in association with the return of bone marrow growth after treatment of hematological malignancies and blood and marrow transplantation.[9] Patients most at risk for engraftment syndrome are women, those with acute leukemia (especially lymphocytic subtype), those who have just had allogeneic blood or marrow transplantation (especially with human leukocyte antigen–mismatched donors), and those who have had transplantation for autoimmune disorders or solid tumors.[9,10] Patients who have had early engraftment after high-dose marrow-ablative treatment are also at risk for engraftment syndrome.

Pathophysiology

Regrowth of bone marrow cells, particularly myelocytes, results in release of inflammatory cytokines that produce vasodilation and capillary leaking similar to sepsis. Lymphocytes and myelocytic precursors engraft the bone marrow earliest, and patients often still appear leukopenic at the onset of symptoms. Patients with engraftment syndrome often present with signs and symptoms similar to infection at a time when their blood counts are still low, and they are equally at risk for engraftment syndrome and severe infection. Therefore, it is extremely difficult to distinguish the two disorders.

Assessment

History
Engraftment syndrome often begins with fever, total-body erythema or rash, and symptoms of respiratory distress,[11] and these symptoms may be the only manifestations. However, many patients exhibit additional signs or symptoms of cytokine effects such as oliguria or hematuria with elevated creatinine, abdominal discomfort with elevated aminotransferases, and gastrointestinal bleeding. The onset of symptoms is rapid, usually occurring over 24 to 48 hours, and symptoms dissipate after the neutrophils engraft and the white blood cell count reaches about 2,500 to 3,000/mm^3.[10,11] Box 48-7 outlines key clinical manifestations that distinguish sepsis and engraftment syndrome.

Diagnostic Studies
There is no clearly definitive diagnostic test that can differentiate engraftment syndrome from sepsis, which it closely resembles. The cornerstones of diagnosis are the constellation of clinical symptoms, subsequent increase in white blood cell count in patients with previous leukopenia, and absence of a positive microbial culture.[10]

Management

Engraftment syndrome is managed supportively and conservatively. Patients are presumed septic and treated with broad-spectrum antimicrobial agents. Acetaminophen and diphenhydramine are administered as needed for erythema and pruritus. Hepatic dysfunction requires cautious monitoring and adjustment of fluids and medication doses as appropriate. IV fluids are used to prevent vasodilatory hypoten-

Table 48-15 • Key Clinical Features of Bone Marrow Suppression

Feature	Anemia	Thrombocytopenia	Leukopenia
Definition	General criteria • Hemoglobin <12 mg% • RBC count <3.0 × 10⁶/mm³ • Hematocrit <32% Specific to types of anemia • Aplastic anemia • Nutritional anemia • Hemolytic anemia	Classified according to severity of thrombocytopenia and risk of bleeding: • Mild <100,000/mm³ • Moderate <50,000/mm³ • Severe <20,000/mm³	Classified according to severity of leukopenia and risk for infection Decreased granulocytes (granulocytopenia) classified by severity of ANC • Mild <1,000/mm³ • Moderate <500/mm³ • Severe <100/mm³ Decreased lymphocytes (lymphocytopenia) classified by severity of absolute lymphocyte count • Mild <250 cells/mm³ • Moderate <100 cells/mm³ • Severe <50 cells/mm³
Pathophysiology Etiology/ contributing factors	General • Bone marrow suppression (e.g., chemotherapy, radiation to axial skeleton) • Nutritional deficits—iron, protein, B vitamins • Medications (estrogens, allopurinal [Zyloprim]) Aplastic anemia • Congenital disorders (e.g., Fanconi's syndrome, maternal ingestion of thiazides) • Viral infection • Medications Nutritional anemia • Iron deficiency • B vitamin deficiency Hemolytic anemia • Immune hemolysis (viral illness, autoimmune disease) • Sickle cell anemia • PNH	• Bone marrow suppression (e.g., chemotherapy, radiation to axial skeleton) • Medications (nonsteroidal anti-inflammatory drugs) • Large-bone IV lines (e.g., IABP) • High metabolic rate (e.g., fevers)	• Bone marrow suppression (e.g., chemotherapy, radiation to axial skeleton) • Nutritional deficits • Medications
Clinical manifestations	• Due to decreased oxygen carrying and tissue delivery: fatigue, oliguria, chest pain, decreased bowel sounds and constipation • Due to decreased body insulation and vascular volume: hypothermia, hypotension, orthostasis • Due to compensation for inadequate oxygen delivery to the tissue: tachycardia, tachypnea, cool extremities	• Due to decreased platelet plugging for normal vascular wear and tear: gum oozing, petechiae, occult blood in urine and stool • Related to inadequate platelet response to injury: ecchymoses, hematomas, bleeding around procedure sites, frank hematuria, or gastrointestinal bleeding	Granulocytopenia • Due to decreased phagocytic properties and recognition of invading microbes: fever, pain at site of potential infection, bacterial and fungal infecting organisms (after 7–10 days of granulocytopenia) • Related to diminished inflammatory response: lack of localized erythema, swelling or exudates Lymphocytopenia • Due to decreased cellular immune responses and recognition of foreign tissue or proteins: tissue anergy to pathogens, (opportunistic and viral infections more common)
Diagnostic tests	General • RBC count • Hematocrit and hemoglobin • RBC morphology Aplastic anemia • Bone marrow aspirate and biopsy	• Platelet count • Bleeding time tests platelet quality to identify whether symptoms may be partly related to platelet function rather than number	• White blood cell count is initial screening tool, but analysis of actual cell count may be helpful • ANC demonstrates the true number of granulocytes available for phagocytic activity

(continued)

Table 48-15 • Key Clinical Features of Bone Marrow Suppression (Continued)

Feature	Anemia	Thrombocytopenia	Leukopenia
	Nutritional anemia • Ferritin level • Transferrin level • Total iron-binding capacity (TIBC) • Folate level • Vitamin B_{12} level Hemolytic anemia • Total and direct bilirubin • Erythrocyte sedimentation rate (ESR) • RBC morphology • Hemoglobin electrophoresis (sickle cell, PNH) • Indium-tagged RBC survival studies		• Absolute lymphocyte count demonstrates the true number of lymphocytes available for recognition of foreign tissue and proteins
Common nursing problems	• Fatigue • Activity intolerance • Hypoxemia • Digestion disorders	• Bleeding • Altered body image	• Infection • Risk for hemodynamic instability
Medical management	• Erythropoietin injections • RBC transfusions • Energy conservation	• Interleukin-1 (Oprelvekin) injections • Platelet transfusions • Bleeding precautions	• Granulocyte colony-stimulating factor (G-CSF) or granulocyte–macrophage colony-stimulating factor (GM-CSF) injections • Broad-spectrum antimicrobial therapy

ANC, absolute neutrophil count; PNH, paroxysmal nocturnal hemoglobinuria; RBC, red blood cell.

sion, but, occasionally, vasoconstricting agents such as phenylephrine are necessary. Rapid-acting IV corticosteroids have been used effectively when clinical symptoms are strongly suggestive of this disorder.[11] Mechanical ventilation and renal replacement therapy are initiated as indicated, with the understanding and presumption that the syndrome is usually very short-lived.

Complications

The long-term outcome for most patients with engraftment syndrome is excellent, and there are no significant clinical sequelae.[11,12] Rarely do patients die or have long-term ischemic organ damage. In situations in which negative sequelae have occurred, it has been difficult to determine whether engraftment syndrome or sepsis was the primary pathophysiological process. For example, patients with a rapid onset and progression of respiratory distress syndrome may die of refractory hypoxemia, yet whether this has been caused by undiagnosed and untreated infection or engraftment syndrome cannot be determined.

LEUKOSTASIS

Leukostasis is a disorder of excess circulating immature white blood cells, resulting in hyperviscosity and microvascular occlusions.[13,14] Cancers such as acute leukemias are the primary cause of leukostasis. The incidence of symptomatic leukostasis in acute

Box 48-7 • Distinguishing Between Engraftment Syndrome and Sepsis

SEPSIS	ENGRAFTMENT SYNDROME
• Fever, variable clinical features • Variable symptom onset • Variable skin manifestations • Dyspnea, often with distinct infiltrates on chest radiography • Thrombocytopenia; occasional mucous membrane bleeding • Hypotension-related oliguria and elevated creatinine • Hypotension-related hepatomegaly, elevated aminotransferases	• Fever, sudden onset, often high and continuous • Sudden symptom onset over 24–48 h near engraftment period • Erythema with or without pruritic total body rash • Dyspnea; bilateral diffuse alveolar infiltrates on chest radiography • Gastrointestinal bleeding • Unprecipitated oliguria, elevated creatinine, hematuria • Unprecipitated hepatomegaly, elevated aminotransferases

leukemia is estimated to be 5% to 30%,[14] and its association with high circulating immature white blood cells confers a poor prognosis. Initial mortality in patients with this syndrome is estimated to be approximately 40%.[13]

Pathophysiology

Excess numbers of circulating white blood cells, such as commonly occur in patients with acute leukemia, can cause a hyperviscosity syndrome that may lead to microcirculatory occlusion with ischemia and vessel rupture. Several types of leukemia can cause elevated white blood cell counts. The immature myelocytes (blasts) found in acute nonlymphocytic leukemia have the greatest propensity for "stickiness" due to adhesion molecules and their interaction with endothelial vessel linings and are most likely to cause leukostasis.[13,15] Risk for leukostasis is considered greatest when the white blood cell count is greater than 100,000/mm³, although significant clinical symptoms may be present even when counts are in the 50,000/mm³ range, especially if the white blood cell count is increasing rapidly or the cells are immature.[13] Vascular occlusion of the lungs and brain is most common, although coronary artery occlusion, renal failure, and splenic or bowel infarctions have been reported.[13,15]

Assessment

History
Patients with leukostasis usually first present with respiratory or neurological symptoms.[12,14] Onset of symptoms is acute (several hours to 1 day). Severe respiratory distress with hypoxemia and inflammatory alveolar infiltrates are the hallmarks of pulmonary involvement. It is difficult to determine the severity of hypoxemia because the immature white blood cell blasts consume the oxygen in the arterial blood gas (ABG) specimen, making the arterial blood oxygen level appear even lower than suspected based on clinical evidence. Oxygen saturation may be low (e.g., 82% to 90%), but ABG oxygen levels may be only 30 mm Hg.[14,16] It is believed that immediate icing and rapid transit may reduce but not eliminate this testing problem. Neurological leukostasis presents as mental status changes with clear focal deficits; vascular occlusions cause thrombotic or embolic strokes.[12]

Diagnostic Studies
Leukostasis may be suspected in high-risk groups, but the diagnosis is primarily made on the basis of clinical manifestations. In many instances, the existence of pathophysiological complications such as infarction or stroke may validate the presumed diagnosis. Patients have specific diagnostic tests performed to assess their presenting symptoms. Chest radiography is often sufficient to diagnosis pulmonary leukostasis. A head computed tomography (CT) scan may reveal neurological leukostasis. Ultrasonography and magnetic resonance imaging (MRI) may also be performed. In pulmonary leukostasis, ABG results are used with a clear understanding of their diagnostic limitations.

Management

In leukostasis, the preferred management is to identify high-risk or early symptomatic patients and perform leukapheresis before the cells cause organ damage. Some clinicians have noted that although leukapheresis does not have an impact on mortality, it does notably affect the number of white blood cells and their influence on end-organ damage.[12,15,17] Therapeutic leukapheresis removes 20,000 to 40,000 white blood cells per treatment, and once- or twice-daily treatments are often required until the white blood cell count is less than 30,000 to 40,000/mm³.[13,17] If leukapheresis cannot be performed immediately, large amounts of IV fluids should be administered to dilute the blood and enhance renal excretion of metabolic toxins. If leukapheresis is still not possible within a 12- to 24-hour period, and the patient's symptoms continue to worsen, exchange transfusions may be necessary.[13,17]

Many patients also receive immediate concomitant chemotherapy to prevent rapid cell regrowth or spontaneous tumor lysis syndrome with renal failure.[14] If possible, it is preferred to complete the necessary leukapheresis cycles before starting chemotherapy; however, many patients are too sick for such treatment. When this occurs, the critical care nurse must administer antimicrobial agents or chemotherapy between leukapheresis or continuous renal replacement therapy (CRRT). Low-dose cranial radiation (100 to 300 Gy) was once believed to stabilize cell membranes and destroy malignant cells, but this practice is now not recommended.[14] Patients with leukostasis receive supportive drug therapy with agents such as antimicrobials, diuretics, bronchodilators, phosphate-binding agents, rasburicase, and allopurinol, which are aimed at stabilizing their symptoms.

It is important to recognize interventions that worsen the hyperviscosity of leukostasis and avoid these actions. Patients with acute leukemia are often anemic, but blood products should be administered with extreme caution and in combination with crystalloid fluids to avoid increased blood viscosity.[14] Diuretics may be given to enhance renal excretion of uric acid associated with tumor cells lysis, but also only in combination with crystalloid fluids to maintain normal vascular osmolarity. Supportive interventions to reduce intracranial hemorrhage may include elevating the head of the bed and administering corticosteroids. Definitive treatment requires administration of chemotherapy directed against the leukemia. Box 48-8 lists nursing interventions aimed at reducing the risk for leukostasis-related complications.

Complications

Even in the face of appropriate, definitive treatment, patients with leukostasis may experience stroke, respiratory failure, bowel infarction, renal failure, or myocardial infarction. In many, some degree of

---

Box 48-8 • NURSING INTERVENTIONS for Leukostasis

- Recognize patients at risk for leukostasis—acute myelocytic leukemia (with circulating blasts), white blood cell count >100,000/mm³, renal dysfunction, dehydration.
- Administer large volumes of intravenous fluids to dilute cells and aid excretion of lysis components.
- Perform cytoreduction with leukapheresis or rapid-acting chemotherapy (e.g., cyclophosphamide) as soon as possible.

- Treat organ system–specific leukostatic symptoms (e.g., elevation of head of bed, bronchodilators).
- Administer agents to reduce effects of tumor lysis: phosphate-binding agents, allopurinol, rasburicase
- Administer blood components cautiously early in the disease when hyperviscosity is problematic.
- Plan assessment interventions aimed at monitoring for ischemia or infarction of the body organs.

---

reversible organ ischemia develops, requiring supportive treatment.[13]

• Anatomical–Structural Complications

CARDIAC TAMPONADE

Cardiac tamponade is the result of accumulation of excess pericardial fluid or the presence of a tumor that compresses the heart. At autopsy, as many as 20% of people with cancer are found to have cardiac or pericardial metastases.[18]

Pathophysiology

The pericardium is a double-walled sac that surrounds the heart and great vessels. A visceral layer lines the surface of the heart, and the parietal layer (or outer layer) moves freely. The pericardium supports the heart in a stable position and provides a frictionless sac for cardiac contractions. The pericardial cavity lies between the two layers and contains 10 to 50 mL of serous fluid.

Neoplastic cardiac tamponade results from the formation and accumulation of excessive amounts of fluid in the pericardial sac. This emergent condition may also be caused by encasement of the heart by tumor or postradiation pericarditis. The severity of the tamponade is in direct proportion to the rate of fluid formation and the volume of fluid accumulated. Slow accumulation may stretch the pericardium so that cardiac contractility is not adversely affected for months. Normal diastolic filling is impaired by elevated pericardial pressures, and stroke volume is reduced. As stroke volume continues to fall, hypotension, compensatory tachycardia, and equalization and elevation of the mean left atrial, pulmonary arterial and venous, right atrial, and vena caval pressures occur. In an attempt to maintain arterial pressure, increase blood volume, and improve venous return, tachycardia and peripheral vasoconstriction develop. If the tamponade goes undiagnosed or untreated, circulatory collapse ensues.

Cancers of the esophagus or lung grow by direct extension into the pericardium, whereas distant primary cancers (e.g., renal cell) metastasize to the pericardium through the bloodstream. Large chest tumors may also cause pericardial effusion due to lymphatic obstruction of pericardial fluid recirculation. The primary tumors most commonly associated with pericardial effusion are tumors of the breast, lung, or esophagus; lymphoma; gastrointestinal carcinomas; melanoma; sarcoma; and leukemia. Radiation pericarditis may be a causative factor, especially if the patient's heart was in the treatment field and if the total dose of radiation to this field exceeded 4,000 rad (40 Gy).[19] Biotherapeutic agents such as interleukin-2 (Aldesleukin) and interferon-α cause increased capillary permeability and clinically significant pericardial effusions.[20]

Assessment

History

Signs and symptoms reflect the rapidity with which the fluid accumulates in the pericardial sac and, in the patient with cancer, are mainly those of right-sided heart failure due to slow accumulation. Signs of tamponade include rapid, weak pulse; distant heart sounds; distended neck veins during inspiration (Kussmaul's sign); pulsus paradoxus (inspiratory decrease in arterial blood pressure of more than 10 mm Hg from baseline); ankle or sacral edema; edema; ascites; hepatosplenomegaly; hepatojugular reflex; lethargy; and altered level of consciousness.[18,19,21] The patient may complain of dyspnea, cough, and retrosternal pain that is relieved by leaning forward. On occasion, a patient with a large effusion experiences epigastric pain, hiccups, hoarseness, nausea, and vomiting.

Diagnostic Studies

A variety of studies are used to determine the presence and severity of cardiac tamponade. A chest film is used to determine the presence of cardiac enlargement, mediastinal widening, or hilar adenopathy. The electrocardiogram (ECG) may show nonspecific abnormalities, including low QRS complex voltage in limb leads, sinus tachycardia, precordial ST-segment elevations, and T-wave changes.[18] Echocardiography is the most sensitive and most specific noninvasive test for the presence of tamponade and is used routinely in most settings.[19] Two distinct echoes may be identified, one from effusion and the other from the posterior heart border. Spaces between these echoes indicate the size of the effusion or the thickness of the pericardium. Catheterization of the right side of the heart reveals pericardial tamponade or constriction but is performed infrequently because echocardiograms are routinely available. Pericardiocentesis gives a positive cytological result in the patient with metastatic cancer.

Management

First, volume expansion is necessary because it increases venous pressure so that it is greater than pericardial pressure, allowing increased venous return and improved cardiac output.[18] Oxygen administration is required, although assisted or mechanical ventilation may increase thoracic pressures, further impeding venous return and worsening the tamponade.

The definitive treatment for pericardial effusion is fluid drainage. Acute or life-threatening symptoms are indications for emergent pericardial drainage by needle or catheter pericardiocentesis (Box 48-9). Without definitive treatment to alleviate the fluid in the pericardium, cardiac arrest occurs. Tamponade is likely to recur in 24 to 48 hours if treatment to prevent pericardial fluid reaccumulation is not initiated quickly.

Factors that clinicians should consider when selecting a therapeutic option include the sensitivity of the primary tumor to specific treatment modalities, previous treatment, and the patient's life expectancy. If effective drugs are available (e.g., as in lymphoma and small cell lung cancer), systemic chemotherapy may be initiated after the patient is clinically stable.[20,22] This treatment may also be effective in patients with leukemia, lymphoma, and breast cancer who have pericardial effusion. In radiosensitive tumors such as lymphoma and breast cancer, radiation therapy may be the treatment of choice. Research has shown that radiation therapy may control more than 50% of malignant pericardial effusions.[23] Insertion of a pericardial catheter guided by fluoroscopy or echocardiography to permit rapid fluid drainage is often the preferred immediate treatment.[23,24] The catheter may remain in place while anticancer therapy begins. Pericardial sclerosis through the pericardial catheter, which is rarely used, can control tamponade by causing adherence of the two pericardial layers and inhibiting fluid accumulation.[23]

In patients with a longer life expectancy and adequate performance status, an inferior pericardiotomy may be performed thoracoscopically. In this procedure, a pleural–pericardial window is created, which provides immediate relief of cardiac compression and tissue specimens for histological diagnosis. Fewer than 5% of patients have recurrence of symptoms after this procedure. Pericardectomy is necessary if radiation-induced pericardial disease is not responsive to conservative medical management. This procedure should not take place if an extensive pericardial tumor is present because surgical morbidity and mortality rates are high.[25]

CAROTID ARTERY RUPTURE

Causes of a carotid artery rupture (or "blowout") are tumor erosion and rupture of the carotid artery. Such rupture results in the loss of large amounts of blood that, without rapid intervention, becomes life-threatening hemorrhage. Patients at risk for this oncological emergency are primarily those with cancer of the head and neck, especially after surgery or radiation, or with a wound infection.[26] Affected patients occasionally have thyroid cancer, lymphoma, or melanoma.[26] Patients with a palpable pulse on top of a tumor, or in close proximity to it, have a greater risk for carotid vessel erosion.[26]

Pathophysiology

Rupture of a carotid artery is likely to occur when that vessel is weakened by invasion of tumor or by surgical manipulation. Other causes of vessel weakness include simultaneous infection or skin flap necrosis.

Assessment

The rupture of the artery may occur suddenly with forceful expulsion of large volumes of blood from the damaged vessel; however, the first sign of erosion or rupture usually is a small trickle of blood from the neck area or unexplained oral bleeding.[26] If the skin over the artery is intact, the patient may have darkened or ecchymotic skin changes, swelling, difficulty swallowing or breathing, retrosternal or high epigastric chest pain, and mental status changes. A unilateral headache or visual disturbance may also signal carotid artery bleeding. Box 48-10 lists the cardinal signs and symptoms of carotid artery rupture.

Box 48-9 • RED FLAG: Signs and Symptoms of Neoplastic Cardiac Tamponade

The life-threatening symptoms listed indicate the need for emergent pericardial drainage.
- Cyanosis, dyspnea with hypoxemia, impaired consciousness, or shock
- Pulsus paradoxus >50% of the pulse pressure
- Decrease >20 mm Hg in pulse pressure
- Central venous pressure >13 mm Hg

Box 48-10 • RED FLAG: Cardinal Signs and Symptoms of Carotid Artery Rupture

- Oozing blood from neck wound
- Unexplained oral bleeding
- Ecchymoses over neck region
- Sudden neck edema
- Retrosternal or epigastric chest pain
- Sense of impending doom, anxiety, or restlessness

Management

Patients identified as high risk for carotid artery rupture may have vascular stents placed during surgery as a preventive measure. In addition, IV access should be in place, and blood should be typed and available for immediate transfusion.[27]

Gauze, irrigation saline, and vascular clamps should be readily available at all times. The first emergency intervention in cases of suspected carotid artery rupture is constant digital pressure with saline-soaked cotton dressing wrapped around the two middle fingers and applied directly to the area over the artery.[27,28] The nurse must not lessen pressure to see whether the bleeding has stopped or attempt to apply a hemostat. Either of these steps increases the likelihood of further blood loss. Maintenance of the airway is essential. Only after the patient is in the operative suite and the operative area has been prepared should the pressure be released. The surgical treatment of choice is ligation of the damaged artery. Embolization or stent placement may be alternatives.[28] Chapter 22 contains a detailed discussion of carotid artery surgery with assessment and nursing care.

Complications

The overall mortality rate of carotid artery rupture is 40% to 60%.[26] About 60% of patients who survive this complication have long-term neurological deficits, the most common of which is hemiparesis. The risk for hemiparesis is reduced by the prevention of shock and replacement of fluid for adequate perfusion of the brain through the opposite internal carotid artery.

HEPATIC VENO-OCCLUSIVE DISEASE

Hepatic veno-occlusive disease, also known as sinusoidal obstruction syndrome, is occlusion of the venous vessels of the liver. The disease is a complication of high-dose radiation therapy and chemotherapy.[29] Its incidence is as low as 5% to 10% in patients receiving some chemotherapy and monoclonal antibody regimens but as high as 30% to 40% in some receiving blood and marrow transplants.[30] Although hepatic veno-occlusive disease is most likely to develop in patients receiving high-dose alkylating agents (e.g., cyclophosphamide, busulfan) or abdominal radiation, it also occurs in patients receiving the leukemic monoclonal antibody gemtuzumab (Mylotarg)[29,31] and oxiliplatin (Arotcarene).[32,33] Other risk factors in patients with cancer are extensive pretreatment, older age, and previous history of hepatitis.[31]

Pathophysiology

Through uncertain mechanisms, etiological agents cause fibrotic changes in the endothelial layer that lines the walls of the veins and sinusoids in the liver, resulting in narrowed and stiff-walled venules that have a tendency for thrombosis. Venous flow through the liver is reduced, and there is congestion and eventual pressure-related hepatic damage.[30]

Assessment

History

The earliest manifestations of hepatic veno-occlusive disease are fluid retention, elevated serum bilirubin, and nonspecific abdominal pain.[30] The onset of these symptoms occurs an average of 8 to 20 days after therapy; the time varies with the causative agent.[30] The clinical course begins primarily as one of portal hypertension with ascites, painful hepatomegaly, and right-sided heart failure; it progresses over 1 to 3 weeks to include hepatic destruction with coagulopathies, thrombocytopenia, hyperammonemia, metabolic alkalosis, increased vagal tone, and hepatorenal failure.[30] Box 48-11 lists early and late clinical findings in hepatic veno-occlusive disease. Most patients with hepatic veno-occlusive disease have mild, reversible disease, and only 10% to 20% have severe, life-threatening manifestations.[30]

Diagnostic Studies

The first and most specific diagnostic test is the elevation of total and indirect bilirubin.[30] Aspartate transaminase (AST; previously known as serum glutamic oxaloacetic transaminase [SGOT]) and alkaline phosphatase also increase early, and when progressive liver failure develops, hepatic aminotransferases also increase. Abdominal ultrasonography confirms hepatic enlargement and is used to rule out causal conditions such as cholestasis and hepatic abscess.[30] The new addition of ultrasonographic Doppler technology can provide more conclusive evidence of hepatic veno-occlusive disease with validation of venous wall turgidity and estimated portal pressures.[30]

In late or severe disease, the platelet count decreases, and coagulation studies such as prothrombin time or partial thromboplastin time are prolonged. A definitive diagnosis may be made only on the basis of liver biopsy. When it is necessary to differentiate hepatic veno-occlusive disease from other clinically similar processes, such as graft-versus-host disease (GVHD), liver biopsy shows venule fibrosis.[34]

Box 48-11 • RED FLAG: Signs and Symptoms of Hepatic Veno-occlusive Disease

Early Findings
- Weight gain
- Fluid retention, edema
- Painful hepatomegaly
- Increased total and direct bilirubin
- Increased aspartate aminotransferase and alkaline phosphatase

Late Findings
- Coagulopathies, thrombocytopenia
- Hyperammonemia
- Metabolic alkalosis
- Hepatorenal syndrome
- Right-sided heart failure
- Elevated aminotransferases
- Increased vagal tone

Management

Because the pathological mechanisms of hepatic veno-occlusive disease are uncertain, therapy is still presumptive and not clearly effective. Once hepatic veno-occlusive disease is suspected, supportive therapies such as balancing fluid administration and diuresis are implemented.[35] Transjugular intrahepatic portosystemic shunt (TIPS) procedures have been used in an attempt to enhance portal blood outflow.[36,37] Patients may require platelet and fresh frozen plasma transfusions, vasopressors, and ammonia-lowering therapies, such as lactulose.[36,38] Researchers have noted modest reports of successful symptom resolution with high-dose methylprednisolone, glutamine with high-dose vitamin E, ursodiol, activated factor VII, defibrotide, and tissue plasminogen activator.[36,35,39] Defibrotide, an oligonucleotide derived from porcine intestinal mucosa that demonstrates simultaneous antithrombotic properties with microvascular protective features, producing minimal hemorrhagic risk, is the most promising and well-studied agent.[36,40] Renal replacement therapy is often required; continuous venovenous hemofiltration is often the preferred method of therapy because of increased vagal tone and a tendency for vasodilatory hypotension. Some experts advocate early implementation to preserve renal function and reduce the need for respiratory support.[36] Before the advent of CRRT, mechanical ventilation to control fluid imbalance–induced respiratory distress was often necessary.

No methods to prevent hepatic veno-occlusive disease have yet proved successful. Results of studies of low-dose heparin (subcutaneously or intravenously), prostaglandin E_1, and defibrotide as potential preventive agents have so far been inconclusive.[36,41,42]

Complications

Patients with mild to moderate hepatic veno-occlusive disease experience complete reversal of the pathological process. It is uncertain whether supportive therapies have any influence on this outcome. Well-controlled studies clearly show that mortality is high in patients with total bilirubin levels greater than 15 to 18 mg/dL, renal dysfunction, high fibrinogen D-dimers, or a hepatic pressure gradient of greater than 20 mm Hg.[31,35,36]

SUPERIOR VENA CAVA SYNDROME

Superior vena cava syndrome (SVCS)—obstruction of the superior vena cava—results in venous blockage that produces pleural effusion and facial, arm, and tracheal edema.[43,44] Severe obstruction may result in impaired cardiac filling and cerebral edema.

Pathophysiology

The superior vena cava is a thin-walled, low-pressure blood vessel in the mediastinal cavity that collects blood from the venous vessels that drain the head and neck and the upper thoracic cavity. The mediastinum is a rigid anatomical structure that contains the trachea, the vertebral column, the sternum and ribs, and the lymph nodes.

Most cases of SVCS result from mediastinal malignancies or involved lymph nodes that cause extrinsic compression or invade the vessel.[43–45] More than 75% of cases are secondary to small cell or squamous cell lung cancers, and 10% to 15% are secondary to mediastinal lymphomas.[43–45] Obstruction of the vessel lumen by a thrombus may also occur; it is most commonly caused by a central venous catheter or a hypercoagulability syndrome due to cancer.[43–45] Box 48-12 summarizes the causes of SVCS.

Assessment

History

Signs and symptoms of SVCS depend on the rapidity of compression of the superior vena cava. If it is compressed gradually and collateral circulation develops, indications of SVCS may be more subtle.[45] Initial symptoms are most prominent in the early morning and include periorbital and conjunctival edema, facial swelling, and Stokes' sign (tightness of the shirt collar). These signs may disappear after the patient has been upright for a few hours. The patient may also complain of visual disturbances and headache. Altered consciousness and focal neurological signs may result from brain edema and impaired cardiac filling. Late signs and symptoms include distention of the veins of the thorax and upper extremities, dysphagia, dyspnea, cough, hoarseness, and tachypnea. All patients, including children, most commonly visit health care providers because of dyspnea.[43,44] Pleural effusions are present in approximately 60% of cases, compounding respiratory symptoms and providing a complex dimension for treatment planning.[46] Most pleural effusions are transudative and related to obstruction of pleural and lymphatic outflow.

Diagnostic Studies

Until recently, diagnostic evaluation of SVCS required multiple tests to validate the location, size, and vena

---

Box 48-12 • Risk Factors for Superior Vena Cava Syndrome

- Chest, neck, or epigastric tumors (e.g., lung cancer, breast cancer, lymphoma, head and neck cancer, thyroid cancer, gastric cancer, esophageal cancer, pancreatic cancer, metastatic renal cell cancer, metastatic colorectal cancer, melanoma)
- Devices in the superior vena cava (e.g., large-bore, multilumen central lines, especially if placed in the subclavian site)
- Hypercoagulability syndromes (disseminated intravascular coagulation, hypercoagulability of malignancy [e.g., mucin-producing adenocarcinomas, brain tumors, Trousseau's syndrome])

cava involvement of tumors or thrombus. Conventional chest CT with IV contrast, venography, angiography, and radionuclide scans were necessary. Currently, the spiral CT scan with contrast, which provides accurate information about tumor location and involvement of the vena cava, may be the only diagnostic test performed.[47,48] However, biopsy or cytological tests may be required to establish a diagnosis in many patients because this syndrome is the presenting symptom at the time of diagnosis of cancer.[45]

Management

The primary treatment of choice for SVCS caused by a tumor is radiation therapy. Dosage depends on the size of the tumor and its radiosensitivity. Radiation therapy is initially given in high daily fractions (total dose of 30 to 50 rad), and symptom relief occurs in 7 to 14 days.[43] Radiation therapy is palliative for SVCS in 70% of patients with lung cancer and for more than 95% of patients with lymphoma.[43] Radiation of the mediastinal, hilar, and supraclavicular lymph nodes and any adjacent parenchymal lesions is appropriate in patients with locally advanced non–small cell lung cancer.

Patients who receive radiation therapy experience increased cough within 3 days of the start of therapy. During the initial 7 to 10 days, secretions are increased because of inflammation, but a dry irritation then develops, resulting in a dry, hacking cough with few secretions but possible bleeding.[43]

Chemotherapy may be the treatment of choice for SVCS in patients with disseminated disease, such as small cell anaplastic carcinoma or lymphoma. The agents used most often include high-dose regimens containing cyclophosphamide, cisplatin or carboplatin, bleomycin, and doxorubicin. The adverse effects of these agents include bone marrow suppression, cardiac toxicity, and renal dysfunction.

Treatment of SVCS caused by a thrombus around a central venous catheter may include antifibrinolytics or anticoagulants and possibly surgical removal of the catheter.[43] In any case, chest and neck central venous catheter placements should be avoided until effective treatment has been delivered.

In some circumstances, the placement of stents or vascular grafts in the superior vena cava provides immediate symptomatic relief while patients receive definitive therapy.[49,50] It is unclear whether long-term anticoagulation is required.

Supportive care is essential. Maintenance of a patent airway is of the highest priority.[43] Because many patients have severe dyspnea, they are unable to lie flat for their radiation therapy, and short-term airway intubation may be necessary. Clinicians may prescribe oxygen therapy, diuretics, steroids, and heparin, and their administration requires careful observation of patient response. If necessary, administration of corticosteroids for 3 to 7 days to decrease the edema associated with the disease and treatment is warranted.[45] The nurse teaches the patient not to bend over and to avoid Valsalva maneuvers. When the patient is in bed, the head should be at least in a semi-Fowler's position. Elevation of the arms on pillows helps alleviate swelling; however, elevation of the legs does not because this increases fluid volume in the torso.

Complications

Several complications may occur in patients with SVCS. Right-sided heart failure is the most common.[43] Such heart failure is usually self-limiting and is treated symptomatically with fluid restrictions, diuretics, and digoxin. Vessel rupture in SVCS when a tumor invades the vena cava is a great risk because the tumor shrinks with treatment. The incidence of vessel rupture is highest in patients with esophageal and lung cancer; peak incidence is 3 to 4 weeks after initiation of therapy.[43] Warning signs of vessel rupture are acute and sudden dyspnea, hypoxia, cough, and vascular collapse. Radiation pneumonitis, an inflammatory response in the radiation field that correlates with breath sound and radiographic changes reflective of alveolar capillary permeability, may occur 2 to 8 weeks after start of therapy in patients who receive chest radiation for SVCS.[43] Treatment of radiation pneumonitis involves corticosteroids and supportive therapy. SVCS recurs in 10% to 30% of patients.[44]

PLEURAL EFFUSION

Pathophysiology

There is normally 30 to 150 mL of fluid between the visceral and parietal pleura that helps maintain a negative pleural pressure to facilitate lung expansion with minimum work of breathing. A pleural effusion is excess accumulation of fluid in the pleural space with subsequent impaired lung expansion and hypoxemia. When lymphatic obstruction (particularly of the thoracic duct), venous congestion, pleural inflammation, or excess capillary permeability occurs, the amount of fluid increases or does not drain properly. Although many nonmalignant conditions (e.g., congestive heart failure, hypothyroidism) may cause pleural effusion, malignant conditions involving lymphatic obstruction or infiltration with malignant cells may also have the same result. Pleural effusions that result from volume overload, capillary permeability, or lymphatic obstruction produce a transudate characterized by the presence of albumin and the absence of cell fragments or enzymes in the pleural fluid.[51] Malignant cell infiltration or pleuritic infection causes pleural inflammation and exudates characterized by the release of red blood cells, white blood cells, and lactate dehydrogenase into the pleural fluid.[51,52] As many as 15% of patients with cancer experience pleural effusions during the course of their disease.[53,54]

Accumulation of pleural fluid leads to increased (more positive) pleural pressure. Higher pleural pressures increase the work of breathing, and collapsed alveoli cause decreased gas exchange and hypoxemia.[51]

Assessment

History
The clinical findings in pleural effusion are related to the two major physiological mechanisms: increased work of breathing and alveolar collapse. Excess pleural pressures decrease lung compliance ("stiff lungs"). Patients feel short of breath and must use their accessory muscles to breathe, and chest excursion on the affected side is reduced. When patients are in an upright position, the force of gravity pulls down the fluid, and breath sounds are diminished to the level of fluid. The pleural fluid takes up space in the chest, impeding lung expansion with consequent alveolar collapse. Symptoms that relate to this pathological process are diminished breath sounds, tracheal shift away from the effusion, and signs of hypoxemia (e.g., dyspnea, anxiety, confusion, oliguria, decreased bowel sounds).[51]

Diagnostic Studies
The first diagnostic test performed to confirm the presence of pleural effusion is an upright chest radiograph.[55] The fluid accumulates in the lower lung, causing a blunted diaphragmatic dome and decreased radiolucence in the lower lung. Fluid accumulation often produces a meniscus of decreased radiolucence and a thickened lateral pleural lining, indicating fluid tracking up the side.[55] After a pleural effusion is confirmed, a cytological evaluation, which involves extraction of a sample of fluid and sending it for fluid chemistry and cytology, is necessary.[52,55] Pleural fluid is categorized as transudative or exudative, which provides clues to the cause of the effusion. Cytological studies confirm the presence or absence of malignant cells; the result influences treatment decisions.

Management

The treatment of pleural effusion depends on the etiological mechanism, rapidity of symptom onset, and degree of respiratory compromise.[54] When pleural effusions are small or have a nonmalignant cause, observation without definitive treatment may be indicated. Aggressive antineoplastic therapy may be indicated when a large tumor causes lymphatic obstruction, heart failure, or pneumonitis that in turn causes pleural effusion.

When malignant cells are present in the pleural fluid, management may be determined by overall treatment goals. Repeated therapeutic thoracenteses are often the preferred initial choice; this assumes that the ultimate cause of the pleural effusion is being treated or that the patient's life expectancy does not warrant more interventional measures.

When the patient's life expectancy is longer, and pleural effusions do not resolve with anticancer therapy and intermittent thoracenteses, treatment includes long-term chest catheter drainage or pleurodesis.[54,56] Long-term pleural drainage via a soft tunneled catheter (e.g., Pleurex catheter) allows patients to have a means of draining excess fluid while remaining at home.[57] When drainage slows and patients become a good candidate for pleurodesis, they are admitted to the hospital for this procedure. Pleurodesis, also called pleural sclerosing, involves intrapleural administration of a chemical (e.g., doxycycline, bleomycin) or a mechanical agent (e.g., talc slurry) to alter the pH of the pleural fluid and cause inflammatory adherence of the visceral and parietal pleura to each other.[56] Sclerosed pleura do not have the normal lubricating pleural fluid, and restrictive lung disease is the long-term consequence. Pleurodesis is successful only about 67% of the time, necessitating the availability of additional treatment options.[54,56] Box 48-13 presents nursing interventions related to the management of pleurodesis.

Pleurectomy is a thoracic surgical procedure that removes the entire pleura. Pleurectomy is effective but can be difficult to perform when long-term inflammation and pleurodesis attempts cause a friable pleura that is not easily separated. Chronic, long-term pleuroperitoneal shunts or implanted access devices have been used, but development of fibrin sheaths on the catheters often causes occlusion. Newer, small-bore chest catheters that permit home drainage of the pleural fluid have recently become available. Box 48-14 summarizes home care considerations for patients with malignant pleural effusions.

Complications

Untreated pleural effusions that continue to accumulate lead to clinically significant alveolar collapse and respiratory failure, which may be caused by loss of gas-exchanging airways or mediastinal shifting with

---

Box 48-13 • NURSING INTERVENTIONS for Pleurodesis

- Be certain pleural drainage from chest tube in previous 24 h is <150 mL.
- Obtain sclerosing agent (bleomycin, doxycycline, or talc slurry) and postsclerosing flush solution (preservative-free sterile water or normal saline or lidocaine [Xylocaine] 1% or 2%).
- Plan to inject sclerosing agent into the chest drainage tube.
- Set up an extra Pleur-Evac with tubing to connect if tubing leaks after injecting sclerosing agent.

- Clamp tubing for 4–6 h after instillation of sclerosing agent.
- Have patient be as mobile as possible, but scheduled body rotation is not necessary to ensure distribution of the agent throughout the pleura.
- Unclamp chest tube and observe drainage (effective 67%–70% of time). If effective, drainage is minimal to absent.
- Assist with removal of chest tube and monitor patient for air tracking and pneumothorax, or reaccumulation of fluid.

Box 48-14 • Oncological Emergencies: Pleural Effusions

Malignant pleural effusions are a common cause of severe debilitating disease and impaired quality of life in patients with end-stage cancer. Effectiveness of pleurodesis is only 65% to 70%; many patients do not achieve resolution of their pleural effusions with standard therapy. Multiple devices such as pleuroperitoneal shunts or access ports inserted into the pleural space have been used to permit home drainage of pleural effusions, with limited success. Newer, small-bore thoracostomy catheters have now been developed that permit these patients to return to their homes with a comfortable chest catheter drainage system. Small-bore thoracostomy tubes are connected to a one-way valve similar to the flutter valve, and a drainage bag that resembles a Foley catheter drainage bag.

From Sahin U, Unlu M, Akkaya A, et al: The value of small-bore catheter thoracostomy in the treatment of malignant pleural effusions. Respiration 68(5):501–505, 2001.

major airway obstruction. Progressive hypoxemia leads to profound respiratory acidosis and ischemic organ failure. Evacuation of an extensive and long-standing pleural effusion may result in re-expansion pulmonary edema or hypotension from fluid shifts.[58]

SPINAL CORD COMPRESSION

Spinal cord compression occurs when tumor cells or collapsed vertebrae in the epidural space exert pressure on the spinal cord, which may result in permanent dysfunction (including paralysis) if not diagnosed and treated promptly. Epidural tumors are found in more than 5% of patients with metastatic disease at autopsy.[59,60] Factors associated with effective local control and long-term survival after spinal cord compression include favorable histologic diagnosis, no visceral metastases, and long-course radiation therapy schedule.[61]

Pathophysiology

Two major pathophysiological mechanisms are likely to result in spinal cord compression: (1) tumors arising within the epidural space through vertebral or lymphatic spread, and (2) bony metastasis causing vertebral collapse with spinal cord and nerve root compression.[60] Permanent neurological damage from proximal tumors may also occur if spinal circulation is compromised such as in prolonged ischemia or hemorrhage.[60,62] Other disorders producing signs and symptoms of cord compression are paraneoplastic syndromes, radiation myelopathy, herpes zoster, pain from a pelvic or long bone metastasis, or cytotoxic drug effects. Table 48-16 presents the tumors most likely to cause cord compression and the location of compression.

Assessment

History

When a primary tumor presses on the spinal cord, signs and symptoms usually develop slowly. Problems develop more rapidly with metastatic disease.

Table 48-16 • Spinal Cord Compression: Etiology and Clinical Presentation

Location of Lesion	Common Malignant Etiologies	Physical Symptoms	Autonomic Symptoms
Cervical spine	• Head and neck cancers • Melanoma	• Radicular pain in the neck, occipital region, and shoulders (pain is often provoked by neck movement) • Quadriplegia • Upper extremity weakness (may be spastic or atrophic) • Sensory loss in area of weakness • Weakness or paralysis of the diaphragm may occur with lesion at or above C4 (may be unilateral or bilateral)	• Hypotension • Bradycardia • Loss of temperature autoregulation • Autonomic hyperreflexia • Gastric hypersecretion and paralytic ileus • Reflex bowel, bladder, and erection • Hoffman's sign (flicking of the middle finger induces flexion of the ipsilateral thumb or index finger)
Thoracic spine	• Breast cancer • Gastric cancer • Lung cancer • Lymphoma • Pancreatic cancer	• Pain (may be local, radicular, or both) • Paraplegia • Sensory loss below the level of the lesion • Reflex abnormalities distal to the lesion	• Venous stasis and associated complications • Reflex bowel, bladder, and penile erection
Lumbar spine	• Ovarian cancer • Renal cell cancer • Prostate cancer	• Bowel and bladder dysfunction • Extensor plantar response	• Venous stasis and associated complications • Reflex bowel, bladder, and penile erection
Cauda equina	• Bladder cancer • Prostate cancer	• Pain (may be local, referred, or radicular) • Sphincter disturbances • Loss of buttock and leg sensation • Lower extremity weakness/paralysis	• Areflexic bowel, bladder, and penile erection

Most patients with spinal cord compression complain of progressive central or radicular back pain that often is aggravated by weight bearing, lying down, coughing, sneezing, or performing the Valsalva maneuver. Sitting relieves the pain.[59]

The earliest neurological symptoms are sensory changes, such as numbness, paresthesia, and coldness.[59,60] Compression occurs most often in the thoracic section of the spinal cord, causing neurogenic bladder with urinary retention and incontinence. Patients may also lose the urge to defecate and be unable to bear down. Men on occasion lose the ability to have or maintain an erection. Metastases to the cauda equina frequently produce impaired urethral, vaginal, and rectal sensations; bladder dysfunction; decreased sensation in the lumbosacral dermatomes; and saddle anesthesia.[59] Box 48-15 describes spinal cord considerations in the older adult.

It is possible to determine the level of cord compression by the patient's report of pain during straight leg raising, neck flexion, or vertebral percussion. The upper limit of the sensory level is usually one or two vertebral bodies below the site of compression.[60] Lessened rectal tone and perineal sensation are observed with autonomic dysfunction. Deep tendon reflexes can be brisk with cord compression and diminished with nerve root compression.[60]

Once patients experience pain, motor weakness and ataxia often follow. They may complain that the arms or legs feel heavy. Some patients lose the ability to sense light touch, pain, and temperature. Over time, weakness may progress to spasm, paralysis, and muscle atrophy; sensations of deep pressure and position may disappear.

Diagnostic Studies

MRI is highly sensitive for neurological tissues and can clearly demonstrate all epidural deposits as well as complete or partial block of the spinal cord.[60,63] Therefore, it is the diagnostic test of choice. A myelogram or CT scan may reveal spinal tumors, but these studies are less sensitive for diagnosing the presence and extent of cord compression. Lumbar puncture, which is used to obtain cerebrospinal fluid, reveals malignant cells in the presence of epidural disease.[60]

Management

Factors considered in the selection of the best therapeutic option are the level of cord compression, the rate of neurological deterioration, and previous use of radiation therapy.[64,65] Corticosteroids decrease peritumoral edema and neurological dysfunction. Dexamethasone, 10 mg as an initial dose, is administered to patients with neurological symptoms before emergency diagnostic procedures are performed and is continued during radiation therapy (4 to 20 mg every 6 hours) and then tapered.[59,65] It is not clear whether such steroid therapy affects final patient outcome.

Radiation therapy is appropriate when the tumor is determined to be radiosensitive and should be initiated as soon as the diagnosis of cord compression has been confirmed.[59,65] Radiation portals include the entire area of blockage and two vertebral bodies above and below this area. More than 50% of patients with rapid neurological deterioration improve with radiation therapy; however, patients with autonomic dysfunction or paraplegia have a poor prognosis with any therapy.[65]

Laminectomy, with or without placement of stabilization rods in the nearby vertebral bodies, may result in immediate decompression of the spinal cord and nerve roots.[66] The posterior approach is preferred but is often difficult because most metastases arise in the vertebral bodies anterior to the spinal cord.[62] The anterior approach is warranted for people with tumors that are believed to be resectable, making the clinical risks worth the aggressive surgical intervention.[66] Postoperative radiation therapy is used to shrink residual tumor, relieve pain, and improve the patient's functional status. Surgery is usually contraindicated if there is a collapsed vertebral body or if there are several areas of cord compression. If there is no previous histological diagnosis of cancer or if infection or epidural hematoma must be ruled out, then laminectomy can be used for both diagnosis and treatment. If high cervical cord compression precludes surgery, a neurologist should stabilize the patient's neck in halo traction to prevent respiratory paralysis. If the patient continues to deteriorate neurologically despite high doses of steroids and radiation therapy, then emergency decompression may be necessary.[65,66] In some people, stabilization of the spine with vertebroplasty represents a less invasive and equally effective short-term resolution for acute cord compression and its associated pain.[64,67] If the tumor is chemosensitive, chemotherapy concurrently with or soon after completion of radiation therapy or surgery may be appropriate. Chemotherapy may also be effective in patients with multiple myeloma who have had previous radiation therapy. Systemic chemotherapy or hormonal therapy may be useful in certain types of tumors, such as lymphoma or prostatic cancer.

Pain management includes the administration of appropriate analgesics, bed rest, and patient support during position changes and transfer. Range-

---

Box 48-15 • CONSIDERATIONS FOR THE OLDER PATIENT: Spinal Cord Compression

Signs and symptoms of spinal cord compression often begin as subtle and nonspecific back pain and sensory changes. The older patient may have concomitant diabetes mellitus or osteoarthritis that produces overlapping symptoms, delaying diagnosis of the oncological complication. In addition, older persons often have bowel and bladder changes causing constipation or urinary incontinence, mimicking the more serious autonomic changes that occur in later spinal cord compression. People at high risk for spinal cord compression, such as those with known bone metastases, should be taught the importance of reporting and having evaluated all back pain and sensory changes, especially in the lower extremities. In spinal cord compression, palpable vertebral tenderness is more often present than with other nononcologic disorders.

of-motion exercises are useful in patients with motor and sensory deficits. Bowel retraining and intermittent urinary catheterization may be necessary. Frequent skin care is essential. Surgical wounds are particularly susceptible to skin breakdown (with possible wound dehiscence) because of limited mobility and the effects of concomitant corticosteroid therapy.

TRACHEOBRONCHIAL OBSTRUCTION

Pathophysiology

Obstruction of the trachea or major branches of the bronchi with tumor results in respiratory distress and hypoxemia. The severity of symptoms depends on the rapidity of obstruction and degree of closure.[68] Tumors most likely to cause airway obstruction are lung cancer and lymphoma, although other metastatic tumors (e.g., head and neck cancer, melanoma, renal or breast cancer) and nonmalignant disorders (e.g., amyloidosis, bronchomalacia) may also cause airway obstruction.[68]

Assessment

History

Patients with tracheobronchial obstruction present with varying degrees of dyspnea depending on the amount and location of the obstruction and the rapidity of onset. Some patients with slowly developing tumors have compensated respiratory acidosis and minimal symptoms even with nearly complete obstruction. Other patients, especially those with lymphoma or small cell lung carcinoma, have rapidly growing tumors and severe symptoms even when the airway is less than 75% obstructed. Stridor is present in tracheal obstruction, and wheezing with unequal chest excursion is seen with bronchial obstruction.[68]

Diagnostic Studies

Bronchoscopy makes it easy to detect tracheal or bronchial obstruction and grade its severity. However, bronchoscopy does not always reveal whether the airways are compressed extrinsically or invaded with tumor. Bronchoscopy is used in conjunction with spiral CT scans to provide a comprehensive description of the obstructive process that is used to guide therapy.[69]

Management

Clinically significant obstruction of the major airways always necessitates immediate treatment, although the therapeutic plan varies according to tumor-specific factors and therapeutic goals. Emergent treatment of airway occlusive-induced hypoxemia or hypercapnia may require nasal inhalation or heliox-based nebulizer treatments. A combination of oxygen and helium that is lighter than pure oxygen, heliox enhances movement of the air beyond the area of obstruction and provides palliative relief until more aggressive operative measures are possible.[70]

Effective treatment for endobronchial tumors includes laser, cautery, photodynamic therapy, and endobronchial brachytherapy. These therapies for tumors invading the major airways are highly successful for prolonging life as well as improving its quality. Most procedures entail use of a rigid bronchoscope under anesthesia, and patients usually experience a rapid recovery with little more than a sore throat and annoying cough for a few days afterward.[69,71–78] Endobronchial brachytherapy involves endotracheal intubation with precisely directed radiation therapy through an endobronchial catheter.[72] In laser therapy, electrocautery, photodynamic therapy, and endobronchial brachytherapy, close observation for airway bleeding is necessary, and clinicians may prescribe cough suppressants or low-dose corticosteroids to reduce the incidence of bleeding.

Airway opening with tracheal or bronchial stents may provide temporary symptomatic relief while definitive anticancer treatment is implemented for palliative relief of symptoms near the end of life. For insertion of an airway stent, a rigid bronchoscope and light anesthesia are necessary, and multiple bronchoscopic procedures to assess or adjust placement are required. The most common problem with stents, especially if placed before shrinking the tumor, is displacement because the airway naturally opens with the reduction of tumor. Displaced stents usually cause severe and sudden respiratory distress and require immediate interventional adjustment. In rare circumstances, or when stenting is not possible, patient positioning to shift the chest tumor off the major airway (e.g., prone positioning) may provide temporary symptomatic relief while cancer therapy is used to shrink the tumor.[79–81]

Complications

Two severe complications that may occur are total airway occlusion and hemorrhage caused by tumor erosion into the nearby pulmonary vessels. Treatment of total obstruction is the same as that of partial obstruction when an improvement in symptoms can be reasonably expected as a result of therapy. Treatment of hemorrhage, when recognized before massive bleeding occurs, may involve embolization. If severe hemorrhage occurs, it is necessary to insert a dual-lumen endotracheal tube and occlude the bleeding lung while ventilating the good lung until surgical repair can be performed. Airway obstruction may also lead to erosion through the airway and accompanying pneumothorax. In these circumstances, supportive therapy such as chest tube insertion may be used but is rarely helpful.

• Metabolic Complications

HYPERCALCEMIA

Hypercalcemia exists when the corrected serum calcium level is above 11 mg/dL (normal range, 8.5 to 10.5 mg/dL).[82] This oncological emergency develops when the bones release more calcium into the extracellular fluid than can be filtered by the kidneys and excreted in the urine.

Pathophysiology

Ninety-nine percent of the calcium in the body is in an insoluble form in the bones. The remaining 1% is freely exchangeable calcium. The calcium of importance is the ionized calcium, which must be maintained within a precise range. Serum calcium levels are regulated by parathyroid hormone and calcitonin. The release of parathyroid hormone from the parathyroid glands stimulates an increase in serum calcium levels, whereas the release of calcitonin produces a decrease in serum calcium levels.[83,84]

Destruction of the bone by metastatic invasion is believed to be the most common cause of malignant hypercalcemia; however, 20% of patients with solid tumors usually associated with hypercalcemia do not show evidence of bony involvement. [85,86] Tumor cells secrete certain humoral substances, such as parathyroid hormone–like substances or osteolytic prostaglandins. In patients with multiple myeloma, the abnormal plasma cells produce osteoclast-activating factor (OAF); however, hypercalcemia does not develop in these patients unless they have inadequate renal function.[87] Patients with adult T-cell lymphoma have severe hypercalcemia related to the ectopic production of OAF, colony-stimulating factor, interferon-γ, and an active vitamin D metabolite.[83,85] Additional causes of hypercalcemia in the presence of malignancy include immobilization, renal insufficiency, high dietary calcium or vitamin D intake, and low phosphate levels.[82,84,88] Box 48-16 lists causes of hypercalcemia in malignancy.

Hypercalcemia develops in as many as 40% to 50% of women with metastatic breast cancer.[88] There is a risk for bone metastasis, and estrogen and antiestrogens stimulate breast cancer cells to produce osteolytic prostaglandins and to increase bone resorption.

Assessment

History

The severity of signs and symptoms of hypercalcemia often correlates with the serum calcium level. Common presenting symptoms include nausea, constipation, polyuria, and mental status changes. Most patients present with somnolence, combativeness, or confusion.[88]

Box 48-16 • Causes of Hypercalcemia in Malignancy

- Bone demineralization due to bone metastases (most common in breast cancer, colorectal cancer, renal cell cancer)
- Tumor production of a parathormone-like substance (thyroid cancer, multiple myeloma, leukemia, lymphoma, gastric cancer, pancreatic cancer, lung cancer)
- Renal insufficiency
- Immobilization
- Dehydration

Diagnostic Studies

Elevated serum calcium and elevated ionized calcium are the hallmark diagnostic findings in hypercalcemia. The serum calcium measurement is often reported as an absolute number without considering that only the calcium bound to albumin is counted. The serum calcium may be corrected for a low albumin by subtracting the patient's albumin from low normal, multiplying this number by a correction factor of 0.8, and adding this number to the reported calcium.[88,89] Serum ionized calcium levels are accurate, but because the normal value is 1.0 mEq/L (±0.02), it is a less sensitive indicator of clinically significant hypocalcemia.

In addition to increased calcium levels, there are also elevations in alkaline phosphatase and immunoreactive parathyroid hormone.[88,89] Serum phosphate and serum potassium are decreased. Symptomatic patients usually have ECGs that show a bradycardia and prolonged PR, QRS, and QT intervals.[82]

Management

Medical management of hypercalcemia involves the use of IV fluids and drug therapy to enhance renal excretion of calcium and to decrease bone resorption. Acute hypercalcemia is initially treated with IV 0.9% normal saline to dilute calcium levels and increase urinary calcium excretion.[90] When hypercalcemia is life-threatening, aggressive hydration (250 to 300 mL/hour) and IV loop diuretics such as furosemide are necessary.

In most patients, treatment with hydration, diuretics, appropriate antitumor therapy, and mobilization is effective. Patients who do not respond to these therapies require hypocalcemic therapy indefinitely. Bisphosphonates are most frequently used. Currently, the most potent bisphosphonate available is zoledronic acid. It is administered as an 8-mg 15-minute IV infusion daily for 3 days unless serum calcium levels decrease before that time.[91] Until recently, the mainstay of bisphosphonate therapy was pamidronate, and some clinicians may still be preferred it. It is usually given as a 90-mg, 24-hour infusion with continued hydration, possibly diuretics, and careful monitoring of calcium levels. However, because of clinical safety and efficacy studies, many clinicians give this dose over 90 to 120 minutes. An FDA-licensed bisphosphonate for prevention of bone breakdown, ibandronate, has recently become available, but its use in hypercalcemia has been limited.[92] In cases unresponsive to bisphosphonates, calcitonin, corticosteroids, or strontium-98 may be useful.[86,90,93]

If possible, patients should ambulate to prevent osteolysis. It is necessary to eliminate constipation, which is usually caused by an increased level of calcium in the blood. Reduced oral intake of calcium or increased salt intake may be of some help. Patients should not take medications such as thiazide diuretics and vitamins A and D because they elevate the calcium level.[86] Close monitoring of fluid status is essential. Patients may receive up to 10 L of IV fluids daily, and the nurse should carefully measure intake and output. In addition, careful observation for overhydration is important. Potassium supplements may be necessary. Hypercalcemia is a common oncological emergency that can be prevented or diminished in a large number of patients with the appropriate education and precautions. Box 48-17 presents a teaching guide for patients with hypercalcemia.

Complications

Permanent renal tubular abnormalities may develop in patients with prolonged hypercalcemia. Sudden death from cardiac dysrhythmias may result from an acute increase in serum calcium. Long-term bisphosphonate use has been associated with severe osteonecrosis of the jaw. Specific risk factors for this complication are not yet unclear.[94]

SYNDROME OF INAPPROPRIATE ANTIDIURETIC HORMONE SECRETION

The syndrome of inappropriate antidiuretic hormone secretion (SIADH) is a clinical disorder characterized by excess stimulation of pituitary excretion of antidiuretic hormone (ADH). Under normal circumstances, the posterior pituitary gland releases ADH in response to changes in plasma osmolality (concentration of solutes) and circulating blood volume. ADH release causes decreased urine production and volume and increased water resorption. SIADH has several specific causes related to cancer and its treatment.[84] The clinical consequences of SIADH and its management strategies are discussed in Chapter 44.

Box 48-17 • TEACHING GUIDE:
Malignancy-Associated Hypercalcemia

Patients at high risk for malignancy-associated hypercalcemia include those with:

- Bone metastases (most common in breast, lung, and colon cancer)
- Lung cancer
- Gastrointestinal cancers (gastric, pancreatic, colon)
- Hematological cancers (leukemia, lymphoma, multiple myeloma)
- Renal (kidney) cancer
- Thyroid cancer

Other factors that increase the risk for developing hypercalcemia include:

- Lack of physical activity
- Low fluid status
- Poor kidney function

Suggestions for prevention of hypercalcemia include:

- Drink at least six to eight glasses of water every day
- Eat salty foods
- Remain physically active
- Limit dairy products and vitamin D–enriched foods such as milk, cheese, and yogurt

Pathophysiology

When thoracic or mediastinal tumors press on major cardiac vessels, the obstruction may impede cardiac output. The posterior pituitary gland perceives this to be a fall in circulatory volume and compensates by inappropriately secreting ADH, which in turn suppresses urinary output. The resulting volume expansion improves cardiac output but leaves the patient with a relative sodium deficiency (dilutional hyponatremia).

In addition to the pressure of thoracic or mediastinal tumors on cardiac vessels, cancers and treatment-related factors can also precipitate SIADH. Small cell lung cancers or mixed cellularity lung cancers, thyroid cancer, and melanoma release an ADH-like substance.[84,95–97] Certain chemotherapeutic agents, such as cyclophosphamide, vincristine, and alemtuzumab, as well as morphine, may stimulate ADH release or potentiate its effects on the kidneys.[84,98] One study views ongoing evidence of SIADH after antineoplastic treatment as a poor prognostic sign, often a subtle indicator of persistent tumor.[99]

Management

Treatment of the underlying malignancy is of primary importance in cancer-related SIADH.[99,100] Clinical evidence of excess ADH is present until the primary tumor stops compressing the major cardiac vessels or producing ADH-like substances. Antineoplastic therapy may include chemotherapy, radiation therapy, or corticosteroids. Fluid intake limited to 500 to 1,000 mL/day should result in a corrected fluid balance in 7 to 10 days.[84,100] Demeclocycline, an antibiotic that inhibits ADH secretion, may be effective; patients with chronic SIADH may receive demeclocycline, 900 to 1,200 mg/day.[84] Adverse effects include diarrhea, nausea, dysphagia, and photosensitivity. New specific vasopressin-receptor antagonists, called vaptens, enhance water diuresis without sodium loss and show promise in the treatment of this disorder.

Diuretics are not necessary except in severe circumstances because they may produce additional electrolyte imbalances. However, the patient who is comatose or convulsing should receive 3% IV hypertonic saline and a potent loop diuretic, such as furosemide.[101] Fluid imbalances and hyponatremia may be severe enough to warrant initiation of mechanical ventilation; the need for this aggressive respiratory support is the most predictive of a mortality rate of 22% to 40%.[99]

TUMOR LYSIS SYNDROME

Tumor lysis syndrome is a metabolic imbalance caused by rapid cancer cell death. Most patients experience this complication 1 to 5 days after initiation of therapy in patients with chemosensitive or radiosensitive tumors. However, there are documented instances of tumor lysis syndrome in rapidly proliferating disease even before treatment initiation.[102–104]

Patients at greatest risk for tumor lysis syndrome are those with bulky tumors having a high growth rate (e.g., acute leukemia or Burkitt's lymphoma) and those with highly radiosensitive or chemosensitive tumors such as small cell lung cancer and most malignant lymphomas. Patients with preexisting renal dysfunction may be at greatest risk owing to their difficulty in clearing the metabolic waste products fast enough to prevent clinical complications. Other patients at high risk are those with Merkel's tumor, hepatoblastoma, and medulloblastoma.[105]

Pathophysiology

Rapid cell death causes the release of intracellular contents (potassium, phosphorus, and nucleic acids) into the circulating serum. The normal filtration mechanisms in the kidneys should immediately detect the levels of metabolic waste products and attempt to excrete them. If production is more rapid than excretion or renal insufficiency is present, accumulation of electrolytes and uric acid occurs in the serum. The most common abnormalities include hyperkalemia, hyperphosphatemia, and hyperuricemia. High phosphorus causes the kidneys to excrete calcium, causing hypocalcemia. Hyperuricemia causes deposition of uric acid crystals in the urinary tract and may lead to renal failure.[105,106]

Assessment

History

Signs and symptoms of tumor lysis syndrome are related to the specific electrolyte imbalances involved and renal dysfunction. Hyperkalemia, hyperphosphatemia, hypocalcemia, hyperuricemia, and acidosis may occur. Box 48-18 lists the typical clinical signs and symptoms associated with the metabolic abnormalities of tumor lysis syndrome.

Diagnostic Studies

The electrolyte panel is used to identify key abnormalities in patients at risk for tumor lysis syndrome. Elevated serum potassium, phosphate, uric acid, blood urea nitrogen (BUN), and creatinine, with low calcium, are reported. Acidosis may be present in patients with severely compromised renal function. The urinary uric acid/creatinine ratio is greater than 1. Renal ultrasonography is used to exclude ureteral obstruction.[107]

Management

Treatment involves recognition of high-risk patients and promoting prevention through aggressive hydration, as well as administration of phosphate-binding agents and allopurinol for at least 48 hours before beginning chemotherapy. It is necessary to avoid agents that block tubular reabsorption of uric acid (e.g., aspirin, radiographic contrast, probenecid, thiazide diuretics). The goal is to keep the serum uric acid level within normal limits. Electrolyte disturbances are specifically treated as needed.[108]

> ## Box 48-18 • RED FLAG: Signs and Symptoms of Tumor Lysis Syndrome
>
> **Hyperkalemia**
> - Peaked T waves on ECG
> - Dysrhythmias (tachycardia, ventricular ectopy/torsade de pointes [especially when potassium >6.8 mEq/L])
> - Muscle flaccidity, weakness
> - Hyperactive bowel sounds, abdominal cramping, diarrhea
>
> **Hyperphosphatemia**
> - Muscle weakness
> - Bone marrow suppression (thrombocytopenia, leukopenia)
> - Bone demineralization with tendency for pathological fractures
> - Renal dysfunction
>
> **Hypocalcemia**
> - Muscle tetany
> - Seizures
> - Short PR and QT intervals on ECG
> - Dysrhythmias (tachycardia, ventricular ectopy/torsade de pointes)
> - Hyperactive bowel sounds, abdominal cramping, diarrhea
>
> **Hyperuricemia**
> - Uric acid crystals in urine
> - Hematuria
> - Oliguria, anuria
> - Flank pain
> - Renal failure
>
> **Acidosis**
> - Tachypnea
> - Hypotension

IV fluids are given to ensure a urine volume of more than 3 L/day. In the past, IV sodium bicarbonate (4 g initially, then 1 to 2 g every 4 hours) has been administered to alkalinize the urine and reduce uric acid crystallization in the kidney tubules. Clinicians are now less likely to initiate alkalinization if the phosphate is high because calcium-phosphate precipitation is equally likely to cause renal failure.[109] To measure urine output more accurately, insertion of a Foley catheter into the bladder is usually necessary. If oliguria or anuria develops, ureteral obstruction must be excluded. Phosphate-binding agents such as aluminum hydroxide are given every 2 to 4 hours in an effort to keep phosphate levels below 4 mg/dL. Concomitant diuresis or medications such as Kayexalate that enhance gastrointestinal excretion of potassium may effectively manage elevated serum potassium levels not prevented with hydration. Allopurinol, a xanthine oxidase inhibitor that blocks uric acid production, is administered in doses ranging from 300 to 900 mg/day. Because it is now available in an IV form given as 200 to 400 mg/m²/day, rapid normalization of uric acid levels is an achievable objective.[103] Its greatest limitation is that it cannot assist in breakdown or clearance of already existing uric acid.[108] Rasburicase

(Elitek), a new agent, acts like the natural enzyme urate oxidase to oxidize uric acid to allantoin for excretion.[110] If diuresis does not occur within a few hours after the initiation of treatment, renal replacement therapy is needed. An initial hemodialysis treatment usually reduces the patient's uric acid levels by 50%, but most patients then receive several additional days of CRRT until electrolyte abnormalities and hyperuricemia resolve.[108,111] A low-calcium dialysate is used to prevent calcium phosphate precipitation. If peritoneal dialysis is used, albumin is added to the dialysate to increase uric acid protein binding and removal.

The focus of nursing care is on careful monitoring of fluid therapy, intake and output, and electrolyte balance. The use of prophylactic allopurinol, aggressive hydration, and early intervention with CRRT has reduced the incidence and severity of tumor lysis syndrome.

• Clinical Applicability Challenges

Case Study

Ms. M., a 50-year-old woman, has newly diagnosed small cell lung cancer involving the right middle lung, lower right mainstem bronchus, and hilar lymph node enlargement, with presumed tumor infiltration due to the large size of the nodes. These results were finalized late last evening, and she is due for an oncology consultation in the morning. Recently, she presented to her primary care practitioner with a 2-month history of fatigue, weight loss, and progressive cough. During the following night, she experienced chest discomfort, palpitations, and profound dyspnea, and her family called emergency medical services.

Emergent assessment reflects a patient in acute cardiopulmonary distress. Vital signs are: heart rate, 142 beats/minute and irregular; respirations, 36 breaths/minute; and blood pressure, 142/88 mm Hg. Oxygen saturation is 86% on room air. Mucous membranes are dry. Bronchial breath sounds and dullness in the right lung base, as well as harsh inspiratory and expiratory wheezes in the anterior right lung, are apparent. The cardiac monitor shows peaked T waves and frequent premature ventricular contractions consistent with possible hyperkalemia. A 12-lead electrocardiogram shows mild nonspecific ischemia in the anterior leads. Laboratory values are: serum calcium, 11.4 mg/dL; serum phosphorus, 6.5 mg/dL; potassium, 6.6 mEq/L; blood urea nitrogen (BUN), 55.0 mg/dL; and creatinine, 2.2 mg/dL.

Immediate treatment of respiratory distress involves administration of oxygen 0.60% by face mask as well as the inhaled bronchodilators metaproterenol (Alupent) and ipratropium bromide (Atrovent). This assists in ventilation and may also temporarily reduce the potassium level. In addition, anterior–posterior and right lateral chest radiographs are obtained to evaluate for bronchial obstruction. Heliox therapy is on standby in case oxygen therapy does not relieve the respiratory distress.

Further treatment includes IV fluids (0.9% sodium chloride 250 mL/hour) to correct volume depletion and electrolyte imbalance. It is unclear as yet whether the patient is demonstrating clear tumor-related hypercalcemia or whether the slightly elevated calcium is related to volume depletion. The high potassium and phosphorus with increased BUN and creatinine suggest "self" tumor lysis due to the high amount of tumor burden. A Foley catheter is inserted, and an accurate intake and output record is maintained. A uric acid level is obtained as treatment for presumed tumor lysis is begun with IV fluids, Kayexalate for reduction of potassium, and aluminum hydroxide to bind with phosphorus. Safety precautions include side rails in the upright position at all times and frequent assessment of her level of consciousness.

After 2 hours of initial stabilization, Ms. M. is admitted to the ICU. After a nephrology consult, renal function improves with fluids and medical therapies. A pulmonologist is consulted for potential bronchial stent placement. However, it believed that lymph nodes impinging on the airway will quickly shrink with therapy and that it would be more effective to start chemotherapy, reserving the stent for later use if needed. Immediate chemotherapy with carboplatin and etoposide with antiemetics are initiated that morning. The patient requires high oxygen by mask and heliox breathing treatments. She also needs 4 days of CRRT initiated 12 hours after administration of day 1 chemotherapy and interrupted for day 3 chemotherapy. She receives hematopoietic growth factors to reduce the severity and length of myelosuppression, particularly given her high risk for postobstructive pneumonia.

After 1 week in the ICU, Ms. M. is transferred to the oncology unit, and her 1-month CT scan shows normalization of hilar lymph nodes and considerable reduction of her primary tumor. She undergoes five additional chemotherapy cycles with partial response of the tumor but significant improvement in her quality of life.

1. In a patient with a known large mediastinal tumor, several oncological emergencies may occur. Describe the emergent conditions Ms. M. experienced in the case study as well as the physiological basis of these emergencies.

2. Patients and families often are surprised by the sudden occurrence of an oncological emergency. Develop a teaching plan for Ms. M. and her family.

3. Explore the psychosocial challenges of treating a patient with newly diagnosed cancer presenting initially in the ICU.

4. A patient with tumor lysis syndrome may have several electrolyte and metabolic disorders. Develop a comparative list of symptoms for each of the different metabolic disorders that shows the overlapping and widely different symptoms.

Review Questions

1. A 37-year-old man was diagnosed with HIV 10 years ago. He has now been admitted to the intensive care unit for *Pneumocystis* pneumonia. He should be placed on which type of precautions:
   a. Enteric
   b. Standard
   c. Droplet
   d. Reverse

2. A woman consented to be tested for HIV. This patient underwent testing 6 months ago, and the test results came back negative for HIV. She was potentially exposed to HIV 11/2 weeks ago. The nurse would expect the HIV test result to come back
   a. positive.
   b. negative.
   c. indeterminate.
   d. reactive.

3. Mr. T. was diagnosed with HIV 8 years ago. He has never received antiretroviral therapy. Recently, his CD4 count was 296 cells/mm^3, and his viral load was 115,000 copies/mL. The nurse would expect which of the following to take place:
   a. Nothing. These values are acceptable, and no treatment is necessary at this time.
   b. Initiate monotherapy with zidovudine to help with immune reconstruction.
   c. Initiate combination therapy consisting of non-nucleoside reverse transcriptase inhibitors (NNRTIs), nucleoside reverse transcriptase inhibitors (NRTIs), and protease inhibitors (PIs).
   d. Initiate combination therapy consisting of three NRTIs.

4. Six months after starting treatment, Mr. T.'s CD4 count is 270 cells/mm^3, and his viral load is 75,000 copies/mL This type of response to antiretroviral therapy is considered
   a. virological failure.
   b. immunological failure.
   c. clinical progression.
   d. immunological reconstruction.

5. A 65-year-old man with head and neck cancer calls the nurse to his room complaining of indigestion and a taste of blood in his mouth. He has a dry, nonproductive cough. He is most likely experiencing
   a. tracheal obstruction.
   b. carotid artery rupture.
   c. cardiac tamponade.
   d. superior vena cava syndrome.

6. Hypercalcemia can be prevented or lessened by which intervention?
   a. Allopurinol
   b. Urinary alkalinization
   c. Increasing fluid intake
   d. Limiting activity

7. A 59-year-old patient with small cell lung cancer is admitted with severe dyspnea and upper body edema. The first diagnostic test performed probably is
   a. chest computed tomography scan.
   b. echocardiogram.
   c. electrocardiogram.
   d. multigated acquisition (MUGA) scan.

8. Patients with acute leukemia are at greatest risk for which of the following complications?
   a. Cardiac tamponade, syndrome of inappropriate antidiuretic hormone secretion
   b. Hypercalcemia, carotid artery rupture
   c. Pleural effusions, superior vena cava syndrome
   d. Cytokine release syndrome, tumor lysis syndrome

References

Human Immunodeficiency Virus Infection

1. Centers for Disease Control and Prevention: Epidemiology of HIV/AIDS-United States, 1981–2005. MMWR Morb Mortal Wkly Rep 55(21):589–592, 2006

2. Huang L, Quartin A, Jones D, Havlir DV: Intensive care of patients with HIV infection. N Engl J Med 355(2):173–181, 2006

3. Centers for Disease Control and Prevention: Revised recommendations for HIV testing of adults, adolescents, and pregnant women in health-care settings. MMWR Morb Mortal Wkly Rep 55(RR14):1–17, 2006

4. Centers for Disease Control and Prevention: HIV/AIDS Surveillance Report 17:1–54, 2006

5. Barlett JG: The stages and natural history of HIV infection. Retrieved February 26, 2007, from http://www.uptodate.com.

6. Centers for Disease Control and Prevention: Twenty-five years of HIV/AIDS—United States, 1981–2006. MMWR Morb Mortal Wkly Rep 55(21):585–589, 2006

7. Centers for Disease Control and Prevention: Guidelines for preventing opportunistic infections among HIV-infected persons: 2002 Recommendations of the U.S. Public Health Service and the Infectious Diseases Society of America. MMWR Morb Mortal Wkly Rep 51(RR-8):1–51, 2002

8. Centers for Disease Control and Prevention: Updated U.S. Public Health Services guidelines for the management of occupational exposures to and recommendations for Postexposure Prophylaxis. MMWR Morb Mortal Wkly Rep 54(RR-9):1–17, 2005

9. Morris A, Luce JM: Human Immunodeficiency virus infection. In Fink MP, Abraham E, Vincent J, Kochanek PM (eds): Textbook of Critical Care, 5th ed. Philadelphia: Elsevier Saunders, 2005, pp 1325–1330

10. Piscitelli SC, Pau AK: AIDS-related medications. In Dolin R, Masur H, Saag MS (eds): AIDS Therapy, 2nd ed. New York: Churchill Livingstone, 2003, pp 940–970

11. Holodniy M, Busch MP: Establishing a diagnosis of HIV infection. In Dolin R, Masur H, Saag MS (eds): AIDS Therapy, 2nd ed. New York: Churchill Livingstone, 2005, pp 3–20

12. Kleinman S, Busch MP, Hall L, et al: False-positive HIV-1 test results in a low-risk screening setting of voluntary blood donation. JAMA 280(12):1080–1085, 1998

13. Barlett J: The 2002 Abbreviated Guide to Medical Management of HIV Infection. Baltimore: Johns Hopkins University, Division of Infectious Diseases, 2002
14. Kaplan JE, Hanson D, Dworkin MS, et al: Epidemiology of human immunodeficiency virus–associated opportunistic infections in the United States in the era of highly active antiretroviral therapy. Clin Infect Dis 30(Suppl 1):S5–S14, 2000
15. Department of Health and Human Services: Guidelines for the use of antiretroviral agents in HIV-1-infected adults and adolescents. 2006, pp 1–113
16. John L, Marra F, Enson M: Role of therapeutic drug monitoring for protease inhibitors. Ann Pharmacother 35:745–754, 2001
17. Madge S, Singh S: The GP's role in HIV and AIDS care. Practitioner 244:772–777, 2000

Oncological Complications and Emergencies

1. Shelton BK: Preventing crises in the patient with cancer. Oncol Nurs Forum 27(6):905–914, 2000
2. Azoulay E, Afessa B: The intensive care support of patients with malignancy: Do everything that can be done. Intensive Care Med 32(1):3–5, 2006
3. Lim Z, Pagliuca A, Simpson S, et al: Outcomes of patients with haematological malignancies admitted to the intensive care unit: A comparative review of allogeneic haematopoeitic stem cell transplantation data. Br J Haematol 136(3):448–450, 2007
4. Shelton BK: Critical care of cancer patients. Crit Care Connect SCCM 4(4):1, 5, 2005
5. Marik PE: Management of patients with metastatic malignancy in the intensive care unit. Am J Hospice Palliat Care 23(6):479–482, 2006
6. Benoit DD, Depuydt PO, Vandewoude KH, et al: Outcome in severely ill patients with hematological malignancies who received intravenous chemotherapy in the intensive care unit. Intensive Care Med 32(1):93–99, 2006
7. Shelton BK, Rome SI, Lewis SL: Nursing assessment: Hematologic system. In Lewis SL, Heitkemper MM, Dirkson SR, et al (eds): Medical-Surgical Nursing: Assessment and Management of Clinical Problems, 7th ed. Philadelphia: Elsevier, 2007, pp 665–683
8. Shelton BK: General toxicity: Myelosuppression and secondary malignancies. In Gobel B, Triest S, Vogel W (eds): Advanced Oncology Certification Review and Resource Manual. Pittsburgh: Oncology Nursing Society Press, in press.
9. Sreedharan A, Bowyer S, Wallace CA, et al: Macrophage activation syndrome and other systemic inflammatory conditions after BMT. Bone Marrow Transplant 37(7):629–634, 2006
10. Gorak E, Geller N, Srinivasan R, et al: Engraftment syndrome after nonmyeloablative allogeneic hematopoietic stem cell transplantation: Incidence and effects on survival. Biol Blood Marrow Transplant 11:542–550, 2005
11. Dai E, Couriel D, Kim SK: Bilateral marginal keratitis associated with engraftment syndrome after hematopoietic stem cell transplantation. Cornea 26(6):756–758, 2007
12. Singh H, Prasad BD, Jagdish S, Batra A: Hyperleukocytosis associated pulmonary leukostasis in acute leukemia. J Assoc Physicians India 54:405–407, 2006
13. Blum W, Porcu P: Therapeutic apheresis in hyperleukocytosis and hyperviscosity syndrome. Semin Thromb Hemost 33(4):350–354, 2007
14. Chang M, Chen T, Tang J, et al: Leukapheresis and cranial irradiation in patients with hyperleukocytic acute myeloid leukemia: no impact on early mortality and intracranial hemorrhage. Am J Hematol 82:976–980, 2007
15. Tan D, Hwang W, Goh YT: Therapeutic leukapheresis in hyperleukocytic leukaemias: The experience of a tertiary institution in Singapore. Ann Acad Med Singapore 34:229–234, 2005
16. Lele AV, Mirski MA, Stevens RD: Spurious hypoxemia. Crit Care Med 33(8):1854–1856, 2005
17. Balint B, Ostojic G, Pavlovic M, et al: Cytapheresis in the treatment of cell-affected blood disorders and abnormalities. Transfus Apheres Sci 35:25–31, 2006
18. Shelton BK: Pericardial effusion and tamponade. In Chernecky C, Murphy-Ende K, Berger B (eds): Acute and Critical Care of Cancer Patients. Philadelphia: Elsevier, 2006
19. Quraishi AR, Khan AA, Kazmi KA, et al: Clinical and echocardiographic characteristics of patients with significant pericardial effusion requiring pericardiocentesis. J Pakistan Med Assoc 55(2):66–70, 2005
20. Imazio M, Demichelis B, Parrini I, et al: Relation of acute pericardial disease to malignancy. Am J Cardiol 95(11):1393–1394, 2005
21. Billikanty S, Bashir R: Images in cardiovascular medicine: Echocardiographic demonstration of electrical alternans. Circulation 113(24):e866–e868, 2006
22. Martionini A, Cipolla CM, Cardinae D, et al: Long-term results of intrapericardial hemotherapeutic treatment of malignant pericardial effusions with thiotepa. Chest 126(5):1412–1416, 2004
23. Becit N, Unlu Y, Ceviz M, et al: Subxiphoid pericardiostomy in the management of pericardial effusions: Case series analysis of 368 patients. Heart 91:785–790, 2005
24. Marcy PY, Bondiau PY, Brunner P: Percutaneous treatment in patients presenting with malignant cardiac tamponade. Eur Radiol 15:2000–2009, 2005
25. Cullinane CA, Paz IB, Smith D, et al: Prognostic factors in the surgical management of pericardial effusion in the patient with concurrent malignancy. Chest 125(4):1328–1334, 2004
26. Frawley T, Begley C: Causes and prevention of carotid artery rupture. Br J Nurs 15(22):1198–1202, 2006
27. Kim H, Lee D, Kim H, et al: Life-threatening common carotid artery blowout: rescue treatment with a newly designed self-expanding covered nitinol stent. Br J Radiol 79:226–231, 2006
28. Frawley T, Begley C: Caring for people with carotid artery rupture. Br J Nurs 15(1):24–28, 2006
29. McKoy JM, Angelotta C, Bennett CL, et al: Gemtuzumab ozogamicin-associated sinusoid obstructive syndrome (SOS): An overview from the research on adverse drug events and reports (RADAR) project. Leuk Res 31(5):599–604, 2007
30. Negrin RS, Bonis PAL: Pathogenesis and clinical features of hepatic veno-occlusive disease following hematopoietic cell transplantation, 2006. Up-to-Date Online 15.2. Retrieved August 20, 2007, from http://www.uptodate.com, last updated 1/31/2006
31. Cheuk DK, Wang P, Lee TL, et al: Risk factors and mortality predictors of hepatic veno-occlusive disease after pediatric hematopoietic stem cell transplantation. Bone Marrow Transplant 40(10):935–944, 2007
32. Arotcarena R, Cales V, Berthelemy P, et al: Severe sinusoid lesions: A serious and overlooked complication of oxiliplatin-containing chemotherapy? Gastroenterol Clin Biol 30(11):1313–1316, 2006
33. Schouten van der Velden AP, Punt CJ, Van Krieken JH, et al: Hepatic veno-occlusive disease after neoadjuvant treatment of colorectal liver metastases with oxiliplatin. Eur J Surg Oncol 34:353–355, 2008
34. Senzolo M, Burra P, Cholongitas E, et al: Digest Liver Dis 39(2):105–116, 2007
35. Senzolo M, Germani G, Cholongitas E, et al: Veno occlusive disease: Update on clinical management. World J Gastroenterol 13(29):3918–3924, 2007
36. Negrin RS: Treatment and prevention of hepatic veno-occlusive disease following hematopoietic cell transplantation, 2005. Up-to-Date Online 15.2. Retrieved August 20, 2007, from http://www.uptodate.com, last updated 9/8/2005
37. Schoppmeyer K, Lange T, Wittekind C, et al: TIPS for veno-occlusive disease following stem cell transplantation. Z Gastroenterol 44(6):483–486, 2006

38. Matsumoto M, Kawa K, Uemura M, et al: Prophylactic fresh frozen plasma may prevent development of hepatic VOD after stem cell transplantation via ADAMTS13-mediated restoration of von Willebrand factor plasma levels. Bone Marrow Transplant 40(3):251–259, 2007

39. Sucak GT, Aki ZS, Yagci M, et al: Treatment of sinusoidal obstruction syndrome with defibrotide: A single-center experience. Transplant Proc 39(5):1558–1563, 2007

40. Ho VT, Linden E, Revta C, Richardson PG: Hepatic veno-occlusive disease after hematopoietic stem cell transplantation: review and update on the use of defibrotide. Semin Thromb Hemost 33(4):373–388, 2007

41. Dignan F, Gujral D, Ethell M, et al: Prophylactic defibrotide in allogeneic stem cell transplantation: Minimal morbidity and zero mortality from veno-occlusive disease. Bone Marrow Transplant 40(1):79–82, 2007

42. Song JS, Seo JJ, Moon HN, et al: Prophylactic low-dose heparin or prostaglandin E1 may prevent severe veno-occlusive disease of the liver after allogeneic hematopoietic stem cell transplantation in Korean children. Korean Med Sci 21(5):897–903, 2006

43. Drews RE: Superior vena cava syndrome. Up-to-Date Online 15.2. Retrieved August 30, 2007, from http://www.uptodate.com, last updated 10/18/2005

44. Rice TW, Rodriguez M, Light RW: The superior vena cava syndrome: Clinical characteristics and evolving technology. Medicine 85(1):37–42, 2006

45. Wilson LD, Detterbeck FC, Yahalom J: Clinical practice: Superior vena cava syndrome with malignant causes. N Engl J Med 356:18, 2007

46. Rice TW: Pleural effusion in SVCS: Prevalence, characteristics, and proposed pathophysiology. Curr Opin Pulmon Med 13(4):324–327, 2007

47. Eren S, Karaman A, Okur A: The superior vena cava syndrome caused by malignant disease: Imaging with multidetector row CT. Eur J Radiol 59(1):93–103, 2006

48. DiGiammarco G, Storto ML, Marano R, Di Mauro M: Superior vena cava syndrome: A 3D CT-scan reconstruction. Eur J Cardiothorac Surg 30:384–385, 2006

49. Wilson P, Bezjak A, Asch M, et al: The difficulties of a randomized study in superior vena caval obstruction. J Thorac Oncol 2(6):514–519, 2007

50. Uberoi R: Quality assurance guidelines for superior vena cava stenting in malignant disease. Cardiovasc Intervent Radiol 29:319–322, 2006

51. Shelton BK, Onners BK: Pleural effusions. In Shelton BK, Ziegfled CF, Olsen MM (eds): Manual of Cancer Nursing. Philadelphia: Lippincott, Williams & Wilkins, 2004, pp 536–547

52. Ryu JS, Ryu ST, Kim YS, et al: What is the clinical significance of transudative malignant pleural effusions? Korean J Intern Med 18(4):230–233, 2003

53. Antunes G, Neville E, Duffy J, Ali N, on behalf of the BTS Pleural Disease Group, a subgroup of the BTS Standards of Care Committee: BTS Guidelines for the Management of malignant pleural effusions. Thorax 58(Suppl II):29–38, 2003

54. Sahn SA: Management of malignant pleural effusions, 2005. Up-to-Date Online 15.2. Retrieved August 20, 2007, from http://www.uptodate.com, last updated 8/24/2006

55. Stark P: Imaging of pleural effusions in adults, 2005. Up-to-Date Online 15.2. Retrieved August 20, 2007, from http://www.uptodate.com, last updated 3/3/2005

56. Heffner JE, Sahn SA: Chemical pleurodesis, 2007. Up-to-Date Online 15.2. Retrieved August 20, 2007, from http://www.uptodate.com, last updated 5/9/2007

57. Murthy SC, Okereke I, Mason DP, Rice TW: A simple solution for complicated pleural effusions. J Thorac Oncol 1(7):697–700, 2006

58. Adegboye VO, Falade A, Osinusi K, Obajimi MO: Reexpansion pulmonary oedema as a complication of pleural drainage. Nigerian Postgrad Med J 9(4):214–220, 2002

59. Lowey SE: Spinal cord compression: An oncologic emergency associated with metastatic cancer: evaluation and management for the home health clinician. Home Health Nurse 24(7):439–448, 2006

60. Schiff D: Clinical features and diagnosis of epidural spinal cord compression, including cauda equine syndrome, 2003. Up-to-Date Online 15.2. Retrieved August 28, 2007, from http://www.uptodate.com, last updated 10/15/2003

61. Rades D, Fehlauer F, Schulte R, et al: Prognostic factors for local control and survival after radiotherapy pf metastatic spinal cord compression. J Clin Oncol 24(21):3338–3393, 2006

62. Acharya S, Ratra GS: Posterior spinal cord compression: Outcome and results. Spine 31(7):E74–E78, 2006

63. Sevaggi K, Abrahm J: Metastatic spinal cord compression: The hidden danger. Nat Clin Pract Oncol 3(6), 2006

64. Byrne TN, Borges LF, Loeffler JS: Metastatic epidural spinal cord compression: Update on management. Semin Oncol 33(3):307–311, 2006

65. Schiff D: Treatment and prognosis of epidural spinal cord compression including cauda equine syndrome, 2007. Up-to-Date Online 15.2. Retrieved August 28, 2007, from http://www.uptodate.com, last updated 4/13/2007

66. Gerber DE, Grossman SA: Does decompressive surgery improve outcome in patients with metastatic epidural spinal-cord compression? Nat Clin Pract Neurol 2(1):10–11, 2006

67. Satre TJ, Mackler L, Birch JT Jr: Clinical inquiries. Who should receive vertebroplasty? J Fam Pract 55(7):637–678, 2006

68. Cohn WE: Anterior mediastinal mass lesions, 2006. Up-to-Date Online 15.2. Retrieved August 24, 2007, from http://www.uptodate.com, last updated 12/12/2006

69. Ernst A, Hearth F, Becker H: Overview of the management of central airway obstruction, 2005. Up-to-Date Online 15.2. Retrieved August 24, 2007, from http://www.uptodate.com, last updated 7/29/2005

70. Feller-Kopman DJ, O'Donnell C: Physiology and clinical use of heliox, 2006. Up-to-Date Online 15.2. Retrieved August 24, 2007, from http://www.uptodate.com, last updated 5/12/2006

71. Asimakopoulos G, Beeson J, Evans J, Maiwand MO: Cryosurgery for malignant endobronchial tumors: Analysis of outcome. Chest 127(6):2007–2014, 2005

72. Collins AS, Garner M: Caring for lung cancer patients receiving photodynamic therapy. Crit Care Nurse 27(2):53–60, 2007

73. Ernst A, LoCicero J III: Photodynamic therapy of lung cancer, 2007. Up-to-Date Online 15.2. Retrieved August 24, 2007, from http://www.uptodate.com, last updated 1/12/2007

74. Finkelstein SE, Summers RM, Nguyen DM, Schrump DS: Virtual bronchoscopy for evaluation of airway disease. Thorac Surg Clin 14(1):79–86, 2004

75. Kamal I, Quadri T, Lane SJ, Cullen JP: The role of endobronchial electrocautery in the management of malignant airway obstruction. Iranian Med J 100(1):148–150, 2006

76. Mathur PN, Colt HG: Endobronchial electrocautery, 2004. Up-to-Date Online 15.2. Retrieved August 24, 2007, from http://www.uptodate.com, last updated 6/30/2004

77. Moghissi K, Dixon K: Bronchoscopic NdYAG laser treatment in lung cancer, 30 years on: An institutional review. Lasers Med Sci 21(4):186–191, 2006

78. Saenghirunvattana S, Buakham C, Masakul N, Saenghirunvattana R: Management of endobronchial cancer using bronchoscopic electrocautery. J Med Assoc Thailand 89(4):459–461, 2006

79. Colt HG, Mathur PN: Airway stents, 2005. Up-to-Date Online 15.2. Retrieved August 21, 2007, from http://www.uptodate.com, last updated 9/21/2005

80. Madden B, Park JE, Sheth A: Medium-term follow-up after deployment of ultraflex expandable metallic stents to manage

endobronchial pathology. Ann Thorac Surg 78(6):1898–1902, 2004

81. Su JM, Wu TC, Wu MF, et al: Management of malignant tracheobronchial stenoses with the use of airway stents. J Chinese Med Assoc 67(9):458–464, 2004

82. Delaney MF, Carey JJ: Hypercalcemia. Cleve Clin J Med 72(12):1075, 2005

83. Agus ZS: Hypercalcemia of malignancy, 2005. Up-to-Date Online 15.2. Retrieved August 21, 2007, from http://www.uptodate.com, last updated 12/29/2005

84. Spinazze S, Schrijvers D: Metabolic emergencies. Crit Rev Oncol Hematol 58:79–89, 2006

85. Agus ZS: Etiology of hypercalcemia, 2006. Up-to-Date Online 15.2. Retrieved August 21, 2007, from http://www.uptodate.com, last updated 11/1/2006

86. Van Poznak C: Hypercalcemia of malignancy remains a clinically relevant problem. CA Cancer J 12(1):21–23, 2006

87. Oyzjobi BO: Multiple myeloma: Arthritis research and therapy. 9(Suppl 1):S4, 2007

88. Agus ZS: Diagnostic approaches to hypercalcemia. Up-to-Date Online 15.2. Retrieved August 21, 2007, from http://www.uptodate.com, last updated 12/29/2005

89. Ijaz A, Mehmood T, Qureshi AH, et al: Estimation of ionized calcium and total calcium and albumin corrected calcium for the diagnosis of hypercalcemia of malignancy. J Coll Physician Surg Pakistan 16(1):49–52, 2006

90. Agus ZS, Berenson JR: Treatment of hypercalcemia, 2006. Up-to-Date Online 15.2. Retrieved August 21, 2007, from http://www.uptodate.com, last updated 11/7/2005

91. Lambrinoudaki I, Christodoulakos IV, Botsis DC: The cardiovascular effects of selective estrogen receptor modulators. Ann N Y Acad Sci 1092:397–402, 2006

92. Guay DR: Ibandronate, an experimental intravenous bisphosphonate for osteoporosis, bone metastases, and hypercalcemia of malignancy. Pharmacotherapy 26(5):655–673, 2006

93. Diskin CJ, Stokes TJ, Dansby L, et al: Malignancy-related hypercalcemia developing on a bisphosphonates but responding to calcitonin. Clin Lung Cancer 8(7):434–435, 2007

94. Landesberg R, Wilson T, Grbic JT: Bisphosphonate-associated osteonecrosis of the jaw: Conclusions based on an analysis of case studies. Dentist Today 25(8):52, 54–57, 2006

95. Sanghera P, El-Modir A: Malignant melanoma and SIADH. Clin Oncol 17(3):199–200, 2005

96. Tai P, Yu E, Jones K, et al: Syndrome of inappropriate antidiuretic hormone secretion (SIADH) in patients with limited stage small cell lung cancer. Lung Cancer 53(2):211–215, 2006

97. Tho LM, Ferry DR: Is the paraneoplastic syndrome of inappropriate antidiuretic hormone secretion in lung cancer always attributable to the small cell variety? Postgrad Med 81:17–18, 2005

98. Kunz JS, Bannerji R: Alemtuzumab-induced syndrome of inappropriate anti-diuretic hormone. Leuk Lymphoma 46(4):635–637, 2005

99. Adam AK, Soubani AO: Outcome and prognostic factors of lung cancer patients admitted to the medical ICU. Eur Respir J 31:47–53, 2008

100. Held-Warmkessel J: Managing critical cancer complications. Nursing 35(1):58–64, 2005

101. Higdon ML, Higdon JA: Treatment of oncologic emergencies. Am Fam Physician 74(11):1873–1880, 2006

102. Reedy A: Targeting tumor lysis syndrome: New therapeutic options. Adv Studies Nurs 4(3):38–40, 2006

103. Fernandez PC, Agus ZS: Tumor lysis syndrome. Retrieved October 2, 2007, from http://www.uptodate.com, last updated 9/2007

104. Secola R: Tumor lysis syndrome: Nursing management and new therapeutic options. Adv Studies Nurs 4(3):41–48, 2006

105. Del Toro G, Morris E, Cairo MS: Tumor lysis syndrome: Pathophysiology, definition, and alternative treatment approaches. Clin Adv Hematol Oncol 3:54–61, 2005

106. Tiu RY, Mountonakis SE, Dunbar AJ, Schreiber MJ Jr: Tumor lysis syndrome. Semin Thromb Hematol 33(4):397–404, 2007

107. Cairo MS, Bishop M: Tumour lysis syndrome: New therapeutic strategies and classification. Br J Haematol 127:3–11, 2004

108. Jeha S: Current and emerging treatment options for patients with tumor lysis syndrome. Adv Studies Nurs 4(3):49–57, 2006

109. Coiffer B, Riouffol C: Management of tumor lysis syndrome in adults. Exp Rev Anticancer Ther 7(2):233–239, 2007

110. Mayne N, Keady S, Thacker M: Rasburicase in the prevention and treatment of tumor lysis syndrome. Intens Crit Care Nurse 24(1):59–62, 2008

111. Agha-Razii M, Amyot SL, Pichette V, et al: Continuous venovenous hemodiafiltration for the treatment of spontaneous tumor lysis syndrome complicated by acute renal failure and severe hyperuricemia. Clin Nephrol 54(1):59–63, 2000

Other Selected Readings

Human Immunodeficiency Virus

Dakin CL, O'Connor CA, Patsdaughter CA: HAART to heart: HIV-related cardiomyopathy and other cardiovascular complications. AACN Clin Issues 17(1):18–29, 2006

Donaldson TA: Immune responses to infection. Crit Care Nurs Clin N Am 19(1):1–8, 2007

Dorsey SG, Morton PG: HIV peripheral neuropathy: Pathophysiology and clinical implications. AACN Clin Issues 17(1):30–36, 2006

Halloran J: Increasing survival with HIV: Impact on nursing care. AACN Clin Issues 17(1):8–17, 2006

Kirton C: ANAC's Core Curriculum for HIV/AIDS Nursing, 2nd ed. Thousands Oaks, CA: Sage, 2003

Shojania KG, McDonald KM, Wachter RM, Owens DK: Closing the quality gap: A critical analysis of quality improvement strategies. Volume 6: Prevention of Healthcare-Associated Infections. Rockville, MD: Agency for Healthcare Research and Quality, 2007

Oncological Complications and Emergencies

Altman A: Tumor lysis syndrome. Semin Oncol 28(2 Suppl 5):3–8, 2001

Azoulay D, Castaing D, Lemoine A, et al: Transjugular intrahepatic portosystemic shunt (TIPS) for severe veno-occlusive disease of the liver following bone marrow transplantation. Bone Marrow Transplant 25(9):987–992, 2000

Baines MJ: Spinal cord compression: A personal and palliative care perspective. Clin Oncol 14(2):135–138, 2002

Brandt JM: Rasburicase: An innovative new treatment for hyperuricemia associated with tumor lysis syndrome. Clin J Oncol Nurs 6:12–16, 2002

Capizzi SA, Kumar S, Huneke NE, et al: Peri-engraftment respiratory distress syndrome during autologous stem cell transplantation. Bone Marrow Transplant 27(12):1299–1303, 2001

Chiles C, Woodward PK, Gutierrez FR, et al: Metastatic involvement of the heart and pericardium: CT and MR imaging, Radiographics 21(2):439–449, 2001

Doane L: Overview of tumor lysis syndrome. Semin Oncol Nurs 18(3 Suppl 3):2–5, 2002

Eke N: Symptomatic spinal cord involvement in prostate cancer. Central African J Med 47(2):49–53, 2001

Gobel BH: Management of tumor lysis syndrome: Prevention and treatment. Semin Oncol Nursing (3 Suppl 3):12–16, 2002

Hardy JR, Huddart R: Spinal cord compression—what are the treatment standards? Clin Oncol 14(2):132–134, 2002

Hashimoto S, Shirato H, Kaneko K, et al: Clinical efficacy of telemedicine in emergency radiotherapy for malignant spinal cord compression. J Digital Imag 14(3):124–130, 2001

Husband DJ, Grant KA, Romaniuk CS: MRI in the diagnosis and treatment of suspected malignant spinal cord compression. Br J Radiol 74:15–23, 2001

Ijaz A, Mehmood T, Qureshi AH, et al: Estimation of ionized calcium, total calcium and albumin corrected calcium for the diagnosis of hypercalcaemia of malignancy. J Coll Physician Surg Pakistan 16(1):49–52, 2006

Janjan N: Bone metastases: Approaches to management. Semin Oncol 28(4 Suppl 11):28–34, 2001

Kaplow R: Pathophysiology, signs, and symptoms of acute tumor lysis syndrome. Semin Oncol Nurs 18(3):6–11, 2002

Kienstra GE, Terwee CB, Dekker FW, et al: Prediction of spinal epidural metastases. Arch Neurol 57(5):690–695, 2000

Lee CT, Yang CC, Lam KK, et al: Hypercalcemia in the emergency department. Am J Med Sci 331(3):119–123

Malcolm GP: Surgical disorders of the cervical spine: Presentation and management of common disorders. J Neurosurg Psychiatry 73(Suppl 1):34–41, 2002

Mor E, Pappo O, Bar-Nathan N, et al: Defibrotide for the treatment of veno-occlusive disease after liver transplantation. Transplantation 72(7):1237–1240, 2001

Myers JS: Oncologic complications. In S. E. Otto (ed): Oncology Nursing, 4th ed. St. Louis: Mosby, 2001, pp 498–581

Naco GJ, von Gunten C: Refractory neuropathic pain from chronic cord compression. J Palliat Care Med 5(3):433–436, 2002

Polverosi R, Vigo M, Baron S, et al: Evaluation of tracheobronchial lesions with spiral CT: Comparison between virtual endoscopy and bronchoscopy. Radiol Med 102(5–6):313–319, 2001

Porcu P, Cripe LD, Ng EW, et al: Hyperleukocytic leukemias and leukostasis: A review of pathophysiology, clinical presentation and management. Leuk Lymphoma 39(1):1–18, 2000

Porcu P, Farag S, Marucci G, et al: Leukocytoreduction for acute leukemia. Ther Apher 6(1):15–23, 2002

Rogers CL, Theodore N, Dickman CA, et al: Selected neurologic complications in the patient with cancer: Brain metastases and spinal cord compression. Crit Care Nurs Clin N Am 12(3):269–279, 2000

Schoeggl A, Reddy M, Matula C: Neurological outcome following laminectomy in spinal metastases. Spinal Cord 40:363–366, 2002

Seol HJ, Chung CK, Kim HJ: Surgical approach to anterior compression in the upper thoracic spine. J Neurosurg 97(3 Suppl):337–342, 2002

Speiser BL: Surgery and permanent ^{125}I seed paraspinal brachytherapy for malignant tumors with spinal cord compression. Int J Radiat Oncol Biol Physics 54(2):505–513, 2002

Warren F, Cohen J, Nesbit G, et al: Management of carotid "blowout" with endovascular stent grafts. Laryngoscope 112:428–433, 2002

Common Hematological Disorders

Debby Greenlaw

Objectives

Based on the content in this chapter, the reader should be able to:

❶ Describe the compensatory mechanisms and their impact on the management of the critically ill patient with anemia.

❷ Discuss assessment findings and nursing care for the patient with neutropenia.

❸ Describe the clinical syndrome of thrombocytopenia and thrombosis in heparin-induced thrombocytopenia.

❹ Explain the anticipated management and treatment rationales for the patient with disseminated intravascular coagulation.

Critically ill patients are at high risk for developing complications from a variety of hematological disorders. Anemia is common in the critical care unit; the causes are multifactorial and include preexisting disease, blood loss from multiple sources, and suppressed erythropoiesis. Critically ill patients are also highly susceptible to overwhelming infections from severe neutropenia as well as hemorrhagic complications secondary to severe thrombocytopenia and other clotting disorders.

This chapter presents an overview of the pathophysiology, assessment, and management of hematologic disorders in the critically ill patient. Red blood cell, white blood cell, platelet, and coagulation disorders are discussed.

• Disorders of Red Blood Cells

POLYCYTHEMIA

Polycythemia Vera

Polycythemia vera is a myeloproliferative disorder of increased red blood cell (RBC) production resulting in a high hematocrit and an increased RBC mass. Increased RBC production causes decreased tissue oxygenation, increased blood viscosity, vascular insufficiency, and risk for thrombosis. As the disease progresses, some patients may develop bone marrow fibrosis, splenomegaly, and pancytopenia. Acute leukemia may develop in a small percentage of these patients.

Secondary Polycythemia

Secondary polycythemia is a disorder of increased RBC production that can develop as a normal response to chronic hypoxia. Conditions causing chronic hypoxia include living at high altitudes, cardiopulmonary disease, sleep apnea, obesity hypoventilation syndrome, and exposure to carbon monoxide. Secondary polycythemia may also result from an inappropriate increase in erythropoietin production as a result of renal disease, or in rare cases, hepatic disease.

Assessment

Arterial and venous thrombosis due to the blood's hyperviscosity is the major concern. The patient with polycythemia is at increased risk for thromboembolic events such as myocardial and cerebral infarction, deep venous thrombosis, and pulmonary embolism.

It is important to review the patient's past medical history for cardiac or pulmonary disease. Also, any past history of arterial or venous thrombosis is pertinent. Smoking history is relevant because cigarette smokers may have high carboxyhemoglobin levels. Patients with polycythemia often complain of itching after a hot shower or bath. Table 49-1 lists additional clinical findings in polycythemia vera.

Management

Serial phlebotomy is the first-line treatment for polycythemia vera. Generally 500 mL of blood is removed weekly until a hematocrit of less than 45% is achieved. Most patients managed by serial phlebotomy develop iron deficiency, which limits their ability to make RBCs and thus decreases the frequency of phlebotomy. The disadvantage of phlebotomy is that it stimulates bone marrow production, which leads to increased numbers of defective, sticky platelets. Antiplatelet aggregating agents, such as aspirin and dipyridamole, do not reduce thrombotic events and may increase the risk for bleeding.

Older patients with vascular disease are at high risk for thrombosis and require bone marrow suppression in addition to phlebotomy. Hydroxyurea is the medication of choice. Long-term therapy with bone marrow–suppressing agents has been associated with an increased risk for acute leukemia, so the potential benefits must be weighed against the anticipated duration of therapy. Measures to prevent thromboembolic complications, such as lower extremity compression devices or facilitating ambulation if the patient's condition permits, should be instituted.

Treatment of secondary polycythemia focuses on correcting the underlying cause with long-term oxygen therapy, smoking cessation, weight loss, or surgical intervention as indicated. If these measures are ineffective, serial phlebotomy to maintain a hematocrit of 45% or less is required.

ANEMIA

Anemia may be seen in the intensive care unit (ICU) as an incidental condition in a patient admitted to the unit for another acute illness or as an acute condition requiring intensive monitoring and intervention. Typically anemias are classified as blood loss, hemolytic (increased destruction of RBCs) or hypoproliferative (decreased production of RBCs). In addition, anemias can be classified by RBC size as microcytic, normocytic, or macrocytic.

Anemia is prevalent in critically ill patients. Nearly 67% of patients admitted to an ICU have hemoglobin levels of 12.0 g/dL or less, and nearly 95% of patients have below-normal hemoglobin levels by ICU day 3.[1,2] Acute blood loss, especially from intraoperative and gastrointestinal hemorrhage, is a frequent cause of anemia in critically ill patients. Phlebotomy for diagnostic tests has been reported to account for approximately 30% to 50% of anemia cases in the ICU. It is estimated that for every 100 mL of blood drawn, there is an associated decrease in hemoglobin of 0.7 g/dL and in hematocrit of 1.9%.[3] Even with a conservative measurement of phlebotomy blood loss of 100 mL/day, the impact is significant, especially in the patient who is hospitalized for several weeks in the ICU.

In addition to blood loss, disseminated intravascular coagulation (DIC) and a variety of hemolytic disorders can decrease the survival of RBCs, causing anemia in the critically ill. Nutritional deficiencies, inflammation, and sepsis all contribute to anemia as well.

Types of Anemia

The following discussion gives a brief review of the different types of anemia. Because the workup and treatment of many of these anemias does not take place in the critical care setting, the discussion is limited. The main focus of the material presented is specific to anemia in the critically ill.

Blood Loss Anemia

Blood loss anemia is probably the most common anemia requiring admission of the patient to the ICU. Blood loss should always be ruled out in any acute anemia. The primary focus of patient management is to identify and treat the underlying source of blood loss.

Stress gastritis can be the source of significant blood loss. This complication is easier to prevent than it is to treat. All critically ill patients should be considered at risk, and prophylactic therapy with H_2-blockers, proton pump inhibitors, or sucralfate should be initiated. Endoscopy may be performed to evaluate for a potential gastrointestinal source of blood loss.

Hemolytic Anemias

Hemolytic anemias result from the destruction of RBCs. They may be congenital or acquired and can vary greatly in the severity of the anemia.

Congenital Hemolytic Anemia The most common types of congenital hemolytic anemias are caused by enzyme defects or RBC membrane defects (Table 49-2).

Table 49-1 • Clinical Findings and Related Causes in Polycythemia Vera	
Clinical Finding	**Cause**
Dizziness, headache	Increased blood viscosity
Thrombosis	Increased blood viscosity, thrombocytosis, platelet defects
Pruritus	Elevated blood levels of histamine and/or increased skin mast cells
Bleeding tendency	Increased RBC/fibrin ratio; engorged capillaries and venules due to increased blood volume
Epigastric distress	Engorgement of gastric mucosa; increased blood histamine levels
Numbness and burning of toes	Peripheral vascular insufficiency
Cardiovascular insufficiency	Impaired tissue oxygenation due to increased blood viscosity

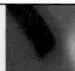

Table 49-2 • Congenital Hemolytic Anemias and Primary Interventions

Type of Defect	Primary Interventions
Enzyme Defects	
Glucose-6-phosphate dehydrogenase	Avoidance of agents that trigger hemolysis; hydration
Pyruvate kinase deficiency	Transfusion; splenectomy
Red Blood Cell Membrane Defects	
Hereditary spherocytosis	Splenectomy; folic acid supplements
Hereditary elliptocytosis	Usually no treatment required; folic acid supplements
Paroxysmal nocturnal hemoglobinuria	Corticosteroids, androgens, recombinant erythropoietin, iron therapy; transfusion as needed; anticoagulation therapy if thrombotic events; possible bone marrow transplantation

Box 49-1 • Substances That May Cause Hemolytic Anemia in Susceptible Individuals

Congenital Hemolytic Anemia (G6PD Deficiency)
- Acetanilid
- Nalidixic acid
- Ciprofloxacin niridazole
- Norfloxacin
- Methylene blue
- Chloramphenicol
- Phenazopyridine
- Vitamin K analogs
- Doxorubicin
- Isobutyl nitrite
- Naphthalene
- Phenylhydrazine
- Pyridium
- Mothballs
- Fava beans (Mediterranean variant of G6PD deficiency)

Acquired Hemolytic Anemia
- Chloramines
- Nitrobenzene
- Isobutyl nitrates
- Aniline dyes
- Arsine gas
- Sodium chlorate
- Potassium chlorate
- Wasp and bee stings
- Spider bites
- Snake bites
- Copper
- Lead
- Paraquat
- Quinine
- Quinidine
- Acetanilid
- Furazolidone
- Isobutyl nitrite
- Nalidixic acid
- Naphthalene
- Niridazole
- Methyldopa
- Levodopa
- Procainamide
- Nonsteroidal anti-inflammatory drugs (NSAIDs)
- Penicillins
- Cephalosporins

Approximately 90% of congenital RBC enzymatic deficiencies are glucose-6-phosphate dehydrogenase (G6PD) and pyruvate kinase deficiencies.[4] Enzyme defects cause the RBCs to lyse when exposed to certain stressful conditions, such as drugs, chemicals, infections, surgery, or pregnancy. Substances to which people with G6PD deficiency may be susceptible are listed in Box 49-1.

Acquired Hemolytic Anemia Acquired hemolytic anemias can be caused by several different factors (Table 49-3). In microangiopathic hemolytic anemia, RBCs are fragmented by vasculitis, collagen vascular disease, abnormal cardiac valves, arteriovenous malformations, thrombotic thrombocytopenic purpura (TTP), or DIC. Patients who experience hypothermia or cold cardioplegia with cardiac surgery may have RBCs with shortened life spans owing to membrane damage. Patients with RBCs recovered from the "cell saver" also experience significant membrane damage and hemolysis. Treatment focuses on removing the causative factor, such as replacing the abnormal heart valve or repairing the arteriovenous shunt. If this is not possible, the patient may be maintained on iron and folate supplements and periodic transfusions of RBCs.

Infectious agents may cause hemolytic anemia indirectly by causing splenomegaly or directly by invading the RBC and destroying its membrane. Malaria is an example of the latter. These patients are treated with transfusion support and anti-infective agents to address the underlying cause.

Abnormally shaped RBCs are frequently noticed in patients with liver disease. These patients may also have congestive splenomegaly, which causes sequestration and destruction of RBCs. In severe hemolysis, splenectomy and supportive RBC transfusions may be required.

Some patients can experience autoimmune hemolytic anemias. Warm autoimmune hemolytic anemia is the most common of these types. Approximately one half of all cases are idiopathic; known causative factors include collagen diseases, lymphoproliferative disorders, and drug reactions (see Box 49-1). Primary therapy is oral glucocorticoids to suppress the immune system. Additional treatments for patients who do not respond to glucocorticoids may include splenectomy, immunosuppressive agents, and intravenous immunoglobulin (IVIG).

Cold-reactive autoimmune hemolytic anemia is a disorder in which exposure to cold triggers complement-fixing immunoglobulin M (IgM) antibodies to attach to RBCs in susceptible people, causing agglutination (clumping) and hemolysis

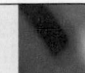

Table 49-3 • Acquired Hemolytic Anemias and Potential Interventions	
Acquired Hemolytic Anemia	Interventions
Microangiopathic	Removal of causative factor; iron and folate supplements; transfusion
Infectious agents	Treatment of underlying infection; transfusion
Liver disease	Splenectomy; transfusion
Autoimmune	
Warm antibody	Glucocorticoids; splenectomy; immuno-suppressive agents; transfusion
Cold-reactive	Avoidance of exposure to cold; transfusion; plasma exchange
Drug-induced	Discontinuation of drug; transfusion

(destruction). Often these patients have an underlying lymphoproliferative disorder; others may have *Mycoplasma pneumoniae* infection, infectious mononucleosis, or hepatitis. If these patients require transfusion, use of a blood warmer and measures to keep the patient warm is recommended. Steroids and splenectomy are ineffective; intervention focuses on avoiding exposure to cold.

Deficiency Anemias

Deficiency anemias include iron-deficiency anemia, megaloblastic anemia, anemia of chronic disease, and aplastic anemia. Table 49-4 lists common interventions for these anemias.

Iron-Deficiency Anemia Iron deficiency is the most common cause of anemia in adults. It is usually caused by chronic blood loss, but it may be due to inadequate iron intake or absorption. It is imperative in chronic blood loss to search for the underlying cause and correct it. Oral iron replacement theory is typically administered; however, in patients with malabsorption disorders or poor tolerance of oral iron, parenteral iron may be considered.

Megaloblastic Anemias Megaloblastic anemias are a group of anemias, most of which are caused by a deficiency of vitamin B_{12} (cobalamin), folate,

Table 49-4 • Common Deficiency Anemias and Primary Interventions	
Type of Anemia	Primary Interventions
Iron-deficiency anemia	Iron supplements; correction of under-lying stressor
Megaloblastic anemia	Vitamin B_{12} replacement; folic acid supplement
Anemia of chronic disease	Transfusion; recombinant erythropoietin (rEPO); correction of underlying disorder
Aplastic anemia	Transfusion; immunosuppression; bone marrow transplantation

Box 49-2 • Drugs That Interfere With Folate Metabolism

- Alcohol
- Methotrexate
- Carbamazepine
- Diphenylhydantoin
- Triamterene
- Trimethoprim
- Pyrimethamine

or both. Drugs that interfere with folate metabolism are listed in Box 49-2. Treatment entails correcting the deficiency.

Vitamin B_{12} is poorly absorbed from the gut; therefore, intramuscular or subcutaneous injection is required. Most patients require maintenance injections monthly for the remainder of their lives. Body stores of folate can be restored with an oral folate supplement given daily for approximately 4 weeks. Once the deficiency is corrected, maintenance therapy is rarely necessary unless underlying factors, such as chronic alcoholism, are present.

Anemia of Chronic Disease Finally, anemia is seen with a number of chronic disorders, such as renal failure, infections, malignancies, and connective tissue diseases including rheumatoid arthritis. Anemia of chronic renal failure generally starts to occur when the creatinine clearance is less than 45 mL/minute and continues to worsen with increasing renal failure. Several mechanisms cause anemia of chronic disease. One factor is suppression of RBC production. Other factors are a decreased RBC survival time and low serum erythropoietin levels. Aspects of anemia in older patients are presented in Box 49-3.

Treatment involves correcting the underlying cause, if possible. Transfusion may be of temporary benefit, although the survival of the transfused red

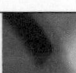

Box 49-3 • CONSIDERATIONS FOR THE OLDER PATIENT: Anemia

Anemia is common in the elderly, and its prevalence increases with age. As with other cells, the body's capacity for red cell replacement decreases with aging, typically with a greater decline seen in men than women. Although most elderly people are able to maintain their hemoglobin and hematocrit levels within a normal range, they are unable to replace their red cells as promptly in situations such as bleeding.

In the elderly, anemia is usually the result of bleeding, infection, malignancy, or chronic disease. Combined deficiencies are common in older adults. Undiagnosed and untreated anemia is associated with decreased functional and self-care abilities and depression. It can also cause neurologic and cognitive disorders, cardiovascular complications, and increased risk for mortality. Orally administered iron is poorly used in older adults.

blood cells is reduced. Recombinant erythropoietin (rEPO) may be the treatment of choice for many people. rEPO is typically given as 50 to 100 units/kg intravenously or subcutaneously 3 times a week, with adjustments based on response. Complications of rEPO therapy are infrequent and are seen mostly in patients on renal dialysis. They may include hypertension, seizures, arteriovenous shunt thromboses, and increased blood viscosity.

Aplastic Anemia In aplastic anemia, there is as deficiency of RBCs as well as white blood cells (WBCs) and platelets (in other words, aplastic anemia is a condition of pancytopenia). In many cases, the cause of aplastic anemia is unknown. Possible factors include drugs, chemicals, viruses, and immunological and congenital disorders (Box 49-4). In some patients, aplastic anemia is thought to result from replacement of normal cells by clones of cells that are incapable of normal hematopoiesis. Clinical features of aplastic anemia are related to the underlying pancytopenia and include anemia, infections, and bleeding.

Severe aplastic anemia is treated with transfusion support, immunosuppressive agents, and bone

---

Box 49-4 • Causative Factors in Aplastic Anemia

Congenital (20% of Cases)
- Fanconi's anemia
- Congenital dyskeratosis
- Shwachman-Diamond syndrome
- Dubowitz's syndrome
- Diamond-Blackfan syndrome
- Familial aplastic anemia

Acquired (80% of Cases)
- Idiopathic
- Irradiation
- Drugs
  Chloramphenicol
  Phenylbutazone
  Quinine derivatives
  Sulfonamides
  Cimetidine
  Gold salts
  Hydantoins
- Chemicals
  Benzene and benzene derivatives
  Insecticides
  Cleaning solvents
- Infections
  Non-A, non-B hepatitis
  Epstein-Barr virus
  Human immunodeficiency virus
  Parovirus
  Mycobacteria
- Immunological
  Graft-versus-host disease
  Systemic lupus erythematosus
  Thymoma
- Pregnancy

---

marrow transplantation. Drugs that stimulate marrow function are of no benefit in this condition. Bone marrow transplantation, preferably from a human leukocyte antigen–matched sibling donor, should be considered for patients younger than 60 years of age. These patients should be considered for immediate transplantation and should not receive any transfusions or drug therapy before transplantation, if possible. Immunosuppressive therapy with antithymocyte globulin, cyclosporine, or methylprednisolone may be of benefit for older patients or those without a compatible donor for bone marrow transplantation.

Assessment

The history of the patient with anemia includes assessment of blood loss (including perioperatively, in the stool, and from the menses) as well as a thorough diet history. General symptoms of anemia include weakness, depressed mood, impaired cognitive function, and easy fatigability. Signs and symptoms indicative of decreased perfusion secondary to anemia are tachycardia, chest pain, dyspnea, and dizziness. Clinical consequences of anemia are impaired tissue oxygenation, impaired organ function, impaired susceptibility to thrombocytopenic bleeding, increased risk for postoperative mortality, increased probability of transfusion, and decreased survival.[3] Anemia in critically ill patients is similar in clinical presentation to the anemia of chronic disease, both of which lead to underproduction of RBCs.

Physical examination findings of anemia include pallor, tachycardia, hypotension, and signs of high-output heart failure. Patients with hemolytic anemia may have splenomegaly, jaundice, and dark urine owing to the excretion of bilirubin. It is necessary to review the intake and output records for fluid balance because hemodilution is common, particularly in the postoperative patient, because of aggressive intravenous hydration. All patients should have a stool guaiac test performed to look for occult gastrointestinal blood loss.

Typically, critically ill patients have low serum iron and total iron-binding capacity with elevated serum ferritin. When the iron studies are abnormal, serum erythropoietin levels are only mildly elevated, with little evidence of a reticulocyte response to endogenous erythropoietin. Further laboratory assessment to evaluate anemia is discussed in Chapter 46.

Management

The treatment of anemia starts with identifying the underlying cause. Iron sulfate, 325 mg by mouth 2 to 3 times per day, may be indicated. Parenteral iron may be administered when the patient is unable to take oral medications, or in the case of malabsorption or severe renal failure. Intramuscular iron injection may be painful and stain the patient's skin. Instead, intravenous injection is recommended. Close patient observation is necessary because severe anaphylactic reactions may occur with this treatment. Vitamin C is often given to aid in the absorption of iron. Folic acid and vitamin B_{12}, if needed, should be considered.

Blood Transfusion

The risk versus benefit of blood transfusion in the critically ill patient continues to be an area of scrutiny and study. In the past, hemoglobin transfusion triggers varied between 7 and 10 g/dL, most often between 8 and 9 g/dL. However, this practice is changing because of a number of factors associated with worse clinical outcomes occurring in patients receiving blood transfusions.

Therapeutic Considerations Currently, it is believed that transfusion of packed RBCs should be reserved for management of severe, active bleeding or for the patient who is experiencing serious symptoms from anemia. In other words, the practice should be to transfuse when the risks of decreased oxygen-carrying capacity outweigh the risks of transfusion, rather than relying on a specific hemoglobin or hematocrit trigger. Recent data suggest that many critically ill patients can tolerate hemoglobin levels as low as 7 g/dL.[2]

The normal compensatory mechanisms in response to the decreased oxygen supply of anemia (increased heart rate, increased cardiac output and index, decreased systemic vascular resistance) may not work efficiently or at all in critically ill patients. This deficit in compensatory mechanisms is particularly relevant in patients with cardiac disease and in those at high risk for myocardial infarction. For example, a patient with coronary stenosis may not have the normal response of vasodilation as a compensatory mechanism to the anemia. Likewise, increased cardiac output may not be achievable in patients with cardiomyopathy or pulmonary edema. Other patients who may have a poor prognosis if not transfused include those with sepsis and higher APACHE II scores.

Complications Complications of blood transfusion may be noninfectious, infectious, or immunologic. A common noninfectious complication of transfusion is volume overload, particularly in the patient with pulmonary edema or cardiomyopathy. Patients can have a transfusion-related acute lung injury (TRALI) resembling acute respiratory distress syndrome (ARDS) with dyspnea, hypoxia, and noncardiogenic pulmonary edema. Febrile reactions are associated with white cell antigens present in units of packed RBCs. Unfortunately, preventable fatal hemolytic reactions result from transfusion of ABO-incompatible blood.

Viral screening of blood products and careful selection of donors have certainly decreased the risk for transfusion transmission of viruses such as human immunodeficiency virus (HIV) and hepatitis C virus. However, there is still a risk posed by donors who donate during the infectious period before they seroconvert. In addition to viral contaminants that can be tested, blood screening methods do not exclude other infectious agents such as hepatitis A virus, human parvovirus B19, cytomegalovirus (CMV), malaria, and disease-causing bacteria.

Multiple published studies report an increased risk for infection associated with transfusions and a mortality rate about twice that seen in nontransfused patients. Taylor and colleagues identified a fivefold increase in risk for health care–associated infections (HAIs) in critically ill patients who received transfusion.[5] For each unit of packed RBCs transfused, the odds of infection increased by a factor of 1.5. These findings were independent of severity of illness and hemoglobin level.

Exposure to the donor's leukocytes in transfusion may trigger an immune system response. Potential adverse outcomes include exacerbation of infections, earlier recurrence of malignancy, impaired wound healing and other postoperative complications, and increased likelihood of mortality.

To avoid some of these complications, consideration may be given to transfusing critically ill patients with leuko-reduced blood. Leuko-reduction is the process of removing WBCs from the blood product by filtration. Leuko-reduced blood is less likely to cause development of antibodies against specific blood types and less likely to cause febrile transfusion reactions. Also, leuko-reduced blood greatly reduces the chance of CMV transmission.

Erythropoietic-Stimulating Proteins

Administration of erythropoietic-stimulating proteins, such as epoetin and darbepoetin, may be a safer method of increasing hemoglobin and reducing the need for transfusion in many patients. Contraindications include uncontrolled hypertension and hypersensitivity to albumin. The optimal effective dose and timing of administration for anemia in critically ill patients have not yet been determined, and this is a topic of ongoing clinical trials.

Nursing Care of the Patient With Anemia

Nursing interventions in all anemias are supportive of treatment protocols and of measures to identify the underlying cause. Other important actions include assessing for adverse effects of replacement therapy and for signs and symptoms indicative of decreased perfusion. If transfusion therapy is prescribed, vigilance in identifying the correct patient and ensuring ABO compatibility is of utmost importance to prevent adverse and potentially fatal outcomes. In addition, measures to decrease metabolic needs and reduce oxygen demand should be instituted, including promotion of a restful environment, adequate pain control, and minimization of agitation. Supplemental oxygen may be needed to assist in maintaining adequate oxygen supply to the tissues.

Critical care nurses are in an ideal position to identify when phlebotomy appears excessive or unnecessary and to question the clinical justification for testing. Strategies to reduce phlebotomy blood loss should be instituted. These include eliminating standing orders for laboratory tests, organizing blood draws to eliminate duplicate testing, consolidating multiple collections, using smaller collection tubes, and using devices that return waste blood to the patient. The frequency of arterial blood gas collection can often be decreased by the use of noninvasive monitoring techniques such as pulse oximetry and capnography.

SICKLE CELL DISEASE

Pathophysiology

Sickle cell disease (SCD) is a chronic hereditary hemolytic anemia that occurs almost exclusively in blacks; however a variety of other ethnicities can be affected. The sickle cell gene results in abnormal hemoglobin, usually hemoglobin S (HbS). When oxygen and pH levels fall, HbS RBCs become elongated, sickle or crescent shaped, and rigid. These sickled cells are unable to pass through small blood vessels, causing inflammation, obstruction of the vessels, and decreased delivery of oxygen that perpetuates the cycle with more sickling. The cells are hemolyzed or destroyed when the body recognizes their abnormal structure.

Clinical Presentation

The most common clinical picture in SCD is painful vaso-occlusive crisis. The crisis begins suddenly, sometimes as a consequence of infection or a change in temperature, or for no identifiable reason. Severe deep pain is present in the long bones of the extremities. Sometimes the abdomen is affected by severe pain resembling an acute abdomen. The pain may be accompanied by fever, malaise, and leukocytosis.

SCD also results in organ damage with microinfarcts of the heart, skeleton, spleen, and central nervous system (CNS). Repeated splenic infarcts result in splenic failure, predisposing the patient to overwhelming infection, especially gram-negative sepsis. Other manifestations of SCD that may be seen in the critical care patient are stroke, cardiac chamber enlargement, pulmonary hypertension, renal failure, and chronic leg ulcers.

Acute chest syndrome is caused by pulmonary infarction from fat embolism; bacterial infections likely contribute to its development as well. Symptoms include chest pain, fever, tachypnea, leukocytosis, and pulmonary infiltrates. Acute chest syndrome is a medical emergency, and if not treated properly, complications such as ARDS may develop.

Management

Treatment of sickle cell crisis includes aggressive intravenous fluid hydration to decrease blood viscosity and maintain renal perfusion. The patient must be evaluated for infection, and if this is suspected, they must be treated promptly with broad-spectrum antibiotics until the causative organism is identified and the therapy can be tailored. Oxygen administration may be needed to maintain adequate tissue perfusion. Anemia is usually well tolerated, and RBC transfusions are not usually required. Patients with SCD take folic acid supplementation and may take hydroxyurea, which helps prevent sickling. Although activity is usually not restricted, the patient may not be able to tolerate exercise because of pain.

The pain experienced by patients in sickle cell crisis is intense. Patients require around-the-clock dosing with a strong narcotic, such as intravenous morphine. Frequent, lower doses of narcotics avoid the erratic levels of analgesia caused by infrequent doses of stronger narcotics. Time-release narcotics and patient-controlled analgesia are two methods of delivering steady doses of pain medication. Patients with sickle cell crisis may not display overt signs of pain, as is typical for patients who experience chronic pain. The patient's report of pain, as well as clinical indicators, should be used in assessing pain.

Nursing care of the patient with sickle cell crisis includes close monitoring for response to interventions to promote tissue perfusion, treat infection, and effectively manage pain. A multidisciplinary approach might include input from pain management experts, social workers, psychiatrists, physical and occupational therapists, orthopedists, and infectious disease specialists.

• Disorders of White Blood Cells

LEUKOPENIA

Leukopenia refers to an abnormally low number of WBCs. The most common type of WBC deficiency is neutropenia, defined as a neutrophil count of less than 1,500 cells/mm³. Severe neutropenia, in which the neutrophil count is less than 200 cells/mm³, is referred to as agranulocytosis. Neutropenia can be seen as a result of a wide variety of conditions (Table 49-5). The most common cause of leukopenia is drug related.

Clinical Presentation

Because the neutrophil is essential to defense against bacterial and fungal infections, patients with neutropenia are susceptible to overwhelming infection and life-threatening sepsis. The risk for infection is related to the severity of the neutropenia. Untreated infections can be rapidly fatal, particularly if the neutrophil count is less than 250/mm³. In severe neutropenia, the usual signs of the inflammatory response to infection may be absent.

Neutrophils provide the first line of defense against organisms that inhabit the skin and gastrointestinal tract. Thus, skin infections and ulcerative lesions of the mouth are common infections in the neutropenic patient. The most frequent site of serious infection is the respiratory tract, a result of bacteria or fungi that frequently colonize the airways.

Assessment

The history should include presence of viral infection or autoimmune diseases such as systemic lupus erythematosus or rheumatoid arthritis. A thorough medication history, including over-the-counter preparations, should be obtained. Patients with neutropenia may present with mouth ulcers, fever, shaking chills, and systemic infection. Physical examination may reveal splenomegaly.

The presence of abnormal RBCs or WBCs suggests a primary bone marrow process. Laboratory studies

Table 49-5 • Causes of Neutropenia

Cause	Mechanism
Accelerated removal (e.g., inflammation and infection)	Removal of neutrophils from the circulation exceeds production
Drug-induced granulocytopenia	
Cytotoxic drugs used in cancer therapy	Depressed bone marrow function with decreased production of all blood cells.
Phenothiazines, propylthiouracil, and others	Toxic effect on bone marrow precursors
Aminopyrine, certain sulfonamides, phenylbutazone, and others	Immune-mediated destruction
Periodic or cyclic neutropenia (occurs during infancy and later)	Unknown
Neoplasms involving bone marrow (e.g., leukemias and lymphomas)	Overgrowth of neoplastic cells, which crowd out granulopoietic precursors
Idiopathic neutropenia that occurs in the absence of other disease or provoking influence	Autoimmune reaction
Felty's syndrome	Intrasplenic destruction of neutrophils

From Porth CM: Essentials of Pathophysiology, 2nd ed. Philadelphia: Lippincott Williams & Wilkins, 2007, p 183.

should include viral serology for hepatitis and HIV, as well as antinuclear antibody (ANA). Bone marrow aspiration and biopsy may be needed if the neutropenia is severe or the cause is not apparent.

Management

Neutropenia is treated by removing or managing the underlying cause if known. If the patient is febrile, appropriate cultures and a chest radiograph should be obtained, followed by immediate broad-spectrum intravenous antibiotic therapy to prevent progression to septic shock and death. Signs and symptoms of infection without fever should also prompt administration of antibiotics in patients with neutropenia. If evidence of infection persists despite adequate antibiotic therapy, antifungal agents may be added to provide coverage for potential *Candida* or *Aspergillus* infections.

If the neutropenia is severe, treatment may include a hematopoietic growth factor (filgrastim, pegfilgrastim, or sargramostim) that stimulates bone marrow production of new neutrophils and enhances the activity of already circulating neutrophils. Additionally, patients with severe neutropenia or those with recurrent or serious infections may benefit from steroids. IVIG may improve the neutrophil count. Transfusions are used cautiously in patients who may require bone marrow transplantation.

NEOPLASTIC DISORDERS

Neoplastic disorders refer to those disorders characterized by new and abnormal growth of cells that may be benign or malignant. The clinical features of neoplastic disorders are determined largely by their site of origin. Lymphoproliferative disorders (disorders in which lymphoid tissue increases by reproducing) may originate in the bone marrow or in the lymph nodes and thymus. Lymphoproliferative disorders of the bone marrow are leukemias and multiple myeloma; lymphoproliferative disorders of the lymph nodes and thymus are lymphomas. Because blood cells circulate throughout the body, these neoplasms are systemically disseminated from the onset.

Lymphoma

Hodgkin's Lymphoma
Hodgkin's lymphoma is a cancer of the lymphatic system, beginning as a malignancy in a single lymph node and then spreading to surrounding lymph nodes. A diagnosis of Hodgkin's disease is confirmed by the presence of abnormal Reed-Sternberg cells in biopsied tissue.

Non-Hodgkin's Lymphoma
Non-Hodgkin's lymphoma (NHL) is a diverse group of malignancies that originate in the lymphoid cells. NHL can occur as a discreet mass, such as a single lymph node, or as a widespread disease that affects multiple organ systems, including the bone marrow.

Clinical Presentation
Symptoms of both types of lymphoma are related to the body area affected by the rapid growth of abnormal lymphoid cells. Constitutional symptoms include fever, fatigue, and weight loss. In the advanced stages, patients may have extensive chest disease and experience increasingly severe dyspnea. Bulky chest disease can cause superior vena cava syndrome. Abdominal disease can cause obstruction of the bowel or the ureters. Bone marrow involvement can lead to decreased production of RBCs, WBCs, and platelets. Extensive involvement of the lymphatic system can lead to impaired immune function and frequent, severe infections. Lymphoma of the CNS can cause headaches, visual disturbances, motor dysfunction, and increased intracranial pressure.

Management

The diagnosis, staging, and treatment of lymphomas are typically performed entirely on an outpatient basis. The care of a critically ill patient with lymphoma is usually for the management of complications that arise from the disease or its treatment. Oncological complications and their management are discussed in detail in Chapters 47 and 48.

Leukemia

The leukemias are malignant neoplasms characterized by rapid proliferation of hematopoietic stem cells, resulting in the accumulation of abnormal (leukemic) cells in the bone marrow and a decreased production of normal blood cells. These abnormal leukemic cells circulate in the blood stream and infiltrate many body organs. Leukemias commonly are classified according to their predominant cell type (lymphoblastic or myelogenous) and whether the condition is acute or chronic. The chronic leukemias are not discussed in this chapter.

Acute Lymphoblastic Anemia

Acute lymphoblastic leukemia (ALL) is a disorder in which a clone of immature lymphocytes proliferates and replaces the normal cells of the bone marrow. The leukemic clones proliferate and infiltrate other normal tissues, such as the liver, spleen, and lymph nodes. Anemia, thrombocytopenia, and granulocytopenia are common. The spleen, liver, thymus, and lymph nodes are usually enlarged.

Acute Myelogenous Leukemia

A malignant disorder of hematopoietic stem cells, acute myelogenous leukemia (AML) causes abnormal production of the myeloid cell lines (erythrocyte, neutrophil, megakaryocyte, and macrophage). The malignant clones proliferate but do not differentiate into mature, functional cells. The blood, bone marrow, or both contain more than 30% immature blast cells. The proliferation of immature cells and bone marrow infiltration results in anemia, neutropenia, and thrombocytopenia. The patient's symptoms are related to these conditions. Splenomegaly is present in approximately one third of patients. Patients may require immediate interventions at the time of diagnosis for infections or anemia, or to achieve hemostasis.

Clinical Presentation

Although ALL and AML are distinct disorders, they typically present with similar clinical features. These manifestations and their pathologic basis are summarized in Table 49-6.

Patients with leukocyte counts greater than 100,000 cells/mm^3 are at risk for leukostasis, a condition in which the high number of blasts increase blood viscosity, develop leukoblastic emboli, and aggregate in the capillaries. Manifestations include headache, confusion, CNS infarcts, acute respiratory insufficiency, and pulmonary infiltrates. Leukostasis requires immediate treatment to lower the blast count rapidly. Initial treatment involves emergent leukapheresis (removal of WBCs from the circulation) along with hydroxyurea. Chemotherapy should be initiated to stop leukemic cell production in the bone marrow.

Management

A discussion of diagnosis and treatment of leukemia is beyond the scope of this text. As in the patient with

---

Table 49-6 • Clinical Manifestations of Acute Leukemia and Their Pathologic Basis*

Clinical Manifestations	Pathologic Basis
Bone marrow depression	
Malaise, easy fatigability	Anemia
Fever	Infection or increased metabolism by neoplastic cells
Bleeding	Decreased thrombocytes
Petechiae	
Ecchymosis	
Gingival bleeding	
Epistaxis	
Bone pain and tenderness upon palpation	Subperiosteal bone infiltration, bone marrow expansion, and bone resorption
Headache, nausea, vomiting, papilledema, cranial nerve palsies, seizures, coma	Leukemic infiltration of central nervous system
Abdominal discomfort	Generalized lymphadenopathy, hepatomegaly, splenomegaly due to leukemic cell infiltration
Increased vulnerability to infections	Immaturity of the white cells and ineffective immune function
Hematologic abnormalities	Physical and metabolic encroachment of leukemia cells on red blood cell and thrombocyte precursors
Anemia	
Thrombocytopenia	
Hyperuricemia and other metabolic disorders	Abnormal proliferation and metabolism of leukemic cells

*Manifestations vary with the type of leukemia.
From Porth CM: Essentials of Pathophysiology, 2nd ed. Philadelphia: Lippincott Williams & Wilkins, 2007, p 189.

lymphoma, the patient with leukemia will typically be seen in the critical care unit as a result of complications of the disorder or its treatment. Refer to discussions of anemia, granulocytopenia, and thrombocytopenia in this chapter, as well as Chapters 47 and 48, for coverage of bone marrow or stem cell transplantation and oncological emergencies.

NURSING CARE OF THE PATIENT WITH A WHITE BLOOD CELL DISORDER

The goals of nursing care of the patient with a WBC disorder are vigilant assessment for and prevention of infection, delivery of therapy, and management of disease and treatment-associated complications. Nursing interventions are guided by the treatment modality (e.g., chemotherapy, radiation, bone marrow transplantation).

Meticulous attention to infection control procedures and vigilant surveillance of invasive lines and equipment are mainstays of care. Attention must be paid during daily oral care to ensure that superinfection with *Candida* or herpesvirus has not developed. Antibacterial mouthwashes decrease the risk for infection. Severe mucositis may require opiates for pain control. Assessment for early indications of infection (e.g., fever, chills, tachycardia, and tachypnea) may allow for prompt and aggressive initiation of pharmacological therapies to reduce morbidity and mortality associated with infection in patients with white blood cell disorders.

Diarrhea may be a side effect of chemotherapy, neutropenia, or secondary causes. *Clostridium difficile* infection must be considered and treated if present. Digital rectal examinations should not be performed on neutropenic patients.

• Disorders of Hemostasis

The term hemostasis refers to the stoppage of blood flow.[6] The hemostatic system is a finely balanced network of coagulation factors and endothelial and platelet components. Hemostasis may be impaired by disruption of numerous interactions in the coagulation pathways or deficiencies or dysfunction in the required components for coagulation. Disorders of hemostasis include hypercoagulable states and bleeding disorders, whether from platelet defects (thrombocytopenia) or coagulation defects. Disorders of hemostasis are often seen in critically ill patients.

PLATELET DISORDERS

Normally, approximately two thirds of platelets are circulating in the blood, and one third are sequestered or stored in the spleen. The life span of circulating platelets is 7 to 10 days. Thrombocytopenia occurs when there is decreased production or increased destruction of platelets, or increased sequestration of platelets in the spleen. Common causes of thrombocytopenia are listed in Table 49-7. The most common causes seen in critical care patients are discussed here. A complete etiological discussion is beyond the scope of this chapter.

Types of Thrombocytopenia

Drug-Induced Thrombocytopenia
The most common cause of thrombocytopenia in hospitalized patients is drug induced. The confirmation of this diagnosis occurs when the thrombocytopenia resolves after withdrawal of the causal medication. Medications commonly associated with

Table 49-7 • Differential Diagnosis of Thrombocytopenia

Decreased Production	Splenic Sequestration	Increased Destruction
Marrow infiltration	Splenic enlargement	Nonimmune
Malignancy	Tumor infiltration	Vascular prostheses
Myelofibrosis	Infection	Disseminated intravascular coagulation
Granulomatous disease		Sepsis
	Splenic congestion	Vasculitis
Marrow failure	Portal HTN or liver disease	Thrombotic thrombocytopenic purpura
Medication		
Chemotherapy		Immune
Aplastic anemia		Autoantibody (idiopathic thrombocytopenic
Severe iron deficiency		purpura)
		Drug-associated*
Infection (HIV, Epstein-Barr virus, TB)		Circulating immune complexes (systemic lupus erythematosus, viral, bacterial sepsis)
Alcohol use		Posttransfusion ab (PLA1)
Nutritional deficiency		
Iron, folate, vitamin B_{12}		

*One of most common causes of thrombocytopenia
From Kwoh C, Buch E, Quartarolo J: The Washington Manual General Internal Medicine Consult. Philadelphia: Lippincott Williams & Wilkins, 2004, p 167.

thrombocytopenia include antineoplastic agents, heparin, H₂-blockers, trimethoprim-sulfamethoxazole, rifampin, vancomycin, amiodarone, and valproic acid; however, this list is not complete.

After antineoplastic agents, heparin is the next most common drug associated with thrombocytopenia. Heparin-induced thrombocytopenia (HIT) is interesting in that thrombosis, rather than bleeding, may accompany the low platelet count. HIT places patients at risk for life- and limb-threatening consequences, including deep venous thrombosis, arterial occlusion, ischemic stroke, limb gangrene, myocardial infarction, and pulmonary embolism.

Generally, full anticoagulation with continuous intravenous heparin carries the greatest risk. However, it is important to be aware that any amount of heparin, whether unfractionated or low molecular weight, can cause HIT. Subcutaneous unfractionated heparin or low–molecular-weight heparin for prophylaxis of deep venous thrombosis, arterial or venous line flushes, heparin-coated catheters, and intermittent heparin during dialysis may lead to HIT. Although HIT typically appears 4 to 14 days after initiation of heparin therapy, it can occur as early as 10 hours after administration if the patient has been exposed to heparin within the previous 100 days (re-exposure) or several days after withdrawal of all forms of heparin.

The hallmark of HIT is a decrease in platelet count to less than 50% of baseline or to less than 150,000/mm³, or the occurrence of an unexplained thromboembolic event. The nurse should always have a low threshold for considering HIT when any unexpected and substantial percentage decline in platelet count occurs during heparin treatment.

Thrombotic Thrombocytopenic Purpura

TTP is an acute disorder with a mortality rate of 30% to 40%. Patients with TTP have absent or decreased levels of platelet-aggregating factor inhibitor, which is normally present in plasma. As a result, platelets become sensitized and clump in blood vessels, causing occlusion.

A presentation of five classic findings suggests TTP. Not every patient exhibits all five findings; however, the first two of the following conditions must be present for the diagnosis to be considered:

▶ Thrombocytopenia and bleeding due to increased consumption of platelets

▶ Microangiopathic hemolytic anemia due to rupture of RBCs as they try to pass through partially occluded blood vessels

▶ Fever, possibly due to hemolysis or vascular infarction of the hypothalamus

▶ Neurologic abnormalities, including fluctuating and often bizarre neurological abnormalities, transient ischemic attacks, strokes, seizures, and coma due to interrupted blood flow to the brain

▶ Renal dysfunction due to obstruction of intraglomerular capillaries and infarction of the renal cortex

Clinical features of TTP are described further in Table 49-8. Initiation of the disease process may be related to endothelial damage, autoimmune disorders, viral and bacterial infections, toxic agents, and genetic predisposition.

Immune Thrombocytopenic Purpura

Immune thrombocytopenic purpura (ITP) is an immune-mediated disorder of platelet destruction. Historically, ITP stood for idiopathic thrombocytopenic purpura because the mechanism of thrombocytopenia was not understood. However, now the pathophysiology of the disease is clearer, and some have suggested that the name autoimmune thrombocytopenic purpura might be more accurate.

There are two distinct forms of ITP. Acute ITP typically occurs in childhood and may resolve spontaneously in several weeks. Autoimmune platelet destruction appears to be stimulated after a viral illness, even mild infections. Chronic ITP usually occurs in adults, more often in women than men. The platelet membrane is coated with an autoantibody (usually IgG), and the sensitized platelets are destroyed in the spleen and liver. Therefore, platelet survival in the circulation is decreased. In at least 50% of patients with ITP, no known causative agent is identified; other patients may have underlying autoimmune, rheumatic, or lymphoproliferative diseases or HIV infection. ITP is diagnosed when other disorders of platelet destruction are ruled out.

Assessment

The history, physical examination, and initial laboratory data help differentiate between the mechanisms of thrombocytopenia.

The patient history includes assessment of symptoms associated with any of the risk factors or associated disorders (see Table 49-8). A patient or family

Table 49-8 • Clinical Manifestations of Thrombotic Thrombocytopenic Purpura (TTP) 	
Abnormality	**Findings**
Thrombocytopenia	Bleeding, ecchymosis, purpura at various sites
Hemolytic anemia	Schistocytes, reticulocytosis, elevated serum lactate dehydrogenase and bilirubin, jaundice, pallor, weakness
Neurological abnormalities	Headache, mental changes, confusion, visual problems, seizures, coma, aphasia, dysphasia, paresthesias
Renal dysfunction	Proteinuria, microscopic hematuria, elevated blood urea nitrogen and creatinine, renal failure
Fever	Persistent elevation of temperature during acute phase
Other	Abdominal pain, malaise, nausea, vomiting, weakness, ECG changes

history of bleeding may help differentiate between acquired and congenital disorders. Critical to the assessment is an accurate medication and alcohol history. Fatigue, fever, weight loss, or night sweats may be associated with infection or malignancy. It is also important to note a history of platelet transfusion.

The physical examination includes a thorough examination of the skin for petechiae and bruising. It is important to also include the oropharynx in this examination, as well as checking the stool for guaiac. Hypotension, tachycardia, and fever are suggestive of sepsis. A fever is also frequently present in TTP. An enlarged spleen suggests splenic sequestration of trapped blood from portal hypertension. In this setting, patients are likely to exhibit signs of liver disease, including jaundice, ascites, and extremity muscle wasting.

Laboratory examination is also significant. Signs and symptoms of low platelets vary depending on the platelet count. Platelet counts greater than $100,000/mm^3$ should result in normal hemostasis. Platelet counts less than $50,000/mm^3$ may lead to prolonged bleeding after procedures, easy bruising, and bleeding from the oral or gastrointestinal mucosa. Platelet counts less than $20,000/mm^3$ are associated with an exponential increase in the risk for bleeding The nurse carefully assesses the patient for petechial rash or spontaneous bleeding such as epistaxis or bleeding gums. Platelet counts less than $10,000/mm^3$ are associated with possible intracranial hemorrhage.

The complete blood count (CBC) with differential is the most important first step to identifying the etiology of thrombocytopenia. It is important to check for accompanying anemia and leukopenia. If pancytopenia is present, bone marrow failure may be the cause of the problem. If this is suspected, a bone marrow biopsy may be performed. The presence of microcytosis or macrocytosis suggests vitamin deficiency. Severely decreased ferritin, folate, or vitamin B_{12} levels also support this as an etiology. The presence of schistocytes on the differential may indicate TTP or DIC.

It is important to rule out artifactual thrombocytopenia caused by clumping of the platelets in a test tube containing ethylenediamine tetra-acetic acid (EDTA; lavender top). A report of platelet clumping should raise this suspicion. If the platelets are clumped, the automatic counter may inaccurately measure the number of platelets resulting in a falsely low count. In this case, the sample should be redrawn in a citrate tube (blue top) or heparinized tube (green top).

Bleeding time is a test of platelet function. When the platelet count drops below $50,000/mm^3$, the bleeding time is significantly prolonged and is not useful. The bleeding time is a helpful test when a patient has mucosal bleeding but a normal platelet count. Evaluating prothrombin time (PT), partial thromboplastin time (PTT), and fibrin degradation products may help identify DIC and distinguish a hemolytic anemia from TTP. Additional studies that may be ordered to assist in determining the underlying etiology include HIV and ANA screening as well as liver function tests.

Management

The initial step in management of thrombocytopenia is to review the patient's medication list, placing on hold any drugs that may be suspected to induce thrombocytopenia. In addition, medications that inhibit platelet function should be avoided, including aspirin, antiplatelet agents, and nonsteroidal anti-inflammatory drugs. Avoidance of trauma is essential and may even preclude the placement of central venous catheters and other invasive procedures. Evaluation of continued blood loss and assessment of daily laboratory data for adequacy of the platelet count and other parameters of hemostasis are important measures.

Patients with mild to moderate thrombocytopenia without bleeding require no treatment. Platelet transfusions are indicated when the platelet count is below $20,000/mm^3$ or in the case of spontaneous bleeding. A single donor unit of platelets is equivalent to six random donor platelets and should increase the platelet count by $30,000/mm^3$. The patient must be monitored for allergic reactions, anaphylaxis, and volume overload.

In sequestration or destruction-mediated thrombocytopenia, the response to platelet transfusion is typically very poor. Transfused platelets are destroyed very quickly by the same mechanism that causes the disease. Platelet transfusion should be used only for major life-threatening bleeding. In these patients, because the platelets may not last long, platelets need to be administered shortly before performing any invasive procedures.

TTP is an emergency because of its extremely high mortality rate. Early recognition and prompt initiation of treatment are imperative to improve patient survival. Acutely ill patients require plasma exchange in which plasmapheresis is used to remove 2 to 3 liters of the patient's plasma, with an equal amount of fresh plasma given as replacement. Plasmapheresis is initiated as quickly as possible and repeated daily until the platelet count is greater than $150,000/mm^3$. This may take 5 to 10 days or more. Plasma exchange is superior to simple plasma infusion. However, because some patients do respond to simple plasma infusions, all patients should be infused immediately with fresh frozen plasma until plasma exchange can be arranged. Antiplatelet agents and prednisone may be used, although the effectiveness of these therapies is controversial. Platelet transfusion is contraindicated even in severe thrombocytopenia because the transfused platelets may aggregate, resulting in myocardial infarction, stroke, coma, or death. Patients with TTP may be "cured," may relapse years later, or may have a chronic relapsing course.

Immunosuppression with corticosteroids is the initial therapy for ITP. Prednisone usually takes a few days before the count begins to rise. When the platelet count is critically low ($<5,000/mm^3$) or the patient shows signs of serious bleeding, prednisone alone may not raise the platelet count rapidly enough. When a rapid increase in the platelet count is needed, IVIG, in addition to steroids, is highly successful. A typical treatment regimen is IVIG at 1 g/kg/day and prednisone 1 mg/kg/day. Patients with chronic ITP who fail to respond to steroids or are steroid dependent may require splenectomy. These patients should receive pneumococcal, meningococcal, and *Haemophilus influenzae* type B vaccines.

COAGULATION DISORDERS

Coagulation disorders can result from deficiencies or impairment of one or more of the clotting factors. These disorders of coagulation may be congenital or acquired. The most common congenital bleeding disorders are von Willebrand's disease and hemophilia A. These disorders are caused by a deficiency in a specific factor. Numerous complications can occur as a result of these bleeding disorders (Table 49-9).

Management of these bleeding disorders involves correcting the coagulation factor deficiency and treating sequelae that occur as a result of abnormal bleeding. Patients with mild hemophilia A and mild von Willebrand's factor deficiency may respond to intravenous or nasal spray administration of desmopressin acetate, a hormone that temporarily stimulates the release of factor VIII to control bleeding. More severe cases of hemophilia A or active bleeding require intravenous infusion of factor VIII concentrate. More severe bleeding in von Willebrand's disease requires factor VIII concentrate that contains von Willebrand's factor. Von Willebrand's factor is also found in cryoprecipitate, and factors VIII and IX are in fresh frozen plasma.

DISSEMINATED INTRAVASCULAR COAGULATION

Pathophysiology

DIC is defined as the inappropriate triggering of the coagulation cascade and a breakdown in the normal feedback mechanisms in the body that allow for the dissolution of clots. Instead of a localized response to tissue damage or vascular injury, there is systemic coagulation activity, resulting in diffuse intravascular fibrin formation and widespread intravascular clotting. Eventually, coagulation factors become depleted as the body attempts to dissolve the newly formed clots. Because of the rapidity of intravascular thrombin formation, clotting factors are used up at a rate exceeding factor replenishment. In essence, there is an imbalance between the natural procoagulant and anticoagulant systems in the body. The result is unregulated thrombin activity, microvasculature thrombi, platelet consumption, and microangiopathic hemolytic anemia.

Activation of coagulation mechanisms also activates the fibrinolytic system. The breakdown of fibrin and fibrinogen results in fibrin degradation products and D-dimers. These products interfere with platelet function and the formation of the fibrin clot. In addition, plasmin can activate the complement and kinin systems, leading to increased vascular permeability, hypotension, and shock. Thus, the patient has a simultaneous, self-perpetuating combination of thrombotic and bleeding activity occurring in response to the precipitating event, as well as the potential for hemodynamic instability (Fig. 49-1).

Etiology

A number of etiologies can lead to the development of DIC. Common to them all is an underlying condition that serves as the initial triggering event for the inappropriate stimulation of clotting. This involves the activation of any of the coagulation pathways. The extrinsic pathway is activated by damage to the endothelial lining of blood vessels. Common causes include surgery, burns, heat stroke, bacterial endotoxin, and malignant tumors. The intrinsic pathway is activated when subendothelial tissue is exposed to the bloodstream and circulating factor XII comes in contact with the exposed tissue. The exposure may follow vascular injury or damage from immune complexes or bacterial endotoxins. The result is clot formation and activation of the coagulation cascade. Endotoxins released by gram-negative bacteria and the resulting sepsis are significant triggers of DIC, accounting for approximately 20% of cases.

Shock or low-flow states can result in metabolic acidosis, tissue ischemia, and necrosis, which may also lead to clot formation. In cancer, a common etiology of DIC, the condition is caused by tumors eroding tissue with subsequent release of thromboplastin or stimulation of factor XII from vascular injury, as well as by the autolysis of tumor cells in rapidly proliferating tumors. In cancers that are able to autolyse (e.g., acute leukemia, Burkitt's lymphoma, small cell lung cancer), the cell fragments that result from the lysis are seen as "foreign bodies" and stimulate clotting. Still other cancers release procoagulants that enhance clotting (e.g., mucin-producing adenocarcinomas, prostate and renal cancer, promyelocytic leukemias, and brain tumors).[7] Box 49-5 outlines some malignant and nonmalignant states of physiological disequilibrium that can be precipitating factors for DIC.

Table 49-9 • Complications in Coagulation Disorders	
Bleeding Site	**Complication**
Abdomen	Hypotension, hypovolemic shock
Muscle	Compartment syndrome
Joint	Hemarthrosis with destruction of bone and cartilage in joint capsule
Intracranial	Increased intracranial pressure
Retropharyngeal	Airway obstruction
Gastrointestinal	Anemia, melena
Urinary tract	Clots in ureters (especially after factor administration)

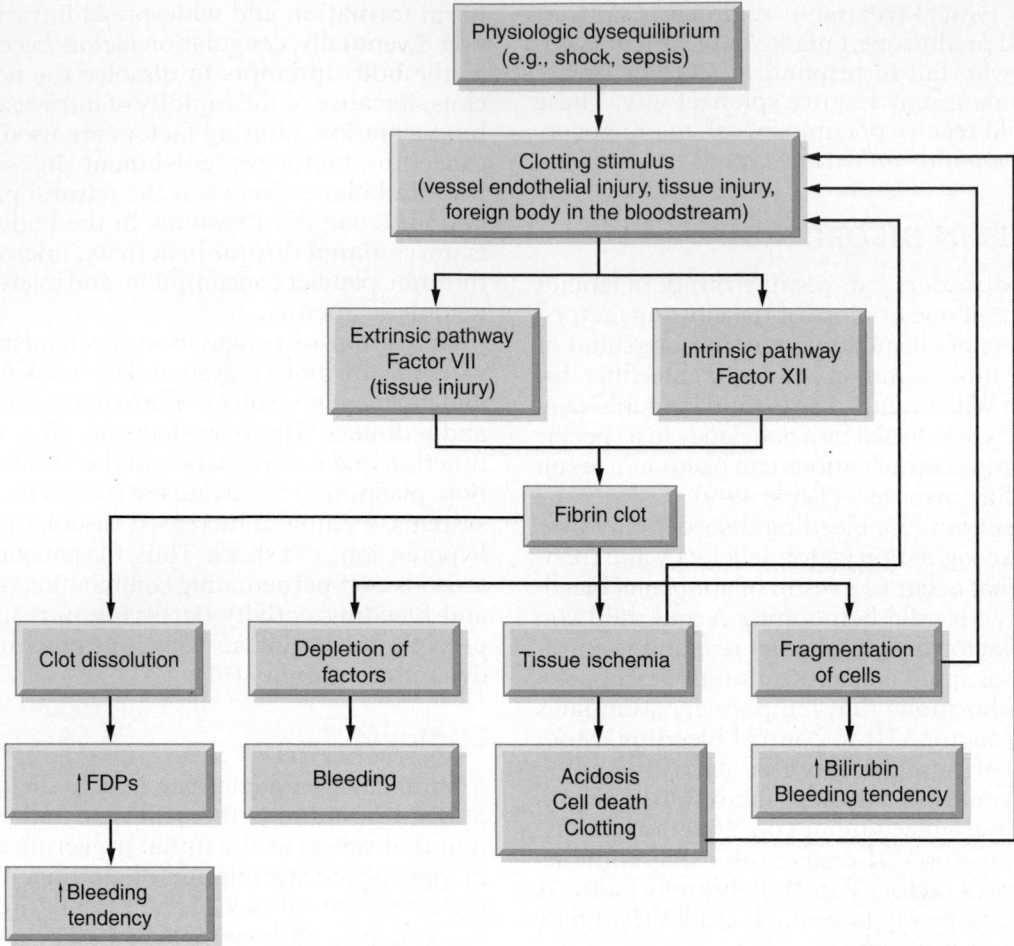

Figure 49-1 • Self-perpetuating cycle of thrombosis and bleeding in disseminated intravascular coagulation (DIC).

Clinical Presentation

Clinical consequences include systemic ischemia from the thrombi formation as well as minor or major hemorrhage from ongoing fibrinolysis and depletion of clotting factors. A patient with DIC is vulnerable to a wide variety of complications resulting from the thrombotic or hemorrhagic disease processes. Thrombosis may result in ischemia or infarction in any organ, with concomitant loss of function. With depletion of clotting factors and platelets, bleeding into subcutaneous tissues, skin, and mucous membranes, or more serious hemorrhage, may result.

Assessment

All critically ill patients are at risk for development of DIC because many are in the state of physiological disequilibrium characterized by hypovolemia, hypotension, hypoxia, and acidosis, all of which have procoagulant effects. In addition, the patient's critical illness may have been triggered by an injury that itself could result in the development of DIC. Increased awareness of DIC as a potentially catastrophic complication in the critically ill patient has resulted in earlier recognition and intervention. The critical care nurse who is armed with knowledge of physiological

norms and who uses a systemic approach to assessment may be the first person to identify the early signs of coagulation dysfunction and its probable trigger.

History and Physical Examination

DIC may be acute in presentation, evidenced by severe clinical deterioration, or chronic in presentation, evidenced by mildly abnormal laboratory values and minimal, varied clinical symptoms. In chronic DIC, thrombosis is the prevalent disorder, and the degree of symptomatology is related to the ability of the liver and bone marrow to compensate for the disorder. Affected patients may have low-grade bleeding if factors become depleted, unexpected thrombotic events (including large vessel thrombi), or both. Chronic DIC must be ruled out in patients with multiple thrombotic sites developing simultaneously, serial thromboses, superficial venous thromboses, or arterial thromboses, especially in the presence of malignancy.[8]

However, most critical care nurses care for patients with acute DIC. It is important to realize that the assessment varies as the disease state evolves. Clinical assessment is organized according to the basic pathological process of DIC: clot formation with resulting emboli and perfusion defects, or unchecked clot dissolution with resultant bleeding. The nurse evaluates the patient for signs and symptoms of inappropriate

Box 49-5 • Selected Disease States Associated With Disseminated Intravascular Coagulation (DIC)

Nonmalignant

- Bacterial infections (gram-negative, gram-positive)
- Viremias (human immunodeficiency virus, cytomegalovirus, hepatitis)
- Burns
- Heat stroke
- Brain injury
- Crush injuries and necrotic tissue
- Obstetrical complications (amniotic fluid embolism, missed abortion, eclampsia, retained dead fetus, abruptio placentae)
- Intravascular hemolysis (hemolytic transfusion reactions, massive blood replacement therapy)
- Acute liver disease
- Intravascular prosthetic devices
- Prolonged low cardiac output states (cardiac failure, prolonged cardiopulmonary bypass, hemorrhagic shock, cardiopulmonary arrest)
- Vasculitis
- Immunological disorders (immune complex disorders, allograft reaction, incompatible blood transfusion)
- Surgery
- Other (snake venom, vascular malformations, fat embolism)

Malignant

- Leukemias (acute promyelocytic, acute myelomonocytic, others)
- Solid tumors (adenocarcinoma, lung cancer, breast cancer, hepatic cancer, colon cancer, prostate cancer, brain cancer)
- Chemoradiation therapy

clotting: cyanosis, gangrene, mental status changes, altered level of consciousness, cerebrovascular accident, pulmonary embolus, bowel ischemia and infarction, and renal insufficiency or failure. Thrombosis may involve both arteries and veins, and clinical examination may reveal demarcation cyanosis (total occlusion of microvessels, most common in digits but may be evident in earlobes). In addition, the nurse evaluates the patient for signs of bleeding: bleeding from the nose, gums, lungs, gastrointestinal tract, surgical sites, injection sites, and intravascular access sites; hematuria; acral cyanosis; petechial rashes; and purpura fulminans. Bleeding is a manifestation of later disease because it is evidence of depletion of clotting factors, bleeding diathesis, or both.

Care of the patient with possible DIC requires constant reassessment and interpretation of findings. For example, the patient with a dull headache is likely to have a thrombotic defect, whereas a sudden and acute headache is more likely to be hemorrhagic. Dyspnea can be from a thrombotic disorder (pulmonary embolism) or from a hemorrhagic disorder (bleeding in the lungs). Either condition may present with hemoptysis and blood with suctioning. Hypotension may result from myocardial infarction (a thrombotic disorder) or cardiac tamponade

(a hemorrhagic disorder). Ischemic bowel is characterized by decreased bowel sounds and a crampy and painful abdomen, with potential gastrointestinal bleeding when the mucosal layer sloughs, whereas gastrointestinal bleeding presents with heme-positive to melanotic stool and hyperactive bowel sounds. Nurses must monitor patients with DIC closely for signs and symptoms of the onset of shock, either hypovolemic or ischemic in origin. When caring for patients at risk for DIC, constant assessment of all body systems and critical thinking are necessary.

Laboratory Studies

Regardless of the inciting event, four basic diagnostic components of DIC can be appreciated: excessive rate of clot formation; increased rate of clot dissolution; consumption of essential clotting factors; and end-organ damage resulting from the excessive clotting process.[9]

Table 49-10 outlines studies that are commonly used to assess DIC. These studies, unfortunately, are neither specific nor sensitive, and results vary throughout the course of the disease. For the average patient, thrombocytopenia occurs as platelets are consumed during the unchecked clotting, followed by hypofibrinogenemia. Normal fibrinogen levels do not preclude DIC because it is an acute-phase reactant. Serial measurements of platelet count, PT, PTT, and fibrinogen levels help gauge disease progression. Peripheral smears may reveal the presence of schistocytes reflecting fragmentation of RBCs moving through clots or partially occluded vessels.

Management

The backbone of therapy for DIC is elimination of the causative agent. The culprit that activates the clotting factors must be eliminated, whether through antibiotic or antifungal therapy for sepsis, antineoplastic therapy, rehydration, increasing oxygenation, or resolution of low-flow states. Unfortunately, some causes (such as burns, crush injury, and brain injury) cannot be as easily eliminated. General treatment principles include avoiding vasoconstriction that may worsen perfusion defects, maintaining adequate fluid volume status, and screening for and eliminating all medications that may enhance bleeding. Attention is also directed to correction of hypotension, hypoxia, and acidosis, all of which have procoagulant effects (Box 49-6).

Patients at risk for development of DIC as a result of sepsis may be given activated protein C (drotrecogin alfa [activated], marketed as Xigris) to slow the development of uncontrolled clotting that may result from the septic process. There are stringent criteria for the use of activated protein C. The argument for use is that with aggressive treatment of the causative agent (sepsis), it may be possible to decrease the rate of clot formation, slow the clotting cascade, and reclaim the balance between clotting and fibrinolysis. This agent has not been investigated for its potential benefit in patients with confirmed DIC.

Heparin therapy may be initiated to minimize further clotting by increasing neutralization of thrombin.

(text continues on page 1308)

Table 49-10 • Laboratory Findings in Acute Disseminated Intravascular Coagulation (DIC)

Test	Normal Value	Value in DIC
Massive Intravascular Clotting		
Platelet count	150,000–400,000/mm³	Decreased
Fibrinogen level	200–400 mg/100 mL	Decreased
Thrombin time	7.0–12.0 sec	Prolonged
Protein C level	4 µg/mL	Decreased
Protein S level	23 µg/mL	Decreased
Secondary Depletion of Essential Clotting Factors		
Prothrombin time (PT)	11–15 sec	Prolonged
Activated partial thromboplastin time (aPTT)	30–40 sec	Prolonged
International normalized ratio (INR)	1.0–1.2 times normal	Prolonged
Excessive/Accelerated Fibrinolysis		
Fibrin degradation products (FDPs)	<10 mg/mL	Increased
D-dimer assay	<50 µg/dL	Increased
Antithrombin III level	89%–120%	Decreased
Clinical Effects of Microvascular Clotting/Cell Destruction		
Schistocytes on peripheral smear		Present
Bilirubin level	0.1–1.2 mg/dL	Increased
Blood urea nitrogen (BUN)	8–20 mg/dL	Increased

Box 49-6 • COLLABORATIVE CARE GUIDE for the Patient With Disseminated Intravascular Coagulation (DIC)

OUTCOMES	INTERVENTIONS
Oxygenation/Ventilation	
Arterial blood gases are within normal limits.	• Monitor pulse oximetry and arterial blood gases. • Validate significant changes in pulse oximetry with co-oximetry arterial saturation measurement. • Transfuse as necessary to increase oxygen carrying capacity. • Turn, cough, deep breathe, and use incentive spirometer q2h.
Breath sounds are clear bilaterally.	• Suction oropharynx and trachea carefully when necessary (see Chapter 25, Box 25-7) • Turn, cough, deep-breathe, and use incentive spirometer q2h.
Circulation/Perfusion	
Patient will achieve/maintain tissue perfusion.	• Monitor tissue perfusion: color, temperature, pulses, capillary refill, level of consciousness, urinary output, and PaO₂. • Monitor vital signs qh–4h based on clinical condition. • Monitor cardiac output, stroke volume, systemic vascular resistance, and pulmonary artery pressures q4h if pulmonary artery catheter in place.
Serum lactate will be within normal limits.	• Monitor lactate qd or more frequently until it is within normal limits. • Administer red blood cells, positive inotropic agents, IV infusions as ordered to increase oxygen delivery. • Assess patient for potential sources of lactate (e.g., ischemic bowel, ischemic distal digits) or decreased ability to clear lactate (liver dysfunction).
Hematological	
Patient will not experience bleeding related to coagulopathies.	• Monitor PT, PTT, complete blood count (CBC), fibrin split products, and fibrinogen levels daily; more frequently if monitoring for acute changes or response to therapy. • Assess q4h for signs of bleeding, including thrombotic and hemorrhagic manifestations. • Quantify degree of bleeding (weigh dressings, count pads, measure bodily drainage; test stool, urine, drains, and emesis for heme).

(continued)

Box 49-6 • COLLABORATIVE CARE GUIDE for the Patient With Disseminated Intravascular Coagulation (DIC) (Continued)

OUTCOMES	INTERVENTIONS
	• Assess individual organs for signs and symptoms of bleeding: crackles, decreased SaO_2 with pulmonary bleeding; visual changes (diplopia, blurred vision, visual field deficit) with retinal thrombosis/hemorrhage; back pain, flank pain, abdominal pain consistent with visceral organ bleeding.
	• Administer blood and coagulation factors as indicated.
	• Maintain strict adherence to bleeding precautions.
	• Avoid invasive procedures and treatments.
	• Avoid medications that inhibit coagulation or promote thrombosis.
	• Apply pressure to puncture sites for 3–5 min, then use pressure dressing.
Fluids/Electrolytes Patient is euvolemic.	• Take daily weights.
	• Monitor intake and output; replace/diurese as required.
	• Maintain IV access and fluid replacement therapy.
Mineral and electrolyte levels are within normal limits.	• Monitor and replace electrolytes Mg and PO_4 daily and PRN.
Mobility/Safety There is no evidence of bruising due to preventable injury.	• Institute bleeding precautions, including padded side rails, no sharp objects at or around bedside, assistance out of bed, and padded self-protective devices (if necessary).
	• Assess for bleeding/bruising q2h or more frequently.
Skin Integrity Skin will remain intact.	• Assess skin q8h and each time patient is repositioned for pressure areas, petechiae, and ecchymosis.
	• Turn q2–4h.
	• Consider pressure relief/reduction mattress, avoid shearing forces.
	• Perform range-of-motion exercises every shift.
	• Use Braden scale to assess risk for skin breakdown.
Nutrition Caloric and nutrient intake meets metabolic requirements per calculation (e.g., basal energy expenditure).	• Provide parenteral feeding if NPO.
	• Assess for gastrointestinal bleeding and report.
	• Consult dietitian or nutritional support service.
Comfort/Pain Control Patient will be as comfortable as possible as evidenced by stable vital signs or cooperation with treatments or procedures.	• Objectively assess comfort/pain using a pain scale.
	• Correlate pain ratings with sites of potential ischemia/infarction/hemorrhage. Notify house officer for correlation.
	• Provide warm compresses to promote vasodilation and decrease ischemic pain as indicated (with MD/NP/PA approval).
	• Provide analgesia and sedation as indicated by assessment.
	• Monitor patient response to medication.
Psychosocial Patient demonstrates decreased anxiety.	• Educate patient and family regarding disease process, actions taken to correct disorder.
	• Provide areas of control to patient and family as possible (e.g., performance of ADLs, visitors)
	• Provide explanations and reassurance before procedures.
	• Consult social services, clergy as appropriate.
	• Provide for adequate rest and sleep.
Teaching/Discharge Planning Patient/significant others understand procedures and tests needed for treatment.	• Prepare the patient and family for procedures, such as blood transfusions and laboratory studies.
	• Educate the patient and family regarding clinical parameters and patient presentation required for safe discharge from unit/hospital.

However, the risk for increased bleeding is always a major concern. In acute DIC, few clinical studies have shown heparin's effectiveness in slowing the coagulation cascade.

Replacement therapy and repletion of clotting factors are the focus of the treatment for significant hemorrhage. Fresh frozen plasma contains components of both the coagulation and fibrinolytic systems and can be given to normalize the International Normalized Ratio (INR). The recommended dose is 10 to 20 mL/kg. Platelet transfusions are usually used only for patients with active bleeding or a platelet count of less than 20,000/mm^3. Cryoprecipitate may be used for patients with plasma fibrinogen levels below 100 mg/dL. A single unit provides 200 mg of fibrinogen, as well as factor VIII, factor XII, and von Willebrand's factor. The usual adult dose is 5 to 10 units, with each unit raising the fibrinogen level by 5 to 10 mg/dL. Depleted antithrombin III (necessary to balance clot production) can be replaced using heat-treated pooled plasma concentrates; this has been shown to shorten the duration of DIC. RBC transfusions, although not useful for repleting coagulation factors, may be given to increase hemoglobin and oxygen-carrying capacity.

Localized bleeding can be minimized when possible. With venipuncture or removal of vascular access from compressible sites, pressure is applied for a minimum of 15 to 30 minutes or until bleeding has stopped. Sites are reassessed frequently for rebleeding because the initial clot may dissolve if the patient is deficient of the factors required to maintain hemostasis. Topical hemostatics may be used to provide superficial hemostasis.

• Clinical Applicability Challenges

Case Study

Mr. C. is a 64-year-old African American man with a known history of coronary artery disease who had an inferior wall myocardial infarction (MI) last month. He presents to the emergency department complaining of chest pain unrelieved by sublingual nitroglycerin. His home medications include aspirin, a statin, and a β-blocker. An initial electrocardiogram (ECG) and troponin are normal. After initiation of oxygen and an intravenous (IV) nitroglycerin drip, his pain is relieved. However, because of his recent MI, he is admitted to the telemetry unit with orders for serial troponins and an ECG in the morning. Admission orders include continuing the aspirin and statin, increasing the dose of β-blockers, and adding low–molecular-weight heparin (LMWH) at 1 mg/kg subcutaneously every 12 hours.

The next afternoon, Mr. C. has had no further chest pain, his troponins have remained normal, and his ECG is unchanged. All the results from his morning laboratory work are within normal limits, with the exception of a mildly low platelet count of 140,000/mm^3. His cardiologist believes that Mr. C. can be discharged home on the increased β-blocker dose with a follow-up in the office next week.

Mr. C. is dressing to go home when he calls the nurse to his room, complaining of chest pain and shortness of breath. The nurse calls for a "stat" ECG and places him on 2 liters of oxygen via nasal cannula. His vital signs are: pulse, 110 beats/minute; respirations, 32 breaths/minute; and blood pressure (BP), 90/64 mm Hg. Auscultation of his chest reveals clear lungs and a tachycardic but regular heart rhythm. The stat ECG remains unchanged from the ECG he had earlier in the morning. The nurse calls Mr. C.'s cardiologist, who requests that the patient be transferred to the intensive care unit (ICU).

On arrival to the ICU, Mr. C. becomes more tachypneic, his oxygen saturation is 85% on 2 L of oxygen, and his BP is now 80/40 mm Hg. His lungs remain clear. He is placed on a 100% non-rebreather mask (NRM). His cardiologist arrives on the unit and orders a 500-mL IV fluid bolus of normal saline. After a second fluid bolus and the NRM, his BP is 96/60 mm Hg, and his oxygen saturation is 95%. He remains dyspneic. He is sent for a stat computed tomography (CT) scan of the chest.

While the patient is in the CT department, the nurse has a chance to review his chart. The nurse notices that Mr. C.'s platelet count on admission was 285,000/mm^3, and this morning had decreased by more than 50% to 140,000/mm^3. About that time, the CT department calls the ICU to report Mr. C. has a pulmonary embolism. The nurse reports both of these findings to the cardiologist. A stat complete blood count is ordered; findings are: hemoglobin, 11.2 g/dL; hematocrit, 32.8%; and platelets, 63,000/mm^3.

The nurse and physician review the medication record for drugs that could affect the platelet count. LMWH is identified as a possibility. The nurse then remembers taking care of Mr. C. when he had his MI last month. She recalls that he was taking LMWH during his hospital stay. Heparin-induced thrombocytopenia (HIT) is strongly suspected. The LMWH is immediately stopped. Instead, a nonheparin anticoagulant (e.g., lepirudin, argatroban, or bivalirudin) is started. Even though Mr. C. has no lower extremity edema or discomfort, a lower extremity venous ultrasound is performed to rule out deep venous thrombosis.

After 2 days of therapy, Mr. C.'s oxygen saturation is 99% on 2 liters of oxygen. His platelet count is substantially higher, although it is still less than 150,000/mm^3. He is transferred out of the ICU and remains on the nonheparin anticoagulant. The next morning, his platelet count is now 159,000/mm^3. He is started on warfarin 5 mg each evening. On day 5 of warfarin therapy, his INR is 2.2. On day 6 of warfarin therapy, his INR is 2.5, and his platelet count is 324,000/mm^3.

The nonheparin anticoagulant is stopped. He is now off oxygen and is ambulatory on the unit without shortness of breath.

Mr. C. is discharged home on his prior medications of aspirin, statin, and the increased dose of β-blocker. He is given a prescription for warfarin, 5 mg daily, and an appointment to have his INR checked in 3 days. In addition to teaching Mr. C. and his wife about warfarin therapy and anticoagulation, the nurse instructs them to inform health care providers that he is not to be given unfractionated heparin or LMWH because of this episode of HIT. The nurse suggests a medical alert bracelet with this information.

1. Mr. C.'s critical care nurse remembers he received LMWH during his previous admission for an acute MI. What is the importance of this history?

2. Mr. C. is treated for HIT before the diagnosis is confirmed by laboratory testing. Why?

3. Despite his thrombocytopenia, Mr. C. is started on anticoagulation. What is the rationale?

Review Questions

1. Mr J. has been diagnosed with polycythemia vera. A common complaint of patients with this disorder is
   a. pruritus after bathing.
   b. frequent nosebleeds.
   c. tingling in the feet.
   d. easy bruising.

2. An appropriate transfusion trigger for a critically ill patient with anemia is
   a. a heme-positive stool.
   b. a hemoglobin less than 8.5 g/dL.
   c. angina with known coronary artery disease.
   d. anticipated frequent laboratory testing.

3. A patient is admitted to the critical care unit with anemia and thrombocytopenia. Which of the following is pertinent to ask when taking the patient's history?
   a. Do you drink any alcohol?
   b. Have you had any unexplained bruises or bleeding?
   c. Have you had fever?
   d. All of the above

4. Ms. S. has been diagnosed with immune thrombocytopenic purpura with a platelet count of 3,000/mm³. Her best treatment option is
   a. platelet transfusion.
   b. prednisone.
   c. intravenous immune globulin and prednisone.
   d. splenectomy.

5. A patient with sickle cell disease is being transferred to the intensive care unit with chest pain, respiratory distress, high fever, and hypotension. The most likely explanation for the patient's symptoms is
   a. acute chest syndrome.
   b. severe symptomatic anemia.

   c. pericarditis.
   d. myocardial infarction.

6. Key to the management of disseminated intravascular coagulation is
   a. heparin.
   b. fresh frozen plasma.
   c. vitamin K.
   d. treatment of the underlying disorder.

References

1. Pearl RG, Pohlman A: Understanding and managing anemia in critically ill patients. Crit Care Nurse 22(12 Suppl):2, 2002
2. Corwin HL, Gettinger A, Pearl RG, et al: The CRIT study: Anemia and blood transfusion in the critically ill—current clinical practice in the United States. Crit Care Med 32(1): 39–52, 2004
3. Shander A, Spence RK, Amin A: The hospitalists' perspective: Evidence-based strategies for inpatient anemia. Medscape. Available at http://www.medscape.com/viewprogram/5481. Released June 30, 2006
4. Conrad ME: Anemia. Emedicine. Available at http://www.emedicine.com/med/topic123.htm. Accessed February 15, 2002
5. Taylor RW, Manganaro L, O'Brien J, et al: Impact of allogenic packed red blood cell transfusion on nosocomial infection rates in the critically ill patient. Crit Care Med 30:2249–2254, 2002
6. Gaspard KJ: Alterations in homeostasis. In Porth CM (ed): Essentials of Pathophysiology. Philadelphia, Lippincott Williams & Wilkins, 2007
7. Ziegfeld C, Shelton BK, Olsen M: Manual of Oncology Nursing. Philadelphia, Lippincott Williams & Wilkins, 2005
8. Messmore HL, Wehrmacher WH: Disseminated intravascular coagulation: A primer for primary care physicians. Postgrad Med 111(3), 2002
9. Geiter H: Disseminated intravascular coagulopathy. Dimens Crit Care Nurs 22(3):108–114, 2003

Other Selected Readings

Bick RL: Disseminated intravascular coagulation. A review of etiology, pathophysiology, diagnosis, and management: guidelines for care. Clin Appl Thromb Hemost 8(1):1–31, 2002
Cleveland K: Argatroban: A new treatment option for heparin-induced thrombocytopenia. Crit Care Nurse 23(6):61–69, 2003
Cooney MF: Heparin-induced thrombocytopenia: Advances in diagnosis and treatment. Critical Care Nurse. 26(6). 30–37, 2006
Distenfeld, A: Sickle cell anemia. Emedicine. Available at http://www.emedicine.com/med/topic2126.htm. Accessed May 2, 2005
Levi MM, Vink R, deJonge E: Management of bleeding disorders by prohemostatic therapy. Int J Hematol 76(Suppl 2):139–144, 2002
Montoya V, Wink D, Sole ML: Adult anemia: Determination of clinical significance. Nurse Practitioner 27(3):38–53, 2002
Rudis MI, Jacobi J, Hassan E, Dasta JF: Managing anemia in the critically ill patient. Pharmacotherapy 24(2):229–247, 2004
Steinberg MH, Farber HW: Sickle Cell Disease. In Wachter RM, Goldman L, Hollander H (eds): Hospital Medicine. Philadelphia, Lippincott Williams & Wilkins, 2005
Vernon S, Preifer GM: Blood management strategies for critical care patients. Crit Care Nurse 23(6):34–41, 2003
Warkentin TE, Greinacher A: Heparin-induced thrombocytopenia: recognition, treatment, and prevention: the Seventh ACCP Conference on Antithrombotic and Thrombolytic Therapy. Chest 126(3 Suppl):311S–37S, 2004
Williams E: Disseminated intravascular coagulation. In Loscalzo J, Schafer AI (eds): Thrombosis and Hemorrhage. Philadelphia, Lippincott Williams & Wilkins, 2003

Integumentary System

PART 12

INTERNET RESOURCES

Topic	Web Page Address
Alberta Burn Rehabilitation Society	www.burnrehab.com
The Alisa Ann Ruch Burn Foundation	www.aarbf.org
American Academy of Wound Management	www.aawm.org
American Burn Association	www.ameriburn.org
American Professional Wound Care Association	www.apwca.org
Burn Prevention Foundation	www.burnprevention.org
Canadian Association of Wound Care	www.cawc.net
Dr. Koop's Online	www.drkoop.com
Medline Plus: Skin Cancer	www.nlm.nih.gov/medlineplus/skincancer.html
National Center for Injury Prevention & Control	www.cdc.gov/ncipc/default.htm
National Pressure Ulcer Advisory Panel	www.npuap.org
Ostomy Wound Management	www.o-wm.com
The Phoenix Society	www.phoenix-society.org
Regranex Gel Information	www.regranex.com
Shriners Hospitals for Children	www.shrinershq.org
Skin Care Physicians Homepage	www.skincarephysicians.com
U.S. Fire Administration	www.usfa.fema.gov/
University of Michigan Trauma Burn Center	www.traumaburn.org
Wound Care Education Institute	www.wcei.net
Wound Care Information Network	www.medicaledu.com
Wound Care Network	www.woundcarenet.com
Wound Care Resource	www.wounds1.com
Wound Care Strategies Homepage	www.woundcarestrategies.com
Wound Ostomy & Continence Nurses Society	www.wocn.org
Wounds: Clinical Research and Practice	www.woundsresearch.com

Anatomy and Physiology of the Integumentary System

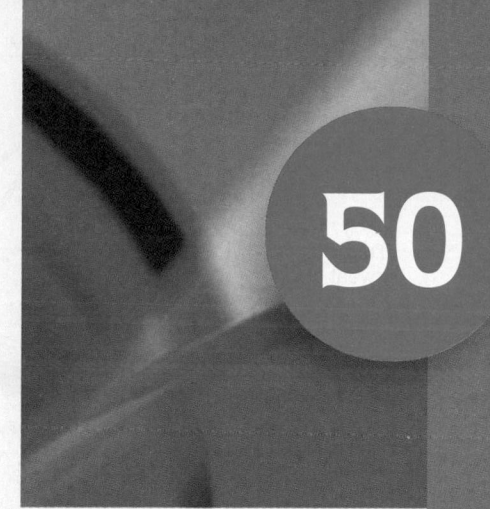

50

Joan M. Davenport

Epidermis
Dermis
Hypodermis
Skin Appendages
    Sweat Glands
    Sebaceous Glands
    Hair
    Nails
Functions of the Skin

Objectives

Based on the content in this chapter, the reader should be able to:

❶ Describe the features of the epidermis, dermis, and hypodermis.

❷ Describe the appendages of the skin and state the purpose of each.

❸ Discuss the homeostatic functions of the skin.

❹ Explain the mechanism of infection resistance afforded by the integument.

The skin is described as protective, sensitive, reparative, and capable of maintaining a person's homeostasis. These physiological features are explored in this chapter as functions of the anatomy of the skin and its appendages. The skin, which covers 1.2 to 2.3 m² of area, is the largest organ of the body and is supplied with one third of the circulating blood volume.[1] The three layers of the skin are the outer epidermis, middle dermis, and underlying hypodermis or subcutaneous tissue. The appendages include the hair, nails, eccrine and apocrine sweat glands, and sebaceous glands. The structures and layers of the skin are shown in Figure 50-1. The functions of the skin include protection, sensation, water balance, temperature regulation, and vitamin production.

• Epidermis

This outer layer of the skin serves to protect underlying structures from invasion by microbes and other foreign substances. The cornified, external layer of the epidermis helps in the body's regulation of water loss. The innermost sublayer blends into the dermis and serves as the basis for the glands, nails, and hair roots. The epidermis does not have vascular supply; it depends on the dermal level for its nourishment.

Melanin and keratin are formed in the inner cellular layer of the epidermis. Melanocytes supply melanin, a pigment for both the skin and hair. This pigment provides the color for the skin and, more important, protects the underlying structures from exposure to ultraviolet light by absorbing and scattering the radiation.[2]

Keratin is a tough protein that makes up hair, nails, and the tough outer epidermal surface. These flattened scales of the skin slough continually and are replaced every 2 to 4 weeks.[3] The epidermis is actually made up of five distinct layers; the keratinocytes move from inner to outer sublayers as they mature. At the top, outermost layer, the keratinocytes are dead and are arranged in various thicknesses depending on the area of the body. In parts of the face there is a thin stratum made up of a layer 15 cells deep. This contrasts with the thicker soles of the feet and palms of the hands, which have at least 100 layers of keratinized cells.[2] It is these tough protein cells that serve to protect the underlying structures of the body.

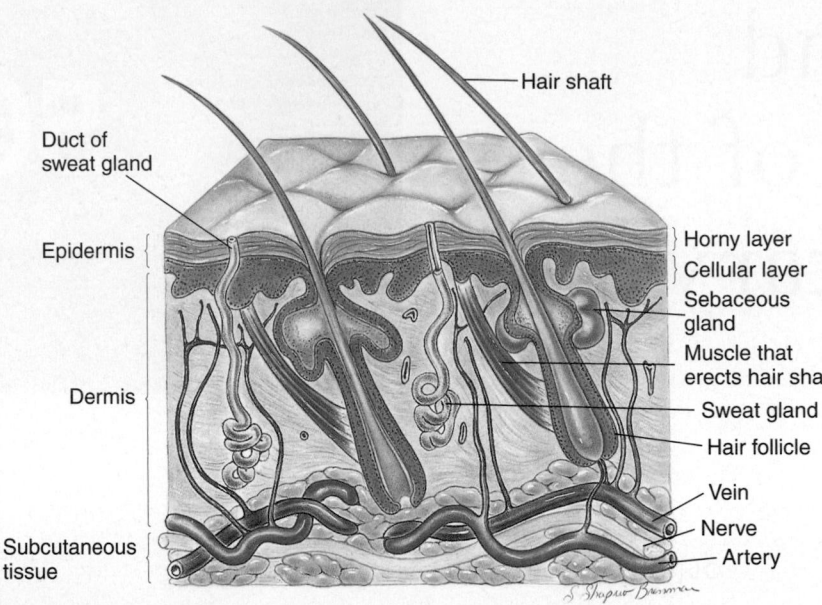

Figure 50-1 • Layers of the skin. (From Bickley LS: Bates' Guide to Physical Examination and History Taking, 9th ed. Philadelphia: Lippincott Williams & Wilkins, 2007, p 121.)

• Dermis

The middle layer of the skin, the dermis, provides support for the outer epidermal layer. It is a very vascular connective tissue; the blood vessels are integral to regulation of body temperature and blood pressure. The arteriovenous anastomoses, under control of the sympathetic nervous system and found in the dermal layer, are able to dilate or constrict in response to environmental conditions of heat and cold and to internal stimulation from anxiety or blood volume loss.

The sensory function of the skin includes receptors for heat, cold, touch, pressure, and pain; these are located in the dermal layer. There is a great variety in the function of the nerve endings. Multiple stimuli are mediated centrally and result in patterned responses.[2]

The dermis is composed of two distinct layers. The papillary dermis, lying just beneath the epidermis, is the more superficial of the two layers. This layer provides the attachment for the epidermis as the epidermal basal cells project into the papillary dermis.[4]

The thicker underlayer of the dermis is the reticular dermis. Collagen is organized in a three-dimensional mesh pattern in this portion of the dermis. It is this mesh arrangement that allows the dermis to stretch with movement. Immune system components of the skin are found in the dermal layer and include macrophages, mast cells, T cells, and fibroblasts.[2]

• Hypodermis

The hypodermis or subcutaneous skin layer consists of connective tissue interspersed with fat. The fat of the hypodermis has the protective functions of heat retention and cushioning the underlying structures. In addition, the fat of the subcutaneous skin layer serves as storage for calories.[5]

• Skin Appendages

The hair, nails, and sebaceous and sweat glands are considered a part of the skin. These structures arise from or extrude through the epidermal or dermal skin layers.

SWEAT GLANDS

Eccrine sweat glands are distributed throughout the surface of the skin. These glands arise from the dermis and open at the skin surface. These specialized glands secrete sweat for the purpose of internal body temperature regulation.

Apocrine sweat glands are not as widespread as the eccrine glands; are larger than eccrine glands; and open through hair follicles of the axillae, nipples, areolae, groin, eyelids, and external ears.[5] Another difference between the two types of sweat glands is that the larger, less abundant apocrine glands secrete an oily substance with a particular odor. This odor is used by animals to recognize the presence of other animals. In humans, the odor, known as body odor, is produced when the secretions come in contact with bacteria and when the fluid begins to decompose.[2,5]

SEBACEOUS GLANDS

The sebaceous glands secrete sebum, a combination of triglycerides, cholesterol, and wax, through the hair follicles. These glands are situated over the entire surface of the skin except for the palms and soles of the feet. Sebaceous glands are inactive until puberty. At this time, they enlarge and are stimulated to secrete sebum by a rise in sex hormones. The sebum serves to keep the skin and hair from drying out.[5] By protecting the outer layer of the epidermis from undue drying, the sebum helps conserve body heat. Table 50-1 sum-

Table 50-1 • Sweat and Sebaceous Glands

Type of Gland	Location	Function
Eccrine sweat glands	All over body Numerous in thick skin Extended from dermis to epidermis	Regulate body temperature Respond to emotional distress Respond to physiological stimuli
Apocrine sweat glands	Axillae Nipples, breasts Anogenital region External ear canal Eyelids	Respond to hormonal influences Respond to emotional distress

Sebaceous glands	All over body except palms of hands,
	    dorsum, and soles of feet
		Produce sebum to lubricate hair
		    and skin

From Allwood J, Curry K: Normal and altered functions of the skin. In Bullock BA, Henze RL (eds): Focus on Pathophysiology. Philadelphia: Lippincott Williams & Wilkins, 2000, p. 842.

marizes the location and function of the eccrine, apocrine, and sebaceous glands.[6]

HAIR

Epidermal cells in the dermis form the hair. Together with the sebaceous gland, the hair follicle forms the pilosebaceous unit. Vellus hair is unobtrusive, soft, and less pigmented than terminal hair. Terminal hair

is darker, coarser, and more obvious. The follicular bulb is the site of vascular papilla, which nourishes and maintains the hair follicle. Hair color is determined by the melanocytes also found at the bulb. Under the sebaceous gland, adjacent to the hair follicle, are the arrector pili muscles. Contraction of the arrector pili causes gooseflesh, a reduction of skin surface area, and reduced surface area for heat loss (Fig. 50-2).

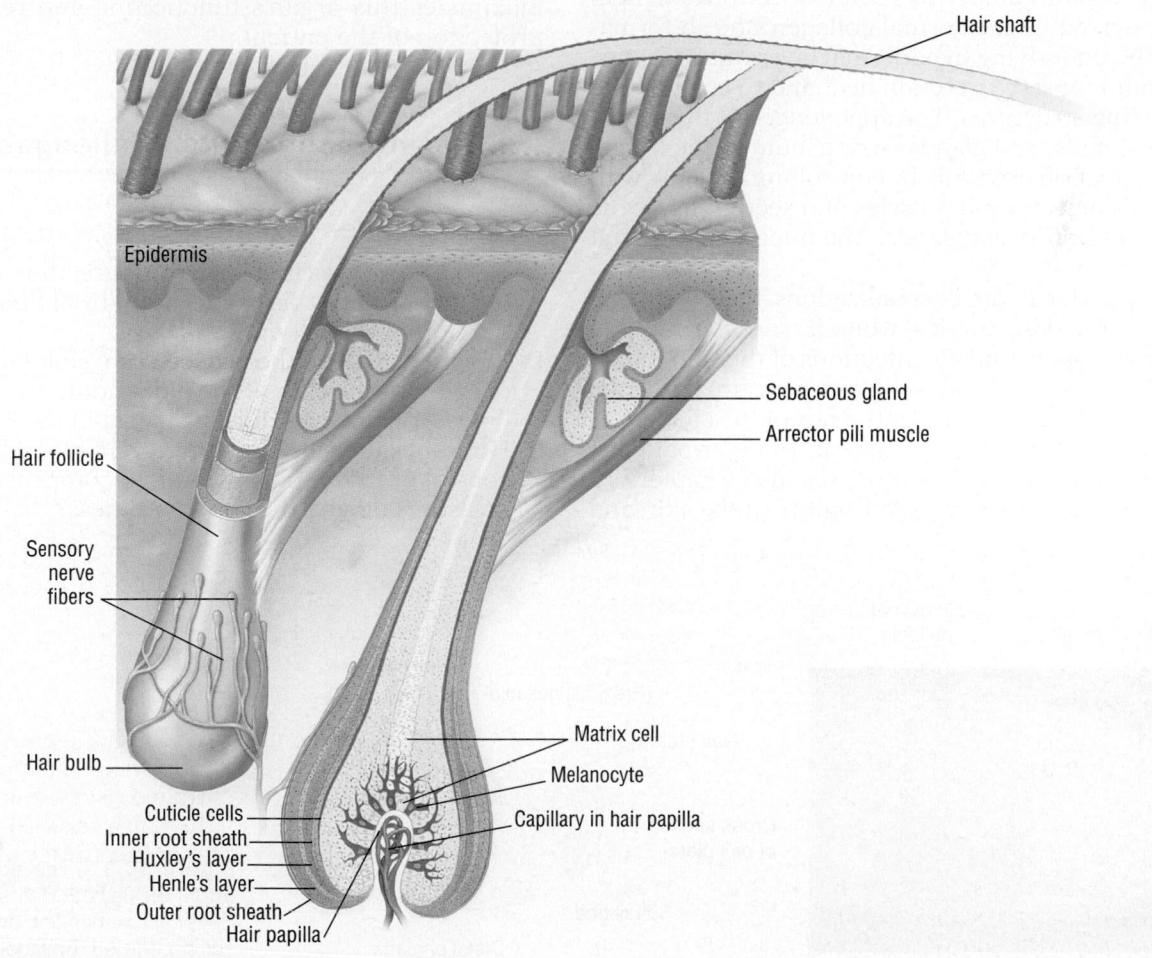

Figure 50-2 • Anatomical structures of hair. (From Anatomical Chart Company: Atlas of Human Anatomy. Springhouse, PA: Springhouse, 2001, p 329.)

NAILS

Hardened plates of epidermal keratin cells grow from a curved groove over the distal dorsal fingertips. These nails serve to protect the fingers and toes and increase physical dexterity. Approximately one fourth of the nail is covered by the proximal nail fold; the cuticle extends from the fold and serves to waterproof the space between the plate and the fold. The lunula is the white, half-moon–shaped edge distal to the cuticle. The angle between the proximal nail fold and the nail plate is expected to be less than 180 degrees (Fig. 50-3).

• Functions of the Skin

The epidermal layer of the integument provides protection against microbes, ultraviolet light, and countless other threats. This tough, hardened outer layer also restricts water loss and thus helps maintain homeostasis. The vascular dermis, with its rich supply of blood vessels, provides blood pressure and temperature regulatory features. Immune functions performed by macrophages, mast cells, T cells, and fibroblasts are also housed in the dermis. Nerve endings here supply receptors for heat, cold, touch, pressure, and pain. The skin's ability to stretch with movement is also provided by the dermal collagen's mesh formation. The underlying hypodermal layer of connective tissue and fat serve to retain heat and to cushion the underlying structures. The appendages of the skin—the hair, nails, and glands—contribute to the homeostatic function primarily by controlling heat loss with the hair's arrector pili muscles and secretions by the sebaceous and sweat glands. The integument is vital to a person's survival.

During critical care hospitalizations, there are many insults to the skin. Surgical wounds, vascular catheter insertions, opportunistic infections of the skin, nutritional compromise, and persistent pressure that leads to reduced blood flow are only a few of the challenges faced by the patient's integument. In older patients, age-related changes (Box 50-1; see also Chapters 12 and 51) leading to increased fragility of the skin and

Box 50-1 • Anatomical and Physiological Changes in the Integumentary System That Occur With Aging

- The skin becomes thinner, and there is a decrease in skin flexibility, placing the person at risk for epidermal tearing.
- The skin loses dermal elasticity, collagen, and mass, resulting in fine wrinkling, looseness, and sagging.
- The number of dermal blood vessels decreases; the vessels become thinner and more fragile, thus increasing the risk for bruising and hemorrhage.
- There is decreased density and activity of the eccrine and apocrine glands and decreased sebum production, resulting in dryness, itching, and decreased perspiration.
- Decreased peripheral circulation leads to slowed nail growth and brittle nails that split easily.
- Reduced hormone levels lead to thinning of the hair and transition from terminal to vellus hair.
- Decreased melanin leads to graying of the hair.
- Sun exposure over a long period of time leads to yellowing and thickening of the skin and the development of old age spots (solar lentigo).

slower healing magnify the effects of these insults. Attention to the skin and appendages by the nurse maximizes this organ's functioning and results in protection of the patient.

• Clinical Applicability Challenges

Short-Answer Questions

1. Patients in the critical care unit are often edematous. How does this excess interstitial fluid affect the skin of the patient?
2. In what ways are the expected physiological changes of the skin of the older adult exacerbated or worsened during critical illness?
3. How does the vascular supply and blood flow control of the skin contribute to compensatory measures during the stress of illness?

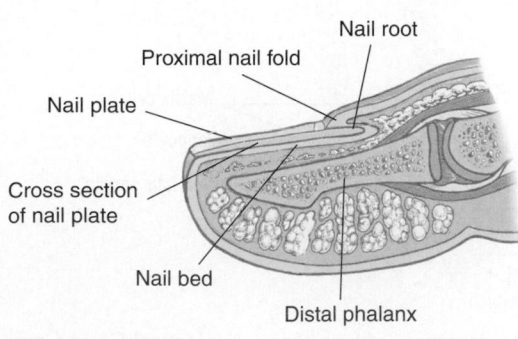

Lateral nail fold Lunula Proximal nail fold

Free edge Nail plate Cuticle

Nail root

Proximal nail fold

Nail plate

Cross section of nail plate

Nail bed

Distal phalanx

Figure 50-3 • The normal nail. (From Bickley LS: Bates' Guide to Physical Examination and History Taking, 9th ed. Philadelphia: Lippincott Williams & Wilkins, 2007, p 123.)

Review Questions

1. The purpose of secretions from the eccrine sweat glands is to
   a. provide an odor to attract and assist with recognition of others.
   b. help with internal body temperature regulation.
   c. lubricate the skin to prevent drying.
   d. assist with arrector pili muscle function.
2. Sebum, the secretion from the sebaceous glands, serves to
   a. protect the skin and hair from drying out.
   b. facilitate the elimination of cholesterol.
   c. maintain the health of melanocytes.
   d. control the arrector pili muscles.
3. The dermal layer of the skin
   a. protects against ultraviolet light exposure.
   b. controls apocrine sweat gland production.
   c. supports the immune system.
   d. serves as a storage for calories.
4. The fat of the hypodermal skin layer is important for
   a. heat retention by the body.
   b. the maintenance of blood supply to the epidermis.
   c. the synthesis of hormones.
   d. the production of macrophages.
5. Melanin is a pigment that provides for skin and hair color. In addition to color, what other purpose does melanin serve?
   a. Melanin also produces keratin.
   b. Melanin absorbs and scatters radiation.
   c. Melanin supports the vascular bed of the dermal layer.
   d. Melanin is thicker over the soles of the feet and palms of the hands to protect these surfaces.

References

1. Bickley LS, Szilagyi PG: The skin. In Bickley LS, Szilagyi PG (eds): Guide to Physical Examination and History Taking, 9th ed. Philadelphia: Lippincott Williams & Wilkins, 2007
2. Simandl G: Structure and function of the skin. In Porth CM (ed): Pathophysiology: Concepts of Altered Health States, 7th ed. Philadelphia: Lippincott Williams & Wilkins, 2005
3. Lewis SM, Heitkemper MM, Dirksen SR: Medical-Surgical Nursing: Assessment and Management of Clinical Problems, 6th ed. St. Louis: Mosby, 2004
4. Nicol NH: Dermatology nursing essentials: Anatomy and physiology of the skin. Dermatol Nurs 17(1):62, 2005
5. Wilson SF, Giddons JF: Skin, hair, and nails. In Wilson SF, Giddons JF (eds): Health Assessment for Nursing Practice, 2nd ed. St. Louis, Mosby, 2002, pp 257–287
6. Nicol HN, Huether, SE, Weber, R: Structure, function, and disorders of the integument. In McCance KL, Huether, SE (eds): Pathophysiology: The Biological Basis for Disease in Adults and Children, 5th ed. St. Louis: Mosby, 2006

Other Selected Readings

American Academy of Dermatology: Agingskinnet. Skincarephysicians.com (2005). Retrieved February 9, 2007, from http://www.skincarephysicians.com/agingskinnet/basicfacts.html
Hayes KVD: Skin wellness and illness. In Condon MC (ed): Women's Health. Upper Saddle River, NJ: Prentice-Hall, 2004
Johnstone CC, Harley A, Hendry C: The physiological basics of wound healing. Nurs Stand 19(43), 2005
Lawton S: Anatomy and function of the skin: Part 1. Nurs Times 102(31), 2006

51

Patient Assessment: Integumentary System

Joan M. Davenport • Janet A. Wulf

History
Physical Examination
  Inspection
  Palpation
Assessment of Pressure Ulcers
Assessment of Skin Tumors

Objectives

Based on the content in this chapter, the reader should be able to:

1 Discuss the health history and physical assessment skills necessary for the critical care nurse to use when evaluating the health of a patient's skin.

2 Explain expected differences in skin color related to racial or skin tone characteristics.

3 Describe and recognize abnormal changes in skin color.

4 Recognize and describe skin lesions resulting from increased vascularity.

5 Describe the significance of rashes related to infection or to allergic reaction.

6 Compare and contrast the pitting and nonpitting edema.

7 Explain the cause of pressure ulcers and the Braden scale used to assess a patient for pressure ulcer development.

8 Discuss the features of malignant skin diseases.

The skin of a critically ill person is exposed to insults ranging from diminished blood flow and the resultant risk for pressure ulceration to rashes from hypersensitivity drug reactions and opportunistic infections. There is often ample opportunity for the critical care nurse to assess the skin—the intimacy involved in providing care to someone who is critically ill, the relative level of undress of the patient, and the attention to detail implicit in critical care nursing make integument assessment an ongoing and vital process.

• History

When caring for patients with skin disorders, it is important to obtain information from the health history (Box 51-1). The information is useful in guiding the physical examination and in determining appropriate interventions.

• Physical Examination

The assessment techniques necessary for an evaluation of the integument involve inspection and palpation.

INSPECTION

Inspection of the general appearance of the skin includes assessment of color; determination of the presence of lesions, rashes, or increased vascularity; and assessment of the condition of the nails and hair.

Color

Skin color is expected to be uniform over the body, except for the areas with greater degrees of vascularity. The genitalia, upper chest, and cheeks may appear pink or have a reddish tone in people with light skin. These same areas may appear darker in people with dark skin. Additional normal variations in skin color include those listed in Table 51-1.

Skin color is determined by the presence of four pigments: melanin, carotene, hemoglobin, and deoxyhemoglobin. The amount of melanin is genetically determined and produces varying degrees of dark skin tone. Carotene, a yellow pigment, is in subcutaneous fat and is most evident in those areas with the most keratin, the palms and soles of the feet. Skin color abnormalities, such as pallor, cyanosis, jaundice, and erythema, manifest differently depending on the person's normal skin tone (Table 51-2).

The degree of oxygenation affects skin color. Hemoglobin, attached to red blood cells, transports

Box 51-1 • Integumentary System Health History

Chief Complaint
- Patient's description of the problem

History of the Present Illness
- Complete analysis of the following signs and symptoms (using the NOPQRST format; see Box 17-1)
- Changes in skin color, pigmentation, temperature, or texture
- Changes in a mole
- Excess dryness or moisture
- Skin itching
- Excess bruising
- Delay in healing
- Skin rash or lesions
- Hair loss or increased growth
- Changes in hair texture
- Changes in nails

Past Health History
- Relevant childhood illnesses and immunizations: impetigo, scabies or lice exposure, measles, chickenpox, scarlet fever
- Past acute and chronic medical problems including treatments and hospitalizations: diabetes, peripheral vascular disease, Lyme disease, Parkinson's disease, immobility, malnutrition, trauma, skin cancers, radiation treatments, HIV/AIDS
- Risk factors: age, ultraviolet sun exposure, tanning beds, exposure to dyes, toxic chemicals, insect bites, contact with some poisonous plants, autoimmune disease, exposure to extremes of temperature
- Past surgeries: skin biopsy
- Past diagnostic tests and interventions: allergy testing
- Medications: aspirin, antibiotics, barbiturates, sulfonamides, thiazide diuretics, oral hypoglycemic agents, tetracycline, antimalarials, antineoplastic agents, hormones, metals, topical steroids

- Allergies and reactions: foods, medications, contrast dyes, latex, soaps
- Transfusions

Family History
- Health status or cause of death of parents and siblings: skin cancer, autoimmune diseases

Personal and Social History
- Tobacco, alcohol, and substance use
- Family composition
- Occupation and work environment: farmers, roofers, creosote or coal workers, furniture repair and refinishing, gardeners
- Living environment: ability for self-care and hygiene, exposure to insects and pests, availability of indoor sleeping in environmental temperature extremes
- Diet
- Sleep patterns
- Exercise
- Cultural beliefs
- Spiritual/religious beliefs
- Coping patterns and social support systems
- Leisure activities
- Sexual activity
- Recent travel

Review of Systems
- Psychiatric/emotional: increased anxiety, nervousness, sleeplessness
- Neurologic: loss or decrease in sensation, numbness, pain or neuropathy, stroke
- Cardiovascular: swelling of extremities, cold extremities, varicose veins
- Gastrointestinal: change in diet, recent weight loss or gain, loss of appetite
- Musculoskeletal: immobility, weakness
- Metabolic: altered glucose levels

---

oxygen to the tissues. A diminished flow of oxyhemoglobin through the cutaneous circulation results in pallor. In people with light skin, the skin appears very pale, without the usual pink undertones. In people with darker skin, pallor manifests as a yellowish-brown or ashen appearance (again, because the usual pink undertones are lost).

As hemoglobin gives up its oxygen to the tissues, the hemoglobin changes to deoxyhemoglobin. When deoxyhemoglobin is present in the cutaneous circulation, the skin takes on a blue cast, and the person is said to be cyanotic.[1] In light-skinned people, cyanosis may be seen as a grayish-blue color, especially in the palms and soles of the feet, the nail beds, the earlobes, the lips, and the mucous membranes. In those with darker skin, cyanosis evidences itself as an ashen-gray color seen most easily in the conjunctiva, oral mucous membranes, and nail beds.[2]

The yellowish hue of jaundice is indicative of liver disease or of hemolysis of red blood cells. In dark-skinned people, jaundice is seen as a yellowish-green color in the sclera, palms of the hands, and soles of the feet. In light-skinned people, jaundice is seen as a yellow coloration of the skin, sclera, lips, hard palate, and underside of the tongue. Bickley and Szilagyi recommend using a transparent slide pressed against the lips to "blanch out the red color," making the yellow of jaundice more easily seen.[1]

Another skin color abnormality is erythema. Erythema manifests as a reddish tone in light-skinned

Table 51-1 • Normal Variations in Skin Color

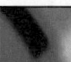

Normal Variation	Description
Moles (pigmented nevi)	Tan to dark brown; may be flat or raised
Stretch mark (striae)	Silver or pink; may be caused by weight gain or pregnancy
Freckles	Flat macules anywhere on the body
Vitiligo	Unpigmented skin area; more prevalent in people with dark skin
Birthmarks	Generally flat marks anywhere on the body; may be tan, red, or brown

Table 51-2 • Skin Color Abnormalities

Skin Color Abnormality	Underlying Cause	Manifestation in Light-Skinned People	Manifestation in Dark-Skinned People
Pallor	Decreased blood flow (decreased oxyhemoglobin flow to tissues)	Excessively pale skin	Yellowish-brown or ashen color to the skin
Cyanosis	Increased deoxyhemoglobin in the cutaneous circulation	Grayish-blue color of the palms and soles of the feet, the nail beds, the lips, the earlobes, and the mucous membranes	Ashen-gray color of the conjunctiva, oral mucous membranes, and nail beds
Jaundice	Increased red blood cell hemolysis, liver disease	Yellow color of the sclera, lips, and hard palate	Yellow-green color of the sclera and palms and soles of the feet
Erythema	Inflammation	Reddish tone	Deeper brown or purple tone

people and a deeper brown or purple tone in dark-skinned people. It is indicative of increased skin temperature caused by inflammation. The process of inflammation increases vascularity of the tissues, and this, in turn, produces the color alteration seen with erythema. Erythema may be expected when associated with a surgical wound, due to the inflammatory process inherent in any tissue trauma. It is also seen in disease processes affecting the skin, such as cellulitis. In either case, the erythema is indicative of inflammation.

Lesions

Skin lesions are variously described by their color, shape, cause, or general appearance (Tables 51-3 and 51-4). They are considered abnormal conditions and arise from many factors. In general, it is important to note the anatomical location, distribution, color, size, and pattern of any abnormal skin lesion (Fig. 51-1). In addition, details about the lesion's borders or edges, as well as whether the lesion is flat, raised, or sunken, should be noted. Finally, the length of time the lesion has been present and any environmental or medication exposure that may be considered contributory should also be noted.[3]

Vascular lesions can be either a normal variation or an abnormal finding. Vascular changes considered to be normal variants include nevus flammeus (port-wine stain), immature hemangioma (strawberry mark), telangiectasis, cherry angioma, and capillary hemangioma (Table 51-5). Abnormal vascular findings include petechiae, purpura, ecchymoses, spider angiomas, and urticaria (hives). These findings may indicate disease or injury and warrant further investigation by the critical care nurse.

Petechiae are purple or red, small (1- to 3-mm) lesions easily seen on light-skinned people and more difficult to see on those with dark skin (Fig. 51-2A). They may be seen on the oral mucosa and in the conjunctiva. They do not disappear when pressure is applied to them.[2] Petechiae result from tiny hemorrhages in the dermal or submucosal layers. Purpura

are very similar to petechiae, only larger. Purpura may appear brownish-red.

Ecchymoses are bruises. They may appear as purple to yellowish-green rounded or irregular lesions and are more easily seen in people with light skin (see Fig. 51-2B). Ecchymoses occur as a result of trauma, when blood leaks from damaged blood vessels into the surrounding tissue.

Spider angiomas are fiery red lesions that are most often located on the face, neck, arms, or upper trunk (see Fig. 51-2C). Spider angiomas are seldom seen below the waist. They have a central body that is sometimes "raised and surrounded by erythema and radiating legs."[1] These lesions are most often associated with liver disease and vitamin B deficiency.[2]

Urticaria is a reddened or white, raised, nonpitting plaque that often occurs as a result of an allergic reaction. The lesion often changes shape and size during the course of the reaction. The edema associated with urticaria is a result of local vasodilation and inflammation, which is followed by transudation of serous vascular fluid into the surrounding tissue.

Rashes

Rashes identified during inspection may indicate infection or a reaction to drug therapy. Some of these rashes are identified by the names listed in Table 51-3. Identifying the type of lesion may help in identifying the cause of the rash. Attention to the development of a rash in association with a change in pharmacotherapy is essential to help identify the occurrence of an allergic hypersensitivity reaction.[4] The development of urticaria is often associated with food or drug reactions. Urticaria usually resolves completely over days to several weeks as the excess local fluid is reabsorbed. These lesions are often pruritic, and patient scratching may precipitate secondary skin abrasions, which can place the patient at risk for localized skin infections.

Skin infections are most often caused by fungi or yeasts and may range from superficial tinea pedis (athlete's foot) to intermediate yeast infections (e.g.,

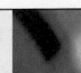

Table 51-3 • Primary Skin Lesions

Type	Description	Examples	Illustration
Macule	<1 cm in diameter, flat, non-palpable, circumscribed, discolored	Brown: freckle, junctional nevus, lentigo, melasma Blue: Mongolian spot, ochronosis Red: Drug eruption, viral exanthema, secondary syphilis Hypopigmented: vitiligo, idiopathic guttate hypomelanosis	*Macule*
Patch	<1 cm in diameter, flat, non-palpable, irregular shape, discolored	Brown: larger freckle, junctional nevus, lentigo, melasma Blue: Mongolian spot, ochronosis Red: Drug-eruption viral exanthema, secondary syphilis Hypopigmented: vitiligo, idiopathic guttate hypomelanosis	*Patch*
Papule	<1 cm in diameter, raised, palpable, firm	Flesh, white or yellow: flat wart, milium, sebaceous hyperplasia, skin tag Blue or violaceous: venous lake, lichen planus, melanoma Brown: seborrheic keratosis, melanoma, dermatofibroma, nevi Red: acne, cherry angioma, early folliculitis, psoriasis, urticaria, and eczema	*Papule*
Nodule	>1 cm, raised, solid	Wart, xanthoma, prurigo nodularis, neurofibromatosis	*Nodule*
Plaque	>1 cm, raised, superficial, flat-topped, rough	Psoriasis, discoid lupus, tinea corporis, eczema, seborrheic dermatitis	*Plaque*

(continued)

Table 51-3 • Primary Skin Lesions (Continued)

Type	Description	Examples	Illustration
Tumor	Large nodule	Metastatic carcinoma, sporotrichosis	Tumor
Vesicle	<1 cm, superficially raised, filled with serous fluid	Herpes simplex, herpes zoster, erythema multiforme, impetigo	Vesicle
Bulla	>1 cm vesicle	Pemphigus, herpes gestationis, fixed drug eruption	Bulla
Pustule	Raised, superficial, filled with cloudy, purulent fluid	Acne, candidiasis, rosacea, impetigo, folliculitis	Pustule
Wheal	Raised, irregular area of edema, solid, transient, variable size	Hives, cholinergic urticaria, angioedema, dermatographism	Wheal

(continued)

Table 51-3 • Primary Skin Lesions (Continued)

Type	Description	Examples	Illustration
Cyst	Raised, circumscribed, encapsulated with a wall and lumen, filled with liquid or semisolid	Digital mucus, epidermal inclusion, pilar	Cyst

From Rhoads J: Advanced Health Assessment and Diagnostic Reasoning. Philadelphia: Lippincott Williams & Wilkins, 2006, pp 81–83.

moniliasis resulting from *Candida albicans* infection) to deep fungal infections (e.g., aspergillosis) that invade the underlying tissues. Most often in the critical care setting, fungal and yeast infections are of the intermediate type and are the result of an opportunistic infection by normal flora. Antibiotics and corticosteroids place the patient at risk for these infections. Candidiasis presents in the groin and under the breasts of female patients with "erythema, a whitish pseudomembrane, and peripheral papules and pustules."[5] Oral candidiasis, also known as thrush, manifests as a whitish coating of the oral mucosa, especially the tongue. This painful condition may produce fissures on the tongue and often restricts a patient's oral intake, further compromising the patient from a nutritional perspective.

Condition of the Hair

The patient's terminal hair is inspected daily, noting the hair's quantity, distribution, and texture. Scalp hair should be resilient and evenly distributed.

Alopecia refers to hair loss and can be diffuse, patchy, or complete. Hair loss in the critical care setting can be associated with pharmacotherapy. Chemotherapy used in oncology treatment produces alopecia. Other drugs, such as heparin, used for a prolonged time may also be responsible for hair loss.[6] Hirsutism or increased facial, body, or pubic hair growth is an abnormal finding in the examination of women and children. Hirsutism has a familial pattern and is associated with menopause, endocrine disorders, and certain pharmacotherapies (e.g., corticosteroids and androgenic medications).[2]

A change in the hair's texture may indicate ongoing health concerns. Hair that is thin and brittle occurs in hypothyroidism. In those with severe protein malnutrition, the hair color may appear reddish or bleached, and the hair texture is described as coarse and dry.[7]

Also not to be overlooked is the presence of infection or infestation of the scalp and hair. The patient's scalp and body hair are inspected regularly

Table 51-4 • Secondary Skin Lesions

Type	Description
Crust	Dried exudates over a damaged epithelium; may be associated with vesicles, bullae, or pustules. Large adherent crust is a scab.
Erosion	Loss of superficial epidermis; does not extend to the dermis; may be associated with vesicles, bullae, or pustules.
Fissure	Crack in the epidermis usually extending into the dermis.
Keloid	Hypertrophied scar tissue; secondary to collagen formation during healing; elevated irregular and red; more common in African Americans.
Lichenification	Thickening and roughening of the skin; accentuated skin markings; may be secondary to repeated rubbing irritation and scratching.
Scale	Skin debris on the surface of the epidermis secondary to desquamated, dead epithelium. Color and texture vary.
Scar	Skin mark left after healing of wound or lesion that represents replacement by connective tissue of the injured tissue. Young scars are red or purple. Mature scars are white or glistening.
Ulceration	Loss of epidermis, extending into dermis or deeper. Bleeding and scarring are possible.

Adapted from Weber J, Kelley J: Health Assessment in Nursing, 3rd ed. Philadelphia: Lippincott Williams & Wilkins, 2006, pp 180–181.

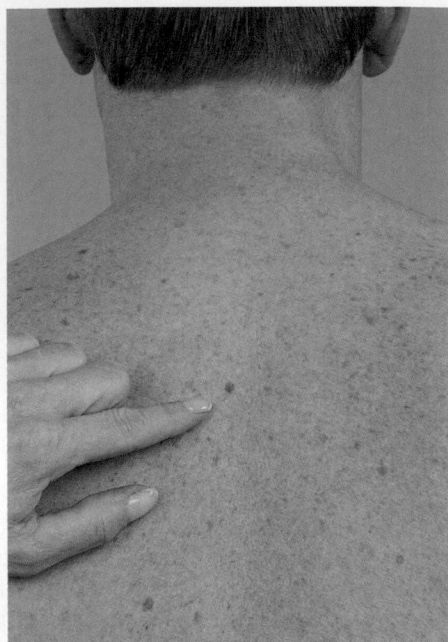

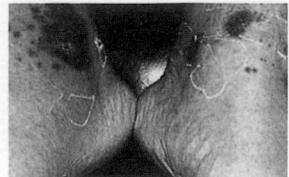
A. Petechiae/purpura

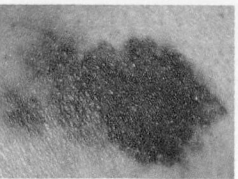
B. Ecchymosis

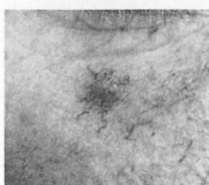
C. Spider angioma

Figure 51-2 • Abnormal vascular lesions. (**A,** from Kelley WN: Textbook of Internal Medicine. Philadelphia: JB Lippincott, 1989. **B,** from Bickley LS: Bates' Guide to Physical Examination and History Taking, 9th ed. Philadelphia: Lippincott Williams & Wilkins, 2003, p 141. **C,** from Marks R: Skin Disease in Old Age. Philadelphia: JB Lippincott, 1987.)

Figure 51-1 • Inspecting for lesions. (From Rhoads J: Advanced Health Assessment and Diagnostic Reasoning. Philadelphia: Lippincott Williams & Wilkins, 2006, p 76.)

for evidence of flaking, sores, lice, louse eggs, and ringworm.[7] During the inspection, the hair is parted in several areas to reveal the underlying scalp (Fig. 51-3).

Condition of the Nails

Nails, like hair, can be overlooked in the rush of critical care nursing; however, a careful inspection as part of the routine assessment can reveal information about the patient's general state of health. The nail bed is very vascular and is an excellent location for assessing the adequacy of the patient's peripheral circulation. The capillary refill test, done by blanching the nail beds and then releasing the pressure, should indicate a return of the pink tones in less than 3 seconds. Nail beds that are bluish or purplish in tint may be indicative of cyanosis; nail beds that are pale may indicate reduced arterial blood flow.

When the angle of the nail is 180 degrees or greater, clubbing is said to be present (see Chapter 24,

Fig. 24-2). Clubbing is attributed to chronic hypoxemia. Other shapes that the nail takes on may provide clues to deficient nutritional states of the patient (Fig. 51-4). A spoon-shaped nail, called koilonychias, is associated with iron-deficiency anemia.

Chronic disease states such as cirrhosis, heart failure, and type 2 diabetes mellitus may affect the nails by producing Terry's nails.[1] These nails are whitish with a distal band of dark reddish-brown color, and the lunulae may not be visible (Fig. 51-5). Bands across the nails, especially in the older adult, may indicate protein deficiency. White spots on the nails are associated with zinc deficiency.[7] Hyperkeratotic, dull, discolored, and distorted nails may be onychomycosis, a fungal infection of the nails seem frequently in critically ill patients. It is more common in toenails than fingernails. Risk factors include diabetes, poor venous and lymphatic drainage, poorly fitting shoes, and increasing age.[8]

PALPATION

The skin is palpated for texture, moisture, temperature, mobility and turgor, and edema (Fig 51-6). In

Table 51-5 • Vascular Lesions: Normal Variations

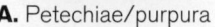

Normal Variation	Description
Nevus flammeus (port-wine stain), immature hemangioma (strawberry mark)	Range from dark red to pale pink in color and are considered birthmarks
Cherry angioma	Small, slightly raised, bright red lesions on the face, neck, and trunk; increase in size and number with advancing age
Capillary hemangioma	Red, irregular patch caused by capillary dilation in the dermis of the skin
Telangiectasis	Irregular, fine red lines caused by permanent dilation of a group of superficial vessels

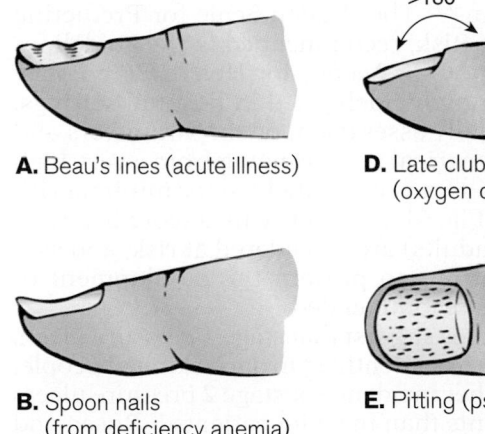

Figure 51-3 • Inspecting the scalp and hair. (From Weber J, Kelley J: Health Assessment in Nursing, 3rd ed. Philadelphia: Lippincott Williams & Wilkins, 2007, p 172. Copyright B. Proud.)

addition, any evidence of discomfort arising from the areas palpated is noteworthy.

Texture

Texture refers to the smoothness of the skin surface. It requires gentle palpation to assess. Rough skin occurs in patients with hypothyroidism.

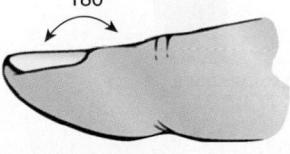
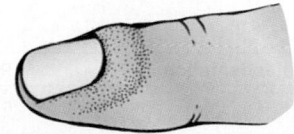

A. Beau's lines (acute illness)

B. Spoon nails (from deficiency anemia)

C. Early clubbing (oxygen deficiency) 180°

D. Late clubbing (oxygen deficiency) >180°

E. Pitting (psoriasis)

F. Paronychia (local infection)

Figure 51-4 • Common nail disorders. (From Weber J, Kelley J: Health Assessment in Nursing, 3rd ed. Philadelphia: Lippincott Williams & Wilkins, 2007, p 185.)

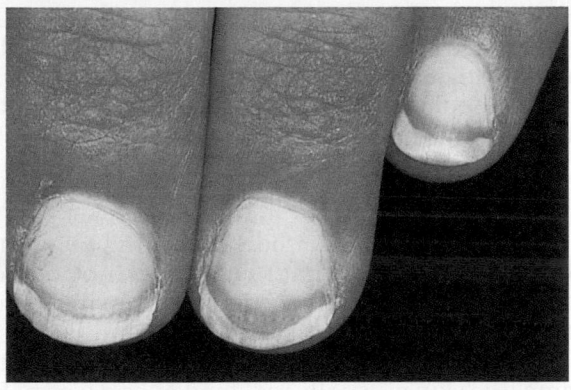

Figure 51-5 • Terry's nails, seen in people with chronic diseases such as cirrhosis, congestive heart failure, and type 2 diabetes mellitus. (From Bickley LS: Bates' Guide to Physical Examination and History Taking, 9th ed. Philadelphia: Lippincott Williams & Wilkins, 2007, p 150.)

Moisture

The skin may be described as dry, oily, diaphoretic, or clammy. Dry skin may be seen in the patient with hypothyroidism. Skin is oily with acne and with increased activity of the sebaceous glands, as in Parkinson's disease. Diaphoresis may be a response to increased temperature or increased metabolic rate. Hyperhidrosis is the term given to excessive perspiration. Bromhidrosis refers to foul-smelling perspiration. Low cardiac output states may produce skin that is referred to as clammy.

Temperature

Temperature is usually assessed with the dorsal surface of the hand to identify the general skin temperature as warm or cool. The skin's temperature can also be used to assess the possibility of reduced blood flow from an arterial insufficiency. In this case, the skin may be noticeably cooler distal to an occluding lesion.

Mobility and Turgor

Mobility and turgor provide information about the health of the skin and may yield information about the patient's fluid volume balance. When assessed

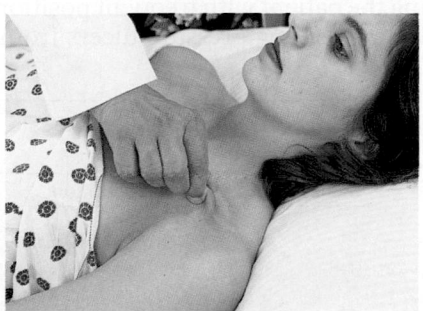

Figure 51-6 • Palpating to assess skin turgor and mobility. (From Weber J, Kelley J: Health Assessment in Nursing, 3rd ed. Philadelphia: Lippincott Williams & Wilkins, 2007, p 171. Copyright B. Proud.)

centrally, over the clavicles, the skin is expected to lift up easily and quickly return into place. Skin mobility may be decreased in scleroderma or in a patient with increased edema. Skin turgor is decreased in the patient with dehydration.[1]

Edema

Edema is classified as either nonpitting or pitting. Nonpitting edema is that which does not depress with palpation. Nonpitting edema is seen in patients with a local inflammatory response and is caused by capillary endothelial damage. In addition to the edema, the skin is usually red, tender, and warm. Pitting edema is usually in the skin of the extremities and in dependent body parts. Pitting edema is identified as edema that retains the depression made when palpated. This type of edema can be further classified by the depth of the depression and, occasionally, by the amount of time it takes the pit to rebound (Table 51-6).

• Assessment of Pressure Ulcers

The development of pressure ulcers in the critically ill patient is a preventable complication. The difficulty arises in the patient with multiple-system dysfunction with concomitant fluid, electrolyte, and nutritional deficiencies. Common pressure ulcer points include the occiput, scapula, sacrum, buttocks, ischium, heels, and toes. Pressure applied by the weight of the body causes a reduction in arterial and capillary blood flow, leading to these ischemic events. Therefore, frequent position changes are required to prevent the development of pressure ulcers. Pressure ulceration on the toes occurs as a result of the pressure of the bed linen on the feet. Dressing devices and wound appliances can place pressure on underlying skin, resulting in reduced blood flow. The back of the neck of the patient with a tracheostomy tube must be assessed because the tube holder may be applied too tightly. The tape securing a nasogastric tube must be regularly removed and the condition of the tip of the nose and nares assessed for changes resulting from pressure from the tube.

Assisting the patient with frequent position changes is crucial in preventing pressure ulcers from develop-

ing. In addition, keeping the skin clean and dry is requisite in the prevention of pressure ulceration. Moisture increases the risk for maceration of the skin and promotes its breakdown. Infectious matter in wound drainage or feces increases the risk that an ulcer will progress and become a major source of sepsis.

Patients with decreased sensation (e.g., from brain or spinal cord injury or from a peripheral neuropathy such as that caused by diabetes) are at greater risk for ulceration because they do not recognize the discomfort from being in one position for extended periods. Similarly, patients with sedation or frequent analgesic dosing are at increased risk for problems related to their immobility. Patients with poor circulation, such as that caused by hypotension, heart failure, or peripheral vascular insufficiency, are also at higher risk because of the underlying possibility of tissue hypoxia. Lack of movement then serves only to accelerate the process of pressure ulcer development.

Identifying those people most at risk for pressure ulcer development is a focus of assessment. Recognizing that there are certain features that increase a patient's risk for development of pressure ulcers allows the critical care nurse to increase surveillance and implement preventive treatment modalities. Problems with sensory perception, moisture, activity, mobility, nutrition, and friction and shearing forces increase the patient's risk for development of pressure ulcers, which are debilitating and expensive to treat. Critically ill patients are among those with the most significant limitations of these parameters, and therefore are at very high risk for the development of pressure ulcers.

Many tools for assessing pressure ulcer risk use a point system.[9,10] The Braden Scale for Predicting Pressure Sore Risk, recommended in the guidelines set forth by the U.S. Agency for Health Care Policy and Research and widely used in hospital settings, requires the daily assessment of six parameters and provides a numerical score ranging from a very high risk score of 6 to a very limited risk or minimal risk score of 23[11] (Fig. 51-7). Adults with a score below 16 (18 for older adults) are considered at risk, and specific interventions to prevent the development of ulceration are recommended.

Recent studies suggest that stage 1 pressure ulcers are less likely to be identified in dark-skinned people, leading to higher incidence of stage 2 pressure ulcers in black patients than in white patients.[12] Rosen and

Table 51-6 • Pitting Edema Scale

Scale	Description	Depth of Indentation	Return to Baseline
4+	Severe	8 mm	2–5 minutes
3+	Moderate	6 mm	1–2 minutes
2+	Mild	4 mm	10–15 seconds
1+	Trace	2 mm	Disappears rapidly

From Rhoads J: Advanced Health Assessment and Diagnostic Reasoning. Philadelphia: Lippincott Williams & Wilkins, 2006, p 253.

Braden Scale
FOR PREDICTING PRESSURE SORE RISK

Patient's Name_____ Evaluator's Name_____

Date of Assessment

SENSORY PERCEPTION Ability to respond meaningfully to pressure-related discomfort	1. Completely Limited: Unresponsive (does not moan, flinch, or grasp) to painful stimuli, due to diminished level of consciousness or sedation. OR limited ability to feel pain over most of body surface.	2. Very Limited: Responds only to painful stimuli. Cannot communicate discomfort except by moaning or restlessness. OR has a sensory impairment which limits the ability to feel pain or discomfort over 1/2 of body	3. Slightly Limited: Responds to verbal commands, but cannot always communicate discomfort or need to be turned. OR has some sensory impairment which limits ability to feel pain or discomfort in 1 or 2 extremities.	4. No Impairment: Responds to verbal commands. Has no sensory deficit which would limit ability to feel or voice pain or discomfort.	
MOISTURE Degree to which skin is exposed to moisture	1. Constantly Moist: Skin is kept moist almost constantly by perspiration, urine, etc. Dampness is detected every time patient is moved or turned.	2. Very Moist: Skin is often, but not always, moist. Linen must be changed at least once a shift.	3. Occasionally Moist: Skin is occasionally moist, requiring an extra linen change approximately once a day.	4. Rarely Moist: Skin is usually dry, linen only requires changing at routine intervals.	
ACTIVITY Degree of physical activity	1. Bedfast: Confined to bed	2. Chairfast: Ability to walk severely limited or nonexistent. Cannot bear own weight and/or must be assisted into chair or wheelchair.	3. Walks Occasionally: Walks occasionally during day, but for very short distances, with or without assistance. Spends majority of each shift in bed or chair.	4. Walks Frequently: Walks outside the room at least twice a day and inside room at least once every 2 hours during waking hours.	
MOBILITY Ability to change and control body position	1. Completely Immobile: Does not make even slight changes in body or extremity position without assistance.	2. Very Limited: Makes occasional slight changes in body or extremity position but unable to make frequent or significant changes independently.	3. Slightly Limited: Makes frequent though slight changes in body or extremity position independently.	4. No Limitations: Makes major and frequent changes in position without assistance.	
NUTRITION Usual food intake pattern	1. Very Poor: Never eats a complete meal. Rarely eats more than 1/3 of any food offered. Eats 2 servings or less of protein (meat or dairy products) per day. Takes fluids poorly. Does not take a liquid dietary supplement. OR is NPO and/or maintained on clear liquids or IVs for more than 5 days.	2. Probably Inadequate: Rarely eats a complete meal and generally eats only about 1/2 of any food offered. Protein intake includes only 3 servings of meat or dairy products per day. Occasionally will take a dietary supplement. OR receives less than optimum amount of liquid diet or tube feeding.	3. Adequate: Eats over half of most meals. Eats a total of 4 servings of protein (meat, dairy products) each day. Occasionally will refuse a meal, but will usually take a supplement if offered. OR is on a tube feeding or TPN regimen which probably meets most of nutritional needs.	4. Excellent: Eats most of every meal. Never refuses a meal. Usually eats a total of 4 or more servings of meat and dairy products. Occasionally eats between meals. Does not require supplementation.	
FRICTION AND SHEAR	1. Problem: Requires moderate to maximum assistance in moving. Complete lifting without sliding against sheets is impossible. Frequently slides down in bed or chair, requiring frequent repositioning with maximum assistance. Spasticity, contractures or agitation leads to almost constant friction.	2. Potential Problem: Moves feebly or requires minimum assistance. During a move skin probably slides to some extent against sheets, chair, restraints, or other devices. Maintains relatively good position in chair or bed most of the time but occasionally slides down.	3. No Apparent Problem: Moves in bed and in chair independently and has sufficient muscle strength to lift up completely during move. Maintains good position in bed or chair at all times.		

Braden Scale Scores 1 = Highly Impaired 3 or 4 = Moderate to Low Impairment Total Points Possible: 23 Risk Predicting Score: 16 or Less	NPO: IV: TPN:	Nothing by Mouth Intravenously Total parenteral nutrition	Total Score

Figure 51-7 • The Braden scale is a widely used screening tool to identify people at risk for pressure ulcers. (Courtesy of Barbara Braden and Nancy Bergstrom. Copyright, 1988. Reprinted with permission.)

colleagues found that an educational intervention for nursing home staff about pressure ulcer prevention eliminated the racial disparity and reduced overall incidence of pressure ulcers.[13]

During assessment of the skin, the nurse must be vigilant for signs of skin breakdown. The formation of pressure ulcers is illustrated in Figure 51-8.

• Assessment of Skin Tumors

Benign nevus and seborrheic keratosis are common, benign skin lesions. The benign nevus or mole appears in the first two to three decades, and its appearance remains unchanged over time. These lesions have clearly defined borders, are uniform in color, and are

Stage I. Skin is unbroken but appears red; no blanching when pressed.

Stage II. Skin is broken, and there is superficial skin loss involving the epidermis alone or also the dermis. The lesion resembles a vesicle, erosion, or blister.

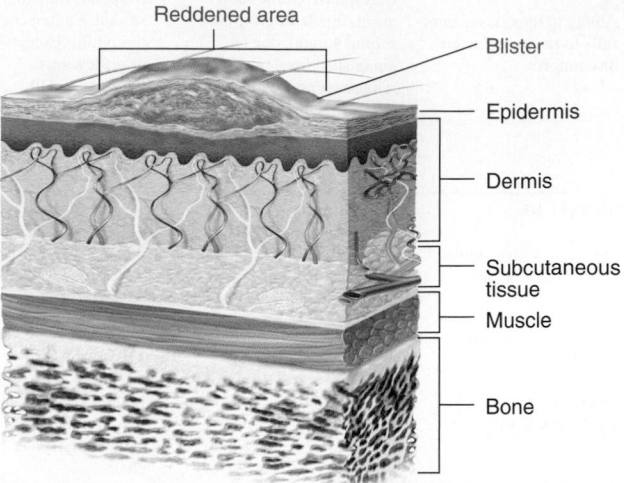

Stage III. Pressure area involves epidermis, dermis, and subcutaneous tissue. The ulcer resembles a crater. Hidden areas of damage may extend through the subcutaneous tissue beyond the borders of the external lesions but not through underlying fascia.

Stage IV. Pressure area involves epidermis, dermis, subcutaneous tissue, bone, and other support tissue. The ulcer resembles a massive crater with hidden areas of damage in adjacent tissue.

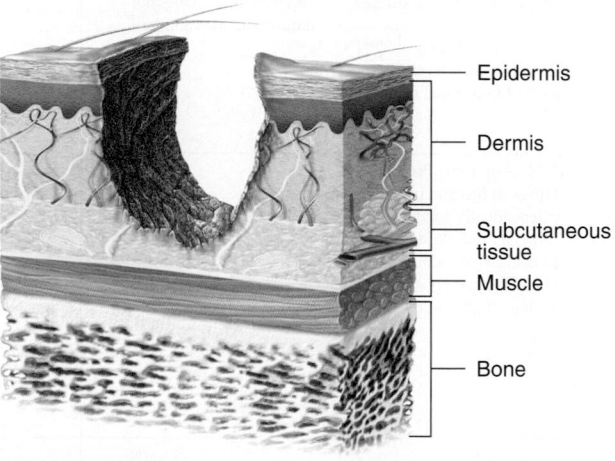
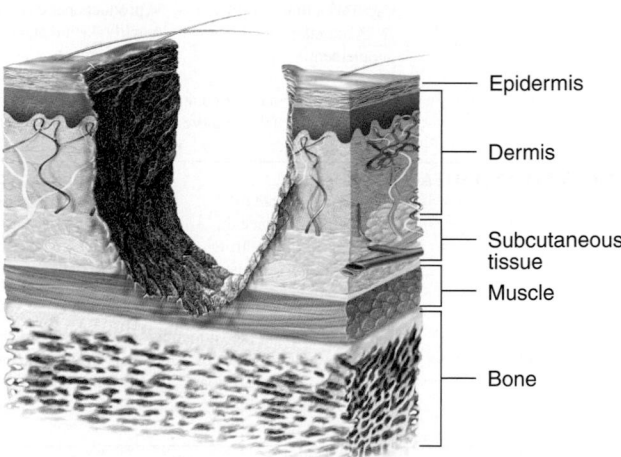

Figure 51-8 • Pressure ulcers: identifying stage. (From Weber J, Kelley J: Health Assessment in Nursing, 3rd ed. Philadelphia: Lippincott Williams & Wilkins, 2007, p 176.)

round or oval in shape. The nevus is periodically assessed for changes because a change may indicate dysplasia of the tissue and the risk for melanoma. Seborrheic keratoses are common, yellow to brown lesions that are described as velvety when touched (Fig. 51-9A). These lesions are often multiple and often symmetrically distributed on the trunk and face. Precancerous lesions (actinic keratoses) are thick, rough patches that develop on sun-exposed areas of the skin, especially in fair-skinned people (see Fig. 51-9B). They are described as dry, scaly, and rough

textured; however, not all actinic keratoses look alike.[14] The color may vary from brown to red to yellowish-black, or they may appear as red bumps or scaly patches. They are often described as feeling like sandpaper. These lesions require attention because there is a risk for development of squamous cell carcinoma.[14]

Skin cancer is the most common type of cancer in the United States. It is estimated that one in five people will be diagnosed with skin cancer in their lifetimes.[15] Basal cell and squamous cell cancers are often

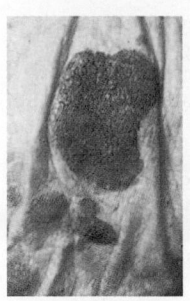 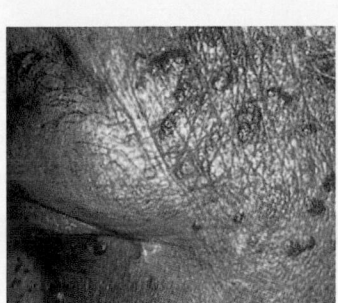 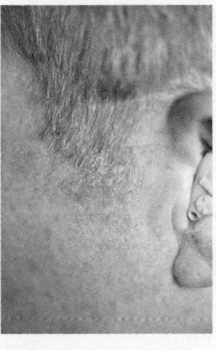 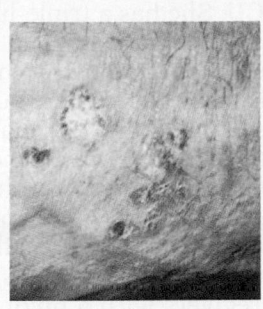 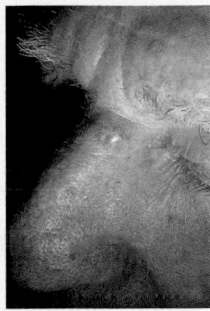

A. Seborrheic keratosis   **B.** Actinic keratosis   **C.** Basal cell carcinoma

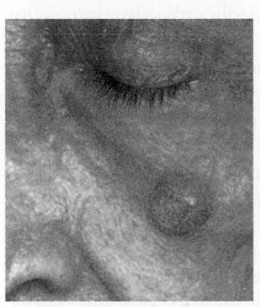 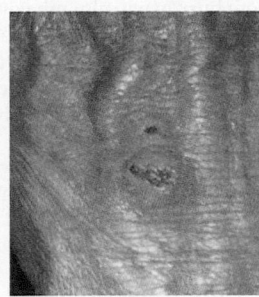 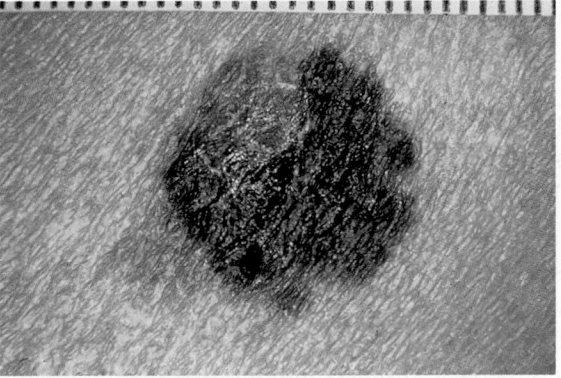

D. Squamous cell carcinoma   **E.** Malignant melanoma

Figure 51-9 • Benign, premalignant, and malignant skin lesions. (**A** and **D** from Hall JC: Sauer's Manual of Skin Diseases, 9th ed. Philadelphia: Lippincott Williams & Wilkins, 2007. **B** and **C** from Bickley LS: Bates' Guide to Physical Examination and History Taking, 9th ed. Philadelphia, Lippincott Williams & Wilkins, 2007, p 142. **E** from the American Cancer Society.)

grouped as nonmelanoma skin cancers. Basal cell carcinomas are found exclusively in light-skinned people and arise from the hair follicles on the head and neck. Prolonged and cumulative exposure to the sun is recognized as the cause of basal cell carcinoma. These tumors are slow growing and rarely metastasize but do cause local skin destruction and disfigurement. Basal cell carcinomas appear with pearly borders, depressed centers, and rolled edges[16] (see Fig. 51-9C).

Squamous cell carcinomas affect the skin and the mucous membranes. Like basal cell cancers, the primary cause is exposure to ultraviolet light. Radiation and tissue damage from scars, ulcers, and fistulas may give rise to squamous cell carcinomas. These cancers can be invasive and are more malignant than basal cell cancers if not treated promptly. As it develops, the carcinoma takes on a hyperkeratotic appearance and may ulcerate and bleed[15] (see Fig. 51-9D).

Malignant melanomas are highly metastatic lesions that come from the melanin-producing cells of the body. The worldwide frequency of malignant melanomas is growing more rapidly than for any other cancer except lung cancer. Those at highest risk include those with fair complexions, those prone to sunburn, and those with a family history of melanoma.[15] The most common location for the development of these lesions is on the trunk in men and on the legs in women. The tumors have irregular borders, are dark brown or black, and are usually larger than 6 mm (see

Fig 51-9E). The American Cancer Society (ACS) recommends a monthly self-assessment for melanoma using the "ABCDs."[17] A is for asymmetry; B is for borders (are they irregular, ragged, notched, or blurred?); C is for color (dark brown or black, red, white, or blue?); and D is for diameter.

Figure 51-9 provides pictures and descriptions of these benign, premalignant, and malignant lesions. While in a critical care setting, it is possible to perform a thorough assessment for suspect skin lesions that may be cancerous, refer the patient to a dermatologist or oncologist, and have treatment initiated much sooner than would otherwise be the case.

• Clinical Applicability Challenges

Case Study

Mrs. H., a 62-year-old widow, has been in the medical-surgical intensive care unit (ICU) for the past 2 weeks after a diagnosis of respiratory failure and pneumonia. Her medical history includes obesity, type 2 diabetes mellitus, and chronic obstructive pulmonary disease. She has been intubated and on mechanical ventilation. She has received continuous enteral feedings through a nasogastric tube, numerous antibiotics, and dopamine for blood pressure support during her first 3 days in the ICU. She has a triple-lumen central venous access catheter.

Mrs. H. is scheduled for a tracheostomy tomorrow, and she will also have a percutaneous gastric feeding tube inserted at that time. She has a continuous bladder catheter and an incontinence fecal bag in place draining liquid stool. Over the past 5 days, she has received a benzodiazepine for sedation at least once per day. Physical therapy consultation was made on day 3, and she is assisted by two caregivers with a pivot to a chair twice each day. Her family visits daily and helps her communicate with a pencil and paper tablet.

1. What factors place Mrs. H. at increased risk for developing pressure ulcers?
2. What are Mrs. H.'s risk factors related to compromised integument that may lead to infection?

Review Questions

1. The patient with the highest risk for pressure ulcers is one that is
   a. postcardiac surgery, ventilated, and sedated, previously ambulatory.
   b. diabetic, sedated, and on a ventilator with low serum albumin.
   c. diabetic, elderly, and ambulatory with assistance.
   d. sedated, on a ventilator, with nasogastric tube feedings.

2. A patient has scratched through the epidermis, leaving bleeding, eroded patches. These lesions would best be described as being
   a. urticaria.
   b. petechiae.
   c. wheals.
   d. excoriation.

3. Jaundice in a dark-skinned patient can best be assessed
   a. by liver function tests.
   b. as a yellowish-brown color in the oral mucosa.
   c. as a yellowish-green color in the sclera, palms of the hands, and soles of the feet.
   d. as an ashen-gray color in the conjunctiva, mucous membranes, and nail beds.

4. Spider angiomas are most often
   a. precancerous lesions.
   b. on the skin of the legs and lower torso.
   c. associated with zinc deficiency.
   d. on the skin of the upper torso, face, and arms.

5. A critical care nurse has the opportunity to perform regular, thorough skin assessments on patients. What signs should be referred for further examination?
   a. White, scaly patches on head and arms
   b. Small ecchymotic patches in an elderly patient
   c. An unpigmented skin area on a dark-skinned patient
   d. Silver or pink striae on torso or limbs

References

1. Bickley LS, Szilagyi PG: The skin. In Bickley LS (ed): Guide to Physical Examination and History Taking, 9th ed. Philadelphia: Lippincott Williams & Wilkins, 2007
2. Wilson SF, Giddons JF: Skin, hair, and nails. In Wilson SF, Giddons JF (eds): Health Assessment for Nursing Practice, 2nd ed. St. Louis: Mosby, 2002
3. Jarvis C: Skin, hair and nails. In Jarvis C (ed): Physical Examination and Health Assessment, 4th ed. St. Louis: Saunders Elsevier, 2004
4. Medsafe: Information for health professionals, prescriber update articles: Drug Hypersensitivity Syndrome. 2003. Retrieved January 30, 2007, from http://www.medsafe.govt.nz/profs/PUarticles/DHS.htm
5. Stawiski MA, Price SA: Cutaneous infections. In Price SA, Wilson LM (eds): Pathophysiology, 6th ed. St. Louis: Mosby, 2003, pp 1087–1096
6. MedlinePlus. Heparin (Systemic). 2006. Retrieved February 5, 2007, from http://www.nlm.nih.gov/medlineplus/druginfo/drug_Ha.html
7. Kozier B, Erb G, Berman AJ, Snyder S: Health assessment. In Kozier B, Erb G, Berman AJ, Snyder S (eds): Fundamentals of Nursing, 7th ed. Upper Saddle River, NJ: Prentice-Hall, 2004, pp 531–629
8. American Pediatric Medical Association: Nail problems. 2007. Retrieved October 18, 2007, from http://www.apma.org/s_apma/doc.asp
9. Bergstrom N, Braden BJ, Laguzza A, et al: The Braden scale for predicting pressure sore risk. Nurs Res 36:205–210, 1987
10. Gosnell DJ: An assessment tool to identify pressure sores. Nurs Res 22(1):55, 1973
11. Agency for Health Care Policy and Research, Panel for the Prediction and Prevention of Pressure Ulcers in Adults: Pressure Ulcers in Adults: Prediction and Prevention. Clinical Practice Guideline no. 3, AHCPR publication no. 92-0047. Rockville, MD: Agency for Health Care Policy and Research, Public Health Service, U.S. Department of Heath and Human Services, 1992
12. Baumgarten M, Margolis, D, van Doorn C, et al: Black/white differences in pressure ulcer incidence in nursing home residents. J Am Geriatr Soc 52:1293–1298, 2004
13. Rosen J, Mittal V, Degenholtz H, et al: Pressure ulcer prevention in black and white nursing home residents: A QI initiative of enhanced ability, incentives and management feedback. Adv Skin Wound Care 19(5)262–269, 2006
14. National Cancer Institute: What you need to know about skin cancer? 2002. Retrieved January 30, 2007, from http://www.cancer.gov/cancertopics/wyntk/skin
15. American Academy of Dermatology. In Skincarephysicans.com. 2005. Retrieved January 31, 2007, from http://www.skincarephysicians.com
16. Huether SE: Structure, function, and disorders of the integument. In McCance KL, Huether SE (eds): The Biological Basis for Disease in Adults and Children, 4th ed. St. Louis: Mosby, 2002, pp 1434–1468
17. American Cancer Society: Detecting skin cancer. 2003. Retrieved January 30, 2007, from http://www.cancer.org

Other Selected Readings

Cuzzell JZ: Wound assessment and evaluation: Pressure ulcer protocol. Dermatol Nurs 15(1):56, 2003
Finch A: Assessment of skin in older people: As the largest organ in the body, the skin can offer valuable information about the general health of an older person. Nurs Older People 15(2):29, 2003
Hayes KVD: Skin wellness and illness. In Condon MC (ed): Women's Health. Upper Saddle River, NJ: Prentice-Hall, 2004
Scott EM, Buckland R: Pressure ulcer risk in the peri-operative environment. Nurs Stand 20(7):74–86, 2005
Strayer SM, Reynolds P: Diagnosing skin malignancy: Assessment of predictive clinical criteria and risk factors. J Fam Pract 53:210, 2003
Worley CA: The new (or at least newer) kids on the block: New technology in wound care. Dermatol Nurs 17(5):377, 380, 2005

Patient Management: Integumentary System

52

Susan Luchka

Objectives

Based on the content in this chapter, the reader should be able to:

❶ Define specific terms related to wounds: *acute wound*, *chronic wound*, *partial thickness*, *full thickness*, *stages of wound healing*.

❷ Explain the normal healing process.

❸ Describe what is meant by *primary intention*, *secondary intention*, and *tertiary intention*.

❹ Describe nursing care for the patient with a wound.

❺ Discuss the influence of nutrition and pharmacotherapeutics on wound healing.

• Types of Wounds

A wound is simply a break in skin integrity. Wounds may be acute or chronic. An acute wound is a wound that follows an orderly, sequential healing process, resulting in an area that has anatomical and functional integrity.[1,2] Acute wounds are caused by surgery or trauma. Conversely, a chronic wound fails to yield an area that has anatomical and functional integrity. Chronic wounds fail to follow an orderly, sequential process due to precipitating factors such as diabetes, pressure, malnutrition, peripheral vascular disease, immune deficiencies, and infection.[1,2] An acute wound may become a chronic wound at any time.

Acute and chronic wounds may be defined as partial- or full-thickness wounds. Partial-thickness wounds involve the epidermis and may involve the dermis. A partial-thickness wound is a shallow wound that is usually moist and painful (because the loss of the epidermis exposes the nerve endings). Full-thickness wounds involve the loss of the epidermis, dermis, and subcutaneous tissue, and they may involve muscle, tendons, ligaments, and bone. A full-thickness wound involves a large amount of tissue loss and appears as a crater or crevice.

Pressure ulcers and leg ulcers are two specific types of wounds that may be seen in the critical care setting. Critically ill patients are at risk for developing pressure ulcers due to hemodynamic factors, disease processes, immobility, and nutritional deficits. Leg ulcers are due to specific disease processes. Both pressure ulcers and leg ulcers may complicate the critically ill patient's overall recovery.

PRESSURE ULCERS

Pressure ulcers are wounds caused by pressure, shearing, and friction. Pressure ulcers start as acute wounds but become chronic in patients with other risk factors. Risk factors for the development of pressure ulcers include prolonged and impaired mobility, incontinence, malnutrition, diabetes, spinal cord injuries, metastatic cancers, decreased level of consciousness, impaired mental status, and peripheral vascular disease.[1,2] A patient teaching guide for pressure ulcers is shown in Box 52-1.

Pressure ulcers are the only type of wound that is staged. Staging occurs when the wound is assessed and documented.

► Stage I is defined as nonblanchable erythema of intact skin. In patients with darker skin, the stage I pressure ulcer may be red, blue, or purple. It may be accompanied by hardness, induration, and edema.

Box 52-1 • TEACHING GUIDE:
Pressure Ulcers

- Pressure ulcers are also known as *pressure sores* or *bed sores*.
- Pressure ulcers occur in people who have trouble moving around easily.
- At first, a pressure ulcer is just a reddened, tender area. If pressure is not relieved, the skin in this area may break down (open up or pull off, forming a blistered area). Pressure ulcers can destroy the underlying muscles, bone, ligaments, and tendons if they are not treated.
- Risk factors for pressure ulcers include difficulty moving around, medical problems (such as diabetes), spinal cord injury, incontinence of urine and stool, surgeries that limit mobility for an extended period (such as hip or knee replacement surgery), poor nutrition, and poor hydration (decreased fluid intake).
- Pressure ulcers occur most frequently over bony prominences (e.g., heels, sacral area, hips, and shoulder blades), but they can occur anywhere on the body where there is constant pressure that is unrelieved.
- Many times, pressure ulcers can be prevented by turning the person in bed at least every 2 h and by placing a pillow under the person's ankles to keep the heels off the bed, thus relieving pressure. A specialty bed may also be used to decrease pressure.
- *Not all pressure ulcers can be prevented.* The person's medical condition, nutrition and hydration status, immune status, and overall health status are all factors that affect the person's risk for developing pressure ulcers.
- Treatment depends on the type of pressure ulcer and the person's health status.

► Stage II involves partial-thickness tissue loss and presents as a blistered or denuded area (a shallow open wound).
► Stage III is a full-thickness wound involving the subcutaneous tissue and presents as a crater.
► Stage IV is also a full-thickness wound involving a large amount of tissue loss. A stage IV wound extends through the subcutaneous tissue and deep into the fascia, involving muscle, bone, ligament, or tendon.

Reverse staging is inappropriate. The tissue that fills in the wound bed is not the same as the tissue that has been lost. Lost muscle or subcutaneous tissue cannot be replaced. Therefore, it is appropriate to document "healing stage IV wound," but it is not appropriate to document "stage IV wound now stage III."

Pressure ulcers covered by eschar are considered unstageable. Eschar prevents the assessment of the wound bed. Documentation is "unstageable, wound covered by eschar." If the wound is débrided, it may then be staged.

The standards of care for pressure ulcers are established by the Agency for Healthcare Research and Quality (AHRQ), formerly known as the Agency for Health Care Policy and Research (AHCPR), committee. The AHRQ is part of the U.S. Department of Health and Human Services. The AHRQ publishes Clinical Practice Guidelines and a patient reference booklet on pressure ulcers. These guidelines are the basis for individual institutions' policies and procedures. The AHRQ guidelines address the economic impact of pressure ulcers and establish the basic standards for assessment, turning, dressings, wound cleansers, treatment of infections, operative repair, quality improvement, and education. In addition, the AHRQ guidelines include a glossary, an extensive reference list, clinical algorithms, and research methodology. The AHRQ guidelines are the gold standard for individual institution guidelines, journal articles, and other publications.

The Wound Ostomy and Continence Nurses Society (WOCN) has expanded the AHRQ standards through evidenced-based practice. The WOCN issues clinical practice guidelines that apply evidence-based practice, new research and drugs, and the original AHRQ standards. WOCN guidelines specific to wound care are:

► Guidelines for Management of Wounds in Patients with Lower Extremity Arterial Disease (2002)
► Guideline for the Prevention and Management of Pressure Ulcers (2003)
► Management of Wounds in Patients with Lower-Extremity Neuropathic Disease (2004)
► The V.A.C. Therapy Clinical Guidelines (2007)

LEG ULCERS

Leg ulcers are chronic wounds seen frequently in critically ill patients with underlying health problems, such as venous stasis ulcers, arterial ulcers, and diabetic foot ulcers. Although patients with leg ulcers may have a high risk for pressure ulcers, leg ulcers are not pressure ulcers and are not staged.

Venous Stasis Ulcers

Venous stasis ulcers are usually found on the medial aspect of the lower leg, superior to the medial malleolus.[1,2] The wound margins are irregular and present as shallow craters, and the wound margins and lower leg may have a ruddy appearance or hemosiderin staining.[1,2] The drainage from venous stasis ulcers may vary from mild to heavy. The primary treatment for venous stasis ulcers is compression therapy using an Unna boot or a multiple-wrap dressing.[1,2] Multiple-wrap dressings have the advantage of continuous compression, which may not be achieved with the Unna boot. The affected leg is elevated above heart level to decrease edema (edema impedes the healing process).

Arterial Ulcers

Arterial ulcers (ischemic ulcers) are usually found on the distal leg, medial malleoli, and dorsal aspect of the foot and toes.[1,2] The wound margins of arterial ulcers are round, smooth (*not* irregular), and frequently described as having a punched-out appearance.[1,2] Arterial ulcers have pale wound beds and may be shallow or deep. The affected leg may be cool to the touch, cyanotic, and pale with minimal hair distribution. The patient experiences increased pain to the affected area if the leg is elevated.[1,2] The primary dressing for arterial leg ulcers is an occlusive dressing. Healing does not occur unless the vascular deficit is addressed surgically.

Diabetic Foot Ulcers

Diabetic foot ulcers are found in patients with diabetes and are frequently not recognized early, owing to the patient's accompanying neuropathy. The primary locations for diabetic foot ulcers are the plantar aspect of the foot, heels, and metatarsals.[1,2] To promote wound healing, a dressing that provides a moist environment is used most often. The ulcer area usually needs débridement and must be assessed carefully for infection. Other treatment modalities include off-loading the patient's weight using special shoes. Osteomyelitis is always a concern in patients with diabetic foot ulcers. Healing is prolonged because of the diabetes. Therefore, it is important to aggressively manage the diabetes to promote an optimal healing environment.

SKIN TEARS

Skin tears (partial-thickness wounds) are acute wounds secondary to the removal of tape or transparent occlusive dressings. Skin tears occur when the skin is thin and fragile. Fragile skin may be due to age, disease process, nutritional status, drug therapy (i.e., steroids), or a combination of these factors. The skin is so fragile that it literally tears as tape or plastic film dressings are removed.

It is a common misconception that plastic film dressings, Steri-Strips, or wound adhesives should be applied to skin tears. Plastic film dressings and Steri-Strips potentiate more skin tears as they are removed or become dislodged. Because it is difficult to approximate the wound margins in a skin tear, wound adhesive frequently drips into the wound bed, prolonging the healing process and promoting infection.

Skin tears are cleansed gently with normal saline (or other institution-approved cleanser). Care is taken not to create a larger skin tear. After the wound area is cleansed, a hydrogel is applied to the wound and covered with a nonadherent dressing. Then the wound is wrapped with Kling or Coban to hold the dressing in place without using tape on the skin. It is important to minimize the use of adhesives in all forms for patients prone to skin tears.

• Wound Healing

CONCEPTS in action **ANIMATI😳N**

PHASES OF WOUND HEALING

Optimal wound healing occurs in a moist (not extremely wet or dry) environment. The wound healing process is composed of three phases (Fig. 52-1).

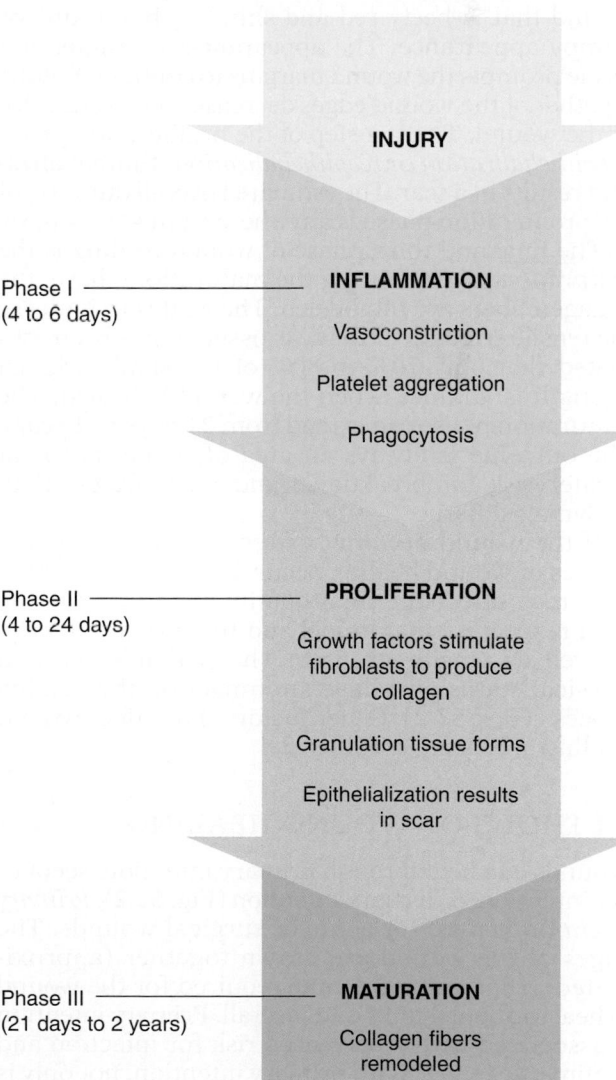

Figure 52-1 • The stages of wound healing.

The first phase is the *inflammatory phase*, which occurs immediately after the wound occurs. At the time of injury, there is immediate vasoconstriction; this is the body's way of controlling bleeding. Once vasoconstriction occurs, platelets collect at the site and deposit fibrin to form a clot. The vasoconstriction is holding the wound together, and the platelets with their fibrin clot formation essentially "plug the hole." Phagocytosis also occurs during the inflammatory phase. Phagocytosis is the release of macrophages at the site of injury to destroy any bacteria that may be present and to remove the wound's cellular debris. This is the body's way of providing the optimal environment for wound healing (i.e., a clean wound bed). It is at this time that growth factors are also present at the site of the injury. Overall, the inflammatory phase is estimated to last between 4 and 6 days. Visual assessment of the wound during the inflammatory phase reveals a wound with erythema, edema, and pain.

The second phase of wound healing is the *proliferation phase*. Growth factors stimulate the fibroblast to produce collagen. Collagen, along with new blood vessels and connective tissue, creates granulation tissue. Visual assessment of the wound at this point reveals a wound that is beefy red and shiny with a grainy or bumpy appearance. The appearance of granulation tissue prompts the wound margins to contract. Pulling together of the wound edges decreases the overall size of the wound. The last step of the proliferation phase is *epithelialization* or *reepithelialization*. Epithelialization results in a scar. The estimated overall duration of the proliferation phase is anywhere from 4 to 24 days.

The final and third phase of wound healing is the *maturation phase*. During the maturation phase, the collagen fibers are remodeled. The goal is to increase the tensile strength of the scar tissue. It has been estimated that only 70% to 80% of the skin's original strength is attained when the wound is healed. The maturation phase can extend from 21 days to 2 years. The outcome is always an area of tissue that is at greater risk for breakdown and more fragile than undamaged tissue.

If the wound becomes extremely wet or dry, the phases of wound healing occur, but at a slower rate. This may affect the final quality of the scar tissue with respect to anatomical and functional integrity as well as tensile strength. The patient's age and physical status also have an impact on the healing process (Box 52-2). Other factors that affect wound healing are listed in Table 52-1.

METHODS OF WOUND HEALING

Wounds can heal through primary intention, secondary intention, or tertiary intention (Fig. 52-2). *Primary intention* is used for acute or surgical wounds. The edges of the wound are drawn together (approximated), shortening the time required for the wound to heal to about 4 to 14 days overall. Primary intention is associated with a decreased risk for infection and minimal scarring. With primary intention, not only is scarring minimal and the risk for infection decreased, but the amount of tissue loss is decreased.

Box 52-2 • CONSIDERATIONS FOR THE OLDER PATIENT: Factors That Affect Wound Healing

- Less subcutaneous tissue
- More fragile skin secondary to age and drug therapy
- Increased number of precipitating risk factors for pressure ulcers
- Increased number of precipitating risk factors for chronic wounds
- Nutrition: less than or more than body requirements
- Decreased ability to care for self with age
- Decreased immune system function
- Decreased pulmonary and cardiovascular function
- Increased potential for incontinence (urine and stool)

Secondary intention is seen most frequently in chronic wounds but can occur in acute wounds, when the wound edges cannot be approximated to each other due to a significant tissue loss. An example of secondary intention is a pressure ulcer or a venous stasis ulcer. The potential for infection is increased because of the inability to approximate the edges, thus leaving the area open to bacteria. Scarring may also be significant, depending on the amount of tissue loss.

The last form of wound repair is *tertiary intention*, which may also be called *delayed primary intention*. Tertiary (delayed primary) intention should not be confused with primary intention. With this type of wound healing, the wound is not closed for a period (usually 3 to 5 days) to allow infection, edema, or both, to resolve. During this time, the wound is packed or irrigated to remove exudate and cellular debris. When the edema and risk for infection have decreased, the wound edges are approximated and the wound is closed as it is in primary intention. Scarring is usually greater than that seen with primary intention but less than that seen with secondary intention.

• Wound Assessment

Wound assessment is done in an orderly, sequential manner (Box 52-3).

The location of the wound is defined as precisely as possibly using anatomical terminology (e.g., "medial aspect of the left lower leg, 10 cm distal to the knee"). Using correct anatomical terminology allows other health care professionals to visualize the location of the wound. Correct location is especially important if the patient has more than one wound.[1–3] Photography may be used, more frequently in chronic wounds than in acute wounds. Factors to consider when using photography are lighting consistency and distance. To portray the wound accurately, room lighting and distance from the wound must be as identical as possible from one photograph to another.

The size of the wound should always be measured in centimeters, millimeters, or both.[2,4] Terminology

Table 52-1 • Factors Affecting Wound Healing

Factors	Rationale	Nursing Interventions
Age of patient	The older the patient, the less resilient the tissues.	Handle all tissues gently.
Handling of tissues	Rough handling causes injury and delayed healing.	Handle tissues carefully and evenly.
Hemorrhage	Accumulation of blood creates dead spaces as well as dead cells that must be removed. The area becomes a growth medium for organisms.	Monitor vital signs. Observe incision site for evidence of bleeding and infection.
Hypovolemia	Insufficient blood volume leads to vasoconstriction and reduced oxygen and nutrients available for wound healing.	Monitor for volume deficit (circulatory impairment). Correct by fluid replacement as prescribed.
Local factors Edema	Reduces blood supply by exerting increased interstitial pressure on vessels.	Elevate part; apply cool compresses.

Inadequate dressing technique
    Too small
    Too tight
	Permits bacterial invasion and contamination
	Reduces blood supply carrying nutrients and oxygen
		Follow guidelines for proper dressing technique.

Nutritional deficits	Protein-calorie depletion may occur. Insulin secretion may be inhibited, causing blood glucose to rise.	Correct deficits; this may require parenteral nutritional therapy. Monitor blood glucose levels. Administer vitamin supplements as prescribed.
Foreign bodies	Foreign bodies retard healing.	Keep wounds free of dressing threads and talcum and powder from gloves.
Oxygen deficit (tissue oxygenation insufficient)	Insufficient oxygen may be due to inadequate lung and cardiovascular function as well as localized vasoconstriction.	Encourage deep breathing, turning, controlled coughing.
Drainage accumulation	Accumulated secretions hamper healing process.	Monitor closed drainage systems for proper functioning. Institute measures to remove accumulated secretions.

Medications
  Corticosteroids
 	
  Anticoagulants
  Broad-spectrum
    and specific antibiotics
	May mask presence of infection by impairing normal inflammatory response
	May cause hemorrhage
	Effective if administered immediately before surgery for specific pathology or bacterial contamination. If administered after wound is closed, ineffective because of intravascular coagulation.
		Be aware of action and effect of medications patient is receiving.

Patient overactivity	Prevents approximation of wound edges. Resting favors healing.	Use measures to keep wound edges approximated: taping, bandaging, splints. Encourage rest.

Systemic disorders
  Hemorrhagic shock
  Acidosis
  Hypoxia
  Renal failure
  Hepatic disease
  Sepsis
	These depress cell functions that directly affect wound healing.	Be familiar with the nature of the specific disorder. Administer prescribed treatment. Cultures may be indicated to determine appropriate antibiotic.

Immunosuppressed state	Patient is more vulnerable to bacterial and viral invasion; defense mechanisms are impaired.	Provide maximum protection to prevent infection. Restrict visitors with colds; institute mandatory hand hygiene by all staff.

Wound stressors
  Vomiting
  Valsalva maneuver
  Heavy coughing
  Straining
	Produce tension on wounds, particularly of the torso.	Encourage frequent turning and ambulation and administer antiemetic medications as prescribed.
		Assist patient in splinting incision.

From Smeltzer SC, Bare BG, Hinkle JL, Cheever KH: Brunner & Suddarth's Textbook of Medical–Surgical Nursing, 11th ed. Philadelphia: Lippincott Williams & Wilkins, 2008, p 541.

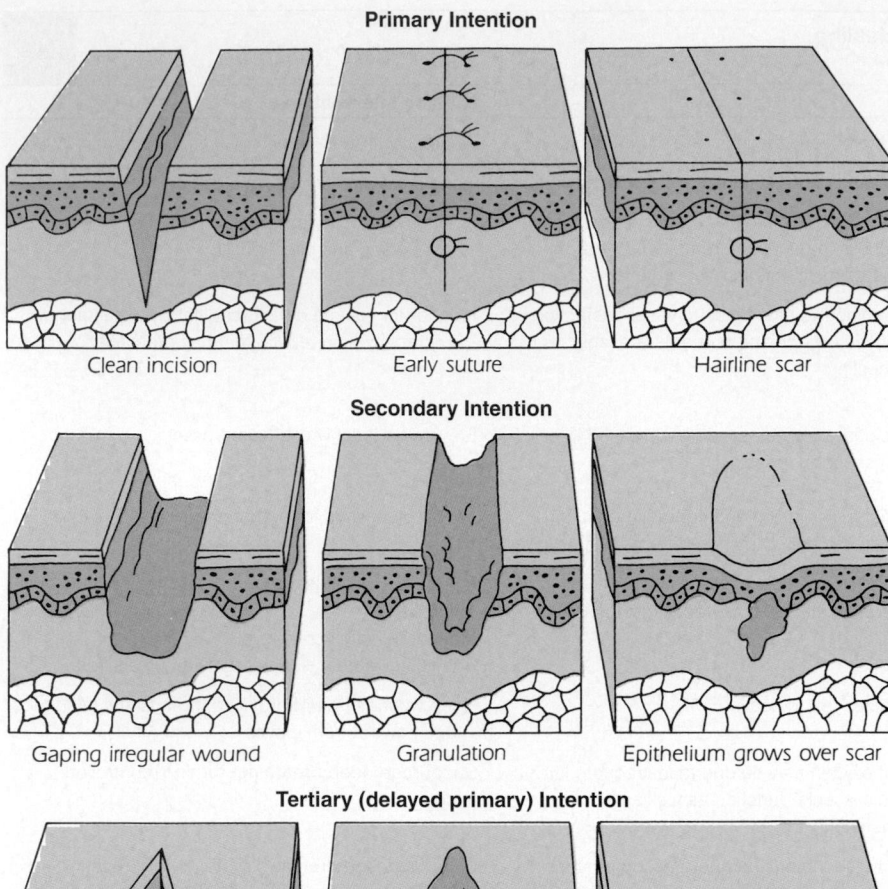

Primary Intention

Clean incision   Early suture   Hairline scar

Secondary Intention

Gaping irregular wound   Granulation   Epithelium grows over scar

Tertiary (delayed primary) Intention

Wound   Increased granulation   Late suturing with wide scar

Figure 52-2 • Types of wound healing: primary intention healing, secondary intention healing, and tertiary intention healing. (From Smeltzer SC, Bare BG, Hinkle JL, Cheever KH: Brunner & Suddarth's Textbook of Medical–Surgical Nursing, 11th ed. Philadelphia: Lippincott Williams & Wilkins, 2008, p 539.)

such as "the size of a half dollar" should be avoided. This leads to inconsistent and inaccurate documentation. Linear measurements of a wound are taken at the greatest length and width perpendicular to each other (Fig. 52-3).

Depth of the wound is measured by placing a sterile swab in the deepest area of the wound and marking the location of the wound's margin on the swab.[2] The sterile swab is dipped in normal saline before inserting it into the wound to minimize the potential of leaving cotton fibers in the wound. After removing the swab, measure from the distal tip of the swab to the area that was marked. Documentation includes the depth in centimeters and also the location where the assessment was made (e.g., "depth 5.8 cm in the distal wound bed in the 0900 clock position") (Fig. 52-4). Clear, concise documentation allows other health care professionals to reassess the wound depth in the same area with each reevaluation.

Undermining and tunneling do not usually occur in acute wounds, but the nurse always assesses the wound for their presence. Undermining occurs when there is the loss of tissue along the wound margins, the "lip of tissue."[2] Tunneling is exactly what it implies, a tunnel opening somewhere in the wound bed. Tunneling can begin in acute wounds in which there are drains. (Note that if tunneling occurs, the wound is not an acute wound but has become a chronic wound.) The process for assessing the direction and depth of tunneling is shown in Figure 52-5.

Determining the tissue type entails visual assessment of the wound bed. The tissue in the wound bed should be beefy red (as opposed to pale). The presence or absence of granulation tissue (shiny red, grainy, or bumpy tissue) is noted. The nurse assesses for necrotic tissue, which presents as black or brown tissue. Slough may also be present in the wound bed. Slough is yellow and stringy in appearance. If the wound bed is not visible, the presence or absence of eschar (scab), sutures, staples, Steri-Strips, wound adhesives, or negative pressure dressings is documented.

Box 52-3 • Wound Assessment

Location: Document the location, using anatomical positions.

Size: Document the size, in centimeters or millimeters. Measure the length from the 1200 to 1800 position. Measure the width from the 0900 to 0300 position.

Depth: Use a sterile swab to determine the depth (see Fig. 52-4).

Undermining or tunneling: Document the presence or absence of undermining or tunneling (see Fig. 52-5).

Tissue type: Describe the wound bed. If the wound bed is not visible, document the presence and condition of the eschar (scab), sutures, staples, or other wound closure.

Drainage: Note the presence or absence of drainage. If drainage is present, describe its odor, color, amount, and consistency.

Wound margins: Describe the wound margins (approximation, condition, and appearance of surrounding tissue).

Drains and tubes: Note the type of drain or tubing, and its location (using anatomical or clock positions).

Condition of dressing: Describe the amount and type of drainage on the dressing, as well as the ease with which the dressing was removed.

Pain: Evaluate on a 0 to 10 scale (or other institution-approved assessment scale). Provide pain relief as needed before, during, and after wound assessment or dressing change.

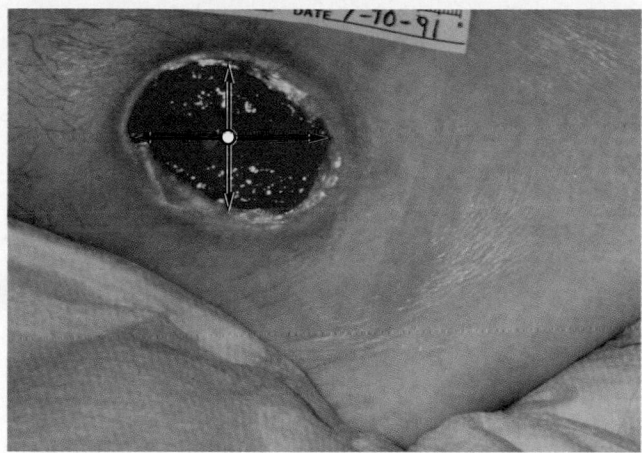

Figure 52-3 • Wound measurement. Linear measurements of a wound should be taken at the greatest length and width perpendicular to each other, as shown. (From Baranoski S, Ayello EA: Wound Care and Essentials Practice Principles, 2nd ed. Philadelphia: Lippincott Williams & Wilkins, 2008, p 84.)

The presence or absence of drainage is also important to note, along with the location of the drainage or exudate (e.g., "drainage/exudate noted at the proximal end of the wound"). The drainage or exudate needs to be assessed for odor, color, consistency, and amount (e.g., "abdominal dressing of multiple 4 × 4's is saturated with serosanguineous drainage every 2 hours").

The wound margins are also assessed when performing a wound assessment. Are the edges well approximated? Is the surrounding tissue clean, dry, reddened, edematous, pale, intact, or blistered? Again, it is important to be as exact as possible to paint an

accurate picture of the wound margins for the next health care professional.

Drains or tubes may be present in or near the wound bed. Drains or tubes are assessed for location, the appearance of the surrounding tissue, and the characteristics of the drainage. Consider the insertion site of a drain or tube as an acute wound in itself!

The dressing is assessed after it is removed. The soiled dressing's condition (e.g., "saturated"), the ease with which the dressing was removed (e.g., "sticking"), and the location and type of drainage on the dressing are described. If the dressing came off without being removed by the nurse, this is noted as well (e.g., "dressing found lying in bed—wound uncovered").

Pain is assessed using an institution-approved standardized scale, such as the 0 to 10 scale. The patient should never be in pain while a wound is being assessed. If the patient experiences pain during wound assessment, the assessment should be stopped, and the patient should be medicated before continuing. Management of pain as it relates to wound

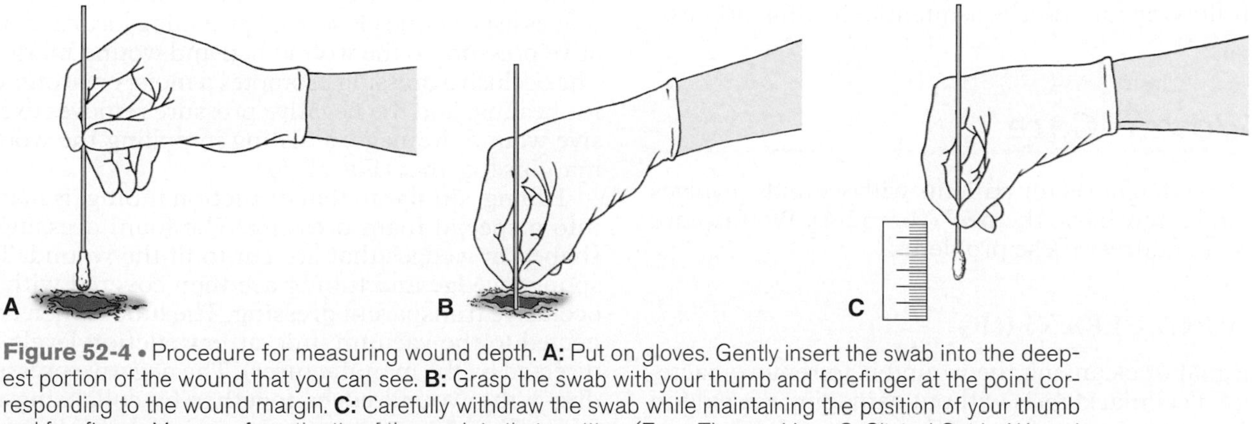

Figure 52-4 • Procedure for measuring wound depth. **A:** Put on gloves. Gently insert the swab into the deepest portion of the wound that you can see. **B:** Grasp the swab with your thumb and forefinger at the point corresponding to the wound margin. **C:** Carefully withdraw the swab while maintaining the position of your thumb and forefinger. Measure from the tip of the swab to that position. (From Thomas Hess C: Clinical Guide: Wound Care, 5th ed. Philadelphia: Lippincott Williams & Wilkins, 2005, p 21.)

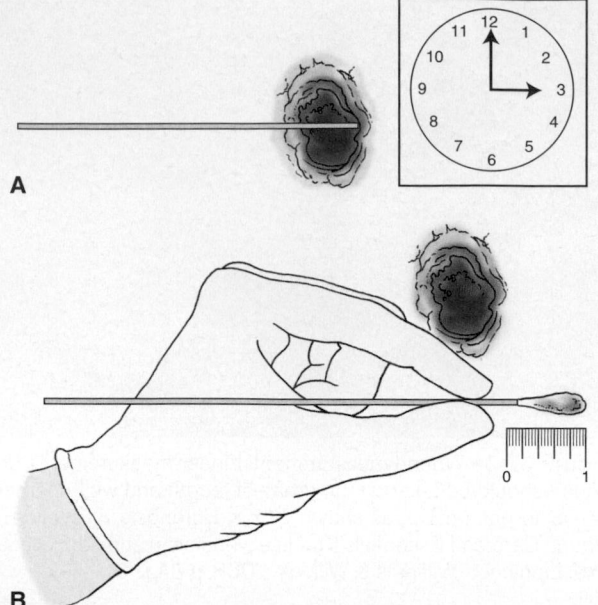

A

B

Figure 52-5 • Procedure for determining the direction and depth tunneling. **A:** To assess the direction of tunneling, put on gloves and insert the swab into the sites where tunneling occurs. Progressing in a clockwise direction, document the deepest sites where the wound tunnels. (Twelve o'clock points in the direction of the patient's head, so in this example, tunneling occurs at 3 o'clock.) **B:** To assess the depth of tunneling, insert the swab into the tunneling areas, and grasp the swab where it meets the wound margin. Remove the swab, place it next to a measuring guide, and document the measurement centimeters. (From Thomas Hess C: Clinical Guide: Wound Care, 5th ed. Philadelphia: Lippincott Williams & Wilkins, 2005, p 23.)

assessment and care is discussed in more detail later in this chapter.

Wound documentation includes all descriptions and measurements, the presence and absence of pain during the procedure, and the type of dressing applied.[1-3] Many institutions use special wound measurement tools, wound assessment tools, and documentation tools (e.g., flow sheets) for wound documentation. The flow sheet format allows the health care provider to track the wound healing process and to identify, early on, those wounds that may not be following an orderly, sequential healing process.

• Wound Care

Nursing diagnosis for patients with wounds revolves around a few basic themes[5] (Box 52-4). Wound care seeks to address these problems.

WOUND CLEANSING

The goal of cleansing the wound is to remove bacteria and cellular debris without damaging the wound bed or granulating tissue. The periwound area must also be cleansed to prevent bacteria from migrating

into it. All wounds are cleansed before reapplying the dressing. Normal saline is the safest wound cleanser. Some commercial cleansers are also safe for the wound bed. Solutions to be avoided when cleansing wounds are povidone-iodine, acetic acid, sodium hypochlorite (Dakin's solution), and hydrogen peroxide. These solutions have been found to be toxic to epithelial cells, thus impeding granulation and wound healing.

Open wounds are cleansed starting in the middle, and moving outward in a circular motion to include the periwound area. Incisions are cleansed from top to bottom, again starting in the middle and moving outward to include the periwound area.

WOUND CLOSURE

The goal of all wound care is ultimately the closure of the wound and restoration of skin integrity. Wound closure is usually promoted by various types of treatments and dressings.

Vacuum-Assisted Wound Closure (Negative Pressure Therapy)

Vacuum-assisted wound closure (VAC) is a system that assists wound closure by providing localized negative pressure to the wound bed and wound margins. The occlusive dressing promotes a moist environment for healing, and the negative pressure removes excessive wound drainage, assisting in pulling the wound margins together (Fig. 52-6).[6]

Tubing, similar to that of suction tubing, is placed into a special foam dressing. The foam dressing is shaped in wedges that are cut to fit the wound. The sponge wedge and tubing are then covered with an occlusive transparent dressing. The tube is then connected to the vacuum unit, at low suction levels (as directed by the manufacturer). The negative pressure draws the wound edges together by collapsing the foam dressing and removing wound fluids while maintaining a moist wound environment that pro-

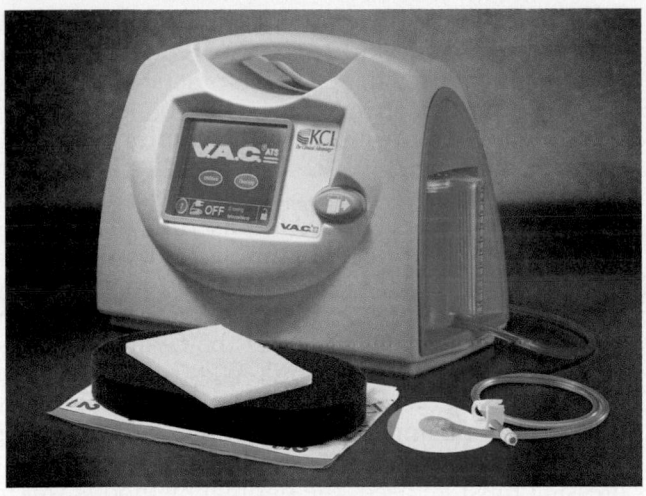
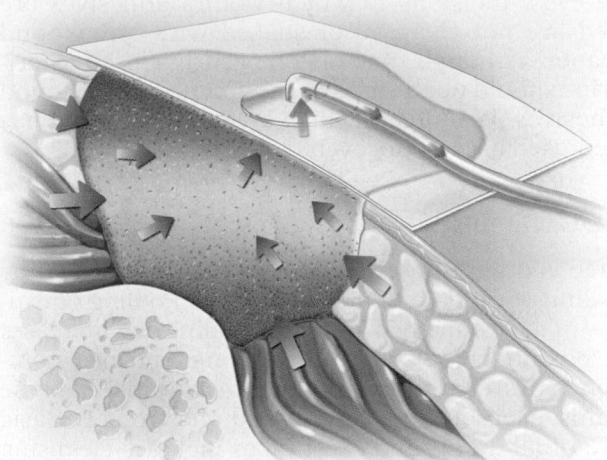

Figure 52-6 • A vacuum-assisted wound (VAC) closure device, such as the V.A.C. ATS device shown here, assists wound closure by providing localized negative pressure to the wound bed and wound margins. (Courtesy of KCI Licensing, Inc., 2007.)

motes healing. If the dressing is not collapsed, there is a leak in the system, and the dressing must be replaced with attention given to the transparent occlusive dressing application. The transparent occlusive dressing must be securely in place to maintain negative pressure in the wound. Dressings have the appearance of being "vacuum packed" when the dressing is secure and occlusive.

With the VAC system, granulation tissue is stimulated, infection and bacterial colonization are decreased, and wound closure occurs in a moist "vacuum" environment. In addition, the VAC system decreases the frequency of dressing changes, thus decreasing patient discomfort and nursing time.[6]

The VAC system can be used in both acute and chronic wounds.[6] The VAC system may be indicated for chronic wounds (including diabetic and nonhealing stage III and IV pressure ulcers); flaps and grafts (both acute surgical wounds); dehisced incisions; acute and traumatic wounds; and burns. Dehisced incisions are ones that are split open along natural or sutured lines. The VAC system should be used with extreme caution in patients with active bleeding, those who are on anticoagulant therapy, or patients with a history of uncontrolled bleeding.[6] The VAC system is contraindicated for any patient with untreated osteomyelitis, necrotic tissue with eschar, malignancies of the wound, or nonenteric and unexplored fistulas. The foam wedge dressing is not to be placed in direct contact with exposed blood vessels, organs, or nerves. VAC sponges must be positioned on viable tissue; therefore, if necrotic tissue or devitalized tissue is present, the wound needs to be débrided before the VAC sponges can be placed. The VAC system may be used in an infected wound but only with appropriate antibiotic therapy.[6] Patients at risk for bleeding must be monitored carefully, and if bleeding occurs, the VAC therapy must be discontinued.[6]

The use of the VAC system continues to increase as clinical case studies show positive patient outcomes in grafts, flaps, and orthopedic surgeries. The use of wound irrigations or instillations (antibiotics or anesthetic agents) in conjunction with this type of wound therapy is another promising area.[7]

VAC therapy also has made an economic impact. It decreases the length of wound healing, nursing labor, supplies, length of stay, complications, and hospital readmission, while it promotes the salvage of limbs.[8] In addition, use of this therapy has an emotional impact that can be directly related to the nursing diagnosis of Disturbed Body Image related to dysfunctional open wounds, scarring, or amputation.[5]

It is the nurse's responsibility to be familiar with the operation and maintenance of the VAC system. Nursing responsibilities include wound assessment and documentation, along with placing the patient on the VAC system, changing the canister, and maintaining the system. The wound should demonstrate progressive healing. If documentation fails to demonstrate progressive wound healing within 30 days, then alternative therapies must be considered.

Sutures, Staples, and Wound Adhesives

Sutures or staples must be cleaned with sterile normal saline or a wound cleanser. Immediately after surgery, the wound needs to be covered with a dry sterile dressing. Frequently after the initial postoperative period, the staples or sutures are left open to air.

Wound adhesives may be used on surgical or traumatic wounds to approximate the wound margins, in which case sutures are used to close the underlying tissue, and the wound adhesive is applied topically to the wound margins as they are drawn together. Wound adhesives are not to be placed in the wound bed (only on the margins) because this may lead to delayed wound healing or infection. The wound adhesive appears like a shiny, clear coating over the incision. Caution is needed when applying wound adhesives because of their liquid status. Wound adhesives may inadvertently spread to other areas. Extreme caution must be exercised when using wound adhesives near the eyes. Incisions in which wound adhesives are used are not cleansed or soaked with any wound cleaner, although they may be gently rinsed. Steri-Strips should not be used in conjunction with wound adhesives. Wounds in which a wound adhesive has been used are left uncovered.

WOUND DRAINAGE

Often, a drain is inserted in the wound to prevent the pooling of exudate in the wound bed. Pooling of exudate in the wound bed decreases healing and increases the potential of infection or tunneling. The most common types of drains are Hemovac drains, Penrose drains, Jackson-Pratt drains, and chest tubes. Basic care of all drains and chest tubes includes cleansing with sterile normal saline and applying a dressing. The dressing stabilizes the drain and prevents the drain insertion site from coming in contact with drainage and other potentially infectious surfaces. Drain and tube insertion sites are never left open to air because of the risk for infection. If drainage from another source may potentially saturate the dressing (over the drain site), the dressing also needs to be occlusive. Drain tubing is stabilized with tape to decrease the potential for inadvertent dislodgment, removal, and pain. Inadvertent removal of a drain potentiates pain and infection, and an acute wound may become a chronic one.

Bacitracin or Neosporin may be applied, although hydrogen peroxide and povidone-iodine (Betadine) ointment are always avoided because they destroy granulation tissue and prolong the healing process. Normal saline causes no damage to the wound bed and is physiologically normal and cost-effective. Some institutions may use prepared wound cleansers. Most wound cleansers have some potential to destroy granulating tissue (compared with normal saline) but are less toxic to granulating tissue than hydrogen peroxide or Betadine. Prepared wound cleansers are improving rapidly, becoming less cytotoxic and more time-efficient and cost-effective.

Impregnated gauzes for packing and various solutions (e.g., Betadine and Dakin's solution) may be used in the event that the wound is infected; however, they should not be used as a routine wound treatment for a prolonged time because they destroy granulating tissue and inhibit the normal healing process. Remember that the use of these products signals that the wound is not an acute wound but has become a chronic wound.

WOUND DRESSINGS

The goal of wound dressings is to protect the wound from infection and promote a moist environment. There are hundreds of dressing products available. The dressing of choice depends on the wound.

Wet-to-Dry Dressings

A wound healing by secondary or tertiary intention is frequently packed with wet-to-dry dressings. The use of wet-to-dry dressings is not recommended. Although wet-to-dry dressings are frequently used in clinical practice, evidence-based practice has shown they are actually detrimental to the wound.[9] Wounds need a moist environment to heal without impediment. Changing a wet-to-dry dressing every 8 or 12 hours leads to the dressing becoming exceptionally dry. Thus, when it is removed, indiscriminate débridement of both necrotic and granulating tissue occurs. This constant débriding of the wound increases the patient's discomfort, promotes infection (due to frequent dressing changes), slows the healing process, and may enlarge the wound. Wet-to-dry dressings affect not only wound healing but also health care costs by prolonging the healing time and increasing nursing labor and supply expenses. If a wet-to-dry dressing must be used, the optimal method is wet to moist, changing the dressing every 4 hours and covering the wet-to-dry dressing with a transparent dressing to promote and maintain a moist wound environment.

Calcium Alginates and Foam Dressings

Wound healing by secondary or tertiary intention may also be promoted with calcium alginates or foam dressings (as opposed to wet-to-dry dressings). Calcium alginates are made from brown seaweed. They come in ropelike or flat pieces that must be "fluffed" and packed into the wound bed. Calcium alginates have an absorptive quality and can hold up to 20 times or more their weight in wound drainage. As the calcium alginate absorbs the wound drainage, its appearance changes from dry, fluffed strands to that of a gel that is easily removed from the wound. Calcium alginates may be covered with a hydrocolloid or a transparent dressing.

Foam dressings have the advantage of being highly absorptive. They are available in various shapes and sizes and are placed over the wounds. When it is time to remove the foam dressing, it is simply lifted off the wound. Minimal trauma occurs to the wound bed and surrounding tissue. Foam dressings, like calcium alginates, provide a moist wound environment.

Contraindications to calcium alginates and foam dressings vary according to the manufacturer. Caution should always be used if the wound is infected.

Hydrocolloids

Hydrocolloids are most frequently used in the care and treatment of stage I and II pressure ulcers. Hydrocolloids are occlusive, self-adhesive, and absorptive, although their absorptive capacity is not as great as that of calcium alginates or foam dressings. The advantage of hydrocolloids is that they need changing only every 3 to 5 days or if they are inadvertently removed. Contraindications to hydrocolloids depend on the manufacturer's recommendations. Again, caution is always used if the wound is infected.

Hydrogels

Hydrogels are most frequently used for dry wounds. They help maintain a moist wound environment, promoting granulation, epithelialization, and autolytic débridement. Hydrogels are water or glycerin based.

Absorptive Wound Dressings

Absorptive dressings vary in construction; they are composed of hydrofibers, cellulose, rayon, or cotton. Absorptive dressings can contain larger amounts of exudates than calcium alginate dressings. Absorptive dressings may be used as primary or secondary dressings.

Silver (Ag) Dressings

Silver dressings are dressings that have been impregnated with silver. They may be topical dressings, such as Acticoat, which has the appearance of a 4 × 4 and is placed against the wound bed, or hydrofiber dressings, such as Aquacel Ag, which is highly absorptive and can be packed into the wound. Many silver dressings may be left in place for prolonged periods of time, which is advantageous for nursing care and patient teaching.

The silver has a bactericidal effect. Before the advent of antibiotics, silver was the treatment of choice for wound infections. The potential for bacteria to develop a resistance to silver is negligible; to date, only one possible case has been reported. Silver dressings work well in conjunction with other medical and pharmacotherapeutic treatments.

Bilayered Dressings

Bilayered dressings are engineered dressings that are applied as "grafts" to wounds that fail to progress with other treatment plans. These graft materials may be composed of fibroblast, collagen, and growth factors depending on the type and brand. They act by giving the (noninfective) chronic wound a "jump start." Examples of these dressings are Apligraf, Integra, and Oasis. They are frequently used on venous stasis ulcers and diabetic foot ulcers or on exposed bone, tendon, or joints. The cost of these graft materials is much more than conventional treatments; however, by "jumpstarting" the process of wound healing, they may actually be more cost-effective in difficult cases.

WOUND DÉBRIDEMENT

At times, both acute and chronic wounds need to be débrided. Débridement is the removal of necrotic (dead) or devitalized tissue. Necrotic or devitalized tissue presents as dark brown, black, yellow, pale, cyanotic, or crusty eschar. To promote optimal wound healing, this tissue needs to be removed from the wound. Débridement may be performed in several ways: autolytic, chemical, mechanical, or laser. Occasionally, a combination of débridement methods may be used throughout the healing process. Combination therapy depends on the type of wound and its location, the patient's status, and physician preference.

Autolytic Débridement

In autolytic débridement, the body breaks down necrotic or devitalized tissue. Hydrocolloid dressings are frequently used to promote autolytic débridement. Autolytic débridement is not the optimal choice in wounds that have large amounts of necrotic tissue. Autolytic débridement takes time for the body to use its own ability to lyse and dissolve necrotic tissue.

Chemical Débridement

Chemical débridement is accomplished using proteolytic enzymes or collagen-based drugs applied topically to the wound. Examples of chemical débridement medications include Collagenase Santyl, Accuzyme, and Panafil. Chemical débridement agents dissolve nonviable tissue. Chemical débridement requires caution because some enzyme agents may destroy healthy tissue while débriding the wound of necrotic and devitalized tissue. Product instructions must be reviewed before use.

Mechanical Débridement

Mechanical débridement can be accomplished by wet-to-dry dressings, whirlpools, or the use of sharps. Although wet-to-dry dressings are an effective method of débridement, care must be taken to change to another method of wound care when the wound bed is débrided. Use of the whirlpool is controversial because although it does débride (but not effectively), the potential for infection is increased with multiple patients using a static number of whirlpools (even though they are cleaned between patients). Use of whirlpools also leaves the wound margins macerated, which increases tissue loss, impeding wound closure. In sharps débridement, using a scalpel or scissors, the wound bed is cleared of all necrotic and devitalized tissue surgically. This surgical procedure may require anesthesia, intravenous conscious sedation, a local anesthetic, or a combination of the three.

Laser Débridement

Laser débridement may also be used to provide a clean wound bed. Currently, laser débridement is not performed as frequently as autolytic, chemical, and mechanical débridement. As technology advances, the use of laser debridement will become more common.

WOUND CULTURES

Routine wound cultures are not recommended unless there are signs and symptoms of infection such as fever, erythema, edema, induration, foul odor, purulent exudates, increased amount of exudate, abscess, cellulitis, discoloration of granulation tissue, friable granulation tissue (bleeds easily), increase or unexpected pain or tenderness, or an elevated white blood cell count. All wounds are considered contaminated and have the potential to become infected. Several methods may be used to culture a wound, including fluid biopsy, wound (tissue) biopsy, and surface culture (culture swab).

A surface culture is usually done first. The wound is cleansed or irrigated with sterile normal saline before swabbing the wound. Exudate and necrotic tissue are not cultured—doing so provides invalid results. After the wound is cleansed, the swab is gently rolled or rotated, starting at the 12-o'clock position and moving in a zigzag pattern from side to side down the wound to the 6-o'clock position.[2] Optimally, there should be 10 points of contact (Fig. 52-7).[2] A colony count of 100,000 organisms/mL indicates an infection that needs to be treated with the appropriate antibiotic.[10] At colony counts of greater than 100,000 organisms/mL, normal wound healing is inhibited, and the wound becomes a chronic wound.[2] Wounds that do not respond to antibiotic treatment need to be recultured. The most appropriate form of culture in this scenario is a wound biopsy. Wounds that contain necrotic tissue or tunneling need both aerobic and anaerobic cultures.

USE OF PRESSURE-RELIEVING DEVICES

Pressure relief is a major component of wound care. A variety of methods may be used, ranging from low to high technology.[1-3,11] Programs that use both high- and low-technology solutions and adapt to meet the patient's needs at various stages in the recovery process tend to be the most successful.

The easiest and most effective treatment for pressure ulcers on the heels is to keep the heels off the bed by placing a pillow under the lower legs (a low-technology, cost-effective treatment). A schedule for turning and positioning the patient is an effective, easily implemented, and cost-effective intervention for relief of pressure. Critically ill patients may require specialty beds that are designed to reduce pressure. Many specialty beds inflate, deflate, alternate pressures, and laterally rotate. In many institutions, patients must meet specific criteria to qualify for specialty beds. To prevent the occurrence of additional pressure ulcers, it is necessary to follow manufacturer's recommendations when positioning patients on specialty beds. Although these beds do relieve some pressure, they do not eliminate all pressure, as turning the patient from side to side does. Another pressure-relieving device is the Vollman-Turner device, which places the patient in the prone position (thus relieving all pressure on the patient's back). The Vollman-Turner device is not a specialty bed; rather, it is a device that is attached to the bed frame. The advantage of the Vollman-Turner device is that only a minimal number of people are needed to turn the patient.

PAIN MANAGEMENT

In all areas of wound care (assessment, cleansing, dressing changes, and positioning), the nurse needs to focus on pain assessment and control. No procedure should occur without assessing for pain and then medicating the patient as needed. Once pain is controlled, the nurse may proceed with the wound care. The choice of pain medication and the delivery method used (e.g., continuous drip, epidural, patient-controlled analgesia pump, local anesthesia) depends on the patient's status.

PHARMACOTHERAPY

Pharmacotherapy in wound care entails the use of pain medications and, in some cases, growth hormones and steroids. Pain medications are used to control pain during wound assessment, cleansing, and dressing changes. Growth hormones (e.g., becaplermin [Regranex Gel 0.01%]) may be used to stimulate wound healing. Regranex is applied topically to the wound in measured doses that are recalculated weekly or biweekly. The gel is spread evenly over the wound and covered with gauze moistened with saline. Topical steroid creams, such as clocortolone pivalate (Cloderm) and doxepin hydrochloride (Prudoxin), may be prescribed for wound care to relieve surface inflammation and pruritus of the wound margins. Chemical débridement agents (discussed earlier) are also considered pharmacotherapy.

Although silver dressings are referred to as antimicrobials, they are considered a dressing and not a pharmacotherapeutic agent. Silver gels such as SilvaSorb can be used instead of a silver dressing. SilvaSorb gel is combined with a hydrogel applied into the wound and is a controlled-release formula.

Xenaderm is a protective ointment composed of balsam Peru, castor oil, and trypsin. This ointment increases blood flow to partial-thickness wounds while acting as a barrier in incontinent patients.

• Care of Specific Wounds

PRESSURE ULCERS

Pressure ulcer treatment depends on the stage of the wound. Stage I and II pressure ulcers are usually treated with hydrocolloid dressings. Stage III and IV pressure ulcers may be dressed using absorptive hydrofiber dressings in the wound bed or with calcium alginates fluffed and placed into the wound bed and then covered with hydrocolloid or occlusive transpar-

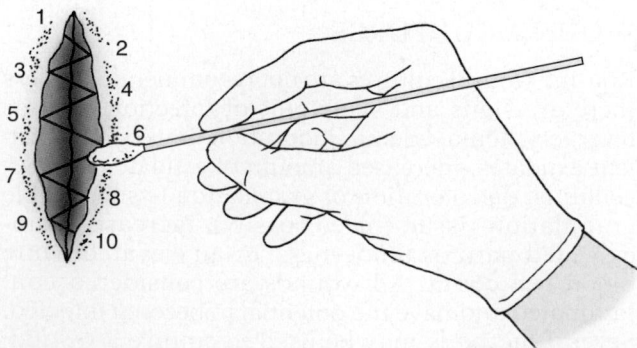

Figure 52-7 • Procedure for collecting a wound culture. The wound edges are swabbed using 10-point coverage. (From Thomas Hess C: Clinical Guide: Wound Care, 5th ed. Philadelphia: Lippincott Williams & Wilkins, 2005, p 104.)

ent dressings. Although they are used, wet-to-dry dressings are not optimal, as previously discussed. Other options for stage III and IV pressure ulcers are foam dressings and the VAC system.

BURNS

Burns are acute wounds, graded as first, second, or third degree, and described as partial or full thickness. Wound care goals in burns are a clean wound, free from infection. Burns are cleaned with sterile normal saline or a mild soap and water. Topical ointments such as bacitracin, polymyxin, or silver sulfadiazine may be applied. After cleansing the wound, a dressing is applied. The type of dressing depends on the type of burn, the amount of tissue involved, institutional policy, and physician preference. A dressing that releases silver into the wound bed when dampened, such as Acticort or Aquacel, is a possibility. Hydrocolloids, calcium alginates, and foam dressings may also be used, depending on the type and location of burn.

Broad-spectrum antibiotic therapy is not used routinely because of the potential for antibiotic resistance. Infection is treated only if it occurs and is documented with positive cultures. The antibiotic chosen is based on sensitivity results. Care of the patient with burns is discussed thoroughly in Chapter 53.

HIGH-VOLUME DRAINING WOUNDS

Some wounds may have high volumes of exudate (drainage). Exudate is the response of the body to the inflammatory phase. Wound drainage is composed of neutrophils, macrophages, cellular debris, proteins, and toxins. High-volume draining wounds generate more drainage than traditional gauze pad dressings can manage, in which case hydrocolloids, calcium alginates, hydrogels, or foam dressings may be used. A composite dressing may also be used. These dressings combine the physical attributes of two or more dressings to enhance the absorptive capability.

If the exudate cannot be controlled with these measures, alternatives must be considered. The goal of wound care in this instance is to contain the drainage and protect the surrounding tissue from breakdown. Frequently, the wound maybe "pouched" or "bagged." The same supplies used for ostomy pouching are used for pouching a wound[2] (Fig. 52-8), or a product designed specifically for pouching high-volume draining wounds may be used. Pouching the high-volume draining wound allows for accurate measurement of output from the wound and protects the surrounding wound margins.

To pouch a wound, the skin is first cleaned with saline or an antibacterial soap and water, then dried. The skin may then be prepared with a protective skin barrier wipe, which protects the skin and enhances the adherence of the wafer. The wound is measured or traced, and a wafer is cut to fit. Stoma paste is applied around the cut-out area to prevent leakage of the drainage onto the skin. A one- or two-piece pouching system may be used. With a one-piece pouching sys-

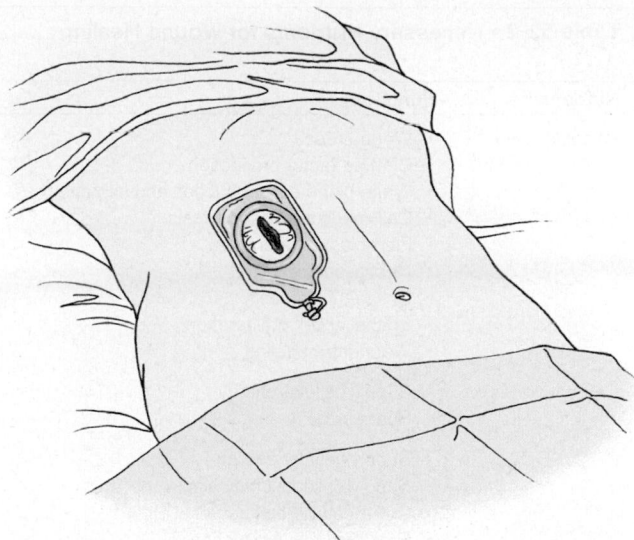

Figure 52-8 • Procedure for "pouching" or "bagging" a high-volume draining wound. (From Thomas Hess C: Clinical Guide: Wound Care, 5th ed. Philadelphia: Lippincott Williams & Wilkins, 2005, p 100.)

tem, the wafer or pouch is applied to the wound. With a two-piece system, the wafer is applied first, and then the pouch is attached. Both systems need a clamp closure device at the end of the pouch. A benefit of a two-piece system is that it allows for pouch removal so that the wound can be assessed without disturbing the wafer. The wound margins need to be assessed for skin breakdown and may be protected by a variety of skin wipes or protective ointments.

• Nutrition and Wound Healing

In critical care, monitoring nutritional status is as important as monitoring hemodynamics. Nutrition needs to be addressed early in the patient's admission to promote the optimal opportunity and environment for healing. One study showed that patients who receive a nutritional assessment within the first 48 hours of admission to the hospital setting have a lower incidence of pressure ulcer development during their hospital stay.[4] Nutrition is paramount in critically ill patients or patients with wounds, whether the wounds are acute or chronic. To heal properly, the body needs adequate carbohydrates, fats, proteins, minerals, calories, vitamins, and hydration (Table 52-2).[1,2,4]

Protein is a basic and key component of all cellular activity. Without proteins, the inflammatory process is impaired, and the risk for infection increases. Proteins also affect oncotic pressure, which predisposes the patient to edema. Wound edema decreases the diffusion of oxygen and nutrients, impeding the healing process even more.

Although protein is a key component in the healing process, other nutrients play major roles. Carbohydrates are the body's fuel source and spare the proteins, so they can be used in cellular construction.

Table 52-2 • Necessary Nutrients for Wound Healing

Nutrient	Function	Results of Deficiency
Proteins	• Wound repair • Clotting factor production • White blood cell production and migration • Cell-mediated phagocytosis • Fibroblast proliferation • Neovascularization • Collagen synthesis • Epithelial cell proliferation • Wound remodeling	• Poor wound healing • Hypoalbuminemia and generalized edema, which slows oxygen diffusion and metabolic transport mechanisms from the capillaries and cell membranes • Lymphopenia • Impaired cellular immunity
Carbohydrates	• Supply cellular energy • Spare protein	• Body uses visceral and muscle proteins for energy
Fats	• Supply cellular energy • Supply essential fatty acids • Cell membrane structure • Prostaglandin production	• Inhibited tissue repair • Use of visceral and muscle proteins for energy
Vitamin A	• Collagen synthesis • Epithelialization	• Poor wound healing • Impaired immunity
Vitamin C	• Membrane integrity • Antioxidant	• Impaired immunity • Poor wound healing • Capillary fragility
Vitamin K	• Normal blood clotting	• Increased risk for hemorrhage and hematoma formation
Iron	• Collagen synthesis • Enhances leukocytic bacterial activity • Hemoglobin synthesis	• Anemia, leading to increased risk for local tissue ischemia • Impaired tensile strength
Zinc	• Cell proliferation • Cofactor for enzymes • Vitamin A utilization	• Impaired collagen cross-linkage • Slow healing • Alteration in taste • Anorexia • Impaired immunity
Copper	• Collagen cross-linkage • Red blood cell synthesis	• Decreased collagen synthesis • Anemia
Pyridoxine, riboflavin, and thiamine	• Energy production • Cellular immunity • Red blood cell synthesis	• Decreased resistance to infection • Impaired wound healing
Arginine	• Increases local wound immune system • Nitrogen-rich (32% nitrogen, whereas the average amino acid is 16% nitrogen) • Precursor to proline, which is converted to hydroxyproline and then to collagen	• Decreased local wound immune system
Glutamine	• Primary fuel for fibroblasts • Preservation of lean body mass	• Less fuel for fibroblasts

From Hess CT: Clinical Guide: Wound Care, 5th ed. Ambler, PA: Lippincott Williams & Wilkins, 2005, p. 28.

Fats maintain cell membrane function and assist with the movement of minerals and fat-soluble vitamins in and out of the cell. Vitamins act as catalysts in the body's chemical reactions and are also needed for protein and cellular replication. Minerals are needed in the body's biochemical reactions and control the movement of fluids into and out of the cell, through the process of osmosis.

An adequate caloric intake is required for a wound to heal. Normal adult caloric intake is 25 to 30–40 kcal/kg/day, and the normal adult protein intake is 0.8 g/kg/day.[1,2] In a critically ill or critically injured patient, caloric and protein intakes must be dramati-

cally increased. Caloric intake requirements increase to 35 to 40 kcal/kg/day, and protein requirements increase to 1.5 to 2 g/kg/day (Table 52-3).[2] Optimal nutritional care for the patient with wounds can be achieved by consulting a dietitian and monitoring laboratory test results along with the patient's basic intake, output, daily weights, anthropometrics, calorie count, and social history.

Serum albumin is of particular interest in that it is a key indicator of protein available for cellular construction and replication. Table 52-4 demonstrates the various albumin requirements at specific ages.[10] In each case, if the albumin level is less than the

Table 52-3 • Nutrient Needs Based on Body Weight

Nutrient	Requirements
Calories	
Normal	25 to 30 kcal/kg/day
Protein-calorie malnutrition (PCM)*	30 to 35 kcal/kg/day
Critically ill or injured*	35 to 40 kcal/kg/day
Protein	
Recommended daily allowance (RDA)	0.8 g/kg/day
PCM	1.5 g/kg/day
Critically ill or injured*	1.5 to 2.0 g/kg/day
Fat	<30% kcal
Water	30 mL/kg body weight or 1 L/1,000 kcal

*Nutrient supplementation required
From Hess CT: Clinical Guide: Wound Care, 5th ed. Ambler PA: Lippincott Williams & Wilkins, 2005, p. 26.

minimal parameter, replacement therapy is needed to provide the optimal wound healing environment. Normal serum albumin is defined as 3.8 to 5 g/dL. In an adult, a serum albumin level of less than 3.5 g/dL necessitates replacement therapy.

Serum total protein levels are also monitored. Normal levels for serum total protein are 6 to 8 g/dL (see Table 52-4).[10] As stated earlier, protein also affects the oncotic pressure, and levels less than 6 g/dL lead to edema. Note that the serum total protein level, like the albumin level, varies according to age.

Along with electrolytes, complete blood count (CBC), serum albumin, and serum total protein, two other laboratory tests that may be assessed are serum transferrin and the total lymphocyte count (TLC). The serum transferrin level is an indicator of the body's ability to transfer iron through the plasma. The normal serum transferrin level is 180 to 260 mg/dL.[10,11] Decreased serum transferrin levels lead to anemia, as demonstrated by the CBC. TLC normal parameters are 1,500 to 3,000 cells/μL.[10] A TLC assists in the assessment of the patient's immune status and may be decreased in states of malnutrition.

Micronutrients, vitamins, and minerals also affect wound healing. Zinc is needed in the structure of collagen and production of protein. Ascorbic acid is also a component of collagen synthesis. Vitamin A plays a role in cellular proliferation and increases the tensile strength of healing wound tissue. Therefore, use of a high-potency daily multivitamin and mineral supplement is recommended for patients with altered skin integrity.[4]

Patients who are on nothing by mouth (NPO) status for longer than 24 to 48 hours are at risk for slowed healing owing to the lack of an adequate supply of protein, carbohydrates, and other nutrients. Nutritional management includes monitoring laboratory test results; documenting intake and output and daily weights; a nutritional assessment by a dietitian; total parental or peripheral parental nutrition or enteral feedings; and calorie counts.

Adequate hydration is paramount to ensure oxygen delivery to the tissues. If the patient is hypovolemic, oxygen transport to the peripheral tissues is impaired. The optimal goal is to maintain hemodynamic stability. (For a thorough discussion of hemodynamic assessment, see Chapter 17.) In the critically ill patient, tissue perfusion must be addressed based on the symptom and cause. For example, if the cardiac output is decreased, systolic blood pressure is decreased, the heart rate is tachycardic, and the pulmonary artery wedge pressure is decreased, the patient is hypovolemic. To improve tissue perfusion for this critically ill patient, fluids are given. The hemoglobin and hematocrit must also be assessed, and if low, the patient should be transfused. By improving hydration and correcting the anemia, the circulating volume and the oxygen-carrying capacity of the blood are increased, thus improving tissue perfusion; this enhances the environment for wound healing.

• Patient Teaching and Discharge Planning

Patient teaching and discharge planning are ongoing processes that occur throughout the patient's hospital stay. Discharge planning for patients with wounds is a multidisciplinary challenge. Multiple factors must be considered if discharge is to be

Table 52-4 • Normal Values for Serum Total Protein and Serum Albumin

Age of Patient	Total Protein	Albumin
Adult	6.0–8.0 g/dL or 60–80 g/L	3.5–5.0 g/dL or 38–50 g/L
10–19 y	6.3–8.6 g/dL or 68–86 g/L	3.7–5.6 g/dL or 37–56 g/L
7–9 y	6.2–8.1 g/dL or 62–81 g/L	3.7–5.6 g/dL or 37–56 g/L
4–6 y	5.9–7.8 g/dL or 59–78 g/L	3.5–5.2 g/dL or 35–52 g/L
1–3 y	5.9–7.0 g/dL or 59–70 g/L	3.4–4.2 g/dL or 34–42 g/L
<5 days	5.4–7.0 g/dL or 54–70 g/L	2.6–3.6 g/dL or 26–36 g/L

From Fischbach FT: A Manual of Laboratory and Diagnostic Tests, 7th ed. Philadelphia: Lippincott Williams & Wilkins, 2004, p. 576.

Box 52-5 • DISCHARGE PLANNING GUIDE: Wound Care

- Determine whether the patient can be discharged home, or whether skilled nursing will be necessary.
- Evaluate the home environment for safety.
- Determine the availability of financial resources for expenses such as dressing supplies and home support.
- Assess the patient's or family member's readiness to learn wound care.
- Determine the type of treatment or wound care. This will be dictated by the type of wound (e.g., stage, acute, chronic, burn).
- Assess the patient's access to transportation to and from the health care provider's office for follow-up.
- Within 48 hours of admission, a nutritional assessment must be completed, and dietary concerns need to be addressed by the nurse and dietitian.
- Self-care deficits must be addressed. A home health nurse or a home health aide may need to follow at discharge if the patient is unable to perform activities of daily living (ADLs). Family members may need instruction in assisting the patient at home.
- Document the location of the wound and instruct the patient and family members on how to perform wound care.
- Assess the patient's psychosocial support system. Referrals to various community programs may be needed.
- Supply the patient and family members with readily available resources to troubleshoot problems (for example, specific instructions about when to call 911, versus the primary care provider's office).

successful (Box 52-5). An important part of discharge planning is ensuring that the patient or a family member knows how to care for the wound after the patient leaves the hospital. Examples of patient teaching guides for wound care are given in Boxes 52-6 and 52-7.

• Clinical Applicability Challenges

Case Study

Ms. B. is a 36-year-old white woman with a history of smoking, hypertension, and obesity (weight: 204.5 kg). While undergoing bariatric surgery, she has an acute inferior and anterior wall myocardial infarction. Subsequently, she is transferred to the intensive care unit, where she has two cardiac arrests. Her abdominal incision dehisces (pulls open, with sutures that are not intact) after the second cardiac arrest.

Currently, Ms. B.'s vital signs are: temperature, 100°F; blood pressure, 92/52 mm Hg; heart rate, 118 beats/minute; and respirations, 14 breaths/minute. Other measurements are: cardiac output, 2.8 L/minute; pulmonary artery wedge pressure, 4 mm Hg; central venous pressure, 0 mm Hg; oxygen saturation, 90%; and urinary output, 10 mL/hour. Currently she is being ventilated with a fraction of inspired oxygen of 55%, tidal volume of 700 mL, synchronized intermittent mandatory ventilation rate of 14, and pressure support of 5 cm H_2O. The following intravenous (IV) fluids are being infused through a right subclavian pulmonary artery catheter: dobutamine, 10 µg/kg/minute; dopamine, 15 µg/kg/minute; nitroglycerin, 22 µg/kg/minute; and a lidocaine drip, 2 mg/minute. In addition, she is receiving magnesium sulfate, 2 g IV for two episodes of torsades de pointes. She responds only to painful stimuli.

1. Discuss Ms. B's potential for skin breakdown. What are the risk factors? Of these risk factors, which can be modified?

Box 52-6 • TEACHING GUIDE: Wound Care (Sutures, Staples, and Wound Adhesives)

Wound Closure
- Sutures are threadlike. They are placed using a needle to pull the skin together. You may see "knots."
- Staples are special surgical staples. They are placed using a special staple gun to pull the skin together.
- Wound adhesives are a type of glue that holds the edges of the skin together.

Patient Activity
- Keep your sutures/staples/wound adhesive clean and dry.
- Wash your hands before you start.
- Do not rub or pull the area.
- Clean the wound gently with mild soap and water and rinse, or use a wound cleanser as directed by your physician. Do not "soak" the sutures/staples/wound adhesive. Gently pat the area dry.
- A dry gauze dressing may be applied to keep your wound clean or pad the area if your clothes rub.
- Wash your hands when you are done.

When To Call Your Physician
- Call if you find any redness, tenderness, pus-type drainage, swelling, missing sutures or staples, or increased pain, or if the area is warm or hot to the touch.
- Call if you have a fever of more than 101°F.
- Call immediately and go to the emergency department if your incision "pulls open."

Medications
- Take your medications as prescribed.
- If you are taking an antibiotic, take all pills prescribed. Do not stop taking them when you feel better!

Safety
- You may drive, climb stairs, work, begin sexual activity, and lift when instructed by the physician.

Box 52-7 • TEACHING GUIDE:
Wound Care (Dry Dressing, Calcium Alginate, Hydrocolloid, or Hydrofiber)

Patient Activity

Always wash your hands before and after changing your dressing.

Dry Dressing
- Change your dressing every day.
- Clean your wound with normal saline, mild soap and water, or a wound cleanser as directed.
- Cover the wound with a dry gauze dressing.

Calcium Alginate

Calcium alginate is a dressing that can be packed (lightly) into your wound. It is made of a special type of seaweed that has healing properties. Calcium alginate looks similar to "angel hair" when "fluffed."
- Change your dressing every 3 days unless otherwise directed by your physician.
- Remove the old dressing (it will appear to be a gelatinous mass, not the fibrous "angel hair" you put in.)
- Clean your wound with normal saline or with a wound cleanser as directed.
- Take the calcium alginate out of the package and gently fluff it (pull it apart slightly so that it has a light, fluffy look).
- Place the fluffed calcium alginate into the wound.
- Cover the wound and calcium alginate with the type of covering you were directed to use.

Hydrocolloid

Hydrocolloid is a thicker type of wound covering that can be placed over open wounds such as bed sores (pressure ulcers). Hydrocolloid may also be placed over a wound in which calcium alginate has been packed. Hydrocolloid comes in various shapes and sizes. It has an adhesive (sticky) side. The adhesive side goes over the wound.
- Change your dressing every 3 to 7 days unless otherwise directed by your physician, or when it comes off.
- Gently peel the old hydrocolloid off, being careful not to peel too quickly or too roughly.
- Clean your wound with normal saline or with a wound cleanser as directed.

- If you are packing the wound with calcium alginate, do it at this time.
- Peel the paper off the adhesive side of the hydrocolloid.
- Place the hydrocolloid adhesive side down over the wound.
- Press gently and smooth the hydrocolloid over the wound.
- Place your hand on top of the hydrocolloid for about 1 minute. This helps the adhesive to stick better.

Hydrofiber

Hydrofiber is a dressing that is absorbent, interacting with wound drainage by forming a soft gel that is easily removed from the wound while maintaining a healing environment. Hydrofiber may or many not have silver added to the dressing. Silver has an antimicrobial effect that helps to keep the wound free of bacteria.
- Change your dressing when it is saturated with drainage, or after 7 days.
- Remove the old dressing (it will appear to be a gelatinous mass).
- Clean your wound with normal saline or with a wound cleanser as directed.
- Take the hydrofiber out of the package and place it in the wound.
- Cover the wound and hydrofiber with the type of covering you were directed to use.

When to Call Your Physician
- Call if you have any redness, tenderness, pus-type drainage, swelling, missing sutures or staples, or increased pain, or if the area is warm or hot to the touch.
- Call if you have a temperature higher than 101°F.

Medications
- Take your medications as prescribed.
- If you are taking an antibiotic, take all pills prescribed. Do not stop taking them when you feel better!

Safety
- You may drive, climb stairs, work, begin sexual activity, and lift when instructed by the physician.

---

2. Develop and prioritize your plan of care for Ms. B.
3. Discuss treatment options for Ms. B's dehisced abdominal wound.

Review Questions

1. A critical care nurse is assessing a patient's abdominal wound and determines it has dehisced. The nurse knows that this is
   a. an acute wound.
   b. a chronic wound.
   c. healing by secondary intention.
   d. healing by delayed primary intention.

2. A critical care nurse is presenting an in-service to peers on wound care. The proliferation phase can best be described as
   a. the phase in which remodeling occurs.
   b. the phase lasting 4 to 6 days, in which phagocytosis and vasoconstriction occur.
   c. the phase in which the goal is to increase tensile strength of the scar tissue.
   d. the phase in which granulation tissue is created.

3. A critical care nurse is caring for a patient who has an abdominal wound that is positive for methicillin-resistant *Staphylococcus aureus*. The most appropriate wound dressing for this patient is
   a. Betadine wet-to-dry every 12 hours.
   b. silver dressing packed into the wound.
   c. hydrogel applied to wound and covered with a hydrocolloid.
   d. calcium alginate, fluffed and packed into the wound every 24 hours.

4. A critical care nurse admits a patient with a diagnosis of septic shock secondary to venous stasis ulcers. The nurse would expect to find wounds that are
   a. pale and punched out with a large amount of exudates.
   b. irregular, shallow craters on the medial aspect of the lower leg.

c. on the medial aspect of the upper leg with minimal exudates.

d. draining clear fluids in small amounts.

5. A critical care nurse is caring for a patient on whom autolytic débridement is being used for a sacral ulcer. An example of autolytic débridement would be

a. application of a hydrocolloid dressing.

b. application of an Apligraf or Oasis dressing.

c. application of a wet-to-dry dressing.

d. application of a proteolytic enzyme and 4 × 4.

References

1. Baranoski S, Ayello EA: Wound Care Essentials: Practice Principles, 2nd ed. Philadelphia: Lippincott, Williams & Wilkins, 2008

2. Thomas Hess C: Clinical Guide: Wound Care, 5th ed. Philadelphia: Lippincott Williams & Wilkins, 2005

3. Hahn JF, Olsen CL, Tomaselli N, et al: Wounds: Nursing care and product selection—Part I. Nursing Spectrum, 2003. Retrieved August 4, 2003, from http://nsweb.nursingspectrum.com/ce/ce80.htm

4. Stefanski, JL, Smith, KJ: The role of nutrition intervention in wound healing. Home HealthCare Management & Practice 18(4):293–299, 2006

5. Ackley BJ, Ladwig GB: Nursing Diagnosis Handbook, 5th ed. St. Louis: Mosby, 2002

6. KCI Licensing, Inc., V.A.C.® Therapy Clinical Guidelines, May 2007

7. Wolvos T: Wound instillation with negative pressure wound therapy. Ostomy Wound Manage 51(2A):215–265, 2005

8. Niezgoda JA, Page JC, Kaplan M: The economic value of negative pressure wound therapy. Ostomy Wound Manage 51(2A):445–475, 2005

9. Ovington LG: Hanging wet to dry dressings out to dry. Adv Skin Wound Care 15(2):79–84, 2002

10. Fischbach FT, Dunning MB III: Nurse's Quick Reference to Common Laboratory and Diagnostic Tests, 4th ed. Philadelphia: Lippincott Williams & Wilkins, 2006

11. Junkin J: Failure to thrive in wounds: Prevention and early intervention. Infect Control 1(2):1–8, 2002

Other Selected Readings

Baranoski S: Raising awareness of pressure ulcer prevention and treatment. Adv Skin Wound Care 19(7):398–405, 2006

Biala K: Case conferencing for wound care patients. Home Healthcare Nurse 20(2):120–126, 2002

Bergstrom N, Allman R Alvarez O, et al: Treatment of Pressure Ulcers Clinical Practice Guideline no. 15. AHCPR publication no. 95-0652. Rockville, MD: U.S. Department of Health and Human Services, 1994

Clever K, Smith G, Bower C, et al: Evaluating the efficacy of a uniquely delivered skin protectant and its effect on the formation of sacral/buttock pressure ulcers. Ostomy Wound Manage 48(12):60–67, 2002

Convatec, Inc. Retrieved July 24, 2003, from http://www.woundcarehelpline.com/conva.edu.htm

Cutting, KF, White, RJ: Criteria for identifying wound infection-revisited. Ostomy Wound Manag 51(1):28–34, 2005

Frantz BA: Chronic wound healing. University of Iowa, Nursing Education, 2003. Retrieved May 15, 2006, from http://coninfo.nursing.uiowa.edu/sites/chronicwounds

Gupta S: Differentiating negative pressure wound therapy devices: An illustrative case study. Wounds 19(1):1–9, 2007

Hahn JF, Olsen CL, Tomaselli N, et al: Wound: Nursing care and product selection—Part II. Nursing Spectrum, 2003. Retrieved May 15, 2006, from http://nsweb.nursingspectrum.com/ce/ce81.htm

Hard TA: Nutrition and wound-care management/prevention. Wound Care Canada 2(2):20–24, 2003

Hogan SL: How to help wounds heal. RN 67(8):26–31, 2004

Kuznar W: Adjunctive approaches aid in acute wound healing. Dermatol Surg (May):58, 2002

Mendez-Eastman S: New advances in wound therapy. 2003. Retrieved April 15, 2003, from http://www.wounds1.com/hero/hero.cfm

National Pressure Ulcer Advisory Panel. 2004. NPUAP staging report. Retrieved May 15, 2006, from http://www.npuap.org/positn6.html

Ovington LG: Dealing with drainage: The what, why and how of wound exudate. Home Healthcare Nurse 20(6):368–374, 2002

Thompson CW: Nutrition and adult wound healing. 2003. Retrieved May 15, 2006, from http://www.nutritioncare.org/listserv/wound%20healing.pdf

Burns and Common Integumentary Disorders

53

Louis R. Stout

Objectives

Based on the content in this chapter, the reader should be able to:

❶ Explore the mechanism of a burn injury.

❷ Describe the pathophysiology of a burn injury.

❸ Review the physiological changes associated with each organ system in relation to a burn injury.

❹ Discuss the initial priorities of caring for a patient with a burn injury.

❺ Formulate a plan of care for a patient who has sustained a burn injury.

❻ Select appropriate wound care coverings for a patient with a burn injury.

❼ Evaluate the collaborative efforts of the burn team in relation to desired outcomes in a patient with a burn injury.

❽ Discuss other types of injured patients who are cared for in the burn unit.

The past two decades have witnessed a significant decline in the number of burn injuries and hospitalizations. Total burn injuries in the United States have decreased more than 50%, from 2.5 million to approximately 1 million per year. Burn injuries account for 700,000 emergency department visits per year, and about 45,000 patients are hospitalized. The average size of a burn is about 14% of the total-body surface area (TBSA).

Of the patients with burns who are hospitalized, about half are treated at specialized burn centers.[1] Burn treatment centers are composed of nurses, physicians, physical therapists, occupational therapists, recreational therapists, nutritionists, psychologists, social workers, and spiritual support staff. The American Burn Association (ABA) has established guidelines for transfer and referral of these patients.

Great strides have been made in the technological and pharmacological care of the burned patient. In the 1940s and 1950s, a patient with a 30% to 40% TBSA burn had a 50% chance of survival (LD_{50}). Over the decades, the survivability increased as the result of penicillin and broad-spectrum antibiotics, the burn center concept, and aggressive nutrition and excision. Today, a patient with a 75% TBSA burn has a 50% chance of survival. The trend toward outpatient management has contributed to the decreased number of hospitalized patients. Acute hospitalization resulting from a burn injury has declined 50% since the 1970s. From 1995 to 2005, the average length of stay for inpatient hospitalization declined from 13 days to 8 days, and the mortality rate decreased from 6.2% to 4.7%.[1]

Despite the dramatic reductions in incidence, an acute burn injury remains the third leading cause of death in children between the ages of 1 and 9 years, although it has decreased to the sixth leading cause of death in the remainder of the population. The advocacy of several national organizations has helped introduce increased fire-resistant products, fire prevention programs, and legislation (e.g., flame-retardant children's sleepwear, smoke alarms, fire suppression systems). Nevertheless, there are an estimated 4,500 fire and burn deaths per year.[1,2] Safety measures for preventing burns are given in Box 53-1.

• Classification of Burn Injuries

Burn injuries are described in terms of causative agent, depth, and severity.

CAUSATIVE AGENT

A burn injury usually results from energy transfer from a heat source to the body. The heat source may be thermal, chemical, electrical, or radiation producing.

Thermal Burns

Thermal burns may be caused by a flame source such as a house fire, a cooking accident, or a fiery explosion. Scald burns from steam or contact with a hot object, such as a cooking pan or hot steel, may also cause thermal injury.

Chemical Burns

Chemical injuries are commonly encountered after exposure to acids and alkali, including hydrofluoric acid, formic acid, anhydrous ammonia, cement, and phenol. Other specific chemical agents that cause chemical burns include white phosphorus, certain elemental metals, nitrates, hydrocarbons, and tar.

Contact time is a critical element in determining the severity of injury. Initiation of hydrotherapy is crucial to limit the effects of the chemical. Regardless of the causative agent, the irrigation must continue once the patient arrives at the emergency department. Time should not be lost attempting to neutralize the acid or alkali; a neutralizing agent may cause further burn injury through additional chemical reactions. For all chemical burns, hydrotherapy treatment should continue until the pain is resolved, this may take 2 to 3 hours or longer. Chemicals to the eyes should be flushed continuously until a full evaluation can be completed by an ophthalmologist.

Electrical Burns

The effects of electricity on the body are determined by seven factors: the type of current, the amount of current, the pathway of the current, the duration of contact, the area of contact, the resistance of the body, and the voltage. Humans are sensitive to very small electric currents because of their highly developed nervous system. Electricity travels the path of least resistance; therefore, tissue, nerves, and muscle are easily damaged, whereas bone is not.

Low-voltage injuries are considered to be caused by 1,000 volts or less. Low-voltage injuries tend to occur at home and involve the hands and oral cavities. The most common cause of low-voltage electric burns of the hand is contact with an extension cord in which the insulating material has worn off, either from wear or misuse. A low-voltage burn of the hand usually consists of a small, deep burn that may involve vessels, tendons, and nerves. Although these burns involve a small area of the hand, they may be severe enough to require amputation of a finger. Low-voltage electricity can also damage the oral cavity, leaving a permanent scar. These injuries occur most frequently in children between the ages of 1 and 2 years. Most are caused by sucking on, or biting, an extension cord socket. Low-voltage current usually follows the path of least resistance (nerves, blood vessels), whereas high-voltage current takes a direct path between entrance and ground. Current is concentrated at its entrance to the body, then diverges centrally, and finally converges before exiting. Unfortunately, the most severe damage to tissue occurs at the sites of contact, which are commonly referred to as the entrance and exit wounds. High-voltage electric entry wounds are charred, centrally depressed, and leathery in appearance, whereas exit wounds are more likely to "explode" as the charge exits.

Box 53-1 • TEACHING GUIDE:
Preventing Burns

Prevent Accidents in the Home
- Never leave children unattended in a bathtub.
- Set your hot water heater no higher than 120°F.
- Never leave candles unattended, and always be sure candles are fully extinguished.
- Exercise caution with foods that are cooked in a microwave.
- Have your furnace serviced once a year.
- Install a carbon monoxide detector.
- Install a smoke detector on each floor of your house; change the batteries twice a year.
- Plan an exit route in your house in the event of a fire and have routine fire drills once a month.
- Exercise caution with cooking. Avoid wearing clothes with sleeves that may dangle and accidentally ignite clothing.
- Keep pot and skillet handles turned in toward the stove.
- Never use the oven as a heating source.
- Never allow children to stand on an open oven door, as this may cause the entire stove to collapse.

Prevent Accidents Outside the Home
- Only a responsible adult should handle fireworks. Never leave fireworks out where children can have access.
- Exercise caution with campfires.
- If an electrical wire is found in a tree, do not touch! Call the local electric company as soon as possible.
- Use sunscreens! Choose a sunscreen with ultraviolet A (UVA) and ultraviolet B (UVB) protection and a sun protection factor (SPF) of 30. Apply every 2 to 3 h.

Should a Burn Occur
- Stop the burning process by removing the source!

Table 53-1 • Characteristics of Burns of Various Depths

Depth	Tissues Involved	Usual Cause	Characteristics	Pain	Healing
Superficial (first-degree)	Minimal epithelial damage	Sun	Dry Blisters after 24 h Pinkish red Blanches with pressure	Painful	About 5 d No scarring
Superficial partial-thickness (second-degree)	Epidermis, minimal dermis	Flash Hot liquids	Moist Pinkish or mottled red Blisters Some blanching	Pain Hyperesthetic	21–28 d Minimal scarring
Deep partial-thickness (second-degree)	Entire epidermis, part of dermis: epidermal-lined hair and sweat glands intact	Above plus hot solids, flame, and intense radiant injury	Dry, pale, waxy No blanching	Sensitive to pressure	30 d to months Late hypertrophic scarring; marked contracture formation
Full-thickness (third-degree)	All of above, and portion of subcutaneous fat; may involve connective tissue, muscle, bone	Sustained flame, electrical, chemical, and steam	Leathery, cracked avascular, white, cherry red, or black	Little pain	Cannot self-regenerate; needs grafting

DEPTH

Many factors alter the response of body tissues to heat. The degree or depth of burn depends on (1) the temperature of the injuring agent, (2) the duration of exposure to the injuring agent, and (3) the areas of the body that are exposed to the injuring agent. Whereas the body can sustain prolonged exposure to moderate temperatures such as a hot tub of water (110°F or 43°C), significant damage can occur in as little as 1 second when the temperature exceeds 150°F (68°C). Hot water heaters are often installed with the setting at 140°F (60°C). A safer setting would be 124°F to 130°F (51°C to 54°C), or as low as 120°F (49°C) in homes with children or elderly family members. Damage to the skin is frequently described according to the depth of injury and is defined in terms of superficial, partial-thickness, and full-thickness injuries, which correspond to the various layers of the skin (Table 53-1; Fig. 53-1).

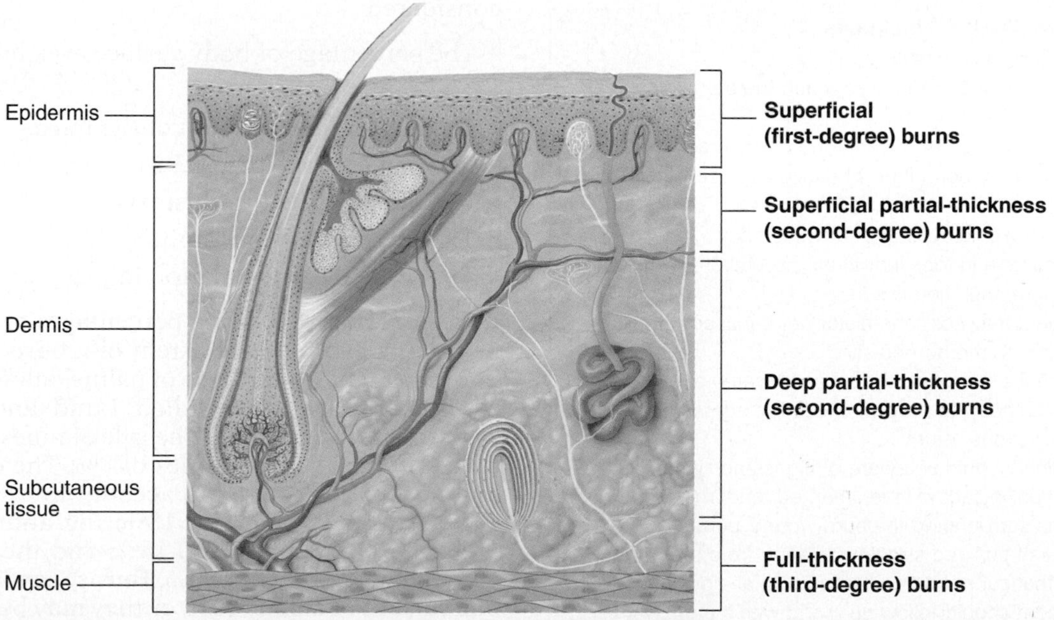

Figure 53-1 • Classification of burns by depth of injury. (From Anatomical Chart Company: Atlas of Pathophysiology. Springhouse, PA: Springhouse, 2001, p 361.)

Superficial Burns

Superficial burn injuries are commonly known as first-degree burns. Superficial burns affect the epidermal layer and heal with minimal intervention. Sunburn is a familiar example of a first-degree superficial burn injury; others may be very brief exposure to hot liquid, flash, flame, or chemical agent. The burned skin is painful at first and later itches because of the stimulation of sensory receptors. Because of the continuous replacement of epidermal epithelial cells, this type of injury heals spontaneously without scarring in 3 to 6 days. Care of superficial burns is minimally supportive and is summarized in Box 53-2.

Partial-Thickness Burns

Partial-thickness burns (second-degree burns) are differentiated into superficial and deep partial-thickness burns. Superficial partial-thickness burns affect the epidermal and superficial dermal layers and usually heal with minimal intervention in 10 to 14 days (see Box 53-2). Deep partial-thickness burns affect the entire epidermal layer and more deep dermal layers. Fluid resuscitation, nutritional status, and the presence of premorbid conditions may affect the healing potential of a deep partial-thickness burn injury.

Box 53-2 • Care of Superficial (First-Degree) Burns and Superficial Partial-Thickness (Second-Degree) Burns

Superficial (First-Degree) Burns
- Apply ice packs or cold compresses.
- No dressing is required.
- Aloe gel with lidocaine can be applied topically as necessary for localized relief.
- Acetaminophen, aspirin, or ibuprofen can be taken as necessary for generalized discomfort.

Superficial Partial-Thickness (Second-Degree) Burns
- If the skin or blister is broken, wash the area with water and mild antiseptic soap.
- Apply a layer of silver sulfadiazine or bacitracin.
- Apply a layer of nonadherent gauze and secure with a gauze roll.
- Dressings should be changed twice a day.
- Wrap fingers and toes individually to prevent "webbing" of healing granulation tissue.
- The patient may continue his or her usual activity depending on the burned site.
- Dependent extremities should be elevated above the level of the heart to prevent excessive edema and promote venous return.
- The patient should be aware of signs and symptoms of infection, including fever, marked tenderness and erythema surrounding the burn wound, purulent drainage of pus, red streaks radiating from the wound, or pain that cannot be controlled with analgesics.
- The patient should follow up in 2 d with a primary care provider.

Deep partial-thickness burn injuries may have some spontaneous healing in 3 to 4 weeks but require surgical intervention (excision and skin grafting) if the burn is of any significant size. Delayed healing may result in scarring and loss of function.

Full-Thickness Burns

Prolonged exposure to flame, a hot object, or chemical agent or contact with high-voltage electricity can result in full-thickness burns (third-degree burns). These burns expose the fat layer, which is composed of poorly vascularized adipose tissue. This layer contains the roots of the sweat glands and hair follicles. All epidermal and dermal elements are destroyed. These burns may appear white, red, brown, or black. Reddened areas do not blanch in response to pressure because the underlying blood supply has been interrupted. Thrombosed blood vessels and capillaries may be visualized. These burns are insensate because the sensory receptors have been completely destroyed, and the patient may feel deep pressure only. In addition, the burns may appear sunken because of the loss of underlying fat and muscle.

The destruction of the hair follicle eliminates the ability of the skin to regenerate. A small wound (<4 cm) may be allowed to heal by granulation and migration of healthy epithelium from the wound margins. However, extensive, open full-thickness wounds leave the patient highly susceptible to overwhelming infection and malnutrition. Wound closure by skin grafting restores the integrity of the skin.

SEVERITY

Burn severity is determined by the extent and depth of the burn and the causative agent, time, and circumstances surrounding the burn injury. To assess the severity of the burn, several factors must be considered:

▶ The percentage of body surface area burned
▶ The depth of the burn
▶ The anatomical location of the burn
▶ The person's age (Box 53-3)
▶ The person's medical history
▶ The presence of concomitant injury
▶ The presence of inhalation injury

Several methods using percentages of TBSA may be used to estimate the extent of a burn (Fig. 53-2). The "rule of nines" or "rule of palms" allows for quick assessment until a detailed Lund and Browder assessment can be done. The rule of nines divides the body into parts in multiples of 9%. The entire head and neck is considered to account for 9% of TBSA; each arm, 9%; each leg, 18%; the anterior trunk, 18%; the posterior trunk, 18%; and the perineum, 1%, making a total of 100%. Burns may involve only one surface of a body part, or they may be circumferential. For example, if only the anterior surface of the arm is burned, then the TBSA is estimated to be

4.5%. However, if the burn circles the entire arm, then the value is 9%. The rule of palms can be used for estimating small scattered burns (e.g., scald or grease burns). The patient's palmar surface (including the fingers) equals 1% of the patient's TBSA.

The Lund and Browder method (see Fig. 53-2) is highly recommended because it corrects for the large head/body ratio of infants and children. Surface measurements are assigned to each body part in terms of the age of the patient. However, because this method of measuring burn size is time consuming, it should be done after resuscitation efforts are well established.

A burn injury may range from a small blister to a massive full-thickness burn. Recognizing the need for a clear description of terms, the ABA has developed the Injury Severity Grading System, which is used to determine the magnitude of the burn injury and to provide optimal criteria for hospital resources for patient care. The severity of burn injury has been categorized into minor, moderate, and major, as outlined in Box 53-4. Minor burn injuries can be treated in the emergency department with outpatient follow-up every 48 hours, until the risk for infection is reduced and wound healing is underway. Patients with moderate, uncomplicated burn injuries or major burn injuries should be referred to a regional burn center and, if appropriate, transferred for specialized care.

• Pathophysiology

LOCALIZED TISSUE RESPONSE

Cellular injury is started when tissues are exposed to an energy source (thermal, chemical, electrical, or radiation). The depth of the thermal injury is demon-strated by the extent of injury down through the layers of skin. Figure 53-3 represents the concentric zones of a burn injury. The zone of coagulation is the area where the most damage has been sustained; temperatures have reached 113°F (45°C). The tissues are black, gray, khaki, or white and have undergone protein coagulation and cell death. This area has lost the ability to recover and requires surgical intervention. The zone of stasis immediately surrounds the zone of coagulation. This area contains cells that are at the most risk during the burn resuscitation. They can recover or become necrotic in the initial 24 to 72 hours, depending on the conditions and course of resuscitation. The zone of hyperemia is the area of increased blood flow in an effort to bring the needed nutrients to the tissue for recovery (*active hyperemia*) and to remove the metabolic waste products (*reactive hyperemia*). This area heals rapidly and has no cell death.

SYSTEMIC RESPONSE

Major changes at the cellular level are responsible for the tremendous systemic response noted in a patient with burns. The localized response causes a coagulation of cellular proteins, leading to irreversible cell injury with local production of complement, histamine, and oxygen free radicals (i.e., byproducts of oxidative processes). Oxygen free radicals alter cell lipids and proteins, affecting the integrity of the cell membrane. This is particularly problematic in the endothelium of the microvascular circulation because disruption of the cell membrane leads to increased vascular permeability.[3] Increased vascular permeability leads to loss of plasma proteins and results in a marked decrease in circulating volume. Complement (particularly C5a) activation and histamine release contribute to the increased vascular permeability by increasing production of oxygen free radicals.[3,4] Increased vascular permeability leads to the formation of interstitial edema, which usually peaks within 24 to 48 hours of injury. It is postulated that the microvasculature takes weeks to restore itself completely to its premorbid state. The pulmonary vasculature is not spared, and pulmonary interstitial edema forms, with intra-alveolar hemorrhages; this initial pulmonary insult is thought to be a precursor to the development of acute respiratory distress syndrome (ARDS).[5]

Systemically, a burn injury causes a release of vasoactive substances such as histamine, prostaglandins, interleukins, and arachidonic acid metabolites. These substances initiate the systemic inflammatory response syndrome (SIRS). The potent mediators and cytokines (nitric oxide, platelet-activating factor [PAF], serotonin, thromboxane A_2, and tumor necrosis factor [TNF]) deplete the intravascular volume, decreasing blood flow to the kidneys and the gastrointestinal tract. If left uncorrected, hypovolemic shock, metabolic acidosis, and hyperkalemia may occur. Intestinal mucosal permeability also markedly increases and can become the primary source of bacterial infection; early enteral feeding is one step to help prevent the translocation of bacteria.[6]

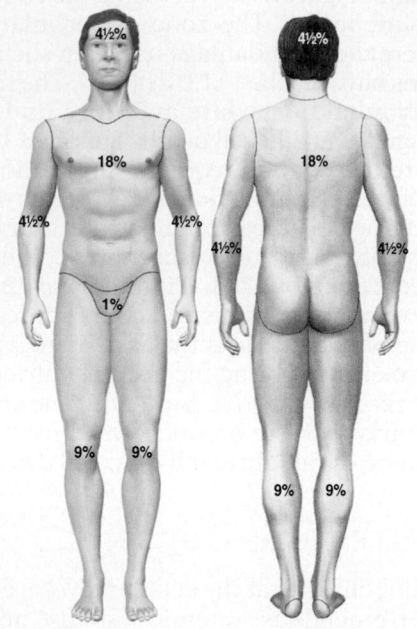

A. Rule of Nines

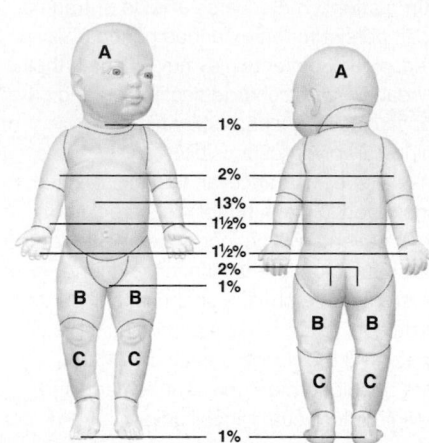

AREA	PERCENT OF BURN					SEVERITY OF BURN		TOTAL PERCENT
	0-1 Year	1-4 Years	5-9 Years	10-15 Years	Adult	2°	3°	
Head	19	17	13	10	7			
Neck	2	2	2	2	2			
Ant. Trunk	13	13	13	13	13			
Post. Trunk	13	13	13	13	13			
R. Buttock	2½	2½	2½	2½	2½			
L. Buttock	2½	2½	2½	2½	2½			
Genitalia	1	1	1	1	1			
R. U. Arm	4	4	4	4	4			
L. U. Arm	4	4	4	4	4			
R. L. Arm	3	3	3	3	3			
L. L. Arm	3	3	3	3	3			
R. Hand	2½	2½	2½	2½	2½			
L. Hand	2½	2½	2½	2½	2½			
R. Thigh	5½	6½	8½	8½	9½			
L. Thigh	5½	6½	8½	8½	9½			
R. Leg	5	5	5½	6	7			
L. Leg	5	5	5½	6	7			
R. Foot	3½	3½	3½	3½	3½			
L. Foot	3½	3½	3½	3½	3½			
Total	Blue areas indicate 2° Red areas indicate 3°			**Total**				

B. Lund and Browder chart

Figure 53-2 • A: The "rule of nines" method for determining percentage of body area with burn injury. **B:** Lund and Browder method for determining percentage of body area with burn injury. (**A,** from Anatomical Chart Company: Atlas of Pathophysiology. Springhouse, PA: Springhouse, 2001, p 361.)

Nitric oxide relaxes smooth muscle and produces vasodilation and hypotension. It may also depress myocardial function and block platelet aggregation and adhesion. PAF initiates neutrophil and white blood cell activation and produces tissue inflammation. PAF increases permeability of vessels, thereby decreasing myocardial contractility, causing vasodilation and hypotension. Some prostaglandins cause vasoconstriction and increased blood flow. A fever may also accompany prostaglandin activation. Sero-

tonin causes vasodilation, hypotension, and increased vessel permeability. Thromboxane A_2 is responsible for inflammation, platelet aggregation, and polymorphonuclear cell adherence. TNF is responsible for numerous cellular responses, including increased formation of oxygen free radicals, which leads to injury of the lungs, gastrointestinal tract, and kidneys; increased cytokine production; initial hyperglycemia followed by hypoglycemia; hypotension; metabolic acidosis; coagulopathy; and activation of the coagulation cascade.

The end results of the local and systemic responses are dramatic, if the burn covers more than 20% of the TBSA. The person with a major burn injury experiences a form of hypovolemic shock known as burn shock (Fig. 53-4). Within minutes of thermal injury, a marked increase in capillary hydrostatic pressure occurs in the injured tissue, accompanied by an increase in capillary permeability. This results in a rapid shift of plasma fluid from the intravascular compartment across heat-damaged capillaries, into interstitial areas (resulting in edema), and to the burn wound itself. The loss of plasma fluid and proteins results in a decreased colloid osmotic pressure in the vascular compartment. As a result, fluid and electrolytes continue to leak from the vascular compartment, resulting in additional edema formation in the burned tissue and throughout the body.

This "leak," which consists of sodium, water, and plasma proteins, is followed by a decrease in cardiac output, hemoconcentration of red blood cells, diminished perfusion to major organs, and generalized body edema. The pathophysiological response after burn injury is biphasic. In the early postinjury (ebb) phase, generalized organ hypofunction develops as a consequence of decreased cardiac output. Peripheral vascular resistance increases as a result of the neurohumoral stress response after trauma. This increases cardiac afterload, resulting in a further decrease in cardiac output. The increase in peripheral vascular resistance (selective vasoconstriction) and the hemoconcentration resulting from plasma fluid loss may cause the blood pressure to appear normal at first. However, if fluid replacement is inadequate, and plasma protein loss continues, hypovolemic shock soon occurs.

In patients receiving adequate fluid resuscitation, the cardiac output usually returns to normal in the latter part of the first 24 hours after burn injury. As plasma volume is replenished during the second 24 hours, the cardiac output increases to hypermetabolic levels (hyperfunction phase) and slowly returns to more normal levels as the burn wounds are closed.[6,7]

In some instances, with burns exceeding 60% of the TBSA, depressed cardiac output does not respond to aggressive volume resuscitation. A myocardial depressant factor capable of depressing ventricular contractility by 60% has been identified. Myocardial depression in the early postburn period may also be the result of reduced coronary blood flow.[4,6]

The response of the pulmonary vasculature is similar to that of the peripheral circulation. However, pulmonary vascular resistance is greater and lasts

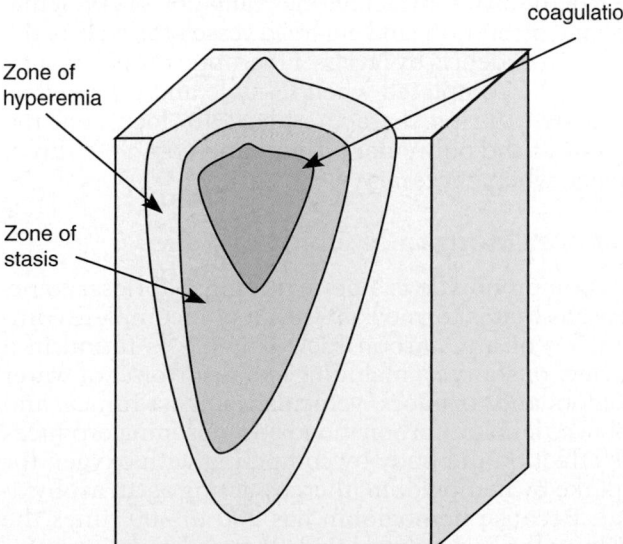

Zone of coagulation

Zone of hyperemia

Zone of stasis

Figure 53-3 • The concentric zones of a burn injury.

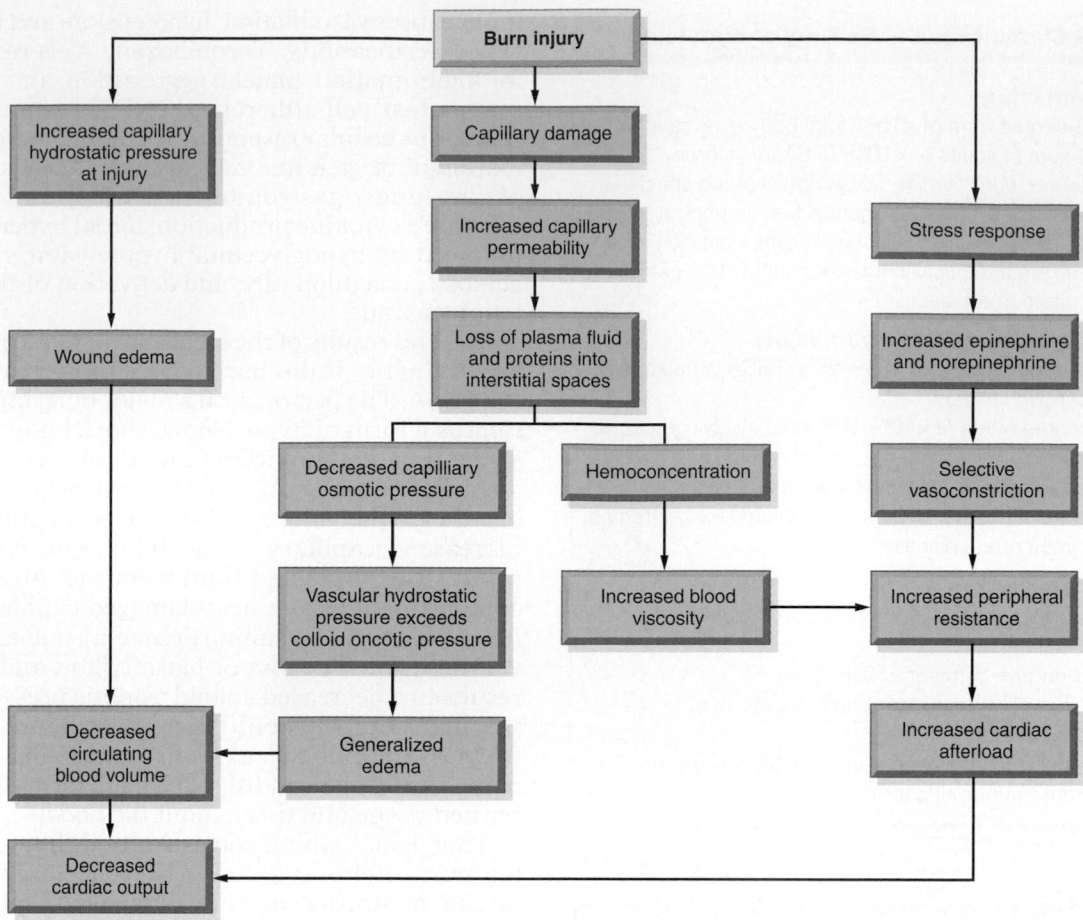

Figure 53-4 • Fluid shifts in burn shock.

longer. Immediately after burn injury, the patient may experience a mild, transient pulmonary hypertension. A decrease in oxygen tension and lung compliance may also be evident.

The loss of fluid throughout the body's intravascular space results in a thickened, sluggish flow of the remaining circulatory blood volume. The effects reach all body systems. This slowing of circulation permits bacteria and cellular material to settle in the lower portions of blood vessels, especially in the capillaries, which results in sludging.

The antigen–antibody reaction to burned tissue adds to circulatory congestion by the clumping or agglutination of cells. Coagulation problems occur as a result of the release of thromboplastin by the injury itself and the release of fibrinogen from injured platelets. If thrombi occur, they may cause ischemia of the affected part and lead to necrosis. Although of limited incidence in patients with burns, the increased coagulation process may develop into disseminated intravascular coagulation.

• Concomitant Problems

PULMONARY INJURY

Pulmonary damage usually appears within 24 to 48 hours of the injury and is secondary to the inhalation of combustible products or may be the result of inhaled superheated air. In an incident involving large amounts of steam, the risk for injury is far greater because water has a heat-carrying capacity 4,000 times greater than air and has the ability to be inhaled deeply in the pulmonary system. Pulmonary injury may also be the result of a systemic process related to SIRS.

Fiberoptic bronchoscopy permits direct visualization of the airways (facilitating evaluation of erythema, edema, ulceration, and enlarged vessels) as well as the removal of debris by lavage. Fiberoptic bronchoscopy should be completed when feasible and repeated as indicated during the acute phase to document the extent of the pulmonary injury and complete direct lavage when necessary.

Carbon Monoxide Toxicity

Carbon monoxide is a nonirritating, odorless, colorless gas that is formed as a result of incomplete combustion of any carbon fuel. This gas is found in a variety of sources, including exhaust from hot water heaters and furnaces, vehicular exhaust fumes, and tobacco smoke. Carbon monoxide poisoning produces its effect on the body by competing with oxygen for uptake by hemoglobin, thereby acting as an asphyxiant. Because hemoglobin has 200 to 300 times the affinity for carbon monoxide than it has for oxygen, carbon monoxide readily displaces the oxygen, leading to the formation of carboxyhemoglobin and a reduction in systemic arterial oxygen content. Carboxyhemoglobin shifts the oxyhemoglobin dissociation curve to the left, further decreasing the ability of the red blood cells to release oxygen to body tissues.[8] This may lead to severe anoxia and related brain injury.

The patient with a clear history of exposure to carbon monoxide is usually found in a closed environment in the presence of combusted gases, such as smoke, automobile exhaust, or fumes from a faulty furnace. The signs of carbon monoxide poisoning depend on the amount of carboxyhemoglobin that is present in the patient's blood (Table 53-2).

When carbon monoxide poisoning is suspected, 100% high-flow oxygen is administered. Carbon monoxide has a half-life of 4 hours if the patient breathes room air and 45 minutes if the patient is breathing 100% oxygen. 100% oxygen should be continued until the carboxyhemoglobin level is less than 15% to 20%. Serial arterial blood gas (ABG) measurements are the most accurate way to assess responsiveness to oxygen therapy. Pulse oximetry is inaccurate when the carboxyhemoglobin level is elevated because pulse oximetry cannot distinguish between oxygen and carbon monoxide on the hemoglobin.

Inhalation Injury

Besides carbon monoxide poisoning, smoke inhalation can result in thermal injury to the airway. Pulmonary damage, primarily as a result of inhalation injury, is historically seen in less than 10% of the total cases but accounts for 20% to 84% of burn mortality and is a significant factor in increasing the hospital length of stay. Three stages of injury have been described:

1. Acute pulmonary insufficiency may occur during the first 36 hours.
2. Pulmonary edema occurs in 5% to 30% of patients with burns between 6 and 72 hours after injury.
3. Bronchopneumonia appears in 15% to 60% of patients with burns 3 to 10 days after injury.

Upper airway injury is the result of inhalation of superheated air, which may cause blisters and edema in the supraglottic area around the vocal cords. This situation may cause airway obstruction and edema. Hoarseness, stridor, dyspnea, carbonaceous sputum, and tachypnea indicate airway compromise, which must be addressed immediately. Early intubation may thwart such disastrous occurrences.

Tracheobronchial and parenchymal lung injuries are usually a result of incomplete combustion of chemicals (e.g., aldehyde, acrolein) and result in a chemical pneumonitis. Inflammatory changes in the trachea and alveoli occur within 24 hours of injury. The pulmonary tree becomes irritated and edematous. The alveoli may collapse, causing a decreased compliance, which leads to atelectasis. ARDS may develop rapidly. However, changes may not become apparent until the second 24 hours. Pulmonary edema is a possibility any time from the first few hours to 7 days after the injury. Subtle changes in the patient's sensorium may indicate hypoxia.

History and physical assessment findings that should alert the nurse to the potential for inhalation injury are given in Box 53-5. Serial ABGs show a decreasing arterial oxygen tension (PaO_2). Usually, the admission chest film appears normal because changes are not reflected until 24 to 48 hours after the burn. A sputum specimen is obtained for culture and sensitivity studies. Laryngoscopy and bronchoscopy may be of value in determining the presence of extramucosal carbonaceous material (the most reliable sign of inhalation injury) and the state of the mucosa (blistering, edema, erythema). More specific confirmation of inhalation injury is achieved with the use of fiberoptic bronchoscopy, which permits direct examination of the proximal airway, and xenon-133 scintigraphy (ventilation–perfusion scanning). Xenon-133 scintigraphy is helpful in establishing a diagnosis of injury to small airways and lung parenchyma.

INFECTION

There is no greater problem for the patient with burns than infection. Loss of the mechanical barrier between the human body and the environment is the first step in the weakening of defenses. All aspects of the immune system, including phagocytosis, soluble mediators of innate immunity such as complement, antibody production, and cellular (T-cell) defense systems, are compromised by severe burn injury. The most common cause of death in patients with burns after the first 7 days is infection.

Actions of the health care team can compromise patient survival. All catheters invading the body, including endotracheal tubes, central venous catheters, and bladder catheters, must be handled

Table 53-2 • Signs and Symptoms of Carbon Monoxide Poisoning	
Carboxyhemoglobin Saturation (%)	Clinical Presentation
10	No symptoms
20	Headache, vomiting, dyspnea on exertion
30	Confusion, lethargy, changes on electrocardiogram (ECG)
40–60	Coma
More than 60	Death

Box 53-5 • RED FLAG: History and Physical Examination Findings Suggestive of Inhalation Injury

- History of incident occurring in a confined area
- Singed nasal hairs
- Burns of the oral or pharyngeal mucous membranes
- Burns in the perioral area or neck
- Carbonaceous sputum
- Change in voice

with as clean a technique as possible. Although the skin and gut are the source of endogenous bacteria, a greater threat to the patient is colonization with antibiotic-resistant pathogens carried by the burn team from other patients. The hands must be washed without fail before and after handling the patient, the patient's bed, or equipment. When dressings are removed and wounds exposed, sterile gloves must be worn. Frequent and meticulous handwashing alone probably prevents infection more than any other single action. Infection control policies vary from burn center to burn center, but the philosophy remains the same: Make every effort to minimize the transmission of bacteria from patient to patient.

Diagnosis of invasive infection in the patients with burns is unusually difficult. Most patients with burns have elevated core temperatures and white blood cell counts. The significance of these signs becomes blunted in the patient with burns. In a patient with burns, a more useful sign of infection is the appearance of sugar in the urine, particularly if this appears paradoxically when the blood sugar level is within normal limits. Hyperglycemia and increased difficulty in controlling the blood sugar in a person with diabetes are signs of threatening sepsis. A drop in the platelet count, particularly in children, is an early warning sign of sepsis. Manifestations of multisystem organ dysfunction, such as hypotension, hypoxia, decreased pulmonary compliance, renal failure, or hepatic dysfunction, are almost certain signs of septic shock.

Qualitative wound cultures done by swabbing the wound yield no new information other than the nature of the bacterial species colonizing the surface of the wound. A biopsy of the burn wound permits a quantitative assay of the number of colony-forming units (CFUs) of bacteria per gram of tissue. Burn wound sepsis is likely if the colony count is greater than 105 CFU/g, and the quantitative culture also allows isolation and identification of the invading organism.

TRAUMA

Concomitant injuries such as fractures and head trauma pose significant risk for the patient with burns. Ensuring adequate airway, breathing, and circulation takes precedence over caring for specific injuries. Cervical spine injuries should be stabilized and cleared. If head trauma is suspected, a computed tomography scan is obtained. The history of the burn injury is critical to assisting with the evaluation of the patient. The burn wounds may mask some of the classic signs of underlying injuries, such as ecchymosis or swelling. The burn event may include events such as an explosion, the patient being thrown or falling, or a motor vehicle crash. Patients with electrical injuries must also be evaluated for fractures secondary to the violent muscular contraction after exposure; special focus should be placed on the cervical spinous process and long bones.

• Assessment and Management

The initial assessment of the patient with burns is like that of any trauma patient. The ABA has identified criteria for referral to a burn center (Box 53-6). Patients with these burns should be treated in a specialized burn facility after initial assessment and treatment at an emergency department. Whether the patient stays at the initial hospital or is transferred to a burn center facility, the resuscitation phase begins immediately after the burn insult has occurred. The primary and secondary surveys are completed before transfer. Proper stabilization of the patient is crucial for successful transfer. As with any major trauma, the first hour is crucial, and the next 24 to 36 hours are also important. The management of fluid balance, the respiratory system, and nutrition are vital, and all systems have a major impact on the patient's survival.

RESUSCITATIVE PHASE
Primary Survey

The following parameters are assessed in the primary survey:

► Airway maintenance with cervical spine protection
► Breathing and ventilation
► Circulation with hemorrhage control
► Disability (assess neurological deficit)
► Exposure (completely undress the patient, but maintain temperature)

Airway

On initial assessment of the patient with burns, the airway must be assessed immediately. The

---

Box 53-6 • Criteria for Referral to a Burn Center

- Partial-thickness burns >10% of total body surface area (TBSA)
- Burns that involve the face, hands, feet, genitalia, perineum, or major joints
- Third-degree burns in any age group
- Electrical burns, including lightning injury
- Chemical burns
- Inhalation injury
- Burn injury in patients with preexisting medical disorders that could complicate management, prolong recovery, or affect mortality
- Concomitant trauma, in which the burn injury poses the greatest risk for morbidity or mortality*
- Children with burns in hospitals without qualified personnel or equipment for the care of children
- Patients with burns who will require special social, emotional, or long-term rehabilitative intervention

*In such cases, if the trauma poses the greater immediate risk, the patient may be initially stabilized in a trauma center before being transferred to a burn unit. Physician judgment is necessary in such situations and should be in concert with the regional medical control plan and triage protocols.

compromised airway may be controlled by a chin lift, jaw thrust, insertion of an oropharyngeal airway in an unconscious patient, or endotracheal intubation. It is crucial not to hyperextend the neck in patients with suspected cervical spine injuries.

Breathing and Ventilation

Ventilation requires adequate functioning of the lungs, chest wall, and diaphragm. To assess for breathing and ventilation, the nurse must listen to the chest and verify breath sounds in each lung, assess adequacy of rate and depth of respiration, administer high-flow oxygen at 15 L/minute using a nonrebreathing mask, and assess for circumferential full-thickness burns of the chest that may impair ventilation.

Circulation

Assessment of the circulation includes a measurement of blood pressure and heart rate. Special attention should be paid to the distal pulses of any extremity with circumferential burns. Intravenous cannulation is performed by inserting two large-bore catheters into the skin that is unburned, if possible. A central venous catheter should be inserted when indicated. Doppler ultrasonography can be used to assess for pulses. Box 53-7 lists risk factors for impaired circulation.

Disability

Typically, the patient with burns is alert and oriented. If not, associated injuries such as inhalation injury, head trauma, substance abuse, or preexisting medical conditions should be considered. The assessment is initiated by determining the patient's level of consciousness using the AVPU (**A**lert, responds to **V**erbal stimuli, responds to **P**ainful stimuli, **U**nresponsive) method.

Exposure

All the patient's clothing and jewelry are removed to complete the primary and secondary survey. After examination, the patient is covered with a clean, dry sheet and warm blankets to prevent evaporative cooling. If possible, intravenous fluids are warmed to 98.6°F (37°C) to 104°F (40°C).

Secondary Survey

The secondary survey is completed after resuscitative efforts are well established and consists of a detailed history and physical examination of the patient as well as a complete history of the accident. Every attempt is made to determine exactly what happened (Box 53-8). A detailed neurological examination is completed, and initial radiographic and laboratory

---

Box 53-8 • Information Obtained During a Secondary Survey

Thermal Burns
- How did the burn occur?
- Did the burn occur inside or outside?
- Did the clothes catch fire?
- How long did it take to extinguish the fire?
- Were there any explosions?
- Was the patient found in a smoke-filled room?
- How did the patient escape?
- Did the patient jump out of a window?
- Were there other people injured or killed at the scene?
- Was the patient unconscious at the scene?
- Was there a motor vehicle crash?
- Was the car severely damaged?
- Was there a car fire?
- Are the purported circumstances of the injury consistent with the burn characteristics (is there possibility of abuse)?

For Scald Injuries
- How did the burn occur?
- What was the temperature of the liquid?
- What was the liquid; how much liquid was involved?
- What was the burn cooled with?
- Who was present when the burn took place?
- Where did the burn take place? Is there possibility of abuse?

Chemical Burns
- What was the agent?
- How did the exposure occur?
- What was the duration of contact?
- Did contamination take place?

Electrical Burns
- What kind of electricity was involved?
- Did the patient lose consciousness?
- Did the patient fall?
- What was the estimated voltage?
- Was cardiopulmonary resuscitation (CPR) administered at the scene?

---

studies are done. Resuscitative measures are ongoing and constantly evaluated.

A complete history and physical examination are the hallmarks of the secondary survey. It is not uncommon for patients to have comorbid diseases. Preexisting diseases such as diabetes, hypertension, asthma, cancer, and stroke should be documented. A medication list is obtained from the patient if possible, or a family member is asked to provide the information. In addition, any allergies, the person's tetanus immunization history, and the time of the person's last meal should be documented. Burn depth and burn size are assessed.

Burn injuries require a global assessment. The following laboratory and diagnostic studies are indicated for patients with burns:

▶ Complete blood count (CBC)

▶ Comprehensive chemistry panel, including blood urea nitrogen

---

Box 53-7 • RED FLAG: Risk Factors for Impaired Circulation

- Decreased sensation
- Progressive worsening of pain
- Paresthesias
- Decreased capillary refill
- Pallor of extremity

► Creatinine level
► Urinalysis
► ABGs with a carboxyhemoglobin
► Electrocardiogram
► Chest radiograph

After the primary and secondary surveys are complete, the burned area is usually covered with a dry sheet. This reduces the risk for infection and keeps the patient warm. Ice can be applied to small superficial burns. If the patient has a high-voltage electrical burn or cardiac changes are noted, continuous cardiac monitoring is provided. If the patient has a chemical burn, the area is immediately flushed with large amounts of water to remove the chemical, and all contaminated clothing is removed and bagged. If the patient is going to be transferred to a burn center, initiation of fluid resuscitation, insertion of a nasogastric tube, and insertion of an indwelling urinary catheter may be carried out during the secondary assessment.

Providing Hemodynamic Support

Therapy for burn shock is aimed at supporting the patient through the period of hypovolemic shock ("burn shock") until capillary integrity is restored. Fluid resuscitation is the primary intervention in the resuscitative phase in the intensive care unit (ICU). Goals in fluid resuscitation are as follows:

► Correct fluid, electrolyte, and protein deficits.
► Replace continuing losses, and maintain fluid balance.
► Prevent excessive edema formation.
► Maintain a urine output in adults of 30 to 50 mL/hour.

Formulas for Fluid Administration

Numerous formulas have been developed for fluid resuscitation (Box 53-9). Each has advantages and disadvantages. They differ primarily in terms of recommended volume administration and salt content. In general, lost crystalloid and colloid solutions must be replaced rigorously. Free water, given as 5% dextrose in water (D_5W) with or without added electrolytes, is regulated so that insensible fluid loss is covered. Lactated Ringer's solution is used as the crystalloid solution because it is a balanced salt solution that closely approximates the composition of extracellular fluid.

The ABA recommends the use of the ABA consensus formula for the resuscitation of patients with burns. The formula is a combination of the modified Brooke formula and the Baxter (commonly called Parkland) formula. The ABA consensus formula requires 2 to 4 mL of lactated Ringer's solution per kilogram of body weight per percentage TBSA burn. The total amount calculated is administered in the first 24 hours after injury. One half is given in the first 8 hours *from the time of the burn,* one fourth is given during the next 8 hours, and the remaining one fourth is given over the next 8 hours. The ABA consensus formula and the other fluid resuscitation formulas are guidelines, and individual patients may require more or less than 2 to 4 mL/kg per percentage TBSA during the first 24 hours. Patients who often require more fluid than the formula predicted include those with electrical injuries, inhalation injuries, delayed resuscitation, prior dehydration at time of injury, and concomitant trauma.

Other formulas contain various amounts of hypertonic saline or colloid. Hypertonic saline resuscitation lowers the amount of fluid that needs to be given to selected patients; however, it can cause severe

---

Box 53-9 • Fluid Resuscitation Formulas

Baxter (Parkland) Formula
• First 24 h: Lactated Ringer's solution (4 mL/kg/% TBSA); half given over first 8 h, remaining half given over next 16 h
• Second 24 h: Dextrose in water, plus potassium- and colloid-containing fluid (0.3–0.5 mL/kg/%TBSA)

Brooke Formula
• First 24 h: Lactated Ringer's solution (1.5 mL/kg/% TBSA) plus colloid solution (0.5 mL/kg/%TBSA); half given over first 8 hours, remaining half given over next 16 h
• Second 24 hours: Lactated Ringer's solution (0.5–0.75 mL/kg/%TBSA), plus 5% dextrose in water (2 L)

Modified Brooke Formula
• First 24 h: Lactated Ringer's solution (2 mL/kg/% TBSA); half given over first 8 hours, remaining half given over next 16 h
• Second 24 h: Colloid solution (0.3–0.5 mL/kg/% TBSA), plus 5% dextrose in water to maintain adequate urine output

Consensus Formula
• First 24 h: Lactated Ringer's solution (2–4 mL/kg/% TBSA in adults; 3–4 mL/kg/%TBSA in children); half given over first 8 h, remaining half given over next 16 h
• Second 24 h: Colloid-containing fluid (0.3–0.5 mL/kg/%TBSA), plus electrolyte-free fluid (in adults) or half-normal saline (in children) to maintain adequate urine output

Dextran Formula
• First 8 h: Dextran 40 in saline (2 mL/kg/h), plus lactated Ringer's solution infused to maintain urine output at 30 mL/h
• Second 8 h: Fresh frozen plasma (0.5 mL/kg/h) for 18 h, plus additional crystalloid to maintain adequate urine output

Evans Formula
• First 24 h: 0.9% normal saline (1 mL/kg/%TBSA), plus colloid solution (1 mL/kg/%TBSA); half given over first 8 h, remaining half given over next 16 h
• Second 24 h: 0.9% normal saline (0.5 mL/kg/% TBSA), plus 5% dextrose in water (2 L)

hypernatremia and must be used cautiously. The argument against colloid administration within 12 hours of injury is that during this time, the diffuse postburn capillary leak allows colloids to extravasate through endothelial junctions. Therefore, colloid administration does not produce any demonstrable oncotic benefit over administration of a crystalloid while the capillary leak is present. The postinjury time at which capillary integrity is restored varies among people but usually is between 12 and 14 hours. Many physicians administer colloids at this point to restore albumin levels to 2.0 to 3.0 mg/dL. Controversy exists over the type of colloid to be administered, with some centers using salt-poor albumin, and others using fresh frozen plasma.

Nonprotein collagens may be used in burn shock resuscitation. Dextran and hetastarch are high–molecular-weight solutions that generate colloid osmotic pressure when given intravascularly. Allergic responses have been reported with dextran, but the risk virtually is eliminated by pretreatment with Promit, a very low–molecular-weight dextran.

Care must be taken to avoid fluid overload and pulmonary edema. This is often difficult because large amounts of fluids are given over a short period during fluid resuscitation immediately after the burn. For example, using the high range of the ABA consensus formula, a male patient weighing 75 kg who received burns over 50% of his body would require up to 15,000 mL of fluid (4 mL × 75 kg × 50% TBSA = 15,000 mL). Of this, 7,500 mL is to be administered during the first 8 hours, and 3,750 mL is to be administered in the second and third 8-hour periods. It is extremely difficult to avoid fluid overload and pulmonary edema when it is necessary to infuse large amounts of fluids so rapidly.

After the first 24 hours after injury, replacing the massive evaporative water loss is a major consideration in fluid management. The primary solution given at this time is D_5W, with the goal of keeping the patient's sodium concentration at 140 mEq/L. The fluid volume depends on the severity of injury, the age of the patient, the physiological status of the patient, and any associated injuries. Consequently, the volume recommended by a resuscitation formula must be modified according to the person's response to therapy (Fig. 53-5).

Urine output is the single best indicator of fluid resuscitation in patients with previously normal renal function. The onset of spontaneous diuresis is

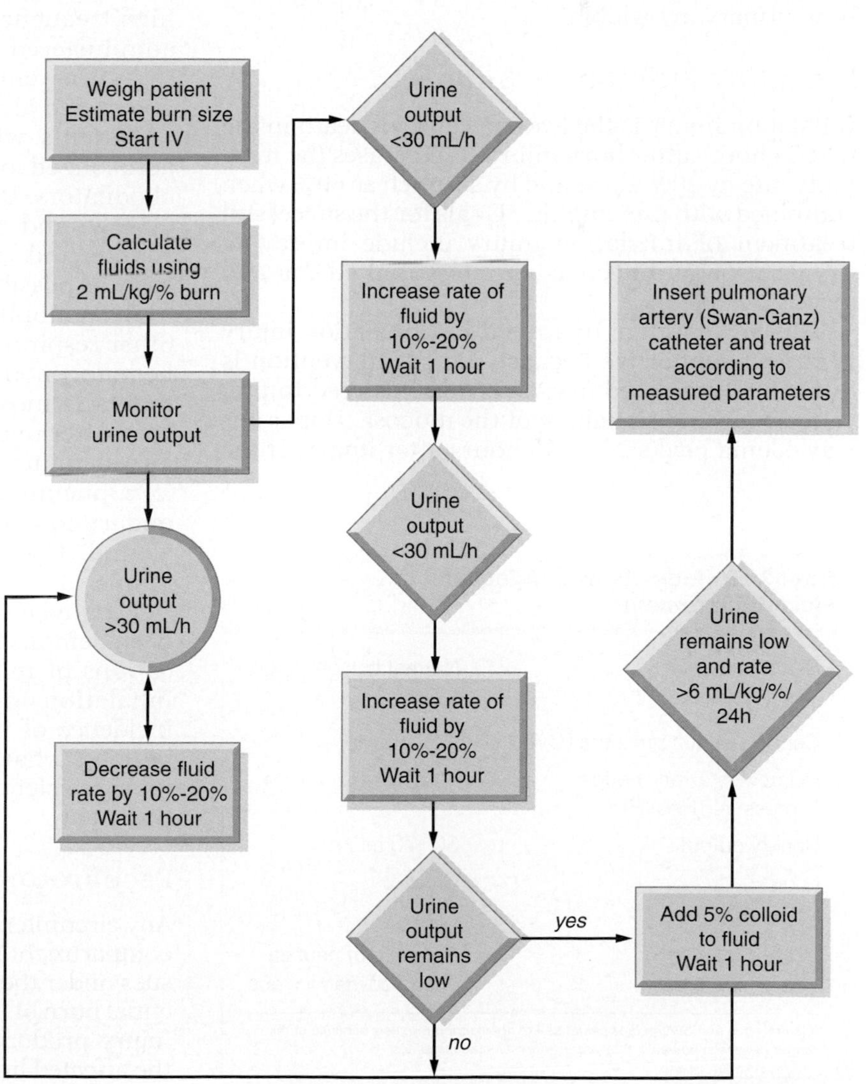

Figure 53-5 • Initial 24-hour fluid management. (From Rue LW, Cioffi WG: Resuscitation of thermally injured patients. Crit Care Nurs Clin North Am 3[2]:186, 1991.)

a hallmark indicating the end of the resuscitative phase. Infusion rates can be decreased by 25% for 1 hour if the urine output is satisfactory and can be maintained for 2 hours; the reduction may then be repeated. It is essential that urinary outputs be maintained within normal limits of 30 to 50 mL per hour (0.5 mL/kg/hour) in the adult. Other indications of adequate fluid replacement are listed in Box 53-10.

Patients are usually weighed daily. A gain of 15% of admission weight may be expected with large fluid resuscitation. Intake and output must be monitored meticulously. Patients who sustain deep muscle injury (i.e., second- or third-degree burns or electrical injuries) are at risk for development of acute renal insufficiency. This renal dysfunction may be the result of inadequate fluid resuscitation, or it may be the consequence of the liberation of the myoglobin and hemoglobin from damaged cells. These compounds, sometimes called hemochromogens, may precipitate in renal tubules, resulting in acute tubular necrosis. Hemochromogens produce a clear reddish-brown color in the urine. Should hemochromogens appear in the urine, acidosis should be corrected promptly and intravenous fluids increased to maintain a brisk urine output (75–100 mL/urine/hour) until the urine returns to its normal clear yellow and there is no urinary myoglobin.

Providing Pulmonary Support

Inhalation injury is the leading cause of death in the first 24 hours after burn injury. It increases the mortality rate by 20% alone and by as much as 60% when combined with pneumonia.[9] Goals for the successful treatment of inhalation injury include improving oxygenation and decreasing interstitial edema and airway occlusion.

The conventional treatment for inhalation injury is largely supportive because direct intervention is difficult. Humidified oxygen is administered to prevent drying and sloughing of the mucosa. Upper airway edema peaks 24 to 48 hours after injury. If the injury is mild or moderately severe, placing the patient in a high Fowler's position and administering aerosolized racemic epinephrine may be sufficient to limit further edema formation. Severe upper airway obstruction may require endotracheal intubation to protect the airway until the edema subsides.

In patients with mild tracheobronchial injury, atelectasis may be prevented by frequent pulmonary toilet, including a high Fowler's position, coughing and deep breathing, chest physiotherapy, repositioning, frequent tracheal suctioning, and incentive spirometry. In patients with more severe inhalation injury, more frequent suctioning may be necessary, and bronchoscopic removal of debris may be appropriate. These patients usually require endotracheal intubation and mechanical ventilatory support. The objective of ventilatory support is to provide adequate gas exchange at the lowest possible inspired oxygen concentration and airway pressure, in an attempt to reduce the incidence of oxygen toxicity and pulmonary barotrauma. The use of volumetric diffusive respiration (VDR) appears to offer advantages over conventional mechanical ventilation.[5,9] In VDR, subtidal volume breaths accumulate and build to a set airway pressure, which is then followed by passive exhalation. Throughout the ventilatory cycle, high-frequency pulsations of air are continuously administered. This method of inspiration appears to aid in ventilation and recruitment of partially obstructed alveoli.

Patients with bronchospasm are treated with aerosolized or intravenously administered bronchodilators. Respiratory parameters are monitored closely, and constant attention is paid to breath sounds and vital signs to detect fluid overload as early as possible.

Bronchopneumonia may be superimposed on other respiratory problems at any time and may be hematogenous or airborne. Airborne bronchopneumonia is most common, with an onset occurring soon after injury. It is often associated with a lower airway injury or aspiration. Hematogenous, or miliary, pneumonia begins as a bacterial abscess secondary to another septic source, usually the burn wound. The time of onset usually is 2 weeks after injury.

Prophylactic antibiotics and steroids have not been demonstrated to prevent the common complications of infection encountered in patients with inhalation injury. New methods to decrease the incidence of nosocomial pneumonia in critically ill patients that are currently under investigation include selective decontamination of the orodigestive tract.

Escharotomy

Any circumferential burn to an arm or leg may mimic compartment syndrome. Edema formation in the tissues under the tight, unyielding eschar of a circumferential burn of a deep partial-thickness or full-thickness injury produces significant vascular compromise in the affected limb.

Box 53-10 • Indications of Adequate Fluid Replacement*

Blood pressure	Normal to high ranges
Pulse rate	<120
Central venous pressure (CVP)	<12 cm H$_2$O
Pulmonary artery wedge pressure (PAWP)	<18 mm Hg
Urinary output	30–70 mL/h
Lungs	Clear
Sensorium	Clear
GI tract	Absence of nausea and adynamic ileus

*Central lines and Swan-Ganz catheters are not inserted routinely because of the danger of sepsis; however, they are used in selected instances.

To minimize the risk for circulatory compromise, the patient's rings, watch, and other jewelry are removed during the initial examination. Elevation and range of motion of the injured extremity may alleviate minimal degrees of circulatory distress. Skin color, sensation, capillary refill, and peripheral pulses are assessed and documented hourly in an extremity with a circumferential burn. Doppler ultrasonography is the most reliable means of assessing arterial blood flow and the need for an escharotomy. In the upper extremity, the radial, ulnar, and palmar arch pulses are checked hourly. In the lower extremity, the posterior tibial and dorsalis pedis pulses are checked hourly. Loss—or a progressive diminution (decrease)—of the ultrasonic signal is an indication for escharotomy.

The escharotomy is carried out as a bedside procedure, using a sterile field and scalpel, an electrocautery device, or both. Taking the patient to the operating room is not necessary and causes unacceptable delay. Local anesthesia is rarely needed because full-thickness injuries are insensate. However, small doses of narcotics and benzodiazepines assist in patient comfort. Patients with this severity of injury are often already intubated and therefore receiving sedatives and analgesics.

The incision should be placed along both the mid-medial and mid-lateral aspect of the extremity and should extend through the eschar down to the subcutaneous fat to permit adequate separation of the cut edges for decompression (Fig. 53-6). The incisions should be made from an area of unburned tissue and extended to unburned tissue if possible. The procedure should be completed with the patient in the anatomically correct position to minimize the risk for damage to major blood vessels and nerve bundles, especially when incisions cross joints.

REPARATIVE PHASE

Once the patient is stabilized, measures are taken to promote healing and prevent infection. As noted earlier, burn wounds can have profound effects on nearly every organ system. Box 53-11 lists nursing diagnoses for patients with burns, and Box 53-12 contains a collaborative care guide for the patient with burns.

Ensuring Optimal Nutrition

Before the unique nutritional needs of patients with burns were fully recognized in the late 1970s, those with severe burn injuries who survived languished in a hospital ward with minimal oral intake until they became severely cachectic. It is currently clear that appropriate nutrition plays a significant role in improving outcome for patients with severe burn injuries.

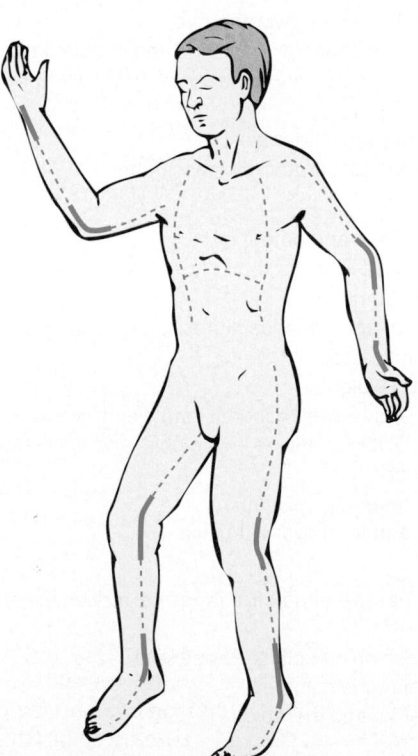

Figure 53-6 • Preferred sites of escharotomy incisions.

Box 5-11 Examples of Nursing Diagnoses and Collaborative Problems for the Burn Patient

- Ineffective Airway Clearance related to impaired cough, oropharyngeal and tracheal swelling, or artificial airway
- Impaired Gas Exchange related to inhalation injury, atelectasis, acute respiratory distress syndrome, or carbon monoxide poisoning
- Ineffective Breathing Pattern related to circumferential chest burn, upper airway obstruction, or acute respiratory distress syndrome
- Impaired Peripheral Tissue Perfusion related to edema or circumferential burn
- Deficient Fluid Volume related to altered capillary permeability, insensible and third-spacing losses
- Risk for Fluid Volume Excess related to fluid resuscitation and subsequent fluid mobilization 3 to 5 d postburn
- Impaired Skin Integrity related to burn injury or surgical interventions
- Hypothermia related to impaired integument
- Imbalanced Nutrition: Less Than Body Requirements related to hypermetabolic response to burn injury, paralytic ileus
- Impaired Urinary Elimination related to indwelling urinary catheter
- Risk for Infection related to loss of integument, invasive procedures, and immunocompromise
- Pain related to exposure of nerve endings, invasive procedures, surgical procedures, and dressing changes
- Ineffective Individual and Family Coping related to altered body image and fear
- Anxiety related to traumatic injury, fear of dying, fear of disfigurement, change in body image, and change in role relationships

Box 53-12 • COLLABORATIVE CARE GUIDE for the Patient With a Burn

OUTCOMES	INTERVENTIONS
Oxygenation/Ventilation Patent airway is maintained. Lung is clear on auscultation.	• Auscultate breath sounds q2–4h and PRN. • Assess for inhalation injury, and anticipate intubation. • Assess quantity and color of tracheal secretions. • Suction endotracheal airway when appropriate (see Collaborative Care Guide for Patient on Ventilator). • Hyperoxygenate and hyperventilate before and after each suction pass.
Peak, mean, and plateau pressures are within normal limits for a patient on a ventilator.	• Monitor airway pressures q1–2 h. • Monitor lung compliance q8h (see Chapter 24). • Administer bronchodilators and mucolytics. • Perform chest physiotherapy q4h. • Monitor airway pressures and lung compliance for improvement after interventions.
There is no evidence of atelectasis or infiltrates.	• Turn side to side q2h. • Consider kinetic therapy or prone positioning. • Take daily chest x-ray.
Arterial blood gases are within normal limits.	• Monitor carboxyhemoglobin and carbon monoxide levels. • Monitor arterial blood gases using cooximeter analysis of arterial saturation. (Pulse oximeter and calculated SaO_2 are inaccurate measures in the presence of carbon monoxide.) • Provide humidified oxygen. • Consider hyperbaric therapy.
Circulation/Perfusion Blood pressure, heart rate, central venous pressure (CVP), and pulmonary artery pressures are within normal limits.	• Assess vital signs q1h. • Assess hemodynamic pressures q1h if patient has pulmonary artery (PA) catheter. • Administer intravascular volume as ordered to maintain preload (see below).
Temperature is within normal limits.	• Monitor temperature q1h. • Maintain a warm environment, and use warming lights or blankets to prevent hypothermia. • Treat fever with antipyretics and cooling blankets.
Perfusion to extremities is maintained; pulses are intact.	• Monitor perfusion using pulse oximetry, Doppler, palpation q1h. • Elevate burned extremities. • Prepare for escharotomy or fasciotomy.

Fluids/Electrolytes
Restore and maintain fluid balance:
    Urine output 30–70 mL/h or 0.5 mL/kg.
    CVP, 8–12 mm Hg; pulmonary artery wedge pressure
    (PAWP), 12–18 mm Hg; blood pressure,
    within normal limits; heart rate, <120 beats/min.
	• Assess intake and output q1h.
	• Give lactated Ringer's 4 mL/kg/% burn, divided into first 24 h postburn.
	• Monitor for spontaneous diuresis, and reduce IV infusion rate as indicated.
	• Take daily weight.

Electrolytes, mineral, and renal function values are within normal limits.	• Monitor and replace minerals and electrolytes. • Monitor BUN, creatinine, myoglobin, and urine electrolytes and glucose. • Monitor neurological status. • Monitor and treat dysrhythmias.
Mobility/Safety Patient is free of joint contractures.	• Provide passive and active range-of-motion exercises q1–2h. • Apply positioning splints as needed.
There is no evidence of complications related to immobility.	• Turn and reposition q2h. • Consider kinetic therapy.

(continued)

Box 53-12 • COLLABORATIVE CARE GUIDE for the Patient With a Burn (Continued)

OUTCOMES	INTERVENTIONS
There is no evidence of infection.	• Consider deep venous thrombosis (DVT) prophylaxis. • Maintain strict sterile technique, and monitor technique of others. • Maintain sterility of invasive catheters and tubes. • Per hospital protocol, change dressings and invasive catheters. Culture wounds, blood, urine, as necessary. • Monitor systemic inflammatory response syndrome criteria: increased white blood cell (WBC) count, increased temperature, tachypnea, tachycardia.
Skin Integrity Unburned skin will remain intact.	• Assess skin q4h and each time patient is repositioned. • Turn q2h. • Consider pressure relief/reduction mattress.
Burns begin healing without complications.	• Treat burns per hospital protocol; apply topical medications and debride as indicated. • Monitor skin graft viability. • Protect grafted areas (e.g., bed cradle, dressings). • Consider air fluidized bed to enhance healing and relieve pressure from burned surface.
Nutrition Caloric and nutrient intake meets metabolic requirements per calculation (e.g., Basal Energy Expenditure).	• Provide parenteral or enteral nutrition within 24 h of injury. • Consult dietitian or nutritional support service to assess nutritional requirements with team. • Monitor protein and calorie intake. • Monitor albumin, prealbumin, transferrin, cholesterol, triglycerides, glucose.
Comfort/Pain Control Patient will have minimal pain, <5 on pain scale, and discomfort.	• Assess pain and discomfort using objective pain scale q4h, PRN, and following administration of pain medication. • Administer analgesics before procedures, and monitor patient response. • Use nonpharmacological pain management techniques (e.g., music, distraction, touch).
Psychosocial Patient demonstrates decreased anxiety.	• Assess vital signs during treatments, discussions, and so forth. • Administer sedatives before treatments/procedures. • Consult social services, clergy, and so forth as appropriate. • Provide for adequate rest and sleep. • Encourage discussion regarding long-term effects of burns, available resources, and coping strategies.
Teaching/Discharge Planning Patient/significant others understand procedures and tests needed for treatment. Significant others understand the severity of the illness, ask appropriate questions, anticipate potential complications.	• Prepare patient/significant others for procedures, such as débridement, escharotomy, fasciotomy, intubation, and mechanical ventilation. • Explain the potential effects of burns and the potential for complications, such as infection, respiratory or renal failure. • Encourage significant others to ask questions related to the management of burns, disfigurement, coping, and so forth.

Although early parenteral feeding has been associated with increased mortality because of an increase in the risk for infection, early enteral feeding has been proposed because it may reduce the translocation of bacteria from the intestinal lumen.[6] Passage of bacteria from the gut into the intestinal lymphatics or portal venous system probably occurs in all healthy people. However, the intestinal edema that accompanies the burn resuscitation period and the immunosuppression that follows make it difficult for the body to clear these microorganisms effectively. Microbial products—either live organisms or cell wall fragments—disseminate through the body, prompting the release of cytokines such as TNF, interleukin-1

(IL-1), and IL-6. These cytokines exacerbate the hypermetabolic response and may initiate SIRS.

The rationale for enteral feeding within the first 24 hours of injury is that the presence of food in the gut lumen reduces the rate of microbial translocation. Although not proved definitively in the clinical setting of patients with burns, safety and simplicity of early feeding have been demonstrated. One approach is to slowly infuse tube feedings through the nasogastric tube at a rate of 10 to 20 mL/hour. Although this clearly does not meet the nutritional needs of adult patients, it is enough to protect the gut mucosa. Long feeding tubes can be placed into the small bowel using endoscopy or fluoroscopy and the rate steadily increased to meet the estimated calculated caloric requirements. The advantages of such tubes are higher and earlier rates of infusion, and continuous feeding of patients during surgical procedures requiring general anesthesia. Patients with minor burns may be able to satisfy their caloric needs and fluid resuscitation through oral intake only.

Despite the theoretical advantages and need for the calories provided by enteral feeding, difficulties exist, and the technique cannot be used in all patients. Patients receive, on average, only 80% of the goal rate for enteral feedings because of frequent interruptions for patient care, including radiological procedures and surgery. This deficit increases when patients develop intestinal ileus, as typically occurs with major infection. Osmotic diarrhea is troublesome, particularly when the patient's feces soil the burn dressings. A variety of techniques combat diarrhea, including replacement of intestinal flora with lactobacillus granules and nonpasteurized yogurt, as well as retardation of small bowel motility with diphenoxylate hydrochloride.

The estimated caloric and protein needs of a patient may be met more reliably with parenteral than enteral feeding. The central venous catheter, which predisposes the patient to invasive infections (particularly infections with *Candida* species), is a disadvantage. Reports suggest that the rate of bacterial translocation is increased with the use of parenteral nutrition compared with enteral nutrition and that infection rates are higher.[6,10] Long-term use of parenteral nutrition alone is associated with hepatobiliary dysfunction, including cholestatic hepatitis and acalculous cholecystitis. Nevertheless, parenteral nutrition can be used for patients who do not tolerate enteral feedings because of paralytic ileus of the intestine or prolonged diarrhea.

Burn injury results in an increase in the metabolic expenditure. Initial investigative work performed in the 1970s demonstrated that some patients with burns needed as many as 7,000 or 8,000 kcal/day to maintain weight. Although patients with burns still become hypercatabolic after injury, they do not become so to the same degree because of changes in management. Because of the effect of earlier enteral feeding and the introduction of procedures that promote early wound closure (early and aggressive excision and grafting and the use of biological dressings), the increase in metabolic rate has diminished; healing does not fully begin until the wounds are closed. Recently, indirect calorimetry has shown that the most severe injuries require no more calories than twice the resting energy expenditure as described in the Harrison-Benedict formula. The resting energy expenditure calculated by the Harrison-Benedict formula is multiplied by a stress factor in direct proportion to the size of the burn (Box 53-13). The stress factor is judged conservatively to avoid overfeeding, which is associated with increased susceptibility to infection. Studies suggest that although indirect calorimetry prevents gross underestimation or overestimation of the patient's caloric needs, in most patients it is probably not superior to estimating their needs from a formula (such as the Harrison-Benedict formula) alone.

Wound repair depends on amino acids, which are the building blocks of proteins. The type of amino acids used in enteral feedings varies. The amino acids arginine and glutamine have immune-enhancing properties, improve nitrogen retention, and maintain lean body mass. Formulas containing arginine supplements have been reported to reduce infections in trauma patients and to reduce length of stay of critically ill patients.

Judging the amount of protein necessary for recovery from burn injuries is difficult. Massive and unquantified loss of protein from the burn wound exudates precludes nitrogen balance studies based on urine excretion alone. Sequential measurements of serum proteins such as transferrin and prealbumin are a better index of the body's response to the amount and type of dietary protein given; however, few clinical studies show a correlation between an increase in serum proteins and improved clinical outcome. It is important to avoid overfeeding of protein because it predisposes patients to sepsis. Amounts of protein greater than 3 g/kg/day in adults are usually not tolerated because of azotemia. Dietary protein should be started at an administration rate of 1.2 g/kg/day and should be increased if there is not a subsequent increase in serum protein markers. A patient's diet

---

Box 53-13 • Stress Factors for Energy Expenditure Related to Burn Size (Harrison-Benedict Equations)

Women: REE = 655 + [4.3 × Wt (lb)]
            + [4.3 × Ht (in)] − [4.7 × age]

Men: REE = 65 + [6.2 × Wt (lb)]
          + [12.7 × Ht (in)] − [6.8 × age]

TBSA	STRESS FACTOR
0–10%	1.4
11–20%	1.5
21–30%	1.6
31–40%	1.7
41–50%	1.8
51–60%	1.9
>60%	2.0

REE, resting energy expenditure.

can also be supplemented with vitamins A and C, and with the trace element zinc, all of which improve wound healing.

Successful weaning of patients from nutritional supplements sometimes occurs earlier than expected. A regular diet with liquid supplements is offered within 24 hours of extubation. The increased thirst of patients with burns is used to encourage the intake of protein-containing solutions, either soy- or milk-based supplements, or protein-containing fruit drinks. Using supplements, patients can take up to 2,000 kcal each day. It is preferable to feed patients or allow them to feed themselves because of the inherent risks of feeding tubes and central lines.

Providing Musculoskeletal Support

Physical and occupational therapy begins on day 1 of a burn injury. Independent of the patient's general condition, injured upper and lower extremities can be elevated to allow adequate venous drainage and reduce edema. Passive exercises are initiated and, if alert and cooperative, the patient should participate in these exercises. Active and passive exercises to maintain joint range of motion are continued throughout hospitalization and the outpatient rehabilitation period.

Two important axioms influence rehabilitation. First, the burn wound will shorten by contraction until it meets an opposing force. Across a flexor surface, this may result in a contracture. Second, the position of comfort is the position of contracture. Range-of-motion exercises prevent tendon shortening and restriction of joint motion by burn scar contractures. As patients begin to recover and participate actively in therapy, exercises are designed to increase muscle strength and endurance. A return to activities of daily living frequently takes months.

An unfortunate consequence of contractures and immobility is heterotopic ossification. Heterotopic ossification develops when there is an abnormal deposition of calcium phosphate crystals in joint spaces or along tendons. Heterotopic ossification restricts the motion of joints, particularly in elbows and knees. Unlike the heterotopic ossification seen in patients with spinal cord injuries, the heterotopic ossification seen in patients with burns does not respond to treatment with etidronate disodium, and early surgical removal is not indicated. Resolution occurs with time in most patients, and few need surgical removal of the ossified crystals in the joints.

Managing Pain

The pain associated with burns is managed aggressively. All narcotics are given intravenously because absorption of the drug is unpredictable when given intramuscularly or subcutaneously secondary to the hypermetabolic response and the fluid shifts. Patients are given anxiolytics for anxiety related to appearance, procedures, and fear. Patient-controlled analgesia (PCA) is ideal for patients who are awake and sufficiently oriented to use the pump. PCA pumps can provide a continuous pain medication, with a "dose" available every 6 to 8 minutes for intermittent pain. The nurse can give the patient a "bolus" dose before procedures such as dressing changes and physical therapy. Recommended narcotics include morphine, fentanyl, and hydromorphone.

Caring for the Wound

Cleansing
The wound protocols of all burn centers and hospitals vary, but the most common wound cleansing involves water and chlorhexidine or saline and povidone-iodine (Betadine). Wounds are cleansed at each dressing change and are observed for signs of infection and rate of healing.

Hydrotherapy is the preferred approach of most burn centers because the warm, flowing water is beneficial to help loosen exudates, clean and assess the wound, and provide range-of-motion exercises. The solutions used vary and may contain salt, povidone-iodine, and bleach. Because the procedure is usually painful, patients should receive an analgesic 20 to 30 minutes before beginning and small, frequent doses throughout as needed. In addition, the patient should receive a complete explanation of, and assistance with, pain-controlling techniques (e.g., imagery, music therapy). Additional support should be offered by providing ongoing explanations of what is to be done and why and by permitting the patient to participate in care as much as possible. Limiting the time the procedure takes is important to the patient's pain tolerance and temperature control. Hydrotherapy should be limited to 20 minutes to prevent extreme chilling, which increases metabolic demand.

Care must be taken to avoid cross-contamination of wounds during bathing procedures. For this reason, many centers no longer immerse patients in Hubbard tanks. Portable shower trolleys with disposable liners can provide hydrotherapy without the risk for contamination. These may be used in a central shower room or in facilities so equipped, or used directly in the patient's room, reducing the risk for transporting the critically ill. Clean or healing wounds should be cleaned separately from contaminated ones.

Application of Topical Antimicrobial Agents
The choice of topical antimicrobial agents depends on the wound depth, location, and condition and on the presence of specific organisms. Common antimicrobial agents used from time of admission to a burn unit include silver sulfadiazine (Silvadene), mafenide acetate (Sulfamylon), 0.5% silver nitrate, nitrofurazone, povidone-iodine, bacitracin, gentamicin, and nystatin (Table 53-3). No single agent is totally effective against all burn wound infections. Treatment is guided by in vitro testing or in vivo results. Eschar and granulating wound surfaces may be cultured 3 times weekly to identify contaminating organisms and determine antibiotic sensitivity.

Silver sulfadiazine is the primary topical agent of choice on admission. The most common adverse reaction is transient leukopenia; therefore, serial

Table 53-3 • Agents for Burn Wound Management

Agent	Advantages	Disadvantages	Nursing Considerations
Mafenide acetate	Broad-spectrum, penetrates eschar	Painful application, acid–base imbalances	Apply twice a day, leave open to air
Silver nitrate	Painless application, broad-spectrum, rare sensitivity	No eschar penetration, discolors wound and environmental surfaces, must be kept moist	Wet-to-wet dressing with nonadhering layer, followed by a gauze layer every 24 h
Silver sulfadiazene	Painless application, broad-spectrum, easy application	May cause transient leukopenia, minimal eschar penetration	Apply a moderate layer and wrap in a gauze dressing every 12 h
Bacitracin	Painless application, nonirritating	No eschar penetration, antimicrobial spectrum not as wide as above agents	Apply a thin layer and nonadhering dressing; if used on face, leave open to air
Mupirocin	Antimicrobial spectrum broader than bacitracin	Expensive	Apply a thin layer and nonadhering dressing; if used on face, leave open to air
Neomycin	Painless application	Antimicrobial spectrum not as wide as above agents	Apply a thin layer and nonadhering dressing; if used on face, leave open to air

CBCs must be monitored. If the white blood count falls below 3,000 cells/mm³, the physician will probably change to another topical agent. When the leukocyte count returns to normal (4,000 to 5,000 cells/mm³), silver sulfadiazine therapy may be reinstituted.

If the colony counts increase, the topical agent of choice is usually mafenide acetate cream, an effective broad-spectrum bacteriostatic agent. Mafenide acetate diffuses through third-degree eschar to the burn wound margin within 3 hours of application. Patient discomfort is common because mafenide acetate may cause a burning sensation as it penetrates the eschar tissue, lasting 20 to 30 minutes after application. This agent inhibits carbonic anhydrase, resulting in metabolic acidosis. This acidosis initially is compensated for by hyperventilation. Oral administration of sodium citrate dihydrate (Bicitra) or intravenous sodium bicarbonate usually corrects this acid–base imbalance.

The application of topical antimicrobial agents inhibits the rate of wound epithelialization and may increase the metabolic rate. Electrolyte imbalances (e.g., sodium leaching by silver nitrate) and acid–base abnormalities may occur. The best topical agents are water soluble because they do not hold in heat and macerate the wound. With the application of any topical agent, it is important to use sterile technique. Antimicrobial creams should be applied to a thickness recommended by the manufacturer and reapplied at the necessary frequency to maintain consistent coverage.

Débridement

Eschar covers the burn wound until it is excised or has separated spontaneously. Small burn wounds may be allowed to separate on their own if the wound shows no signs or symptoms of infection, the patient is hemodynamically stable, or the situation does not allow for excision. In theory, burn wound management is simple. It calls for débridement of the eschar and skin graft closure before the eschar

becomes infected. However, the sometimes serious systemic complications of burn injury, such as hypovolemia and sepsis, may delay this course of action significantly.

Mechanical Débridement Mechanical débridement may be accomplished using forceps and scissors to gently lift and trim loose necrotic tissue. Another form of mechanical débridement is dressing the wound with coarse gauze in the form of wet-to-dry or wet-to-wet dressings. Wet-to-dry dressings consist of layers of moistened coarse mesh gauze. As the inner layer dries, it adheres to the wound, entrapping exudate and wound debris. The dressing should be removed at a 90-degree angle, and every effort should be made to avoid damaging fragile, newly granulating tissue. As the wound forms increasing amounts of granulation tissue, wet-to-wet dressings may be used to prevent desiccation and trauma. These dressings remain moist until the next dressing change. The dressing should be removed by first gently lifting from the edges toward the center of the wound, and then removing the dressing at a 180-degree angle. This procedure prevents detachment of newly formed epithelial tissue.

Enzymatic Débridement Enzymatic débridement involves the application of a proteolytic substance to burn wounds to shorten the time of eschar separation. Travase and Elase are the most commonly used agents. The wound is first cleaned and débrided of any loose necrotic material. The agent is then applied directly to the wound bed and covered with a layer of fine-mesh gauze. A topical antimicrobial agent is applied next, and the entire area is covered with saline-soaked gauze. The dressing is changed 2 to 4 times per day.

Enzymatic débridement has the advantage of eliminating the need for surgical excision; however, certain complications must be considered. Hypovolemia may occur as a result of excessive fluid loss through the wound. Hence, no more than 20% TBSA should be treated in this manner. Cellulitis and maceration of normal skin may occur around the wound periphery, and patients often complain of a burning sensation lasting 30 to 60 minutes after enzyme application.

Surgical Débridement In surgical excision, the wound is excised to viable bleeding points while minimizing the loss of viable tissue. Early excision has contributed significantly to the survival of people with major burns. The open burn causes hypermetabolism and a stress response that is not corrected until wound closure occurs. Surgical excision should be done as soon as the patient is hemodynamically stable, usually within 72 hours.

After excision is complete, hemostasis must be achieved. This may be accomplished by topical thrombin sprayed on the wound or application sponges soaked in a 1:10,000 epinephrine solution. After removal of necrotic tissue, the exposed underlying structures must be dressed with a temporary or permanent covering to provide protection and prevent infection.

Grafts

The ideal substitute for lost skin is an autograft of similar color, texture, and thickness from a close location on the body. Sheets of the patient's epidermis and a partial layer of the dermis are harvested from unburned locations using a dermatome. These grafts, referred to as split-thickness skin grafts, can be applied to the wound as a sheet graft or mesh grafts.

Grafts must be inspected frequently to ensure that fluid is not collecting underneath them. Fluid accumulation is prevented by rolling a cotton-tipped applicator over the graft to express any trapped fluid. The sheet graft should be "pie-crusted" to allow for the expression of fluid through the closest opening; this avoids rolling the fluid to the edge of the graft, increasing the risk for dislodging the grafted tissue. After adherence has begun, usually after 24 hours, the fluid may be removed with a very small-gauge needle (26-gauge) to avoid disrupting the adherence of graft.

In a sheet graft, the harvested skin is applied to the surgically excised area. It is usually covered with a petroleum-based gauze dressing. Over exposed areas such as the face and hands, a sheet graft gives a more natural appearance than a mesh graft.

In a mesh graft, the harvested skin is slit, and the graft is then placed on the burn site. The slits (or interstices) allow the skin to expand, providing for greater coverage and drainage and facilitating draping over uneven surfaces. Mesh grafts frequently have to be expanded to obtain maximal coverage from each piece of autograft. An expansion ratio of 1:3 or 1:4 is often practical. Sometimes ratios such as 1:6 or 1:7 are used to cover large burns when donor tissue is limited. With these larger ratios, the expanded autograft is covered with either cadaver skin allografts or synthetic skin (Biobrane, Winthrop Pharmaceuticals). In addition to physically stabilizing the fragile mesh, the cover decreases evaporation, heat loss, and bacterial contamination.

Dressings are used after surgery to immobilize the grafted area and prevent shearing and dislodging of the graft. Postoperative dressings also provide a degree of compression to minimize hematoma and seroma formation, but they may be a source of vascular compression in the extremities. Pulse checks distal to the dressings are documented every 4 hours for 24 hours after surgery. The dressings are usually left in place until the third postoperative day. Until that time, the dressings are moistened every 6 hours with a solution containing normal saline and polymyxin. The antibiotic solution keeps the fragile meshed grafts moist and protects against infection. On postoperative day 3, the dressings are removed and evaluated by the physician, who determines the success of the grafting. This is expressed in terms of percentages. The grafted area is then covered with a nonadherent dressing and a gauze layer, which are secured with a gauze roll. All components of the dressing are moistened with the antibiotic solution.

Donor site care can vary with a variety of products used at burn centers and sometimes between burn surgeons. The donor site is covered during surgery with a single layer of fine-mesh gauze (e.g., Scarlet Red, Biobrane, Acticoat). Most products are kept in place until separation from the donor site begins. Positioning to prevent pressure on the site and to allow for drying is important. Daily inspection of the donor site is essential to detect early signs of infection or cellulitis.

A new technique that involves the growth and subsequent graft placement of cultured epithelial autografts has become an important adjunct to permanent coverage of extensive burn wounds. Biopsies are taken from unburned skin, and cells are cultured in the laboratory. Sheets of cultured epithelial cells are attached to petroleum jelly gauze and applied to the wound. The cultured cells are highly fragile, and the surgeon may elect to place the patient in traction for increased protection of the grafted tissue. After 7 to 10 days, the petroleum jelly gauze is removed, and a nonadherent dressing is applied to prevent mechanical trauma.

Providing Psychological and Familial Support

Providing psychological support for the newly admitted patient with burns and the family is not the least of the many tasks facing the critical care nurse. The patient most often is awake and alert, although anxious and overwhelmed by the suddenness and magnitude of injuries. With high anxiety levels and lack of knowledge pertaining to burns, the family approaches the burn unit with fear, hesitancy, and sometimes hysteria. The physical appearance of the patient and the high-technology atmosphere of the burn unit are frightening. Preparing the family for the initial visit by explaining what to expect and escorting them to the bedside is extremely important. Visitors often are overwhelmed on the first visit and stand silently with increasing feelings of anxiety and hopelessness. Burn injuries are dramatic and are psychologically traumatic for the patient and for those who witnessed the accident. Counseling for the patient and the family begins on the day of admission. Families require constant support, and the burn team should plan weekly family meetings to discuss the patient's care plan and progress. This is often the all-important basis for establishing a trusting relationship for the long months of rehabilitation ahead. The trusting relationship that is established initially provides a strong base for patient and family teaching and rehabilitation in the months to follow. Critically ill patients with burns are likely to experience a series of small gains combined with intermittent setbacks, and this pattern does not stop until the burn wounds are closed, which can be 2 to 3 months after injury. The family needs to be informed and provided with the means to care for their own physical and psychological needs. Families of patients who were transferred from a great distance and who lack nearby support systems find the entire situation particularly stressful. The need to provide support for families cannot be overemphasized.

Patients with burns often become depressed and withdrawn, asking to be left alone and not to be made uncomfortable. The nurse should respond by making certain expectations of the patient clear. That is, the nurse should make it clear to the patient that he or she is to feed himself or herself, go to the bathroom, or do as much as his or her physical condition permits, while communicating to the patient that the situation is not hopeless and that recovery is expected.

The best way to handle regression in a patient with burns is to acknowledge it. First, the nurse must accept the fact that the patient may be unable to cope on an adult level and that the patient may be unstable emotionally and physically. Second, the nurse must devise ways to help the patient cope on an appropriate level. Interventions that usually help include following a regular schedule so that the patient knows what is expected, rewarding the patient for adult behavior, and permitting the patient as much control and choice as possible.

It is not uncommon for severely burned patients, and sometimes family members, to transfer their fears to a specific caregiver (physician, nurse, therapist) and to complain that they are being treated unjustly or unkindly. Working with a psychiatric liaison nurse may help the burn survivor recognize and deal with his or her fears more effectively and help the caregiver support the patient by responding therapeutically.

Hallucinations, confusion, and combativeness are common in severely burned patients for physical and mental reasons. Exhaustion, pain, and medications may distort reality and produce schizophrenic behavior.

Although the patient tends to concentrate on the present, the family members look to the future and want to know what to expect. Information about the patient's condition and treatments should be shared with them using an honest and open approach.

REHABILITATIVE PHASE

Patients with extensive burns require many months for recovery and rehabilitation. Physical and psychological rehabilitation measures are begun in the ICU and continued throughout the recovery period.

Physical Rehabilitation

The diet of the patient with burns should remain high in protein until all wounds have healed. As healing takes place, the diet should be tapered to meet normal caloric requirements. The patient with burns may become accustomed to eating frequently and in large amounts. After healing is complete, metabolism returns to normal, and weight will be gained if eating habits are not controlled properly.

Prevention of Scarring and Contractures

Once regarded as inevitable, hypertrophic scarring and joint contractures are now largely preventable. Preventive measures start when the person is admitted to the hospital and continue for at least 12 months or until the scar is fully mature.

These preventive measures (i.e., positioning the body and helping the patient perform range-of-motion exercises) are not new to the nurse. Positioning the body with the extremities extended is extremely important. Although tightly flexed positions are preferred by patients for comfort, they result in severe contractures. The range-of-motion exercises should be carried out with each dressing change or more often if indicated. Special splints are used to maintain arm, legs, and hands in extended, yet functional, positions. Later, when the wounds have healed sufficiently, the person is custom-fitted for a special pressure garment. By applying continuous uniform pressure over the entire area of the burn, the garment prevents hypertrophic scarring. The garment must be worn almost 24 hours a day for approximately 1 year. The smooth elastic garment forms a shield that permits the person to wear normal clothing and resume ordinary activities much sooner.

Healed and grafted skin is dry and tight. Itching is a major patient complaint as healing occurs. Massaging a mild, nonirritating lotion into the healed skin provides lubrication, aids in range of motion, and promotes circulation.

Psychological Rehabilitation

The burn survivor may have many psychological issues once discharge is nearing. The patient may have post-traumatic stress disorder, anxiety, depression, or a combination of these. To ensure that these issues are effectively managed, the multidisciplinary team caring for the patient with burns must include mental health professionals.

• Other Types of Injuries Treated in Burn Centers

Burn center referrals are not limited to the traditional burn injuries (thermal, chemical, electrical, or radiation). Patients with disease processes that primarily involve the integumentary system have had better outcomes in burn centers because the unit is structured with the high levels of necessary resources for patient care. Patients who are referred to burn centers may have such conditions as toxic epidermal necrolysis syndrome (TENS), erythema multiforme minor, and extensive Stevens-Johnson syndrome, as well as diseases that may result in the loss of large amounts of tissue, such as necrotizing fasciitis, staphylococcal scalded skin syndrome, bullous pemphigoid, or pemphigus vulgaris. Patients with significant cold injuries may also be routinely referred to regional burn centers in some areas of the country.

TOXIC EPIDERMAL NECROLYSIS SYNDROME

TENS is a superficial, exfoliative dermatitis that has been related to multiple sources, the most common being an adverse reaction to medications, the staphylococcal toxin, or viral infections. The source may be undeterminable. TENS can involve the entire mucosal surface of the body to include the oral mucosa and conjunctiva as well as the vaginal or urethral linings. The immediate concern is the oral lesions and the possible occlusion of the respiratory system; intubation may be indicated as a supportive measure. The definitive diagnosis is made by sending a biopsy from the involved tissue for microscopic examination where an epidermal split is observed at the junction of the epidermis and dermis.

Patients with TENS are often described by the percentage of their body surface area that is currently open, requiring fluid and electrolyte replacement for evaporative water loss through the open wounds. This disease is similar in its effects to the body as a partial-thickness injury seen with a thermal burn. The lesions in TENS tend to be hypersensitive and extremely painful, with the nerve endings exposed to the environment. If the soles of the feet are involved, ambulation is extremely painful and may lead to debilitation if physical activity is not maintained. Nutritional support is also important to assist with the healing process; the insertion of a small-bore feeding tube may be indicated if caloric intake cannot be maintained secondary to oral lesions.

To increase patient survival, patients with TENS should be admitted to a burn center because of the complexity of wound care and the need for meticulous infection control standards. Historically, these patients have been treated with silver nitrate dressings, but more recently, a variety of products such as Acticoat or biological dressings have been used. The primary concern of wound care is that the dressings remain moist, not wet, at all times to decrease the desiccation of the dermal layer. Steroids are not indicated, and antibiotics used only for specific infections.

NECROTIZING FASCIITIS

Necrotizing fasciitis is an infection of the soft tissue that presents a diagnostic and therapeutic challenge. The source is often polymicrobial; the pathogens enter the tissue through an open wound and spread rapidly in the extracellular space between the subcutaneous tissue and the fascia. Diagnosis may be difficult initially because the external cutaneous damage may not be readily appreciated and the signs and symptoms may be diffuse. Early diagnosis is paramount, with timely and radical surgery being the definitive intervention. Necrotic tissue must be completely excised and explored to clean tissue borders. Broad-spectrum antibiotics are started preoperatively, and culture and Gram stain are used to provide guidance for the antibiotic regimen. Local and systemic infection must be completely controlled before wound closure is addressed.[11]

As in burn injuries, infection control is the primary component of wound management in necrotizing fasciitis. The need for extensive excision of tissue to the depth of the fascial compartments can result in extreme contractures and the loss of the protective mechanisms of the subcutaneous tissue (e.g., protection from shearing and blunt forces, fat storage, temperature regulation).[11]

COLD INJURIES

Environmental exposure without appropriate protection may result in a cold injury. Although these injuries are more common in temperatures below freezing, their onset may occur also at relatively moderate temperatures depending on the length of the exposure and the person's condition at the time. Injuries may range from a localized frostbite to systemic lowering of the body's core temperature with hypothermia.

Frostbite is most often seen of the fingers, toes, and nose because they tend to be the most exposed to the environment with outdoor activity, and circulation is the most difficult to maintain in the microvasculature. Mild cases involve only the skin and subcutaneous tissues, whereas the more severe cases involve deeper structures. The symptoms range from numbness and itching to paresthesia and decreased motion.[3] With prolonged exposure, the intracellular and extracellular fluids of the body tissue become chilled and may eventually form ice crystals, impeding the blood flow to the area and leading to tissue destruction.

Tissue should not be rewarmed until the patient is in a controlled environment where the warmth can then be maintained. Rewarming the tissue also contains risks because this may release a shower of microemboli. In addition, it is also extremely painful. Purplish or bluish blisters are left intact, whereas clear or white blisters are débrided, similar to burn blisters. To preserve functional length, amputation is discouraged until definitive demarcation occurs, which can take weeks to months.[3,12]

• Clinical Applicability Challenges

Case Study

Mr. M. is a 29-year-old man who was in an industrial fire caused by an indoor explosion where he is employed. He was able to get out of the structure unassisted. An ambulance transports Mr. M. to the emergency department of the nearest hospital, where he arrives 45 minutes after the fire. The size of the burn is estimated to be 60% of total-body surface area (TBSA).

Mr. M. is a well-nourished, well-developed man who has been in relatively good health. He denies using tobacco products or recreational drugs but reports drinking 1 case of beer per week for the past 3 years. There is no history of significant past medical or surgical history; family history indicates no significance of hypertension, cardiac or renal disease, diabetes, or cancer. He is married and has no children.

Since the accident, Mr. M. states that his voice has become very hoarse. Physical assessment notes burns to the face with singed nasal and facial hairs, circumferential burns to bilateral upper extremities, the anterior torso, portions of the posterior torso, and scattered areas to bilateral lower extremities, as well as carbonaceous sputum in the mouth. He reports that his preburn weight was 154 lb (70 kg).

For airway protection and based on facial burns, Mr. M. is intubated, and a nasogastric tube is inserted. Intravenous catheters are placed in bilateral upper extremities, and an indwelling urinary catheter is inserted. Tetanus immunization is given prophylactically. Analgesics are given in small, frequent doses intravenously as indicated for pain.

The regional burn center is contacted and transport arranged. Mr. M. is wrapped in clean, dry dressings and airlifted. He is further wrapped in wool blankets for additional insulation to maintain body temperature while being transported. A copy of all documentation is sent with him. When Mr. M. arrives 3 hours after the accident, he is admitted directly. The airway is confirmed, and pulses are immediately assessed with a focus on the upper extremities secondary to the circumferential burns; pulses are present in all distal extremities but slightly diminished in bilateral upper extremities.

Mr. M.'s initial vital signs are: heart rate, 144 beats/minute; blood pressure, 108/58 mm Hg; respirations (assisted via the ventilator with a set rate), 12 breaths/minute; and temperature, 96.8°F (36.0°C). Breath sounds are auscultated with coarse rhonchi. Heart sounds are normal and at a fast rate. The cardiac monitor demonstrates sinus tachycardia without ectopy. An arterial line and central line are placed in the left femoral artery and vein, respectively. Admission laboratory studies are sent. A chest x-ray is taken. Distal pulses on extremities with circumferential burns are assessed at least every hour. The upper extremities are checked more frequently because the pulses are diminished, and these are confirmed with Doppler ultrasound when not palpable. Bronchoscopy is performed, revealing carbonaceous material to the bilateral upper airways with reddening throughout; the bilateral lower airways appear to be uninjured. Lastly, a continuous infusion of fentanyl and midazolam is given for analgesic relief and sedation, with additional dosing as indicated.

When resuscitation is well underway, the Lund-Browder chart is completed, and a burn size of 44% TBSA is calculated. Full-thickness burns (third-degree) account for 36% of the injuries; the texture is leathery, and the surface is dry with thrombosed vessels. Mr. M. denied pain in these areas when touched or being exposed to the air before being intubated. The remaining partial-thickness burns are reddened, moist, and weeping serous fluid where thin-walled blisters have ruptured. The patient reported that these were very painful to palpation. To determine estimated fluid requirements in the first 24 hours from the time of the burn, the burn resuscitation formula is calculated:

$$(2 \text{ mL lactated Ringer's}) \times (\text{body weight } [\text{kg}])$$
$$\times (\text{TBSA burned } [\%]) = 24 \text{ hours fluid}$$
$$2 \times 70 \times 44 = 6,160 \text{ mL}$$

First 8 hours (from the time of the burn)
$$= 3,080 \text{ mL, or } 385 \text{ mL/hour}$$

Next 16 hours $= 3,080$ mL, or 193 mL/hour

Mr. M. had received 750 mL at the transferring facility and 350 mL while in transport, which means that he needs an additional 1,980 mL of fluid in first 8 hours from the time of the burn. It is now 3 hours since the time of the burn, so the fluid is divided for the remaining 5 hours, or 396 mL/hour. Since the placement of the urinary catheter, urine output has been 180 mL, or an average of 60 mL/hour; although this is currently adequate, it will be closely monitored because it has been trending down.

Mr. M. is taken to the shower room, and all wounds are manually débrided. Shower time is minimized to reduce the risk for hypothermia, a significant contributor to the mortality of trauma patients. The following topical agents are applied: silver sulfadiazine (Silvadene) cream to all partial-thickness and full-thickness burns, bacitracin ophthalmic around eyes and bacitracin ointment to the rest of face, and mafenide acetate (Sulfamylon) cream to the ears. The patient is placed on a pressure relief mattress to decrease the incidence of decubitus, with particular concern for the occiput, sacrum, and heels. The head of the bed is elevated to 30 degrees, and the bilateral upper extremities are placed in airplane slings to elevate hands and abduct the axilla.

Selected initial laboratory results are as follows: sodium, 143 mEq/L; potassium, 3.5 mEq/L; chloride, 107 mEq/L; blood urea nitrogen, 19.0 mg/dL; creatinine, 0.9 mg/dL; white blood count, 18,100 cells/mm^3; and hematocrit, 47.6%. Urine outputs for hours 6 and 7 from the time of the burn are 23 mL and 17 mL, respectively, and the intravenous rate of fluid administration is increased by 20% to 475 mL/hour.

Nine hours after the burn, Mr. M.'s forearms are tight and edematous, and pulses in the upper extremities are no longer present per Doppler. Fluid resuscitation appears controlled; the patient is not hypotensive, with a blood pressure of 112/63 mm Hg. The heart rate has decreased within the expected range (128 beats/minute), and urinary output is adequate (43 mL last hour). Escharotomies are performed to the medial and lateral aspects of both arms and the dorsum of the hands. Pulses are immediately palpable at the conclusion of this procedure. A small-bore feeding tube is placed, and a nutrient-dense tube feeding is started and increased slowly as tolerated.

Albumin 5% is added to Mr. M.'s fluid resuscitation during the second 24 hours at 39 mL/hour (0.3 mL/70 kg/44% TBSA for 30%–49% TBSA burn). The burn wounds are to be cleansed twice a day with 4% chlorhexidine gluconate (Hibiclens) soap. Alternating solutions are applied to all burn wounds except the face, with mafenide acetate (Sulfamylon) in the morning and silver sulfadiazine (Silvadene) in the evening. Mafenide acetate is always applied to the ears, with bacitracin to the face and bacitracin ophthalmic around the eyes. Nursing and rehabilitative personnel provide passive range of motion to all major joints frequently, with particular attentiveness to the hands.

Mr. M. is taken to the operating room on postburn day 3 for a full excision and grafting. It is estimated that every patient with burns will require one surgical procedure for every 10% TBSA burned. The donor sites are the areas of bilateral thighs that were not burned and the bilateral calves. These are covered with fine mesh (Xeroform) gauze. The arms, right thigh, and posterior torso are covered with 3:1 autograft and wrapped with a veil dressing and 5% Sulfamylon solution–moistened gauze. The posterior torso is bolstered to protect from shearing forces. The dressings are moistened every 6 hours and whenever necessary to avoid tissue desiccation. To maximize donor tissue, the anterior torso is excised and covered with the template Integra to close the wounds. The dorsum of the hands are covered with a split-thickness sheet graft and left open, and the palms are covered with Integra. The hands are splinted in a position of function. The sheet graft is observed hourly for the first 24 hours postoperatively; blebs are rolled to ensure that grafts adhere. After this time, small hematomas are aspirated via a tuberculin syringe. Donor sites are elevated on leg nets to expose to the air. Heat lamps are used at low settings to assist with drying.

Mr. M. is weaned from the ventilator postoperatively and extubated the morning of postburn day 5. Aggressive pulmonary toileting is initiated to reduce the risk for pneumonia. He is started on vancomycin for burn wound cellulitis, which is stopped after 5 days when resolved. He is assisted to the bedside chair on postoperative day 5 (postburn day 8), and diet is advanced as tolerated. He is assisted to the standing table on postoperative day 9 (postburn day 12). When he is tolerating 50% of his daily caloric needs orally, enteral feeds are changed to only night feeds and stopped when he is tolerating more than 75%. He begins ambulating on postoperative day 11 (postburn day 14) and is transferred to the ward.

Mr. M. returns to the operating room on four more occasions for additional excision and grafting procedures and to cover the Integra templates when donor sites are ready for reharvesting. His wounds are healing with minimal graft loss and without difficulty. On postburn day 49, he is discharged to an inpatient rehabilitation facility with compression garments, for continued strengthening and stretching of contracted tissue. He is discharged from rehabilitation on postburn day 64. He is seen in the outpatient burn clinic for periodic follow-up and is readmitted to the burn center 6 months after the burn for surgical intervention of contracted tissue.

1. Discuss the clinical rationale for performing prophylactic intubation of Mr. M. before transport versus waiting to see if he develops respiratory compromise.

2. How do you perform a neurovascular assessment in a patient who is intubated?

3. How does the use of alcohol relate to potential complications for the fluid resuscitation of Mr. M.?

4. Discuss the pathophysiological effect of circumferential burns on the peripheral perfusion of Mr. M.

5. Discuss why only the partial-thickness (second-degree) and full-thickness (third-degree) burns are considered, and not the superficial (first-degree) burns, when calculating the TBSA for fluid replacement.

6. Discuss the potential complications of under-resuscitation of patients with burns as well as the over-resuscitation.

Review Questions

1. A 33-year-old man who was in a house fire and jumped from the two-story building is transported to the emergency department. Burn size is estimated at 55% total-body surface area. He responds to painful stimuli, but respirations are being assisted by the bag-valve-mask and oxygen. What action takes priority in the initial assessment of this patient with burns?
   a. Medicate the patient for pain
   b. Consider endotracheal intubation
   c. Contact the regional burn center and dress the burn wounds in clean, dry dressings for transport
   d. Stop the burning process

2. A 27-year-old woman presents with a chemical burn on her right hand. What is your first intervention?
   a. Tell her to write with her left hand while you contact poison control to determine the best neutralizing agent
   b. Begin irrigating the wound with copious amounts of water
   c. Elevate the extremity and perform passive range of motion
   d. Apply ice to the injured area

3. A male patient sustains a burn at 8:00 a.m. The partial-thickness and full-thickness burns cover 50% total-body surface area (TBSA), and he weighs 80 kg. How much fluid should be infused by 4:00 p.m. using the formula (2 mL × weight [kg] × TBSA [%])?
   a. 8,000 mL
   b. 6,000 mL
   c. 4,000 mL
   d. 2,000 mL

4. What is the leading cause of death for patients with burns in the first 24 hours?
   a. Infection
   b. Hypoxemia
   c. Compartment syndrome
   d. Contractures

5. Which of the following is best defined as a decrease in arterial oxygen levels?
   a. Hypoxemia
   b. Hypercapnia
   c. Hypotension
   d. Hyperactivity

6. A male patient has sustained burns to his face and neck, entire right arm, and the upper half of his anterior torso. Using the "rule of nines" method, what is the percentage of his burn injury?
   a. 23%
   b. 27%
   c. 36%
   d. 45%

7. All of the following patients require more fluid than the fluid resuscitation formula would predict *except*
   a. a 36-year-old electrician who made contact with a high-voltage power line.
   b. a 25-year-old camp counselor who is burned by a camp fire and is immediately transported to a nearby burn center.
   c. a 22-year-old man exposed to a thermal flash while preparing food after a night of consuming large amounts of alcohol.
   d. a 47-year-old woman whose bathrobe caught fire and who did not seek treatment until the following morning.

8. What is the nursing priority for a patient who has suffered a circumferential burn to the left upper extremity?
   a. Check the pulse with an ultrasound device of extremity with diminished pulses.
   b. Elevate the extremity to the level of the heart.
   c. Débride the burn wounds and apply topical antimicrobial creams.
   d. Encourage the patient to complete active range-of-motion exercises at least hourly.

9. All of the following are signs of adequate fluid resuscitation *except*
   a. urine output between 30 and 50 mL per hour (0.5–1.0 mL/kg/hour).
   b. appropriate level of consciousness consistent with analgesia or sedation.
   c. an increase in the hematocrit level.
   d. vital signs consistent with the hypermetabolic response.

10. Urinary output is maintained at 75 to 100 mL/hour in a high-voltage electrical injury patient to prevent acute tubular necrosis. Acute tubular necrosis is a result of which of the following events?
    a. Cellular destruction
    b. Interstitial edema
    c. Hypoxemia
    d. Abdominal compartment syndrome

11. Which of the following areas sustains the most severe destruction with exposure to a burn source?
    a. The zone of stasis
    b. The zone of hyperemia
    c. The zone of coagulation
    d. The zone of contraction

References

1. American Burn Association. Available at: http://www.ameriburn.org
2. Kochanek KD, Murphy SL, Anderson RN, Scott C: Deaths: Final data for 2002. Natl Vital Stat Rep 53(5):1–116, 2004
3. Cohen R, Moelleken BRW: Disorders due to physical agents. In Tierney LM, Papadakis MA, McPhee SJ (eds): Current Medical Diagnosis and Treatment, 44th ed. New York: McGraw-Hill, 2005
4. Kramer GC, Lund T, Beckum OK: Pathophysiology of burn shock and burn edema. In Herndon DN (ed): Total Burn Care, 3rd ed. Philadelphia: Saunders, 2007, pp 93–106
5. Gibran NS, Heimbach DM: Management of the patient with thermal injuries. In Wilmore DW, et al (eds): ACS Surgery: Principles and Practice. New York: WebMD, 2005
6. LaBorde PJ: Management of patients with burn injury. In Smeltzer SC, Bare BG (eds): Brunner and Suddarth's Textbook of Medical-Surgical Nursing, 10th ed. Philadelphia: Lippincott Williams & Wilkins, 2004, pp 1703–1745
7. Warden GD: Fluid resuscitation and early management. In Herndon DN (ed): Total Burn Care, 3rd ed. Philadelphia: Saunders, 2007, pp 107–118
8. Van Meter KW: Carbon monoxide poisoning. In Tintinalli JE, Kelen GD, Stapcznski JS (eds): Emergency Medicine: A Comprehensive Study Guide, 6th ed. New York: McGraw-Hill, 2004
9. Cancio LC, Pruitt BA: Inhalation injury. In Tsokos GC, Atkins JL (eds): Combat Medicine: Basic and Clinical Research in Military, Trauma, and Emergency Medicine. Totowa, NJ: Humana Press, 2002, pp 325–349
10. Hart DW, Wolf SE, Chinkes DL, et al: Effects of early excision and aggressive enteral feeding on hypermetabolism, catabolism, and sepsis after severe burn. J Trauma 54(4):755–764, 2003
11. Fagan S, Spies M, Hollyoak M, et al: Exfoliative and necrotizing diseases of the skin. In Herndon DN (ed): Total Burn Care, 3rd ed. Philadelphia: Saunders, 2007, pp 554–565

12. American Burn Association: Advanced Burn Life Support Course. Chicago: Author, 2005

Other Selected Readings

Ahrns K: Trends in burn resuscitation: Shifting the focus from fluids to adequate endpoint monitoring, edema control, and adjuvant therapies. Crit Care Nurs Clin North Am 16(1):75–98, 2004

Bishop JF: Burn wound assessment and surgical management. Crit Care Nurs Clin North Am 16(1):145–178, 2004

Flynn MB: Nutritional support of the burn-injured patient. Crit Care Nurs Clin North Am 16(1):139–144, 2004

Honari S: Topical therapies and antimicrobials in the management of burn wounds. Crit Care Nurs Clin North Am 16(1): 1–12, 2004

LaBorde P: Burn epidemiology: The patient, the nation, the statistics, and the data resources. Crit Care Nurs Clin North Am 16(1):13–26, 2004

Merrel P, Mayo D: Inhalation injury in the burn patient. Crit Care Nurs Clin North Am 16(1):27–38, 2004

Merz J, Schrand C, Mertens D, et al: Wound care of the pediatric burn patient. AACN Clin Issues 14(4):429–441, 2003

Montgomery RK: Pain management in burn injury. Crit Care Nurs Clin North Am 16(1):39–50, 2004

Ruth-Sahd L, Gonzales M: Multiple dimensions of caring for a patient with acute necrotizing fasciitis. Dimens Crit Care Nurs 25(1):15–21, 2006

Santucci S, Gobara S, Santos C, et al: Infections in a burn intensive care unit: Experience of seven years. J Hosp Infect 53(1):6–13, 2003

Sicoutris CP, Holmes JH: Fire and smoke injuries. Crit Care Nurs Clin North Am 18(3):403–418, 2006

Smith M, Doctor M, Boulter T: Unique considerations in caring for a pediatric burn patient: A developmental approach. Crit Care Nurs Clin North Am 16(1):99–108, 2004

Supple K: Physiologic response to burn injury. Crit Care Nurs Clin North Am 16(1):109–118, 2004

Multisystem Dysfunction

PART 13

INTERNET RESOURCES

Topic	Web Page Address
The Agency for Toxic Substances and Disease Registry	www.atsdr.cdc.gov
Alcoholics Anonymous	www.alcoholics-anonymous.org
The American Academy of Clinical Toxicology	www.clintox.org
American Association for the Surgery of Trauma	www.aast.org
American Association of Poison Control Centers	www.aapcc.org
The American College of Medical Toxicology	www.acmt.net
American Society for Microbiology	www.asm.org
American Trauma Society	www.amtrauma.org
Association for Professionals in Infection Control and Epidemiology	www.apic.org
Association of Rehabilitation Nurses	www.rehabnurse.org
British Trauma Society	www.trauma.org/bts/
Community Anti-Drug Coalitions of America	www.cadca.org
The Eastern Association for the Surgery of Trauma	www.east.org
Emergency Nurses Association	www.ena.org
Infectious Disease Society of America	www.idsociety.org
International Council on Alcohol, Drugs and Traffic Safety	www.icadts.org
International Society for Biomedical Research on Alcoholism	www.isbra.com
Johns Hopkins Division of Infectious Diseases Antibiotic Guide	www.hopkins-abxguide.org
National Association of Orthopaedic Nurses	www.orthonurse.org
Orthopaedic Trauma Association	www.ota.org
Society of Critical Care Medicine	www.sccm.org
Society of Trauma Nurses	www.traumanurses.org
Toxicology Data Network	www.toxnet.nlm.nih.gov
Trauma Association of Canada	www.traumacanada.org
The U.S. Department of Educations's Higher Education Center for Alcohol and Other Drug Abuse and Violence Prevention	www.edc.org/hec

Shock, Systemic Inflammatory Response Syndrome, and Multiple Organ Dysfunction Syndrome

Karen L. Johnson • Kiersten Henry

Objectives

Based on the content in this chapter, the reader should be able to:

❶ Describe common pathophysiological processes involved in the generalized shock response.

❷ Compare and contrast the etiology and clinical manifestations of the major types of shock.

❸ Explain the anticipated medical management and rationale for treatment of the various shock states.

❹ Describe patients at risk for development of shock and complications associated with the various shock states.

❺ Discuss nursing management principles for patients with shock, systemic inflammatory response syndrome, and multiple organ dysfunction syndrome.

• Pathophysiology of Shock

Under normal conditions, the body provides sufficient oxygen to the cells to meet metabolic needs. Under stress, the body consumes oxygen more rapidly, and compensatory mechanisms are initiated to meet the increased demands of the body and restore oxygen and perfusion to cells. These compensatory mechanisms are the same, regardless of the clinical condition causing the cellular hypoperfusion. Clinical conditions that result in cellular hypoperfusion are often referred to as shock states.

Although shock states have different causes and different presentations, researchers have gradually concluded that some features, such as hypoperfusion, hypercoagulability, and activation of the inflammatory response, are common to all shock states. Moreover, it has become clear that once a shock state develops, the subsequent course may have more to do with the physiological response to shock, including activation of the sympathetic nervous system, the inflammatory response, and the immune system, rather than with the initial cause of the shock. These findings have led to a unified theory of shock as a derangement of compensatory mechanisms that results in further circulatory and respiratory hypofunction with subsequent multiple organ damage.

TISSUE OXYGENATION AND PERFUSION

Oxygenation of all organs and tissues is directly related to the ability of the body to provide oxygen to the blood and transport the oxygenated blood to cells. The pulmonary system provides for the diffusion of oxygen into the blood through the process of respiration (ventilation [partial pressure of arterial carbon dioxide, or $PaCO_2$] and oxygenation [partial pressure of arterial oxygen, or PaO_2]). The cardiovascular system assists in the transport of the oxygenated blood to the cells for metabolism; hemoglobin in the blood acts as the carrier for the oxygen (arterial oxygen saturation [SaO_2]). Typically, cells consume about 25% of the oxygen delivered; this utilization of oxygen is referred to as oxygen consumption (VO_2). The body's ability to provide oxygen to the cells is called oxygen delivery (DaO_2). Chapter 17 reviews how these oxygen parameters are calculated.

Under normal conditions, VO_2 is independent of DaO_2. This means that when cells need to consume additional oxygen to produce energy, they can extract the necessary amount required to produce energy in the form of adenosine triphosphate (ATP). However, during times of physiological stress, VO_2 becomes dependent on DaO_2. Initial respiratory, endocrine, and circulatory compensatory mechanisms respond to the cells' need for oxygen by increasing elements of DaO_2. If additional oxygen is required, and the cells cannot extract the oxygen, they must use anaerobic metabolism to produce ATP. Anaerobic metabolism is not an efficient method of energy production, and the ATP produced is insufficient to meet cellular demands. Moreover, anaerobic metabolism produces lactic acid as a byproduct, increasing the amount of acid that must be eliminated. If oxygen continues to be insufficient to meet cellular demands for energy, cell death ensues. As more cells die, tissues and organs eventually become progressively dysfunctional.

During shock states, oxygen is consumed at a much greater rate than it is delivered, but it is difficult to predetermine the amount of oxygen the cells will require. To meet the increased need for cellular VO_2, the DaO_2 must be increased. Although it is not possible to manipulate cellular VO_2 directly, many nursing interventions can be implemented to manipulate and increase DaO_2. In shock states, the primary goal is to maximize DaO_2 to meet cellular oxygen requirements in an ongoing effort to prevent tissue and cell death and maintain end-organ perfusion.

COMPENSATORY MECHANISMS

Cellular perfusion depends on the synergy of multiple physiological processes. The pulmonary, endocrine, and circulatory systems maintain an intricate balance of oxygen exchange and delivery to the cells by generation of an adequate oxygenated blood supply and cardiac output (Fig. 54-1). The autonomic nervous system assists in the orchestration of this delicate balance.

During states of hypoxia, activated compensatory mechanisms increase the depth and rate of respiration. The cardiovascular system increases cardiac output to increase oxygen delivery to the cells. During states of low perfusion (low blood pressure), compensatory mechanisms are initiated and result in increases in heart rate, systemic vascular resistance (SVR), preload, and cardiac contractility in an effort to restore appropriate circulatory volume. Chapter 16 provides a discussion of these terms. The fall in systemic blood pressure activates a series of neurohormonal responses aimed at reestablishing sufficient cardiac output and perfusion to vital organs. The fall in blood pressure results in decreased stimulation of baroreceptors and eventually an increase in sympathetic response.

Continued sympathetic stimulation causes an increased heart rate and contractile force, increasing the cardiac output. Arteriolar vasoconstriction (increased SVR) increases blood pressure and also shunts blood from less vital organs such as the stomach and intestines to vital organs such as the heart, lungs, and brain. The preload and subsequently the cardiac output are increased by venoconstriction. The kidneys respond to sympathetic stimulation and local hypoperfusion by activating the renin–angiotensin system, which also increases vasoconstriction of the arterioles and veins, increasing cardiac output and SVR. Activation of the renin–angiotensin system also stimulates the adrenal cortex to release aldosterone, which acts on the kidney to conserve sodium and water, increasing circulating volume. A drop in blood pressure also causes the pituitary gland to release antidiuretic hormone, which also increases vascular tone and stimulates water and sodium retention by the kidney, further increasing preload. An increase of preload (from multiple sources) increases cardiac output, thereby increasing blood pressure. Collective compensatory responses act together to increase the body's circulating volume, blood pressure, and cardiac output to provide perfusion and oxygen to the cells (Fig. 54-2).

The goal in treating patients in shock states is to reestablish perfusion and oxygenation adequate to the needs to the cells as quickly as possible. Early recognition of signs of shock and ongoing assessments guide therapeutic interventions. The nurse plays a key role in the ongoing assessment of shock. The patient's clinical presentation depends on the cause of the shock state and degree of compensation. Clinical assessment parameters should be evaluated frequently to establish effectiveness of interventions and progression of shock state. Traditional assessment parameters include altered level of consciousness, tachypnea (PaO_2, $PaCO_2$, SaO_2), tachycardia, hypotension, decreased urine output, and metabolic acidosis (base deficit and serum lactate levels), which are commonly found in all states of hypoperfusion. Recent advances in technology provide methods for earlier assessment

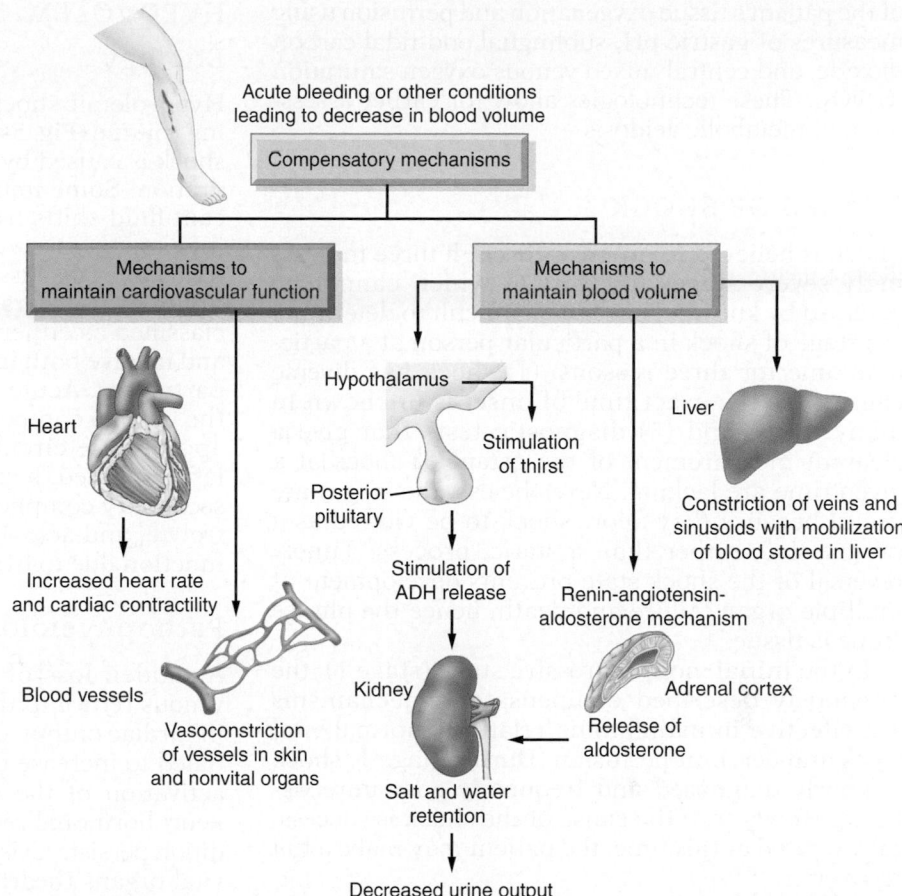

Figure 54-1 • Compensatory mechanisms used to maintain circulatory function and blood volume in hypovolemic shock. ADH, antidiuretic hormone. (From Porth CM: Essentials of Pathophysiology: Concepts of Altered Health States [2nd Ed], p 432. Philadelphia, Lippincott Williams & Wilkins, 2007.)

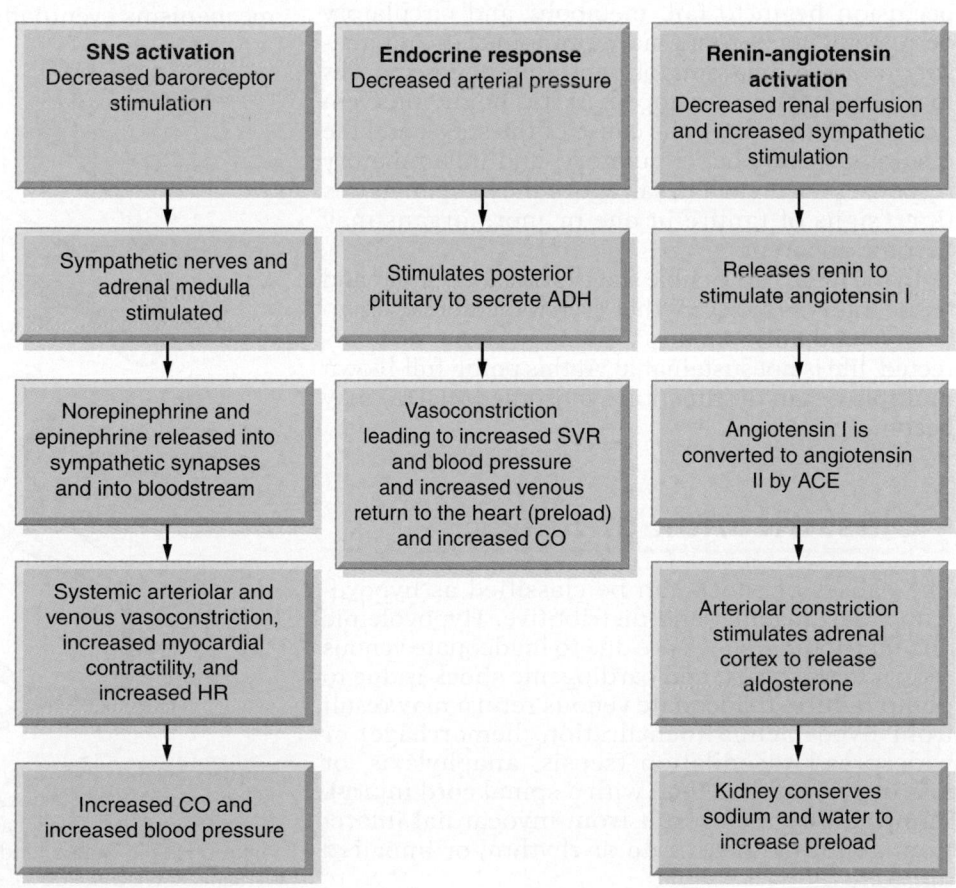

Figure 54-2 • Compensatory mechanisms in shock. ACE, angiotensin-converting enzyme; ADH, antidiuretic hormone; CO, cardiac output; HR, heart rate; SNS, sympathetic nervous system.

of the patient's tissue oxygenation and perfusion using measures of gastric pH, sublingual end-tidal carbon dioxide, and central mixed venous oxygen saturation ($Sc\overline{v}O_2$). These technologies allow for earlier assessment of metabolic acidosis.

STAGES OF SHOCK

Shock is believed to progress through three increasingly severe stages, the last of which cannot be reversed by known means. It is difficult to determine the stage of shock in a particular person at a particular time for three reasons: (1) shock has diverse causes, (2) the exact time of onset is unknown in many cases, and (3) diagnostic tests that give a clearcut measurement of the extent of shock at a given time are lacking. Nevertheless, the stages are useful because they allow shock to be viewed as a progressive, rather than a static, process. Timely reversal of the shock state prevents development of multiple organ failure and death, hence the phrase "time is tissue."[1]

In the initial, nonprogressive stage (stage 1), the previously described compensatory mechanisms are effective in maintaining relatively normal vital signs and cerebral perfusion. During stage 1, shock is poorly diagnosed and frequently goes unrecognized. However, if the cause of the shock is successfully treated at this time, the patient may make a full recovery.

In the intermediate, progressive phase (stage 2), compensatory mechanisms that maintain normal perfusion begin to fail, metabolic and circulatory derangements become more pronounced, and activation of the inflammatory and immune responses may become fully developed. At this point, interventions that target both the cause of the shock and the resultant metabolic, circulatory, and inflammatory responses may result in salvage of the patient. At this time, signs of failure in one or more organs may become apparent.

In the final, irreversible stage (stage 3), cellular and tissue injury is so severe that even if metabolic, circulatory, and inflammatory derangements are corrected, life is not sustainable. At this point, full-blown multiple organ dysfunction syndrome (MODS) may become evident.

• Classification of Shock

The causes of shock can be classified as hypovolemic, cardiogenic, and distributive. Hypovolemic and distributive shock are due to inadequate venous return to the heart, and cardiogenic shock is due to pump failure. Inadequate venous return may result from hypovolemia (dehydration, hemorrhage) or widespread vasodilation (sepsis, anaphylaxis, or loss of sympathetic tone with a spinal cord injury). Pump failure may result from myocardial infarction, abnormal heart rate or rhythm, or impaired diastolic filling.[1]

HYPOVOLEMIC SHOCK

Etiology

Hypovolemic shock is a result of inadequate circulating volume (Fig. 54-3). Most commonly, hypovolemic shock is caused by sudden blood loss or severe dehydration. Some injuries, such as burns, cause significant fluid shifts from the intravascular space to the interstitial space, resulting in hypovolemia. See Chapter 53 for a discussion of care of patients with burns. Volume disorders in critically ill patients may be classified as either depletion or expansion disorders and involve both intracellular and extracellular compartments. Acute fluid volume loss does not allow the normal compensatory mechanisms to restore an appropriate circulating volume rapidly enough. If left untreated, hypovolemia may lead to a variety of secondary complications, such as hypotension, electrolyte, and acid–base disturbances, and organ dysfunction due to hypoperfusion (Fig. 54-4).

Pathophysiology

A sudden loss of intravascular volume decreases venous return to the heart and results in a reduction in cardiac output. Compensatory mechanisms are initiated to increase the circulating volume through the activation of the sympathetic nervous system and neurohormonal responses (see Fig. 54-1). If the condition persists, existing blood volume is shunted to the vital organs (heart, lungs, and brain), causing hypoperfusion to such organs as the liver, stomach, and kidneys. If volume is not replaced, compensatory mechanisms eventually become ineffective. The fail-

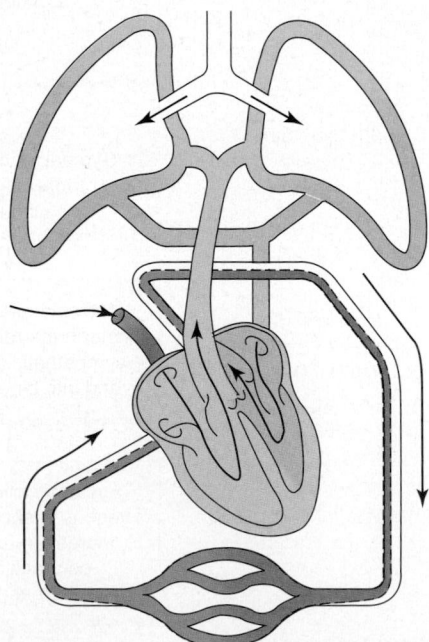

Figure 54-3 • Hypovolemic shock is caused by diminished blood volume with decreased filling of the circulatory system. (From Porth CM: Essentials of Pathophysiology: Concepts of Altered Health States [2nd Ed], p 431. Philadelphia, Lippincott Williams & Wilkins, 2007.)

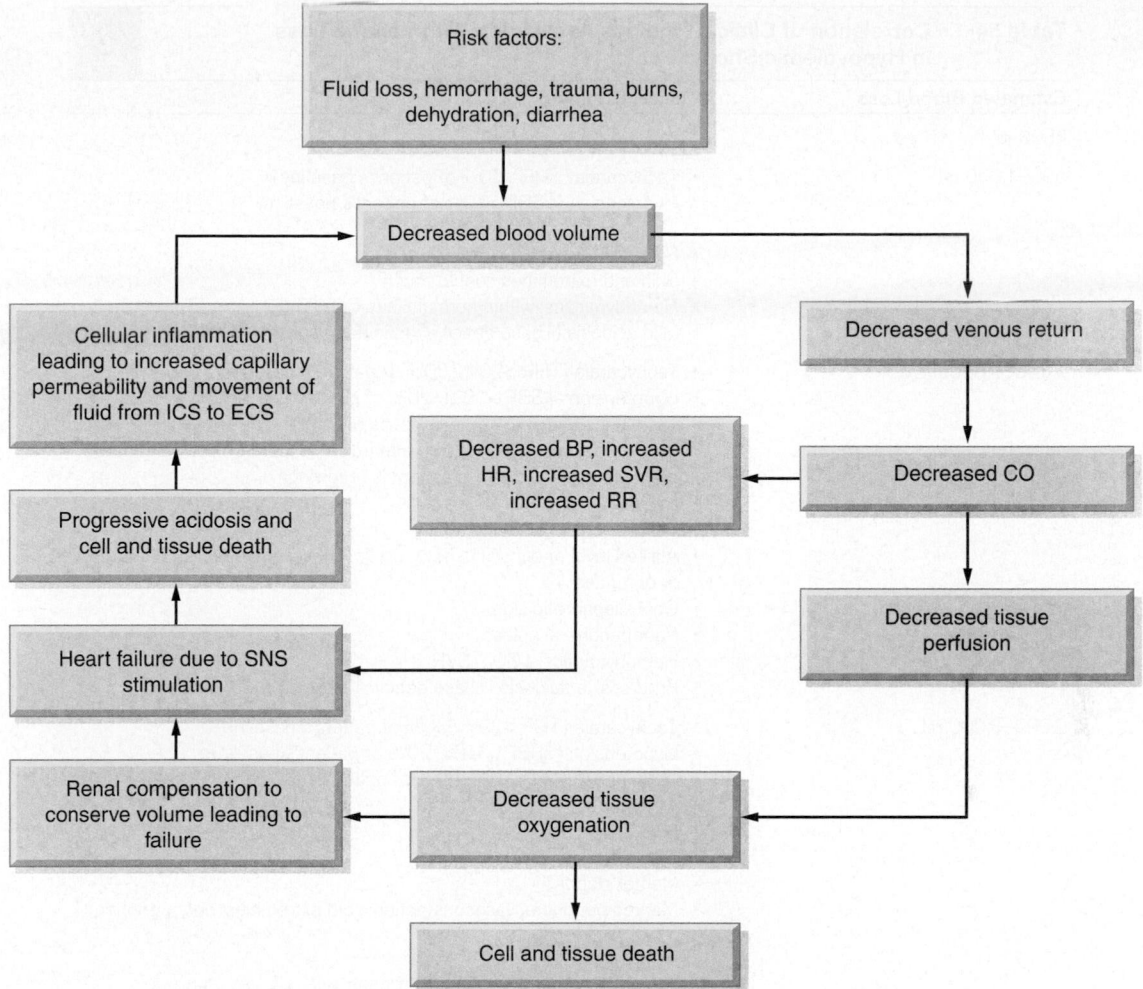

Figure 54-4 • Hypovolemic shock. BP, blood pressure; CO, cardiac output; ECS, extracellular space; HR, heart rate; ICS, intracellular space; RR, respiratory rate; SNS, sympathetic nervous system; SVR, systemic vascular resistance.

ure of the compensatory mechanisms to restore adequate circulating volume causes cellular hypoperfusion and inability to meet cellular oxygen requirements for metabolism. The cells must use anaerobic metabolism in an effort to meet their ATP requirements, resulting in lactic acidosis.

Failed compensatory mechanisms, which were initiated to restore cardiac output, eventually cause the myocardium to fatigue. Sympathetic stimulation to increase heart rate, contractility, and SVR escalates the workload of the heart. Ejection of a higher volume of blood against a higher SVR requires production of more oxygen and energy. Such stress on the heart causes an increase in myocardial metabolism and myocardial oxygen consumption ($M\dot{v}O_2$). The continued lack of circulating volume prevents appropriate oxygen delivery to the heart, creating a vicious cycle. Inability of the circulatory system to provide end-organ perfusion with enough oxygen forces conversion to anaerobic metabolism to meet cellular energy needs. Anaerobic metabolism cannot provide enough ATP to meet energy demands; thus, ischemic damage may ensue.

If the situation continues, end-organ failure may occur (see Fig. 54-4).

Assessment

Clinical findings are directly related to the severity and acuity of volume loss (Table 54-1). Some patients, especially older patients or those who have chronic diseases, have more subtle compensatory responses, which may be overlooked. Box 54-1 lists considerations in older patients. Serial assessments of physical and laboratory findings may uncover trends that guide treatment and prevent vascular collapse.

History

A thorough history of the patient's presenting problem may reveal risk factors for hypovolemic shock. Patients experiencing significant blood loss because of gastric hemorrhage or liver or splenic rupture from trauma require a rapid replacement of circulating blood volume to prevent the consequences of hypovolemia. Both very young and older patients are at greater risk for hypovolemia that may be caused

Table 54-1 • Correlation of Clinical Findings Associated With Volume Loss in Hypovolemic Shock

Estimated Blood Loss	Clinical Findings
<500 mL	None
500–1,000 mL	• Tachycardia (↑HR >20% of patient's baseline) • Hypotension (↓SBP >10% of patient's baseline) • ↓Urine output • Pulses weaker • Skin and extremities cool to touch • Hemodynamics: within normal limits CO, ↑SVR • Mild acidosis (↑base deficit, ↑lactic acid, ↓gastric pH)
1,000–2,000 mL	• Tachycardia (↑HR >20%–30% of patient's baseline) • Hypotension (↓SBP >10%–20% of patient's baseline) • Tachypnea (↑RR >10% of patient's baseline) • Oxygen saturation may not be altered dependent on the percentage of exogenous oxygen the patient is receiving • $S\bar{v}O_2$ <60% • ↓Urine output (<30 mL/h) • Altered level of consciousness: restlessness, agitation, confusion, or obtunded • Cool, diaphoretic skin • Poor peripheral pulses • Hemodynamics: ↓CO, ↑SVR • Progressive acidosis (↑base deficit, ↑lactic acid, ↓gastric pH)
2,000–3,000 mL	• Tachycardia (↑HR >20%–30% of patient's baseline) • Hypotension (↓SBP >10%–20% of patient's baseline) • Tachypnea (↑RR >10%–20% of patient's baseline) • ↓Oxygen saturation • $S\bar{v}O_2$ <55%–60% • Oliguria → anuria • Mental stupor • Marked peripheral vasoconstriction: cold extremities, poor peripheral pulses, pallor • Hemodynamics: ↓CO, ↑SVR • Severe acidosis (↑base deficit, ↑lactic acid, ↓gastric pH)

SBP, systolic blood pressure; SVR, systemic vascular resistance; CO, cardiac output; RR, respirations; HR, heart rate.

by severe dehydration or other medical illness, rather than trauma.[1,2]

Physical Findings

Patients with hypovolemic shock have the following signs and symptoms caused by poor organ perfusion[3,4]:

► Altered mentation, ranging from lethargy to unresponsiveness

► Rapid and deep respirations, which gradually become labored and shallower as the patient's condition deteriorates

► Cool and clammy skin, with weak and thready pulses

► Tachycardia due to activation of the sympathetic nervous system

► Hypotension, seen with loss of more than 30% of total blood volume

► Decreased urine output; urine is dark and concentrated because the kidneys are conserving fluid

Laboratory Studies

Useful laboratory studies include determinations of serum lactate, arterial pH, and base deficit to assess the presence of anaerobic metabolism. Test results can be used to measure the effectiveness of fluid replacement therapy. A serum lactate level that remains elevated for 24 to 48 hours is a poor prognostic indicator. Metabolic laboratory studies and electrolyte determinations assist with adjustment of fluid and electrolytes. Serial hemoglobin and hematocrit determinations and coagulation panels may be drawn to assess the need for blood product replacement. However, the hemoglobin and hematocrit may not directly reflect the severity of blood loss due to either hemoconcentration caused by dehydration or hemodilution caused by intravenous (IV) fluid therapy.

Management

Management focuses on restoring circulating volume and resolving the cause of volume loss. Composition of volume replacement therapy depends on what was lost. Crystalloid solutions are used primarily as first-line therapy. Isotonic solutions, such as lactated Ringer's solution or 0.9% normal saline solution, are preferred over hypotonic solutions (5% dextrose solution). Blood products and other colloid solutions (albumin and synthetic volume expanders) may be used to assist in the resuscitation process, especially if blood loss is the primary cause. The use of packed red

Box 54-1 • CONSIDERATIONS FOR THE OLDER PATIENT: Response to Shock States

As a person ages, normal physiological changes may limit the ability of the body to respond efficiently to shock states. The nurse should be aware of physiological changes of aging and monitor closely for changes in the older patient's baseline assessment(s). The patient's medical history indicates other chronic disease states that further compromise normal physiological changes seen with aging.

Cardiovascular system: Increased dysrhythmias, increased atrial size and irritability, left ventricular myocardial thickening leading to decreased compliance and lower ejection fraction; thickened heart valves that interfere with forward flow; decreased response to sympathetic nervous system; decreased sensitivity of baroreceptors; generalized stiffening of arterial vessels, including aorta

Pulmonary system: Decreased tidal volume and respiratory muscle strength, decreased alveolar surface area, increased dead space at end expiration, decreased elastic recoil of lungs, increased resting respiratory rate, increased risk for infection as a result of decreased number of cilia, blunted response to hypoxemia, decreased gag and cough reflex leading to increased risk for infection, aspiration

Hematological system: Decreased ability of bone marrow to produce cells (red blood cells, white blood cells, platelets), increased anemia, decreased immune function (decreased production of T and B lymphocytes) leading to increased infections, lower baseline temperature, gradual changes in temperature in the elderly versus spikes (101.3°F [38.5°C]), increased risk for adverse drug reactions

Table 54-2 • Complications of Volume Resuscitation

Fluid Type	Complications
Crystalloid and colloid	Dilutional coagulopathy
	Dilutional thrombocytopenia
	Hypothermia
	Increased hemorrhage
	Decreased blood viscosity
	Pulmonary edema
	Intracranial hypertension (patients with traumatic brain injury)
Packed red blood cells	Acidosis (banked blood has pH 6.9–7.1)
	Left shift on the oxyhemoglobin dissociation curve (banked blood is deficient in 2,3-DPG)
	Hyperkalemia
	Immunologic and infectious complications

inhibit adequate oxygenation, further compromising oxygen delivery to the tissues. Fluids should also be warmed during infusion to limit the negative effects of hypothermia.[3] Lower extremities may be elevated to prevent distal venous pooling and enhance blood return to the heart.[6] Frequent documentation of vital signs, heart rate, respiratory rate and depth, oxygen saturation, urine output, and mentation, as well as laboratory results and interventions, is essential.

Complications

Complications associated with hypovolemic shock depend on the length of time and severity of the hypotensive crisis. Complications may range from renal damage to cerebral anoxia and death.

CARDIOGENIC SHOCK

Etiology

Cardiogenic shock is actually extreme congestive heart failure and therefore results from loss of critical contractile function of the heart. Usually, cardiogenic shock is diagnosed by the presence of systemic and pulmonary hemodynamic alterations, which result from inadequate cardiac output and tissue perfusion. Typically, this occurs when greater than 40% of ventricular mass is damaged. The most common cause of cardiogenic shock is an extensive left ventricular myocardial infarction. In-hospital mortality rates have declined as a result of early revascularization procedures, defined as the capability to perform cardiac catheterization, percutaneous coronary intervention, and open heart surgery.[7] Although cardiogenic shock may develop within a few hours after the onset of myocardial infarction symptoms, it often occurs after hospitalization. Other causes of cardiogenic shock include papillary muscle rupture, ventricular septal rupture, cardiomyopathy, acute myocarditis, valvular disease, and dysrhythmias.

Box 54-2 shows independent predictors for development of cardiogenic shock. Patients with all five risk factors have a greater than 50% chance of developing

blood cells is of utmost importance if hypotension is due to hemorrhage, and they may be useful in other hypovolemic states.

The use of colloids in the early phase of fluid replacement is controversial. During shock, a state of increased capillary membrane permeability causes a shift of intravascular volume into the extravascular space. However, in some cases, colloids may enter the extravascular space, further shifting fluids from the intravascular space to the extravascular space and thereby worsening the hypovolemia. The existing research trials do not show a reduction in mortality or other complications of resuscitation with the use of colloids.[5] Table 54-2 summarizes some of the known complications of fluid resuscitation.

Nursing management of hypovolemic shock focuses on the restoration of circulating volume through volume administration. Obtaining and maintaining adequate IV access is essential. Ideally, large-bore (16-gauge or larger) IV catheters are inserted in the antecubital space or central venous system to assist with the rapid infusion of fluids. Care must be taken to administer fluids as rapidly as possible without compromising the pulmonary system. Fluids given too rapidly may cause pulmonary congestion and

> **Box 54-2 • RED FLAG: Factors for Inpatient Development of Cardiogenic Shock**
>
> - Increased age (elderly)
> - Left ventricular ejection fraction <35% on hospital admission
> - Large myocardial infarction
> - History of diabetes mellitus
> - Previous myocardial infarction

cardiogenic shock. Research indicates that mortality rates for patients who present with cardiogenic shock compared with those in whom it develops in the hospital are similarly high. Identifying patients at risk for development of cardiogenic shock and formulating strategies for prevention are extremely important.

Pathophysiology

Cardiogenic shock is caused by loss of ventricular contractile force, which results in decreased stroke volume and decreased cardiac output (Fig. 54-5). Neuroendocrine compensatory mechanisms, which are discussed in detail in the section on hypovolemic shock, are activated to increase preload through retention of sodium and water (see Fig. 54-1). Vasoconstriction also increases afterload (SVR). Ventricular filling pressures increase because of the increased preload, but lack of contractility prevents complete ejection. The ventricle becomes distended, further impairing effective contraction, and cardiac output continues to decrease. Compensatory mechanisms continue the vicious cycle of elevated ventricular filling pressures and SVR in combination with an

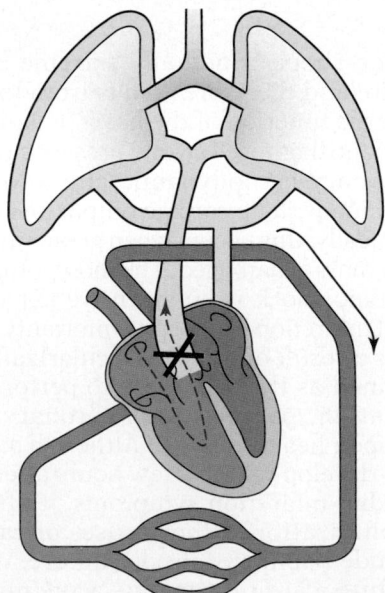

Figure 54-5 • Cardiogenic shock is caused by the loss of ventricular contractile force, which results in decreased stroke volume and decreased cardiac output. (From Porth CM: Essentials of Pathophysiology: Concepts of Altered Health States [2nd Ed], p 433. Philadelphia, Lippincott Williams & Wilkins, 2007.)

inability of the heart to eject an adequate volume of blood into circulation (Fig. 54-6). Blood pools in the pulmonary circulation, resulting in pulmonary congestion. Pulmonary capillaries are under increased pressure and leak fluid into the interstitium and alveoli, preventing the diffusion of oxygen from alveoli into the pulmonary capillaries and reducing oxygen tension in the blood.

The body's cells become ischemic because of the decreased cardiac output, adding to an already tenuous state of myocardial functioning by further stimulating compensatory mechanisms to increase perfusion to the cells. Increased sympathetic stimulation increases the heart rate even more, further escalating myocardial oxygen demands and compounding the crisis. Associated hypotension prevents adequate oxygenation of myocardial tissue, exacerbating the anaerobic metabolism of the myocardial tissue and further decreasing the contractile state of the heart. These stressors placed on the failing heart may result in extension of a myocardial infarction.

Assessment

Patients admitted with the diagnosis of myocardial infarction require close monitoring. Assessment parameters are similar to the signs and symptoms of congestive heart failure but are more extreme. Assessment findings should be followed over time to allow the nurse to perceive the subtle changes that signal the beginning of cardiogenic shock.

History

A thorough history provides the information necessary to predict patients at risk for development of cardiogenic shock. Cardiogenic shock frequently occurs in people who have suffered an extensive myocardial infarction, have an admission ejection fraction of less than 35%, have diabetes mellitus, or are elderly (see Box 54-2). These patients in particular should be closely monitored; the existence of the predisposing factors should alert the clinician to assess for the initial phases of shock, allowing for rapid, lifesaving intervention. It is important to rule out other causes of decreased cardiac output before initiating therapy. Patients with acute myocardial infarction may require rapid revascularization with thrombolytics (see Chapter 21), percutaneous coronary intervention (see Chapter 18), or cardiac surgery (see Chapter 22).[8]

Physical Findings

Clinical manifestations associated with cardiogenic shock are outlined in Box 54-3. In addition to the signs and symptoms listed in the box, patients with cardiogenic shock often experience recurrent chest pain, which is suggestive of infarct extension. Other clinical findings are directly related to the decrease in cardiac output.

Laboratory Studies

Presence of elevated myocardial tissue markers, accompanied by progressive hemodynamic compromise and clinical deterioration, is often a hallmark of extensive myocardial necrosis, which may precipitate cardiogenic shock. Laboratory studies suggestive of

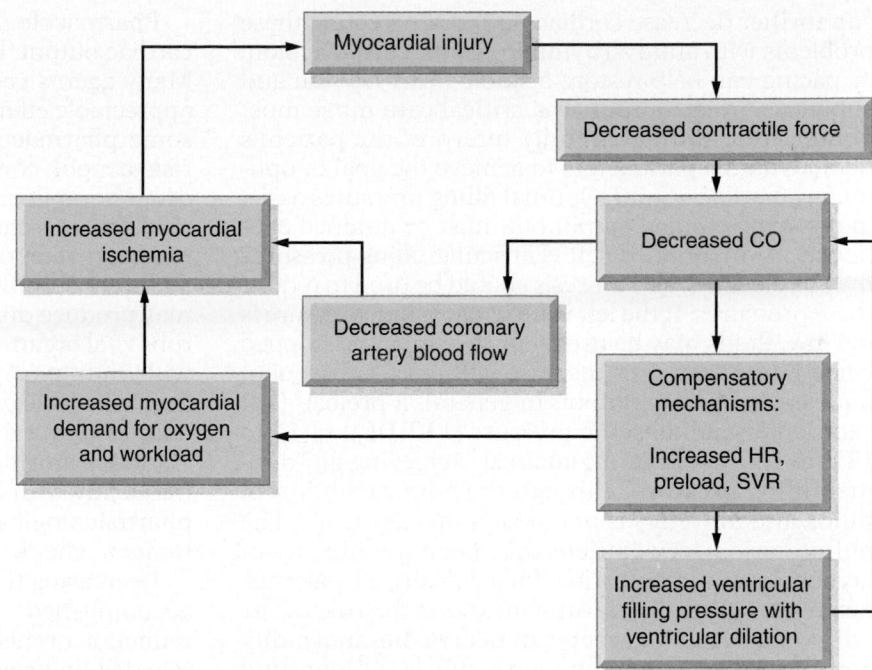

Figure 54-6 • Cardiogenic shock. CO, cardiac output; HR, heart rate; SVR, systemic vascular resistance.

myocardial tissue death reveal a continuous release of myocardial bands of creatine phosphokinase (MB-CPK) and cardiac troponin I into the circulation. These cardiac markers are released by dying cardiac cells into the bloodstream. Each marker has a time course for its peak level indicative of myocardial injury. Brain natriuretic peptide (BNP), another cardiac marker that may be assessed by laboratory analysis, is produced and released by the ventricle in

response to pressure overload. An elevated BNP does not correlate with myocardial ischemia; however, it may provide information about the patient's ventricular compliance, providing additional data that may place the patient at higher risk for cardiogenic shock after a myocardial infarction.[9]

Management

Management is aimed at increasing myocardial oxygen delivery, maximizing cardiac output, and decreasing left ventricular workload. The first goals of treatment are to correct reversible problems, protect the ischemic myocardium, and improve tissue perfusion. Early treatment is imperative to preserve myocardial muscle. Reversing the hypoxemia and acidosis can improve the response to other therapies. Fluids should be managed to provide adequate filling pressure without overdistention of the ventricle. Left ventricular filling pressures are often elevated; therefore, diuresis or nitrate infusion may be indicated to achieve optimal preload. Electrolytes, specifically potassium, calcium, and magnesium, may need to be replaced to provide optimal conditions for the damaged myocardial muscle.

Nursing management for the patient with cardiogenic shock is centered on conserving myocardial energy and decreasing the workload of the heart. Use of narcotic analgesics and sedatives to minimize the sympathetic nervous system response can increase venous capacitance and decrease resistance to ejection. Narcotics also relieve ischemic pain. Increasing the oxygen concentration of inspired air is a simple but important step, but may require initiation of mechanical ventilation. Nurses need to provide physical care and periods of rest to minimize myocardial energy expenditure.

Dysrhythmias often occur with acute myocardial infarction, ischemia, or acid–base imbalances and

---

Box 54-3 • Clinical Manifestations of Cardiogenic Shock

Hemodynamic findings
Systolic blood pressure <90 mm Hg
Mean arterial pressure <70 mm Hg
Cardiac index <2.2 L/min/m²
Pulmonary artery wedge pressure >18 mm Hg

Noninvasive findings
Thready, rapid pulse
Narrow pulse pressure
Distended neck veins
Arrhythmias
Chest pain
Cool, pale, moist skin
Oliguria
Decreased mentation

Pulmonary findings
Dyspnea
↑Respiratory rate
Inspiratory crackles, possible wheezing
Arterial blood gases show ↓ in PaO₂
Respiratory alkalosis

Radiographic findings
Enlarged heart
Pulmonary congestion

can further decrease cardiac output. Correcting these problems with antidysrhythmic agents, cardioversion, or pacing can help restore a stable heart rhythm and enhance cardiac output. The critical care nurse must obtain, follow, and carefully interpret the patient's hemodynamic parameters to achieve the goal of optimizing cardiac output. Optimal filling pressures assist in restoring cardiac output but must be attained cautiously. As mentioned, left ventricular filling pressures may be elevated, and diuresis should be used to reduce these pressures. If the left ventricular filling pressure is too low, fluids may be used, but they must be stopped when filling pressures increase without a subsequent increase in cardiac output. In general, a preload (left ventricular end-diastolic pressure [LVEDP]) of 14 to 18 mm Hg should be maintained. Achieving an "optimal filling pressure" through the administration of fluids and diuretics is not always an easy task.[8] The pulmonary artery catheter has been a mainstay of hemodynamic monitoring for critically ill patients; however, current literature questions the role of the pulmonary artery catheter in decreasing morbidity and mortality in patients with shock.[10] Slow fluid administration or diuresis requires a diligent assessment of the effectiveness of the interventions. Invasive measures of fluid status may be used in patients with pulmonary artery catheters, whereas noninvasive measures such as blood pressure, mental status, and urine output may be used in other patients.[8,10]

Pharmacological agents can be used to augment cardiac output, but they too must be used cautiously. Many agents can increase $M\dot{v}O_2$ without having an appreciable effect on cardiac output. Decisions to use some pharmacological agents are based on overall risk–benefit considerations. The sympathomimetic drugs norepinephrine and epinephrine hydrochloride may enhance cardiac output by increasing contractility, heart rate, or SVR but increase cardiac work. In addition, stimulation of β_2 receptors by epinephrine may produce dilation in peripheral vascular beds that robs vital organs of blood. Therefore, this agent is used with caution. Agents with positive inotropic effects that have little activity on vascular tone, such as low-dose dopamine hydrochloride, dobutamine hydrochloride, amrinone, and milrinone, are used more frequently with favorable results.[1,11–13] Table 54-3 lists pharmacological agents used in the treatment of patients in shock states.

Decreasing the workload of the left ventricle can be accomplished through pharmacological afterload reduction or mechanical support devices. It is recommended that vasodilators, such as sodium nitroprusside, nitroglycerin, or angiotensin-converting enzyme inhibitors, be administered to reduce SVR and LVEDP in an effort to increase cardiac output and improve left ventricular function.[8] Mechanical support for the failing ventricle includes the intra-aortic balloon pump and left ventricular assist device. Both devices reduce

Table 54-3 • Pharmacologic Agents Used in the Treatment of Shock*

Drug Category	Heart Rate	Effects on Contractility	Systemic Venous Resistance	Nursing Considerations
Vasoconstrictors				
Dopamine (Intropin)	↑	↑↑	↑	Hemodynamic effects are dose dependent
Epinephrine (Adrenaline)	↑↑	↑↑	↑	May induce ventricular dysrhythmias; May exacerbate $M\dot{v}O_2$ demands; β_2 Activity may dilate peripheral beds
Norepinephrine (also known as levarterenol [Levophed])	↑	↑	↑↑↑	Monitor peripheral circulation closely; may increase $M\dot{v}O_2$
Phenylephrine (Neo-synephrine)			↑↑	May induce dysrhythmias
Vasopressin (Pitressin)		↑	↑↑	Monitor peripheral circulation closely; may increase $M\dot{v}O_2$
Vasodilators				
Sodium nitroprusside (Nipride)	↑		↓↓	Hemodynamic effects are dose dependent; adjust dosage slowly
Nitroglycerine (Tridil)	↑		↓	Hemodynamic effects are dose dependent; adjust dosage slowly; tolerance may develop
Angiotensin-converting enzyme (ACE) inhibitors	↑		↓	
Inotropic Agents				
Amrinone (Inocor)	↑	↑	↓	May exacerbate $M\dot{v}O_2$ demands
Milrinone (Primacor)	↑	↑↑	↓	May exacerbate $M\dot{v}O_2$ demands; Monitor for tachyarrhythmias
Dobutamine (Dobutrex)	↑	↑↑	↓	May exacerbate $M\dot{v}O_2$ demands; Monitor for tachyarrhythmias

$M\dot{v}O_2$, myocardial oxygen consumption.
*All agents should be administered through a great vein (central access) and using a volumetric pump.

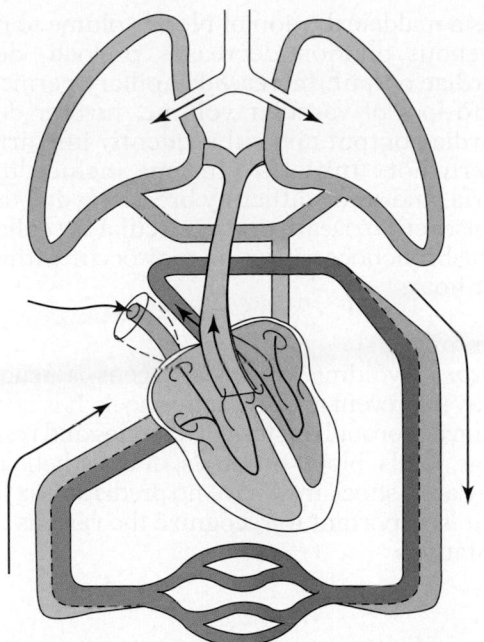

Figure 54-7 • Distributive shock states are caused by decreased venous return as a result of displacement of blood volume away from the heart due to enlargement of the vascular compartment and loss of blood vessel tone. (From Porth CM: Pathophysiology: Concepts of Altered Health States [7th Ed], p 413. Philadelphia, Lippincott Williams & Wilkins, 2007.)

the workload of the left ventricle by supplementing pumping ability (see Chapter 18).

DISTRIBUTIVE SHOCK STATES

Distributive shock states can be caused by anaphylaxis (anaphylactic shock), loss of sympathetic tone (neurogenic shock), or sepsis (septic shock). The underlying mechanism is decreased venous return as a result of displacement of blood volume away from the heart due to enlargement of the vascular compartment and loss of blood vessel tone (Fig. 54-7). Loss of blood vessel tone occurs as a consequence of a loss of sympathetic innervation to blood vessels (neurogenic shock) or because of the presence of vasodilating substances in the blood (anaphylactic and septic shock). Distributive shock states can occur in a variety of settings, although the most common is sepsis.[1]

Anaphylactic Shock

Anaphylaxis results from an allergic reaction to a specific allergen that evokes a life-threatening hypersensitivity response. Recent epidemiologic evidence suggests that 59% of reported cases of anaphylactic shock are due to insect venoms, 18% to drugs, and 10% to food.[14] If left untreated, vascular collapse occurs, resulting in greatly decreased tissue perfusion. Prompt intervention is critical.

Etiology

Antigens, the substances that elicit the response, can be introduced through injection or ingestion, or through the skin or respiratory tract. Substances capable of evoking anaphylaxis in humans include a multitude of factors (Box 54-4).

Anaphylaxis may be either immunoglobulin E (IgE) or non-IgE mediated. Non-IgE responses occur without the presence of IgE antibodies and are called anaphylactoid reactions. It is thought that direct activation of mediators causes this response. Anaphylactoid reactions are commonly associated with nonsteroidal anti-inflammatory drugs (NSAIDs), including aspirin. If there has been an anaphylactoid reaction to one agent, restrictions should include all NSAIDs because any of them could elicit a second reaction.

IgE-mediated anaphylaxis occurs as a result of the immune response to a specific antigen. The first time the immune system is exposed to the antigen, a very specific IgE antibody is formed and circulates in the blood. When a second exposure to this antigen occurs, the antigen binds to this circulating IgE, which then activates mast cells and basophils, triggering release of histamine, prostaglandins, leukotrienes, and other biochemical mediators that initiate anaphylaxis.

Box 54-4 • RED FLAG: Agents Commonly Implicated in Anaphylactic and Anaphylactoid Reactions

Antibiotics	Penicillin and its synthetics, cephalosporins, erythromycin, streptomycin, tetracyclines
Anti-inflammatory agents	Salicylates, aminopyrine, ibuprofen, naproxen, and others
Narcotic analgesics	Morphine, codeine
Other medications	Protamine, chlorpropamide, parenteral iron, iodides, thiazide diuretics
Anesthetics	Procaine, lidocaine, cocaine, thiopental
Anesthetic adjuncts	Succinylcholine, tubocurarine
Blood products	Red blood cell, white blood cell, and platelet transfusions; gamma globulin
Immune sera	Rabies, tetanus, diphtheria antitoxin, snake and spider antivenom
Diagnostic agents	Iodinated radiocontrast agents
Venoms	Bees, wasps, hornets, spiders, snakes, jellyfish
Hormones	Insulin, corticotropin, pituitary extract
Enzymes and other biologicals	Acetylcysteine, pancreatic enzyme supplements
Extracts used in desensitization	Food, pollen, venoms
Foods	Eggs, fish, shellfish, milk, nuts, legumes
Textiles	Latex

Pathophysiology

The antibody–antigen reaction causes antibody-specific mast cells and basophils to secrete substances such as histamine, leukotrienes, eosinophil chemotactic substance, heparin, prostaglandins, neutrophil chemotactic substance, and platelet-activating factor 2 (Fig. 54-8). These substances, particularly histamine, prostaglandins, and leukotrienes, cause systemic vasodilation, increased capillary permeability, bronchoconstriction, coronary vasoconstriction, and urticaria (hives). Platelet-activating factor 2 is thought to be crucial in the development of anaphylactic shock and is implicated in the development of hypotension and cardiovascular dysfunction, but its mechanism of action is not clearly understood.[15] Some of the other substances precipitate a continued downward spiral by causing myocardial depression, inflammation, excessive mucus secretion, and peripheral vasodilation. The diffuse arterial vasodilation creates a maldistribution of blood volume to tissues, and venous dilation decreases preload, decreasing cardiac output. Increased capillary permeability leads to loss of vascular volume, further decreasing cardiac output and subsequently impairing tissue perfusion. Initial symptoms include itching, urticaria, and some difficulty breathing due to bronchoconstriction. Death due to circulatory collapse or extreme bronchoconstriction may occur within minutes or hours.

Assessment

History Avoiding known allergens is usually the best way to prevent anaphylactic shock. It is necessary to obtain a thorough history of allergies and responses to drugs, foods, blood products, or anesthetic agents. Anaphylactic shock may have no predisposing factors. Thus, it is important to recognize the various clinical presentations.

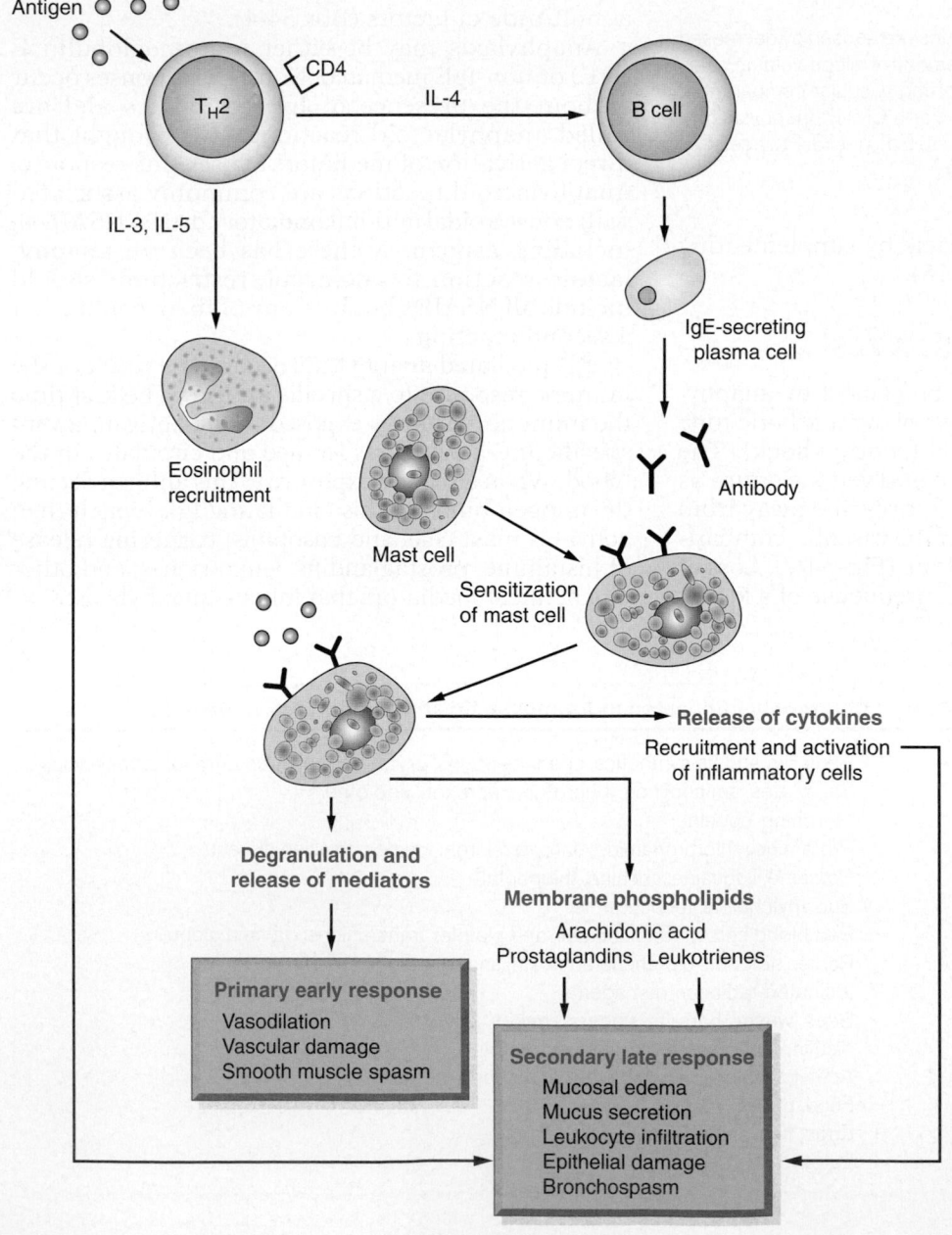

Figure 54-8 • IgE-mediated hypersensitivity reaction. IL-3, interleukin 3; IL-4, interleukin 4; IL-5, interleukin 5. (From Porth CM: Concepts of Altered Health States [7th Ed], p 413. Philadelphia, Lippincott Williams & Wilkins, 2005.)

Physical Findings The earlier the symptoms of anaphylaxis appear after exposure to the antigen, the more severe the response. Initially, generalized erythema, urticaria, and pruritus may occur in response to the antigen. Other symptoms may include anxiety and restlessness, dyspnea, wheezing, chest tightness, a warm feeling, nausea and vomiting, angioedema, and even abdominal pain. As the episode progresses, severe respiratory manifestations, such as laryngeal edema or severe bronchoconstriction with stridor, may develop. Hypotension from vasodilation soon occurs and leads to circulatory collapse. As circulatory collapse or hypoxia due to severe bronchoconstriction progresses, the level of consciousness deteriorates to unresponsiveness.

Management
Early recognition and treatment of anaphylaxis is essential. Therapeutic goals include removal of the offending antigen, reversal of effects of the biochemical mediators, and restoration of adequate tissue perfusion. Regardless of the cause of the anaphylactic reaction, treatment depends on clinical symptoms. If the symptoms are mild, immediate therapy includes oxygen and subcutaneous or IV administration of an antihistamine, such as diphenhydramine, to block the effects of histamine, and possibly an epinephrine injection to reverse the vasodilation and bronchoconstriction[16,17] (Box 54-5). For adults, rapid infusion (over 1 to 3 minutes) of normal saline IV is given for severe hypotension or if the patient does not respond promptly to epinephrine.[16] Other pharmacotherapy includes corticosteroids, bronchodilators, and, if necessary, vasoconstrictors and positive inotropic agents to combat circulatory collapse.

Nursing care involves maintaining an adequate airway and monitoring patient response to the antigen. The nurse also monitors respirations, heart rate, blood pressure, and level of anxiety, and institutes comfort measures related to the dermatological manifestations. If the agent causing the anaphylaxis is unknown, evaluation for allergies and future risk for anaphylaxis should be completed. Patient education regarding prevention and treatment is critical for any person who experiences a significant anaphylactic or anaphylactoid reaction.

 Box 54-5 • Epinephrine Dosage in Anaphylaxis (Adults)

If IV access is not available:
- Epinephrine, 0.01 mg/kg (maximum, 0.5 mg) into anterolateral thigh (absorption is greatest here)
- Proceed to obtain IV access.

If IV access is available:
- Epinephrine, 1 mg in 100 mL (10 µg/mL; 1:100,000) IV by infusion pump
- Initiate infusion at 30–100 mL/h (5–17 µg/min) and titrate to response aiming for lowest effective infusion rate.
- Stop infusion rate 30 min after signs and symptoms have resolved.

Neurogenic Shock
Neurogenic shock results from loss or disruption of sympathetic tone, which causes peripheral vasodilation and subsequent decreased tissue perfusion. The disturbance of sympathetic tone may be caused by any event that disrupts the sympathetic nervous system. The most common cause of neurogenic shock is a spinal cord injury above the level of T6. Other causes include spinal analgesia, emotional stress, pain, drugs, or other central nervous system problems. (Refer to Chapter 37 for a thorough discussion of spinal cord injury and neurogenic shock.)

Septic Shock
Septic shock is a complex and generalized process that involves all organ systems. Sepsis, severe sepsis, and septic shock represent progressive stages of the same illness. In 1991, the Society of Critical Care Medicine and the American College of Chest Physicians established universal definitions for the term sepsis and other associated clinical conditions.[18] These organizations wished to promote earlier detection of and intervention for these states, improve outcomes, and standardize the terminology used in research protocols to make the information derived easier to disseminate and apply to practice. In 2002, a second consensus conference was held to modify the existing definitions for accuracy, reliability, and clinical utility of the diagnosis of sepsis[19] (Box 54-6).

Etiology
In the United States, there are approximately 750,000 new episodes of sepsis each year. The incidence is increasing for several reasons: an aging population, infection with antibiotic-resistant organisms, more immunocompromised patients, and patients who undergo high-risk surgery.[20] Severe sepsis has a mortality rate of 25% to 30%,[21] and septic shock has a mortality rate of 40% to 70%.[22] Risk factors for the development of septic shock include host factors and treatment-related factors (Box 54-7). Approximately one in four patients in the intensive care unit (ICU) with sepsis worsen to severe sepsis or shock, and the risk for this progression is greatest in the first 10 days of diagnosis.[23] Risk factors for progression from sepsis to systemic inflammatory response syndrome (SIRS) are listed in Box 54-8.

Septic shock is initiated by an infection. Infections may be due to invading gram-negative or gram-positive bacteria, fungi, and viruses. In many patients, multiple causative organisms are identified. Bacteria may be introduced through the pulmonary system, urinary tract, or gastrointestinal system; through wounds; or through invasive devices. Both gram-negative and gram-positive organisms may directly stimulate the inflammatory response and other aspects of the immune system that activate cytokines, complement, and coagulation systems.

Pathophysiology
Septic shock is the culmination of complex interactions among invading microorganisms and immune,

Box 54-6 • Clinical Terminology: Sepsis and Organ Failure

Definitions developed by the Consensus Conferences of the Society of Critical Care Medicine and American College of Chest Physicians.

Bacteremia: The presence of viable bacteria in the blood.

Hypotension: A systolic blood pressure of <90 mm Hg or a reduction of >40 mm Hg from baseline in the absence of other causes for hypotension.

Infection: Microbial phenomenon characterized by an inflammatory response to the presence of micro-organisms or the invasion of normally sterile host tissue by those organisms.

Multiple organ dysfunction syndrome: Presence of altered organ function in an acutely ill patient such that homeostasis cannot be maintained without intervention.

Sepsis: The systemic response to infection. This systemic response is manifested by two or more of the following conditions as a result of infection:

- Temperature >38°C or <36°C (100.4°F or 96.8°F)
- Heart rate >90 beats/minute
- Respiratory rate >20 breaths/minute or $PaCO_2$ <32 mm Hg (<4.3 kPa)
- WBC count >12,000 cells/mm^3, <4,000 cells/mm^3, or >10% immature (band) forms

The **PIRO mnemonic** may be used to diagnose and track the progression of sepsis:

- **P**atient predisposition and response to infection based on genetics

- **I**nfection
- **R**esponse to inflammation
- **O**rgan dysfunction

Severe sepsis: Sepsis associated with organ dysfunction, hypoperfusion, or hypotension. Hypoperfusion and perfusion abnormalities may include, but are not limited to, lactic acidosis, oliguria, or an acute alteration in mental status.

Septic shock: Sepsis with hypotension, despite adequate fluid resuscitation, along with the presence of perfusion abnormalities that may include, but are not limited to, lactic acidosis, oliguria, or an acute alteration in mental status. Patients who are on inotropic or vasopressor agents may not be hypotensive at the time that perfusion abnormalities are measured.

Systemic inflammatory response syndrome: The systemic inflammatory response to a variety of severe clinical insults. The response is manifested by two or more of the following conditions:

- Temperature >38°C or <36°C (>100.4°F or <96.8°F)
- Heart rate >90 beats/minute
- Respiratory rate >20 breaths/minute or $PaCO_2$ <32 mm Hg (<4.3 kPa)
- WBC count >12,000 cell/mm^3, <4,000 cells/mm^3, or >10% immature (band) forms

Adapted from Levy MM: Definitions of sepsis revisited: Results of the SSSM/ESICM/ACCP/ATS consensus conference. In Levy MM, Vincent JL (eds): Sepsis: Pathophysiologic Insights and Current Management. Chicago: Society of Critical Care Medicine, 2003, pp 39–42.

inflammatory, and coagulation systems, which results in a proinflammatory and procoagulation state.[24] In response to the presence of microorganisms, macrophages and helper (CD4+) type 1 helper T (Th1) cells secrete proinflammatory cytokines, such as tumor necrosis factor-α and interleukin-1β. In addition to activating neutrophils that kill microorganisms, these

proinflammatory cytokines also injure endothelial cells. Once injured, endothelial cells release mediators that cause endothelial cells to lose their tight junctions between each other, resulting in increased vascular permeability. Protein-rich fluid moves from the vascular space into the interstitial spaces of tissues, including the lungs. The release of anti-inflammatory cytokines also occurs. Th2 cells secrete the anti-inflammatory cytokines interleukin-4 and interleukin-10, which balance the proinflammatory response. But in some patients, these proinflammatory

Box 54-7 • RED FLAG: Risk Factors for the Development of Septic Shock

Host Factors
- Extremes of age
- Malnutrition
- General debilitation
- Chronic debilitation
- Chronic illness
- Drug or alcohol abuse
- Neutropenia
- Splenectomy
- Multiple organ failure

Treatment-Related Factors
- Use of invasive catheters
- Surgical procedures
- Traumatic or thermal wounds
- Invasive diagnostic procedures
- Drugs (antibiotics, cytotoxic agents, steroids)

Box 54-8 • RED FLAG: Risk Factors for Progression From Sepsis to Systemic Inflammatory Response Syndrome

- Systolic blood pressure < 110 mm Hg
- Temperature > 38.2°C
- Sodium > 145 mmol/L
- Platelets < 150 × 10^9/L
- Bilirubin > 30 μmol/L
- Mechanical ventilation
- Presence of infection
  - Primary bacteremia
  - Aerobic gram-negative bacilli
  - Gram-positive cocci
  - Peritonitis
  - Pneumonia

cytokines fail to shut down or control the proinflammatory cytokines, and the "out of control" proinflammatory response activates the coagulation cascade.

Another important aspect of sepsis is the imbalance between procoagulant and anticoagulant factors. Procoagulant factors increase, and anticoagulant factors decrease[25] (Fig. 54-9). Endotoxins stimulate endothelial cells to release tissue factor, which then activates factors Va and VIIIa of the coagulation cascade. As a result, thrombin converts fibrinogen to fibrin. Fibrin binds to platelet plugs that have adhered to damaged endothelial cells. This forms a stable fibrin clot. These clots form throughout the microvasculature and cause additional injury and ischemia to distal tissues. Normally, anticoagulant factors (protein C, protein S, antithrombin III, tissue factor pathway inhibitor) modulate coagulation,[25] as shown in Figure 54-9. Thrombin binds with thrombomodulin on a specific receptor on endothelial cells. This binding "activates" protein C. Activated protein C then inactivates factors V and VIII and inhibits the synthesis of plasminogen-activator inhibitor, which then allows plasmin to break down the fibrin-platelet clots.[25] Unfortunately, sepsis lowers the levels of these anticoagulant factors, and the net result is a procoagulant state. Recognition that the proinflammatory and procoagulant responses result in a loss of homeostasis of almost every organ system is key to understanding of sepsis.

Cardiovascular Alterations

In general, septic shock is associated with three major pathophysiological effects on the cardiovascular system: vasodilation, maldistribution of blood flow, and myocardial depression.

Proinflammatory cytokines stimulate the release of nitric oxide (NO) from endothelial cells. NO is a potent vasodilator and causes widespread vasodilation. This vasodilation is often resistant to vasopressor agents.[26] Because of this vasodilation, there is decreased venous return to the heart, decreased cardiac output, and decreased systemic vascular resistance.

Other inflammatory mediators, including tumor necrosis factor-α and endothelin, cause vasoconstriction in other vascular beds. This situation of mixed vasodilation and vasoconstriction produces maldistribution of blood flow, particularly in the microcirculation. Such maldistribution also occurs as inflammatory mediators and endotoxins damage endothelial cells. This initiates the coagulation cascade within the microvasculature. Small clots form, causing hypoxia to cells distal to the obstruction. This is pivotal to the progression from sepsis to septic shock, SIRS, MODS, and death.

In septic shock, evidence of depressed myocardial performance occurs in the form of decreased ventricular ejection fraction, dilation of the ventricles, and a flattening of the Frank-Starling curve after fluid

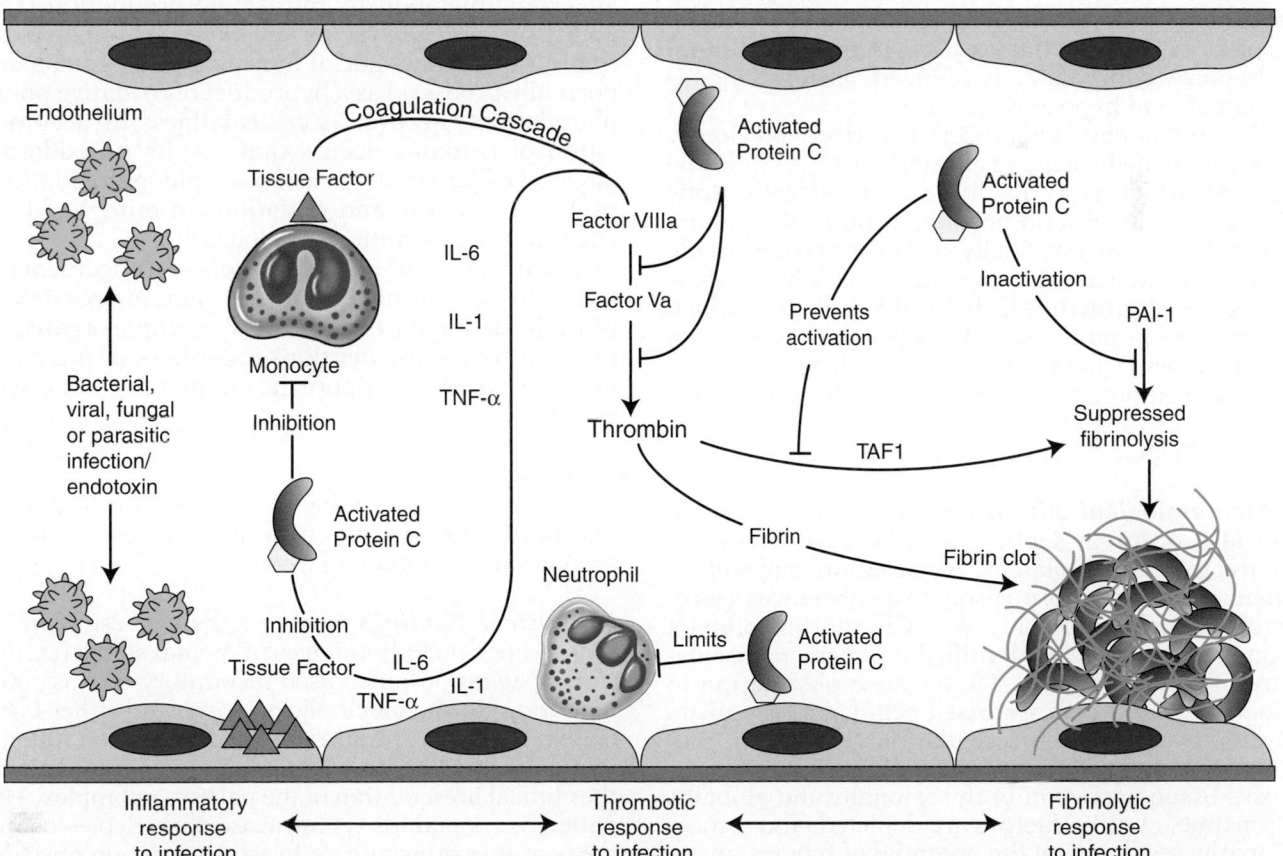

Figure 54-9 • Inflammatory/immune response in septic shock. IL-1, interleukin 1; IL-6, interleukin 6; TNF-α, tumor necrosis factor-α; TAFI; thrombin-activated fibrinolysis inhibitor; PAI-1, plasminogen activator inhibitor-1. (Copyright © 2001, Eli Lilly and Company. All rights reserved. Reprinted with permission from Eli Lilly and Company.)

resuscitation.[6] This myocardial depression is not caused by myocardial ischemia but rather by myocardial depressant factors released as part of the inflammatory cascade and the generation of NO. Lactic acidosis, which decreases myocardial responsiveness to catecholamines, may also be partly responsible. Whatever the mechanism, the heart demonstrates impaired contractility and ventricular performance.

Early in septic shock, it is believed that the heart is hyperdynamic, with high cardiac output and low SVR. However, evidence indicates that even at this stage, the heart is performing less than optimally. Later, as circulating cardiac depressants increase, the heart becomes hypodynamic, with low cardiac output and increased SVR. Hemodynamic parameters, including $Sc\overline{v}O_2/S\overline{v}O_2$ and measures of metabolic acidosis, should be followed over time to recognize early and progressive cardiac failure.

Pulmonary Alterations Events initiated by activation of the inflammatory response and its mediators affect the lungs both directly and indirectly. Activation of the sympathetic nervous system and release of epinephrine from the adrenal medulla produce bronchodilation. However, this may be overridden by activity of cytokines, and the net result is bronchoconstriction. More important, inflammatory mediators and activated neutrophils cause capillary leak into the pulmonary interstitium, resulting in interstitial edema, areas of poor pulmonary perfusion (shunting), pulmonary hypertension, and increased respiratory work. As fluid collects in the interstitium, pulmonary compliance is reduced, gas exchange is impaired, and hypoxemia occurs.

The pulmonary alterations described previously may culminate in acute respiratory distress syndrome (ARDS), which is frequently associated with septic shock. Continued fluid accumulation in the pulmonary interstitium may finally spill over into the alveoli, producing alveolar infiltrates that provide fertile areas for bacterial growth. Mechanical ventilation, which is common in patients with ARDS, may provide an avenue of entry for lung infections. Therefore, a secondary pneumonia may develop, possibly caused by a different organism than that which produced the sepsis. See Chapter 27 for more information about ARDS.

Hematological Alterations Platelet abnormalities also occur in septic shock because endotoxin indirectly causes platelet aggregation and subsequent release of more vasoactive substances (serotonin and thromboxane A_2). Circulating platelet aggregates have been identified in the microvasculature of septic patients. These cause obstruction to blood flow and compromised cellular metabolism. Overactivation of the coagulation cascade without the counterbalance of adequate fibrinolysis compromises tissue perfusion both regionally and globally. Over time, clotting factors are depleted, and a coagulopathy results, with the potential of progressing to disseminated intravascular coagulation (DIC).

Metabolic Alterations Septic shock induces a hypermetabolic state characterized by an increase in resting energy consumption, extensive protein and fat catabolism, negative nitrogen balance, hyperglycemia, and hepatic gluconeogenesis.[27] Excessive catecholamine release stimulates gluconeogenesis and insulin resistance, which both result in hyperglycemia in critically ill patients who do not have diabetes. Cells are progressively unable to use glucose, protein, and fat as energy sources. Hyperglycemia that is resistant to insulin therapy is a frequent finding in early shock. Eventually, all glycogen energy stores are depleted, cells lack ATP, and cellular pumps fail, progressing to tissue and organ death.

In response to lack of effect of insulin, proteins break down, as shown by high blood urea nitrogen and urinary nitrogen excretion. Muscle protein is broken down to amino acids, some of which are used as energy sources for the Krebs cycle or as substrates for gluconeogenesis. In later stages of shock, the liver is unable to use the amino acids because of its own metabolic dysfunction. Amino acids then accumulate in the bloodstream.

As shock progresses, adipose tissue is broken down (lipolysis) to furnish the liver with lipids for energy production. Hepatic triglyceride metabolism produces ketones, which circulate to peripheral cells that can use them in the Krebs cycle for ATP production. However, as liver function decreases, triglycerides are not broken down; they collect in the mitochondria, inhibiting the Krebs cycle and resulting in increased anaerobic metabolism and lactate production. The ability of cells to extract or use oxygen is impaired as a result of mitochondrial dysfunction. Oxidants are normally produced as a byproduct of oxidative phosphorylation. However, in critical illness, an accumulation of oxidants occurs that results in oxidative stress. Oxidative stress causes lipid peroxidation, protein oxidation, and mutations in mitochondrial DNA, thus contributing to cell death.

The net effect of these metabolic derangements is that cells become energy starved. This energy deficit is implicated in the emergence of multiple organ failure that frequently develops regardless of interventions designed to support the circulatory and organ systems.

Assessment

A thorough understanding of the mediator responses that occur during sepsis aids in the assessment and evaluation of response to treatment.

Physical Findings Some of the earliest signs of septic shock include changes in mental status (confusion or agitation), increased respiratory rate as compensation for the metabolic acidosis, and either fever or hypothermia. Because of the exaggerated inflammatory response with release of vasoactive mediators, the clinical presentation of the patient is complex. The patient is edematous yet intravascularly depleted, and areas of microthrombi and vasoconstriction obstruct perfusion. As fluid replacement occurs, the leaking capillary beds shift the fluid interstitially, requiring more fluid resuscitation, which may further exacerbate interstitial edema. Because of the inappropriate systemic activation of the coagulation system, clotting factors are depleted, and spontaneous bleeding may occur. Perfusion imbalances cause ischemia in some vascular beds, such as the splanchnic circulation, skin, and extremities, which may lead to necrosis. Cardiac output may be unusually high, but it is insufficient to maintain adequate perfusion due to circulating myocardial depressant factors. Compensatory mechanisms, such as activation of the sympathetic nervous system, continue to increase cardiac output. However, inflammatory mediators prevent necessary vasoconstriction, and the SVR remains inappropriately low, thereby perpetuating the hypoperfusion crisis.

As sepsis progresses and organ hypoperfusion persists, cells in hypoperfused organs begin to die, and the organs begin to fail. This may lead to MODS.

Laboratory Studies Laboratory and diagnostic studies that may be helpful in the identification of sepsis are summarized in Box 54-9. Despite the use of such testing, the early diagnosis of sepsis and septic shock is usually made on the basis of patient risk factors and clinical findings (see Box 54-7).

Management

Septic shock requires a prompt, aggressive, multidisciplinary team approach with monitoring and treatment facilities found in an ICU. The primary goals of treatment are to maximize oxygen delivery above cellular oxygen consumption requirements and to halt the exaggerated inflammatory response. The treatment of sepsis involves early, goal-directed therapy. Initiating therapy promptly (ideally within the first 6 hours), with specific hemodynamic goals for resuscitation, has been shown to slow the decompensation of patients in a septic state and decrease the risk for cardiovascular collapse.[28] The Surviving Sepsis Guidelines,[29] developed in 2003 by an international team, outline the evidence-based care of patients with sepsis (Table 54-4).

Prevention Because diagnosis of sepsis is so complex and mortality from septic shock so high, it is imperative that preventive infection control measures be in place. Defense mechanisms may be impaired, and protection from hospital-acquired (nosocomial) infections is essential. The estimated cost of treating nosocomial infections is nearly $5 billion dollars per year,[30] and nosocomial infection increases the length of the ICU stay by 4.3 to 15.6 days.[31] Therefore, a critical aspect of nursing care involves adherence to aseptic techniques, thorough handwashing, and a continuing awareness of multiple sites and causes of infection. Sources of equipment-related infections are listed in Box 54-10.

Identification and Treatment of Infection Identification of the infecting organism and use of appropriate antibiotic treatment are of utmost importance. Before the causal organism has been identified, empiric broad-spectrum antibiotic therapy is initiated, usually with multiple antibiotics with coverage against gram-negative and gram-positive bacteria and anaerobes. However, once the infectious organism has been isolated, antibiotic therapy should be changed so that specific antibiotics effective against that organism are used to try to minimize development of antibiotic resistance. Other definitive measures to alleviate the cause of sepsis might include resection or drainage of purulent tissues or secretions.[29]

However, antimicrobial treatment of sepsis is not sufficient to treat the generalized inflammatory reactions seen with septic shock. Supportive measures establish and maintain adequate tissue perfusion, and other therapies aim to block or interfere with the action of the various mediators implicated in shock. Aspects of supportive care include the following:

▶ Restoring intravascular volume
▶ Maintaining an adequate cardiac output
▶ Ensuring adequate ventilation and oxygenation
▶ Restoring balance between coagulation and anticoagulation
▶ Providing an appropriate metabolic environment

Restoration of Intravascular Volume Adequate volume replacement is important for reversing hypotension. Patients may require several liters or more of fluid because of mediator-induced vasodilation and capillary leak. Fluid replacement should be guided by hemodynamic parameters, urine output,

(text continues on page 1398)

Box 54-9 • Physiological Data Helpful in Diagnosing Sepsis

- Cultures: blood, sputum, urine, surgical or nonsurgical wounds, sinuses, and invasive lines; positive results are not necessary for diagnosis.
- CBC: WBCs usually will be elevated and may decrease with progression of shock.
- Sequential multiple analysis-7 (SMA-7): hyperglycemia may be evident, followed by hypoglycemia in later stages.
- Arterial blood gases: metabolic acidosis with possibly compensating respiratory alkalosis ($PaCO_2$ <35 mm Hg) is present in sepsis, with mild hypoxemia (PaO_2 <80 mm Hg)
- CT scan may be needed to identify sites of potential abscesses.
- Chest and abdominal radiographs may reveal infectious processes.
- $S\overline{v}O_2$ pulmonary artery catheter will assist in the assessment of oxygen delivery and consumption needs of the tissues and cells.
- Lactate level: decreasing levels of lactate in the serum indicates aerobic metabolism is able to meet cellular energy requirements. Elevated levels indicate inadequate perfusion and anaerobic metabolism to meet cellular energy requirements.
- Base deficit: elevated levels indicate inadequate perfusion and anaerobic metabolism.
- $EtCO_2$: may detect early indications of inadequate regional and global tissue perfusion

Table 54-4 • Surviving Sepsis Campaign Guidelines

Collaborative Care Focus	Surviving Sepsis Guidelines	Interventions and Patient Care Considerations
Oxygenation, ventilation	**Mechanical Ventilation** • For patients requiring mechanical ventilation, a tidal volume of 6 mL/kg should be used. • Permissive hypercapnia may be tolerated in patients with elevated plateau pressures and tidal volumes. • A minimum amount of positive end-expiratory pressure should be used to prevent lung collapse at end expiration. • Prone position should be considered in patients with ARDS requiring high levels of FiO_2 or plateau pressure. • The head of bed should be raised to at least 45 degrees unless contraindicated to prevent ventilator-associated pneumonia • A weaning protocol should be in place to promote ventilator weaning in patients who are arousable, hemodynamically stable, who do not have life-threatening conditions, and who are not requiring high levels of FiO_2 or ventilatory support.	• Maintain a patent airway. • Auscultate breath sounds q2–4h and PRN. • Suction endotracheal airway when appropriate (see Collaborative Care Guide for Patient on Mechanical Ventilation, Chapter 25). • Hyperoxygenate and hyperventilate before and after each suction pass. • Monitor pulse oximetry and end-tidal CO_2. • Monitor arterial blood gases as indicated by changes in noninvasive parameters. • Monitor intrapulmonary shunt (Qs/Qt and PaO_2/FiO_2). • Monitor airway pressures q1–2h. • Consider kinetic therapy. • Obtain a daily chest x-ray (see Box 27-5, Collaborative Care Guide for Patient with ARDS, Chapter 27).

Circulation, perfusion	**Initial Resuscitation**
	• Resuscitation should begin as soon as sepsis is identified.
	• Fluid resuscitation may consist of natural or artificial colloids or crystalloids.
	• Lactate level may be used to confirm hypoperfusion in patients who are not hypotensive.
	• Goals of resuscitation in the initial 6-h period after identifying sepsis should include:
	  • Central venous pressure (CVP): 8–12 mm Hg
	  • Mean arterial pressure ≥ 65 mm Hg
	  • Urine output ≥0.5 mL/kg/h
	• Monitor $S\overline{v}O_2$, if <70% with CVP 8–12 mm Hg, initiate the following:
	  • Transfuse packed red blood cells to achieve a hematocrit of ≥30%
	  • Consider dobutamine infusion (to a maximum of 20 µg/kg/min)
	
	Ongoing Hemodynamic Management
	• A fluid challenge may be given to patients with suspected hypovolemia.
	• Vasopressors should be considered for patients unresponsive to fluid challenges (inadequate blood pressure and organ perfusion).
	  • Either dopamine or norepinephrine may be used.
	  • Low-dose dopamine should not be used for renal protection as a part of the treatment for severe sepsis.
	  • Vasopressin may be considered in patients with refractory shock despite adequate fluid resuscitation and high-dose dopamine and/or norepinephrine.
	• Inotropic therapy may be initiated for patients with low cardiac output despite adequate fluid resuscitation.
	  • Dobutamine may be used to increase cardiac output.
	  • Patients with hypotension should also receive a vasopressor to maintain mean arterial pressure.
		• Administer intravascular fluids and vasopressors as ordered.
		
		• Monitor serum lactate level on admission and then a least once daily.
		• Consider monitoring gastric mucosal pH as an indicator of systemic vascular perfusion.
		
		• Assess vital signs hourly.
		• Assess hemodynamic pressures hourly if patient has a pulmonary artery catheter in place.
		• Monitor $S\overline{v}O_2$ via venous blood gases or $S\overline{v}O_2$ catheter.
		• Administer red blood cells or inotropic agents as ordered to increase oxygen delivery.
		
		• Monitor for response to fluid challenge with increases in blood pressure or urine output.
		• Monitor for evidence of intravascular volume overload.
		• Vasopressors should be administered through central venous access whenever possible.
		• For patients on vasopressors, an arterial catheter should be placed as soon as possible for accurate monitoring of blood pressures.
		
		• Monitor cardiac output and cardiac index per hospital protocol.
		• Monitor hemoglobin and hematocrit.

(continued)

Table 54-4 • Surviving Sepsis Campaign Guidelines (Continued)

Collaborative Care Focus	Surviving Sepsis Guidelines	Interventions and Patient Care Considerations
	• Blood products: After the initial resuscitation is complete, administer red blood cells only when the hemoglobin is <7 g/dL. • The target hemoglobin is 7–9 g/dL for patients without significant coronary artery disease, acute hemorrhage, or lactic acidosis. • Erythropoietin is not recommended for anemia related to severe sepsis but may be used for anemia of other etiologies (such as renal failure). • Routine use of fresh frozen plasma is not routinely used to correct altered coagulation without the presence of bleeding.	• During transfusion, observe for signs of transfusion reaction.
Sedation, analgesia, and neuromuscular blockade	• A sedation protocol should be in place, using a standardized sedation scale for patient evaluation. • Intermittent bolus sedation or continuous sedation is recommended.	• Monitor sedation level per sedation scale. • Continuous infusions of sedative agents should be interrupted daily for assessment of patient status while awake, with subsequent retitration to the prescribed level of sedation.
Steroid therapy	• Intravenous corticosteroids (hydrocortisone) for 7 d in three or four divided doses are recommended in patients with septic shock who require vasopressor therapy despite fluid resuscitation.	• Monitor for elevated glucose levels, gastric ulcers, and other complications of steroid administration.
Fluids, electrolytes, and glycemic control	• Blood glucose: After initial stabilization, blood glucose should be maintained at <150 mg/dL. • Renal replacement therapy with venous hemofiltration or intermittent hemodialysis should be used for patients in acute renal failure who are not hemodynamically unstable.	• Monitor intake and output q1h. • Monitor electrolytes daily and PRN. • Replace electrolytes as ordered. • Monitor blood urea nitrogen (BUN), creatinine, serum osmolality, and serum electrolytes daily. • Monitor fluid balance and hemodynamic stability of patients receiving renal replacement therapy.
Identifying and treating the cause of sepsis	• Cultures should be obtained before antimicrobial therapy is initiated. At least two cultures should be obtained: • At least one culture drawn percutaneously • At least one culture from each vascular access device inserted >48 h prior • Culture other sites as indicated (urine, cerebrospinal fluid, wounds, respiratory secretions, or other body fluids). • The source of infection (i.e., necrotic tissue, abscesses, or infected vascular access devices) should be removed or treated. • Intravenous antibiotics should be started within the first hour of recognizing severe sepsis (after cultures are obtained). • Initial therapy should include medications with activity against the like pathogen, with consideration of patterns of resistance in the hospital and community.	• Obtain urine, sputum, and blood cultures as ordered. • Obtain wound and central vascular line tip cultures as ordered. • Administer antibiotics as ordered. • Monitor serum antibiotic levels. • Obtain infectious disease consult. • Monitor systemic inflammatory response syndrome criteria: increased white blood cells, increased temperature, tachypnea, and tachycardia.
Preventing new infection	• The antimicrobial regimen should be reassessed in 48–72 h when culture results are obtained.	• Adjust antibiotics based on culture results. • Use strict aseptic technique during procedure, and monitor technique of others. • Maintain sterility of invasive catheters and tubes. • Per hospital protocol
Recombinant human activated protein C	• Recombinant activated protein C (drotrecogin alfa) is recommended for patients at high risk for death (APACHE II score ≥25, sepsis-induced multiple organ failure, septic shock, or sepsis-induced acute respiratory distress syndrome). • Use only in patients with no absolute contraindication related to bleeding risk.	• Discontinue 2 h before procedures with a risk for bleeding. • Consider resuming recombinant activated protein immediately after minimally invasive procedures • Consider resuming 12 h after major procedures.

(continued)

Table 54-4 • Surviving Sepsis Campaign Guidelines (Continued)

Collaborative Care Focus	Surviving Sepsis Guidelines	Interventions and Patient Care Considerations

Deep venous thrombosis (DVT) prophylaxis	• Patients with sepsis should receive prophylaxis against DVT.
	  • Low-dose unfractionated heparin or low-molecular-weight heparin is preferred.
	  • For patients with a contraindication to heparin administration, mechanical therapy should be used (graduated compression device or intermittent compression device).
	  • For patients at high risk, both pharmacological and mechanical prophylaxis should be considered
		• Monitor for signs and symptoms of deep venous thrombosis (redness, swelling, tenderness, or pain in calf).

Stress ulcer prophylaxis	• All patients with sepsis should receive stress ulcer prophylaxis. • The preferred agents are H_2 blockers (cimetidine, famotidine, nizatidine, ranitidine).	• Monitor for signs and symptoms of peptic ulcer disease (abdominal pain, gastrointestinal bleeding).
Consideration for limitation of support	• Communicate likely outcomes and realistic goals of treatment to patients and family. • Consider less aggressive support or withdrawal of support if in the best interest of the patient.	• Consult social services, clergy, and palliative care team as appropriate. • Provide for adequate rest and sleep.

Adapted from Dellinger RP, Carlet JM, Masur H, et al: Surviving Sepsis Campaign guidelines for management of severe sepsis and septic shock. Crit Care Med 32(3):858–871, 2004.

and indicators of metabolic acidosis (end-tidal carbon dioxide, base deficit, lactic acid levels). Patients usually require pulmonary artery and arterial catheterization for close monitoring. Invasive catheters that also monitor venous oxygen saturation ($Sc\overline{v}O_2$ or $S\overline{v}O_2$) are helpful in guiding fluid resuscitation.[29] A downward trend in the markers of metabolic acidosis is a good indicator of improvement in tissue perfusion.

The use of crystalloid or colloid fluids for fluid replacement is controversial in clinical practice (see Management, Hypovolemic Shock). The underlying condition and response to fluid administration help determine which fluids should be used. Blood products may be administered even in the absence of bleeding to enhance the delivery of oxygen to cells. Administering the fluid and closely monitoring the response to fluid therapy are important nursing responsibilities (see Table 54-4).

Maintenance of Adequate Cardiac Output In the early phase of septic shock, cardiac output may be normal or elevated. However, the cardiac output is not adequate to maintain tissue oxygenation and perfusion because of decreased SVR and peripheral vasodilation. As septic shock progresses, cardiac output begins to decrease because of cardiac dysfunction. Therefore, maintenance of cardiac output is an essential therapeutic goal.

If adequate volume replacement does not improve tissue perfusion, vasoactive drugs are administered to support circulation. The Surviving Sepsis Campaign Guidelines recommend that the catecholamines dopamine and norepinephrine (Levophed) be used as first-line vasopressors for patients in septic shock.[29] Low-dose dopamine is no longer recommended because it increases renal blood flow but does not provide renal protection for patients in shock states.[6] Vasopressin is recommended as a second-line agent for patients with shock refractory to fluid resuscitation and high-dose catecholamine therapy.[29] A vasoconstrictor that functions independently of catecholamines, vasopressin is thought to increase the sensitivity of vascular smooth muscle to the effects of dopamine and norepinephrine.[32] For patients with a low cardiac output or $S\overline{v}O_2$ despite fluid resuscitation, dobutamine may be added as an inotropic agent[29] (see Table 54-4).

Maintenance of Adequate Ventilation and Oxygenation Maintaining a patent airway, augmenting ventilation, and ensuring adequate oxygenation in the patient with septic shock usually require endotracheal intubation and mechanical ventilation. Because of the ARDS-like picture, positive end-expiratory pressure frequently is necessary to aid oxygenation (for nursing management issues on ventilation, see Chapter 25).

Assessment of circulatory support, ventilation, and oxygenation is essential. The patient's DaO_2 and VO_2 needs are evaluated frequently. The goal is to maximize DaO_2 to ensure that VO_2 remains independent

Box 54-10 • RED FLAG: Equipment-Related Sources of Infections

Intravascular catheters
Endotracheal/tracheostomy tubes
Indwelling urinary catheters
Surgical wound drains
Intracranial monitoring devices and catheters
Orthopedic hardware
Nasogastric tubes
Gastrointestinal tubes

of DaO$_2$. Aerobic metabolism is maintained, and tissue energy needs are satisfied through the delivery of adequate oxygen to the cells.

Restoration of Balance Between Coagulation and Anticoagulation There has been intense investigation of drugs aimed directly at the bacterial toxins and mediators implicated in the inflammatory response seen in sepsis and SIRS. Drotrecogin alfa (activated) (Xigris), a form of human recombinant activated protein C, is now recommended for patients at high risk for death from sepsis[29] (see Table 54-4). This agent reestablishes homeostasis of coagulation and fibrinolysis that is lost in septic shock states (see Fig. 54-9), and research has shown that it reduces morbidity and mortality in patients with severe sepsis.[21] Further studies will evaluate the best use of this agent[33]; it has antithrombotic and profibrinolytic properties that preclude its use in patients with high risk for bleeding. Nursing considerations for a patient receiving drotrecogin alfa (activated) include close monitoring of the patient for signs of bleeding.[34]

Maintenance of Appropriate Metabolic Environment The many and varied metabolic derangements associated with septic shock necessitate frequent monitoring of hematological, renal, and hepatic function. Nutritional stores are depleted, and the patient requires supplemental nutrition to prevent malnutrition and to optimize cellular function. Enteral nutrition is the preferred route of nutritional support because it maintains the integrity of the gastrointestinal tract, decreases infection, and decreases mortality in patients with a septic or hypotensive event.[35] Intolerance of enteral feeding may necessitate the use of total parenteral nutrition (TPN), but ideally, a small amount of enteral nutrition can still be delivered. Recent research suggests that specific nutrients typically found in enteral nutrition and some in TPN may help support the immune system during states of stress. Essential nutrients for immune support include glutamine, arginine, omega-3 fatty acids, and nucleotides.[36] Immunological formulas supplemented with arginine are widely used to enhance immune function in critically ill surgical patients. However, their use in patients with SIRS, sepsis, and MODS is controversial, and further research is needed to determine the safety and efficacy of immunonutrition.[37] (See Chapter 40 for a discussion of nutritional support.)

• Systemic Inflammatory Response Syndrome

Assessment of the severity of shock is often difficult. It has become clear that progressive shock states involve systemic activation of the inflammatory response, with resultant damage to tissues and organs (see Stages of Shock). Efforts have been made to identify patients in whom this systemic reaction is occurring, with the thought that prompt, effective intervention might prevent progression of the shock to the irreversible stage.

The term SIRS has been developed to describe patients in whom the inflammatory response is fully and systemically activated, no matter what the underlying cause of shock.

ETIOLOGY

SIRS is manifested by two or more conditions listed in Box 54-6. SIRS may frequently occur in patients with septic shock, but it may be caused by any type of shock. Moreover, in cases of SIRS that occur as the result of progression of septic shock, the infecting organism may be undetectable by the time SIRS is identified because of previous antibiotic therapy. Therefore, blood cultures are negative in many patients. SIRS should be suspected in any patient with shock or any condition that might lead to shock.

PATHOPHYSIOLOGY

Normally, the inflammatory response is an essential, tightly regulated, and controlled protective mechanism of local response to invasion by microorganisms or to local tissue damage. However, in SIRS, this usually local inflammatory response becomes a systemic response that results in an unregulated inflammatory response with widespread involvement of endothelial cells and a generalized activation of inflammation and coagulation.

In response to mediators released by macrophages, such as tumor necrosis factor-α or IL-1, blood vessels dilate and become leaky, discharging coagulation factors and fibrinogen into the immediate area and resulting in local activation of the coagulation cascade. Fibrin, the end product of the coagulation cascade, walls off this area and isolates it from the rest of the body. Mediators also attract phagocytic white blood cells (WBCs) to the area and activate the complement cascade. The combination of activity of WBCs and complement proteins may result in elimination of the invading microorganism.

The endothelial cells that line blood vessels are central players in the development of a local inflammatory response. Important functions of endothelial cells include providing an anticoagulant surface and controlling permeability of vessels.[38] In a local inflammatory response, endothelial cells near the site of inflammation become activated as a result of mediators released by injured tissue cells. The activated endothelial cells express cell surface proteins that attract platelets and neutrophils. A procoagulant endothelial surface is formed in the area. WBCs, platelets, and activated endothelial cells themselves release vasodilating compounds such as NO, histamine, and bradykinin. These compounds and other substances also promote leakiness of local vessels, resulting in local extravasation of plasma with coagulation factors.

In SIRS, the inflammatory response is systemic; it occurs throughout the body. The result is overwhelming, unregulated inflammation with uncontrolled coagulation, widespread leakiness of vessels with maldistribution of circulating volume, and unbalanced oxygen supply and demand. Endothelial cells become activated in many vessels throughout the body, resulting in widespread extravasation of fluid into the interstitial compartment and systemic activation of the immune system and coagulation cascade. There is substantial extravascular fluid accumulation and widespread microthrombi in vessels and in the interstitium. The combination of intravascular coagulation and low circulating volume results in decreased perfusion of vital organs, increasing the likelihood of MODS and death.

Events surrounding the complex interactions of the mediators of SIRS remain an active area of clinical research. Several mediators are believed to play a key role in the maldistribution of blood flow and oxygen delivery and consumption imbalance associated with SIRS and sepsis. Table 54-5 lists these key mediators and summarizes their activity.

Management of SIRS is similar to that of septic shock. Therapies are aimed at tissue perfusion and adequate oxygenation.

• Multiple Organ Dysfunction Syndrome

MODS is defined as a progressive physiological failure of several organ systems in acutely ill patients such that homeostasis cannot be maintained without intervention.[27] MODS represents another point in the continuum of shock. A consequence of the inability to maintain end-organ perfusion and oxygenation, MODS results in injury and organ failure (inability of an organ to maintain function). For example, the inability of the pulmonary system to oxygenate the blood adequately through ventilation and gas exchange is considered pulmonary failure.

ETIOLOGY

Table 54-6 gives the mortality rate from MODS according to the number of organ systems involved. The etiology of MODS is unknown. Systemic inflammatory mediators found in SIRS (see Table 54-5) may play a role in the etiology of MODS. In addition, a loss of integrity of mucosal barrier function may liberate bacterial toxins from the gut. These toxins circulate systemically, damaging multiple organs. Finally, tissue hypoxia caused by microvascular thromboses probably also contributes to MODS.

PATHOPHYSIOLOGY

Several mechanisms may contribute to the pathophysiology of MODS; it appears to result from a cascade of bacterial factors, endothelial injury, inflammatory mediators, disturbed hemostasis, and microcirculatory failure.[27] Damage to organs may be primary or secondary and cause organ failure. A primary insult refers to a direct injury to an organ that results in organ dysfunction. For example, severe blunt chest trauma injures the lungs and may cause ARDS. Secondary insult is due to mechanisms operable in shock states. For example, a wound infection

may cause sepsis, but the resultant septic shock or SIRS may cause ARDS. (ARDS is discussed in Chapter 27.) Typically, the first organs to manifest signs of dysfunction are the lungs, heart, and kidneys. Liver failure tends to occur later because the liver has a considerable compensatory capacity. If the shock state persists, eventually all vital organs fail, and death occurs. It is paramount that interventions increase end-organ perfusion and oxygenation and lessen the inflammatory response during the clinical management of shock states.

The concept of MODS reflects that no organ is independent of any other. Therefore, failure of a particular organ makes the failure of a second or third organ more likely. Moreover, restoration of function to the organ system that failed first may not save the patient because organ systems that subsequently failed may be damaged beyond repair.

Organ dysfunction may occur in the following sequence. The lungs are typically the first organ system to fail. They are particularly vulnerable to failure because the capillary beds act as a filter that is exposed to cytokines, mediators, and activated neutrophils. Leaky capillaries create interstitial edema, which impairs pulmonary gas exchange. The cardiovascular system includes abnormalities of cardiac output (dysrhythmias, myocardial depression) as well as abnormalities in the peripheral vascular system, including hypotension unresponsive to fluid administration, increased capillary permeability, edema, and maldistribution of blood flow. The most common hematologic dysfunction is thrombocytopenia, which is due to increased consumption of platelets, sequestration of platelets in the vasculature, and impaired thrombopoiesis as a result of bone marrow suppression. This increases the risk for DIC. (See Chapter 49 for a discussion of DIC.) Neurologic dysfunction can be manifested by altered levels of consciousness, confusion, and psychosis. The dysfunction may be secondary to poor cerebral perfusion or an increase in metabolic substances that are neurotoxic (ammonia), or they can be due to electrolyte imbalances or prolonged sedation. Renal dysfunction can occur secondary to poor renal perfusion or intrarenal causes such as nephrotoxic drugs or prolonged ischemia to renal tubular cells. Progressive liver dysfunction results in hepatic failure. Hepatic failure affects multiple body systems because the liver has so many functions, including synthesis of albumin, clotting factors, and drug metabolism.

ASSESSMENT

Early recognition and management of MODS is essential to prevent escalating mortality rates.[27] The nurse assesses the patient's vital signs for signs of SIRS (see Box 54-6), including hypotension, tachycardia, tachypnea, hypothermia, and hyperthermia. Signs of organ failure should be identified early. Multiple scoring systems exist to determine the extent of MODS, but to date there has not been uniform acceptance of one tool over another. The Sepsis-Related Organ Failure Assessment (SOFA) system[39] is presented

Table 54-5 • Mediators of the Inflammatory/Immune Responses (IIR)

Mediator	Description of Activity	Clinical Response
Endotoxin	• Activates complement system and coagulation cascades • Activates macrophages, which release TNF and IL-1	• Increased microvascular permeability, vasodilation, third-spacing, microthrombi formation • Inflammatory response
Tumor necrosis factor (TNF)	• Released by monocyte–macrophages • Multiple effects locally and systemically • Stimulates other mediator activity	• Hypotension, tachycardia, myocardial depression, tachypnea, hyperglycemia, metabolic acidosis, third-spacing, fever, microvascular vasoconstriction
Interleukin-1 (IL-1)	• Released by monocyte–macrophages • Stimulates leukocytosis • Triggers production of acute phase proteins and release of amino acids from skeletal muscle • Activates procoagulant activity • Decreases vascular responsiveness to catecholamines	• Increased white blood cells • High urinary nitrogen excretion and muscle wasting • Elevated coagulation laboratory values • Decreased SVR, which is not as responsive to low dosages of vasopressor or synthetic catecholamine agents
Interleukin-6 (IL-6)	• Released by monocytes, helper T cells and macrophages • Increases inflammatory response • B-cell stimulation and differentiation • Synergistic with IL-1	• Fever • Antibody secretion
Complement cascade	• Inflammatory process • Opsonization and lysis of foreign particles and cells • Stimulates neutrophils (and oxygen radicals) and IL-1 • Degranulation of mast cells and basophils	• Edema formation, vasodilation, vascular permeability, third-spacing • All effects of IL-1
Platelet aggregating factor (PAF)	• Released by mast cells, basophils, macrophages, neutrophils, platelets, and damaged endothelium • Increases platelet aggregation • Increases neutrophil adhesion • Increases vascular permeability and bronchoconstriction • Negative inotropic effects on the heart	• Microthrombi formation interfering with perfusion • Third-spacing • Bronchoconstriction, rhonchi and wheezes, increased pulmonary airway pressures • Decreased heart contractility and force, which is not as responsive to low dosages of vasopressor and inotropic agents
Arachidonic acid metabolites (AA)	• Stimulation of AA causes the release of metabolites prostaglandins (PG), thromboxanes (TX), and leukotrienes (LT) • PGF and TXA2 cause pulmonary hypertension, vasoconstriction, and platelet activation and aggregation • PGE, PGD, and prostacyclin cause vasodilation and decreased platelet aggregation • Leukotrienes increase neutrophil chemotaxis, vascular constriction, and vascular permeability • Increase gastric permeability to gram-negative bacteria • Inhibits leukocyte adhesion and platelets	• Oxygenation and ventilation difficulties, increased airway resistance, wheezing • Third-spacing and edema formation • Vasolidation, increased capillary permeability, and hypotension
Oxygen radicals	• Generate metabolites (O_2^-, H_2O_2, OH^-) during the respiratory burst of the neutrophils • Damage cell structure and interfere with cell activities • Damage endothelial cells, which stimulate the coagulation system • Increase permeability	• Inflammatory response, edema formation, fever • Microthrombi formation • Third-spacing

in Table 54-7. Other scoring systems include the Acute Physiology and Chronic Health Evaluation (APACHE)[40] and the Mortality Probability Models (MPM) systems.[41] Nursing diagnoses for shock states, SIRS, and MODS are shown in Box 54-11.

MANAGEMENT

Nurses play a key role in preventing, recognizing, and managing patients with MODS.[27] Prevention strategies include enforcement of measures to prevent

Table 54-6 • Mortality Rates From Multiple Organ Dysfunction Syndrome According to the Number of Organ Systems Involved

Number of Failing Systems	Mortality (%)
0	0.8
1	6.8
2	26.2
3	48.5
4	68.8
5	83.3

From Irwin RS, Rippe JM: Irwin and Rippe's Intensive Care Medicine, 5th ed. Philadelphia: Lippincott Williams & Wilkins, 2003, p. 1837.

Box 54-11 • Nursing Diagnoses for the Patient With Shock States, Systemic Inflammatory Response Syndrome, and Multiple Organ Dysfunction Syndrome

- Ineffective Tissue Perfusion
- Altered Cardiac Output
- Deficient Fluid Volume and Electrolytes
- Ineffective Breathing Pattern
- Impaired Gas Exchange
- Impaired Spontaneous Ventilation
- Impaired Physical Mobility
- Imbalanced Nutrition: Less Than Body Requirements
- Acute Pain
- Fear and Anxiety

nosocomial infections, such as proper positioning (head of bed elevated during mechanical ventilation), oral care, turning and skin care, invasive catheter care, and wound care.[34]

Unfortunately, no specific medical treatment for MODS, other than supportive care, is available. Treatment directed at specific organ systems has not been shown to result in improved survival in patients with MODS. This may reflect the interdependence of organ systems and the systemic character of MODS. However, there is evidence that early identification of patients with a high likelihood of developing MODS and early normalization of $S\bar{v}O_2$, arterial lactate concentration, base deficit, and pH lead to a more benign hospital course with decreased inpatient mortality.[28] These data, which require confirmation, point out the systemic nature of MODS. Other treatments that target the inflammatory nature of SIRS or MODS include drotrecogin alfa (Xigris) and corticosteroid administration after appropriate adrenal studies are completed[29] (see Table 54-4).

• Clinical Applicability Challenges

Case Study

Mr. B., a 63-year-old man, is brought to the emergency department in an ambulance after being struck by a car at a local shopping center. He has suffered no loss of consciousness, and the car was reported to be traveling at a slow rate of speed. His past medical history is significant for chronic obstructive pulmonary disease (COPD) and a cholecystectomy 5 years ago. Home medications include an albuterol/ipratropium bromide (Combivent) inhaler. He currently works as a security officer at a local high school and lives with his wife. He drinks 1 to 2 beers per week, has smoked one pack of cigarettes per day for the past 30 years, and denies illicit drug use.

Table 54-7 • Sepsis-Related Organ Failure Assessment (SOFA) Scoring System

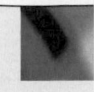

Organ System	SOFA Score			
	1	2	3	4
Respiration Partial pressure of oxygen/fraction of inspired oxygen (mm Hg)	<400	<300	<200 with respiratory support	<100
Coagulation Platelets × 10³ mm³	<150	<100	<50	<20
Liver Bilirubin (mg/dL)	1.2–1.9	2.0–5.9	6.0–11.9	>12
Cardiovascular Hypotension	MAP <70 mm Hg	Dopamine ≤5 or dobutamine any dose	Dopamine >5 or epinephrine ≤0.1 or norepinephrine ≤0.1	Dopamine >15 or epinephrine >0.1 or norepinephrine >0.1
Central nervous system Glasgow Coma Scale score	13–14	10–12	6–9	<6
Renal Creatinine (mg/dL) or urine output	1.2–1.9	2.0–3.4	3.5–4.9 or <500 mL/day	>5.0 or <200 mL/day

MAP, mean arterial pressure.
From Irwin RS, Rippe JM: Irwin and Rippe's Intensive Care Medicine, 5th ed. Philadelphia: Lippincott Williams & Wilkins, 2003, p 1836.

⊞ EVIDENCE-BASED PRACTICE HIGHLIGHT: SEVERE SEPSIS

Excerpted from: American Association of Critical-Care Nurses Practice Alert

Expected Practice:

- Assess all patients and immediately notify physician when a patient presents with risk factors for sepsis, which includes documented or suspected infection and 2 or more of the following SIRS criteria.
  - Heart rate > 90 beats per minute
  - Temperature < 36°C (96.8°F) or > 38°C (100.4 F)
  - Respiratory rate > 20 breaths per minute or $PaCO_2$ < 32 mm Hg or mechanical ventilation
  - White blood cell count > 12,000/mm³ or < 4,000 mm³ or <10% mature neutrophils
- Obtain serum lactate measurements.
- Obtain blood cultures as well as cultures from all potential sites of infection prior to initiating broad-spectrum antibiotics.
  - Evaluate for and remove other potential sources of infection (ie, obviously infected invasive devices).
- Administer fluids to maintain mean arterial pressure at > 65 mm Hg, central venous pressure (CVP) 8–12 mm Hg and central venous or mixed venous oxygen saturation >70%.
- Administer vasopressors if necessary to achieve a mean arterial blood pressure of 65 mm/Hg if fluid replacement is not successful.
- Obtain cortisol stimulation test and start continuous low-dose steroid infusion.
- Maintain cardiac output at normal physiologic levels.
- Maintain blood glucose levels at < 150 mg/dL.
- Consider administration of human recombinant activated protein C (drotrecogin alfa activated) for patients at risk for dying and presenting with septic shock, sepsis with multiple organ failure and sepsis induced acute respiratory distress syndrome.

Supporting Evidence:

- More than 750,000 cases of severe sepsis occurred annually (year 2000) and mortality ranges from 28%–50% with an overall hospital mortality of about 30%.[1] Sepsis (infection and 2 of the 4 SIRS criteria) can rapidly progress to severe sepsis (infection + organ dysfunction + SIRS criteria) to septic shock (persistent tissue hypoxia with vasopressors on board) within 24 hours.[1-4] Treatment should be initiated regardless of where the patient is located within the hospital. A prospective randomized study of 263 emergency department patients diagnosed with severe sepsis or septic shock showed that patients treated aggressively with a goal direction towards tissue oxygenation within the first 6 hours of presentation had a 16% improvement in mortality. Another small retrospective study showed a decrease in mortality in patients identified with signs of severe sepsis and treated within the first 6 hours.[3,5,6] (Level V)
- Serum lactate levels can be elevated in the setting of a normal or increased cardiac output. The measurement of serum lactate can reflect occult decreases in global tissue perfusion and as such may be an indicator of organ dysfunction. The presence and the clearance rate of lactate are associated with increases in patient morbidity and mortality.[3,7] (Level IV)

- Early administration of appropriate antibiotics decreases mortality in patients with Gram positive and negative bacteremias. Empiric broad spectrum antibiotics should be initiated prior to identification of the infecting organism and reassessed after 48–72 hours based on culture results and clinical data.[8]
- According to the Surviving Sepsis Campaign guidelines, during the first 6 hours of treatment the goal is to achieve and maintain a CVP of 8–12 mm Hg or 12–15 mm Hg for patients receiving mechanical ventilation and a MAP of at least 65 mm Hg. with fluid resuscitation.[7] Dobutamine is identified as the medication of choice to increase cardiac output to normal levels or to improve lactate clearance when cardiac output is not being measured. Two large clinical trials did not show a benefit from increasing CO above physiologic normal levels in order to increase oxygen delivery to the tissues.[9-11] Available data do not support the use of low dose dopamine for renal protection.[12] (Level V evidence)
- Colloids have not been shown to be of more benefit than crystalloid for fluid resuscitation. One large randomized controlled trial compared 4% albumin with normal saline in the treatment of patients requiring volume resuscitation found no significant difference in mortality between the groups. Several literature reviews have concluded that choice of fluids does not appear to change outcomes.[13,14] (Level V)
- In the setting of hypotension fluid replacement should be optimized before vasopressors are started. No high-level evidence exists to identify the most appropriate vasopressor to use for the treatment of septic shock and selection is based on multiple clinical parameters. However, in the Surviving Sepsis Campaign Guidelines for the Management of Severe Sepsis and Septic Shock, norepinephrine or dopamine are identified as the initial vasopressors of choice to increase vascular tone and blood pressure.[7]
- Two meta analyses concluded that administration of high dose corticosteroids are of no benefit or may be detrimental to patients with septic shock.[15,16] (Level VI) In vasopressor dependent shock, the addition of low-dose exogenous cortisol has been shown to improve the uptake of the patients own and the exogenously administered sympathetic stimulants when serum cortisol levels are low.[17] (Level IV)
- Maintaining glucose levels within normal range (80–110 mg/dL) but at least < 150 mg/dL has been shown to decrease morbidity and morality in a surgical population but did not focus on septic patients. Maintaining glucose levels < 150 mg/dL showed reduced morbidity but not mortality in critically ill medical patients with sepsis.[18,19] (Level V)
- In a large double blind study, human recombinant activated protein C (drotrecogin alfa activated) decreased mortality by 6% in patients with severe sepsis and decreased mortality by 13% for patients at high risk for death (ie, patients having an APACHE II score of 25 or greater).[20,21] (Level V)

(continued)

⊞ EVIDENCE-BASED PRACTICE HIGHLIGHT: SEVERE SEPSIS (Continued)
Excerpted from: American Association of Critical-Care Nurses Practice Alert

AACN Grading of Evidence System
Level I: Manufacturer's recommendations only

Level II: Theory based, no research data to support recommendations; recommendations from expert consensus group may exist

Level III: Laboratory data, no clinical data to support recommendations

Level IV: Limited clinical studies to support recommendations

Level V: Clinical studies in more than one or two patient populations and situations to support recommendations

Level VI: Clinical studies in a variety of patient populations and situations to support recommendations.

References:
1. Angus DC, Linde-Zwirble WT, Lidicker J, et al: Epidemiology of severe sepsis in the United States: analysis of incidence, outcome, and associated costs of care. Crit Care Med. 29:1303–1310, 2001
2. Ahrens T, Tuggle D: Surviving severe sepsis: early recognition and treatment. Crit Care Nurse 24(Suppl):2–13, 2004
3. Rivers E, Bryant N, Havstad S, et al: Early goal-directed therapy in the treatment of severe sepsis and septic shock. N Engl J Med 345:1368–1387, 2001
4. Rivers E, McIntyre L, Morro DC, Kandis KR: Early and innovative interventions for severe sepsis and septic shock: Taking advantage of a window of opportunity. Can Med Assoc J 173:1054–1065, 2005
5. McIntyre LA, Fergusson DA, Cebert PC, et al: Are delays in the recognition and initial management of patients with severe sepsis associated with hospital mortality? Crit Care Med 31(Suppl):A75, 2003
6. Engoren M: The effect of prompt physician visits on intensive care unit mortality and cost. Crit Care Med 33:727–733, 2005
7. Dellinger RP, Carlet JM, Masur H, et al: Surviving Sepsis Campaign guidelines for management of severe sepsis and septic shock. Crit Care Med 32:858–870, 2004
8. Bochud P-Y, Bonten M, Marchetti O, Calandra T: Antimicrobial therapy for patients with severe sepsis and septic shock: An evidence-based review. Crit Care Med 32(11 Suppl):S495–S512, 2004
9. Hayes MA, Timmins AC, Yau EH, et al: Elevation of systemic oxygen delivery in the treatment of critically ill patients. N Engl J Med 330:1717–1722, 1994
10. Gattinoni L, Brazzi L, Pelosi P, et al: A trial of goal-oriented hemodynamic therapy in critically ill patients. N Engl J Med 333:1025–1032, 1995
11. Beale RJ, Hollenberg SM, Vincent JL, Parrillo JE: Vasopressor and inotropic support in septic shock: An evidence-based review. Crit Care Med 32(11 Suppl):S455–S465, 2004
12. Bellomo R, Chapman M, Finfer S, et al: Low-dose dopamine in patients with early renal dysfunction: A placebo-controlled randomized trial. Lancet 356:2139–2143, 2000
13. Finfer S, Bellomo R, Boyce N, et al: A comparison of albumin and saline for fluid resuscitation in the intensive care unit. N Engl J Med 350:2247–2256, 2004
14. Vincent JL, Herwig G: Fluid resuscitation in severe sepsis and septic shock: An evidence-based review. Crit Care Med 32(11 Suppl):S451–S454, 2004
15. Lefering R, Neugebaruer EA: Steroid controversy in sepsis and septic shock: A meta analysis. Crit Care Med 23:1294–1303, 1995
16. Cronin L, Cook DJ, Carlet J, et al: Corticosteroid treatment for sepsis: A critical appraisal and meta-analysis of the literature. Crit Care Med 1430–1439, 1995
17. Annane D, Sebille V, Charpentier C, et al: Effect of treatment with low doses of hydrocortisone and fludrocortisone on mortality in patients with septic shock. JAMA 288:862–871, 2002
18. Van den Berghe G, Wouters, et al: Intensive insulin therapy in the critically ill patients. N Engl J Med 345:1359–1367, 2001
19. Van den Berghe G, Wilmer A, Hermans G, et al: Intensive insulin therapy in the medical ICU. N Engl J Med 354:449–461, 2006
20. Bernard GR, Vincent JL, Laterre PF, et al: Recombinant human protein C worldwide evaluation in severe sepsis (PROWESS) study group: Efficacy and safety of recombinant human activated protein C for severe sepsis. N Engl J Med 344:699–709, 2001
21. Bernard GR, Margolis BD, Shanies HM, et al: Extended evaluation of recombinant human activated protein C United States trial (ENHANCE USA): A single-arm phase 3B multicenter study of drotrecogin alfa (activated) in severe sepsis. Chest 125:2206–2216, 2004

On physical examination, Mr. B. is pale and diaphoretic, with diminished pulses in his feet (capillary refill of 4 seconds). His pelvis is found to be unstable on palpation, and he complains of pain in his pelvis that he rates as a 7 on a scale of 1 to 10. Although he is conscious, he is confused to place and time. Two 18-gauge intravenous (IV) lines are started in the bilateral antecubital spaces. A fluid bolus of 2 liters of lactated Ringer's is administered. Vital signs on admission are: temperature, 97.5°F (36.4°C); respiration rate, 24 breaths/minute; heart rate, 156 beats/minute; and blood pressure, 78/42 mm Hg. A Foley catheter is inserted, and 18 mL of concentrated urine is obtained.

Laboratory values are hemoglobin, 7.3 g/dL; hematocrit, 23.7%; white blood cell (WBC) count, 6.8 mm³; glucose, 114 mg/dL; sodium, 148 mEq/L; potassium, 4.1 mEq/L; blood urea nitrogen, 32 mg/dL; creatinine, 1.1 mg/dL; magnesium, 1.8 mg/dL; calcium, 8.7 mg/dL; and lactate, 7.7 mmol/L. Arterial blood gases (ABGs) show metabolic acidosis. Computed tomography (CT) scans show an open-book pelvic fracture. Cervical spinal damage and other traumatic injuries are ruled out with radiography and patient assessment.

Mr. B. is admitted to the ICU with a diagnosis of pelvic fracture with associated hemorrhage. Serial hemoglobin and hematocrit are monitored, revealing ongoing acute blood loss anemia. A double-lumen central venous catheter is inserted for fluid resuscitation and monitoring of CVP. Over the course of 16 hours, Mr. B. requires 8 units of packed red blood cells to achieve a hematocrit of >28%, and 4 additional liters of lactated Ringer's to maintain a CVP of >8 mm Hg. Fluids are warmed using an in-line fluid warmer to prevent hypothermia. Mr. B. is taken to surgery the following morning for repair of bleeding and stabilization of the fracture. Estimated blood loss in surgery is 2 liters. After surgery, he is returned to the ICU on a mechanical ventilator.

On postoperative day 1, Mr. B. is hemodynamically stable with a hematocrit of 32%, CVP of 13 mm Hg, mean arterial pressure (MAP) of 78 mm Hg, heart rate of 86 beats/min, temperature of 98.9°F (37.2°C), and serum lactate level of 2.2 mmol/L. He is recovering from his hypovolemic shock. Morphine is used for pain control, and prophylaxis against deep venous thrombosis and peptic ulcer disease is initiated. IV fluids are administered at 75 mL/hour. He is placed on a ventilator weaning protocol, but attempts to wean are unsuccessful secondary to his COPD. He remains in the ICU, with daily ventilator weaning trials.

On the morning of postoperative day 4, Mr. B. is successfully extubated and placed on 4 liters nasal cannula. He is tolerating a liquid diet, and plans are made for transfer to the trauma-surgical unit in the morning. Later that afternoon, his family reports that he has suddenly become irritable and is pulling at his IV lines and Foley catheter. Vital signs are: temperature, 102.0°F (38.9°C); respiration rate, 34 breaths/min; heart rate, 128 beats/min; and blood pressure, 86/52 mm Hg. Blood and urine are sent for culture. Mr. B. is electively reintubated, and CVP monitoring is reinstated. The initial CVP is 4 mm Hg. Fluid resuscitation is initiated using boluses of lactated Ringer's. Despite an increase in CVP to 10 mm Hg, the MAP remains 59 mm Hg. A norepinephrine infusion is started at 1.0 µg/kg/min, with orders to titrate to a MAP greater than 70 mm Hg. ABGs reveal a metabolic acidosis and a serum lactate of 5.6 mmol/L. Broad-spectrum antibiotic therapy is initiated. The WBC count increases to 12.4/mm³, and preliminary blood cultures are positive for gram-negative rods. Antibiotic therapy is adjusted appropriately.

Mr. B. remains hypotensive (MAP ≤ 65 mm Hg) despite doses of norepinephrine up to 20 µg/min. A vasopressin infusion is initiated at 2 units/hour. Despite titration, his MAP remains ≤ 65 mm Hg. A venous blood gas is obtained, revealing an S$\overline{v}$O₂ of 62%. A dobutamine infusion is started at 5 µg/kg/min. Recombinant activated protein C is not initiated secondary to the patient's recent trauma and bleeding. Anti-inflammatory therapy is started with low-dose corticosteroids.

Mr. B. is not responsive to pain and is unable to follow commands. His family receives regular updates concerning his condition during meetings with the interdisciplinary health care team. On postoperative day 6, Mr. B. continues to require high doses of vasopressor and inotropic therapy and has developed ARDS. In collaboration with the health care team, the family makes the decision to initiate a "do not resuscitate order," and the norepinephrine, vasopressin, and dobutamine infusions are sustained at their existing rates without any further increases. Later that day, he develops sustained ventricular tachycardia that progresses to ventricular fibrillation. Mr. B. passes away with his family at his side.

1. Compare and contrast medical and nursing management interventions for hypovolemic and septic shock.

2. Discuss the serum lactate level as a measure of tissue perfusion and prognostic indicator in shock states.

3. Discuss the care of Mr. B. in the context of the Surviving Sepsis Campaign Guidelines (see Table 54-4). Was evidence-based care provided to this patient?

Review Questions

1. Compensatory mechanisms in response to shock states result in:
   a. Decreased urine output
   b. Vasodilation of blood vessels
   c. Decreased heart rate
   d. Decreased cardiac output

2. Which of the following classifications best describes septic shock?
   a. Hypovolemic shock
   b. Cardiogenic shock
   c. Vasodilatory shock
   d. Anaphylactic shock

3. Which of the following is not a common pathophysiological manifestation seen in patients with hypovolemic shock?
   a. Altered mentation
   b. Rapid and deep respirations
   c. Cool and clammy skin
   d. Bradycardia

4. Which of the following is a clinical manifestation of cardiogenic shock?
   a. Pulmonary artery wedge pressure less than 18 mm Hg
   b. Pulmonary artery wedge pressure greater than 18 mm Hg
   c. Cardiac index greater than 2.2 L/min/m²
   d. Systemic vascular resistance less than 1,000 dynes/sec/cm⁵

5. What is the initial therapy of choice for the treatment of anaphylactic shock?
   a. Epinephrine
   b. Rapid infusion of normal saline
   c. Dobutamine
   d. Norepinephrine

6. Which of the following drugs is given in septic shock to reestablish homeostasis of coagulation and fibrinolysis?
   a. Aspirin
   b. Tissue plasminogen activator (t-PA)
   c. Streptokinase
   d. Drotrecogin alfa (activated) (Xigris)

7. Which of the following patients meets the criteria to have MODS?
   a. A 65-year-old man with chronic obstructive pulmonary disease (COPD) who requires mechanical ventilation and enteral tube feedings
   b. A 42-year-old woman with end-stage renal disease who requires hemodialysis every day
   c. A 28-year-old man with septic shock who requires continuous renal replacement therapy and mechanical ventilation
   d. A 70-year-old man with diabetes who recently had coronary artery bypass surgery

References

1. Holmes CL, Walley KR: The evaluation and management of shock. Clin Chest Med 24;775–789, 2003
2. Frakes M, Evans T: Major pelvic fractures. Crit Care Nurse 24(2):18–30, 2004
3. Shafi S, Kauder DR: Fluid resuscitation and blood replacement in patients with polytrauma. Clin Orthop 422:37–42, 2004
4. Wilson M, Davis DP, Coimbra R: Diagnosis and monitoring of hemorrhagic shock during the initial resuscitation of multiple trauma patients: a review. J Emerg Med 24(4):413–422, 2003
5. Wills BA, Nguyen MD, Loan HT, et al: Comparison of three fluid solutions for resuscitation in dengue shock syndrome. N Engl J Med 353(9):877–889, 2005
6. Bridges EJ, Dukes S: Cardiovascular aspects of septic shock: Pathophysiology, monitoring, and treatment. Crit Care Nurse 25(2):14–42, 2005
7. Babaev A, Frederick PD, Pasta DJ, et al: Trends in management and outcomes of patients with acute myocardial infarction complicated by cardiogenic shock. JAMA 294:448–454, 2005
8. Antman EM, Anbe DT, Armstrong PW, et al: ACC/AHA guidelines for the management of patients with ST-elevation myocardial infarction. A report of the Am Coll of Cardiol/Am Heart Assoc Task Force on Practice Guidelines (Committee to revise the 1999 guidelines). Bethesda (MD): American College of Cardiology, American Heart Association, 2004
9. Gordon C, Rempher K: Brain natriuretic peptide: Implications for heart failure management. AACN Clin Issues 14: 532–542, 2003
10. Richard C, Warszawski J, Anguel N, et al: Early use of the pulmonary artery catheter and outcomes in patients with shock and acute respiratory distress syndrome. JAMA 290(20):2713–2720, 2003
11. Albright TN, Simmerman MA, Selcman CH: Vasopressin in the cardiac surgery intensive care unit. Am J Crit Care 11(4): 326–330, 2002
12. Holmes C: Vasoactive drugs in the intensive care unit. Curr Opin Crit Care 11:413–417, 2005
13. Kee VR: Hemodynamic pharmacology of intravenous vasopressors. Crit Care Nurse 23(4):79–81, 2003
14. Helbling A, Humi T, Meuller UR, Pichler WJ: Incidence of anaphylaxis with circulatory symptoms: A study over a 3 year period comparing 940,000 inhabitants of the Swiss Conton Bern. Clin Exp Allergy 34:285–290, 2004
15. Cauwels A, Janssen B, Buys E, et al: Anaphylactic shock depends on PI3K and eNOS-derived NO. J Clin Invest 116:2244–2251, 2006
16. Brown SGA, Blackman KE, Stenlake, V, Hiddle RJ: Insect sting anaphylaxis: Prospective evaluation and treatment with intravenous adrenaline and volume resuscitation. Emerg Med J 21:149–154, 2004
17. Brown SGA: Cardiovascular aspects of anaphylaxis: Implications for treatment and diagnosis. Curr Opin Allergy Clin Immunol 5:359–364, 2005
18. American College of Chest Physicians/Society of Critical Care Medicine: Consensus conference: Definitions for sepsis and multiple organ failure and guidelines for use of innovative therapies in sepsis. Crit Care Med 20:864–874, 1992
19. Levy MM, Fink MP, Marshall JC: 2001 SCCM/ESICM/AACP/ATS/SIS International sepsis definitions conference. Crit Care Med 31:1250–1256, 2003
20. Martin GS, Mannino DM, Eaton S, Moss H: The epidemiology of sepsis in the United States from 1979 through 2000. N Engl J Med 348:1546–1554, 2003
21. Bernard GR, Vincent JL, Laterre PF, et al: Efficacy and safety of recombinant human activated protein C for severe sepsis. N Engl J Med 344:699–709, 2001
22. Annane D, Aegerter P, Jars-Guincestre MC, Guidet B: Current epidemiology of septic shock: the CUB-Kea Network. Am J Respir Crit Care Med 168:165–172, 2003
23. Alberti C, Burn-Buisson C, Chevret S, et al: Systemic inflammatory response and progression to severe sepsis in critically ill infected patients. Am J Resp Crit Care Med 171:461–468, 2005
24. Hotchkiss RS, Karl IE: The pathophysiology and treatment of sepsis. N Engl J Med 348:138–150, 2003
25. Russell JA: Management of sepsis. N Engl J Med 355:1699–1713, 2006
26. Sessler CN, Sheparher W: New concepts in sepsis. Curr Opin Crit Care 8:465–472, 2002
27. Ely EW, Kleinpell RM, Goyette RE: Advances in the understanding of clinical manifestations and therapy of severe sepsis: An update for critical care nurses. Am J Crit Care 12:120–135, 2003
28. Rivers, E, Nguyen, B, Havstad, S, et al: Early goal-directed therapy in the treatment of severe sepsis and septic shock. N Engl J Med 345(19):1368–1377, 2001
29. Dellinger RP, Carlet JM, Masur H, et al: Surviving Sepsis Campaign guidelines for management of severe sepsis and septic shock. Crit Care Med 32(3):858–871, 2004
30. Houghton D: Antimicrobial resistance in the intensive care unit: Understanding the problem. AACN Clin Issues 13(3):410–420, 2002
31. Chen, YY, Chou Y, Chou P: Impact of nosocomial infection on cost of illness and length of stay in intensive care units. Infect Cont Hosp Ep 26(3):281–287
32. Lee, CS. Management of catecholamine-refractory septic shock. Crit Care Nurse 26(6):17–23, 2006
33. Bernard GR: Drotrecogin alfa (activated) for the treatment of severe sepsis. Crit Care Med 31(1 Suppl):S85–S93, 2003
34. Kleinpel R: Advances in treating patients with severe sepsis: role of drotrecogin alpha (activated). Crit Care Nurse 23 (3): 16–29, 2003
35. Heyland DK, Lukan JK, McClave SA: The role of nutritional support in sepsis. In Vincent J-L, Carlet J, Opal SM (eds): The sepsis text. Boston: Kluwer, 2002, pp 480–490
36. Zarzaur BL, Kudsk KA: The place of immunonutrition. In Vincent J-L, Carlet J, Opal SM (eds): The sepsis text. Boston: Kluwer, 2002, pp 769–785
37. Stechmiller JK, Childress B, Porter T: Arginine immunonutrition in critically ill patients: A clinical dilemma. Am J Crit Care 13:17–23, 2004
38. Schulman CS: New thoughts on sepsis: the unifier of critical care. Dimens Crit Care Nurse 22(1): 20–30, 2003
39. Vincent JL, et al: The SOFA (Sepsis-Related Organ Failure Assessment) score to describe organ dysfunction/failure. On behalf of the Working Group on Sepsis-Related Problems of

the European Society of Intensive Care Medicine. Intens Care Med 22:707–710, 1996

40. Knaus WA, et al: APACHE II: A severity of disease classification system. Crit Care Med 13:818–828, 1985

41. Lemeshow SD, Teres D, Klar J, et al: Mortality Probability Models (MPM II) based on an international cohort of intensive care unit patients. JAMA 270:2478–2486, 1993

Other Selected Readings

Ahrens T: Sepsis: Stopping and insidious killer. Am Nurse Today 2(1):36–40, 2007

Ahrens T: Hemodynamics in sepsis. AACN Adv Crit Care 17(4): 435–445, 2006

Cottingham C: Resuscitation of traumatic shock: A hemodynamic review. AACN Adv Crit Care 17(3):317–326, 2006

Dellinger RP: Cardiovascular management of septic shock. Crit Care Med 31:946–955, 2003

Dettenmeier P, Swindell B, Stroud M, et al: Role of activated protein C in the pathophysiology of severe sepsis. Am J Crit Care 12:518–526, 2003

Ely EW, Kleinpell R, Goyette RE: Advances in the understanding of clinical manifestations and therapy of severe sepsis: An update for critical care nurses. Am J Crit Care 12:120–135, 2003

Gessner P: The effects of vasopressin on the renal system in vasodilatory shock. Dimens Crit Care Nurs 25(1):1–9, 2006

Goodrich C: Endpoints of resuscitation: What should we be monitoring? AACN Adv Crit Care 17(3):306–316, 2006

Giuliano KK: Continuous physiologic monitoring and the identification of sepsis: What is the evidence supporting current clinical practice? AACN Adv Crit Care 17(2):215–223, 2006

Giuliano KK: Physiologic monitoring for critically ill patients: Testing a predictive model for the early detection of sepsis. Am J Crit Care 16(2):122–131, 2007

Kee VR: Hemodynamic pharmacology of intravenous vasopressors. Crit Care Nurs 23(4):79–82, 2003

King JE: Sepsis in critical care. Crit Care Nurs Clin North Am 19(1): 77–86, 2007

Kleinpell R: Advances in treating patients with severe sepsis. Crit Care Nurse 23(3):16–28, 2003

Kleinpell R, Graves B, Ackerman M: Incidence, pathogenesis, and management of sepsis: An overview. AACN Adv Crit Care 17(4): 385–393, 2006

Krau SD: Making sense of multiple organ dysfunction syndrome. Crit Care Nurs Clin North Am 19(1):87–98, 2007

Lee C: The role of exogenous arginine vasopressin in the management of catecholamines-refractory septic shock. Crit Care Nurse 26(6):17–24, 2006

Nguyen HB, Rivers EP, Abrahamian FM, et al: Severe sepsis and septic shock: Review of the literature and emergency department management guidelines. Ann Emerg Med 24:28–54, 2006

Papathanassoglou E, Giannakopoulou M, Bozas E: Genomic variations and susceptibility to sepsis. AACN Adv Crit Care 17(4): 394–422, 2006

Picard KM, O'Donoghue SC, Young-Kershaw DA, Russell KJ: Development and implementation of a multidisciplinary sepsis protocol. Crit Care Nurs 26(3):43–54, 2006

Powers J, Jacobi J: Pharmacologic treatment related to severe sepsis. AACN Adv Crit Care 17(4):423–432, 2006

Tazbir J: Sepsis and the role of activated protein C. Crit Care Nurse 24(6):40–45, 2004

Wood S, Lavieri MC, Durkin T: What you need to know about sepsis. Nursing 2007 37(3):46–52, 2007

55

Trauma

Carla A. Aresco

Objectives

Based on the content in this chapter, the reader should be able to:

❶ Compare and contrast mechanisms of trauma injury.

❷ Describe phases of initial assessment and related care of the trauma patient.

❸ Discuss the assessment of patients with thoracic, abdominal, musculoskeletal, and maxillofacial trauma.

❹ Contrast the response of solid and hollow abdominal organs to trauma.

❺ Explain the management and nursing care of patients with thoracic, abdominal, musculoskeletal, and maxillofacial trauma.

❻ Describe early and late complications of trauma and the impact of these complications on mortality.

Trauma is defined by the *American Heritage Dictionary* as "a wound, especially one produced by sudden physical injury."[1] Injury is defined by the National Committee for Injury Prevention and Control as "unintentional or intentional damage to the body resulting from acute exposure to thermal, mechanical, electrical, or chemical energy or from the absence of such essentials as heat or oxygen."[2] Unintentional injuries include motor vehicle crashes (MVCs), poisonings, falls, drownings, fires, and burns. Intentional injuries (e.g., suicide attempts, assaults, and homicides) include injuries from poisoning, hanging, drowning, firearms, cutting, and jumping. This chapter specifically discusses mechanical injury.

Trauma is one of the leading causes of critical illness and death in the United States. In 2001, the number of injury-related deaths was second only to those caused by heart disease. In 2000, unintentional injury was the fifth leading cause of death. At present, MVCs are the leading cause of injury in the United States. One third of all trauma patients seen at level I trauma centers are admitted to critical care units, where they have a mean stay of 5 days. With the increasing age and comorbidities of patients, the risk for trauma morbidity and death is increased.[3]

• Mechanism of Injury

Knowing the mechanism of injury is important because this information can help explain the type of injury, predict the eventual outcome, and identify common injury combinations.[4] In addition, an injury may exist in a trauma patient without the classic signs. The mechanism of injury may indicate the need for additional diagnostic workup and reassessment.

The mechanism of injury is related to the type of injuring force and the subsequent tissue response. Injury occurs when the force deforms tissues beyond their failure limits. Wounds vary depending on the injuring agent. The effect of injury also depends on personal and environmental factors, such as the person's age and sex, the presence or absence of underlying disease process, and the geographic region.

Force may or may not be penetrating. The injury delivered from force depends on the energy delivered and the area of contact. In penetrating injury, the concentration of force is to a small area. In blunt or nonpenetrating injury, the energy is distributed over a large area. The predominant feature affecting the impact is speed, or acceleration:

$$\text{Force} = \text{mass} \times \text{acceleration}$$

BLUNT INJURY

Mechanisms of blunt injury include MVCs, falls, assaults, and contact sports. Multiple injuries are common with blunt trauma, and these injuries are often more life-threatening than penetrating injuries because the extent of the injury is less obvious and the diagnosis can be more difficult.

Blunt injury is caused by a combination of forces. These forces include acceleration, deceleration, shearing, crushing, and compressive resistance:

▶ Acceleration is an increase in the velocity (or speed) of a moving object.

▶ Deceleration, on the other hand, is a decrease in the velocity of a moving object.

▶ Shearing occurs across a plane when structures slip relative to each other.

▶ Crushing occurs when continuous pressure is applied to a body part.

▶ Compressive resistance is the ability of an object or structure to resist squeezing forces or inward pressure.

In blunt trauma, it is the direct impact that causes the greatest injury. Injury occurs when there is direct contact between the body surface and the injuring agent. Indirect forces are transmitted internally with dissipation of energy to the internal structure. The extent of injury from an indirect force depends on transference of energy from an object to the body. Injury occurs as a result of energy released and the tendency for the tissues to be displaced on impact.[4] Acceleration–deceleration injuries are the most common causes of blunt trauma.

In an MVC, the vehicle size and design change injury patterns. Small cars are involved in more crashes per mile and cause more deaths than larger vehicles. Before the crash, the occupant and the car are traveling at the same speed. During the crash, both the occupant and the car decelerate to zero, but not necessarily at the same rate. There are actually three collisions involved in one crash. The first is the car with another object; the second is the occupant's body with the interior of the car; and the third is the internal tissues with the rigid body surface structure. For example, rapid deceleration in an MVC can cause direct injury to tissue. Subsequently, injury occurs as internal organs impinge on bony internal

structures and cause major vessels to undergo stretching and bowing.

Wearing shoulder and lap restraints reduces the incidence and severity of injury by reducing the force with which a person strikes a surface, thereby preventing the occupant from striking multiple surfaces and being ejected from the vehicle[4] (Fig. 55-1). The occupant's position in the vehicle also makes a difference in the blunt injury received. When a vehicle strikes a pedestrian, it is important to visualize the size of the vehicle and the size of the pedestrian. The area of impact can vary depending on these factors (Fig. 55-2).

PENETRATING INJURY

Penetrating trauma refers to an injury produced by foreign objects penetrating the tissue. The severity of the injury is related to the structures damaged. The mechanism of injury is caused by the energy created and dissipated by the penetrating object into the surrounding areas.[4] The amount of tissue damaged by a bullet is determined by the amount of energy that transfers into the tissue along with the amount of time it takes for the transfer to occur. It is important to note that the external appearance of the wound does not reflect the extent of internal injury.[5]

Velocity determines the extent of cavitation and tissue damage (Fig. 55-3). Low-velocity missiles localize the injury to a small radius from the center of the tract and have little disruptive effect. They cause little cavitation and blast effect, essentially only pushing the

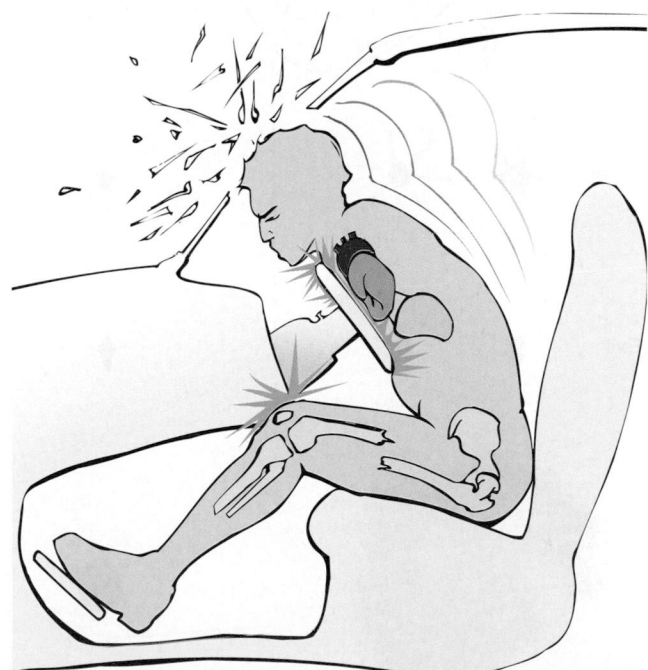

Figure 55-1 • In a motor vehicle crash, if the driver is not wearing a seat belt, damage may occur in various sections of the body. Common injuries occur to the skull, scalp, face, sternum, ribs, heart, liver, or spleen. Bones of the pelvis and lower extremities also may be damaged.

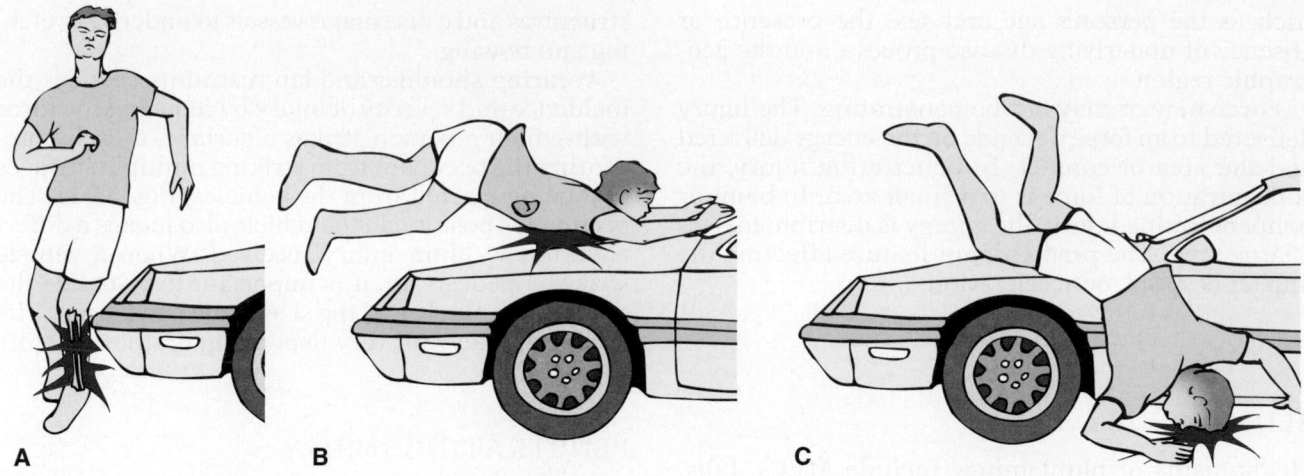

Figure 55-2 • Pedestrians may be hurt critically when hit by a moving vehicle. **A:** A common injury is the fracture of the tibia and fibula at the time of impact. **B:** Impact when the pedestrian strikes the hood of the car may cause fractured ribs and a ruptured spleen. **C:** Injuries to the head and additional fractures of the extremities may occur as the pedestrian rolls off the braking car or is thrown by the impact.

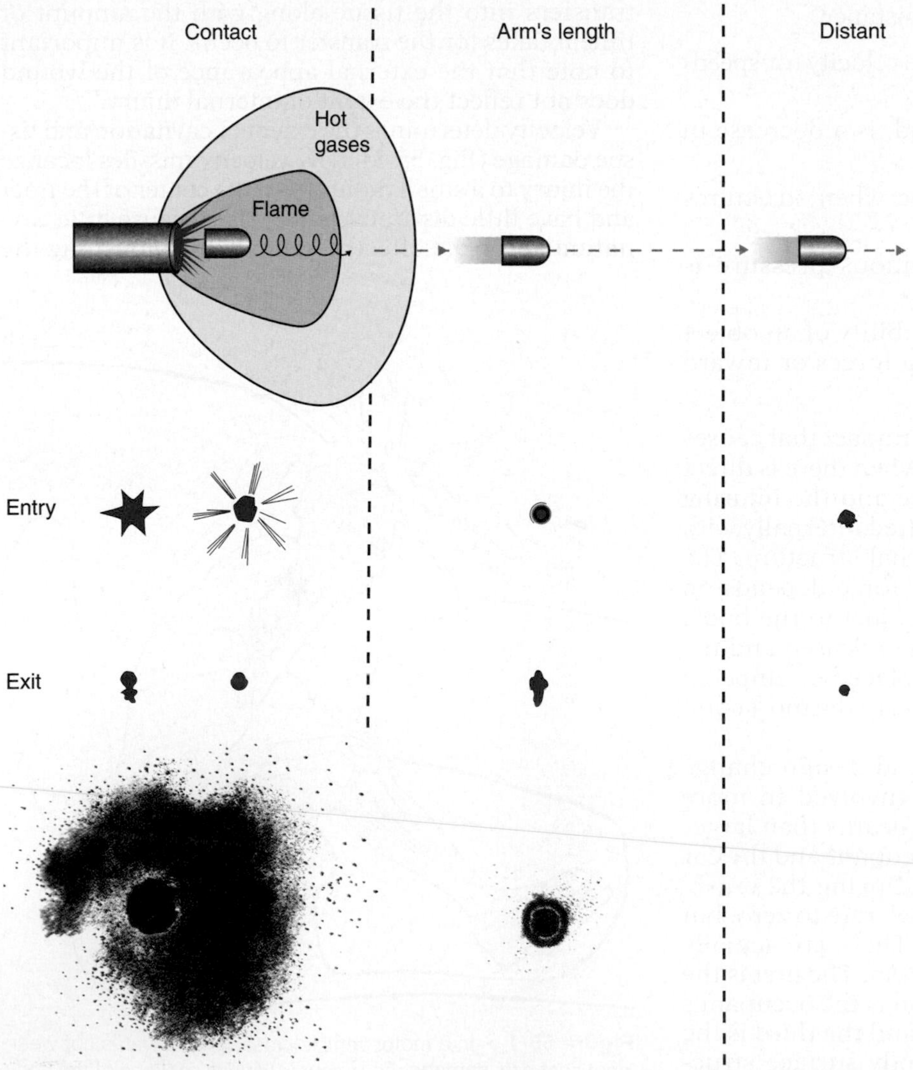

Contact

Arm's length

Distant

Hot gases

Flame

Entry

Exit

Figure 55-3 • Diagrammatic views of the effects of gunshot wounds on the body surface. Kinetic energy is dependent on the distance from which the weapon is fired and the tissue involved. Entry and exit wounds are shown when in direct contact, at arm's reach, and at a distance. The bottom illustrations show entry wounds of .22 rifle at 5-cm range (*left*) and at 20-cm range (*right*). The drilled-in entry wound and faint power markings are indicated.

tissue aside. High-velocity missiles can cause more serious injury because of the amount of energy and cavitation produced. The damage depends on three factors: the density and compressibility of the tissue injured, the missile's velocity, and the fragmentation of the primary missile. High-velocity bullets compress and accelerate tissue away from the bullet, causing a cavity to form around the bullet and its entire tract.

Shotguns are short-range, low-velocity weapons that use multiple lead pellets encased in a larger shell for ammunition. Each pellet is a missile (Fig. 55-4). It is important to obtain a brief description of the mechanism of gunshot injuries, including the weapon, the ammunition, and ballistics. This essential information is used to guide the assessment of patients who sustain injuries from these weapons. All trauma patients must be undressed and inspected for entrance and exit wounds during the assessment process.

A stab wound or impalement is a low-velocity injury. The main injury determinants are length, width, and trajectory of the penetrating object and the presence of vital organs in the area of the wound. Although the injuries tend to be localized, deep organs and multiple body cavities can be penetrated.

• Initial Assessment and Management

When a trauma patient is brought to the emergency department or the trauma resuscitation unit, it is imperative to obtain a thorough history of the preceding events. This initial evaluation aids in assessment and treatment and can decrease morbidity and

mortality. During this initial assessment, it is important to obtain as much detail as possible about the circumstances surrounding the injury, including the mechanism of injury. To facilitate initial assessment, intervention, and triage of the trauma victim, the American College of Surgeons (ACS) Committee on Trauma has developed guidelines. These guidelines provide an organized, standardized approach to the initial assessment of trauma patients, increasing the speed of the primary assessment and minimizing the risk that injuries will be overlooked.

PREHOSPITAL MANAGEMENT

The trauma patient has a greater chance of a positive outcome if admission to a trauma center and definitive care are initiated within 1 hour of injury. Care begins in the prehospital arena and is continued throughout the hospital stay. Many current studies discuss the prehospital management of trauma patients and seem to conclude that the principal factor influencing prehospital care is the transport time to the trauma center. Although prehospital providers have guidelines and protocols to follow in various situations, trauma practitioners appear to have reached a consensus; they have decided that few interventions should be provided if transport time is short and more interventions if transport time is longer.[3,6] Many regionalized systems have a mandated ambulance destination policy that instructs the emergency medical system providers to transport seriously injured patients to the designated trauma center, often bypassing a nondesignated facility.[3]

The advanced trauma life support guidelines state that the emphasis for assessment and management

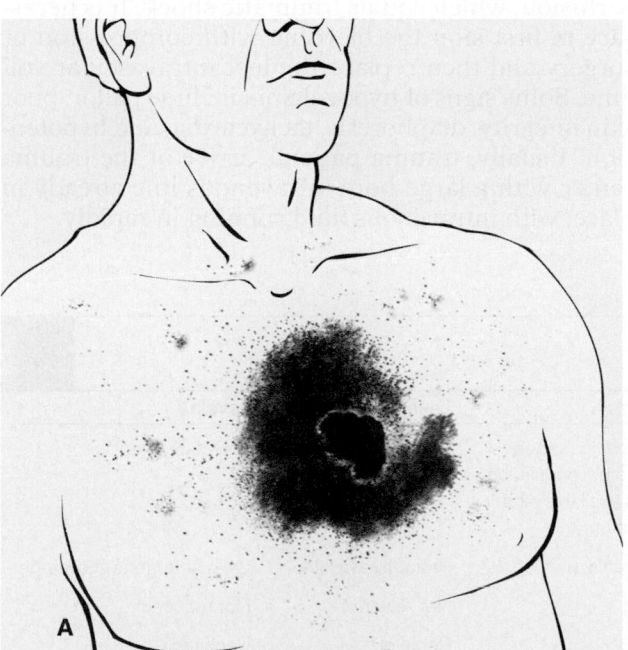

A

B

Figure 55-4 • Damage is caused by shotguns at two different distances. **A:** At close range, opening is extensive and is surrounded by blood splatters and powder burns. **B:** At medium range (8–10 feet), the larger entry wound is surrounded by individual pellet wounds.

in the prehospital phase should be placed on maintaining the airway, ensuring adequate ventilation, controlling external bleeding and preventing shock, maintaining spine immobilization, and transporting the patient immediately to the closest appropriate facility.[3,7] The prehospital priority of maintaining adequate airway, breathing, and circulation (ABCs) may be difficult because of the mechanism of injury. It is imperative that cervical spine immobilization be maintained at all times during airway management and transport to definitive care. After assessing and managing the ABCs, the trauma patient's neurological status is assessed, including level of consciousness and pupil size and reaction. Once this primary assessment is complete, a secondary assessment is performed to determine any other injuries.

The prehospital providers must consider the facility that will receive the patient (Table 55-1). Transporting the patient to a level I facility allows definitive care to be initiated earlier in the process, thereby reducing patient mortality. Trauma systems have been designated to get the "right patient to the right resources in the right time frame."[8] Creation of trauma centers and trauma programs has a positive effect on outcomes in severely injured patients.[9] Transport of the patient to a lesser facility for "stabilization," followed by transport to the definitive care setting later on, is associated with higher patient mortality. For select severe injuries, level I trauma centers have significantly better survival and functional outcomes than level II, III, or IV centers.[9]

Research has shown that injury-related mortality is significantly reduced with organized systems of trauma care, including prehospital care, acute care, and rehabilitation.[10] Inclusive trauma systems have been designed to care for all injured patients and involve all acute care facilities to the extent that their resources allow.[10]

IN-HOSPITAL MANAGEMENT

In-hospital patient management entails a rapid primary evaluation and resuscitation of vital functions, a more detailed secondary survey, a tertiary survey to identify specific injuries, and initiation of definitive care. Table 55-2 shows the process, commonly referred to as the "ABCDEs" of trauma care. According to the ACS, adhering to this sequence allows for the efficient identification of life-threatening conditions.[7] Optimal care of the trauma patient includes a preplanned emergency phase involving a predetermined response team with defined roles and expectations. This is necessary so that multiple procedures can be performed simultaneously. The team leader is a physician. It is the leader's responsibility to assess the patient, order and interpret the diagnostic studies, and prioritize the diagnostics and therapeutic concerns.[3]

Primary Survey

During the primary survey, each priority of care is dealt with in order. The patient's assessment does not continue to the next phase until each preceding priority is effectively managed. For example, if a patient does not have a patent airway, breathing and ventilation cannot be established. Therefore, it is during this initial phase that life-threatening injuries are identified and managed. So, if the patient does not have a patent airway, endotracheal intubation, chest tube insertion, and central line access may be initiated and intravenous fluid and blood products may be administered to maintain life-sustaining vital signs before moving on to the next phase of the evaluation. Initial radiographs and procedures are dependent on the findings in the primary survey. However, chest, abdomen, and pelvis films are generally completed at this time.[3]

Assessing the patient for evidence of hypovolemia is essential. Blood loss can result from an external injury, associated with obvious bleeding, or from an internal injury, where bleeding may not be obvious. Any of these injuries can lead to inadequate tissue perfusion, which equals traumatic shock. It is necessary to first stop the bleeding with compression or surgery and then replace the lost intravascular volume. Some signs of hypovolemia include pallor, poor skin integrity, diaphoresis, tachycardia, and hypotension. Usually, trauma patients arrive at the trauma center with a large-bore intravenous line already in place, with intravenous fluid running in rapidly.

Table 55-1 • Trauma Center Designation

	Level I	Level II	Level III	Level IV
Admission requirements	1,200 patients per year; 20% with an Injury Severity Score (ISS) ≥15 or 35 patients per surgeon with an ISS ≥15	Varies depending on geographical area, population, resources available, and system maturity	No requirement	No requirement
Surgeon availability	24-h in-house attending surgeon	Rapidly available	Promptly available	24-h emergency coverage
Research center	Required	Not required	Not required	Not required
Education, prevention, and outreach	Required	Required	Required	Required

From Scalea TM, Boswell SA: Initial management of traumatic shock. In McQuillan KA, Von Rueden KT, Hartsock RL, et al. (eds): Trauma Nursing, 3rd ed. Philadelphia: WB Saunders, 2002.

Table 55-2 • Initial Assessment and Management of the Patient With Trauma

Parameter	Assessment	Interventions
Airway	Air exchange Airway patency	Jaw thrust, chin lift Removal of foreign bodies Suctioning Oropharyngeal or nasopharyngeal airway Endotracheal intubation (orally or nasally) Cricothyrotomy
Breathing	Respirations (rate, depth, effort) Color Breath sounds Chest wall movement and integrity Position of trachea	Supplemental oxygen Ventilation with bag–valve device Treatment of life-threatening conditions (e.g., tension pneumothorax)
Circulation	Pulse, blood pressure Capillary refill Obvious external bleeding Electrocardiogram	Hemorrhage control: direct pressure, elevate extremity, pneumatic antishock garment Intravenous therapy: crystalloids, blood transfusion Treatment of life-threatening conditions (e.g., cardiac tamponade) Cardiopulmonary resuscitation
Disability	Level of consciousness Pupils	—
Exposure	Inspection of body for injuries	—

During the resuscitation period, an electrocardiogram (ECG) is performed. The patient is placed on a monitor with pulse oximetry and end-tidal carbon dioxide monitoring. A Foley catheter and a nasogastric or orogastric tube are placed, and blood work is sent to the laboratory for evaluation. Blood work includes evaluation of electrolytes, hemoglobin and hematocrit, blood type and crossmatch, and arterial blood gases (ABGs), if the patient is believed to have a high level of injury.

The nurse also assesses the patient for hypothermia. The trauma patient is often subjected to environmental factors, which, along with his or her altered physiological state and possible wet clothing, predispose the patient to hypothermia. Measures such as the infusion of room-temperature intravenous fluids or exposure of the patient's body to inspect for injuries can exacerbate hypothermia. Warm fluids and blankets are used whenever possible to increase body temperature or maintain normothermia.

Secondary Survey

Once the primary survey is completed, a more detailed secondary survey is initiated. This survey begins at the head and works down to the patient's feet. Non–life-threatening injuries are revealed during this survey. During this time, a plan is developed and the appropriate diagnostic tests (e.g., radiographs, ultrasound studies, computed tomography [CT] scans, angiographic studies) are ordered. This is also the time when a more detailed patient history can be obtained, as well as important information regarding the mechanism of injury. The nurse asks the field providers for information regarding the incident because the patient may not be able to speak or may not remember the event. Family and friends might be helpful in providing additional information about the patient.

Questions the nurse asks before or during the trauma patient's arrival to the hospital include the following:

▶ Was the person involved in an MVC? Was the person wearing a restraining device? If the person was hit by a vehicle, was the person on foot or on a bike? What kind of vehicle was involved? Where was the person at the time of impact? What was the speed, point of impact, type of impact? Was there a fatality at the scene?

▶ Is blunt or penetrating trauma the main concern?

▶ Did the patient fall? How far? Was the fall off a ladder, or down a flight of stairs?

Based on the information obtained from field providers or family members of the patient, other injuries may be suspected, and further investigation may be warranted. This is especially true in intubated, comatose, or paralyzed patients who are unable to verbalize their complaints. The nurse continuously reassesses the trauma patient because injuries often go undetected.

Tertiary Survey

The tertiary survey is completed on all trauma patients admitted to the intensive care unit (ICU). It is necessary to identify all of the patient's injuries completely. To do this, another head-to-toe examination is completed, an assessment of the patient's response to resuscitation is made, films are reviewed with radiology, laboratory values are reviewed, and every effort is made to obtain or complete a preinjury medical history. Delays in injury identification are common. However, if the injury is found within 24 hours of admission, it is not considered a missed injury.[3]

Fluid Resuscitation

Most trauma patients have a fluid volume deficit that must be corrected. The goal of fluid resuscitation is to maintain perfusion to the vital organs, especially the heart and the brain, by restoring circulating volume.[11] It is essential to have adequate intravascular volume and oxygen-carrying capacity to transport needed nutrients to the tissues.[8] Fluid administration is one of the most basic concepts in resuscitation and is also a part of the daily routine of medically managed patients in the hospital.[12] To guide fluid resuscitation, the nurse uses the physical assessment and hemodynamic parameters. Two factors affect the choice of fluid: how the volume loss occurred, and which solutes need to be replaced.[11] It is important to address the underlying problem causing the loss of fluids, electrolytes, or both. With aggressive fluid resuscitation, many patients have total-body edema and ascites. The two main complications of aggressive fluid resuscitation are hypothermia and coagulopathy.[3]

Crystalloids

Typically, crystalloids are used in the trauma patient. Crystalloids contain water and other electrolytes that are premixed into the fluid. These electrolytes include sodium, potassium, and chloride. Crystalloids closely mimic the body's extracellular fluid and can be used to expand both intravascular and extravascular fluid volume.[11] There tends to be a larger requirement for crystalloid replacement compared with the amount of blood lost.[12] Crystalloids can be further broken down by their tonicity. The tonicity is based on the amount of sodium in the solution. Crystalloids can be classified as isotonic, hypotonic, and hypertonic (Table 55-3).

Hypertonic saline has been shown to enable a more rapid restoration of cardiac function with a smaller volume of fluid. It is supplied either in a 3%, 7.5%, or 23.4% sodium chloride (NaCl) solution. As little as 4 mL/kg, if given rapidly, may have the same hemodynamic effect as several liters of isotonic crystalloid. Hypertonic saline has the effect of shifting water into the plasma. This water comes from the red blood cells, interstitial space, and tissue.[11] The result is a rapid increase in blood volume, which supports and improves hemodynamics. Hypertonic saline increases the mean arterial pressure and cardiac output, which then leads to peripheral vasodilation.

The initial management of trauma patients often requires the infusion of 2 L of isotonic crystalloid as rapidly as possible, while trying to achieve a normal heart rate and blood pressure.[12] However, research has shown that the infusion of crystalloids in patients with hypotension can cause more harm by displacing a hemostatic clot, only to cause more bleeding.[6,8,13] The infusion of crystalloid also further dilutes the patient's hemoglobin and can increase intraperitoneal blood loss.

Colloids

Colloids can also be given to resuscitate a trauma patient. Colloids, such as albumin, dextran, and hetastarch, create oncotic pressure, which encourages fluid retention and movement of fluid into the intravascular space. Colloids have a longer duration of action because they are larger molecules and stay in the intravascular compartment longer.[11] They are also more efficient in expanding plasma volume, use a smaller volume, and increase colloid osmotic pressure.[12] Proponents of colloid use have argued that less volume of fluid is necessary to achieve hemodynamic stability and that the fluid is retained in the intravascular space longer. Despite possible advantages, there is no clear evidence that colloids are superior to crystalloids for resuscitation of the trauma patient. Potential complications, such as anaphylaxis and coagulopathy, have been reported with certain colloids. These potential adverse affects, together with higher costs, make colloids less desirable than crystalloids for use in resuscitation of trauma patients.

Blood Products

Blood products are considered an excellent resuscitation fluid.[12] Red blood cells increase oxygen-carrying capacity and allow for volume expansion. It is well known that the maintenance of adequate oxygen delivery is critical in the bleeding trauma patient; therefore, packed red blood cells are the mainstay of treatment.[13] Blood also stays in the intravascular space for longer periods of time compared with the other resuscitation fluids.[12] Although there is some concern about blood-borne pathogens and transfusion reactions, it is essential to understand the advantages offered by blood transfusion.

Blood should be transfused when patients are hemodynamically unstable or are showing signs of tissue hypoxia despite crystalloid infusion. Cross-matched blood is preferred but may not be available if emergent transfusion prohibits type and cross-matching of the patient's blood. O-negative blood is the preferred type of uncrossmatched blood, especially in women of childbearing age. O-positive blood may be used in male and postmenopausal female

Table 55-3 • Intravenous Fluid 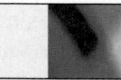	
Isotonic	• Example: 0.9 normal saline • Equivalent to the tonicity of the human body • Causes minimal shifts between intracellular and extracellular fluid
Hypotonic	• Example: 5% dextrose in water (D_5W) • Tonicity is less than that of human body • May cause swelling, pulls into extracellular space
Hypertonic	• Example: 3% saline • Tonicity is more than that of human body • Pulls fluid into the intravascular space

Modified from American Association of Critical-Care Nurses: Clinical Reference for Critical-Care Nursing, 4th ed. Aliso Viejo, CA: American Association of Critical-Care Nurses, 1998.

patients. If the patient requires large amounts of blood, transfusion of fresh frozen plasma and platelets is initiated. It is important to replace coagulation factors and platelets not contained in blood. In the event of massive blood transfusions, the risk for acute respiratory distress syndrome (ARDS) and disseminated intravascular coagulation (DIC) is heightened. An extended period of hypotension increases the possibility of renal failure.

Autotransfusion is another common modality used in the hemorrhaging trauma patient. Obviously, the nature of trauma prevents patients from donating their own blood, as they may in an elective surgery. However, sometimes blood is salvaged. Most often, blood is saved from a chest tube underwater seal device. A cell saver is connected into the system, and the blood from the wound collects there. Once full, the cell saver is disconnected from the underwater seal device, and this blood is then transfused into the patient using a macroaggregate filter.

Blood Substitutes

Blood substitutes have been developed but have not been approved for use in all countries. These agents do not require crossmatching and do not carry the risk for blood-borne pathogen transmission. Blood substitutes have a long shelf life and are not immunosuppressive. Blood substitutes have oxygen-carrying capacity and oxygen dissociation capability of natural hemoglobin, and in addition, they have the ability to maintain hemodynamic stability and intravascular perseverance.[13] Some examples of blood substitutes are perfluorocarbons and hemoglobin solutions.[13]

Damage Control

Damage-control surgery is defined as "rapid termination of an operation after control of life-threatening bleeding and contamination followed by correction of physiologic abnormalities and definitive management." It is designed to avoid or correct the lethal triad of hypothermia, acidosis, and coagulopathy before definitive management can be performed. Uncontrolled bleeding and iatrogenic interventions ultimately result in hypothermia, coagulopathy, and acidosis. Each of these exacerbates the other, causing a spiraling cycle with death as the ultimate result.[14]

Damage control involves using a staged approach to patients with multiple injuries. The stages are as follows:

▶ Stage 1: stop hemorrhage; control contamination and closure methods to close wounds temporarily

▶ Stage 2: correct physiologic abnormalities in the ICU by warming and ensuring adequate resuscitation as well as correcting coagulopathy

▶ Stage 3 (final stage): definitive operative management

The philosophy of damage control is to abbreviate surgical interventions before the development of irreversible physiologic end points.[14] Traditionally, damage control was used for abdominal trauma, but it is now used for all types of trauma that require immediate surgery.

Definitive Care

Increasingly, trauma care consists of nonoperative management of stable patients. Traditionally, solid organ injuries, both blunt and penetrating, were treated with surgery. Today, many trauma surgeons are choosing nonoperative management for their patients whenever possible. Ever more sophisticated techniques for visualization of internal structures, such as CT, ultrasonography, and angiography, have reduced the need for immediate surgical exploration in many cases. Without question, CT has improved accuracy and high sensitivity and specificity. It provides more information to aid in diagnosing injuries that may have been missed without it. Using CT to discharge a patient earlier, or clear him or her for an earlier surgery with another service, makes sense from a patient care and economic perspective.[15] In addition, many of these techniques can be used for management, as well as diagnosis. For example, angiographic interventions may be used to embolize a hemorrhaging internal vessel, obviating the need for invasive surgical intervention. Patients who are treated nonoperatively require frequent assessment and are admitted to the ICU to facilitate this.

To observe the patient effectively, the nurse must be aware of potential injuries and associated signs and symptoms. Examples of nursing diagnoses and collaborative problems are given in Box 55-1. Attention is also given to the management of preexisting medical conditions and the identification of injuries missed during treatment of life-threatening problems. Once again, knowledge regarding the mechanism of injury is necessary. Finally, the patient is monitored for the

---

Box 55-1 — Examples of Nursing Diagnoses and Collaborative Problems for the Person With Trauma

- Deficient Fluid Volume related to hemorrhage, third-spacing
- Impaired Gas Exchange related to pulmonary trauma, respiratory complications (e.g., acute respiratory distress syndrome [ARDS], pain)
- Impaired Tissue Integrity related to trauma, surgery, invasive procedures, immobility
- Anxiety related to critical illness, fear of death or disfigurement, role changes within social setting, or permanent disability
- Risk for Ineffective Tissue Perfusion: Multiple organs related to decreased cardiac output, decreased oxygenation, decreased gas exchange
- Risk for Infection related to trauma, invasive procedures
- Pain related to trauma
- Impaired bowel elimination related to intra-abdominal trauma, ileus, or both
- Increased Risk for Ineffective Family and Individual Coping related to trauma

development of complications. The critical care nurse must be aware of potential complications and related risk factors associated with various injuries. Certain situations, such as prolonged extrication, prolonged hypothermia, respiratory or cardiac arrest, massive fluid resuscitation, or massive blood transfusions, suggest an increased likelihood of severe injuries and a greater chance of complications and death after trauma. A Collaborative Care Guide for the patient with multisystem trauma is given in Box 55-2.

• Assessment and Management of Specific Injuries

Although this section discusses traumatic injuries related to specific areas of the body, the nurse must keep in mind that head-to-toe assessment is required for each trauma patient. Physical assessment of each organ system is indicated, as described in previous chapters throughout this text.

Box 55-2 • COLLABORATIVE CARE GUIDE for the Patient With Multisystem Trauma

OUTCOMES	INTERVENTIONS
Oxygenation/Ventilation	
The patient will maintain a patent airway.	• Auscultate breath sounds. • Perform frequent assessments. • Intubate if needed. • Provide supplemental oxygen PRN.
The patient will maintain an SaO_2 ≥95% and have adequate ABGs.	• Provide pulmonary toilet (chest physiotherapy and incentive spirometry). • Intubate. • Monitor ABGs.
The patient will be able to take deep breaths and will be free of anxiety.	• Use mechanical ventilation if necessary to support adequate ventilation. • Provide adequate pain medication to promote deep breathing (patient-controlled analgesia [PCA], epidural, around-the-clock medications) • Medicate before pain increases. • Use antianxiety drugs as necessary.
Circulation/Perfusion	
The patient will maintain an adequate blood pressure, heart rate, and respiratory rate.	• Monitor respiratory rate and depth. • Use ECG monitor. • Administer intravenous (IV) fluids and packed red blood cells to ensure adequate intravascular volume and oxygen-carrying capacity. • Administer medications, such as vasoactive and inotropic agents, after intravascular volume is restored. • Install pulmonary artery catheter/A-line. • Assess skin color and capillary refill time.
The patient will not experience deep venous thrombosis.	• Use prophylactic anticoagulants unless contraindicated. • Apply antiembolic stockings. • Use pneumatic compression devices.
Fluids/Electrolytes	
The patient will maintain an adequate intake and output.	• Monitor blood pressure, heart rate, central venous pressure, pulmonary capillary wedge pressure, IV fluid • Use Foley catheter to monitor urine output. • Consider insensible fluid loss in output. • Monitor laboratory values.
The patient will maintain electrolyte balance.	• Replace electrolytes PRN. • Monitor ECG.
Mobility/Safety	
The patient's range of motion will be maintained.	• Consult Physical/Occupational Therapy. • Use splints PRN. • Do range-of-motion exercises every 8 h. • Out of bed as tolerated.

(continued)

Box 55-2 • COLLABORATIVE CARE GUIDE for the Patient With Multisystem Trauma (Continued)

OUTCOMES	INTERVENTIONS
Skin Integrity The patient will not experience skin breakdown.	• Monitor skin every 4 h. • Turn patient every 2 h and PRN. • Use pressure-relieving devices. • Remove splints to monitor skin. • Provide prescribed wound care. • Monitor wound for evidence of infection.
Nutrition The patient will maintain an adequate calorie intake to meet metabolic needs.	• Arrange dietary/nutrition consult. • Use total parenteral nutrition (TPN)/lipids if enteral nutrition contraindicated. • Tube feeds: encourage enteral nutrition when possible. • Check prealbumin and electrolytes. • Monitor for weight loss.
Comfort/Pain Control The patient will maintain a pain score of less than 5.	• Administer adequate pain medication. • Use PCA/epidural PRN. • Arrange pain consult if needed. • Use sedation as needed. • Monitor vital signs.
Psychosocial The patient will maintain as much control as possible.	• Inform patient of procedures. • Establish a schedule with the patient if possible. • Provide an alternate means of communication if necessary, such as lip reading, writing, and a communication board.
The patient and family will cope effectively with the traumatic event.	• Provide repeated information. • Encourage use of appropriate coping. • Encourage use of support systems. • Arrange social work consult.
Teaching/Discharge Planning The patient will be involved in discharge planning.	• Discuss discharge with patient. • Allow patient to make decisions if possible.
The patient will understand injuries and complications of injuries.	• Provide discharge instructions accordingly with injury. • Provide patient with list of injuries.

THORACIC TRAUMA

Thoracic injuries range from simple abrasions and contusions to life-threatening insults to the thoracic viscera. Although these injuries are associated with a high mortality rate, most can be managed with simple chest tube insertion, mechanical ventilation, aggressive pain control, and other supportive care.[16] Great vessel injuries or disruption to the heart usually result in immediate death. Early deaths (30 minutes to 3 hours after injury) are related to cardiac tamponade, tension pneumothorax, aspiration, or airway obstruction.[17]

Immediate life-threatening injuries require evaluation and treatment during the primary survey. Examples of these include airway obstruction, tension pneumothorax, cardiac tamponade, open pneumothorax, massive hemothorax, and flail chest (Fig 55-5). Potentially life-threatening injuries such as thoracic aortic disruption, tracheobronchial disruption, myocardial contusion, traumatic diaphragm tear, esophageal disruption, and pulmonary contusion should be addressed during the secondary survey.[17]

In thoracic injury, the first priority is always airway management. This includes immediate airway control as well as adequate oxygenation and protection from aspiration. Airway obstruction may be the result of another injury or the primary problem.[17] The most common causes of airway obstruction are the tongue, avulsed teeth, dentures, secretions, and blood. Other causes of airway obstruction include injuries to the trachea, thyroid cartilage, or cricoid.[17]

Tracheobronchial Trauma

Injuries to the trachea or bronchi can be caused by blunt or penetrating trauma and frequently are accompanied by esophageal and vascular damage. Ruptured

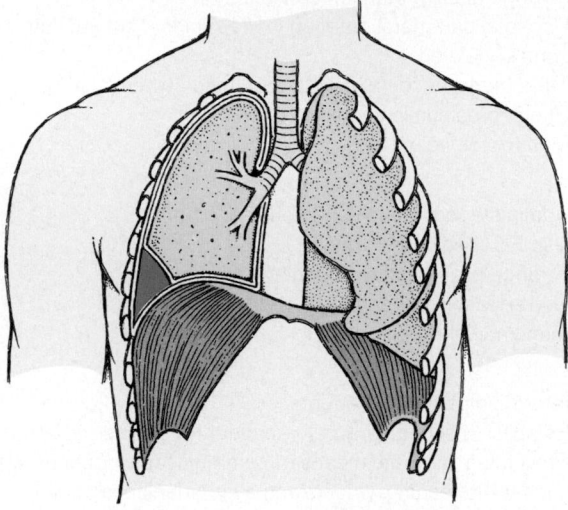

A. Tension pneumothorax

B. Hemothorax

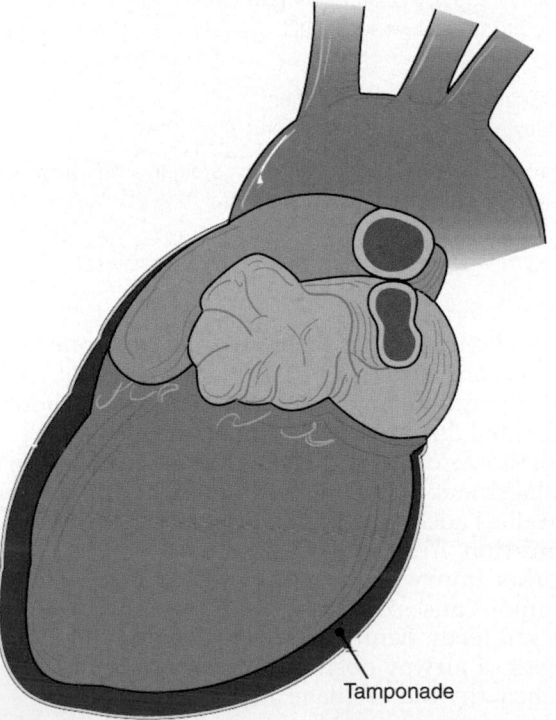

Tamponade

C. Cardiac tamponade

Figure 55-5 • **A:** Tension pneumothorax. **B:** Hemothorax. **C:** Cardiac tamponade. (**B,** Courtesy of Neil O. Hardy, Westpoint, Conn. **C,** Courtesy of LifeART image © 2007 Lippincott Williams & Wilkins. All rights reserved.)

bronchi often are present in association with upper rib fractures and pneumothorax. Severe tracheobronchial injury has a high mortality rate; however, with continued improvements in prehospital care and transport, more of these patients are surviving.

Airway injuries often are subtle. Presenting signs include dyspnea (occasionally the only sign), hemoptysis, cough, subcutaneous emphysema, anxiety, hoarseness, stridor, air hunger, hypoventilation, use of accessory muscles, sternal and subscapular retractions, diaphragm breathing, apnea, and cyanosis. Cyanosis may be a late sign. Often trauma patients are anemic and do not have enough hemoglobin to develop cyanosis.[17] A chest radiograph can alert the physician to a possible injury; however, diagnosis usually is made with bronchoscopy or during surgery. Tracheobronchial injury is considered whenever a persistent air leak accompanies a pneumothorax.

Small lung lacerations or pleural tears can be managed conservatively with mechanical ventilation delivered through an endotracheal tube or tracheostomy. Larger injuries may require surgical repair. Simultaneous independent lung ventilation, where each lung is ventilated separately (each with a dedicated ventilator), may also be used.

Nursing care involves the assessment of oxygenation and gas exchange, along with appropriate pulmonary care. During the first few days, the physician may perform a bronchoscopy to visualize the repair site and provide more effective secretion removal. Pneumonia is a potential short-term complication, whereas tracheal stenosis may occur later.

Bony Thorax Fractures

Rib fractures, sternal fractures, and flail chest are thoracic fractures commonly seen in trauma patients. They occur when the applied force exceeds the strength of the thoracic cage.[16] Rib fractures are common injuries. They are clinically significant as (1) markers of serious intrathoracic and abdominal injuries, (2) sources of significant pain, and (3) predictors of pulmonary deterioration.[16] With rib fractures, the most common associated thoracic injuries are pneumothorax, hemothorax, and pulmonary contusion, and the most frequently injured abdominal organs are the liver and the spleen.[16] The greatest concerns for nurses caring for patients with such injuries are pain, ineffective ventilation, and secretion control. Ribs 1 and 2 are usually protected by the clavicle, scapula, humerus, and surrounding muscles. If these ribs are fractured, it often signifies high-impact trauma and other injuries, such as to the aorta, the thorax, and the spine, are very likely and should be investigated. Ribs 3 through 9 are most commonly fractured in blunt trauma. If these ribs are fractured, there are often associated underlying lung injuries. Fractures of the lower ribs can also be associated with injury to the liver or other abdominal structures. Sternal fractures are associated with blunt trauma.

Flail chest is an injury that involves multiple rib fractures. These fractures can be anterior, posterior, or lateral, and usually a sternal fracture is present as well. The stability of the thorax is disrupted, and the rib cage no longer moves in unison. The diagnosis of flail chest is made on the basis of a fracture of two or more ribs, in two or more separate locations, causing an unstable segment. This creates a free-floating segment of rib or sternum.[17] The injured area does not respond to the action of the respiratory muscles; rather, it moves in accordance with the changes in intrapleural pressure. The flail segment movement is paradoxical, hence the term paradoxical breathing. The flail segment causes a decrease in the normal negative pressure of the chest, thereby decreasing ventilation and causing some degree of hypoxia. The flail segment follows pleural pressure instead of respiratory muscle activity. As the patient's pulmonary status worsens, the paradoxical movement of the flail segment increases.[17] Initially, muscular splinting may mask the injury until the patient becomes fatigued.[16]

Initial management of patients with bony thorax fractures includes airway management, pain management, and oxygen therapy to maintain adequate saturation. The nurse must consider the underlying structures and the possible injury to them. Treatment of flail chest includes turning the patient with the injured side down to improve oxygenation. This is often difficult because of the need to maintain cervical spine immobilization. Other treatment modalities include internal splinting, accomplished by placing the intubated patient on positive-pressure ventilation. Sometimes surgical repair is performed, especially if a thoracotomy is necessary for other reasons. Surgical repair may help decrease the need for prolonged mechanical ventilation.

Pleural Space Injuries

For the purpose of this chapter, the term pleural space injuries is used in reference to pneumothorax (intrapleural air collection), hemothorax (intrapleural blood collection), and hemopneumothorax (interpleural air and blood collections). Pleural space injuries are caused by disruption of an intrathoracic structure that allows air or blood to build up in the pleural layers, thereby leading to a decrease in negative intrathoracic pressure. Sometimes air and blood continue to build up in the pleural cavity, causing increased tension, which leads to a tension pneumothorax or a tension hemothorax. Either blunt or penetrating trauma may result in a pleural space injury.

The mechanism of injury may lead the nurse to suspect a pleural space injury. For example, an unrestrained driver whose chest hits the steering wheel has a great potential for this injury. When assessing the patient, respiratory distress may be evident along with altered ventilation, which leads to impaired gas exchange. Impaired gas exchange may be evidenced by restlessness, anxiety, tachypnea, decreased oxygenation, poor color, and diaphoresis. The nurse continuously reassesses the patient because even if the original injury is small, it can expand, causing a life-threatening emergency.

Chest radiography is usually used to diagnose pleural space injuries. Sometimes if the pneumothorax is less than 20% of the chest cavity, it may not be seen initially on chest film. A chest CT scan often shows the smaller pleural space injuries.

Treatment of pleural space injuries includes appropriate management of the patient's airway, ventilation, and oxygenation. A large-bore chest tube, such as a 40-French tube, is often inserted to reexpand the lung and drain the air or blood. This tube is inserted in the fourth or fifth intercostal space at the mid-axillary line. For trauma patients with a simple pneumothorax, a chest tube may be placed in the second intercostal space at the mid-clavicular line. Once the tube is inserted, it is attached to an underwater seal system and then attached to suction. The effects of treatment are assessed by chest radiograph, physical examination, and noting of improved oxygenation. Often there is an air leak in the underwater seal system of the chest tube drainage device that ceases within a few days.

The nurse monitors the amount of blood that drains into the chest tube drainage device. Drainage of more than 200 mL/hour for 2 consecutive hours may indicate a missed injury or the need for further exploration and should be reported.[17]

A massive hemothorax is defined as 1.5 to 4 L of intrathoracic blood loss and truly constitutes a life-threatening injury. A massive hemothorax is often caused by severe thoracic injuries, and the source of bleeding is a large systemic blood vessel or mediastinal structure. Patients with massive hemothorax often arrive at the emergency department or trauma resuscitation unit in cardiopulmonary arrest. These patients require immediate thoracotomy to control bleeding. The patients who are not in cardiopulmonary arrest present with signs of hypovolemic shock (see Chapter 54), dyspnea, tachypnea, and cyanosis. Initial management of these patients includes treatment of the shock state. Two large-bore intravenous lines should be established and resuscitation fluid administered. The amount of fluid administered depends on the patient's response.[17]

A left massive hemothorax is more common than a right one and is often associated with aortic rupture.[17] The chest cavity is large enough to hold most of the patient's circulating blood volume. Because of this, the bleeding stops only when the pressure in the pleural cavity is equal to or greater than the pressure in the damaged vessel. Placement of a chest tube in a patient with massive hemothorax could lead to exsanguination by eliminating the tamponade caused by a closed chest injury. If a chest tube is inadvertently placed, it should be clamped until exploratory thoracotomy can be performed.

Tension pneumothorax is a life-threatening condition that requires immediate recognition. It may be the result of a primary injury to the thorax or a delayed complication related to tracheobronchial injury or mechanical ventilation. Tension pneumothorax is caused by air entering the pleural space and becoming trapped without an exit. A one-way valve closed system is formed. This causes a compression of one or more of the intrathoracic structures (trachea, heart, lungs, and great vessels) and prohibits them from functioning adequately. The outcome is ventilation failure, compromised venous return, and insufficient cardiac output.[18]

Tension pneumothorax is often difficult to diagnose in the trauma patient because of other injuries the patient may have, as well as the presence of a shock state. It may not be diagnosed until the patient has decompensated. The nurse may notice that it is difficult to ventilate the patient, despite an open airway. There is often a drop in the patient's oxygenation. Other signs of tension pneumothorax include chest asymmetry, tracheal shift, neck vein distention (unless the patient is hypovolemic), decreased breath sounds on the affected side, and evidence of decreased cardiac output (e.g., decreased blood pressure and poor tissue perfusion).

Treatment of tension pneumothorax requires immediate decompression of the trapped air. This is done initially by placing a 14- or 16-gauge needle into the pleural space, usually between the second to fourth anterior intercostal space. An immediate rush of air should escape, and the patient's ventilation should improve. Supplemental oxygen is provided to the patient before decompression. After emergent decompression, the needles are changed to chest tubes. This is done to allow the lungs to expand as well as to prevent a reoccurrence. Last, additional assessment is necessary to determine the cause of tension pneumothorax. The nurse must continue to assess and reassess the patient.

Pulmonary Contusion

A pulmonary contusion is a bruising of the lung parenchyma, often caused by blunt trauma. It is the most common lung injury and can be potentially lethal.[17,18] It is often apparent on the chest radiograph and CT as an "ill defined, patchy, ground glass density regions of opacification in mild contusion to widespread areas of consolidation in more severe injury."[18] CT is more sensitive in diagnosing pulmonary contusions; it may take up to 6 hours for the pulmonary contusion to show up on chest radiograph.[18] However, the presence of a scapular fracture, rib fractures, or a flail chest should lead to the suspicion of a possible underlying pulmonary contusion. In fact, pulmonary contusion should be anticipated in any patient who sustains significant high-energy blunt chest trauma.[16] The most common mechanism for pulmonary contusion is MVCs.

Pulmonary contusion occurs when rapid deceleration ruptures capillary cell walls, causing hemorrhage and extravasation of plasma and protein into alveolar and interstitial spaces. This results in atelectasis and consolidation, leading to intrapulmonary shunting and hypoxemia. Presenting signs and symptoms include dyspnea, rales, hemoptysis, and tachypnea. Severe contusions also result in increasing peak airway pressures, hypoxemia, and respiratory acidosis. Pulmonary contusion may mimic ARDS; both are poorly responsive to high fractions of inspired oxygen (FiO_2). ARDS is discussed in detail in Chapter 27. The greater the degree of pulmonary contusion, the greater degree of ventilatory impairment.[17]

Treatment of pulmonary contusion is supportive. Patients with a mild contusion require close observation with frequent ABG measurements or pulse oximetry monitoring. Additional nursing interventions include frequent respiratory assessment, pulmonary care, and pain control. Chest physiotherapy and continuous epidural analgesia also may be beneficial. An oximetric pulmonary artery catheter and arterial line usually are placed to facilitate monitoring of ABGs, hemodynamics, and respiratory parameters (oxygen delivery, oxygen consumption, intrapulmonary shunt).

Severe pulmonary contusion may require ventilatory support with positive end-expiratory pressure (PEEP). Although alveolar ventilation improves as PEEP is added, blood flow to alveoli may diminish, leading to an increased intrapulmonary shunt. To optimize tissue perfusion and oxygenation, each change in PEEP requires assessment of the status of the shunt, oxygen delivery, and other indicators of tissue perfusion (cardiac output, blood pressure, and urine output). Adequate pain control is necessary and may require epidural or intrapleural infusions of analgesics or an intracostal nerve block. In severe cases of respiratory compromise, increased sedation or paralysis may be indicated to decrease energy expenditure and oxygen requirements. A rotation bed also may be considered to promote pulmonary toilet and respiratory gas exchange. Positioning the patient with the injured side up is beneficial in the case of a severe unilateral contusion. In rare instances, when the patient is not responding to traditional mechanical ventilation, prone positioning and high-frequency jet ventilation may be used. Another mode of ventilation commonly used is airway pressure-release ventilation.

Fluid management also is important. Intake and output, daily weights, central venous pressure, and pulmonary artery and capillary wedge pressures are monitored to guide fluid administration. Medications may need to be more concentrated to compensate for excess fluid intake, and diuretics may be required periodically. Severe fluid restriction is not indicated. Instead, fluid balance should be maintained at a normal level (euvolemia) to support optimal cardiac output and oxygen delivery. The contused lung should show radiographic signs of improvement within 72 hours. The presence of persistent infiltrates may indicate complications, such as pneumonia or superimposed ARDS. Long-term sequelae include prolonged reduced functional residual capacity, dyspnea, and fibrosis.

Blunt Cardiac Injuries

Blunt cardiac injuries encompass a wide spectrum of clinical manifestations ranging from asymptomatic myocardial bruise to cardiac rupture and death.[19] These injuries include cardiac wall rupture, valvular disruption, coronary artery dissection, and cardiac contusions. Table 55-4 describes the blunt cardiac injury classification according to the sequelae of the injury. There are few clinical signs and symptoms of blunt cardiac injury. Chest pain is usually the most common, and others secondary to thoracic injuries

Table 55-4 • Blunt Cardiac Injury (BCI) Classification According to the Sequelae of the Injury	
Classification	Description
1	BCI with cardiac free wall rupture
2	BCI with septal rupture
3	BCI with coronary artery injury
4	BCI with cardiac failure
5	BCI with complex dysrhythmias
6	BCI with minor electrocardiographic or cardiac enzymes abnormalities

From Schultz JM, Trunkey DD: Blunt cardiac injury. Crit Care Clin 20:57–70, 2004.

often occur (e.g., dyspnea, chest wall ecchymosis, flail chest).[19]

Cardiac contusions, the most common form of blunt cardiac injuries, are usually caused by blunt trauma as the heart hits the sternum during rapid deceleration. A contusion can also develop if the heart is compressed between the sternum and the spine. Symptoms vary from none (common) to severe congestive heart failure and cardiogenic shock. Complaints of chest pain must be evaluated carefully after trauma. Nonspecific ECG changes, which can include any type of dysrhythmia, are frequently seen. A dysrhythmia always indicates a cardiac contusion until proven otherwise. Atrial dysrhythmias and conduction disturbances may be seen with right-sided cardiac injuries; ventricular disturbances are more likely after left-sided cardiac injuries.

A cardiac contusion is suspected when there is a history of severe anterior blunt trauma and the patient has chest wall bruising and fractures of the ribs or sternum. A 12-lead ECG is performed to detect any electrical abnormalities. Most patients with cardiac contusions have ECG abnormalities on admission. However, there is no correlation between the complexity of the dysrhythmia and the degree of the cardiac contusion.[20] These patients are placed on continuous cardiac monitoring, and blood is drawn for cardiac isoenzyme and troponin studies. Although cardiac enzymes lack specificity in terms of diagnosis, they are used to guide therapy.[19]

Controversy exists over the standard of care for patients with cardiac contusion.[19] Because there is no standard in diagnosing this injury, there is also no standard in treatment. Continuous monitoring must be done to evaluate for symptomatic dysrhythmias, especially ventricular irritability and conduction defects. Echocardiography or multigated angiography may be helpful in determining any muscle defect or damage. In general, patients are treated to relieve their symptoms.

Penetrating Cardiac Injury

In most cases, a penetrating injury to the heart results in prehospital death. The mortality rate is 50% to 85%. Those who survive do so because of cardiac tamponade.[17] Cardiac tamponade and hypovolemic shock are the common presenting signs.[17] The right ventricle is injured most often because of its anterior location. Occasionally, small stab wounds to the ventricles seal themselves because of the thick ventricular musculature. Treatment of hemodynamically stable patients remains controversial. In some instances, monitoring with serial CT scanning or with pericardial and pleural ultrasound is acceptable. In other cases, surgery to create a thoracoscopic pericardial window may be necessary to aid in the diagnosis of ongoing hemorrhage and to drain pericardial fluid collections.[17] In the presence of ongoing hemorrhage and shock, lost blood volume is replaced, and the patient is immediately transported to the operating room for a median sternotomy and exploration. In severe cases, a thoracotomy in the emergency department may be required as a life-saving measure.

After surgical repair, a pulmonary artery catheter and arterial line are placed to facilitate careful hemodynamic monitoring. Vasopressors or inotropic agents may be necessary to maintain adequate blood pressure and cardiac output. Fluid and electrolyte balance, along with cardiac rhythm, must be monitored closely. Heart sounds are assessed to detect murmurs, indicating valvular or septal defects, and for signs of congestive heart failure. Chest and mediastinal tube drainage are recorded frequently. Fresh frozen plasma and platelets are administered, as indicated, to correct coagulopathies. Complications include continued hemorrhage and postcardiotomy syndrome.

Cardiac Tamponade

Cardiac tamponade, known as both a symptom and injury, can result from both penetrating and blunt trauma. It is a life-threatening injury that needs to be immediately assessed and treated. Cardiac tamponade is caused by blood filling the pericardium and compressing the heart, causing decreased cardiac filling, which leads to reduced cardiac output and eventually shock. Bleeding into the pericardial sac (hemopericardium) or a small pericardial rupture may or may not cause cardiac tamponade, depending on the amount of pressure in the pericardium.[17,21]

The pericardial sac normally holds about 25 mL of fluid, which serves to cushion and protect the heart. Only a small amount of pericardial blood (50 to 100 mL) is necessary to increase intrapericardial pressure. Continued bleeding increases the pressure rapidly, and the patient presents with signs and symptoms of cardiac tamponade.

Classic symptoms include decreased blood pressure, muffled heart sounds, and increased central venous pressure manifested by distended neck veins (Beck's triad). Another key sign to cardiac tamponade is pulsus paradoxus, "an inspiratory systolic fall in arterial pressure of 10 mm Hg or more during normal breathing."[17] This is caused by a fall in cardiac output. Because these signs may be obscured in the hypovolemic trauma victim, patients with a history of precordial trauma must be treated with a high index of suspicion. Diagnosis of cardiac tamponade is not easy. An echocardiogram is most useful in the diagnosis and is readily available.[17] Treatment of cardiac tamponade includes airway control, oxygenation, hemodynamic support, and rapid transport to a definitive care center. The rapid transfusion of intravenous fluids increases venous pressure and ultimately improves cardiac output as well as provides the needed time to prepare for interventions.[17] Ultimately, the treatment of cardiac tamponade is drainage of blood from the pericardial sac. This is the only life-sustaining intervention.[17] Nursing management of a patient with cardiac tamponade includes airway protection and ventilatory support, hemodynamic support, and assistance with interventions provided to the patient.

Aortic Injuries

Aortic disruption is the leading cause of immediate death from blunt trauma.[17,22] Disrupting the blood flow in the aorta inhibits perfusion to vital organs and extremities. The location and size of the disruption determine its significance.[17] Blunt aortic injury is usually associated with sudden deceleration or compression forces. MVCs are the primary causes of this injury. The on-scene mortality rate is 70% to 90%, and the majority of surviving patients die before reaching the hospital. If patients do reach the hospital and their injury is quickly identified, they have a 40% to 70% survival rate.[22] Aortography is the gold standard for diagnosis of aortic injuries, although transesophageal echocardiography and chest CT play an increasingly important role.[22]

There are three common locations of vessel rupture. Because the thoracic aorta is very mobile, the tears occur at points of fixation. The most common is at the aortic isthmus, just distal to the left subclavian artery, where the vessel is attached to the chest wall by the ligamentum arteriosum. The two other sites of rupture are in the ascending aorta, where the aorta leaves the pericardial sac, and at the entry to the diaphragm. The inner layers of the vessel tear on impact from deceleration. The outer layers remain intact and balloon out into a pseudoaneurysm. A partial circumferential hematoma may also be tamponaded by surrounding tissues. Both of these mechanisms may prolong survival, but only for a limited time.

An understanding of the injury history can raise the suspicion of aortic injury. Penetrating mediastinal injuries or thoracic injuries caused by blunt trauma should raise suspicion. Other injuries that may raise suspicion include first or second rib fractures, high sternal fractures, clavicular fractures at the sternal margin, and massive left-sided hemothorax.

Loss of effective blood transport because of major vessel rupture is the main physiological problem associated with aortic rupture. The goal of assessment is to identify evidence of poor perfusion beyond the aortic lesion. Many patients are asymptomatic on presentation. Findings associated with aortic injuries are given in Box 55-3.

A supine chest radiograph is obtained to aid in diagnosis of an aortic injury. After spinal injury has been ruled out, an upright chest radiograph may be obtained as well. If a widened mediastinum is detected

> **Box 55-3 • RED FLAG: Signs and Symptoms of Aortic Injuries**
>
> - Pulse deficit in any area, particularly lower extremities or left arm
> - Hypotension unexplained by other injuries
> - Upper extremity hypertension relative to lower extremities
> - Interscapular pain or sternal pain
> - Precordial or interscapular systolic murmur caused by turbulence across the disrupted area
> - Hoarseness caused by hematoma pressure around the aortic arch
> - Respiratory distress or dyspnea
> - Lower extremity neuromuscular or sensory deficit
>
> *Adapted from Sherwood SF, Hartsock RL: Thoracic injuries. In McQuillan KA, Von Rueden KT, Hartsock RL, et al (eds): Trauma Nursing, 3rd ed. Philadelphia, WB Saunders, 2002, pp 543–590.*

on radiograph, additional evaluation is necessary for definitive management. Although an aortic tear is sometimes seen on CT scan, aortography is the study used for definitive diagnosis.[17,22]

A positive aortogram indicates the need for surgical repair. The torn aorta may require end-to-end anastomosis or, more commonly, the placement of a synthetic graft. Cardiopulmonary bypass may be necessary for repair of the ascending aorta or the aortic arch. However, repair of the descending thoracic aorta is usually accomplished during aortic cross-clamping. Because this maneuver occludes distal blood flow, it is imperative that the cross-clamp time be as short as possible (preferably less than 30 minutes). To prevent leakage from the repair site, vasodilators may be administered after surgery to reduce afterload. After replacement of intravascular volume, a vasopressor may be added to support adequate blood pressure. Nursing care focuses on hemodynamic monitoring with a pulmonary artery catheter and titrating medications to maintain optimal blood pressure. Autotransfusion may also be necessary.

Complications are related to the level of the tear and the extent of altered perfusion. Hypoperfusion and resulting damage to organs below the level of the laceration can result from the injury itself or from prolonged cross-clamping during repair. Serious complications resulting from prolonged cross-clamp time include renal failure, bowel ischemia, lower extremity weakness, or permanent paralysis of the lower extremities. Other sequelae, such as ARDS or DIC, can be a consequence of hemorrhagic shock and multiple blood transfusions.

ABDOMINAL TRAUMA

Abdominal trauma can be caused by both blunt and penetrating injuries. Abdominal injuries can rapidly lead to death secondary to hemorrhage, shock, and sepsis.[5] Missed abdominal injuries are a frequent cause of trauma deaths.[23] Compared with penetrating trauma, blunt abdominal trauma is associated with more fatalities, because many of the injuries are "hidden" and often more obvious but less severe injuries lead to a delay in diagnosis.[5] Deaths that occur more than 48 hours after abdominal injury are due to sepsis and its complications.[24] In intra-abdominal trauma, rarely does single-organ or single-system injury occur.

The abdomen contains both solid and hollow organs. The solid organs include the liver, spleen, pancreas, and kidneys. The hollow organs include the intestines, stomach, gallbladder, and urinary bladder.[5] Clinicians divide the abdomen into three main regions to facilitate description of the location of the injury. The three areas are:

▶ The peritoneal area, which includes the diaphragm, liver, spleen, stomach, transverse colon, and the portion covered by the bony thorax

▶ The retroperitoneal area, which includes the aorta, vena cava, pancreas, kidney, ureters, and parts of the duodenum and colon

▶ The pelvis, which includes the rectum, bladder, uterus and the iliac vessels

MVCs are the most common cause of blunt abdominal trauma, although assaults, falls, pedestrian–motor vehicle collisions, and industrial accidents also contribute to blunt abdominal injuries. These injuries occur as the result of compressive, crushing, shearing, and deceleration forces.[23] Diagnosis of blunt abdominal trauma can be difficult, especially if there are multisystem injuries. If the patient has abdominal tenderness or guarding, hemodynamic instability, lumbar spine injury, pelvic fracture, retroperitoneal or intraperitoneal air, or unilateral loss of the psoas shadow on radiograph, visceral damage should be suspected.

Blunt trauma is likely to cause serious damage to solid organs, and penetrating trauma most often damages the hollow organs. The compression and deceleration of blunt trauma leads to fractures of solid organ capsules and parenchyma, whereas hollow organs can collapse and absorb the force. However, the bowel, which occupies most of the abdominal cavity, is prone to injury by penetrating trauma. In general, solid organs respond to trauma with bleeding. Hollow organs rupture and release their contents into the peritoneal cavity, causing inflammation and infection.[5]

Stab wounds, impalements, and gunshot wounds can cause penetrating trauma. Injury patterns differ depending on the mechanism. If the mechanism of penetrating trauma is a stab wound, knowledge of the size, shape, and length of the instrument used is helpful in determining the extent of intra-abdominal damage. However, it is estimated that only half of stab wounds enter the abdomen, which means that compared with gunshot wounds, stab wounds are less destructive and have a decreased morbidity and mortality.[5,23] Impalement is considered a "dirty" wound. "Dirty" wounds can result in high mortality secondary to the infection that is caused by bacterial contamination and subsequent multisystem organ failure. Gunshot wounds (missile injuries) are difficult to evaluate. The amount of major vessel disruption and multiple organ involvement are predictors of mortality. The velocity and amount of energy dispersed by the bullet often determine the extent of injury. A bullet can rebound off organs or bones, changing its trajectory and causing massive internal damage to organs and vessels. The blast effect from bullets can also cause significant intra-abdominal injury.

Abdominal trauma requires continual assessment. Unrecognized abdominal trauma is a frequent cause of preventable death.[5,7,23] The nurse must be organized and methodical in the approach to patient assessment. The nurse needs to understand the mechanism of injury as well as the patient's complaints to perform an adequate assessment and identify potentially life-threatening abdominal injuries. It is important to remember that in blunt trauma, the validity of the physical examination alone is questionable. It is often unreliable because of use of alcohol, illicit drugs, analgesics, or narcotics or a decreased level of consciousness. In penetrating trauma, the physical examination tends to be more reliable.[23]

Usually, a primary survey is completed, and the patient is resuscitated before the abdomen is assessed. During the secondary survey, the abdomen is assessed and reassessed, and laboratory and diagnostic tests are performed. An orogastric or nasogastric tube and a Foley catheter are placed during the secondary survey phase.

Often, diagnosis of penetrating trauma requires local wound exploration. However, it is important to note the site of the injury because wound exploration depends on mechanism and location. If the injury is in the anterior abdominal region (anterior costal margins to the inguinal creases between the anterior axillary lines), the likelihood that the peritoneum has been penetrated is low. If the injury is in the thoracoabdominal region (fourth intercostal space anteriorly and seventh intercostal space posteriorly to inferior costal margins), exploration is not recommended because there is an increased risk for tension pneumothorax. The patient requires a laparoscopy, thoracoscopy, or exploratory laparotomy. Exploration tends to be difficult in flank or back wounds. The patient usually requires a triple contrast CT.[23]

Diagnostic testing may include focused abdominal sonography for trauma (FAST), diagnostic peritoneal lavage (DPL), a chest radiograph (to determine gross abnormalities as well as any organ displacement), and an abdominal CT scan. Many trauma centers are performing FAST on all trauma patients. This is an ideal diagnostic study because it is portable, fast, and reproducible.[23] It is performed by placing an ultrasound probe over various areas on the abdomen to determine whether free fluid is located in those areas. The areas evaluated are Morison's pouch in the right upper quadrant, the pericardial sac, the splenorenal region in the left upper quadrant, and the pelvis (pouch of Douglas). If the results of FAST are positive and the patient is hemodynamically unstable, an exploratory laparotomy is performed.

A DPL is a quick diagnostic procedure that is used during the resuscitation phase of care in hemodynamically unstable trauma patients to diagnose intra-abdominal bleeding (Box 55-4). Other indications for use may include:

1. Unexplained hypotension, decreased hematocrit, or shock
2. Equivocal results of abdominal examination
3. Altered mental status caused by brain injury or alcohol or drug intoxication
4. Spinal cord injury
5. Distracting injuries, such as major orthopedic fractures or chest trauma[24]

If the results of DPL are positive and the patient is hemodynamically unstable, an exploratory laparotomy is performed.

There are several contraindications to performing a DPL. These include morbid obesity, third-trimester pregnancy, advanced cirrhosis, a history of coagulopathy, and a history of multiple abdominal surgeries.[24] There is an increased risk for omental laceration and visceral or vascular perforation if DPL is performed in patients with these findings.

Box 55-4 • Diagnostic Peritoneal Lavage (DPL)

Indications
- Blunt abdominal injury with:
    Altered mental status
    Unexplained hypotension, decreased hematocrit, shock
    Equivocal results of abdominal examination
    Spinal cord injury
    Distracting injuries (e.g., orthopedic fractures, chest trauma)
- Penetrating abdominal trauma (if exploration is not indicated)

Possible Contraindications
- History of multiple abdominal operations
- Third-trimester pregnancy
- Advanced cirrhosis of the liver
- Morbid obesity
- Known history of coagulopathy

Technique
1. Insert lavage catheter into peritoneal cavity through 1- to 2-cm incision.
2. Attempt to aspirate peritoneal fluid.
3. Infuse normal saline or Ringer's lactate by gravity.
4. Turn patient from side to side (unless contraindicated).
5. Allow fluid to run back into bag by gravity.
6. Send specimens to laboratory.

Positive Results
- 10–20 mL gross blood on initial aspirate
- Greater than 100,000 red blood cells/mm³
- Greater than 500 white blood cells/mm³
- Elevated amylase level
- Presence of bile, bacteria, or fecal matter

When performing DPL, it is important to first ensure that the patient has a Foley catheter and an orogastric or nasogastric tube in place to decompress the stomach and the bladder. Decompression of the stomach and bladder guards against accidental perforation when the lavage catheter is placed. Once the Foley catheter and an orogastric or nasogastric tube are placed, the lavage catheter is inserted into the peritoneal space. If less than 10 mL of frank blood is returned, a liter bag of warm crystalloid (lactated Ringer's solution or 0.9% normal saline) is infused into the peritoneum. After the infusion is complete, the intravenous bag is placed in a dependent position to allow the fluid to exit the abdomen by gravity. A sample of the fluid is then sent to the laboratory for evaluation.

CT scans are now being used more often in trauma patients. In blunt trauma, the CT scan has become the mainstay of diagnosis for abdominal injury, with a 92% to 97% sensitivity and 98% specificity.[5] Often, the CT scan is performed with both intravenous and oral contrast to visualize the organs and note any disruption. The CT scan allows visualization of the peritoneal, retroperitoneal, and pelvic areas and permits estimation of the amount of fluid in these areas. CT scans are also used to grade solid organ injuries. Limitations to the use of CT include penetrating trauma, the amount of time required to perform the study, the need to transport the patient out of the resuscitation area, and the requirement that the patient must be hemodynamically stable and have limited movement during the study.

Trauma to the Esophagus and Diaphragm

Esophageal injury is the "most rapidly fatal injury," with an 18% mortality rate.[17] This rate increases significantly when the diagnosis is delayed or missed; death is likely if the diagnosis is delayed.[5,17] Penetrating trauma is the most likely cause of esophageal injury, and usually the cervical esophagus is where the injury occurs. The clinical symptoms are subtle. Presenting symptoms that should lead to a suspicion of esophageal injury include a hemothorax or pneumothorax without rib fractures.

Diagnosis includes CT scan of the chest, abdomen, and pelvis with and without contrast. Esophagoscopy, flexible endoscopy, and swallow studies are also performed. Treatment for esophageal injury is surgical repair. The patient is kept NPO with a nasogastric tube to continuous suction, and antibiotic therapy is initiated. Nursing considerations include paying close attention to the airway of the patient, ventilation, oxygenation, and hemodynamic support.[5,17]

Diaphragm rupture is more common in blunt injury than in penetrating injury. Such rupture occurs more frequently on the left side because there the diaphragm is not protected by the liver.[17] Injury is often secondary to the rising and falling associated with respiration. If a diaphragm rupture is suspected, it is necessary to look for both thoracic and abdominal injury.[5] It is not uncommon to see abdominal contents in the thorax, which subsequently causes bowel strangulation in approximately 30% of patients.[24] Respiratory compromise may also be seen because of impairment of lung capacity and displacement of normal lung tissue.[17]

The clinical picture of diaphragm rupture depends on the size and site of injury. This injury is often difficult to diagnose because there is minimal bleeding and the patient is often asymptomatic. Clinical findings may include marked respiratory distress, dyspnea, decreased breath sounds on the affected side, positive bowel sounds in the thorax, palpation of abdominal contents when inserting a chest tube, and paradoxical movement of the abdomen when breathing.[5,17]

Chest radiography is the initial modality used to diagnose diaphragm rupture. However, it is often normal or nonspecific. The presence of abdominal contents in the chest denotes an injury. If an injury is suspected, an ultrasound and CT scan should be performed.[5] DPL may be falsely negative. The only definitive treatment for diaphragm rupture is surgical repair.[17]

Trauma to the Stomach and Small Bowel

Significant gastric injury is rare. Small bowel injuries are much more common. Although frequently damaged by penetrating trauma, the small bowel can also burst when subjected to blunt trauma. The multiple convolutions occasionally form a closed loop, which can rupture when subjected to increased pressure caused by impact with a steering wheel or seat belt. The bowel's mobility around fixed points (such as the ligament of Treitz) predisposes it to shearing injuries with deceleration.

Blunt small bowel or gastric injury can present with blood in the nasogastric aspirate or hematemesis. Physical signs often are absent, and CT findings may be subtle and nonspecific. Close observation is required; often, the diagnosis is not made until peritonitis develops. Penetrating injuries usually cause positive results on DPL. Although a mild bowel contusion can be managed conservatively (gastric decompression and withholding oral intake), surgery usually is necessary to repair penetrating wounds or bowel rupture.

Postoperative decompression with a gastric tube is maintained until bowel function returns. In most cases, a feeding jejunostomy tube is placed distal to the repair site, and tube feedings can be initiated early in the postoperative course. As the concentration and rate of feedings are advanced slowly, frequent assessment for signs of intolerance (distention, vomiting) is essential.

Because the stomach and small bowel contain an insignificant amount of bacteria, the risk for sepsis is small after rupture of these organs. If the injury goes unrecognized, there is a risk for sepsis. On the other hand, the acidic gastric juice is irritating to the peritoneum and may cause peritonitis. Potential complications related to stomach and small bowel trauma are listed in Box 55-5. Some of these conditions may necessitate additional surgical procedures.

> **Box 55-5 • RED FLAG: Complications Related to Stomach and Small Bowel Trauma**
>
> - Intolerance to tube feedings
> - Peritonitis
> - Postoperative bleeding
> - Hypovolemia caused by third-spacing
> - Development of a fistula or obstruction

Trauma to the Duodenum and Pancreas

The pancreas and duodenum are discussed together because these retroperitoneal organs are closely related anatomically and physiologically. A great deal of force is necessary to injure these organs because they are well protected deep in the abdomen. Most injuries are related to penetrating trauma. Injuries to adjacent organs almost always are present. The retroperitoneal location makes these injuries difficult to diagnose with DPL. An abdominal CT scan is very useful in this instance. Signs and symptoms may include an acute abdomen, increased serum amylase levels, epigastric pain radiating to the back, nausea, and vomiting.

Small lacerations or contusions may require only the placement of drains, whereas larger wounds need surgical repair. Most pancreatic injuries require postoperative closed-suction drainage to prevent fistula formation. Distal pancreatectomy and Roux-en-Y anastomosis are two procedures commonly performed for injuries to the body and tail of the pancreas. Occasionally, the spleen also must be removed because of its multiple vascular attachments to the pancreas. Damage to the head of the pancreas is associated with duodenal injury and severe hemorrhage because of the close proximity of vascular structures. Surgical procedures used in these cases include pancreaticoduodenectomy, Roux-en-Y anastomosis, and, on rare occasions, total pancreatectomy.

Postoperative nursing assessment and care are similar for the various procedures. Patency of drains must be maintained, and the patient must be monitored for the development of fistulas, the most common complication. Skin protection is important if a cutaneous fistula does develop because of the high enzyme content of pancreatic fluid. Assessment of fluid and electrolyte balance is also important because a pancreatic fistula results in fluid loss, along with loss of potassium and bicarbonate. Pancreatic stimulation can be decreased by administering parenteral hyperalimentation or jejunal feedings instead of an oral diet. The onset of diabetes mellitus is rare unless a total pancreatectomy is performed.

Primary repair or resection with reanastomosis is sufficient to manage most penetrating duodenal injuries. A duodenostomy tube may be placed for decompression and a jejunostomy tube for feeding. Blunt trauma to the duodenum can cause an intramural hematoma, which may lead to duodenal obstruction. The diagnosis is made with a diatrizoate

(Gastrografin) upper gastrointestinal study. A complete obstruction usually requires surgical drainage of the hematoma.

Trauma to the Colon

Usually, injury to the colon results from penetrating trauma. The nature of the injury most often dictates surgical exploration (exploratory laparotomy). Primary repair is the treatment of choice for lacerations of the colon.[25] In some situations, such as injury to the left colon or when there is massive blood loss, an exteriorized repair or colostomy is required. A cecostomy tube may be placed for colon decompression. Subcutaneous tissue and skin of the incision site are often left open to decrease the chance of wound infection. The colon has a high bacteria count; spillage of the contents predisposes the patient to intra-abdominal sepsis and abscess formation.

Postoperative nursing care focuses on prevention of infection. Dressing changes are necessary for open incisions, and prophylactic antibiotics may be used. In the case of an exteriorized colon repair, resection and end-to-end anastomosis is performed, and the repair site is exteriorized to facilitate identification of a leak. The exteriorized colon must be kept moist and covered with a nonadherent dressing or bag to protect the integrity of the sutures. Because sepsis is a major complication of colon injuries, a series of radiographic and surgical procedures may be required to locate and drain abscesses.

A teaching guide for patients who have undergone a laparotomy can be found in Box 55-6.

Trauma to the Liver

After the spleen, the liver is the most commonly injured abdominal organ. Both blunt and penetrating trauma can cause hepatic injuries. Fractures of the right lower ribs increase suspicion for a liver injury. Presenting signs and symptoms may include right upper quadrant pain, rebound tenderness, hypoactive or absent bowel sounds, or signs of hypovolemic shock. Box 55-7 presents the liver injury scale.

Hemodynamically stable patients with liver injuries may be managed nonoperatively. In this case, serial CT scans are performed to verify bleeding cessation. However, in many cases, the patient's unstable clinical condition dictates the need for surgery. Hepatic trauma can cause a large blood loss into the peritoneum, but bleeding may stop spontaneously. In some instances, bleeding vessels may be ligated or embolized. Small lacerations are repaired, whereas larger injuries may require segmental resection or débridement. In the case of uncontrollable hemorrhage, the liver is packed. After packing, the abdomen may be closed or simply covered and left open. An additional surgical procedure is required within the next few days to remove the packing and repair the laceration. Large liver injuries also need postoperative drainage of bile and blood with closed-suction drains.

After surgery, coagulopathies may be present. Incomplete hemostasis also is a possibility and must

---

Box 55-6 • TEACHING GUIDE:
After a Laparotomy

Patient Activity
- No tub baths or showers while the staples/stitches are in place.
- If you are tired, rest.
- Only lift what you can easily lift with one hand.
- You may eat your normal diet.
- Take your temperature once a day at the same time and write it down.
- Maintain a normal schedule with your bowel movements.
- If you become constipated, drink more fruit juices.
- Do not drive until you have your doctor's permission.

Wound Care
- It is important to keep the staple/stitch line clean.
- Monitor your wound closely.
- Cleanse the area once a day. To do this, you will need 4" × 4" gauze pads and a solution of half peroxide/half saline.
- Wash your hands.
- Open the gauze pad and leave it on the paper.
- Pour a small amount of the peroxide/saline solution on the center of the pad while it is laying on the paper.
- Pick up the pad, pulling all four corners together without touching the center.
- Wipe over the stitches/staples from top to bottom, covering them well with the solution. It is normal to see bubbles when cleaning with this solution. Wipe the area only once with a single gauze pad.
- Repeat.
- Allow the area to dry.
- Tape a gauze pad over the stitch/staple line to prevent rubbing or irritation caused by a belt or waistband.

Signs of Infection
- Swelling around the site
- Increased redness
- Increased tenderness
- Warmth around the site
- Wound edges separating
- Increased drainage
- Foul-smelling drainage
- Change in color of drainage
- Temperature of 101°F or higher
- Vomiting, diarrhea, or constipation

---

be differentiated from coagulopathy-induced bleeding. Severe bleeding resulting from incomplete hemostasis requires clot removal, packing, and additional repair. With a coagulopathy, bleeding arises from numerous sites, whereas with incomplete hemostasis, the bleeding is mainly from the surgical site.

Nursing care of patients with liver injuries includes the replacement of blood products while monitoring the hematocrit and coagulation studies. Assessment of the character and amount of tube drainage, along with fluid balance, also is essential. Potential complications of liver injury include hepatic or perihepatic abscess, biliary obstruction or leak, sepsis, ARDS, and DIC. In 6 to 8 weeks, the physical examination should

Box 55-7 • Liver Injury Scale

Hematomas
- **Grade I hematomas:** subcapsular and nonexpanding; involving <10% of surface area
- **Grade II hematomas:** subcapsular, <1 cm intraparenchymal hematoma; involving 10%–50% of surface area
- **Grade III hematomas:** expanded and subcapsular, involving >50% of surface area, or ruptured and actively bleeding; intraparenchymal ≥2 cm or expanding
- **Grade IV hematomas:** ruptured parenchyma with active bleeding

Lacerations
- **Grade I lacerations:** capsular tear <1 cm deep and nonbleeding
- **Grade II lacerations:** actively bleeding capsular tear 1–3 cm deep without trabecular vessel involvement
- **Grade III lacerations:** >3 cm deep
- **Grade IV lacerations:** involving 25%–50% hepatic lobe parenchymal disruption
- **Grade V lacerations:** involving >50% hepatic lobe parenchymal disruption; vascular injury includes retrohepatic vena cava and juxtahepatic venous injuries
- **Grade VI lacerations:** vascular hepatic avulsion

From Eckert KL: Penetrating and blunt abdominal trauma. Crit Care Nurse Q 28(1):41–59, 2005.

Box 55-8 • Splenic Injury Scale

Hematomas
- **Grade I hematomas:** involving <10% of surface area; subcapsular and nonexpanding
- **Grade II hematomas:** subcapsular; involving 10%–50% of surface area or <1 cm intraparenchymal hematoma
- **Grade III hematomas:** expanding, subcapsular, and ruptured, with active bleeding, involving >50% of surface area; subcapsular hematoma ≥2 cm or expanding intraparenchymal
- **Grade IV hematomas:** involving ruptured parenchyma with active bleeding

Lacerations
- **Grade I lacerations:** nonbleeding capsular tear <1 cm deep
- **Grade II lacerations:** actively bleeding capsular tear 1–3 cm deep without trabecular vessel involvement
- **Grade III lacerations:** >3 cm deep or involving trabecular vessels
- **Grade IV lacerations:** including hilar vessel with >25% devascularization
- **Grade V lacerations:** involving completely shattered spleen; hilar vascular injury with total devascularization of the spleen

From Eckert KL: Penetrating and blunt abdominal trauma. Crit Care Nurse Q 28(1):41–59, 2005.

be improved. To prevent rebleeding, patients should not participate in contact sports until a repeat CT scan shows healing of the injury.[5]

Trauma to the Spleen

The spleen is the most commonly injured abdominal organ, usually as a result of blunt trauma. Because of its vascularity, the spleen has a tendency to lose blood rapidly.[5] Presence of left lower rib fractures increases suspicion for a splenic injury. Presenting signs and symptoms include left upper quadrant pain radiating to the left shoulder (Kehr's sign), hypovolemic shock, and the nonspecific finding of an increased white blood cell count. DPL or abdominal CT is usually necessary for diagnosis. Box 55-8 provides the splenic injury scale.

Adults with minor injuries and most children are treated nonoperatively with observation (serial abdominal examinations, serial hematocrits) and gastric decompression. Because the spleen and stomach are both in the left upper quadrant, decompression of the stomach reduces pressure on the injured spleen. Preferred surgical treatment is splenorrhaphy, although in some cases splenectomy is necessary. Splenic autotransplantation, a fairly new procedure, consists of implanting splenic fragments into pockets of omentum after splenectomy. Splenic autotransplantation may be performed after severe injuries to retain the normal splenic immune functions.[26]

Early complications include recurrent bleeding, subphrenic abscess, and pancreatitis resulting from surgical trauma. Rupture of an expanding subscapular hematoma or pseudoaneurysm may present days or weeks after an initial normal examination.[5] Late complications consist of thrombocytosis and overwhelming postsplenectomy sepsis (OPSS). Because the spleen plays an important role in the body's response to infection, a splenectomy predisposes the patient to an increased risk for infection. This risk is especially high among children and highest in those younger than 2 years of age. Pneumococcus, an encapsulated microorganism resistant to phagocytosis, is the organism that most often infects patients after splenectomy. OPSS frequently begins with the onset of pneumococcal pneumonia, which progresses to a fulminant sepsis. Postsplenectomy patients can increase their immunity toward pneumococcal infections by receiving a polyvalent pneumococcal vaccine (Pneumovax). Complications of OPSS include adrenal insufficiency and DIC. OPSS has a high incidence and mortality rate, especially within 1 year of surgery. Patient and family teaching should focus on information about signs and symptoms of infection. Splenic autotransplantation may prove beneficial in decreasing the incidence of OPSS.

Trauma to the Kidneys

Injury to the kidney may lead to a "free" hemorrhage, contained hematoma, or the development of an intravascular thrombus. Sudden deceleration injury can cause the kidney to move, avulsing smaller renal vessels or tearing the renal artery intima, which also may lead to vessel thrombosis. Blunt and penetrating trauma can also cause a laceration or contusion of the renal parenchyma or rupture of the collecting system. Lower rib or lumbar vertebral fractures, along with liver and spleen injuries, should raise suspicion of an associated renal injury. Signs and symptoms, when present, consist of hematuria, pain, a flank hematoma, or ecchymosis over the flank.[5] Because the bleeding is retroperitoneal, it can be difficult to detect. A helical CT scan, ultrasound, or an intravenous pyelogram (less commonly used) usually provides the diagnosis.

Renal injuries are classified based on their severity. Many renal injuries can be managed conservatively with observation and bed rest until gross hematuria resolves. However, in some instances (mainly for vascular injury), surgical repair or nephrectomy is necessary.

Postoperative assessment and support of renal function are imperative. Optimal fluid balance must be maintained. Low-dose dopamine may be ordered to promote renal perfusion. Major complications consist of arterial or venous thrombosis and acute renal failure. Other complications include bleeding, perinephric abscess, the development of a urinary fistula, and late onset of hypertension.

Trauma to the Bladder

The bladder can be lacerated, ruptured, or contused, most often as the consequence of blunt trauma (usually because of a full bladder at the time of injury).[5] Bladder injuries frequently are associated with pelvic fractures. Gross hematuria is typically noted with bladder rupture. Presence of blood at the urethral meatus, a scrotal hematoma, or a displaced prostate gland requires examination for urethral injuries with a CT scan or conventional cystography before the insertion of a urinary catheter.[5]

A bladder injury can cause intraperitoneal or extraperitoneal urine extravasation. Extraperitoneal extravasation, usually associated with pelvic fractures, can often be managed with urinary catheter drainage. However, intraperitoneal extravasation (associated with a high-force injury) requires surgery. This injury has a high mortality rate because of associated injuries that occur secondary to the force involved.[5] A suprapubic cystostomy tube may be placed. Complications are infrequent, but infection due to the urinary catheter or sepsis from extravasation of infected urine can occur. Patients may complain of an inability to void or of shoulder pain (caused by urine extravasation into the peritoneal space).

MUSCULOSKELETAL INJURIES

Although musculoskeletal injuries take a long time to heal and can often result in lifelong disability, they are usually not considered life-threatening unless there is a traumatic amputation or pelvic fracture. Routinely, the musculoskeletal assessment is done in the secondary survey after hemodynamic stabilization. These injuries do require prompt recognition and stabilization to promote optimal recovery and function.

There are approximately 33 million musculoskeletal injuries per year, including 20 million fractures, dislocations, and sprains, with approximately 8,000 deaths.[27] Although there are a variety of causes of trauma-related musculoskeletal injuries, the major ones include MVCs; falls; industrial, farming, and home accidents; and assaults. Musculoskeletal injuries are often associated with other injuries to the body.

It is important to understand the circumstances surrounding, and the mechanism involved in, musculoskeletal trauma. Force might be applied to one area, but the transferred energy and distribution of force may cause injury somewhere else. For example, in a person who falls off a two-story building and lands on his or her feet, one would expect to find calcaneus or ankle fractures, but the transference of energy may also cause a pelvic or lumbar spine fracture. Obviously, if the patient is conscious, he or she can verbalize his or her pain. However, many times, fractures and sprains go unrecognized because the patient is not able to verbalize and communicate the location of his or her pain.

As in all trauma patients, initial assessment begins with the primary survey. Once this is complete and the patient is hemodynamically stable, the secondary assessment is conducted. When trauma patients are admitted to the resuscitation unit, cervical spine, chest, and pelvis films are obtained first. Sometimes thoracic and lumbar spine films are obtained, depending on the mechanism of injury. The initial pelvic film tells the nurse whether the patient has a life-threatening pelvic fracture. If this is the case, immobilization of the pelvis should be maintained to prevent exsanguination. Immobilization of the pelvis is achieved with a C-clamp, external fixator, pelvic binder, or sheets wrapped tightly around the patient to attempt to stop the bleeding.

During the secondary survey, if limb swelling, ecchymosis, or deformity is noted, that extremity should be immobilized. Proper films are ordered to determine the extent of the injury. The nurse tests the extremities for capillary refill (less than 2 seconds is normal), pulses, crepitus, muscle spasm, movement, sensation, and pain.

The most common studies used to diagnose musculoskeletal injuries are plain radiographs, CT, and magnetic resonance imaging (MRI). When obtaining radiographs, it is important to get two views of the affected area. It is also important to assess the joint above and below the injured area. If the affected area is in a place that is difficult to visualize on plain films, a CT scan usually gives a better picture. An MRI also gives more specific detail about the area surrounding the injury and about the injury itself.

There are many types of musculoskeletal injuries, including fractures, fracture–dislocations, amputations, and trauma to the soft tissue (i.e., skin, muscle, tendons, ligaments, and cartilage). Fracture classification is based on type, cause, and anatomical location. Several fracture types are shown in Figure 55-6. If the skin is broken at the fracture site, the injury is considered to be an "open" fracture. If the skin is

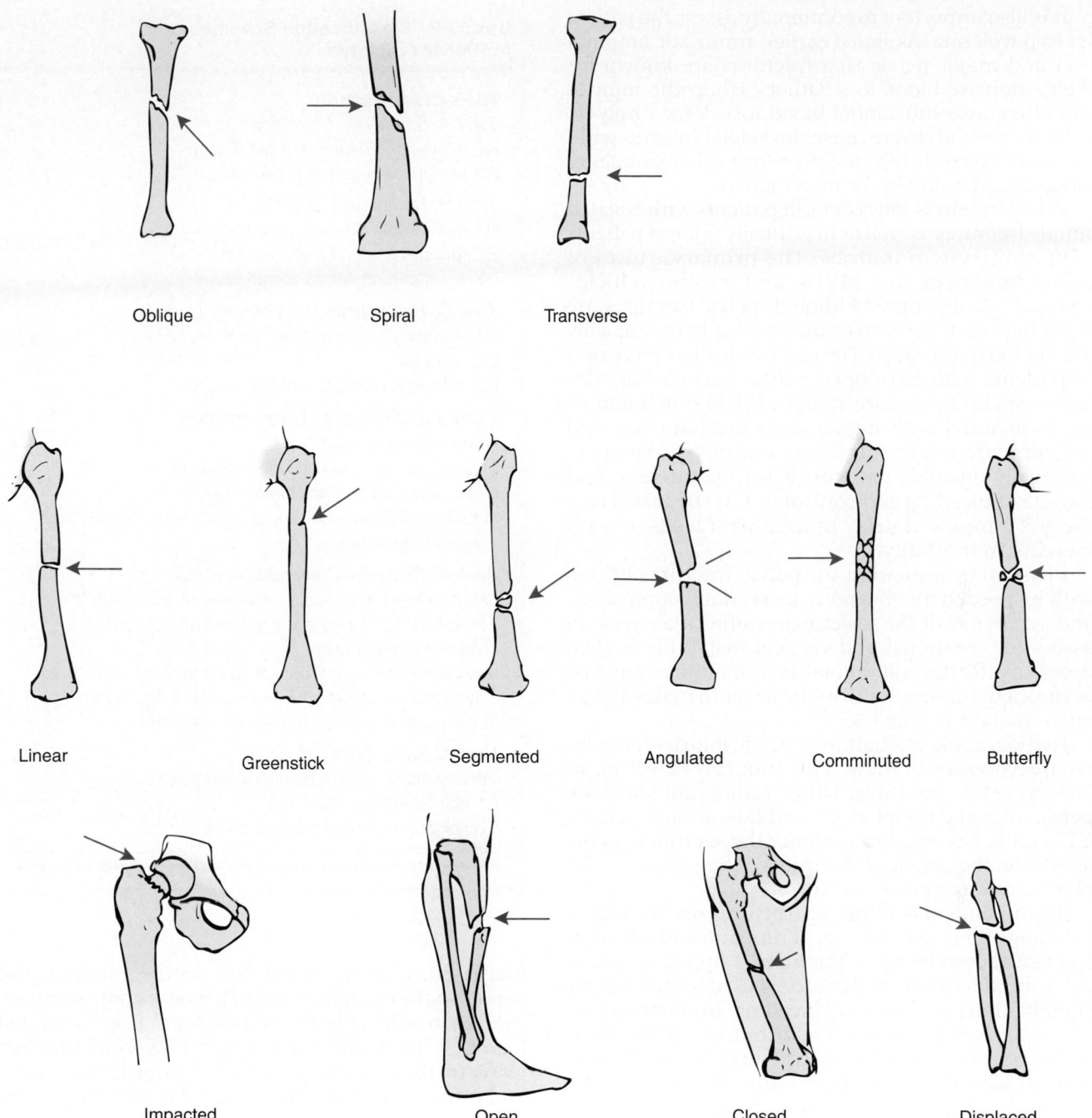

Oblique   Spiral   Transverse

Linear   Greenstick   Segmented   Angulated   Comminuted   Butterfly

Impacted   Open   Closed   Displaced

Figure 55-6 • There are many different types of fractures.

intact, the injury is said to be a "closed" fracture. An open fracture is further classified as grade I, II, or III, depending on the tissue damage involved.

Dislocation occurs when the articulating surfaces of a joint are no longer in contact because of joint disruption. Joint mobility may be restricted. There may also be associated vascular or nerve injury with dislocations. Ligamentous injury usually accompanies dislocations because ligaments stretch or tear at the time of dislocation.

Amputations are classified according to the amount of tissue, nerve, and vascular damage. A cut or guillotine amputation has clean lines and well-defined edges, whereas a crush amputation has more soft tis-

sue damage and the edges are not as well defined. An avulsion amputation occurs when a force stretches and tears away tissues, causing nerves and vessels to be torn in different areas than the bone.

As with any injury, musculoskeletal trauma requires continuous assessment. It is not uncommon for vascular or neurological compromise, or both, to develop in patients with musculoskeletal injury. Any musculoskeletal injury involving bone or soft tissue can cause neurological or vascular compromise because nerves and blood vessels are located in such close proximity to the bones and muscles. The nerves and muscles are very sensitive to impaired circulation and compression.

It is also important to continually assess the patient for hypovolemia. As stated earlier, traumatic amputation and major pelvic ring fractures are known for their extensive blood loss. Other orthopedic injuries can also cause substantial blood loss. Very rarely do patients sustain severe musculoskeletal injuries without other systemic injuries; therefore, other sources of blood loss should also be investigated.

Pelvic fractures may occur in patients with isolated simple fractures as well as in critically injured patients with multisystem injuries. The primary causes of pelvic fractures are MVCs and motor vehicle–pedestrian collisions.[28] Although pelvic fractures are thought to contribute to traumatic death, they usually are not the main cause. The risk for death is increased in patients who have open pelvic fractures or who have been hit by a motor vehicle. Pelvic ring fractures are associated with high-energy mechanisms, and patients often have soft tissue injury.[29] In hemodynamically unstable patients, it is imperative to find the site of bleeding and control it. It is suggested that every 3 minutes of delay in treatment leads to a 1% increase in mortality.[30]

Physical examination for pelvic fractures begins with inspection for abrasions, lacerations, contusions, and symmetry of the lower extremities. Palpation to assess for rotational and vertical instability is then necessary. Rectal and vaginal examinations should be performed to assess for a urethral tear in males and an open fracture in females.[28,29]

Radiographic evaluation of pelvic injuries includes an anteroposterior view. This film can detect up to 90% of pelvic fractures. Other radiographs include pelvic inlet and outlet views and lateral sacral views. CT scan is also used to evaluate the sacroiliac joints as well as the extent of the injury.[29] See Box 55-9 for classification of pelvic fractures.

Treatment goals of pelvic fractures are to control bleeding and to prevent loss of function and infection (sepsis) caused by open fractures.[31] Application of a pelvic binder or external fixator is used for temporary stabilization and to control bleeding. Embolization is also indicated for hemorrhage control.[32] Permanent orthopedic repair of pelvic fractures is usually performed within 24 to 72 hours after injury when the patient is adequately resuscitated and hemodynamically stable. This can be accomplished with either internal or external fixation.[28]

Infection is common in open injuries. Ideally, patients with musculoskeletal trauma are brought to the operating room within 6 hours of injury for a washout of the affected area. Sometimes antibiotic prophylaxis is started; however, this practice is controversial. A tetanus booster is given if indicated to all patients with open injuries.

Other serious complications of musculoskeletal injuries include compartment syndrome, deep venous thrombosis (DVT), pulmonary embolus, and fat embolus syndrome.

Compartment Syndrome

Compartment syndrome occurs when the pressure within the fascia–enclosed muscle compartment is

---

Box 55-9 • Classification Schemes for Pelvic Fractures

Tile's Classification

Type A, Stable
A1, without involvement of pelvic ring
A2, with involvement of pelvic ring

Type B, Rotationally Unstable
B1, open book
B2, ipsilateral lateral compression
B3, contralateral lateral compression

Type C, Rotationally and Vertically Unstable
C1, rotationally and vertically unstable
C2, bilateral
C3, with associated acetabular fracture

Young and Burgess Classification

Lateral Compression (LC)
I, Sacral compression on side of impact
II, Iliac wing fracture on side of impact
III, LCI or LCII injury on side of impact with contralateral open-book injury

Anterior Posterior Compression (APC)
I, slight widening of pubis symphysis or anterior part of sacroiliac joint with intact anterior and posterior sacroiliac ligaments
II, widened anterior part of sacroiliac joint with disrupted anterior and intact posterior sacroiliac ligaments
III, complete disruption of the sacroiliac joint

Vertical Shear (VS)
Vertical displacement anteriorly and posteriorly
Combined mechanism (CM)
Combination of other injury patterns

From Frakes MA, Evans T: Major pelvic fractures. Crit Care Nurse 24(2):18–32, 2004.

---

increased, causing blood flow to the muscles and nerves in the compartment to become compromised, thereby resulting in tissue ischemia. It is suspected based on mechanism of injury.[33] This ischemia then leads to tissue damage, which compromises nerve and muscle function. A prolonged elevation of compartmental pressure leads to death of the muscles and nerves involved.[33] Intracompartmental pressures that exceed 30 to 50 mm Hg can cause significant muscle ischemia.[33]

Patients with higher diastolic pressures are able to tolerate higher tissue pressures without ischemic damage. Fasciotomy is recommended when the compartment pressure approaches 20 mm Hg below the diastolic pressure. Hypotensive trauma patients may experience significant muscle ischemia at lower compartment pressures.[33]

Patients with compartment syndrome complain of increased pain in the affected area. The lower leg is the most common location of compartment syndrome.[33] The pain is described as being "out of proportion" to the injury. The most reliable early sign of compartment syndrome is decreased sensation. The compartment involved is firm, and the patient eventually has paresthesia. Pallor and pulselessness are late signs of compartment syndrome. When the compartment syndrome has progressed to the point that the patient is showing late signs, loss of the affected extremity is threatened. The nurse must constantly monitor the affected extremity and compare it with the nonaffected extremity. If any of the signs or symptoms of compartment syndrome are present, the orthopedic or general surgeon should be notified immediately so that compartment pressures can be measured. If it is deemed that the compartment pressures are high, a fasciotomy is performed to release the pressure and save the extremity.

Deep Venous Thrombosis

DVT is a significant risk for all trauma patients, especially those with musculoskeletal injuries. It is known as a common, life-threatening complication of major trauma. The danger of DVT is that it may progress to pulmonary embolus. The administration of low-dose heparin or low–molecular-weight heparin and the use of intermittent pneumatic compression devices are recommended to prevent DVT.

The pathophysiology of DVT, and later pulmonary embolus, is related to Virchow's triad:

1. Venous stasis from decreased blood flow, decreased muscular activity, and external pressure on the deep veins
2. Vascular damage or concomitant pathological state
3. Hypercoagulability[34]

The nurse assesses for signs and symptoms of DVT on a regular basis. These include the presence of Homans' sign (calf pain on dorsiflexion of the foot), swelling of the affected area, tachycardia, fever, and distal skin color and temperature changes. If these signs or symptoms are found, they should be reported immediately. Sometimes an acute pulmonary embolus is the first indication of DVT.

Pulmonary Embolus

A pulmonary embolus occurs when a blood clot dislodges from the vein, travels through the heart, and lodges in the pulmonary artery, obstructing blood flow. Sudden onset of dyspnea is the classic sign of a pulmonary embolus, but signs and symptoms vary, depending on the size of the clot and the number of vessels occluded. Signs and symptoms may include a decline in oxygenation, substernal chest pain, hypovolemic relative shock, tachypnea, shortness of breath, anxiety, a feeling of impending doom, a low-grade fever, an altered level of consciousness, and a pale, dusky, or cyanotic skin color.

Fat Embolism Syndrome

Fat emboli are fat globules in the lung tissue and peripheral circulation after a long bone fracture or major trauma. Fat emboli may or may not cause systemic symptoms. Fat embolism syndrome is a serious (but rare) manifestation of fat emboli that involves progressive respiratory insufficiency, thrombocytopenia, and a decrease in mental status. It usually occurs within 72 hours of injury. Clinical indications of this syndrome include tachypnea, dyspnea, cyanosis, tachycardia, and fever.[34] Nurses should be aware of the potential for fat embolism syndrome and monitor the patient for hypoxemia with pulse oximetry. The patient's neurological status is also monitored for signs of a decreasing mental status.

MAXILLOFACIAL TRAUMA

Despite laws that mandate lower speed limits and the use of air bags and seat belts, the incidence of maxillofacial trauma remains high because the face is unprotected during rapid deceleration.[35-37] The degree of maxillofacial injury is directly related to the force at impact when the face makes contact with a stationary object. As the force increases, the amount of energy that is dispersed increases, causing an increase in injury. Penetrating injury is less common than blunt injury in patients with maxillofacial trauma.

As with any trauma patient, initial management priorities remain airway, breathing, and circulation. The trauma team cannot be distracted from these priorities by obvious deformities that may be associated with maxillofacial injuries. Maxillofacial trauma can cause airway obstruction and death if airway and breathing are not adequately and urgently established. When the primary survey is completed, an adequate assessment of the maxillofacial injuries is performed. Figure 55-7 shows diagnosis of maxillae fractures according to Le Fort's classification.

When assessing for maxillofacial injuries, the nurse assesses soft tissues as well as bony structures. The nurse inspects the face for symmetry and then palpates systematically to observe for any movement of bony structures. Cranial nerves are assessed. Often, maxillofacial injuries coincide with head injuries, reinforcing the importance of a thorough neurological examination (see Chapter 33). Any midface fractures that communicate through the orbit require a thorough ocular assessment and frequent reassessment.

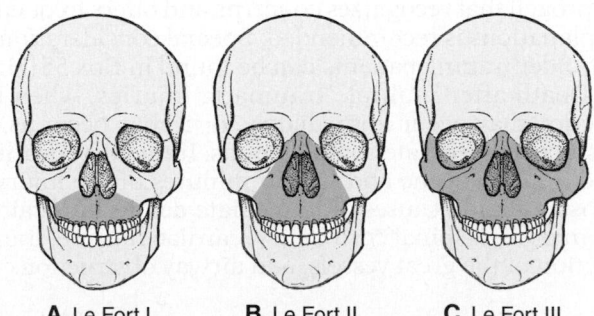

A. Le Fort I   **B.** Le Fort II   **C.** Le Fort III

Figure 55-7 • Le Fort fractures. **A:** Le Fort I: Transverse disarticulation of the maxillary dentoalveolar process from the remaining basal bone of maxilla and midface. **B:** Le Fort II: Pyramidal fracture involving entire maxilla and nasal complex. **C:** Le Fort III: Complete craniofacial-midface disassociation. (Courtesy of Neil O. Hardy, Westpoint, Conn.)

Most maxillofacial injuries involve the soft tissue. In any soft tissue injury, there is potential for contamination. Therefore, each patient's immunization to tetanus is assessed. If needed, a tetanus booster is given. All wounds are assessed for dirt, grease, particles, and other contaminants. Many wounds require an operation for washout to débride the tissue and clean the area. These injuries are usually not life-threatening and are treated in the appropriate order. However, even a small abrasion to a person's face can lead to a lifetime of disfigurement; therefore, all injuries must be attended to appropriately.

As stated earlier, in any type of trauma, but especially in maxillofacial trauma when the patient's airway may be compromised, it is imperative to assess and maintain an adequate airway for the patient continuously. Loss of an artificial airway (e.g., inadvertent removal of the endotracheal tube) can be life-threatening because of soft tissue swelling. It is also essential to assess for and treat hypovolemia secondary to hemorrhage from facial arteries. Epistaxis may also occur with any fracture that communicates with the nose. The nurse continuously assesses the patient's neurological status and reports any abnormalities. The patient's pain and anxiety must be assessed and treated. Many patients with maxillofacial injuries are robbed of their senses. They may be unable to see, smell, taste, or speak secondary to their injury. This is an anxiety-provoking situation; patients require continuous reassurance and medication as necessary. Many maxillofacial injuries require multiple surgeries before the patient is definitively treated.

• Complications of Multiple Trauma

Complications associated with multiple trauma are numerous (Box 55-10). Because most trauma patients are in the ICU when these complications develop, the nurse plays an essential role in detecting, preventing, and treating these sequelae.

The unexpected nature of trauma tends to amplify fear and anxiety. Therefore, nursing care must also provide psychosocial support for the seriously injured patient and his or her family. A multidisciplinary approach that recognizes concerns and offers frequent explanations is recommended. Special considerations for older trauma patients can be found in Box 55-11.

Death after multiple traumatic injuries, when it occurs, may occur immediately, or it may occur as a result of early or late complications. Immediate deaths occur at the scene and within minutes of the injury. Most common causes of immediate deaths are brainstem or high spinal cord injury, cardiac rupture, transection of the great vessels, and airway obstruction.

EARLY COMPLICATIONS

Severe head injuries and hemorrhage are the early complications of multiple trauma most often responsible for causing death within hours of the injury, usually in the emergency department or operating

Box 55-10 • RED FLAG: Delayed Complications of Multiple Trauma

Hematologic
- Hemorrhage, coagulopathy, disseminated intravascular coagulation (DIC)

Cardiac
- Dysrhythmia, heart failure, ventricular aneurysm

Pulmonary
- Atelectasis, pneumonia, emboli (fat or thrombotic), acute respiratory distress syndrome (ARDS)

Gastrointestinal
- Peritonitis, adynamic ileus, mechanical bowel obstruction, acalculous cholecystitis, anastomotic leak, fistula, bleeding

Hepatic
- Liver abscess, liver failure

Renal
- Hypertension, myoglobinuria, renal failure

Orthopedic
- Compartment syndrome

Skin
- Wound infection, dehiscence, skin breakdown

Systemic
- Sepsis

room. Often, death at this stage can be prevented with quick assessment, resuscitation, and management of injuries.

Management of head injuries is discussed in Chapter 36. To prevent exsanguination, hemorrhage must be controlled and volume resuscitation begun with the infusion of crystalloids and blood. Patients may require emergent surgical ligation or packing, or embolization by angiography. Massive hemorrhage complicated by hypothermia, metabolic acidosis, and coagulopathy is highly lethal.

LATE COMPLICATIONS

Late complications of multiple trauma include hypovolemic shock, infection and septic shock, ARDS, and multiple organ dysfunction syndrome (MODS).

Hypovolemic Shock

Massive hemorrhage or continued bleeding because of incomplete hemostasis or an undiagnosed injury can lead to hypovolemic shock and eventually decreased organ perfusion. The various organs respond differently to the decrease in perfusion caused by hypovolemia. Multiple blood transfusions are often necessary, further increasing the likelihood of ARDS and MODS.

Infection and Septic Shock

Another frequent and potentially serious complication of multiple trauma is infection. The risk for infection

Box 55-11 • CONSIDERATIONS FOR THE OLDER PATIENT: Trauma

- Trauma is the seventh most frequent cause of death among the elderly.
- The older person is injured less frequently than the younger person; however, when an older person does sustain injuries, the injuries are more likely to be life-threatening.
- The injuries occurring in the elderly population tend to be less severe but are associated with a greater risk for death.
- Falls are the most prominent cause of trauma in the older person.
- Constant monitoring is essential with the older trauma patient.
- Providers should have a decreased threshold for invasive monitoring with an elderly patient, secondary to predisposing conditions and past medical history.
- Management considerations are as follows:
    Consider cervical osteoarthritis when intubation is necessary.
    Pain management should be more local if possible (e.g., epidural catheter, nerve block).
    Fluid management should be done cautiously. Older adults require adequate rapid fluid replacement without excess. Consider a pulmonary artery or central venous pressure line for guidance in fluid replacement.
    Older adults tend to become hypothermic more quickly than younger people. Use warm fluid and warming devices as indicated.

Adapted from Atwell SL: Trauma in the elderly. In McQuillan KA, Von Rueden KT, Hartsock RL, et al (eds): Trauma Nursing, 3rd ed. Philadelphia: WB Saunders, 2002, pp 772–787.

is increased after close-range shotgun blasts, high-velocity penetrating injuries, penetrating wounds to the colon, prolonged surgery, multiple blood transfusions, and injury to multiple organs. Other risk factors include advanced age, underlying immunosuppression, and a history of diabetes mellitus.

Infections can range from a minor wound infection to fulminant sepsis syndrome and septic shock. In septic shock, the release of toxins causes dilation of vessels, leading to venous pooling that results in a decreased venous return. Initially, cardiac output increases to compensate for decreased systemic vascular resistance. Eventually, the compensatory mechanisms fail, and cardiac output falls along with blood pressure and organ perfusion (i.e., septic shock).

The source of infection must be found and eradicated to treat sepsis effectively. The nurse must watch for the sometimes subtle indicators of sepsis. Hyperthermia or hypothermia and altered mental status are often present early in the septic process, as well as tachycardia, tachypnea, and an increase in the white blood cell count. These findings should prompt further assessment to detect a possible infectious source.

When sepsis is suspected, cultures are obtained, antibiotics are prescribed, radiological studies are done, and exploratory surgery frequently is performed.

Intra-abdominal abscess is a frequent cause of sepsis. Some abscesses can be drained percutaneously, whereas others require surgery. After the surgical drainage of an abdominal abscess, the incision is left open with drains in place to allow healing and prevent recurrence. Other sources of infection are invasive lines, the urinary tract, and the lungs. Pneumonia is a common cause of sepsis in trauma patients. Risk factors for pneumonia include advanced age, aspiration, underlying pulmonary disease, thoracic or abdominal surgery, and prolonged intubation.

Hemodynamics are altered and metabolic demands are increased during sepsis. The typical patient exhibits elevated cardiac output, decreased systemic vascular resistance, and increased oxygen consumption. Hemodynamics must be supported and a balance between oxygen delivery and oxygen consumption maintained. Research suggests that early nutritional support decreases the development of sepsis and MODS. Enteral feeding should be used whenever possible because it is associated with a lower incidence of sepsis than total parenteral nutrition.

Acute Respiratory Distress Syndrome

ARDS is a local inflammatory response of the capillary-alveolar membrane to systemic up-regulation.[38] It is distinguished by an acute onset of severe hypoxemia accompanied by "characteristic" radiographic changes in the absence of cardiogenic pulmonary edema.[38] ARDS is thought to be the first step on the pathway to death. Because pulmonary physiology is extremely sensitive, the respiratory system is generally the first system to demonstrate that the patient is failing.[38]

Sepsis may predispose the patient to ARDS (see Chapter 27). In addition to sepsis, specific injuries (e.g., head trauma, pulmonary contusion, multiple major fractures), massive blood transfusions, aspiration, and pneumonia can also increase the likelihood of ARDS. With a mortality rate of about 50% to 80%, ARDS is characterized by hypoxemia with shunting, decreased lung compliance, tachypnea, dyspnea, and the appearance of diffuse bilateral pulmonary infiltrates.

Treatment of ARDS is multifaceted. Initially, therapy is aimed at treatment of the primary cause. Fluid and hemodynamic management, management of infection, adequate nutrition, mechanical ventilation, and supportive oxygen delivery are incorporated in the therapeutic regimen.

Systemic Inflammatory Response Syndrome

Systemic inflammatory response syndrome (SIRS) describes a pathophysiologic response to a cascade of events precipitated by shock, which usually occurs after trauma. A controlled inflammatory response takes place designed to heal wounds and ward off infection. Continuous stimulation or severe infection may result in sustained inflammation—SIRS. The result is an imbalance of cellular oxygen supply and demand, causing an oxygen extraction deficit.[8]

Multiple Organ Dysfunction Syndrome

Sixty percent of trauma patients have clinical signs of sepsis without an apparent bacterial source.[8] Many factors have been associated with the development of MODS, including hemorrhage, massive blood transfusion, hypovolemic shock, and sepsis. Characterized by the failure of two or more organs, MODS accounts for many late deaths in trauma patients. Usually, the lungs are the first organs to fail (heralded by the onset of ARDS), followed by the liver, gastrointestinal tract, and kidneys.[39,40]

Liver failure can result from initial damage, vascular compromise, shock, or sepsis. Jaundice is a common indicator of deteriorating liver function, although other causes, such as post-traumatic biliary obstruction, must be ruled out. Liver function tests are diagnostic. Liver failure can lead to a decreased level of consciousness, abnormal clotting study results, and hypoglycemia (see Chapter 41).

Gastrointestinal failure manifests with hemorrhage from stress ulcers requiring blood transfusion. Prophylactic neutralization of gastric acid can minimize the risk for bleeding (see Chapter 41).

Renal failure can be precipitated by a renal injury, ischemia, radiographic contrast material, rhabdomyolysis, hypovolemia (due to hemorrhage, third spacing), or sepsis. Initial signs include increasing blood urea nitrogen and serum creatinine levels. Renal failure may be polyuric or oliguric. Dialysis may be necessary (see Chapter 30).

Cardiovascular failure, DIC, metabolic changes (e.g., hyperglycemia, metabolic acidosis), and central nervous system changes, ranging from confusion to obtundation, also may be evident in MODS (see Chapter 49 for a discussion of DIC).

• Clinical Applicability Challenges

Case Study

Mr. W., a 17-year-old man, is admitted to the trauma resuscitation unit after being involved in an MVC. He was the driver and was wearing his seat belt. His car was broadsided. He was intubated at the scene. On arrival at the emergency department, he is unresponsive, and his vital signs are: blood pressure, 100/70 mm Hg; heart rate, 110 beats/min; and respiratory rate, 12 breaths/minute (on ventilator). Oxygen saturation is 100%.

After the primary and secondary survey and initial radiographs, Mr. W. is taken for a computed tomography scan. At this time, his only apparent injury appears to be a brain injury. He is transferred to the intensive care unit (ICU), where a tertiary survey is completed and managed appropriately according to the brain injury protocol. Despite the efforts taken in the ICU, his intracranial pressure continues to rise. He eventually goes to the operating room for a decompressive craniectomy.

After the operation, the nurse notices that Mr. W.'s ventilator requirements are increasing, his urine output is beginning to decrease, and his abdomen is firm. A bladder pressure of >30 cm H_2O is obtained. This time, because he is not stable, the operating room "comes to him," and a damage-control surgery to treat the abdominal compartment syndrome is performed.

Mr. W.'s myoglobins continue to increase, and increased pressures in all four leg compartments are now noticeable. Four compartment fasciotomies on the patient's legs are performed. He is also placed on dialysis to prevent further renal failure from rhabdomyolysis.

After several weeks in the ICU and rehabilitation, Mr. W. woke up and returned to his baseline (status before the accident).

1. After reviewing this case study, what additional information would be helpful to gather to determine the plan of care for Mr. W.?

2. What expectations would the bedside nurse have when caring for a patient who has just had damage-control surgery?

3. When caring for an intubated patient with a head injury, how does the bedside nurse handle the complication of compartment syndrome?

Review Questions

1. A 45-year-old man presents to the trauma resuscitation unit after a gunshot wound to the abdomen. He has a temperature of 93°F and a pH of 7.15. What is the third condition that may be a sign of death in the trauma patient?
   a. Hypovolemia
   b. Tachycardia
   c. Coagulopathy
   d. Sepsis

2. A woman arrives in the intensive care unit after a 30-foot fall. Initial computed tomography scans reveal multiple orthopedic fractures, including a right humerus fracture, pelvic fracture, and bilateral calcaneus fractures. The patient's chart mentions no other injuries. After assessing the patient, the nurse finds her to be short of breath. After listening to breath sounds, the nurse thinks bowel sounds can be heard in the patient's chest. What is the next step?
   a. Call the physician.
   b. Order an immediate chest radiograph.
   c. Continue to monitor the patient.
   d. Do nothing.

3. A man arrives in the intensive care unit after an operation for abdominal compartment syndrome. This surgery was a damage-control procedure to stop hemorrhaging. What is the next step?
   a. Monitor the patient's vital signs and watch for postoperative bleeding.
   b. Explain the procedure to the patient and family.
   c. Watch for signs of postoperative infection.

d. Continue to resuscitate the patient and continuously monitor the patient for hypothermia, acidosis, and coagulopathy.

4. A man involved in a motor vehicle crash with multiple injuries has been in the intensive care unit for approximately 2 weeks. When doing the morning assessment, the nurse notes that the patient's oxygenation requirement has increased, that he needs more ventilator support, and that his oxygen saturation is decreasing. What complication with this patient should concern the nurse?
   a. Acute respiratory distress syndrome
   b. Deep venous thrombosis
   c. Pulmonary embolism
   d. Fat embolus

5. A 21-year-old woman is admitted to the floor after being assaulted. Her injuries are primarily facial. She has Le Fort's fractures of her face and soft tissue swelling; because her eyes are swollen, she is unable to see. What does the nurse need to provide to this patient?
   a. Stimulation (e.g., lights, noise, TV)
   b. Contact with a social worker
   c. A quiet, safe environment in which the patient feels safe and is able to have her questions answered and concerns addressed
   d. Nothing; the patient is conscious and is able to ask for what she needs

6. A 30-year-old man is involved in a motorcycle crash. Barely conscious, he is intubated secondary to a decrease level of consciousness. He complains of excruciating hip pain. His blood pressure is 90/50 mm Hg, and as his primary survey is completed, his blood pressure is decreasing and his heart rate is increasing without any obvious signs of bleeding. Initial films show a LCIII pelvic fracture. What is the next step?
   a. Continue to monitor the patient because there is no obvious signs of bleeding.
   b. Call orthopedics immediately and notify the operating room of a potential orthopedic surgery.
   c. Call the pain team to adequately medicate this patient for his hip pain.
   d. Increase IV fluid to attempt to correct his blood pressure.

References

1. The American Heritage Dictionary, 2nd ed. Boston: Houghton Mifflin, 1991
2. National Safety Council: Accident Facts, 2000. Chicago: National Safety Council, 2000
3. Richards CF, Mayberry JC: Initial management of the trauma patient. Crit Care Clin 20:1–11, 2004
4. Weigelt JA, Klein JD: Mechanism of injury. In McQuillan KA, Von Rueden KT, Hartsock RL, et al (eds): Trauma Nursing, 3rd ed. Philadelphia, WB Saunders, 2002, pp 149–172
5. Eckert KL: Penetrating and blunt abdominal trauma. Crit Care Nurse Q 28(1):41–59, 2005
6. Salomone JP, Ustin JS, McSwan NE, Feliciano DV: Opinions of trauma practitioners regarding prehospital interventions for critical injured patients. J Trauma 58(3):509–517, 2005
7. American College of Surgeons' Committee on Trauma: Advanced Trauma Life Support: Program for Physicians. Chicago: American College of Surgeons, 1997
8. Kelley DM: Hypovolemic shock an overview. Crit Care Nurse Q 28(1):2–19, 2005
9. Demetriades D, Martin M, Salim A, et al: The effect of trauma center designation and trauma volume on outcome in specific severe injuries. Ann Surg 242(4):512–519, 2005
10. Utter GH, Major RV, Rivara FP, et al: Inclusive trauma systems: Do they improve triage or outcomes of the severely injured? J Trauma 60(3):529–537, 2006
11. Diehl-Oplinger L, Kaminsk MF: Choosing the right fluid to counter hypovolemic shock. Nursing 34(3):52–54, 2004
12. Rizoli SB: Crystalloids and colloids in trauma resuscitation: A brief overview of the current debate. J Trauma 54(5):s82–s88, 2003
13. Soudry E, Stein M: Prehospital management of uncontrolled bleeding in trauma patients: Nearing the light at the end of the tunnel. Isr Med Assoc J 6:486–489, 2004
14. Schreiber MA: Damage control surgery. Crit Care Clin 20:101–118, 2004
15. Salim A, Sangthong B, Martin M, et al: Whole body imaging in blunt multisystem trauma patients without obvious signs of injury: Results of a prospective study. Arch Surg 141(5):468–475, 2006
16. Wanek S, Mayberry JC: Blunt thoracic trauma: Flail chest, pulmonary contusion, and blast injury. Crit Care Clin 20:71–81, 2004
17. Yamamoto L, Schroeder C, Beliveau C: Thoracic trauma the deadly dozen. Crit Care Nurse Q 28(1):22–40, 2005
18. Miller LA: Chest wall, lung and pleural space trauma. Radiol Clin North Am 44:213–224, 2006
19. Schultz JM, Trunkey DD: Blunt cardiac injury. Crit Care Clin 20:57–70, 2004
20. Bansal MK, Maraj S, Chewaproug D, Amanullah A: Myocardial contusion injury: Redefining the diagnostic algorithm. Emerg Med J 22:465–469, 2005
21. Sherwood SF, Hartsock RL: Thoracic injuries. In McQuillan KA, Von Rueden KT, Hartsock RL, et al (eds): Trauma Nursing, 3rd ed. Philadelphia: WB Saunders, 2002, pp 543–590
22. Holdgate A, Dunlop S: Review of branch aortic injuries in blunt chest trauma. Emerg Med Aust 17:49–56, 2005
23. Montonye JM: Abdominal injuries. In McQuillan KA, Von Rueden KT, Hartsock RL, et al (eds): Trauma Nursing, 3rd ed. Philadelphia: WB Saunders, 2002, pp 591–619
24. Todd SR: Critical concepts in abdominal injury. Crit Care Clin 20:119–134, 2004
25. Miller PR, Fabian TC, Croce MA, et al: Improving outcomes following penetrating colon wounds: Application of a clinical pathway. Ann Surg 235(6):775–781, 2002
26. Zhang H, Chen J, Kaiser G, et al: The value of partial splenic autotransplantation in patients with portal hypertension: A prospective randomized study. Arch Surg 137(1):89–93, 2002
27. Walsh C: Musculoskeletal injuries. In McQuillan KA, Von Rueden KT, Hartsock RL, et al (eds): Trauma Nursing, 3rd ed. Philadelphia: WB Saunders, 2002, pp 646–689
28. Frakes MA, Evans T: Major pelvic fractures. Crit Care Nurse 24(2):18–32, 2004
29. Wardle NS, Haddad FS: Pelvic fractures and high energy traumas. Hosp Med 66(7):396–398, 2005
30. Heetveld MJ, Harris I, Schlaphoff G, et al: Hemodynamically unstable pelvic fracture: Recent care and new guidelines. World J Surg 28:904–909, 2004
31. Kataoka Y, Maekawa K, Nishimaki H, et al: Iliac vein injuries in hemodynamically unstable patients with pelvic fracture caused by blunt trauma. J Trauma 58:704–710, 2005
32. Krieg JC, Mohr M, Ellis TJ, et al: Emergent stabilization of pelvic ring injuries by controlled circumferential compression: A clinical trial. J Trauma 59:659–664, 2005

33. Malinoski DJ, Slater MS, Mullins RJ: Crush injury and rhabdomyolysis. Crit Care Clin 20:171–192, 2004

34. Walsh C: Musculoskeletal injuries. In McQuillan KA, Von Rueden KT, Hartsock RL, et al (eds): Trauma Nursing, 3rd ed. Philadelphia: WB Saunders, 2002, pp 646–689

35. Robertson BC, McQuillan KA: Maxillofacial injuries. In McQuillan KA, Von Rueden KT, Hartsock RL, et al (eds): Trauma Nursing, 3rd ed. Philadelphia: WB Saunders, 2002, pp 462–483

36. Cox D, Vincent DG, McGuin G, et al: Effect of restraint systems on maxillofacial injury in frontal motor vehicle collisions. J Oral Maxillofac Surg 62:571–575, 2004

37. Brookes CN: Maxillofacial and ocular injuries in motor vehicle crashes. Ann R Coll Surg Engl 86:149–155, 2004

38. Michaels AJ: Management of post traumatic respiratory failure. Crit Care Clin 20:83–99, 2004

39. Robertson BC, McQuillan KA: Maxillofacial injuries. In McQuillan KA, Von Rueden KT, Hartsock RL, et al (eds): Trauma Nursing, 3rd ed. Philadelphia: WB Saunders, 2002, pp 462–483

40. Khadaroo RG, Marshall JC: ARDS and the multiple organ dysfunction syndrome: Common mechanisms of a common systemic process. Crit Care Clin 18(1):127–141, 2002

Other Selected Readings

Blank-Reid C: A historical review of penetrating abdominal trauma. Crit Care Nurs Clin North Am 18(3):387–402, 2006

Bridges E: Blast injuries: Triage to critical care. Crit Care Nurs Clin North Am 18(3):333–348, 2006

Clements PT, Garzon L, Milliken TF: Survivors' guilt following sudden traumatic loss: Promoting early intervention in the critical care setting. Crit Care Nurs Clin North Am 18(3):359–370, 2006

Day M: What you need to know about facial fractures. ED Insider Fall: 4–9, 2006

DePalma JA, Fedorka P, Simko LC: Quality of life experienced by severely injured trauma survivors. AACN Clin Issues 14(1):54–63, 2003

Epstein CD, Peerless J, Martin J, Malangoni M: Oxygen transport and organ dysfunction in the older trauma patient. Heart Lung 31(5):315–326, 2002

Fort CW: How to combat three deadly trauma complications. Nursing 2003 33(5):58–64, 2003

Frawley PM, Cowan J: Airway pressure release ventilation: The future of trauma ventilatory support? J Trauma Nurs 9(3):75–82, 2002

Gaylord KM: The psychosocial effects of combat: The frequently unseen injury. Crit Care Nurs Clin North Am 18(3):349–358, 2006

Guzzo JL, Bochicchio GV, Napolitano LM, et al: Prediction of outcomes in trauma: Anatomic or physiologic parameters? J Am Coll Surg 201(6):891–897, 2005

Kobziff L: Traumatic pelvic fractures. Orthop Nurs 25(4):235–241, 2006

McCabe S: Substance use and abuse in trauma: Implications for care. Crit Care Nurs Clin North Am 18(3):371–387, 2006

Morse JM, Pooler C: Patient-family-nurse interactions in the trauma-resuscitation room. Am J Crit Care 11(3):240–249, 2002

Pudelek B: Geriatric trauma: Special needs for a special population. AACN Clin Issues 13(1):61–72, 2002

Richmond TS, Thompson HJ, Kauder D, et al: A feasibility study of methodological issues and short-term outcomes in seriously injured older adults. Am J Crit Care 15(2):158–165, 2006

Richmond TS, Kauder D, Hinkle J, Shults J: Early predictors of long-term disability after injury: Am J Crit Care 12(3):197–205, 2003

Thompson HJ, Bourbonniere M: Traumatic injury in the older adult from head to toe. Crit Care Nurs Clin North Am 18(3):419–432, 2006

Wetzel RC, Burns RC: Multiple trauma in children: Critical care overview. Crit Care Med 30(Suppl 11):S486–S477, 2002

Drug Overdose and Poisoning

Eric R. Schuetz • Julie Schuetz

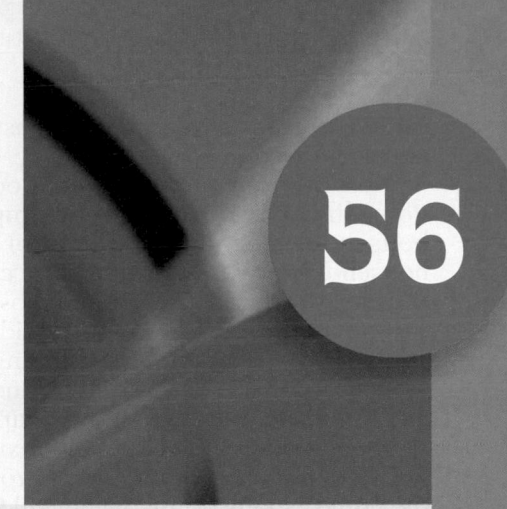

56

Objectives

Based on the content in this chapter, the reader should be able to:

❶ Explain the initial assessment and management of acutely poisoned or overdosed patients.

❷ Describe the groups of symptoms that may help identify the drugs or toxins to which a patient may have been exposed.

❸ Compare and contrast methods used to prevent absorption and enhance elimination of a drug or toxin.

❹ Formulate a plan of care for the poisoned patient.

In 2004, more than 2.4 million exposures to various drugs and toxins were reported to the American Association of Poison Control Centers. Of these exposures, 1,183 resulted in death. The largest age group of human exposures was children younger than 6 years (57.7%); however, the largest age group for fatalities was adults (89.8%).[1] The types of toxic exposure reported to poison control centers are diverse: herbal remedies purchased at health food stores, snake and arthropod envenomations, alcohol or drugs, fumes emitted by faulty furnaces, poisonous plants, and industrial hazardous material spills or releases.

Because of clinical experience and new research information, therapy for toxic exposure changes rapidly. Health care professionals may find it challenging to keep abreast of the most advanced therapy. Fortunately, phone consultation with poison control centers offers rapid access to this information. A local poison control center can be reached nationwide by calling 1-800-222-1222. The services of a local poison control center are a useful resource for both health care professionals and the public. Nurses, pharmacists, and physicians with specialized training in clinical toxicology staff such centers.

This chapter presents general guidelines for the assessment and management of the acutely poisoned or overdosed patient. It lists commonly observed poisonings and contains a collaborative care guide for the patient with cocaine toxicity. The chapter ends with a section discussing prevention through patient teaching.

• The Poisoned or Overdosed Patient

Poisonings and drug overdoses can cause quick physical and mental changes in a person. Bystanders usually are the ones who must initiate care and call a poison control center or emergency number. Commonly observed poisonings or drug overdoses are caused by (but certainly not limited to) acetaminophen, amphetamines, benzodiazepines, carbon monoxide, cocaine, fluorinated hydrocarbons, lysergic acid diethylamide (LSD), methanol, opiates, salicylates, and tricyclic antidepressants. These particular substances and care of the toxic patient exposed to them are described later in the chapter.

POISONING

The most common routes of exposure in poisoning are inhalation, ingestion, and injection. Toxic chemical reactions can compromise cardiovascular, respiratory, central nervous, hepatic, gastrointestinal (GI), and renal systems.

Most exposures to toxic fumes occur in the home. Poisoning may result from the improper mixing of household cleaning products or malfunctioning household appliances that release carbon monoxide. Burning wood, gas, oil, coal, or kerosene also produces carbon monoxide. Carbon monoxide gas is colorless, odorless, tasteless, and nonirritating, which makes it especially dangerous. Prevention and patient teaching are discussed at the end of this chapter.

The ingestion of poisons and toxins occurs in various settings and in different age groups. Poisoning in the home usually occurs when children ingest household cleaners or medicines. Improper storage of these items contributes to such accidents. Plants, pesticides, and paint products are also potential household poisons. Because of mental or visual impairment, illiteracy, or a language barrier, older adults may ingest incorrect amounts of medications. In addition, poisoning may occur in the health care environment when medications are administered improperly.

Similarly, poisoning can also occur in the health care environment when a medication normally given only by the subcutaneous or intramuscular route is given intravenously, or when the incorrect medication is injected. Poisoning by injection can also occur in the setting of substance abuse, as when a heroin addict inadvertently injects bleach or too much heroin.

SUBSTANCE ABUSE AND OVERDOSE

Admission of most poisoned patients to a critical care unit is for an intentional or suspected suicidal overdose. As part of their histories, these patients frequently have mental illness, substance abuse problems, or both. Often, withdrawal symptoms and syndromes complicate the assessment of potential toxidromes. A toxidrome is a group of signs and symptoms (syndrome) associated with overdose or exposure to a particular category of drugs and toxins.

Commonly abused substances are nicotine, alcohol, heroin, marijuana, narcotic analgesics, amphetamines, benzodiazepines, and cocaine. Some children and adolescents turn to common household substances because they are readily available. People who attempt to manage stress through substance abuse require a comprehensive treatment program to address their coping and adaptation problems.

• Assessment

A health care facility's systematic approach to the assessment of the poisoned or overdosed patient includes performing triage, obtaining the patient's history, performing a physical examination, and conducting laboratory studies.

TRIAGE

Although some type of triage usually is performed at the scene or by an emergency response team, triage is always the first step performed in the emergency department. Two essential questions to be considered in the triage evaluation are:

1. Is the patient's life in immediate danger?
2. Is the patient's life in potential danger?

If the patient's life is in immediate danger, the goals of immediate treatment are patient stabilization and evaluation and management of airway, breathing, and circulation (ABCs).

HISTORY

A history of the patient's exposure provides a framework for managing the poisoning or overdose. Key points include identifying the drugs or toxins, the time and duration of the exposure, first aid treatment given before arrival at the hospital, allergies, and any underlying disease processes or related injuries. This information may be obtained from the patient, family members, friends, rescuers, or bystanders. In some cases, family or police may need to search the patient's home for clues. Clothing and personal effects may supply additional information.

PHYSICAL EXAMINATION

A quick but thorough physical examination is essential. Preliminary examination results lead to the in-depth evaluation and serial assessment of affected systems (actual or anticipated). As noted previously, a toxidrome is a group of signs and symptoms associated with overdose or exposure to a particular category of drugs and toxins. Recognizing the presence of a toxidrome may help identify the toxins or drugs to which the patent was exposed, and the crucial body systems that may be involved. Table 56-1 lists four common toxidromes with their signs and symptoms and common causes.

LABORATORY STUDIES

Relevant clinical laboratory data are vital to the assessment of the poisoned or overdosed patient. Tests that provide clues to the agents taken by the patient include electrolytes, hepatic function, urinalysis, electrocardiography, and serum osmolality tests. A serum level measurement of acetaminophen is obtained in all patients who have overdosed because acetaminophen is a component of many prescription and over-the-counter preparations. In the event of an acetaminophen overdose, the result of the level is plotted against the time since ingestion on the Rumack-Matthew nomogram (Fig. 56-1). Serum level measurements are also available for carbamazepine, iron, ethanol, lithium, aspirin, and valproic acid and may be obtained if these agents are suspected in an overdose.

• Management

Management of the poisoned or overdosed patient seeks to prevent absorption of and further exposure to the agent. After triage to determine the status of

Table 56-1 • Toxidromes

Toxidrome	Signs/Symptoms	Common Causes
Anticholinergic	Delirium; dry, flushed skin; dilated pupils; elevated temperature; decreased bowel sounds; urinary retention; tachycardia	Antihistamines, atropine, Jimson weed
Cholinergic	Excessive salivation, lacrimation, urination, diarrhea, and emesis; diaphoresis, bronchorrhea, bradycardia, fasciculations, central nervous system depression, constricted pupils	Organophosphate insecticides (e.g., Malathion, Diazinon); carbamate insecticide (e.g., carbaryl, propoxur)
Opioid	Central nervous system depression, respiratory depression, constricted pupils, hypotension, hypothermia	Opiates (e.g., codeine, morphine, propoxyphene, heroin), diphenoxylate (e.g., diphenoxylate/atropine sulfate [Lomotil])
Sympathomimetic	Agitation, tachycardia, hypertension, seizures, metabolic acidosis	Amphetamines, cocaine, theophylline, caffeine

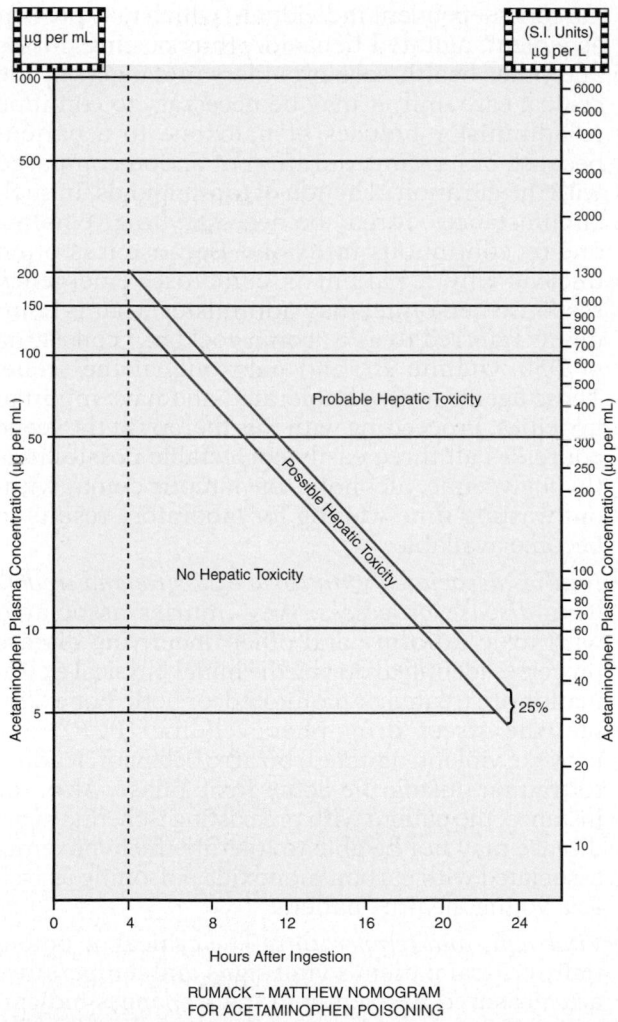

RUMACK – MATTHEW NOMOGRAM
FOR ACETAMINOPHEN POISONING

CAUTION FOR USE OF THIS CHART
1) The time coordinates refer to time of ingestion.
2) Serum levels drawn before 4 hours may not represent peak levels.
3) The graph should be used only in relation to a single acute ingestion.
4) The lower solid line is 25% below the standard nomogram and is included to allow for possible errors in acetaminophen plasma assays and estimated time from ingestion of an overdose.

Figure 56-1 • Semilogarithmic plot of plasma acetaminophen levels versus time. (From Rumack BH, Matthew HJ: Acetaminophen poisoning and toxicity. Pediatrics 55:871–876, 1975.)

the patient's ABCs, the patient must be stabilized. Treatment begins with first aid at the scene and continues in the emergency department and often in the intensive care unit (ICU). Advanced general management involves further steps to prevent absorption and enhance elimination of the agent. For instance, antidotes, antivenins, or antitoxins may be administered. The health care team must further support vital functions and monitor and treat multisystem effects. Patient and family teaching to prevent future exposures is another part of the nurse's management strategy. Nursing diagnoses for the poisoned or overdosed patient are listed in Box 56-1.

STABILIZATION

Stabilization of patients includes performing the steps summarized in Box 56-2, which are also discussed in the following list:

▶ *Airway.* Nasotracheal or endotracheal intubation may be necessary to adequately maintain and protect the patient's airway.

▶ *Breathing.* Mechanical ventilation may be necessary to support the patient. Many drugs and toxins,

Box 56-1 Examples of Nursing Diagnoses and Collaborative Problems for the Poisoned or Overdosed Patient

- Ineffective Breathing patterns related to overdose of medication
- Decreased Cardiac Output related to ingestion of poisonous substance
- Impaired Verbal Communication related to overdose of medication
- Acute Confusion related to overdose of medication.
- Impaired Gas Exchange related to carbon monoxide poisoning
- Swallowing, Impaired related to poisoning
- Dysrhythmias related to overdose of medication

> **Box 56-2 • NURSING INTERVENTIONS for the Stabilization of the Poisoned or Overdosed Patient**
>
> - Assess, establish, and maintain the airway.
> - Evaluate respiratory effort.
> - Maintain adequate circulation.
> - Monitor cardiac function.
> - Maintain or correct acid–base balance and electrolyte homeostasis.
>
> - Assess mentation.
> - Identify injuries and disease processes that increase risk.
> - Measure vital signs and temperature frequently to track changes.

such as heroin, depress the respiratory drive. Patients therefore may require ventilator assistance until the drugs or toxins are eliminated from the body.

▶ *Circulation.* Complications range from shock caused by fluid loss to fluid overload. These are often related to the patient's hydration status and the ability of the cardiovascular system to adjust to drug- or toxin-induced changes. For example, rattlesnake envenomations often cause third-spacing of fluid into the area of the bite, leading to intravascular hypovolemia. As a consequence, the patient develops hypotension, which usually responds to aggressive intravenous (IV) fluid therapy. Some toxic drug ingestions impair myocardial contractility, and fluid overload may result because of the heart's inability to pump effectively. In these cases, fluid balance needs to be carefully controlled. Invasive monitoring (e.g., central venous pressure, pulmonary artery catheter, Foley catheter with urometer) and drug therapy may be necessary to prevent or minimize complications such as pulmonary edema.

▶ *Cardiac function.* Many drugs and toxins cause cardiac conduction delays and dysrhythmias. The history of the drugs or toxins involved may not be reliable or even known, especially when patients are found unconscious or have attempted suicide. In these cases, continuous cardiac monitoring and 12-lead electrocardiograms help detect cardiotoxic effects.

▶ *Acid–base balance and electrolyte homeostasis.* Electrolyte abnormalities and metabolic acidosis frequently occur, which may require serial measurements of electrolytes and arterial blood gases (ABGs), as well as other specific laboratory tests. For example, serial measurements of electrolytes, ABGs, and salicylate levels are the means of evaluating aspirin toxicity. Aspirin, in large ingestions, may form a solid mass in the GI tract, called a concretion, instead of breaking apart and dissolving. As a result, absorption is delayed, and the development of toxic effects, such as hypokalemia, metabolic acidosis, and respiratory alkalosis, may not be observed for several hours.

▶ *Mentation.* Many factors can affect the patient's mental status. Hypoglycemia and hypoxemia are two that can be life-threatening but easily addressed by administering oxygen and IV dextrose until laboratory results are available. Patients with chronic alcoholism also are at special risk for Wernicke-Korsakoff syndrome, which is characterized by ataxia and altered mentation. Early IV or intramuscular administration of thiamine (vitamin B$_1$) may prevent exacerbation of the syndrome. Naloxone (Narcan) is a narcotic antagonist that reverses narcotic-induced central nervous system (CNS) and respiratory depression. It is often initially given to comatose patients. However, it must be given cautiously because it can precipitate withdrawal in narcotic-dependent individuals, which may present as violent, agitated behavior, thus placing nurses and other health care providers in danger. In the critical care unit, it may be necessary to continue to administer boluses of naloxone to a patient because of its short duration of action compared with the duration of action of most opioids. In such circumstances, it may be necessary to give naloxone by continuous infusion.[2] Because it is often unclear why a patient is comatose, emergency response personnel may administer what is commonly referred to as a "coma cocktail," consisting of D50, vitamin B$_1$, and naloxone, at the scene. These agents are well tolerated and have minimal toxicities. Proceeding with this therapy at the scene addresses all three easily correctable possibilities (hypoglycemic, alcoholic, or narcotic coma) without wasting time waiting for laboratory results to become available.

▶ *Injuries associated with toxic exposure and underlying disease processes.* Any injuries associated with toxic exposure and other underlying disease processes identified during the initial physical examination are treated or monitored, or both. For example, the street drug phencyclidine (PCP) may provoke violent, agitated, bizarre behavior, leading to trauma during the acute toxic phase. Also, for instance, the patient with preexisting ischemic heart disease may not be able to tolerate the hypoxemia associated with carbon monoxide poisoning as well as a young, healthy patient.

▶ *Vital signs and temperature.* The critical or potentially critical patient's vital signs and temperature are measured frequently to track changes indicating additional problems.

INITIAL DECONTAMINATION

First aid may be given by a bystander, health care provider, or emergency response team, or in the emergency department. The physicochemical properties of the agent and the amount, route, and exposure time help determine the type and extent of management required. Decontamination methods for ocular, dermal, inhalation, and ingestion exposures follow.

Ocular Exposure

Many substances can accidentally splash into the eyes. When this happens, the eyes must be flushed to remove the agent. Immediate irrigation with lukewarm water or normal saline is recommended. Continuous flooding of the eyes with a large glass of water or low-pressure shower should be done for 15 minutes. The patient should blink the eyes open and closed during the irrigation. If necessary, the pH of the eyes can be tested. If the pH is abnormal, irrigation should continue until the pH normalizes. An ophthalmologic examination is needed if ocular irritation or visual disturbance persists after irrigation.

Dermal Exposure

When dermal exposure occurs, the patient should flood the skin with lukewarm water for 15 to 30 minutes. Most companies that produce or use chemical agents have showers for this purpose. The patient should remove any clothing that may have been contaminated. After standing under running water for the allotted time, the patient should then wash the area gently with soap and water and rinse thoroughly.

Some toxins may require further decontamination. For example, three separate soap-and-water washings or showers are recommended to decontaminate organophosphate pesticides (e.g., Malathion or Diazinon). Protective clothing should be worn to reduce the risk for toxicity while handling contaminated clothing or assisting with skin decontamination.

Although it may seem logical to apply an acid to neutralize a base exposure and a base to neutralize an acid exposure, this can be quite dangerous. Neutralization is the reaction between an acid and a base in which the H^+ of the acid and the OH^- of the base react to produce H_2O (water) and heat. The heat produced by this reaction is significant enough to cause burns. Therefore, neutralizing the skin after a dermal exposure is not recommended.

Inhalation Exposure

A person who has experienced an inhalation exposure should be moved to fresh air as quickly as possible. The responder must also protect himself or herself from the airborne toxin. Further evaluation is needed if the patient experiences respiratory irritation or shortness of breath. Large-scale exposures or those that occur at the workplace may require consultation with a HAZMAT team, a group of individuals specially trained to manage exposures to hazardous materials.

Ingestion Exposure

Milk or water dilutes ingested irritants such as bleach or caustics such as drain cleaner. After such an inges-tion, adults should drink 8 ounces of milk or water, and children should drink 2 to 8 ounces (based on their size). Further evaluation is necessary after dilution if there is mucosal irritation or burns. Because of the risk for aspiration, ingestions should not be diluted when they are accompanied by seizures, depressed mental status, or loss of the gag reflex. Again, neutralization is not used because of the risk for thermal burn.

GASTROINTESTINAL DECONTAMINATION

Gastric lavage, adsorbents, cathartics, and whole-bowel irrigation are used to prevent absorption of, and forestall toxicity from, almost all drugs and a variety of toxins. The American Academy of Pediatrics no longer recommends the use of emetics (such as syrup of ipecac) for GI decontamination.

Gastric Lavage

Gastric lavage is a method of GI decontamination. Fluid (usually normal saline) is introduced into the stomach through a large-bore orogastric tube and then drained in an attempt to reclaim part of the ingested agent before it is absorbed. A small-bore nasogastric tube is ineffective for lavage because particulate matter, such as tablets or capsules, is too large to pass through the tube. If airway protection is necessary, the patient should be intubated before lavage begins.

As noted, a large-bore orogastric tube (36- to 40-French in adults and 16- to 28-French in children) is used to evacuate particulate matter, including whole tablets and capsules. For the lavage, the patient is positioned in the left lateral decubitus position, with the head lower than the feet. Before beginning, the tube should be coated with a jelly lubricant such as hydroxyethylcellulose. The position of the tube must be confirmed after passing, either by aspirating and checking the pH of the aspirate, or by insufflation of air, while listening over the stomach. The lavage is accomplished by attaching a funnel or syringe to the end of the tube and instilling aliquots of 150 to 200 mL (50 to 100 mL in children) of 100°F (38°C) saline into the stomach. Placing the funnel and tube below the patient allows the fluid to return by gravity. This procedure is repeated until clear fluid returns or 2 L of fluid has been used. The contents of the stomach can then be collected for drug or toxin identification.

Complications of gastric lavage include esophageal perforation, pulmonary aspiration, electrolyte imbalance, tension pneumothorax, and hypothermia (when cold lavage solutions are used). Lavage is contraindicated in cases of ingestion of caustics or hydrocarbons with a high aspiration potential. Because of the associated risks and the lack of clear evidence supporting its use, gastric lavage should be used only if the patient has ingested a life-threatening amount of a substance and the procedure is undertaken within an hour of the ingestion.[3]

Adsorbents

An adsorbent is a solid substance that has the ability to attract and hold another substance to its surface ("to adsorb"). Activated charcoal is an effective nonspecific adsorbent of many drugs and toxins. Activated charcoal adsorbs, or traps, the drug or toxin to its large surface area and prevents absorption from the GI tract. Box 56-3 identifies both drugs and toxins that are adsorbed effectively by activated charcoal and those not adsorbed effectively.

Activated charcoal is a fine, black powder that is given as a slurry with water, either orally or by nasogastric or orogastric tube, as soon as possible after the ingestion. Commercially available activated charcoal products may be mixed with 70% sorbitol to decrease grittiness, increase palatability, and serve as a cathartic. The usual dose that is given is one 50-g bottle. Administration of more than one dose is controversial and usually is limited to overdoses of large quantities of aspirin, valproic acid, and theophylline. Activated charcoal is used cautiously in patients with diminished bowel sounds and is contraindicated in patients with bowel obstruction.[3]

Cathartics

A cathartic is a substance that causes or promotes bowel movements. The use of cathartics alone in the management of poisoning is not an acceptable means of GI decontamination. In theory, cathartics decrease the absorption of drugs and toxins by speeding their passage through the GI tract, thereby limiting their contact with mucosal surfaces. Magnesium citrate or 70% sorbitol often is used. Currently, however, there is no clinical evidence that shows that a cathartic can reduce the bioavailability of drugs or improve the outcome of poisoned patients.[3] Data regarding the effectiveness of mixing cathartics with activated charcoal are not yet available. Clearly, more research needs to be done in this area of clinical practice.[3]

Whole-Bowel Irrigation

The goal of whole-bowel irrigation is to give large volumes of a balanced electrolyte solution rapidly (1 to 2 L/hour) to flush the patient's bowel mechanically without creating electrolyte disturbances. Used as a bowel preparation for colonoscopy, it is also used as a GI decontamination procedure for patients who have ingested bags or vials of narcotics to avoid arrest, for drug smugglers who pack their GI tracts with narcotics (either orally or rectally), and for patients who have overdosed on modified-release pharmaceuticals.

Commercial products used in whole-bowel irrigation include GoLYTELY and Colyte. Both products are dispensed as powders and are given after adding water. Whole-bowel irrigation is contraindicated in the patient with bowel obstruction or perforation.[3]

ENHANCED ELIMINATION OF THE DRUG OR TOXIN

The pharmacological and kinetic characteristics of a drug or toxin greatly influence the severity and length of the clinical course in the acutely poisoned or overdosed patient. The absorption rate, body distribution, metabolism, and elimination must be considered when choosing methods to eliminate the drug or toxin from the body. There are six methods of enhanced elimination:

1. Multiple-dose activated charcoal
2. Alteration of urine pH
3. Hemodialysis
4. Hemoperfusion
5. Chelation
6. Hyperbaric oxygenation (HBO) therapy

Multiple-Dose Activated Charcoal

Administering multiple doses of activated charcoal can result in greater adsorption of certain drugs such as aspirin, valproic acid, and theophylline. Multiple-dose activated charcoal is given orally, by nasogastric tube, or by orogastric tube every 2 to 6 hours. Complications of multiple-dose activated charcoal include aspiration and bowel obstruction.[3]

Alteration of Urine pH

Alkalinizing the patient's urine enhances excretion of drugs that are weak acids by increasing the amount of ionized drug in the urine. This form of enhanced elimination is also termed ion trapping. The urine is

---

Box 56-3 • Adsorption of Drugs and Toxins by Activated Charcoal

Drugs and Toxins Well Adsorbed by Activated Charcoal
- Acetaminophen
- Amphetamines
- Antihistamines
- Aspirin
- Barbiturates
- Benzodiazepines
- β blockers
- Calcium channel blockers
- Cocaine
- Opioids
- Phenytoin
- Theophylline
- Valproic acid

Drugs and Toxins Not Well Adsorbed by Activated Charcoal
- Acids
- Alkalis
- Alcohols
- Iron
- Lithium
- Metals

alkalinized by administering a continuous IV infusion of 1 to 3 ampules of sodium bicarbonate per 1 liter of fluid. Urine alkalinization is frequently used in patients experiencing a salicylate overdose. Complications of alkalinization include cerebral or pulmonary edema and electrolyte imbalances.

Urine acidification is no longer recommended because of low drug clearance and the risk for complications such as rhabdomyolysis.

Hemodialysis

Hemodialysis is the process of altering the solute composition of blood by removing it from an artery, diffusing it across a semipermeable membrane (between the blood and a salt solution), then returning it into a vein. It is used in moderate to severe intoxications to remove a drug or toxin rapidly when more conservative methods (e.g., gastric lavage, activated charcoal, antidotes) have failed or in patients with decreased renal function. Hemodialysis requires consultation with a nephrologist and specially trained nurses to perform the procedure and monitor the patient. Low molecular weight, low protein binding, and water solubility are factors that make a drug or toxin suitable for hemodialysis. Drugs and toxins that may be removed by hemodialysis include ethylene glycol (commonly found in antifreeze), methanol, lithium, salicylates, and theophylline.[4]

Hemoperfusion

Hemoperfusion removes drugs and toxins from the patient's blood by pumping the blood through a cartridge of adsorbent material, such as activated charcoal. An advantage of hemoperfusion over hemodialysis is that the total surface area of the dialyzing membrane is much greater with the hemoperfusion cartridges. As in hemodialysis, drugs that have high tissue-binding characteristics and a large volume distributed outside the circulation are not good candidates for hemoperfusion because little drug is found in the blood. Although rarely used in the poisoned and overdosed population, hemoperfusion has been used successfully in patients experiencing a theophylline overdose.[4]

Chelation

Chelation involves the use of binding agents to remove toxic levels of metals from the body, such as mercury, lead, iron, and arsenic. Examples of chelating agents are dimercaprol (BAL in oil), calcium disodium edetate (EDTA), succimer (DMSA), and deferoxamine. Concerns about the toxicity of the chelators; their tissue distribution characteristics; and the stability, distribution, and elimination of the chelator–metal complex make chelation a complicated procedure.

Hyperbaric Oxygenation Therapy

In HBO therapy, oxygen is administered to a patient in an enclosed chamber at a pressure greater than the pressure at sea level (e.g., 1 atmosphere absolute).

This therapy has been used in carbon monoxide and methylene chloride poisonings (methylene chloride is metabolized to carbon monoxide in the body). The result is enhanced elimination of carbon monoxide: in room air, the half-life of carbon monoxide is 5 to 6 hours; in 100% oxygen, it is 90 minutes; and in an HBO chamber, it is 20 minutes. Another use of HBO therapy is the treatment of diving sickness (the "bends"). However, the small number of HBO chambers and lack of around-the-clock staffing limit the wide use of this therapy.

Complications of HBO therapy include pressure-related otalgia, sinus pain, tooth pain, and tympanic membrane rupture. Confinement anxiety, convulsions, and tension pneumothorax also have been observed in patients receiving HBO therapy.[5]

ANTAGONISTS, ANTITOXINS, AND ANTIVENINS

In pharmacology, an antagonist is a substance that counteracts the action of another drug. Although the general public often believes there is an antidote for every drug or toxin, the opposite is closer to the truth. There are, in fact, very few antidotes. Antidotes for specific intoxications are listed in Table 56-2.

Antitoxins neutralize a toxin. For instance, botulism antitoxin trivalent (equine) is available through the Centers for Disease Control and Prevention to counteract the effects of botulism.

Antivenins are antitoxins that neutralize the venom of the offending snake or spider. There are several antitoxins; each is active against a specific venom. For example, antivenin Crotalidae polyvalent (equine) is active against venoms of the family Crotalidae, which are pit viper snakes native to North, Central, and South America. Because this agent is derived from horse serum (and therefore recognized as "foreign" by the human immune system), significant side effects, such as anaphylactic or anaphylactoid reactions, are common. Recently approved by the U.S. Food and Drug Administration (FDA) is Crotalidae polyvalent immune Fab (CroFab), a product that is produced using a purification process that removes the Fc fragment and leaves only the Fab fragments of the immunoglobulins. Typically, this process results in a product that causes fewer reactions in humans. Antivenin (*Latrodectus mactans*; equine) is available for black widow spider bites as well as for envenomations by the eastern and Texas coral snake (*Micrurus fulvius*; equine). However, there are many venomous snakes and spiders for which no antivenin exists. Envenomation from one of these species is treated with symptomatic and supportive care.[8]

CONTINUOUS PATIENT MONITORING

Seriously poisoned or overdosed patients may require continued monitoring for hours or days after exposure. Physical examination, the use of diagnostic tools, and careful assessment of clinical signs and symptoms provide information about the patient's progress and

Table 56-2 • Antidotes for Specific Drugs and Toxins	
Drug/Toxin	**Antidote**
Acetaminophen	N-acetylcysteine (Mucomyst [PO], Acetadote [IV])
Anticholinergics	Physostigmine (Antilirium)
Benzodiazepines	Flumazenil (Romazicon)
β-blocking agents	Glucagon
Calcium channel blockers	Glucagon, calcium chloride
Carbon monoxide	Oxygen
Cyanide	Lilly Cyanide Antidote Kit: amyl nitrite, sodium nitrite, and sodium thiosulfate
Digoxin	Digoxin-specific fab fragments (Digibind)
Ethylene glycol	Fomepizole (Antizol)[6], ethanol
Methanol	Fomepizole (Antizol)[7], ethanol
Nitrites	Methylene blue
Opioids	Naloxone (Narcan)
Organophosphate insecticides	Atropine, pralidoxime

direct medical and nursing management. Diagnostic tools include the following:

▶ *Electrocardiography.* Electrocardiography can provide evidence of drugs causing dysrhythmias or conduction delays (e.g., tricyclic antidepressants).

▶ *Radiology.* Many substances are radiopaque, or can be visualized using a contrast-enhanced computed tomography (CT) scan (e.g., heavy metals, button batteries, some modified-release tablets or capsules, aspirin concretions, cocaine or heroin containers). Chest radiographs provide evidence of aspiration and pulmonary edema.

▶ *Electrolytes, ABGs, and other laboratory tests.* Acute poisoning can cause an imbalance in a patient's electrolyte levels, including sodium, potassium, chloride, carbon dioxide content, magnesium, and calcium. Signs of inadequate ventilation or oxygenation include cyanosis, tachycardia, hypoventilation, intercostal muscle retractions, and altered mental status. Such signs should be evaluated by pulse oximetry and ABG measurements. Seriously poisoned patients require routine screening of electrolytes, ABGs, creatinine, and glucose; complete blood count; and urinalysis.

▶ *Anion gap.* The anion gap is a simple, cost-effective tool that uses common serum measurements, such as sodium, chloride, and bicarbonate, to help evaluate the poisoned patient for certain drugs or toxins. The anion gap represents the difference between unmeasured anions and cations in the blood. Using measured anions and a cation, the anion gap is calculated using the following formula:

$$[Na] - ([Cl] + [HCO_3]) = \text{anion gap}$$

The normal value for the anion gap is approximately 8 to 16 mEq/L. An anion gap that exceeds the upper normal value can indicate metabolic acidosis caused by an accumulation of acids in the blood. Drugs, toxins, or medical conditions that can produce an elevated anion gap include iron, isoniazid (INH), lithium, lactate, carbon monoxide, cyanide, toluene, methanol, metformin, ethanol, ethylene glycol, salicylates, hydrogen sulfide, strychnine, diabetic ketoacidosis, uremia, seizures, and starvation. Although these substances and processes can cause an elevated anion gap, a normal anion gap alone does not preclude a toxic exposure.

▶ *Osmolal gap.* The osmolal gap is the difference between the measured osmolality (using the freezing point depression method) and the calculated osmolality. The calculated osmolality is derived using laboratory values for the major osmotically active substances in the serum, such as sodium, glucose, and blood urea nitrogen (BUN). Like the anion gap, it is a simple, cost-effective tool for evaluating the poisoned patient for certain drugs or toxins. The calculated osmolality (using serum electrolyte values) is defined as follows:

$$2(Na^+) + \frac{glucose}{18} + \frac{BUN}{2.8} = \text{calculated osmolality}$$

The osmolal gap is then calculated as follows:

Measured osmolality − calculated osmolality
= osmolal gap

An osmolal gap that exceeds 10 mOsm is abnormal. Toxins that can cause an elevated osmolal gap include ethanol, ethylene glycol, and methanol. If an ethanol level is known, it can be factored into the following equation:

$$2(Na^+)+\frac{glucose}{18}+\frac{BUN}{2.8}+\frac{BAL}{4.6}$$
$$= \text{calculated osmolality}$$

where BAL is the blood alcohol level measured in milligrams per deciliter.

▶ *Toxicology screens.* A toxicology screen is a laboratory analysis of a body fluid or tissue to identify drugs or toxins. Although saliva, spinal fluid, and hair may be analyzed, blood or urine samples are used more frequently. The number and type of drugs assessed by toxicology screens vary. Each screen tests for specific drugs or agents. For example, drug abuse screens usually identify several common street or prescription drugs, whereas a coma panel detects common drugs that cause CNS depression. Comprehensive screens include many drugs (ranging from antidepressants to cardiac drugs to alcohols) and are more expensive. A number of factors limit the role of toxicology screens in managing poisonings or overdoses. The test sample must be collected while the drug or toxin is in the body fluid or tissue used for testing. For example, cocaine is a rapidly metabolized drug; however, its metabo-

lite, benzoylecgonine, can be detected in the urine for several hours after cocaine use. Also, a toxicology screen with a negative result does not necessarily mean that no drug or toxin is present, but rather that none of the drugs or toxins for which a patient has been screened is present. For example, γ-hydroxybutyrate (GHB) is not included in toxicology screens because it is rapidly metabolized to small, unmeasurable molecules. The sample must also be properly collected, and there must be a laboratory near enough to obtain results quickly. For many smaller, rural laboratories, these tests are taken by a courier service or mailed to a larger laboratory, and the results are not available for several days. In these situations, the value of the test for managing the immediate overdose or poisoning needs to be considered.

Patient care in some of the more common poisonings and overdoses is summarized in Table 56-3. Clinical manifestations are included in the table. Management of the patient who is toxic with cocaine is summarized in Box 56-4.[12]

(text continues on page 1451)

Table 56-3 • Common Patient Care in Poisonings and Overdoses

Drug/Substance	Clinical Presentation and Assessment	Intervention

Acetaminophen (APAP):
Common OTC antipyretic and analgesic
Often sold as a component of combination drugs for pain, cough, cold, and sleep
Examples: OTC remedies such as Tylenol, Tylenol Extended Relief, Tempra, Liquiprin, Panadol, Excedrin PM (diphenhydramine-APAP) and in controlled-substance combination drugs such as oxycodone-APAP (Percocet), codeine-APAP (Tylenol #3), hydrocodone-APAP (Vicodin)
Acetaminophen toxicity: Hepatotoxicity and occasionally renal dysfunction, 1–3 d postingestion
	• Phase 1 (up to 24 h postingestion): anorexia, nausea, malaise
	• Phase 2 (24–48 h postingestion): clinical picture improves, increase in AST, ALT, and total bilirubin, prolongation of prothrombin time
	• Phase 3 (72–96 h postingestion): peak hepatotoxicity usually observed
	• Coagulopathies
	• Jaundice
	• AST and ALT may rise into the 10,000–20,000 IU/L range and return to normal without the patient experiencing long-term sequelae
	• Chronic toxicity well described in the medical literature
		Prevention of absorption:
		• Activated charcoal
		
		Laboratory:
		• Draw acetaminophen level at 4 h (or later if patient presents late to the health care facility), plot level on the Rumack-Matthew nomogram (see Fig. 56-1) to determine whether antidote is indicated.
		• Monitor daily AST, ALT, total bilirubin, BUN, creatinine, and prothrombin time in patients with a toxic acetaminophen level.
		
		Treatment:
		• Antidote: N-acetylcysteine (NAC)
		• Oral: NAC, Mucomyst
		  • Loading dose: 140 mg/kg orally
		  • Maintenance doses: 70 mg/kg orally every 4 h for a total of 17 maintenance doses
		  • Dilute NAC (20% solution) 3:1 with a soft drink or juice
		  • Repeat any dose not retained 1 h, may need large doses of antiemetics to control vomiting[9]
		• IV: Acetadote
		  • Loading dose: 150 mg/kg in 200 mL of D5W IV over 60 min
		  • First maintenance dose: 50 mg/kg in 500 mL of D5W IV over 4 h
		  • Second maintenance dose: 100 mg/kg in 1000 mL of D5W IV over 16 h[10]
		• Supportive care

Amphetamines Group of drugs used therapeutically for narcolepsy, short-term treatment of obesity, and attention-deficit disorder	• Flushing • Diaphoresis • Restlessness	Prevention of absorption: • Activated charcoal

(continued)

Table 56-3 • Common Patient Care in Poisonings and Overdoses (Continued)

Drug/Substance	Clinical Presentation and Assessment	Intervention
As drugs of abuse, used for ability to stimulate central nervous system to combat fatigue or produce a "high" Prescription amphetamines and related agents: methylphenidate (Ritalin), dextroamphetamine (Dexedrine), mixed salts of amphetamine (Adderall) Street names: speed, uppers, crank, E, X, ecstasy, ice, crystal	• Talkativeness • Irritability • Confusion • Panic • Seizures • Intracranial hemorrhage • Hypertension • Tachycardia • Chest pain • Myocardial infarction • Cardiac arrhythmias • Palpitations • Peripheral vasoconstriction • Nausea • Vomiting • Chronic amphetamine toxicity may lead to the development of paranoia or hallucinations • IV abusers may also have complications such as hepatitis, sepsis, abscesses, and HIV infection	Laboratory: • Monitor electrolytes and acid–base status • Urine drug screen may detect amphetamines Treatment: • External cooling measures for hyperthermia • Benzodiazepines to control agitation • Severe hypertension controlled with IV nitroprusside (Nipride), other drugs suggested • Supportive care
Benzodiazepines Antianxiety agents, anticonvulsants, muscle relaxants, and sedatives Examples: alprazolam (Xanax), clonazepam (Klonopin), diazepam (Valium), lorazepam (Ativan), midazolam (Versed) Primarily cause CNS and respiratory depression. Due to their low order of toxicity, fatalities unlikely unless ingested with other CNS depressants	• Respiratory depression • Airway protection/gag reflex • Lethargy • Coma • Confusion • Slurred speech • Ataxia	Prevention of absorption: • Activated charcoal Laboratory: • Urine drug screen may detect benzodiazepines. Treatment: • Flumazenil reverses CNS and respiratory depression; due to risk in unmasking controlled seizures, flumazenil is contraindicated in the face of simultaneous potential seizure causing overdose.[10] • Supportive care
Carbon Monoxide Colorless, odorless gas that is a component of automobile exhaust, natural gas or propane furnace emissions, cigarette smoke, wood stove emissions, and pollution Methylene chloride, a component found in some paint strippers, is metabolized in the body to carbon monoxide after inhaled or ingested It displaces oxygen from the hemoglobin, leading to hypoxia It is absorbed rapidly by inhalation and combines readily with hemoglobin due to a greater affinity than oxygen Fetal carboxyhemoglobin levels are possibly 10%–15% greater than the maternal carboxyhemoglobin level	• Flulike symptoms • Headache • Nausea • Vomiting • Syncope • Fatigue • Weakness • Lack of concentration • Irritability • Chest pain, especially in people with underlying cardiovascular disease • Occasionally, irreversible changes in memory and personality • Fetotoxicity • People usually report feeling better when not in the area of the carbon monoxide; for example, if the exposure is occurring in the home because of a faulty furnace, the person will often report a decrease or resolution of symptoms when away from the home	Prevention of absorption: • Fresh air Laboratory: • Carboxyhemoglobin levels Treatment: • 100% oxygen until all signs and symptoms resolve • Thorough neurological examination • Hyperbaric oxygen therapy (HBO) to decrease half-life; however, due to lack of available HBO chambers, use is limited and efficacy not well documented by research • Supportive care

(continued)

Table 56-3 • Common Patient Care in Poisonings and Overdoses (Continued)

Drug/Substance	Clinical Presentation and Assessment	Intervention
Cocaine Common street drug that produces a temporary feeling of well-being for the user Routes of exposure: IV, snorting, smoking Street names: crack, rock, coke, snow, blow Toxic effects related to the rapid onset of CNS and cardiac stimulation	• Tachycardia • Hypertension • Cardiac arrhythmias • Chest pain • Myocardial infarction • Aortic dissection • Bowel infarction • Hyperthermia • Anxiety • Seizures • Tactile hallucinations ("cocaine bugs") • Cerebral hemorrhage • Cerebral infarction • Rhabdomyolysis • Rapid onset of toxic effects • In pregnant women, abruptio placentae or abortion possible • Chronic snorting, nasal septal perforation If clinical presentation is inconsistent with cocaine alone, possibly adulterants, substitutes, co-ingestants, or withdrawal	Prevention of absorption (for ingested packets): • Activated charcoal • Whole-bowel irrigation Laboratory: • Urine drug screen to detect metabolite of cocaine: benzoylecgonine • Cardiac enzymes as indicated to rule out myocardial infarction Treatment: • Benzodiazepines such as diazepam (Valium) usually control hyperactivity, hypertension, tachycardia, anxiety, hyperthermia, and seizures • Phenobarbital may be necessary if seizures not controlled with benzodiazepines • Life-threatening hyperthermia may be reduced by external cooling measures • Cardiac monitoring and serial 12-lead electrocardiogram are used to evaluate arrhythmias and myocardial ischemia[11] • Monitor for other organ ischemia or infarction • Provide supportive care
Halogenated Hydrocarbons Agents used as propellants and refrigerants Freon, dichlorodifluoromethane (freon 12), and trichloromonofluoromethane (freon 11) included in this category Exposures to leaking household air conditioners are usually minor, causing transient eye, nose, and throat irritation; dizziness; and palpitations More concentrated exposures such as in industrial spills or deliberate abuse ("huffing") associated with possible fatal ventricular arrhythmias (due to myocardial sensitization to catecholamines) and pulmonary edema	• Eye, nose, and throat irritation • Cough • Dizziness • Disorientation • Palpitations • Bronchial constriction • Pulmonary edema • Ventricular arrhythmias • Frostbite possible with dermal exposures	Prevention of absorption: • Fresh air Laboratory: • No specific laboratory tests Treatment: • Quiet environment • Cardiac monitoring • Frostbite: complete rewarming • Supportive care
Heroin Common street drug that produces a temporary euphoria in the user Routes of exposure: IV, snorting Street names: dope, smack, junk	• Miosis • Decreased respiratory drive • Decreased level of consciousness • "Nodding"	Prevention of absorption: • Not applicable Laboratory: • As clinically indicated • Serum toxicology screen Treatment: • Careful administration of naloxone • Referral to substance abuse counselor
LSD Common name for psychedelic drug lysergic acid diethylamide Common drug of abuse since its rise in popularity in the 1960s Street drug: available in tablet, capsule, sugar cubes, or as a substance on blotting paper known as "blotter acid" One source of LSD is ingestion of morning glory seeds	• Anxiety • Impaired color perception • Impaired judgment • Paranoia or ideas of persecution • Time distortions • Blood pressure normal • Tachycardia • Tachypnea	Prevention of absorption: • Activated charcoal • Cathartic Laboratory: • Urine drug screen Treatment: • Acute anxiety may be managed with IV or oral diazepam (Valium)

(continued)

Table 56-3 • Common Patient Care in Poisonings and Overdoses (Continued)

Drug/Substance	Clinical Presentation and Assessment	Intervention
In addition to the psychedelic experience, may result in physical effects and behavior-related trauma during the acute toxic phase	• Slight temperature elevation • Flashbacks (transient recurrences of a psychedelic experience) possible after a period of abstinence, may recur for years • Trauma due to behavioral changes associated with LSD use	• A quiet, nonstimulating environment may be useful while trying to help the patient who is experiencing a bad reaction • Evaluate for evidence of trauma • Provide supportive care
Methanol Highly toxic antifreeze and solvent Available forms: most windshield washer fluids, Sterno canned heat, and components of some paints, gasoline additives, and shellacs Toxic effects: life-threatening acidosis and irreversible blindness, caused by the toxic metabolite, not the methanol itself	• Blurred vision • Decreased visual acuity • Subjective description of vision as if walking in a snowstorm • Retinal edema • Hyperemia of the optic disk • Headache • Vertigo • Lethargy • Confusion • Coma • Nausea • Vomiting • Abdominal pain • Metabolic acidosis	Prevention of absorption: • Syrup of ipecac • Gastric lavage • Activated charcoal and cathartic are of little value Laboratory: • Methanol level drawn 1 h postingestion • Serial electrolytes • If using ethanol therapy, serial glucose and blood ethanol level monitored every hour initially Treatment: • Treatment is aimed at preventing the formation of toxic metabolites with either Antizol (4-methylpyrazole: 4-MP) or ethanol • Hemodialysis usually indicated for methanol levels >50 mg/dL, visual changes, renal failure, or refractory acidosis • Folic acid administration to assist with oxidation of the toxic metabolite formic acid to carbon dioxide • Supportive care
Salicylates Group of drugs used primarily for anti-inflammatory, antipyretic, and analgesic properties Common sources: aspirin, some formulations of Alka-Seltzer, Aspergum, PeptoBismol, sunscreens, liniments such as Icy Hot, and oil of wintergreen (methylsalicylate) Life-threatening metabolic acidosis, cerebral edema, and pulmonary edema from salicylism Aspirin ingestions difficult to manage due to the formation of a mass of aspirin in the gastrointestinal tract called a concretion Concretion formation leads to delayed absorption and therefore delayed toxicity Chronic salicylism more common in older adults and easily missed due to lack of careful history taking Higher salicylate levels tolerated with acute overdose as opposed to chronic toxicity	• Tinnitus • Tachypnea • Pulmonary edema • Confusion • Lethargy • Seizures • Cerebral edema • Respiratory alkalosis coupled with metabolic acidosis (initially) • Hypokalemia • Platelet dysfunction • Hypothrombinemia • Gastrointestinal hemorrhage • Nausea • Vomiting • Hyperthermia • Dehydration	Prevention of absorption: • Syrup of ipecac • Gastric lavage • Multiple-dose activated charcoal • Single-dose cathartic Laboratory: • Serial salicylate levels • Serial electrolytes • Arterial blood gas as indicated • Hematological and coagulation studies Treatment: • IV hydration • Urinary excretion is enhanced by urine alkalinization (urine pH = 7.5–8.0); IV fluid is usually D_5W with 20–40 mEq KCl and two to three ampules of sodium bicarbonate per liter to infuse at a rate of 2–3 mL/kg/h to achieve equal urine output (Note: It is difficult to alkalinize the urine without a normal serum potassium level) • Potassium is replaced intravenously as needed • Monitor onset of cerebral or pulmonary edema; chest radiograph is taken as needed • Hemodialysis is indicated for renal failure, cerebral edema, pulmonary edema, refractory acidosis, chronic salicylate level >50 mg/dL, or acute salicylate level >100 mg/dL postingestion • Provide supportive care Note: Treatment is based on serial salicylate levels and clinical presentation; each case is individually assessed and managed

(continued)

Table 56-3 • Common Patient Care in Poisonings and Overdoses (Continued)

Drug/Substance	Clinical Presentation and Assessment	Intervention
Tricyclic Antidepressants (TCA) Class of drugs prescribed for depression and chronic pain Examples: amitriptyline (Elavil), clomipramine (Anafranil), desipramine (Norpramin), doxepin (Adapin, Sinequan), imipramine (Tofranil), nortriptyline (Pamelor, Aventyl), protriptyline (Vivactil), and trimipramine (Surmontil)	• Tachycardia • Ventricular arrhythmias (including ventricular tachycardia and ventricular fibrillation) • Cardiac conduction delays (e.g., QRS >100 msec) • Hypotension • Agitation • Sedation • Seizures • Coma • Dry, flushed skin • Decreased gastrointestinal motility • Urinary retention • Metabolic acidosis	Prevention of absorption: • Syrup of ipecac contraindicated because of the rapid onset of sedation or seizures • Gastric lavage • Activated charcoal • Cathartic Laboratory: • Serum TCA levels not clinically useful in managing overdoses • Urine drug screen for TCAs • Serial electrolytes and arterial blood gases as indicated Treatment: • Prepare for rapid onset of cardiovascular collapse • Seizures may be treated initially with intravenous benzodiazepines (diazepam, lorazepam), and, if necessary, phenytoin (Dilantin) and phenobarbital • Ventricular arrhythmias may initially be controlled with systemic alkalinization (keeping blood pH +7.45–7.55 using intravenous boluses of sodium bicarbonate or intubation and hyperventilation); ventricular arrhythmias not controlled with systemic alkalinization may be controlled with lidocaine or bretylium (Bretylol); do not use procainamide (Pronestyl) or quinidine due to effects on cardiac conduction similar to those of TCAs • Cardiac conduction delays (e.g., QRS >100 msec) also are treated with systemic alkalinization as outlined in previous point; conduction delays not responsive to systemic alkalinization may be treated with phenytoin • Hypotension may be addressed initially with Trendelenburg position and IV fluids; if necessary, follow with dopamine infusion; norepinephrine (Levophed) may be necessary • Provide supportive care

ALT, alanine aminotransferase; AST, aspartate aminotransferase; OTC, over the counter.

 Box 56-4 • COLLABORATIVE CARE GUIDE for the Patient With Cocaine Toxicity

OUTCOMES	INTERVENTIONS
Oxygenation/Ventilation Arterial blood gases are within normal limits.	• Monitor pulse oximetry and arterial blood gases. • Validate significant changes in pulse oximetry with co-oximetry arterial saturation measurement.
Respiratory rate and depth are within normal limits.	• Monitor q15min, then q1h. • Prepare for intubation and mechanical ventilation (see Collaborative Care Guide for the Patient on a Ventilator).
Circulation/Perfusion Blood pressure, heart rate are within normal limits. Patient is free of dysrhythmias. There is no evidence of myocardial dysfunction, such as altered electrocardiogram (ECG) or cardiac enzymes.	• Monitor vital signs q15min then q1h. • Provide continuous ECG monitoring. • Monitor 12-lead ECG daily and PRN. • Monitor cardiac enzymes, magnesium, phosphorus, calcium, and potassium as ordered. • Assess for chest pain. • Monitor ECG for dysrhythmias and changes consistent with evolving myocardial infarction.

(continued)

Box 56-4 • COLLABORATIVE CARE GUIDE for the Patient With Cocaine Toxicity (Continued)

OUTCOMES	INTERVENTIONS
Patient is euthermic.	• Assess temperature q15–30min, then q1h. • Provide a cool environment, and institute cooling strategies (e.g., hypothermia blanket, tepid sponge bath), as indicated.
Fluids/Electrolytes Patient's urine output >30 mL/h (or >0.5 mL/kg/h). There is no evidence of electrolyte imbalance or renal dysfunction.	• Take intake and output q1h. • Administer fluids and diuretics to maintain intravascular volume and renal function per order. • Monitor electrolytes daily and PRN. • Replace electrolytes as ordered. • Monitor BUN, creatinine, serum osmolality, and urine electrolytes daily.
Mobility/Safety There is no evidence of seizure activity. Patient does not harm self.	• Monitor for seizure activity. • Administer anticonvulsants. • Assess anticonvulsant levels qd if indicated. • Maintain calm, quiet environment. • Institute seizure precautions. • Institute fall precautions. • Assess need for physical or chemical restraint to protect from self-injury. • Monitor agitation and administer sedation when appropriate. • Evaluate risk for suicide and take measures to protect patient.
Skin Integrity There is no evidence of skin breakdown.	• Document skin integrity q8h. • Turn and reposition q2h. • Use Braden Scale to assess risk for skin breakdown.
Nutrition Caloric and nutrient intake meet metabolic requirements per calculation (e.g., Basal Energy Expenditure).	• Provide parenteral or enteral nutrition if patient is NPO. • Consult dietitian or nutritional support service. • Monitor protein and calorie intake. • Monitor albumin, prealbumin, transferrin, cholesterol, triglycerides, glucose.
Comfort/Pain Control Patient will have minimal discomfort related to withdrawal from cocaine and other substances.	• Obtain toxicology screen to identify other substances used by the patient. • Treat drug withdrawal and overdose symptoms promptly and with appropriate intervention (e.g., remove from circulation, administer antidote, administer methadone).
Psychosocial Patient and family acknowledge substance abuse.	• Assess patient and family response to overdose. • Support healthy coping behaviors. • Consult substance abuse counselor and social worker. • Encourage patient discussion regarding use of illegal drugs, support system, financial concerns, and readiness for substance abuse treatment.
Teaching/Discharge Planning Patient and family have information about treatment and self-help resources. Patient and family each have a plan for follow-up care.	• Assess patient and family knowledge and understanding of substance abuse. • Provide literature and explanations to patient and family regarding substance abuse, treatment, relapse, legal issues, and self-help groups. • Refer family to self-help resources. • If patient agrees, initiate referral for substance abuse rehabilitation. • Coordinate referral with patient, family, and social worker to address other possible issues (e.g., housing, financial issues, long-term care planning).

Box 56-5 • TEACHING GUIDE:
Prevention of Childhood Poisoning

- Keep all medications and toxic products in original containers in a locked cabinet out of the reach of children.
- Read labels carefully before using drugs or toxic products.
- Use toxic chemical products in a well-ventilated area.
- Do not mix common household cleaning products.
- Identify any poisonous house plants, and keep seeds, bulbs, leaves, and fruits of such plants away from children.
- Do not treat medicines as candy.
- Measure and give medicine in well-lit areas to avoid error.
- Use child-resistant containers when available.
- Recap containers immediately after measuring dose.
- Destroy all old medications in a safe way, such as flushing them down the toilet.
- Keep Poison Control Center telephone numbers posted by the phone.
- Do not take medications in front of children.
- Keep all household products and drugs in original containers. Never put chemicals in empty food or drink containers.

PATIENT TEACHING

One of the interventions the nurse can perform in the emergency department or ICU is preventive teaching. All patients (and parents of pediatric patients) who have survived a toxic encounter should be taught how to prevent such an incident from recurring. Parents of young children need information on child-proofing their home. Teaching information related to the prevention of childhood poisoning is given in Box 56-5. Family teaching guidelines for lead poisoning are included in Box 56-6. Finally, a summary of

Box 56-6 • TEACHING GUIDE:
Lead Poisoning

- Lead is commonly found in old homes, in paint, plumbing, and dinnerware.
- Lead is excreted more slowly than it is absorbed, leading to a buildup of lead in the body.
- Accumulation of lead in high levels is frequently missed through lack of blood lead level screening, and not detected until effects such as learning disabilities are diagnosed.
- Children can be tested for lead by their health care providers.
- The local health department can provide lead poisoning treatment and information about lead abatement programs.

Box 56-7 • CONSIDERATIONS FOR THE
OLDER PATIENT: Accidental Poisoning

- Poison Control Centers receive many calls from or related to older adults regarding accidental poisonings.
- Telephone numbers for the health care provider and the Poison Control Center should be in a readily accessible place.
- The older population uses more medicine than any other age group.
- Older people may be more susceptible to the effects of drugs.
- When questions arise concerning drugs, a responsible adult should not hesitate to call a health care provider.
- The patient should not change the dose or discontinue taking prescription drugs without first consulting the physician or nurse.
- It is not wise to double medication when a pill is forgotten. The patient should seek the advice of his or her physician, nurse, or pharmacist.
- Medications and alcohol should not be mixed without first checking with the pharmacist for possible interactions.
- The pharmacist can provide large-print labels.
- A medication calendar or diary will help the older person keep track of the dosing schedule.
- Pill dispensers are helpful for the patient who has to take a variety of pills or who has trouble remembering the prescribed schedule.
- When a drug is discontinued, the remaining medication should be thrown away.

poison prevention for the older patient can be found in Box 56-7.

In addition, carbon monoxide detectors alert families to problems in their homes. Utility companies and local health and fire authorities can help identify and remove sources of fumes.

• Clinical Applicability Challenges

Case Study

Mr. S., a 48-year-old, 176-lb (80-kg) man, was brought to the emergency department by emergency medical services (EMS). The patient's family had called EMS to the scene after a suspected suicidal overdose. Mr. S. was uncooperative, refusing to answer questions, but seemingly alert. His initial vital signs were: blood pressure, 140/90 mm Hg; pulse, 120 beats/minute; and respirations, 30 breaths/minute and nonlabored. His pupils were equal and reactive to light. His skin was warm and dry. EMS started an intravenous (IV) line with lactated Ringer's solution at a keep vein open (KVO) rate, and initial blood draws were performed. The family reported that the patient had recently stopped taking his medications for bipolar disorder, and had taken approximately 200 aspirin tablets within the last hour.

On initial examination in the emergency department, the patient's vital signs were: blood pressure, 142/92 mm Hg; pulse, 132 beats/minute; respirations, 30 breaths/minute; and temperature, 99°F (37.2°C). The patient complained of feeling tired and nauseous. His pupils remained normal, and all reflexes were intact. A nasogastric tube was placed, some stomach contents were withdrawn, and 50 g of activated charcoal was instilled. Within minutes, he vomited.

The nurse in the emergency department called the poison control center, which initially recommended an antiemetic to control the nausea and vomiting, instillation of a second 50-g dose of activated charcoal, cardiac monitoring, seizure precautions, measurement of arterial blood gases (ABGs), and serial (every 2 hours) measurements of the patient's blood salicylate and electrolyte levels. IV hydration with fluids containing 2 to 3 ampules of sodium bicarbonate and 40 mEq of potassium chloride was also recommended. In addition, a blood acetaminophen level was recommended to rule out the possibility of co-ingestion.

The initial salicylate level drawn by EMS approximately 1 hour after ingestion was 30 mg/dL. The patient's acetaminophen level was less than 10 µg/mL. His initial basic metabolic panel levels were: sodium, 142 mEq/L; potassium, 4.0 mEq/; chloride, 100 mEq/L; carbon dioxide, 14 mEq/L; blood urea nitrogen (BUN), 10 mg/dL; creatinine, 0.9 mg/dL; and glucose, 140 mg/dL. His ABGs were: pH, 7.48; PCO_2, 20 mm Hg; PO_2, 85 mm Hg; and bicarbonate, 12 mEq/L. The patient had received 10 mg of IV metoclopramide (Reglan) and was able to tolerate a second 50-g dose of activated charcoal by nasogastric tube, without vomiting. IV fluids had been changed to 5% dextrose in water (D_5W) with 2 ampules of sodium bicarbonate and 40 mEq of potassium chloride at 15 mL/hour. Mr. S. was admitted to the intensive care unit (ICU) for continued treatment and monitoring.

While Mr. S. was in the ICU, the second salicylate level came back at 88 mg/dL (drawn approximately 3.5 hours after ingestion). The nurse in the ICU called the poison control center with this information and asked for further recommendations. The poison control center recommended another 50-g dose of activated charcoal and a renal consultation to consider hemodialysis. An abdominal computed tomography scan to look for a possible concretion was also recommended.

Repeated laboratory studies obtained on arrival in the ICU included measurements of the patient's salicylate level, basic metabolic panel levels, and ABGs. The third salicylate level drawn approximately 7 hours after ingestion was 122 mg/dL.

Basic metabolic panel levels were: sodium, 144 mEq/L; potassium, 3.6 mEq/L; chloride, 110 mEq/L; carbon dioxide, 20 mEq/L; BUN, 10 mg/dL; creatinine, 1.0 mg/dL; and glucose, 152 mg/dL. His ABGs were pH, 7.50; PCO_2, 34 mm Hg; PO_2, 88 mm Hg; and bicarbonate, 16 mEq/L. The patient remained lethargic and tachycardic at 120 beats/minute with a respiratory rate of 16 breaths/minute. A nephrology consultation resulted in the placement of an intravascular catheter for hemodialysis to allow better management of the high salicylate level and more rapid correction of the electrolyte and ABG abnormalities. The abdominal CT scan failed to show a concretion. In the ICU, Mr. S. continued to receive 50-g doses of activated charcoal every 4 hours for a total of three doses. He began passing activated charcoal rectally in combination with stool. The fourth salicylate level drawn approximately 10 hours after ingestion was 120 mg/dL, and hemodialysis was initiated. The patient received one 4-hour run of hemodialysis and experienced a significant improvement in symptoms. His salicylate level after hemodialysis was 20 mg/dL, with normal measurements of electrolytes and ABGs. Supportive care continued, and he was discharged on the third hospital day.

1. What are some of the body systems affected by a salicylate (aspirin) overdose? Discuss the effects and the implications for monitoring and treatment.

2. How is an aspirin overdose different from an acetaminophen overdose? Discuss the differences in timing of the levels and the need for different levels of patient monitoring.

3. Why is the administration of activated charcoal, even comparatively late in the clinical course, so important in the management of an aspirin overdose? Discuss the changes in absorption seen in aspirin overdose.

4. Why would intubation and artificial respiration be potentially lethal to a patient who is experiencing a salicylate overdose? Discuss the acid–base changes seen and what affect they could have on the availability of aspirin to diffuse into major organ systems such as the brain, heart, and lungs.

5. What role does hemodialysis have in the management of a patient with an aspirin overdose? At what point is it advisable or necessary to call nephrology for a consult?

Review Questions

1. The nurse is receiving a 25-year-old woman from emergency medical transport who is a suspected overdosed patient. What are the first concerns in the approach to the patient?
   a. Name, age, and sex
   b. Airway, breathing, and circulation
   c. Product, quantity, and time since ingestion
   d. Level of consciousness, degree of orientation, vital signs

2. A 19-year-old woman who is 6 months pregnant has recently taken a large quantity of prenatal vitamins with iron. The physician asks the nurse to administer 50 g of activated charcoal to the patient. What is the proper response to such a request?
   a. Administer the activated charcoal as ordered.
   b. Call the pharmacy for clarification of the dose of 50 g.
   c. Call the patient's provider of prenatal care to ask about the effects on the fetus.
   d. Question the physician's use of activated charcoal to adsorb iron.

3. Which toxidrome is described by the patient with the following clinical presentation: coma, constricted pupils, respiratory depression, and hypotension?
   a. Anticholinergic
   b. Cholinergic
   c. Opioid
   d. Sympathomimetic

4. A 25-year-old man is suffering from an acute overdose; he took a full bottle of his son's homeopathic teething tablets. The nurse, who is asked to plan for the man's care, requests that the physician order an acetaminophen level. When asked for a rationale, the nurse's answer should include the following:
   a. There may be acetaminophen in the teething tablets.
   b. Teething tablets frequently contain acetaminophen.
   c. Homeopathic products frequently contain acetaminophen.
   d. If acetaminophen was co-ingested, liver injury would precede manifest symptoms.

References

1. American Association of Poison Control Centers: 2004 Toxic exposure surveillance system poisoning data. Retrieved June 06, 2006, from http://www.aapcc.org
2. Sporer KA: Acute heroin overdose. Ann Intern Med 130: 584–590, 1999
3. American Academy of Clinical Toxicology, European Association of Poison Centers and Clinical Toxicologists: Position statements. J Toxicol Clin Toxicol 35:699–762, 1997
4. Goldfrank L, Flomenbaum N, Lewin N, et al: Toxicologic Emergencies, 7th ed. New York: McGraw-Hill Medical, 2002, pp 58–67
5. Ford M, Delaney K, Ling L, et al: Clinical Toxicology. Philadelphia: WB Saunders, 2001, pp 661–665
6. Brent J, McMartin K, Phillips S, et al: Fomepizole for the treatment of methanol poisoning. N Engl J Med 344:424–429, 2001
7. Brent J, McMartin K, Phillips S, et al: Fomepizole for the treatment of ethylene glycol poisoning. N Engl J Med 340:832–838, 1999
8. Haddad L, Shannon M, Winchester J: Clinical Management of Poisoning and Drug Overdose, 3rd ed. Philadelphia: WB Saunders, 1998, pp 343–347
9. Wright RO, Anderson AC, Lesko SL, et al: Effect of metoclopramide dose on preventing emesis after oral administration of N-acetylcysteine for acetaminophen overdose. J Toxicol Clin Toxicol 37:35–42, 1999
10. Product Information: Acetadote ® injection. Nashville: Cumberland Pharmaceuticals, 2006
11. Barnett R, Grace M, Boothe P, et al: Flumazenil in drug overdose: Randomized, placebo-controlled study to assess cost effectiveness. Crit Care Med 27:78–81, 1999
12. Tanen DA, Graeme KA, Curry SC: Crack cocaine ingestion with prolonged toxicity requiring electrical pacing. J Toxicol Clin Toxicol 38:653–657, 2000
13. Hoffman RS: Cocaine overdose: Clinical manifestations and treatment. J Toxicol Clin Toxicol 38:181–182, 2000

Other Selected Readings

Brent J, Wallace KL, Burkhart KK, et al: Critical Care Toxicology, Philadelphia: Elsevier-Mosby, 2005
Fenton JJ: Toxicology: A Case-Oriented Approach. Boca Raton: CRC Press, 2002
Flomenbaum NE, Goldfrank LR, Hoffman RS, et al: Goldfrank's Toxicologic Emergencies, 8th ed. New York: McGraw-Hill Medical, 2006
Ford MD, Delaney KA, Ling LJ, et al: Clinical Toxicology. Philadelphia: WB Saunders, 2001
Klasssen CD: Casarett and Doull's Toxicology: The Basic Science of Poisons, 6th ed. New York: McGraw-Hill Medical, 2001
Olson KR: Poisoning and Drug Overdose, 5th ed. San Francisco: McGraw-Hill Medical, 2006
Wexler P: Encyclopedia of Toxicology, 2nd ed. Oxford, UK: Elsevier, 2005

Appendix 1

ACLS Guidelines

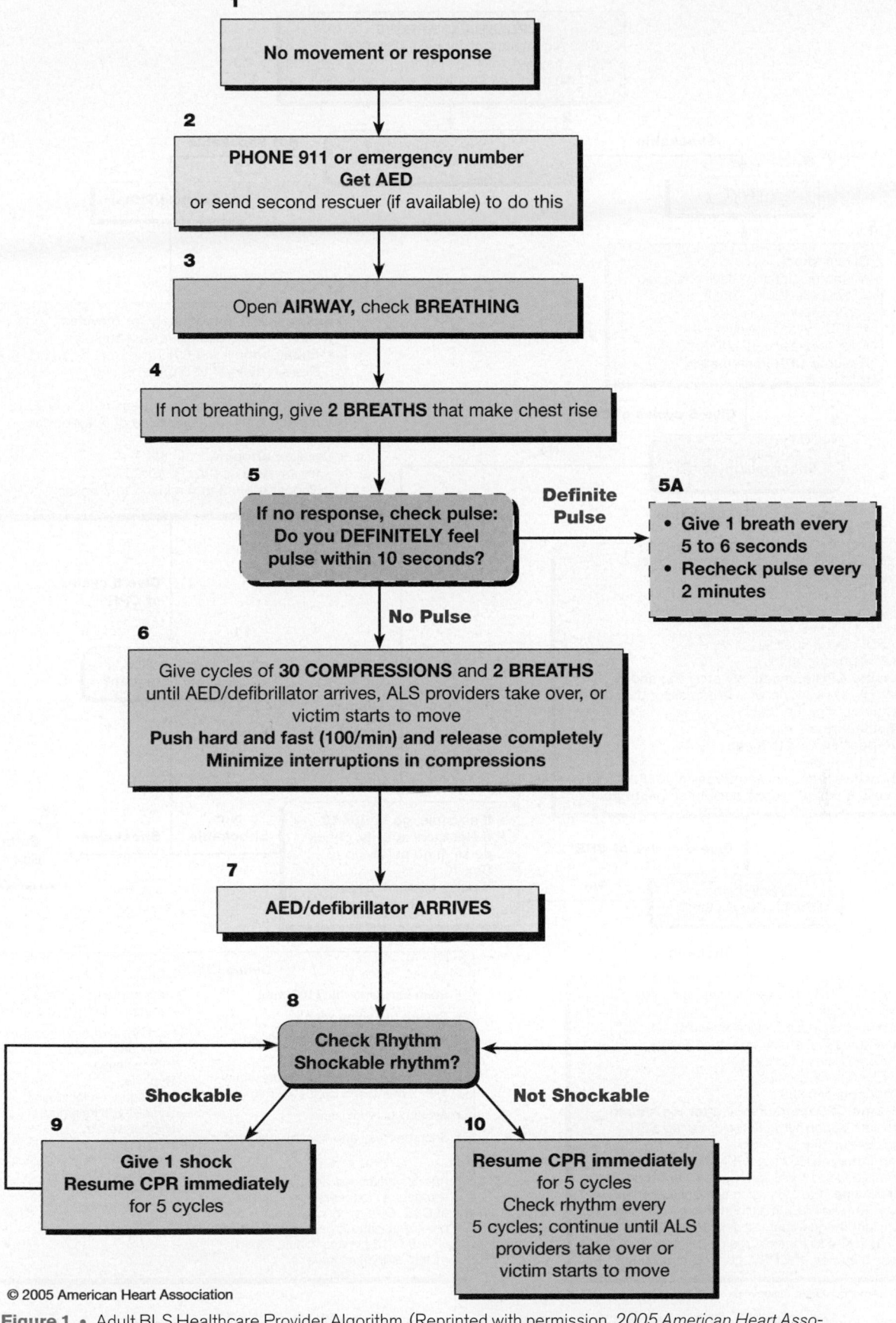

1
No movement or response

2
PHONE 911 or emergency number
Get AED
or send second rescuer (if available) to do this

3
Open AIRWAY, check BREATHING

4
If not breathing, give 2 BREATHS that make chest rise

5
If no response, check pulse:
Do you DEFINITELY feel
pulse within 10 seconds?

Definite Pulse

5A
• Give 1 breath every
  5 to 6 seconds
• Recheck pulse every
  2 minutes

No Pulse

6
Give cycles of 30 COMPRESSIONS and 2 BREATHS
until AED/defibrillator arrives, ALS providers take over, or
victim starts to move
Push hard and fast (100/min) and release completely
Minimize interruptions in compressions

7
AED/defibrillator ARRIVES

8
Check Rhythm
Shockable rhythm?

Shockable

Not Shockable

9
Give 1 shock
Resume CPR immediately
for 5 cycles

10
Resume CPR immediately
for 5 cycles
Check rhythm every
5 cycles; continue until ALS
providers take over or
victim starts to move

© 2005 American Heart Association

Figure 1 • Adult BLS Healthcare Provider Algorithm. (Reprinted with permission. *2005 American Heart Association Guidelines for Cardiopulmonary Resuscitation and Emergency Cardiovascular Care, Part 4: Adult Basic Life Support. Circulation. 2005; 112(suppl IV): IV-1-IV-111.* © 2005, American Heart Association, Inc.)

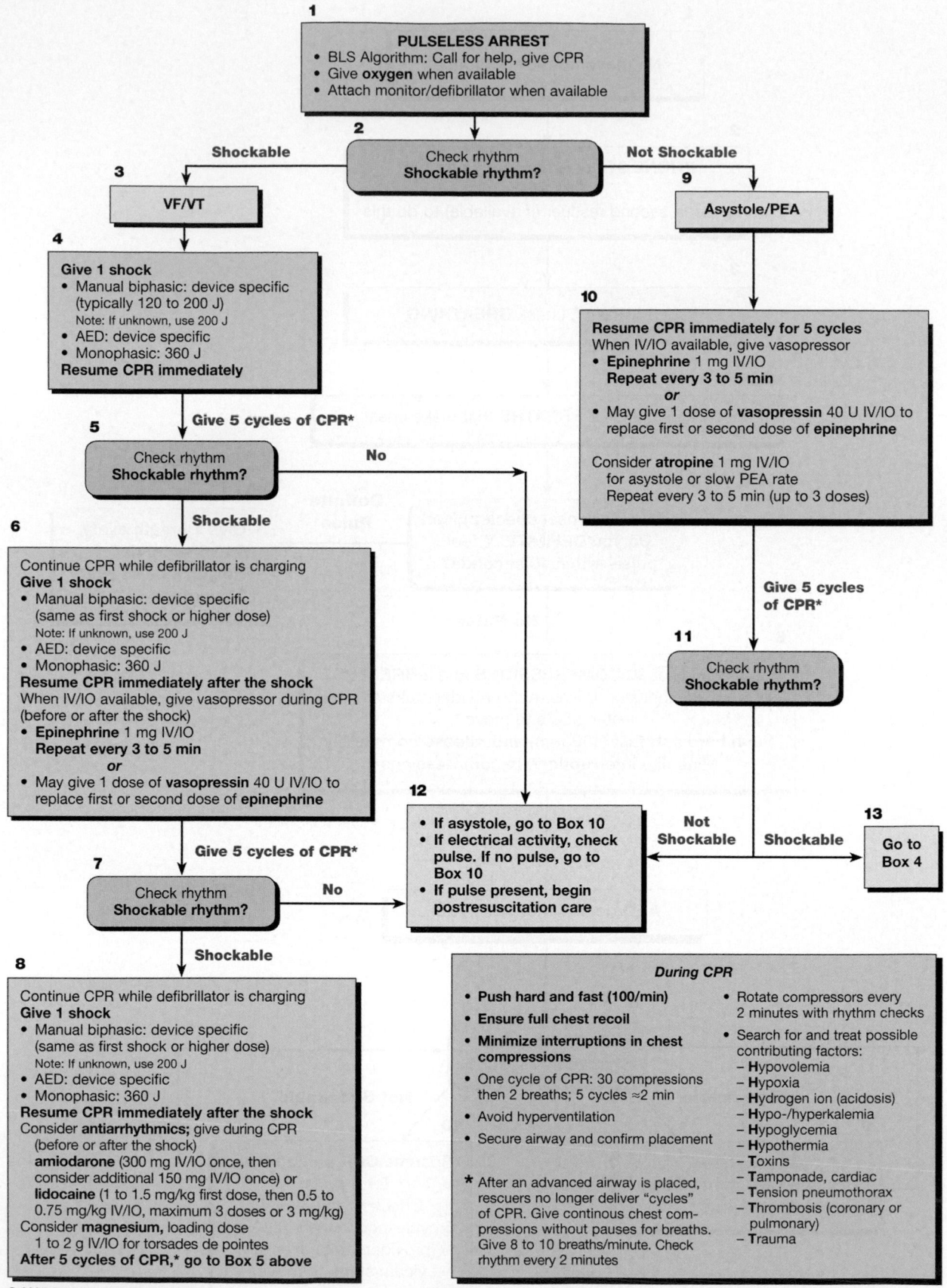

1 — PULSELESS ARREST
- BLS Algorithm: Call for help, give CPR
- Give **oxygen** when available
- Attach monitor/defibrillator when available

2 — Check rhythm
Shockable rhythm?

Shockable → **3 — VF/VT**

Not Shockable → **9 — Asystole/PEA**

4
Give 1 shock
- Manual biphasic: device specific (typically 120 to 200 J)
  Note: If unknown, use 200 J
- AED: device specific
- Monophasic: 360 J
Resume CPR immediately

Give 5 cycles of CPR*

5 — Check rhythm
Shockable rhythm?

No →

Shockable ↓

6
Continue CPR while defibrillator is charging
Give 1 shock
- Manual biphasic: device specific (same as first shock or higher dose)
  Note: If unknown, use 200 J
- AED: device specific
- Monophasic: 360 J
Resume CPR immediately after the shock
When IV/IO available, give vasopressor during CPR (before or after the shock)
- **Epinephrine** 1 mg IV/IO
  Repeat every 3 to 5 min
  or
- May give 1 dose of **vasopressin** 40 U IV/IO to replace first or second dose of **epinephrine**

Give 5 cycles of CPR*

7 — Check rhythm
Shockable rhythm?

No →

Shockable ↓

8
Continue CPR while defibrillator is charging
Give 1 shock
- Manual biphasic: device specific (same as first shock or higher dose)
  Note: If unknown, use 200 J
- AED: device specific
- Monophasic: 360 J
Resume CPR immediately after the shock
Consider **antiarrhythmics**; give during CPR (before or after the shock)
  amiodarone (300 mg IV/IO once, then consider additional 150 mg IV/IO once) or
  lidocaine (1 to 1.5 mg/kg first dose, then 0.5 to 0.75 mg/kg IV/IO, maximum 3 doses or 3 mg/kg)
Consider **magnesium,** loading dose 1 to 2 g IV/IO for torsades de pointes
After 5 cycles of CPR,* go to Box 5 above

10
Resume CPR immediately for 5 cycles
When IV/IO available, give vasopressor
- **Epinephrine** 1 mg IV/IO
  Repeat every 3 to 5 min
  or
- May give 1 dose of **vasopressin** 40 U IV/IO to replace first or second dose of **epinephrine**

Consider **atropine** 1 mg IV/IO for asystole or slow PEA rate
  Repeat every 3 to 5 min (up to 3 doses)

Give 5 cycles of CPR*

11 — Check rhythm
Shockable rhythm?

Not Shockable → / Shockable →

13 — Go to Box 4

12
- If asystole, go to Box 10
- If electrical activity, check pulse. If no pulse, go to Box 10
- If pulse present, begin postresuscitation care

During CPR
- **Push hard and fast (100/min)**
- **Ensure full chest recoil**
- **Minimize interruptions in chest compressions**
- One cycle of CPR: 30 compressions then 2 breaths; 5 cycles ≈2 min
- Avoid hyperventilation
- Secure airway and confirm placement

* After an advanced airway is placed, rescuers no longer deliver "cycles" of CPR. Give continous chest compressions without pauses for breaths. Give 8 to 10 breaths/minute. Check rhythm every 2 minutes

- Rotate compressors every 2 minutes with rhythm checks
- Search for and treat possible contributing factors:
  – **H**ypovolemia
  – **H**ypoxia
  – **H**ydrogen ion (acidosis)
  – **H**ypo-/hyperkalemia
  – **H**ypoglycemia
  – **H**ypothermia
  – **T**oxins
  – **T**amponade, cardiac
  – **T**ension pneumothorax
  – **T**hrombosis (coronary or pulmonary)
  – **T**rauma

© 2005 American Heart Association

Figure 2 • ACLS Pulseless Arrest Algorithm. (Reprinted with permission. *2005 American Heart Association Guidelines for Cardiopulmonary Resuscitation and Emergency Cardiovascular Care, Part 4: Adult Basic Life Support. Circulation. 2005; 112(suppl IV): IV-1-IV-111.* © 2005, American Heart Association, Inc.)

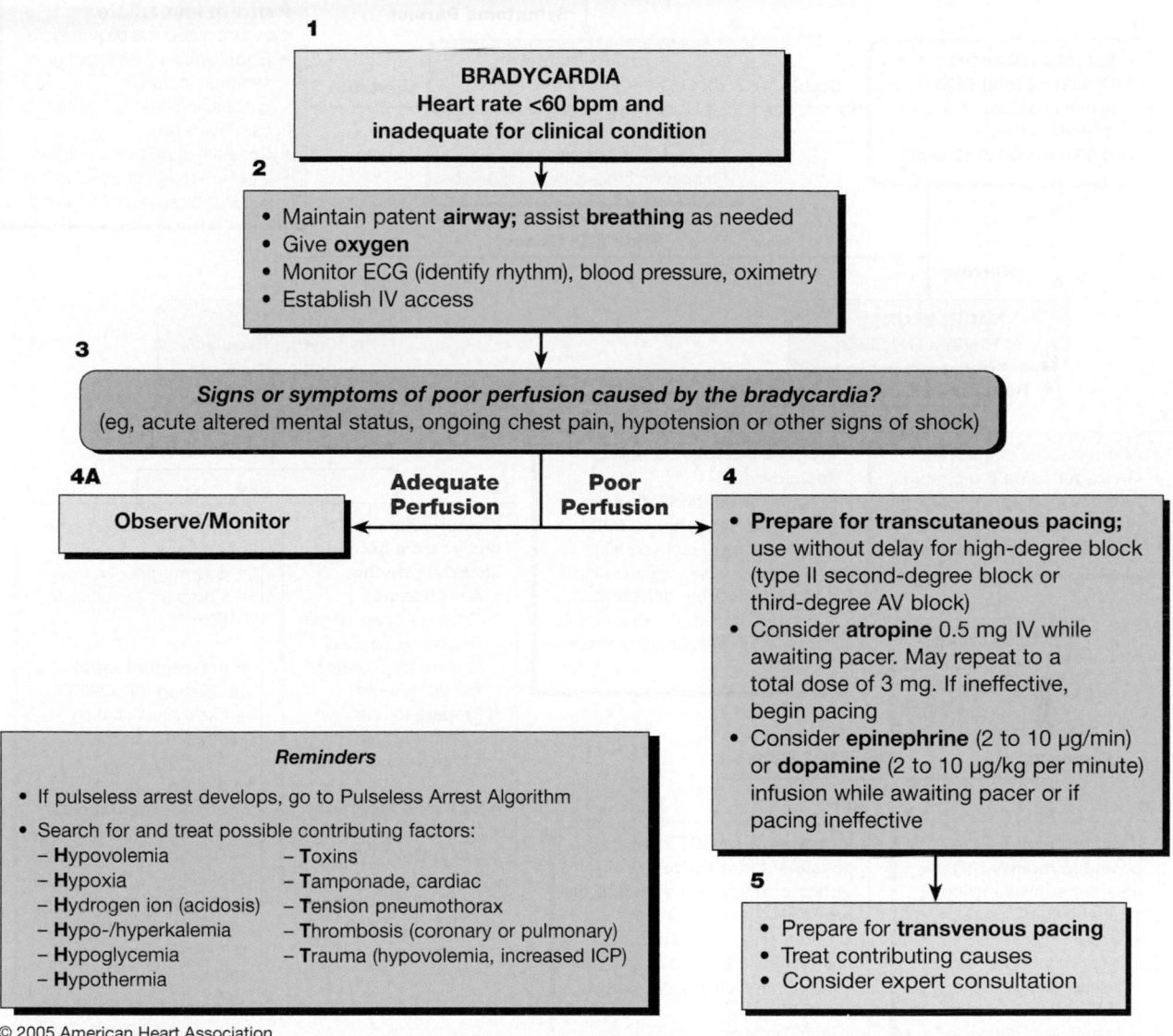

1

BRADYCARDIA
Heart rate <60 bpm and
inadequate for clinical condition

2
- Maintain patent **airway;** assist **breathing** as needed
- Give **oxygen**
- Monitor ECG (identify rhythm), blood pressure, oximetry
- Establish IV access

3
Signs or symptoms of poor perfusion caused by the bradycardia?
(eg, acute altered mental status, ongoing chest pain, hypotension or other signs of shock)

4A   **Adequate**   **Poor**   **4**
                       Perfusion   **Perfusion**

Observe/Monitor

4
- **Prepare for transcutaneous pacing;** use without delay for high-degree block (type II second-degree block or third-degree AV block)
- Consider **atropine** 0.5 mg IV while awaiting pacer. May repeat to a total dose of 3 mg. If ineffective, begin pacing
- Consider **epinephrine** (2 to 10 µg/min) or **dopamine** (2 to 10 µg/kg per minute) infusion while awaiting pacer or if pacing ineffective

5
- Prepare for **transvenous pacing**
- Treat contributing causes
- Consider expert consultation

Reminders
- If pulseless arrest develops, go to Pulseless Arrest Algorithm
- Search for and treat possible contributing factors:
  - **H**ypovolemia
  - **H**ypoxia
  - **H**ydrogen ion (acidosis)
  - **H**ypo-/hyperkalemia
  - **H**ypoglycemia
  - **H**ypothermia
  - **T**oxins
  - **T**amponade, cardiac
  - **T**ension pneumothorax
  - **T**hrombosis (coronary or pulmonary)
  - **T**rauma (hypovolemia, increased ICP)

© 2005 American Heart Association

Figure 3 • Bradycardia Algorithm. (Reprinted with permission. *2005 American Heart Association Guidelines for Cardiopulmonary Resuscitation and Emergency Cardiovascular Care, Part 4: Adult Basic Life Support. Circulation. 2005; 112(suppl IV): IV-1-IV-111.* © 2005, American Heart Association, Inc.)

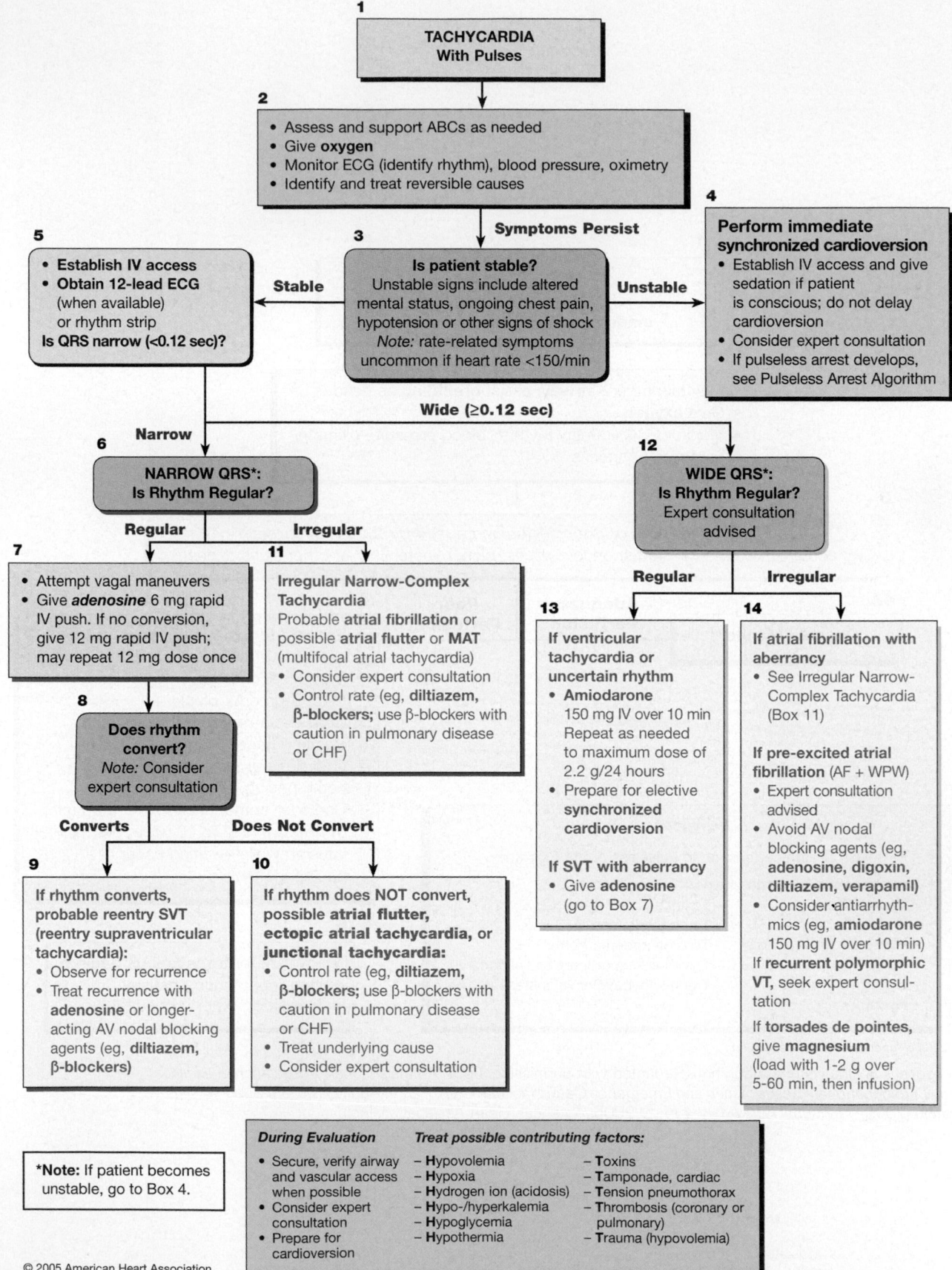

1
TACHYCARDIA
With Pulses

2
- Assess and support ABCs as needed
- Give **oxygen**
- Monitor ECG (identify rhythm), blood pressure, oximetry
- Identify and treat reversible causes

Symptoms Persist

3
Is patient stable?
Unstable signs include altered mental status, ongoing chest pain, hypotension or other signs of shock
Note: rate-related symptoms uncommon if heart rate <150/min

Stable

Unstable

4
Perform immediate synchronized cardioversion
- Establish IV access and give sedation if patient is conscious; do not delay cardioversion
- Consider expert consultation
- If pulseless arrest develops, see Pulseless Arrest Algorithm

5
- Establish IV access
- Obtain 12-lead ECG (when available) or rhythm strip
Is QRS narrow (<0.12 sec)?

Narrow

Wide (≥0.12 sec)

6
NARROW QRS*:
Is Rhythm Regular?

Regular

Irregular

7
- Attempt vagal maneuvers
- Give *adenosine* 6 mg rapid IV push. If no conversion, give 12 mg rapid IV push; may repeat 12 mg dose once

11
Irregular Narrow-Complex Tachycardia
Probable **atrial fibrillation** or possible **atrial flutter** or **MAT** (multifocal atrial tachycardia)
- Consider expert consultation
- Control rate (eg, **diltiazem, β-blockers;** use β-blockers with caution in pulmonary disease or CHF)

8
Does rhythm convert?
Note: Consider expert consultation

Converts

Does Not Convert

9
If rhythm converts, probable reentry SVT (reentry supraventricular tachycardia):
- Observe for recurrence
- Treat recurrence with **adenosine** or longer-acting AV nodal blocking agents (eg, **diltiazem, β-blockers)**

10
If rhythm does NOT convert, possible **atrial flutter, ectopic atrial tachycardia,** or **junctional tachycardia:**
- Control rate (eg, **diltiazem, β-blockers;** use β-blockers with caution in pulmonary disease or CHF)
- Treat underlying cause
- Consider expert consultation

12
WIDE QRS*:
Is Rhythm Regular?
Expert consultation advised

Regular

Irregular

13
If ventricular tachycardia or uncertain rhythm
- **Amiodarone** 150 mg IV over 10 min Repeat as needed to maximum dose of 2.2 g/24 hours
- Prepare for elective **synchronized cardioversion**

If SVT with aberrancy
- Give **adenosine** (go to Box 7)

14
If atrial fibrillation with aberrancy
- See Irregular Narrow-Complex Tachycardia (Box 11)

If pre-excited atrial fibrillation (AF + WPW)
- Expert consultation advised
- Avoid AV nodal blocking agents (eg, **adenosine, digoxin, diltiazem, verapamil)**
- Consider antiarrhythmics (eg, **amiodarone** 150 mg IV over 10 min)

If **recurrent polymorphic VT,** seek expert consultation

If **torsades de pointes,** give **magnesium** (load with 1-2 g over 5-60 min, then infusion)

During Evaluation
- Secure, verify airway and vascular access when possible
- Consider expert consultation
- Prepare for cardioversion

Treat possible contributing factors:
- **H**ypovolemia
- **H**ypoxia
- **H**ydrogen ion (acidosis)
- **H**ypo-/hyperkalemia
- **H**ypoglycemia
- **H**ypothermia

- **T**oxins
- **T**amponade, cardiac
- **T**ension pneumothorax
- **T**hrombosis (coronary or pulmonary)
- **T**rauma (hypovolemia)

*Note: If patient becomes unstable, go to Box 4.

© 2005 American Heart Association

Figure 4 • ACLS Tachycardia Algorithm. (Reprinted with permission. *2005 American Heart Association Guidelines for Cardiopulmonary Resuscitation and Emergency Cardiovascular Care, Part 4: Adult Basic Life Support. Circulation. 2005; 112(suppl IV): IV-1-IV-111.* © 2005, American Heart Association, Inc.)

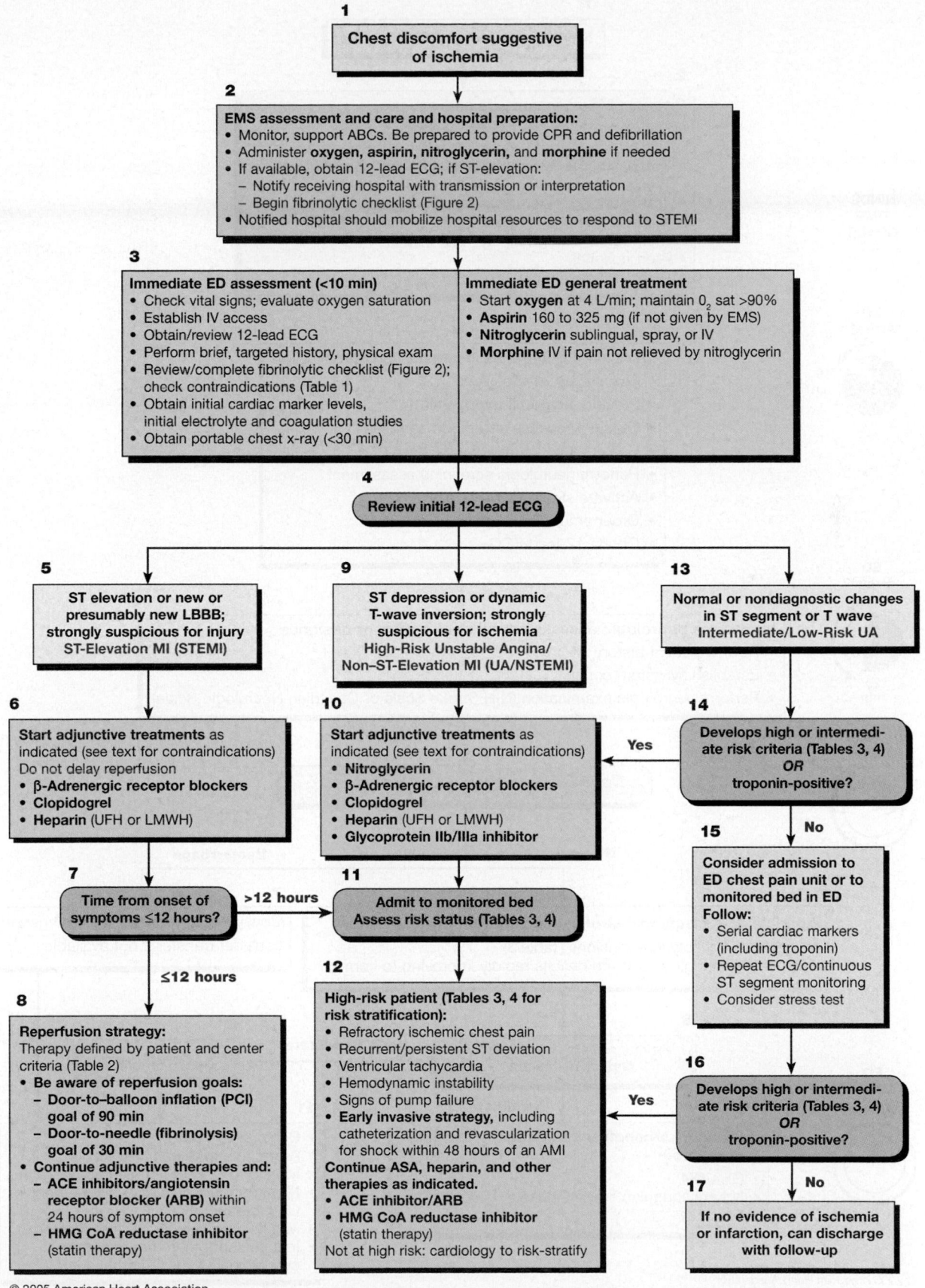

1
Chest discomfort suggestive of ischemia

2
EMS assessment and care and hospital preparation:
- Monitor, support ABCs. Be prepared to provide CPR and defibrillation
- Administer **oxygen, aspirin, nitroglycerin,** and **morphine** if needed
- If available, obtain 12-lead ECG; if ST-elevation:
  – Notify receiving hospital with transmission or interpretation
  – Begin fibrinolytic checklist (Figure 2)
- Notified hospital should mobilize hospital resources to respond to STEMI

3
Immediate ED assessment (<10 min)
- Check vital signs; evaluate oxygen saturation
- Establish IV access
- Obtain/review 12-lead ECG
- Perform brief, targeted history, physical exam
- Review/complete fibrinolytic checklist (Figure 2); check contraindications (Table 1)
- Obtain initial cardiac marker levels, initial electrolyte and coagulation studies
- Obtain portable chest x-ray (<30 min)

Immediate ED general treatment
- Start **oxygen** at 4 L/min; maintain O_2 sat >90%
- **Aspirin** 160 to 325 mg (if not given by EMS)
- **Nitroglycerin** sublingual, spray, or IV
- **Morphine** IV if pain not relieved by nitroglycerin

4
Review initial 12-lead ECG

5
ST elevation or new or presumably new LBBB; strongly suspicious for injury ST-Elevation MI (STEMI)

9
ST depression or dynamic T-wave inversion; strongly suspicious for ischemia High-Risk Unstable Angina/ Non–ST-Elevation MI (UA/NSTEMI)

13
Normal or nondiagnostic changes in ST segment or T wave Intermediate/Low-Risk UA

6
Start adjunctive treatments as indicated (see text for contraindications) Do not delay reperfusion
- **β-Adrenergic receptor blockers**
- **Clopidogrel**
- **Heparin** (UFH or LMWH)

10
Start adjunctive treatments as indicated (see text for contraindications)
- **Nitroglycerin**
- **β-Adrenergic receptor blockers**
- **Clopidogrel**
- **Heparin** (UFH or LMWH)
- **Glycoprotein IIb/IIIa inhibitor**

14
Develops high or intermediate risk criteria (Tables 3, 4) OR troponin-positive?

Yes →

7
Time from onset of symptoms ≤12 hours?

>12 hours →

11
Admit to monitored bed Assess risk status (Tables 3, 4)

15
Consider admission to ED chest pain unit or to monitored bed in ED Follow:
- Serial cardiac markers (including troponin)
- Repeat ECG/continuous ST segment monitoring
- Consider stress test

No ↓

≤12 hours ↓

8
Reperfusion strategy:
Therapy defined by patient and center criteria (Table 2)
- **Be aware of reperfusion goals:**
  – Door-to–balloon inflation (PCI) goal of 90 min
  – Door-to-needle (fibrinolysis) goal of 30 min
- **Continue adjunctive therapies and:**
  – ACE inhibitors/angiotensin receptor blocker (ARB) within 24 hours of symptom onset
  – HMG CoA reductase inhibitor (statin therapy)

12
High-risk patient (Tables 3, 4 for risk stratification):
- Refractory ischemic chest pain
- Recurrent/persistent ST deviation
- Ventricular tachycardia
- Hemodynamic instability
- Signs of pump failure
- **Early invasive strategy,** including catheterization and revascularization for shock within 48 hours of an AMI
Continue ASA, heparin, and other therapies as indicated.
- **ACE inhibitor/ARB**
- **HMG CoA reductase inhibitor** (statin therapy)
Not at high risk: cardiology to risk-stratify

16
Develops high or intermediate risk criteria (Tables 3, 4) OR troponin-positive?

Yes →

No ↓

17
If no evidence of ischemia or infarction, can discharge with follow-up

© 2005 American Heart Association

Figure 5 • Acute Coronary Syndromes Algorithm. (Reprinted with permission. *2005 American Heart Association Guidelines for Cardiopulmonary Resuscitation and Emergency Cardiovascular Care, Part 4: Adult Basic Life Support. Circulation. 2005; 112(suppl IV): IV-1-IV-111.* © 2005, American Heart Association, Inc.)

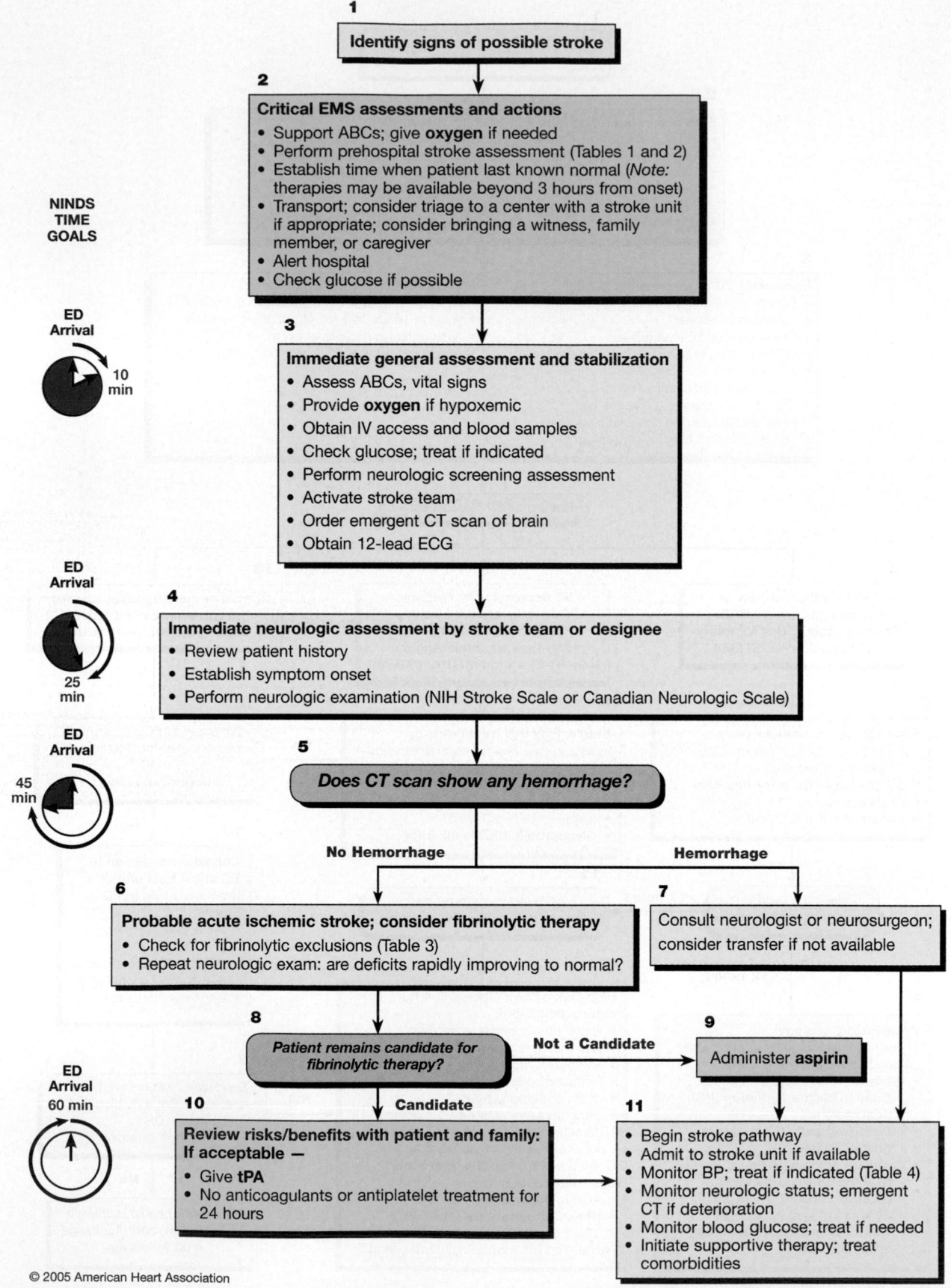

1

Identify signs of possible stroke

NINDS TIME GOALS

2

Critical EMS assessments and actions
- Support ABCs; give **oxygen** if needed
- Perform prehospital stroke assessment (Tables 1 and 2)
- Establish time when patient last known normal (*Note:* therapies may be available beyond 3 hours from onset)
- Transport; consider triage to a center with a stroke unit if appropriate; consider bringing a witness, family member, or caregiver
- Alert hospital
- Check glucose if possible

ED Arrival 10 min

3

Immediate general assessment and stabilization
- Assess ABCs, vital signs
- Provide **oxygen** if hypoxemic
- Obtain IV access and blood samples
- Check glucose; treat if indicated
- Perform neurologic screening assessment
- Activate stroke team
- Order emergent CT scan of brain
- Obtain 12-lead ECG

ED Arrival 25 min

4

Immediate neurologic assessment by stroke team or designee
- Review patient history
- Establish symptom onset
- Perform neurologic examination (NIH Stroke Scale or Canadian Neurologic Scale)

ED Arrival 45 min

5

Does CT scan show any hemorrhage?

No Hemorrhage   Hemorrhage

6

Probable acute ischemic stroke; consider fibrinolytic therapy
- Check for fibrinolytic exclusions (Table 3)
- Repeat neurologic exam: are deficits rapidly improving to normal?

7

Consult neurologist or neurosurgeon; consider transfer if not available

8

Patient remains candidate for fibrinolytic therapy?   Not a Candidate →

9

Administer **aspirin**

ED Arrival 60 min

Candidate ↓

10

Review risks/benefits with patient and family: If acceptable —
- Give **tPA**
- No anticoagulants or antiplatelet treatment for 24 hours

11
- Begin stroke pathway
- Admit to stroke unit if available
- Monitor BP; treat if indicated (Table 4)
- Monitor neurologic status; emergent CT if deterioration
- Monitor blood glucose; treat if needed
- Initiate supportive therapy; treat comorbidities

© 2005 American Heart Association

Figure 6 • Goals for Management of Patients with Suspected Stroke Algorithm. (Reprinted with permission. *2005 American Heart Association Guidelines for Cardiopulmonary Resuscitation and Emergency Cardiovascular Care, Part 4: Adult Basic Life Support. Circulation. 2005; 112(suppl IV): IV-1-IV-111.* © 2005, American Heart Association, Inc.)

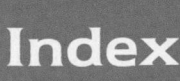

Note: Page numbers followed by b indicate boxed material; those
followed by f indicate figures; those followed by t indicate tables.